The Cornea

SECOND EDITION

Edited by

HERBERT E. KAUFMAN, M.D.

Boyd Professor of Ophthalmology and Pharmacology and Experimental Therapeutics; Head, Department of Ophthalmology, and Director, LSU Eye Center, Louisiana State University Medical Center School of Medicine, New Orleans

BRUCE A. BARRON, M.D.

Professor of Ophthalmology, LSU Eye Center, Louisiana State University Medical Center School of Medicine, New Orleans

MARGUERITE B. McDONALD, M.D., F.A.C.S.

Clinical Professor of Ophthalmology, Tulane University Medical Center, New Orleans; Director, Refractive Surgery Center of the South, Eye, Ear, Nose, and Throat Hospital, New Orleans

With a foreword by

CLAES H. DOHLMAN, M.D., PH.D.

Professor and Chairman Emeritus, Department of Ophthalmology, Harvard Medical School, Boston; Chief Emeritus, Department of Ophthalmology, Massachusetts Eye and Ear Infirmary, Boston

BUTTERWORTH–HEINEMANN

Boston • Oxford • Johannesburg • Melbourne • New Delhi • Singapore

Every effort has been made to ensure that the drug dosage schedules within this text are accurate and conform to standards accepted at time of publication. However, as treatment recommendations vary in the light of continuing research and clinical experience, the reader is advised to verify drug dosage schedules herein with information found on product information sheets. This is especially true in cases of new or infrequently used drugs.

Recognizing the importance of preserving what has been written, Butterworth-Heinemann prints its books on acid-free paper whenever possible.

Butterworth-Heinemann supports the efforts of American Forests and the Global ReLeaf program in its campaign for the betterment of trees, forests, and our environment.

Library of Congress Cataloging-in-Publication Data

The cornea / [edited by] Herbert E. Kaufman, Bruce A. Barron, Marguerite McDonald. -- 2nd ed.

p. cm.

Includes bibliographical references and index.

ISBN 0-7506-9928-0

1. Cornea--Diseases. 2. Cornea--Pathophysiology. I. Kaufman, Herbert E. (Herbert Edward), 1931- . II. Barron, Bruce A. III. McDonald, Marguerite B.

[DNLM: 1. Corneal Diseases--therapy. 2. Corneal Diseases--diagnosis. 3. Corneal Diseases--physiopathology. WW 220 C8125 1997]

RE336.C63 1997

617.7'19--dc21

DNLM/DLC

for Library of Congress 97-25706

CIP

British Library Cataloguing-in-Publication Data

A catalogue record for this book is available from the British Library.

The publisher offers special discounts on bulk orders of this book.

For information, please contact:

Manager of Special Sales

Butterworth-Heinemann

313 Washington Street

Newton, MA 02158-1626

Tel: 617-928-2500

Fax: 617-928-2620

For information on all Butterworth-Heinemann publications available, contact our World Wide Web home page at: http://www.bh.com

10 9 8 7 6 5 4 3 2 1

Printed in the United States of America

The Cornea

To those, past and present, who have contributed to our knowledge of the cornea

Contents

Contributing Authors

Luis G. Alcaraz-Micheli, M.D.
Director, Photorefractive Surgery Committee, Clínica de Cirugía Ambulatoria Dr. Luis A. Vázquez, Inc., Mayagüez, Puerto Rico
7. Bacterial Conjunctivitis

Penny A. Asbell, M.D.
Professor of Ophthalmology, Mount Sinai School of Medicine and Medical Center, New York
7. Bacterial Conjunctivitis; 44. Intrastromal Corneal Ring

Dmitri T. Azar, M.D.
Associate Professor of Ophthalmology, Harvard Medical School, Boston; Director, Corneal, External Disease and Refractive Surgery Services, Massachusetts Eye and Ear Infirmary, Boston
30. Phototherapeutic Keratectomy

Keith H. Baratz, M.D.
Assistant Professor of Ophthalmology, Mayo Medical School, Rochester, Minnesota; Consultant in Ophthalmology, Mayo Clinic, Rochester
11. Varicella-Zoster Viral Infections

Bruce A. Barron, M.D.
Professor of Ophthalmology, LSU Eye Center, Louisiana State University Medical Center School of Medicine, New Orleans
34. Penetrating Keratoplasty; 36. Prosthokeratoplasty

Roger W. Beuerman, Ph.D.
Professor of Ophthalmology, Psychiatry, and Anatomy, LSU Eye Center, Louisiana State University Medical Center School of Medicine, New Orleans
1. Structure and Function of the Cornea

John R. Bierly, M.D.
Assistant Professor of Ophthalmology, University of Kentucky College of Medicine, Lexington
13. Nonherpetic Viral Infections

Guy J. Boswall, M.D.
Staff Department of Surgery, Queen Elizabeth Hospital, Charlottetown, Prince Edward Island, Canada
27. Corneal Changes from Contact Lenses

William M. Bourne, M.D.
Joseph E. and Rose Marie Green Professor in Visual Sciences, Department of Ophthalmology, Mayo Clinic, Rochester, Minnesota
33. Corneal Preservation for Penetrating Keratoplasty

Thomas J. Byrd, M.D.
Proprietor, Holland Eye Center, Lincoln Park, Michigan; Staff Ophthalmologist, Henry Ford Wyandotte Hospital, Wyandotte, Michigan
46. Corneal Topography

John W. Chandler, M.D.
Attending Ophthalmologist, St. Joseph Hospital, Bellingham, Washington
25. Corneal Trauma

Deepak Chitkara, M.B.Ch.B., D.O., F.R.C.Ophth.
Consultant Ophthalmic Surgeon, Walton Hospital, Liverpool, United Kingdom
40. Principles of Excimer Laser Photoablation

Y. Ralph Chu, M.D.
Attending Physician, Department of Ophthalmology, Phillips Eye Institute, Minneapolis; Attending Physician,

Department of Ophthalmology, St. Paul Ramsey Hospital, St. Paul
38. Astigmatic Keratotomy

Michael Cobo, M.D.
Former Associate Professor of Ophthalmology, Duke University School of Medicine, Durham, North Carolina
11. Varicella-Zoster Viral Infections

Elisabeth J. Cohen, M.D.
Professor of Ophthalmology, Jefferson Medical College of Thomas Jefferson University, Philadelphia; Co-Director, Cornea Service, Wills Eye Hospital, Philadelphia
26. Corneal Changes from Ocular Surgery

Douglas J. Coster, M.D.
Professor of Ophthalmology, Flinders University of South Australia, Adelaide, Australia; Chairman of Ophthalmology, Flinders Medical Centre, Adelaide
28. Surgical Procedures to Restore the Corneal Epithelium

Oliver H. Dabezies, Jr., M.D.
Clinical Professor of Ophthalmology, Tulane University School of Medicine, New Orleans; Staff Member, Department of Ophthalmology, Eye, Ear, Nose, and Throat Hospital, New Orleans
27. Corneal Changes from Contact Lenses

Chandler Dawson, M.D.
Professor of Ophthalmology, Francis I. Proctor Foundation for Research in Ophthalmology, University of California, San Francisco, School of Medicine
14. Chlamydial Infections

David A. DiLoreto, M.D., F.A.C.S.
Director of Oculoplastic Surgery, LSU Eye Center, Louisiana State University Medical Center School of Medicine, New Orleans
6. Surgical Management of Eyelid Abnormalities

John F. Doane, M.D.
Clinical Faculty, Department of Ophthalmology, Kansas University Medical Center, Kansas City; Refractive Surgeon, Eye Care, Inc., Independence, Missouri
43. Laser-Assisted In Situ Keratomileusis

Peter C. Donshik, M.D., F.A.C.S.
Clinical Professor and Chief, Division of Ophthalmology, University of Connecticut Health Center, Farmington; Ophthalmologist, Hartford Hospital, Hartford
27. Corneal Changes from Contact Lenses

Donald J. Doughman, M.D.
Professor of Ophthalmology, University of Minnesota Medical School, Minneapolis; Professor of Ophthalmology, Fairview-University Hospitals, Minneapolis
27. Corneal Changes from Contact Lenses

Raj Dugel, M.D.
Attending Physician, Department of Ophthalmology, Little Company of Mary Hospital, Torrance, California
23. Immunologic Disorders of the Cornea and Conjunctiva

William H. Ehlers, M.D.
Assistant Clinical Professor of Ophthalmology, Department of Surgery, University of Connecticut Health Center, Farmington; Ophthalmologist, John Dempsey Hospital, Farmington; Ophthalmologist, Hartford Hospital, Hartford
27. Corneal Changes from Contact Lenses

R. Linsy Farris, M.D.
Professor of Clinical Ophthalmology, Harkness Eye Institute, Columbia University, College of Physicians and Surgeons, New York; Director of Ophthalmology, Harlem Hospital Center, New York
5. Abnormalities of the Tears and Treatment of Dry Eyes

Macie Finkelstein, M.D.
Assistant in Ophthalmology, Massachusetts Eye and Ear Infirmary, Boston
24. Corneal Tumors

C. Stephen Foster, M.D., F.A.C.S.
Director of Ophthalmology, Immunology Service, Massachusetts Eye and Ear Infirmary, Boston; Professor of Ophthalmology, Harvard Medical School, Boston
3. Basic Ocular Immunology

Bradley P. Gardner, M.D.
Ophthalmologist, Idaho Eye Center, Idaho Falls
21. Pterygium; 29. Conjunctival Flaps

Bryan M. Gebhardt, Ph.D.
Professor of Ophthalmology and Microbiology, LSU Eye Center, Louisiana State University Medical Center School of Medicine, New Orleans
10. Herpes Simplex Viral Infections

Kenneth Goins, M.D.
Assistant Professor of Ophthalmology, The University of Chicago, Pritzker School of Medicine, Chicago
11. Varicella-Zoster Viral Infections

Kenneth A. Greenberg, M.D.
Lecturer in Ophthalmology, Columbia Presbyterian Medical Center, New York; Associate Attending Physician, Department of Ophthalmology, Danbury Hospital, Danbury, Connecticut
41. Photorefractive Keratectomy for Myopia

Warren Hamilton, M.D.
Chairman, Department of Surgery, North Okaloosa Medical Center, Crestview, Florida
31. Inlay Lamellar Keratoplasty

David R. Hardten, M.D.
Assistant Clinical Professor of Ophthalmology, University of Minnesota Medical School, Minneapolis; Attending Surgeon, Department of Ophthalmology, Phillips Eye Institute, Minneapolis; Attending Surgeon, Department of Ophthalmology, St. Paul Ramsey Medical Center, St. Paul
38. Astigmatic Keratotomy

Jack Hartstein, M.D.
Professor of Clinical Ophthalmology and Director of Contact Lens Clinics, Washington University School of Medicine, St. Louis
27. Corneal Changes from Contact Lenses

Michael J. Hodkin, M.D.
Anterior Segment Surgeon, Eye Center Group, Muncie, Indiana
35. Complications of Penetrating Keratoplasty

Frederick A. Jakobiec, M.D., D.Sc.
Henry Willard Williams Professor of Ophthalmology, Chairman of Ophthalmology, and Professor of Pathology, Harvard Medical School, Boston; Chief of Ophthalmology, Massachusetts Eye and Ear Infirmary, Boston
24. Corneal Tumors

Herbert E. Kaufman, M.D.
Boyd Professor of Ophthalmology and Pharmacology and Experimental Therapeutics; Head, Department of Ophthalmology, and Director, LSU Eye Center, Louisiana State University Medical Center School of Medicine, New Orleans
10. Herpes Simplex Viral Infections

Stephen C. Kaufman, M.D., Ph.D.
Assistant Professor of Health Research, Clinical Assistant Professor of Ophthalmology, LSU Eye Center, Louisiana State University Medical Center School of Medicine, New Orleans
45. Phakic Intraocular Lenses

Stephen D. Klyce, Ph.D.
Professor of Ophthalmology and Anatomy, LSU Eye Center, Louisiana State University Medical Center School of Medicine, New Orleans; Adjunct Professor of Biomedical Engineering, Tulane University, New Orleans
1. Structure and Function of the Cornea; 27. Corneal Changes from Contact Lenses; 46. Corneal Topography

Jay H. Krachmer, M.D.
Professor and Chairman of Ophthalmology, University of Minnesota Medical Center, Minneapolis
18. Epithelial and Stromal Dystrophies; 19. Endothelial Dystrophies

Andrew W. Lawton, M.D.
Associate Professor of Ophthalmology, Tulane University School of Medicine, New Orleans
2. Structure and Function of the Eyelids and Conjunctiva

Thomas J. Liesegang, M.D.
Professor of Ophthalmology, Mayo Clinic Jacksonville, Jacksonville, Florida
8. Bacterial Keratitis; 9. Fungal Keratitis

Richard L. Lindstrom, M.D.
Clinical Professor of Ophthalmology, University of Minnesota Medical School, Minneapolis; Attending Surgeon and Medical Director, Center for Teaching and Research, Phillips Eye Institute, Minneapolis
38. Astigmatic Keratotomy

Jeffery Machat, M.D., F.R.C.S.C.
National Medical Director, The Laser Center, Inc., Toronto, Ontario
43. Laser-Assisted In Situ Keratomileusis

Naoyuki Maeda, M.D.
Assistant Professor of Ophthalmology, Osaka University Medical School, Suita, Osaka, Japan
46. Corneal Topography

Leo J. Maguire, M.D.
Associate Professor of Ophthalmology, Mayo Medical School, Rochester, Minnesota
22. Ectatic Corneal Degenerations

Alice Y. Matoba, M.D.
Associate Professor of Ophthalmology, Baylor College of Medicine, Houston; Chief of Ophthalmology Service, Houston Veterans Affairs Medical Center, Houston
12. Epstein-Barr Viral Infections

James P. McCulley, M.D.
Professor and Chairman of Ophthalmology, University of Texas Southwestern Medical School, Dallas; Chairman and Chief of Service, Department of Ophthalmology, Zale Lipshy University Hospital, Dallas; Chairman and Chief of Service, Department of Ophthalmology, Parkland Memorial Hospital and Children's Medical Center, Dallas
4. Meibomianitis

Marguerite B. McDonald, M.D., F.A.C.S.
Clinical Professor of Ophthalmology, Tulane University Medical Center, New Orleans; Director, Refractive Surgery Center of the South, Eye, Ear, Nose, and Throat Hospital, New Orleans
32. Onlay Lamellar Keratoplasty; 39. Epikeratophakia for Aphakia and Myopia; 40. Principles of Excimer Laser Photoablation

Corey A. Miller, M.D.
Associate Clinical Professor of Ophthalmology, University of Utah School of Medicine, Salt Lake City; Chairman, Division of Ophthalmology, LDS Hospital, Salt Lake City
18. Epithelial and Stromal Dystrophies; 19. Endothelial Dystrophies

Mary Beth Moore, M.D.
Department of Ophthalmology, Kaiser Permanente Medical Group, Sacramento, California
15. Parasitic Infections

John F. Morgan, M.D., F.R.C.S.(C.)
Professor Emeritus of Ophthalmology, Queens University, Kingston, Ontario, Canada
27. Corneal Changes from Contact Lenses

Keith S. Morgan, M.D.
Clinical Professor of Ophthalmology, Louisiana State University Medical Center School of Medicine, New Orleans
39. Epikeratophakia for Aphakia and Myopia

Marc G. Odrich, M.D.
Assistant Professor of Clinical Ophthalmology, Columbia University College of Physicians and Surgeons, New York; Director of Refractive Surgery, E.S. Harkness Eye Institute, Columbia Presbyterian Medical Center, New York
41. Photorefractive Keratectomy for Myopia

H. Bruce Ostler, M.D.
Former Clinical Professor, Francis I. Proctor Foundation, University of California Medical Center, San Francisco
13. Nonherpetic Viral Infections

Carolyn M. Parrish, M.D.
Ophthalmologist in Private Practice, Nashville
25. Corneal Trauma

Alex Poon, M.B.B.S., F.R.A.C.O., F.R.A.C.S.
Senior Registrar, Melbourne University Department of Ophthalmology, Royal Victorian Eye and Ear Hospital, Melbourne, Victoria, Australia
42. Photoastigmatic Refractive Keratectomy

Christopher J. Rapuano, M.D.
Associate Professor of Ophthalmology, Jefferson Medical College of Thomas Jefferson University, Philadelphia; Associate Surgeon, Cornea Service, Wills Eye Hospital, Philadelphia
26. Corneal Changes from Ocular Surgery

Mark A. Rayfield, Ph.D.
Assistant Chief for International Laboratory Activities, Retrovirus Diseases Branch, Centers for Disease Control and Prevention, Atlanta
10. Herpes Simplex Viral Infections

Jeffrey B. Robin, M.D.
Clinical Associate Professor of Ophthalmology, Case Western Reserve University School of Medicine, Cleveland
23. Immunologic Disorders of the Cornea and Conjunctiva

Steven B. Robin, M.D.
Assistant Professor of Ophthalmology, University of Minnesota Medical School, Minneapolis; Staff Ophthalmologist, Ramsey Clinic/St. Paul Ramsey Medical Center, St. Paul
23. Immunologic Disorders of the Cornea and Conjunctiva

Allan Richard Rutzen, M.D.
Assistant Professor of Ophthalmology, University of Maryland School of Medicine, Baltimore; Assistant Professor of Ophthalmology, University of Maryland Medical Systems, Baltimore
15. Parasitic Infections

Ward E. Shine, Ph.D.
Assistant Professor of Ophthalmology, University of Texas Southwestern Medical School, Dallas
4. Meibomianitis

Stephen G. Slade, M.D., F.A.C.S.
Clinical Faculty, Department of Ophthalmology, University of Texas Medical School, Houston
43. Laser-Assisted In Situ Keratomileusis

Walter J. Stark, M.D.
Professor of Ophthalmology, Johns Hopkins University School of Medicine, Baltimore; Director, Cornea Service, The Wilmer Ophthalmological Institute, Johns Hopkins Hospital, Baltimore
30. Phototherapeutic Keratectomy

Raymond M. Stein, M.D., F.R.C.S.C.
Assistant Professor of Ophthalmology, University of Toronto Faculty of Medicine, Ontario; Chief of Ophthalmology, Scarborough General Hospital, Toronto, Ontario
27. Corneal Changes from Contact Lenses

Alan Sugar, M.D.
Professor of Ophthalmology, W.K. Kellogg Eye Center, University of Michigan Medical School, Ann Arbor
20. Corneal and Conjunctival Degenerations

Joel Sugar, M.D.
Professor of Ophthalmology and Director of Cornea Service, University of Illinois College of Medicine, Chicago
17. Metabolic Disorders of the Cornea

Hugh R. Taylor, M.D., F.R.A.C.S., F.R.A.C.O., F.A.C.S., F.A.A.O.
Ringland Anderson Professor of Ophthalmology, University of Melbourne, Melbourne, Victoria, Australia; Director of Eye Services, Corneal Unit, Royal Victorian Eye and Ear Hospital, Melbourne, Victoria, Australia
42. Photoastigmatic Refractive Keratectomy

William M. Townsend, M.D.
Professor and Chairman of Ophthalmology, University of Puerto Rico School of Medicine, San Juan; Attending Physician, Department of Surgery, Auxilio Motuo Hospital, San Juan, Puerto Rico
16. Congenital Anomalies of the Cornea; 21. Pterygium

Edward W. Trudo, M.D.
Clinical Assistant Professor of Surgery, Uniformed Services University of the Health Sciences, Bethesda, Maryland; Clinical Fellow, Cornea Service, The Wilmer Ophthalmological Institute, Johns Hopkins Hospital, Baltimore
30. Phototherapeutic Keratectomy

George O. Waring III, M.D., F.A.C.S., F.R.C.Ophth.
Professor of Ophthalmology and Director of Refractive Surgery, Emory University School of Medicine, Atlanta; Professor of Ophthalmology, Emory University Hospital, Atlanta
37. Radial Keratotomy

Steven E. Wilson, M.D.
Director of the Eye Laser Center and Professor of Cell Biology, Neurobiology, and Anatomy, The Cleveland Clinic Foundation, Health Sciences Center of the Ohio State University, Cleveland
33. Corneal Preservation for Penetrating Keratoplasty

Thomas O. Wood, M.D.
Clinical Professor of Ophthalmology, University of Tennessee, Memphis College of Medicine
31. Inlay Lamellar Keratoplasty

Foreword

A century ago, the cornea was considered an inert tunic that could be clouded by trauma or "disease"—the latter from unidentifiable causes. As on most other medical frontiers, progress in understanding the cornea has since increased rapidly. Particular milestones have been the introductions of keratoplasty, the slit lamp, antibiotics, steroids, antivirals, and many other additions that collectively make up our present armamentarium. This ever-expanding mass of knowledge has, only during the last few decades, resulted in the emergence of the management of corneal diseases as a distinct subspecialty and has required the creation of ever larger and more detailed textbooks by multiple authors. This treatise, edited by Drs. Kaufman, Barron, and McDonald, is for the moment the most comprehensive of its kind and is now in its second edition. Due to his vast research contributions to the field, Dr. Kaufman is a most suitable lead editor. His co-editors and other contributors are also known experts in their particular subjects, guaranteeing the high quality of this book. It is highly recommended as a reference for ophthalmology departments and individual practices alike.

Claes H. Dohlman, M.D., Ph.D.

Preface

Ten years have passed since the first edition of *The Cornea* was published. Since then, numerous advances have been made in the understanding and treatment of corneal disorders. Laboratory techniques once considered exotic are now commonplace, and previously theoretical technologies are now taken for granted. The second edition of *The Cornea* has been updated, revised, reorganized, and expanded to include these advances. To accomplish this, a multitude of authors who are experts in their fields have contributed their wealth of knowledge. The format has been improved: Gone are the color plates; color figures are presented where cited in the text.

The goal of the second edition of *The Cornea* is the same as that of the first edition: to provide a pragmatic approach to the diagnosis and treatment of corneal disorders based on state-of-the-art knowledge and expert experience. We believe that this approach is more useful to our readers than a less selective compendium of encyclopedic information without a distinct point of view. In this second edition, we hope to provide a comprehensive overview of the cornea—basic science, pathology, and treatment—as we see it today and into the next millennium.

Herbert E. Kaufman, M.D.
Bruce A. Barron, M.D.
Marguerite B. McDonald, M.D., F.A.C.S.

Acknowledgments

The editors would like to acknowledge and thank Paula Gebhardt for editorial assistance, Jerry Sewell for medical illustration, and Maxine Haslauer for medical photography.

I

Basic Science

1

Structure and Function of the Cornea

STEPHEN D. KLYCE AND ROGER W. BEUERMAN

The cornea is a unique portion of the outer, fibrous ocular tunic that is transparent and serves a refractive function while maintaining a mechanically tough and chemically impermeable barrier between the eye and the environment. In concert with the evolutionary development of vision, the cornea became structurally and functionally specialized to achieve the required optical properties. It evolved as an avascular structure that meets its oxygen requirements largely from the atmosphere via the anterior corneal surface and most of its additional nutritional requirements from the aqueous humor via the posterior corneal surface. Some of the protective functions and optical properties of the cornea are derived from adjacent tissues, such as the conjunctiva and lacrimal glands, which provide secretions that are spread over the cornea by the blinking action of the eyelids, resulting in a smooth anterior corneal surface. The mechanical strength of the cornea is provided by its collagen matrix, which is different from that of skin or the contiguous sclera and which requires the presence of mechanisms that regulate hydration to maintain transparency. For protection, the cornea is endowed with exquisitely sensitive nerves. In contrast to skin, where nerves have anatomically complex endings, the cornea relies on free nerve endings because specialized neural receptors would compromise corneal transparency.

This chapter focuses on the basic anatomy and physiology of the cornea to provide a foundation for understanding both corneal diseases and current and potential medical and surgical approaches to their treatment.

ANATOMY

Gross Anatomy

The eye is composed of three concentric tunics: an outer fibrous shell, a middle uveal tract, and an inner neuroretina. The cornea makes up one-sixth of the outer tunic; the sclera makes up the other five-sixths. The cornea is a clear transparent tissue that joins the opaque sclera at the corneoscleral limbus.

Although the cornea is circular when viewed from the posterior surface, it is oval when viewed from the anterior surface because of a more prominent limbus superiorly and inferiorly. The average diameters of the cornea are 12.6 mm horizontally and 11.7 mm vertically.

The anterior surface of the cornea is not uniformly curved. The central one-third of the cornea is called the optical zone and is approximately spherical. The average radius of curvature of the anterior surface centrally is 7.8 mm. As the major refractive surface of the eye, the anterior surface of the cornea provides approximately 48 diopters of power. The peripheral cornea is flattened, more so nasally than temporally. The posterior surface of the cornea is more spherical than the anterior surface. Therefore, the central cornea is thinner (520 μm) than the peripheral cornea (650 μm or more).

Microscopic Anatomy

The cornea can be divided into five layers: the epithelium, Bowman's layer, stroma, Descemet's membrane, and the endothelium (Figure 1-1). Although the preocular tear film is not part of the cornea, it is intimately associated with the cornea anatomically and functionally and is also described below.

Tear Film

The surface of the cornea must be kept moist to prevent damage to the epithelium, and this moisture must be evenly spread across the anterior membranes of the epithelial cells to prevent local drying. For the cornea to func-

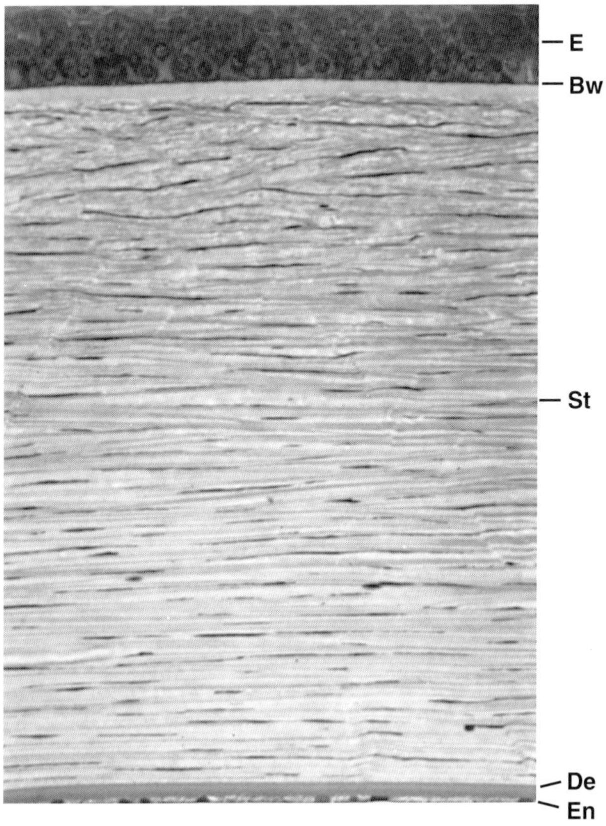

FIGURE 1-1 The cornea is a layered structure consisting of the epithelium (*E*), Bowman's layer (*Bw*), stroma (*St*), Descemet's membrane (*De*), and the endothelium (*En*).

tion as an optical lens, smoothing of the epithelial surface is needed because reticulations 0.5 μm high and 0.3 μm wide on the epithelial surface are a potential source of image degradation[1] (Figure 1-2). This moisture and smoothing are provided by the preocular tear film, in conjunction with the spreading function of the eyelids during blinking.

The tear film is 7 μm thick. There are two structurally identifiable layers: a thin (0.5 μm) anterior lipid layer derived from meibomian gland secretions and a thick (6 μm or more) aqueous layer into which a mucin-rich glycocalyx extends. The lipid layer retards evaporation from the preocular tear film, which prevents drying between blinks.

Aqueous tears are supplied primarily by the lacrimal gland located in the superior temporal orbit[2] at a rate of approximately 1.2 μl/min.[3] Normally, tears flow through the puncta and canaliculi to the nasolacrimal sac, which drains to the inferior nasal meatus via the nasolacrimal duct. Tears also leave the eye by evaporation and conjunctival absorption. Although the ocular surface is a good barrier against diffusion of polar and physically large substances, water can move, within limits, back and forth between the ocular interior and the tears, which to some extent can offset the effects of evaporation. The rate of evaporation, which is approximately 3 μl/hr at 30 percent relative humidity,[4] is significantly reduced in humid environments and increases in dry environments. Evaporation has the potential to elevate tear film osmolarity. In normal humans, the osmolarity may be as high as 318 mOsm,[5] which is 10 to 15 mOsm higher than the osmolarity of the aqueous humor.

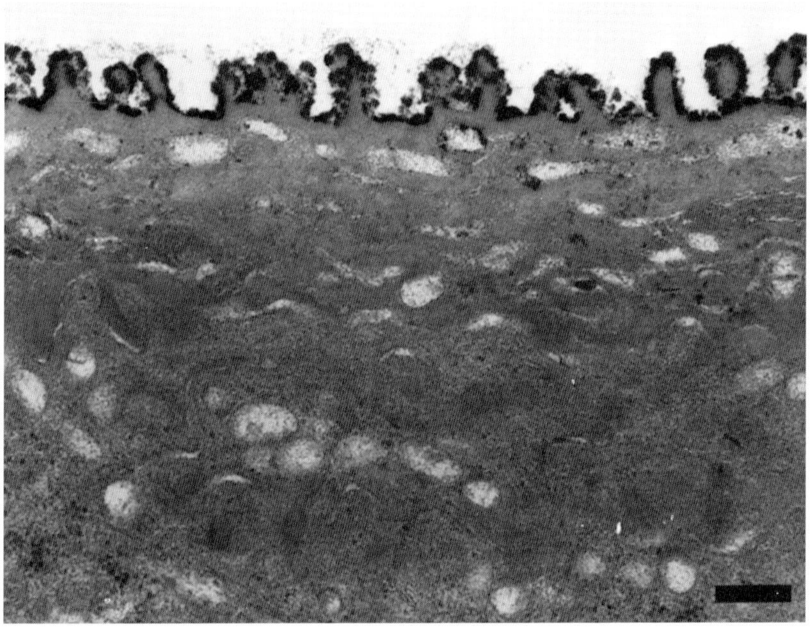

FIGURE 1-2 Electron micrograph of the epithelial surface and microprojections of the outer membrane. The mucoid substances of the tear film have dried onto the surface and are seen as electron-dense deposits. The actual thickness of the tear film extends beyond the height of the microprojections. (Bar, 0.3 μm.)

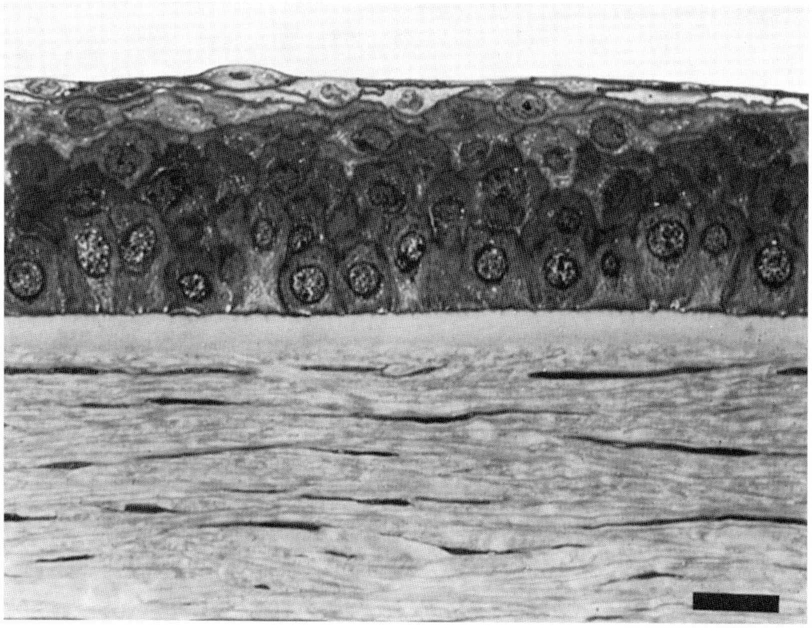

FIGURE 1-3 Light micrograph of the central corneal epithelium and anterior portion of the stroma. As the cells mature, they move anteriorly, forming the superficial cell layer. At this power, it is evident that the cytoplasm of the superficial cell layer contains fewer stainable structures, compared with the cytoplasm of the cells in the other layers of the epithelium. (Bar, 20 μm.)

The tear mucin is secreted by conjunctival goblet cells. It had been thought that mucin was compacted and absorbed onto the epithelial surface to form an anchoring layer for the tear film. However, it is more likely that mucin associates with the epithelial surface glycocalyx rather than interacting directly with epithelial surface membranes, forming a several-microns-thick hydrophilic coating on the corneal surface (see Figure 1-2), which may extend throughout the tear film. Such a layer has been best demonstrated by Nichols et al.[6]

Epithelium

The nonkeratinized, stratified squamous epithelium of the cornea consists of four to six layers of cells and represents 10 percent of the corneal thickness.[7] The epithelium is divided morphologically into three layers: the superficial or squamous cell layer, the middle or wing cell layer, and the deep or basal cell layer (Figure 1-3). The basal cells are the only epithelial cells that undergo mitosis. The daughter cells thus formed push anteriorly and change their shape, conforming to the contiguous wing cells, which are defined by the way they overlap onto the apices of the underlying basal cells. As the cells continue to move anteriorly, they become the superficial cells, after which they disintegrate and are shed into the tear film in a process known as desquamation. The superficial cells represent the highest level of differentiation and are, chronologically, the oldest epithelial cells. The epithelium turns over approximately every 7 days.[8] At the limbus, the corneal epithelium graduates into transitional epithelium and then into conjunctival epithelium[9] (Figure 1-4).

Superficial Cells Although the superficial cells of the epithelium ultimately undergo cellular disintegration and desquamation, they have unique specializations that maintain the tear film and the barrier that separates the extracellular space of the cornea from the tears. There are usually two layers of superficial cells. The cells are polygonal in shape and 40 to 60 μm in diameter. Confocal microscopic views of human corneal epithelium confirm the regular appearance of the superficial cells and permit direct observation of departures from the hexagonal arrangement in vivo (Figure 1-5). At the nucleus, superficial cells are 4 to 6 μm thick; peripherally, they are only 2 μm thick. The surface membranes of these cells are distinctive in two respects: they have microscopic projections (microvilli, reticulations, and microplicae) and the outer leaflet is thickened and supports an extensive fibrillar glycocalyx, also called the buffy coat. The increased surface area that results from folding of the surface membrane increases the adherence of the mucin layer of the tear film to the glycocalyx. The thickened outer leaflet and the fine filaments that emerge into the tear film may also play a role in the mechanism of adherence of the tear film to the superficial cells.[10] Light-, medium-, and dark-appearing superficial cells are distinguished by scanning electron microscopy, depending on the amount and pattern of microplicae[11-13] (Figure 1-6). Light cells are the youngest of the superficial cells, those that are newly arrived at the surface; dark cells are hypermature and are about to desquamate. Dark cells pos-

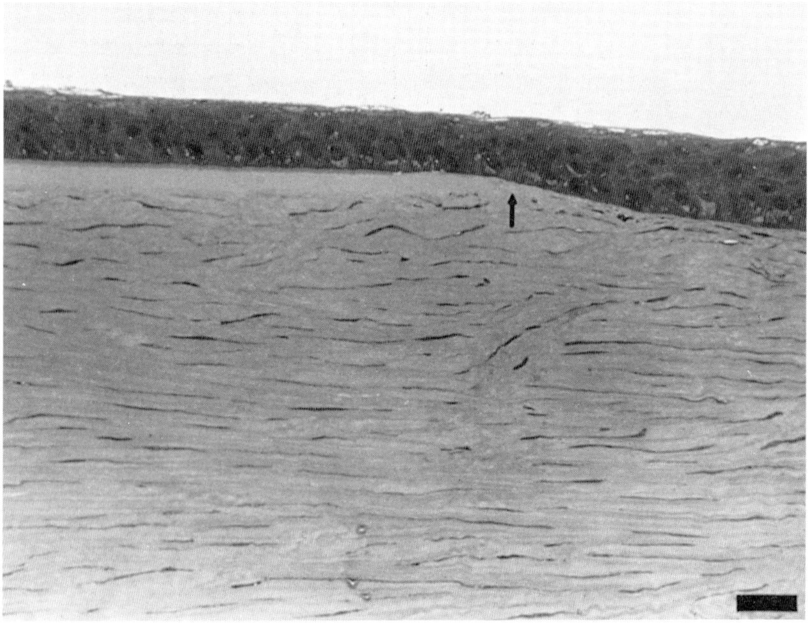

FIGURE 1-4 The termination of Bowman's layer (arrow) marks the transition of the corneal epithelium seen on the left side of the micrograph to the thicker and less organized conjunctival epithelium on the right. (Bar, 50 μm.)

sess few surface features; their surface is less rough than that of light cells.

During the process of superficial cell replacement, tear film continuity is preserved by the emergence of the underlying cell before the loss of the superficial cell (Figure 1-7). Holes form and deepen in the membrane of the superficial cell, eventually exposing the surface membrane of the underlying cell.[11,13] At the same time, junctional arrangements of the superficial cell with those of the underlying cell are broken. Normal superficial cells have many desmosomal attachments, which provide lateral mechanical stability (Figure 1-8A). During desquamation, the desmosomes are broken or dissolved. The newly exposed surface of the underlying cell develops typical surface projections and is covered by the tear film. Formation of a hole in the tear film, which may occur when desquamation is uneven, may lead to the development of dry spots and, eventually, dellen.[14] Abnormal desquamation is associated with a dull, dry corneal surface and is accompanied by a breakdown of the epithelial barrier function.

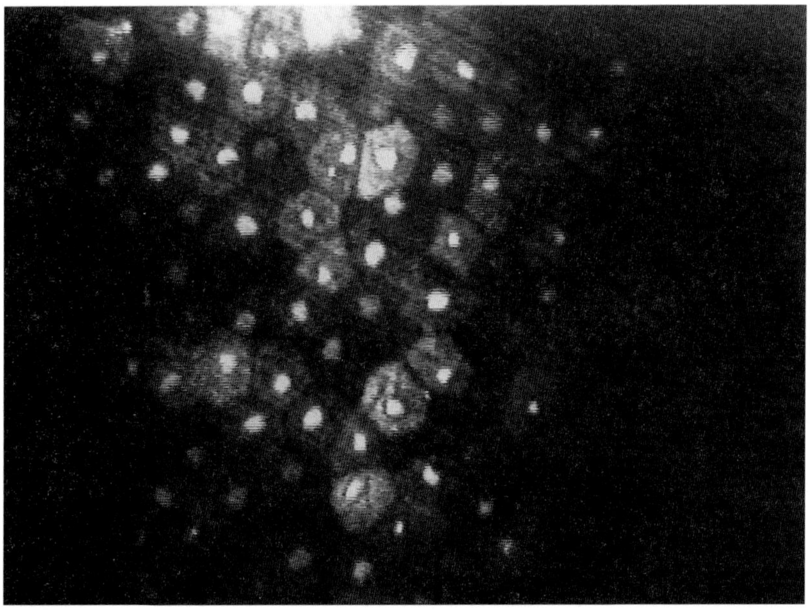

FIGURE 1-5 Confocal micrograph of the corneal epithelium. The corneal surface shows a regular arrangement of cells with some suggestion of differences in the surface reflectivity similar to what would be expected with scanning electron microscopy. (Original magnification × 230.)

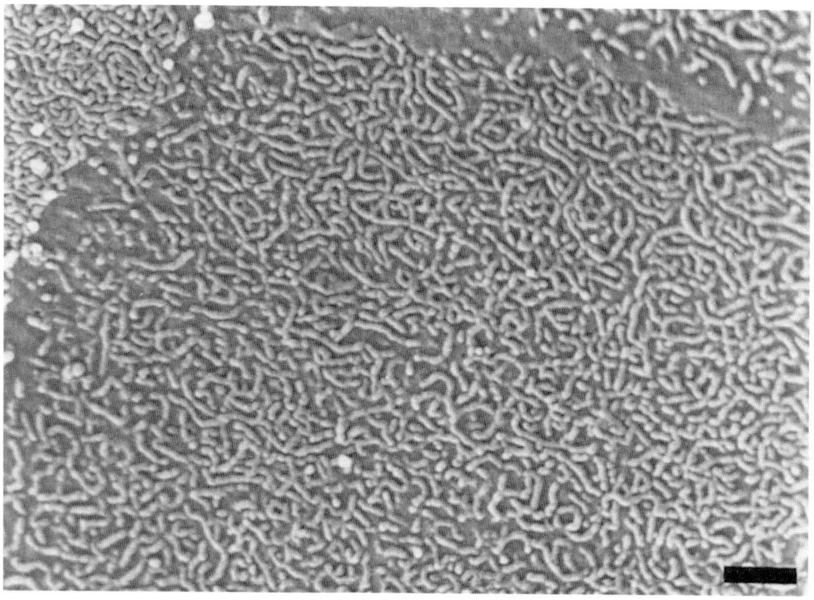

FIGURE 1-6 Projections of the outer membrane of the surface cells into the tear film, readily seen by scanning electron microscopy, are indicative of younger cells. Lateral borders of neighboring surface cells overlap, as seen at the top and left. (Bar, 5 μm.)

An important property of the superficial cell layer is the junctional complex formed with laterally adjacent cells. This complex consists of ribbon-like tight junctions that surround the entire cell[15] (Figure 1-8B). The joining of adjacent superficial cells at their lateral borders in this manner prevents the movement of substances from the tear film into the intercellular spaces of the epithelium. Tight junctions also resist the flow of fluid through the epithelial surface. If aqueous humor passes into the stroma because of either a damaged endothelium or high pressure within the eye, it is trapped within the epithelium, resulting in epithelial edema and bullae.

The junctional complex is the anatomic representation of the barrier property of the epithelium and is the anatomic substrate of the paracellular (between cells) pathway measured in electrophysiologic studies.[16] A clinical test to determine whether this barrier is intact uses dyes, such as fluorescein, which are instilled into the conjunc-

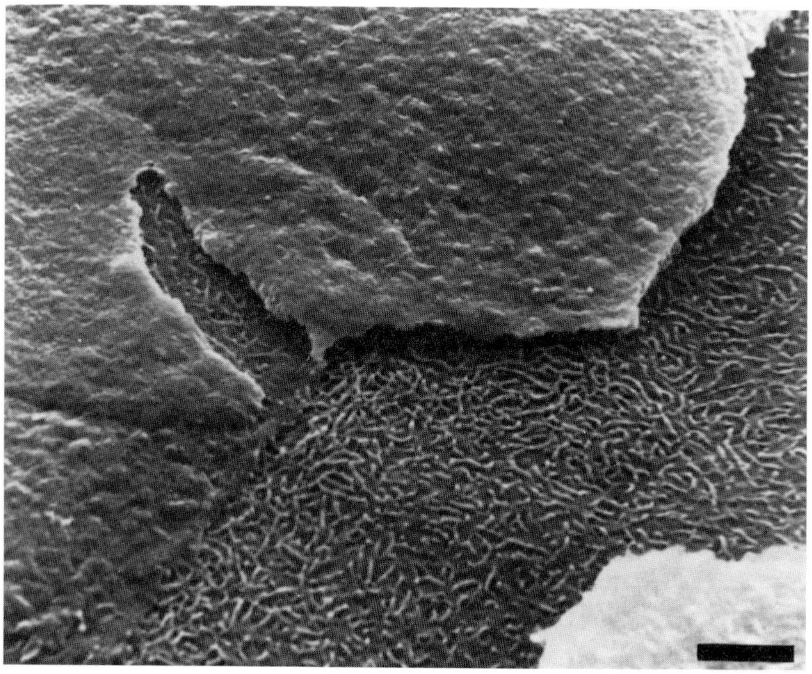

FIGURE 1-7 Scanning electron micrograph illustrating a late stage in the process of normal desquamation. The free surface of the underlying cell is emerging from beneath the smooth-surfaced cell it will replace. (Bar, 5 μm.)

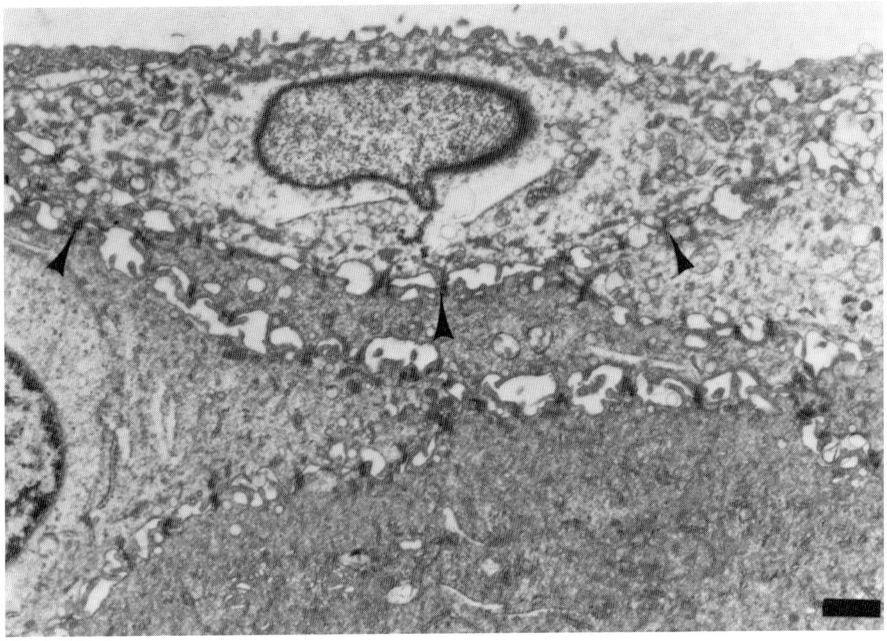

A

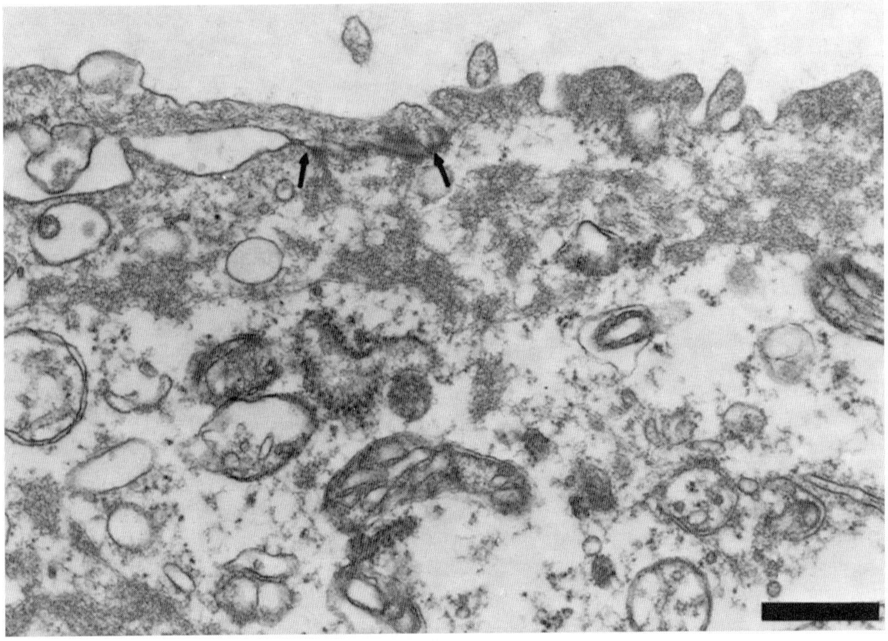

B

FIGURE 1-8 Electron micrographs illustrating the structure of the most superficial cells and their relation to cells that are subjacent. **(A)** The few cellular constituents and homogeneous chromatin of the nucleus are typical of the outermost cells. Although the free outer surface in contact with the tears is thrown into microprojections, surfaces in contact with other cells are tightly bound by many desmosome contacts (arrowheads). (Bar, 1 μm.) **(B)** At their margins, the superficial cells form focal tight junctions (arrows) that restrict the passage of substances from the tears into the extracellular space of the epithelium. (Bar, 0.5 μm.)

tival sac. The normal epithelial surface stains little or not at all. Rubbing the corneal surface under the closed eyelids damages the fragile surface cells, resulting in punctate staining.[17] Diabetic patients have increased surface staining, which suggests that the barrier property of the epithelium is impaired, although the cause is unknown.[18] Several factors, such as rapid or abnormal epithelial cell loss or the inability to form tight junctions, could lead to surface staining in diabetic patients.

The superficial cells have few organelles. Although these cells have a limited life span, the maintenance of the glycocalyx probably requires some synthetic source.[19] Generally, the surface cells are nucleated; however, the nuclei may disintegrate before desquamation. The relatively lucent

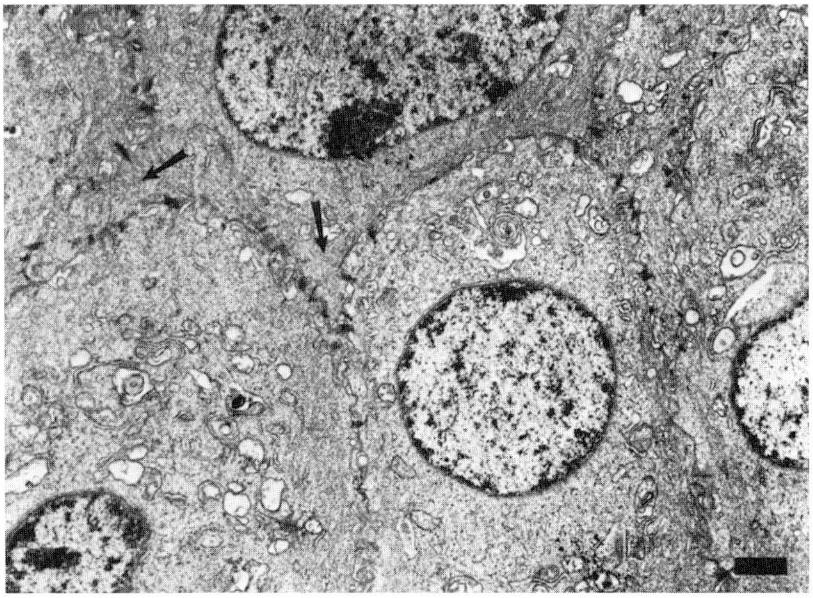

FIGURE 1-9 Lateral projections (arrows) that overhang the dome-like apices of the basal cells (bottom) give the wing cell its characteristic appearance and name. (Bar, 1 μm.)

cytoplasm of the superficial cells is the result of a paucity of the fibrillar material that is seen in greater abundance in the wing and basal cells; however, the cytoplasm does contain some free ribosomes and fragments of cisternae of endoplasmic reticulum. The Golgi complex, which is considered necessary for the export of synthesized proteins, is generally poorly developed. The mitochondria are small and the cristae are sparse.[9] Some tonofilaments are associated with the desmosomes. More interesting is the presence of a layer of actin filaments, also called microfilaments, that lie parallel to and just beneath the cell membrane. The microvilli and microplicae have cores of actin filaments, which may allow some movement of the surface projections.[20] Collapse of the actin network could be a prelude to the smooth surface appearance of hypermature cells.

Wing Cells The wing cell layer reveals the foreshortening that occurs during the transition from basal cells to superficial cells (Figure 1-9). Nuclei in this region are round or somewhat elongated in a direction parallel to the surface. At their periphery, the cells are extensively interdigitated and joined by desmosomal junctions and gap junctions (Figure 1-10A). Mats of tonofilaments fill the wing cell cytoplasm, along with a few microtubules (Figure 1-10B). The tonofilaments are also known as intermediate filaments because of their diameter (about 8 nm), which is intermediate between the diameters of the microfilaments and the microtubules. These filamentous bands may spread across the cell and help maintain its shape. Tonofilaments often loop through the inner placode of the desmosomes, possibly contributing to their structural properties. Other cell organelles, such as mitochondria, are also present in the wing cells, but not in large numbers.

Basal Cells The columnar basal cells are 18 to 20 μm high and 8 to 10 μm in diameter. They represent the germinative layer of the epithelium and possess many more cytoplasmic organelles than the more anterior layers (Figure 1-11). The mitochondria are small and are found in moderate numbers around the nuclei and in the posterior portion of the basal cells. The cristae of the mitochondria are irregular and laminated. Although the Golgi complex is prominent during embryonic development, it is much less so in the mature epithelium and is usually found anterior to the nucleus (Figure 1-12). The Golgi complex is closely associated with the endoplasmic reticulum and, sometimes, an area of continuity can be found. The cytoplasm of the basal cell has large numbers of glycogen granules, which represent a source of stored metabolic energy to be used in times of epithelial stress, such as wound healing. Scattered ribosomes and segments of rough endoplasmic reticulum complete the usual array of organelles. The mats of tonofilaments, which are arrayed in both of the major dimensions of the cell, and the microtubules make up an elaborate cytoskeleton. Actin filaments are seen along the cytoplasmic side of the membrane and may be important for cell migration in the healing of abrasions during which these cells may become motile.[20] At the lateral borders, the basal cells are extensively interdigitated and joined together in places by zonula adherens and gap junctions. At their posterior surface, the cells are flat and rest on the basal lamina, to which they are attached by hemidesmosomes (Figures 1-13 and 1-14).

Basal Lamina and Bowman's Layer

Light microscopy of the human cornea demonstrates a wide, 8- to 12-μm band of amorphous material along

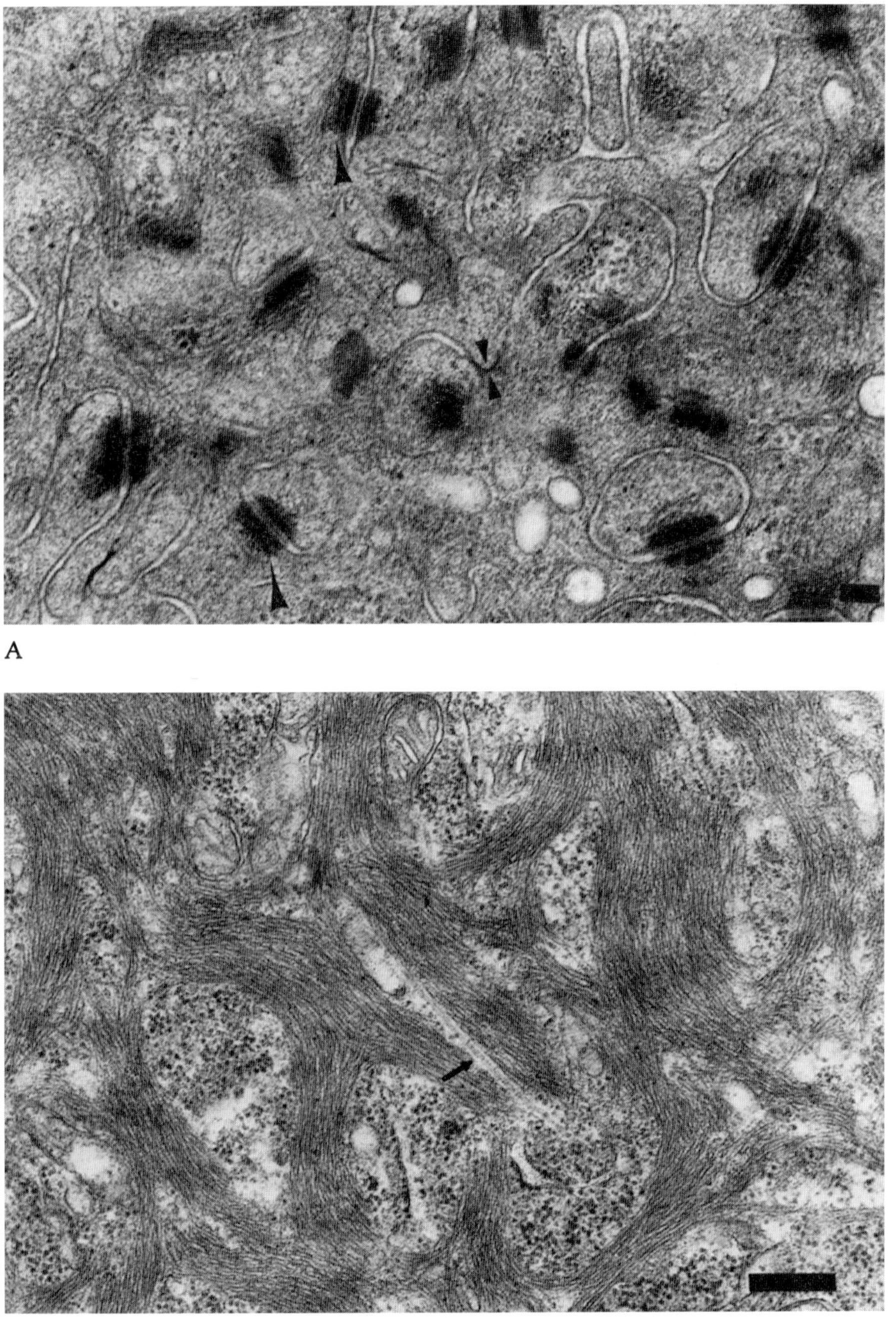

A

B

FIGURE 1-10 **(A)** A horizontal section at the level of the wing cell overlap with basal cells shows the elaborate interdigitation of the processes of adjacent cells. Desmosomes (arrowheads) provide mechanical stability, whereas gap junctions (double arrowheads) are involved in intercellular communication. (Bar, 0.1 μm.) **(B)** An intracellular network of fibrils is responsible for maintaining the three-dimensional structure of the wing cell. Extensive mats of tonofilaments and a microtubule (arrow) are shown in this electron micrograph. (Bar, 0.1 μm.)

the anterior surface of the stroma. Bowman's layer (or membrane, as it has been referred to) does not regenerate after injury and is often thought to be involved in re-epithelialization of the cornea. However, that role can be ascribed more appropriately to the thin basement membrane, as it was termed by light microscopists, that lies anterior to Bowman's layer. The differentially staining band immediately below the basal epithelium, seen by light microscopy, is not identical to the basal lamina seen by electron microscopy. The former also includes material subjacent to the basal lamina that may consist of breakdown products from the basal lamina.

The basal lamina has two important functions: it forms the scaffold for the organization of the epithelium and it is a boundary that separates the epithelium from the stroma.[21] The electron microscopic structure of the basal lamina consists of an anterior clear zone, the lamina lucida, and a more obvious posterior dense zone, the lamina densa (see Figures 1-13 and 1-14). The basal lamina is an extracellular secretory product of the basal epithelial cells and is produced not only during embryonic development but also throughout adult life, although the rate of secretion is slow. The absence of the basal lamina can result in the ingrowth of epithelial cells into Bowman's layer or the anterior stroma. In the other direction, however, cells of vascular origin and Langerhans cells are able to penetrate both Bowman's layer and the basal lamina and invade the epithelium[22,23]; how this is accomplished is not understood. Clinically, various disease entities related to chronic epithelial defects are probably disorders of the basal lamina. The corneal epithelium may be present as a sheet, but it does not adhere to the underlying stroma without the basal lamina as an intermediary. The mechanism of adherence of the basal lamina to the stroma is not clear; however, anchoring filaments that radiate into the stromal collagen are probably involved.[24] Biochemical analysis of anchoring filaments has shown them to have a periodicity appropriate for type VII collagen and antibodies to this material are localized to the basal lamina.[25,26] Increased age and thickening of the basal lamina have been found to be associated with disruption of the anchoring filaments.[27] Studies on the corneas of diabetic patients have shown that the primary loss of adhesion occurs at the anchoring filaments.[28]

A study comparing basal lamina thickness in a series of corneas from diabetic patients with that from a group of age-matched normals[29] found that thickening of the basal lamina was associated with diabetes but not with age, race, sex, or duration of diabetes. Alvarado et al[27] found a linear increase in the thickness of the basal lamina with age in 45 corneas ranging in age from 17 weeks of gestation to 93 years. The lamina densa increased by approximately 40 percent from fetal life to early childhood, reaching 128 nm in these specimens. Although the number of older corneas was small, regression analysis indicated an increase of about 3 nm/yr. Multilaminar regions of basal lamina occurred more frequently in corneas from individuals older than 45 years of age, and every specimen from donors older than 60 years of age had areas of basal lamina reduplication. Reduplication has been suggested to be the result of repeated cell injury,[30] and it is reasonable to suppose that environmental stress over an extended period leads to increased production of basal lamina in older corneas. In multilaminar basal lamina, the anchoring filaments may extend only to the next deeper band of basal lamina, never coming into contact with stromal collagen. Thus, the epithelium is not tightly attached to the underlying cornea, and the cornea is susceptible to the consequences of poor or delayed epithelial healing. In this regard, it is interesting that epithelium removed from diabetic patients during vitrectomy often includes thickened or reduplicated basal lamina,[31,32] indicating that the basal lamina is poorly attached to the stroma (Figure 1-15).

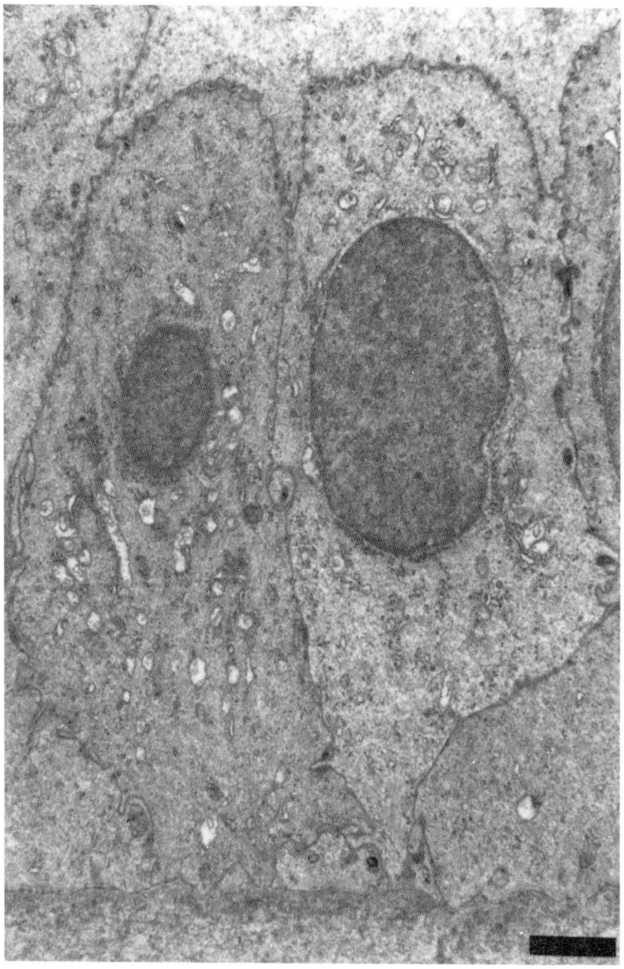

FIGURE 1-11 The nucleus is usually located in the anterior part of the basal cell, whereas the cytoplasm posteriorly is filled with cytoplasmic organelles, mitochondria, and components of the cytoskeleton. (Bar, 3 μm.)

Until recently, very little was known about the biochemical composition of the basal lamina; however, some of the constituents have now been identified and have been shown to have clinical importance in the understanding of corneal disease. The use of monoclonal antibodies to components of the extracellular matrix has furthered our understanding of basal lamina substructure. Generally, the biochemical structure is similar to that of the basal lamina of skin. Type IV collagen, which is probably found in the primary structural molecules of all adult basal lamina,[24] is present throughout the lamina densa.

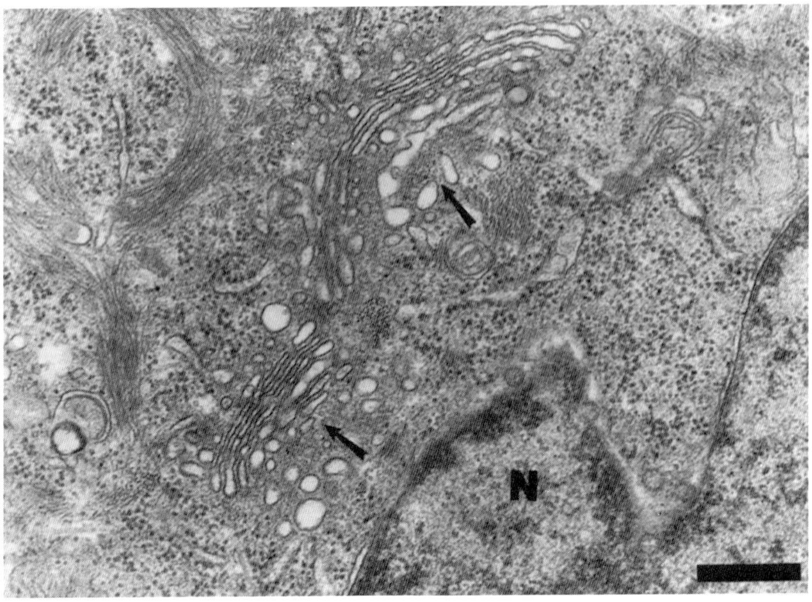

FIGURE 1-12 The Golgi complex (arrows) of the basal cell is relatively compact in that the lamellae are not numerous; however, its presence indicates the active metabolic status of these cells. In the adult, as shown here, the Golgi complex is located anterior to the nucleus (*N*). Note the many glycogen granules and the tonofilaments (upper left). (Bar, 0.5 μm.)

Laminin, a glycoprotein, is found in both the lamina densa and lamina lucida.[24,33] Fibronectin and fibrin are components of normal human basal lamina (Figure 1-16). Corneas of patients with keratoconus stain poorly for fibrin, which may signal part of the destruction of basal lamina seen in this disease.[34] Bullous pemphigoid antigen is found in the lamina lucida in skin and cornea.[35,36]

Biochemical resolution and identification of additional proteins made by both the epithelium and the keratocytes (collectively called extracellular matrix proteins) have added complexity to our understanding of interactions in the cornea. Fibronectin, which was one of the first members of this family to be identified, was found to increase in the anterior stroma after wounding.[37,38] Other extracellular matrix proteins are tenascin, vitronectin, and laminin. These proteins bind to cellular receptors called integrins and serve to regulate cellular responses to the environment.[39,40] The integrins that appear on the cell surface differ in the normal and wound-healing states. Specific complexes of integrins bind to the various extracellular matrix proteins, including those found along the basal lamina.

Bowman's layer is a layer of randomly arrayed collagen fibrils that merge into the more organized anterior

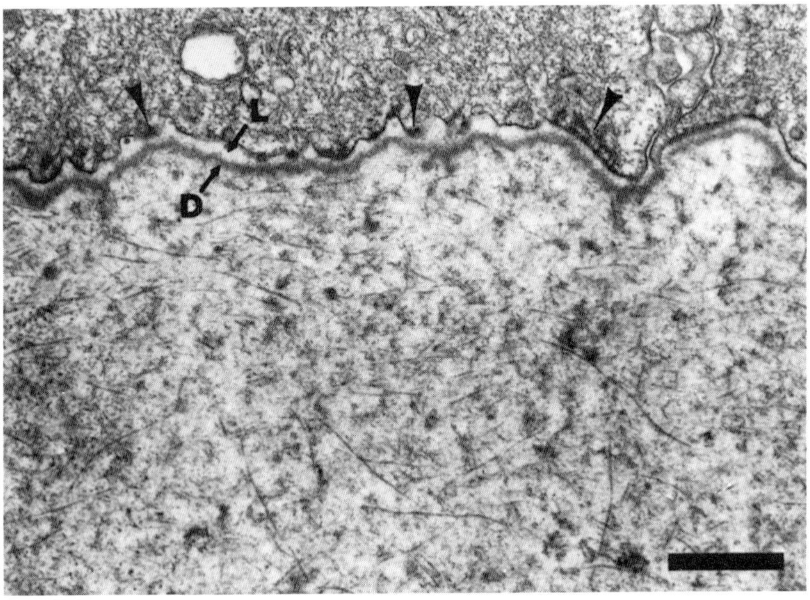

FIGURE 1-13 Along their flattened posterior membranes, the basal cells are secured to the corneal surface by mechanical junctions, the hemidesmosomes (arrowheads). The strength of the mechanical attachment is primarily based on the large number of sites. This structural complex must be severed during wound healing and postmitotic anterior migration. Note the two layers of the basal lamina: lamina lucida (*L*) and lamina densa (*D*). The collagen fibrils of Bowman's layer (bottom) are randomly arranged. (Bar, 1 μm.)

stroma (Figures 1-13 and 1-17). The diameter of the collagen fibrils in Bowman's layer is approximately two-thirds the diameter of the collagen fibrils in the stroma. Ridges form in this fibrillar network under conditions of hypotony; the resultant uneven epithelial topography can be demonstrated by fluorescein staining.[41] Bowman's layer is attached to the stroma by collagen fibrils that insert into Bowman's layer and become part of the anterior stromal lamellae. High-voltage electron microscopy of the interface between Bowman's layer and stroma has shown paired fibrils 30 nm in diameter crossing from Bowman's layer into stroma.[42] If these fibrils could be shown to be continuous with the anchoring filaments, a true ultrastructural basis for epithelial adhesion could be described. Unmyelinated axons penetrate Bowman's layer irregularly across the corneal surface to provide epithelial innervation.[43] Bowman's layer is prominent in primates; although other mammals have a suggestion of a similar zone, it is very thin. Bowman's layer functions as a dome-like structure that is anchored to the limbus. Because of this, attempts to change the refractive power of the cornea by inserting lenses or gels into the stroma to alter the anterior corneal curvature have been relatively unsuccessful. Instead of altering the shape of Bowman's layer, these lenses and gels alter the shape of the less resistant posterior cornea. It is difficult, if not impossible, to change the shape of Bowman's layer, and hence the anterior corneal curvature, without first cutting through it and the underlying anterior stromal lamellae.

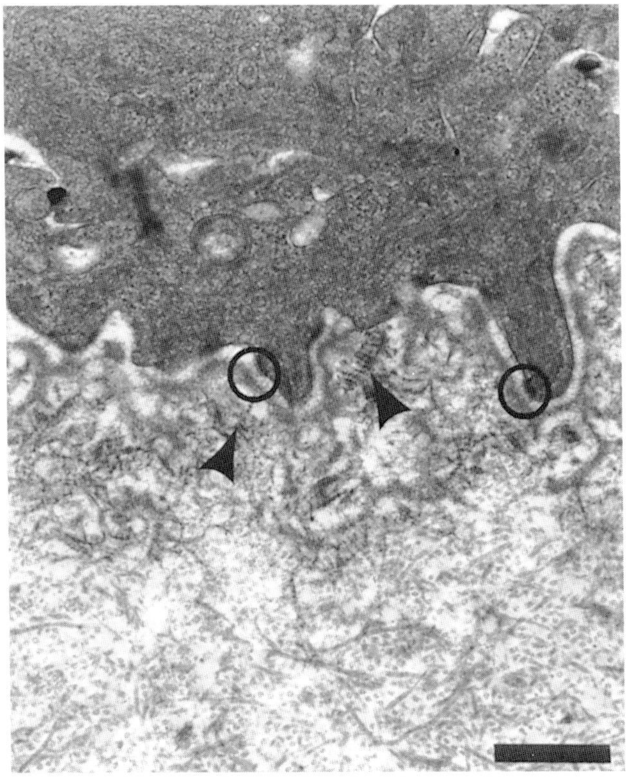

FIGURE 1-14 The hemidesmosome complex (circles) comprises intracellular and extracellular densities joined by fibrils. Additionally, densely staining fibrils, called anchoring filaments (arrowheads), leave the basal lamina and merge into the collagen of Bowman's layer, securing the attachment. (Bar, 0.5 μm.)

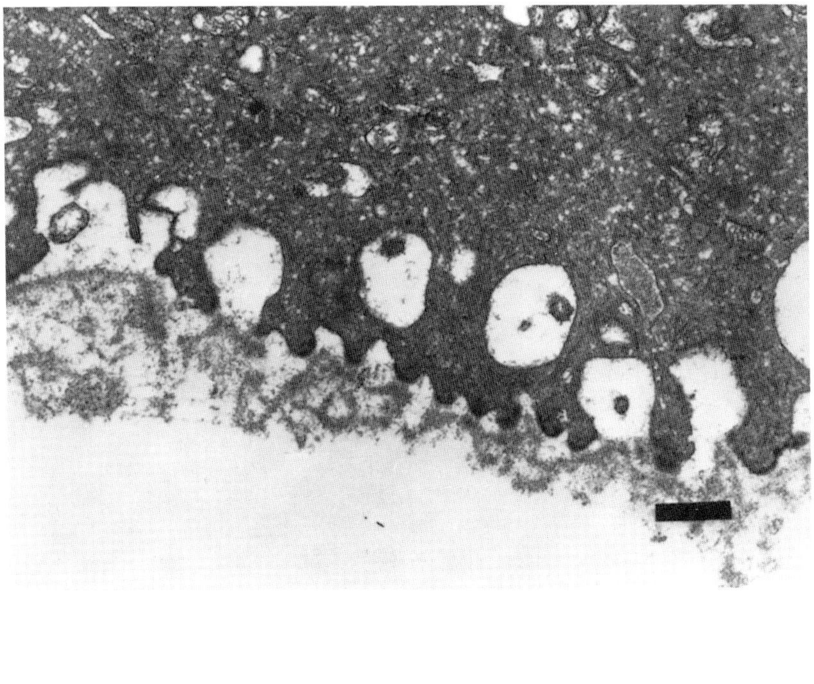

FIGURE 1-15 Electron micrograph illustrating early reduplication of basal lamina in a 59-year-old patient with diabetes. The epithelium was removed during vitrectomy. Vertical aggregates of basal lamina material extend from the unilaminar band beneath the epithelium. However, the hemidesmosome attachment sites onto the basal lamina are not disrupted. (Bar, 0.5 μm.)

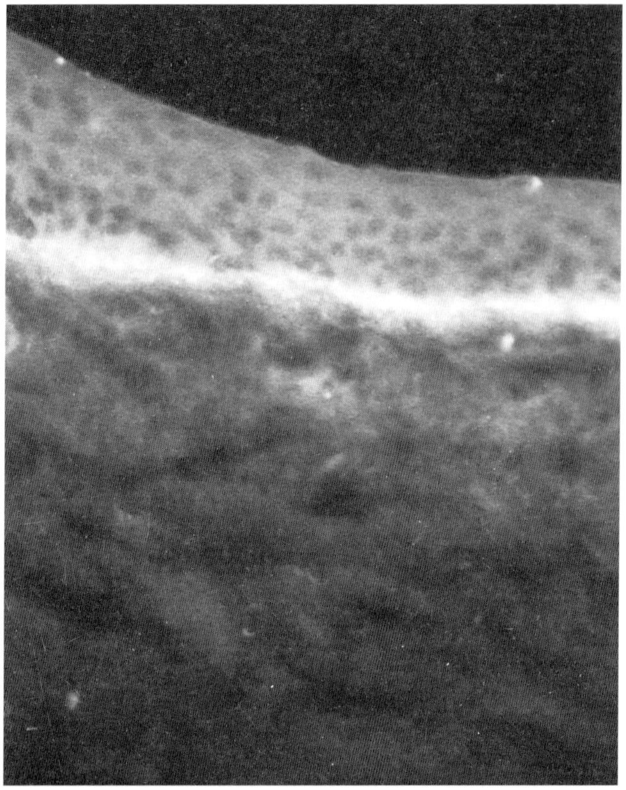

FIGURE 1-16 Indirect immunofluorescence demonstrating fibronectin in the basal lamina beneath the epithelium. Bowman's layer does not fluoresce. The basal lamina may be a sandwich of several types of molecules that, in combination, bond epithelial cells onto the stroma. When antibodies against type IV collagen or laminin are used in this procedure, localization is also seen in the basal lamina.

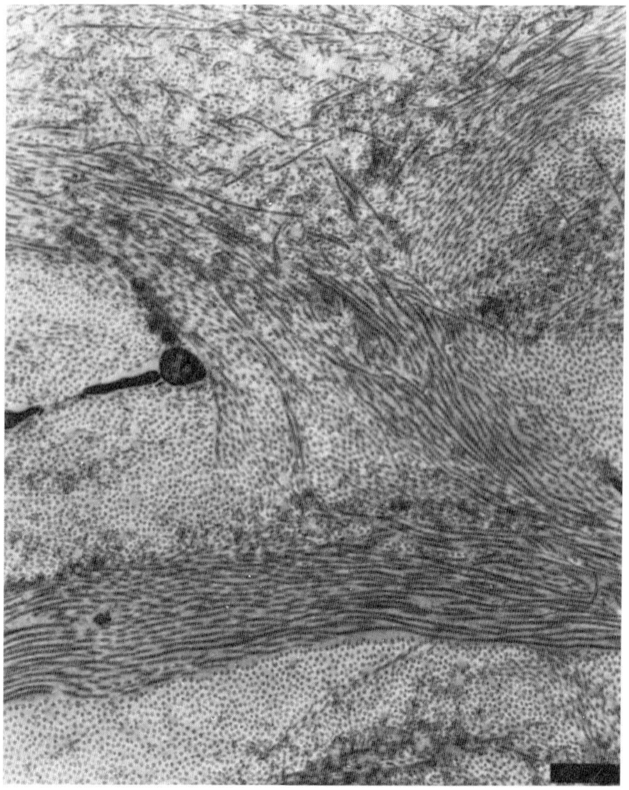

FIGURE 1-17 Random fibrils of Bowman's layer (top) are embedded in a matrix, which must be intercalated with the underlying collagen lamellae. The apparent mechanisms for this attachment reside in the physicochemical forces applied to collagen fibrils projecting into Bowman's layer. (Bar, 0.5 μm.)

Stroma

Stacked lamellae of collagen fibrils are the most obvious morphologic characteristic of the stroma, which constitutes about 90 percent of the corneal thickness. The layered arrangement is more regular in the posterior stroma than in the anterior stroma, where the lamellae are narrow and interleaved (Figure 1-18). Conventional histopathologic study often reveals artifactual spaces between lamellae caused by dislocation during processing. The cellular density in the stroma is low, with many keratocytes scattered throughout, primarily between lamellae. Nerve axons and their associated Schwann cells are found in the anterior and middle third of the stroma.

Collagen constitutes about 71 percent of the dry weight of the cornea and is the structural macromolecule providing tissue transparency and mechanical resistance to intraocular pressure.[34,44] In the quiescent cornea, both procollagen and collagen are secreted at a low basal rate; however, in the initial phase of healing of corneal wounds, collagen secretion may be greatly increased.[45] Although there is some disagreement about which collagen types are found in the corneas of various species, there is agreement that type I collagen predominates.[46] Additionally, there is strong evidence that types III and V collagen are found in the human cornea.[47]

The collagen fibrils, which are packed in parallel arrays,[48] make up the 300 to 500 lamellae of the stroma. The lamellae extend from limbus to limbus and are oriented at various angles to one another, less than 90 degrees in the anterior stroma but nearly orthogonal in the posterior stroma.[44] A random cross-sectional electron micrograph of the stroma, therefore, reveals some fibrils cut nearly perpendicularly and other fibrils cut tangentially (Figure 1-19). On electron microscopy, the fibrils appear to have uniform diameters; however, various studies have found mean diameters ranging from 22 to 32 nm.[49,50] At high magnification, the fibrils appear to have several small filaments, which may be the precursor subunits. In longitudinal view, the fibrils have a macroperiodicity of 64 nm, which is constant throughout the cornea. There is little variation in fibril size at different depths in the central cornea.

The collagen fibrils are surrounded by a polyanionic extracellular matrix, which may be important in maintaining the fairly constant separation distance of 60 nm between the centers of the fibrils.[1] The primary glycosaminoglycans of the stroma are keratan sulfate and chondroitin sulfate, which occur in a ratio of 3:1.[51] In culture, human keratocytes can be induced to produce dermatan sulfate and heparan sulfate, which may be analogous to wound healing.[52] Some regional differences may exist in the distribution of these substances. The concentration of keratan sulfate appears to be greatest in the central anterior stroma and least peripherally, where the concentration of chondroitin sulfate is increased. There is a rough correlation between the increase in the diameter of collagen fibrils (60 to 70 nm) peripherally and the decrease in keratan sulfate.[53]

The extracellular matrix interacts with the individual collagen fibrils. The physical basis for this is not clear, but it is probably not covalent binding. Electron microscopy, particularly after staining with ruthenium red, shows fine strands radiating from collagen fibrils in cross section. Electron microscopy after extraction of extracellular matrix material shows a loss of these radiating strands. Extraction of extracellular matrix material, which may occur in corneal edema, could result in a change in the interfibrillar distance and a decrease in the swelling response.

The keratocytes occupy 3 to 5 percent of the stromal volume. Their function is to maintain the collagen fibrils and extracellular matrix by a constant synthetic activity. Keratocytes in the normal cornea usually lie between collagen lamellae. The cell body contains a large nucleus (Figure 1-20). Although the cytoplasm is not extensive, free ribosomes, rough endoplasmic reticulum, and a prominent Golgi complex can be seen. Slender processes, which may taper to only one to several microns in cross section, leave the nuclear region at all angles (Figure 1-21A). Although these spatially extensive processes may penetrate into the collagen lamellae, they do not normally extend through the lamellae. However, within the lamellar plane, the tips of the processes sometimes touch those of a neighboring keratocyte and form a tight junction. The junctional interactions with neighboring keratocytes are believed to be important in the regulation of cell function.[54] Adjacent to the outer leaflet of the keratocyte membrane, small fibrillar bundles of recently synthesized collagen can be seen. Basal lamina-like material aggregates in patches around keratocytes, particularly in the peripheral cornea.[1] In some pathologic situations, particularly in endothelial dystrophy, and in refractive surgical procedures in which an impermeable material is placed in the stroma, keratocytes produce large amounts of basal lamina and basal lamina-like material that can result in opacities.[1] Keratocytes undergo extensive cellular transformation in response to wounding or acute edema, entering a fibroblastic state. The processes become less numerous, but in the vicinity of the wound, new keratocyte processes extend toward the damaged area (Figure 1-21B). Keratocytes, as well as epithelial cells, also have receptors for several growth factors. The action of growth factors on these cells may be important in the response of the cells to wounding.[54,55]

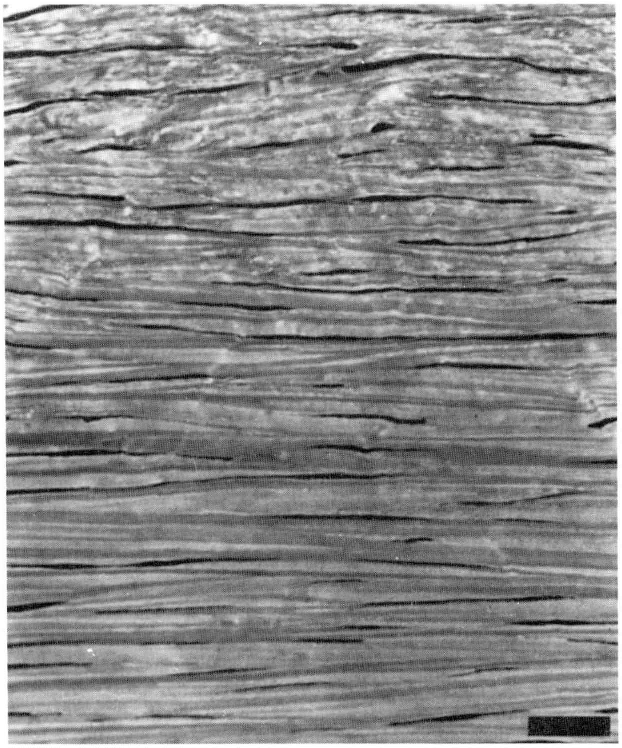

FIGURE 1-18 Light micrograph depicting the organization of the stromal lamellae. Anteriorly, the lamellae are interleaved, but in the middle and posterior thirds of the stroma, the lamellae are more compact. Keratocyte cell bodies largely reside at the interface of adjacent lamellae. (Bar, 50 μm.)

Descemet's Membrane

Descemet's membrane is the thick basal lamina secreted by the endothelium (Figure 1-22). It is composed of an anterior banded layer and a posterior nonbanded layer (Figure 1-23). Secretion of Descemet's membrane begins at approximately 4 months of gestation; the banding appears in the anterior layer before birth. Descemet's

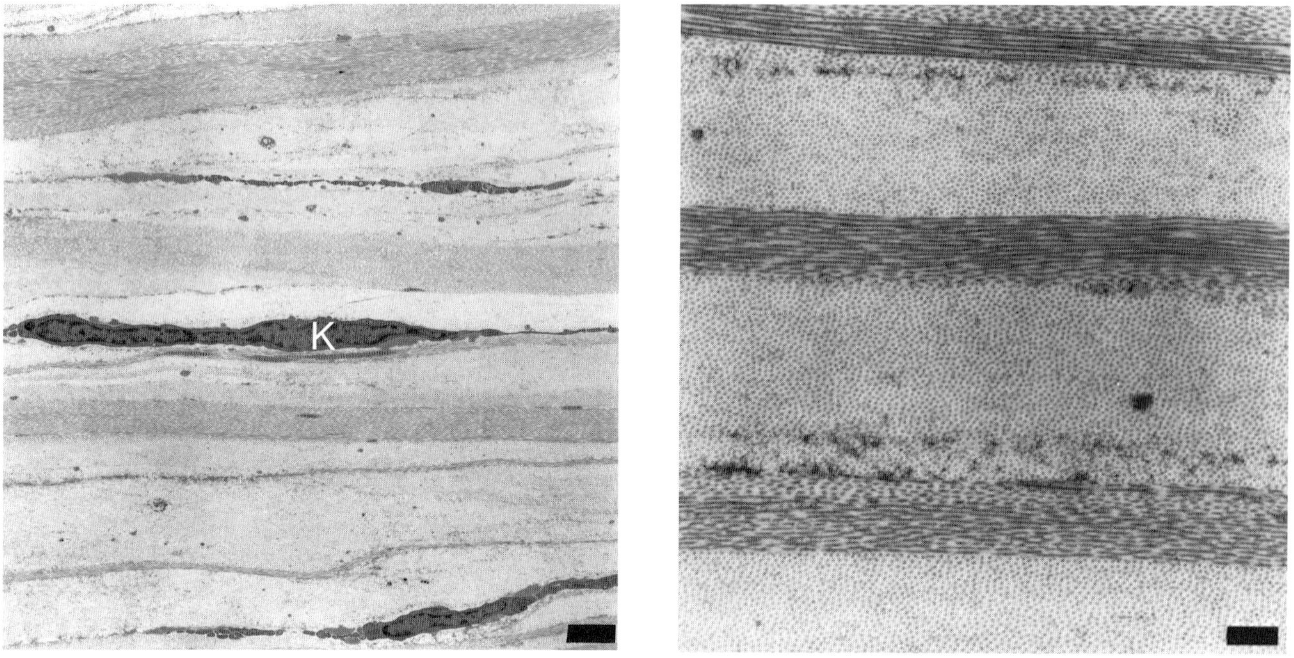

A B

FIGURE 1-19 **(A)** Electron micrograph demonstrating the alternating orientation of collagen lamellae in the midcentral stroma. *K,* keratocyte cell body. (Bar, 2 μm.) **(B)** Higher-power electron micrograph illustrating the regular arrangement of individual collagen fibrils within various lamellae. Each fibril is composed of several smaller subunits. (Bar, 0.5 μm.)

membrane increases in thickness during life, but this accumulation appears to be limited to the nonbanded posterior layer.[56] In a series of corneas from individuals 10 to 80 years of age, the 3-μm thickness of the banded anterior layer did not vary significantly.[56] In contrast, the thickness of the posterior layer in the same population increased from 2 to 10 μm with age.

Descemet's membrane is loosely attached to the stroma. Obvious mechanical attachment sites have not been seen by conventional electron microscopy, sug-

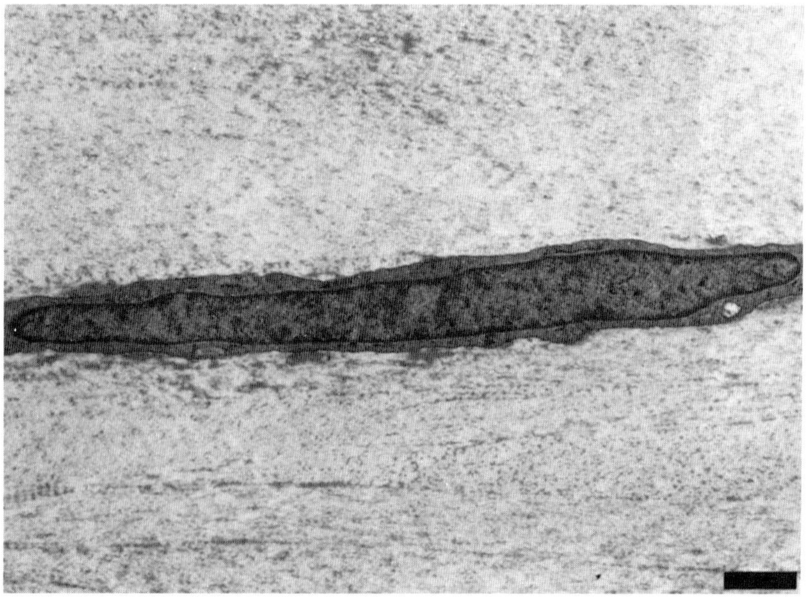

FIGURE 1-20 In the quiescent state, the keratocyte nucleus fills the cell body. The usual organelles are found in the cytoplasm. The cell body represents a region of decreased mechanical strength between adjacent collagen lamellae because it prevents exchange of fibrils between lamellae. Rupture of lamellae may be initiated at these sites, and leaching of the polyanionic material into the spaces is followed by water, creating edema. (Bar, 0.5 μm.)

FIGURE 1-21 By mounting the cornea flat after gold chloride staining, the spatial organization of keratocyte processes can be appreciated. (A) The micrograph is from a normal rabbit cornea and the cell processes are nearly symmetrical about the cell body. (B) The keratocytes in the vicinity of a stromal wound (to the left) elongate and become fibroblastic. (Bar, 100 μm.)

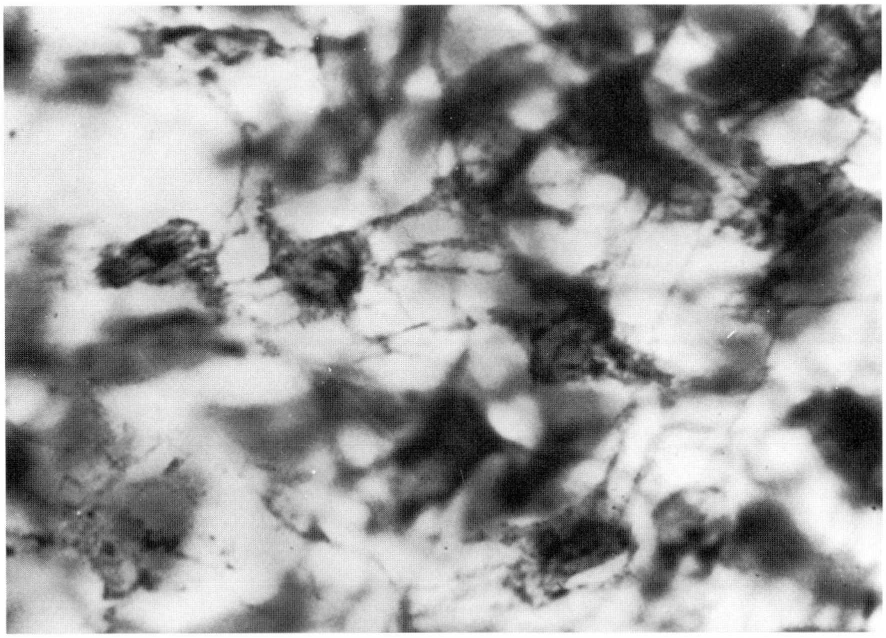

A

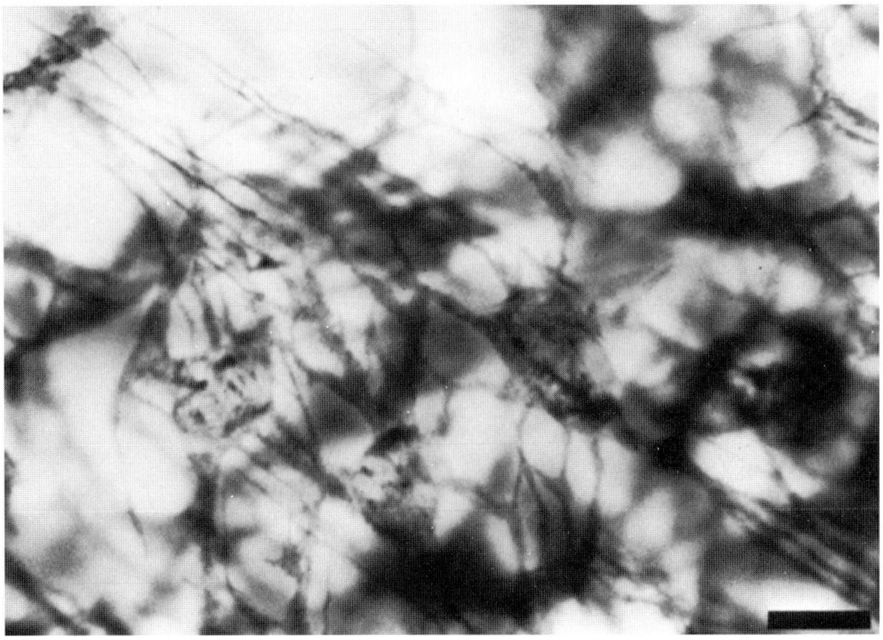

B

gesting that intraocular pressure may play a role in attachment. However, high-voltage electron microscopy has shown short, densely staining fibrils extending from the stroma into Descemet's membrane a few tenths of a micron.[42]

When sectioned in the plane of the cornea, the banded anterior layer reveals a hexagonal array of collagen bundles; in cross section, the bundles of collagen have intervals of 110 nm. Antibodies to basal lamina components, fibronectin, and type IV collagen recognize Descemet's membrane, and a characteristic railroad track appearance is seen[34] (Figure 1-24). This pattern of staining is caused by naturally occurring zones in Descemet's membrane. If endothelial cells are stimulated to produce excess amounts of basal lamina material, focal thickenings of Descemet's membrane, called *guttae*, develop.

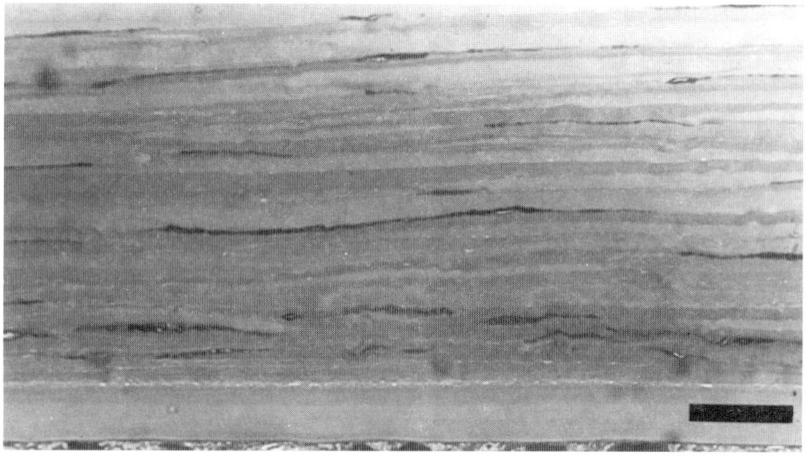

FIGURE 1-22 Light micrograph of the posterior central cornea illustrating posterior stroma, Descemet's membrane, and the single cell layer of endothelium. (Bar, 25 μm.)

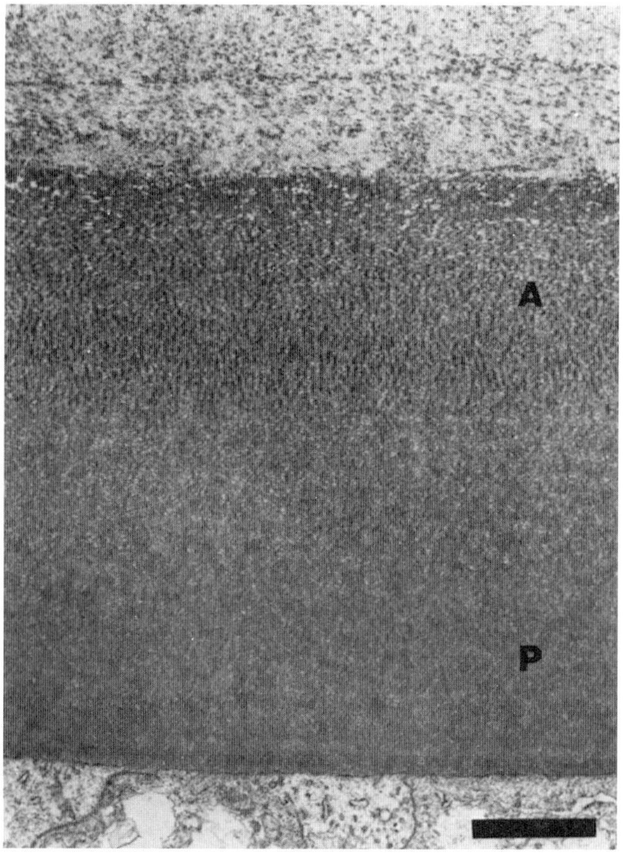

FIGURE 1-23 Electron micrograph of Descemet's membrane illustrating the banded anterior layer (*A*) and the nonbanded posterior layer (*P*), which increases in thickness with age. Endothelial cells lie on Descemet's membrane with no special mechanical junctions. (Bar, 1 μm.)

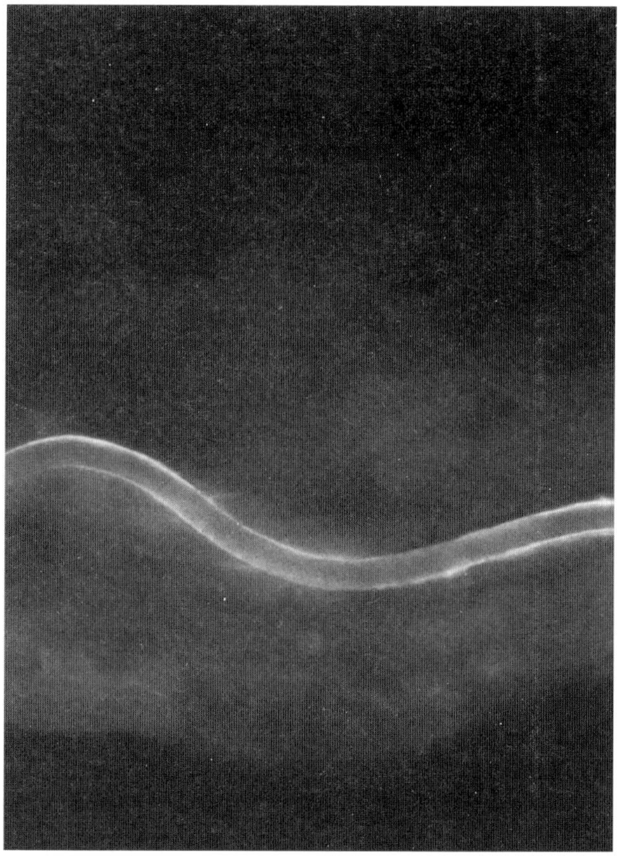

FIGURE 1-24 Immunofluorescence of Descemet's membrane showing the location of type IV collagen along the anterior and posterior portions producing a characteristic "railroad track" appearance. Antibodies to laminin result in a similar staining pattern.

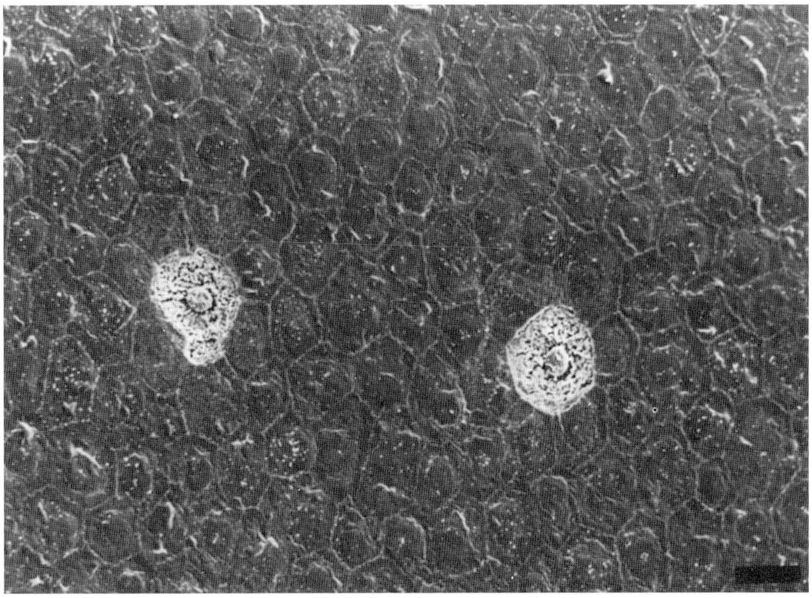

FIGURE 1-28 Spontaneous endothelial cell death, depicted here, results in large cell formation. Neighboring endothelial cells spread out, maintaining overall cellularity but decreased cell density. (Bar, 20 μm.)

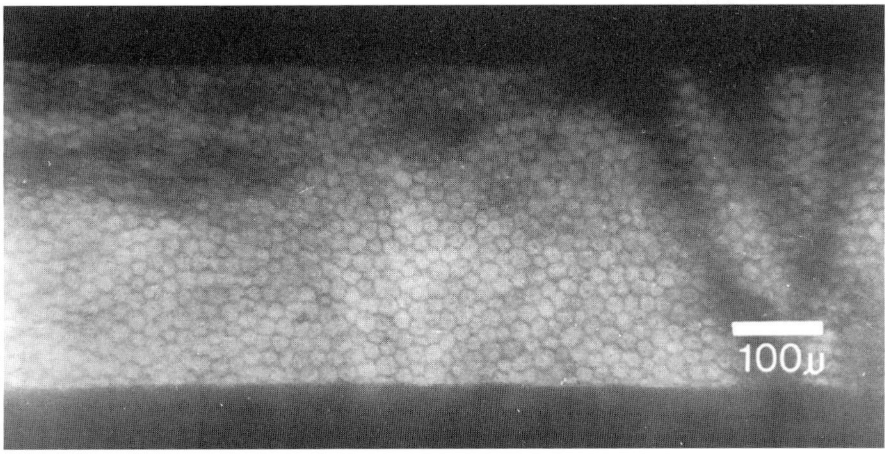

A

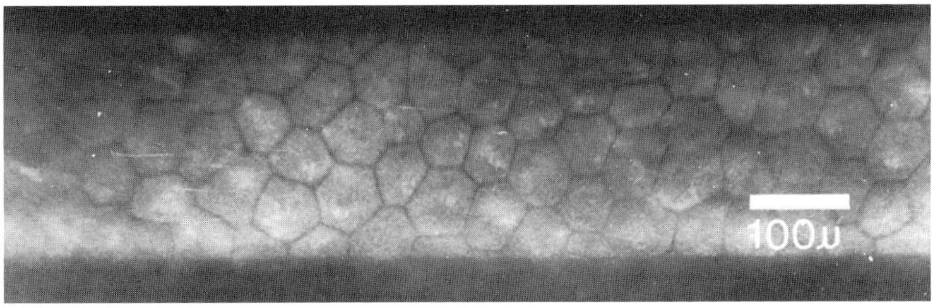

B

FIGURE 1-29 **(A)** Specular photomicrograph of the corneal endothelium of a 28-year-old patient. The cell density is approximately 2,800 cells/mm^2. The dark bands are artifacts from applanation. **(B)** Endothelial cell density of approximately 400 cells/mm^2 in a clinically successful corneal graft. Note the large cell size, pleomorphism, and polymegethism. (Courtesy of Bruce A. Barron, M.D., New Orleans, LA.)

As endothelial cells enlarge to compensate for losses, one might anticipate a gradual decrease in endothelial stromal dehydration function. Such is the case in early Fuchs' dystrophy, in which stromal edema is associated with decreased cell density and increased endothelial fluorescein permeability.[66] However, in patients with cell densities as low as 615 cells/mm^2 after penetrating keratoplasty, stromal edema was absent and endothelial fluorescein permeability was reduced compared with normal cornea.[67] Fluorescein traverses cell layers predominantly through paracellular pathways. The density of ATPase pump sites, located in the lateral membranes of endothelial cells and quantified by binding to radioactive ligands, is significantly decreased in dystrophic corneas, compared with normal corneas.[68] One can conclude from the above findings that a reduction in endothelial cell density alone is not sufficient to cause stromal edema. However, when the barrier property of the endothelium is compromised, as occurs with cornea guttata, the corneal dehydrating mechanism is overwhelmed by ion and water leakage into the stroma through damaged paracellular pathways.

In summary, there is a critical density of endothelial cells (400 to 700 cells/mm^2) below which endothelial decompensation occurs, with progressive stromal edema and eventual epithelial edema. Stromal edema, which is associated with endothelial pathologic states, can occur with higher cell densities and is the probable result of disruption of the paracellular pathways, as in early Fuchs' dystrophy.

When endothelial cells are subjected to stress, and especially when some cells are lost, the remaining cells may lose their regular hexagonal shape and become irregular in shape (pleomorphism) and size (polymegethism). These changes can occur with age, after trauma, and in long-term contact lens wearers. The significance of pleomorphism and polymegethism is unclear, but there is evidence that a cornea with these changes cannot withstand additional trauma as well as a normal cornea. Contact lens wearers can develop small blebs in the endothelium shortly after a contact lens is inserted. These blebs are transient and are probably caused by the osmotic effects or low pH resulting from lactic acid accumulation.

Intercellular Junctions

In the preceding descriptions of the corneal epithelium and endothelium, several types of cell junctions were mentioned, including tight junctions, desmosomes, hemidesmosomes, and gap junctions. These cell junctions can be grouped into several functional types: mechanical, electrical, and barrier junctions. Many of the tissue properties ascribed to the corneal epithelium are dependent on cell junctions. Cell division does not proceed normally when these junctions are compromised. Apical membranes of cells exposed to an environment from which access to the extracellular space is to be limited are specialized for tight junctions. Thus, the anterior membrane of the superficial epithelial cells (see Figure 1-8B), as well as the posterior membrane of the endothelial cells (see Figure 1-27), forms a barrier by the fusion of the outer leaflets of the cell membranes of adjacent cells. The tight junctions of the superficial epithelial cells close the extracellular space to the flow of ions, foreign substances, and disease vectors. Nonphysiologic conditions such as high concentrations of ions open tight junctions, allowing direct communication between the extracellular space and the external environment. These junctions can reform rapidly when conditions become more physiologic.[69] The tight junctional complexes are larger in the endothelium,[15] although the integrity of the barrier is greater in the epithelium. Large areas of membrane fusion are also found throughout the epithelium and between the lateral interdigitations of endothelial cells; these zones of tight junctions may be as long as 0.5 μm and may have a mechanical function in stabilizing adjacent cells.

The most obvious mechanical junctions in the epithelium are desmosomes and hemidesmosomes. Desmosomes are spot-like and may be 0.2 to 0.5 μm in diameter (see Figure 1-10A). In contrast, hemidesmosomes may develop as an aggregate and become more spot-like after normal cell turnover begins. Desmosomes have parallel cell membranes that are separated by the usual intercellular space of 220 Å. The intercellular space is filled with an electron-dense material, a glycoprotein, that does not impede the movement of substances. In pathologic conditions characterized by drying of the epithelial surface, desmosomes become more obvious and the number of tonofilaments increases.[1] Epithelial edema causes an increase in the intercellular space and, consequently, a loss in cell size. Under these conditions, desmosomes continue to maintain some intercellular attachments.

The hemidesmosome-basal lamina complex is responsible for adherence of the epithelium to the underlying cornea[70,71] (see Figure 1-14). This complex includes several components that are only now beginning to be analyzed, although it is clear that they may all contribute to adhesion. Fibrils that leave the membrane of the basal cell appear to attach the hemidesmosomes to the dense band of basal lamina (lamina densa). However, fibrillar aggregates that leave the lamina densa and are spatially correlated with hemidesmosomes probably attach the basal lamina to the stroma.[72] These fibrils have been suggested to be type VII collagen and have a characteristic banding pattern.[71,73]

Gap junctions (see Figure 1-10A) do not impede the flow of materials within the extracellular space, although the extracellular space is narrowed to 100 Å or less. Gap junctions consist of arrays of packed tubules that connect the cytoplasm of adjacent cells and allow the passage of small molecules and ions from cell to cell. Cells at all levels of the corneal epithelium are joined by gap junctions, although these junctions are often not seen by transmission electron microscopy. Electron microscopic detection of these structures depends on how the tissue is prepared.[69,74] Studies of membranes using the replica technique have shown that epithelial cell gap junctions vary in area and are larger at the basal cell level.[15] Basal cells are the most metabolically active cells in the epithelium, although it is not clear whether this factor is directly related to gap junction size. Endothelial cells also have many gap junctions with variable areal geometry.[62]

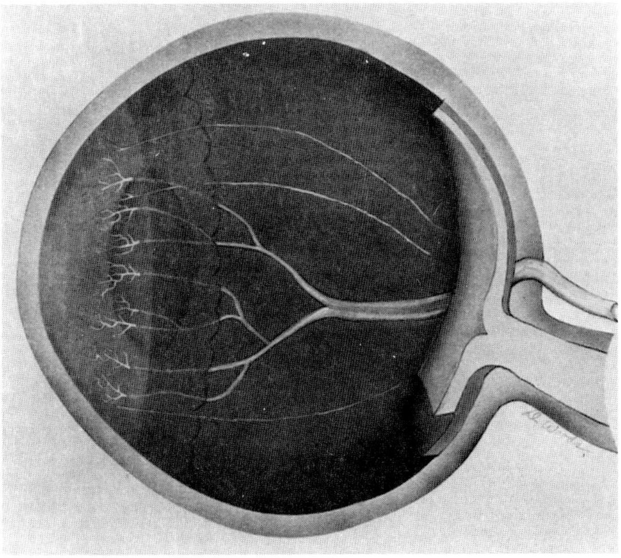

FIGURE 1-30 Artist's rendition illustrating the manner in which discrete nerve bundles entering the globe posteriorly branch within the globe, providing symmetrical circumferential innervation of the anterior segment. A large ciliary nerve is shown entering the scleral foramen. Intraocular pressure results in expansion of the nerve bundle in the scleral plane and prevents formation of ridges in the retina.

Corneal Innervation

The anterior segment of the eye is innervated by neural processes from at least three ganglia: the trigeminal (semilunar), the superior cervical, and the ciliary. The cornea has two major nerve supplies: sensory innervation by fibers from the ophthalmic division of the trigeminal nerve (5th cranial nerve) whose cell bodies lie in the trigeminal ganglion, and sympathetic innervation by fibers whose cell bodies lie in the superior cervical ganglion. In terms of quantity, the number of corneal sensory axons is greater than the number of sympathetic axons.

The nasociliary nerve, which arises from the ophthalmic division of the trigeminal ganglion, leaves the medial superior border of the trigeminal ganglion and enters the orbit through the superior orbital fissure. This nerve is identifiable as it passes through the superior orbital fissure, where it runs inferiorly and somewhat temporally to the superior rectus muscle, and then just over the top of the optic nerve. The nasociliary nerve branches before it penetrates the sclera, so that one to three long ciliary nerves may pierce the sclera several millimeters from the optic nerve. Immediately on entering the sclera, the geometry of the nerve changes, with flattening in the scleral plane (Figure 1-30). The nerves travel in the suprachoroidal space, where they branch several times to form a loose network. Within the suprachoroidal space, there is branching and possible exchange between the axons of the long ciliary nerves and those of the short ciliary nerves. There are as many as 12 to 16 circumferentially arranged branches at the corneoscleral limbus that contain a mixed population of fibers of sympathetic as well as sensory origin. Recurrent branches around the circumference innervate the conjunctiva bordering the limbus, as well as the limbal corneal epithelium.

After entering the cornea, nerve trunks run in a quasiradial direction through the middle third of the stroma, branch anteriorly, and form a dense subepithelial plexus. From the subepithelial plexus, the nerves penetrate Bowman's layer and supply terminal endings to the corneal epithelium[75] (Figure 1-31).

The subject of adrenergic or sympathetic axons within the cornea has caused considerable controversy. Although early studies showed that sensory fibers from the ophthalmic division of the trigeminal nerve entered the cornea early in the first trimester of gestation, a similar study by Ehinger and Sjöberg[76] showed that adrenergic fibers were first found in the cornea during the second trimester. These authors were especially interested in whether there are adrenergic terminals in the epithelium, but they found very few. More terminals were found forming a plexus around the limbus in conjunction with the developing vascularization of that area. Some evidence suggests that occasional adrenergic nerves are found in the adult cornea. Toivanen et al[77] demon-

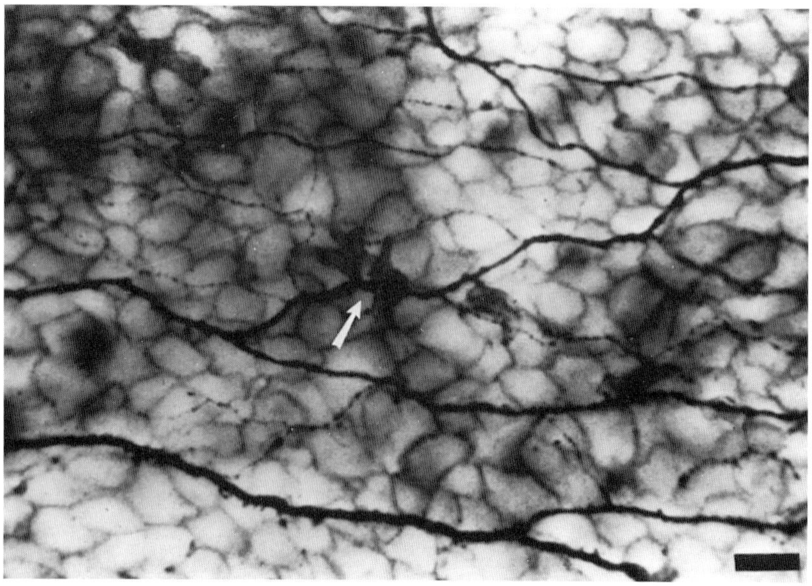

FIGURE 1-31 Human cornea stained by the gold chloride method and mounted flat. Parallel axon terminals are seen within the basal epithelial cell layer. Cell outlines of the basal cells are seen, as well as dendritic cells (arrow). (Bar, 20 μm.) (Courtesy of Bernd Schimmelpfennig, M.D., Zurich, Switzerland.)

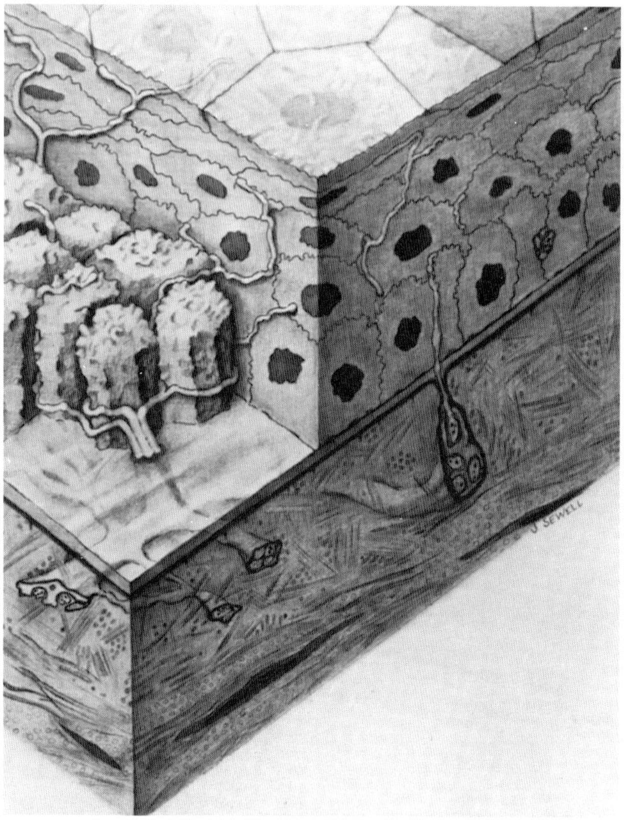

FIGURE 1-32 Artist's rendition of the mode of innervation of the human corneal epithelium. Schwann cells accompany the unmyelinated axons up to the base of the epithelium.

strated histochemically that a few sympathetic axons can be seen in the stroma of the adult human cornea. Neuroanatomic mapping techniques, such as the horseradish peroxidase-labeled wheat germ agglutinin lectin (WGA-HRP) procedure, which has been used to examine the rabbit cornea,[78] show that classic histochemical techniques grossly underestimate the density of adrenergic fibers in the cornea.

The course of the nerves through Bowman's layer can be seen by light microscopic examination, because the accompanying Schwann cells are visible. Scanning electron microscopic examination of sodium hydroxide-treated corneas reveals pores in the anterior surface of Bowman's layer with diameters of 0.5 to 1 μm that may represent the path of the nerves as they enter the epithelium.[79] As the nerves continue anteriorly into the epithelium, they lose their Schwann cell covering and become tightly wrapped by processes of the epithelial cells (Figures 1-32 and 1-33). The term "free nerve ending" is old and is based on light microscopic observations in the late 19th century. Within the epithelium, the nerves are more properly referred to as axon terminals; they represent the sensory receptors. There are leash arrangements that may arise from one axon, branching into several processes that elongate through the basal cell layer approximately parallel to the epithelial surface. In normal corneas, from three to seven axons within a leash arrangement can run for several hundred microns. Rising from these elongated neural processes are randomly displaced axon terminals that innervate all layers of the epithelium. Some axon ter-

FIGURE 1-33 Nerve endings invade the epithelium by penetrating the epithelial basal lamina. An intraepithelial axon terminal (arrowhead), as shown here, is closely surrounded by processes of epithelial cells. Terminals like this one are also referred to as "free nerve endings." The round profiles of several neural mitochondria are seen within the terminal. (Bar, 0.5 μm.)

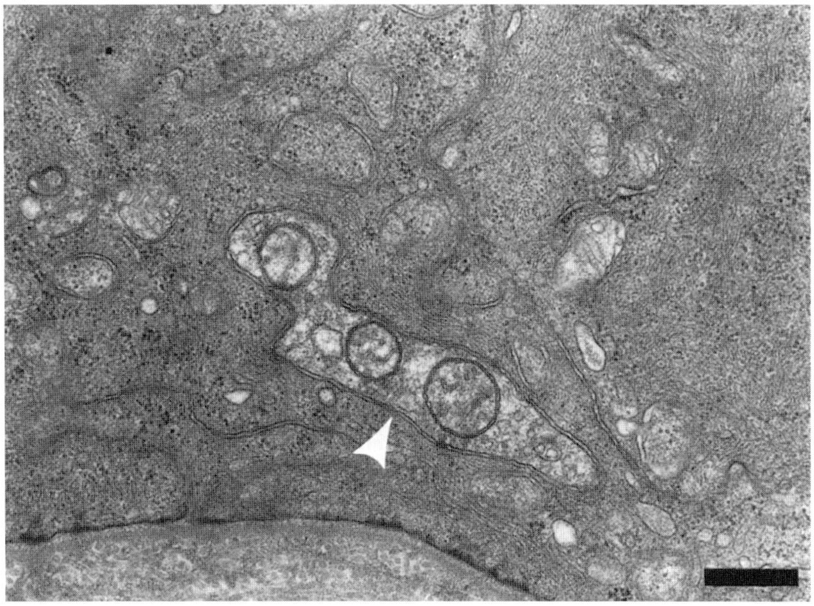

minals wander anteriorly to within one cell layer of the surface of the cornea.

In addition to the classic neurotransmitters, acetylcholine and norepinephrine, corneal nerves may contain one or more peptides, which may have roles in the regulation and maintenance of the cornea. However, only substance P has been positively identified in human corneas, presumably in the trigeminal axons[80] (Figure 1-34). Corneas with decreased sensation are subject to trauma, and the loss of corneal innervation may adversely affect the normal blinking mechanism. Pathologic changes in corneal sensation may be indicative of certain diseases. For example, decreased corneal sensation is of diagnostic value in ocular herpetic infections.[81] Also, diabetic patients have significantly decreased corneal sensation, which has been related to the progress of the disease.[18]

Corneal nerves can be seen with a slit lamp microscope if the light is tangential to the surface of the cornea. At the limbus and for several millimeters cen-

FIGURE 1-34 Immunohistochemical localization of substance P in axons of the subepithelial plexus. (Courtesy of Timo Tervo, M.D., Helsinki, Finland.)

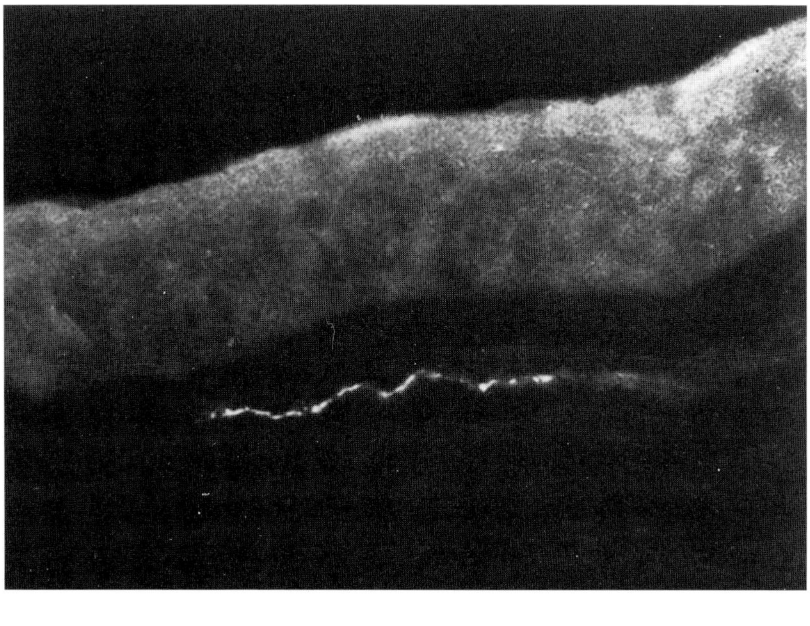

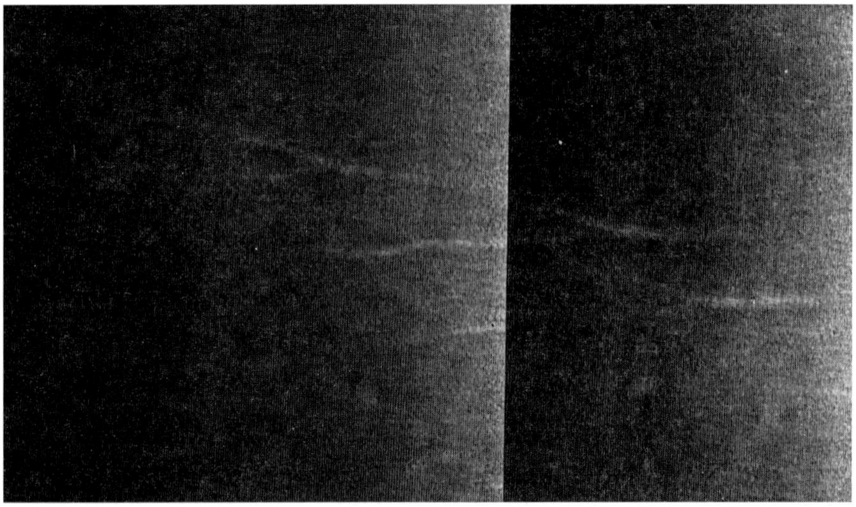

FIGURE 1-35 Confocal micrograph of the intraepithelial nerve endings in a normal human cornea. These nerves are unmyelinated at this level of organization. (Original magnification × 230.)

trally, the structure of the nerve is similar to that of other peripheral nerves. More recently, the development of the confocal microscope has permitted the direct observation of intraepithelial nerve terminals (Figure 1-35). This microscope should be of use in understanding the types of nerve rearrangements that may be associated with contact lens wear and pathologic conditions such as diabetes.

Several layers of cells envelop the axon bundles. The endoneurial collagen fibrils, which run longitudinally with the nerve bundle, are of different diameters than the stromal collagen. In some disease entities, such as multiple endocrine neoplasia, the corneal nerves are thickened, possibly as a result of abnormally large amounts of connective tissue. Thickened nerves are also associated with leprosy. Although this thickening has often been attributed to increased myelination, the actual cause is related to degeneration of the axons and Schwann cells. The fine anterior plexus cannot be observed by clinical means and must be assessed indirectly by psychophysical testing, which is usually carried out with an esthesiometer.[81] Decreased sensation associated with atypical corneal lesions is often indicative of herpetic infection. Corneal sensation is also decreased in patients with leprosy, diabetes, and other conditions, as in the area around a corneal ulcer. Neurotrophic keratitis is typified by epithelial decompensation and may occur as a result of surgical injury to the ophthalmic division of the trigeminal nerve. After penetrating keratoplasty, there is only limited reinnervation of the donor stroma even after several years, because the regenerating host nerves are unable to penetrate the scar of the keratoplasty wound. However, the more limited damage from operations such as epikeratophakia permits a better quality of graft innervation.[82] Lesions of the cornea associated with trauma or surgery are often extremely painful, possibly because there is a loss of specificity and exaggerated responsiveness of the nerve terminals to stimulation.[83]

EMBRYOLOGY

At birth, the cornea is relatively large compared with the rest of the globe. Most of the growth in the size of the cornea occurs from the age of 6 months to 1 year. The adult size (1.3 cm^2) is attained between the first and second years.

From an evolutionary point of view, the cornea has progressed to provide the appropriate optical properties as well as protection for the contents of the globe. In the development of the cornea from primitive to advanced vertebrates, the anterior refractive surface has become more refined in its optical properties, which has allowed more precise vision but has also made the cornea susceptible to environmental stress.[84] Outer layers composed of specialized skin in lower vertebrates, such as the lamprey, have given way to eyelids in mammals. The refracting surface is found in amphibians, and a structure similar to Bowman's layer is seen in reptiles.[85] The avian cornea is structurally most similar to the primate cornea, as only these two have Bowman's layer.

Information about human corneas at particular gestational times has been augmented by studies of other mammalian eyes. Many of the developmental processes of the cornea in humans are similar to those of the chicken, extensive studies of which have formed the basis for most of our experimental information in this area.[86,87]

Early Development

Formation of the human cornea begins at approximately 5 to 6 weeks of gestation (8- to 10-mm stage).[88] After the surface ectoderm invaginates into the optic cup, producing the lens vesicle, and the surface layers separate, the lens vesicle detaches from the overlying surface ectoderm. At this early stage, a faint amorphous line just beneath the surface ectoderm shows the formation of basal lamina. By this time, the ectodermal layer over the developing cornea can be referred to as epithelium.

The incipient corneal stroma is composed of a layer of loose collagen fibrils between the developing epithelium and the anterior surface of the lens.[36] The stroma remains acellular before fibroblast invasion[35,89] but has many short, small collagen fibrils. Mesenchymal cells, located at the perilimbic cell mass, begin to form the corneal endothelium at approximately 6 weeks of gestation.[87,89] For successful corneal development, the lens must be present; its loss before mesenchymal invasion results in microphthalmos and an opaque cornea.[88] Also, the origin of the cornea differs from that of the sclera. The sclera develops from vascular mesenchymal connective tissue, whereas the primitive cornea is formed by neural-crest-derived mesenchymal cells.[90–93]

At about 40 days of gestation, the cornea consists of an epithelial layer, an acellular matrix of collagen fibrils, and an endothelial layer. This setting prepares the way for the migration of the corneal fibroblasts (future keratocytes). These cells are now believed to be derived from neural crest at the perilimbal area.[86,91,94] However, it was once thought that the stroma is formed by cells of mesodermal origin.[95] Studies using monoclonal antibodies to neuronal proteins have shown that keratocytes in the posterior stroma and endothelial cells stain intensely.[96] These results corroborate the idea that the posterior keratocytes and the endothelium may be not of mesodermal origin, but rather of neural crest origin. Explanations of developmental disorders of the endothelium may be better understood by recognizing the cells of origin. The acellular stroma expands, possibly as a result of hydration of increasing amounts of extracellular matrix material.[87] Migratory waves of cells from the perilimbal region result in layers of fibroblasts within the stroma. It is presumed that the short fibril matrix of the acellular stroma provides a substrate for this migration.

Initially, the endothelium is formed by a strand of cells with contiguous and overlapping processes and, often, wide intercellular gaps. Focal tight junctions at the apical surface, as well as various other types of junctions along the lateral membranes, slowly develop. The endothelial cells begin to lay down their basement membrane, Descemet's membrane, which can be distinguished at 4 months of gestation. At birth, the endothelial layer is about 10 μm thick and Descemet's membrane is 0.7 μm thick.[56] Descemet's membrane continues to increase in thickness postnatally, with additional material being laid down at the rate of 1 μm/decade.[56]

Within the developing epithelium, apical tight junctions are seen. Also, gap junctions joining lateral surfaces of the cells are present, as well as desmosomes, which are more numerous toward the epithelial surface. Ozanics et al[89,97] documented the development of the monkey cornea, with particular emphasis on the membrane junctional arrangements between adjacent epithelial cells. Shortly after the cuboidal epithelial cells form, they develop into a more organized, but still irregular, columnar layer. At 28 days of gestation in the nonhuman primate, the cuboidal epithelial cells rest on a thin basal lamina with sparse fibrils in the underlying space. The cytoplasm of the epithelial cells contains very few filaments.

Late Development

Up to the third month of gestation, the epithelium is exposed to amniotic fluid. At about this time, the eyelids meet and adhere, not separating again until the sixth month. Glycogen granules appear in great numbers in the epithelial cells around the time the eyelids close over the surface of the cornea. The epithelium continues to develop during the prenatal stages. At birth, the epithelium is composed of only four layers; the adult complement (four to six layers) is reached by 5 to 6 months of age.

Shortly after the closure of the eyelids, the stroma is invaded by neural processes, which can be identified at the basal surface of the epithelial layer by approximately the end of the first trimester. Nerve endings invade the epithelium by penetrating the epithelial basal lamina. Hemidesmosomes, initially faint condensations along the plasma membrane, begin to form along the basal cell membrane shortly after the beginning of the second trimester. The appearance of filaments within the epithelial cytoplasm marks the development of more mature hemidesmosomes. The basal lamina is present in the second trimester in humans and grows by slow deposition during life to reach thicknesses of more than 0.2 μm in some individuals.[25] Nerve terminals containing both dense core vesicles and clear vesicles are seen during this time. According to the study of Ozanics et al[89] in the nonhuman primate, most of the dense core vesicles are of the large size and their origins are unclear. Also, the type of neurotransmitter contained in these vesicles has not been definitely identified, although it may be substance P.[98]

Corneal epithelial cells are capable of collagen synthesis. Embryonic basal cells have an extensive Golgi complex located beneath the nucleus.[99,100] In the nonhuman primate, the epithelium may contribute to the development of Bowman's layer. Because the density of Bowman's layer seems to be greatest near the basal lamina, it is generally accepted that Bowman's layer originates from the epithelium. However, others have suggested that Bowman's layer is the remnant of the primary acellular stroma. In development, an acellular zone remains in the anterior stroma. Randomly distributed, small-diameter (20 nm) fibrils mark the location of Bowman's layer. This layer is composed of types I and V collagen, which are synthesized by the epithelium along with type IV collagen. The endothelium secretes Descemet's layer beginning at about the fourth month of gestation.[90] As described earlier, this is a true basement membrane. However, the anterior layer shows 110-nm bands at 5 months of gestation[56] and is about 3 μm thick at birth. Immunohistochemical studies of type VIII collagen in the developing eye have described positive staining fibers in Descemet's membrane in the late second or the third trimester.[101] The tight junction formation of the apical membranes of the endothelial cells may continue to develop after birth; however, some physiologic studies of permeability do not correlate well with the presence of these junctions.[102]

At the beginning of the second trimester, the fibrocytes in the stroma have widely extended endoplasmic reticulum, which contains granules or finely flocculent electron-dense material. These cells also have a prominent Golgi complex and vesicles that enclose compact fibrillar masses, suggested to be collagen fibrils. Extracellular aggregates of collagen fibrils begin to appear in parallel arrays within small groups around the cell body. During the first trimester of development, collagen fibrils have cross-sectional diameters of 44 to 62 nm. However, the periodicity is not observable at this time. Elastic fibrils with diameters of 17 nm are situated among the irregularly arranged collagen fibrils. The fibrocytes are the predominant source of collagen synthesis within the stroma, although assembly into collagen fibrils occurs extracellularly. The layers of fibrocytes increase, presumably through mitosis. During the prenatal period, the fibrocytes develop various types of contacts with other cells, forming both tight junctions and gap junctions. Toward the end of the third trimester, the corneal collagen fibrils have well-defined fine cross bandings with macroperiods distinguishable by electron microscopy.

METABOLISM AND NUTRITION

The cells of the cornea are actively involved in the maintenance of the functions of molecular synthesis and volume regulation, and much of the energy for these processes is derived from the catabolism of glucose by both aerobic and anaerobic pathways. The bulk of the glucose used (105 $\mu g/cm^2/hr$)[103] is derived from the aqueous humor; negligible amounts enter the cornea from the tears and the limbus.[44] Glucose reserves are present in the form of epithelial glycogen granules, which serve as a source of energy during periods of metabolic stress (hypoxia and injury). At such times, glycogenolysis provides a short-term metabolic buffer, maintaining adequate cell glucose levels. Corneal refractive surgical procedures that chronically reduce glucose supply to the anterior cornea will be successful as long as the metabolic needs of the anterior cornea are adequately met (Figure 1-36).

The corneal catabolism of glucose yields energy in the form of ATP by the oxygen-dependent Krebs cycle and by anaerobic glycolysis[104] (Figure 1-37). The hexose monophosphate shunt uses a fraction of available glucose for the production of reduced triphosphopyridine used for cell synthetic activities, and it produces ribose-5-phosphate, which re-enters the glycolytic pathway. The extent to which each pathway contributes to total corneal glucose utilization and ATP production is controversial.

Both direct and indirect entry of glucose into the anaerobic glycolytic pathway result in the formation of pyruvate, which is converted either to CO_2 in the Krebs cycle or to lactate by lactic acid dehydrogenase. Corneal membranes are highly permeable to CO_2, and the endothelium apparently has an active carbonic anhydrase system so that elimination of this metabolic by-product from the cornea is not a problem. In fact, the corneal generation of CO_2 may provide substrate for the endothelial ionic transport of HCO_3^-, which is thought to be the principal factor underlying the regulation of corneal stromal hydration (see below). By contrast, the elimination of lactate is not as easily accomplished. The barrier properties of the superficial corneal epithelial cells preclude the transfer of significant amounts of corneal lactate to the tears.[103,105] Instead, lactate must be removed by diffusion across the stroma and endothelium into the aqueous humor.

Normally, the corneal uptake of glucose from the aqueous humor is balanced by the loss of corneal lactate. How-

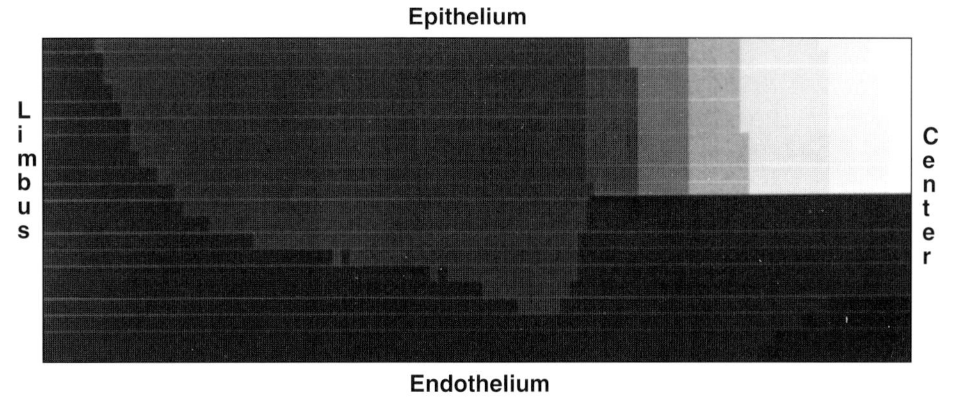

FIGURE 1-36 Example of the influence of a 5.5-mm–diameter impermeable membrane implant at mid-depth in stroma (black bar, mid-right) on stromal glucose concentration obtained by computer simulation. Highest concentration of glucose (5.7 mM) is represented by black, with concentration intervals shown by gray series through white (0.7 mM). The simulation calculated the effects of epithelial and stromal glucose consumption and the limbal and endothelial diffusional contribution to stromal glucose, as well as facilitated glucose transport by the endothelium. Note glucose depletion anterior to the implant, glucose accumulation posterior to the implant centrally, and the effect of the limbal supply.

ever, when the corneal oxygen supply is diminished, and perhaps during other forms of corneal metabolic stress, entry of pyruvate into the Krebs cycle is reduced, and the rate of lactate production increases. The resulting increase in the corneal concentration of lactate has several consequences. Epithelial edema can occur, altering the cellular refractive index and producing the Sattler's veil phenomenon (increased glare and halos surrounding bright lights).[106] Stromal edema accompanying hypoxia is a consequence of excess osmotic solute load presented by lactate accumulation.[105] Finally, localized stromal acidosis[107] caused by increased metabolic lactate production may alter endothelial morphology and function.[63] All these changes can compromise the optical properties of the cornea.

The normal metabolism of the corneal cells also requires a constant supply of amino acids, vitamins, and other constituents. As with glucose, the principal source of these molecules is the aqueous humor. If these needs are not met or the supply is significantly reduced over a long time, for example, by a large, nutrient-impermeable implant,[108] anterior corneal necrosis can occur. Although the cornea has some tolerance for interruption of the normal nutrient supply, neither the limbus nor the tears can provide sufficient nutrients to maintain corneal function when the aqueous humor is deficient, as during ciliary body shutdown.[109]

Oxygen is the single known corneal metabolic requirement not met by the aqueous humor[110] (Figure 1-38). Normally, a substantial portion of the oxygen used by the cornea is derived by diffusion from the tear film. Tight-fitting contact lenses made from materials with a low oxygen permeability can reduce oxygen tension below critical levels, resulting in epithelial and/or stromal edema,[111] as well as morphologic alterations in the corneal endothelium.[63] These are well-documented observations, which have not always correlated well with theoretical analyses of oxygen diffusion and tension profiles in tears, cornea, and aqueous humor. Part of the confusion arises from the technical difficulty of measuring tissue oxygen tension. The oxygen tension measured in the anterior chamber of the rabbit eye, for example, ranges from 20 to 80 mmHg. It is clear from calculations that if the rabbit (or human) aqueous humor oxygen tension were 80 mmHg or more, sufficient oxygen should be available to the cornea for normal function without additional supply from the tears.[112] In rabbit experiments, corneal edema cannot be induced by tear hypoxia unless the oxygen tension of the aqueous humor is less than 40 mmHg.[105,113] Given these arguments and the results of measurements in human eyes,[114] it is likely that in humans, oxygen tension in the aqueous humor is normally 30 to 40 mmHg. With such values, the corneal edema observed in humans in nitrogen atmosphere experiments[111] and under tight-fitting,

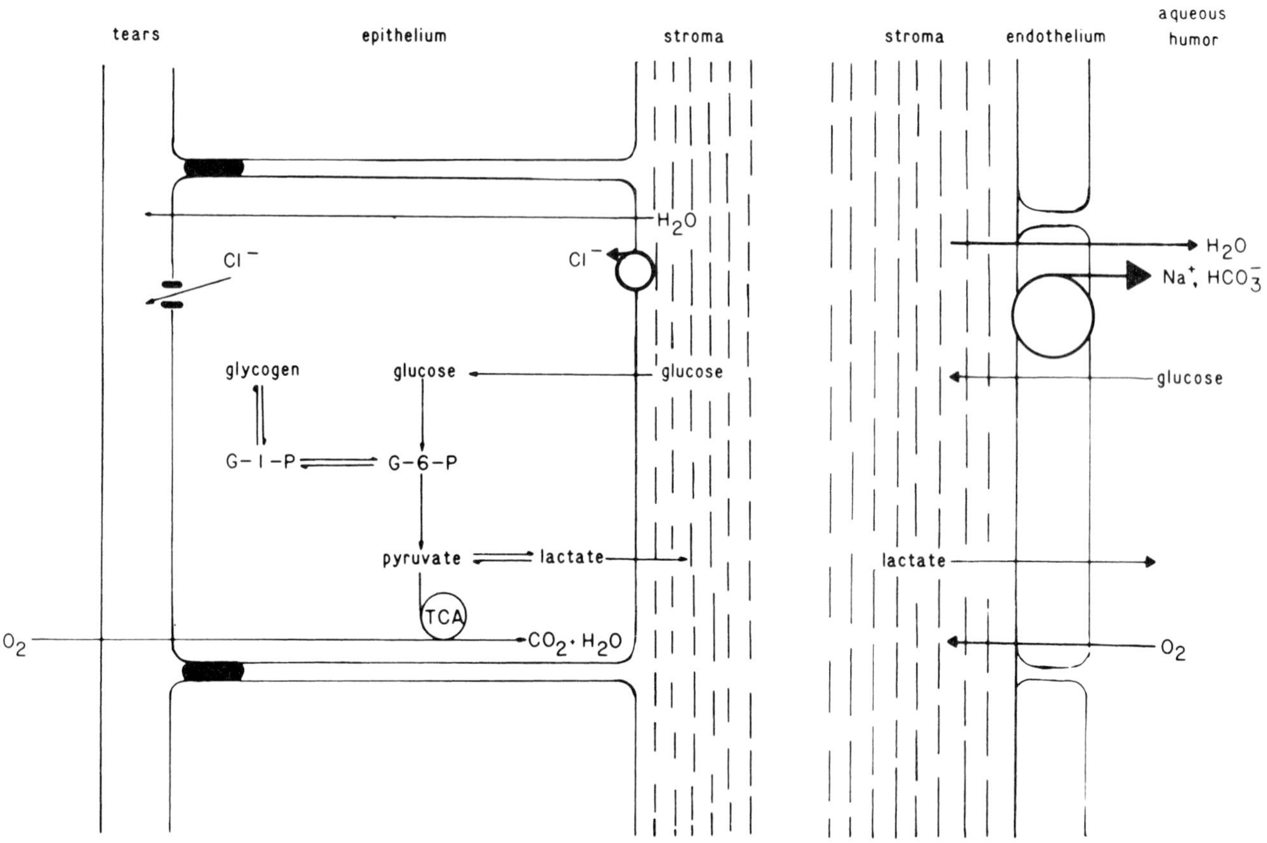

FIGURE 1-37 Processes contributing to corneal edema during hypoxia. Barrier properties: epithelium, with its apical tight junctions, retards fluid exchange with the tears, whereas flows across the endothelium are less restricted. Ion transport mechanisms: epithelial Cl^- secretion and endothelial Na^+ and HCO_3^- secretion combat edema by reducing the stromal osmotic pressure. Metabolic aspects: under normoxic conditions, the corneal cells produce lactate, nearly all of which exits the cornea by diffusion into the anterior chamber. When the oxygen supply from the atmosphere is restricted, additional amounts of lactate are formed, increasing the osmotic load to the stroma, which, in turn, causes stromal swelling. *TCA,* tricarboxylic acid (Krebs) cycle. (Reprinted with permission from P Rosenthal, SD Klyce: Contact lens induced corneal edema. In OH Dabezies (ed): Contact Lenses. The CLAO Guide to Basic Science and Clinical Practice. Grune & Stratton, Orlando, FL, 1984.)

oxygen-impermeable contact lenses[115] is consistent with theoretical analyses.[105]

The partial pressure of oxygen in the tears normally ranges from 155 mmHg (with the eyelids open) to 55 mmHg (with the eyelids closed).[116] The cornea is approximately 5 percent thinner during waking hours than during sleep. This difference is a result of evaporation from the tear film when the eyelids are open, producing slight tear hypertonicity and subsequent corneal dehydration,[117,118] and is not caused by a reduction in the availability of oxygen under closed eyelids. The cornea can tolerate sustained exposure to oxygen levels down to 25 mmHg in the tear film before edema is induced.[119] During sleep, some oxygen is provided to the anterior cornea by diffusion from the eyelid vasculature, whereas during waking hours a surplus is available from the atmosphere.

In terms of adequate corneal oxygenation, the successful tolerance of contact lenses depends on several factors. Daily-wear, oxygen-impermeable hard lenses are well tolerated if the lens is small in diameter and fitted so that the blink action of the eyelids assists in the exchange of tears under the lens; with oxygenated tears from the periphery, adequate oxygen delivery is achieved. However, larger-diameter extended-wear soft lenses must have sufficient oxygen permeability so that the critical oxygen level is met by diffusion through the contact lens. This requirement is most taxing during sleep, when the available oxygen tension at the contact lens surface is reduced (from 155 mmHg to 55 mmHg).

Extended-wear contact lenses also have other effects on corneal metabolism. Most important, extended wear of a contact lens alters the microenvironment of the corneal surface epithelium, eliminating its normal exposure to the environment (evaporation, mechanical eyelid abrasion), as well as denying full access to normal tear components. Well-documented metabolic consequences of extended-wear lenses include reductions in corneal sensation,[120] glucose utilization,[121] mitotic activity,[122] and epithelial oxygen consumption.[123] The corneal epithelium functions as a primary barrier against infection. It is not surprising, then, that extended-wear lenses, by altering epithelial metabolism, compromise this barrier function and permit ulcerative processes.[124,125]

In summary, metabolites derived primarily from the aqueous humor provide essential nutrition to the cornea. The single exception to this rule is that a certain necessary proportion of corneal oxygen is obtained from the tears. Contact lens wear can alter this pattern and, in certain situations, the resulting alteration in epithelial metabolism can lead to complications.

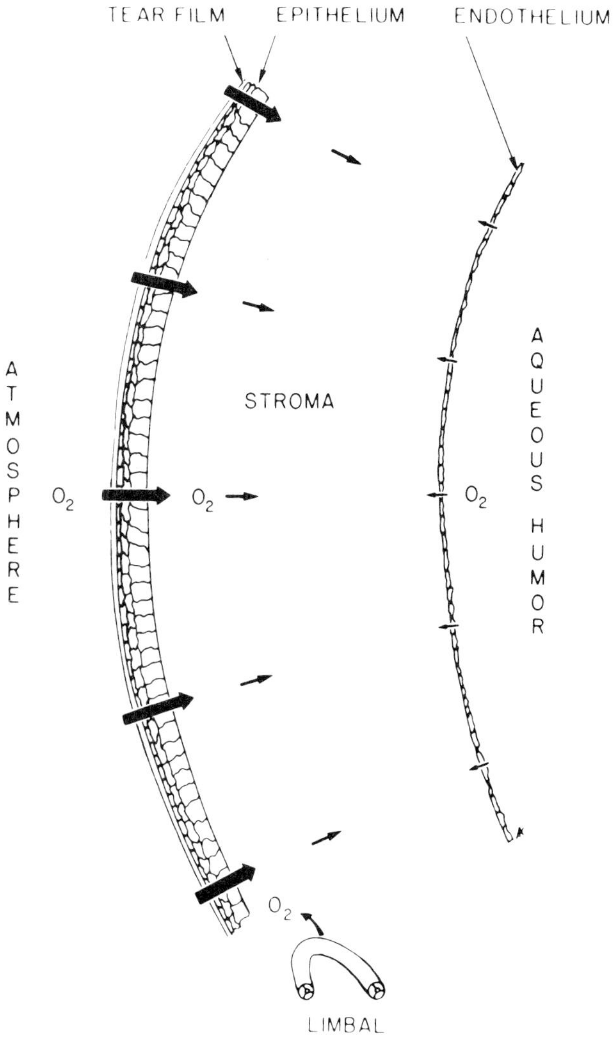

FIGURE 1-38 Conceptual scheme of oxygen supply to the cornea. Although some oxygen enters the cornea from the limbus and aqueous humor, the anterior cornea derives essential amounts from the tears. (Reprinted with permission from SD Klyce, RL Farris, OH Dabezies: Corneal oxygenation in contact lens wearers. In OH Dabezies (ed): Contact Lenses. The CLAO Guide to Basic Science and Clinical Practice. Grune & Stratton, Orlando, FL, 1984.)

PHYSIOLOGY

Epithelium

The primary function of the corneal epithelium is that of a barrier. This section reviews some of the features of this barrier and describes the ion transport systems and the neuropharmacology of the control mechanisms involved in these transport systems.

Active Na^+ Transport

Corneal ion transport systems have been intensely studied since it was recognized that metabolism-linked processes are responsible for the control of corneal hydration. A tears-to-stroma transport of Na^+ has been demonstrated in the rabbit and frog.[126-132] This absorptive transport of Na^+ presents somewhat of an anomaly inasmuch as an inward solute transport to the stroma would increase its osmotic pressure and presumably favor stromal edema. It has been proposed[133,134] that an increase in the stromal content of Na^+ might neutralize the anionic groups of the glycosaminoglycans and reduce or prevent their ability to swell. However, in both rabbits[131] and humans,[135] when factors such as corneal resting potential and other ion transport systems are taken into account, the net flow of Na^+ across the epithelium is from stroma to tears. It is not anomalous for an ion to be actively transported in one direction and to obtain a net flow of that ion in the opposite direction when one considers the total analysis of epithelial structure and properties, which include parallel pathways for ion movements, asymmetries in membrane ion permeabilities, and active ion transport systems.[136]

Nevertheless, the corneal epithelium contains an active Na^+ transport system directed from tears to stroma. The presence of the specific energy-supplying enzyme for Na^+ transport, Na^+/K^+ ATPase, has been demonstrated histochemically.[137] The activity of this enzyme can be enhanced severalfold by reacting the superficial epithe-

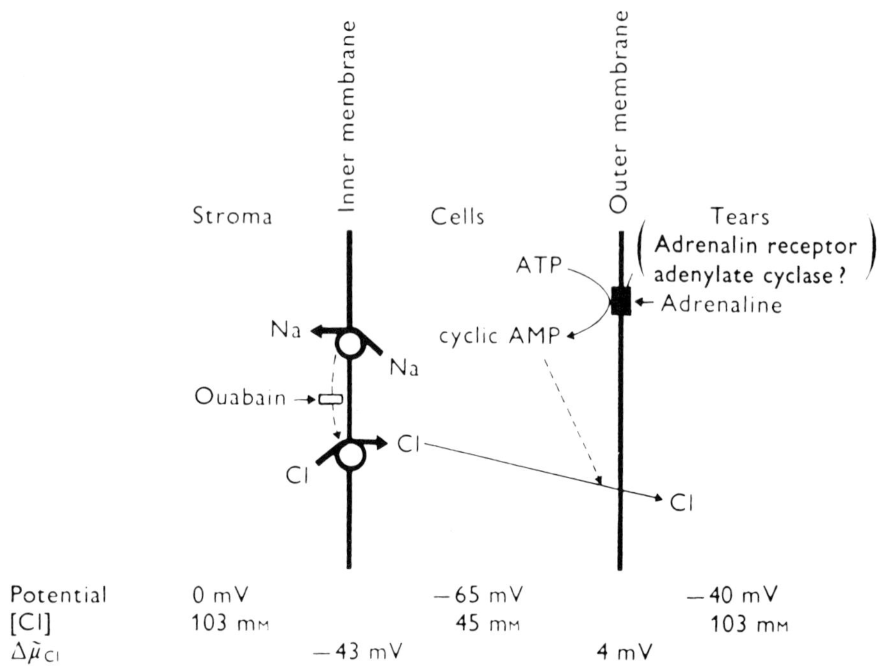

FIGURE 1-39 Model for the action of epinephrine (adrenaline) in the stimulation of epithelial Cl⁻ transport. Electrical potentials and Cl⁻ concentrations, [Cl], for the stroma, epithelial cells, and tears are listed, as well as the Cl⁻ electrochemical potential gradients ($\Delta\tilde{\mu}_{Cl}$) across the outer and inner membranes. (Reprinted with permission from SD Klyce, RKS Wong: Site and mode of adrenaline action of chloride transport across the rabbit corneal epithelium. J Physiol 266:777, 1977.)

lial cell membrane with amphotericin B or Ag^+.[138,139] Normally, the superficial epithelial cell membrane restricts the entry of Na^+. However, both amphotericin B and Ag^+ create cation channels in this membrane, which greatly increases intracellular Na^+ concentration and the rate of absorptive Na^+ transport. In this situation, the stroma swells in accord with the added osmotic load.[139] The epithelial Na^+ transport system is inhibited by ouabain, a specific inhibitor of Na^+/K^+ ATPase.

The transepithelial transport of Na^+ is most likely secondary to the Na^+/K^+ exchange activity of the deeper epithelial membrane, which maintains the high K^+ and low Na^+ characteristic of the cells. The Na^+/K^+ ATPase activity of the epithelial surface is less than that of the basolateral membranes, which accounts for the directionality of transepithelial Na^+ transport. The small amount of Na^+ that leaks into the cells across the apical membrane is more efficiently removed by the basolateral membrane Na^+/K^+ exchange mechanism.

Active Cl⁻ Transport

The corneal epithelium transports Cl⁻ in a secretory direction (i.e., from stroma to tears).[129,140,141] Corneal epithelial transport of Cl⁻ is regulated by the β-adrenergic receptor/adenylate cyclase complex. Stimulation of Cl⁻ transport is accompanied by an elevation of intracellular cyclic AMP and can be accomplished by the addition of membrane-permeable forms of cyclic AMP.[129] Catecholamines, such as epinephrine, stimulate Cl⁻ secretion, unless blocked by β-adrenoreceptor antagonists, such as propranolol or timolol. This stimulation is enhanced by theophylline, which is a compound that inhibits phosphodiesterase and slows the breakdown of cyclic AMP.

Net Na^+ absorptive transport and net Cl⁻ secretory transport can occur simultaneously only under special experimental conditions, such as are found with the short-circuit current technique. In the living eye, the epithelium generates an electrical potential of about 30 mV, tear side negative, and in this situation, the net movement of NaCl across the epithelium appears to be in the stroma-to-tears direction.[131]

Microelectrodes have been used to analyze the site of action of epinephrine in the stimulation of Cl⁻ transport. In the transport of ions across epithelial cells, there is an energy-consuming translocation of the transported ion at one epithelial surface and a passive diffusional translocation of the same ion at the opposite surface. In the rabbit cornea, the active step in Cl⁻ transport appears to be Cl⁻ uptake by the epithelial cells from the stroma in conjunction with a passive diffusional barrier at the corneal surface, which limits the exit of Cl⁻ from the superficial epithelial cells to the tear film. The action of epinephrine in the regulation of the overall net secretion of Cl⁻ appears to be the formation of functional Cl⁻ conductance channels in the apical membrane of the superficial epithelial cells[142] (Figure 1-39).

The presence of active Cl⁻ secretory transport in the epithelium raises the possibility that the epithelium might

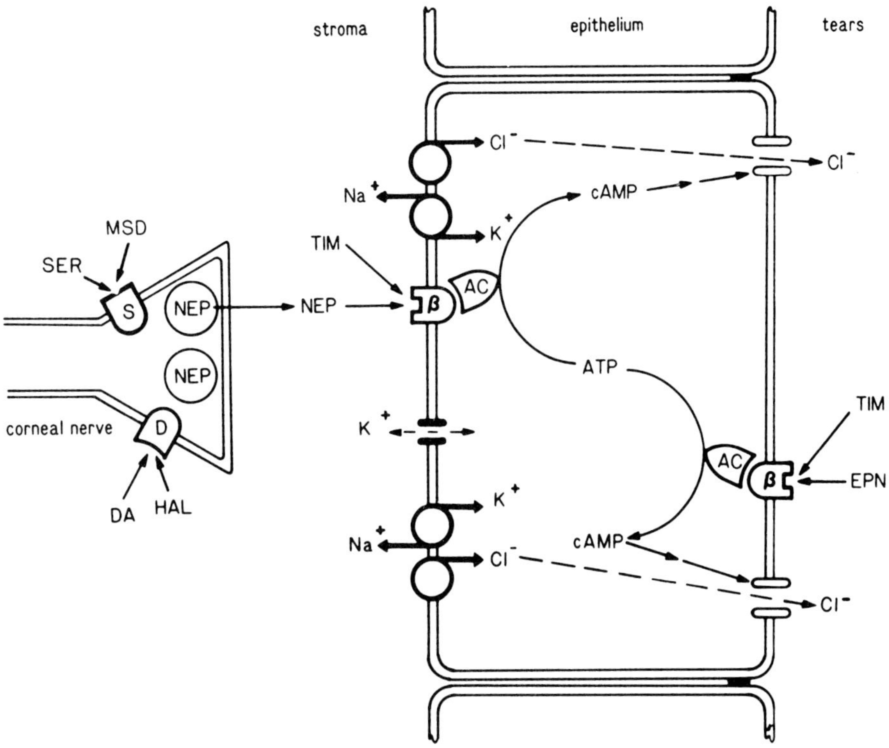

FIGURE 1-40 Scheme for the neuroregulation of Cl⁻ transport in the corneal epithelium. It is proposed that serotonin and dopamine can evoke the release of norepinephrine from the sympathetic nerve fibers in the cornea. In turn, norepinephrine may activate adenylate cyclase via the β-adrenoreceptor to increase cell levels of cyclic AMP and, finally, to increase the chloride conductance of the apical epithelial membrane. *EPN,* epinephrine; *NEP,* norepinephrine; *TIM,* timolol; *SER,* serotonin; *MSD,* methysergide; *DA,* dopamine; *HAL,* haloperidol; β, β-adrenoreceptor; *S,* serotonin receptor; *D,* dopamine receptor; *AC,* adenylate cyclase. (Reprinted from SD Klyce, CE Crosson: Transport processes across the rabbit corneal epithelium: a review. Curr Eye Res 4:323, 1985 by permission of Oxford University Press.)

participate in the regulation of stromal hydration in addition to its role as a diffusion barrier. In the frog, Cl⁻ secretion by the epithelium produces significant stromal dehydration.[143,144] Epithelial fluid secretion has also been identified in the rabbit,[145] where stromal thinning at a rate of 1.3 μm/hr is observed. Epithelial fluid transport in the primate has not been reported, although, as mentioned above, Cl⁻ secretion has been demonstrated.

The presence of catecholamine-activated β-adrenergic receptors as a control mechanism for epithelial function has been confirmed in several studies. The population of these receptors is dynamic; their density decreases after topical administration of epinephrine[146] and increases after superior cervical ganglionectomy,[147] a manipulation that would be expected to deplete the normal supply of corneal catecholamines. Other sources of catecholamines, such as the tears and the aqueous humor, that might activate corneal β-adrenergic receptors have been considered, but concentrations of epinephrine in these compartments are minute, owing in part to the cellular activity of monoamine oxidase, the principal enzyme responsible for the catabolism of catecholamines. Additionally, anatomic evidence presented above underscores the role of sympathetic fibers as the likely physiologic source of catecholamines in the cornea.

Other epithelial regulatory receptors have been identified, again using Cl⁻ transport as a measure of functional response. Both serotonin[148] and dopamine[149] stimulate Cl⁻ secretion in the rabbit cornea via mechanisms inhibited by specific receptor antagonists. Serotonin increases cyclic AMP in the epithelium[150] and evokes membrane conductance changes similar to those of epinephrine, including increased Cl⁻ conductance in the outer membrane of the superficial cells.[151] The specificity of the serotonin and dopamine responses became suspect when it was found that timolol blocks their activity, especially since timolol has been found to crossreact with other receptor types, although it is nonselective and blocks both β_1- and β_2-adrenoreceptors. Additionally, it was shown that the corneas of animals that had undergone superior cervical ganglionectomy[147] and pure subcultures of corneal epithelium[152] lack responsiveness to serotonin. On this basis, it was suggested that the serotonin receptors and, potentially, the dopamine receptors are located on the sympathetic fibers themselves[153] (Figure 1-40). In this scheme, activation of serotonin or dopamine receptors located on the sympathetic fibers causes the release of catecholamines (presumably norepinephrine), which, in turn, activates epithelial β-adrenoreceptors. Such a mechanism explains the apparent anomalous timolol antagonism to the serotonin response, as well as the disappearance of serotonin receptors in epithelial subculture. It does not alter the earlier notion that the β-adrenoreceptors are located on the epithelial membranes themselves, in that the responses to catecholamines in cultured cells remain intact.[152]

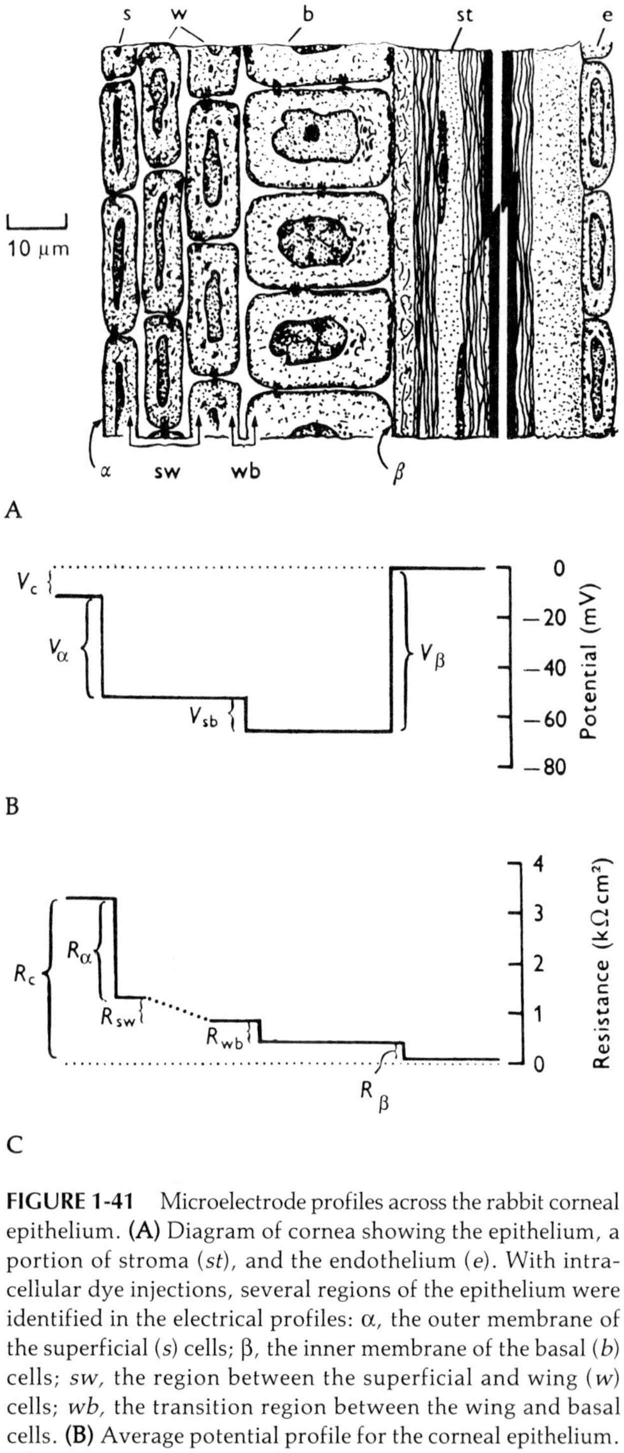

FIGURE 1-41 Microelectrode profiles across the rabbit corneal epithelium. **(A)** Diagram of cornea showing the epithelium, a portion of stroma (*st*), and the endothelium (*e*). With intracellular dye injections, several regions of the epithelium were identified in the electrical profiles: α, the outer membrane of the superficial (*s*) cells; β, the inner membrane of the basal (*b*) cells; *sw,* the region between the superficial and wing (*w*) cells; *wb,* the transition region between the wing and basal cells. **(B)** Average potential profile for the corneal epithelium. **(C)** Average resistance profile for the corneal epithelium. Note the large resistance of the outer membrane of the superficial cell. (Reprinted with permission from SD Klyce: Electrical profiles in the corneal epithelium. J Physiol 226:407, 1972.)

This section has emphasized the neuropharmacology of specific corneal membrane receptors to detail a model for a sequence of events linked to epithelial Cl^- transport, which, on its own merit, provides some understanding of epithelial function. However, it should be emphasized that activation of the β-adrenoreceptor increases cell levels of cyclic AMP, which is a rather common second messenger in terms of cell signaling, and that the assay of one specific function (Cl^- transport) may reveal only one aspect of receptor activation in this tissue. Other functional modalities are likely to be controlled via this receptor, such as cell proliferation[152] during epithelial repair, corneal immunologic response, and recurrence of herpes simplex viral disease.[154,155]

Electrophysiology and Ion Pathways

One of the most useful clinical tools in the assessment of the barrier properties of the corneal epithelium is the topical application of fluorescein. Normally, the corneal epithelium is impermeable to this anionic molecule. As a result, normal areas stain little or not at all, whereas areas with epithelial defects stain intensely. The location of this barrier and the membrane events associated with epithelial transport systems have been examined by means of intracellular measurements of electrical potential and ion activities with microelectrodes.

Intracellular microelectrode recordings in the corneal epithelium have been reported in frogs, rabbits, and cats.[7,16,139,142,156–162] Such work has led to several general conclusions, which are summarized in Figure 1-41. As with other cells, corneal epithelial cells have negative intracellular potentials, which are an expression of the fact that most cells maintain a high ratio of K^+ to Na^+ by means of the ubiquitous Na^+/K^+ exchange pump, which assists in the regulation of individual cell volume. The negative intracellular potential is also related to the relatively high K^+ permeability of most cell membranes. In such a situation, K^+, which is favored to diffuse out of the cell, creates a Nernst diffusion potential across the cell membrane oriented so that the cell interior remains electrically negative.

Measurement of the electrical potential profile across the epithelial cell membranes reveals three major steps (see Figure 1-41). Starting on the tear side, the microelectrode records a negative potential of 30 mV as the superficial epithelial cell is penetrated. No additional change in potential is recorded until the microelectrode penetrates the basal cell layer, whereupon the potential becomes 5 to 10 mV more negative. Normally, the superficial epithelial cells have the same intracellular potential as the deeper wing cells because of the presence of many ion-conducting desmosomes between these cells. The small step in potential between the deep wing and the basal cell layers indicates less electrical coupling between cells at this site. As the microelectrode penetrates the posterior membrane of the basal cell, the potential becomes more positive. The level of this potential is similar to the electrical potential in the aqueous humor inasmuch as transendothelial potential is small. The difference between stromal potential and tear potential is equal to transepithelial potential and is similar in magnitude to values measured in vivo (10 to 35 mV).[16,163]

During the measurement of the electrical potential profile of the epithelium, it is possible to measure the resistance of the cell membranes (see Figure 1-41). Sixty percent of total corneal resistance to ion flow is ascribed to the outer membranes of the superficial epithelial cells. This places the major barrier to corneal permeation of polar (charged) substances at the superficial epithelial cells, a site that is vulnerable to trauma. The measurement also implies that the parallel route for epithelial ion permeation, the paracellular pathway, is of low permeability. The site of the resistive barrier in the paracellular pathway is thought to be the continuous tight junctions present between the superficial epithelial cells (see Figure 1-8B). Despite the fact that the epithelial cell layer is continually regenerated, the barrier remains intact; before a superficial cell desquamates, the underlying cells reorganize to establish tight junctions with adjacent cells to maintain the electrical potential.

The effectiveness of the tight junctions as an ionic diffusion barrier can be measured with microelectrode experiments, and estimates of the cellular pathway resistance to ion permeation can be made.[162] The outer membrane of the superficial cell, in the absence of factors that stimulate ion transport, is twice as good a barrier to ion flow as the tight junction. Considered on the basis of actual surface areas represented by membranes and by junctions, this ratio increases by at least two orders of magnitude. Hence, the tight junctions in the corneal epithelium offer a significant barrier to ion diffusion across the epithelium, but, area for area, the tight junctions are more permeable than the cell membranes they surround.

Stroma

The corneal stroma is primarily an extracellular compartment with keratocytes and nerves accounting for only 5 percent and 0.01 percent of its volume, respectively. The activities* of the major diffusible ions (K^+, Na^+, and Cl^-) are similar in the stroma and the aqueous humor. Although the concentrations of K^+ and Na^+ are higher in the stroma than in the aqueous humor, their effective concentrations (activities) are reduced by physicochemical factors such as ion binding by anionic sites on stromal molecules. The fluid pressed from a swollen stroma, which contains equilibrium activities of stromal ions, has essentially the same ionic composition as aqueous humor. Hence, although the concentration of Na^+ and K^+ may collectively be 35 mEq/L higher in the stroma than in the aqueous humor,[164] the combined activity of these ions, and hence their effective osmolarity, is probably less in the stroma than in the aqueous humor. This concept is necessary to make the chemical ion concentrations measured in the stroma consistent with the current theory of corneal hydration control discussed below.

The negative charges of glycosaminoglycans (10 to 50 mEq/L) are primarily responsible for the abundance of Na^+ and K^+ in the stroma.[165-167] When the stroma swells, the diameter of the collagen fibrils remains constant; swelling takes place in the ground substance, which is rich in glycosaminoglycans, and leads to an increased spatial separation of the collagen fibrils.[168] Several factors influence the swelling force generated by the ground substance: long-range electrostatic repulsive forces between negative charges on the glycosaminoglycans, excess cations required to preserve ionic charge neutrality (Donnan effect), mechanical limitations in the corneal structure that prevent swelling beyond a certain limit,[169] and chemical effects such as change in pH and total ionic strength. For corneal stroma, the major forces involved in stromal swelling appear to be long-range electrostatic repulsion and the Donnan effect (see ref. 44 for a more complete discussion of this issue).

In addition to imparting the underlying force for stromal swelling, the glycosaminoglycan component of the stromal ground substance has other effects on the nature of stromal swelling. Glycosaminoglycans form polymeric macromolecules, which in turn associate with protein cores to form megamolecular complexes within the ground substance. These complexes increase the viscosity of the fluid within the ground substance in a stromal hydration-dependent fashion. Fatt and Goldstick[170] pointed out an important feature of fluid flow in tissues such as stroma: the ability of fluid to flow (to even out differences in hydration) is greatest in tissue that has near-normal hydration and less for swollen or dehydrated tissue—nature's apparent mechanism to preserve homeostasis in the internal environment (Figure 1-42). For example, as the stroma is dehydrated below normal conditions, the driving force for fluid flow (swelling pressure gradient) increases exponentially (Figure 1-43), whereas the stromal hydraulic fluid conductivity decreases as a power function of hydration (Figure 1-44). Because of these properties, normal corneal thickness is

* The activity of an ion is equal to the product of its activity coefficient and its concentration. Gradients in ion activity (not concentration) determine osmotic and diffusional consequences related to flows of solute and solvent across membranes.

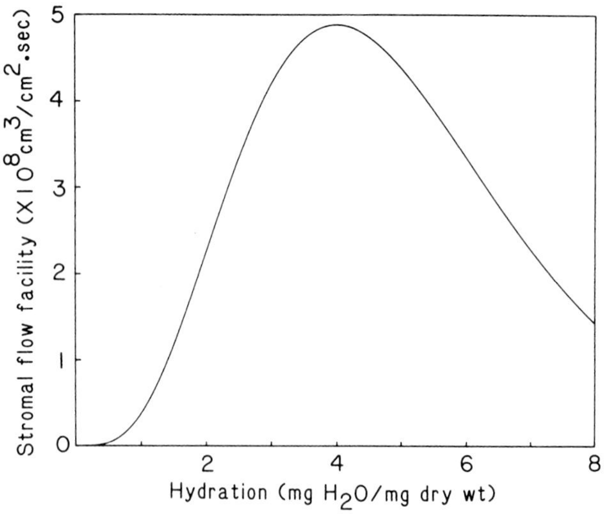

FIGURE 1-42 Plot of stromal fluid flow facility as a function of stromal hydration. Note that fluid flows are most rapid when stromal hydration is normal (3.45).

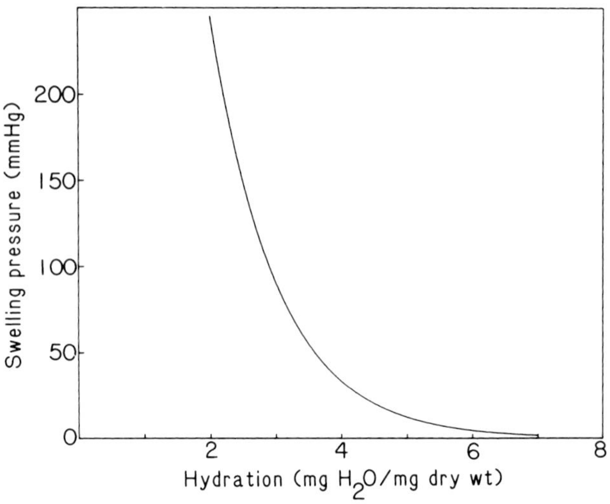

FIGURE 1-43 Stromal swelling pressure for various stromal hydrations. In vivo, average stromal hydration is 3.45 and the swelling pressure is 55 mmHg. Swelling pressure is the driving force that causes fluid to flow from moist stroma to drier regions. The swelling pressure may be very high beneath a corneal delle, but the delle may persist because evaporative loss of fluid through a tear film defect may exceed the rate at which fluid may be replaced by viscous flow from neighboring stromal regions.

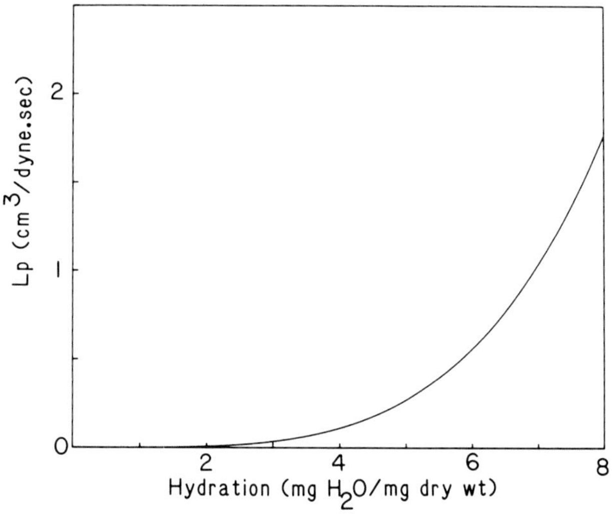

FIGURE 1-44 Plot of stromal hydraulic fluid conductivity (Lp) as a function of stromal hydration.

responsive to subtle changes in the environment, as demonstrated by the 5 percent thinning during waking hours, yet local dry spots or dellen can persist in the anterior stroma while the surrounding tissue is normally hydrated.

It is important to emphasize that the stroma is normally maintained in a relatively dehydrated state, in comparison to its ability to swell. The stroma consists of 78 percent water, which is equivalent to a ratio of 3.45 parts water (by weight) to 1 part solid material. Thus, the hydration is 3.45. The ability of the stroma to swell decreases as its hydration increases. This relationship has been carefully measured for corneal stroma by placing disks of stroma between layers of rigid porous glass in a saline solution. The force necessary to prevent stromal swelling at various hydrations has been termed the *swelling pressure* (SP); these measurements show a near exponential drop with increasing stromal hydration (see Figure 1-43). At normal hydration (3.45), the stromal swelling pressure is approximately 80 g/cm^2 or 55 mmHg.[171,172] This is the amount of force that corneal membranes must create to counterbalance stromal swelling in the living cornea and is equivalent to a stromal osmotic deficit of 2 to 3 mOsm.

It has been proposed that the swelling pressure of stroma as measured in vitro is not an adequate measure of the situation in the living cornea. It was suggested that measurements of swelling pressure determined with excised stroma could be misleading because the conditions normally present in the living eye have been altered. However, Hedbys and co-workers[173] implanted fine saline-filled cannulas into the central stroma of living rabbits and showed that a negative pressure in the cannula was necessary to prevent the stroma from drawing fluid continuously from the tube. The equilibrium suction that prevented this fluid loss was termed the stromal imbibition pressure (IP) and was found to be related to the stromal swelling pressure (SP) by the simple relation

$$IP = IOP - SP \quad (1)$$

In the absence of intraocular pressure (IOP) effects, the imbibition pressure measured in vivo was identical to the swelling pressure measured in vitro.

The pressure of swelling in the normal cornea in vivo was confirmed by a second approach by Klyce and colleagues,[174] who inserted thin, high-water-content hydrogel disks into intralamellar stromal pockets and found that, after the eyes stabilized, the disks were thinner by the amount previously predicted on the basis of stromal swelling pressure. The in vivo cannulation and gel implant experiments confirm the notion that the tendency of the stroma to swell in vivo is the same as was indicated by earlier in vitro experiments.

Ytteborg and Dohlman[175] explored the clinical significance of Equation 1 and showed that when the intraocular pressure exceeds the swelling pressure, subepithelial edema ensues. This dynamic relationship has clinical implications. Stromal swelling pressure is normally 50 to 60 mmHg; the intraocular pressure in glaucoma rarely exceeds this value. However, as noted above, stromal swelling pressure drops off exponentially with stromal edema, so that mild stromal edema combined with mild intraocular pressure elevation can lead to positive stromal imbibition pressure, which, because of the barrier properties of the epithelium, can lead to the collection of subepithelial fluid. Table 1-1 relates the appearance of epithelial edema to intraocular pressure and corneal thickness.

TABLE 1-1
Epithelial Edema: Critical Corneal Thickness Versus Intraocular Pressure

Intraocular Pressure (mmHg)	*Corneal Thickness[a] (μm)*
5	824
10	737
15	687
normal → 20	651
25	623
30	600
35	581
40	564
45	549
50	536
55	524 ← normal
60	513
65	503
70	494
75	485

[a]Calculated from thickness = 0.0875 - $\log_e$(IOP/1810)/8. At normal thickness, intraocular pressure may rise to 55 mmHg without epithelial edema. At normal intraocular pressure, the cornea should be able to swell up to 650 μm without epithelial edema.

The stromal experiments led to another important topic in stromal physiology, which deals with how intraocular pressure distributes itself across corneal thickness in terms of stress factors on the structural tunic. This has an important bearing on current problems in refractive surgery.[176] Intraocular pressure normally commutes through the stroma and is dissipated by stress on the anteriormost stromal lamellae. Several implications of this concept are discussed below. It is, however, important to emphasize that when anterior stromal lamellae are cut, they can no longer bear the stress of intraocular pressure, which is then transferred to the deeper, intact lamellae.[176]

There is a linear relationship between central corneal thickness (q), expressed in millimeters, and stromal hydration (H), expressed as the ratio of the weight of water in the tissue to the dry tissue weight:

$$H = 8q - 0.7 \quad (2)$$

It has been shown experimentally that the hydration of the anterior stroma is less than that of the posterior stroma.[177] This is usually taken to mean that there are differences in the types or concentrations of glycosaminoglycans at these different locations. However, such a gradient can be predicted by computer simulation on the basis of dissimilarities in the permeability properties between the epithelium and endothelium alone, even in the absence of tear film evaporation.[178]

The stroma requires continuous maintenance by its keratocytes to sustain its macromolecular composition and consequent organization. Normally, keratocytes, although having all the anatomic features consistent with synthetic activity, appear to be quiescent in terms of mobility. In fact, however, keratocytes are quite responsive to changes in their environment. They can mobilize to repopulate stromal areas devoid of keratocytes and may rapidly degenerate below areas where trauma to the epithelium has occurred,[179] although this phenomenon is the subject of controversy.[180]

Endothelium

This section summarizes the features of endothelial physiology that contribute to the maintenance of corneal hydration and transparency.

Endothelial Ion Transport Mechanisms

The specific ion transport mechanisms associated with the endothelial stromal dehydrating mechanism have been sought for several years. Initial studies reported that ouabain inhibits fluid transport by the rabbit corneal endothelium in vitro.[181] It was found that ouabain inhibits Na^+/K^+ ATPase, which is normally associated with the regulation of cell volume; this suggested that active Na^+ transport is intimately involved in the endothelial fluid transport function. However, whether Na^+ transport is simply a necessary prerequisite for normal cell function or whether it is the primary mechanism for endothelial fluid transport awaited further experimental demonstration. In association with its high ionic permeability, the corneal endothelium has a low electrical resistance.[182] This leaky property made classic tracer experiments to demonstrate net ion transport mechanisms technically difficult.[183] However, with advances in technology, the endothelium was shown to transport bicarbonate from the stroma to the aqueous humor in amounts sufficient to explain the simultaneous isotonic transport of fluid.[184,185] Subsequently, the transport of sodium ions in the same direction was inferred.[186] Although the specific details of these transport mechanisms are as yet unclear, several different schemes appear in the literature,[187-189] indicating dependency of the transport system on both sodium and bicarbonate but not chloride.

How the transport of solute by the endothelium brings about the transport of fluid across the endothelium is not clear. It is generally agreed that the basic mechanism for the corneal endothelial fluid pump is the transport of solute(s) from some sequestered volume into the aqueous humor. On a theoretical basis, a model of corneal hydration dynamics that used the stroma as this sequestered volume was remarkably accurate in its ability to predict the corneal response to a variety of environmental and metabolic perturbations.[105,178] However, it has been clearly shown that the endothelial fluid pumping capability remains intact despite the removal of most[190-192] or all[190] of the corneal stroma.[190-192] Hence, whether this sequestered volume may be the endothelial extracellular space, or the endothelial cells themselves, remains unclear.[138,187-196]

In summary, the corneal endothelium secretes bicarbonate and sodium into the aqueous humor, and this transport system creates an osmotic gradient that balances the swelling tendency of the corneal stroma.

Endothelial "Fluid Pump"

As originally proposed,[190] the concept of an endothelial "fluid pump" was used to explain many independent experimental observations that the corneal endothelium can transfer fluid from a swollen stroma to the aqueous humor by means of an energy-consuming mechanism. Implicit in this concept was the underlying principle that flow of water across the endothelium occurred in predictably non–energy-consuming fashion in response to osmotic gradients established by membrane ion transport systems, a fundamental principle that has dominated general physiologic volume regulation teachings for decades. However, until recently, the ionic basis for the driving force(s) behind the endothelial volume regulatory property has been elusive. Corneal endothelial fluid transport studies led to increasing acceptance of the idea that the corneal endothelium pumps fluid as a primary metabolic process. This, in turn, led to generalized terminology and less than ideal concepts, including the notion of endothelial "fluid pump" and "fluid leak" balance in the maintenance of corneal hydration. It is emphasized that this terminology is, at best, misleading. As discussed above, the endothelium has specific membrane ion transport complexes whose collective actions lead to the passive secondary movement of water. The active membrane transport of water has never been demonstrated in any tissue. Hence, the terms "fluid pump" and "fluid leak" poorly represent the ionic mechanisms that underlie the ability of the endothelium to regulate stromal volume. The ability of the endothelium to transport fluid is well documented by experiments that show this transport to be consistent with observed active ion transport processes. An endothelium that becomes "leaky" in the process of trauma or aging leaks both ions and water. It is probable that ion leakage is a more important factor than water leakage in the explanation of why the cornea swells during endothelial decompensation.

In summary, the term "fluid pump" was originally developed to describe experimentally observed stromal dehydration capabilities. However, the driving force for this process is now known to be based on ion transport mechanisms, not the energy-consuming transfer of fluid itself across the corneal endothelium.

CONTROL OF CORNEAL HYDRATION

Several hypotheses have been proposed to explain the control of corneal hydration. Several components of corneal physiology are involved in this process (Figure 1-45). Underlying each of the hypotheses is the fact that stromal imbibition pressure (IP) must be counteracted to prevent swelling. In the past, it was suggested that although the cornea is surrounded by fluid, it would not swell if the cell membranes were impermeable to either water[197] or salt.[171,198] Although both the epithelial and endothelial cell membranes have defined barrier properties, neither membrane is impermeable to water or electrolytes.[199] The effect of evaporation from the tear film has also been suggested as a major source for the control of corneal hydration[200] and, as mentioned above, the

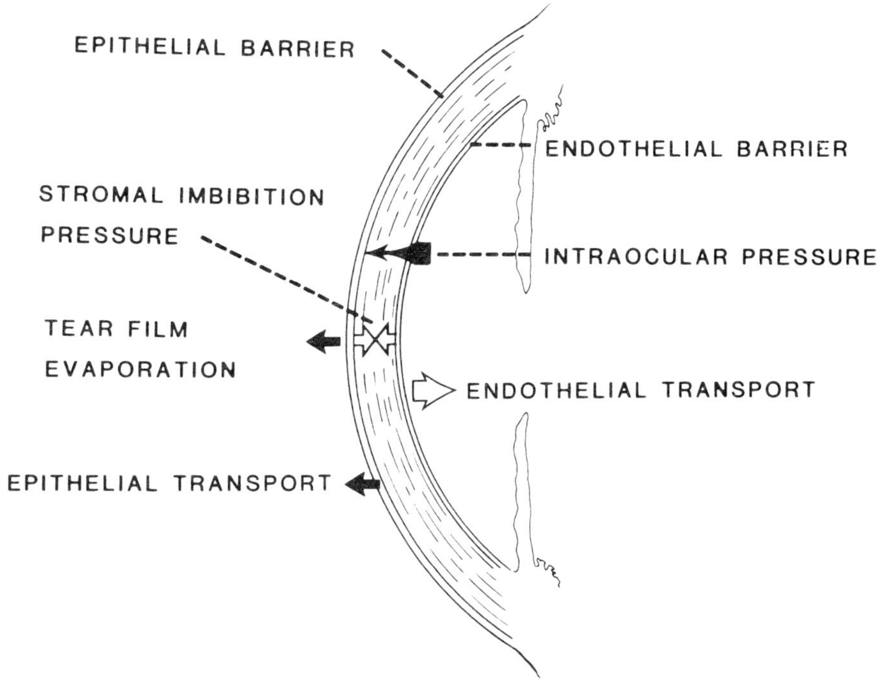

FIGURE 1-45 Factors and forces involved in the control of corneal stromal hydration. Intraocular pressure and stromal imbibition pressure are forces that promote water accumulation in the stroma. Ion transport pumps in the corneal membranes reduce the osmotic pressure of the stroma such that the semipermeable membrane properties of the epithelium and endothelium balance the forces promoting edema.

cornea is 5 percent thinner during waking hours than during sleep.[118,201] However, an isolated cornea, bathed by identical media on both sides, can maintain near-normal thickness for up to 30 hours,[202] which argues against a major role for evaporation in the control of hydration. The intraocular pressure has also been considered in this respect, and although the corneal thickness varies with changes in intraocular pressure, these changes are not sufficient to explain the control of normal corneal hydration. Additionally, isolated corneas maintain near-normal thickness in the absence of intraocular pressure.

These factors may not normally be paramount in the control of stromal hydration, but they are important properties of the dynamics of the control of corneal hydration. Disruption of the lipid layer of the tear film leads to evaporation from the epithelial surface, which can lead to dellen formation. High postoperative intraocular pressure can promote more rapid clearing of a corneal graft by accelerating the movement of fluid through the anterior corneal surface, thereby thinning the cornea. However, elevated intraocular pressure can also cause epithelial edema, as well as stromal swelling, in certain refractive surgical procedures,[176] and the barrier properties of the epithelium and endothelium are also important factors in the control of corneal hydration.

Maurice[199] first proposed that because the corneal membranes are not impermeable to solute or water, they could prevent corneal edema if ions were actively transported out of the stroma as fast as they leaked in by passive means (solvent drag, diffusion). Such a process would, in essence, lead to the sustaining of an osmotic gradient (2 to 3 mOsm) between the corneal stroma and the external solutions, which would balance the swelling pressure of the stroma. This stromal solute deficit is 1 percent or less of the aqueous humor osmolarity and is, therefore, difficult to detect with freezing point depression measurements.[203] However, Davson[204] and Harris and Nordquist[205] convincingly demonstrated that corneal hydration is closely linked to the metabolic activity of corneal membranes: corneas swelled when refrigerated at temperatures that slowed metabolic processes and returned to normal thickness when warmed to body temperature. The temperature reversal phenomenon, as it has come to be known, is mediated by the corneal endothelium and inhibited by ouabain.[206] Studies involving the temperature reversal phenomenon have provided much information on the functional characteristics of the corneal endothelium in terms of the ability of the corneal endothelium to transport fluid from the stroma into the aqueous humor. Implicit in the term fluid pump, as applied here, is that it is the active transport of one or more ions by a cell layer that causes osmotic gradients to occur and water to flow across membranes in accordance with the laws of thermodynamics, as discussed above.

Because corneal epithelial and endothelial ion transport processes have been fairly well described and because the water flow properties of the stroma have also been characterized, it has been possible to combine these proper-

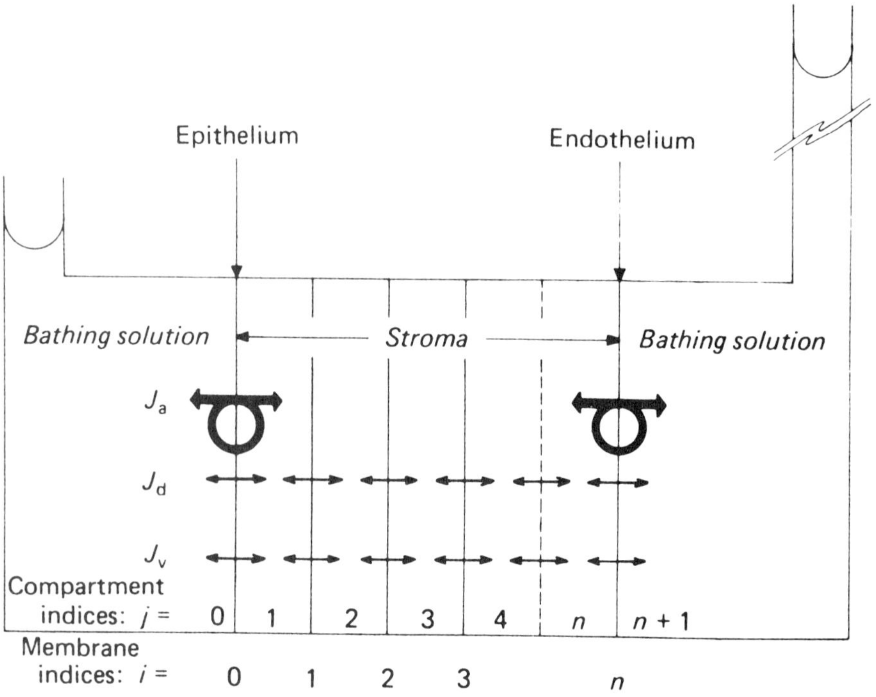

FIGURE 1-46 Model for the simulation of corneal hydration dynamics. Schematic representation of corneal model. Flows of volume (J_v), and solute, both active (J_a) and passive (J_d), can be calculated across the series of n + 1 membranes, where n is determined by stability criteria for a given calculation. The thicknesses of the stromal compartments, hence the relative positions of the membranes, are permitted to vary in time. (Reprinted with permission from SD Klyce, SR Russell: Numerical solution of coupled transport equations applied to corneal hydration dynamics. J Physiol 292:107, 1979.)

ties into models that describe the dynamics of corneal hydration to evaluate the relative contributions of the factors shown in Figure 1-46.

Fluid flow (J_v) across a membrane is equal to the difference between the hydrostatic pressure gradient (ΔP) and the osmotic gradient ($\Delta\pi$) multiplied by the membrane water permeability (Lp):

$$J_v = Lp(\Delta P - \Delta\pi) \tag{3}$$

This equation states that an increase in hydrostatic pressure on one side of a membrane and/or an increase in osmotic pressure on the other side of the membrane produces a flow rate controlled by the water permeability of the membrane. With regard to fluid flow into the cornea across the endothelium, Equation 3 intentionally implies that intraocular pressure and stromal imbibition pressure both drive fluid into the stroma, whereas ion pumps that remove solute from the stroma osmotically counter this flow. When the net fluid flow is zero, as is nearly the case for the healthy cornea, the hydrostatic pressure gradient across the endothelium (IOP – SP) is equal to the osmotic gradient (reduced stromal solute).

To complete this model, flows of solute must be considered. Solutes diffuse across membranes at a rate equal to their solute permeability (ω) times their concentration gradient, ΔC_s. Solutes are also transported actively across corneal membranes, and this may be expressed by the term J_a. Finally, it has been shown that in many membranes (such as the highly permeable corneal endothelium), the bulk flow of fluid carries solute with it, which adds a third term to net solute flow (J_s). This relationship can be written

$$J_s = (1 - \sigma)\bar{C}_s J_v + \omega RT\Delta C_s + J_a \tag{4}$$

$$\text{net solute flow} = \text{solvent drag} + \text{diffusion} + \text{active transport}$$

where σ, the reflection coefficient, is a membrane property related to the extent that bulk fluid flow across a membrane can drag along solute, $\bar{C}_s$ is the average solute concentration on each side of the membrane, and RT is the product of the gas constant and the temperature. In the normal case, where the stroma is not changing in thickness, Equation 4 would predict that $J_s = J_v = 0$, where the active transport of solute (J_a) out of the stroma just balances the diffusional leak ($\omega RT\Delta C_s$) of solute into the stroma, which is the basis of Maurice's original pump-leak hypothesis.

Equations 3 and 4 form the basis for our understanding of the contribution of various factors (see Figure 1-45) in corneal hydration control. As noted above, it is easy to state that the endothelial pump controls normal hydration, but this simplification does not help us to understand the causes of edema, especially when factors other than endothelial decompensation are involved. These equations have been used in their simplest form to provide a quantitative method to help evaluate the cause of corneal stromal edema. Yet in the model described, simplicity has been preserved in that the corneal membranes are considered to be homogeneous, which makes it possible to determine the unknowns experimentally without using indirect inference or best guesses.

The epithelial and endothelial corneal membranes are characterized by Equations 3 and 4, whereas the stroma is characterized by reduced forms of these equations. There is no active transport of solute within the stroma and no volume transport owing to osmotic gradients across the stroma. Whereas the concentration of solutes across the stroma is fairly uniform as a result of a relatively high stromal permeability (only two times less than free diffusion in aqueous medium), the flow of water is far more restricted. Hence, to allow for the steep gradients that can arise (corneal dellen are a good example), the corneal stroma is subdivided into layers in the model (see Figure 1-46).

In this approach, no assumptions were made as to the permeability coefficients (σ, ω, Lp) for the corneal epithelium or endothelium. These were determined by fit to experiments that measured the response of corneal thickness to small changes in the osmolarity of the tear-side bathing solution. Permeability coefficients for solute and water across the stroma were taken directly from the precise work of Fatt and Goldstick.[170] Table 1-2 summarizes the results of these determinations and compares them with previous measurements and to solute permeabilities measured with tracers.[131,178,181,184,185,207-213]

The model was tested rigorously against well-documented experimental observation. A comparison between a temperature reversal experiment and model prediction is shown in Figure 1-47A. The fit is not precise, but it substantiates the notion that if the cornea is considered simply as two thin ion-transporting membranes bounding the stroma, temperature reversal can be predicted with reasonable accuracy. Ouabain completely inhibits endothelial fluid transport. Setting the model's endothelial solute pump equal to zero led to a calculated stromal swelling indistinguishable from the rate reported experimentally (Figure 1-47B). Several other reactions of the cornea to experimental manipulations support this approach.[177,178] Additionally, this model has been used to provide evidence supporting the thesis that stromal edema after hypoxia of the tear film is the result of stromal accumulation of lactate,[107] an osmotically active by-product of anaerobic respiration.

There are limitations to the scope of the model. For example, the model gives a value for permeability of the endothelium to small solutes such as NaCl that is several times higher than the value measured for NaCl isotope fluxes. However, the model, as well as traditional isotope flux measurements, does not consider that the endothelium is heterogeneous (has cellular and paracellular pathways), and this could be the source of the discrepancy

TABLE 1-2
Corneal Membrane Permeability

Epithelium				Endothelium				
σNaCl	*Lp*[a]	*ωRT*[b]	J_a[c]	*σNaCl*	*Lp*[a]	*ωRT*[b]	J_a[c]	*Reference*
—	—	0.016 (Na)	—	—	—	2 (Na)	—	Maurice (1953)[207]
1[d]	6.9	—	—	0.6	15.8	—	—	Mishima and Hedbys (1967)[208]
1[d]	6.5	—	—	0.6[d]	13.8	—	—	Stanley et al (1966)[209]
—	—	—	—	—	—	2.1 (urea)	—	Trenberth and Mishima (1968)[181]
0.8	0.4	—	—	0.4	1.4	—	—	Green and Green (1969)[210]
—	—	—	—	—	—	2.2 (Cl)	—	Kim et al (1971)[211]
—	—	0.014 (Cl)	<0.03[e]	—	—	—	—	Klyce (1975)[131]
—	—	—	—	—	—	—	3.9 (HCO_3)	Hodson and Miller (1976)[184]
—	0.9	—	—	—	3	—	—	Green and Downs (1976)[212]
—	—	—	—	0.6[d]	8	—	—	Fischbarg et al (1977)[213]
—	—	—	—	—	—	—	12.9 (HCO_3)	Hull et al (1977)[185]
0.79	6.1	0.019 (NaCl)	<0.08e	0.45	42	8 (NaCl)	4.7	Klyce and Russell (1979)[178]

[a] $\times 10^{-12}$ cm³/dyne · sec.
[b] $\times 10^{-5}$ cm/sec.
[c] $\times 10^{-10}$ mole/cm² · sec.
[d] Assumed values.
[e] Basal epithelial transport rate (Cl secretion unstimulated).
Source: Adapted from SD Klyce, SR Russell: Numerical solution of coupled transport equations applied to corneal hydration dynamics. J Physiol 292:107, 1979.

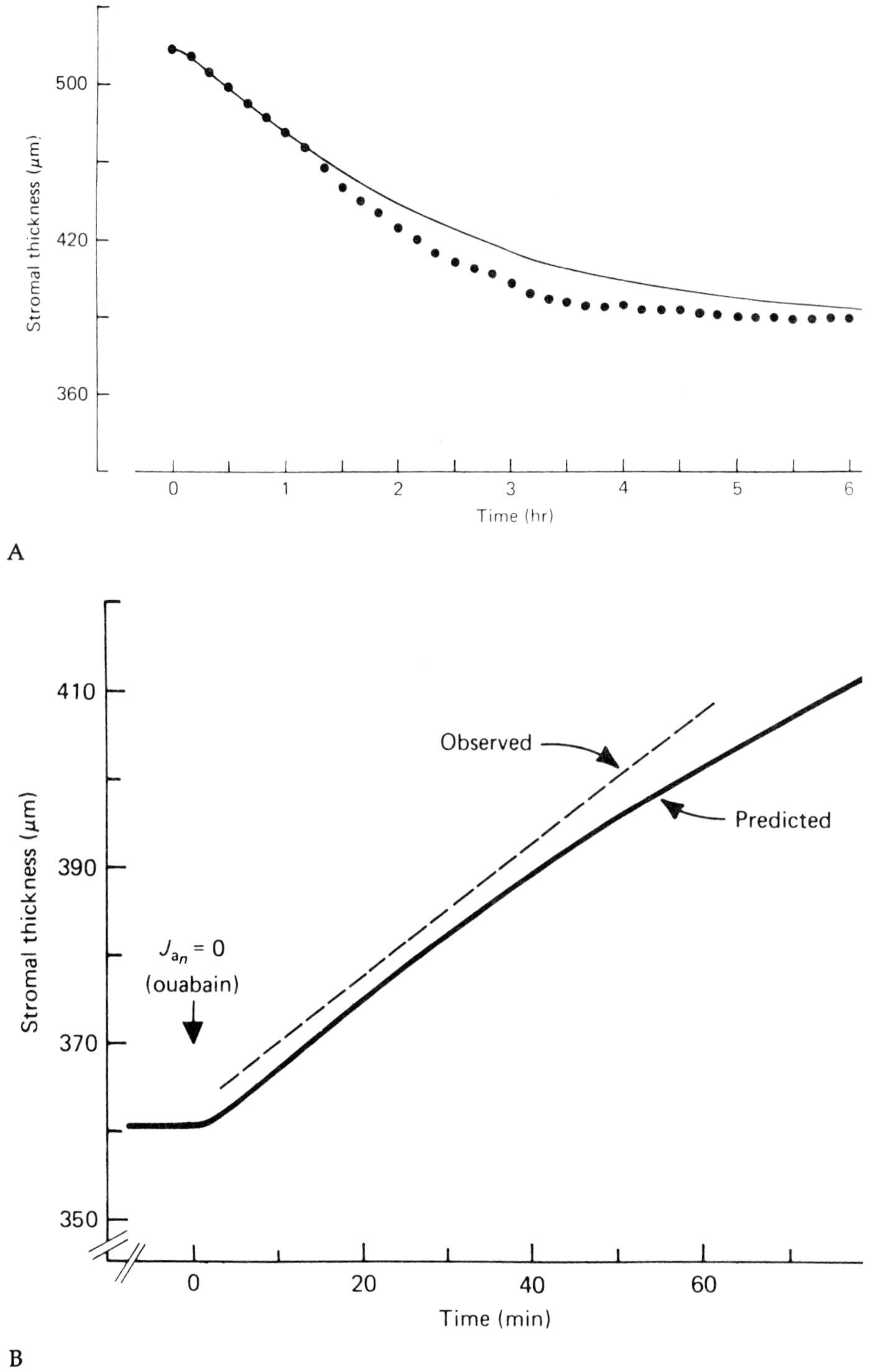

FIGURE 1-47 **(A)** Fit to a "temperature reversal" experiment. The continuous line is the calculated stromal thickness after swelling the bare stromal surface with Ringer's solution and subsequently blocking it with oil. Experimental data (•) were obtained with an automatic specular microscope.[202] **(B)** The calculated effect of ouabain inhibition on stromal thickness. The continuous line is the calculated (predicted) response with the endothelial solute pump set to zero at the arrow. The experimentally observed rate determined by Mishima et al[113] is indicated by the dashed line. (Reprinted with permission from SD Klyce, SR Russell: Numerical solution of coupled transport equations applied to corneal hydration dynamics. J Physiol 292:107, 1979.)

between the two measurements. One measurement is a functional description of permeability, in terms of effect, and the other is a physical measurement with isotopes, also without regard for endothelial heterogeneity.[214] The second limitation is that the model relies on sequestration of solute in the corneal stroma to explain osmotic fluid transport by the endothelium. This assumption preserves simplicity (enabling unique determination of unknowns) and is quite successful in matching the model to many experimental observations in terms of corneal hydration dynamics, but it is apparently not accurate, in that the corneal endothelium can transport fluid when the bulk of the stroma has been removed,[190,191] as well as in a monolayer in tissue culture.[193] Because this simple model fits so well with many other whole corneal responses to environmental manipulations, it is unlikely that the endothelial transport characteristics determined in special situations, which emphasize its separate capabilities, will alter our understanding of the fundamental contributions of the endothelium to the control of corneal hydration.

It is important to emphasize in this section that the pump-leak hypothesis, as originally proposed[199] for the control of corneal hydration, implied that normal corneal thickness and the prevention of corneal edema are the result of active transport of solute out of the stroma, creating the necessary osmotic deficit for the osmotic prevention of stromal fluid imbibition. Further work has confirmed that it is solute that is transported by direct cell metabolic energy expense and not fluid. Fluid (water plus solutes dragged along) follows osmotic gradients established by ion transport processes. There is no substantial evidence to support the notion that fluid per se is actively transported in the cornea. Transcellular fluid transport in the cornea, as elsewhere, is secondary to osmotic gradients established by ion transport pumps.

OPTICAL PROPERTIES

As the major refractive element of the eye, the cornea must fulfill the criteria for optical lenses: adequate smoothness, spherical shape, and internal transparency. The anterior and posterior surfaces of the human cornea are nearly spherical, particularly in the central region, which is most important in the attainment of good visual acuity. As the cornea thickens toward the periphery, the anterior surface becomes flatter, resulting in a lower peripheral surface power.[215] This can be illustrated by videokeratography[215-218] (see Ch. 46).

The total refractive power of the cornea is the sum of the refractive powers across three interfaces: air/tear, tear/cornea, and cornea/aqueous humor. The formula for calculating the power of a given interface is

$$P_s = \frac{n_2 - n_1}{r} \qquad (5)$$

where P_s is the refractive power of the surface in diopters, n_1 and n_2 are the refractive indices of the first and second media, respectively, and r is the radius of curvature (in meters) of the surface. The indices of refraction of air (1.000), tears (1.336), cornea (1.376), and aqueous humor (1.336) are well established. In the normal adult, the average central anterior corneal radius of curvature is 7.8 mm (range, 7.0 to 8.8 mm), whereas the average posterior corneal radius of curvature is 6.5 mm. Hence, the power of the air/tear interface is (1.336 - 1.000)/0.078 or +43.1 diopters, the power of the tear/cornea interface is +5.1 diopters, and the power of the cornea/aqueous humor interface is -6.2 diopters. The total corneal power for the average eye is, therefore, +42.0 diopters. This value represents the most common total corneal power, although emmetropes can have a range of powers from +38 to +48 diopters without pathology.

The total power of the combination of air, tears, cornea, and aqueous humor can thus be expressed as a single dioptric power. This calculation, however, ignores the possibility of changes that may be introduced by alterations in corneal thickness or the refractive index of the cornea (which changes with corneal edema). Clinically, these factors are difficult to measure; therefore, in many optical calculations (such as intraocular lens formulas and contact lens fitting), the assumption is made that the power contributions of a specific cornea are those of the normal cornea. In contrast, the curvature of the air/tear interface can be measured precisely with the keratometer, which calculates the power of the tear surface using the curvature and a constant that combines the individual contributions of the corneal surfaces. This semiempirical constant is the Keratometric Index; it most commonly has a value of 337.5 ([1.3375 - 1.0000] × 1000), although there may be some variation in the numbers used by manufacturers of keratometers and keratoscopes. Based on the Keratometric Index, the dioptric power of a cornea with an average central radius of curvature of 7.8 mm would be 337.5/7.8, or 43.3 diopters. The dioptic power calculated by Equation 5 is different from that calculated by the Keratometric Index; the former calculation is a simplification and does not account for variations in corneal refractive index and thickness, whereas the latter calculation is empirical.

The optical performance of the cornea can be degraded by tissue scarring and edema. These problems can best be understood by a summary of the physical basis for stromal transparency. Dry collagen has a refractive index of 1.550; ground substance has a refractive index of 1.354.[219] Commonly, such disparity in refractive indices produces light scatter, and the tissue appears white, as in the sclera. On the basis of the observation that the collagen fibrils within the stromal lamellae are arranged in what appears to be a perfect crystalline lattice (see Figure 1-19), it was proposed that corneal transparency is maintained because light scattered by individual fibers is cancelled by destructive interference with scattered light from neighboring fibers.[219] However, Goldman and Benedek[220] and others[221,222] recognized that refractive elements in tissues whose dimensions are small (less than 2,000 Å) compared with the wavelength of light (approximately 5,000 Å) should not scatter as much light as might be predicted by the crystalline lattice theory. Accordingly, the normal stroma scatters light minimally because its collagen fibrils are uniformly small in diameter (approximately 300 Å) and closely spaced (approximately 550 Å), whereas the opaque sclera contains collagen fibrils with diameters ranging from 250 to 4,800 Å. Furthermore, the quasiregular arrangement of stromal collagen fibrils appears to be an unnecessary requirement for transparency. In humans, Bowman's layer is 8 to 12 μm thick and its constituent collagen fibrils are irregularly arranged; nevertheless, it is relatively transparent. According to the Goldman-Benedek criterion, the stroma should remain relatively transparent as long as the dimensions of spatial fluctuations in refractive index remain less than 2,000 Å. As the stroma swells, it expands the ground substance, which increases the spacing between collagen fibrils. As the spacing increases and the degree of short-range fibril order decreases, large fluctuations in refractive index occur, and light scattering ensues. This criterion has also been applied to suggest the origin of light scattering in the human corneal epithelium.[223]

CORNEAL PERMEABILITY/DRUG DELIVERY

The pharmacokinetics of topical ocular drugs are important to the treatment of ocular disease. The epithelial surface retards the diffusion of water-soluble (hydrophilic) substances through both the apical superficial cell membranes and the paracellular pathways between cells, which are occluded by a continuous band of tight junctions. Lipid-soluble (lipophilic or hydrophobic) substances, however, permeate cell membranes with ease but are immiscible in the aqueous layer of the tear film. Some solubility in both water and lipid, therefore, is necessary for topical drugs to penetrate the cornea.

Several techniques have been used to facilitate drug penetration. A drug applied topically to the eye is almost immediately diluted by the tears. Maintaining a useful concentration of the drug in the precorneal tear film for minutes rather than seconds can dramatically increase drug penetration. Soft contact lenses soaked in various drugs (to absorb the drug) and placed on the eye (to hold the drug on the surface of the cornea) have been used in the past[224]; however, this technique never became very practical. The same principle has been used with collagen shields, and collagen shields soaked in antibiotics have become valuable in the treatment of corneal ulcers and in providing prophylactic antibiotics after surgery.[225-227]

Drugs may be incorporated into carriers such as microscopic liposomes or lipid micelles that are small enough to be suspended in the tears. This approach offers the potential for increasing contact time with the surface of the cornea and provides the opportunity for fusion with epithelial cell membranes and consequent dispensing of the contents of the carriers into the cells. Another possibility is the entrapment of drug molecules in the interstices of the matrix of small pieces of collagen, which can be suspended in a vehicle and applied like eye drops. Water-soluble drugs are washed out of the collagen matrix relatively rapidly by the tears, so this system does not substantially extend their contact time. However, poorly water-soluble drugs form suspensions within the collagen and are slowly released as the collagen dissolves. In this way, drugs such as cyclosporine, which are difficult to administer because of poor penetration, may become practical for topical use on the eye.

Special solvents have been used to dissolve and administer drugs. Various oils, such as cod liver oil, dissolve cyclosporine, but the drug preferentially remains dissolved in the oil, and total penetration may be limited. Other solvents, such as dimethylsulfoxide, penetrate the lipid membrane readily but are toxic, which makes them of little use.

The addition of groups that make the drug lipid soluble and are then hydrolyzed off the drug to restore the active compound are commonly used in ophthalmology. Such drugs are called prodrugs; they are not active in themselves and require biotransformation to the parent compound before therapeutic activity is seen. For example, dipivefrin is a prodrug of epinephrine formed by the diesterification of epinephrine and pivalic acid. The addition of the pivaloyl groups to the epinephrine enhances its lipophilic character and, as a consequence, its penetration into the anterior chamber. After the facilitated penetration of the lipid-soluble ester has taken place, the drug is converted to epinephrine inside the eye. This type of conversion of a lipid-soluble compound to an active drug has also been applied to a variety of other drugs.

An alternative approach to enhancing the corneal penetration of topical medication involves increasing corneal surface permeability using agents such as tetracaine, which has been shown to disrupt the epithelial paracellular junctional complexes.[228] The major disadvantage of this approach is that before the epithelial tight junctions re-form, tear-borne pathogens could also enter the eye, causing secondary infection. In the past, other substances that damage the lipid membrane have been used in this way. For example, carbachol, which penetrates poorly under normal circumstances, can become a useful drug in combination with a relatively high concentration of the detergent/preservative benzalkonium chloride, which minimally damages the epithelial cell membrane and facilitates drug penetration.

Iontophoresis, the use of a charged electrode to repel charged drug and drive it into the cornea, has been studied for many years but has never gained wide use.[225,226]

Acknowledgments
We are grateful to Dr. Craig E. Crosson for his contributions to the description of epithelial ion transport processes.

This work was supported in part by USPHS grants EY03311, EY04074, and EY02377 from the National Eye Institute, National Institutes of Health, Bethesda, Maryland, and by the Louisiana Lions Eye Foundation.

We also thank the National Disease Research Interchange (NDRI) for providing the human corneas used to illustrate this chapter.

REFERENCES

1. Kuwabara T: Current concepts in anatomy and histology of the cornea. Contact Intraocular Lens Med J 4:101, 1978
2. Records RE: Tear film. p. 47. In Records RE (ed): Physiology of the Human Eye and Visual System. Harper & Row, New York, 1979
3. Mishima S, Gasset A, Klyce SD, et al: Determination of tear volume and tear flow. Invest Ophthalmol 5:264, 1966
4. Rolando M, Refojo M: Tear evaporimeter for measuring water evaporation rate from the tear film under controlled conditions in humans. Exp Eye Res 36:25, 1983
5. Benjamin WJ, Hill RM: Human tears: osmotic characteristics. Invest Ophthalmol Vis Sci 24:1624, 1983
6. Nichols BA, Chiappino ML, Dawson CR: Demonstration of the mucous layer of the tear film by electron microscopy. Invest Ophthalmol Vis Sci 26:464, 1985
7. Ehlers N: Some comparative studies on the mammalian corneal epithelium. Acta Ophthalmol (Copenh) 48:821, 1970
8. Hanna C, Bicknell DS, O'Brien J: Cell turnover in the adult human eye. Arch Ophthalmol 65:695, 1961
9. Teng CC: The fine structure of the corneal epithelium and basement membrane of the rabbit. Am J Ophthalmol 51:278, 1961
10. Nichols B, Dawson CR, Togni B: Surface features of the conjunctiva and cornea. Invest Ophthalmol Vis Sci 24:570, 1983
11. Pfister RR: The normal surface of corneal epithelium: a scanning and electron microscopic study. Invest Ophthalmol 12:654, 1973
12. Hoffman F: The surface of epithelial cells of the cornea under the scanning electron microscope. Ophthalmic Res 3:207, 1972
13. Hazlett LD, Wells P, Spann B, et al: Epithelial desquamation in the adult-mouse cornea. A correlative TEM-SEM study. Ophthalmic Res 12:315, 1980
14. Pfister R, Renner M: The histopathology of experimental dry spots and dellen in the rabbit cornea: a light microscopy and scanning and transmission electron microscopy study. Invest Ophthalmol Vis Sci 16:1025, 1977
15. McLaughlin BJ, Caldwell RB, Sasaki Y, et al: Freeze-fracture quantitative comparison of rabbit corneal epithelial and endothelial membranes. Curr Eye Res 4:951, 1985
16. Klyce SD: Electrical profiles in the corneal epithelium. J Physiol 226:407, 1972
17. Kikkawa Y: Normal corneal staining with fluorescein. Exp Eye Res 14:13, 1972
18. Schultz RO, Peters MA, Sobocinski K, et al: Diabetic keratopathy as a manifestation of peripheral neuropathy. Am J Ophthalmol 96:368, 1983
19. Ito S: Form and function of the glycocalyx on free cell surfaces. Philos Trans R Soc Lond [Biol] 268:55, 1974
20. Gipson IK, Anderson RA: Actin filaments in normal and migrating corneal epithelial cells. Invest Ophthalmol Vis Sci 16:161, 1977
21. Vracko R, Benditt EP: Basal lamina: the scaffold for orderly cell replacement. Observations on regeneration of injured skeletal muscle fibers and capillaries. J Cell Biol 55:406, 1972
22. Segawa K: Electron microscopic studies on the human corneal epithelium: dendritic cells. Arch Ophthalmol 72:650, 1964
23. Gillette TE, Chandler JW, Greiner JV: Langerhans cells of the ocular surface. Ophthalmology 89:700, 1982
24. Madri JA, Pratt BM, Yurchenco PD, et al: The ultrastructural organization and architecture of basement membrane. p. 6. In Porter R, Whelan J (eds): Basement Membranes and Cell Movement, CIBA Foundation Symposium. Vol. 108. Pitman Press, London, 1984
25. Sakai LY, Keene DR, Morris MP, Burgeson RE: Type VII collagen is a major structural component of anchoring fibrils. J Cell Biol 103:1577, 1986
26. Tisdale AS, Spurr-Michaud SJ, Rodrigues M, et al: Development of the anchoring structures of the epithelium in rabbit and human fetal corneas. Invest Ophthalmol Vis Sci 29:727, 1988
27. Alvarado J, Murphy C, Juster R: Age-related changes in the basement membrane of the human corneal epithelium. Invest Ophthalmol Vis Sci 24:1015, 1983
28. Azar DT, Spurr-Michaud SJ, Tisdale AS, Gibson IK: Altered epithelial-basement membrane interactions in diabetic corneas. Arch Ophthalmol 110:537, 1992
29. Taylor HR, Kimsey RA: Corneal epithelial basement membrane changes in diabetes. Invest Ophthalmol Vis Sci 20:548, 1981
30. Vracko R: Basal lamina layering in diabetes mellitus: evidence for accelerated rate of cell death and cell regeneration. Diabetes 23:94, 1974
31. Kenyon K, Wafai Z, Michels R, et al: Corneal basement membrane abnormality in diabetes mellitus. ARVO abstract. Invest Ophthalmol Vis Sci 17(suppl):245, 1978

32. Packer L, Packer A, Harrison L, et al: Relationship between ultrastructure of diabetic corneal epithelium and postvitrectomy epithelialization. ARVO abstract. Invest Ophthalmol Vis Sci 26(suppl):93, 1985
33. Madri JA, Roll J, Furthmay H, et al: Ultrastructural localization of fibronectin and laminin in the basement membrane of the murine kidney. J Cell Biol 86:682, 1980
34. Newsome DA, Foidart JM, Hassell JR, et al: Detection of specific collagen types in normal and keratoconus corneas. Invest Ophthalmol Vis Sci 20:738, 1981
35. Masutani M, Ogawa H, Taneda A, et al: Ultrastructural localization of immunoglobulins in the dermoepidermal junction of patients with bullous pemphigoid. J Dermatol 5:107, 1976
36. Millin JA, Golub BM, Foster CS: Human basement membrane components of keratoconus and normal corneas. Invest Ophthalmol Vis Sci 27:604, 1986
37. Tervo K, van Setten G-B, Beuerman RW, et al: Expression of tenascin and cellular fibronectin in the rabbit cornea after anterior keratectomy. Invest Ophthalmol Vis Sci 32:2912, 1991
38. Ruoslahti E: Fibronectin and its receptors. Annu Rev Biochem 57:375, 1988
39. Bourdon MA, Ruoslahti E: Tenascin mediates cell attachment through an RGD-dependent receptor. J Cell Biol 108:1149,1989
40. Tervo K, Tervo T, van Setten G-B, Virtanen I: Integrins in human corneal epithelium. Cornea 10:461, 1991
41. Bron AJ, Tripathi RC: Anterior corneal mosaic. Further observations. Br J Ophthalmol 53:760, 1969
42. Binder PS, Rock ME, Schmidt KC, Anderson JA: High-voltage electron microscopy of normal human cornea. Invest Ophthalmol Vis Sci 32:2234, 1991
43. Matsuda H: Electron microscopic study on the corneal nerve with special reference to its endings. Jpn J Ophthalmol 12:163, 1967
44. Maurice DM: The cornea and sclera. p. 1. In Davson H (ed): The Eye. Vol. 1B. Vegetative Physiology and Biochemistry. 3rd Ed. Academic Press, Orlando, FL, 1984
45. Cintron C, Schneider H, Kublin C: Corneal scar formation. Exp Eye Res 17:251, 1973
46. Freeman IL: Collagen polymorphism in mature rabbit cornea. Invest Ophthalmol Vis Sci 17:171, 1978
47. Newsome DA, Gross J, Hassell JR: Human corneal stroma contains three distinct collagens. Invest Ophthalmol Vis Sci 22:376, 1982
48. Hamada R, Giraud JP, Graft B, et al: Étude analytique et statistique des lamelles, des keratocytes, des fibrilles de collagène de la région centrale de la cornée humaine normale. Arch Ophtalmol (Paris) 32:563, 1972
49. Giraud JP, Pouliquen Y, Offret G, et al: Statistical morphometric studies in normal human and rabbit corneal stroma. Exp Eye Res 21:221, 1975
50. Hogan MJ, Alvarado JA, Weddell E: Histology of the Human Eye. WB Saunders, Philadelphia, 1971
51. Praus R, Brettschneider I: Glycosaminoglycans in embryonic and postnatal human cornea. Ophthalmic Res 7:542, 1975
52. Yue BYJT, Baum JL, Silbert JE: Synthesis of glycosaminoglycans by cultures of normal human corneal endothelial and stromal cells. Invest Ophthalmol Vis Sci 17:523, 1978
53. Borcherding MS, Blacik LJ, Sittig RA, et al: Proteoglycans and collagen fibre organization in human corneoscleral tissue. Exp Eye Res 21:59, 1975
54. Assouline M, Chew SJ, Thompson HW, Beuerman R: Effect of growth factors on collagen lattice contraction by human keratocytes. Invest Ophthalmol Vis Sci 33:1742, 1992
55. Lopez JG, Chew SJ, Thompson HW, et al: EGF cell surface receptor quantitation on ocular cells by an immunocytochemical flow cytometry technique. Invest Ophthalmol Vis Sci 33:2053,1992
56. Johnson DH, Bourne WM, Campbell RJ: The ultrastructure of Descemet's membrane. I. Changes with age in normal corneas. Arch Ophthalmol 100:1942, 1982
57. Alaerts ML: Aspects de l'endothelium cornéen au biomicroscope. Bull Soc Belge Ophtalmol 122:320, 1959
58. Wolf J: The secretory activity and the cuticle of the corneal endothelium. Doc Ophthalmol 25:150, 1968
59. Sperling S, Jacobsen SR: The surface coat on human corneal endothelium. Acta Ophthalmol (Copenh) 58:96, 1980
60. Svedbergh B, Bill A: Scanning electron microscopic studies of the corneal endothelium in man and monkeys. Acta Ophthalmol (Copenh) 50:321, 1972
61. Gallagher B: Primary cilia of the corneal endothelium. Am J Anat 159:475, 1980
62. Kreutziger GO: Lateral membrane morphology and gap junction structure in rabbit corneal endothelium. Exp Eye Res 23:285, 1976
63. Zantos SG, Holden BA: Transient endothelial changes soon after wearing soft contact lenses. Am J Optom Physiol Optics 54:856, 1977
64. Maurice DM: Cellular membrane activity in the corneal endothelium of the intact eye. Experientia 24:1094, 1968
65. Laing RA, Sandstrom MA, Liebowitz HM: In vivo photomicrography of corneal endothelium. Arch Ophthalmol 93:143, 1975
66. Burns RR, Bourne WM, Brubaker RF: Endothelial function in patients with cornea guttata. Invest Ophthalmol Vis Sci 20:77, 1981
67. Bourne WM, Brubaker RF: Decreased endothelial permeability in transplanted corneas. Am J Ophthalmol 96:362, 1983
68. McCartney MD, Robertson DP, Wood TO, McLaughlin BJ: ATPase pump site density in human dysfunctional corneal endothelium. Invest Ophthalmol Vis Sci 28:1955, 1987
69. Staehelin LA: Structure and function of intercellular junctions. Int Rev Cytol 39:191, 1974
70. Khodadoust AA, Silverstein AM, Kenyon KR, et al: Adhesion of regenerating corneal epithelium. The role of basement membrane. Am J Ophthalmol 65:339, 1968
71. Brewitt H, Reale E: The basement membrane complex of the human corneal epithelium. Albrecht von Graefes Arch Klin Exp Ophthalmol 215:223, 1981
72. Gipson IK, Grill SM, Spurr SJ, et al: Hemidesmosome formation in vitro. J Cell Biol 97:849, 1983

73. Robert L, Jungua S, Moczar M: Structural glycoproteins of the intercellular matrix. Front Matrix Biol 3:113, 1976
74. Brightman MW, Reese TS: Junctions between intimately apposed cell membranes in the vertebrate brain. J Cell Biol 40:468, 1969
75. Rózsa AJ, Beuerman RW: Density and organization of free nerve endings in the corneal epithelium of the rabbit. Pain 14:105, 1982
76. Ehinger B, Sjöberg N-O: Development of the ocular nerve supply in man and guinea-pig. Z Zellforsch 118:579, 1971
77. Toivanen M, Tervo T, Partanen M, et al: Histochemical demonstration of adrenergic nerves in the stroma of human cornea. Invest Ophthalmol Vis Sci 28:398, 1987
78. Klyce SD, Jenison GL, Crosson CE, et al: Distribution of sympathetic nerves in the rabbit cornea. ARVO abstract. Invest Ophthalmol Vis Sci 27(suppl):354, 1986
79. Komai Y, Ushiki T: The three-dimensional organization of collagen fibrils in the human cornea and sclera. Invest Ophthalmol Vis Sci 32:2244, 1991
80. Tervo K, Tervo T, Eranko L, et al: Substance P-immunoreactive nerves in the human cornea and iris. Invest Ophthalmol Vis Sci 23:671, 1982
81. Beuerman RW, McCulley JP: Comparative clinical assessment of corneal sensation with a new anesthesiometer. Am J Ophthalmol 86:812, 1978
82. Koenig SB, Berkowitz RA, Beuerman RW, et al: Corneal sensitivity after epikeratophakia. Ophthalmology 90:1213, 1983
83. Beuerman RW, Rózsa AJ, Tanelian DL: Neurophysiological correlates of posttraumatic acute pain. p. 73. In Fields HL, Dubner R, Cervero F (eds): Advances in Pain Research and Therapy. Vol. 9. Raven Press, New York, 1985
84. Walls GL: The Vertebrate Eye and Its Adaptive Radiation. Cranbrook Institute of Science, Bloomfield Hills, MI, 1942
85. Thomas CI: The Cornea. Charles C. Thomas, Springfield, Il, 1955
86. Hay ED, Revel JP: Fine structure of the developing avian cornea. Monogr Dev Biol 1:1, 1969
87. Hay ED: Development of the vertebrate cornea. Int Rev Cytol 61:263, 1980
88. Zinn KM, Mockel-Pohl S: Fine structure of the developing cornea. Int Ophthalmol Clin 15:19, 1975
89. Ozanics V, Rayborn M, Sagun D: Observations on the morphology of the developing primate cornea: epithelium, its innervation and anterior stroma. J Morphol 153:263, 1977
90. Wulle KG: Electron microscopy of the fetal development of the corneal endothelium and Descemet's membrane of the human eye. Invest Ophthalmol 11:897, 1972
91. Johnston MC, Noden DM, Hazelton RD, et al: Origins of avian ocular and periocular tissues. Exp Eye Res 29:27, 1979
92. Coulombre J, Coulombre A: Corneal development. V. Treatment of five-day-old embryos of domestic fowl with 6-diazo-5-oxo-L-norleucine (DON). Dev Biol 45:291, 1975
93. Pei YF, Rhodin JAG: The prenatal development of the mouse eye. Anat Rec 168:105, 1971
94. Johnston MC, Bhakdinarouk A, Reid AC: An expanded role of the neural crest in oral and pharyngeal development. p. 37. In Bosma JF (ed): Fourth Symposium on Oral Sensation and Perception. US Government Printing Office, Washington, DC, 1974
95. Warwick R: Eugene Wolff's Anatomy of the Eye and Orbit. WB Saunders, Philadelphia, 1976
96. Adamis AP, Molnar ML, Tripathi BJ, et al: Neuronal-specific enolase in human corneal endothelium and posterior keratocytes. Exp Eye Res 41:665, 1985
97. Ozanics V, Rayborn M, Sagun D: Some aspects of corneal and scleral differentiation in the primate. Exp Eye Res 22:305, 1976
98. Hökfelt T, Kellerth JO, Nilsson G, et al: Experimental immunohistochemical studies on the localization and distribution of substance P in cat primary sensory neurons. Brain Res 100:235, 1975
99. Hay ED, Dodson JW: Secretion of collagen by corneal epithelium. I. Morphology of the collagenous products produced by isolated epithelia grown on frozen-killed lens. J Cell Biol 57:190, 1973
100. Dodson JW, Hay ED: Secretion of collagen by corneal epithelium. II. Effect of the underlying substratum on secretion and polymerization of epithelial products. J Exp Zool 189:51, 1974
101. Tamura Y, Konomi H, Sawada H, et al: Tissue distribution of type VIII collagen in human adult and fetal eyes. Invest Ophthalmol Vis Sci 32:2636, 1991
102. Stiemke MM, McCartney MD, Cantu-Crouch D, Edelhauser HF: Maturation of the corneal endothelial tight junction. Invest Ophthalmol Vis Sci 32:2757, 1991
103. Riley MV: Glucose and oxygen utilization by the rabbit cornea. Exp Eye Res 8:193, 1969
104. Rosenthal P, Klyce SD: Contact lens induced corneal edema. p. 15.1. In Dabezies OH (ed): Contact Lenses. The CLAO Guide to Basic Science and Clinical Practice. Grune & Stratton, Orlando, FL, 1984
105. Klyce SD: Stromal lactate accumulation can account for corneal edema osmotically following epithelial hypoxia in the rabbit. J Physiol 321:49, 1981
106. Lambert SR, Klyce SD: The origins of Sattler's veil. Am J Ophthalmol 91:51, 1981
107. Bonanno JA, Polse KA: Corneal acidosis during contact lens wear: effects of hypoxia and CO_2. Invest Ophthalmol Vis Sci 28:1514, 1987
108. Brown SI, Dohlman CH: A buried corneal implant serving as a barrier to fluid. Arch Ophthalmol 73:635, 1965
109. Berkowitz RA, Klyce SD, Kaufman HE: Aqueous hyposecretion after penetrating keratoplasty. Ophthalmic Surg 15:323, 1984
110. Klyce SD, Farris RL, Dabezies OH: Corneal oxygenation in contact lens wearers. p. 14.1. In Dabezies OH (ed): Contact Lenses. The CLAO Guide to Basic Science and Clinical Practice. Grune & Stratton, Orlando, FL, 1984
111. Polse KA, Mandell RB: Critical tension at the corneal surface. Arch Ophthalmol 84:505, 1970
112. Fatt I: Steady-state distribution of oxygen and carbon dioxide in the in vivo cornea. Exp Eye Res 7:413, 1968
113. Mishima S, Kaye GI, Takahashi GI, et al: The function of the corneal endothelium in the regulation of corneal hydra-

tion. p. 207. In Langham ME (ed): The Cornea, Macromolecular Organization of a Connective Tissue. Johns Hopkins Press, Baltimore, 1969
114. Hamano H, Kawabe H, Mitsunaga S: Reproducible measurement of oxygen permeability (Dk) of contact lens materials. CLAO J 11:221, 1985
115. Smelser GK, Chen DK: Physiology changes in cornea induced by contact lenses. Arch Ophthalmol 53:676, 1955
116. Efron N, Carney LG: Oxygen levels beneath the closed eyelid. Invest Ophthalmol Vis Sci 18:93, 1979
117. Mishima S, Maurice DM: The oily layer of the tear film and evaporation from the corneal surface. Exp Eye Res 1:39, 1961
118. Mishima S, Maurice DM: The effect of normal evaporation on the eye. Exp Eye Res 1:46, 1961
119. Mandell RB, Farrell R: Corneal swelling at low atmospheric oxygen pressures. Invest Ophthalmol Vis Sci 19:697, 1980
120. Strughold H: The sensitivity of cornea and conjunctiva of the human eye and the use of contact lenses. Am J Optom Arch Am Acad Optom 30:625, 1953
121. Kilp H, Heisig-Salentin B, Framing D: Metabolites and enzymes in the corneal epithelium after extended contact lens wear. The effects of contact lenses on the normal physiology and anatomy of the cornea: symposium summary. Curr Eye Res 4:738, 1985
122. Hamano H, Hori M, Hamano T, et al: Effect of contact lens wear on the mitosis of corneal epithelial cells and the amount of lactate in aqueous humor. Jpn J Ophthalmol 27:451, 1983
123. Holden BA, Vannas A, Nilsson K, et al: Epithelial and endothelial effects from the extended wear of contact lenses. The effects of contact lenses on the normal physiology and anatomy of the cornea: symposium summary. Curr Eye Res 4:739, 1985
124. Schein OD, Glynn RJ, Poggio EC, et al: The relative risk of ulcerative keratitis among users of daily-wear and extended-wear soft contact lenses: a case-control study. N Engl J Med 321:773, 1989
125. Poggio EC, Glynn RJ, Schein OD, et al: The incidence of ulcerative keratitis among users of daily-wear and extended-wear soft contact lenses. N Engl J Med 321:779, 1989
126. Donn A, Maurice DM, Mills NL: Studies on the living cornea in vitro. I. Method and physiologic measurements. Arch Ophthalmol 62:741, 1959
127. Donn A, Maurice DM, Mills NL: Studies on the living cornea in vitro. II. The active transport of sodium across the epithelium. Arch Ophthalmol 62:748, 1959
128. Green K: Ion transport in isolated cornea of the rabbit. Am J Physiol 209:1311, 1965
129. Klyce SD, Neufeld AH, Zadunaisky JA: The activation of chloride transport by epinephrine and Db cyclic-AMP in the cornea of the rabbit. Invest Ophthalmol 12:127, 1973
130. Van der Hayden C, Weekers JF, Schoffeniels E: Sodium and chloride transport across the isolated rabbit cornea. Exp Eye Res 20:89, 1975
131. Klyce SD: Transport of Na, Cl, and water by the rabbit corneal epithelium at resting potential. Am J Physiol 228:1446, 1975
132. Candia OA, Askew WA: Active sodium transport in the isolated bullfrog cornea. Biochim Biophys Acta 163:262, 1968
133. Langham ME, Hart RW, Cox J: The interaction of collagen and mucopolysaccharides. p. 157. In Langham M (ed): The Cornea. Macromolecular Organization of a Connective Tissue. Johns Hopkins Press, Baltimore, 1969
134. Green K: Relation of epithelial ion transport to corneal thickness hydration. Nature 217:1074, 1968
135. Fischer FH, Schmitz L, Hoff W, et al: Sodium and chloride transport in the isolated rabbit cornea. Pflugers Arch 373:179,1978
136. Friedman MH: Mathematical modeling of transport in structured tissues: corneal epithelium. Am J Physiol 234:F215, 1978
137. Kaye GI, Tice LW: Studies on the cornea. V. Electron microscopic localization of adenosine triphosphate activity in the rabbit cornea in relation to transport. Invest Ophthalmol 5:22, 1968
138. Shapiro MP, Candia OA: Corneal hydration and metabolically dependent transcellular passive transfer of water. Exp Eye Res 15:659, 1973
139. Klyce SD, Marshall WS: Effect of Ag^+ on the electrophysiology of the rabbit corneal epithelium. J Membr Biol 66:133, 1982
140. Zadunaisky JA: Active transport of chloride in frog cornea. Am J Physiol 211:506, 1966
141. Wiederholt M: Physiology of epithelial transport in the human eye. Klin Wochenschr 58:975, 1980
142. Klyce SD, Wong RKS: Site and mode of adrenaline action of chloride transport across the rabbit corneal epithelium. J Physiol 266:777, 1977
143. Zadunaisky JA, Lande MA: Active chloride transport and control of corneal transparency. Am J Physiol 221:1837, 1971
144. Candia OA: Fluid and Cl transport by the epithelium of the isolated frog cornea. ARVO abstract. Invest Ophthalmol Vis Sci 15(suppl):12, 1976
145. Klyce SD: Enhancing fluid secretion by the corneal epithelium. Invest Ophthalmol Vis Sci 16:968, 1977
146. Candia OA, Neufeld AH: Topical epinephrine causes a decrease in density of β-adrenergic receptors and catecholamine-stimulated chloride transport in rabbit cornea. Biochim Biophys Acta 543:403, 1978
147. Klyce SD, Beuerman RW, Crosson CE: Alteration of corneal epithelial transport by sympathectomy. Invest Ophthalmol Vis Sci 26:434, 1985
148. Klyce SD, Palkama KA, Neufeld AH, et al: Neural serotonin stimulates chloride transport in the rabbit corneal epithelium. Invest Ophthalmol Vis Sci 23:181, 1982
149. Crosson CE, Beuerman RW, Klyce SD: Dopamine modulation of active ion transport in rabbit corneal epithelium. Invest Ophthalmol Vis Sci 25:1240, 1984
150. Neufeld AH, Ledgard SE, Jumblatt MM, et al: Serotonin-stimulated cyclic AMP synthesis in the rabbit corneal epithelium. Invest Ophthalmol Vis Sci 23:193, 1982
151. Marshall WS, Klyce SD: Cellular mode of serotonin action on Cl^- transport in the rabbit corneal epithelium. Biochim Biophys Acta 778:139, 1984

152. Jumblatt MM, Neufeld AH: β-Adrenergic and serotonergic responsiveness of rabbit corneal epithelial cells in culture. Invest Ophthalmol Vis Sci 24:1139, 1983
153. Klyce SD, Crosson CE: Transport processes across the rabbit corneal epithelium: a review. Curr Eye Res 4:323, 1985
154. Hill JM, Shimomura Y, Kwon BS, et al: Iontophoresis of epinephrine isomers to rabbit eyes induced HSV-1 ocular shedding. Invest Ophthalmol Vis Sci 26:1299, 1985
155. Hill JM, Shimomura Y, Dudley JB, et al: Timolol induces HSV-1 ocular shedding in the latently infected rabbit. Invest Ophthalmol Vis Sci 28:585, 1987
156. Kikkawa Y: The intracellular potential of the corneal epithelium. Exp Eye Res 3:132, 1964
157. Fee JP, Edelhauser HF: Intracellular electrical potentials in the rabbit corneal epithelium. Exp Eye Res 9:233, 1970
158. Akaike N, Hori M: Effect of anions and cations on membrane potential of rabbit corneal epithelium. Am J Physiol 219:1811, 1970
159. Akaike N: The origin of the basal cell potential in frog corneal epithelium. J Physiol 219:57, 1971
160. Klyce SD: Electrophysiology of the corneal epithelium. Ph.D. Thesis, Department of Physiology, Yale University, New Haven, CT, 1971
161. Festen CMAW, Slegers JFG: The influence of ions, ouabain, propranolol and amiloride on the transepithelial potential and resistance of rabbit cornea. Exp Eye Res 28:413, 1979
162. Marshall WS, Klyce SD: Cellular and paracellular pathway resistances in the "tight" Cl^--secreting epithelium of the rabbit cornea. J Membr Biol 73:275, 1983
163. Maurice DM: Epithelial potential of the cornea. Exp Eye Res 6:138, 1967
164. Otori T: Electronic content of the rabbit corneal stroma. Exp Eye Res 6:356, 1967
165. Friedman MH, Green K: Swelling rate of corneal stroma. Exp Eye Res 12:239, 1971
166. Hodson S: Why the cornea swells. J Theor Biol 33:419, 1971
167. Elliot GF, Goodfellow JM, Woolgar AE: Swelling studies of bovine corneal stroma without bounding membranes. J Physiol 298:453, 1980
168. Kanai A, Kaufman HE: Electron microscopic studies of swollen corneal stroma. Ann Ophthalmol 5:178, 1973
169. Ehlers N: Variations in hydration properties of the cornea. Acta Ophthalmol (Copenh) 44:461, 1966
170. Fatt I, Goldstick TK: Dynamics of water transport in swelling membranes. J Colloid Sci 20:434, 1965
171. Cogan DG, Kinsey VE: The cornea. V. Physiologic aspects. Arch Ophthalmol 28:661, 1942
172. Hedbys BO, Dohlman CH: A new method for the determination of the swelling pressure of the corneal stroma in vitro. Exp Eye Res 2:122, 1963
173. Hedbys BO, Mishima S, Maurice DM: The imbibition pressure of the corneal stroma. Exp Eye Res 2:99, 1963
174. Klyce SD, Dohlman CH, Tolpin DW: In vivo determination of corneal swelling pressure of the corneal stroma. Exp Eye Res 11:220, 1971
175. Ytteborg J, Dohlman CH: Corneal edema and intraocular pressure. II. Clinical results. Arch Ophthalmol 74:477, 1965
176. McPhee TJ, Bourne WM, Brubaker RF: Location of the stress-bearing layers of the cornea. Invest Ophthalmol Vis Sci 26:869, 1985
177. Wilson G, O'Leary DJ, Vaughn W: Differential swelling in the compartments of the corneal stroma. Invest Ophthalmol Vis Sci 25:1105, 1984
178. Klyce SD, Russell SR: Numerical solution of coupled transport equations applied to corneal hydration dynamics. J Physiol 292:107, 1979
179. Pedroza L, Beuerman RW, Klyce SD, et al: Keratocyte degeneration following epithelial abrasion. ARVO abstract. Invest Ophthalmol Vis Sci 27(suppl):31, 1986
180. Crosson CE: Cellular changes following epithelial abrasion. p. 3. In Beuerman RW, Crosson CE, Kaufman HE (eds): Healing Processes in the Cornea. Portfolio Publishing Company, The Woodlands, TX, 1989
181. Trenberth SM, Mishima S: The effect of ouabain on the rabbit corneal endothelium. Invest Ophthalmol 7:44, 1968
182. Lim JJ, Fischbarg J: Electrical profiles of rabbit corneal endothelium as determined from impedance measurements. Biophys J 36:677, 1981
183. Ussing HH: The distinction by means of tracers between active transport and diffusion. Acta Physiol Scand 19:43, 1949
184. Hodson S, Miller F: The bicarbonate ion pump in the endothelium which regulates the hydration of the rabbit cornea. J Physiol 263:563, 1976
185. Hull DS, Green K, Boyd M, Wynn HR: Corneal endothelium bicarbonate transport and the effect of carbonic anhydrase inhibitors on endothelial permeability and fluxes and corneal thickness. Invest Ophthalmol Vis Sci 16:883, 1977
186. Lim JJ, Ussing HH: Analysis of presteady-state Na^+ fluxes across the rabbit corneal endothelium. J Membr Biol 65:197, 1982
187. Fischbarg J, Hernandez J, Liebovitch LS, et al: The mechanism of fluid and electrolyte transport across corneal endothelium: critical revision and update of a model. Curr Eye Res 4:351, 1985
188. Wiederholt M, Jentsch TJ, Keller SK: Electrical sodium-bicarbonate symport in cultured corneal endothelial cells. Pflugers Arch 405:S167, 1985
189. Kuang KY, Xu M, Koniarek JP, Fischbarg J: Effects of ambient bicarbonate, phosphate and carbonic anhydrase inhibitors on fluid transport across rabbit corneal endothelium. Exp Eye Res 50:487, 1990
190. Maurice DM: The location of the fluid pump in the cornea. J Physiol 221:43, 1972
191. Fischbarg J, Lim JJ, Bourget J: Adenosine stimulation of fluid transport across rabbit corneal endothelium. J Membr Biol 35:95, 1977
192. Hodson S, Miller F, Riley M: The electrogenic pump of rabbit corneal endothelium. Exp Eye Res 24:249, 1977
193. Narula P, Xu M, Kuang KY, et al: Fluid transport across cultured bovine corneal endothelial cell monolayers. Am J Physiol 262:C98, 1992
194. Fischbarg J, Montoreano R: Osmotic permeability across corneal endothelium and antidiuretic hormone-stimulated

toad urinary bladder structures. Biochim Biophys Acta 690:207, 1982
195. Liebovitch LS, Weinbaum S: A model of epithelial water transport—the corneal endothelium. Biophys J 35:315, 1981
196. Wigham C, Hodson S: The movement of sodium across short-circuited rabbit corneal endothelium. Curr Eye Res 4:1241, 1985
197. Leber T: Studies on fluid exchange in the eye. Albrecht von Graefes Arch Ophthalmol 19:87, 1873
198. von Bahr G: Measurements of the effect of solutions of different osmotic pressure on the thickness of the living cornea. Trans Ophthalmol Soc UK 68:515, 1948
199. Maurice DM: The permeability to sodium ions of the living rabbit cornea. J Physiol 112:367, 1951
200. Friedman MH: Unsteady transport and hydration dynamics in the in vivo cornea. Biophys J 13:890, 1973
201. Mandell RB, Fatt I: Thinning in the human cornea on awakening. Nature 208:292, 1965
202. Klyce SD, Maurice DM: Automatic recording of corneal thickness in vitro. Invest Ophthalmol 15:550, 1976
203. Brubaker RF, Kupfer C: Microcryoscopic determination of the osmolarity of interstitial fluid in the living rabbit cornea. Invest Ophthalmol 1:653, 1962
204. Davson H: The hydration of the cornea. Biochem J 59:24, 1955
205. Harris JE, Nordquist LT: The hydration of the cornea. I. The transport of water from the cornea. Am J Ophthalmol 40:100, 1955
206. Mishima S, Trenberth SM: Permeability of the corneal endothelium to nonelectrolytes. Invest Ophthalmol 7:34, 1968
207. Maurice DM: The permeability of the cornea. Ophthalmic Lit 7:3, 1953
208. Mishima S, Hedbys BO: The permeability of the corneal epithelium and endothelium to water. Exp Eye Res 6:10, 1967
209. Stanley JA, Mishima S, Klyce SD: In vivo determination of endothelial permeability to water. Invest Ophthalmol 5:371, 1966
210. Green K, Green MA: The permeability to water of rabbit corneal membranes. Am J Physiol 217:635, 1969
211. Kim JH, Green K, Martinez M, Paton D: Solute permeability of the corneal endothelium and Descemet's membrane. Exp Eye Res 12:231, 1971
212. Green K, Downs SJ: Corneal membrane water permeability as a function of temperature. Invest Ophthalmol 15:304, 1976
213. Fischbarg J, Warshavsky CR, Limm JJ: Pathways for hydraulically and osmotically-induced water flows across epithelia. Nature 266:71, 1977
214. Friedman MH: The effect of membrane heterogeneity on the predictability of fluxes, with application to the cornea. J Theor Biol 61:307, 1976
215. Mandell R, as cited in Duke-Elder S, Abrams D (eds): System of ophthalmology. p. 130. Ophthalmic Optics and Refraction. Vol. V. CV Mosby, St. Louis, 1970
216. Klyce SD: Computer-assisted corneal topography: high resolution graphical presentation and analysis of keratoscopy. Invest Ophthalmol Vis Sci 25:1426, 1984
217. Maguire LJ, Singer DE, Klyce SD: Graphic presentation of computer-analyzed keratoscope photographs. Arch Ophthalmol 105:223, 1987
218. Rabinowitz YS, Wilson SE, Klyce SD: Color Atlas of Corneal Topography. Interpreting Videokeratography. Igaku-Shoin, New York, 1993
219. Maurice DM: The structure and transparency of the cornea. J Physiol 136:263, 1957
220. Goldman JN, Benedek GB: The relationship between morphology and transparency in the nonswelling corneal stroma of the shark. Invest Ophthalmol 6:574, 1967
221. Benedek GB: Theory of transparency of the eye. Appl Optics 10:459, 1971
222. Farrell RA, McCally RL, Tatham PER: Wavelength dependencies of light scattering in normal and cold swollen rabbit corneas and their structural implications. J Physiol 233:589, 1973
223. Goldman JN, Benedek GB, Dohlman CH, et al: Structural alterations affecting transparency in swollen human corneas. Invest Ophthalmol 7:501, 1968
224. Waltman SR, Kaufman HE: Use of hydrophilic contact lenses to increase ocular penetration of topical drugs. Invest Ophthalmol 9:250, 1970
225. Shofner RS, Kaufman HE, Hill JM: New horizons in ocular drug delivery. Ophthalmol Clin North Am 2:15, 1989
226. Friedberg ML, Pleyer U, Mondino BJ: Device drug delivery to the eye: collagen shields, iontophoresis, and pumps. Ophthalmology 98:725, 1991
227. Mondino BJ: Collagen shields. Am J Ophthalmol 112:587, 1991
228. Burstein NL, Klyce SD: Electrophysiological and morphological effects of ophthalmic preparations on the rabbit corneal epithelium. Invest Ophthalmol Vis Sci 16:899, 1977

2

Structure and Function of the Eyelids and Conjunctiva

ANDREW W. LAWTON

The eyelids and conjunctiva act as a physical barrier, protecting the cornea from environmental trauma. These structures also contribute to and properly distribute the tear film, serve as a source of immunologic mediators that combat infection, supply epithelial cells and blood vessels for corneal healing, and, albeit undesirably, augment tissue rejection. This chapter discusses the normal anatomy, histology, and physiology of the eyelids and conjunctiva.[1-3] Chapters 4, 5, 6, 7, 10, 11, 13, 14, 15, 20, 21, and 23 contain information concerning pathologic conditions of the eyelids and conjunctiva that affect corneal homeostasis.

EYELID AND CONJUNCTIVAL MORPHOLOGY

The eyelid comprises four layers. Anteriorly to posteriorly, these layers are (1) skin, (2) orbicularis muscle and levator aponeurosis, (3) fibrous tissue and smooth muscle, and (4) conjunctiva (Figure 2-1). The four layers meet at the margin of the eyelid.

The eyelid margin is separated by the punctum into ciliary (lateral) and lacrimal (nasal) portions. An important anatomic feature of the eyelid margin is the gray line, which is the surface marking of the most superficial portion of the orbicularis muscle, the muscle of Riolan.[4] Located immediately anterior to the meibomian gland orifices, the gray line divides the eyelid into the anterior lamella (skin and muscle) and the posterior lamella (tarsus and conjunctiva) and is an important landmark for eyelid surgery.

Immediately posterior to the meibomian gland orifices, at the mucocutaneous junction, the keratinized epithelium of the skin and the nonkeratinized epithelium of the conjunctiva meet. Normally, keratinization does not extend beyond the mucocutaneous junction. If keratinization occurs on the conjunctival surface or if keratin is turned inward by an entropion, however, the cornea may be severely damaged.

Skin and Associated Appendages

The skin of the eyelid is tightly attached only at the medial and lateral canthi. Elsewhere, it is thin and loosely attached, permitting easy distension by fluid or blood. Such stretching may lead to blepharochalasis syndrome, which is a complex of ptosis, lateral canthal laxity, and redundant skin.[5] With age, the eyelids may develop involutional laxity and redundant skin, referred to as dermatochalasis.

The upper eyelid crease is created by fibrous attachments from the levator aponeurosis to skin; a similar crease is created in the lower eyelid by connections from the sheath of the inferior rectus muscle to skin. Many other complex attachments between eyelid structures and orbital tissues exist.[6]

As elsewhere on the body, the skin of the eyelids consists of the epidermis and dermis. The epidermis is keratinized stratified squamous epithelium. It is composed of multilaminar keratinocytes that can be divided into the basal layer; malpighian, or prickle cell layer; granular cell layer; and keratin or superficial layer (Figure 2-2). The basal layer is a single layer of slightly elongated cuboidal cells. Normally, these cells are the only source of mitotic activity for the epidermis. The malpighian, or prickle cell layer, contains polygonal cells that have no visible evidence of keratinization. During formalin fixation, the cells shrink and expose their desmosomes (intercellular junctions), hence the term *prickle.* The granular cell layer consists of cells that are more flattened than those found in the malpighian layer. These cells are distinguished by the

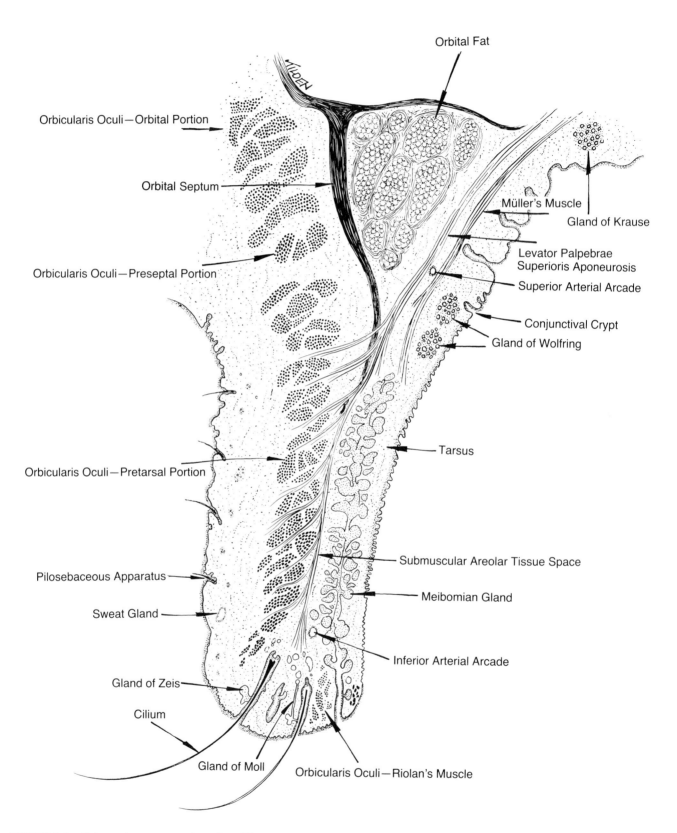

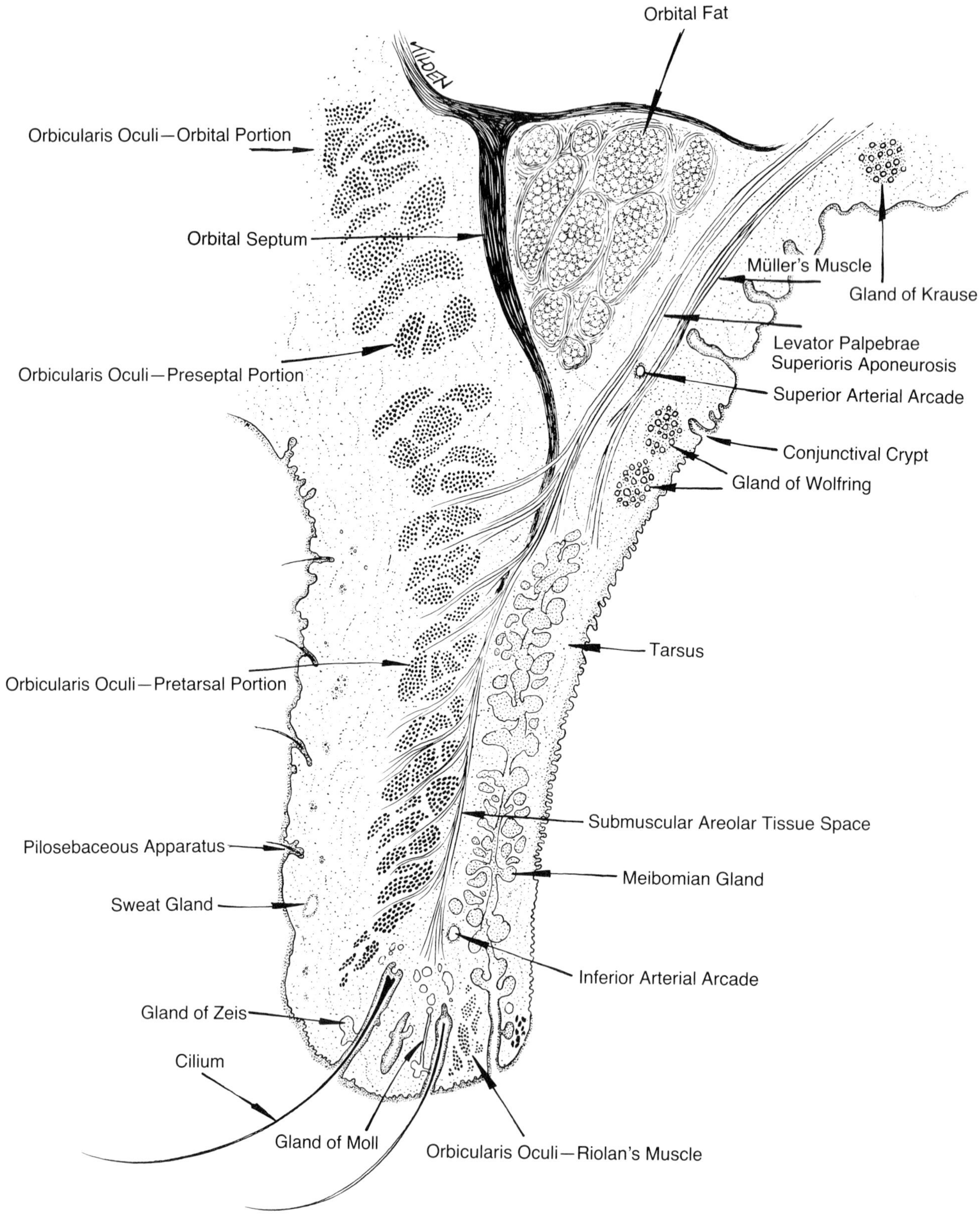

FIGURE 2-1 Schematic representation of eyelid anatomy.

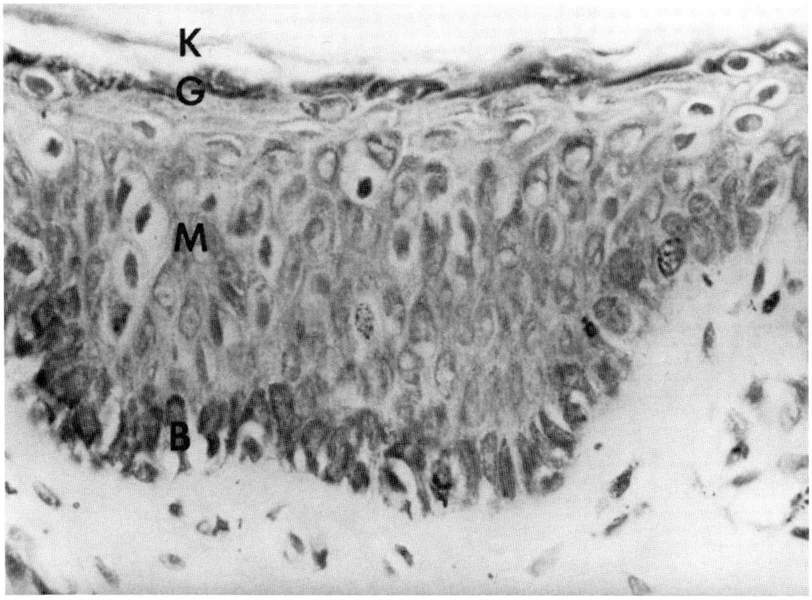

FIGURE 2-2 The epithelium of the eyelid skin is composed of four layers: the basal layer (*B*), the malpighian layer (*M*), the granular layer (*G*), and the keratin layer (*K*).

presence of keratohyalin granules. The most superficial layer is the keratin layer, where all that remains are flattened, fully keratinized cells that have lost their nuclei. The keratin acts as a physical barrier, protecting the underlying tissues from most chemical and infectious agents.

Admixed with the keratinocytes is a group of cell types characterized by their dendritic appearance. This group includes melanocytes, Langerhans cells, and Merkel cells. Melanocytes, which are found in the basal layer, produce melanin that is subsequently transferred to keratinocytes. Melanin forms a cap over the epithelial nuclei, which filters ultraviolet light and protects against chromosomal damage. Langerhans cells are scattered diffusely throughout the epidermis, where they aid the immune system by processing and presenting antigens to lymphocytes. These cells stain positively for the immunologic markers CD1 and HLA-DR and are difficult to locate without immunohistochemical staining techniques. Merkel cells may appear singly or in groups. Located at the basal layer of rete ridges and epidermal appendages,[7] Merkel cells can be differentiated from melanocytes and Langerhans cells only with immunohistochemical staining techniques; they have staining characteristics similar to those of neuroendocrine cells. The function of Merkel cells is not clear, although ultrastructural studies indicate evidence of phagocytic activity. Clusters of Merkel cells in complex with myelinated nerve fibers, particularly between successive eyelashes at the eyelid margin, indicate a possible function as touch receptors.

The dermis of the eyelids is unusually supple and loose and contains broad bundles of collagen and moderate amounts of elastin and reticulin fibers. The dermis tends to disappear at the eyelid margin, eyelid crease, and attachments of the skin to the palpebral ligaments. A thin layer of fat separates the dermis from the orbicularis muscle. The dermis contains many skin appendages. Because the lining of these structures and the epidermis are contiguous, the appendages should be considered as extensions of the epidermis. The epidermal appendages of the eyelids are essentially identical to those found elsewhere in the skin.

Hair, which is diffuse on the eyelids, is most prominent at the eyelid margins as eyelashes, or cilia. Eyelash follicles are buried within the eyelids and can be found as deep as the anterior tarsus (Figure 2-3). The follicles are lined by keratinized stratified squamous epithelium. Eyelashes have a normal life span of about 5 months; they take about half that long to reach normal length after epilation. Unlike other hairs, eyelashes lack erector pili muscles. The eyelashes assist in protection of the cornea from foreign bodies, trapping them like a sieve.

Sebaceous glands empty via ducts into the space surrounding each eyelash. A hair and its associated sebaceous glands are called a pilosebaceous unit. Sebaceous glands associated with the eyelashes are known as the glands of Zeis. Like other sebaceous glands, the glands of Zeis are classified as holocrine glands, because the cells discharge their lipid content by disintegration of the entire cell. The lipid lubricates the eyelashes and skin. Sebaceous cell carcinoma rarely originates in the glands of Zeis.

Eccrine and apocrine sweat glands are found in the eyelids. The cells of eccrine sweat glands discharge their secretion without disrupting the cell membrane. Eccrine sweat glands have three types of cells: (1) clear cells that contain

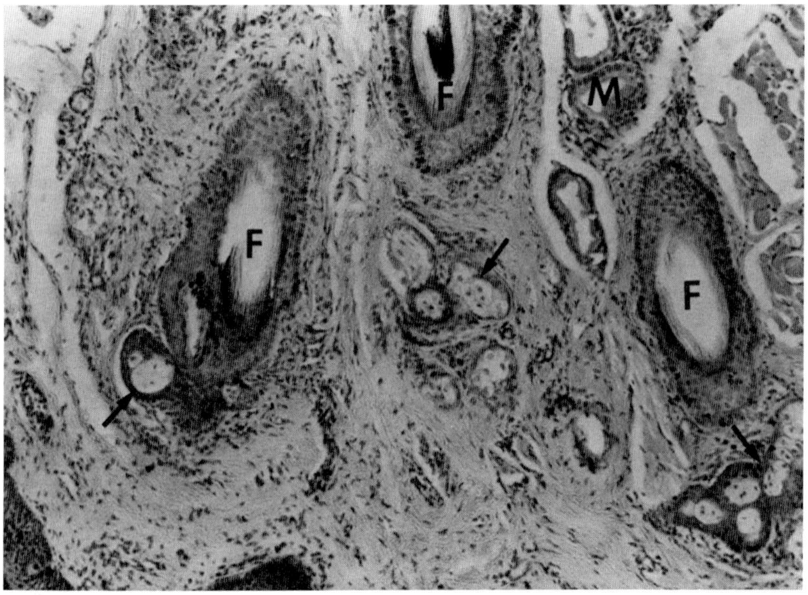

FIGURE 2-3 Anterior portion of the eyelid showing the skin at the lower left. Eyelash follicles (*F*), with associated glands of Zeis (arrows), are seen. The glands of Moll (*M*) are seen in the upper right corner.

glycogen, (2) granular cells that contain mucopolysaccharides, and (3) peripheral myoepithelial cells. The cells form acini that empty into a duct connected to the surface of the skin (Figure 2-4). The watery secretion of eccrine sweat glands is used to cool the skin surface by evaporation.

Apocrine sweat glands, known as glands of Moll, lie deep within the eyelid, often posterior to the orbicularis muscle, near the eyelid margin (Figure 2-5). These glands have an inner layer of secretory cells and an outer layer of myoepithelial cells. Apocrine cells secrete by an apocrine, or decapitation, method; the apical portion of the secretory cell is cast off along with the secretory product. Although no clear function has been attributed to the glands of Moll, elsewhere in the body apocrine sweat glands secrete pheromones.

Orbicularis Oculi Muscle and Levator Aponeurosis

The orbicularis oculi muscle forms an elliptical array of striated muscle around the eyelids and is arbitrarily divided into pretarsal, preseptal, and orbital components.[8] The pretarsal and preseptal components are densely adherent to the skin at the medial and lateral canthi. Riolan's muscle is the portion of the orbicularis muscle that follows the eyelid margin circumferentially. It is separated from the rest of the pretarsal portion of the orbicularis muscle by the eyelash follicles and the glands of Moll. The orbital portion of the orbicularis muscle extends superiorly onto the forehead to cover the frontalis and corrugator muscles and inferiorly to overlie the levator muscles of the upper lip and nasal ala. Laterally, the orbicularis muscle spreads over part of the masseter muscle. The nerve supply for the orbicularis muscle comes from the facial (7th cranial) nerve.

Spontaneous and voluntary blinking are produced by contraction of the orbicularis muscle. Under normal circumstances, humans blink spontaneously approximately 15 to 20 times per minute. Involuntary blinking is normally instigated by corneal irritation via the trigeminal (5th cranial) nerve secondary to corneal drying or mechanical irritation, bright light via the optic nerve, and loud noise via the auditory nerve. Blinking serves to redistribute the tear film and clear metabolic wastes and foreign material from the tears.

The physical action of blinking requires coordination of the nucleus of the facial nerve with the nuclei of the trigeminal and abducens (6th cranial) nerves. For blinking to be effective, the levator palpebrae superioris muscle must relax as the orbicularis muscle contracts. The superior rectus muscle and lateral rectus muscle also contract to elevate the globe, producing Bell's phenomenon. Spontaneous blinking involves solely the pretarsal orbicularis muscle fibers; voluntary blinking triggers all three orbicularis components. Contractions of the orbicularis muscle begin laterally and flow medially, forcing the tear film toward the puncta and into the canalicular system. When the orbicularis muscle relaxes, the retreating eyelid margin pulls the tear film over the cornea through fluid surface tension.

The levator palpebrae superioris muscle originates at the orbital apex. By the time it reaches the upper eyelid, it has converted from striated muscle to a dense fibrous

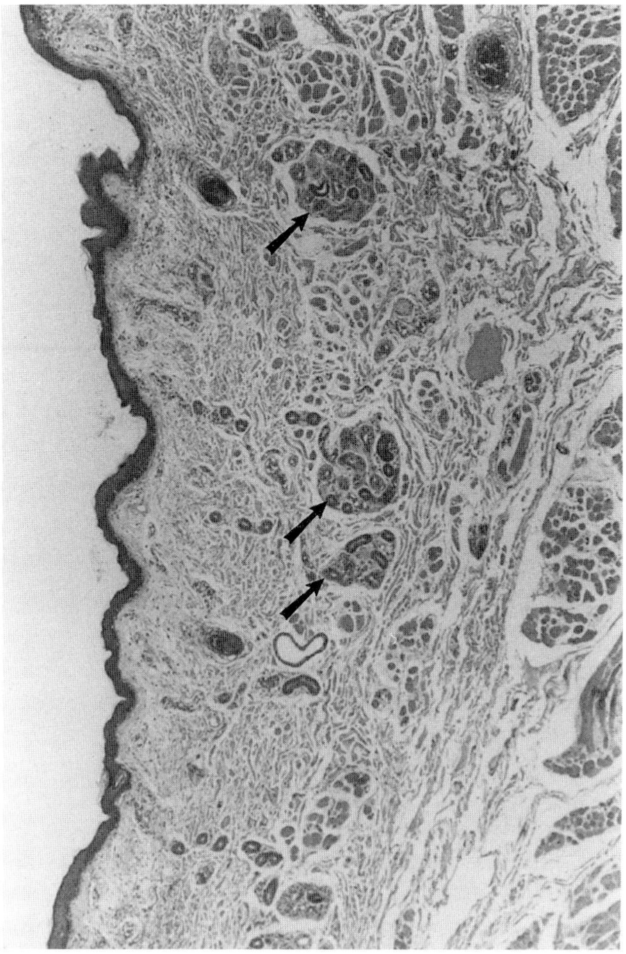

FIGURE 2-4 Anterior portion of the eyelid showing several sweat glands (arrows).

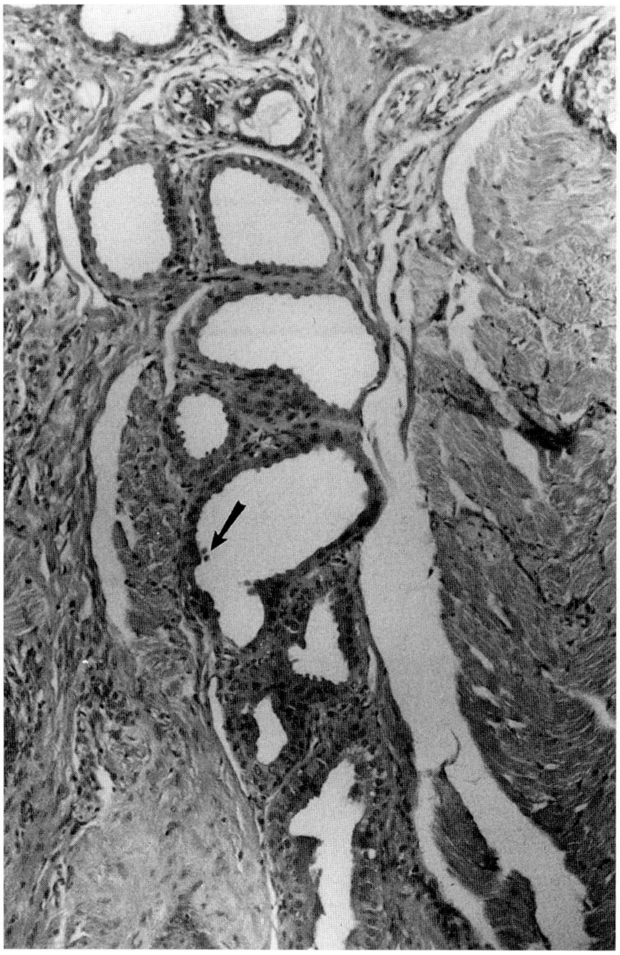

FIGURE 2-5 Glands of Moll demonstrating apocrine mechanism of secretion (arrow).

aponeurosis. The aponeurosis passes between the orbicularis muscle and tarsus; it sends tight attachments (the superior transverse or Whitnall's ligament) anteriorly into the orbicularis muscle and skin and posteriorly into the tarsus. The levator aponeurosis is shaped like a fan, with medial and lateral horns. Approximately 1 cm from its insertion, the aponeurosis combines with the anterior margin of the superior transverse ligament to act as a check ligament for the upper eyelid. The levator palpebrae superioris muscle is supplied by the superior branch of the oculomotor (3rd cranial) nerve. There is no muscular equivalent of the levator palpebrae superioris muscle in the lower eyelid, although the capsulopalpebral head of the inferior rectus muscle (formed by an extension of the inferior rectus tendon and the sheath of the inferior oblique muscle) inserts into the inferior edge of the lower tarsus.

Fibrous Tissue and Müller's Muscle

The tarsal plates are composed of dense fibrous tissue with relatively uniform collagen fibers 60 to 70 nm in diameter[1]; they do not contain cartilage. Elastic fibers and fibroblasts are interspersed among the collagen fibers. Both the superior and inferior tarsi are flat and semilunar in shape. They are 1 mm in thickness and measure approximately 29 mm horizontally. The superior tarsus averages 10 mm in height, and the inferior tarsus is between 3.8 and 4.5 mm in height.[8] The medial and lateral tarsal margins are loosely attached to the canthal tendons.

The tarsi contain modified sebaceous glands, known as meibomian glands, the ducts of which run perpendicular to and open onto the eyelid margins (Figure 2-6). There are 30 to 40 meibomian glands in the upper eyelid and 20 to 30 in the lower eyelid. Meibomian glands

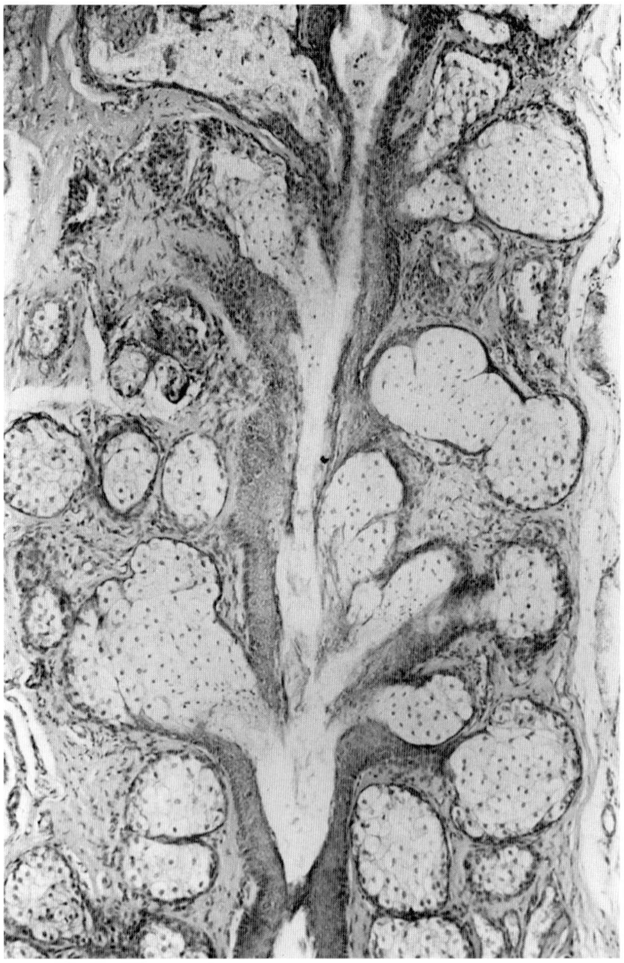

FIGURE 2-6 Meibomian gland with several alveoli emptying into a central duct.

can be readily visualized by transillumination of the eyelids. Although meibomian glands are not associated with hair follicles, they are similar in structure to sebaceous glands elsewhere in the body.

Between 10 and 15 lobules of secretory cells, the alveoli, arise laterally from each central meibomian duct. As with all sebaceous glands, the alveoli consist of a thin peripheral layer of relatively cuboidal cells that rapidly fill their cytoplasm with large lipid droplets. The secretions are discharged into the central duct by a holocrine method.

The ducts of the meibomian glands are lined by keratinized, stratified squamous epithelium. The lipid secretions of the meibomian glands differ from those of most sebaceous glands in that they contain more cholesterol and less triglycerides and fatty acids.[9,10] Meibomian secretions contribute to the outer layer of the tear film, decreasing evaporation of aqueous tears and behaving as a surfactant to provide a smooth focusing surface for the cornea. If a meibomian duct is obstructed, the resultant granulomatous inflammation is clinically evident as a chalazion. Sebaceous cell carcinoma most commonly originates in the meibomian glands. Meibomian gland dysfunction is discussed in Chapter 4.

The fibrous layer of the eyelids also contains accessory lacrimal glands. Some are located at the edge of the tarsal plates (glands of Wolfring); others are found in the fornices (glands of Krause). The accessory lacrimal glands lack a capsule and are composed of acini of eccrine cells that surround a central duct. The interstitial fibrous tissue contains scattered lymphocytes and plasma cells that are responsible for the production and secretion of immunoglobulins, including IgA.

The canalicular system drains tears from the eyes. It is lined by an unusually thick, nonkeratinized stratified squamous epithelium. Each upper and lower punctum leads into a 0.5-mm–diameter segment of canaliculus that is perpendicular to the eyelid margin. Each canaliculus widens to form an ampulla, then makes a right-angled turn toward the medial canthus. Within approximately 8 mm, the superior and inferior canaliculi either fuse into a common canaliculus or enter the lacrimal sac separately. Occlusion of the lacrimal drainage system generally occurs at the distal end of the lacrimal sac in adults or at the distal end of the nasolacrimal duct in children.

The orbital septa are the primary barriers that prevent an eyelid infection (preseptal cellulitis) from spreading to the orbit (orbital cellulitis). The septa also confine intraorbital hemorrhage, potentially increasing orbital tension and damaging the globe or optic nerve. The orbital septa arise from the arcus marginalis, which is dense fibrous tissue at the junction of the periorbita and periosteum of the skull.[7] The orbital septa may originate several millimeters inferior to the temporal orbital margin and produce a potential space, called the *recess of Eisler*. The superior orbital septum inserts into the levator aponeurosis at the level of the upper eyelid crease; the inferior orbital septum inserts into the capsulopalpebral head of the inferior rectus at the level of the lower eyelid crease. In Asian eyelids, the superior orbital septum inserts more inferiorly, yielding a lower or absent eyelid crease.

Loose bundles of smooth muscle, called *Müller's muscle*, insert into the superior margin of the upper tarsus and the inferior margin of the lower tarsus and travel posterior to the orbital septa. They act as retractors in both the upper and lower eyelids. Müller's muscle originates in the levator aponeurosis superiorly and the capsulopalpebral head inferiorly. Innervation is provided

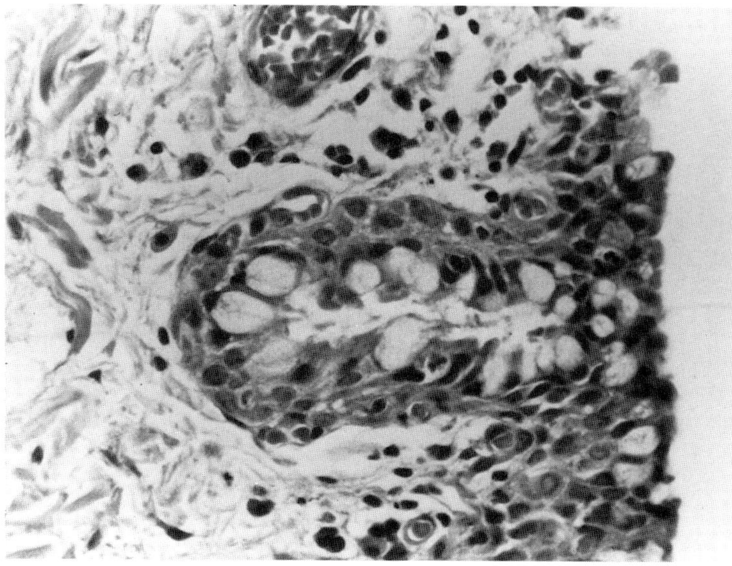

FIGURE 2-7 Conjunctival infolding (crypt or pseudogland of Henle) with several clear goblet cells.

by sympathetic fibers that arise from the superior cervical ganglion and travel to the eyelids via branches of the ophthalmic artery. If sympathetic input is interrupted, the resultant Horner syndrome produces upper eyelid ptosis and lower eyelid elevation, which gives the appearance of enophthalmos.

The levator palpebrae superioris muscle and aponeurosis, orbicularis muscle, and Müller's muscle strike a delicate balance, maintaining an appropriate interpalpebral fissure between blinks. Too large an interpalpebral fissure, as seen in Graves orbitopathy, can lead to corneal desiccation. Too narrow an opening, as seen with 3rd cranial nerve paresis or Horner syndrome, may result in obstruction of the visual axis. Relative inadequacy of tone of the orbicularis muscle may lead to lagophthalmos and corneal exposure, particularly during sleep.

Conjunctiva

The conjunctiva arises at the mucocutaneous junction, covers the posterior surface of the eyelids (palpebral conjunctiva), reflects in the cul-de-sac (forniceal conjunctiva), and covers the globe up to the limbus (bulbar conjunctiva). The bulbar and forniceal conjunctiva are loosely attached to underlying tissues whereas the palpebral conjunctiva is tightly attached. Fluid can collect beneath the tissues and distend the conjunctiva; this phenomenon is termed *chemosis*. The vestige of the nictitating membrane of animals can be seen medially as the plica semilunaris. The caruncle at the medial canthus represents a blend of conjunctiva and skin; it is covered by conjunctival epithelium but has epidermal appendages in its substantia propria. The surface area of the palpebral conjunctiva is expanded by many infoldings. These infoldings, when cut in cross section, suggest the acini of glands, yielding the name *crypts* or *pseudoglands of Henle* (Figure 2-7). Conjunctival crypts are more numerous nasally and in the plica semilunaris.

The conjunctival epithelium consists of nonkeratinized stratified columnar epithelium with admixed columnar goblet cells. At the limbus, the conjunctival epithelium converts to stratified squamous epithelium. Papillary arrangements at the limbus are known as the palisades of Vogt. The thickness of the conjunctival epithelium varies regionally; in women, its maturation can vary during the menstrual cycle.[11] The flattened surface cells of the conjunctival epithelium demonstrate many microvilli and are coated by a glycocalyx and mucin[12,13] (Figure 2-8). Keratinization of the conjunctival epithelium is always pathologic and can occur in conditions such as vitamin A deficiency (Bitot spot), superior limbic keratoconjunctivitis, pemphigoid, Stevens-Johnson syndrome, and keratoconjunctivitis sicca.

Although conjunctival epithelial cells can slide over a corneal epithelial defect and transdifferentiate into normal-appearing corneal epithelial cells,[14] the ability to heal a corneal epithelial defect and to maintain a normal cycle of corneal epithelial cell turnover depends on the presence of epithelial stem cells at the limbus, thought to be represented by areas of thickened epithelium between the palisades of Vogt[15,16] (see Ch. 28). Damage to the limbal epithelium either from disease or mechanical injury can significantly retard the epithelial healing process.[17-19]

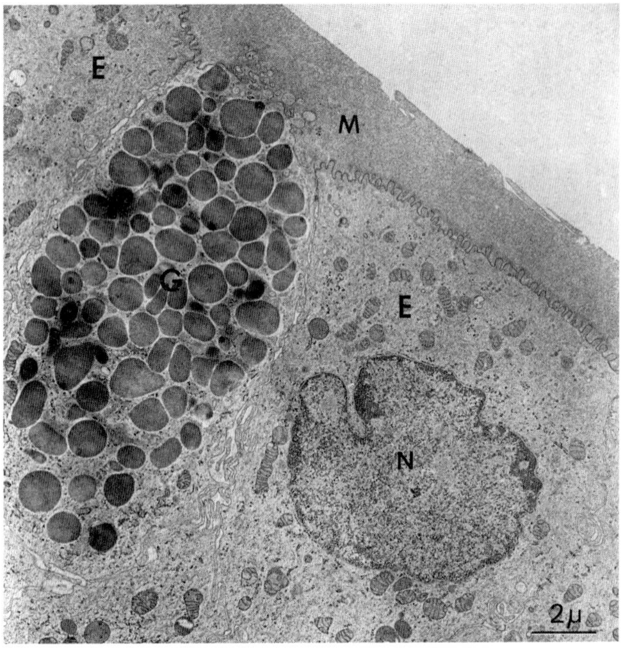

FIGURE 2-8 Transmission electron micrograph of the forniceal conjunctiva. The surface epithelial cells (*E*) have many microvilli. A goblet cell (*G*) secretes mucin (*M*), which covers the anterior surface of the conjunctiva, smoothing out the irregularities. *N*, nucleus. (Reprinted with permission from BA Nichols, ML Chiappino, CR Dawson: Demonstration of the mucous layer of the tear film by electron microscopy. Invest Ophthalmol Vis Sci 26:464, 1985.)

Goblet cells constitute approximately 10 percent of the conjunctival epithelial cell population; they are scattered in the conjunctival epithelium, especially in the fornices, plica semilunaris, and caruncle. They are absent at the limbus. Goblet cells secrete mucin, which is dispersed over the surface of the globe and, by its hydrophilic nature, decreases the surface tension of the tear film.[20,21] This allows even distribution of tears over the ocular surface.[13] Two types of goblet cells are identifiable in the conjunctiva.[21] Type I cells are found in the forniceal conjunctiva and secrete by an apocrine method. Type II cells are found diffusely throughout the conjunctiva and secrete by a merocrine method, which involves discharge of the secretory product from an intact cell. Goblet cells may be significantly decreased in various disorders, including keratoconjunctivitis sicca, Stevens-Johnson syndrome, pemphigoid, and chemical injury.[22]

The conjunctival epithelium contains nonepithelial cells similar to those in the skin. Melanocytes are present basally, and Langerhans cells are scattered throughout.[23,24] The concentration of Langerhans cells is highest in individuals younger than 20 years and older than 40 years.[24] Conjunctival Langerhans cells may play a major role in corneal graft rejection.[25] Lymphocytes are also present in conjunctival epithelium; cytotoxic/suppressor T cells (CD8 cells) predominate.[20]

The substantia propria of the conjunctiva plays an important role in ocular immune mechanisms.[23,24] The lymphocytic population is predominantly helper/inducer T cells; however, the number of cytotoxic/suppressor T cells may increase in disease states, such as ocular rosacea.[26] Only scattered B cells and macrophages are present. The number of helper/inducer T cells and macrophages increases with age. Aggregates of lymphocytes with germinal centers in the conjunctiva are abnormal and are referred to clinically as follicles. Although no Langerhans cells are present in the substantia propria, $CD1^-/HLA\text{-}DR^+$ phagocytic cells can be found. Mast cells within the substantia propria may increase significantly in allergic states[27]; tear levels of tryptase secreted by mast cells have been used as a measure of atopic activity.[28]

VASCULAR SUPPLY AND LYMPHATIC DRAINAGE

For the most part, blood supply to the eyelids and palpebral conjunctiva is from the terminal branches of the ophthalmic artery (internal carotid artery distribution). The blood supply is supplemented by divisions of the facial artery (external carotid artery distribution). The anterior ciliary arteries supply blood to the bulbar conjunctiva and limbal region. These arterial beds freely anastomose, however. The eyelids and conjunctiva drain to both the orbital and facial venous systems. Communication with the ophthalmic vein means that eyelid infections can lead to cavernous sinus thrombosis.

A rich lymphatic plexus is present in the eyelids and conjunctiva. The lymphatics of the outer two-thirds of the upper eyelid and the outer one-third of the lower eyelid drain into the preauricular nodes. The lymphatics of the inner two-thirds of the lower eyelid and the inner one-third of the upper eyelid drain into the submandibular nodes (Figure 2-9).

INNERVATION

The orbicularis muscle is innervated by branches of the facial nerve that enter laterally and posteriorly. The levator palpebrae superioris muscle is supplied by the superior branch of the oculomotor nerve. Sympathetic fibers arising in the superior cervical ganglion project to Müller's

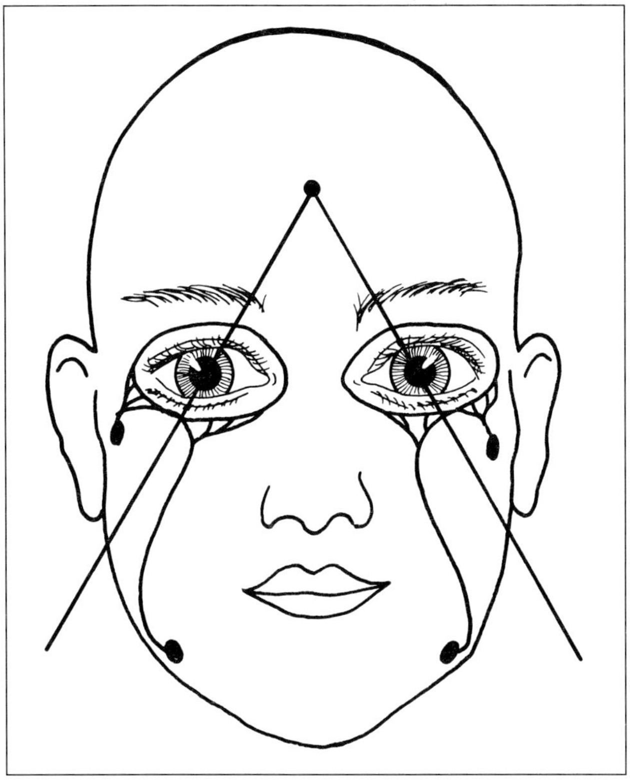

FIGURE 2-9 Lymphatic drainage of the conjunctiva and eyelids.

muscle. Sensation in the upper eyelid is mediated by the supraorbital branch of the ophthalmic division of the trigeminal nerve; sensation in the lower eyelid is mediated predominantly by the infraorbital branch of the maxillary division of the trigeminal nerve. Sensory nerves tend to run between the orbicularis muscle and tarsus. The conjunctiva is innervated by the ophthalmic division of the trigeminal nerve.

REFERENCES

1. Jakobiec FA, Iwamoto T: The ocular adnexa. p. 290. In Fine BS, Yanoff M (eds): Ocular Histology. 2nd Ed. Harper & Row, New York, 1979
2. Spencer WH, Zimmerman LE: Conjunctiva. p. 109. In Spencer WH (ed): Ophthalmic Pathology. 3rd Ed. WB Saunders, Philadelphia, 1985
3. Font RL: Eyelids and lacrimal drainage system. p. 2141. In Spencer WH (ed): Ophthalmic Pathology. 3rd Ed. WB Saunders, Philadelphia, 1986
4. Wulc AE, Dryden RM, Khatchaturian T: Where is the gray line? Arch Ophthalmol 105:1092, 1987
5. Bergin DJ, McCord CD, Berger T, et al: Blepharochalasis. Br J Ophthalmol 72:863, 1988
6. Koornneef L: Eyelid and orbital fascial attachments and their clinical significance. Eye 2:130, 1988
7. Kivela T, Tarkkanen A: The Merkel cell and associated neoplasms in the eyelids and periocular region. Surv Ophthalmol 35:171, 1990
8. Jelks GW, Jelks EB: The influence of orbital and eyelid anatomy on the palpebral aperture. Clin Plast Surg 18:183, 1991
9. Andrews JS: The meibomian secretions. Int Ophthalmol Clin 13:23, 1973
10. McCulley JP, Dougherty J: Classification of chronic blepharitis. Ophthalmology 89:1173, 1982
11. Kramer P, Lubkin U, Potter W, et al: Cyclic changes in conjunctival smears from menstruating females. Ophthalmology 30:3, 1990
12. Nichols B, Dawson CR, Togni B: Surface features of the conjunctiva and cornea. Invest Ophthalmol Vis Sci 24:570, 1983
13. Nichols BA, Chiappino ML, Dawson CR: Demonstration of the mucous layer of the tear film by electron microscopy. Invest Ophthalmol Vis Sci 26:464, 1985
14. Shapiro MS, Friend J, Thoft RA: Corneal re-epithelialization from the conjunctiva. Invest Ophthalmol Vis Sci 21:135, 1981
15. Thoft RA: The role of the limbus in ocular surface maintenance and repair. Acta Ophthalmol (Copenh) 67(suppl):91, 1989
16. Dua HS, Forrester JV: The corneoscleral limbus in human corneal epithelial wound healing. Am J Ophthalmol 110:646, 1990
17. Tseng SCG: Concept and application of limbal stem cells. Eye 3:141, 1989
18. Huang AJW, Tseng SCG: Corneal epithelial wound healing in the absence of limbal epithelium. Invest Ophthalmol Vis Sci 32:96, 1991
19. Chen JJY, Tseng SCG: Abnormal corneal epithelial wound healing in partial-thickness removal of limbal epithelium. Invest Ophthalmol Vis Sci 32:2219, 1991
20. Wanko T, Lloyd BJ, Matthews J: The fine structure of human conjunctiva in the perilimbal zone. Invest Ophthalmol 2:285, 1964
21. Streuhl KP, Knorr M: The second, mucus-secreting system of the conjunctiva: ultrastructural findings. Fortschr Ophthalmol 87:492, 1990
22. Ralph RA: Conjunctival goblet cell density in normal subjects and in dry eye syndromes. Invest Ophthalmol 14:299, 1975
23. Sacks EH, Wieczonek R, Jakobiec FA, Knowles DM: Lymphocytic subpopulations in the normal human conjunctiva: a monoclonal antibody study. Ophthalmology 93:1276, 1986
24. Chen CC, Nussenblat RB, Ni M, et al: Immunohistochemical markers in the normal human epibulbar conjunctiva from fetus to adult. Arch Ophthalmol 106:215, 1988
25. Ross J, Callahan D, Kunz H, Niederkorn J: Evidence that the fate of class II-disparate corneal grafts is determined

by the timing of class II expression. Transplantation 51:532, 1991
26. Hoang-Xuan T, Rodriguez A, Zaltas MM, et al: Ocular rosacea: a histologic and immunopathologic study. Ophthalmology 97:1468, 1990
27. Morgan SJ, Williams JH, Walls AF, et al: Mast cell numbers and staining characteristics in the normal and allergic human conjunctiva. J Allergy Clin Immunol 87:111, 1991
28. Butrus SI, Ochsner KI, Abelson MB, Schwartz LB: The levels of tryptase in human tears: an indicator of activation of conjunctival mast cells. Ophthalmology 97:1678, 1990

3

Basic Ocular Immunology

C. STEPHEN FOSTER

The concept that individuals can be altered in such a way that they can be protected against disease dates back to the 11th century in China, where crusts from smallpox lesions were first inhaled and later introduced into skin punctures in an effort to prevent lethal smallpox infections. The efficacy of these procedures formed the basis for similar experiments in England by Lady Montagu[1] and Edward Jenner.[2] By 1880, when Koch[3] discovered the tubercle bacillus and described the delayed (type IV) hypersensitivity reaction, the foundations of experimental medicine were being laid. Pasteur's research at this time resulted not only in the development of the germ theory of disease but also in experiments in immunization with both killed and attenuated microorganisms.[4]

By 1900, the information available regarding protective responses of an organism against foreign material (especially microorganisms) was substantial enough to provide the basis for two schools of thought. Metchnikoff, Arthus, von Pirquet, Swartzmann, and others thought that cellular responses were important in protective and allergic responses. Ehrlich, Landsteiner, Kabat, and others believed that soluble (humoral) biochemical products (later to be called antibodies) were the important protective elements. We now realize that both schools were correct in their beliefs: the cellular and the humoral elements of the immune system are both important, and further, each system is intimately intertwined with the other.

IMMUNE MECHANISMS

Immunology is the study of immunity and the immune response. The word *immunity* is derived from the Latin *immunis,* which means "free from." It is the state of being protected from infectious and other harmful agents. There are two types of immunity: natural immunity and acquired immunity.

Natural Immunity

Natural immunity has no specificity and no memory, two features that are characteristic of acquired immunity. The eyelids, intact ocular surface, and tear flow provide natural immunity for the eye. Certain components of the tears, such as fatty acids, mucin, lysozyme, neutrophils, macrophages, and complement components, also provide natural protection. Macrophages and natural killer cells are early-response, primitive natural immunity cells that provide immediate defense against foreign antigens without specific recognition, without central processing, and without memory.

Acquired Immunity

What is generally meant when speaking of immunity is protection acquired by the organism in processes known collectively as the immune response. The immune response has three components: the afferent arc, central processing, and the efferent arc (Figure 3-1). In the afferent arc, immunocompetent cells are exposed to an antigen. Specific recognition of the antigen by the immunocompetent cells occurs, resulting in sensitization. In central processing, immunocompetent cells produce antibodies or mature into immunocompetent effector cells. In the efferent arc, an attack is mounted against the antigen by the antibodies and/or immunocompetent cells.

Acquired immunity is specific, retains memory of prior antigenic encounter, and is capable of differentiating between self and nonself. The forces that hold antigen and antibody or antigen and cell-receptor sites together are

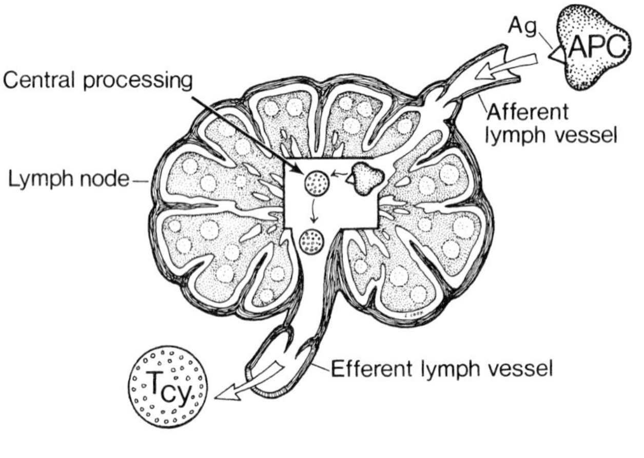

FIGURE 3-1 Immune response components. The afferent arc of the immune response begins when antigen (*Ag*) is bound to an antigen-presenting cell (*APC*) with subsequent migration of that APC to the central processing station (e.g., lymph node). Central processing occurs within the node, with proper presentation of the antigen to other cells of the immune system. The efferent arc of the immune response occurs when immunocompetent antigen-specific effector cells (T_{cy}) migrate from the central processing station to the area of immunologic interest.

not ionic or covalent bonding forces, but rather coulombic, hydrophobic, van der Waals, and hydrogen-bonding forces. These are relatively weak forces and depend on close approximation of the involved molecules, which can occur only if the electron cloud shapes of the respective molecules are highly complementary. This accounts for the high degree of specificity in acquired immunity.

Immunologic memory is evident when an organism encounters a particular antigen for a second or subsequent time. The second immune response is accelerated compared with the first immune response. Specific antibodies and/or effector cells are produced more rapidly (Figure 3-2). This rapid secondary or anamnestic response results from persistence of certain memory cells formed as a result of the organism's first encounter with the specific antigen. These memory cells, on subsequent encounter with that specific antigen, rapidly swing into action and amplify the development of the immune response.

The survival of an organism depends on a fail-safe mechanism by which the immune system recognizes and discriminates between self and nonself. Failure to do so leads to an immune response against self, with resultant damage to the organism.

COMPONENTS OF THE IMMUNE SYSTEM

Antigens

A variety of biologic molecules can act as antigens. An antigen incites a specific immune response. The result may be production of a specific antibody and/or production of specifically sensitized lymphocytes. Proteins and complex polysaccharides are generally excellent antigens, especially if they possess little or no symmetry. In general, a given antigen molecule has several antigenic determinants, called *epitopes.* An epitope is a relatively small section of a molecule whose electron cloud configuration provides the proper noncovalent force relationships necessary for reacting specifically with the binding site, or paratope, of an antibody molecule. Larger molecules are better antigens than smaller molecules, because they have more epitopes that may be recognized

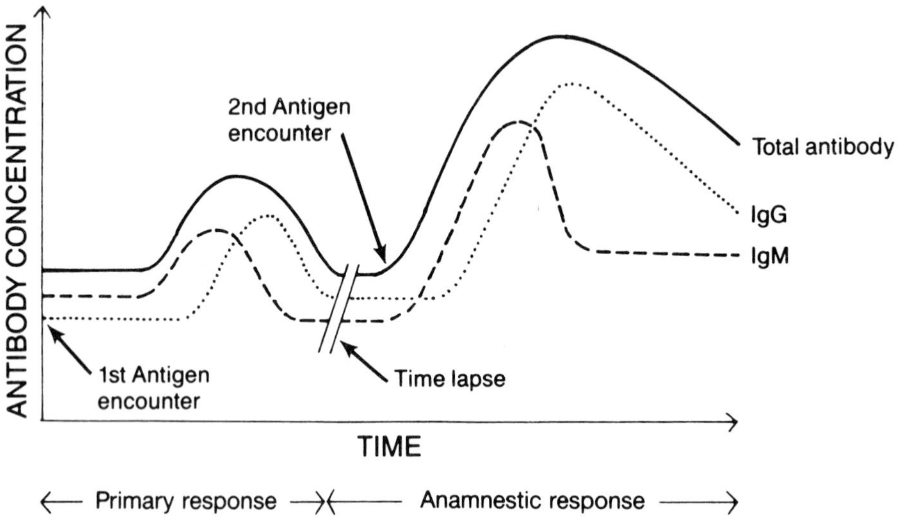

FIGURE 3-2 Anamnestic response. The primary response, depicted here as specific antibody formation, begins to be detectable after some delay following initial antigen presentation. On subsequent encounter with the same antigen, however, antibody production is rapidly detectable, and the total amount of antibody is greater than that after the primary antigenic encounter. This anamnestic response stems largely from the persistence of long-lived memory cells.

as foreign by the organism's immune system. A hapten is a small molecule that, in and of itself, does not elicit an immunogenic (antigenic) response but can elicit such a response when attached to a larger antigenic molecule, usually a protein.

Antibodies

An antibody is an immunoglobulin produced in response to an antigen. An antibody binds to or reacts specifically with that antigen. Immunoglobulins are composed of four polypeptide chains linked by disulfide bonds. Two of the polypeptide chains are longer than the other two and hence are designated heavy or H-chains; the two shorter chains are designated light or L-chains (Figure 3-3). A heavy chain has a molecular weight of approximately 50,000; a light chain, approximately 25,000.

If the heavy and light chains of many different immunoglobulin molecules are analyzed, it becomes apparent that the amino acid sequences in certain regions are similar. These regions are termed *constant regions* and are designated C_H for the constant region of heavy chains and C_L for the constant region of light chains. There are also certain regions that are different. These regions are termed *variable regions* (V_H and V_L). Additionally, certain regions are extremely variable and are termed *hypervariable regions.* The hypervariable regions are the specific areas that bind to an antigen.

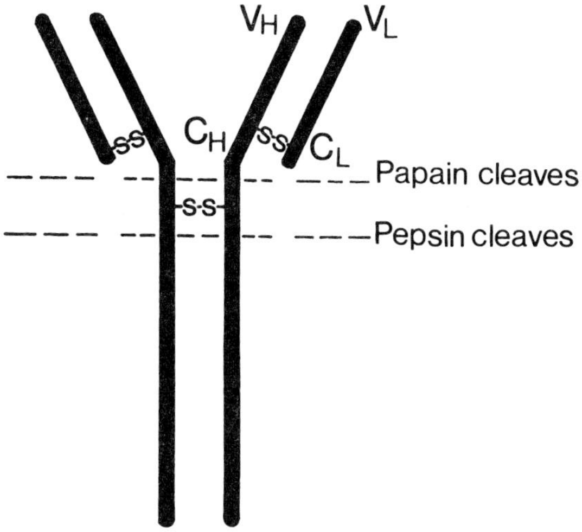

FIGURE 3-3 An immunoglobulin molecule comprises two heavy and two light chains joined by disulfide bonds. Constant and variable regions of both the heavy and the light chains are labeled C_H, V_H, C_L, and V_L, respectively.

A diagrammatic representation of a typical immunoglobulin molecule is shown in Figure 3-4. The molecule can be

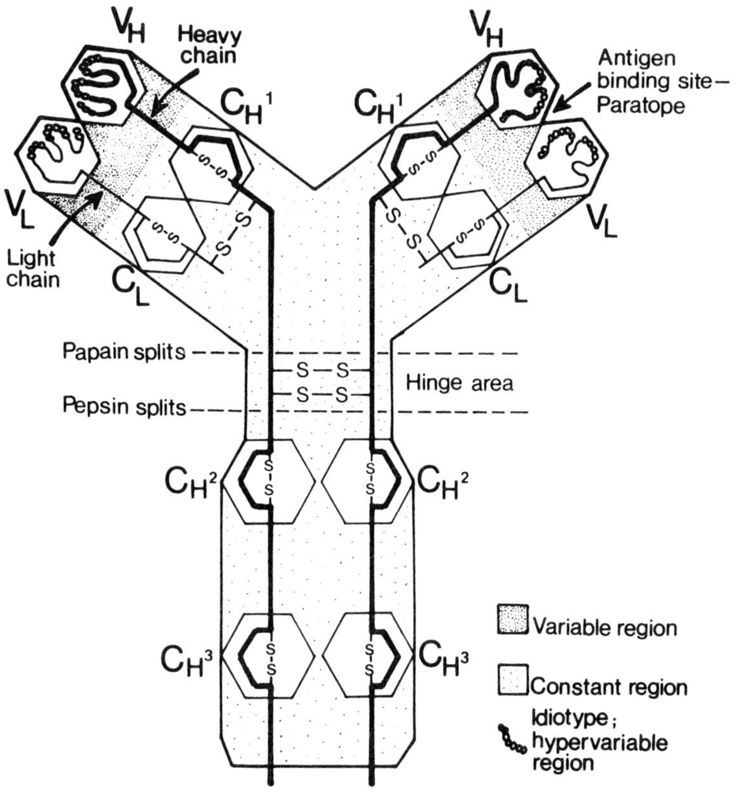

FIGURE 3-4 Schematic representation of an immunoglobulin molecule. The constant regions (C_L, C_H) comprise amino acid sequences that are strikingly constant and homogeneous from immunoglobulin to immunoglobulin. The variable regions (V_L, V_H) contain considerably fewer identical amino acid residues, molecule to molecule. A small region in this variable region, the hypervariable region, is the antigen binding site, or paratope.

TABLE 3-1
Characteristics of the Five Immunoglobulin Classes

Characteristic	*Classes* IgG	IgA	IgM	IgD	IgE
Molecular weight	160,000	170,000	900,000	185,000	200,000
Electrophoretic mobility	γ	Slow β	Between β and γ	Between β and γ	Slow β
Typical serum form	Monomer	Dimer	Pentamer	Monomer	Monomer
Secretory form	Monomer	Dimer with secretory piece	Pentamer	—	Monomer
Heavy chain designation	γ	α	μ	δ	ε
Percentage of total immunoglobulin	80	13	6	1	0.002
Concentration in normal serum (mg/ml)	8–16	1.5–3.5	0.5–2.0	0–0.5	0.00015–0.00045

split into three fragments by papain digestion. The two identical fragments, each composed of an intact light chain and a piece of heavy chain, are called *Fab fragments*, and the remaining pieces of the heavy chains together are called the *Fc fragment*. Fab stands for fragment antigen binding; Fc stands for fragment crystallizable. The immunoglobulin molecule binds antigen with its Fab portion; this binding site is called the *paratope*. The Fc portion of the molecule is involved with biologic attachments and functions other than antigen binding (e.g., attachment to cell membranes, passage through the placental barrier, and fixation of complement).

Five classes of immunoglobulins are found in humans, and each contains a different type of heavy chain. The five classes are designated IgG, IgA, IgM, IgD, and IgE, depending on the type of heavy chain. Two types of light chains are found throughout the immunoglobulin classes: κ- and λ-light chains. Immunoglobulin-producing B cells produce either κ-chain or λ-chain antibody, but not both.

Table 3-1 shows characteristics of the five classes of immunoglobulins. Tables 3-2 and 3-3 show the biologic properties and functions of the immunoglobulins. The structure of IgM is shown in Figure 3-5 and that of IgA as it occurs in the serum is shown in Figure 3-6. The subunits of these pentameric and dimeric molecules are joined by a protein called the *J-chain*. Secretory IgA, found, for example, in tears, is further stabilized by a protein called secretory piece, which is acquired during IgA passage across mucosa (Figure 3-7). Immunoglobulin variants within a given class and within a given individual are shown in Table 3-4. Table 3-5 shows estimated levels of immunoglobulins in the eye. Some ocular structures, including conjunctiva and cornea, are rich in IgG and IgA.

TABLE 3-2
Biologic Properties of the Five Immunoglobulin Classes

Property	*Classes* IgG	IgA	IgM	IgD	IgE
Complement fixation	+	–	+	–	–
Placental transfer	+	–	–	–	–
Synthetic rate (g/day/70 kg)	2.3	2.7	0.4	0.03	[a]
Half-life (days)	23	6	5	3	3

[a] Too small to measure.

TABLE 3-3
Major Functions of the Five Immunoglobulin Classes

IgG	*IgA*	*IgM*	*IgD*	*IgE*
Functions				
Toxin neutralization	Toxin neutralization	Toxin neutralization	Cell-surface receptor	Reagin
Opsonization	Opsonization	Opsonization		
Bacteriolysis	Agglutination	Bacteriolysis		
Agglutination		Agglutination		
Disease participation				
Serum sickness	Autoantibody	Serum sickness		Atopy
Immune complex disease		Immune complex disease		Anaphylaxis
Autoantibody		Autoantibody		

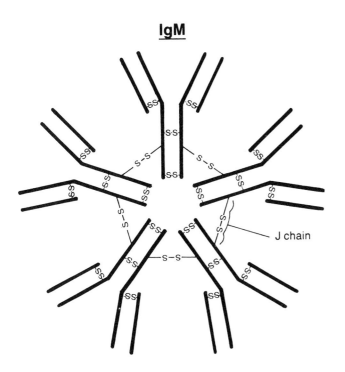

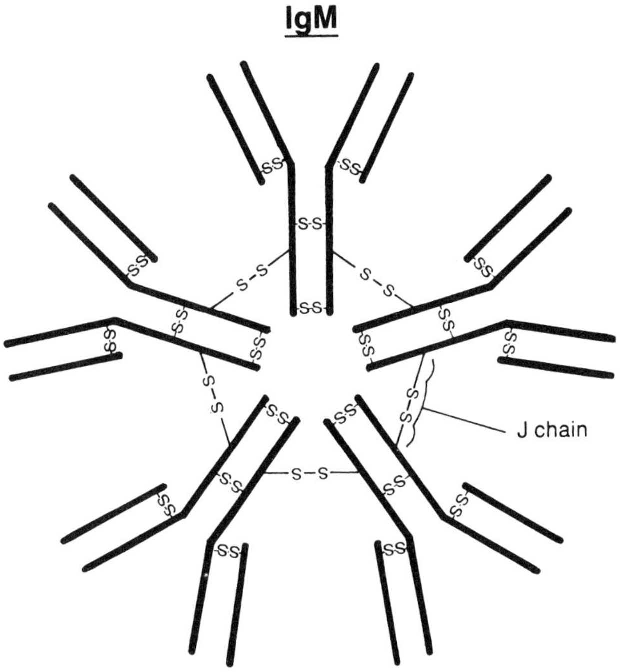

FIGURE 3-5 Schematic representation of IgM. This pentamer, made up of five basic immunoglobulin units, is formed by the joining together of the subunits through an amino acid chain known as the J-chain, which also possesses disulfide bonds.

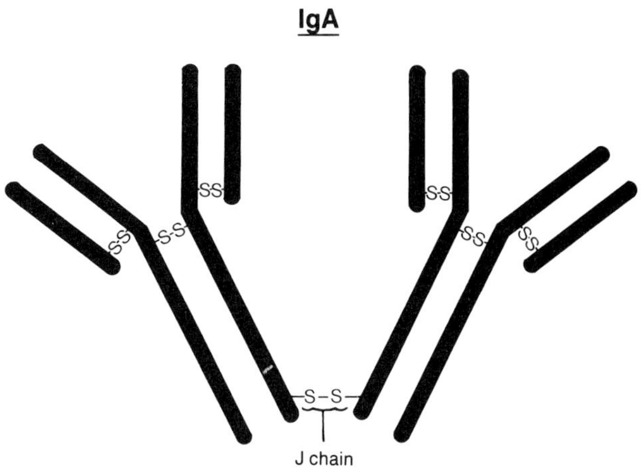

FIGURE 3-6 Schematic representation of IgA, as it appears in serum. IgA typically exists predominantly as a dimer, with the two immunoglobulin units joined to each other by a J-chain.

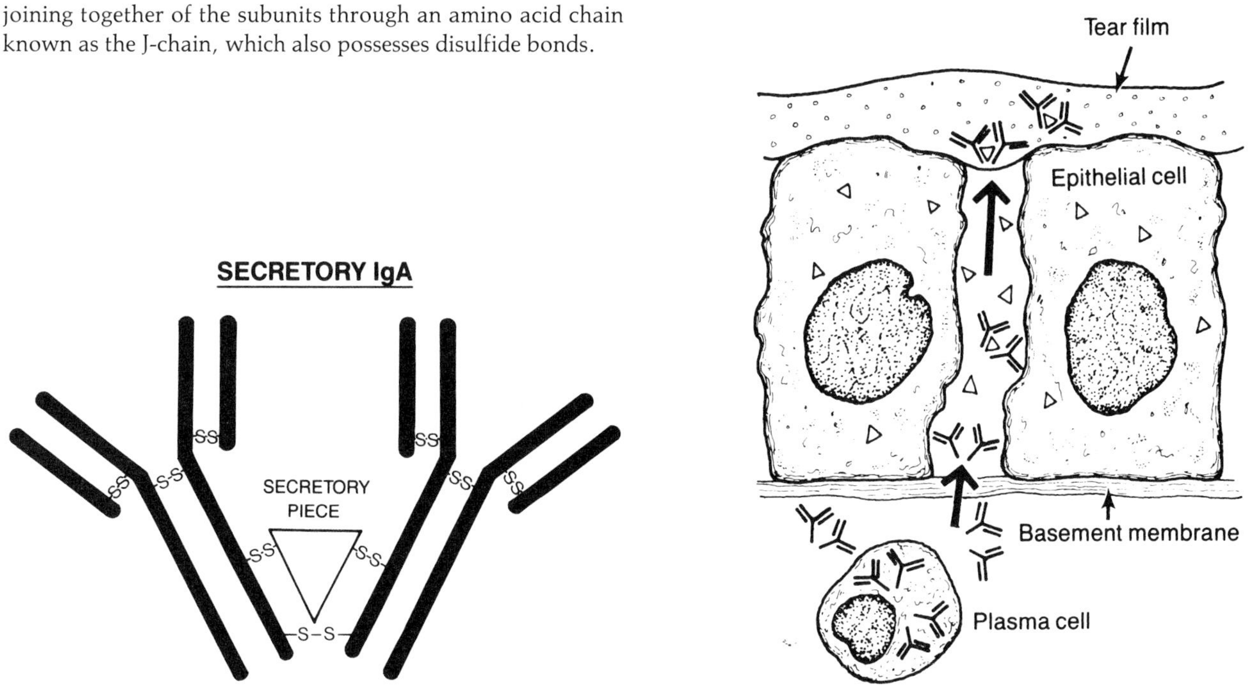

A B

FIGURE 3-7 (A) Schematic representation of secretory IgA. This form of IgA is found predominantly in external secretions, such as milk, saliva, tears, and respiratory and gastrointestinal mucus. It is a dimeric form; its monomers are joined by a J-chain, with further stabilization by a secretory piece, which is a protein secreted by mucosal epithelium. (B) Schematic representation of the production and incorporation of secretory piece into IgA during its transit across the lacrimal gland epithelium, with subsequent appearance of secretory IgA in the tear film.

TABLE 3-4
Immunoglobulin Variants

Type of Variation	*Distribution*	*Variant*	*Location*	*Examples*
Isotypic	All variants present in serum of a normal individual	Classes	C_H	IgM, IgE
		Subclasses	C_H	IgA, IgA_2
		Types	C_L	
		Subtypes	C_L	
		Subgroups	V_H/V_L	
Allotypic	Allelic forms; not present in all individuals	Allotypes	Mainly C_H/C_L, sometimes V_H/V_L	GM groups
Idiotypic	Individually specific to each immunoglobulin molecule	Idiotypes	Variable region	—

Source: Adapted from IM Roitt: Essential Immunology. Blackwell Scientific Publications, Oxford, 1984.

TABLE 3-5
Estimated Levels of Immunoglobulin in the Eye[a]

	Levels of Immunoglobulin (μg/mg wet weight)	
Part of Eye	*IgG*	*IgA*
Sclera	1.0	0.15
Cornea	6.0	0.75
Conjunctiva	3.5	1.5
Choroid	3.0	1.0
Iris	1.0	—
Ciliary body	0.4	0.5
Retina	—	—
Aqueous	0.4	0.01
Vitreous	—	—

[a]Calculations based on average normal serum concentrations (see Table 3-1) and estimates of approximate amount of IgG and IgA in various tissues of the eye.
Source: Adapted from MR Allansmith: The Eye and Immunology. CV Mosby, St. Louis, 1982.

It should be emphasized that the IgA/IgG ratio is dramatically reversed in tears, compared with serum, a fact that may have important implications for protection of the ocular surface.

Over the past 50 years, several theories have been proposed to explain how antibodies are synthesized. For many years, it was thought that the antigen acts as a template, with the ability to "instruct" a lymphocyte to produce antibodies specific for that antigen. A later theory, the selection or germ line theory, held that lymphocytes, as a group, already have the ability to produce antibodies against all the possible antigens and that each individual lymphocyte is specific for one of these potential antigens. When the proper lymphocyte encounters its particular antigen, it undergoes a blastogenic transformation and proliferates into a clone of cells, all of which synthesize the same specific antibody.

Roitt[5] used the analogy of a customer wanting to purchase a new suit. In terms of the instructional theory, the customer (antigen) presents himself personally to the tailor (lymphocyte) to be fitted for the suit (antibody). In the selection theory, the customer goes to the tailor and is supplied with a suit from a stock of 10,000 ready-to-wear suits.

Today, knowledge gained from advances in molecular biology suggests that the truth contains a combination of these theories. It appears that in various species there are between 50 and 300 gene fragments in the DNA that encode for immunoglobulin light and heavy chains. It further appears that the mechanisms that generate antibody diversity include recombination of these gene fragments into single genes, variations in DNA base pairs at the junctions of the variable and joining regions, and somatic point mutations in the variable regions.[7] Thus, it seems that, by extension of Roitt's analogy, what the tailor actually has is a collection of patterns for sleeves, lapels, pockets, and pants, and when the customer appears, the appropriate pieces are put together to make a coherent pattern, from which the suit is made.

In reality, an organism produces a family of antibodies reactive against an encountered antigen. This occurs because most antigens are complex molecules that have more than one epitope but also occurs even when a discrete hapten is used as the priming antigenic determinant. This results in a family of antibodies composed of individual antibody molecules that have different affinities for the stimulating antigen. A phenomenon may occur in which two different antigens share some degree of similarity of molecular structure, and one may mimic the other so that the antibody produced in response to immunization with one antigen may actually have stronger affinity for the other antigen. This may explain why, although our repertoire of antibodies is large, it is not so large as to require most of our genetic material to encode for all possible antibodies.

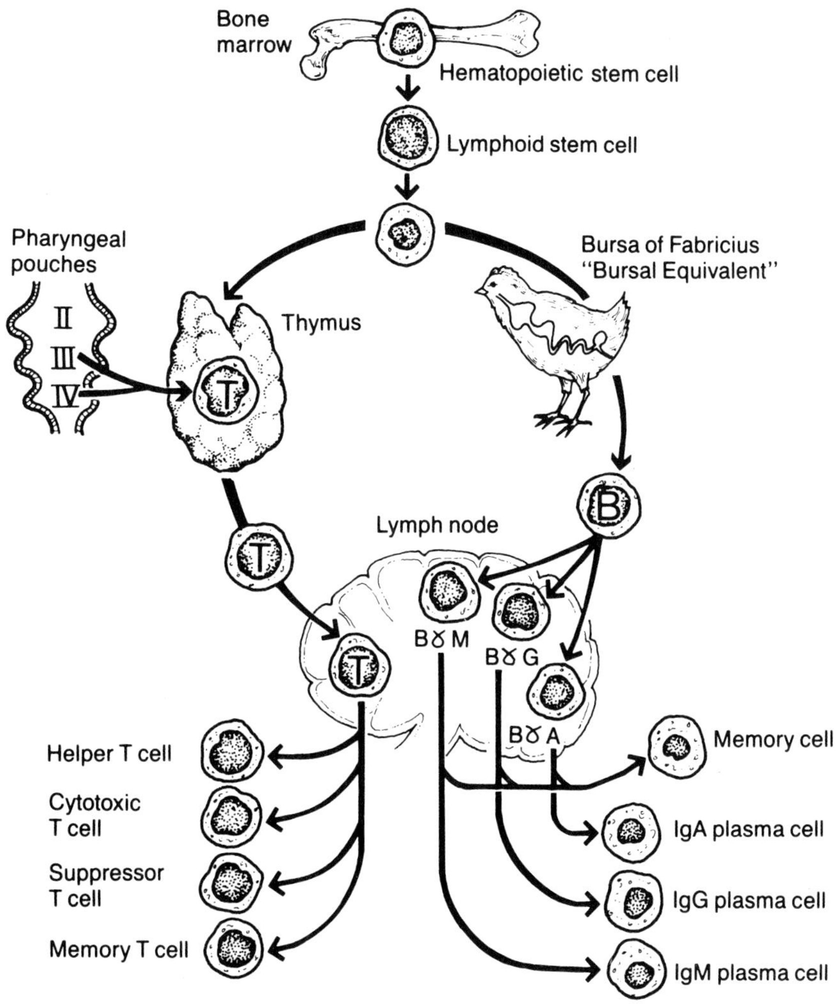

FIGURE 3-8 Development of the immune system. Pluripotential hematopoietic stem cells may differentiate through varying lines to mature blood elements. One line of development for lymphoid stem cells is through influence of the bursal equivalent, with subsequent end-stage differentiation into B cells and eventually into antibody-producing plasma cells. An alternative route of differentiation occurs after influence by the thymus gland, with subsequent development of an array of T cells possessing a variety of functions.

Cellular Components

The major cellular components of the immune system are T cells (classically and in oversimplified terms, the cells responsible for cell-mediated immunity), B cells (classically, the cells responsible for humoral immunity), null cells, and antigen-presenting cells.

Undifferentiated bone marrow stem cells produce immature lymphocytes (Figure 3-8). These lymphocytes may be affected by certain influences in the bone marrow or in the thymus. Lymphocytes acted on by the thymus are called T cells; they develop specific characteristics and functions that make them unique and distinct from lymphocytes not acted on by the thymus. The influences affecting the differentiation of lymphocytes into T cells probably include the hormone thymosin. T cells retain immunologic memory, help B cells produce antibodies, become effector cytotoxic cells, and suppress or modulate the efferent arc of the immune response.

The influences in the bone marrow that are responsible for the differentiation of lymphocytes into B cells are less well understood. In the chicken, immature lymphocytes migrate to and are affected by the bursa of Fabricius.[8] The human equivalent of the bursa of Fabricius is the bone marrow. B cells retain immunologic memory, become antibody-producing cells, and eventually differentiate into plasma cells.

The cell membranes of T cells and B cells differ substantially in their reaction to certain chemicals, antibodies, and other cells (Table 3-6). For example, human T cells have receptors on their cell membranes for sheep erythrocytes. The biologic significance of this receptor is unknown; however, it has been used as a marker for identifying T cells. The sheep red blood cell rosetting technique allows identification of T cells in a lympho-

TABLE 3-6
Cell-Surface Receptors of Lymphocytes

Receptor	Cell Type: T cells	B cells	K cells	NK cells
Thy-1(θ)	+	–	–	–
Sheep erythrocyte	+	–	–	–
Surface immuno-globulin	–	+	–	–
C3b complement	–	+	–	–
Fc of IgG	–	+	+	–
Epstein-Barr virus	–	+	–	–
Measles	+	–	–	–

Abbreviations: K, killer; NK, natural killer.

TABLE 3-7
Cluster of Differentiation (CD) Surface Glycoproteins and the Cells of the Immune System on Which They Are Found

CD Glycoprotein	Cell Type
CD1	Langerhans cells
CD3	T cells
CD4	Helper T cells (T_H)
CD7	Natural killer (NK) cells, T cells
CD8	Cytotoxic T cells (T_{Cy})/suppressor T cells (T_S)
CD14	Monocytes
CD16	NK cells
CD19	B cells
CD22	B cells
CD25	Interleukin-2 (IL-2) receptor
CD33	Monocytes
CD45	All leukocytes
CD45RA	Most T cells, B cells, and NK cells
CD45RO	Activated/memory T cells
CD71	Proliferating cells

cyte preparation (Figure 3-9). More modern technology involving the use of monoclonal antibodies to identify cell surface glycoproteins unique to various types of leukocytes (cluster of differentiation or CD determinants) has replaced this technique for T-cell identification (Table 3-7). B cells have membrane receptors for the Fc portion of antibody molecules. In addition, B cells have membrane-bound immunoglobulin molecules on their surfaces, and fluorescein-labeled antibody can be used to identify B cells (Figure 3-10). T cells do not have membrane receptors for the Fc portion of antibody molecules or surface immunoglobulins.

B Cells

B cells are derived from bone marrow stem cells that have been affected by the bursal equivalent (bone marrow cells in the endosteal region) under which influence the cells acquire immunocompetence (i.e., the ability to respond to a single antigenic determinant or to a configuration closely resembling this determinant). Precursor B cells, or pre-B cells, lack surface receptors for antigen but have cytoplasmic immunoglobulin heavy chains of the μ class

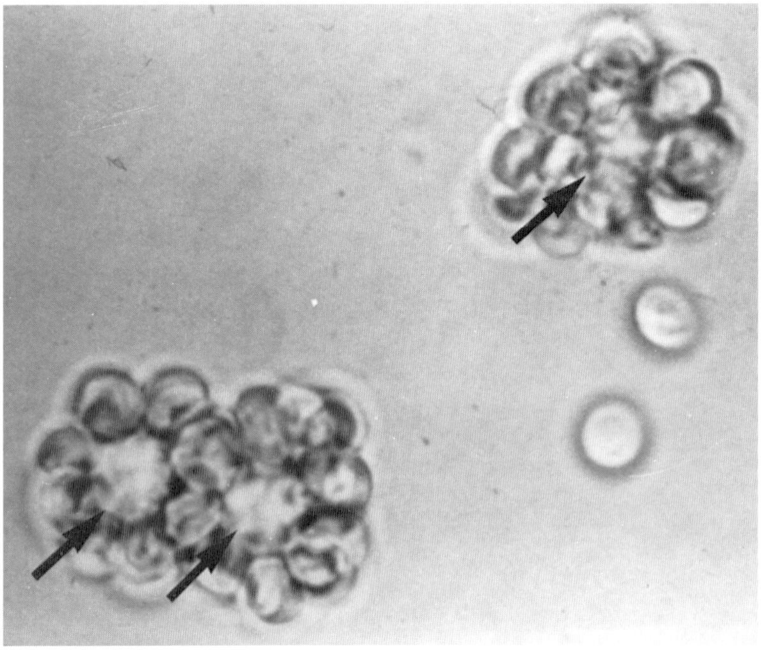

FIGURE 3-9 Lymphocyte preparation after incubation with sheep erythrocytes. Note the three T cells (arrows) that have formed rosettes by adherence of sheep erythrocytes to their cell surfaces. Also note the two lymphocytes that have not formed rosettes; these are non–T cells and may be B cells or null cells.

FIGURE 3-10 Immunofluorescence microscopy of B cells. The conjunctival specimen has been incubated with antiserum to human IgA. B cells expressing surface IgA have "fixed" the fluorescein-labeled anti-IgA antibody molecules and, by fluorescence microscopy, one can see the cluster of these B cells in this specimen of human conjunctiva.

and express the CD45 (or B220) cell-surface glycoprotein. With maturation and the influence of interleukin, surface membrane immunoglobulin of the IgM class appears, as do small amounts of class II antigen (see below). As B-cell maturation proceeds, surface IgD appears, class II antigen on the cell-surface membrane increases, and receptors for complement components appear. Mature B cells express a variety of glycoproteins on their surfaces (Figure 3-11), including specific receptors (immunoglobulins) for specific antigens. Binding of antigen to such receptors results in B-cell activation if certain additional factors are present (see below). Specific B cells respond to specific antigenic stimulation by blastogenic transformation, antibody synthesis, and eventual evolution to end-stage plasma cells and memory cells.

B cells initially produce IgM specific for an antigenic determinant and subsequently switch from IgM synthesis to IgG synthesis. Most of the cells of a clone of antibody-producing B cells become end-stage plasma cells, which ultimately die. Some of the B cells, however, revert to small lymphocytes and become memory cells.

Two major B-cell subsets have been defined in the mouse (Figure 3-12). One subset expresses a surface membrane glycoprotein called Lyb5. $Lyb5^-$ B cells lack the Lyb5 surface membrane glycoprotein. $Lyb5^+$ B cells respond to both type 1 (thymic-dependent) antigens and type 2 (thymic-independent) antigens (Figure 3-13). $Lyb5^-$ B cells require helper T-cell interaction during antigen presentation by an antigen-presenting cell for activation, proliferation, differentiation, and antibody production and secretion to occur. $Lyb5^-$ B cells do not respond to type 2 antigens, and they respond poorly to B-cell mitogens. It is clear that various B-cell subsets exist, including B cells responsible for antigen presentation and B cells involved in modulation or suppression of immune reactions.

T Cells

T cells are lymphocytes derived from bone marrow stem cells that have been acted on by the thymus gland. They

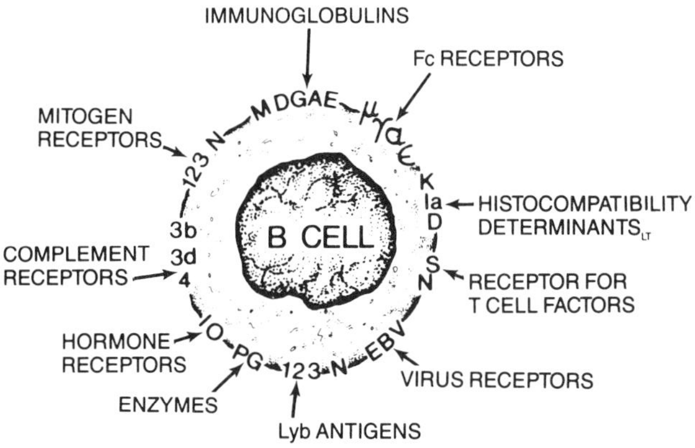

FIGURE 3-11 Cell membrane–surface determinants and receptors on a B cell. On a mature B cell, the immunoglobulin being produced by the B cell will be detectable, as will Fc receptors for the particular heavy chain being produced by the B cell. B cells also possess receptors for Epstein-Barr virus, T-cell stimulatory factors, certain complement components, mitogens, and hormones.

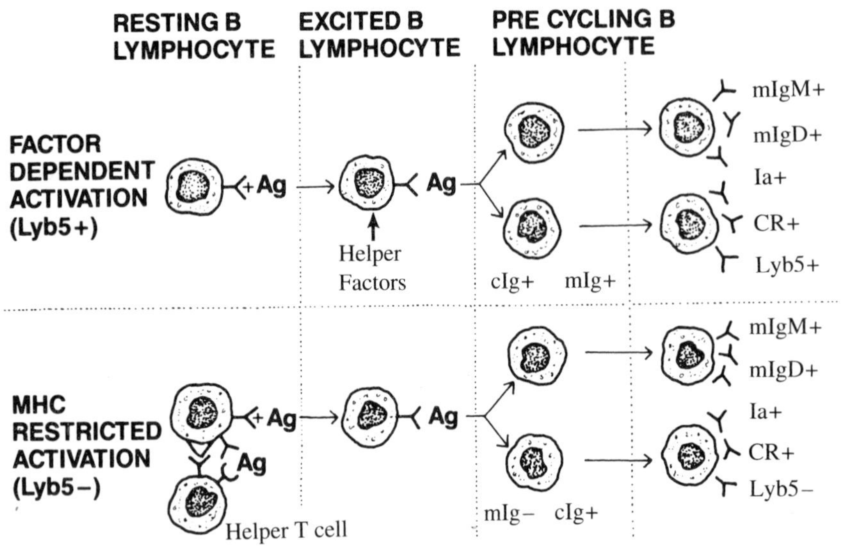

FIGURE 3-12 Schematic representation of the maturation of Lyb5$^+$ and Lyb5$^-$ B cells. *cIg*, cytoplasmic immunoglobulin; *mIg*, membrane immunoglobulin; *mIgM*, membrane IgM; *mIgD*, membrane IgD; *Ia*, surface protein; *CR*, complement receptors; *MHC*, major histocompatibility complex; *Ag*, antigen.

are responsible for cell-mediated immunity. T cells can be classified into several subsets. Helper T cells enable B cells to respond appropriately to specific antigen and to begin specific antibody production. They also facilitate other T-cell subset reactions to antigen. Suppressor T cells exert an opposite action on B cells and possibly exhibit modulating suppressor-type activity on other classes of lymphocytes, including other T cells.

Recently, progress has been made in identifying cell-surface antigenic differences between T-cell subsets. It is now possible, for example, with the use of monoclonal antibodies, to identify cell-surface determinants specific for helper T cells and others that are specific for suppressor T cells. Disturbances in the T-cell subset ratios have been noted in several diseases (Table 3-8). Certain disease states, including states of atopy characterized by extremely high IgE levels, may result from a defect in the suppressor T cells such that the B cells responsible for producing an immunoglobulin (e.g., IgE) are not correctly modulated and hence exhibit unbridled production of the immunoglobulin. As these methods and investi-

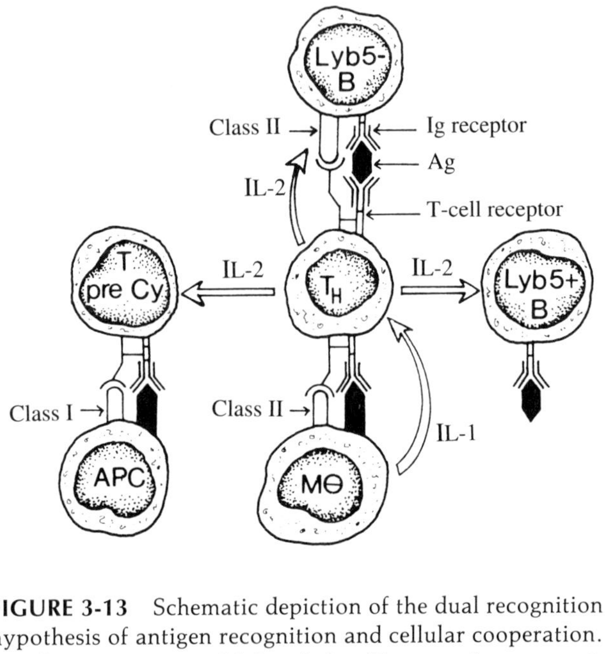

FIGURE 3-13 Schematic depiction of the dual recognition hypothesis of antigen recognition and cellular cooperation. Simultaneous antigen (*Ag*) and class II autoantigen recognition by a helper T cell (T_H) and Lyb5$^-$ B cell results in elaboration of interleukin-2 (*IL-2*) by the helper T cell, with subsequent stimulation of the Lyb5$^-$ B cell to lymphocytic proliferation and immunoglobulin production. In contrast, the Lyb5$^+$ B cell requires only stimulation by the interleukin-2 liberated by the helper T cell after antigen presentation to this helper T cell. *APC*, antigen-presenting cell; *Mθ*, macrophage; *T pre Cy*, precytotoxic T cell.

TABLE 3-8
Disorders with Abnormal Helper T-Cell/Suppressor T-Cell Proportions

Systemic lupus erythematosus
Sarcoidosis
Pemphigoid
Behçet's disease
Progressive systemic sclerosis
Multiple sclerosis
Graft-versus-host disease
Acquired immunodeficiency syndrome

gations are extended and refined, more subsets may be identified and characterized.

Null Cells

Other subpopulations of lymphocytes have been described, including killer cells and natural killer cells. Killer cells (K cells) do not have surface antigens characteristic of B or T cells but do have surface receptors for the Fc region of immunoglobulin. The origin of K cells is obscure, and K-cell activity may be a property of several cell types. K-cell activity involves interaction of the K-cell surface receptor with the Fc region of immunoglobulin molecules that are bound to antigen on the target cell, with subsequent lysis of the target cell. In addition to this antibody-dependent cell-mediated cytotoxicity (ADCC), K cells are involved in immunologic removal of cellular antigens when the target cell is too large to be phagocytized.

Natural killer cells (NK cells) are lymphocytes present in all normal individuals. They arise in the bone marrow from the promonocyte/macrophage precursor line. They are small, nonadherent, and nonphagocytic and lack detectable surface immunoglobulin or cell-surface markers typical of either B or T cells. Their unique cell-surface glycoprotein has been designated CD16. With no primary or prior antigenic contact, NK cells spontaneously destroy transformed tumor cells, virus-infected cells, and possibly cells in transplanted tissues. Although the exact biologic significance of NK cells is unclear, they are an important component of the immune surveillance system and provide one of the earliest defense responses to foreign antigen.

Antigen-Presenting Cells

Antigen-presenting cells are the fourth cellular component critical to the development of acquired immunity. Antigen presentation by antigen-presenting cells to the other cells of the immune system is the first event in the afferent arc or sensitization phase of an acquired immune response. Table 3-9 shows the classic antigen-presenting cells and their distinguishing surface and intracellular characteristics. Macrophages are the pre-eminent antigen-presenting cells and arise from pluripotential bone marrow stem cells. Macrophages phagocytize foreign protein (antigen), degrade it, and provide an appropriate receptor substrate on which antigen and lymphocyte can be properly introduced. They also elaborate a soluble mediator called *interleukin-1*, which promotes the response of helper T cells. Other mononuclear cells, including B cells, can serve as antigen-presenting cells.

Langerhans cells are of hematopoietic origin and are present in skin and mucosa, including the conjunctiva. The peripheral corneal epithelium also contains Langerhans cells. Stimulation of the central cornea (e.g., by trauma, infection, or surgery) results in migration of these cells to the site of stimulation. Langerhans cells have HLA-DR (class II) antigens and cell-surface receptors for the third component of complement (C3) and for the Fc portion of IgG. Langerhans cells function not only in antigen presentation but, as do macrophages, also in other aspects of inflammatory reactions through the release of enzymes and monokines (cytokines produced by monocytes).

TABLE 3-9
Characteristics of Human Antigen-Presenting Cells

Characteristics	*Monocyte/ Macrophage*	*Langerhans Cell (Skin and Mucosa)*	*Dendritic Cell (Spleen)*
Cell surface			
Ia antigen	+	+	+
Fc receptor	+	+	–
C3 receptor	+	+	–
Intracellular			
Esterase	+	+	–
ATPase	+	+	–
Peroxidase	+	–	–
Birbeck granule	–	+	–

The cellular elements of the immune system reside in the blood, bone marrow, thymus, lymph nodes, and in specialized areas of other tissues. The gut-associated lymphoid tissue, the mammary-associated lymphoid tissue, and the conjunctival-associated lymphoid tissue are examples of these specialized areas. The cells also exist at any site of immunologic activity. The cells may change form under stimulating conditions. For example, a macrophage exposed to a stimulus that typically produces a delayed hypersensitivity reaction may transform into an epithelioid cell or may fuse with other macrophages to form a giant cell.

IMMUNOREGULATION

The major components of the immune system have just been described. The immune system is considerably more complex than this, however, and involves other cell types and proteins. The cellular cooperation that occurs in an immune response (Figure 3-14) is a complex symphony, the primary conductor of which is the genetic material on chromosome 6 in the region known as the *major histocompatibility complex* (Figure 3-15). These genes have different names in different species. In the mouse, the major histocompatibility complex is called the *H-2 com-*

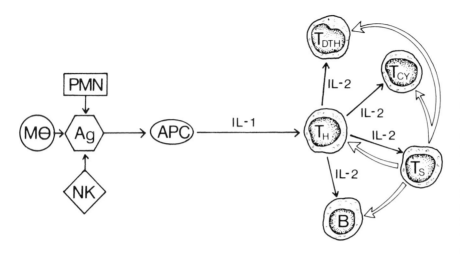

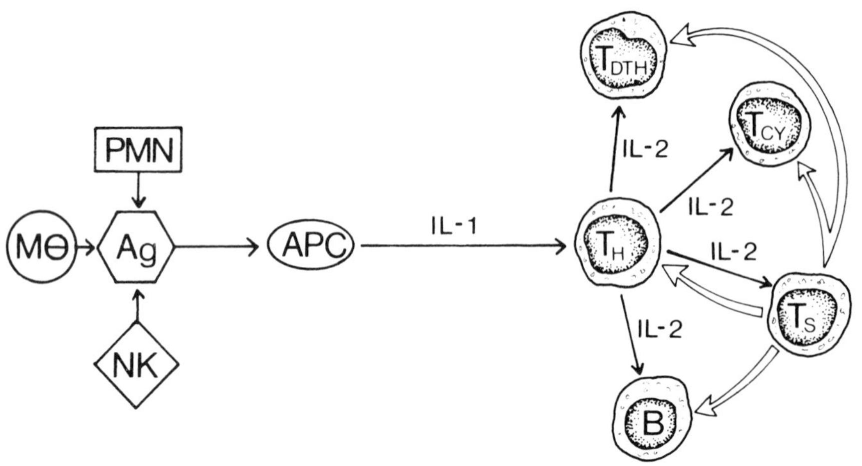

FIGURE 3-14 Cellular cooperation. Small amounts of antigen (*Ag*) may be eliminated quickly through the "natural" immune system, represented here by polymorphonuclear leukocytes (*PMN*), macrophages (*Mθ*), and natural killer cells (*NK*). Antigen not eliminated quickly by this system is "processed" by an antigen-presenting cell (*APC*) with presentation to other immunocompetent cells in the central processing station of the organism. The elaboration of interleukin-1 (*IL-1*) results in helper T-cell (T_H) proliferation and secretion of interleukin-2 (*IL-2*), which then activates all the other subsets of immunocompetent lymphocytes, suppressor T cells (T_S), and cytotoxic T cells (T_{cy}). T_{DTH}, T cells that mediate delayed-type hypersensitivity; *B*, B cell.

plex and is located on chromosome 17. In humans, the major histocompatibility complex is called the *HLA antigen (human leukocyte antigen) system.* The products of the major histocompatibility complex are important in the differentiation between self and nonself. In addition, it is possible that products of these genes may help exogenous factors cause disease more readily.

In humans, the HLA antigens are glycoproteins with a molecular weight of 44,000. There is a smaller polypeptide moiety (molecular weight 15,000), which is a β_2-microglobulin, associated with the larger molecule. These antigens are components of the cell membrane of nucleated cells (Figure 3-16), secured by hydrophobic forces but capable of moving (capping) along the membrane.

To date, 161 distinct HLA antigens have been identified and accepted by international authorities: 27 HLA-A, 59 HLA-B, 10 HLA-C, 26 HLA-D, 24 HLA-DR, 9 HLA-DQ, and 6 HLA-DP.[9] HLA antigens are divided into two major classes. Class I includes HLA-A, HLA-B, and HLA-C antigens. Class II includes HLA-D, HLA-DR, HLA-DQ, and HLA-DP antigens. HLA antigen distribution varies among racial groups. Certain HLA antigen combinations seem to appear in some groups of individuals more frequently than would be expected from chance. This phenomenon is termed *linkage disequilibrium.* HLA-A1 and HLA-B8 are in linkage disequilibrium in the white population. A1 has a frequency of 0.19 and B8 a frequency of 0.16 in this population. The expected frequency of their appearing as a combination in the same individual is 0.03 (0.19 × 0.16), but the actual frequency is 0.128.

Various HLA antigens have been associated with a variety of diseases, including ocular diseases (Table 3-10). HLA-B27 has been associated with anterior uveitis in whites. Other HLA antigens of ocular interest are the association of HLA-B8 in anterior uveitis in black Americans, HLA-B5 in Behçet's disease, HLA-B7 in the pre-

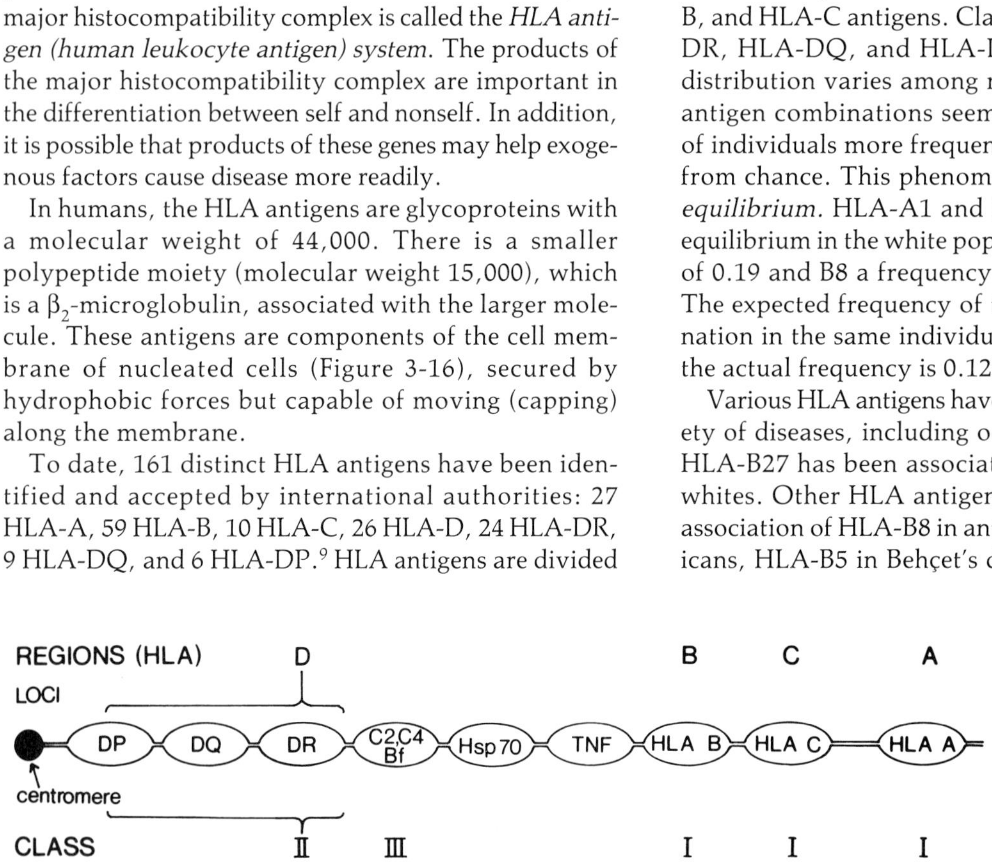

FIGURE 3-15 Major histocompatibility complex. The genes responsible for encoding for the synthesis of human leukocyte (*HLA*) antigen glycoproteins are present on chromosome 6. Class I antigens are encoded by loci *A*, *B*, and *C*; class II antigens, or *D* antigens, by loci *DP*, *DQ*, and *DR*.

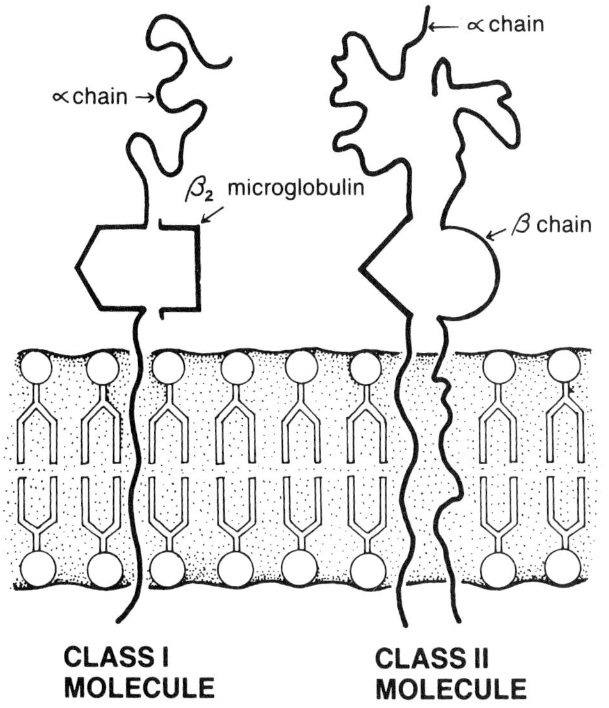

FIGURE 3-16 Diagrammatic representation of class I and class II HLA antigens expressed on the surface membrane of a cell.

sumed ocular histoplasmosis syndrome, HLA-A29 in birdshot retinochoroidopathy, and HLA-DQW7 in ocular cicatricial pemphigoid.

Lymphocytes can regulate the immune response in a variety of ways. One of the most important ways is by secretion of proteins (lymphokines). Lymphokines are nonimmunoglobulin proteins. At least 60 have been described. They exert effects on a variety of cells, host and foreign, leukocytic and nonleukocytic. For example, separate chemotactic factors for neutrophils, eosinophils,

TABLE 3-10
Association Between HLA Type and Ocular Disease

Ocular Disease	*HLA Antigen*
Uveitis	
Whites	B27
Japanese	No association
Juvenile onset	No association
Bilateral: black Americans	B8
Behçet's disease: Japanese, French, Turks, Swiss	B5
Presumed ocular histoplasmosis	B7
Birdshot retinochoroidopathy	A29
Ocular cicatricial pemphigoid	DQW7

basophils, macrophages, and lymphocytes may be produced. Other lymphokines that retain these cells in an area of immunologic interest (e.g., macrophage inhibiting factor and leukocytic inhibiting factor) are also secreted. Still other lymphokines may activate a particular cell type with respect to its function (e.g., macrophage activating factor) or with respect to proliferation (e.g., lymphocyte mitogenic factor). Table 3-11 lists many of the currently known lymphokines and other cytokines and some of their target cells.

The adult human immune system can be rather simply described as a system of approximately 10^{20} antibody molecules and 10^{12} lymphocytes that react to antigenic determinants (or epitopes) and, by so doing, protect the organism from infectious and other harmful agents. Attempts to describe the immune system more precisely become complicated very quickly. Since the studies by Pasteur and by Metchnikoff in the late 1800s, many observations of immune responses have been made, and many theories have been postulated in an attempt to explain these observations.

One theory that explains observed immunologic phenomena and correctly predicts current findings is the immunologic network theory of Jerne.[10] The following principles and observations are important to the development and understanding of Jerne's network theory.

An antibody molecule produced in response to an epitope possesses unique amino acid sequences in its hypervariable region that are responsible for specifically reacting with that epitope. This region is the antibody combining site, or paratope.

The paratope can itself act as an epitope. That is, the organism's own immune system can recognize this region in its own antibody molecule and respond by lymphocyte proliferation and by antibody production. The epitope-like region of an antibody molecule is termed an *idiotope,* and the antibody produced against it is termed an *anti-idiotypic antibody*. Jerne[10] suggested that idiotypes form the central basis of a complex immunologic network.

The essence of the immune system is the regulation of lymphocyte responses. Lymphocyte-mediated immunity can be modulated by anti-idiotypic antibodies, anti-idiotypic suppressor T cells, anti-allotypic antibodies, and anti-allotypic suppressor T cells. The predictions of Jerne's hypothesis have largely been validated experimentally. The antibody response to an antigen may be accompanied by anti-idiotypic antibody production. Both idiotype-bearing and anti-idiotype-bearing lymphocytes are activated during an immune response to an antigen. T and/or B cells of the appropriate idiotype may suppress the production of idiotypic antibody.

TABLE 3-11
Cytokines and Their Target Cells

Cytokine	*Secreted by*	*Cells Affected*
IL-1	Macrophages, fibroblasts, natural killer cells, neutrophils, B cells	Helper T cells, natural killer cells, neutrophils, basophils, LC, B cells
IL-2	Helper T cells, cytotoxic/suppressor T cells	Helper T cells, delayed-type hypersensitivity T cells, cytotoxic/suppressor T cells, macrophages, B cells, natural killer cells
IL-3	Mast cells, helper T cells	Mast cells, basophils, B cells, helper T cells
IL-4	Helper T cells (T_H, T_{H2})	Macrophages, natural killer cells, mast cells, B cells, helper T cells
IL-5	Helper T cells	Eosinophils, B cells, helper T cells
IL-6	Macrophages, fibroblasts, helper T cells, mast cells	B cells, helper T cells
	Fibroblasts, adherent bone marrow cells	Pre-B cells, thymocytes, neutrophils
IL-7	Fibroblasts, helper T cells	Helper T cells, fibroblasts, B cells
IL-8	Fibroblasts	Helper T cells
IL-9	Helper T cells	Mast cells, helper T cells
IL-10	Helper T cells (T_{H2}), cytotoxic/suppressor T cells	T cells
IL-11	B cells	B cells
TGF-β	Macrophages	Macrophages
IFN-α	Macrophages	Helper T cells
IFN-β	Fibroblasts	Helper T cells, fibroblasts
IFN-γ	Natural killer cells, helper T cells	Macrophages, natural killer cells
TNF-α	Macrophages	Helper T cells
TNF-β	Cytotoxic/suppressor T cells	Helper T cells
GM-CSF	Macrophages, mast cells, null cells, helper T cells	Stem cells, helper T cells

Abbreviations: IL, interleukin; TGF, transforming growth factor; IFN, interferon; TNF, tumor necrosis factor; GM-CSF, granulocyte macrophage-colony stimulating factor; LC, Langerhans cell.

Herzenberg and Black[11] described another type of immunoregulatory lymphocyte network based on allotypy. Allotypes represent allelic forms of immunoglobulin molecules, analogous, for example, to blood types. All the immunoglobulins in a given individual are the same allotype. Allotypes occur mainly in the constant region of the antibody molecule and are unrelated to the antibody combining site.

There are allotype-specific helper T cells that help B cells bearing a specific allotype. There are suppressor T cells that specifically suppress these allotype-specific helper T cells and thereby indirectly suppress the allotype-specific B cells.

This network of lymphocytes is organized, then, around allotypes and is independent of antigen specificity. Because of its lack of antigen specificity, it could be expected to interact with many lymphocyte sets functionally limited in an idiotype network.

There may also be lymphocyte networks based on immunoglobulin class (e.g., helper T cells and suppressor T cells specific for IgE B cells), and there may also be lymphocyte networks organized around determinants of the major histocompatibility complex.

COMPLEMENT CASCADE

The classic complement system, comprising separate components designated C1 to C9, was first described as the complementary factors in serum necessary to participate with specific antibody for lysis of cells. An alternative entry pathway into the cascade of reactions of the complement components was subsequently discovered, and the factors in this alternative pathway (properdin convertase, properdin, factor D, and factor B) were eventually defined (Figure 3-17). Although cell lysis is the classic result of complement participating in immunologic reactions, it appears to be of little consequence in ocular diseases. Much more important is the action of the split products from the complement cascade: C3a, C5a, and C6,7a. These products are chemoattractive for neutrophils and macrophages, and the action of these cells, when they are attracted to sites of complement activity in the eye, produces the devastating consequences of this component of the inflammatory response. Additional consequences may also result from the interaction of the complement system with the clotting and the kinin systems (Figure 3-18).

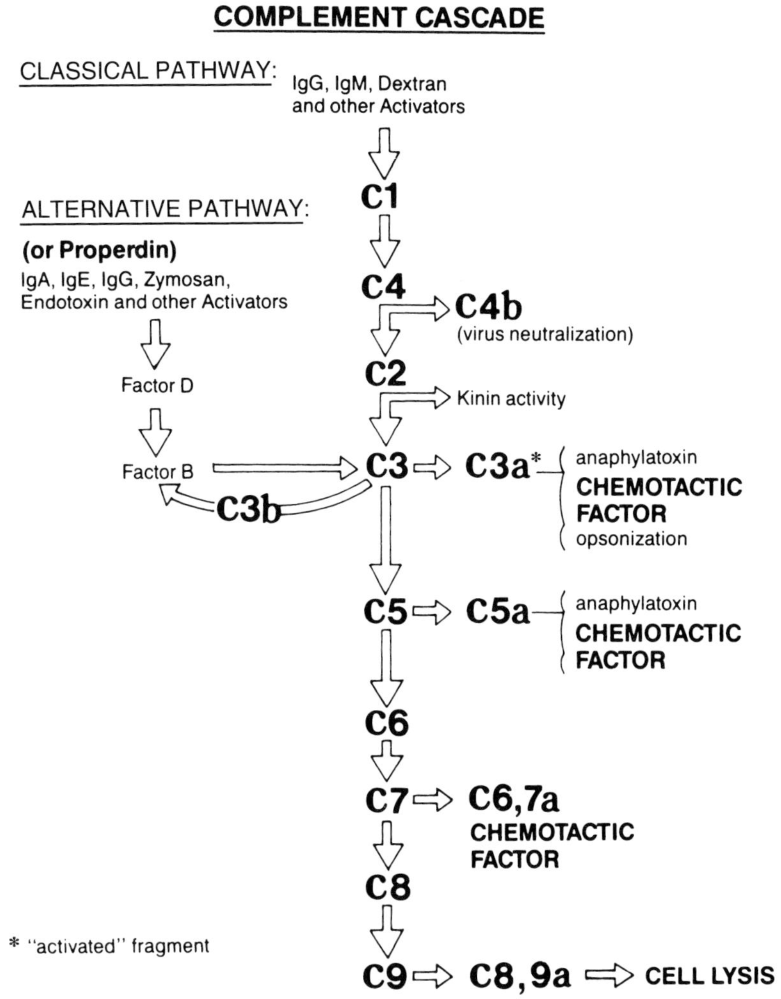

FIGURE 3-17 Schematic representation of the complement cascade. Regardless of the stimulus that results in activation of either the classic or the alternative pathway, the central pivotal point is the third component of complement (C3), with subsequent activation of the remaining five components. Note also that the C3a and C5a split products of the cascade, as well as C6,7a, are highly chemotactic and can have a variety of effects on production of inflammatory phenomena above and beyond the cell lysis action of the final complement C8,9a component.

Complement components C6 and C3b can participate in activation of the clotting system, and Hageman factor activation activates plasminogen, which leads to plasmin formation. This can have two significant effects on ocular inflammation: plasmin can activate collagenase, and it can, through the kallikrein-kinin system, enhance C1 activity, ultimately resulting in further recruitment of inflammatory cells through the actions of C3a and C5a.

Another action of C3a and C5a plays a less well-known role in ocular inflammation. These complement fragments possess anaphylatoxin activity (i.e., they cause degranulation of mast cells). It is important to recognize that mast cells intimately participate in inflammatory reactions other than classic allergic (type I) reactions, without participation of IgE. The products of inflammation that are liberated from degranulating mast cells include histamine, heparin, serotonin, prostaglandins, platelet-activating factor, and leukotrienes (LT), including LTB (a family of chemotactic factors, among which are eosinophil chemotactic factor and chemotactic factors for macrophages and for neutrophils), LTC (slow-reacting substance of anaphylaxis), LTD, and LTE (a potent mediator of increased vascular permeability) (Figure 3-19).

The importance of understanding the relationships of the various cell types of inflammation and their mediators to each other and to the cells and structures of the eye cannot be overemphasized. For example, who could have imagined 25 years ago that some drugs that lower intracellular cyclic AMP, such as echothiophate iodide and practolol, might play a role in the development of chronic conjunctival inflammation with resultant subepithelial fibrosis and, as a consequence, chronic pseudopemphigoid? Or who could have suspected that a mast cell stabilizing agent, cromolyn sodium, could play a beneficial corticosteroid-sparing role in some patients with vernal keratoconjunctivitis? It is clear that one who thinks

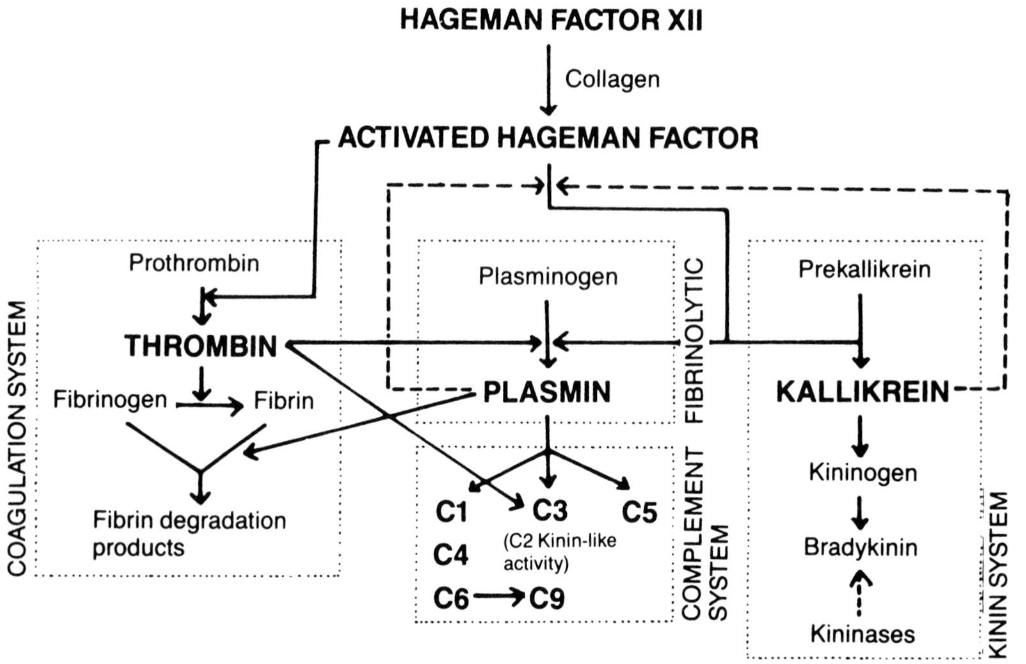

FIGURE 3-18 Schematic representation of interaction between the complement, clotting, and kinin inflammatory systems.

of mechanisms and who studies an inflammatory disease carefully will be better prepared to develop a thoughtful therapeutic strategy than one who simply reaches for the corticosteroid eye drops.

PATHOLOGIC IMMUNE MECHANISMS

The immune response of an organism to an antigen may be either helpful or harmful. If the immune response is excessive or inappropriate, tissue damage to the host may occur. Gell et al[12] described four types of hypersensitivity reactions, all of which can occur in the eye (Table 3-12). The necessary constituents for these reactions are already present or can be readily recruited into ocular tissues. Immunoglobulins, complement components, inflammatory cells, and inflammatory mediators can, under certain circumstances, be found in ocular fluids (tears, aqueous humor, and vitreous) and in the ocular tissues, adnexa, and orbit. Unfortunately, these tissues, especially the ocular tissues, can be rapidly damaged by inflammatory reactions, with irreversible alterations in structure and function. For this reason, a prompt and thorough work-up of ocular inflammation and rapid

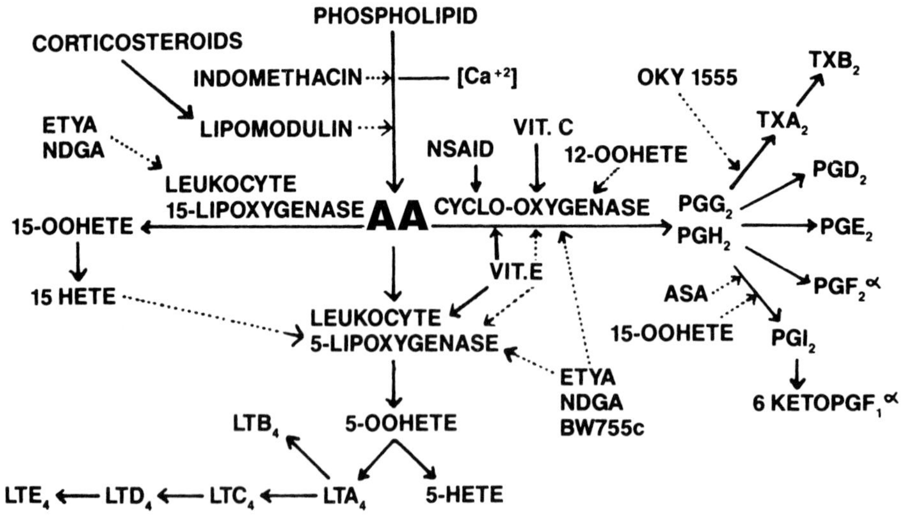

FIGURE 3-19 Flow diagram of arachidonic acid metabolism. Arachidonic acid is generated through two major enzymatic degradative pathways: the 15-lipoxygenase and cyclooxygenase pathways. The predominant product of the cyclooxygenase pathway is the prostaglandin family, and the predominant product of the lipoxygenase pathway is the leukotriene family of inflammatory mediators.

TABLE 3-12
Ocular Diseases According to Type of Hypersensitivity Reaction

Type of Hypersensitivity	*Possible Ocular Disease*
Type I	Hay fever conjunctivitis
	Acute allergic conjunctivitis
	Chronic allergic conjunctivitis
	Atopic keratoconjunctivitis
	Vernal keratoconjunctivitis
	Giant papillary conjunctivitis
Type II	Cicatricial pemphigoid
	Pemphigus vulgaris
	Dermatitis herpetiformis
Type III	Stevens-Johnson syndrome
	Erythema nodosum
	Sjögren's syndrome
	Reiter syndrome
	Ocular lesions associated with connective tissue diseases
	Ocular lesions associated with vasculitis
Type IV	Contact dermatitis/conjunctivitis
	Phlyctenulosis
	Vernal keratoconjunctivitis
	Giant papillary conjunctivitis
	Herpes simplex virus disciform keratitis
	Corneal graft rejection

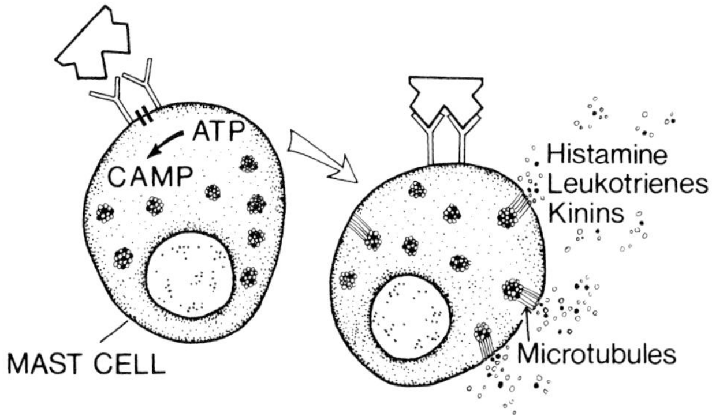

FIGURE 3-20 Type I hypersensitivity reaction. Antigen-binding IgE affixed to the mast cell membrane results in increased cyclic AMP. Tubulin subunits aggregate into microtubules, with degranulation of vasoactive amines as the end result.

treatment are necessary in patients with ocular inflammatory diseases.

Type I Hypersensitivity (Immediate Hypersensitivity)

Antigens commonly associated with type I reactions include dust, pollens, danders, microbes, and drugs. The antibodies responsible for type I reactions are homocytotropic antibodies, which are primarily IgE but may include IgG_4 as well. The mediators of type I reactions include histamine, serotonin, leukotrienes (including slow-reacting substance of anaphylaxis), kinins, and other vasoactive amines. Examples of type I reactions include anaphylactic reactions to insect bites or to penicillin injections, allergic asthma, hay fever, and hay fever conjunctivitis. Some hypersensitivity reactions have a type I reaction as one of several components. Examples of these more complex clinical entities include eczema, atopic blepharokeratoconjunctivitis, and vernal keratoconjunctivitis.

A type I reaction involves the binding of antigen to two adjacent IgE molecules that are already attached to the cell membrane of either a mast cell or a basophil (Figure 3-20). The simultaneous binding of antigen to two adjacent IgE molecules results in a change in the cell membrane, which results in a change in the level of activity of adenylate cyclase. Conversion of ATP to cyclic AMP is increased, and the intracellular level of cyclic AMP increases. Cyclic AMP then activates cytoplasmic cyclic AMP-dependent protein kinase, which presumably acts to phosphorylate cell proteins. This leads to the aggregation of tubulin into microtubules, which then participate in the degranulation of vasoactive amines.[13] It is interesting that pharmacologic agents that elevate cyclic AMP (e.g., β-adrenergic receptor agonists, prostaglandins of the E_1 class, and the phosphodiesterase inhibitors caffeine, theobromine, and theophylline) inhibit mast cell degranulation. This apparent paradox appears to result from the fact that nonspecific cyclic AMP may have an inhibitory effect on degranulation by leaving the cell depleted of cyclic AMP-dependent protein kinases at a critical time in response to immunologic challenge or by phosphorylation of an inhibitory protein. Carefully performed experiments indicate that a monophasic rise in cyclic AMP is essential to the degranulation process, and as in other systems, this elevation in cyclic AMP is responsible for the activation of two protein kinase isoenzymes. Winslow and Austen[13] have emphasized that although other apparently essential biochemical steps, such as uncovering a serine esterase, methylation of membrane phospholipid, and increased calcium influx, are noted, the earliest signal for the cascade of events that ultimately results in degranulation is the IgE-Fc receptor-initiated, transmembrane-coupled activation of adenylate cyclase and the subsequent cytoplasmic cyclic AMP-dependent activation of type I and II protein kinases.

The classic diagnosis of type I reactions required the passive transfer of the reaction, in a method known as the Prausnitz-Kustner reaction. Intradermal injection of the patient's serum into a volunteer was followed by injection of the presumed offending antigen at the same site. A positive Prausnitz-Kustner reaction occurred when local flare and wheal formation followed the antigen injection. This method for proving type I reactions is not used today. Circumstantial evidence for making the diagnosis of a type I reaction includes a typical history, the symptom of itching, the development of elevated IgE levels in serum or other body fluids, and eosinophilia.

Therapy for type I reactions includes avoidance of the offending antigen, inhibition of mediator release, inhibition of mediator action, generalized suppression of inflammation, and desensitization. Avoidance of the offending antigen is frequently not practical. However, an often neglected yet important component of the therapeutic plan for a patient with a type I reaction is an environmental control program. A careful environmental history and meticulous attention to environmental details can make the difference between relative stability and progressive inflammatory attacks that ultimately produce blindness (e.g., severe atopic blepharokeratoconjunctivitis). Elimination of pets, carpeting, feather pillows, and quilts and installation of air-conditioning and air-filtering systems are therapeutic strategies that should not be overlooked.

Until recently, at least for ocular type I reactions, methods for inhibiting histamine mediator release were not available. Theoretically, any substance that elevates cyclic AMP levels in mast cells or basophils, or that interferes with microtubule function (and hence with degranulation), should be effective in controlling type I reactions. Some substances affecting these systems are epinephrine, theophylline, and isoproterenol. One of the more effective of the drugs that affect the cyclic AMP system is cromolyn sodium (Crolom). This drug is useful in the treatment of allergic asthma in patients with high serum IgE levels. Topical administration of a 4-percent solution was also found to be safe and effective in the treatment of vernal keratoconjunctivitis.[14] Lodoxamide 0.1 percent eye drops (Alomide) and nedocromil sodium (Tilovist) are significant second-generation mast cell stabilizing agents that have recently become available for treatment of allergic eye disease. Lodoxamide has been approved for ocular use in the United States for the treatment of vernal keratoconjunctivitis, and nedocromil sodium has been approved in several European countries for ocular allergy. Both medications represent advances in efficacy and convenience, because twice-a-day dosing is often sufficient to accomplish the desired clinical effect. Lodoxamide may have stabilizing effects on eosinophils as well as mast cells, and both drugs appear to have a beneficial effect on the level of pro-inflammatory cytokines present in ocular tissues under treatment. No comparisons between the two agents have yet been performed.

Mediator action is inhibited by H_1 antihistamines. Their efficacy in the treatment of ocular hay fever and vernal keratoconjunctivitis is marginal at best, but when one is planning a multipronged approach to type I reactions, antihistamines should be part of the program. Systemic antihistamines are more effective in controlling type I ocular disease than are topical antihistamines. Recently, topical 0.1 percent olopatadine (Patanol), which is both an inhibitor of histamine release and a relatively selective H_1-receptor antagonist, has become available in the United States.

Corticosteroids are commonly used for the treatment of type I ocular reactions. They have direct effects on all inflammatory cells, including eosinophils, mast cells, and basophils. Corticosteroids are extremely effective, but the risks of chronic topical corticosteroids must be weighed against their benefits.

Desensitization immunotherapy can provide an important additional component to the therapeutic plan for a patient with type I hypersensitivity. Proper desensitization immunotherapy is difficult to perform. If done correctly, however, it can be helpful (Figure 3-21). Patients with vernal keratoconjunctivitis who are sensitive to house dust mite antigen have benefited from this approach. Immunotherapy with this antigen stimulates the production of IgG-blocking antibody and may result in the generation of specific suppressor T cells and reduction in sensitivity to the antigen.

Type II Hypersensitivity

Type II reactions require the participation of complement-fixing antibodies (IgG_1, IgG_3, or IgM) and complement. Antigens that stimulate such a reaction include exogenous antigens, such as microbes, or endogenous antigens. The mediators for tissue damage in type II reactions include complement, as well as macrophages and other leukocytes that liberate their enzymes. The mechanism of tissue damage involves antibody binding to the cell membrane and complement fixation to the bound antibody with resultant cell membrane lysis (Figure 3-22) and/or facilitation of phagocytosis. Additionally, macrophages are called to the site of disease activity, and because they have receptors for complement and for the Fc portion of the antibody, they participate efficiently in the phagocytosis of the involved cell. Killer cells may cause direct damage to the

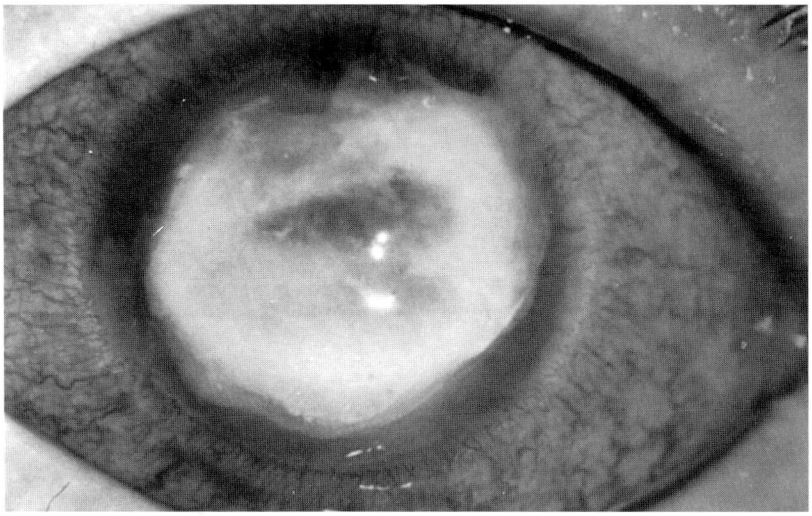
A

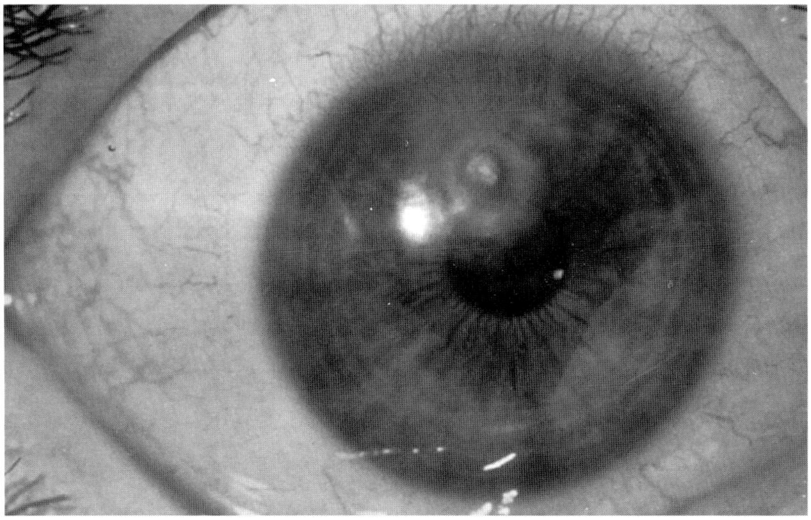
B

FIGURE 3-21 **(A)** Atopic blepharokeratoconjunctivitis with corneal ulceration. **(B)** Same eye. With appropriate systemic and topical therapy, the atopic blepharokeratoconjunctivitis resolved and visual acuity improved from hand motions to 20/80.

involved cell through antibody-dependent cell-mediated cytotoxicity.

The definitive diagnosis of type II reactions requires the demonstration of fixed antitissue antibodies at the disease site (Figure 3-23), as well as demonstration in vitro of killer cell activity against the tissue. No ocular disease has been definitively proved to represent a type II reaction, but several candidates, including ocular cicatricial pemphigoid, exist.

Therapy for type II reactions is extremely difficult. Immunosuppressive therapy has, in general, been the mainstay in treating diseases caused by type II reactions. Experience with cicatricial pemphigoid has been especially gratifying in this regard. Bilateral cases of severe activity, progressing to end-stage disease, have been brought under control with various chemotherapeutic agents[15] (Figure 3-24).

Type III Hypersensitivity (Immune Complex Diseases)

Type III reactions, or immune complex diseases, require participation of complement-fixing antibodies (IgG_1, IgG_3, or IgM), as in type II reactions. The antigens participating in such reactions may be soluble diffusible antigens, microbes, drugs, or endogenous antigens. Mediators of tissue damage include antigen-antibody-complement complexes, macrophages, and neutrophils (Figure 3-25).

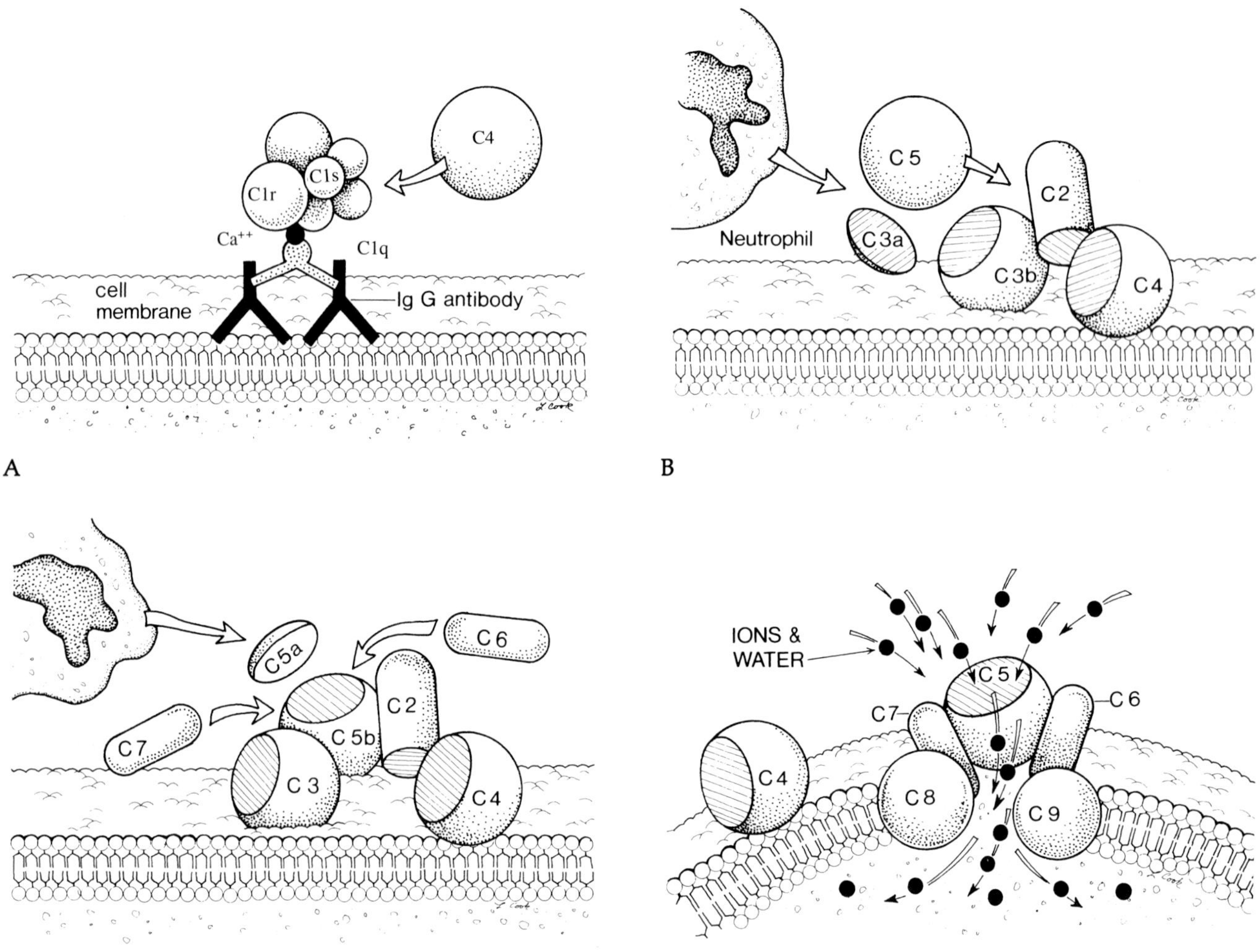

FIGURE 3-22 Type II reaction. **(A)** Cell membrane affixes complement-fixing antibody. In this case, IgG affixes the C1q component of complement, with subsequent fixation of C1r and C1s. C4 is then added to this complex. **(B)** The cascade continues, with incorporation of C2, C3, and C5 into the complex and the liberation of C3a, which is chemotactic for neutrophils. **(C)** The C6 and C7 components are added, and another chemotactic factor, C5a, is liberated. **(D)** The classic end result of the addition of the components C8 and C9 into the complex is the formation of a hole in the cell membrane with subsequent influx of ions and water and resultant osmotic lysis of the cell.

The injection of antigen into the skin of a previously sensitized host with circulating antibodies results in an edematous, hemorrhagic, and eventually necrotic lesion. This reaction, known as the active Arthus reaction, is considered to be one of the classic lesions obtained as a result of the deposition of immune complexes in the skin. A direct passive Arthus reaction can be demonstrated if antibody is injected intravenously in a normal recipient, followed by injection of the antigen intradermally. Initially, there is an accumulation of neutrophils within the capillary and venule walls. Immunofluorescence techniques show the deposition of antigen, antibody, and complement within the blood vessel walls. It appears that neutrophils, and later other cells, are responsible for the tissue damage. The classic condition ascribed to type III hypersensitivity is serum sickness (immune complex disease). After the injection of a foreign protein, vascular, cardiac, joint, cutaneous, and renal lesions can occur. Evidence suggests that immune complexes are the cause of this disease. The peak disease period begins just after immune complexes are formed and ends as they disappear.

The definitive diagnosis of type III reactions requires demonstration of antigen-antibody-complement complexes

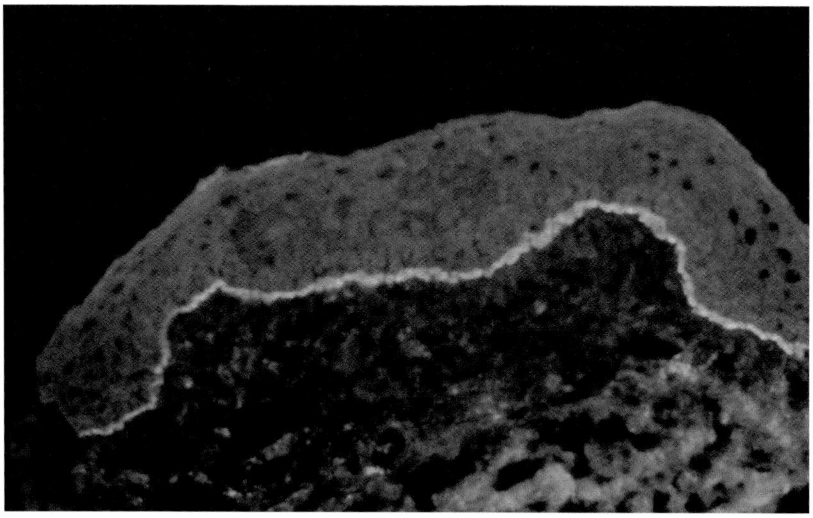

FIGURE 3-23 Immunofluorescence microscopy of human conjunctiva. The patient had suspected ocular cicatricial pemphigoid. The conjunctival biopsy specimen was processed for fluorescence microscopy and incubated with an antiserum against human IgA. Note the continuous, linear, bright staining of the epithelial basement membrane zone.

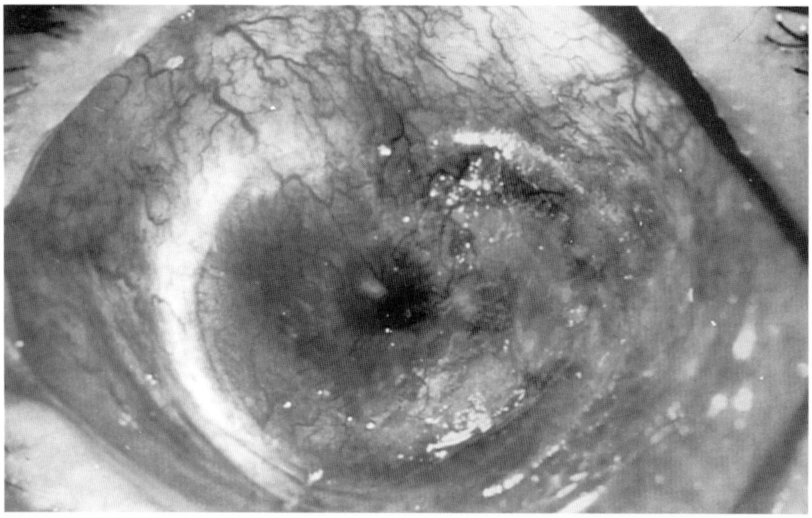

A

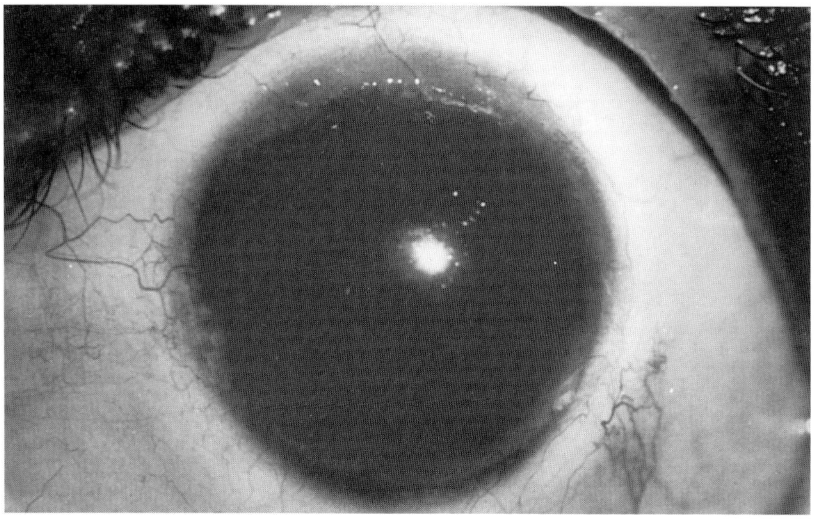

B

FIGURE 3-24 **(A)** Ocular cicatricial pemphigoid with advanced keratopathy, corneal scarring, and corneal neovascularization. The patient was on topical corticosteroid therapy but had no cytotoxic immunosuppressive treatment. **(B)** The disease process has been controlled with systemic cyclophosphamide and prednisone. No topical ocular therapy was used except for topical lubricants. Visual acuity improved from counting fingers at 4 ft to 20/70.

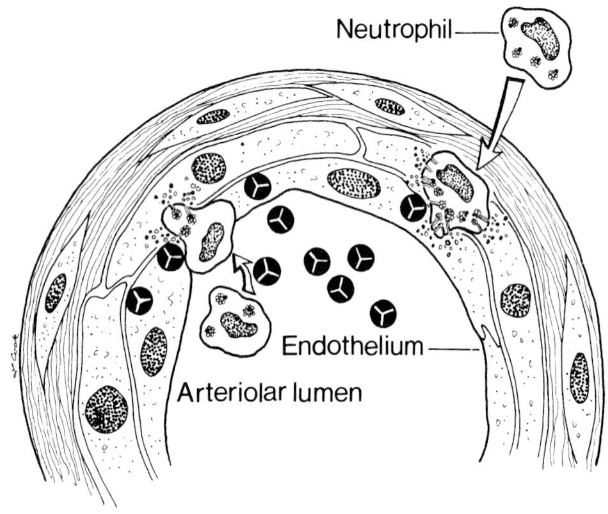

FIGURE 3-25 Type III reaction. In this diagram, circulating immune complexes comprising antigen, antibody, and complement are present in an arteriolar lumen. They easily traverse the endothelial lining but become entrapped at the level of the endothelial basement membrane. The immune complexes are highly chemotactic for phagocytic cells; attempted phagocytosis of these lodged complexes by such cells results in the liberation of proteolytic, collagenolytic, and hydrolytic enzymes that produce fibrinoid necrosis of the vessel.

at the site of tissue injury (Figure 3-26) and possibly isolation of the offending antigen from the immune complexes. Circumstantial evidence for type III reactions is a reduced level of complement in body fluids.

Circulating immune complexes have been described in patients with intraocular inflammatory diseases, but the possible role of the complexes in ocular tissue damage is unclear. Many investigators have assumed that the obstructive retinal vasculitis characteristic of some diseases, such as Behçet's disease, is immune complex mediated.

Therapy for type III reactions consists predominantly of corticosteroids and/or immunosuppressive agents. The development of a treatment plan depends on correct diagnosis and analysis of the mechanism. These goals, in turn, depend on a detailed history, careful examination of the patient, appropriate laboratory studies, and immunopathologic analysis of affected tissue. Randomly selected immunosuppression for idiopathic ocular inflammatory diseases amounts to negligent patient care.[16] Thus, patients with retinal vasculitis of unknown cause that is responsive to high-dose prednisone should not be treated with other immunosuppressive agents when they become cushingoid from chronic prednisone therapy unless a specific diagnosis of a disease typically responsive to immunosuppressive agents can be established or a significant body of evidence of extraocular immune complex involvement can be amassed.

When properly used, cytotoxic immunosuppression can be both sight saving and life saving, as in cases of Wegener's granulomatosis (Figure 3-27), rheumatoid arthritis with peripheral ulcerative keratitis or necrotizing scleritis (Figure 3-28), and polyarteritis nodosa[17] (Fig-

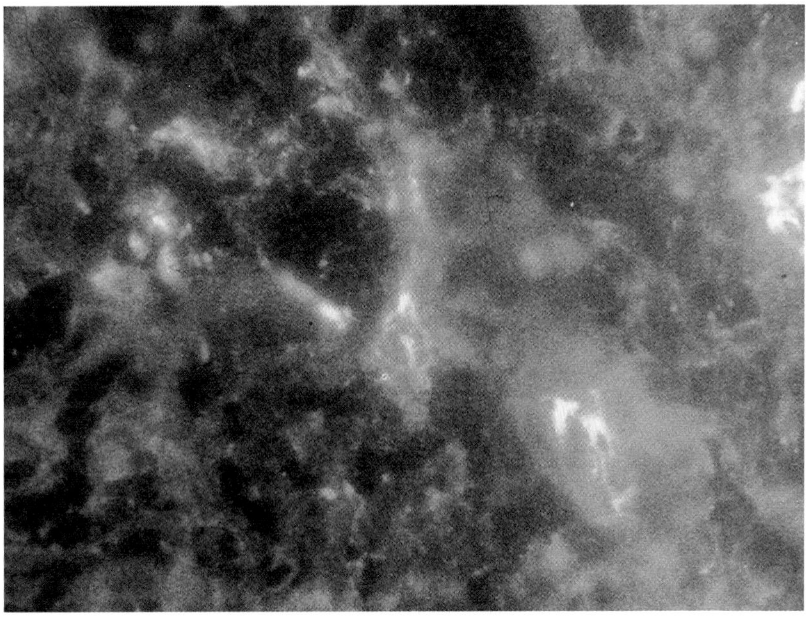

FIGURE 3-26 Immunofluorescence microscopy of a conjunctival biopsy specimen demonstrating vasculitis, with immunoreactant deposition in vascular walls. The immunoreactant detected in this specimen was IgG.

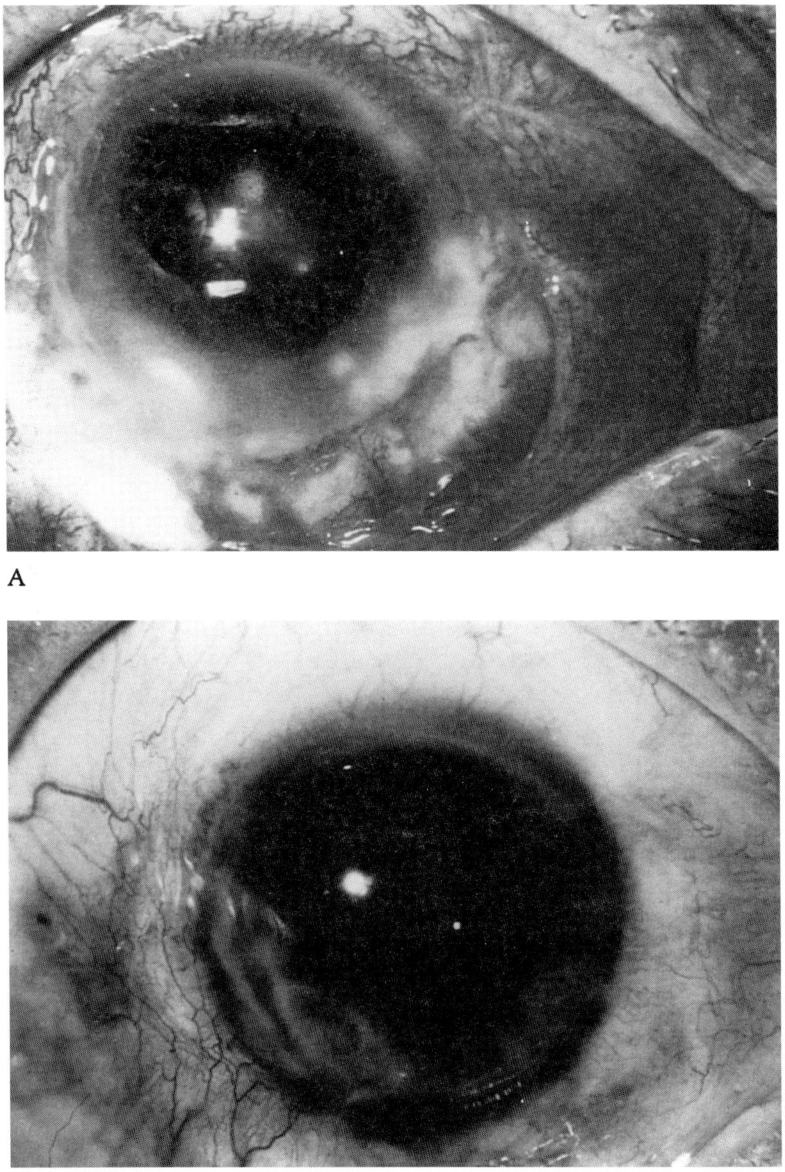

A

B

FIGURE 3-27 **(A)** Peripheral ulcerative keratitis and necrotizing scleritis, unresponsive to topical and systemic corticosteroids, multiple keratectomies, conjunctival resections, and the use of cyanoacrylate tissue adhesive. Ultimately, the diagnosis of Wegener's granulomatosis was made. The patient was treated for 1 year with systemic cyclophosphamide, after which therapy was discontinued. **(B)** The involved eye 2 years after cessation of treatment. Visual acuity was 20/20, and there was no evidence of recurrent ocular inflammatory disease.

ure 3-29). Cytotoxic immunosuppression may or may not be necessary to save both the sight and the life of a patient with Behçet's disease.[18] Making the correct diagnosis and analyzing the severity and the mechanism may allow one to treat successfully with less toxic drugs, such as colchicine. Progressive, bilateral Mooren's ulcer, although not lethal, shares immunopathologic features of many classic type III diseases and has a well-documented history, in its bilateral form, of unresponsiveness to all therapy except systemic immunosuppression.[19]

Type IV Hypersensitivity (Delayed Hypersensitivity)

Type IV reactions are reactions to specific antigens mediated by cells and not by antibodies. The antigens may be microbes, transplant antigens, or endogenous antigens. The central cell in these reactions is the T cell. The rate-limiting step in type IV reactions is the time needed for the development of antigen-specific responder T cells. The development of T-cell memory depends on antigen

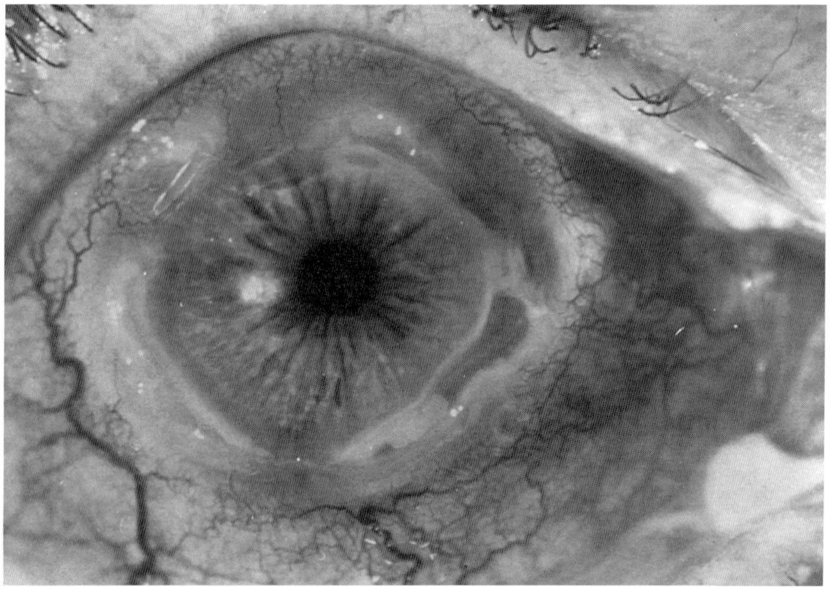

A

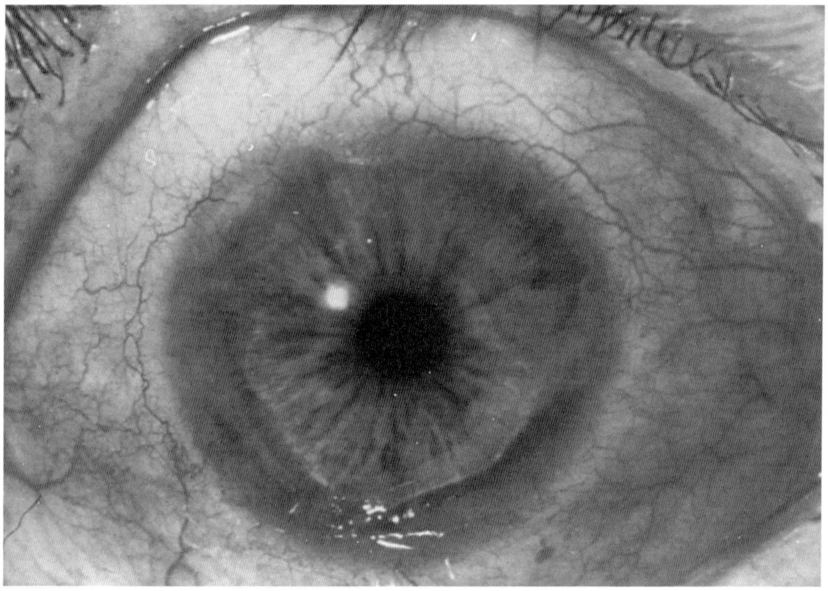

B

FIGURE 3-28 **(A)** Peripheral ulcerative keratitis. The peripheral corneal ulceration recurred multiple times after local conjunctival excisions, ulcer debridement, cyanoacrylate tissue adhesive, and soft contact lens therapy. The patient had rheumatoid arthritis and was subsequently shown to have vasculitis. **(B)** Control of the underlying vasculitis and the progressively destructive ocular inflammatory disease was achieved with systemic cyclophosphamide therapy.

presentation from macrophages. Once this cell-mediated immune memory has been established, the sensitized T cells, in response to renewed contact with the specific sensitizing antigen, can produce a variety of effects, including direct cytotoxicity against cells bearing the offending antigen and elaboration of lymphokines, which then have various secondary effects (Figure 3-30). Lymphokines may be involved in direct cytotoxicity of cells with which they come into contact, generalized inflammatory processes, recruitment and activation of macrophages that then participate in cell destruction and phagocytosis, and recruitment of other inflammatory cells, including natural killer cells and other T cells. Type IV hypersensitivity can be transferred to a naive host by transfer of T cells or by transfer factor, a lymphokine produced by T cells that is capable of transferring the same information as the cells carry. The demonstration of a type IV reaction requires more elaborate techniques than that of a type II or III reaction. One way is to show the presence of delayed skin responses to specific anti-

FIGURE 3-29 **(A)** Diffuse intense scleritis. Aggressive systemic work-up disclosed underlying polyarteritis nodosa. **(B)** Initial therapy with prednisone was tapered because of subsequent development of steroid myopathy. Central nervous system involvement with polyarteritis nodosa occurred, and successful control of both the ocular and systemic manifestations of this disease was achieved with systemic cyclophosphamide therapy.

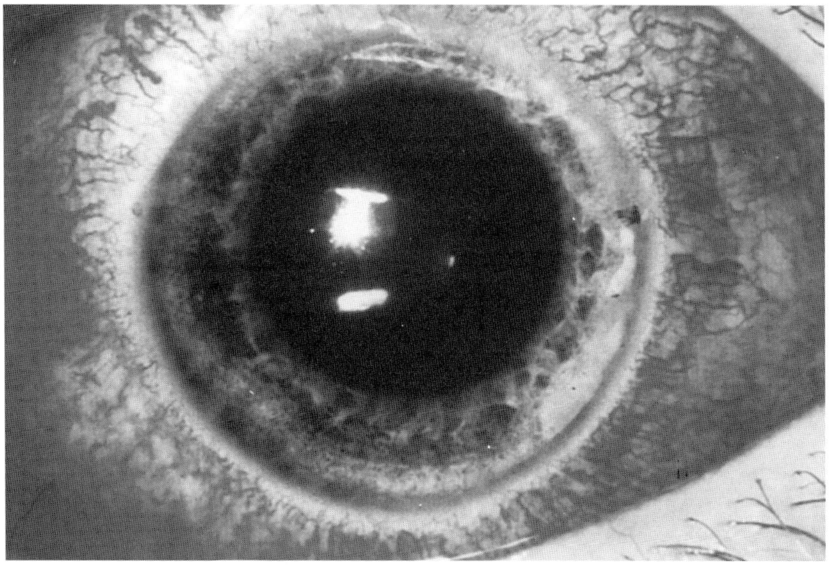

A

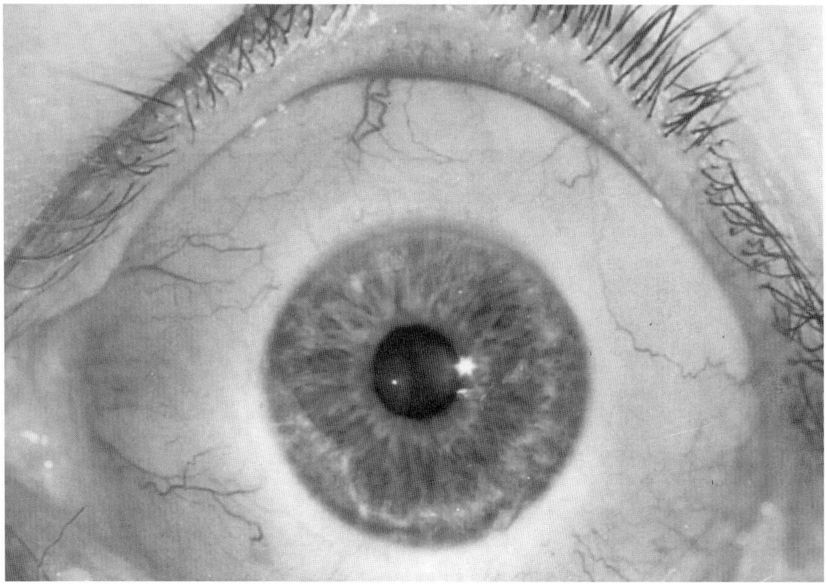

B

gens. These skin responses appear 24 to 48 hours after intradermal injection of an antigen to which the recipient has been previously sensitized. The basic histologic finding is an infiltration of mononuclear cells, predominantly lymphocytes. One way to demonstrate a type IV reaction in vitro is to measure the proliferative (blastogenic) responses of lymphocytes when cultured in the presence of sensitizing antigens. This is considered the in vitro equivalent of the in vivo anamnestic response. Another in vitro method involves demonstration of the ability of previously sensitized lymphocytes to kill other cells bearing the immunizing antigens. Therapy for type IV reactions may involve corticosteroids or immunosuppressive agents.

IMMUNOLOGIC TOLERANCE

Immunologic tolerance is the specific inhibition of immune responses to an antigen after previous exposure to that antigen. Antigens that can act as tolerogens (i.e., antigens to which an animal can be tolerized) may be

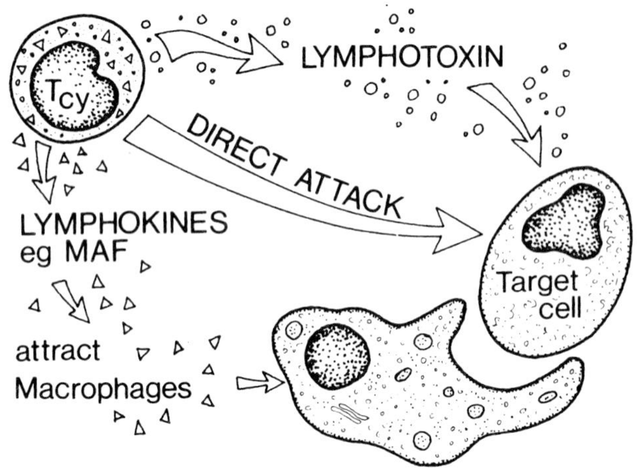

FIGURE 3-30 Type IV reaction. A sensitized cytotoxic T cell (T_{cy}) may have an effect on the specific target cell through one of three routes: direct attack on the target cell; liberation of a lymphokine known as lymphotoxin, which produces a direct effect on the cell; liberation of other lymphokines, such as macrophage activating factor (*MAF*), which may recruit other cells that secondarily attack and destroy the target cell.

soluble or particulate. The concept of immunologic tolerance is the key to a major characteristic of acquired immunity: the ability to discriminate between self and nonself. The normal immune system tolerates its own antigens through active immunologic mechanisms. Escape from this state of self-tolerance results in autoimmune disease.

Many factors influence the development of immunologic tolerance. Host factors (genetic constitution, immunologic maturity, state of immunocompetence), the nature of the antigen, the dose of the antigen, the dose schedule of the antigen, and the route of antigen presentation all influence the development of either tolerance or an immune response.

Immunologic tolerance may result from two main mechanisms: central unresponsiveness caused by lymphocyte clonal deletion, and peripheral unresponsiveness produced by regulatory mechanisms involving suppressor T cells and/or antibodies. In central unresponsiveness, a clone of immunocompetent cells specific for reactions relevant to the antigen-inducing tolerance (tolerogen) is either irreversibly inhibited or destroyed. This form of immunologic unresponsiveness is inducible most easily in the immature organism and involves predominantly B cells. Clonal inactivation or deletion is especially easy to produce when the developing B cell expresses only IgM surface-membrane receptors. As the B-cell system matures and IgD surface receptors begin to appear, induction of central unresponsiveness becomes difficult. Experimental maneuvers resulting in elimination of the surface IgD receptors on mature lymphocytes (e.g., through the use of antiserum specific for IgD) again render the organism tolerizable through central unresponsiveness or clonal deletion.

Antibody-mediated unresponsiveness may occur through a continuous consumption mechanism whereby a never-ending supply of specific antibody continually reacts with antigen, with subsequent harmless elimination of the immune complexes formed. Similar effects may occur through antibody competition with lymphocyte receptors for any available antigen. Blocking factors or enhancing antibodies may result in immunologic tolerance through interaction with antigenic determinants in such a way that these determinants are masked and hence unavailable for subsequent reactions with the immune system. Blocking factors may also interact with host lymphocyte-surface receptors, thereby inducing inactivation of the relevant clones of lymphocytes for a particular antigen.

Autoantibodies in the form of anti-idiotypic antibodies play a critical role in immunoregulation and, therefore, in immunologic tolerance. Antibodies may effectively delete a clone of relevant lymphocytes through antibody-dependent cell-mediated cytotoxicity or through surface-antigen binding and lymphocyte inactivation.

Finally, suppression of various aspects of the immune system can occur through suppressor T cells and soluble factors from suppressor cells. Active suppression of helper T cells and/or B cells is a source of immunoregulation and of immunologic tolerance.

Autoimmunity develops when an organism escapes from the normal state of tolerance to its own tissue antigens to the abnormal state of responding to self as nonself. Specific defects in immunoregulation have been characterized in a variety of autoimmune diseases, including suppressor T-cell defects in systemic lupus erythematosus and in atopy. The possibilities are complex, and the details of specific immune defects in various diseases are discovered only with enormous difficulty.

The issue of immunologic tolerance is especially provocative with regard to the eye. Scientists have long been fascinated by the special immunologic privilege of the cornea and anterior chamber. In the 1940s, Medawar[20] hypothesized that tolerance of foreign antigens in these sites is the result of avascularity and hence the inability of the central processing stations of the immune system to "see" the foreign antigens. This notion of afferent arc blockade persisted for nearly 30 years. We now know, however, that foreign antigens placed in these sites are recognized quickly, with rapid development of systemic immune responses. Antigen encounter in these ocular sites results in the rapid elaboration of suppressor T cells that actively mediate tolerance to the stimulatory antigen. This suppressor T-cell–induced tolerance is antigen specific and is adoptively transferable.[21-23] This phenomenon—constant low-dose antigen presentation via an aqueous-vascular route, resulting in suppressor T-cell modulation of the immune response—may explain the high degree of tolerance for corneal transplants.

IMMUNOMODULATION

Two ocular diseases, hay fever conjunctivitis and phacoantigenic uveitis, satisfy all the Koch-type postulates for proving that they are immune disorders: (1) the relevant antigens have been identified; (2) the abnormal immune responses to those antigens have been defined; (3) the diseases have been produced in experimental models; and (4) passive transfer of the disease models has been accomplished. The understanding of the immunopathogenesis of hay fever conjunctivitis has enabled scientists to design therapeutic strategies that are more specific than the traditional approach of generalized suppression of inflammation with corticosteroids. Application of the Koch-type postulates to the study of other ocular diseases has just begun. Circumstantial evidence strongly suggests that a defect in immunoregulation plays a role in several ocular diseases (Table 3-13).

Until recently, a discussion such as this would have dealt, in a rather simplistic way, with immunosuppression. New knowledge of immunoregulation renders such an approach inappropriate. Our current understanding of immunoregulation is summarized in Figure 3-14. It is clear that a deficient immune response, to *Candida* for example, may occur because of (1) defective B-cell function; (2) excessive suppressor T-cell and/or B-cell activity; (3) defective suppressor T-cell function (causing production of autoantibodies that may attack B cells, helper T cells, neutrophils, macrophages, and natural killer cells); and/or (4) defective activity of one or more components of the natural immune system, such as monocytes, macrophages, other antigen-presenting cells, neutrophils, or natural killer cells.

TABLE 3-13
Ocular Diseases in which a Defect in Immunoregulation Plays a Role

Recurrent herpes simplex keratitis
Mooren's corneal ulcer
Keratoconjunctivitis sicca
Vernal keratoconjunctivitis
Idiopathic uveitis
Sympathetic ophthalmia
Ocular tumors (retinoblastoma, malignant melanoma)
Optic neuritis
Vogt-Koyanagi-Harada syndrome
Behçet's disease
Cicatricial pemphigoid
Stevens-Johnson syndrome
Reiter syndrome
Atopic keratoconjunctivitis
Ocular lesions in association with
Connective tissue diseases
Vasculitic diseases, including Wegener's granulomatosis
Sarcoidosis
Inflammatory bowel disease
Multiple sclerosis
Acquired immunodeficiency syndrome

Drugs that are immunosuppressive under some circumstances can be immunostimulatory under others. For example, suppression of excessive suppressor T-cell function will eliminate inappropriate suppression; the clinical result is enhanced immune function, or immunostimulation. Similarly, immunostimulation produced by desensitization immunotherapy with antigen extract can result in enhanced suppressor T-cell activity. Clinically, the result appears to be decreased immunoreactivity to the relevant antigen (i.e., immunosuppression).

Immunopotentiation

True stimulation of immune activity (as opposed to reduction of suppressor function or inhibitory phenomena) may be accomplished through specific or nonspecific means. Specific immunostimulation, either active (by means of a specific vaccine) or passive (by transfer of specific immune cells or serum), has found little use to date in ophthalmology. For example, treatment of localized herpes zoster ophthalmicus with hyperimmune herpes zoster globulin has not been more efficacious than treatment with systemic and topical corticosteroids and acyclovir.

Nonspecific enhancement of immune function may be accomplished by a variety of agents. Immunization with bacillus Calmette-Guerin (BCG), *Bordetella pertussis,* or *Corynebacterium parvum* causes a generalized increase in activity of the immune system. Macrophage activity, T- and B-cell function, and natural killer cell activity may all be enhanced by these agents under certain conditions. Such agents have been used in cancer immunotherapy, both systemically and by injection into tumors after systemic sensitization to the agent.

Levamisole, thymosin, thymopoietin (TP 5), and facteur thymique serique (FTS) are examples of reagents that act more specifically on selected populations of immune cells. Levamisole appears to stimulate mature lymphocytes and monocytes. It has been used with some success in Behçet's disease and rheumatoid arthritis, but its efficacy in patients with recurrent herpes simplex keratitis has been disappointing. In many respects, levamisole mimics thymopoietin, although the latter also triggers differentiation of immature precursor cells, particularly of T cells.

Thymopoietin enhances tumor rejection by promoting generation of cytotoxic T cells. It also corrects some of the cell-mediated immune defects in patients with systemic lupus erythematosus by shifting the predominant T-cell population from immature autoreactive T cells to mature T cells with relatively normal suppressor functions. The result is clinical remission of disease. Facteur thymique serique has similar effects.

Interferon and interferon inducers have also been used as nonspecific immunostimulatory agents. Interferon enhances natural killer cell activity and directly inhibits cellular and viral replication. It has been used successfully in the treatment of cancer and recurrent viral papillomas.

Immunosuppression

Although the use of pharmacologic and biological agents to inhibit the immune response dates back at least half a century, we know little about their mechanisms of action. Frequently, we cannot even be certain that a particular agent is in fact suppressing the immune response rather than merely suppressing inflammation. By definition, immunosuppressive agents suppress the development of at least one type of immune response. Table 3-14 lists some common immunosuppressive agents.

TABLE 3-14
Immunosuppressive Agents

Class	*Generic Name*	*Brand Name*	*Manufacturer*
Purine analogues	6-Mercaptopurine	Purinethol	Glaxo Wellcome
	Azathioprine	Imuran	Glaxo Wellcome
	Thioguanine	Tabloid	Glaxo Wellcome
Alkylating agents	Cyclophosphamide	Cytoxan	Bristol-Myers Squibb Oncology
	Chlorambucil	Leukeran	Glaxo Wellcome
	Nitrogen mustard	Mustargen	Merck & Co.
Folic acid analogues	Methotrexate	Methotrexate	Lederle
Antibiotics	Mitomycin C	Mutamycin	Bristol-Myers Squibb Oncology
	Actinomycin		
	Doxorubicin	Adriamycin	Pharmacia & Upjohn
	Azaserine		
	Puromycin		
	Cyclosporine	Sandimmune	Novartis
Biological agents	Antilymphocyte serum		
	Antithymocyte antibodies		
	Antimacrophage serum		
	Phytohemagglutinin		
	L-Asparaginase		
	Ribonuclease		
	Monoclonal antibodies to lymphocyte subsets		
	Interferon-γ-1b	Actimmune	Genentech
	Lymphocyte immune globulin, antithymocyte globulin	Atgam	Upjohn
	Muromonab-CD3	Orthoclone OKT3	Ortho Biotech
Pyrimidine analogues	Cytosine arabinoside	Cytosar-U	Pharmacia & Upjohn
	Bromodeoxyuridine		
	5-Fluorouracil	Fluorouracil	Roche
		Efudex	Roche
		Fluoroplex	Allergan
Corticosteroids			
Ionizing radiation			
Miscellaneous	Vinblastine	Velban	Lilly
	Vincristine	Oncovin	Lilly
	Colchicine	ColBENEMID	Merck & Co.
		Colchicine	Lilly

A feature common to many of the agents listed in Table 3-14 is their ability to interfere with the synthesis of nucleic acids and proteins. This interference is commonly assumed to be the mechanism of immunosuppression; because lymphocytes stimulated by antigens proliferate, they are exquisitely sensitive to drugs that interfere with nucleic acid or protein synthesis. However, the effect of immunosuppressive agents cannot be explained solely by this mechanism.[24] Considering the complexity of the idiotypic-anti-idiotypic immunoregulatory network of T-cell subsets, B-cell subsets, and macrophage subsets, it seems that the pioneers in the study of immunosuppression were fortunate to discover dosages that produced enough differential effect on subsets of helper and cytotoxic cells to produce immunosuppression.

Purine Analogues

Purine analogues, such as 6-mercaptopurine and azathioprine, interfere with the synthesis of purines and, as a result, with DNA, RNA, and protein synthesis. These drugs must be converted, predominantly in the liver, to active metabolites, such as thioinosinic acid. They inhibit purine formation and purine nucleotide interconversion reactions, as well as the function of coenzymes (e.g., coenzyme A), thereby inhibiting DNA and RNA synthesis. These agents or their metabolites are incorporated into DNA and RNA, but that is probably not the locus of their suppressive effect.

At clinical, nontoxic doses, purine analogues have little effect on humoral immunity. Immunoglobulin levels and specific antibody responses are relatively unaffected. However, in experimental systems, high doses of purine analogues given within 48 hours of antigen priming can suppress the antibody response and, when given in conjunction with high doses of antigen, can induce temporary tolerance to the antigen.

Purine analogues appear to exert a relatively selective effect on T cells. They depress recirculating T cells that are in the process of homing, suppress development of monocyte precursor cells, inhibit participation of killer cells in antibody-mediated cytotoxicity reactions, suppress mixed lymphocyte reactions in vitro, and inhibit delayed hypersensitivity reactions. In renal transplant patients, for example, the suppression is only partial; these patients consistently show lymphocyte responsiveness (proliferation, lymphokine production, cytotoxicity, and cytotoxic antibody) to donor antigen in vitro.

Purine analogues, most notably azathioprine, are used extensively in graft recipients, and they prolong renal, skin, lung, and cardiac transplants. They have also been used in the treatment of pemphigus vulgaris, bullous pemphigoid, rheumatoid arthritis, and Crohn's disease.

Complications of therapy with azathioprine include hepatotoxicity, bone marrow suppression (with resultant anemia, leukopenia, thrombocytopenia, and secondary infection), anorexia, nausea, vomiting, gastrointestinal distress, diarrhea, rash, fever, and arthralgia.

Alkylating Agents

Cyclophosphamide, the most potent of the therapeutic alkylating agents, is used extensively for immunosuppression. All alkylating agents act through nucleophilic substitution reactions, and such reactions with DNA probably account for the immunosuppressive activity of these agents. Breaks occur in single-stranded DNA. When these breaks are repaired, phosphodiester bonds form and result in defective cell function. Cross-linking reactions occur between DNA strands, between DNA and RNA, and between these molecules and cell proteins, generally resulting in death of the affected cell.

Similarly to most other immunosuppressive agents, cyclophosphamide is not immunosuppressive in its native state. Phosphoramidase, present in high concentrations in liver microsomes, catalyzes the conversion of the drug to its active form.

At clinical doses, alkylating agents are cytotoxic for lymphocytes. The effect on B and T cells appears to be equal, except that high doses enhance the effect on B cells. Cyclophosphamide has a potent effect on B cells and antibody responses when given with, or even up to 4 days after, antigen encounter. It suppresses secondary antibody responses in previously sensitized patients. Cyclophosphamide is effective in inhibiting delayed-type hypersensitivity reactions and is as effective as azathioprine in the treatment of liver, cardiac, bone marrow, skin, and pulmonary graft rejections. It is the only immunosuppressive agent that can induce immunologic tolerance to particulate antigen. The pharmacokinetics and the kinetics of the development of such tolerance are complex. The drug must be given 24 to 48 hours after antigen priming. It is likely that the tolerance is mediated predominantly by suppressor T cells that develop after antigen priming. However, at least in the experimental murine model, low-dose cyclophosphamide therapy can eliminate suppressor T cells that actively mediate tolerance, resulting in a release from tolerance and the expression of immunoreactivity in the form of delayed hypersensitivity reaction to the antigen. The dose and route of administration of cyclophosphamide are critical to its effect on lymphocyte subsets, which makes the use of the drug in nonclinical settings difficult. Cyclophosphamide inhibits monocyte precursor development but has little effect on fully developed macrophages. It is used extensively in the treatment of Wegener's granulomatosis, rheumatoid arthritis, polyarteritis nodosa, bullous pemphigoid, and malignancies.

Complications of cyclophosphamide therapy include bone marrow suppression, anorexia, nausea, vomiting, hemorrhagic cystitis, gonadal suppression, alopecia, and interstitial pulmonary fibrosis.

Folic Acid Analogues

Methotrexate, a folic acid analogue, binds to dihydrofolate reductase and blocks the conversion of dihydrofolic acid to tetrahydrofolic acid. This interferes with thymidine synthesis and hence with DNA synthesis and cell division. Methotrexate has little effect on resting cells but has pronounced effects on rapidly proliferating cells. Methotrexate affects both B and T cells and can inhibit humoral and cellular responses. The drug is excreted unchanged in the urine. Folinic acid can reverse the metabolic block produced by methotrexate.

Methotrexate is used in the treatment of cancer and psoriasis. Complications include bone marrow suppression, cirrhosis, hepatic atrophy, ulcerative stomatitis, nausea, vomiting, diarrhea, interstitial pneumonitis, malaise, fatigue, secondary infection, rash, cystitis, nephritis, headache, blurred vision, drowsiness, and sterility.

Antibiotics

Cyclosporine is a fungal metabolite, originally isolated from cultures of *Trichoderma polysporum* by Sandoz Laboratories (now Novartis) as part of a screening program of fungal products with antifungal activity. This undecacyclic peptide is also produced by *Cyclindrocarpon lucindum.* Borel et al[25] found that this agent had potent immunosuppressive properties. Subsequent work in experimental models showed the drug to be immunosuppressive and capable of suppressing graft rejections.

The mechanism of action of cyclosporine is not completely understood, but the best available evidence suggests that the drug interferes with receptors on the surface membranes of certain T cells (particularly helper T cells) that recognize DR antigens (antigens present on the cells, most notably antigen-presenting cells, including macrophages). DR antigens participate in the production of interleukin-2 (IL-2) by helper cells by rendering IL-2-producing T cells sensitive to interleukin-1 (IL-1) (see Figure 3-14). Cyclosporine's interference with T-cell receptors for DR antigens results in a block of helper T-cell response to IL-1 and thus blocks IL-2 production and/or IL-2 release from helper T cells. Cyclosporine may also inhibit IL-1 release from antigen-presenting cells, such as macrophages.

The suppressive effect of cyclosporine on T cells is relatively selective and occurs early in the phase of T-cell subset interactions. The drug decreases antibody production to T-cell-dependent antigens, inhibits cytotoxic activity generated in mixed lymphocyte reaction, and prolongs skin, kidney, and heart allografts in experimental animals and humans. It may also prevent or mitigate graft-versus-host disease and may prolong the survival of other transplanted organs, such as pancreas and cornea.

Complications associated with cyclosporine include an apparent increase in the incidence of B-cell lymphomas, interstitial pneumonitis, opportunistic infections, particularly from herpes simplex virus, *Candida, Pneumocystis,* renal toxicity, and hypertension.

Biologic Agents

Heterologous antisera to leukocytes relevant to immune reactions have been used for immunosuppression experimentally since 1956 and clinically in humans for more than two decades. Antiserum prepared against human lymphocytes has been the most extensively studied and widely used agent. Various antilymphocyte serum (ALS) preparations have been used; the most potent are usually obtained after immunization of horses with human thymus or thoracic duct cells. The highest immunosuppressive activity usually appears in the IgG fraction of horse serum 2 to 4 weeks after immunization. Newer monoclonal antibody products specific for eliminating T cells from humans are more predictable and are currently used in some instances for treating patients with allograft rejection.

The effects of intravenous administration of such antisera include leukopenia (highly immunosuppressive preparations of antilymphocyte serum markedly reduce the number of T cells); depletion of thymus-dependent areas in the spleen and other lymphoid tissue; inhibition of delayed hypersensitivity reactions; prolonged survival of skin, renal, cardiac, liver, and lung grafts; and suppression of primary and secondary antibody responses if the antiserum is given before antigen priming. Antilymphocyte serum has been used in humans predominantly for organ transplantation in conjunction with corticosteroid and cytotoxic drug therapy (usually azathioprine). Its efficacy is well established. Its toxicity includes anaphylaxis, passive cutaneous anaphylaxis, and, possibly, lymphoproliferative tumor enhancement.

The issue of a causal relationship between the administration of immunosuppressive agents and the development of malignant disease has been controversial, particularly for patients with no malignant disease or major defect in immunosurveillance before immunosuppressive therapy. Patients should be informed, however, that such a relationship may exist and that if it does, the risk of developing a malignancy may be a function of the dose and duration of immunosuppressive therapy.

TABLE 3-15
Ocular Conditions Treatable by Immunosuppression

Idiopathic anterior uveitis
Idiopathic chronic cyclitis
Peripheral uveitis (pars planitis)
Sympathetic ophthalmia
Behçet's disease
Thyroid exophthalmos
Peripheral ulcerative keratitis associated with Wegener's granulomatosis
Peripheral ulcerative keratitis and scleritis associated with polyarteritis nodosa, rheumatoid arthritis, or systemic lupus erythematosus
Cicatricial pemphigoid
Mooren's corneal ulcer

Immunosuppressive Agents in Ophthalmology

Until recently, cytotoxic agents were used only rarely for nonlethal disorders. As experience has accumulated and dosage schedules have been refined, the applications have been extended to the treatment of diseases that appear to involve immunoregulatory abnormalities unresponsive to more conventional therapies. The use of cytotoxic agents for the treatment of ocular disease, however, is still uncommon. Some progressively destructive ocular conditions for which successful systemic immunosuppressive therapy has been reported are listed in Table 3-15.

Definitive evaluation of the therapeutic efficacy of cytotoxic agents in ocular diseases is complicated by two problems: (1) activity in the natural course of many of these diseases waxes and wanes and (2) the relative rarity of many of the diseases makes a properly designed, controlled, randomized, double-masked clinical trial impractical, even with multi-institutional collaboration. Current evaluation of these agents is based on inferential interpretation of uncontrolled, unmasked therapeutic trials. However, the evidence indicates that systemic cytotoxic therapy is an important alternative for patients with a progressively destructive ocular disease that appears to involve inappropriate immunoreactivity or defective immunoregulation, and that is unresponsive to other, more conventional therapies. Because all the cytotoxic drugs are potentially dangerous, this therapy should be managed by a physician with expertise in the use of these drugs.

The experience in the Immunology Service of the Massachusetts Eye and Ear Infirmary has confirmed the reports of others about the apparent efficacy of cyclophosphamide, chlorambucil, cyclosporine, azathioprine, and methotrexate in cases of intractable idiopathic uveitis. Patients are generally maintained on immunosuppressive doses of either cyclophosphamide (1 to 2 mg/kg) or azathioprine (1 to 3 mg/kg) in conjunction with daily prednisone (60 to 200 mg) until disease activity begins to subside. The daily dose of prednisone is then tapered and eventually switched to an alternate-day dose if disease activity continues to diminish. The dose of the cytotoxic agent is adjusted according to disease activity, bone marrow tolerance, and side effects. Depression of the white blood cell count to less than 3,500 cells/mm^3, the neutrophil count to less than 1,500 cells/mm^3, or platelets to less than 75,000/mm^3 should be avoided. Until the patient is on a stable, controlling, tolerable drug dose, complete blood and platelet counts are obtained every 2 weeks and every month thereafter. Urinalyses are performed monthly, with special concern for evidence of microscopic hematuria.

Idiopathic uveitis patients are maintained on cytotoxic therapy for at least 4 months after resolution of cellular inflammation in the eye. The therapy can often be tapered and finally discontinued without recrudescence of the uveitis.

Combined cytotoxic/prednisone therapy is effective for the uveitis and retinal vasculitis of Behçet's disease. Cyclophosphamide (or chlorambucil) and azathioprine are particularly useful. The addition of colchicine to the regimen significantly enhances the therapeutic response and decreases the ultimate cytotoxic drug dose required for disease control. However, these patients require long-term (many years) maintenance immunosuppressive therapy to prevent a recurrence of the disease.

The results of cytotoxic therapy for other forms of intractable uveitis, including chronic cyclitis, peripheral uveitis, and sympathetic ophthalmia, have been favorable. Patients with Vogt-Koyanagi-Harada syndrome appear to benefit from both azathioprine and cyclosporine.

The use of cytotoxic agents in the treatment of ocular lesions associated with connective tissue diseases is discussed in Chapter 23. Medical and surgical therapy for such ocular lesions is rarely permanently successful. Cytotoxic therapy in patients with destructive ocular lesions associated with rheumatoid arthritis, systemic lupus erythematosus, polyarteritis nodosa, and Wegener's granulomatosis is essential not only to halt the ocular destruction but also, frequently, to preserve the patient's life.[26]

In 1979, the first successful use of systemic immunosuppressive agents for therapy for progressive Mooren's ulcer was reported.[27] The efficacy of this approach has subsequently been confirmed in eight additional patients.[19] Although our understanding of the cause and immunopathology of Mooren's ulcer is incomplete, cytotoxic immunosuppression is a legitimate therapeutic alternative for patients with progressive Mooren's ulcer that is unresponsive to other therapies.

Many patients with cicatricial pemphigoid have slow but progressive conjunctival cicatrization that is unresponsive to any form of medical or surgical therapy and culminates in bilateral blindness. Although the disease may respond to systemic dapsone or to high-dose corticosteroids, the most consistently effective therapy is systemic cytotoxic immunosuppression. Both cyclophosphamide and azathioprine are effective.[15,28]

Future Directions

One of the newer immunomodulating therapeutic strategies on the horizon deserves mention. Over the past 15 years, hybridoma technology and lymphocyte immunobiology have been combined to develop a variety of highly specific monoclonal antibodies that react with individual cell-surface membrane moieties expressed on various subsets of lymphocytes. Preliminary reports suggest that such reagents may have important therapeutic potential. Thus, renal graft rejection may be reversed by intravenous therapy with monoclonal antibodies directed against all T cells. The potential for increased selectivity in therapy directed against T-cell subsets is even more exciting. Furthermore, cloning of autoreactive cells in vitro is now possible, so that the antigens or other factors controlling such cells can be identified and therapeutic strategies developed. It is even possible that clones could be modified in such a way that reintroduction into the patient would stimulate appropriate suppressor cells that would specifically inhibit the abnormal reactivity. These kinds of more selective immunomodulation will clearly offer major therapeutic advantages over our current approach of generalized immunosuppression.

REFERENCES

1. Voltaire: Lettres philosophiques. p. 25. In Paul WE (ed): Fundamental Immunology. Raven Press, New York, 1984
2. Jenner E: An Inquiry into the Causes and Effects of the Variolae Vaccine, a Disease, Discovered in Some Western Countries of England, Particularly Gloucestershire, and Known by the Name of Cowpox. Sampson Low, London, 1798
3. Koch R: Die Aetiologie der Tuberculose. Berl Klin Wochenschr 19:221, 1882
4. Pasteur L: Prevention of rabies. CR Acad Sci Paris 1885–86
5. Roitt IM: Essential Immunology. Blackwell Scientific Publications, Oxford, 1984
6. Allansmith MR: The Eye and Immunology. CV Mosby, St. Louis, 1982
7. Millstein C: From antibody structure to immunological diversification of immune responses. Science 231:1261, 1986
8. Cooper MD, Peterson RDA, South MA, Good RA: The functions of the thymus system and the bursa system in the chicken. J Exp Med 123:75, 1966
9. Bodmer JG, Marsh SGE, Albert ED, et al: Nomenclature for factors of the HLA system, 1991. Immunobiology 187:51, 1993
10. Jerne N: Towards a network theory of the immune system. Ann Inst Pasteur Immunol 125:373, 1974
11. Herzenberg LA, Black SJ: Regulatory circuits and antibody responses. Eur J Immunol 10:1, 1980
12. Gell PGH, Coombs RA, Lackmann P (eds): Clinical Aspects of Immunology. 3rd Ed., Sect. 4. Blackwell Scientific Publications, Oxford, 1974
13. Winslow CM, Austen KF: Enzymatic regulation of mast cell activation and secretion by adenylate cyclase and cyclic AMP-dependent protein kinases. Fed Proc 41:22, 1982
14. Foster CS, The Cromolyn Sodium Collaborative Study Group: Evaluation of topical cromolyn sodium in the treatment of vernal keratoconjunctivitis. Ophthalmology 95:194, 1988
15. Foster CS, Wilson LA, Ekins MB: Immunosuppressive therapy for progressive ocular cicatricial pemphigoid. Ophthalmology 89:340, 1982
16. Foster CS: Ocular manifestations of the non-rheumatic acquired collagen vascular diseases. p. 264. In Smolin G, Thoft RA (eds): The Cornea: Scientific Foundations and Clinical Practice. Little, Brown, Boston, 1983
17. Foster CS: Immunosuppressive therapy in external ocular inflammatory disease. Ophthalmology 87:140, 1980
18. Foster CS, Regan CJ: Retinal vascular diseases. II. Management. Int Ophthalmol Clin 26:55, 1985
19. Foster CS: Systemic immunosuppressive therapy for progressive bilateral Mooren's ulcer. Ophthalmology 92:1436, 1985
20. Medawar PB: Immunity to homologous grafted skin. III. The fate of skin homografts transplanted to the brain, to subcutaneous tissue, and to the anterior chamber of the eye. Br J Exp Pathol 29:58, 1948
21. Wetzig RP, Foster CS, Greene MI: Ocular immune response. I. Priming of A/J mice in the anterior chamber with azobenzinearsenate-derivatized cells induces second order-like suppressor T cells. J Immunol 128:1753, 1982
22. Foster CS, Wetzig RP: Immune reactions in the eye. Surv Immunol Res 1:93, 1982
23. Foster CS, Campbell R, Monroe J, et al: Ocular immune response. II. Priming of A/J mice in the vitreous induces either enhancement of or suppression of subsequent hapten-specific DHT responses. J Immunol 136:2787, 1986
24. Bach JF: The Mode of Action of Immunosuppressive Agents. Elsevier North Holland, Amsterdam, 1975
25. Borel JF, Feuer C, Magnee C, Stahelin H: Effects of the new anti-lymphocytic peptide Cyclosporin A in animals. Immunology 32:1017, 1977
26. Foster CS, Forstot SL, Wilson LA: Mortality rate in rheumatoid arthritis patients developing necrotizing scleritis or peripheral ulcerative keratitis. Effects of systemic immunosuppression. Ophthalmology 91:1253, 1984
27. Foster CS, Kenyon KR, Greiner J, et al: The immunopathology of Mooren's ulcer. Am J Ophthalmol 88:149, 1979
28. Foster CS: Cicatricial pemphigoid. Trans Am Ophthalmol Soc 84:527, 1986

II

Clinical Science

4

Meibomianitis

JAMES P. MCCULLEY AND WARD E. SHINE

Inflammation of the meibomian glands and other ocular structures, including the ciliary portion of the eyelid, conjunctiva, and cornea, as a result of meibomian gland dysfunction causes common abnormalities that can be perplexing for both the patient and the ophthalmologist. Little has been written to clarify these abnormalities, and that which has been written has often added to the confusion. Meibomianitis is often not recognized as being a distinct entity; all types of meibomianitis are frequently grouped under one diagnostic heading, and there is no standard nomenclature.

Meibomianitis can be localized, as in a posterior hordeolum, chalazion, and localized or spotty meibomianitis secondary to anterior (ciliary) blepharitis or conjunctivitis; generalized with little inflammation of the meibomian glands themselves but with marked symptoms and moderate conjunctival inflammation, as in meibomian seborrhea; or generalized with moderate to marked inflammation of the meibomian glands with significant conjunctival and corneal involvement, as in meibomian conjunctivitis or meibomian keratoconjunctivitis. Rarely, a suppurative process involves the meibomian glands. Each of these entities (Table 4-1) is discussed separately.

LOCALIZED MEIBOMIANITIS

Posterior (Internal) Hordeolum

A posterior hordeolum is an acute infection of a meibomian gland. It may be thought of as an acneiform lesion of the eyelid of an infectious nature; the most common offending agent is *Staphylococcus*.[1] A posterior hordeolum may occur in conjunction with acute or chronic blepharitis or in an eyelid that appears otherwise normal.

The onset is typically abrupt, with moderate pain. The entire eyelid may be edematous and erythematous. The hordeolum may be identified by palpation of a localized area of tenderness within the involved eyelid or, when more advanced, by the presence of a yellowish nodule seen through the tarsal conjunctival surface after the eyelid is everted (Figure 4-1). The hordeolum may have more localized inflammatory signs from the onset, in which case the diagnosis is less difficult. The eyelid margin surrounding the orifice of the involved meibomian gland is usually inflamed. Secretions within the orifice are either nonexpressible or purulent when expressed. There is rarely a palpable tender preauricular lymph node. Posterior hordeola may be single or multiple, and may involve one or all eyelids. Recurrences are not uncommon, especially if there is an associated, inadequately treated, chronic blepharitis or conjunctivitis. A posterior hordeolum rarely progresses to orbital cellulitis or has an associated cavernous sinus thrombosis.[2,3]

Treatment of a posterior hordeolum should include the search for and, if necessary, the management of underlying blepharitis or conjunctivitis. Hot compresses (two to four times a day, depending on severity), lid scrubs with mild shampoo, and appropriate local antibiotics should be included in all treatment regimens.

A hot compress may be prepared by holding a clean washcloth under hot water until it reaches a temperature that will effectively heat the eyelid without burning the skin. The cloth is applied to the affected eyelid for 5 to 10 minutes and is kept warm by reheating it under the hot water. Hot compresses dilate the surrounding blood vessels and heat the meibomian lipid secretions that are plugging the involved gland. Many components of these secretions have a melting point near body temperature[4] and solidify when the temperature drops below this level,

TABLE 4-1
Classification of Meibomianitis

Localized
Posterior (internal) hordeolum
Chalazion
Localized or spotty meibomianitis secondary to anterior (ciliary) blepharitis or conjunctivitis
Generalized
Meibomian seborrhea
Meibomianitis/meibomian conjunctivitis/meibomian keratoconjunctivitis
Suppurative meibomianitis

as occurs in a dilated meibomian acinus or duct. Heating liquefies the stagnant secretions and makes drainage through the meibomian orifice more likely.

Cellular and sebaceous debris often builds up along the anterior eyelid margin and eyelashes. Hot compresses raise the temperature above the melting point of the lipid component of the debris, making it easier to remove with lid scrubs. A mild shampoo, such as one of the baby shampoos, aids in removal of the debris and lowers the bacterial count on the eyelids. The same washcloth used for the hot compress can be used to apply the shampoo and to scrub the anterior eyelid and eyelashes. Prepackaged eyelid cleansers/scrubs are also available from a number of suppliers.

After the lid scrub, an appropriate antibiotic ointment should be rubbed onto the anterior eyelid along the lash line. The same antibiotic ointment or an antibiotic eye drop, which may be better tolerated, can be placed in the inferior fornix. Cultures with antibiotic sensitivity determination can be helpful in the selection of an antibiotic. However, such relatively elaborate diagnostic procedures are often impractical and, in the absence of such testing, selection can usually be based on typical sensitivity patterns of staphylococci isolated from eyelids. Both *S. aureus* and *S. epidermidis* are usually sensitive to bacitracin, erythromycin, chloramphenicol, and aminoglycosides, but are frequently resistant to sulfonamides and tetracycline.[5] Treatment should be continued until there is total resolution of the hordeolum.

With appropriate treatment, most posterior hordeola resolve without surgical intervention. A posterior hordeolum often ruptures spontaneously and drains through the conjunctival surface. Occasionally, it drains through the duct and orifice of the involved meibomian gland or through the skin surface. The infectious component may occasionally resolve, leaving a sterile nodule with minimal inflammation and the clinical and pathologic appearance of a chalazion. If a posterior hordeolum does not drain spontaneously, it can be incised and drained through the conjunctival surface. If it has progressed to a chalazion, incision and curettage may be necessary. However, if a posterior hordeolum resolves to the point of leaving only a small asymptomatic nodule, it may be left alone.

Chalazion

A chalazion is a localized, sterile, inflammatory process that involves individual meibomian glands (Figure

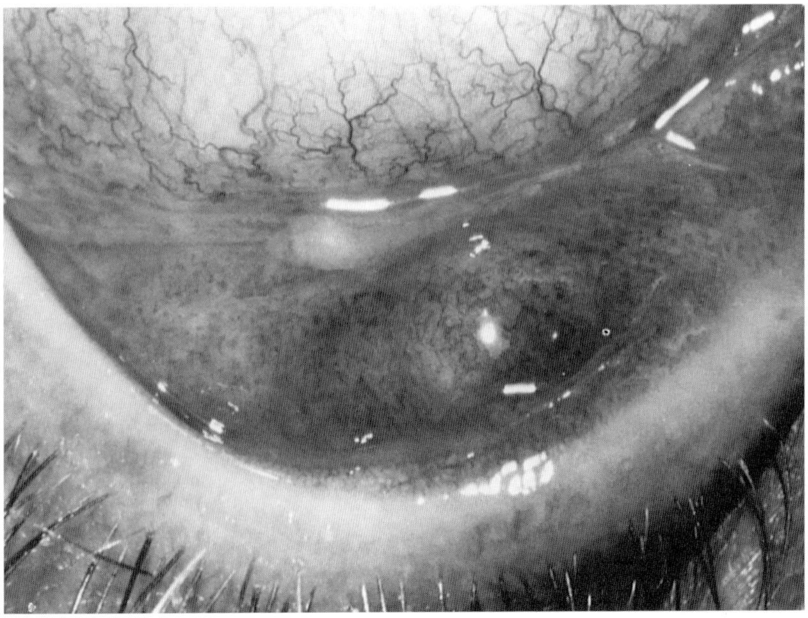

FIGURE 4-1 Posterior (internal) hordeolum pointing on the conjunctival surface with surrounding conjunctival inflammation.

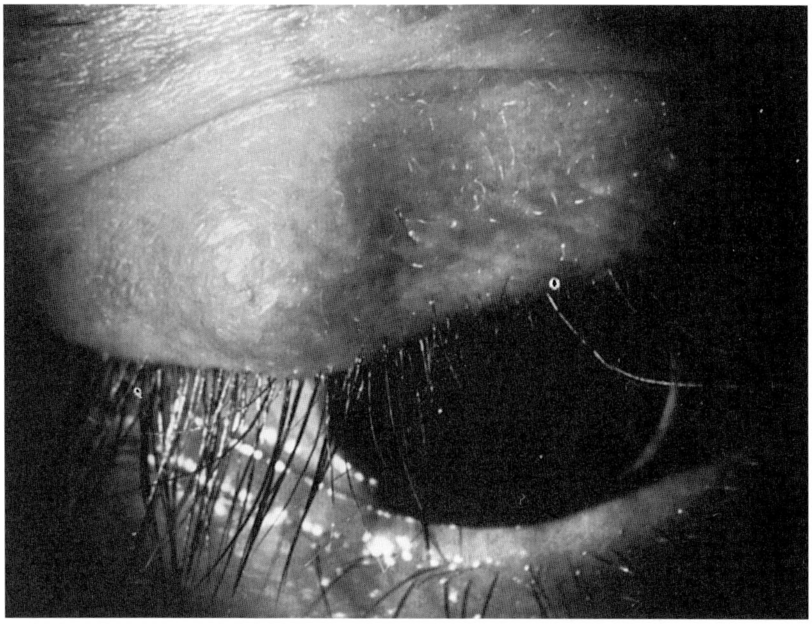

FIGURE 4-2 Anterior view of a chalazion. There is a visible bump in the eyelid and minimal associated inflammation.

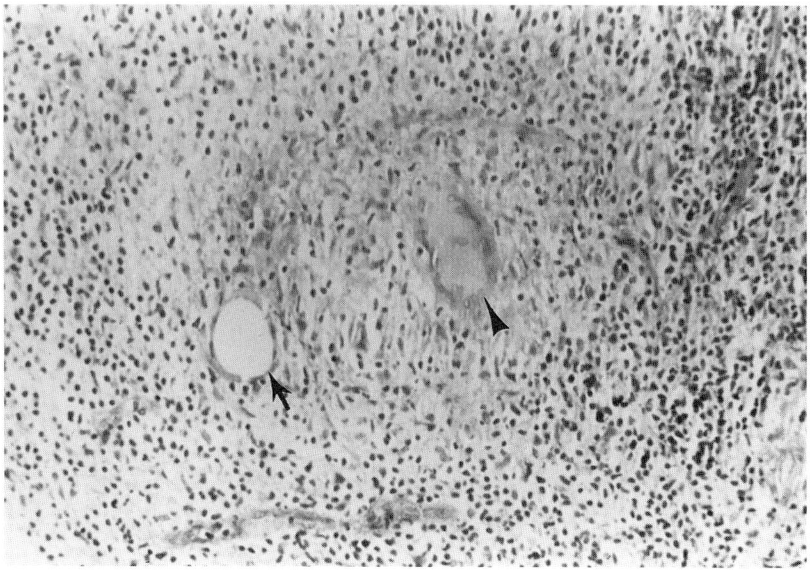

FIGURE 4-3 Histologic appearance of a chalazion. The vacuole (arrow) marks the site where fat from the meibomian glands was dissolved during processing. A multinucleated giant cell is indicated by the arrowhead.

4-2). It may occur as single or multiple lesions. Occasionally a chalazion develops from a posterior hordeolum, but more commonly it develops de novo. The cause is unknown, but the lesion itself appears to be a granulomatous reaction to retained meibomian secretions that extravasate into the surrounding tissue (Figure 4-3). Concomitant chronic blepharitis may be present, but the eyelids may be otherwise normal in appearance. The orifice of the involved meibomian gland usually has minimal surrounding inflammation. The secretions within the gland are stagnant and difficult or impossible to express. The underlying tarsal conjunctiva is initially edematous and congested, and may develop papillary hypertrophy. Recurrences are not uncommon, especially if there is a poorly controlled chronic blepharitis.

The onset and progression are usually slow and have few associated symptoms. There is little or no discomfort or surrounding inflammation of the eyelid. The most common complaint is cosmetic or, if the chalazion is in the upper eyelid, related to induced corneal astigmatism from pressure on the cornea.

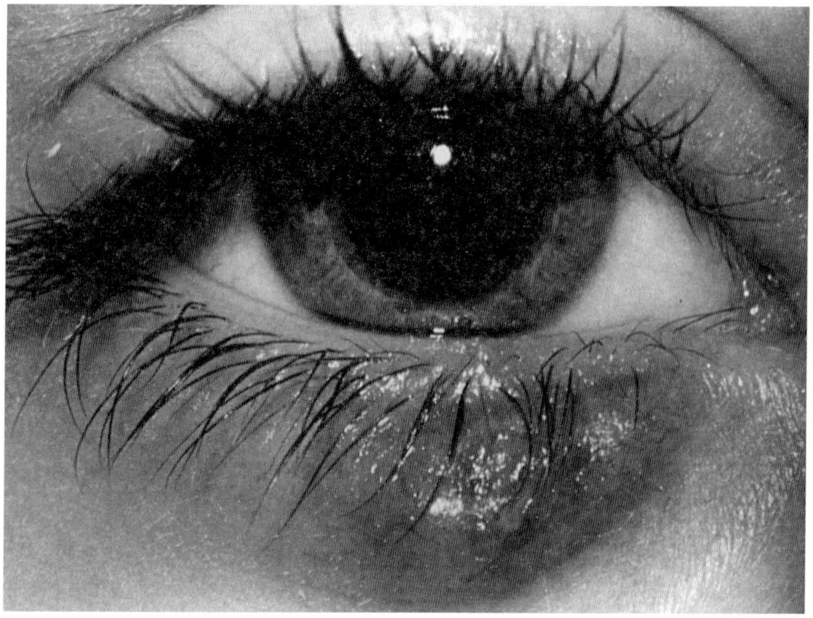

FIGURE 4-4 Extension of a chalazion anteriorly with spread in subcutaneous tissue stimulating an inflammatory response.

A chalazion usually increases in size and then stabilizes, shrinks a variable amount (even to the point of complete resolution), or spontaneously drains. Although drainage is more common through the conjunctival surface, it occasionally occurs through the duct or into the subcutaneous tissue anterior to the tarsus, resulting in the formation of a subcutaneous granuloma (Figure 4-4). If a chalazion forms in the duct of a meibomian gland or progresses toward the orifice along the duct, granulomatous tissue can extend above the eyelid margin. A chalazion may rarely have a suppurative course.

Initially, treatment should be similar to that for a posterior hordeolum, with attention to underlying blepharitis, if present. Local antibiotics are not necessary unless there is a concomitant infection. Hot compresses are applied two to four times a day. Immediately after the hot compress, the eyelid, especially the area involved by the chalazion, is massaged gently in an attempt to evacuate stagnant secretions to prevent further chalazion formation and to encourage drainage along the duct of the involved gland. Too vigorous massage of the chalazion, however, can cause further extravasation of meibomian secretions into the surrounding tissue, with resultant spread of the granulomatous inflammation. Lid scrubs are used to remove debris buildup along the anterior eyelid margin and eyelashes.

If the chalazion does not resolve, it may be left alone if it is not chronically inflamed and does not cause a cosmetic defect or induce astigmatism. If it continues to cause problems, it should be incised and curetted, usually from the conjunctival surface, but occasionally from the skin surface if it is pointing anteriorly. Granulomatous tissue that extends above the eyelid margin or under the conjunctiva may be shaved off.

If there is a tendency to develop recurrent chalazia and there is underlying blepharitis, the blepharitis should be controlled. If there is no underlying blepharitis, but a tendency to develop recurrent chalazia, hot compresses, eyelid massage, and lid scrubs once or twice a day will keep the meibomian secretions from stagnating and help to prevent recurrences.

Localized or Spotty Meibomianitis Secondary to Anterior Blepharitis or Conjunctivitis

Inflammation of the meibomian glands may result from spillover of anterior blepharitis or conjunctivitis. The resultant meibomianitis may be localized, spotty,[6,7] or generalized. All three forms of meibomianitis are discussed below under generalized meibomianitis, because the pathophysiology is similar whether the involvement is localized or generalized.

GENERALIZED MEIBOMIANITIS

Meibomian Seborrhea

Meibomian seborrhea is characterized by excessive meibomian secretions with little associated inflammation.[8,9] The most prominent, and usually the only sign of inflammation is bulbar conjunctival hyperemia. Excess secretions accumulate within the meibomian glands and are easily expressed in copious amounts. The secretions are usually liquid and are relatively clear or occasionally yellowish in appearance. Solidification of the secretions within the meibomian ducts is uncommon unless the meibomian glands themselves are inflamed. Once inflammation begins to play a major role, one is no longer dealing with meibomian seborrhea but with meibomianitis. Meibomian seborrhea probably represents the noninflamed point in the spectrum of meibomian dysfunction. Meibomianitis, meibomian conjunctivitis, and meibomian keratoconjunctivitis represent the superimposition of inflammation on a background of excessive meibomian secretions.

Meibomian seborrhea has been described and referred to as "seborrheic meibomianitis," which is a misnomer because there is no inflammation. It has also been grouped with series reporting seborrheic blepharokeratoconjunctivitis,[10] a term that is confusing because of the more accepted use of the term *seborrheic blepharitis* to identify blepharitis of a seborrheic nature involving the anterior (ciliary) portion of the eyelid. A more appropriate term to identify patients with meibomianitis and associated keratoconjunctivitis is *meibomian keratoconjunctivitis,*[7,11,12] with or without the use of a preceding seborrheic descriptor (e.g., seborrheic meibomian keratoconjunctivitis).

It is assumed that meibomian seborrhea is the result of overproduction of secretions by the meibomian glands; however, this has not been proved.[8,9] Although the theory of overproduction seems most likely, the abnormality could possibly be one of a relatively slow rate of flow.

Furthermore, it has not been established that excessive normal meibomian secretions alone cause disease. It is, therefore, possible that the signs and symptoms found in patients with apparent excessive meibomian secretions are caused by a biochemical alteration in the meibomian secretions. Alterations in several free fatty acids have been found in meibomian secretions from patients with meibomian gland abnormalities, compared with the composition in normal individuals and in patients with other types of blepharitis.[13] The presence of foam in the tear meniscus is suggestive of excessive fatty acid soaps, but this awaits verification. Patients with meibomian seborrhea who have been evaluated dermatologically have been found to have associated generalized sebaceous gland dysfunction.[7,14]

The diagnosis of meibomian seborrhea is based on the clinical appearance of excessive, easily expressible meibomian secretions, a foamy tear meniscus, minimal inflammation, and a moderate to marked burning that is most prominent in the morning.[7,9] Symptoms are often out of proportion to objective findings; therefore, meibomian seborrhea is one of the more commonly overlooked diagnoses in what is euphemistically called the "chronic itchy-burnies."

Even when the correct diagnosis is made, there is a common error on the part of the patient and the ophthalmologist alike, which leads to confusion, frustration, and dissatisfaction with one another. It is often not appreciated that meibomian seborrhea is a chronic condition for which there is no known cure and that treatment must be continued indefinitely and directed toward controlling the condition instead of curing it.

When the secretions are easily expressible, simple eyelid massage on a daily basis (best done in the morning after the secretions have been relatively stagnant overnight) is sufficient to control the condition and prevent the complications of hordeola, chalazia, and meibomianitis. If the secretions are somewhat solidified and difficult to express, the application of a hot compress before eyelid massage is recommended. As previously mentioned, heat raises the temperature of the lipid secretions, making them more fluid and easily expressed. As a qualitative biochemical alteration has been found in the meibomian secretions,[13,15] it may eventually be possible to neutralize the abnormal free fatty acids directly.

Meibomianitis/Meibomian Conjunctivitis/Meibomian Keratoconjunctivitis

Generalized inflammation of the meibomian glands may be primary or secondary to an inflammatory process of the anterior eyelid or conjunctiva.

Primary Meibomianitis

The most prominent and consistent feature of meibomianitis is stagnation of the meibomian secretions, with dilation of the acini and ducts of the meibomian glands (Table 4-2). This is readily seen either through the tarsal conjunctiva with the slit lamp biomicroscope or by transilluminating the eyelid with a fiberoptic light source and photographing the glands with special photographic techniques.[16,17] Solidification of the secretions near the orifices of the glands leads to the formation of semisolid or solid plugs (Figure 4-5). These plugs may contribute further to stagnant buildup of secretions within the glands. Hyperkeratinization of ductal epithelium may also contribute to stagnation of secretions within the glands.[17] By pressing on the tarsus, one may express many of the secretions; however, it is often impossible to express secretions if the eyelids are severely involved. Normal fluid meibomian secretions are clear; stagnant secretions that are semisolid are white or occasionally yellow. This coloration

TABLE 4-2
Ocular Signs in Meibomianitis

Sign	*Frequency (%)*
Anterior eyelid	
Crusting	60
Decreased eyelashes	60
Margin irregularity	45
Scaling	40
Inflammation of eyelash base	25
Trichiasis	5
Conjunctiva	
Hyperemia	100
Papillary hypertrophy	100
Rose bengal staining	100
Redundancy	50
Concretions	25
Tear film	
Rapid break-up time	100
Foam	60
Prominent interference patterns	60
Debris	55
Meibomian glands	
Solidified plugs	100
Dilated (prominent) glands	100
Pouting orifices	35
Distorted orifices	25
Cornea	
Superficial punctate keratopathy	100
Scarring	15
Decreased sensation	15

does not necessarily indicate the presence of inflammatory cells, because normal clear secretions develop a similar appearance if they are allowed to solidify at room temperature. Solidification of the secretions, with resultant turbidity and associated difficulty in expression, is a prominent feature of meibomianitis and is not typically seen in uncomplicated meibomian seborrhea. In meibomianitis, a tubule of white or yellow material several millimeters long can occasionally be expressed.

Once the meibomian glands have been involved to the point that the secretions are stagnant and solidified, there is inflammation involving the meibomian glands, as well as anterior (ciliary) blepharitis, conjunctivitis, and keratitis.[7,11,12] Signs of inflammation along the anterior eyelid margin are usually present but are mild and variable in their characteristics, and represent spillover of the more posteriorly located inflammation.

The tarsus may be thickened, depending on the severity and chronicity of the inflammation. The tarsus and conjunctiva surrounding the orifices of the meibomian glands are inflamed to a variable degree. The orifices may be flush with the eyelid margin or may be elevated and have a pouting appearance. There may be diffuse erythema with or without telangiectatic changes along the eyelid margin; telangiectatic changes occur in chronic cases. Conjunctival changes represent a nonspecific inflammatory process characterized by hyperemia of the bulbar conjunctiva and papillary hypertrophy of the tarsal conjunctiva.

In meibomianitis the tear film is unstable, as represented by a rapid tear film break-up time, which helps to account for the frequency of superficial punctate keratopathy

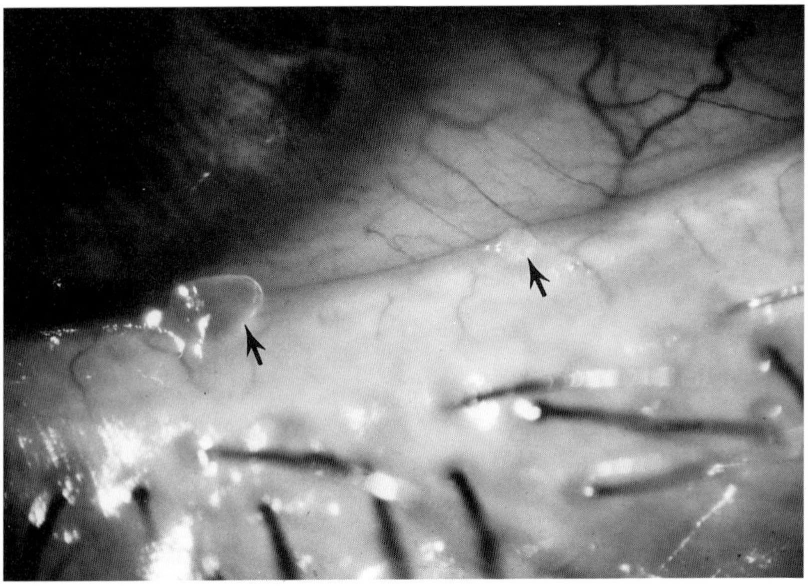

FIGURE 4-5 Large solidified secretions (arrows) plugging meibomian gland orifices.

found in the inferior third of the cornea and in the interpalpebral fissure by means of rose bengal staining.[7,11,12] Foam and debris are commonly seen in the tear film, as are prominent interference patterns. An abnormality in the lipid layer of the tear film can account for many of the symptoms and signs of meibomianitis, but the exact nature of the abnormality is unknown. One hypothetical mechanism is the inability of the lipids to form a monolayer over the tear film, leading to excessive evaporation and hypertonicity of the tears. The problem is apparently not a deficiency in the amount of lipids, which would be accompanied by a diminution of the interference patterns. Neither is the problem related to an excess of lipids, because fresh secretions expressed from deep within the glands tend to stabilize the tear film. This suggests that there is some qualitative abnormality of the tear film lipids, but not the fresh lipids, that results in the characteristic tear film instability.

Meibomianitis almost always occurs in patients who have evidence of more generalized sebaceous gland dysfunction, such as seborrheic dermatitis, acne rosacea, or seborrhea sicca (dry dandruff).[7,10,11,14,18] In patients who present to the ophthalmologist, meibomianitis is usually a more prominent feature than dermatitis, whereas meibomianitis is often not prominent in those who present to the dermatologist. However, if a patient presents with symptoms and signs of meibomianitis but does not have a dermatologic diagnosis, it cannot be assumed that dermatitis does not exist. Such patients should be referred for a dermatologic work-up, because control of the dermatologic disease will aid in the control of the meibomianitis.

The typical clinical course of meibomianitis is one of a chronic waxing and waning inflammatory process involving primarily the tarsus and its glands, with a variable amount of anterior blepharitis, conjunctivitis, and keratitis. Marked exacerbations are not uncommon and may be accompanied by the development of posterior hordeola or chalazia.

Symptoms are variable and nonspecific (Table 4-3). By the time patients seek ophthalmic care, symptoms have usually been present for years. Often symptoms are of a mild nature and patients accept them as a way of life. Another common situation is characterized by the patient who has complained repeatedly to ophthalmologists, who have either not recognized the primary abnormality or not understood the chronicity of the disease and the fact that it is a condition that usually must be controlled and not cured. Other patients accept chronic mild symptoms as normal and seek professional help only during exacerbations or when hordeola or chalazia occur. These patients frequently discontinue treatment when symptoms and signs reach a less bothersome level, only to have the symptoms and signs increase, and, in time, again reach a level that necessitates medical care.

TABLE 4-3
Ocular Symptoms in Meibomianitis

Symptom	*Frequency (%)*
Mattering/crusting	80
Hyperemia	80
Foreign body sensation	65
"Styes"/chalazia	60
Blurred vision	45
Tearing	40
Burning	40
Itching	30
Dryness	25
Swelling	25
Eyelid scaling	20
Irritation	15
Photophobia	5

The two major components of meibomian secretions are waxes and cholesterol esters; cholesterol, free fatty acids, triglycerides, and phospholipids are present in lesser amounts.[4,7] Secretions from one subgroup of normal individuals, however, do not contain cholesterol esters. Several unsuccessful attempts have been made in the past to identify a biochemical alteration in the meibomian secretions in patients with meibomianitis.[10,18] The lack of success may be attributable to the small numbers of patients studied and the incomplete analysis of the secretions; only thin-layer chromatography was done. More extensive studies using both thin-layer and gas-liquid chromatography of meibomian secretions from patients with meibomian seborrhea and meibomianitis have identified increases in minor free fatty acids, which could contribute to the disease process.[13] These free fatty acids may be produced from many of the lipid components found in meibomian secretions.

It is suggested that excessive free fatty acids can contribute to the nonspecific inflammation and symptoms of irritation and burning that accompany meibomianitis.[9] Free fatty acids not only can destabilize the tear film but also are known to be directly toxic to cells. Free fatty acids are irritating to the skin[19-21]; however, they have not been shown to be irritating to ocular and eyelid surfaces, although this is likely. Foam along the eyelid margin has been attributed to fatty acid soaps or other fats in the tear film,[22] but this has not been substantiated.

Other abnormalities in the lipid constituents of meibomian secretions from patients with meibomianitis have been established. Meibomian secretions from patients with meibomianitis differ from those from normal individuals in certain waxes, cholesterol esters,[23] and specific fatty acids obtained from these esters.[24] Meibomian secretions from patients with meibomianitis always contain cholesterol esters, whereas those from normal individuals may or may not.[25] Unsaturated fatty acids are associated with the presence of these esters.

Many of the lipid constituents of meibomian secretions have melting points near or above body temperature; therefore, minimal cooling of the secretions, as occurs in dilated meibomian glands, results in solidification. Biochemical shifts of the secretions to compounds with higher melting points would also contribute to solidification, for example, branched to unbranched fatty acids, unsaturated to saturated fatty acids, short-chain to long-chain fatty acids, or cholesterol esters to cholesterol.

Biochemical abnormalities of the meibomian secretions may occur through several mechanisms: a basic defect in the secretions, an alteration in stagnant secretions as a result of excessive activity by an endogenous enzyme located within the ducts of the gland, and/or an alteration of stagnant secretions by bacterial enzymes near the gland orifice or in the tear film.

No single bacterium has been found in all cases of meibomianitis, and there is general agreement that meibomianitis is not primarily a bacterial disease. Rarely do bacteria invade the meibomian glands to the degree that suppurative meibomianitis develops.[26] Cultures of the eyelid and conjunctiva in patients with meibomianitis yield a variety of bacteria (Table 4-4). The three most frequently isolated bacteria,[5,7,11,12] *Propionibacterium acnes,*[27,28] *S. epidermidis,*[28-30] and *S. aureus,*[28,31] have all been shown to produce a lipase that splits free fatty acids from triglycerides. Other bacterial enzymes that may contribute to meibomianitis are fatty wax esterase and cholesterol esterase. *S. aureus* isolated from patients with meibomianitis uniformly produces all three enzymes. *P. acnes* frequently produces a triglyceride lipase and a fatty wax esterase, but does not produce a cholesterol esterase. *S. epidermidis* frequently produces all three enzymes but is less uniform in its production than *S. aureus. S. epidermidis* isolated from patients with meibomian gland abnormalities has greater enzymatic activity than *S. epidermidis* isolated from normal individuals or patients with blepharitis who do not have meibomian gland abnormalities.[32] The activity of any or all three of these enzymes could significantly contribute to the disease process in meibomianitis and could account for the increase in free fatty acids. Low-dosage oral tetracycline effectively inhibits the production of some of these lipase enzymes.[15]

TABLE 4-4
Bacteria Isolated in Primary Meibomianitis

	Frequency Positive (%)	
Bacterium	*Eyelids*	*Conjunctiva*
Aerobic		
Staphylococcus epidermidis	90–95	80–90
Corynebacterium spp.	50	5
Staphylococcus aureus	15–20	7–10
Streptococcus spp.	Infrequent	Infrequent
Micrococcus spp.	Infrequent	Infrequent
Proteus spp.	Infrequent	Infrequent
Bacillus spp.	Infrequent	Infrequent
Neisseria spp.	Infrequent	Infrequent
Moraxella spp.	Infrequent	Infrequent
Anaerobic		
Propionibacterium acnes	95–100	75
Propionibacterium spp. (not *acnes*)	15–20	10–15
Gram-positive anaerobic cocci	10–15	5–10

In summary, it has been suggested that there is a population of patients with a predisposition to develop abnormalities of sebaceous glands,[7,11,12,14] such as seborrheic dermatitis or acne rosacea, including abnormalities of the meibomian glands (e.g., meibomian seborrhea or meibomianitis). The progression from excessive secretions without significant inflammation (meibomian seborrhea) to stagnant solidified secretions with significant associated inflammation (meibomianitis, meibomian conjunctivitis, meibomian keratoconjunctivitis) may occur as a result of a biochemical alteration in the meibomian secretions within the ducts and/or in the lipid layer of the tear film. The biochemical alteration may occur secondary to bacterial enzymes produced by several different bacteria, thus accounting for the variability in bacterial isolation (Figure 4-6).

The first goal in the treatment of primary meibomianitis, with its almost universal findings of mild anterior blepharitis, conjunctivitis, and keratitis, is to make the patient understand that this is a chronic disease for which no cure is currently known, and that treatment is indefinite and directed at controlling the disease. The recognition of dermatologic abnormalities and their appropriate treatment can aid greatly in the control of the ocular problems. This often requires the participation of a dermatologist, especially in patients with significant acne rosacea. The lack of understanding on the part of the ophthalmologist and effective communication to the patient of the natural history of chronic meibomianitis and the lack of attention to associated dermatologic abnormalities represent two of the biggest obstacles to the effective management of these patients.

Initially, hot compresses should be applied for 5 to 10 minutes, two to four times a day. Effective heating of

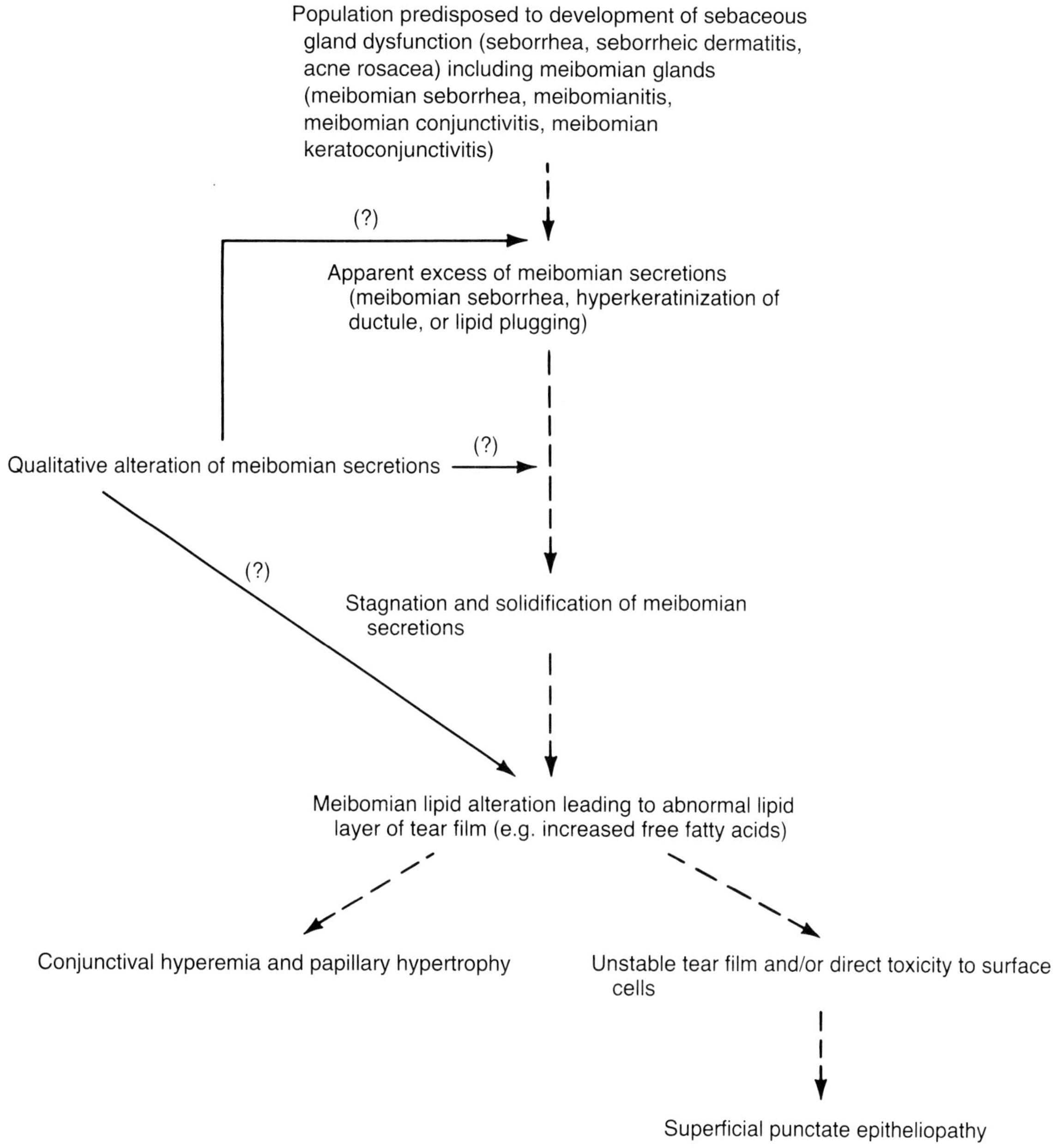

FIGURE 4-6 Proposed pathophysiologic pathway in the development of chronic meibomian keratoconjunctivitis.

the stagnant, solidified secretions within the meibomian glands raises the secretions to a temperature above their melting point. Once the secretions are in a liquid state, massaging the eyelids will help evacuate the glands and establish a more normal secretion flow. There are a number of massage techniques. One technique has the patient place an index finger just outside the eyelash line, look down when massaging the upper eyelid, look up when massaging the lower eyelid, and then rub in a circular pattern while exerting sufficient pressure. It is difficult to describe how much pressure to exert, but it can easily be demonstrated. The force required is usually greater than the patient anticipates. The massage should be repeated in adjacent areas until the full horizontal extent of all four eyelids is covered. The previously applied heat will also loosen crusting and mattering of the anterior eyelid surface and eyelashes, and will make the debris more easily removed by scrubbing with a mild baby shampoo. The shampoo also decreases the bacterial flora of the anterior eyelids and adjacent skin.

Although topical antibiotics are thought to be beneficial, their effect is uncertain. If cultures and antibiotic sensitivities are available, they can be used in the selection of an appropriate antibiotic. Anaerobic cultures and sensitivities are not routinely done; however, the presence of *P. acnes* in almost 100 percent of eyelid cultures and 75 percent of conjunctival cultures of patients with meibomianitis and its almost uniform sensitivity to chloramphenicol, tetracycline, and erythromycin may aid in antibiotic selection. As indicated above, isolated *S. aureus* and *S. epidermidis* are usually sensitive to bacitracin and aminoglycosides, but not to sulfonamides or tetracycline. However, it should be re-emphasized that bacterial sensitivity is usually related to growth. With *S. epidermidis,* the inhibition of lipase production by tetracycline appears to be more important than inhibition of bacterial growth.[15]

Topical corticosteroids can be used in the initial phase of therapy[33,34]; however, their use is usually unnecessary and unwise, unless the disease is severe. Cataracts, glaucoma, and opportunistic infections can occur in patients who use topical corticosteroids. Also, with the control of the inflammatory component of the disease with corticosteroids, patients often reach a greater level of comfort than can be maintained with appropriate long-term therapy, which may lead to further dissatisfaction and lack of acceptance of the chronic disease state.

Local maneuvers are usually sufficient to bring meibomianitis under control; however, the addition of systemic tetracycline is usually required to control meibomian keratoconjunctivitis.[7,34-37] The initial dosage is 250 mg orally four times a day given on an empty stomach. The mechanism of action of oral tetracycline is not through its antibiotic activity alone.[37] The mechanism may be the same in meibomianitis as that proposed in the treatment of acne vulgaris and acne rosacea: stabilization of the lipid (sebaceous or meibomian) secretions by inhibition of bacterial enzymes, such as lipase.[38-41] The dosage of tetracycline is tapered gradually over several months and may be discontinued in many patients, although chronic low-dosage maintenance levels (250 mg/day) are required to control the meibomianitis in others. Tetracycline should not be used in children or pregnant women.

With treatment, the anterior blepharitis, conjunctival hyperemia, superficial punctate keratopathy, and meibomianitis improve markedly within 2 to 3 months. A longer time is required for regression of the papillary hypertrophy of the tarsal conjunctiva. After successful treatment of meibomianitis, meibomian glands take on a more normal appearance, usually like that of meibomian seborrhea with excessive secretions and without the stagnant solidified plugs (Figure 4-7).

Once this point has been reached, treatment has just begun. The meibomianitis with its conjunctivitis or keratoconjunctivitis has been controlled but not cured. Now, the goal is to find the minimal amount of treatment that controls the tendency to develop meibomian keratoconjunctivitis. A minimum includes continued control of associated dermatologic disease, hot compresses, eyelid massage, and lid scrubs once or twice a day. Morning application of the last three procedures is the most important, because the secretions collect and stagnate overnight. The use of long-term, low-dosage oral tetracycline may be required in severely affected patients. Rarely will long-term topical antibiotics be beneficial, but if antibiotics are used, they should be alternated so as to discourage the emergence of resistant organisms.

There is a high incidence (25 to 50 percent) of associated keratoconjunctivitis sicca in patients with meibomianitis or chronic blepharitis. It is often not possible to make the diagnosis until the meibomianitis or blepharitis is under control. Once the diagnosis is made, however, appropriate therapy for keratoconjunctivitis sicca should be added.

The use of oral vitamin A in the treatment of meibomianitis has been suggested, but its benefits have not been substantiated. The use of 13-*cis*-retinoic acid has been evaluated in severe cases of acne vulgaris.[42-44] This or similar compounds may prove useful in the management of chronic meibomianitis or meibomian seborrhea. In the future, inhibition of bacterial lipolytic enzymes may become possible. Additional meibomian or tear lipid biochemical abnormalities may be identified, and it might become possible to directly neutralize the offending compound, for instance, to bind free fatty acids.

Secondary Meibomianitis

The diagnosis of secondary meibomianitis is made on the basis of signs of the primary inflammatory process (e.g., anterior staphylococcal blepharitis, seborrheic blepharitis,[7] or conjunctivitis) and changes in the meibomian glands and their secretions. In the past, meibomianitis secondary to anterior blepharitis or conjunctivitis was attributed to invasion of the meibomian glands by *Staphylococcus,*[45] but later investigations indicated that this is not the case.[4,5] Purulent material is rarely found in meibomian glands and almost always represents staphylococcal invasion of the glands.[26,45] It is possible that *Staphylococcus* plays a role in some cases; however, the mechanism may be more complex and similar to that mentioned above for

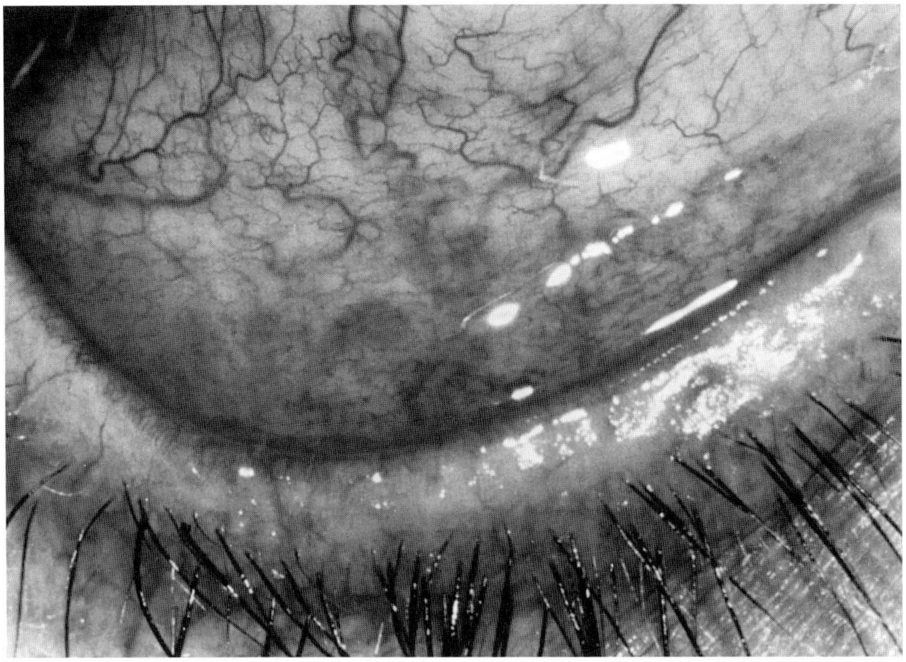

A

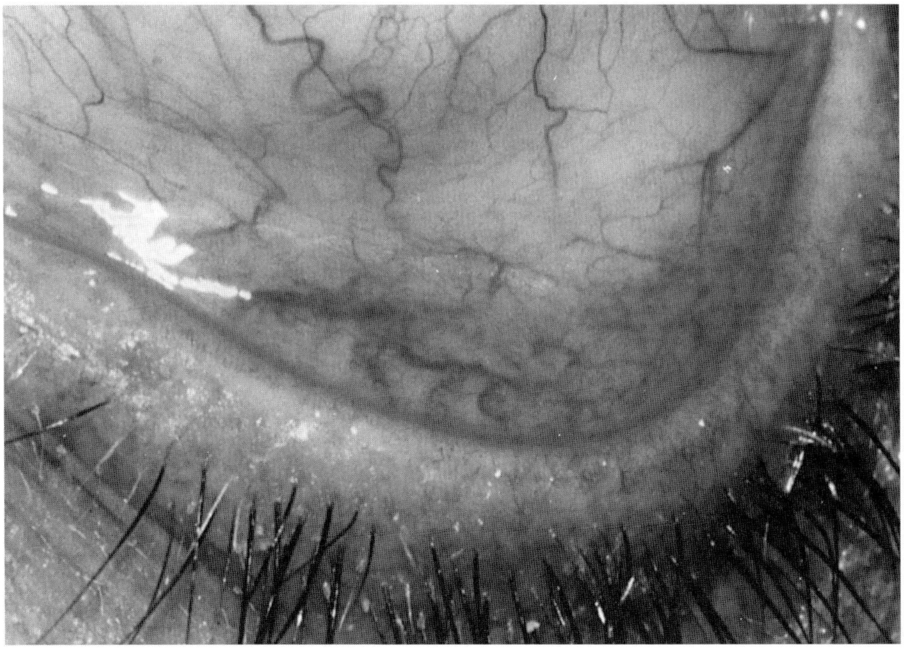

B

FIGURE 4-7 Meibomian keratoconjunctivitis. **(A)** Before treatment: minimal anterior (ciliary) blepharitis, conjunctival papillary hypertrophy, and stagnant solidified meibomian secretions plugging meibomian gland orifices with associated inflammation. **(B)** After treatment: resolution of inflammatory response but continued appearance of meibomian seborrhea with apparent excess secretions dilating uninflamed meibomian glands.

primary meibomianitis. The more common appearance in secondary meibomianitis is one of stagnant secretions dilating the glands and ducts, with plug formation near the orifices representing solidification of the secretions. Inflammation is seen, with thickening of the tarsus, erythema, and telangiectatic changes along the entire eyelid margin. Variable anterior eyelid inflammation, tarsal conjunctival papillary hypertrophy, inferior superficial punctate keratopathy, and diffuse rose bengal staining of the conjunctiva and cornea in the interpalpebral fissure are frequently found.

Treatment of secondary meibomianitis is directed at the primary process plus the mechanical and hygienic maneuvers listed above for primary meibomianitis.

Suppurative Meibomianitis

Suppurative meibomianitis has been mentioned above. It appears to be rare in developed countries since the advent of antibiotics and is therefore not discussed in any further detail.

REFERENCES

1. Duke-Elder S: System of Ophthalmology. Vol. XIII. The Ocular Adnexa. p. 242. CV Mosby, St. Louis, 1974
2. Vittadini A: Un caso letde di sellicemia stafiloccica consecutiva ad orizaiols meibomians. Boll Oculist 12:683, 1933
3. Gozberk R: Sur un cas de septicemie a staphylocoques consecutive a une miebomite suppurée. Ann Oculist (Paris) 175:159, 1938
4. Stevens AJ: The meibomian secretions. Int Ophthalmol Clin 13:23, 1973
5. Dougherty JM, McCulley JP: Comparative bacteriology of chronic blepharitis. Br J Ophthalmol 68:524, 1984
6. Thygeson P: Etiology and treatment of blepharitis. Arch Ophthalmol 36:445, 1946
7. McCulley JP, Dougherty JM, Deneau DF: Classification of chronic blepharitis. Ophthalmology 89:1173, 1982
8. Elschnig Von P: Beitrag zur Aetiologie und Therapie der chronischen Conjunctivitis. Dtsch Med Wochenschr 34:1133, 1908
9. Thygeson P, Kimura SJ: Chronic conjunctivitis. Trans Am Acad Ophthalmol Otolaryngol 67:494, 1963
10. Keight CG: Seborrheic blepharo-kerato-conjunctivitis. Trans Ophthalmol Soc UK 87:85, 1967
11. McCulley JP, Sciallis GF: Meibomian keratoconjunctivitis. Am J Ophthalmol 84:788, 1977
12. McCulley JP, Sciallis GF: Meibomian keratoconjunctivitis: oculodermal correlates. Contact Intraocular Lens Med J 9:130, 1983
13. Dougherty JM, McCulley JP: Analysis of the free fatty acid component of meibomian secretions in chronic blepharitis. Invest Ophthalmol Vis Sci 27:52, 1986
14. McCulley JP, Doughety JM: Blepharitis associated with acne rosacea and seborrheic dermatitis. Int Ophthalmol Clin 25:159, 1985
15. Dougherty DM, Silvany RE, Meyer DR: The role of tetracycline in chronic blepharitis: inhibition of lipase production in staphylococci. Invest Ophthalmol Vis Sci 32:2970, 1991
16. Tapie R: Étude biomicroscopique des glandes de meibomius. Ann Oculist 210:637, 1977
17. Jester JF, Rife L, Nu D, et al: In vivo biomicroscopy and photography of meibomian glands in a rabbit model of meibomian gland dysfunction. Invest Ophthalmol Vis Sci 22:660, 1982
18. Cory CC, Hinks W, Burton JL, Shuster S: Meibomian gland secretions in the red eyes of rosacea. Br J Dermatol 88:25, 1973
19. Kellum RE: Acne vulgaris-studies in pathogenesis: relative irritancy of free fatty acids from C_2 to C_{16}. Arch Dermatol 97:722, 1968
20. Ray T, Kellum RE: Acne vulgaris-studies in pathogenesis: free fatty acid irritancy in patients with and without acne. J Invest Dermatol 57:6, 1971
21. Fulton JE Jr: Lipases: their questionable role in acne vulgaris. Int J Dermatol 15:732, 1976
22. Norn MS: Foam at outer palpebral canthus. Acta Ophthalmol (Copenh) 41:531, 1963
23. Osgood JK, Dougherty JM, McCulley JP: The role of wax and sterol esters in meibomian keratoconjunctivitis. Invest Ophthalmol Vis Sci 30:1958, 1989
24. Dougherty JM, Osgood JK, McCulley JP: The role of wax and sterol ester fatty acids in chronic blepharitis. Invest Ophthalmol Vis Sci 32:1932, 1991
25. Shine WE, McCulley JP: The role of cholesterol in chronic blepharitis. Invest Ophthalmol Vis Sci 32:2272, 1991
26. Duke-Elder S: System of Ophthalmology. Vol. XIII. The Ocular Adnexa. p. 249. CV Mosby, St. Louis, 1974
27. Kellum RE, Stranfeld K: Triglyceride hydrolysis by *Corynebacterium acnes* in vitro. J Invest Dermatol 52:255, 1969
28. Dougherty JM, McCulley JP, Chan F, et al: Chronic blepharitis: new perspectives. ARVO abstract. Invest Ophthalmol Vis Sci 20(suppl):109, 1981
29. Reisner RM, Puhvel M: Lipolytic activity of *Staphylococcus albus.* J Invest Dermatol 53:1, 1969
30. Troller JA, Rozeman MA: Isolation and characterization of a staphylococcal lipase. Appl Microbiol 20:480, 1970
31. Van Bijsterveld OP: Lipolytic activity of *Staphylococcus aureus* from different sources. J Med Microbiol 9:225, 1976
32. Dougherty JM, McCulley JP: Bacterial lipases and chronic blepharitis. Invest Ophthalmol Vis Sci 27:486, 1986
33. Aragones JV: The treatment of blepharitis: a controlled double blind study of combination therapy. Ann Ophthalmol 5:49, 1973
34. Leibowitz HM, Pratt M, Flagstad IJ, et al: Human conjunctivitis. II. Treatment. Arch Ophthalmol 94:1752, 1976
35. Marmion VJ: Tetracycline in the treatment of ocular rosacea. Proc R Soc Med 62:11, 1969
36. Knight AG, Vickers CFH: A follow up of tetracycline-treated rosacea. Br J Dermatol 93:577, 1975
37. Brown SI, Shahinian L: Diagnosis and treatment of ocular rosacea. Ophthalmology 85:779, 1978
38. Weaber K, Freedman R, Eudy WW: Tetracycline inhibition of a lipase from *Corynebacterium acnes.* Appl Microbiol 21:639, 1971
39. Ishidata M, Sakaguchi T: Metal chelate compounds of tetracycline derivatives. I. Aureomycin. Pharmacol Bull (Tokyo) 3:147, 1955
40. Vavrecka M, Petrasek R, Poledne R: The effect of tetracycline antibiotics on fat metabolism. Prog Biochem Pharmacol 3:468, 1967
41. Freinkel RK, Strauss JS, Yip SY, Pochi PE: Effect of tetra-

cycline on the composition of sebum in acne vulgaris. N Engl J Med 373:850, 1965
42. Peck GL, Olsen TG, Yoder FW, et al: Prolonged remissions of cystic and conglobate acne with 13-*cis*-retinoic acid. N Engl J Med 300:329, 1979
43. King K, Jones DH, Daltrey DC, Cunliffe WJ: A double-blind study of the effects of 13-*cis*-retinoic acid on acne, sebum excretion rate and microbial population. Br J Dermatol 107:583, 1982
44. Mathers WD, Shields WJ, Sachdev MS, et al: Meibomian gland morphology and tear osmolarity: changes with Accutane therapy. Cornea 10:286, 1991
45. Thygeson P: Complications of staphylococcic blepharitis. Am J Ophthalmol 68:446, 1969

5

Abnormalities of the Tears and Treatment of Dry Eyes

R. LINSY FARRIS

Any statement about abnormal tear function implies a thorough knowledge of normal tear function. This, however, is not the case. At the present time, many aspects of normal tear function are poorly understood. Research is currently under way to define the characteristics of normal tears. Only when normal tear function has been fully elucidated will the treatment of tear abnormalities and ocular surface diseases be better understood.

This chapter reviews the qualitative and quantitative aspects of normal tears, relates tear abnormalities to corneal disease, and describes the treatment of abnormalities of the tears.

NORMAL TEARS

Tears are composed of several substances, including electrolytes, proteins, lipids, enzymes, and various metabolites[1] (Table 5-1). The tear film consists of three layers: a mucin layer, produced by conjunctival goblet cells; an aqueous layer, produced by the main and accessory lacrimal glands; and a lipid layer, produced by the meibomian glands and the glands of Moll and Zeis. The anatomy and physiology of these layers are described in Chapter 1.

The normal tear volume is approximately 6.2 μl.[2] The average rate of tear production is approximately 1.2 μl/min (range, 0.5 to 2.2 μl/min), which represents a turnover rate of 16 percent of the normal tear volume per minute. The normal rate of water evaporation from the ocular surface is approximately 0.14 μl/min at 30 percent relative humidity.[3]

The distinction between basal and reflex tears has come under scrutiny.[4] It is generally now thought that all significant tear flow results from reflex secretion. The responsiveness of the lacrimal glands to different stimuli results in considerable variation in tear production and in the concentration of tear constituents.[5] Decreases in this responsiveness may explain the decreased tear flow associated with aging.[6,7] Decreased tear flow in patients after large-incision cataract surgery is most likely the result of decreased stimulation following partial denervation of the cornea caused by the surgical incision.

TEAR ABNORMALITIES

Abnormalities of the tears may result from a variety of causes. A correct diagnosis, with all aggravating factors taken into account, will direct practitioners in the search for the most beneficial forms of therapy for a particular patient. Abnormalities of the tears may have their origins in abnormal tear volume, tear surfacing, tear wetting, tear base, and/or tear lipids. The classification of tear abnormalities in terms of one or more of these underlying mechanisms provides the rationale for therapy.

Quantitative Abnormalities

Deficient Tear Volume

Deficient tear volume, which is the most common tear abnormality,[6–12] can be caused by decreased tear secretion and/or increased tear evaporation. Congenital disorders associated with lacrimal hyposecretion include aplasia or hypoplasia of the lacrimal gland, familial dysautonomia (Riley-Day syndrome),[13–15] anhidrotic ectodermal dysplasia, familial sensory neuropathy with anhidrosis,[16] multiple endocrine neoplasia, Holmes-Adie syndrome (pupillotonia, hyporeflexia, and segmental hypohidrosis), and neuroparalysis.[17] Acquired lacrimal

TABLE 5-1
Composition of Tear Fluid

Component	*Concentration in Tears*
Protein	6–20 g/L
Prealbumin	Small fraction
Lysozyme	1–2 g/L
Lactoferrin	—
Transferrin	—
Ceruloplasmin	—
IgA	10–100 mg%
IgG	Very low concentration
IgE	26–144 ng/ml
Complement	1:4
Glycoproteins	0.05–3 g/L (hexosamine concentration)
Antiproteinases	Much lower than in serum
α_1-antitrypsin (α_1-at)	0.1–3 mg%
α_1-antichymotrypsin (α_1-ach)	1.4 mg%
inter-α-trypsin inhibitor	0.5 mg%
α_2-macroglobulin (α_2-M)	3–6 mg%
Enzymes	
Glycolytic and tricarboxylic acid cycle enzymes	Very low levels
Lactate dehydrogenase	Highest in tears
Lysosomal enzymes	2–10 times levels in serum
Amylase	Similar to level in urine
Peroxidase	10^3 units/L
Plasminogen activator	—
Collagenase	Only with corneal ulceration
Lipids	
Cholesterol	200 mg% (same as blood)
Meibomian lipids: hydrocarbons, wax esters, cholesterol esters, triglycerides, diglycerides, monoglycerides, free fatty acids, free cholesterol, and phospholipid	—
Metabolites	
Glucose	0.2 mmol/L
Lactate	1–5 mmol/L
Pyruvate	0.05–0.35 mmol/L
Urea	Equivalent to amounts in plasma
Catecholamines	0–1.5 μg/ml
Dopamine	To 280 μg/ml
Epinephrine	—
Norepinephrine	—
Dopa	—
Histamine	10 mg/ml
Prostaglandin F	75 pg/ml
Electrolytes	
Na^+	80–170 mmol/L
K^+	6–42 mmol/L
Ca^{2+}	0.3–2.0 mmol/L
Mg^{2+}	0.3–1.1 mmol/L
Cl^-	106–138 mmol/L
HCO_3^-	26 mmol/L
Osmotic pressure	305 mOsm/L
pH	7.45 (7.14–7.82)

Source: Adapted from NJ Van Haeringen: Clinical biochemistry of tears. Surv Ophthalmol 26:84, 1981.

hyposecretion may develop as a result of senile or idiopathic lacrimal gland atrophy, or in association with autoimmune disorders such as rheumatoid arthritis, lupus erythematosus, and polyarteritis nodosa.[18-20] Other systemic disorders associated with lacrimal hyposecretion include hematopoietic disorders (e.g., lymphoma, thrombocytopenic purpura, hypergammaglobulinemia, and Waldenström's macroglobulinemia), Hashimoto's thyroiditis, celiac disease, chronic hepatobiliary disease, pulmonary fibrosis, and sarcoidosis. Localized lacrimal disorders that cause hyposecretion include benign lymphoepithelial lesion (Mikulicz's disease),[21] graft-versus-host disease, postinflammatory atrophy, and viral dacryoadenitis.[22-24] Hyposecretion can also be induced by irradiation, mechanical trauma (including surgical excision of the lacrimal gland), and chemical burns.

Sjögren's syndrome is an inflammatory disease of the lacrimal and exocrine glands, and is probably of autoimmune origin.[18,25,26] In 1933, Sjögren described this syndrome in patients who had at least two of the following three conditions: keratoconjunctivitis sicca, xerostomia, and arthritis. It is now recognized that the third criterion, arthritis, may be replaced with any of the connective tissue diseases. The combination of keratoconjunctivitis sicca and xerostomia has been classified as primary Sjögren's syndrome; the presence of a connective tissue disease makes it secondary Sjögren's syndrome. Functional studies of the reticuloendothelial system Fc receptors in patients with Sjögren's syndrome revealed decreased clearance of immune complexes, indicating a possible mechanism of exocrine gland injury caused by the deposition of these complexes, and consequent immunologic insult.[27,28] In a study of 32 patients with dry eyes, but with no clinical evidence of connective tissue disease, Forstot et al[29] found that 59 percent had a positive antinuclear antibody, 59 percent had a positive rheumatoid factor, and 31 percent had SS-A and/or SS-B autoantibodies. An even higher percentage of positive serologic tests was obtained from 15 patients with dry eyes and dry mouth.[19] Pflugfelder et al[30] reported autoantibodies in 82 percent of patients with dry eyes. In contrast to these studies, Farris et al[31] found a lower prevalence of positive antinuclear antibody (36 percent), positive rheumatoid factor (8 percent), and SS-A or SS-B autoantibodies (1 to 3 percent) in 77 patients diagnosed with dry eyes on the basis of history, symptoms, and clinical examination, who also had symptoms of dry mouth and/or arthritis. Sjögren's syndrome, as indicated by the presence of serum antibodies, appears to have a lower incidence in dry eye patients than previously thought.

Many systemic drugs influence tear production,[32,33] in that secretions of the lacrimal gland are controlled primarily by parasympathetic nerve fibers traveling in the 7th cranial nerve. Sympathetic nerve fibers in the lacrimal gland and in blood vessels may also play a role, since they control blood flow, which influences tear production. Antimuscarinic drugs, such as atropine and scopolamine, reduce tear secretion by 50 to 80 percent. Antihistamines also diminish tear secretion by their atropine-like action. Other medications, including sedatives, tricyclic antidepressants, nasal decongestants, antitussives, analgesics, antidiarrheals, and diuretics,[34] diminish the secretion of tears. Practolol, a β-adrenergic receptor blocker, decreases tear secretion and lowers tear lysozyme content, often causing severe dry eyes in patients who use the drug for long-term therapy of heart disease, hypertension, or cardiac dysrhythmias.[35,36] Timolol, a topical β-adrenergic receptor blocker effective in the treatment of glaucoma, can produce ocular symptoms of burning and punctate keratopathy.[37] One study demonstrated decreased Schirmer test results in 25 percent of patients using timolol.[38]

A high rate of tear evaporation may decrease tear volume.[39,40] The relative contribution of tear evaporation to tear dynamics in patients with dry eyes is greater than normal,[41] and in some patients appears to increase as tear production decreases. The cause, which is unknown, may be an unstable tear film resulting in a more rapid tear film break-up time.[3]

Typically, there is an onrush of patients with dry eye symptoms to ophthalmologists' offices in early summer, when air conditioners are turned on and large volumes of air are circulated without replacement of moisture. Dry eye symptoms may also be worse in the winter, when furnaces are turned on and the humidity decreases. Individuals who work in closed spaces, such as office buildings or airplanes, are particularly susceptible to dry eye symptoms. Infrequent blinking and staring also lead to excessive evaporation and decreased tear volume.[40] Frequently, the deficient tear volume caused by these conditions is masked by excessive tearing, which is a compensatory response that is more noticeable to patients than their dry eye symptoms.

Excess Tear Volume

Excess tear volume may be the result of either impaired drainage or excessive tear production. Impaired drainage occurs from blockage of the drainage system at some point between the puncta and the opening of the nasolacrimal duct. Impaired drainage from the inferior marginal tear strip and lacrimal lake into the puncta is a physiologic block, and usually occurs in older patients with lax eyelids and malposition of the puncta.[42,43] Thirty μl of tears may accumulate in the inferior fornix before overflow across the eyelid margin occurs, causing epiphora.

Hypersecretion of tears may result from excessive stimulation from the efferent portion of the tear reflex arc,

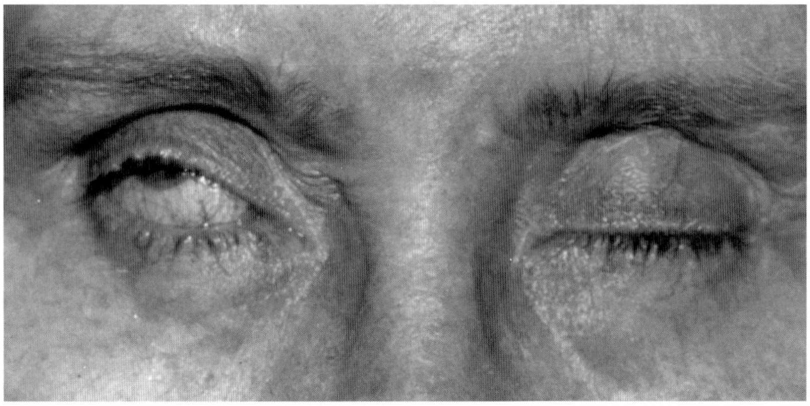

FIGURE 5-1 Lagophthalmos following upper eyelid blepharoplasty. Note the incomplete closure of the eyelids of the right eye. The inferior cornea is exposed in this patient despite a good Bell's reflex.

which receives afferent input from the nasal mucosa, eyelids, eyelashes, conjunctiva, cornea, retina, and the emotional centers.[17,44,45] Some specific causes of neurogenic lacrimal hypersecretion are visual irritation by bright light, accommodative strain, blepharospasm that causes stretching of the trigeminal nerve, toxic neuritis of the trigeminal nerve, trigeminal neuralgia, nasal polyps, chronic ethmoiditis, the eruption of wisdom teeth, and aberrant neural regeneration that develops following injury, disease, or surgery in the vicinity of the lacrimal nucleus. Thyroiditis and syphilis also can be associated with excess lacrimation.[40]

Air contaminants, such as paint fumes, fumes from freshly manufactured or cleaned fabrics, and fumes from printer's ink, are some of the irritants that cause excessive tearing. These irritants, like the preservatives in topical ocular medications, are more toxic in patients with dry eyes than in normal individuals because they are not diluted by normal tear flow. In response to such irritants, individuals tend to wipe their eyes frequently, thus stimulating the conjunctiva and producing even greater irritation. Cigarette smoke is another common irritant that causes reflex tearing and alteration of the tear film. Basu et al[46] found that after 10 minutes of exposure to cigarette smoke, tear film break-up time in 14 young volunteers was reduced 30 to 40 percent, compared with break-up time after exposure to filtered air. Smog and household detergents containing formaldehyde, acrolein, sulfur dioxide, peroxyacetylnitrate, and peroxybenzoylnitrate also cause excessive tearing.

Drugs or allergies may increase lacrimation, either directly or indirectly, and, in addition, may produce changes in the drainage system that impede tear drainage.[47-49] Muscarinic, sympathomimetic, and antihypertensive drugs, including reserpine, hydralazine, and diazoxide, have been reported to increase tear production.[50] Miscellaneous drugs, including marijuana,[51] fluorouracil,[52] nitrofurantoin, sulfathiazole,[53] and histamine[54] have the same effect. Although one would not consider using these drugs for the primary purpose of increasing tear production, their concomitant use with dry eye therapy may explain the decreased symptomatic relief when these drugs are discontinued.

Finally, as described above, a deficiency in tear volume may cause drying and irritation of the cornea and conjunctiva, which, in turn, may lead to the overproduction of tears.[2,4] Not infrequently, as tear production decreases, the eye dries and tear flow is periodically stimulated in a manner such that epiphora can paradoxically be the presenting symptom of dry eyes.

Qualitative Abnormalities

Abnormal Tear Surfacing

Tear surfacing refers to the ability of tears to be spread across the corneal and conjunctival surfaces.[55] The eyelids are primarily responsible for spreading the tears to keep the ocular surface moistened. Inadequate tear surfacing may be caused by lagophthalmos (Figure 5-1), which occurs in some individuals during sleep, and in others secondary to facial nerve palsy, symblepharon formation, or disease of the eyelid margin.[11] The edge of a contact lens, conjunctival swelling after surgery, pingueculae, pterygia, cosmetic eyelid surgery, ptosis surgery, and a retinal encircling band that has slipped anteriorly are examples of conditions that can interfere with proper surfacing of the tear film by the eyelids, and thus lead to localized tear film abnormalities and thinning of the cornea (dellen formation) (Figure 5-2). In addition, thyroid ophthalmopathy produces a wide interpalpebral fissure, abnormal eye movements, and impaired eyelid function. Any condition that causes exophthalmos impairs the movement of the eyelids and leads to inadequate surfacing, increased evaporation of the tear film, and impaired dis-

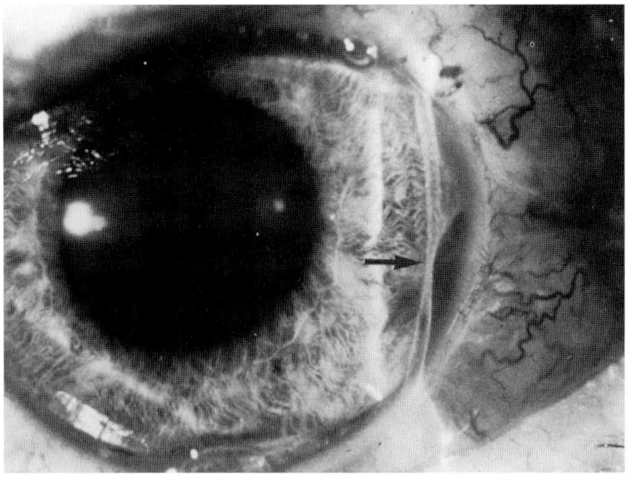

FIGURE 5-2 Corneal delle. Note the thinning of the slit beam near the limbus (arrow). The adjacent conjunctival chemosis led to disruption of the tear film in this area, causing formation of the delle.

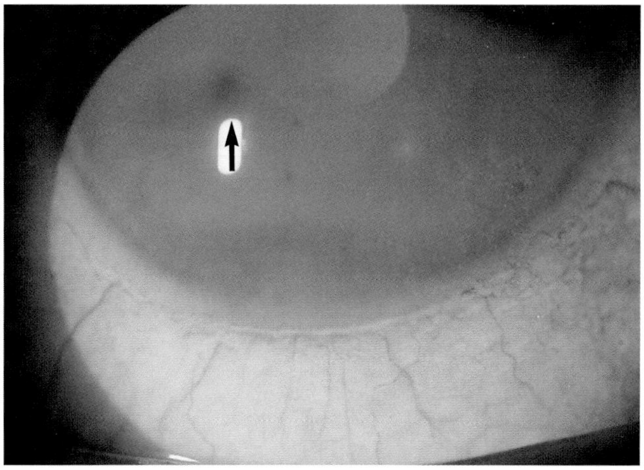

FIGURE 5-3 Tear film break-up time. After instillation of fluorescein, the patient is asked to keep the eyelids open, and the time of appearance of the first dry spot (arrow) is the tear film break-up time. (Courtesy of Michael B. Limberg, M.D., San Luis Obispo, CA.)

tribution of the tears across the ocular surface.[40] Abnormal blinking may be caused by concentrated use of the eyes, contact lenses that produce discomfort on blinking, general anesthesia, the use of sedatives, neurologic disorders such as 5th or 7th cranial nerve paralysis, and autonomic disorders such as parkinsonism.[56] Areas of drying resulting from deficiencies in the lipid layer of the tear film lead to localized excessive evaporation of the tear film and thinning of the cornea.

Abnormal Wetting by Tears

The wetting ability of normal tears is defined as the ability to spread out in a thin, continuous layer over the ocular surface.[57] Inadequate wetting is evident when dry spots occur in the tear film soon after a blink.[58] The interval between a blink and the appearance of such dry spots is called the tear film break-up time and is determined by staining the tears with fluorescein, asking the patient not to blink, and then counting the seconds until dry spots appear (Figure 5-3). Although there is some disagreement about normal values,[57,59] a tear film break-up time of 10 seconds or more is considered normal.[60]

The mucin content of tears is important in permitting adequate wetting.[61-63] Conjunctival goblet cells produce a large proportion of the mucin content of tears, although studies have demonstrated no direct correlation between tear mucin content and the density of conjunctival goblet cells.[64]

Mucin is present in tears in two forms: a dissolved form in tear fluid and an undissolved form that collects in the inferior fornix[65,66] (Figure 5-4). Visible mucus may be a degraded form of mucin that has minimal wetting abilities and may actually worsen a dry eye state by preferential absorption of moisture from the epithelial cells.[66]

Excess mucus is frequently observed in tears as a result of either excessive mucin production or inadequate rinsing secondary to deficient aqueous tear volume.[67,68] Increased production of visible mucus often occurs in inflamed eyes with infections or allergies, and in eyes with foreign bodies, sutures, or contact lenses. Strands

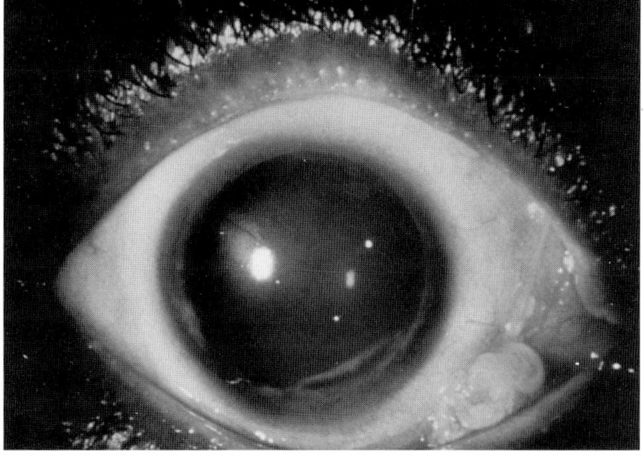

FIGURE 5-4 Large mucin strand in the inferior fornix in a patient with Sjögren's syndrome. Note the area of midperipheral corneal thinning associated with rheumatoid arthritis.

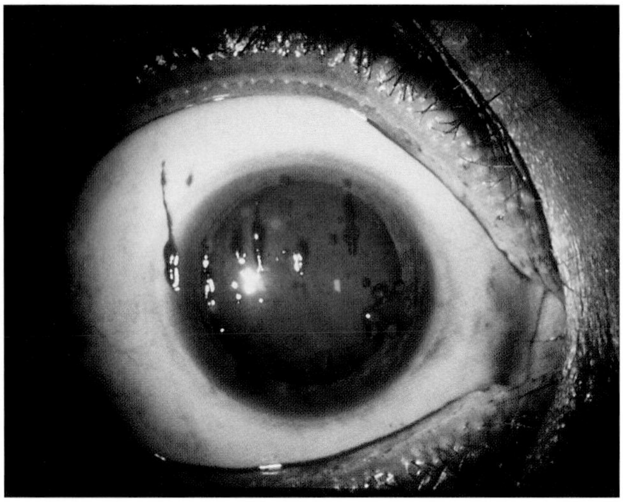

FIGURE 5-5 Filaments associated with dry eyes (rose bengal stain).

of mucus and degenerated corneal epithelial cells attached to the cornea appear as filaments (Figure 5-5).[69] Excess mucus may harden and act as a foreign body, interfering with vision and providing a rich medium for microbial proliferation. Repeated removal of excess mucus from the surface of the eye or inferior fornix by the patient can damage the ocular surface and cause a further increase in mucus production.[70]

Mucin deficiency occurs in a variety of diseases that destroy conjunctival goblet cells. Avitaminosis A, ocular pemphigoid, erythema multiforme (Stevens-Johnson syndrome), trachoma, chemical burns, and the use of certain topical medications, such as phospholine iodide, decrease the goblet cell population. The result of mucin deficiency is a shortened tear film break-up time and reduced wetting of the ocular surface, even in the presence of an adequate tear volume.[62]

Abnormal Tear Base

The superficial cells of the corneal epithelium form the base of the tear film.[71] Defects in this cell layer decrease attachment of the tear film in localized areas, producing inadequate wetting and dry spots.[63] Corneal erosions, corneal dystrophies that affect the epithelium, and corneal scars are common causes of an abnormal tear base.[72] In such cases, restoration of the corneal epithelium and basement membrane over a long period must occur before the wetting properties of the surface return to normal.[73-75] In some cases, scraping or a superficial keratectomy may be necessary to provide a surface that is suitable for adherence of the tear film.[76]

Vitamin A deficiency causes an inadequate tear base by producing keratinization of the conjunctiva, decreased goblet cells, and superficial punctate keratopathy.[77] Vitamin A therapy produces rapid improvement in these ocular surface abnormalities. Chemical burns destroy the normal ocular surface, sometimes permanently, so that the normal tear film cannot be re-established.[78]

Abnormal Tear Lipids

The lipids in the tear film originate mainly from the meibomian secretions,[79] which are produced in sufficient quantity in normal eyes to completely resurface the preocular tear film with every blink.[80] Destruction of the meibomian glands may result in excessive evaporation of tears in association with corneal thinning.[81,82] Deficiencies in tear film lipids are encountered clinically after frequent and prolonged use of eye washes or eye drops. Excess tear lipids commonly occur in patients with excessive meibomian secretions associated with acne and blepharitis (see Ch. 4).[83] Excess lipids decrease the wetting ability of the tears by contaminating the corneal surface with hydrophobic material.[58] Both quality and quantity are important in determining the ability of lipid to spread evenly over the surface of the tear film and to retard evaporation. Meibomianitis, as well as chemical burns, pemphigoid, and Stevens-Johnson syndrome, all of which induce meibomian gland and lipid abnormalities, result in rapid tear evaporation and signs of dry eyes.

DRY EYES

Clinical Signs and Symptoms

Symptoms of dry eyes range from heightened eye awareness to severe pain; signs range from a decreased tear meniscus to corneal ulceration[84,85] and perforation (Figure 5-6). The full spectrum of symptoms includes heaviness of the eyelids, blurred and fluctuating vision, excess ropy mucus, burning, itching, scratchiness, foreign body sensation, photophobia, tearing, and pain. A high index of suspicion for tear abnormalities will prevent misdiagnosing this common cause of such symptoms.

Dry eyes can be responsible for a variety of clinical signs. Decreased visual acuity that varies with blinking is one of the first signs encountered. Although eye redness may vary initially from none to severe, the eyes quickly become red while being examined. The inferior marginal tear strip is small, reflecting a deficient tear volume, but this sign may be missed if it is not checked before visual acuity is tested or lights are shined into the eye. Therefore, observation of the inferior marginal

FIGURE 5-6 **(A)** Corneal ulcer and **(B)** corneal perforation in patients with dry eyes. The inferior location is typical.

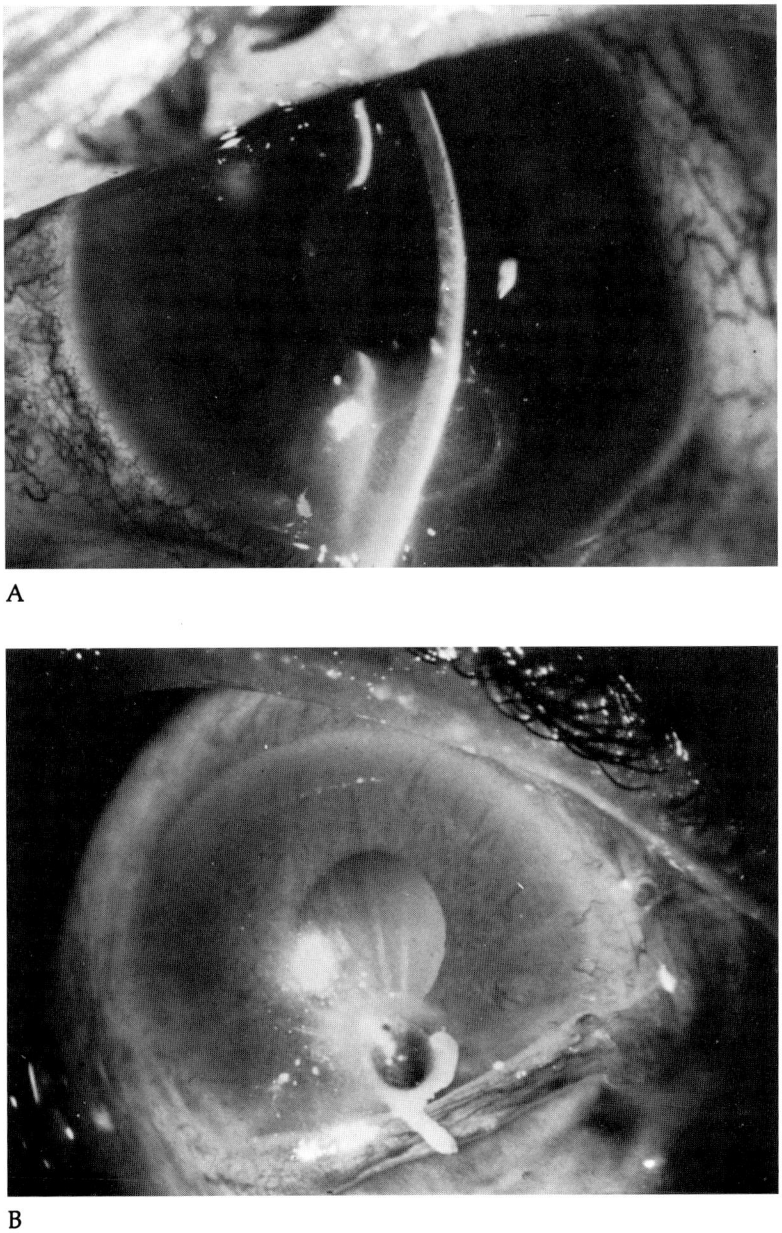

tear strip is the first step in looking for clinical signs of dry eyes, and is best done through a slit lamp that is not turned on, with the use of overhead room lighting. When the slit lamp is turned on, the presence of excess debris in the tear film or a viscous appearance of the tear film is usually observed within a few seconds. The tear film often contains mucus strands. It is also common for the eyelid margins to display excessive foam, debris, and oils.

The cornea and conjunctiva in the interpalpebral area are examined to detect localized elevations and signs of corneal drying. The central corneal thickness is reduced in patients with dry eyes, and measurement of the central corneal thickness may aid in the early diagnosis of this disorder.[86] The eyelids are examined for blepharitis and meibomianitis, which are commonly associated with dry eyes. The upper eyelid is everted to look for papillae and follicles of the upper tarsal conjunctiva.

Fluorescein is instilled into the inferior fornix by gently touching the inferior palpebral conjunctiva with a fluorescein strip moistened with one drop of saline without preservatives. It is important to instill approximately the same amount of fluorescein into each eye so that one can observe the amount of fluorescence, which is an indi-

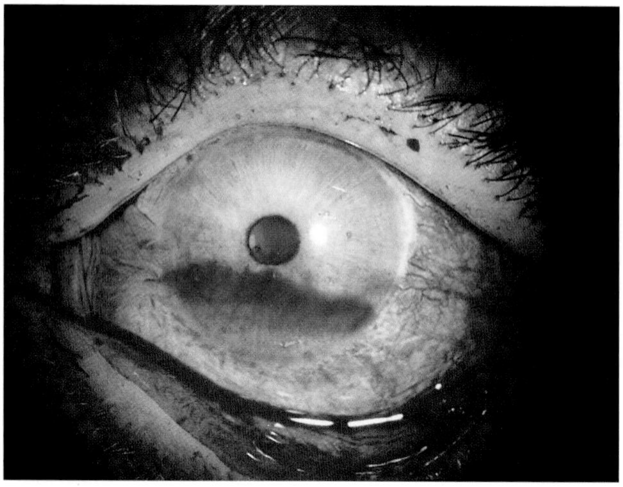

FIGURE 5-7 Rose bengal staining in the interpalpebral area in a patient with dry eyes.

rect measure of the aqueous tear volume. When the tear volume is deficient, hypofluorescence is likely.[87] The conjunctiva and cornea are examined for staining. The tear film break-up time is measured by asking the patient to blink and then to keep the eyelids open while the examiner counts the seconds until the appearance of a dry spot. A break-up time of 10 seconds or longer is considered normal.[60]

If fluorescein staining is not observed, rose bengal staining should be done (Figure 5-7). Conventionally, rose bengal stain was thought to stain devitalized epithelial cells; however, one study suggested that rose bengal staining occurs wherever there is poor protection of the surface epithelium by the tear film, and that a dysfunctional mucin layer, rather than lack of cell vitality, gives rise to staining.[88] Rose bengal is also useful in identifying filaments.

The remainder of the eye examination is carried out in the usual fashion, noting particularly the eyelid position, eyelid action, and conditions of the media that might cause increased glare or light sensitivity.

Diagnostic Tests for Dry Eyes

Several diagnostic tests are available to aid the clinician in the diagnosis of keratoconjunctivitis sicca, including measurement of tear osmolarity, lysozyme, and lactoferrin; fluorescein and rose bengal staining; the Schirmer test; and impression cytology. Galen and Gambino[89] demonstrated the limits of a normal range with diagnostic tests. A referent value concept is provided, which makes testing more meaningful by indicating the predictive value. A variety of tear tests have been compared in normal and diseased populations using the referent value concept.[90]

An established sequence of tests is desirable to prevent one test from interfering with another. Tests to determine the resting state of tears should be done before tests that cause reflex tearing.[91] The effects of eye medications should be eliminated by having the patient discontinue all ocular ointments at least 4 days before testing and ocular drops at midnight the night before.

Measurement of tear osmolarity is a sensitive test for dry eyes.[92] A small sample of tears from the inferior marginal tear strip is collected with a glass micropipette before reflex tears dilute the sample. Tear osmolarity is measured in a freezing point nanoliter osmometer. A value of 312 mOsm/L or greater is considered diagnostic of dry eyes. Tear osmolarity has been shown to be more than 90 percent sensitive and 95 percent specific for dry eyes.[93,94]

Lysozyme is an enzyme produced by the main and accessory lacrimal glands that reduces the local concentration of susceptible bacteria by attacking the mucopeptides of their cell walls.[95] Lactoferrin, another tear protein, has bacteriostatic properties, presumably because of its ability to make certain metals unavailable to microorganisms.[96] Both tear lysozyme and lactoferrin concentrations are decreased in dry eyes. Tear lactoferrin levels less than 90 mg/dl raise the suspicion of a lacrimal gland deficiency capable of producing dry eyes. Although the test is neither sensitive (35 percent) nor specific (70 percent) as a diagnostic test for keratoconjunctivitis sicca,[93] it is helpful in determining the bacterial resistance of tears.

The Schirmer test (Figure 5-8), introduced in 1903, is a readily available clinical test of lacrimal secretion, and is most useful in demonstrating the ability of the lacrimal gland to produce reflex tears.[97,98] The Schirmer test without anesthetic is extremely specific (90 percent) when a cut-off value of 1 mm/min of wetting is used.[93] However, many patients with dry eyes are missed because of the insensitivity (25 percent) of the test. Attempts have been made to measure basal tear secretion by anesthetizing the conjunctiva and cornea with topical anesthetic before inserting a Schirmer filter paper strip. For this procedure, it is important to dry the fornix after the anesthetic is instilled and before the filter paper strip is inserted. Although a 40 percent mean reduction in test values was obtained in one study, abnormally low test values of 0 to 3 mm of wetting in 5 minutes were obtained in 15 percent of normal volunteers.[99] Administration of an anesthetic prior to Schirmer testing does not completely anesthetize the conjunctiva. Therefore, reflex tearing is not completely suppressed; the initial reflex tearing after insertion of the Schirmer

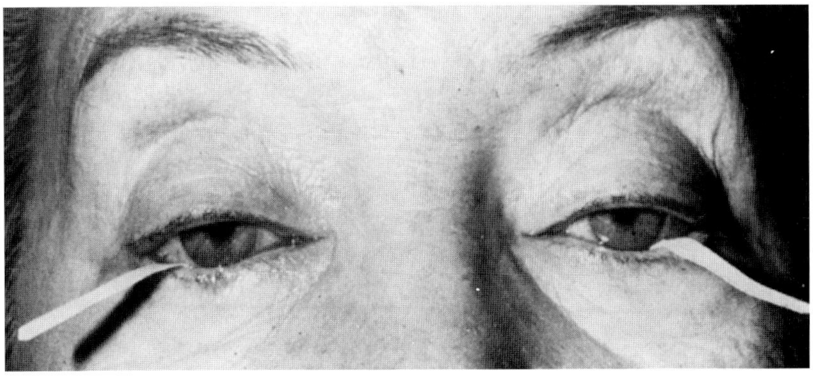

FIGURE 5-8 For the Schirmer test, filter paper strips are placed at the junction of the middle and lateral third of the inferior fornix.

strip is merely dampened.[100] Although the results of the Schirmer test have been reported to be inconsistent,[101] the test remains a simple, fast, and inexpensive way of assessing tear production.

Impression cytology was introduced in ophthalmology by Egbert et al in 1977,[102] and involves pressing and removing cellulose acetate paper on the ocular surface and staining the adherent cell layer. Impression cytology has demonstrated a decreased concentration of conjunctival goblet cells and an increased cytoplasm/nucleus ratio in conjunctival epithelial cells in patients with dry eyes.[103,104]

Comparison of the results of diagnostic tests in patients with dry eyes and normal subjects reveals considerable overlap of basal tear volumes, the results of Schirmer tests with and without anesthetic, rose bengal staining, and concentrations of lysozyme and lactoferrin in basal and reflex tears. The Schirmer test without anesthetic and rose bengal staining are the most specific tests (90 percent), but suffer from low sensitivity (25 percent and 58 percent, respectively). The most sensitive tests are tear osmolarity (90 percent sensitivity) and determinations of percent increases in lactoferrin concentration from basal to reflex tears (96 percent sensitivity).[89,93]

Treatment

The primary goals in the treatment of dry eyes are to relieve discomfort, provide a smooth optical surface, and prevent structural damage to the cornea.[105] Treatment of underlying diseases, avoidance of inciting causes, and frequent instillation of solutions that do not present the risk of toxicity or allergy seem, for the present, to be the most successful forms of therapy. Consideration must be given to adverse reactions that can be caused by some preservatives or vehicles used in such solutions. Patients with dry eyes are particularly susceptible to preservatives because the preservatives are not diluted by normal tear flow. There are very few circumstances that warrant asking patients to use medications that make them more uncomfortable. Excessive use of eye drops can disturb the tear film and increase evaporation, resulting in exacerbation of symptoms.[106]

Treatment of Underlying Diseases and Avoidance of Inciting Causes

A patient's history may reveal the cause of dry eyes, and appropriate treatment should begin with the elimination of this cause. Any systemic diseases associated with dry eyes should be treated.

It is particularly important that ophthalmologists be aware of the systemic disorders that are frequently associated with dry eyes.[107] Lymphoma and autoimmune disorders should be considered first. Appropriate referral for diagnosis and management is extremely rewarding in such cases. The lacrimal gland appears to be quite sensitive to antigen-antibody reactions, and may reflect a general condition that is manifested in other organ systems. It has been reported that dry eyes occur at a greater frequency in men infected with the human immunodeficiency virus (HIV) than in the general population (21 percent vs. 1 percent).[108] A similar increased incidence was noted also in HIV-infected females.[109] Decreased lactoferrin levels in the tears and increased bacterial flora on the eyelids were also found in HIV-positive patients.[110]

Systemic drugs that decrease tearing should be eliminated whenever possible. In many patients with systemic disorders that would become worse without these medications, the dry eyes must be treated by other means. Systemic drugs that increase tearing have not been widely employed.

As noted earlier, excessive tearing, which may be induced by a variety of agents, can produce dry eyes as a result of increased evaporation caused by dilution of the normal superficial lipid layer of the tears. Also, the tear film break-up time decreases as a result of the dilution of mucin that occurs during excessive tearing. Treatment of an allergic condition by elimination of the antigen or by the use of antihistamines improves symptoms and allows the establishment of a normal tear film. However, the identification and elimination of the causative antigen is sometimes difficult. Therefore, the use of suppressive medications, such as decongestants containing vasoconstrictors and antihistamines, cromolyn,[111] ketorolac, or mild corticosteroids, may be required periodically.

Eyelid and eyelash abnormalities frequently play a role in producing tear film deficiencies. The meibomian secretions of fair-skinned individuals appear to be different from those of other individuals and have some component or characteristic that makes them more apt to cling to the eyelid margins and more difficult to remove. Meibomian secretions are primarily lipid; abnormal lipids lessen the wetting properties of the tear film. Improvement of eyelid hygiene can produce dramatic improvement in dry eye symptoms and in the appearance of the tear film. Excessive meibomian secretions that cling to the eyelashes must be removed daily with warm compresses and lid scrubs (see Ch. 4). Small amounts of topical corticosteroid ointment applied after these eyelid treatments reduce inflammation and may increase patients' acceptance of the hygienic methods required to eliminate excessive meibomian secretions.[112] Systemic tetracycline may be necessary to control lipid abnormalities of the eyelids and tear film.

Oily scales of seborrhea are commonly associated with excessive and abnormal meibomian secretions, so attention must also be given to areas adjacent to the eyelid where sebaceous glands are concentrated, particularly the nasolabial folds and between the eyebrows. The use of antiseborrhea shampoos and creams is frequently necessary to clear up this skin condition.

Localized eyelid, conjunctival, and corneal abnormalities that create a disruption of the tear film should be treated. Trichiasis and verrucae on the eyelid border may produce local defects in the tear film and impair the tear surfacing function of the eyelids. Ptosis surgery or the anterior displacement of an encircling band after retinal detachment surgery can also interfere with eyelid function. Pterygia, pingueculae, and corneal scars produce elevations on the ocular surface that also lead to localized defects in the tear film. Adjacent to these elevations, areas of corneal thinning or dellen formation may arise from localized increases in the rate of evaporation caused by defects in the tear film.[113]

Dry air is a frequent cause of dry eyes and should be eliminated with the use of a humidifier. Direct air currents should be avoided.

Artificial Tears

Several attempts have been made to produce an artificial tear that emulates human tears,[114–117] and many artificial tear products are on the market (Table 5-2). The goals of therapy with artificial tears are to provide moisture, surface wetting, comfort, and retention of the solution for as long as possible. Artificial tear solutions usually contain a polymer that thickens the solution. Polyvinyl alcohol is one such polymer.[118] Lipid-containing eye drops have been reported to improve the tear film break-up time, but none can deliver lipid in a practical way to form a continuous monolayer of lipid on the surface of the tear film.[119] In the past, artificial tears were thick and viscous; they were retained for long periods and they soothed irritated surfaces, but with continued use, these solutions dried on the eyelid margins and formed concretions.[120,121] In an attempt to avoid concretions and to provide more moisture, artificial tears of low viscosity were developed.[122] Recent studies demonstrating that patients with dry eyes have a hypertonic tear film led to the development of hypotonic artificial tear solutions.[92,123]

Preservatives are used in artificial tear solutions to prevent bacterial contamination and to allow longer shelf life after the container is opened. A variety of preservatives have been used. The most common ones are thimerosal, chlorhexidine, phenylmercuric acetate, chlorobutanol, paraben, and benzalkonium chloride. Several artificial tears also contain ethylenediaminetetraacetic acid (EDTA). Patients may develop contact sensitivity to eye drops or other medications containing these compounds.[49] The increased incidence of such allergies in soft contact lens wearers led to the use of new preservatives and the development of preservative-free lens care systems.[124,125]

Preservatives may cause toxic reactions in patients who use artificial tears frequently.[126,127] Nonpreserved artificial tears can be useful to these patients.[128] Some patients prefer to make their own artificial tear mixtures from a combination of herbs and spring water, but this practice should be discouraged. Sterility is of great concern because *Pseudomonas* and *Acanthamoeba* are contaminants of spring or tap water, and even distilled water may not be sterile.

Viscoelastic Substances

One percent sodium hyaluronate diluted to 0.1 percent with saline has been used as an artificial tear solution.[129–132] Sodium hyaluronate is a viscoelastic substance that coats surfaces and binds water, thus providing a mucin-like addition to the tear film. Chondroitin sulfate 1 percent, a mixture of 0.38 percent chondroitin sulfate and 0.3 percent sodium hyaluronate, and methylcellulose have also been used to treat dry eyes.[133,134] Patients with severe dry eyes appeared to prefer a solution containing chondroitin sulfate to a solution containing sodium hyaluronate, but none of the viscoelastic solutions was

TABLE 5-2
Constituents of Medications for Dry Eyes

Trade Name	*Manufacturer*	*Ingredients*	*Preservatives*
Drops			
Adsorbotear	Alcon	Hydroxymethylcellulose 0.4% Povidone 1.67% with water-soluble polymers	Thimerosal 0.004% Edetate disodium 0.1%
AKWA Tears	Akorn	Polyvinyl alcohol 1.4% Sodium chloride Mono- and dibasic sodium phosphates Edetate disodium Purified water	Benzalkonium chloride 0.01%
AquaSite	CIBA Vision	Polyethylene glycol 400, 0.2% Dextran 70, 0.1% Polycarbophil Purified water Sodium chloride Edetate disodium Sodium hydroxide to adjust pH	None
AquaSite multidose	CIBA Vision	Polyethylene glycol 400, 0.2% Dextran 70, 0.1% Polycarbophil Purified water Sodium chloride Edetate disodium Sodium hydroxide to adjust pH	Sorbic acid 0.2%
Bion Tears	Alcon	Water-soluble polymeric system containing Dextran 70, 0.1% and hydroxypropyl methylcellulose 2910, 0.3% Sodium chloride Potassium chloride Sodium bicarbonate Magnesium chloride Calcium chloride Zinc chloride Purified water Hydrochloric acid and/or sodium hydroxide and/or carbon dioxide to adjust pH	None
Celluvisc	Allergan	Carboxymethylcellulose sodium 1.0% Calcium chloride Potassium chloride Purified water Sodium chloride Sodium lactate	None
Collyrium Fresh	Wyeth Labs	Tetrahydrozoline HCl 0.05% Glycerin 1.0% Edetate disodium 0.1% Boric acid Hydrochloric acid Sodium borate	Benzalkonium chloride 0.01%
Dry Eye Therapy	Bausch & Lomb	Glycerin 0.3% Calcium chloride Magnesium chloride Purified water Potassium chloride Sodium chloride Sodium citrate Sodium phosphate Zinc chloride	None

TABLE 5-2 *(continued)*

Trade Name	*Manufacturer*	*Ingredients*	*Preservatives*
HypoTears	IOLAB	Polyvinyl alcohol 1% Polyethylene glycol 400, 1% Dextrose Edetate disodium Purified water	Benzalkonium chloride 0.01%
HypoTears PF	IOLAB	Polyvinyl alcohol 1% Polyethylene glycol 400, 1% Dextrose Edetate disodium Purified water	None
Isopto Alkaline	Alcon	Hydroxypropyl methylcellulose 2910, 1% Mono- and dibasic sodium phosphates Sodium citrate Sodium chloride Purified water	Benzalkonium chloride 0.01%
Isopto Tears	Alcon	Hydroxypropyl methylcellulose 2910, 0.5% Mono- and dibasic sodium phosphates Sodium citrate Sodium chloride Purified water	Benzalkonium chloride 0.01%
Isopto Plain	Alcon	Hydroxypropyl methylcellulose 2910, 0.5% Mono- and dibasic sodium phosphates Sodium citrate Sodium chloride Purified water	Benzalkonium chloride 0.01%
Liquifilm Forte	Allergan	Polyvinyl alcohol 3.0% Edetate disodium Mono- and dibasic sodium phosphates Purified water Sodium chloride Hydrochloric acid or sodium hydroxide to adjust pH	Thimerosal 0.002%
Liquifilm Tears	Allergan	Polyvinyl alcohol 1.4% Purified water Sodium chloride Hydrochloric acid or sodium hydroxide to adjust pH	Chlorobutanol 0.5%
Moisture Drops	Bausch & Lomb	Hydroxypropyl methylcellulose 0.5% Povidone 0.1% Glycerin 0.2% Boric acid Edetate disodium Potassium chloride Sodium borate Sodium chloride	Benzalkonium chloride 0.01%
Murocel	Bausch & Lomb	Methylcellulose 1% Boric acid Propylene glycol Purified water Sodium borate Sodium chloride	Methylparaben 0.023% Propylparaben 0.01%
OcuCoat	Lederle	Dextran 70, 0.1% Hydroxypropyl methylcellulose 2910, 0.8% Mono- and dibasic sodium phosphates Potassium chloride Sodium chloride Dextrose Purified water May also contain hydrochloric acid and/or sodium hydroxide to adjust pH	Benzalkonium chloride 0.01%

TABLE 5-2 *(continued)*

Trade Name	*Manufacturer*	*Ingredients*	*Preservatives*
OcuCoat PF	Lederle	Dextran 70, 0.1% Hydroxypropyl methylcellulose 2910, 0.8% Mono- and dibasic sodium phosphates Potassium chloride Sodium chloride Dextrose Purified water May also contain hydrochloric acid and/or sodium hydroxide to adjust pH	None
Refresh	Allergan	Polyvinyl alcohol 1.4% Povidone 0.6% Purified water Sodium chloride Hydrochloric acid or sodium hydroxide to adjust pH	None
Refresh Plus Cellufresh formula	Allergan	Carboxymethylcellulose sodium 0.5% Calcium chloride Magnesium chloride Potassium chloride Purified water Sodium chloride Sodium lactate Hydrochloric acid or sodium hydroxide to adjust pH	None
Tears Naturale	Alcon	A water-soluble polymeric system containing Dextran 70, 0.1%, and hydroxypropyl methylcellulose 2910, 0.3% Potassium chloride Sodium chloride Edetate disodium Purified water Hydrochloric acid and/or sodium hydroxide to adjust pH	Benzalkonium chloride 0.01%
Tears Naturale II	Alcon	A water-soluble polymeric system containing Dextran 70, 0.1% and hydroxypropyl methylcellulose 2910, 0.3% Sodium borate Potassium chloride Sodium chloride Purified water Hydrochloric acid and/or sodium hydroxide to adjust pH	Polyquaternium-1, 0.001%
Tears Naturale Free	Alcon	A water-soluble polymeric system containing Dextran 70, 0.1% and hydroxypropyl methylcellulose 2910, 0.3% Sodium borate Potassium chloride Sodium chloride Purified water Hydrochloric acid and/or sodium hydroxide to adjust pH	None
Tears Plus	Allergan	Polyvinyl alcohol 1.4% Povidone 0.6% Sodium chloride Purified water Hydrochloric acid and/or sodium hydroxide to adjust pH	Chlorobutanol 0.5%
Tears Renewed	Akorn	Hydroxypropyl methylcellulose 2906, 0.3% Dextran 70, 0.1% Sodium chloride	Benzalkonium chloride 0.01%

TABLE 5-2 (*continued*)

Trade Name	*Manufacturer*	*Ingredients*	*Preservatives*
		Potassium chloride Edetate disodium Hydrochloric acid and/or sodium hydroxide to adjust pH Purified water USP	
Ultra Tears	Alcon	Hydroxypropyl methylcellulose 2910, 1% Mono- and dibasic sodium phosphates Sodium citrate Sodium chloride Purified water	Benzalkonium chloride 0.01%
Ointments			
AKWA Tears Ointment	Akorn	White petrolatum Mineral oil	None
DuoLube	Bausch & Lomb	White petrolatum 80% Mineral oil 20%	None
Duratears Naturale	Alcon	White petrolatum Anhydrous liquid lanolin Mineral oil	None
HypoTears	IOLAB	White petrolatum Light mineral oil	None
Lacri-Lube NP	Allergan	White petrolatum 57.3% Mineral oil 42.5% Lanolin alcohols	None
Lacri-Lube S.O.P	Allergan	White petrolatum 56.8% Mineral oil 42.5% Lanolin alcohols	Chlorobutanol
Tears Renewed	Akorn	White petrolatum Light mineral oil	None
Refresh PM	Allergan	White petrolatum 56.8% Mineral oil 41.5% Lanolin alcohols Purified water Sodium chloride	None
Inserts			
Lacrisert Sterile Ophthalmic Insert	Merck & Co.	Hydroxypropyl cellulose 5 mg	None

preferred by a majority of dry eye patients over a polyvinyl alcohol artificial tear solution.[132,134]

Ointments

Some patients find that instillation of an ointment with a petroleum base prevents dryness of the eyes. However, such ointments contain minimal amounts of moisture, and thus may have little value other than providing lubrication and preventing adhesion between the eyelids and the conjunctiva. In some cases, the drying may be so severe that the ointment acts as a foreign body and produces irritation rather than relief. Moreover, ointments remain in contact with the ocular surface longer than do solutions, and sensitivity to preservatives may be more of a problem with ointments than with solutions. Ointments without preservatives are available. Many patients object to the use of ointments during waking hours because they are unsightly and cause blurred vision. Therefore, ointments are most easily accepted and commonly used at bedtime.

Artificial Tear Inserts

Polymer inserts without preservatives (Lacrisert) have been developed that slowly dissolve in the presence of adequate moisture. In the eye, these inserts provide continuous release of polymer.[135–138] However, many patients with dry eyes do not have sufficient tears to melt an insert and must rely on continued use of artificial tears for this purpose. A trial of the tear insert in the office before prescribing is helpful to determine whether the patient shows improvement. Some dexterity is required to insert the

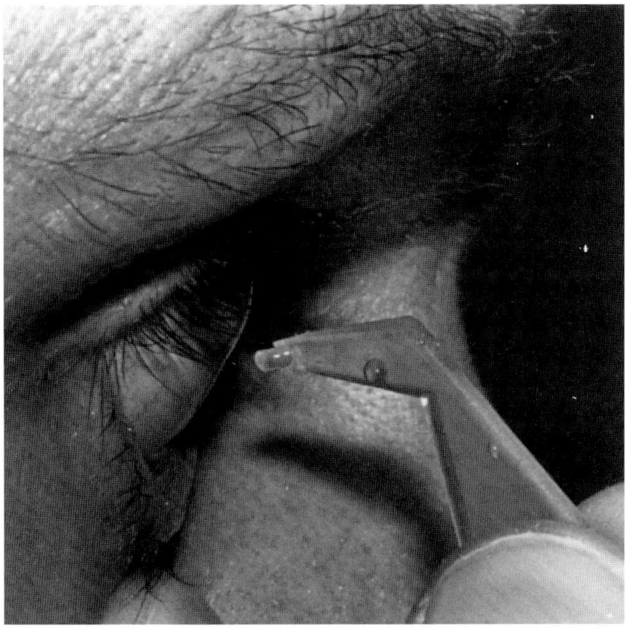

FIGURE 5-9 Lacrisert in applicator about to be applied to inferior fornix. (Reprinted with permission from HE Kaufman: Keratitis sicca. Int Ophthalmol Clin 24:133, 1984.)

tear inserts properly; the patient must be taught how to handle them and how to make sure that they are in the proper position in the inferior fornix[139] (Figure 5-9). The polymer inserts may be used once or twice daily in addition to artificial tears.

Punctal Occlusion

Occlusion of the lacrimal puncta prevents tear drainage, which preserves the natural tears and prolongs the effect of artificial tears that are instilled.[105] However, there is evidence that tear drainage automatically decreases as tear volume decreases, so the effectiveness of this mode of therapy may be more theoretical than actual.[2] The reported results of punctal occlusion vary: in one series of 30 patients with tear deficiencies, 33 percent showed improvement[140]; in another series of 32 patients, improvement was noted in all patients.[141] Although no difficulties with epiphora were reported in the studies, this possibility merits some concern. Temporary occlusion by silicone plugs[142,143] (Figure 5-10), sutures (Figure 5-11), tissue adhesive,[144] or light cautery seems desirable before deep canalicular cauterization[141] or excision[145] is used to effect permanent occlusion. Collagen plugs do not totally occlude the lacrimal drainage system, and fail to predict epiphora after permanent occlusion in some patients.[146] Five types of complications have been reported with silicone plugs: insertion of the plug too far into the canaliculus, spontaneous loss of the plug into the canaliculus, extrusion of the plug, scarring of the punctum, and ocular surface irritation.[147–149]

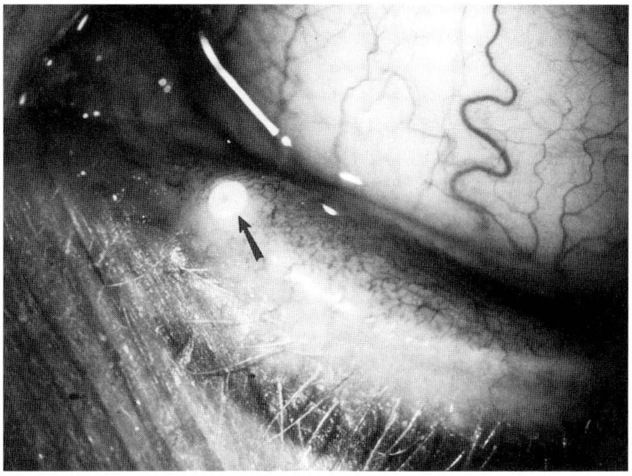

FIGURE 5-10 Punctal plug (arrow).

Punctal occlusion with cautery is done by inserting the tip of a hand-held cautery through the punctum to the full depth of the vertical canaliculus and cauterizing the canaliculus and punctum (Figure 5-12). Deep cauterization of the canaliculus is superior to superficial cauterization of the punctum when permanent punctal occlusion is desired because the incidence of reopening of the punctum is lower with the deep method.[150] Thermal destruction of the punctum with an argon laser (laser punctoplasty) produces only superficial closure and is considerably more expensive and less effective than deep cauterization with a hand-held cautery.[151]

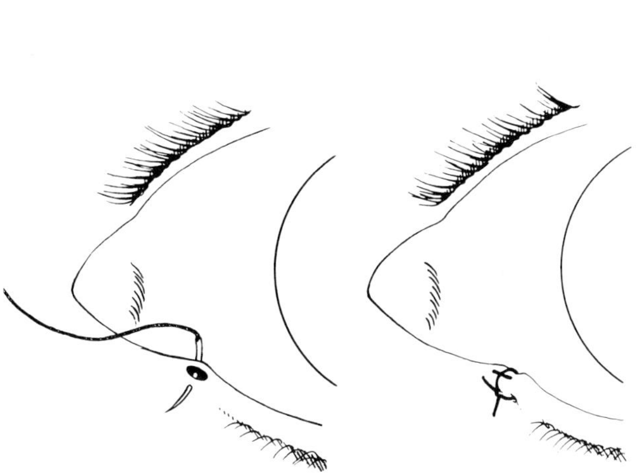

FIGURE 5-11 In testing for the usefulness of punctal occlusion in a given patient, a suture is placed through the punctum, temporarily occluding it. (Reprinted with permission from HE Kaufman: Keratitis sicca. Int Ophthalmol Clin 24:133, 1984.)

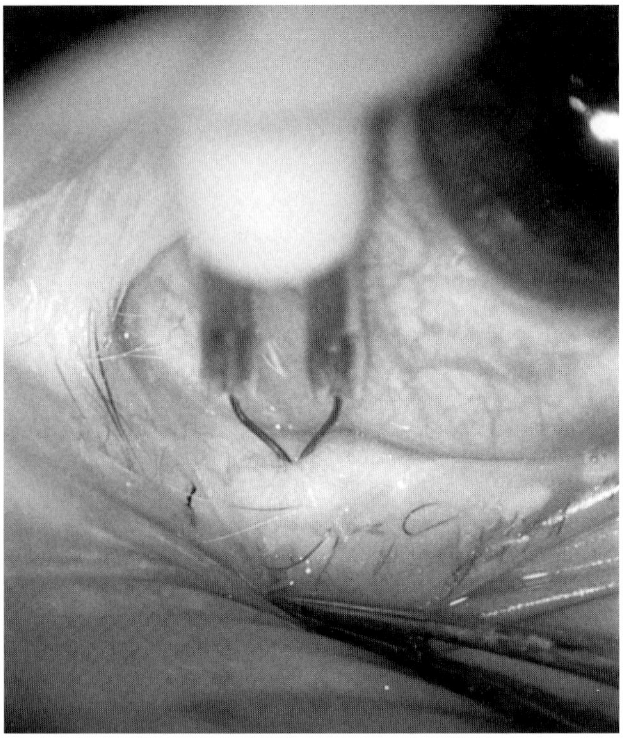

FIGURE 5-12 Punctal occlusion with a hand-held cautery. The tip of the cautery is inserted into the punctum and canaliculus. The cautery is turned on as it is withdrawn.

Moist Chambers

The wearing of a clear plastic bubble over the eye prevents evaporation of tears, but unfortunately, leads to the accumulation of condensation, so that vision is impaired.[152] Holes can be made in the plastic bubble, or a pair of moist chamber spectacles can be constructed with enough clearance from the face to prevent condensation. The major difficulty is finding an optician who is willing to take the time to fashion such moist chamber spectacles, although methods for their construction have been published.[153–155] Swimmer's goggles coated with an antifogging substance have also been used for this purpose.[156] In addition to preventing evaporation, the bubbles or goggles eliminate exposure of the eyes to air currents that increase evaporation. Although these devices are somewhat less than optimal cosmetically, most patients obtain some relief from their use. They are especially valuable in patients with lagophthalmos.

Mucolytic Agents

In the presence of deficient tear volume, mucin accumulates as strands and blobs in the precorneal tear film, corneal filaments or plaques, and enlarged strands in the inferior fornix.[67,68] *N*-Acetylcysteine in 5 to 20 percent concentrations is effective in dissolving excess mucin and rendering the cornea more wettable because of its ability to break the disulfide cross-linkage of mucin.[8] Some patients complain of excessive burning on instillation of the medication, although others use it two to four times a day with great relief. The use of *N*-acetylcysteine on the ocular surface has not been approved by the Food and Drug Administration, and pharmacists are therefore frequently reluctant to dispense the medication, which comes with a convenient dropper for use by pulmonary patients who instill it in atomizers or humidifiers. It is easily contaminated and, when diluted half and half with preserved artificial tears, may not be protected by the preservative. Systemic and topical bromhexine hydrochloride has been reported as an improved mucolytic agent for the treatment of dry eyes, but its effectiveness has not been confirmed.[157,158]

Parotid Duct Translocation

Thirty years ago, attempts were made to relieve dry eyes by translocating the parotid duct to the inferior fornix, thereby providing parotid secretions as a replacement for tears.[159–161] Although there are considerable chemical differences between parotid gland secretions and tears, the moisture provided prevents drying. Unfortunately, the parotid gland frequently secretes more fluid than is required by the eye, and the rate of secretion increases during eating.[162] In addition, some patients do not benefit from this procedure for long because of the eventual development of Sjögren's syndrome in the salivary glands as well as in the lacrimal glands. Recent studies have shown, however, that there is considerable variation in the association of lacrimal and salivary gland disease in Sjögren's syndrome. Therefore, translocation of the salivatory duct may be worth reconsidering in view of this new information.

Artificial Tear Pumps

Battery-powered infusion pumps the size of a cigarette pack have been developed to treat severe dry eyes.[163] A similar device delivers artificial tears to the lower fornix through an implanted small-bore plastic tube that enters at the patient's ear and comes through the lower eyelid into the fornix.[164] These devices are cumbersome and easily contaminated, but they provide continuous, low-dose delivery during waking hours. Spectacles with tear reservoirs in the temples that empty through connecting tubes directly into the lacrimal lake in response to gravitational or periodic head movements have been constructed, but have never been widely used.

Contact Lenses

Hard contact lenses may be beneficial to patients with dry eyes by stimulating reflex tearing and thus increasing the volume of tears.[165] Hard scleral contact lenses may be even more beneficial because they cover more of the cornea and conjunctiva, and thus prevent evaporation from a large portion of the ocular surface.[166] Soft contact lenses may have the same benefit, and in addition, provide a moist covering of the entire cornea that prevents some of the surface erosions indicated by staining.[167] A lens with a high water content is considered by some to be less desirable than one with a low water content because a larger supply of tears is required to keep up with the evaporation from the surface of the hydrophilic high-water-content lens material.[168]

Contact lens wear by patients with dry eyes is risky and can cause severe problems,[167,169,170] and there is no place for the use of contact lenses alone for the treatment of dry eyes. Concomitant use of artificial tear drops and frequent check-ups are essential. Alertness to possible allergic or toxic reactions to the preservatives used in contact lens solutions and cleaning systems is important, because patients with dry eyes are prone to the development of both toxic and allergic reactions. A heat disinfection system that includes no preservatives, or a chemical cleaning and storage system with preservatives known to produce only a low incidence of allergic or toxic reactions, is preferred. Daily-wear disposable contact lenses, which have recently become available, provide another alternative.

Staging of Dry Eye Therapy

A variety of therapeutic options are available for treating dry eyes, as discussed in the preceding sections. An approach is recommended in which the treatment is advanced in stages according to the severity of the condition and its response to each level of therapy.[91] Various causes of dry eyes should be explored, and any underlying or associated eye disorders treated. For mild dry eyes, artificial tears are recommended three or four times a day. Less expensive multidose artificial tears that contain a preservative are usually satisfactory. For moderate dry eyes, artificial tears without preservatives should be used as often as every 2 hours. Spectacles may be worn to block drying air currents. For severe dry eyes, punctal occlusion should be done, temporarily at first. Preservative-free artificial tears are continued as necessary. For extremely severe dry eyes, Lacriserts may be used along with preservative-free artificial tears and punctal occlusion. Low-water-content soft contact lenses may be worn, but carry the attendant risk of infection. Moist chamber spectacles are useful in patients who do not respond to these measures.

Reassurance

One of the most important aspects in the treatment of dry eyes is the need to reassure patients that their vision will be preserved despite some continued discomfort. These patients require time and patience on the part of the physician, in the attention they receive as they describe their symptoms, the care with which the eye examination is performed, and the explanations they are given about their condition.[171]

An emotional component is commonly apparent in the description of symptoms associated with tear abnormalities. Frequently, the severity of the reported symptoms is out of proportion to the clinical signs. It is possible that subclinical disease produces symptoms that cannot be detected by present methods of slit lamp examination and tear film evaluation. It is equally possible that patients become distressed when they are told that their disease is chronic. Patients may rapidly develop an attitude of hopelessness about their condition that is made worse by the feeling that the physician seems not to care.

Patients should be informed in the beginning that they have a chronic condition. Furthermore, they should be told that dry eyes usually do not progressively worsen and that symptoms will probably respond to treatment. It is also important that patients be encouraged to return for regular follow-up care, and that they be permitted to come in when their symptoms worsen unexpectedly. It is certainly possible to overmedicate patients with dry eyes with antibiotics and corticosteroids that interfere with the normal healing process required to repair desquamated surface epithelium. Patients who have corneal ulcers or severe scarring in association with dry eyes may have been exposed to excessive medication or their eye condition may not have been given proper attention, as a result of either their own neglect or that of a physician. A primary goal in the treatment of dry eyes should be to keep the patient out of trouble. Once patients understand and accept their condition, they are better able to maintain an acceptable level of comfort with artificial tear preparations and to control their environment as much as possible in order to minimize exacerbation of their condition by external factors.

REFERENCES

1. Van Haeringen NJ: Clinical biochemistry of tears. Surv Ophthalmol 26:84, 1981
2. Mishima S, Gassett A, Klyce SD, et al: Determination of tear volume and tear flow. Invest Ophthalmol 5:264, 1966
3. Mathers WD, Binarao G, Petroll M: Ocular water evaporation and the dry eye. A new measuring device. Cornea 12:335, 1993
4. Jordan A, Baum JL: Basic tear flow. Does it exist? Ophthalmology 87:920, 1980

5. Stuchell RN, Farris RL, Mandel ID: Basal and reflex human tear analysis. II. Chemical analysis: lactoferrin and lysozyme. Ophthalmology 88:858, 1981
6. Jones LT: The lacrimal secretory system and its treatment. Am J Ophthalmol 62:74, 1966
7. Farris RL, Stuchell RN, Mandel ID: Basal and reflex human tear analysis. I. Physical measurements: osmolarity, basal volumes, and reflex flow rate. Ophthalmology 88:852, 1981
8. Farris RL: Tear analysis in contact lens wearers. CLAO J 12:106, 1986
9. deRoetth A, Sr: Lacrimation in normal eyes. Arch Ophthalmol 49:185, 1953
10. Dohlman CH, Lemp AM, English FP: Dry eye syndromes. Int Ophthalmol Clin 10:215, 1970
11. Jones DB: Prospects in the management of tear-deficient states. Trans Am Acad Ophthalmol Otolaryngol 83:OP693, 1977
12. Holly FJ, Lemp MA: Tear physiology and dry eyes. Surv Ophthalmol 22:69, 1977
13. Riley CM, Day RL, Greeley D, et al: Central autonomic dysfunction with defective lacrimation. Pediatrics 3:468, 1949
14. Liebman SD: Riley-Day syndrome: long-term ophthalmologic observations. Trans Am Ophthalmol Soc 66:95, 1968
15. Mondino BJ, Brown SI: Hereditary congenital alacrima. Arch Ophthalmol 94:1478, 1976
16. Duke-Elder S: System of Ophthalmology. Vol. III, Part 2. Congenital Deformities. CV Mosby, St. Louis, 1963
17. Walsh FB, Hoyt WF: Clinical Neuro-Ophthalmology. Vol. 1. Williams & Wilkins, Baltimore, 1969
18. Manthorpe R, Frost-Larson K, Isager H, et al: Sjögren's syndrome. Allergy 36:139, 1981
19. Forstot JZ, Forstot SL, Greer RO, Tan EM: The incidence of Sjögren's sicca complex in a population of patients with keratoconjunctivitis sicca. Arthritis Rheum 25:156, 1982
20. Baum JL: Systemic diseases associated with tear deficiencies. Int Ophthalmol Clin 13:157, 1973
21. Font RL, Yanoff M, Zimmerman LE: Benign lymphoepithelial lesion of the lacrimal gland and its relationship to Sjögren's syndrome. Am J Clin Pathol 18:365, 1967
22. Shearn MA: Sjögren's syndrome. p. 213. In Smith LH (ed): Major Problems in Internal Medicine. Vol. 2. WB Saunders, Philadelphia, 1971
23. Duke-Elder S: System of Ophthalmology. Vol. XIII, Part 2. The Ocular Adnexa. CV Mosby, St. Louis, 1974
24. Jack ML, Jack GM, Sale GE, et al: Ocular manifestations of graft-vs-host disease. Arch Ophthalmol 101:1080, 1983
25. Sjögren H, Block KK: Keratoconjunctivitis sicca and the Sjögren syndrome. Surv Ophthalmol 16:145, 1971
26. Fox RI, Howell FV, Bone RC, Michelson P: Primary Sjögren's syndrome: clinical and immunopathologic features. Semin Arthritis Rheum 14:77, 1984
27. Hamburger MI, Moutsopoulos HM, Lawley TJ, et al: Sjögren's syndrome: a defect in reticuloendothelial system Fc-receptor-specific clearance. Ann Intern Med 91:534, 1979
28. Moutsopoulos HM (moderator): NIH conference: Sjögren's syndrome (sicca syndromes): current issues. Ann Intern Med 92:212, 1980
29. Forstot SL, Forstot JL, Peebles CL, et al: Serologic studies in patients with keratoconjunctivitis sicca. Arch Ophthalmol 99:888, 1981
30. Pflugfelder SC, Wilhelmus KR, Osato MS, et al: The autoimmune nature of the aqueous tear deficiency. Ophthalmology 93:1513, 1986
31. Farris RL, Stuchell RN, Nisengard R: Sjögren's syndrome and keratoconjunctivitis sicca. Cornea 10:207, 1991
32. Fraunfelder FT: Drug Induced Ocular Side Effects and Drug Interactions. Lea & Febiger, Philadelphia, 1976
33. Kaden I, Mayers M: Systemic associations of dry-eye syndrome. Int Ophthalmol Clin 31:69, 1991
34. Bergmann MT, Newman BL, Johnson NC Jr: The effect of a diuretic (hydrochlorothiazide) on tear production in humans. Am J Ophthalmol 99:473, 1985
35. Mackie IA, Seal DV: Tear fluid lysozyme concentrations: guide to practolol therapy. Br J Med 4:732, 1975
36. Mackie IA, Seal DV, Pescod JM: Beta-adrenergic receptor blocking drugs: tear lysozyme and immunological screening for adverse reaction. Br J Ophthalmol 61:354, 1977
37. McMahon CD, Shaffer RN, Haskins HD, et al: Adverse effects experienced by patients taking timolol. Am J Ophthalmol 88:736, 1979
38. Bonomi L, Zavarese G, Noya E, et al: Effects of timolol maleate on tear flow in human eyes. Albrecht von Graefes Arch Klin Exp Ophthalmol 213:19, 1980
39. Mishima S, Kubota Z, Farris RL: The tear flow dynamics in normal and in keratoconjunctivitis sicca cases. Excerpta Medica International Congress Series No. 222. Proceedings of the XXI International Congress, Mexico, March 1970
40. Gilbard JP, Farris RL: Ocular surface drying and tear film osmolarity in thyroid eye disease. Acta Ophthalmol (Copenh) 61:108, 1983
41. Tsubota K, Yamada M: Tear evaporation from the ocular surface. Invest Ophthalmol Vis Sci 33:2942, 1992
42. Doane MG: Interaction of eyelids and tears in corneal wetting and the dynamics of the normal human eyeblink. Am J Ophthalmol 89:507, 1980
43. Lemp MA, Weiler HH: How do tears exit? Invest Ophthalmol Vis Sci 24:619, 1983
44. Botelho SY, Hisada M, Fuenmayor N: Functional anatomy of the lacrimal gland in the cat. Origin of secretomotor fibers in the lacrimal nerve. Arch Ophthalmol 76:581, 1966
45. Frey WH, Desota-Johnson D, Hoffman C, et al: Effect of stimulus on the chemical composition of human tears. Am J Ophthalmol 92:559, 1981
46. Basu PK, Pimm PE, Shephard RJ, et al: The effect of cigarette smoke on the human tear film. Can J Ophthalmol 13:22,1978
47. Theodore FH, Schlossman A: Ocular Allergy. Williams & Wilkins, Baltimore, 1958
48. Grob D, McGehee H: Strong cholinesterase inhibitor (TEPP) produces excess lacrimation. Bull Johns Hopkins Hosp 84:532, 1949

49. Wilson RM: Adverse external ocular effects of topical ophthalmic medications. Surv Ophthalmol 24:57, 1979
50. Bogdanski DF, Sulser F, Brodie BB: Comparative action of reserpine, tetrabenazine and chlorpromazine on central parasympathetic activity: effects on pupillary size and lacrimation in rabbit and salivation in dog. J Pharmacol Exp Ther 132:176,1961
51. Dawson WW, Jimenez-Antillon CF, Perez JM, et al: Marijuana and vision—after ten years use in Costa Rica. Invest Ophthalmol Vis Sci 16:689, 1977
52. Hammersley J, Luce JK, Florentz TR, et al: Excessive lacrimation from fluorouracil treatment. JAMA 225:747, 1973
53. Bohigian GM: Management of infections associated with soft contact lenses. Ophthalmology 86:1138, 1979
54. Bertaccini G, Impicciatore M, Mossini F: Action of some N-methyl derivatives of histamine on salivary and lacrimal secretion of the cat. Biochem Pharmacol 21:3076, 1972
55. Lemp MA, Holly FJ, Iwata S, et al: The precorneal tear film. I. Factors in spreading and maintaining a continuous tear film over the corneal surface. Arch Ophthalmol 33:39, 1970
56. McEwen WK: Secretion of tears and blinking. p. 341. In Davson H (ed): The Eye. Academic Press, Orlando, FL, 1969
57. Holly FJ, Patten JT, Dohlman CH: Surface activity determination of aqueous tear components in dry eye patients and normals. Exp Eye Res 24:479, 1977
58. Holly FJ: Tear film physiology. Am J Optom Physiol Opt 57:252, 1980
59. Vanley GT, Leopold IH, Gregg TH: Interpretation of tear film breakup. Arch Ophthalmol 95:445, 1977
60. Lemp MA, Hamill JR: Factors affecting tear film breakup in normal eyes. Arch Ophthalmol 89:103, 1973
61. Lemp MA, Dohlman CH, Holly FJ: Corneal desiccation despite normal tear volume. Ann Ophthalmol 2:258, 1970
62. Lemp MA, Dohlman CH, Kuwabara T, et al: Dry eye secondary to mucus deficiency. Trans Am Acad Ophthalmol Otolaryngol 75:1223, 1971
63. Holly FJ, Lemp MA: Wettability and wetting of corneal epithelium. Exp Eye Res 11:239, 1971
64. Friend J, Kiorpes T, Thoft RA: Conjunctival goblet cell frequency after alkali injury is not accurately reflected by aqueous tear mucin content. Invest Ophthalmol Vis Sci 24:612, 1983
65. Iwata S, Kabasawa I: Fractionation and chemical properties of tear mucoids. Exp Eye Res 12:360, 1971
66. Chao CCW, Vergnes JP, Brown SI: Fractionation and partial characterization of macromolecular components from human ocular mucus. Exp Eye Res 36:139, 1983
67. Norm MS: Mucous thread in inferior conjunctival fornix. Quantitative analysis of the normal mucous thread. Acta Ophthalmol (Copenh) 44:33, 1966
68. Norm MS: Mucous flow in the conjunctiva. Rate of migration of the mucous thread in the inferior conjunctival fornix towards the inner canthus. Acta Ophthalmol (Copenh) 47:129, 1969
69. Zaidman GW, Geeraets R, Paylor RR, Ferry AP: The histopathology of filamentary keratitis. Arch Ophthalmol 103:1178, 1985
70. McCulley JP, Moore MB, Matoba AY: Mucus fishing syndrome. Ophthalmology 92:1262, 1985
71. Dohlman CH: The function of the corneal epithelium in health and disease. Invest Ophthalmol 10:383, 1971
72. Kenyon KR: Anatomy and Pathology of the Ocular Surface. Little, Brown, Boston, 1979
73. Matsuda H, Smelser GK: Epithelium and stroma in alkali-burned corneas. Arch Ophthalmol 89:396, 1973
74. Pfister RR: The normal surface of corneal epithelium: a scanning electron microscopic study. Invest Ophthalmol 12:654, 1973
75. Kenyon KR, Fogle JA, Stone DL, et al: Regeneration of corneal epithelium basement membrane following thermal cauterization. Invest Ophthalmol Vis Sci 16:292, 1977
76. Fogle JA, Kenyon KR, Stark WJ, et al: Defective epithelial adhesion in anterior corneal dystrophy. Am J Ophthalmol 79:925, 1975
77. Sommer A: Effects of vitamin A deficiency on the ocular surface. Ophthalmology 90:592, 1983
78. Pfister RR: The effects of chemical injury on the ocular surface. Ophthalmology 90:601, 1983
79. Tiffany JM: Individual variations in human meibomian lipid composition. Exp Eye Res 27:289, 1978
80. Chew CKS, Jansweijer C, Tiffany JM, et al: An instrument for quantifying meibomian lipid on the lid margin: the meibometer. Curr Eye Res 12:247, 1993
81. Mishima S, Maurice DM: Oily layer of tear film and evaporation from corneal surface. Exp Eye Res 1:39, 1961
82. Mathers WD: Ocular evaporation in meibomian gland dysfunction and dry eye. Ophthalmology 100:347, 1993
83. McCulley JP, Sciallis GF: Meibomian keratoconjunctivitis. Am J Ophthalmol 84:788, 1977
84. Hemady R, Chu W, Foster CS: Keratoconjunctivitis sicca and corneal ulcers. Cornea 9:170, 1990
85. Ormerod LD, Fong LP, Foster CS: Corneal infection in mucosal scarring disorders and Sjögren's syndrome. Am J Ophthalmol 105:512, 1988
86. Høvding G: The central corneal thickness in keratoconjunctivitis sicca. Acta Ophthalmol (Copenh) 70:108, 1992
87. Soper JW: Method of diagnosing deficiency of aqueous tears. Contact Lens Spectrum Jan:34, 1983
88. Feensta RPG, Tseng SCG: What is actually stained by rose bengal? Arch Ophthalmol 100:984, 1992
89. Galen RS, Gambino SR: Beyond Normality. John Wiley & Sons, New York, 1975
90. Farris RL, Gilbard JP, Stuchell RN, et al: Diagnostic tests in keratoconjunctivitis. CLAO J 9:23, 1983
91. Farris RL: Staged therapy for the dry eye. CLAO J 17:207,1991
92. Gilbard JP, Farris RL, Santamaria J: Osmolarity of tear microvolumes in keratoconjunctivitis sicca. Arch Ophthalmol 96:677, 1978
93. Lucca JA, Nunez JN, Farris RL: A comparison of diagnostic tests for keratoconjunctivitis sicca: lactoplate, Schirmer, and tear osmolarity. CLAO J 16:109, 1990

94. Farris RL: Tear osmolarity—a new gold standard? p. 495. In Sullivan DA (ed): Lacrimal Gland, Tear Film, and Dry Eye Syndromes. Plenum, New York, 1994
95. Smolin G: The defence mechanism of the outer eye. Trans Ophthalmol Soc UK 104:363, 1985
96. Broekhuyse RM: Tear lactoferrin: a bacteriostatic and complexing protein. Invest Ophthalmol 13:550, 1974
97. Baum J: Discussion of Farris RL, Stuchell RN, Mandel ID: Basal and reflex human tear analysis. Ophthalmology 88:862, 1981
98. Cho P, Yap M: Schirmer Test. I. A review. Optom Vis Sci 70:152, 1993
99. Lamberts DW, Foster CS, Perry HD: Schirmer test after topical anesthesia and tear meniscus height in normal eyes. Arch Ophthalmol 97:1082, 1979
100. Clinch TE, Benedetto DA, Felberg NT, et al: Schirmer's test. A closer look. Arch Ophthalmol 101:1383, 1983
101. Cho P, Yap M: Schirmer Test. II. A clinical study of its repeatability. Optom Vis Sci 70:157, 1993
102. Egbert PR, Lauber S, Maurice DM: A simple conjunctival biopsy. Am J Ophthalmol 84:798, 1977
103. Rolando M, Terragna F, Giordano G, Calabria G: Conjunctival surface damage distribution in keratoconjunctivitis sicca. Ophthalmologica 200:170, 1990
104. Nelson JD, Wright JC: Conjunctival goblet cell densities in ocular surface disease. Arch Ophthalmol 102:1049, 1984
105. American Academy of Ophthalmology: Punctal occlusion for the dry eye. Ophthalmology 99:639, 1992
106. Rolando M, Refojo MF, Kenyon KR: Increased tear evaporation in eyes with keratoconjunctivitis sicca. Arch Ophthalmol 101:557, 1983
107. Whaley K, Buchanan WW: Clinical Immunology. Vol. 1. WB Saunders, Philadelphia, 1981
108. Lucca JA, Farris RL, Bielory L, Caputo AR: Keratoconjunctivitis sicca in male patients infected with human immunodeficiency virus type 1. Ophthalmology 97:1008, 1990
109. Lucca JA, Kung JS, Farris RL: Keratoconjunctivitis sicca in HIV-1 infected female patients. p. 521. In Sullivan DA (ed): Lacrimal Gland, Tear Film, and Dry Eye Syndromes. Plenum, New York, 1994
110. Comrie-Smith SE, Nunez J, Hosmer M, Farris RL: Tear lactoferrin levels and ocular bacterial flora in HIV positive patients. p. 339. In Sullivan DA (ed): Lacrimal Gland, Tear Film, and Dry Eye Syndromes. Plenum, New York, 1994
111. Esty D, Rice NSC, Jones BR: Disodium cromoglycate (Intal) in the treatment of vernal keratoconjunctivitis. Trans Ophthalmol Soc UK 91:491, 1971
112. Allansmith MR: The chronically red eye. Audio Dig 21(8), 1983
113. Lemp MA: Surfacing Abnomalities. Little, Brown, Boston, 1973
114. Barsam PC, Sampson WG, Freedman GL: Treatment of the dry eye and related problems. Ann Ophthalmol 4:122, 1972
115. Lemp MA: Artificial tear solutions. Int Ophthalmol Clin 13:221, 1973
116. Lemp MA, Holly FJ: Ophthalmic polymers as ocular wetting agents. Ann Ophthalmol 4:15, 1972
117. Holly FJ: Surface chemical evaluation of a novel lipid containing tear substitute. Contacto 26:9, 1983
118. Krishna N, Brown F: Polyvinyl alcohol as an ophthalmic vehicle. Am J Ophthalmol 57:99, 1964
119. Rieger G: Lipid-containing eyedrops: a step closer to natural tears. Ophthalmologica 201:206, 1990
120. Swan KC: Use of methylcellulose in ophthalmology. Arch Ophthalmol 33:378, 1945
121. Swanson A, Jeter D, Tucker P: Ophthalmic vehicles. II. Comparison of ointment and polyvinyl alcohol 1.4%. Ophthalmologica 160:265, 1970
122. Flannery LM, Block JH: Mucus substitutes for the dry eyed contact lens wearer. Contact Lens Soc Am J 4:36, 1970
123. Gilbard JP, Kenyon KR: Tear diluents in the treatment of keratoconjunctivitis sicca. Ophthalmology 92:646, 1985
124. Wilson LA, McNatt J, Reitschel R: Delayed hypersensitivity to thimerosal in soft contact lens wearers. Ophthalmology 88:804, 1981
125. Mondino BJ, Salamon S, Zaidman GW: Allergic and toxic reactions in soft contact lens wearers. Surv Ophthalmol 26:337, 1982
126. Wilson FM: Adverse external ocular effects of topical ophthalmic therapy: an epidemiologic, laboratory, and clinical study. Trans Am Ophthalmol Soc 81:854, 1983
127. Pfister RR, Burstein N: The effects of ophthalmic drugs, vehicles, and preservatives on corneal epithelium: a scanning electron microscope study. Invest Ophthalmol 15:246, 1976
128. Berdy GJ, Ableson MB, Smith LM, George MA: Preservative-free artificial tear preparations. Assessment of corneal epithelial toxic effects. Arch Ophthalmol 110:528, 1992
129. Polack FM: Treatment of keratitis sicca with sodium hyaluronate (Healon). Poster exhibit. American Academy of Ophthalmology, Chicago, IL, November 1983
130. DeLuise VP, Peterson WS: The use of topical Healon tears in the management of refractory dry-eye syndrome. Ann Ophthalmol 16:823, 1984
131. Polack FM, McNiece MT: The treatment of dry eyes with Na hyaluronate (Healon). Cornea 1:133, 1982
132. Nelson JD, Farris RL: Sodium hyaluronate and polyvinyl alcohol artificial tear preparations. A comparison in patients with keratoconjunctivitis sicca. Arch Ophthalmol 106:484, 1988
133. Hammer ME, Burch TG: Viscous corneal protection by sodium hyaluronate, chondroitin sulfate, and methylcellulose. Invest Ophthalmol Vis Sci 25:1329, 1984
134. Limberg MB, McCaa C, Kissling GE, Kaufman HE: Topical application of hyaluronic acid and chondroitin sulfate in the treatment of dry eyes. Am J Ophthalmol 103:194, 1987
135. Bloomfield SE, Dunn MW, Mujata T, et al: Soluble artificial tear inserts. Arch Ophthalmol 95:247, 1977
136. Leopold IH, Burns PR: Symposium on Ocular Therapy. John Wiley & Sons, New York, 1977
137. Werblin TP, Rheinstrom SD, Kaufman HE: The use of slow-release artificial tears in the long-term management of keratitis sicca. Ophthalmology 88:78, 1981

138. Guatheron PD, Lotli VJ, LeDouarec JC: Tear film breakup time prolonged with unmedicated cellulose polymer inserts. Arch Ophthalmol 97:1944, 1979
139. Kaufman HE: Keratitis sicca. Int Ophthalmol Clin 24:133, 1984
140. Henderson JW: Keratoconjunctivitis sicca: a review with a survey of 121 additional cases. Am J Ophthalmol 33:197, 1950
141. Tuberville AW, Frederick WR, Wood TO: Punctal occlusion in tear deficiency syndromes. Ophthalmology 89:1170, 1982
142. Freeman JM: The punctum plug: evaluation of a new treatment for the dry eye. Trans Am Acad Ophthalmol Otolaryngol 79:874, 1975
143. Willis RM, Folbert R, Krachmer JH, Holland EJ: The treatment of aqueous-deficient dry eye with removable punctal plugs. A clinical and impression-cytologic study. Ophthalmology 94:514, 1987
144. Patten JT: Punctal occlusion with N-butyl cyanoacrylate tissue adhesive. Ophthalmic Surg 7:24, 1976
145. Putterman AM: Canaliculectomy in the treatment of keratitis sicca. Ophthalmic Surg 22:478, 1991
146. Glatt HJ: Failure of collagen plugs to predict epiphora after permanent punctal occlusion. Ophthalmic Surg 23:292, 1992
147. Nelson CC: Complications of Freeman plugs. Arch Ophthalmol 109:923, 1991
148. Maguire LJ, Bartley GB: Complications associated with the new smaller size Freeman punctal plug. Arch Ophthalmol 107:961, 1989
149. Levenson JE, Hofbaver J: Problems with punctal plugs. Arch Ophthalmol 107:493, 1989
150. Knapp ME, Freuh BR, Nelson CC, Musch DC: A comparison of two methods of punctal occlusion. Am J Ophthalmol 108:315, 1989
151. Vrabec MP, Elsing SH, Aitken PA: A prospective, randomized comparison of thermal cautery and argon laser for permanent punctal occlusion. Am J Ophthalmol 116:469, 1993
152. Guibor P: Expo bandage-bubble. Trans Am Acad Ophthalmol Otolaryngol 79:OP415, 1975
153. Sarver DE, Runacre P, Godfrey CM: Moisture chamber spectacles. A practical guide to their construction. Arch Ophthalmol 97:1347, 1979
154. Davis RH, Van Orman EW: Making moist-chamber spectacles. Am J Ophthalmol 94:256, 1982
155. Hart DE, Simko M, Harris E: How to produce moisture chamber eyeglasses for the dry eye patient. Am Optom Assoc 65:517, 1994
156. Poirier RH, Ryburn RM, Israel CW: Swimmer's goggles for keratoconjunctivitis sicca. Arch Ophthalmol 95:1405, 1977
157. Tiburtius H, Merker HJ: A new treatment for reduced tear production. Klin Monatsbl Augenheilkd 162:535, 1973
158. Grosse Ruyken FJ: A method of treating conjunctivitis sicca and Sjögren's disease with a secretolytic. Klin Monatsbl Augenheilkd 162:540, 1973
159. Katsuelson AB, Zhak EM: Surgical therapy of xerophthalmia by transplantation of parotid duct into conjunctival sac. Vestn Oftalmol 30:3, 1951
160. Lao YS: Transplantation of parotid duct into the conjunctival sac for the treatment of xerophthalmia, with report of a case. Chin Med J [Engl] 73:223, 1955
161. Bennett JE: The management of total xerophthalmia. Arch Ophthalmol 81:667, 1969
162. Nicholas JP Jr, Brown FA: Management of the epiphora following parotid duct transposition for xerophthalmia. Arch Ophthalmol 68:529, 1962
163. Dohlman CH, Doane MG, Reshmi CS: Mobile infusion pumps for continuous delivery of fluid and therapeutic agents to an eye. Ann Ophthalmol 3:126, 1971
164. Doane MG: Mechanical devices. Int Ophthalmol Clin 13:239, 1973
165. Farris RL: Contact lenses and the dry eye. Int Ophthalmol Clin 34:129, 1994
166. Gould HL: Management of the dry eye using scleral lenses. Ear Nose Throat Mon 48:133, 1970
167. Gassett AR, Kaufman HE: Therapeutic uses of hydrophilic contact lenses. Am J Ophthalmol 69:252, 1970
168. Baldone JA, Kaufman HE: Extended wear contact lenses. Ann Ophthalmol 15:595, 1983
169. Gassett AR, Kaufman HE: Hydrophilic lens therapy of severe keratoconjunctivitis sicca and conjunctival scarring. Am J Ophthalmol 71:1185, 1971
170. Lemp MA: Is the dry eye contact lens wearer at risk? Yes. Cornea 9(suppl):S48, 1990
171. Harris E (ed): The Sjögren's Syndrome Handbook. Sjögren's Syndrome Foundation, New York, 1989

6

Surgical Management of Eyelid Abnormalities

DAVID A. DILORETO

Eyelid position and function are integral components of the normal corneal protective mechanisms. Early recognition and correction of eyelid abnormalities are of paramount importance in the successful diagnosis and treatment of corneal disease. Failure to do so can lead to the misdiagnosis and inappropriate and/or incomplete treatment of corneal disease. Eyelid surgery may be undertaken in conjunction with the medical and surgical treatment of corneal disease or as an adjuvant procedure. In general, eyelid malposition should be corrected before corneal surgery is performed.

SURGICAL PRINCIPLES

Preoperative Evaluation

A thorough clinical assessment of the eyelids includes examination of the eyelid margins for eyelash malposition and aberrant eyelash growth, as well as inspection for eyelid malposition and signs of lagophthalmos. Increased eyelid laxity is common in the elderly, and a test of eyelid and canthal laxity can identify many patients who are at risk of ocular exposure following ocular surgery. External photography of the eyelids is useful in documenting clinically detected eyelid abnormalities before surgical correction.

Preoperative evaluation should include a careful drug history. Medications with antiplatelet or anticoagulant properties should be discontinued at least 7 days before elective surgery.

Surgical Instrumentation

Eyelid surgery is generally done on an outpatient basis, often in the office setting. Although traditional ophthalmic instrumentation has been adapted for ophthalmic plastic surgery, the specialization of intraocular microsurgery has resulted in many ophthalmic instruments that are poorly suited for eyelid surgery. Large needle holders are ideal for the needle sizes commonly used in ophthalmic plastic surgery. Forceps for grasping eyelid skin include 0.5-mm Castroviejo forceps and Adson forceps. Skin hooks and fine rakes are useful for retraction, and a Desmarres lid retractor should be included in each set. Direct acting scissors, such as small Metzenbaum or Stevens scissors, should be available, as well as spring-action Westcott scissors. Lacrimal probes are useful for intubating the canaliculi to avoid damage when operating on the medial eyelid. Loupe magnification or a surgical microscope assists in identification of eyelid structures.

Intraoperative Care

The facial skin should be cleansed with povidone-iodine solution or an appropriate antibacterial scrub that is compatible with the ocular surface. Draping with a headwrap and split sheet allows exposure of the entire face, which is most comfortable for the patient. Plastic globe conformers are useful in protecting the eye during eyelid surgery. Gelatin sponges soaked in balanced salt solution can be used to keep the cornea moist. Traction sutures are routinely placed through the central aspect of the eyelid margin to permit eyelid traction. Skin incisions should be planned to minimize unnecessary disfigurement. In general, incisions placed in natural eyelid creases and folds are best.

The amount of bleeding encountered in eyelid surgery is typically negligible. Nonetheless, the ophthalmic surgeon accustomed to intraocular procedures may find the control of eyelid bleeding frustrating. Useful methods for controlling bleeding include local infiltration of anesthetics that contain epinephrine, which should be done 15 to 20 minutes before surgery for maximal vasoconstrictive effects. Unipolar electrocautery with specialized guarded needle tips, bipolar electrocautery with forceps, and cautery with high-temperature battery-powered disposable cautery units are all suited for the coagulation of bleeding tissue. Cotton-tipped applicators, cotton pledgets, or dry neurosurgical cotton sponges are more useful than cellulose sponges in removing blood from the surgical field. In cases of particularly troublesome bleeding, direct compression with microfibrillar collagen or thrombin-soaked gelatin may be required.

Several sutures are commonly used in ophthalmic plastic surgery. Monofilament 5-0 or 6-0 sutures with conventional cutting or tapered three-quarters circle needles are used to close the skin. Silk is also well suited for skin closure, but requires early removal to avoid milia formation. Absorbable sutures for skin closure include rapidly absorbing plain gut and chromic gut suture. These sutures decay variably; however, if they are lubricated with ointment three or four times a day they absorb more predictably. They are particularly useful in small children and patients in whom suture removal would be troublesome or inconvenient. Subcutaneous tissues such as muscle can be sutured with 5-0 or 6-0 absorbable polyglactin or chromic gut suture. Because there is little subcutaneous tissue in the eyelids, the suture knots should be buried when this tissue is sutured to help avoid wound complications.

The tarsus is a crucial structure in maintaining the contour of the eyelid and the integrity of the eyelid margin. Its preservation is essential to prevent recurrences of eyelid malposition. Careful approximation of the tarsus is therefore important. Generally, suture placement through partial thickness tarsus avoids suture exposure on the conjunctival surface, with its potentially significant corneal morbidity. The use of a spatula needle facilitates tarsal closure. Conjunctival closure, if performed, should be done with plain gut sutures and the knots should be buried away from the ocular surface.

Postoperative Care

Postoperative dressings following eyelid surgery should include topical antibiotic ointment suitable for ophthalmic use and nonocclusive eye pads to allow early recognition of visual dysfunction from postoperative hemorrhage. Collagen shields or bandage soft contact lenses are applied in patients at risk of corneal epithelial disruption. Eye pads soaked in chilled saline are useful for controlling postoperative pain, edema, and ecchymosis; the pads should be changed every 20 minutes while the patient is awake for the first 48 hours after surgery. In the absence of concomitant intraocular surgery, a metal shield is required only at bedtime. Patients may resume careful face cleansing and hair washing 24 hours after surgery.

Monofilament skin sutures are typically removed 5 to 7 days postoperatively and silk sutures 3 to 4 days postoperatively. Wounds are often secured with Steri-Strips for 2 days after suture removal.

Postoperative discomfort is variable, but most patients require little more than 500 mg of acetaminophen three times a day. Eyelid ecchymosis resolves within 10 to 14 days, although subtle swelling may persist for several weeks.

BASIC SURGICAL TECHNIQUES

Predictable assurance of optimal surgical results requires adherence to general principles and the skilled use of basic techniques. The corneal surgeon undertaking the surgical correction of eyelid abnormalities will find immediate use for many of the following techniques. In combination with proper patient selection and adequate preoperative evaluation, these techniques may eliminate the need for many secondary procedures.

Tarsorrhaphy

The surgical management of many corneal disorders provides unique opportunities for the use of reliable tarsorrhaphy techniques. Narrowing of the palpebral fissure decreases the exposed ocular surface and improves tear function by decreasing the rate of evaporation. Selection of the appropriate procedure requires determination of the length of time the tarsorrhaphy will be needed.

A temporary tarsorrhaphy can be created by suturing the eyelid margin,[1] injecting botulinum-A toxin into the upper eyelid,[2] or gluing the eyelid margins with cyanoacrylate glue.[3] Whatever the method, a temporary closure should not permanently alter the eyelids. Horizontal 5-0 nylon mattress sutures placed anteriorly through the skin, orbicularis muscle, and tarsus and exiting the eyelid margin posteriorly at the level of the meibomian gland orifices provide stable eyelid immobilization (Figure 6-1). Care is taken to place the sutures far enough posteriorly so that the eyelashes will not roll posteriorly when the sutures are tied. Rubber or plastic bolsters are used to prevent the sutures from eroding through the skin. The sutures should be tied in a bow knot so that they can be untied and retied to allow examination of the cornea. Topical ocular medications can be applied to the medial canthal area and allowed to trickle onto the eye; the patient should not attempt to open the tar-

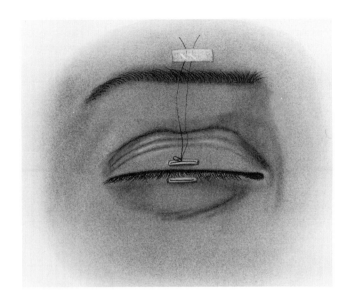

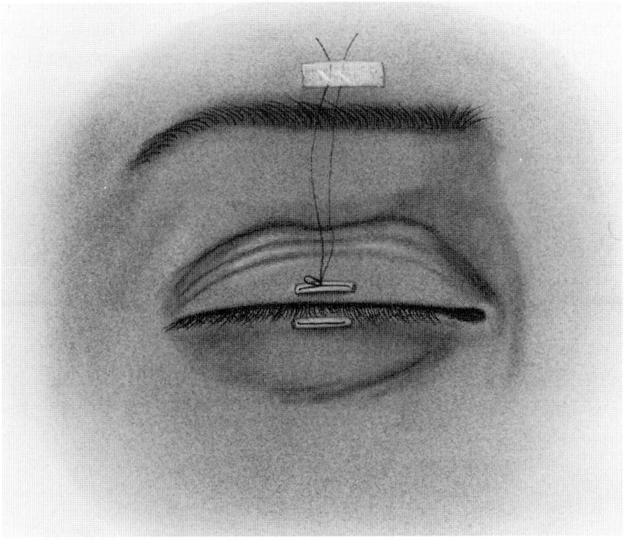

FIGURE 6-1 Temporary tarsorrhaphy created by a centrally placed horizontal mattress suture tied in a bow knot. The ends of the suture are taped to the skin above the eyebrow.

sorrhaphy. A temporary tarsorrhaphy is indicated as long as the corneal epithelium is healing, and can be left in place for as long as 1 month, if necessary. If the cornea does not improve, the tarsorrhaphy should be removed and other treatment modalities used.

A permanent tarsorrhaphy should be performed with full awareness of the potential for disturbance of the eyelid margins. The degree of effective closure is evaluated by lightly squeezing the upper and lower eyelids together, laterally or medially, and noting the minimal closure that gives satisfactory cosmetic and functional results. An effective permanent lateral tarsorrhaphy can be created by dividing the upper and lower eyelids at the gray line, beginning at the lateral canthal angle and extending medially (Figure 6-2). Each eyelid is then separated into an anterior and posterior lamella for a distance of approximately 5 mm vertically. The epithelium of the eyelid margins is excised and the posterior lamellae are sutured together with 5-0 chromic gut. The anterior lamellae are sutured with 6-0 nylon. This permanent tarsorrhaphy is potentially reversible without troubling distichiasis.[4]

Persistent medial ocular exposure following a lateral tarsorrhaphy can be corrected with a medial tarsorrhaphy or canthoplasty. The upper and lower eyelids are divided at the gray line from the lacrimal puncta to the medial commissure. Perforation of the canaliculi can be avoided by placement of lacrimal probes. The epithelium of the eyelid margins is excised and a layered closure of the posterior and anterior lamellae is completed as described above.

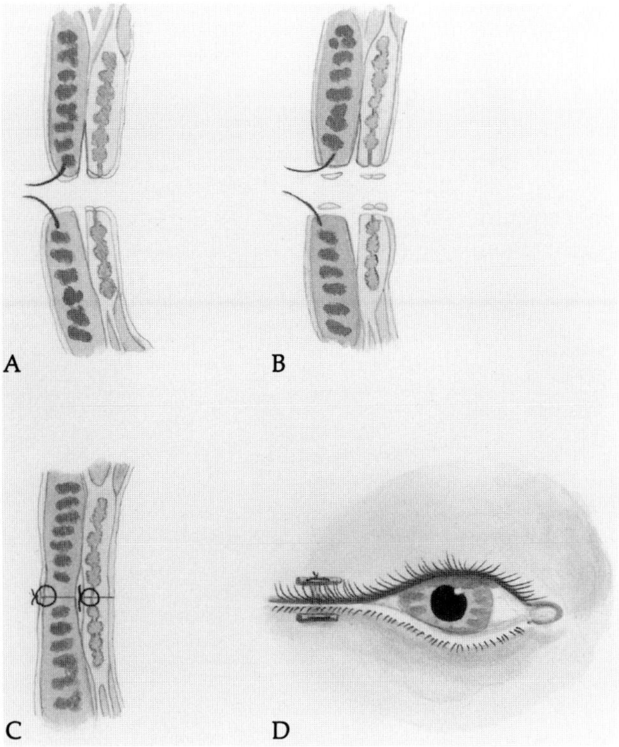

FIGURE 6-2 Permanent lateral tarsorrhaphy. (A) The eyelid margins are split at the gray line. (B) The epithelial coverage of the eyelid margins is removed. (C & D) The anterior and posterior lamellae are approximated with sutures.

Closure of Eyelid Margin Defects

Closure of full-thickness eyelid margin defects requires precise anatomic approximation (Figure 6-3). Tarsal approximation with 6-0 absorbable sutures is a prerequisite in avoiding troublesome rotation or notching of the eyelid margin. These sutures are placed through partial thickness tarsus so that they do not rub against the ocular surface. The eyelid margin is closed with 6-0 nonabsorbable sutures placed through identifiable marginal structures such as the meibomian gland orifices, gray line, and lash line. The ends of these sutures are left long so that they can be drawn anteriorly away from the eye and secured by the sutures used to close the skin. Skin sutures are removed in 5 to 7 days and eyelid margin sutures in 10 to 14 days.

Skin Grafts

Autogenous full-thickness skin grafts may be useful in scar revision, repair of cicatricial ectropion, and eyelid reconstruction.[5] The significant contraction of split-thickness skin grafts and their poor color match to facial skin preclude their use in eyelid surgery. Postauricular skin,

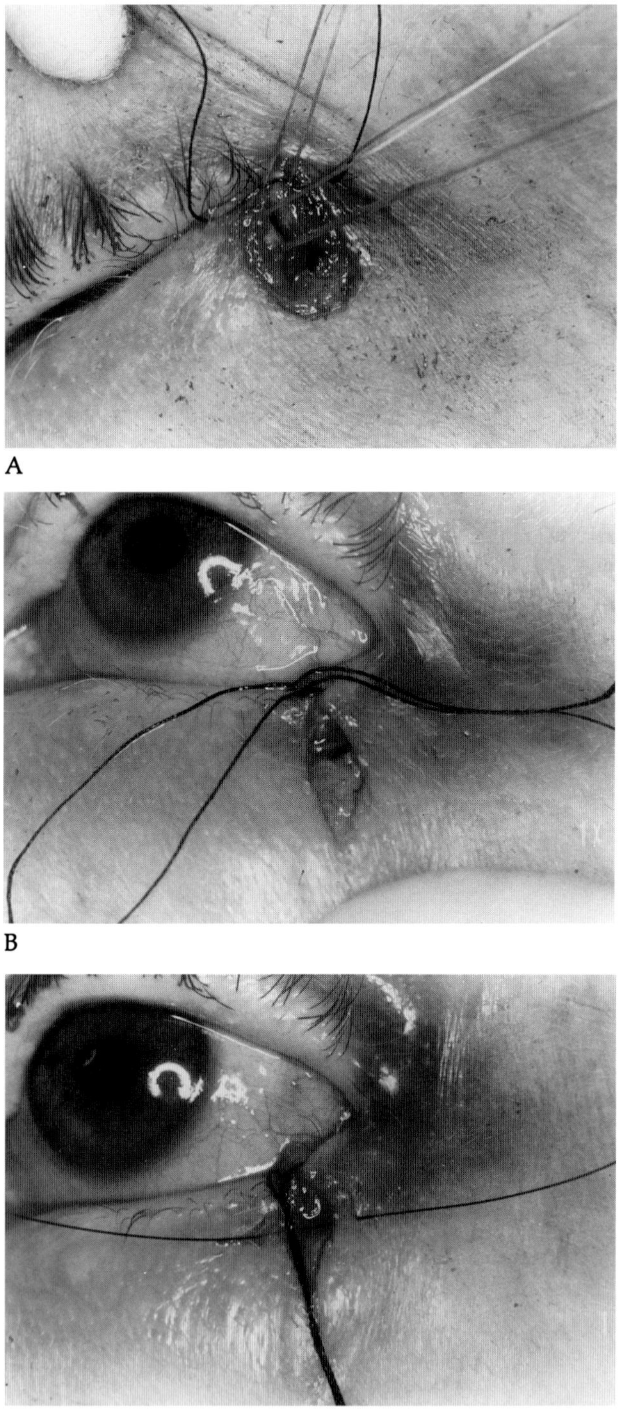

FIGURE 6-3 Closure of full-thickness eyelid margin defect. (A) Tarsal approximation with absorbable sutures. A silk suture has been placed through the eyelid margin to aid in proper approximation of the tissue. (B) Eyelid margin closure with silk sutures. (C) The eyelid margin sutures are left long and secured by the sutures used to close the skin.

preauricular skin, and excessive upper eyelid skin are good choices for full-thickness skin grafting of the eyelids. The recipient bed should be free of oozing blood. A sterile paper template is useful in outlining the shape and size of the recipient site and in obtaining an appropriate graft. A full-thickness skin graft can shrink by approximately 25 percent; therefore, the graft should be oversized accordingly. The graft should be meticulously debrided of subcutaneous tissue to eliminate a potential barrier to vascularization. The graft is sutured in place with interrupted nonabsorbable sutures, and a compressive bolus dressing is applied. In some cases, a suture placed through the eyelid margin (Frost suture) is useful to keep the operated area stretched during the initial postoperative period. Graft sutures are removed 5 to 7 days postoperatively; Steri-Strips are then applied for 2 days. The patient is instructed to avoid sun exposure and to use sun block for 6 to 8 weeks after surgery to minimize irregular pigmentation of the graft.

Tissue Flaps

By definition, tissue flaps have at least one pedicle and, unlike full-thickness skin grafts, do not depend on the recipient bed for vascularization.[6] They may include subcutaneous tissue or muscle and are useful when reconstuction requires deep volume or when blood supply is compromised, such as in irradiated tissues.

Tissue flaps are classified according to whether their blood supply is random or axial. Flaps with random blood supply are more frequently used in the eyelid, where a rich blood supply provides segmental, anastomotic, or axial arteries for vascularization. Among the flaps with random blood supply useful in correction of cicatricial ectropion are Z-plasty,[7] rhomboid flaps,[8] V-Y myocutaneous island flaps,[9] and palpebral pedicle flaps.[10] Flaps with axial blood supply receive their blood supply through a direct cutaneous artery lying within the muscle layer of the flap. Median forehead flaps[11] and nasolabial flaps are common examples of this type of flap used in eyelid surgery.

Mucous Membrane Grafts

Severe cicatricial entropion from trachoma, cicatrizing mucocutaneous diseases, or loss of conjunctiva following tumor resection may require reconstruction with mucous membrane grafts. Full-thickness mucous membrane grafts can be obtained from the lip, cheek, or hard palate.[12] Hard palate mucosa is particularly useful in mucous membrane grafting of the palpebral surface of the eyelid.[13,14] To facilitate removal of an oral mucosal graft, the mucosa is injected with lidocaine and epinephrine. The donor site is outlined and the graft is excised with a knife and removed with sharp and blunt dissection. Full-thickness mucous membrane grafts should be approximately 50 percent larger than the recipient site. Submucosal fat is removed from the graft. Typically, lip and cheek donor sites are closed with interrupted chromic gut sutures. Hard palate donor sites are left open and allowed to granulate. Meticulous postoperative oral hygiene aids in prompt healing. A running 7-0 nylon suture is useful in securing the graft to adjacent conjunctiva. Bandage soft contact lens coverage of the cornea avoids suture or knot irritation. Redundant mucous membrane grafts can be trimmed 6 to 8 weeks postoperatively if needed.

Cartilage Grafts

Replacement or reconstruction of the tarsus may be required in extensive reconstruction following eyelid trauma, tumor removal, or in the treatment of cicatricial entropion or lower eyelid retraction. A tarsoconjunctival composite graft from the contralateral eyelid may be selectively employed when a small area of reconstruction is required.[15,16] When significant or total reconstruction of the posterior lamella is required, a nasal septum chondromucosal composite graft is used as donor tissue.[17]

Auricular cartilage is an excellent source of cartilage, and a graft with dimensions of 10 mm vertically by 35 mm horizontally is easily obtained.[18] The cartilage of the scaphoid fossa can be safely removed with little fear of distorting the ear as long as the helix and antihelix are undisturbed. Figure 6-4 shows the approach to harvesting an auricular cartilage graft from the scaphoid fossa. An anterior incision is placed at the base of the helix and the skin is undermined anteriorly to expose the scaphoid fossa cartilage. Perichondrium lies immediately under the skin. The perichondrium on the anterior surface is incised; the perichondrium on the posterior surface is left intact. Meticulous hemostasis is required to avoid hematoma formation. The skin is closed with nonabsorbable sutures. Topical antibiotics are applied to the skin incision. The natural concavity of scaphoid fossa cartilage can be enhanced by scoring the concave surface to increase its curvature. The graft is secured to the tarsus with 5-0 absorbable sutures and the eyelid is immobilized postoperatively with a Frost suture if needed.

Conchal cartilage can be contoured in grafting of the lower eyelid but produces more local morbidity and should be reserved for secondary consideration.[19]

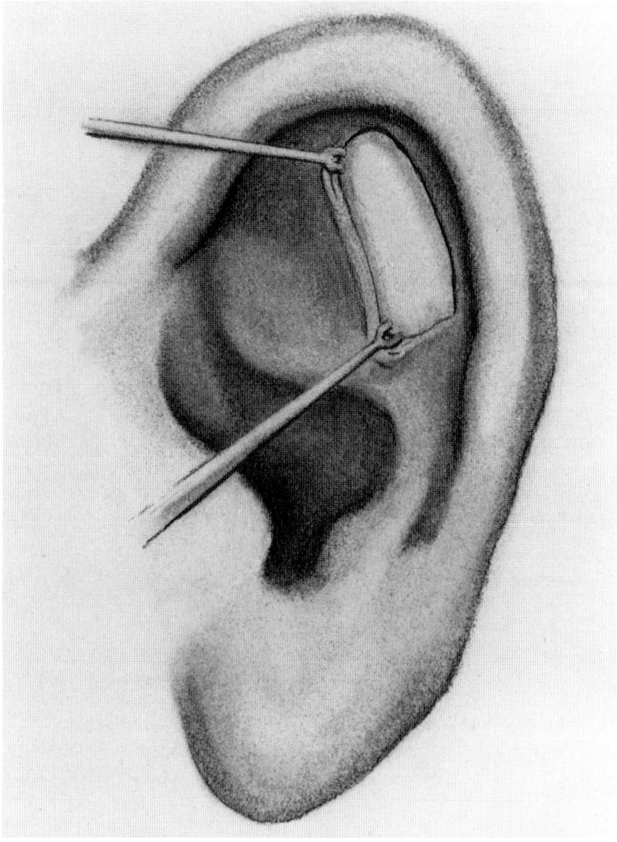

FIGURE 6-4 An auricular cartilage graft is readily harvested through an anterior approach to the scaphoid fossa. The autogenous tissue is useful as a tarsal substitute and in the correction of lower eyelid retraction.

Eyelid Implants

Weakness of the orbicularis muscle from paralytic lagophthalmos is most commonly encountered following facial nerve palsy. Implantation of gold weight implants to correct lagophthalmos of the upper eyelid has gained wide acceptance.[20] (Commercially available gold implants may be obtained from MedDev Corporation, Palo Alto, CA.) The implants range in weight from 0.6 to 2.4 g. The proper weight that permits improved closure without significant mechanical ptosis is chosen preoperatively. The implant may be taped or glued to the eyelid skin to permit preoperative evaluation. Division of the required weight into two implants rather than one large implant reduces unsightly bulk (Figure 6-5).

Implants are placed through an incision in the superior eyelid crease (Figure 6-6). The orbital septum is divided and the tarsus identified. Positioning holes in the implant permit suturing to the tarsus with absorbable sutures. Clo-

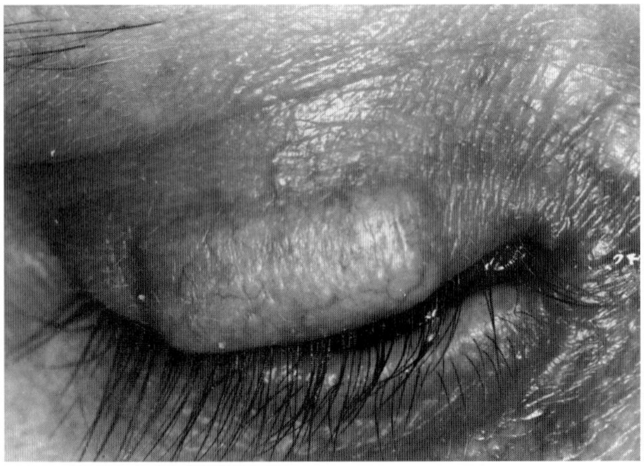

FIGURE 6-5 Bulky gold weight implant in the upper eyelid for the correction of paralytic lagophthalmos. Division of the required weight into two lighter implants would have reduced the thickness and improved the cosmetic appearance.

sure of the orbicularis muscle with absorbable sutures and the eyelid skin with nonabsorbable sutures is done. Intraoperative encapsulation of the implant with a porous polymer, such as Gore-Tex, may reduce the potential for extrusion by facilitating tissue ingrowth through the pores in the polymer.

Patients should be counseled on the possibility of developing ptosis when tired. Late complications include exposure or extrusion of the implant. Removal of the implant is easily performed through an eyelid crease incision if required.

SURGICAL MANAGEMENT OF EYELID ABNORMALITIES

Abnormal Eyelash Position

Trichiasis

Trichiasis is the acquired posterior orientation of previously normal eyelashes. It is a common cause of eyelid-induced corneal disease and may occur in many clinical settings. The correction of trichiasis requires an understanding of its etiology. For example, if the eyelid margin position is abnormal following trauma or surgery, this must be corrected. Cicatricial conjunctival changes must be sought in all cases of trichiasis. The extent and location of trichiasis must be carefully determined. A localized area of trichiasis will be present in most patients, but diffuse or extensive trichiasis may be encountered. Chronic blepharoconjunctivitis is found in many cases and should be treated medically. If a cicatricial mucous membrane disease, such as cicatricial pemphigoid, is present, appropriate medical therapy should be instituted as described in Chapter 23.

Epilation Epilation of eyelashes is a temporizing measure but may be useful in patients with single or focal trichiasis that requires only intermittent therapy. Invariably, the eyelashes regrow. If on repeated examination trichiasis recurs in the same location, repeated epilation may be a satisfactory solution. If the abnormal eyelashes recur intermittently in a diffuse pattern, a search for palpebral conjunctival disease, such as scarring from chronic blepharoconjunctivitis or cicatricial pemphigoid, should be undertaken.

Electrolysis of focal trichiasis results in significant rates of recurrence. Additionally, thermal injury of the eyelid may produce cicatricial changes of the eyelid margin.

Argon laser ablation of eyelash follicles for focal trichiasis has been undertaken with encouraging results.[21,22] Multiple repeated applications of the laser are discouraged because of the possibility of thermal injury.

Cryotherapy When focal trichiasis is recurrent and troublesome or diffuse trichiasis is found in the absence of entropion, cryotherapy can be a highly effective treatment. Eyelash and hair follicles are more sensitive to the effects of freezing than are other epithelial cells and connective tissues such as muscle and blood vessels.[23] Pigmented cells are also more sensitive to the effects of freezing. Normal and abnormal eyelashes can be destroyed by freezing the eyelash follicles to $-20°$ to $-30°C$. Temperatures below $-30°C$ may produce more extensive damage to nonepithelial structures and cause eyelid necrosis. Both the rate of freezing and the depth of freezing are important parameters in eyelash destruction. Although both liquid nitrogen and nitrous oxide probes are effective in eyelash destruction, the rate and the depth of freezing are more predictable with nitrous oxide probes. The predictabil-

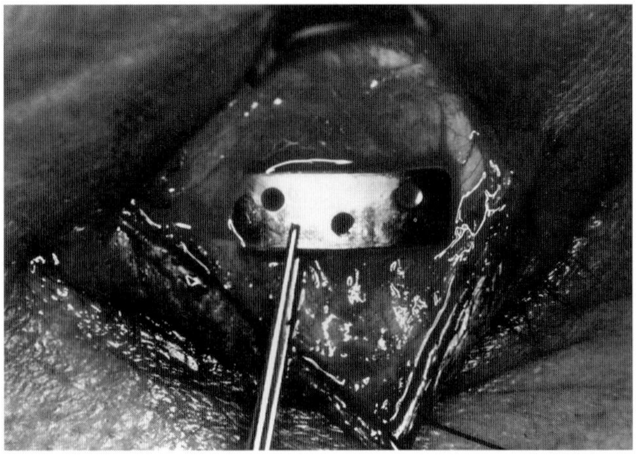

FIGURE 6-6 Transcutaneous implantation of a gold weight in the upper eyelid.

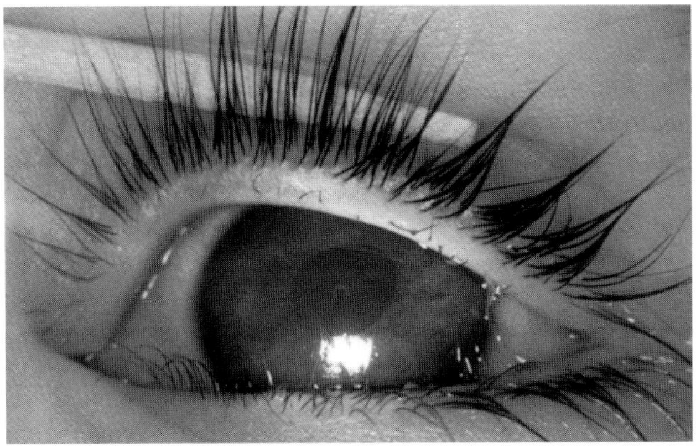

FIGURE 6-7 A young boy with typical congenital distichiasis. Note the incomplete row of eyelashes exiting just posterior to the meibomian gland orifices.

ity of eyelash destruction is higher when a probe specifically designed for eyelash destruction is used.[24] However, other ophthalmic probes, such as retinal probes, can be used if eyelash probes are unavailable.[25]

The procedure is performed under local infiltrative anesthesia with an epinephrine-containing anesthetic. The vasoconstrictive effect of epinephrine reduces the blood supply to the treated tissue and thus enhances the rate of freezing. A thermocouple is generally not required with a nitrous oxide probe. The probe is placed 2 mm below the eyelid margin on the conjunctival surface. Thirty seconds of freezing is required to reach adequate tissue temperatures. When a nitrous oxide probe designed for the treatment of trichiasis is used, a single application is adequate. Use of ophthalmic probes requires a double freeze-thaw method.[26] The treated eyelashes are epilated. Patients are re-examined at 4 to 6 weeks to determine the effectiveness of the therapy. Some loss of skin pigmentation and thinning of the eyelid margin are to be expected.[27] The depigmentation may be unacceptable to some patients and should be discussed preoperatively. A second treatment may be considered if areas of recurrence are found. Fine, pale, or lanugo-like eyelashes do not respond well to cryotherapy and its use should be avoided in such cases.

Microscopic Dissection Isolated or focal trichiasis for which cryotherapy is contraindicated or unsuccessful may be treated with microscopic dissection of eyelash follicles. Vertical incisions are made in the tarsal conjunctival surface and the eyelash and its follicle are resected. The resected site is allowed to heal by secondary intention. This treatment is appropriate for idiopathic localized trichiasis, congenital distichiasis, and traumatic defects of the eyelid margin. Full-thickness resection of the involved eyelid margin may be appropriate when cryotherapy-resistant, pale lanugo eyelashes are present and significant eyelid laxity exists. In the lower eyelid, complete excision of the lash-bearing eyelid margin is possible, with recession of the anterior lamella if entropion is present.[28]

Distichiasis

Distichiasis is a rare condition in which a second row of eyelashes arises from the orifices of metaplastic meibomian glands (Figure 6-7). It may be a congenital, dominantly inherited disorder (in which case all four eyelids are involved) or acquired.[29] Congenital distichiasis may be asymptomatic in infants and thus go undetected until childhood, at which time photophobia or ocular discharge are common complaints. The simplest treatment is to destroy the row of distichiatic eyelashes without creating cicatricial changes of the eyelid margin or destroying normal eyelashes. This can be achieved in various ways, one of which is to split the eyelid into anterior and posterior lamellae and apply cryotherapy to the posterior lamella with a double freeze-thaw cycle. The lamellae are then resutured with absorbable sutures. This procedure may result in significant thinning of the posterior lamella, with the possibility of secondary entropion.

Microscopic dissection and excision of the distichiatic eyelashes may be effective in selected cases. If extensive areas of the eyelid margin are involved, a mucous membrane graft may be placed after the posterior lash-bearing margin is removed.

The treatment of distichiasis is frustrating and regrowth of some eyelashes is to be anticipated. A bandage soft contact lens is useful in reducing symptoms related to recurrence before secondary treatment is undertaken. This delay allows growth of additional areas of recurrent eyelashes to be observed and reduces the frequency of surgical intervention.

Abnormal Eyelid Position

Entropion

Involutional or cicatricial causes may result in the posterior displacement of the eyelid margins with resulting trichiasis and keratitis.

Involutional Entropion Involutional entropion typically involves the lower eyelid and is more recalcitrant to definitive surgical therapy than involutional ectropion. A combination of factors is proposed for the development of involutional entropion, including horizontal eyelid laxity, disinsertion of the lower eyelid retractors, and superior overriding of the preseptal orbicularis muscle during eyelid closure.[30] The rapid and frequent ocular irritation produced by entropion results in repeated eyelid closure and hypertrophy of the orbicularis muscle.

Nearly 100 procedures have been described to correct entropion, attesting to the high rate of recurrence after surgery.[31] Suture entropion repair (Quickert sutures) is a useful office procedure for temporary relief,[32] and is illustrated in Figures 6-8 and 6-9. Recently, the use of combined surgical approaches has greatly increased the rate of success in entropion repair.[33] Using the combined approach described in Figures 6-10 and 6-11, the author has observed no recurrence of entropion in 92 lower eyelids of 61 patients. Complications were uncommon; skin necrosis in the lateral canthal region occurred in two patients, but no subsequent ectropion or fistula formation was seen.

Cicatricial Entropion Cicatricial entropion of the eyelids results from conjunctival disease and should be differentiated into two types—one with focal scarring involving the eyelid margin, frequently seen in chronic blepharoconjunctivitis and herpes zoster ophthalmicus, and the other with more generalized scarring of the tarsus and conjunctiva, as seen in trachoma, Stevens-Johnson syndrome, and cicatricial pemphigoid. If possible, surgical correction is best undertaken when medical therapy has resulted in inactivation of the underlying disease.

A variety of surgical approaches have been described for the treatment of cicatricial entropion. Those procedures that are designed to overcome the force of posterior tarsoconjunctival scarring by tightening the anterior eyelid structures are generally successful in mild cicatricial entropion involving the entire horizontal extent of the eyelid. When more advanced disease occurs or when eyelid scarring is focal, these procedures either fail or produce significant deformity of uninvolved areas of the eyelid. Significant posterior scarring, particularly in the presence of tarsal obliteration, such as occurs in Stevens-Johnson syndrome and cicatricial pemphigoid, requires vertical lengthening of the posterior eyelid lamella.[34] Composite grafts, including chondromucosal grafts from the nasal septum or single-tissue grafts such as oral mucosa and ear cartilage, are routinely used (Figure 6-12). Additional procedures include the use of bipedicle tarsoconjunctival advancement flaps with eyelid margin rotation[35] (Figure 6-13).

Focal scarring of the eyelid margins may follow chronic blepharoconjunctivitis. Typically, the patient develops entropion and trichiasis of the extreme medial and lateral portions of the upper eyelid as a result of the tapering or absence of the tarsus in these areas. Entropion may recur in these regions following anterior lamellar tightening procedures. Rotating the involved segment of eyelid margin and buttressing it with a free tarsoconjunctival graft obtained from the superior tarsal border is an effective means of correcting this problem[36] (Figure 6-14).

Ectropion

Lower eyelid ectropion results from either laxity of the tarsoligamentous sling with eversion of the eyelid margin or shortage of eyelid skin from scarring or congenital malformation.

Involutional Ectropion Involutional ectropion is best corrected by full-thickness horizontal shortening of the lower eyelid performed in the lateral canthal region[37,38] (Figure 6-15). This allows correction of the basic anatomic

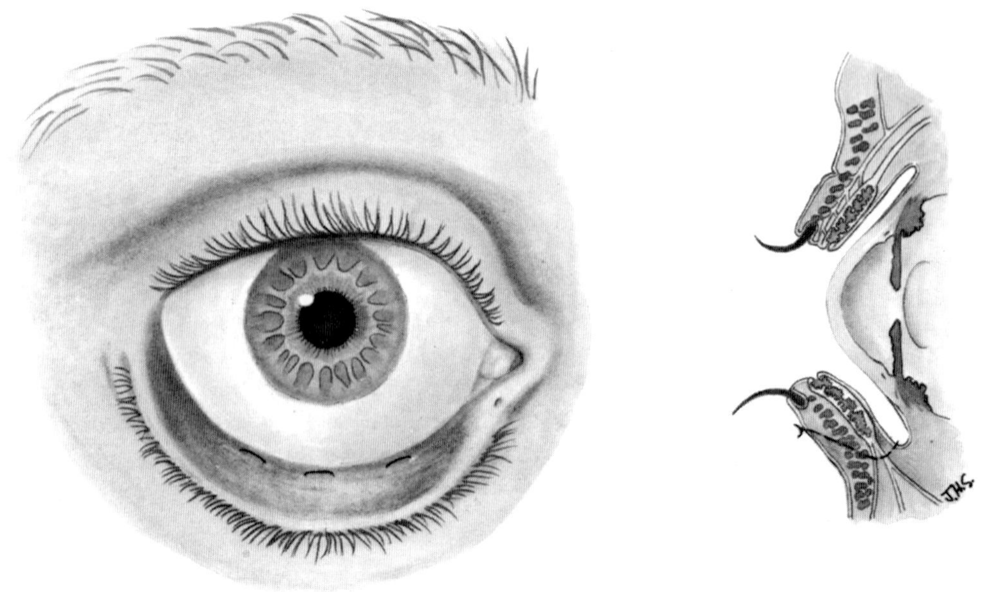

FIGURE 6-8 Placement of Quickert sutures is performed with horizontal mattress sutures (5-0 chromic) entering the eyelid transconjunctivally in the inferior fornix and exiting the skin 2 mm inferior to the lash line. This effects a plication of the lower eyelid retractors and everts the eyelid.

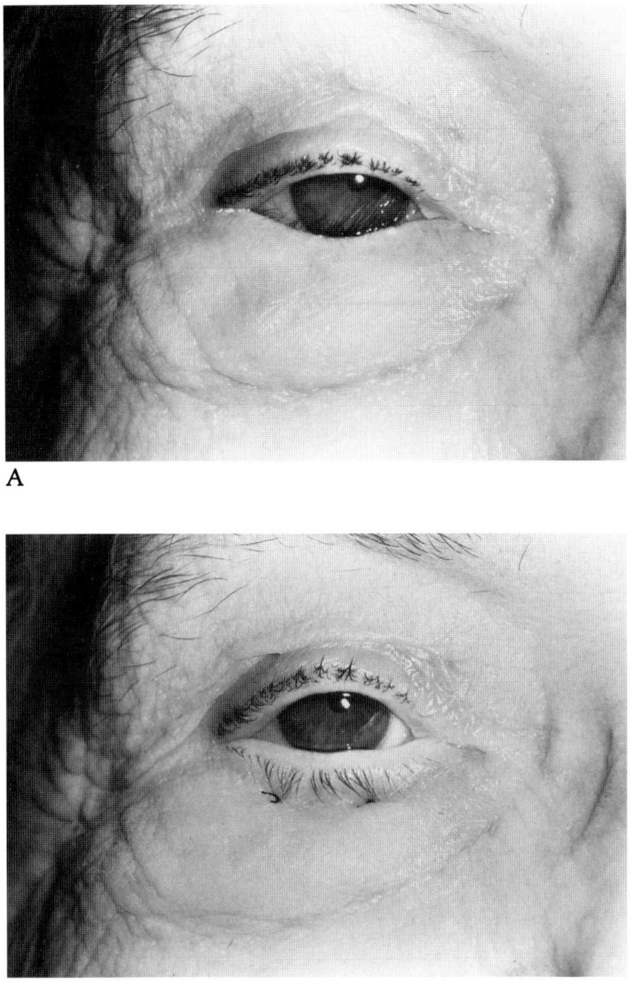

FIGURE 6-9 **(A)** Involutional entropion with spastic inward turning of the eyelid margin and eyelashes. **(B)** Quickert sutures produce effective correction that may persist for many months after suture absorption.

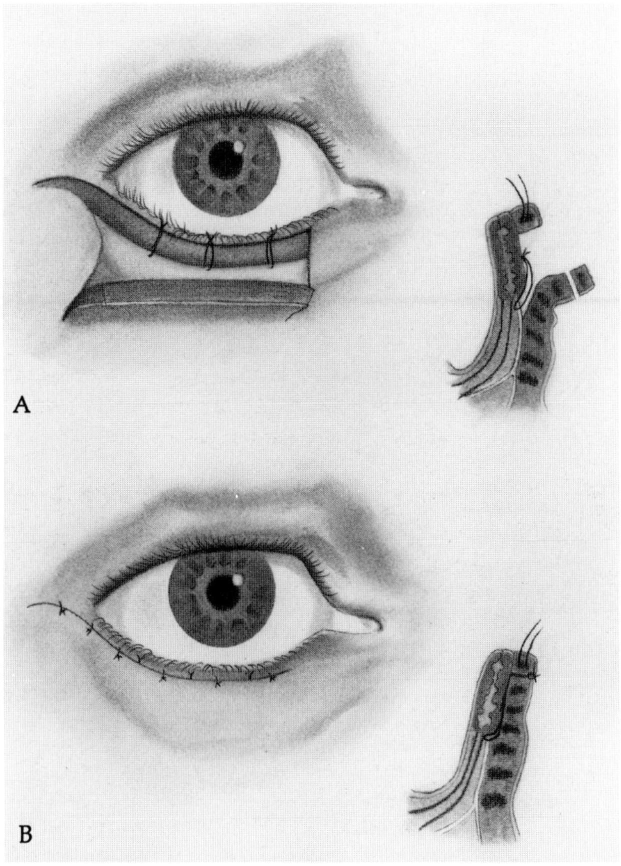

FIGURE 6-10 Involutional entropion is commonly associated with disinsertion of the lower eyelid retractors. Successful correction of this entropion is best performed by combining reinsertion of the eyelid retractors with additional procedures such as skin-muscle resection and full-thickness horizontal eyelid shortening. **(A)** A subciliary incision is made and the lower eyelid retractors are reinserted onto the anterior tarsal plate with absorbable sutures. **(B)** A skin-muscle resection can then be performed prior to closing the subciliary incision.

abnormality while preserving the tarsus, which has a long-term stabilizing effect on the eyelid margin.[39] After horizontal shortening of the eyelid, a lateral canthoplasty is completed by suturing the cut tarsal remnant to the inner aspect of the lateral orbital rim with a nonabsorbable suture on a small half-circle needle placed in a double-armed fashion.[40] Placement at the inner aspect of the lateral orbital rim avoids excessive lateral displacement of the lateral canthal angle. Eyelid height and contour are checked intraoperatively and care is taken to avoid lowering the lateral canthal angle. Medial laxity of the lower eyelid can be detected preoperatively by displacing the eyelid laterally. If the punctum is displaced farther than the nasal limbus with the eye in primary position, a medial tightening procedure is combined with the full-thickness horizontal shortening and lateral canthoplasty. Transcutaneous plication of the anterior limb of the medial canthal tendon or transconjunctival resection of the lower eyelid retractors is used to facilitate the correction of medial laxity (Figure 6-16). The latter is preferred if punctal eversion is present.[41] Upper eyelid ectropion is uncommon, but may be seen in the floppy eyelid syndrome.[42]

Cicatricial Ectropion Ectropion of the lower eyelid resulting from cicatricial changes, as in sun-damaged skin, for example, may necessitate vertical lengthening of the anterior lamella with local flaps or skin grafts in addition to scar lysis or revision. This disorder is found congenitally in some infants with facial clefts and in trisomy 21.

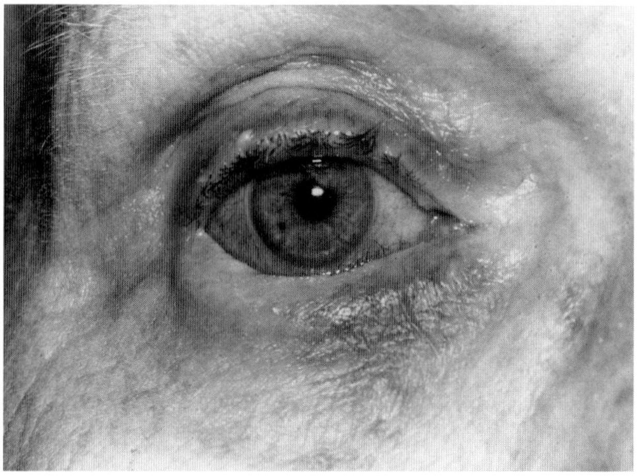

A

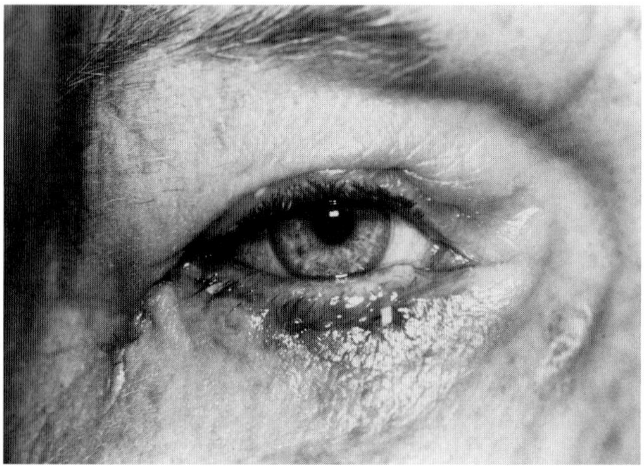

B

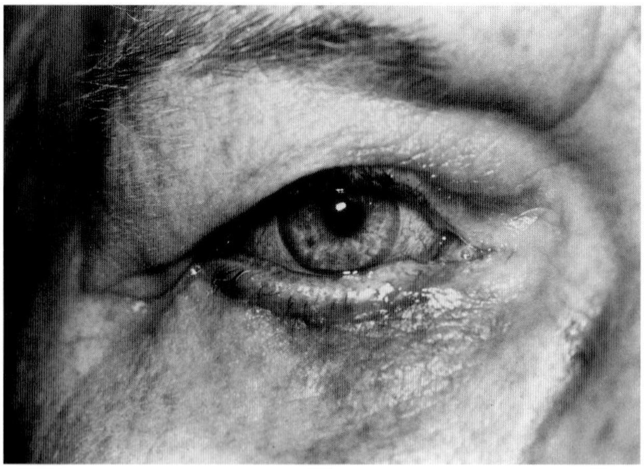

C

FIGURE 6-11 **(A)** Preoperative involutional entropion with trichiasis and keratitis. **(B)** One week after combined repair involving rotation and full-thickness horizontal shortening of the eyelid margin. **(C)** One month after suture removal.

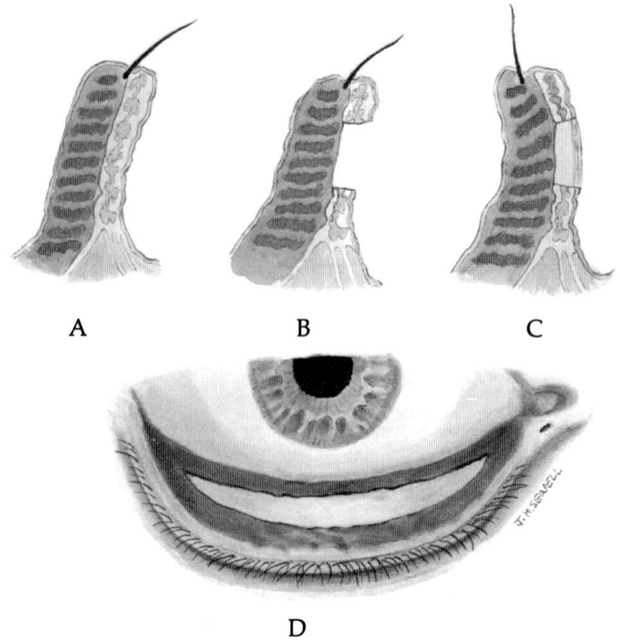

FIGURE 6-12 In severe cicatricial entropion, when the cicatricial changes are not near the eyelid margin, a full-thickness mucous membrane or composite cartilage and mucous membrane graft is placed at the midtarsal region of the posterior lamella of the eyelid. **(A)** Preoperative appearance. **(B)** Incision in the posterior lamella. **(C)** Placement of the graft. **(D)** Postoperative appearance of the inferior fornix and tarsal conjunctival surface.

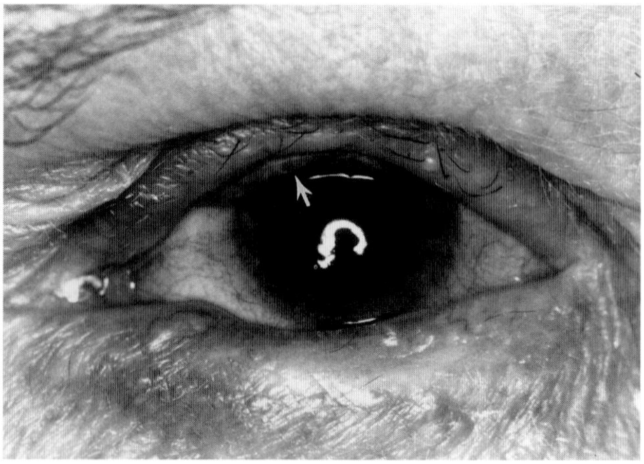

FIGURE 6-13 Cicatricial entropion of the upper eyelid has been corrected with marginal rotation and advancement of a bipedicle tarsoconjunctival flap (arrow) to the eyelid margin. Slight overcorrection buttresses the formerly trichiatic lashes away from the cornea.

Lagophthalmos and Retraction

A variety of diseases may impair the ability to fully close the eyelids. Even small amounts of lagophthalmos may produce significant corneal epitheliopathy. If the corneal epithelial changes resulting from lagophthalmos are unresponsive to medical therapy, surgical correction is undertaken. The treatment is directed at the anatomic abnormality that is producing lagophthalmos. Generally, lagophthalmos resulting from upper eyelid dysfunction is more severe and produces more rapid corneal epitheliopathy than lower eyelid abnormalities.

Paralytic Lagophthalmos Paralytic lagophthalmos following facial nerve paralysis results from weakness and atrophy of the orbicularis muscle, and occurs with concomitant lower eyelid ectropion and often significant lower facial weakness and tissue laxity. An unusual variety of surgical procedures and devices have been used historically to correct this problem, but all are associated with high rates of recurrence. While cross-nerve transfers and free nerve grafts may result in some reanimation of the lower face, they rarely rejuvenate the orbicularis muscle. The current treatment of choice is the implantation of gold weights in the upper eyelid[43] with combined correction of the lower eyelid ectropion[44] (Figure 6-17).

Cicatricial Lagophthalmos Post-traumatic eyelid deformities resulting from soft tissue lacerations and burns are a significant cause of cicatricial lagophthalmos. In addition, bony facial trauma involving the midface may result in lagophthalmos from cicatrization of the orbital septum. If scarring or shortage of skin results in vertical shortening of the eyelids, either focally or across their entire horizontal extent, the surgical options include scar revision with or without the use of skin grafting to vertically lengthen the eyelids. Full-thickness skin grafts are the most suitable source of autogenous tissue to vertically lengthen eyelid skin. Following surgery, the eyelids are immobilized with a suture tarsorrhaphy or Frost suture, and compressive bolsters are applied to the grafts.

Lagophthalmos resulting from thyroid orbitopathy is the result of progressive fibrosis of the levator palpebrae superioris muscle of the upper eyelid and capsulopalpebral fascia of the lower eyelid. Surgical procedures that lengthen these structures are therefore used. In the upper eyelid, recession of the levator aponeurosis can be performed transcutaneously, with intraoperative adjustment of the eyelid height and contour (Figure 6-18). When a significant amount of upper eyelid retraction occurs (greater than 4 mm), the levator aponeurosis can be lengthened further with the implantation of a tissue spacer between the tarsus and recessed edge of the levator aponeurosis. A variety of auto-

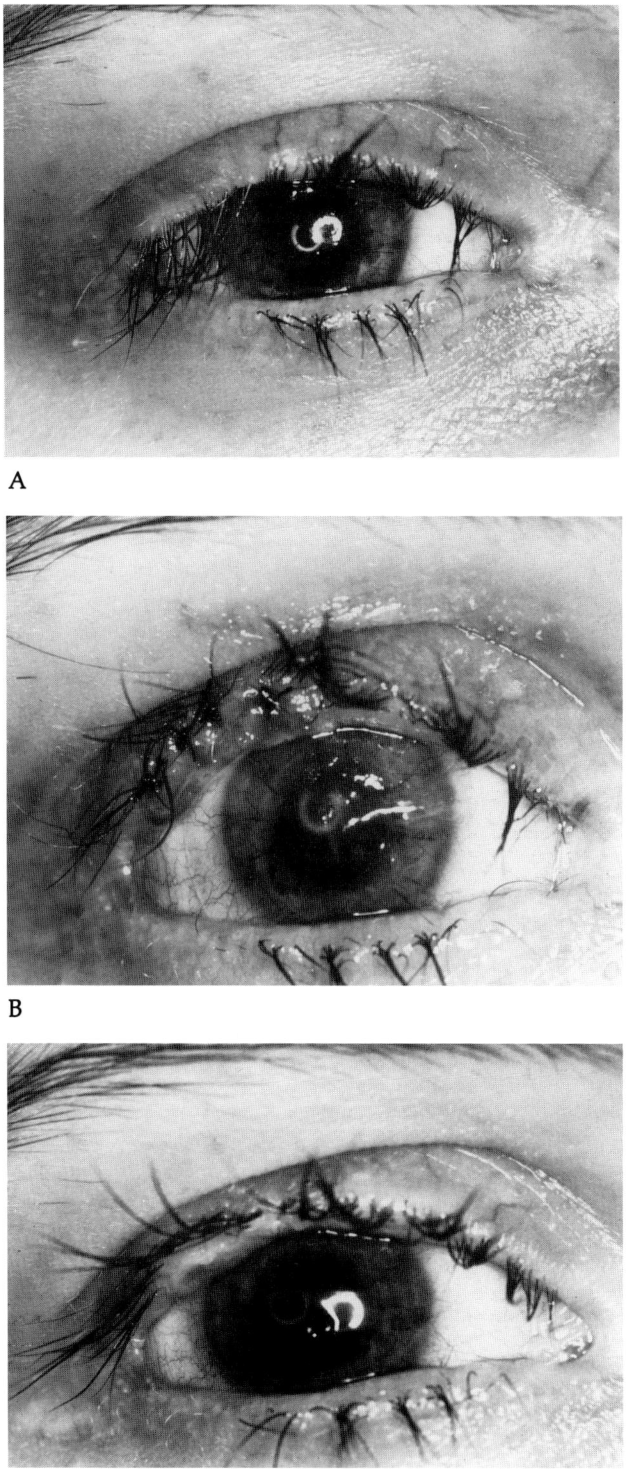

A

B

C

FIGURE 6-14 **(A)** Cicatricial entropion with focal involvement of the lateral eyelid margin and trichiasis. The eye has had penetrating keratoplasty. **(B)** Rotation of the involved segment of the eyelid margin with a free tarsoconjunctival composite graft. **(C)** One month after surgery.

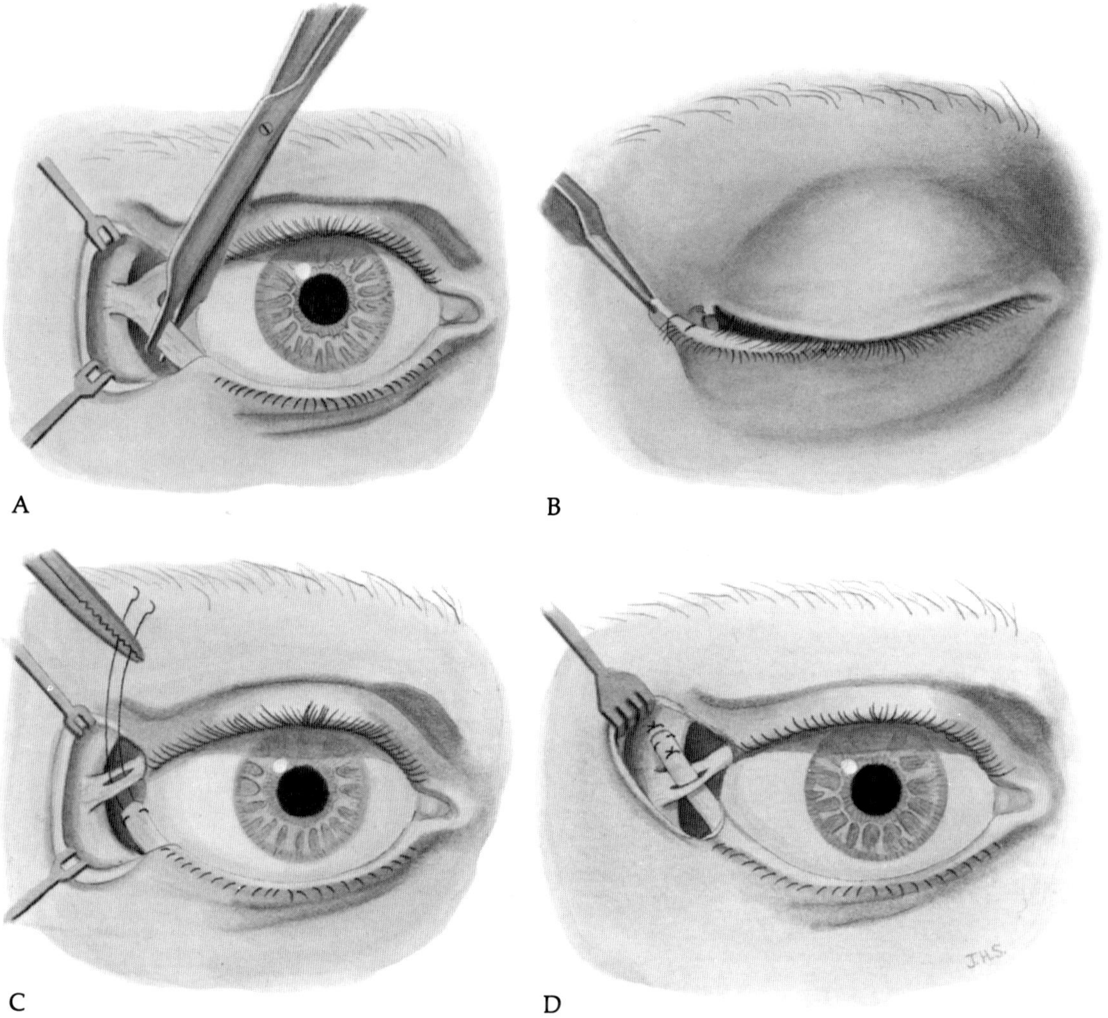

FIGURE 6-15 Lateral canthal tightening procedure. **(A)** The inferior crus of the lateral palpebral tendon is severed near its insertion onto the lateral orbital tubercle. This is achieved by cutting all the tissues between the conjunctiva and the skin surface. **(B)** After the inferior crus of the lateral palpebral tendon is severed, the eyelid margin is pulled laterally and superiorly. The amount of horizontal shortening of the eyelid that is required to achieve adequate horizontal tightening can now be determined. The eyelid margin that will be buried beneath the skin surface is de-epithelialized. The de-epithelialized portion of the eyelid includes tarsus, capsulopalpebral fascia, postorbicularis fascia, and orbicularis muscle. **(C & D)** The de-epithelialized lateral portion of the lower eyelid is passed through the superior crus of the lateral palpebral tendon and sutured to the periosteum of the lateral orbital rim with a permanent 5-0 or 6-0 suture. An even greater amount of horizontal tightening can be achieved by incising the periosteum at the insertion of the lateral palpebral tendon and attaching the de-epithelialized portion of the eyelid more posteriorly through the elevated periosteal flap. The most common error in lateral canthal tightening is failure to approximate the lateral portion of the lower eyelid adequately against the globe. In relatively enophthalmic eyes, the de-epithelialized portion of the lower eyelid must be reattached posteriorly behind the insertion of the superior crus of the lateral palpebral tendon.

genous, alloplastic, and homograft materials have been used for this purpose. When eyelid retraction is minimal, transconjunctival incision and recession of Müller's muscle can also vertically lengthen the upper eyelid.

Elevation of the lower eyelid for the eyelid retraction of thyroid orbitopathy invariably requires the implantation of a spacer between the recessed capsulopalpebral fascia and inferior tarsal border. Auricular cartilage harvested from the scaphoid fossa of the ear can be easily contoured to serve as a spacer.[45] The relative rigidity of this cartilage, in comparison with that of eyebank sclera or autogenous fascia, makes it an ideal material. Immo-

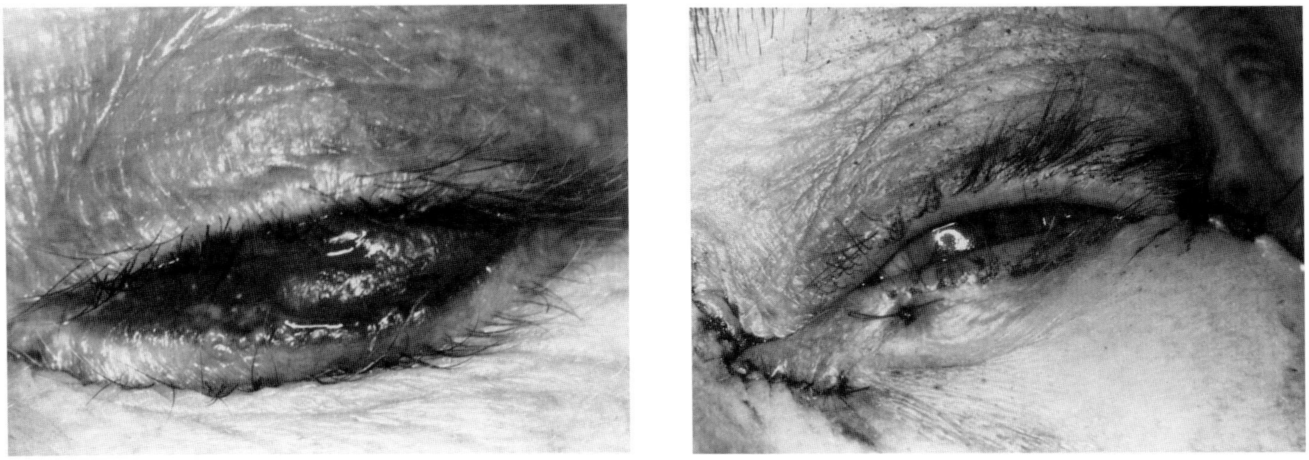

A B

FIGURE 6-16 **(A)** Extensive involutional ectropion with lateral and medial canthal laxity. The lower eyelid retractors have disinserted, everting the tarsus and exposing the tarsal conjunctiva. **(B)** Immediate postoperative result following combined surgical correction by lateral tarsal strip, plication of the anterior limb of the medial canthal tendon, and shortening of the eyelid retractors.

bilization of the eyelid for several days postoperatively is useful in enhancing results.

Occasionally, dysfunction of the orbital septum results from scar contraction following facial fracture repair. If adequate lower eyelid skin is present, the lower eyelid retractors are recessed through a transconjunctival approach and the scarred orbital septum is excised. Dissection must be performed to the level of the inferior orbital rim and onto the anterior maxilla. An ear cartilage graft is then placed as a spacer and the eyelid is placed on stretch. Injectable long-acting corticosteroids are used to reduce scar recurrence and shortening of the septum.

Proptosis Thyroid orbitopathy or orbital tumors may initially present with lagophthalmos, eyelid swelling and fullness, or diplopia. In advanced cases, severe corneal exposure may result from inadequate eyelid closure over proptotic eyes. When ocular exposure is prolonged, conjunctival dehydration increases, and secondary edema and prolapse may ensue. Moisture chambers or a temporary tarsorrhaphy may be required (Figure 6-19). The tarsorrhaphy technique should permit regular observation of the eye for neurologic monitoring.

If exposure worsens, surgery may be necessary. Transcutaneous release of the levator aponeurosis and Müller's

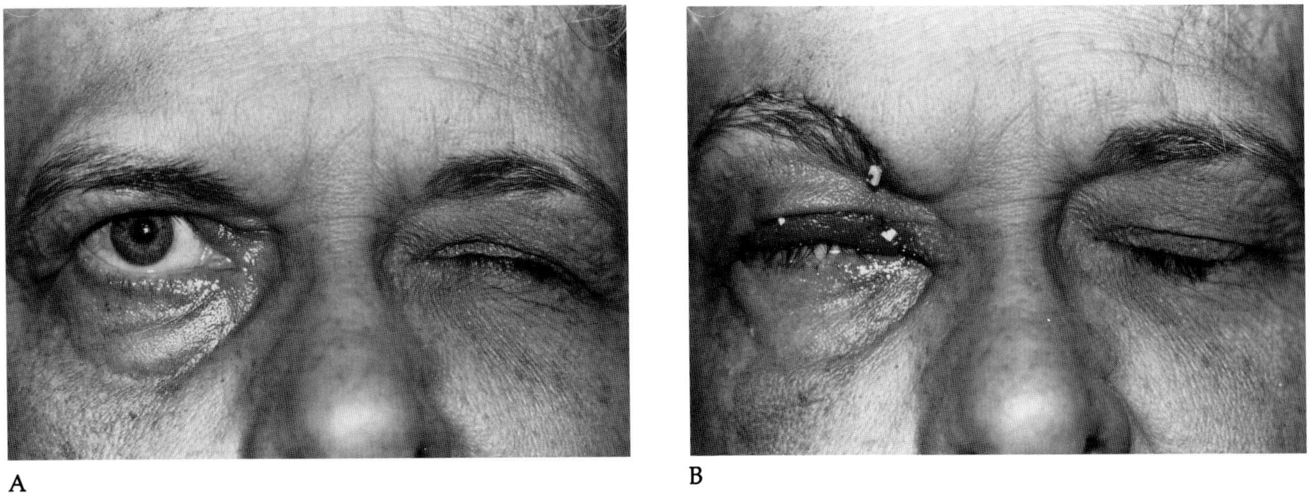

A B

FIGURE 6-17 **(A)** Right facial nerve palsy following acoustic neuroma resection. Paralytic lagophthalmos with inability to close the right eyelids. **(B)** Implantation of a gold weight in the upper eyelid, combined with ectropion correction, and direct browpexy produced improved eyelid closure. A small amount of lagophthalmos is still present.

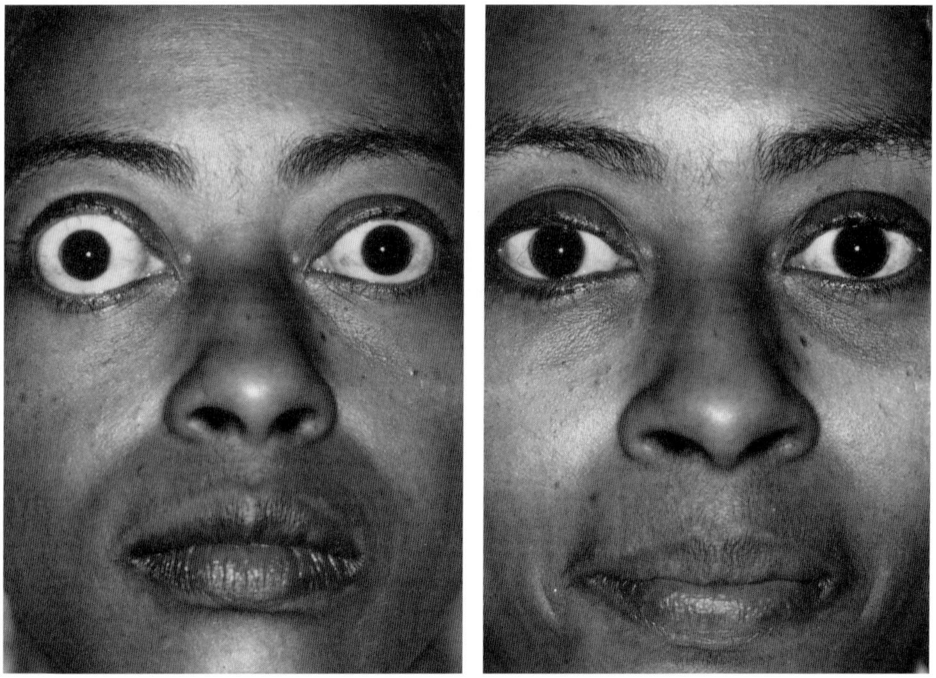

A B

FIGURE 6-18 (A) Thyroid orbitopathy with upper eyelid retraction and superior scleral show. (B) Recession of the upper eyelid retractors lowered the eyelids and produced more functional and cosmetically acceptable eyelids.

muscle can provide eyelid closure and ocular protection, if necessary, in combination with a tarsorrhaphy. If appropriate, orbital decompression is undertaken.

Blepharoptosis

Blepharoptosis of the upper eyelids is rarely associated with corneal abnormalities. In some cases of ptosis, filamentary keratitis may be seen. Induced astigmatic changes are of greater consequence in congenital ptosis because of their potential amblyogenic effect. Early surgical correction is warranted in such cases.

Ptosis repair may result in lagophthalmos. This is particularly pronounced with the use of frontalis slings for the correction of ptosis caused by poor levator function. In children, the chronic low-grade exposure is well tolerated and rarely becomes a problem. In adults, significant corneal morbidity may be associated with induced lagophthalmos. Adults suffering from chronic progressive external oph-

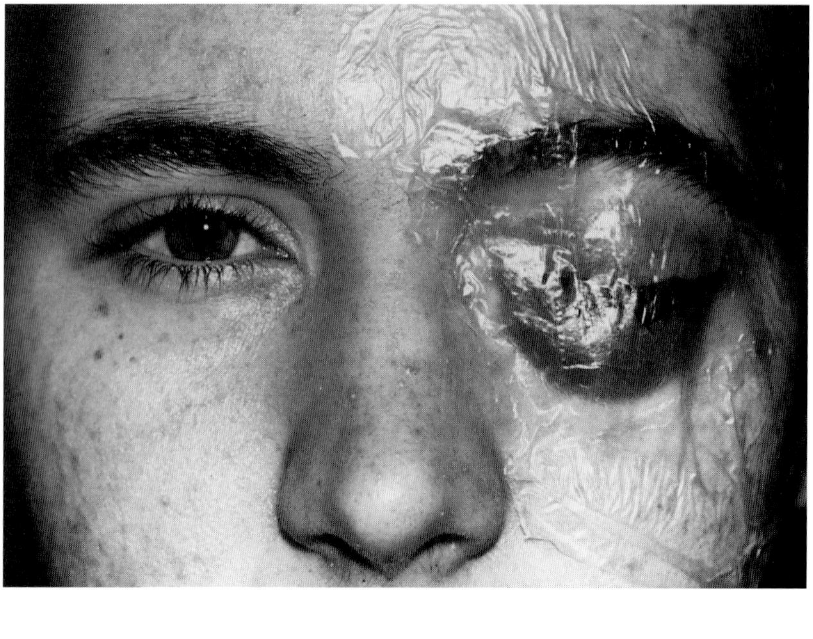

FIGURE 6-19 Moisture chamber created with Tegaderm for treatment of severe conjunctival chemosis associated with high-flow traumatic orbital arteriovenous malformation. The prolapsed conjunctiva could eventually be repositioned.

thalmoplegia or myasthenia gravis may require a frontalis sling for correction of disabling ptosis. The orbicularis muscle weakness encountered in these disorders compounds the problem of lagophthalmos. A useful and functional result can be obtained by minimally elevating the upper eyelid to the level of the superior pupillary border. At the same time, the lower eyelid can be elevated by recessing the lower eyelid retractors and placing an ear cartilage graft at the inferior tarsal border. The vertical height of the graft should exceed 8 mm and should permit the lower eyelid to cover the inferior limbus and cornea. During the immediate postoperative period, ocular irritation should be treated with artificial tears, lubricants, a moisture chamber, or a bandage soft contact lens. Patients should be instructed in the manual closure of the eyelids if necessary.

Eyelid Trauma

Trauma, thermal burns, or herpes zoster ophthalmicus may cause extensive tissue necrosis and loss of eyelid structures. Extensive eyelid reconstruction may be required in several staged procedures. If possible, surgery should be delayed until acute inflammatory signs have resolved. Vigorous treatment with topical ocular lubricants, a moisture chamber, or a tarsorrhaphy is often necessary. Lysis of symblepharon bands and repositioning of exposed conjunctiva should be undertaken promptly. Placement of a bandage soft contact lens and a symblepharon ring may be required. Following acute care and before definitive reconstruction, gentle massage, corticosteroid injections, and topical ocular lubrication may be considered.

REFERENCES

1. Koenig SB, Harris GJ: Temporary suture tarsorrhaphy after penetrating keratoplasty. Cornea 10:121, 1991
2. Kirkness CM, Adams GWA, Dilly PN, Lee JP: Botulinum toxin A-induced protective ptosis in corneal disease. Ophthalmology 95:473, 1988
3. Donnenfeld ED, Perry HD, Nelson DB: Cyanoacrylate temporary tarsorrhaphy in the management of corneal epithelial defects. Ophthalmic Surg 22:591, 1991
4. Stamler JF, Tse DT: A simple and reliable permanent lateral tarsorrhaphy. Arch Ophthalmol 108:125, 1990
5. Hughes WL: Reconstructive Surgery of the Eyelids. CV Mosby, St. Louis, 1943
6. Patrinely JR, Marines HM, Anderson RL: Skin flaps in periorbital reconstruction. Surv Ophthalmol 31:249, 1987
7. Davis WE, Boyd JH: Z-plasty. Facial Plast Surg 23:875, 1990
8. Borges AF: Choosing the correct Limberg flap. Plast Reconstr Surg 62:542, 1978
9. Chan STS: A technique of undermining a V-Y subcutaneous island flap to maximize advancement. Br J Plast Surg 41:62, 1988
10. Adenis JP, Serra F: Bipalpebral sliding flap in the repair of inner and outer canthal defects. Br J Ophthalmol 70:135, 1986
11. Dortzbach RK, Hawes MJ: Median forehead flap in reconstructive procedures of the eyelids and exenterated socket. Ophthalmic Surg 12:257, 1981
12. Hartman DC: Conjunctival Surgery. p. 204. In Hughes WL (ed): Ophthalmic Plastic Surgery. American Academy of Ophthalmology, Rochester, 1964
13. Bartley GB, Kay PP: Posterior lamellar eyelid reconstruction with a hard palate mucosal graft. Am J Ophthalmol 107:609, 1989
14. Cohen MS, Shorr N: Eyelid reconstruction with hard palate mucosa grafts. Ophthal Plast Reconstr Surg 8:183, 1992
15. Stephenson CM, Brown BZ: The use of tarsus as a free autogenous graft in eyelid surgery. Ophthal Plast Reconstr Surg 1:43, 1985
16. Hawes MJ: Free autogenous grafts in eyelid tarsoconjunctival reconstruction. Ophthalmic Surg 18:37, 1987
17. Leone C: Nasal septal cartilage for eyelid reconstruction. Ophthalmic Surg 4:68, 1973
18. Baylis HI, Rosen N, Neuhaus RW: Obtaining auricular cartilage for reconstructive surgery. Am J Ophthalmol 93:709, 1982
19. Jackson IT, Dubin B, Harris J: Use of contoured and stabilized conchal cartilage grafts for lower eyelid support. Plast Reconstr Surg 83:636, 1989
20. Jobe R: A technique for lid loading in the management of the lagophthalmos of facial palsy. Plast Reconstr Surg 53:29, 1977
21. Berry J: Recurrent trichiasis: treatment with laser photocoagulation. Ophthalmic Surg 19:36, 1979
22. Huneke JW: Argon laser treatment for trichiasis. Ophthal Plast Reconstr Surg 8:50, 1992
23. Wilkes DI, Fraunfelder FT: Principles of cryosurgery. Ophthalmic Surg 12:46, 1979
24. Sullivan JH, Beard C, Bullock JD: Cryosurgery for the treatment of trichiasis. Ophthalmic Surg 10:42, 1977
25. Hecht SD: Cryotherapy of trichiasis with use of the retinal cryoprobe. Ann Ophthalmol 9:1501, 1977
26. Bartley GB, Bullock JD, Olsen TG, Lutz PD: An experimental study to compare methods of eyelash ablation. Ophthalmology 94:1286, 1987
27. Wingfield DR, Fraunfelder FT: Possible complications secondary to cryotherapy. Ophthalmic Surg 10:47, 1977
28. Wojno TH: Lid splitting with lash resection for cicatricial entropion and trichiasis. Ophthal Plast Reconstr Surg 8:287, 1992
29. Stewart WB: Trichiasis, distichiasis, entropion. Trans Pac Coast Otoophthalmol Soc Annu Meet 61:113, 1980
30. Hawes MJ, Dortzbach RK: Microscopic anatomy of the lower eyelid retractors. Arch Ophthalmol 100:1313, 1982

31. Wies FA: Spastic entropion. Trans Am Acad Ophthalmol Otolaryngol 59:503, 1955
32. Quickert M, Rathbun E: Suture repair of entropion. Arch Ophthalmol 85:304, 1971
33. Carroll RP, Allen SE: Combined procedure for repair of involutional entropion. Ophthal Plast Reconstr Surg 7:123, 1991
34. Callahan A: Correction of entropion from Stevens-Johnson syndrome. Arch Ophthalmol 94:1154, 1976
35. Baylis HI, Silkiss RZ: A structurally oriented approach to the repair of cicatricial entropion. Ophthal Plast Reconstr Surg 3:17, 1987
36. Shorr N, Christenbury JD, Goldberg RA: Tarsoconjunctival grafts for upper eyelid cicatricial entropion. Ophthalmic Surg 19:316, 1988
37. Benger RS, Frueh BR: Involutional ectropion: a review of the management. Ophthalmic Surg 18:136, 1987
38. Bick MW: Surgical management of orbital tarsal disparity. Arch Ophthalmol 75:386, 1966
39. Tenzel RR, Buffam FV, Miller GR: The use of the "lateral tarsal sling" in ectropion repair. Can J Ophthalmol 12:199, 1977
40. Anderson RL, Gordy DD: The tarsal strip procedure. Arch Ophthalmol 97:2192, 1979
41. Nowinski TS, Anderson RL: The medial spindle procedure for involutional medial ectropion. Arch Ophthalmol 103:1750, 1985
42. Moore MB, Harrington J, McCulley JP: Floppy eyelid syndrome. Ophthalmology 93:184, 1986
43. Goldberg SM: Reanimation of the paretic eyelid using gold weight implantation: a new approach and prospective evaluation. Ophthal Plast Reconstr Surg 7:93, 1991
44. Lisman RD, Smith B, Baker D, Arthurs B: Efficacy of surgical management for paralytic ectropion. Ophthalmology 94:671, 1987
45. Baylis HI, Perman KI, Felt DR, Sutcliffe RT: Autogenous auricular cartilage grafting for lower eyelid retraction. Ophthal Plast Reconstr Surg 1:23, 1985

7

Bacterial Conjunctivitis

PENNY A. ASBELL AND LUIS G. ALCARAZ-MICHELI

Bacterial conjunctivitis is a common infection that occurs worldwide. Many bacteria are capable of causing conjunctivitis; the distribution varies with geography, season, and patient age[1-7] (Table 7-1). The severity of the infection depends on the virulence of the particular organism, the ability of the organism to produce toxins, and the immunologic status of the patient.[8-13] In most cases, the infection is self limited.

A significant number of bacteria may, at some time, be isolated from the conjunctivas of healthy individuals who have no signs of infection.[2,14] To infect the conjunctiva, bacteria must first overcome one or more of the ocular defense mechanisms. The eyelids and the conjunctival and corneal epithelium act as mechanical barriers against infection. The constant flushing of the tears, the sweeping action of the eyelids, and the mucus secretions of the ocular surface inhibit bacterial adhesion. β-Lysin, lactoferrin, and lysozyme, which have intrinsic nonspecific antibacterial activity, are present in the tears. In addition, all components of the complement system are available in the tears, as are immunoglobulins, although only IgA is present in significant quantities.[15-18]

The normal microbial flora of the ocular surface are an additional line of defense against infection. Again, geographic region, as well as patient age and hygiene, affect the specific types of organisms present, but in most cases the normal flora consist of *Staphylococcus epidermidis* and diphtheroids.[19-22] These bacteria inhibit colonization of the eye by more virulent organisms by releasing substances with antimicrobial activity.[23] Fungi are part of the normal flora in only 7 percent of the population.[24]

CLINICAL MANIFESTATIONS

Bacterial conjunctivitis is generally classified as hyperacute, acute, or chronic, based on the severity and duration of the infection. In addition, it can be classified by etiologic agent, by age of the patient (e.g., neonatal conjunctivitis), and/or by the presence or absence of an ocular membrane or pseudomembrane.[25]

Hyperacute Bacterial Conjunctivitis

Neisseria species are the organisms most often found in cases of hyperacute bacterial conjunctivitis; the most frequently involved species is *N. gonorrhoeae.* Gonococcal conjunctivitis is an oculogenital disease that usually is caused by autoinoculation from the urogenital region.[26,27] To identify the source, patients with gonococcal conjunctivitis should be asked about signs of urethritis and prostatitis and about possibly infected sexual contacts. Gonorrhea is most common in sexually active adolescent and young adult males. In 1995, 58 percent of 395,493 cases of gonorrhea reported to the Centers for Disease Control and Prevention occurred in people 15 to 24 years of age.[28] Although the incidence of gonorrhea is high, the incidence of gonococcal conjunctivitis is relatively low. It is estimated that there is only one case of gonococcal conjunctivitis for every 700 to 800 cases of gonorrhea.[29]

Gonococcal conjunctivitis generally begins with conjunctival hyperemia and foreign body sensation. There is rapid progression, with eyelid edema, erythema, and tenderness, as well as severe conjunctival chemosis and a copious purulent discharge (Figure 7-1). Painful

TABLE 7-1
Bacterial Pathogens Associated with Categories of Conjunctivitis

Hyperacute conjunctivitis	
	Neisseria gonorrhoeae[a]
	Neisseria meningitidis
Acute conjunctivitis	
	Staphylococcus aureus
	Streptococcus pneumoniae
	Haemophilus influenzae
Chronic conjunctivitis	
	Staphylococcus aureus[a]
	Staphylococcus epidermidis
	Moraxella lacunata[a]
	Streptococcus pyogenes
	Proteus mirabilis
	Klebsiella pneumoniae
	Serratia marcescens
	Escherichia coli
	Branhamella (formerly *Neisseria*) *catarrhalis*

[a] More frequently encountered pathogens.

preauricular lymphadenopathy is often present and pseudomembranes may also develop. Bilateral infection occurs in about 40 percent of cases,[27,30] but in many cases the progression of the infection is so rapid that patients seek medical help before the fellow eye becomes involved.[31–33]

Because *Neisseria* can penetrate intact corneal epithelium, involvement of the cornea is common (34 to 60 percent of cases[27,30]) and occurs fairly early in the infection.[10,31,33] The degree of corneal involvement varies, ranging from punctate keratitis to perforation (Figure 7-2). The most common corneal finding is anterior stromal infiltrates at the limbus.[30] Corneal perforation can occur as early as 24 hours after onset of the infection, but may occur at any time. The intense polymorphonuclear leukocytic reaction found in gonococcal keratoconjunctivitis is probably responsible for the corneal necrosis. Anterior chamber inflammation may be seen in the presence of keratitis.[34]

In suspected cases of gonococcal conjunctivitis, the conjunctiva should be scraped to obtain material for Gram staining and culture. Gram staining shows numerous polymorphonuclear leukocytes with intracellular gram-negative diplococci (Figure 7-3). For culture, the conjunctival discharge is inoculated onto chocolate agar and chocolate agar that contains selective antibiotics (modified Thayer-Martin medium). Although cultures are useful to confirm the diagnosis and to permit antibiotic sensitivity testing, treatment should not be delayed while the results are awaited.[34]

Gonococcal ocular infections are systemic infections, and systemic antibiotics are the mainstay of treatment. It is imperative to consult the most recent literature when dealing with gonococcal infections because the organism can develop resistance to a variety of antibiotics. The Centers for Disease Control and Prevention currently recommends treating gonococcal ocular infections with a single dose of intramuscular ceftriaxone (1 g for adults).[34–38] Oral norfloxacin is also effective against gonococcus.[31] Lavage of the conjunctiva is recommended to remove toxic conjunctival discharge. Topical antibiotics alone are insufficient therapy for gonococcal ocular infections, but they do deliver a high concentration of medication to the anterior segment and provide ther-

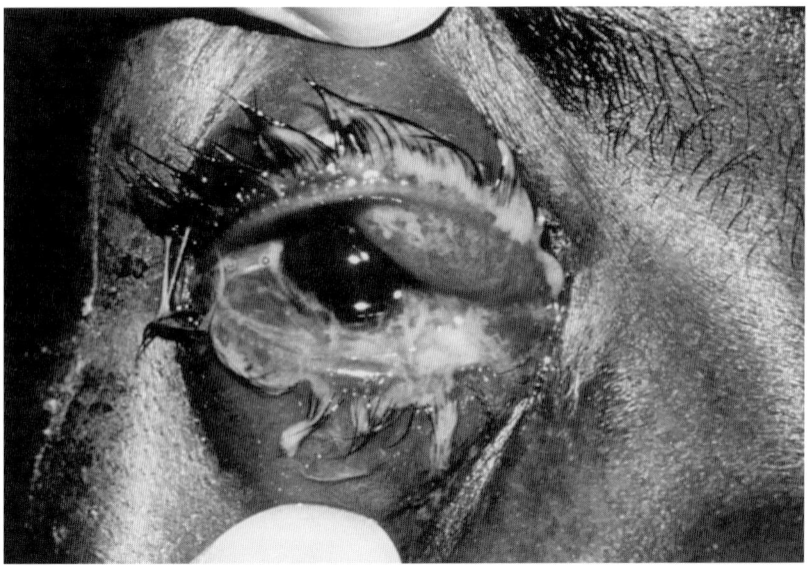

FIGURE 7-1 Hyperacute conjunctivitis caused by *Neisseria gonorrhoeae.* (Courtesy of Mark J. Mannis, M.D., Sacramento, CA.)

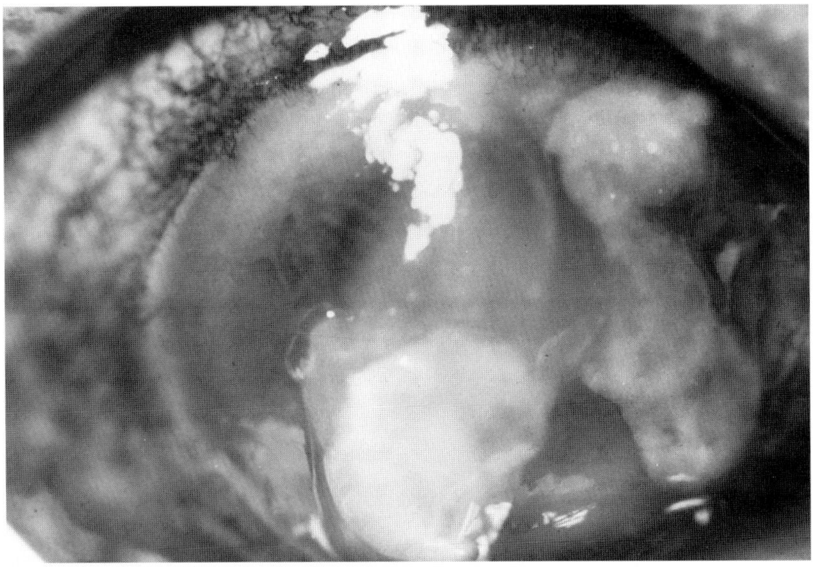

FIGURE 7-2 Gonococcal keratitis.

apeutic coverage for other potential causes of keratitis while the etiologic agent is being confirmed in the laboratory. Also, they are relatively safe. Although some have questioned the requirement for topical antibiotics,[30,34,39] we give topical erythromycin, gentamicin, or bacitracin ointment four times a day.[34]

Coinfection with *Chlamydia* must be considered in every patient with a gonococcal infection in that both are sexually transmitted diseases. As many as 12 percent of neonates with gonococcal urethritis, and 63 percent of women with gonococcal cervicitis have a coexistent chlamydial infection.[40–45] Until a rapid, inexpensive, and accurate test for chlamydial infection is available, adults with gonorrhea should be treated presumptively for chlamydial infection with doxycycline 100 mg orally twice a day for 7 days, or tetracycline 500 mg orally four times a day for 7 days.[34,38] Tetracyclines (including doxycycline) are contraindicated in young children and pregnant or nursing women. Azithromycin (1 g orally as a single dose) is an alternative treatment for chlamydial infections.

Conjunctivitis caused by *N. meningitidis* is similar to that caused by *N. gonorrhoeae,* although corneal involvement is less severe.[45] *N. meningitidis* usually affects younger patients and the clinician must be aware of the possibility of septicemia and meningitis.[3,4] *N. meningitidis* has been isolated from the oropharynx of apparently normal individuals who have no signs of infection.[4,46] As

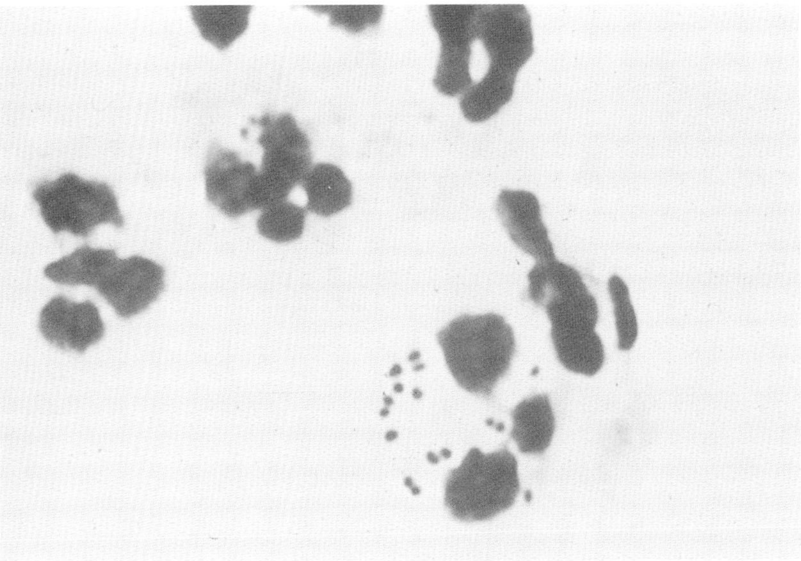

FIGURE 7-3 Gram stain of conjunctival discharge from gonococcal conjunctivitis showing a polymorphonuclear leukocytic reaction with intracellular diplococci. (Reprinted with permission from PA Tarantino, BA Barron: Sexually transmitted diseases of the eye. Ocular Infect Dis 1:59, 1994.)

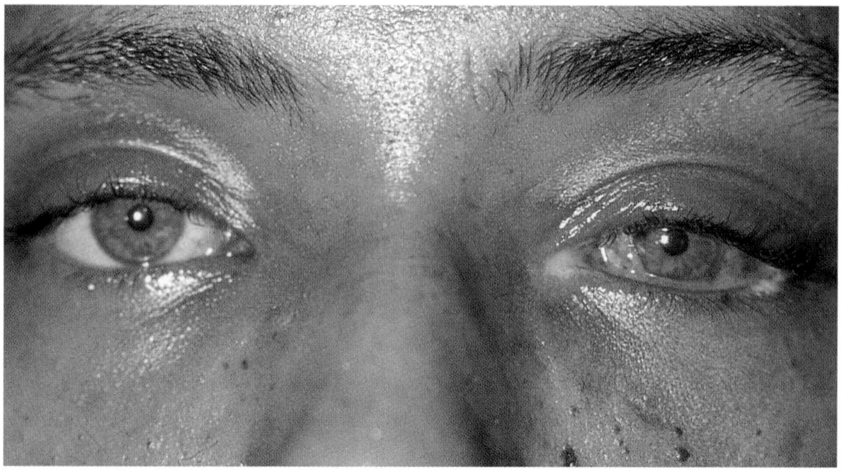

FIGURE 7-4 Acute bacterial conjunctivitis in the left eye characterized by slight eyelid edema, a mucopurulent discharge, and conjunctival hyperemia.

with gonococcal conjunctivitis, treatment with systemic and topical antibiotics is recommended.[6]

Acute Bacterial Conjunctivitis

Most patients with acute bacterial conjunctivitis develop tearing, irritation, and conjunctival hyperemia. Mattering of the eyelids in the morning and a mucopurulent discharge are also frequent signs (Figure 7-4). Infection of one eye may precede infection of the other by 1 to 2 days. Preauricular lymphadenopathy is not common. Although cultures may show the causative organisms, they are generally not needed unless the severity of the infection jeopardizes the eye or there is no response to empiric treatment.[47]

The most common causes of acute bacterial conjunctivitis are *Staphylococcus aureus, Streptococcus pneumoniae,* and *Haemophilus influenzae.*

Staphylococcus aureus

The most frequently isolated organism in acute bacterial conjunctivitis is *S. aureus,* which may, however, be part of the normal ocular microbial flora.[1] Morphologically, *S. aureus* is a gram-positive coccus that grows in clusters. Its virulence is related to its ability to elaborate toxins and enzymes injurious to tissues. *S. aureus* conjunctivitis may last for 7 to 10 days or may run a protracted course and become a chronic infection, particularly if the bacteria colonize the ocular adnexa. Blepharitis, marginal keratitis, and phlyctenulosis are manifestations of chronic staphylococcal infection (see below).[9,48,49]

S. epidermidis is also a gram-positive coccus that grows in clusters and is part of the normal microbial flora of the eye. Some strains produce toxins and enzymes and can give a clinical picture similar to that caused by *S. aureus* infection.[50]

Streptococcus pneumoniae

S. pneumoniae is an encapsulated, gram-positive, obligate aerobic coccus that may be isolated from asymptomatic carriers. Conjunctivitis caused by *S. pneumoniae* is usually self limited and lasts for 9 to 10 days. The infection is most commonly seen in children who live in cold climates.[25,33]

Haemophilus influenzae

H. influenzae is a small, gram-negative coccobacillus and is probably the most common cause of bacterial conjunctivitis in young children.[51] *Haemophilus* conjunctivitis lasts for 10 to 14 days. In addition to ocular irritation and conjunctival hyperemia, petechial hemorrhages may occur in the conjunctiva.

Particular attention should be given to the systemic status of any patient with *Haemophilus* conjunctivitis, since *H. influenzae* has been associated with septicemia, arthritis, meningitis, and otitis media.[52] In neonates, *Haemophilus* conjunctivitis is a potentially fatal infection.[53] Fever, leukocytosis, and hypotonia or irritability in the child are ominous signs of meningeal involvement. Some patients, especially children younger than 3 years of age, may develop a bluish discoloration of the eyelids or cheek, which is a distinctive sign of preseptal or orbital cellulitis.[54] *H. influenzae* type B is isolated in these cases.[55] Treatment with systemic antibiotics is advised in children and in patients with preseptal or orbital cellulitis.

A fulminant pediatric disease, Brazilian purpuric fever, has been associated with *H. influenzae* biogroup aegyptius. In this condition, septicemia, vascular collapse, and hypotension develop after the resolution of an episode of conjunctivitis. Most cases of Brazilian purpuric fever have been reported in areas of Brazil and Australia.[56,57]

Chronic Bacterial Conjunctivitis

By definition, chronic conjunctivitis lasts for more than 4 weeks. A variety of microorganisms, topical medications (especially topical aminoglycosides), chemicals, and cosmetics can cause chronic conjunctivitis (Table 7-2). Although the signs and symptoms of chronic bacterial conjunctivitis vary greatly, they are usually insidious and consist of redness, foreign body sensation, and mattering of the eyelids with scanty secretions. Patients with chronic bacterial conjunctivitis should be evaluated for a source of infection. Because the chronicity of the disease may be related to colonization of the ocular adnexa by bacteria, careful examination of the eyelids, eyelashes, and lacrimal drainage system is also essential.[25]

TABLE 7-2
Causes of Chronic Conjunctivitis

Bacterial infection
Staphylococcus
Moraxella
Nonbacterial infection
Chlamydia (trachoma/adult inclusion disease)
Parinaud's oculoglandular syndrome
Molluscum contagiosum
Toxic reactions
Medications
Cosmetics
Oculodermal disease
Seborrhea
Acne rosacea
Pemphigoid
Psoriasis
Local adnexal eye disease
Keratitis sicca
Chronic meibomianitis
Allergy
Atopic conjunctivitis
Vernal conjunctivitis

The most frequently isolated bacterium is *S. aureus*[9]; however, several others can cause chronic conjunctivitis, including *S. epidermidis, Moraxella lacunata, Proteus mirabilis, Serratia marcescens, Branhamella catarrhalis,* and *Capnocytophaga ochrachea.*

Staphylococcus aureus

S. aureus produces at least 25 biologically active substances, which accounts for its many pathologic manifestations.[58] α-, β-, γ- and δ-Hemolysin, epidermolytic toxin, and several enterotoxins have been isolated from *S. aureus.*[59] However, most of the ocular damage is believed to be through the action of the dermatonecrotic factor or α toxin.[60-62]

Patients complain of conjunctival hyperemia, mattering of the eyelids in the morning, and occasional discharge. The eyelids may demonstrate collarettes, telangiectasis, trichiasis, madarosis (loss of eyelashes), and recurrent hordeola. Although these signs are not pathognomonic of chronic *S. aureus* infection, they are very suggestive. Superficial punctate keratitis in the inferior third of the cornea is also characteristic.

Chronic *S. aureus* infection may present as phlyctenular conjunctivitis or as catarrhal infiltrates or ulcers (see Ch. 23). Phlyctenules (Figure 7-5) are nodular lesions near

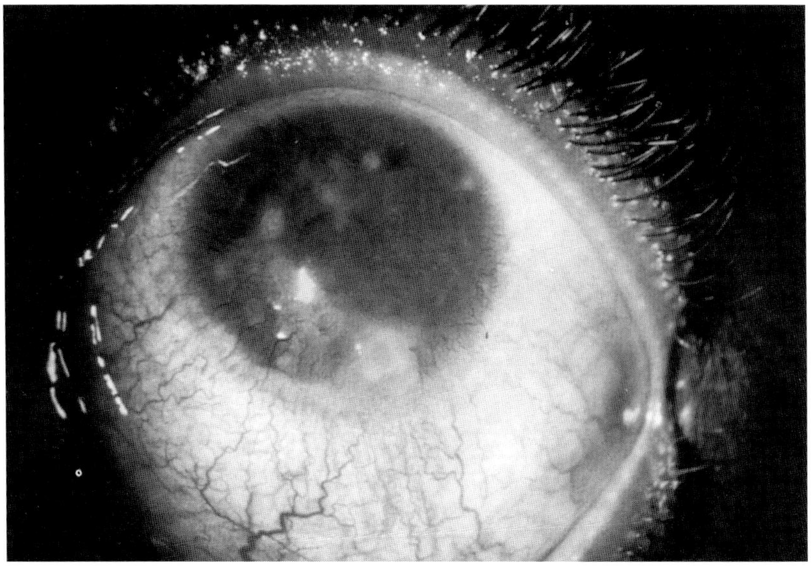

FIGURE 7-5 Phlyctenules caused by chronic staphylococcal infection.

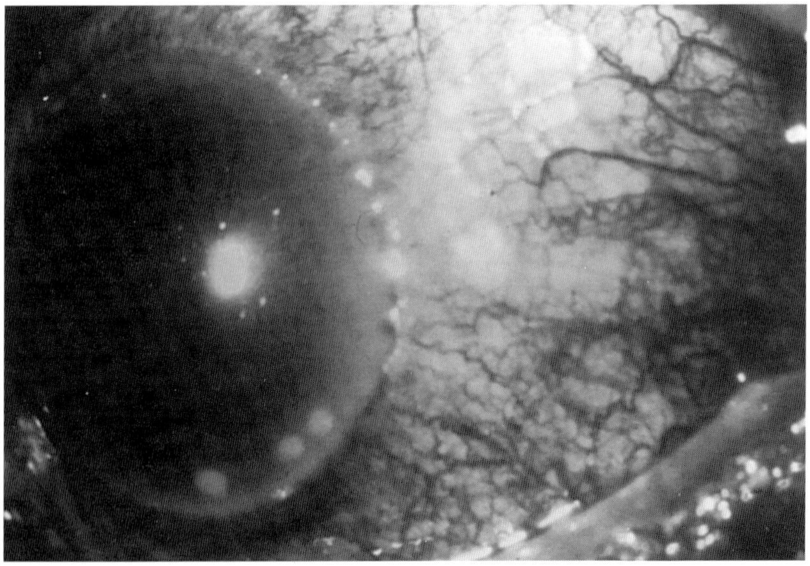

FIGURE 7-6 Catarrhal (marginal) infiltrates caused by chronic staphylococcal infection.

the limbus that may later spread toward the cornea or bulbar conjunctiva. They usually last 1 to 2 weeks. Catarrhal infiltrates or ulcers occur in the peripheral cornea. There is typically a 1- to 2-mm area of uninvolved cornea between the lesion and the limbus (Figure 7-6), although vessels sometimes grow over the area toward the infiltrate. Several marginal catarrhal ulcers may coalesce to form a ring ulcer. Cultures of material from phlyctenules and catarrhal ulcers grow no organisms; the lesions are believed to be caused by an immunologic reaction against microbial toxins and not by direct bacterial invasion.[60,61,63,64]

Treatment for chronic staphylococcal conjunctivitis consists of topical antibiotic preparations supplemented by eyelid hygiene (warm compresses and eyelid scrubs) to eliminate the offending organism.[61] In severe cases, a short course of topical corticosteroids may be helpful.[64]

Staphylococcus epidermidis

Many strains of *S. epidermidis* produce a wide variety of exotoxins that result in ocular signs indistinguishable from those found with *S. aureus.*[50]

Moraxella lacunata

M. lacunata is an encapsulated, aerobic, gram-negative diplobacillus commonly found in the normal respiratory tract. It is associated with chronic angular blepharitis, which is recognized by the characteristic maceration of the skin of the medial and lateral canthal regions (Figure 7-7).

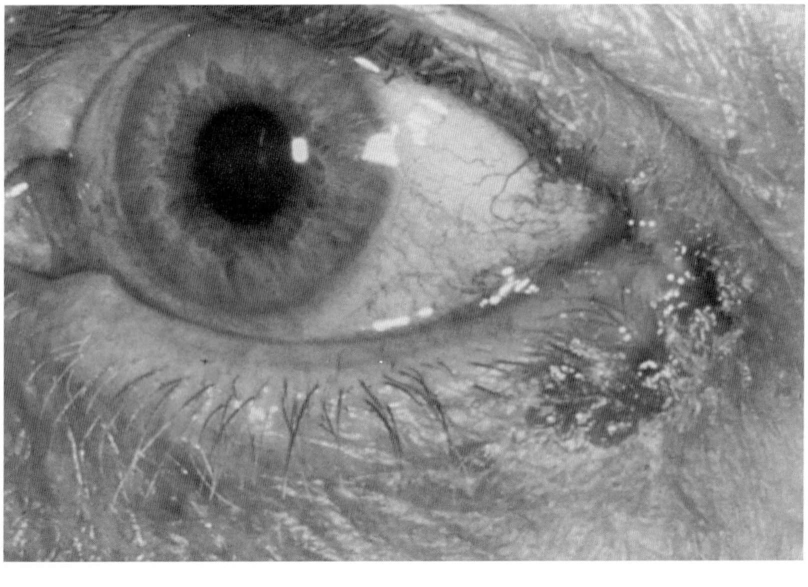

FIGURE 7-7 Angular blepharitis caused by *Moraxella lacunata.*

Proteases elaborated by *Moraxella* are thought to cause these lesions.[65] A similar condition can be found with *S. aureus* blepharitis.

Membranous and Pseudomembranous Conjunctivitis

The characteristic finding of membranous or pseudomembranous conjunctivitis is an accumulation of fibrinocellular material. When the material is organized into a membrane, it adheres firmly to the underlying epithelium; removal is difficult and is accompanied by bleeding. In contrast, a pseudomembrane consists of loose material with no attachment to the epithelium; it is easily removed with no bleeding or scarring.

Corynebacterium diphtheriae, Streptococcus pyogenes, S. pneumoniae, and *S. aureus* are frequently associated with the formation of both membranes[25] and pseudomembranes.[26] *Neisseria* has also been involved in the formation of pseudomembranes.[26]

Bacteria are not the only organisms capable of inducing membrane and pseudomembrane formation. Adenoviruses and herpes simplex virus can cause membranous conjunctivitis. Noninfectious causes include chemical burns, Stevens-Johnson syndrome, cicatricial pemphigoid, and ligneous conjunctivitis.

Neonatal Bacterial Conjunctivitis

The reported incidence of conjunctivitis in neonates varies from 2 to 12 percent.[7,66,67] In many cases, the disease is self limited. Nevertheless, the physician should recognize those cases in which severe damage to the eye or systemic involvement may occur. There are a variety of causes of neonatal conjunctivitis (Table 7-3). In this section, the discussion is limited to bacterial neonatal conjunctivitis; chlamydial neonatal conjunctivitis is discussed in Chapter 14.

Gonococcal ophthalmia neonatorum (Figure 7-8) was once a serious public health problem; however, since the introduction of the Credé prophylaxis (instillation of silver nitrate eye drops), the incidence has dropped from 0.2 percent to 0.013 percent.[67] (Interestingly, chemical conjunctivitis from the silver nitrate now accounts for a significant portion of

TABLE 7-3
Causes of Neonatal Conjunctivitis

Chemical
- Silver nitrate

Infections
- Chlamydial (inclusion conjunctivitis)
- Bacterial
  - *Neisseria gonorrhoeae*
  - *Staphylococcus aureus*
  - *Streptococcus pneumoniae*
  - *Haemophilus* spp.
  - *Pseudomonas aeruginosa*
  - *Escherichia coli*
  - *Proteus* spp.
  - *Klebsiella pneumoniae*
  - *Serratia marcescens*
  - *Enterobacter* spp.

Viral
- Herpes simplex (type 1 or 2[a])

Fungal
- *Candida albicans*

[a] Most commonly encountered.

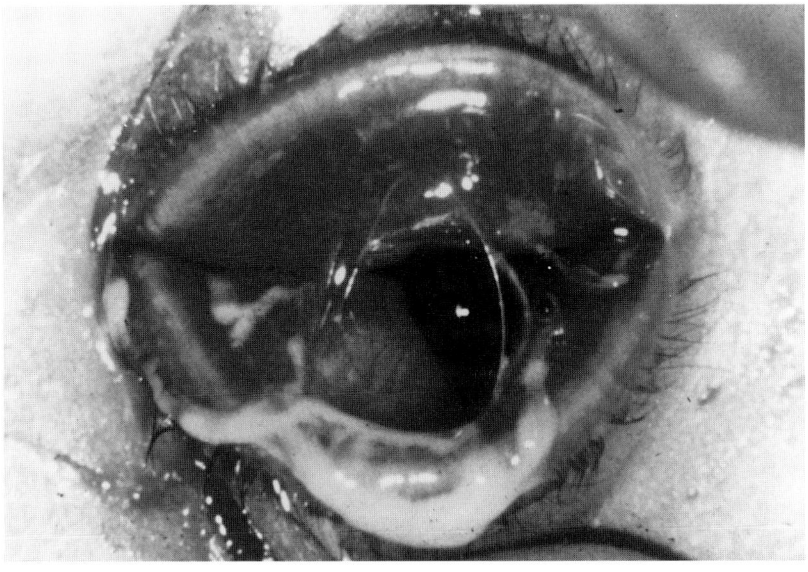

FIGURE 7-8 Gonococcal ophthalmia neonatorum.

neonatal conjunctivitis.) Today, the bacterial disease is seldom seen in developed countries, where prophylaxis is generally mandatory; application of 1 percent silver nitrate drops, 0.5 percent erythromycin ointment, or 1 percent tetracycline ointment immediately after or at least within 1 hour after birth usually prevents the infection.[38]

The causative agent, *Neisseria,* is probably acquired from the genital tract during vaginal delivery. The infected neonate presents with conjunctival hyperemia, eyelid edema, and a severe mucopurulent discharge, usually beginning 48 to 96 hours after birth. Bilateral infection is common. Corneal involvement is seen early in the infection, and, as in the case of adult gonococcal keratoconjunctivitis, corneal perforation may occur. Gram staining of the conjunctival discharge reveals numerous polymorphonuclear leukocytes with intracellular gram-negative diplococci. In the past, the diagnosis of gonococcal ophthalmia neonatorum was based on the time of onset of the conjunctivitis (Table 7-4). However, this criterion is no longer recommended because the time of onset is extremely variable and thus cannot be used as a reliable diagnostic tool. Proper diagnosis is made with the help of the laboratory.[7,20,66]

Current recommendations by the Centers for Disease Control and Prevention for the management of gonococcal ophthalmia neonatorum include evaluation for disseminated gonococcal infection and treatment with systemic antibiotics (ceftriaxone 25 to 50 mg/kg/day intravenously or intramuscularly in a single daily dose for 7 days—10 to 14 days if meningitis is present).[38] Frequent irrigation keeps the eye free of debris and possible toxins. As with gonococcal ocular infections in adults, antibiotic therapy recommendations change frequently with the development of new drugs, and it is important to stay abreast of the literature in this area.[36,37]

Many other gram-negative bacteria can cause neonatal conjunctivitis, including *Escherichia coli, Klebsiella, B. catarrhalis,* and *Enterobacter.* Fatal neonatal infections with *Haemophilus* and *Pseudomonas* that initially presented as conjunctivitis have been reported.[53,68] Preseptal and orbital cellulitis with meningitis can occur with *Haemophilus.* Rarely, *Pseudomonas* conjunctivitis may progress to panophthalmitis and septicemia with devastating results, especially in premature infants.[67]

Gram-positive organisms frequently isolated in neonatal conjunctivitis include *S. aureus, S. epidermidis, Streptococcus viridans,* and *S. pneumoniae.*[20] Colonization of the nasal and pharyngeal mucosa occurs in the neonate soon after birth,[69] and invasion of organisms from the upper respiratory tract may result in infection of the conjunctiva.

GENERAL PRINCIPLES OF TREATMENT

As we have stated above, bacterial conjunctivitis is often self limited, and cultures and sensitivities are seldom needed. Usually, a short course of broad-spectrum topical antibiotics provides adequate treatment. Polymyxin B-neomycin-gramicidin, trimethoprim-polymyxin B, gentamicin, and tobramycin solutions, as well as erythromycin and tetracycline ointments, are effective.[70–73] Aminoglycosides are particularly effective against gram-negative bacteria. Fluoroquinolones (ciprofloxacin and

TABLE 7-4
Clinical Features of Neonatal Conjunctivitis

Causative Agent	*Onset*[a]	*Discharge*	*Corneal Involvement*
Silver nitrate	24 hr	Purulent[b]	Epithelial keratopathy Corneal scarring
Chlamydia	5–14 days	Purulent	Fine epithelial keratopathy Micropannus
Neisseria gonorrhoeae	2–5 days	Purulent	Marginal/central ulcer Ring abscess Perforation
Staphylococcus aureus	≥5 days	Mucopurulent	Epithelial keratopathy
Streptococcus pneumoniae	≥5 days	Purulent	Epithelial keratopathy Ulcer
Haemophilus spp.	≥5 days	Purulent	Rare epithelial keratopathy
California spp.	≥5 days	Purulent, hyperacute	Rare
Herpes simplex	0–15 days	Mucoid, watery	Dendritic epithelial keratitis Stromal keratitis
Candida	≥5 days	—	Occasional marginal ulcer

[a] Onset is extremely variable and cannot be used reliably as a diagnostic criterion.
[b] In severe cases only.

norfloxacin) provide excellent coverage against a wide variety of bacteria.[72,74] Chloramphenicol ointment also has excellent broad-spectrum coverage, but fatal cases of aplastic anemia have been reported with topical use.[75]

If the severity of the infection endangers the integrity of the eye, or if there is poor or no response to empiric antibiotic therapy, cultures and antibiotic sensitivities are mandatory, and therapy is adjusted based on the results. In hyperacute bacterial conjunctivitis, parenteral antibiotics are essential, in addition to cultures and antibiotic sensitivities. Conjunctivitis accompanied by symptoms or signs of systemic infection requires the administration of systemic antibiotics as quickly as possible.

Chronic bacterial conjunctivitis is usually caused by bacterial colonization of the ocular adnexa, rather than by direct infection of the conjunctiva. Therefore, the role of eyelid hygiene in the treatment of chronic blepharoconjunctivitis cannot be overemphasized.

The clinician should be aware of other entities that resemble chronic bacterial conjunctivitis. When the conjunctivitis fails to improve with conventional treatment, cultures and epithelial cytology should be performed. Attention should be given to the tear film and eyelid function. Toxic reactions to topical medications can mimic chronic bacterial conjunctivitis. In these cases, all topical medications should be discontinued. The possibility of malignancy, such as sebaceous cell carcinoma, should be considered in chronic blepharoconjunctivitis that is unresponsive to treatment. Recently, there has been a resurgence of tuberculosis; although rare, there are reports of primary conjunctivitis caused by *Mycobacterium tuberculosis*.[76,77]

REFERENCES

1. Seal DV, Barrett SP, McGill JI: Aetiology and treatment of acute bacterial infection of the external eye. Br J Ophthalmol 66:357, 1982
2. Perkins RE, Kundsin RB, Pratt MV, et al: Bacteriology of normal and infected conjunctiva. J Clin Microbiol 1:147, 1975
3. Monaga FA, Domingo P, Barquet N, et al: Invasive meningococcal conjunctivitis. JAMA 264:333, 1990
4. Barquet N, Gasser I, Domingo P, et al: Primary meningococcal conjunctivitis: report of 21 patients and review. Rev Infect Dis 12:838, 1990
5. Limberg MB: A review of bacterial keratitis and bacterial conjunctivitis. Am J Ophthalmol 112 (suppl):2S, 1991
6. Vichyanond P, Brown Q, Jackson D: Acute bacterial conjunctivitis: bacteriology and clinical implications. Clin Pediatr 25:506, 1986
7. Rapoza PA, Quinn TC, Kiessling LA, Taylor HR: Epidemiology of neonatal conjunctivitis. Ophthalmology 93:456, 1986
8. Leibowitz HM, Pratt MV, Flagstad IJ, et al: Human conjunctivitis. I. Diagnostic evaluation. Arch Ophthalmol 94:1747, 1976
9. Thygeson P, Kimura SJ: Chronic conjunctivitis. Trans Am Acad Ophthalmol Otolaryngol 67:494, 1963
10. Watt PJ: Pathogenic mechanism of organisms virulent to the eye. Trans Ophthalmol Soc UK 105:26, 1986
11. Easty DL: The eye in immunodeficiency disorders. p. 135. In Cavanagh HD (ed): The Cornea: Transactions of the World Congress on the Cornea III. Raven Press, New York, 1988
12. McGill JI: Bacterial conjunctivitis. Trans Ophthalmol Soc UK 105:37, 1986
13. Hansel TT, O'Neill DP, Yee ML, et al: Infective conjunctivitis and corneal scarring in three brothers with sex linked hypogammaglobulinemia (Bruton's disease). Br J Ophthalmol 74:118, 1990
14. Seal DV: Bacterial classification and diagnosis. Trans Ophthalmol Soc UK 105:2, 1986
15. Bron AJ, Seal DV: The defenses of the ocular surface. Trans Ophthalmol Soc UK 105:18, 1986
16. Lamberts DW: Physiology of the tear film. p. 38. In Smolin G, Thoft RA (eds): The Cornea: Scientific Foundations and Clinical Practice. 2nd Ed. Little Brown, Boston, 1987
17. Friedman MG: Antibodies in human tears during and after infection. Surv Ophthalmol 35:151, 1990
18. Franklin RM: The ocular secretory immune system: a review. Curr Eye Res 8:599, 1989
19. Srinivasan M: Dermatomycosis in South India. p. 135. In Cavanagh HD (ed): The Cornea: Transactions of the World Congress on the Cornea III. Raven Press, New York, 1988
20. Prentice MJ, Hutchinson GR, Taylor-Robinson D: A microbiological study of neonatal conjunctivae and conjunctivitis. Br J Ophthalmol 61:601, 1977
21. Rubenfield RS, Cohen EJ, Prentsen JJ, Laibson PR: Diphtheroids as ocular pathogens. Am J Ophthalmol 108:251, 1989
22. Locatcher-Khorazo D, Seegal BC: The bacterial flora of the healthy eye. p. 13. In Locatcher-Khorazo D, Seegal BC (eds): Microbiology of the Eye. CV Mosby, St. Louis, 1972
23. Halbert SP: Inhibitory properties of the ocular flora. p. 24. In: Basic and Clinical Science Course. American Academy of Ophthalmology, San Francisco, CA, 1991–1992
24. Wilson FM: External disease and the cornea. p. VIII:48 In: Basic and Clinical Science Course. American Academy of Ophthalmology, San Francisco, CA, 1991–1992
25. Mannis MJ: Bacterial conjunctivitis. Ch. 5. In Tasman W, Jaeger EA (eds): Clinical Ophthalmology. Vol. 4. JB Lippincott, Philadelphia, 1990
26. Ostler HB: Oculogenital disease. Surv Ophthalmol 20:233,1976
27. Wan WL, Farkas GC, May WN, Robin JB: The clinical characteristics and course of adult gonococcal conjunctivitis. Am J Ophthalmol 102:575, 1986
28. Centers for Disease Control and Prevention: Summary of notifiable diseases, United States, 1995. MMWR 44(53):1, 1996

29. Hausen T, Burns RP, Allen A: Gonorrheal conjunctivitis, an old disease revisited. JAMA 195:1156, 1966
30. Ullman S, Roussel TJ, Culbertson WW, et al: *Neisseria gonorrhoeae* keratoconjunctivitis. Ophthalmology 94:525, 1987
31. Kestelyn P, Bogaerts J, Stevens AM, et al: Treatment of adult gonococcal keratoconjunctivitis with oral norfloxacin. Am J Ophthalmol 108:516, 1989
32. Kenny JF: Meningococcal conjunctivitis in neonates. Clin Pediatr 26:473, 1987
33. Arffa RC: Conjunctivitis. I. Follicular, neonatal and bacterial. p. 103. In: Grayson's Diseases of the Cornea. 3rd Ed. CV Mosby, St. Louis, 1991
34. Ullman S, Roussel TJ, Forster RK: Gonococcal keratoconjunctivitis. Surv Ophthalmol 32:199, 1987
35. Tarantino PA, Barron BA: Sexually transmitted diseases of the eye. Ocular Infec Dis 1:59, 1994
36. American Academy of Pediatrics: Prophylaxis and treatment of neonatal gonococcal infections. Pediatrics 65:1047, 1980
37. Lepage P, Bogaerts J, Kestelyn P, Meheus A: Single-dose cefatoxine intramuscularly cures gonococcal ophthalmia neonatorum. Br J Ophthalmol 72:518, 1988
38. Centers for Disease Control and Prevention: Sexually transmitted diseases treatment guidelines. p. i. MMWR S8:38, 1989
39. Haimovici R, Roussel TJ: Treatment of gonococcal conjunctivitis with single-dose intramuscular ceftriaxone. Am J Ophthalmol 107:511, 1989
40. Bransen L, D'Costa L, Ronald AR, et al: Single-dose kanamycin therapy of gonococcal ophthalmia neonatorum. Lancet 2:1234, 1984
41. Fransen L, Nsanze H, Klauss V, et al: Ophthalmia neonatorum in Nairobi, Kenya: the roles of *Neisseria gonorrhoeae* and *Chlamydia trachomatis.* J Infect Dis 153:862, 1986
42. Hilton AL, Richmond SJ, Milne JD, et al: *Chlamydia* A in the female genital tract. Br J Vener Dis 50:1, 1974
43. Judson FN: The importance of coexisting syphilitic, chlamydial, mycoplasmal, and trichomonal infections in the treatment of gonorrhea. Sex Transm Dis 6:112, 1979
44. Oriel JD, Reeve P, Thomas BJ, Nicol CS: Infection with *Chlamydia* group A in men with urethritis due to *Neisseria gonorrhoeae.* J Infect Dis 131:376, 1975
45. Singal SS, Reichman RC, Graman PS, et al: Isolation of *Chlamydia trachomatis* from men with urethritis: relative value of one vs. two swabs and influence of concomitant gonococcal infection. Sex Transm Dis 13:50, 1986
46. Mangiaracine AB, Pollen A: Meningococcic conjunctivitis. Arch Ophthalmol 31:284, 1944
47. American Academy of Ophthalmology: Conjunctivitis: Preferred Practice Patterns; Conjunctivitis. San Francisco, CA, 1991
48. Locatcher-Khorazo D, Sullivan N, Gutierrez E: *Staphylococcus aureus* isolated from normal and infected eyes. Arch Ophthalmol 77:370, 1967
49. Mahajan VM: Acute bacterial infections of the eye: their aetiology and treatment. Br J Ophthalmol 67:191, 1983
50. Mondino BJ, Adamu S: Ocular immune response to *Staphylococcus epidermidis.* p. 431. In Cavanagh HD (ed): The Cornea: Transactions of the World Congress on the Cornea III. Raven Press, New York, 1988
51. Trottier S, Stenberg K, Von Rosen IA, Svanborg C: *Haemophilus influenzae* causing conjunctivitis in day-care children. Pediatr Infect Dis J 10:578, 1991
52. Bodor FF: Systemic antibiotics for treatment of the conjunctivitis-otitis media syndrome. Pediatr Infect Dis J 8:287, 1989
53. Wong SL, Ng TL: *Haemophilus influenzae* in the neonate: report of two cases and review of the English literature. J Pediatr Child Health 27:113, 1991
54. Londer L, Nelson DL: Orbital cellulitis due to *Haemophilus influenzae.* Arch Ophthalmol 91:89, 1974
55. Feingold M, Gellis SS: Cellulitis due to *Haemophilus influenzae* type B. N Engl J Med 272:788, 1965
56. Harrison LH, da Silva GA, Pittman M, et al: Epidemiology and clinical spectrum of Brazilian purpuric fever. Brazilian purpuric fever study group. J Clin Microbiol 27:599, 1989
57. Wild BE, Pearman JW, Campbell PB, et al: Brazilian purpuric fever in western Australia [letter]. Med J Aust 150:344, 1989
58. Okumoto M: Microbiology. p. 141. In Smolin G, Thoft RA (eds): The Cornea: Scientific Foundations and Clinical Practice. 2nd Ed. Little, Brown, Boston, 1987
59. Wadstrom T: Biological properties of extracellular proteins from staphylococcus. Ann NY Acad Sci 236:343, 1974
60. Thygeson P: Marginal corneal infiltrates and ulcers. Trans Am Acad Ophthalmol Otolaryngol 51:198, 1946
61. Mondino BJ: Inflammatory disease of the peripheral cornea. Ophthalmology 95:463, 1988
62. Thygeson P: Bacterial factors in chronic catarrhal conjunctivitis. Trans Am Acad Ophthalmol Otolaryngol 18:373, 1937
63. Hogan MJ, Diaz-Bonnet V, Okumoto M, Kimura SJ: Experimental staphylococcic keratitis. Invest Ophthalmol 1:267, 1962
64. Ficker L, Ramakrishnan M, Seal D, Wright P: Role of cell-mediated immunity to staphylococci in blepharitis. Am J Ophthalmol 111:473, 1991
65. Van Bijsterveld OP: Bacterial proteases in *Moraxella* angular conjunctivitis. Am J Ophthalmol 72:181, 1971
66. Winceslaus T, Goh BT, Dunlop EM, et al: Diagnosis of ophthalmia neonatorum. Br Med J 295:1377, 1987
67. Burns RP, Rhodes DH: *Pseudomonas* eye infection as a cause of death in premature infants. Arch Ophthalmol 65:517, 1961
68. Milne LM, Isaacs D, Crook PJ: Neonatal infection with *Haemophilus* species. Arch Dis Child 63:83, 1988
69. Torrey JC, Reese MK: Initial aerobic flora of newborn infants; selective tolerance of the upper respiratory tract for bacteria. Am J Dis Child 69:208, 1945
70. The Trimethoprim-Polymyxin B Sulphate Ophthalmic Ointment Study Group: Trimethoprim-polymyxin B sulphate ophthalmic ointment versus chloramphenicol ophthalmic ointment in the treatment of bacterial conjunctivitis—a

review of four clinical studies. J Antimicrob Chemother 23:261, 1989
71. Lohr JA, Austin RD, Grossman M, et al: Comparison of three topical antibiotics for acute bacterial conjunctivitis. Pediatr Infect Dis J 7:628, 1988
72. Jacobson JA, Call NB, Kasworn EM, et al: Safety and efficacy of topical norfloxacin versus tobramycin in the treatment of external ocular infections. Antimicrob Agents Chemother 32:71, 1988
73. Trimethoprim-polymyxin B for bacterial conjunctivitis. Med Lett Drugs Ther 32:71, 1990
74. Leibowitz HM: Antibacterial effectiveness of ciprofloxacin 0.3% ophthalmic solution in the treatment of bacterial conjunctivitis. Am J Ophthalmol 122 (suppl):29S, 1991
75. Brodsky E, Biger Y, Zeidan Z, Schneider M: Topical application of chloramphenicol ointment followed by fatal bone marrow aplasia. Isr J Med Sci 25:54, 1989
76. Chandler AC, Locatcher-Khorazo D: Primary tuberculosis of the conjunctiva. Arch Ophthalmol 71:202, 1964
77. Archer D, Bird A: Primary tuberculosis of the conjunctiva. Br J Ophthalmol 51:679, 1967

8

Bacterial Keratitis

THOMAS J. LIESEGANG

Microbial keratitis is the most common serious ocular infection, and appears to be increasing in incidence. A variety of bacteria, fungi, viruses, and parasites can cause microbial keratitis. The organisms most commonly reported vary from one geographic region to another, depending on the prevalence and type of pre-existing corneal disease, the prevalence and style of contact lens wear, the climate, the soil, and the pattern of patient referrals. There is a shifting scene in microbial keratitis documented by comparative studies over the past several decades[1–11] (Table 8-1). Previously, pneumococcus was the most frequently isolated organism. Now opportunistic commensals are common, and in some regions, *Pseudomonas* is the most frequently isolated bacterial organism. Anaerobic bacteria and protozoa are being reported with increasing frequency. Until 1950, fungal keratitis occurred sporadically. Today it is more frequent, although the incidence varies from region to region. The concept of an ocular pathogen is outmoded; given optimal conditions, any organism can cause keratitis.

The ophthalmologist must distinguish microbial keratitis from other inflammatory conditions of the cornea.[12] There are no specific clinical signs pathognomonic of an infection. When the diagnosis is suspected on clinical examination, laboratory studies are required to identify the causative agent. Based on clinical suspicion, the results of initial laboratory studies, and a knowledge of the likely responsible organism, therapy is initiated. Therapy may be modified later depending on the clinical response and the laboratory results. With an advanced infection or a severe host inflammatory response, devastating complications may occur that result in structural alterations of the eye, such as corneal thinning, corneal perforation, or scleral extension of the infection, and can require surgical intervention.

This chapter describes the pathogenesis, clinical and laboratory features, and medical and surgical management of bacterial keratitis, including ulcerative keratitis and interstitial keratitis. Fungal keratitis is discussed in Chapter 9; viral keratitis in Chapters 10, 11, 12, and 13; chlamydial keratitis in Chapter 14; and parasitic keratitis in Chapter 15.

BACTERIAL ULCERATIVE KERATITIS

Organisms

Bacteria can be divided into two major groups based on the structure of the cell wall. Gram-negative organisms have a thin peptidoglycan layer adjacent to the cytoplasmic membrane and a cell wall containing large amounts of lipoprotein and lipopolysaccharide. Gram-positive organisms have a much thicker peptidoglycan layer, which results in a wall that tends to be more resistant to physical forces. Some bacteria produce endospores, which are highly refractile bodies formed within the vegetative bacterial cell that allow bacteria to survive adverse environmental conditions such as heat and dryness. Mycobacteria have long-chain fatty acids (mycolic acids) in their cell walls and resist decolorization by strong organic solvents, and hence are acid fast.

Because of the large variety of bacteria that can cause keratitis (Table 8-2), it is helpful to divide them into four groups, as suggested by Jones[13]: the Micrococcaceae (*Staphylococcus, Micrococcus*), the *Streptococcus* species, the *Pseudomonas* species, and the Enterobacteriaceae (*Citrobacter, Klebsiella, Enterobacter, Serratia, Proteus*). Eighty-seven percent of cases of bacterial keratitis are caused by organisms in these four groups.[13]

TABLE 8-1
Microbial Keratitis Series (Geographic Comparison)

	Miami[2]	Miami[3]	Boston[4]	Boston[5]	New York[6]	Philadelphia[7]	Southern California[8]	Nepal[9]	Africa[10]	India[11]
Study period	1969–77	1982–86	1977–81	1982–85	1956–79	1978–84	1972–83	1985–87	1981–82	1981–82
No. of patients	663	658	673	397	677	116	227	405	120	674
Culture negative (%)	44	47	NR	52	27	46	18	20	75	55
Contact lens–related (%)	6	30	28	34	NR	100	8	0	0	0
Organism										
Staphylococcus spp. (%)	19	18	43	31	49	34	51	25	61	56
Streptococcus spp. (%)	12	8	18	21	11	12	28	37	35	2
Pseudomonas spp. (%)	20	29	14	15	8	52	19	11	6	21
Enterobacteriaceae (%)	10	17	20	22	16	10	12	7	12	5
Fungi (%)	36	17	NR	5	1	2	10	17	3	12

Abbreviations: NR, not reported.

TABLE 8-2
Classification of Bacteria Important in Microbial Keratitis

- Gram-positive cocci (aerobic)
  - Micrococcus
    - *Staphylococcus aureus*
    - *Staphylococcus epidermidis*
  - Streptococcus
    - *Streptococcus pneumoniae*
    - α-, β-, and nonhemolytic streptococci
    - Enterococcus
- Gram-positive bacilli (aerobic)
  - *Bacillus* (*B. cereus, B. subtilis*)
  - *Corynebacterium* (*C. diphtheriae, C. xeroses*)
  - *Listeria monocytogenes*
- Gram-negative bacilli (aerobic)
  - *Pseudomonas* (especially *P. aeruginosa*)
  - *Acinetobacter*
  - *Azotobacter*
  - Enterobacteriaceae
    - *Klebsiella*
    - *Serratia*
    - *Proteus*
    - *Citrobacter*
    - *Enterobacter*
    - *Escherichia*
    - *Erwinia*
- Gram-negative diplococci (aerobic)
  - *Neisseria*
- Gram-negative diplobacilli (aerobic)
  - *Moraxella*
- Gram-negative coccobacilli (aerobic)
  - *Haemophilus*
- Gram-positive filaments
  - *Mycobacterium* (nontuberculous)
  - *Nocardia*
- Gram-positive cocci (anaerobic)
  - *Peptococcus*
  - *Peptostreptococcus*
- Gram-positive bacilli (anaerobic)
  - *Propionibacterium acnes*
  - Actinomyces (branching filaments)
  - *Clostridium* (rare)
- Gram-negative bacilli (anaerobic)
  - *Fusobacterium*
  - *Bacteroides*
  - *Capnocytophaga*
- Gram-negative cocci (anaerobic)
  - *Veillonella*
- Spirochaetales
  - *Treponema*
  - *Borrelia*
  - *Leptospira*

Pneumococcus *(Streptococcus pneumoniae)* was the predominant cause of bacterial keratitis in the past, especially when the keratitis was associated with chronic dacryocystitis. In most large series, gram-positive organisms continue to be the predominant cause of bacterial keratitis.[4,8] Although *Streptococcus* species are still frequently seen in the northeastern and western United States, *Staphylococcus aureus* is now the most common cause of bacterial keratitis in the northern and northeastern United States and in Canada, both in previously normal corneas and in previously compromised corneas.[4] In series from New York City[6] and southern California,[8] *S. aureus* is the most common cause of bacterial keratitis, followed by *Moraxella, P. aeruginosa,* and *S. pneumoniae.*[6] In London,[14] the most common causes are *S. aureus, S. pneumoniae, Pseudomonas,* and *Moraxella.*

P. aeruginosa is assuming predominance as a cause of bacterial keratitis.[15] It is more common than *S. aureus* in the southern United States.[2,16] *Pseudomonas* keratitis is frequently reported in otherwise healthy patients in association with daily-wear[2] or extended-wear[17-22] soft contact lenses, as a contaminant in the hospital environment, in fluorescein solutions, in cosmetics, and in any fluid that contains minute elements. *Pseudomonas* keratitis is also seen in burn patients, semicomatose or comatose patients, patients with corneal exposure, patients on mechanical respiratory assistance, and patients infected with human immunodeficiency virus (HIV). *Pseudomonas* and *Streptococcus* are the main pathogens in previously healthy eyes in the southern United States.

In two series of children with microbial keratitis, *Pseudomonas* was the most common organism in children under the age of 3 years, whereas *S. aureus, S. pneumoniae,* and *P. aeruginosa* were the most common organisms in older children.[23,24] Medical disease was a frequent concomitant and initiating factor of microbial keratitis and because of the difficulty in delivering medical therapy in children, surgical intervention was frequently necessary.

Moraxella, a gram-negative, boxcar-shaped diplobacillus, is seen mainly in malnourished, alcoholic, or immunocompromised patients,[25,26] but has also been reported in healthy patients.[27]

The indigenous bacteria of the eyelids and conjunctiva *(Staphylococcus epidermidis, Corynebacterium,* and *Propionibacterium* species) are being isolated with increasing frequency in some series. Although their precise role in corneal disease cannot be determined, they have been increasingly implicated as primary pathogens or as participants in polymicrobial keratitis[2,28] as well as in endophthalmitis. Organisms less frequently associated with keratitis include the Enterobacteriaceae[29] *(Serratia,*[30] *Proteus), Azotobacter,*[31] *Neisseria gonorrhoeae,* and *Neisseria meningitidis.*[32] *Bacillus cereus* is a large, aerobic, gram-positive rod that is a pathogen with an extremely virulent course following foreign body injury.[33,34] *Listeria monocytogenes* is a gram-positive organism and has been isolated from corneal infections in animal handlers and farmers.[35]

Non-spore-forming anaerobic bacteria are the major residents of the skin, oral cavity, gastrointestinal tract, and other mucous membranes, and can contribute to the pathogenesis of keratitis and other ocular infections.[36] They can also cause a smoldering iritis after cataract extraction. The organisms usually become invasive under predisposing host conditions. Anaerobic infections should be suspected after human or animal bites, if there is extensive necrosis of tissue, or if there is gas formation in tissues or a foul discharge. The most frequent anaerobic organisms are *Peptostreptococcus, Peptococcus, Propionibacterium, Bacteroides,* and *Fusobacterium.* With the use of specialized media for detection, anaerobic bacteria may become increasingly recognized as a cause of keratitis.[28,37,38] The spore-forming anaerobic bacteria (e.g., *Clostridium perfringens)* rarely cause keratitis.[39]

Due to the emergence of multiple drugs to treat tuberculosis, the number of atypical mycobacterial infections has increased.[40-46] These organisms are acid-fast, aerobic motile mycobacteria that are usually saprophytic in the environment. They differ from typical *Mycobacterium tuberculosis* in some of their biochemical characteristics. Runyon's classification divides the atypical mycobacteria into four groups based on growth rate, pigment production, catalase activity, and virulence in laboratory animals (Table 8-3).

TABLE 8-3
Atypical Mycobacteria Groups (Runyon)

Group	*Characteristics*	*Reported in Microbial Keratitis*
I	Photochromogenic[a] Slow growers	*M. marinum*
II	Scotochromogenic[b] Slow growers	*M. gordonae* *M. flavescens*
III	Nonphotochromogenic[c] Usually slow growers	*M. avium-intracellulare* *M. triviale*
IV	Rapid growers	*M. fortuitum* *M. chelonae*

[a] Produces pigment in light.
[b] Produces pigment in light or dark.
[c] Does not produce pigment.

Several different species of atypical mycobacteria have been documented by culture in cases of infectious keratitis. *M. fortuitum, M. chelonae* (formerly *M. chelonei*), *M. avium-intracellulare, M. marinum, M. gordonae, M. triviale,* and *M. flavescens* have all been isolated from corneal infections, although *M. chelonae* has accounted for the majority of corneal ulcers in recent years.

Cell wall studies indicate that *Actinomyces* and *Nocardia* resemble bacteria more than fungi, despite their filamentous character.[33] These bacteria replicate by spores or by fragmentation of filaments. All are gram-positive; *Nocardia* is acid fast. Corneal infections with these organisms are uncommon.[47,48]

Pathogenesis

The cornea is an avascular structure constantly bathed in a tear film that contains microorganisms. Both the eyelids and the tear film are natural barriers to infection.[49] The eyelids provide a physical barrier to exogenous organisms and deter adherence of organisms to the ocular surface. The tear film provides mechanical lubrication to wash away organisms, and also contains antimicrobial substances, including lymphocytes, immunoglobulins (IgA, IgG, IgD, and IgE), lysozyme, lactoferrin, betalysin, orosomucoid, ceruloplasmin, and complement components. The cornea has a protective coating of two layers of mucosubstances: an adherent glycocalyx and a mucin layer produced by goblet cells. Intact corneal epithelial cells also form a barrier against infection.

Most bacterial corneal infections occur as a result of trauma or contact lens wear, or in patients with compromised local or systemic defense mechanisms[8] (Table 8-4). Local conditions that predispose to bacterial keratitis include defects in the tear film (dry eyes, lacrimal obstruction); blepharitis and malposition of the eyelids and eyelashes (entropion, trichiasis); difficulty in eyelid closure (lagophthalmos and exposure); defects in the integrity and adherence of the corneal epithelium (bullous keratopathy, corneal abrasion, chemical injury, contact lens wear, viral keratitis); and absence of corneal innervation (neurotrophic keratitis). Topical corticosteroids, antiviral medications, contaminated ocular medications,[50] and anesthetics impair the immune mechanisms. Systemic conditions associated with decreased immunity to corneal infection include alcoholism, debilitating diseases, central nervous system and psychiatric disturbances, immunosuppressive therapy, extensive burns, and acquired immunodeficiency syndrome (AIDS).[8] Nosocomial bacterial keratitis occurs more commonly in comatose patients with respiratory infections. Inoculation of the cornea from the perineum is suggested in cases of *E. coli, Enterobacter,* or *Proteus* keratitis. Personal hygiene must be addressed in patients with such infections; otherwise, repeated inoculation and bacterial keratitis are likely to recur.

TABLE 8-4
Mechanisms Contributing to Risk of Microbial Keratitis

- Local
  - Trauma
  - Contact lens wear
  - Tear dysfunction
    - Dry eyes
    - Lacrimal obstruction
  - Eyelid dysfunction
    - Blepharitis
    - Entropion, ectropion
    - Trichiasis
    - Lagophthalmos
    - Cicatricial pemphigoid
  - Corneal disease or damage
    - Epithelial disease
    - Bullous keratopathy
    - Corneal abrasion
    - Keratomalacia
    - Chemical injury
    - Herpes simplex, herpes zoster
    - Corneal exposure
    - Corneal surgery
  - Corneal innervation
    - Neurotrophic keratitis
  - Conjunctivitis
    - Especially with *Neisseria, Corynebacterium, Haemophilus, Listeria,* and *Shigella* spp.
  - Topical drugs
    - Preservatives
    - Anesthetics
    - Corticosteroids
    - Antivirals
- Systemic
  - Extensive burns
  - Alcoholism
  - Debilitating disease, malnutrition
  - Rheumatoid arthritis
  - Diabetes mellitus
  - Drug addiction
  - Acquired immunodeficiency syndrome
  - Mucous membrane disease (e.g., Stevens-Johnson syndrome)
  - Systemic immunosuppressive therapy
  - Chronic neurologic abnormality

Because of its prominent location, the cornea is predisposed to injury and structural alterations. The immediate precipitating event in bacterial keratitis is usually an epithelial defect produced by trauma, contact lens wear, or a chronic corneal disorder. Chronic corneal disorders, such as dry eyes, lagophthalmos, and trichiasis, must be recognized and treated if recurrent bacterial keratitis is to be prevented. Organisms invade the epithelium and stroma from the patient's tear film or as a contaminant of a foreign body, irrigating solution, fluorescein, or contact lens. The glycocalyx of injured corneal epithelial cells may promote adhesion of bacteria and facilitate invasion of bacteria into the corneal stroma. The site of entry may be subtle, for example, a mascara brush injury, an abrasion from a fingernail or vegetable matter, or an abrasion from a contact lens. Rarely, there may be invasion of organisms into the cornea from the anterior chamber in endophthalmitis or from hematogenous dissemination during sepsis.

Contact lenses cause corneal hypoxia, increase corneal temperature, and decrease tear flow over the corneal surface with a subsequent decrease in the cleansing function of the tear film and eyelids. Soft contact lenses cause microtrauma to the corneal epithelium and become coated with mucus and proteins within a few hours of placement on the cornea, which enhances the adherence of bacteria to the lens or to the corneal epithelium.[51-59] Hard contact lenses and daily-wear, extended-wear, disposable, and bandage soft contact lenses all increase the risk of microbial keratitis.[7,18-22,51,60-69] Corneal hypoxia is exacerbated if contact lenses are worn overnight. The relative risk of microbial keratitis is 9 to 15 times higher in patients who wear contact lenses overnight than in patients who wear them exclusively on a daily-wear basis.[62,70] The risk of microbial keratitis with soft contact lenses, especially when worn as extended-wear lenses, is high in aphakic eyes.[71] Disposable soft contact lenses, especially when worn overnight, may have an even higher risk of keratitis.[68,72] Other factors associated with microbial keratitis and contact lens wear include poor contact lens hygiene, history of smoking, contaminated contact lenses and contact lens solutions, and trauma at the time of insertion and removal of the lens.[11,73,74] Failure of patients to follow standard recommendations for contact lens care is widespread and of major epidemiologic importance.[75] *P. aeruginosa* and *Staphylococcus* are the most common causes of bacterial keratitis associated with contact lens wear. Bandage soft contact lenses are associated with a high incidence of polymicrobial infections and infections with commensal organisms.[61] More specifically, *Pseudomonas* is associated with cosmetic soft contact lenses (especially extended-wear lenses); *Staphylococcus, Streptococcus,* and *Serratia* are associated with bandage soft contact lenses.[5] Microbial keratitis not associated with contact lens wear has a broader range of causative organisms.

There is a bimodal distribution of predisposing factors for bacterial keratitis. In younger patients, predisposing factors are ocular trauma and contact lens wear; in older patients, predisposing factors are chronic corneal disease (such as keratitis sicca), mucosal scarring disorders, herpes simplex viral keratitis, surgical trauma, bullous keratopathy, and entropion.[17] Diabetes mellitus, rheumatoid arthritis, chronic alcoholism, dementia, and blood dyscrasia may be identified in patients with bacterial keratitis, although systemic host defenses are usually normal. Up to one-half of bacterial ulcers may be iatrogenic or associated with postsurgical complications.[5] Clustered cases of bacterial keratitis have been identified in premature infants, burn patients, comatose patients, tracheotomized patients, surgical patients, and patients with acquired immunodeficiency syndrome. The estimated annual incidence of ulcerative keratitis in contact lens wearers, given the current pattern of contact lens wear, is estimated to be 4.1 per 10,000 daily-wear soft contact lens users; 20.9 per 10,000 extended-wear soft contact lens users; 2 per 10,000 polymethyl methacrylate contact lens users; and 4.0 per 10,000 rigid gas-permeable contact lens users.[62,70] Wearers of disposable lenses may have an even higher rate.[67,76]

Patients who have undergone penetrating keratoplasty are particularly at risk of microbial keratitis because of frequent use of topical corticosteroids, hypesthesia of the graft, persistent epithelial defects, loosening of sutures, trichiasis, and bandage soft contact lens wear.[77-82] The chronic use of antibiotics allows the emergence of resistant organisms, which complicates the clinical scenario. Up to 12 percent of patients develop a corneal infection after penetrating keratoplasty[83]; such infection tends to occur in the first year after surgery and severely worsens the visual prognosis.[83-86] Gram-positive cocci are most commonly seen, although fungal and polymicrobial infections can occur. The use of contact lenses increases the risk of infection with gram-negative bacilli. Infectious crystalline keratopathy is usually caused by *Streptococcus,* although it can be caused by several other organisms. It presents with slowly progressive needle-like stromal opacities, and is most frequently associated with penetrating keratoplasty; organisms are probably introduced through the suture needle tract.

The primary determinant of the severity of bacterial keratitis is the virulence of the invading organism. Secondary determinants include the previous health of the cornea and the host response. The pathogenicity of the organism is related to its ability to adhere to the edge or base of an epithelial defect and to invade the stroma despite host defenses.[87] The adherence of *S. aureus, S. pneumoniae,* and *P. aeruginosa* to the edge of an epithelial defect is significantly higher than that of other bacteria, and may account for their frequent isolation.[88,89] In gram-positive bacteria, membrane appendages, called fibrillae, are responsible for the adherence of the organism to epithelial cells; in gram-negative bacteria, fimbriae (pili) and a glycocalyx (slime envelope) may be responsible for adherence.[90] With *P. aeruginosa,* adherence may be related to the influence of local calcium or magnesium levels on the pili.[91,92] The adherence of *P. aeruginosa* and *N. gonorrhoeae* is aided by a glycocalyx that enables the bacteria to stick to susceptible cells and to each other, thereby producing aggregates of organisms that resist phagocytosis and allow penetration and invasion into the cornea.[93] The biofilm of *P. aeruginosa* also allows rapid adherence of the organism even to new contact lenses,[53,94,95] with subsequent attachment to epithelial defects.[96,97] Receptors on epithelial cells or the basement membrane may also enhance adherence of *Pseudomonas.*[97–99] *Staphylococcus, Moraxella,* and *Candida* can actively adhere to soft contact lens deposits.[98–100] The coating that forms on contact lenses may facilitate this adherence.[101] The polymer slime secreted by some bacteria can enhance their pathogenicity by inhibiting phagocytosis and decreasing their nutritional requirements.[100] *N. gonorrhoeae, Corynebacterium diphtheriae, Shigella, Listeria,* and *Haemophilus aegyptius* (Koch-Weeks bacillus) are unique in that they may initiate infection without antecedent epithelial ulceration. *Neisseria* penetrates epithelial cells with the aid of a protease, and the virulence of certain strains may be related to protease concentration.[102]

The protective capsules of some bacteria may negate the antimicrobial properties of lysozyme. The capsular polysaccharides of pneumococcus inhibit phagocytosis. The tubercle bacillus can resist destruction by enzymes that inactivate other digestive enzymes.

Specialized bacterial enzymes aid in the penetration of the organisms into the stroma and in the degradation of corneal substance. Multiple toxins are released, including the α, β, γ, and δ toxins of *Staphylococcus;* the A, B, and C toxins of *Pseudomonas;* and other enzymes, including proteases, coagulases, collagenases, nucleases, fibrinolysins, lipases, and hemolysins. Some substances (exotoxins) are released by actively multiplying bacteria; others (endotoxins) are released only after the death of the organisms, and can persist and continue to digest corneal stroma long after the organisms die.

Most exotoxins are thermolabile and have antigenic properties.[103,104] *S. aureus* produces at least 30 different biologically active substances and four immunologically distinct toxins.[105] Coagulase-positive strains are the most pathogenic, and elaborate other extracellular enzymes, such as staphylokinase, lipase, hyaluronidase, DNase, coagulase, and lysozyme. *S. epidermidis* also produces damaging toxins.[106] Streptococcal toxins include streptolysin O and S, erythrogenic toxin, and the enzymes hyaluronidase, streptodornase, and streptokinase. *S. pneumoniae* is inherently invasive without toxin production, but the invasiveness may be aided by collagenase activity.[107] The α toxin of *Clostridium perfringens (C. welchii)* is a phospholipase that digests cell membranes. A protease has been identified as a major pathogenic factor in *Serratia* keratitis.[108] *Pseudomonas* produces exotoxin A that inhibits cellular protein synthesis and impairs phagocytosis. The toxin is found in 90 percent of *Pseudomonas* strains, although it is not necessary for initiation of corneal damage.[109] The cornea-destroying enzyme of *P. aeruginosa* was originally thought to be a collagenase, but has since been demonstrated to be a proteoglycanase.[108] Proteoglycanases break down the protective ground substance around collagen.[110,111] Collagenases attack the terminal peptide of native collagen and, thereby, liberate amino acids. Proteoglycanase and collagenase are both metallodependent and are inhibited by sodium edetate in vitro. Bacterial proteases attack peptide bonds, dissolve elastin, and act as nonspecific collagenases in vitro. Hemolysins (predominantly phospholipases) are elaborated by staphylococci, pneumococci, and *Pseudomonas,* and lyse erythrocytes and other cells.[112,113] Some of these toxins may have antibacterial activity that inhibits the coexistence of other organisms.[112,114] The specific toxins of *Bacillus cereus* are probably responsible for the fulminating nature of ocular infections caused by this organism.[104]

Endotoxins are lipopolysaccharides contained within the cell wall of gram-negative bacteria, and are released only when the organism dies. Endotoxin can cause corneal ring infiltrates, which consist of polymorphonuclear leukocytes within the corneal stroma that are attracted by the alternative complement pathway and chemotaxis through properdin activation.[115,116] Although ring infiltrates occur in gram-negative, fungal, viral, and *Acanthamoeba* keratitis and are thought to represent antigen-antibody precipitates (immune rings), the role of the immune response in suppurative keratitis has not been completely established.

Host-derived enzymes also play a prominent role in bacterial keratitis. The important contribution of host-derived enzymes in the pathogenesis of *Pseudomonas* keratitis has been demonstrated.[117,118] Following invasion, there is stimulation and release of chemotactic substances that initiate polymorphonuclear leukocyte migration from the limbus.[119] The stimulus for these substances may be the organisms themselves, lymphocytes, antigen-antibody complexes, or complement. Polymorphonuclear leukocytes are important in host defenses, but are also implicated in the destruction of corneal collagen and ground substance. The microbial killing power of polymorphonuclear leukocytes is

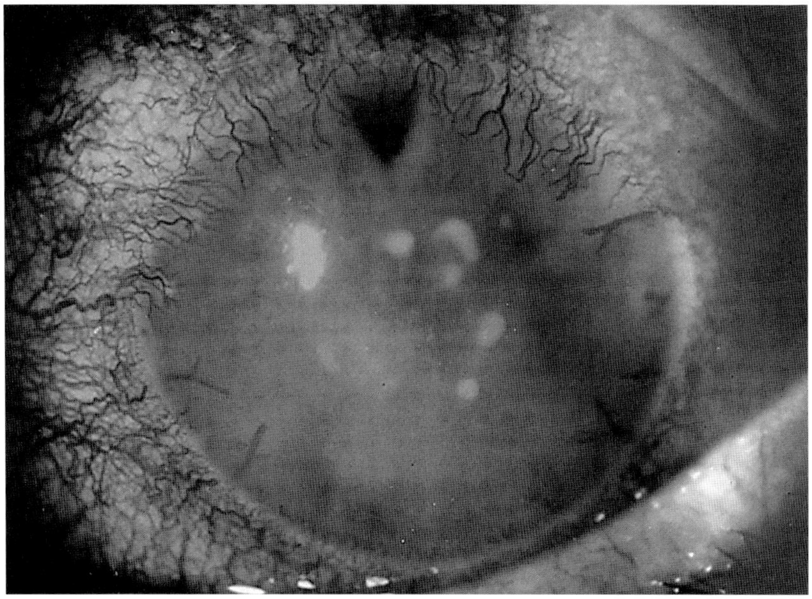

FIGURE 8-1 Multifocal *Staphylococcus aureus* keratitis in a contact lens wearer. Note the circular arrangement of the infiltrates.

accomplished either through degranulation of cytoplasmic organelles that fuse with the membrane of the primary phagosome or through the respiratory burst, that is, a series of metabolic events that follow stimulation of phagocytes.[120]

Polymorphonuclear leukocytes produce toxic oxygen metabolites, such as hydrogen peroxide, and superoxide anions that may contribute to progressive corneal destruction. The extent of visual impairment relates directly to the degree of this inflammatory cell infiltration, phagocytosis, cell death, release of proteolytic enzymes, and damage to the endothelium. Damaged or migratory epithelial cells and polymorphonuclear leukocytes elaborate proteoglycanase and collagenase, which contribute to further structural damage.[93] The extent of damage produced by polymorphonuclear leukocytes is evident from animal experiments in which the leukocytes are suppressed by cyclophosphamide; the resultant decrease in polymorphonuclear leukocytes causes a milder course with better final resolution.[121] Work on mutant strains of *Pseudomonas* that lack exotoxin A and elastase may aid in determining the relative importance of toxins, enzymes, and polymorphonuclear leukocytes.[109]

Corticosteroids and antibiotics can also interfere with the normal chemotactic response. Corticosteroids may enhance the invasion of saprophytic organisms, but may also alter the clinical signs of infection.[122] The use of sublethal antibiotics may also mask the typical features of bacterial keratitis. The toxicity of various therapeutic agents may in itself produce a clinical picture that simulates corneal infection.

Clinical Features

There are no symptoms pathognomonic of bacterial keratitis or biomicroscopic signs that distinguish the responsible bacteria, although several bacteria produce a distinctive clinical appearance. The presenting clinical features are determined by the prior status of the cornea, previous therapy, virulence of the organism, duration of the infection, and the host's response.

Nonspecific symptoms of bacterial keratitis include decreased vision, photophobia, pain, redness, conjunctival and eyelid edema, and discharge. In a previously healthy cornea, the presence of an epithelial defect with mucopurulent exudate adherent to the defect, suppuration of the stroma underlying the defect, diffuse cellular infiltration of the adjacent stroma, and anterior chamber inflammation constitute strong evidence for an infectious process. Additionally, eyelids that are stuck together in the morning and white cells in the tear film are important clinical clues in diagnosing bacterial keratitis. When a bacterial infection occurs under a contact lens, it is often multifocal and tends to form a circle around the pupillary edge, perhaps in one of the transition zones of the optics of the contact lens (Figures 8-1 and 8-2). Iris inflammation and hyperemia vary in intensity. Miosis and synechiae may occur and, with progression, hypopyon, increasing stromal edema, radiating folds in Descemet's membrane as stromal substance is lost (Figure 8-3), and corneal neovascularization occur.

The clinical symptoms and signs are different in a patient with a previously altered cornea. The signs may be difficult to interpret in view of prior corneal inflammation,

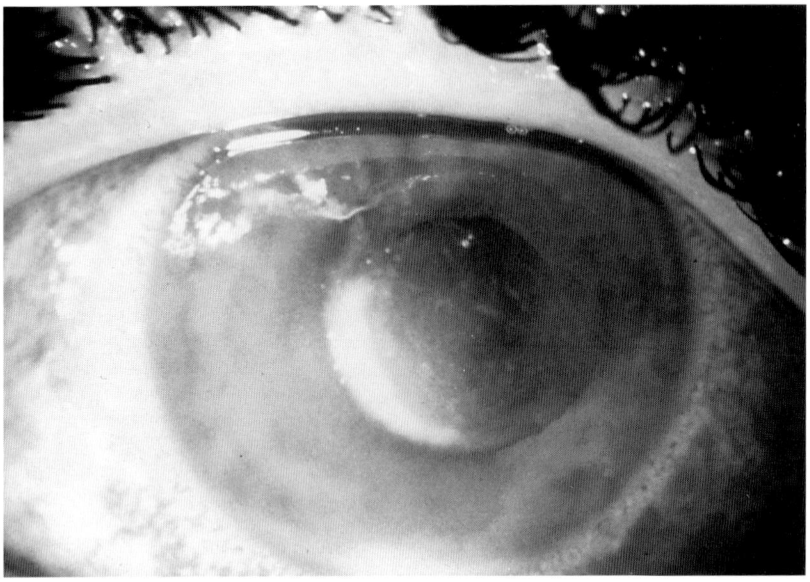

FIGURE 8-2 Arcuate *Pseudomonas* keratitis and hypopyon in a contact lens wearer. The area of infection corresponds to the area of contact lens touch.

iritis, and structural abnormalities. In such patients, an infection should be suspected in the presence of increasing pain, redness, an increase in epithelial and stromal ulceration, an increase in anterior segment inflammation, or any sudden deterioration in the clinical state.

Other factors may alter the clinical presentation. Antecedent treatment with corticosteroids may enhance the likelihood of invasion by opportunistic organisms and also alters the clinical signs of infection. Corticosteroids and immunosuppressive agents impede host defenses by inhibiting chemotaxis and ingestion by phagocytes, blocking degranulation, interfering with lysosomal levels, and reducing the production of phagocytes. Topical corticosteroids also establish the potential for resurgence of stromal inflammation and necrosis if they are abruptly discontinued during the initial management of the infection, which can confuse the initial response to treatment. Topical antibiotics can reduce various inhibitory substances by suppressing normal conjunctival flora and lead to secondary invasion by saprophytic organisms. Partial suppression of bacterial replication by sublethal antibiotics can diminish the suppurative process, mask the typical features of infection, and produce atypical features. Additionally, the toxicity of certain topical drugs,

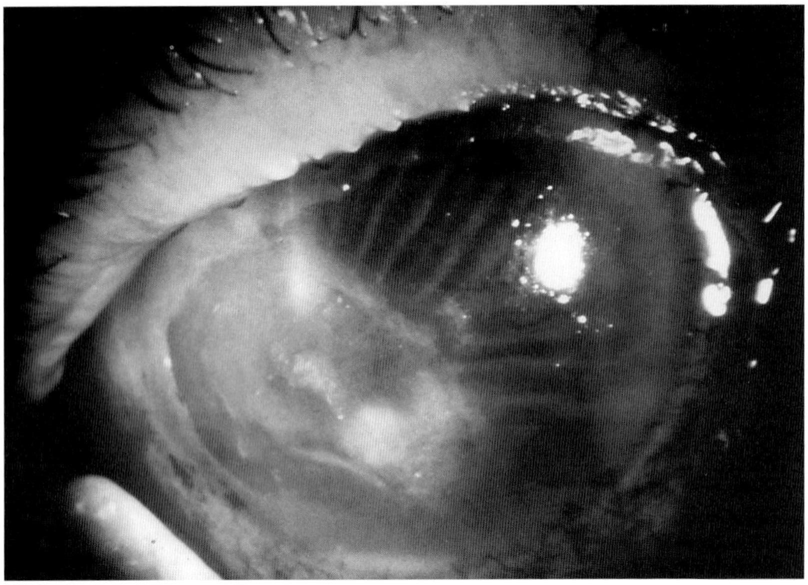

FIGURE 8-3 Bacterial keratitis and hypopyon in a patient with pseudophakic bullous keratopathy. Note the radiating folds in Descemet's membrane, which indicate loss of stromal substance in the area of the ulcer.

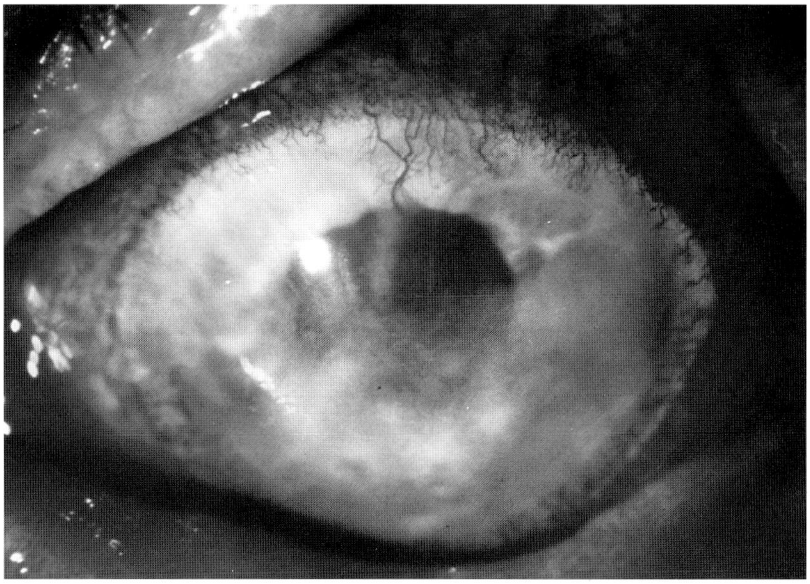

FIGURE 8-4 Patient with corneal abrasion treated with topical gentamicin for several weeks because of failure to re-epithelialize. The patient responded well to withdrawal of gentamicin, confirming that this was a toxic corneal response.

such as aminoglycosides (Figure 8-4), anesthetics (Figure 8-5),[123,124] idoxuridine, and amphotericin B, can simulate corneal infection by causing epithelial and stromal ulceration, multiple focal suppurative infiltrates, and anterior chamber inflammation.

Clinical acumen and experience are essential to distinguish microbial keratitis from nonmicrobial insults to the cornea.[12] The differential diagnosis is particularly difficult in cases of contact lens wear, herpes simplex viral keratitis (Figure 8-6), indolent or neurotrophic ulcers, peripheral marginal infiltration from multiple causes, toxic or chemical keratopathy, and any disease characterized by persistent epithelial defects or anterior stromal ulceration. Keratitis sicca is particularly associated with significant toxicity from potent topical medications, which can lead to stromal lysis and perforation even in the absence of cellular infiltration.

At the initial presentation, the severity of the process should be judged and recordings made of objective parameters that can be remeasured for comparison during subsequent examinations to better monitor the clinical course. The size of the epithelial and stromal ulceration can be measured in two meridians with the variable slit beam of the slit lamp microscope. Photographs may be more

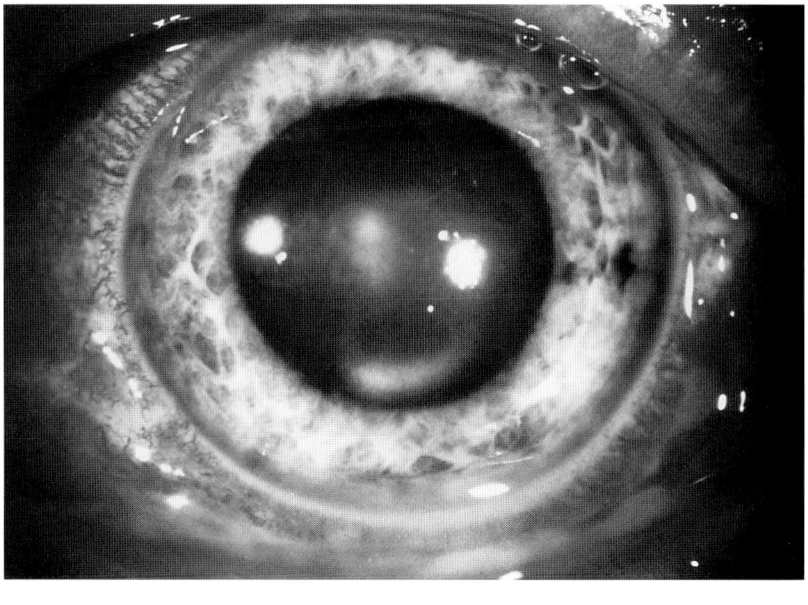

FIGURE 8-5 Large corneal infiltrate caused by proparacaine abuse.

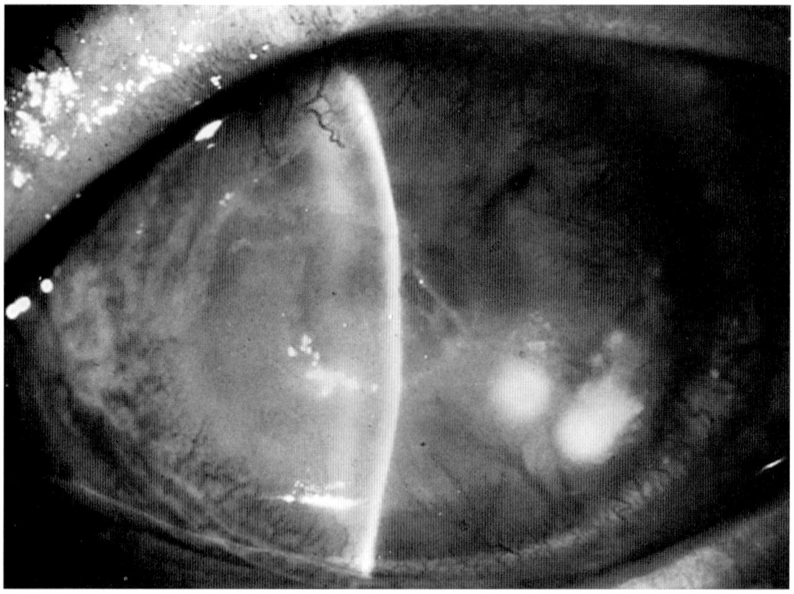

FIGURE 8-6 Multifocal herpes simplex stromal keratitis, the clinical appearance of which may be difficult to distinguish from other causes of microbial keratitis.

valuable, but are difficult to produce in a short time. Features to consider in judging severity are the area and depth of stromal ulceration, suppuration and edema, stromal thickness, amount of scleral suppuration, amount of anterior chamber inflammation, glaucoma, and the rate of progression of the disease. The following grading system is useful in judging the severity of the disease process and provides a guide to the aggressiveness of therapy: mild disease (focal superficial suppuration) (Figure 8-7); moderate disease (large suppurative inflammation that is limited to the superficial two-thirds of the cornea) (Figure 8-8); and severe disease (extensive area of suppuration that involves the posterior third of the cornea, accompanied by a ring abscess, scleral suppuration, or threatened perforation)[125] (Figure 8-9). There may also be a large hypopyon, hyphema, extensive synechiae, and glaucoma. A more complex and detailed grading system has been proposed by several authors.[126,127]

Some characteristic features of certain corneal pathogens are noteworthy, although they are not pathognomonic and should not be used in lieu of smears and cultures for diagnosis or treatment.[128,129] Gram-positive cocci tend to cause

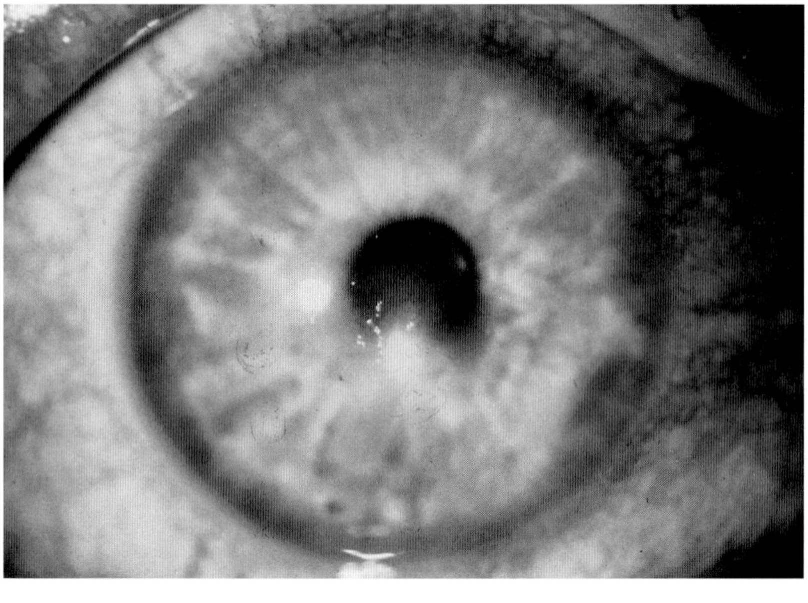

FIGURE 8-7 Mild bacterial keratitis caused by *Staphylococcus aureus.* There is a small focal superficial corneal abscess.

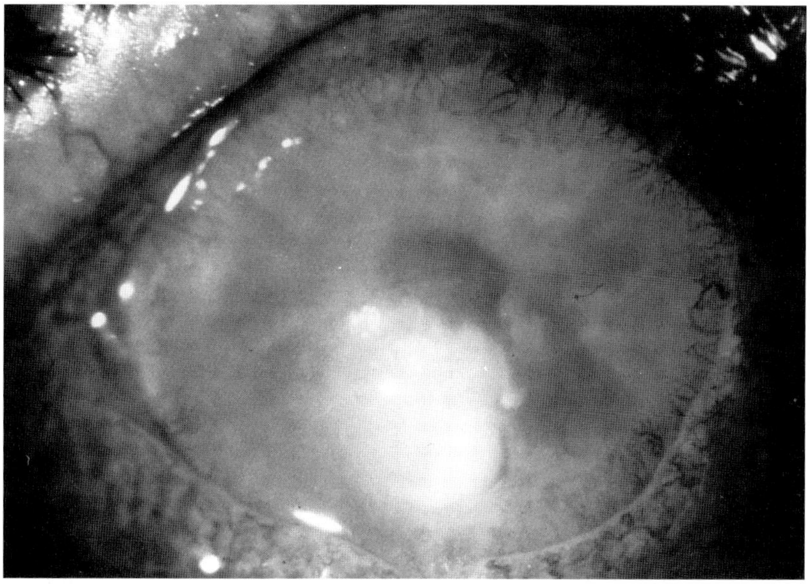

FIGURE 8-8 Moderate bacterial keratitis caused by *Pseudomonas aeruginosa*. The central infiltration and suppurative ulceration are confined to the superficial two-thirds of the cornea. There is also diffuse corneal edema.

localized, round or oval, gray-white ulcers that have distinct borders and minimal surrounding epithelial edema and stromal infiltrate.[130] The ulcer rarely involves the entire corneal surface. *Streptococcus* progresses rapidly, whereas *Staphylococcus* progresses more slowly and is frequently indolent. A distinct, indolent non-inflammatory-appearing crystalline keratopathy has been reported in association with a nutritional variant of *Streptococcus viridans*,[131–137] although other organisms, such as *Haemophilus aphrophilus*,[138] *S. epidermidis*,[139] *Peptostreptococcus*, *Alternaria*, and *Candida*, have also been isolated[140,141] (Figure 8-10). Infectious crystalline keratopathy typically occurs after penetrating keratoplasty and is associated with epithelial defects, corneal ulceration, loose sutures, contact lens wear, topical corticosteroids, and suture manipulation. This chronic corneal infection is characterized by interlamellar plaques of organisms in the absence of inflammatory cells. There is a possible role of intracorneal glycocalyx deposition or increased exopolysaccharide formation from streptococci in infectious crystalline keratopathy.[137,142] Appropriate intensive topical antibiotic therapy may fail to eradicate the infection.[143]

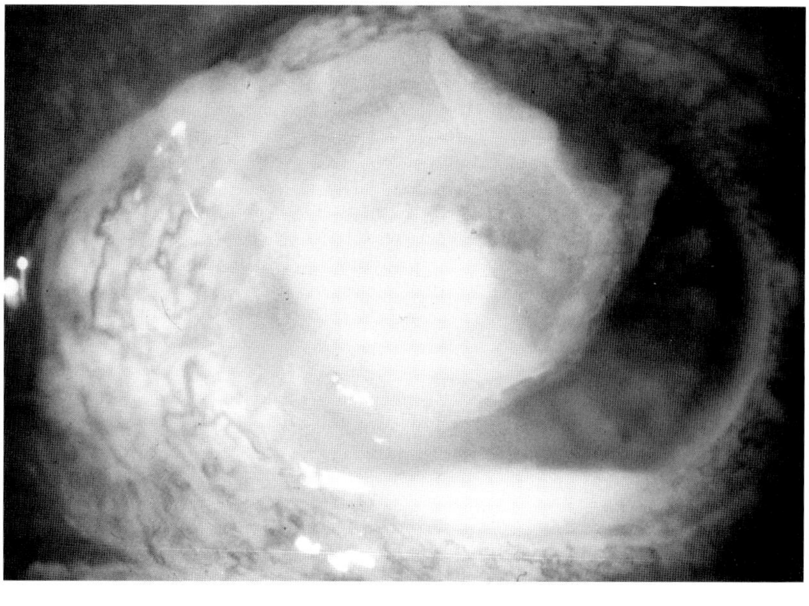

FIGURE 8-9 Severe bacterial keratitis caused by *Streptococcus pneumoniae*. The central infiltration and suppurative ulceration are deep and are accompanied by a hypopyon. Stromal necrosis is extensive.

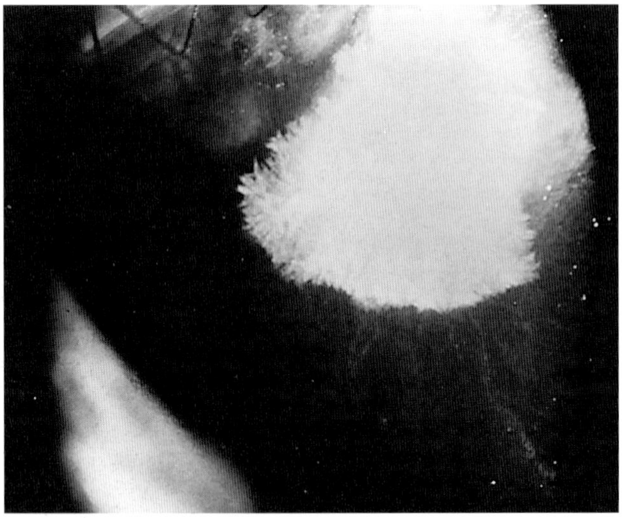

A

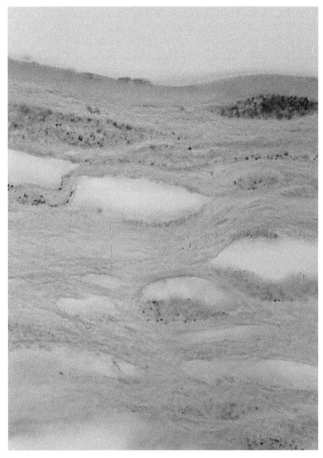

B

FIGURE 8-10 **(A)** Infectious crystalline keratopathy in a corneal graft 3 months after penetrating keratoplasty. The patient was on topical corticosteroids. Note the crystal-like edges of the infiltrate. **(B)** A corneal biopsy revealed interlamellar clusters of gram-positive cocci beneath an intact Bowman's layer. Inflammatory cells are absent (Brown-Brenn stain).

In *S. pneumoniae* ulceration, the classic picture is a deep, oval, central stromal ulcer with undermining edges following trauma (Figure 8-11). The ulcer has a serpiginous edge of activity, which advances on one edge while healing on the opposite edge. There is also increasing dense stromal abscess formation with radiating folds in Descemet's membrane and moderate stromal edema. Hypopyon is a common feature, with fibrin deposition on the endothelium underlying the ulcer. Perforation is possible. β-Hemolytic streptococci also tend to cause a severe corneal infection.

Staphylococcal blepharitis may be associated with hypersensitivity marginal infiltrates or ulcerations (see Chs. 7 and 23). *S. aureus* central ulcers are frequently superinfections in compromised corneas, especially in association with herpes zoster, atopic dermatitis, acne rosacea, or contact lens wear. Prior corneal disease can frequently cause the ulcer to have an atypical appearance. Typically, however, *S. aureus* causes an oval, yellow-white suppurative ulcer with a deep, dense stromal abscess (Figure 8-12). The surrounding cornea is clear, although there may be a wide area of fine cellular infiltration throughout the stroma that is sometimes sharply limited in depth. A large hypopyon or endothelial fibrin plaque is usually present and is larger than expected, based on the area of ulceration. *S. epidermidis* presents with a more indolent ulceration and infiltration, but can also lead to intrastromal abscess formation and perforation (Figure 8-13).

P. aeruginosa produces perhaps the most distinctive bacterial corneal infection. It presents with a rapidly progressive central or paracentral, broad, shallow ulcer with copious mucopurulent, yellowish green exudate that adheres tenaciously to the gray ulcer surface and

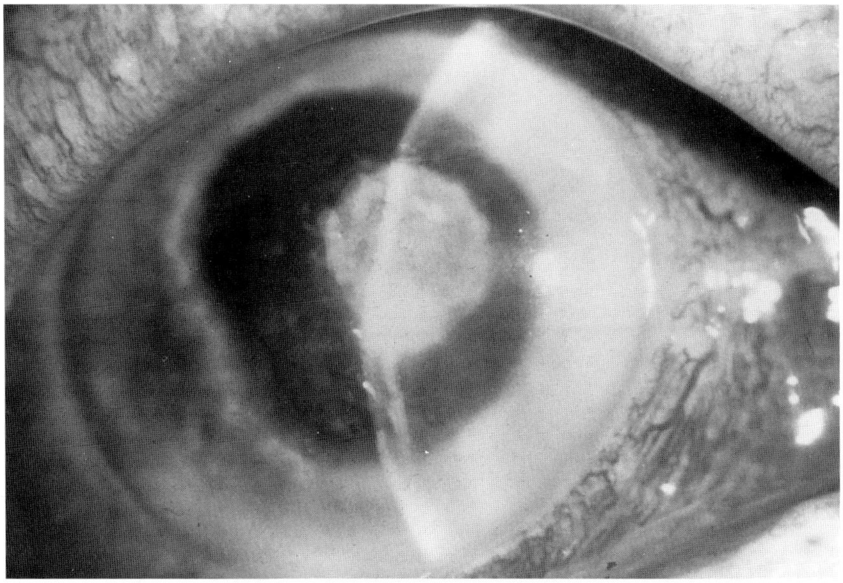

FIGURE 8-11 Central corneal ulcer caused by *Streptococcus pneumoniae.*

covers the conjunctiva (Figure 8-14). The remaining cornea has a ground-glass appearance, with loss of transparency or a diffuse graying of the epithelium (inflammatory epithelial edema) away from the ulcer site. The ulcer can progress rapidly (with or without treatment) to a stromal abscess that can spread concentrically and symmetrically to form a ring ulcer accompanied by a large hypopyon. Perforation is a distinct threat.[144]

There are several clinical types of *Pseudomonas* keratitis. The most common is caused by a corneal-virulent strain that has the potential for rapid destruction of the stroma and early descemetocele formation (liquefactive necrosis), with the risk of perforation within a day. This virulence is attributed to the production of a proteoglycanolytic enzyme[110] rather than a collagenase, in addition to a protease, elastase, exotoxin A, hemolysin, and endotoxin.[145] Another type of *Pseudomonas* keratitis behaves in a more indolent fashion and the organism probably does not elaborate the same destructive enzymes. A third type of *Pseudomonas* keratitis is a granular epithelial keratopathy seen in association with extended-wear contact lenses[146] (Figure 8-15).

Ulcers caused by other gram-negative bacteria lack such discriminating features. *Proteus* can behave like

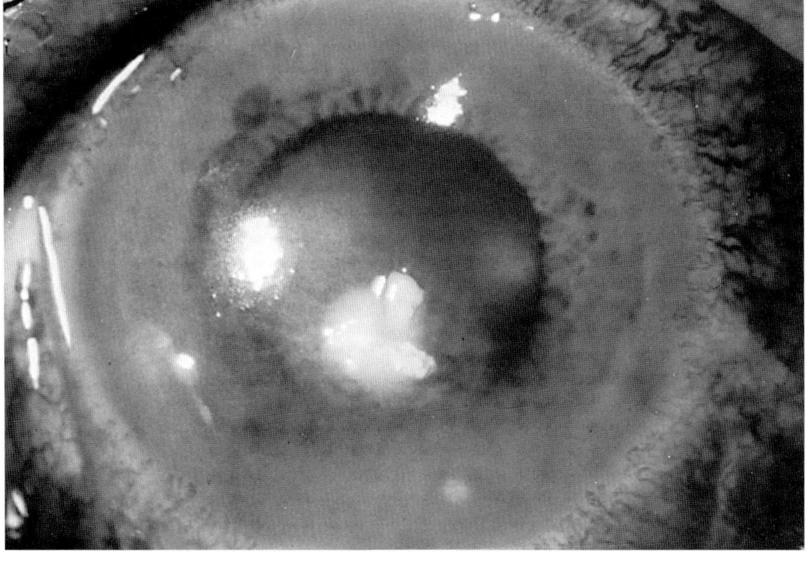

FIGURE 8-12 *Staphylococcus aureus* keratitis in a patient with herpes zoster neurotrophic keratitis. There is a small, deep stromal abscess, with minimal surrounding edema.

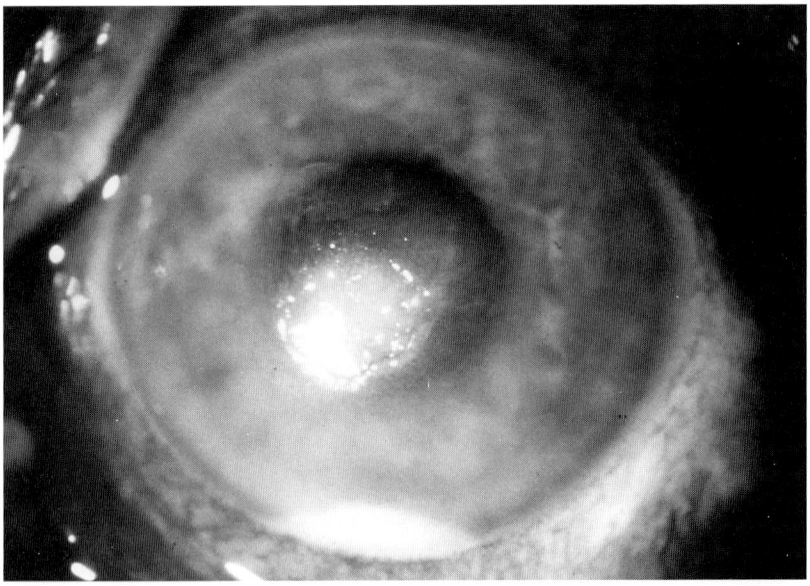

FIGURE 8-13 An indolent superficial central corneal ulcer and hypopyon caused by *Staphylococcus epidermidis.*

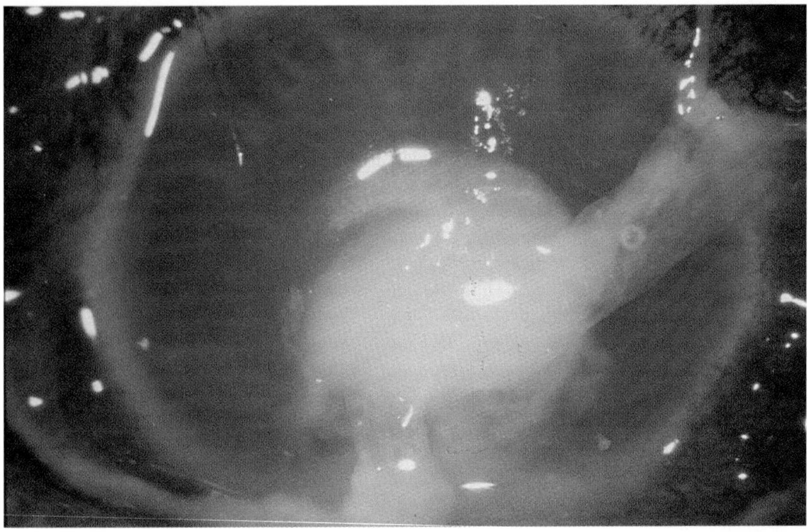

FIGURE 8-14 *Pseudomonas aeruginosa* keratitis in a soft contact lens wearer. There is copious mucopurulent greenish discharge with underlying shaggy superficial ulceration and diffuse epithelial edema of the peripheral cornea. The same organism was grown from the contact lens case.

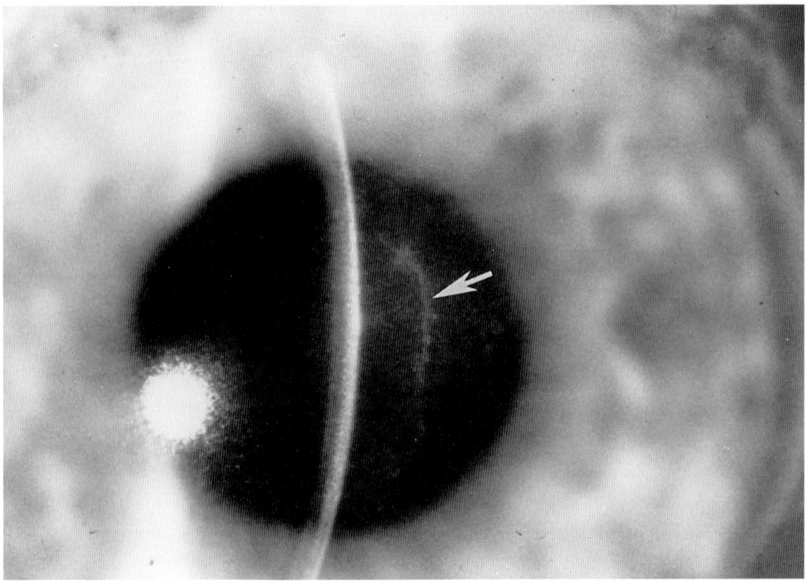

FIGURE 8-15 A ground-glass, granular epithelial keratopathy with an intact epithelium (arrow) in a patient using extended-wear soft contact lenses. Scrapings and cultures confirmed *Pseudomonas aeruginosa* infection.

FIGURE 8-16 **(A)** An elderly man with multiple medical problems maintained on a respirator in an intensive care unit. With exposure, he developed bilateral *Serratia marcescens* corneal ulcers. **(B)** Close-up of the left eye shows the corneal ulcer.

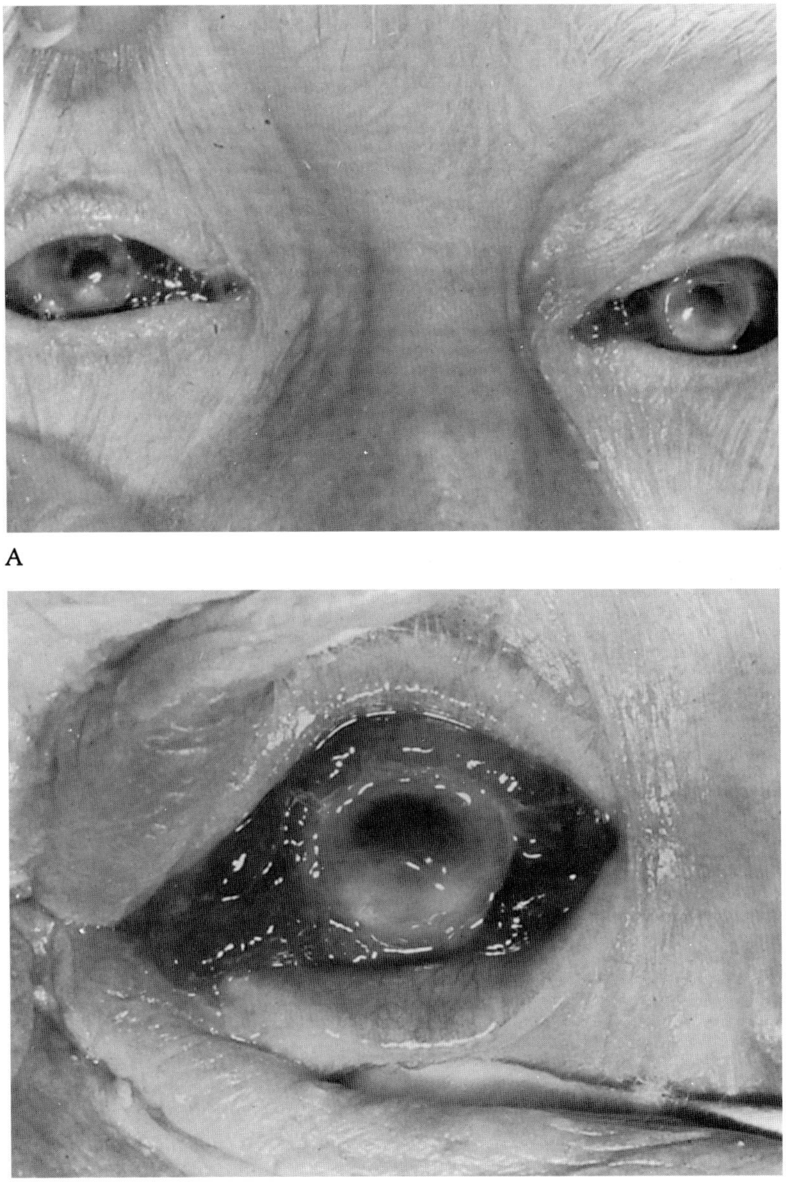

A

B

Pseudomonas. In the absence of a history of trauma, *Klebsiella* is more likely to invade a cornea that has chronic epithelial disease. *Serratia marcescens,* originally throught to be a saprophyte, is now recognized as an opportunistic corneal pathogen (Figure 8-16) and is frequently isolated from contact lens cases.[30] There are no distinguishing features of *Serratia* keratitis. *Moraxella lacunata* (previously *Moraxella liquefaciens*) usually produces a shallow, irregular, indolent gray-white ulcer inferiorly in the paracentral or paralimbal cornea (Figure 8-17). The ulcer can progress to the deep cornea, with hypopyon formation. In some instances *M. lacunata* is extremely aggressive and can lead to perforation.[25,147] Although *M. lacunata* is usually associated with alcoholics, diabetics, and debilitated patients, other *Moraxella* species can be seen in nonalcoholics in the presence of a pre-existing epithelial defect.[27] *Azotobacter* is a recognized cause of keratitis and is frequently mistaken for *Moraxella* in the laboratory. There are no distinctive clinical features of *Azotobacter* keratitis.[31] *Neisseria* should be suspected in the presence of a hyperacute conjunctivitis with chemosis and a copious purulent discharge (Figure 8-18).

Bacillus cereus is a large, aerobic, gram-positive rod that is extremely virulent and causes a rapid and devas-

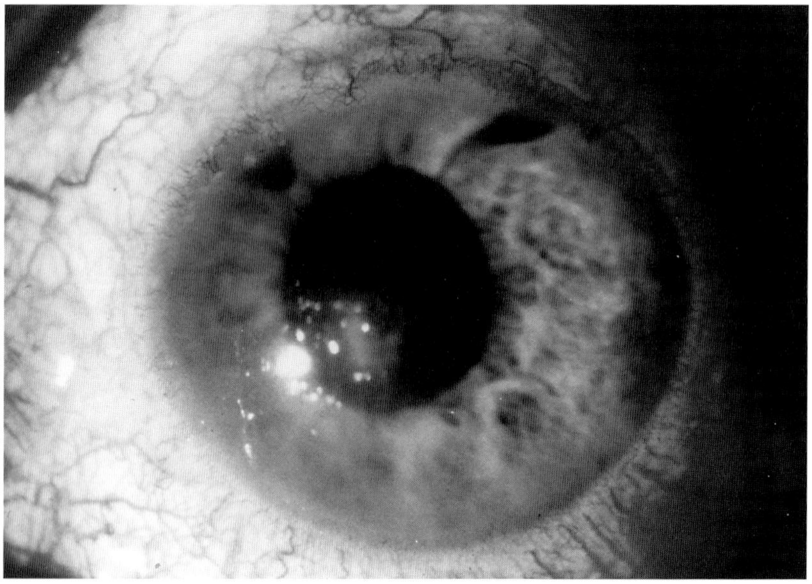

FIGURE 8-17 A shallow indolent ulceration in a patient wearing an aphakic soft contact lens. *Moraxella lacunata* was cultured.

tating keratitis. A distinctive feature is the presence of a ring infiltrate in the cornea remote from the site of a corneal injury, with rapid progression to abscess formation, corneal perforation, and intraocular toxicity associated with the elaboration of specific intradermal vascular permeability exotoxins.[34] Ring abscesses of the cornea have distinctive clinical appearances and are associated with *Proteus, P. aeruginosa, B. cereus,*[148] *Streptococcus,*[149] and *Listeria monocytogenes.*[150] They most frequently occur following penetrating injury at the limbus (Figure 8-19).

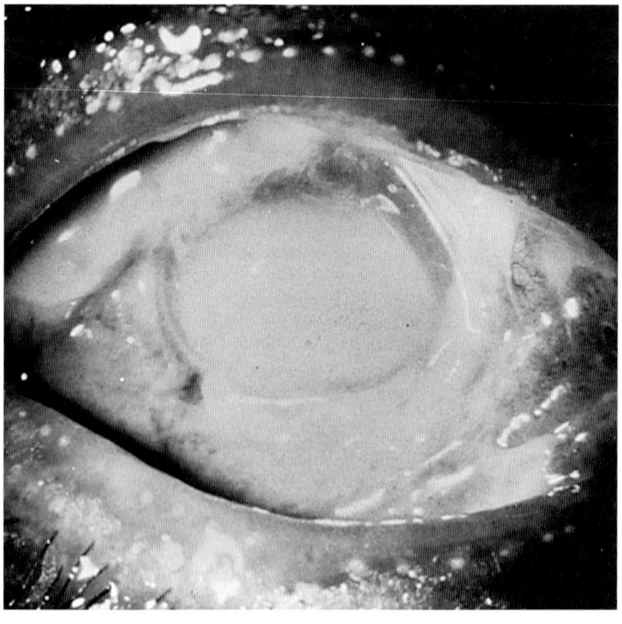

FIGURE 8-18 Gonococcal keratitis. Note the extensive ulceration and copious discharge.

There are no distinct clinical features produced by non-spore-forming anaerobic bacteria.[28,37] These diverse gram-positive and gram-negative rods may become invasive under favorable conditions, such as modification of the host by trauma, extensive surgery, or therapy with corticosteroids or antibiotics. Organisms isolated include *Peptococcus, Peptostreptococcus,* and *Propionibacterium;* they may be present in mixed infections. The spore-forming *Clostridium* can produce a distinctive air bubble in the corneal stroma under the epithelium or in the anterior chamber.[39]

In atypical mycobacterial keratitis, there is usually a history of a corneal foreign body, corneal surgery, contact lens wear, or prior corneal disease, especially herpes simplex viral keratitis (Figure 8-20). Most patients do not have systemic disease, although acquired immunodeficiency syndrome and other immunocompromising disorders are risk factors. There is usually a delay from days to months between the trauma and the onset of a distinct keratitis. The keratitis is slowly progressive, like an indolent ulcer, or it may have a course of remissions and recurrences.[40] Corticosteroid use may exacerbate the infection.[151] The early stage is characterized by a central, shallow, grayish white midstromal plaque surrounded by thin radiating lines that give the cornea a cracked-windshield appearance. The infiltrate remains central but can be superficial or deep with irregular edges. Occasional satellite

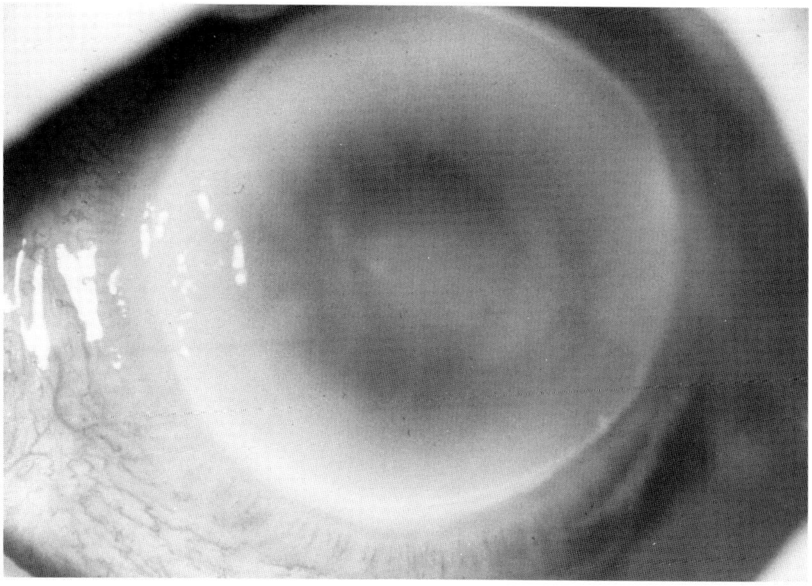

FIGURE 8-19 A ring abscess of the cornea. A β-hemolytic *Streptococcus* was cultured.

lesions are present. Anterior chamber inflammation is usually mild.

Corneal ulceration by *Nocardia, Actinomyces,* and *Streptomyces* is usually indolent and may simulate fungal keratitis, with hyphal edges, satellite lesions, and elevated epithelial lesions (Figure 8-21). Other unusual organisms infecting the cornea may be traceable to marine waters (*Vibrio vulnificus*)[152] or dog bites or scratches,[153] or may be associated with poor oral hygiene.[154-157]

Under appropriate circumstances, indolent corneal ulcers can be caused by almost any bacteria.[158,159] The severity of the disease is modified by the particular strain of the organism, the size of the inoculum, host susceptibility and immune response, antecedent therapy, and the duration of the infection.

Histopathology

Bacterial corneal ulcers pass through distinct histopathologic stages, from progressive infiltration to active ulceration, regression, and finally healing.[160] In the first stage (progres-

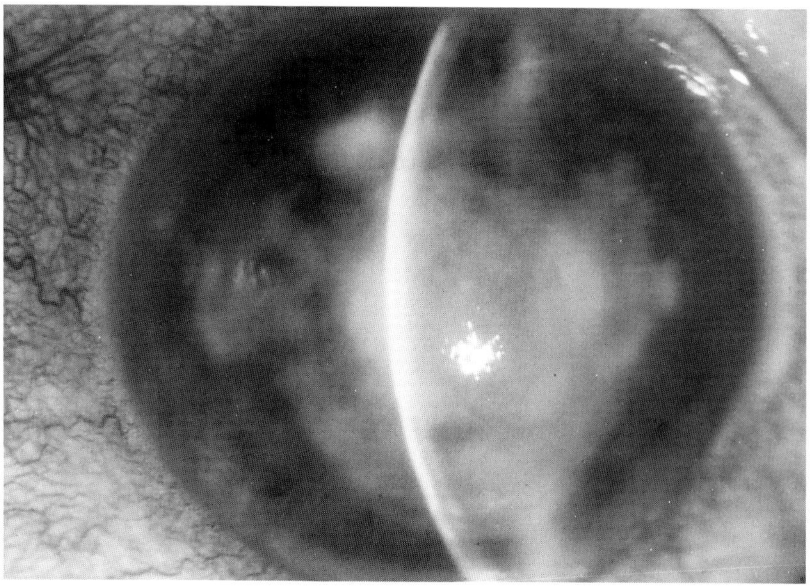

FIGURE 8-20 Atypical mycobacterial keratitis in a patient with a history of recurrent herpes simplex stromal keratitis. Patients with herpetic eye disease are at risk of developing other infections of the cornea.

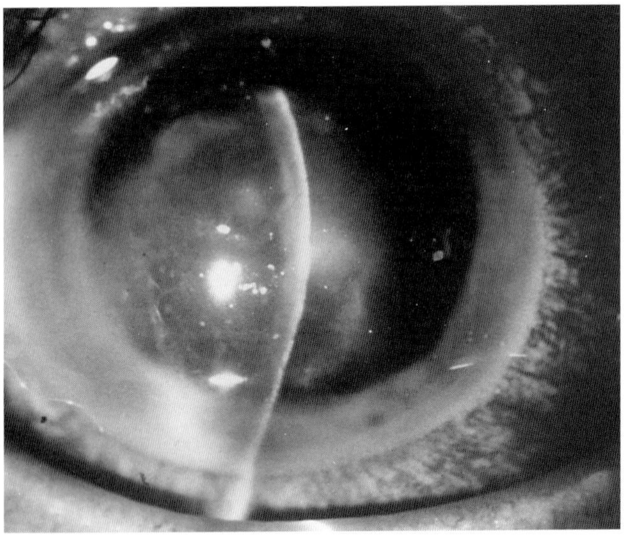

FIGURE 8-21 A shaggy central corneal infection with slightly elevated epithelium in a marine biologist. *Nocardia* was cultured.

sive infiltration) there is adherence and entry of bacteria, followed by invasion into the stroma. The adherence of certain bacteria, such as *P. aeruginosa* and *N. gonorrhoeae,* is aided by a glycocalyx, or slime envelope. Bacteria multiply by binary fission. The host mounts a polymorphonuclear leukocytic and lymphocytic infiltrative response into the epithelium and stroma, which gives the clinical appearance of a yellow or white corneal opacity with overlying epithelial edema or sloughing. There is multiplication of bacteria, with production and diffusion of enzymes and toxins.

In the second stage (active ulceration), the clinical picture varies with the virulence of the organism and toxin production. Symptoms of pain, photophobia, and decreased visual acuity are prominent. There is necrosis and subsequent sloughing of the epithelium and stroma, which creates a demarcated defect, infiltration of polymorphonuclear leukocytes, and edema of the adjacent epithelium and stroma, as illustrated in many of the previous figures. The necrotic base of the ulcer is surrounded by heaped-up tissue. Anterior chamber inflammation may progress to a large hypopyon. The ulcer may penetrate deeper into the cornea and lead to formation of a descemetocele (Figure 8-22). Descemet's membrane is resistant to bacterial invasion, but corneal perforation can occur. A flat anterior chamber with iris prolapse, subluxation of the lens, cataract formation, and/or endophthalmitis is the aftermath of uncontrolled progression. The ulcer may also progress peripherally toward the sclera.

The natural host defense mechanisms dominate the third stage (regression). Humoral and cellular immune defenses combine with antimicrobial therapy to limit proliferation of the bacteria, kill the bacteria, and allow phagocytosis of the bacteria and the cellular debris. It is important to recognize that necrotic corneal tissue heals extremely slowly, and rapid improvement in the clinical appearance of the ulcer cannot be expected. A distinct line of demarcation may develop as the ulcer and stromal infiltration round up their edges. Vascularization of the cornea may occur, especially in indolent ulcers (Figure 8-23).

In the final stage (healing), there is continuous removal of residual debris and repair of structural alterations. Histiocytes and keratocytes transform into fibroblasts.

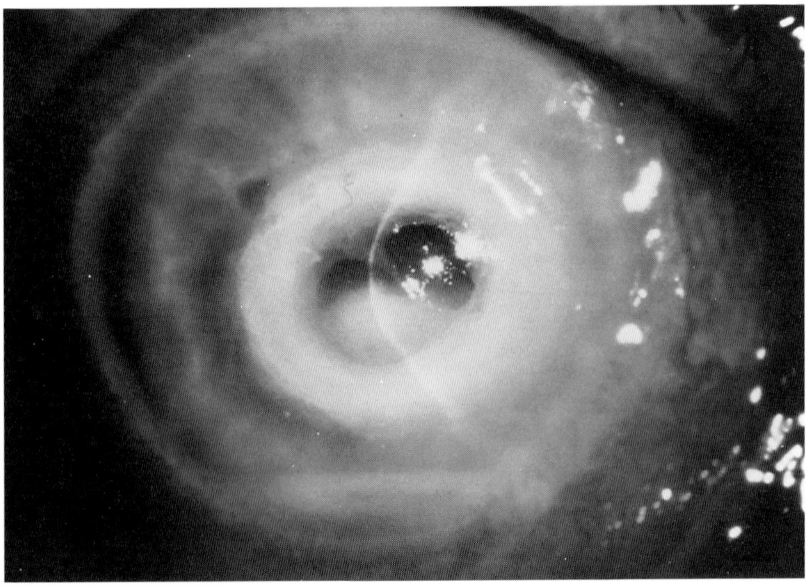

FIGURE 8-22 Active ulceration stage. A clear anteriorly bulging descemetocele is surrounded by a circular dense stromal infiltrate in a patient with herpes zoster neurotrophic keratitis and *Staphylococcus epidermidis* keratitis. There is an accompanying hypopyon.

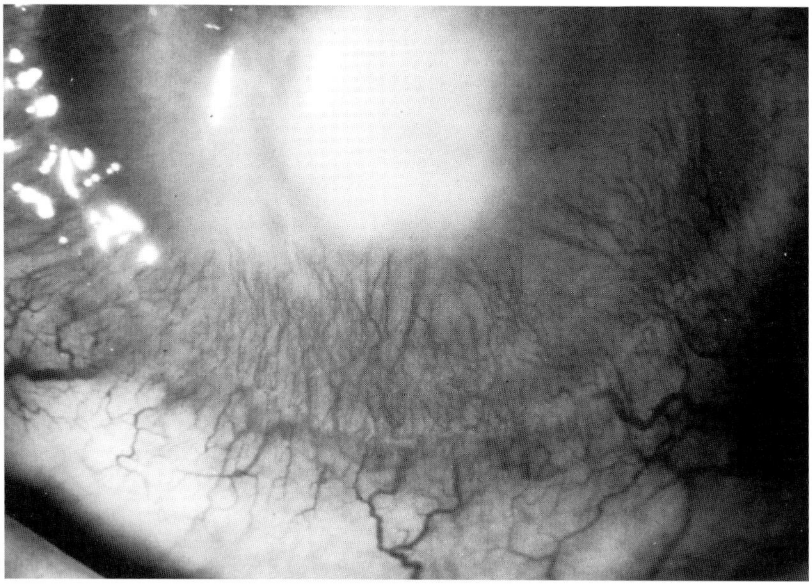

FIGURE 8-23 Regressive stage. Peripheral corneal vascularization approaching the area of a healing corneal abscess caused by *Pseudomonas aeruginosa.*

Corneal vascularization occurs in an attempt to fill in the defect. Bowman's layer does not regenerate, but is replaced with fibrous tissue. The epithelium heals slowly over this irregular base. The thinned stroma may again thicken as new lamellae are added, but depressions and facets may remain (Figure 8-24). Vascularization tends to disappear, leaving ghost vessels. White scarring varies in amount and becomes more translucent with time.

If the ulcer has progressed to corneal perforation, the iris may plug the corneal defect and bring intraocular vascularization directly to the ulceration site. The cornea may heal with an adherent leukoma as telltale evidence of the perforation.

Laboratory Techniques

Taking into account the history of predisposing ocular and systemic diseases and observing the biomicroscopic features, the ophthalmologist judges the severity of the keratitis and the likelihood of microbial infection com-

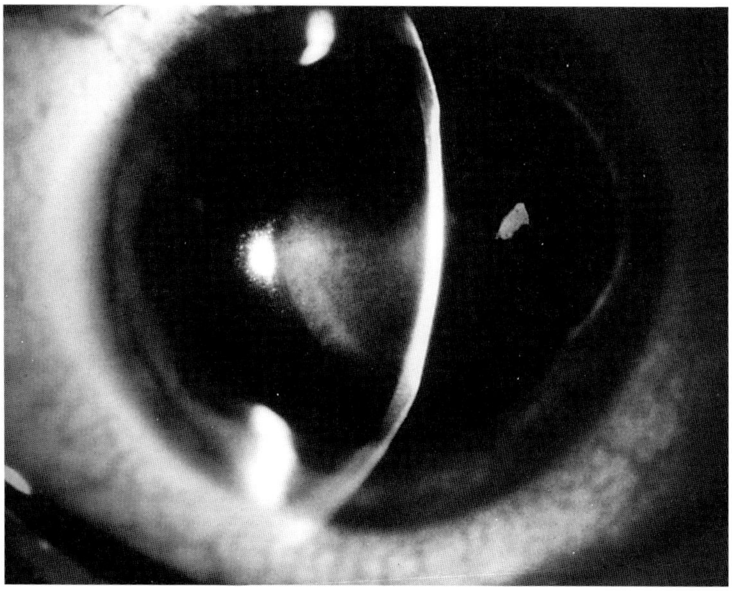

FIGURE 8-24 Healing stage. A thinned cornea after a healed corneal ulcer caused by *Pseudomonas aeruginosa.*

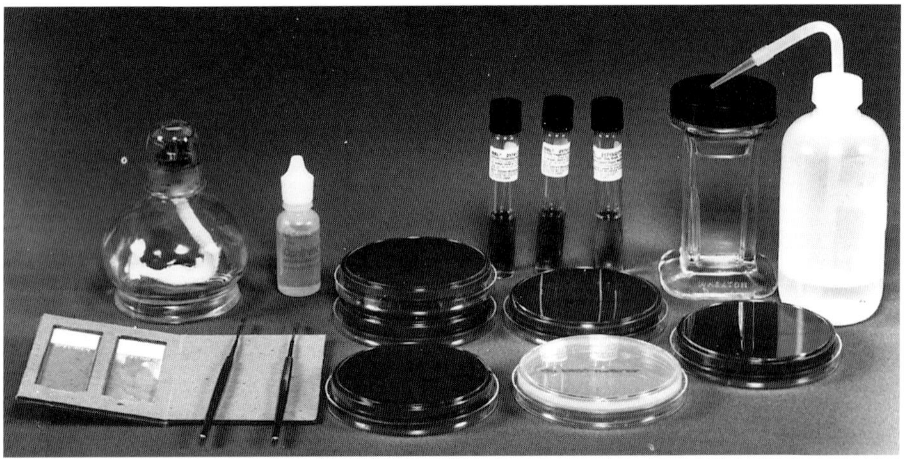

A

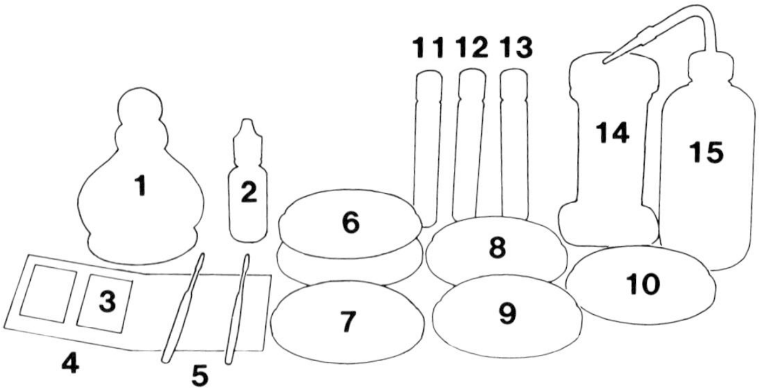

B

FIGURE 8-25 **(A)** Specialized culture media, slides, spatulas, alcohol lamp, anesthetic, and absolute methanol fixative needed for scrapings, smears, and cultures of the eyelid, conjunctiva, and cornea. **(B)** Schematic representative of the equipment and materials shown in A.

1) Alcohol lamp
2) Topical anesthetic
3) Frosted glass slides
4) Glass slide holder
5) 2 Kimura spatulas
6) 2 Blood agar plates
7) Chocolate agar plate
8) Anaerobic plate
9) Sabouraud agar plate
10) Blood agar plate for eyelid and conjunctival cultures
11) Thioglycolate broth
12) Brain-heart infusion broth
13) Trypticase soy broth
14) Coplin staining jar
15) Methyl alcohol (95%) for fixation

pared with a nonmicrobial process. The timing of laboratory studies and the initiation of treatment are based on this information.

Laboratory evaluation of corneal scrapings is important if there is suspicion of microbial keratitis. The same thorough methodology should be applied to all cases of suspected microbial keratitis to encourage recovery of all potential organisms. The proper strategy must include methodology for the likely responsible agents: aerobic bacteria, anaerobic non-spore-forming bacteria, filamentous fungi, and yeasts. Standard laboratory procedures are satisfactory in the recovery of most organisms. Under special circumstances, more selective culture media may be indicated. The practice of treating severe corneal ulcers without appropriate cultures will delay the recognition and effective treatment of several unique forms of microbial keratitis.[161,162]

The ophthalmologist and clinical microbiology laboratory should establish a routine method for obtaining and maintaining standard materials and media for the collection, transport, and culture of the material from corneal scrapings.[164,165] A special tray in the office or hospital with an attached instruction card for guidance is ideal (Figure 8-25).

Although cotton-tipped or polyester applicators are adequate to obtain conjunctival cultures or to inoculate broths, the isolation of organisms from the eyelid and conjunctiva is enhanced by the use of calcium alginate swabs. Corneal material is best obtained under the magnification of a slit lamp microscope. The rounded flexible tip of a Kimura platinum spatula is ideal for scraping the cornea (Figure 8-26), and it cools rapidly after heat sterilization in an alcohol lamp flame. If this type of spatula is not available, large-gauge disposable needles work well. The use of a calcium alginate swab in place of a platinum spatula or a Bard-Parker blade for culturing corneal ulcers was successful in a series of cases of bacterial and fungal keratitis.[165] Proparacaine hydrochloride (0.5 percent) is less antiseptic than other topical anesthetics, and is the preferred anesthetic for obtaining corneal scrapings.

It is imperative to obtain multiple samples from all representative areas of the ulcer because the depth and extent of viable, morphologically distinct organisms vary with a

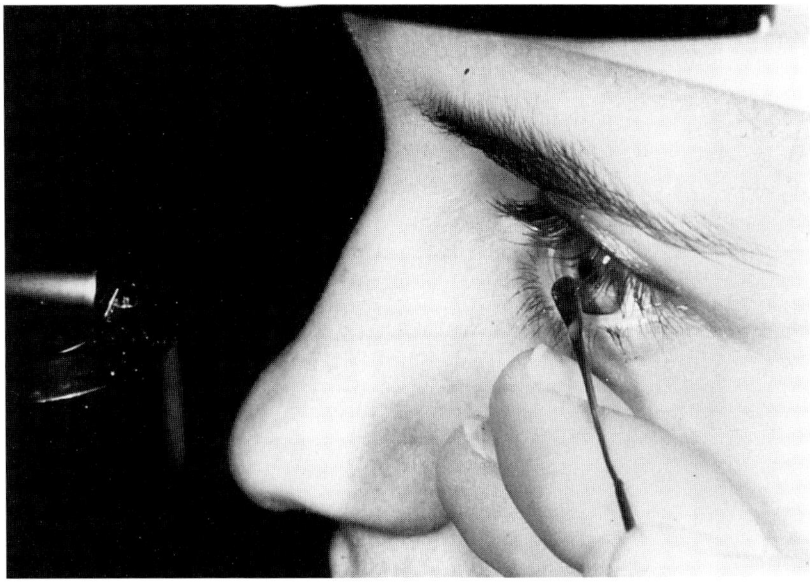

FIGURE 8-26 Patient at the slit lamp microscope for scraping of the cornea with a Kimura spatula.

number of factors. *S. pneumoniae* is more readily found at the active edge of an ulcer, whereas *Moraxella* is more likely to be present in the ulcer crater. Multiple studies have shown the inability to recover organisms from all samples on all culture media.[2,166] Success in recovery and confidence in interpretation are directly related to the number of scrapings done. In certain instances, however, there may not be enough material to inoculate all media, in which case the clinician may have to limit the selection of culture media.

A razor blade, microsurgical scissors, or small trephine may be required to obtain adequate corneal fragments in the absence of surface suppuration or in the presence of a deep ulcer or abscess.[167] The fragments are best inoculated into thioglycolate broth and brain-heart infusion (BHI) broth. Part of a fragment can also be crushed with a spatula onto a glass slide for microscopic examination with routine stains.

The hypopyon that can accompany bacterial keratitis is composed of inflammatory cells and usually contains no organisms because bacteria usually do not penetrate Descemet's membrane. An anterior chamber paracentesis to obtain aqueous humor for smear or culture is contraindicated in most circumstances because of the risk of introducing organisms into the eye. Paracentesis may be considered, however, in the presence of deep disease, in the absence of sufficient material from superficial scrapings, or in the case of suspected entry of organisms into the anterior chamber.[168,169]

Stains

Gram and Giemsa staining of corneal smears should be done routinely in cases of suspected microbial keratitis. They are of value in the initial management because they confirm the presence of a microorganism and distinguish bacteria from fungi; they may also provide clues to suggest a specific subgroup of organisms.[170] In order to use the smear to direct initial antimicrobial therapy, there should be an adequate sample from the suppurative process, careful staining techniques should be followed, and a painstaking evaluation of the slides should be performed. Prior use of antimicrobial agents, an insufficient sample, excessive heat fixation, mechanical damage to the cell wall, poor staining techniques, and failure to examine the whole slide make the smears less reliable.

Smears are prepared by scraping the ulcer and gently transferring the material on the spatula onto a glass slide over an area approximately 1 cm in diameter. An etched or wax pencil circle on the slide circumvents needless searching under the microscope. Gelatin-coated glass slides are preferred for the modified methenamine silver stain.[171] Prompt flooding or immersion of the slide in methanol (95 percent) or cold acetone in a Coplin jar for 5 to 10 minutes is preferable to heat fixation because it reduces the likelihood of alteration of the morphology and staining characteristics of the organisms. At least two samples should be obtained for Gram and Giemsa stains, and an extra slide held for possible special stains (periodic acid–Schiff, calcofluor, Gomori methenamine silver, acid fast).

The 5-minute Gram stain is preferred over the 15-second stain. Gram stain classifies bacteria into two major groups on the basis of differences in the cell wall, although the exact mechanism is not known. Gram-positive bacteria retain the gentian violet-iodine complex and appear blue-purple. Gram-negative bacteria lose the gentian violet-iodine complex by decolorization with acid alcohol and appear pink when counterstained with safranin.

In several large series, Gram stain has shown an accuracy of 55 to 66 percent in detecting the organism in bacterial keratitis.[2,4,6,170] In one series, Gram stain correctly identified the staining properties and morphology of the responsible organism in 75 percent of single-organism infections and 37 percent of polymicrobial infections (61 percent overall).[13] Frequently, only small numbers of organisms are present in the smear, and are therefore difficult to find and identify. Bacteria are usually present in areas that contain large numbers of polymorphonuclear leukocytes and necrotic epithelial cells. Often, fewer organisms are seen in Gram stain of corneal smears in gram-negative bacterial keratitis than in gram-positive bacterial keratitis. Decolorization is an important step to ensure that bacteria get the correct Gram stain reaction. Gram-negative organisms may appear gram positive in thick, underdecolorized areas of the smear. Indigenous bacteria in the tear film may occasionally be detected in corneal smears, but these are usually seen as rare, randomly scattered, extracellular organisms. Practice and experience are necessary to distinguish some of the artifacts that may accompany Gram stain, such as stain deposits, carbon particles, talcum powder, sodium chloride crystals, and melanin granules.[172] Precipitated gentian violet can look like gram-positive cocci. Occasionally, yeast will multiply in neglected gentian violet. Since the stain is often not made up daily and artifacts are possible, interpretation should serve as a guide but not as the sole determinant of therapy. The Gram stain appearances of various bacteria are listed in Table 8-5 and illustrated in Figures 8-27 through 8-33.

Giemsa stain is one of several Romanowsky-type stains that use eosin, methylene blue, and azure dyes. The Giemsa stain highlights DNA in the nuclei of human cells and cytoplasmic RNA in lymphocytes. It is primarily intended to distinguish various types of inflammatory cells and intracytoplasmic inclusions. In microbial keratitis, it can distinguish bacteria from fungi. Giemsa stain renders bacteria dark blue, and occasionally provides better morphologic detail than Gram stain (Figure 8-34). The stain is absorbed by the protoplasm of fungal hyphae, which generally appear purple or blue. Pseudohyphae stain dark blue. Branching septate hyphal fragments are 2 to 6 μm wide, and budding yeasts or pseudohyphae are 2 to 4 μm wide. The stain should be prepared fresh daily to ensure the appropriate distinguishing colors. It may also be of value in distinguishing noninfectious keratitis by the type of inflammatory cells.

Acridine orange is a chemofluorescent dye that stains fungi and bacteria yellow-orange against a green background when the pH is acidic and a fluorescence microscope is used (Figure 8-35). It may be more sensitive than Gram or Giemsa stain; slides stained with acridine orange can be restained with these conventional stains.[173,174]

TABLE 8-5
Gram Stain Morphology of Bacteria

Organism	*Gram Stain Morphology*
Staphylococcus	Gram-positive cocci singly or in pairs, rarely clusters; usually extracellular
Streptococcus	Gram-positive cocci in short chains, singly, or in pairs; slightly smaller than *Staphylococcus*
Streptococcus pneumoniae	Gram-positive encapsulated bullet-shaped diplococci with flattened ends together
Corynebacterium	Gram-positive pleomorphic slender rods sometimes club-shaped or in Chinese-letter formations
Pseudomonas	Gram-negative slender straight rods frequently few in number
Neisseria	Gram-negative kidney-bean diplococci within epithelial and polymorphonuclear leukocytes; many associated polymorphonuclear leukocytes
Haemophilus	Gram-negative small pleomorphic rods or coccobacilli frequently in pairs
Moraxella	Gram-negative large rectangular rods in pairs end-to-end
Enterobacter	Gram-negative rods with variable sizes depending on genus
Actinomyces	Gram-positive branching filaments sometimes fragmented into coccoid or pleomorphic forms[a]
Nocardia	Gram-positive branching filaments sometimes fragmented into coccoid or pleomorphic forms[b]
Mycobacterium	Gram-positive pleomorphic rods[c]
Bacillus	Large gram-positive symmetrical rods of uniform shape and size; spores not usually seen in scraping

[a] Filaments not acid fast.
[b] Some filaments acid fast.
[c] Most acid fast.

The carbolfuchsin or Ziehl-Neelsen stain is helpful in identifying *Mycobacterium, Nocardia,* and *Actinomyces.* The principle of this stain is based on the resistance of mycobacterial species and certain strains of *Nocardia* to decolorization by strong mineral acids after staining with basic carbolfuchsin. This resistance is a feature of intact cells that contain a specific lipid unsaponifiable wax fraction. Preferably, slides are fixed by heat before staining. In the Kinyoun method, fixation is done with detergents. The stain is helpful in distinguishing members of Actinomycetales; for example, *Mycobacterium* is acid fast, *Nocardia* is variable, and *Actinomyces* is not acid fast. *Mycobacterium* can be distinguished morphologically from *Nocardia,* which is a delicate, branching filamentous organism. Also, the fluorochrome stain and fluo-

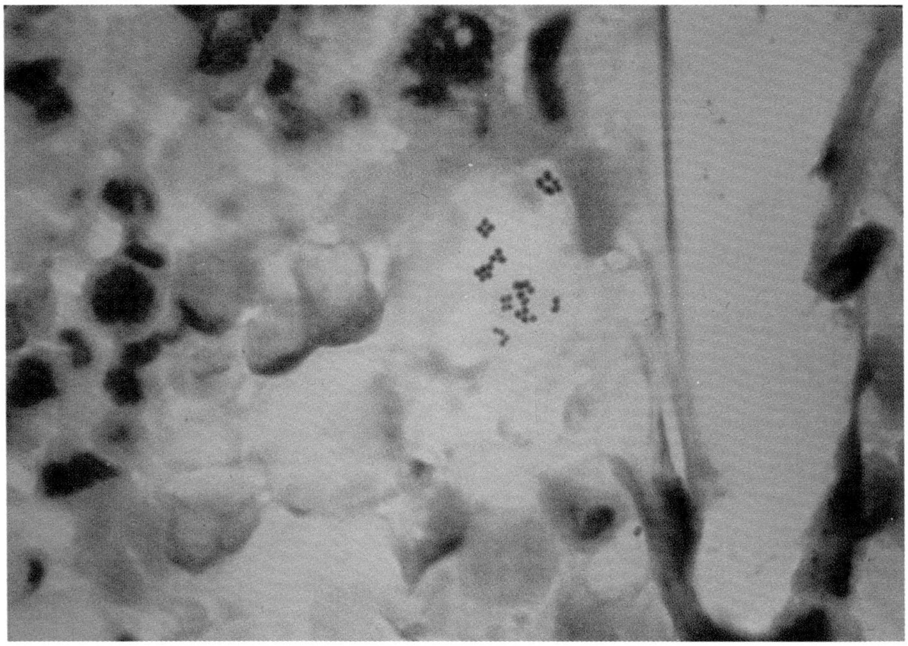

FIGURE 8-27 Gram stain of a corneal scraping showing gram-positive cocci in clusters adjacent to polymorphonuclear leukocytes. Cultures grew *Staphylococcus aureus.*

rescein-conjugated lectins are available for identification of *Mycobacterium;* the rhodamine-auramine fluorochrome dye binds to *Mycobacterium* and *Nocardia,* and can be viewed by fluorescence microscopy.

A number of other stains are available to increase the sensitivity of detecting bacteria.[175,176] The practicality of many of these stains is hampered by the limited quantity of specimen. Fluorescein-conjugated monoclonal antibodies or lectins improve the sensitivity and specificity of the microscopic identification of bacteria. Bacterial antigens can be detected by a number of immunologic techniques, including direct immunofluorescence, immunoelectrophoresis, agglutination, and immunoassay. The detection of microbial DNA with DNA probes offers an exquisite approach to rapid diagnosis. Detection of bacterial metabolites by gas chro-

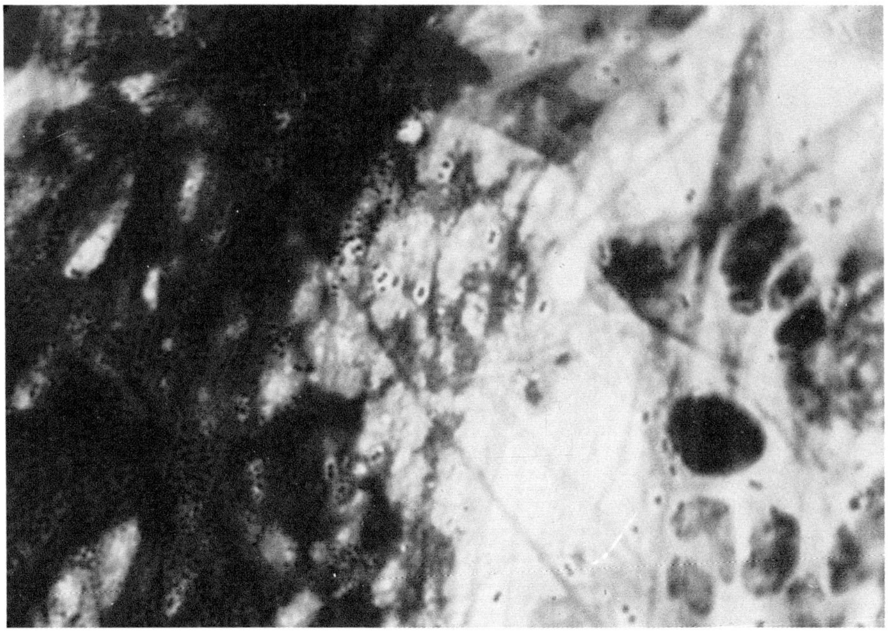

FIGURE 8-28 Gram stain of a corneal scraping with multiple inflammatory cells and gram-positive, encapsulated bullet-shaped diplococci. Cultures grew *Streptococcus pneumoniae.*

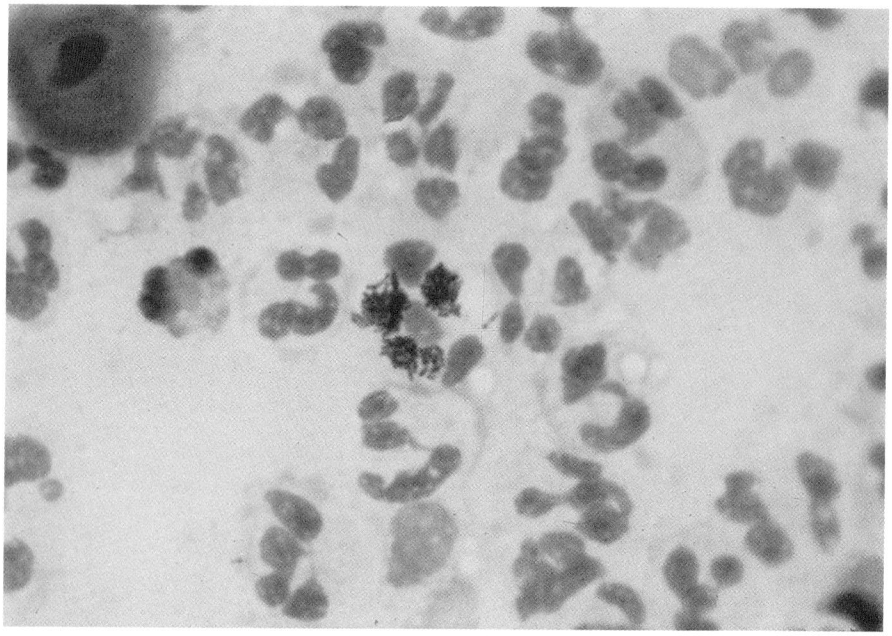

FIGURE 8-29 Gram stain of a corneal scraping with multiple polymorphonuclear leukocytes and clustered gram-positive pleomorphic slender rods in various shapes. Cultures grew *Corynebacterium.*

matography and the polymerase chain reaction technique is highly sensitive.

The *Limulus* lysate test is a simple, rapid, and relatively reliable method for the detection of endotoxin produced by gram-negative bacteria in material obtained by corneal scrapings.[2,177,178] It can also be used to detect endotoxin in contact lens solutions.[179] Circulating cells (amebocytes) in the coelomic fluid of the horseshoe crab, *Limulus polyphemus,* gel in the presence of lipopolysaccharide present in the cell wall of gram-negative bacteria. The crab's response to gram-negative bacterial infection is disseminated intravascular coagulation, and gel formation is a sensitive indicator of bacterial lipopolysaccharides. Corneal scrapings should be emulsified in rehydrated amebocyte lysate reagent in a test tube, which is incubated along with a control tube. A positive reaction for endotoxin is indicated by

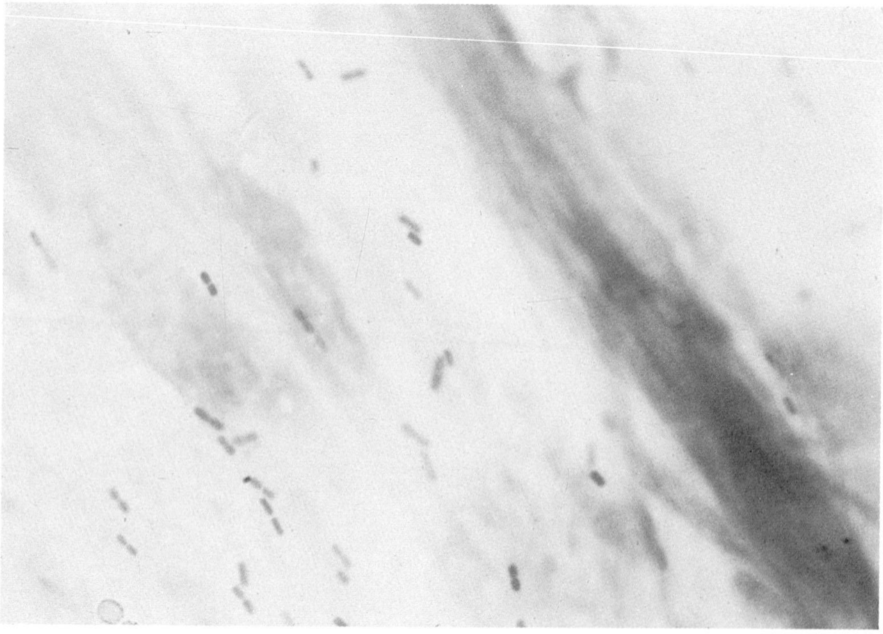

FIGURE 8-30 Gram stain of a corneal scraping showing large boxcar-shaped gram-negative diplobacilli. Cultures grew *Moraxella lacunata.*

FIGURE 8-31 Gram stain of a corneal scraping showing multiple slender and slightly pleomorphic gram-negative rods with multiple polymorphonuclear leukocytes. Cultures grew *Proteus mirabilis.*

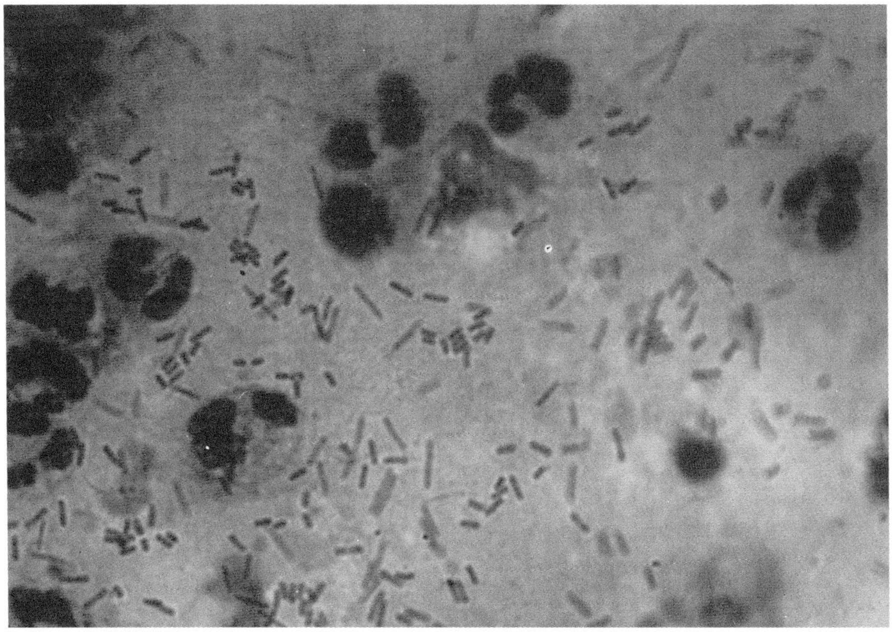

the formation of a clot that adheres to the bottom of the reagent tube. In one series, the *Limulus* lysate test was effective in identifying gram-negative endotoxin in 30 cases, with no false-positive or false-negative results.[2]

Cultures

Culture Media Media can be nonselective (free of inhibitors and able to support the growth of most organisms in the clinical laboratory) or selective (containing dyes or antimicrobial agents that inhibit all but specific groups of organisms). Enrichment media are used to recover a limited number of bacteria from a specimen with other commensal organisms. Differential media contain factors that allow differentiation of colonies of bacteria based on specific culture characteristics of those organisms.

FIGURE 8-32 Gram stain of a corneal scraping showing multiple polymorphonuclear leukocytes and gram-negative diplococci both intra- and extracellularly. Cultures grew *Neisseria gonorrhoeae.*

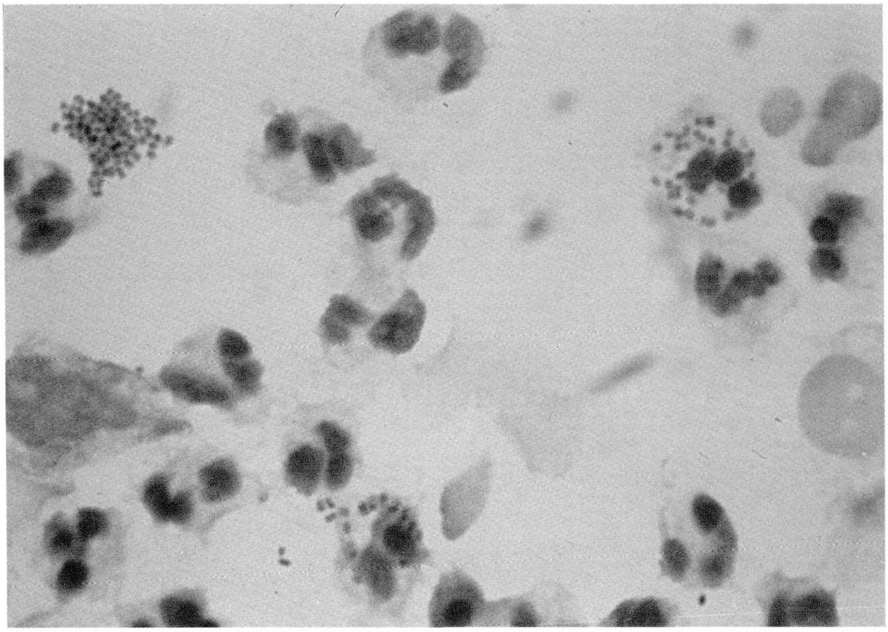

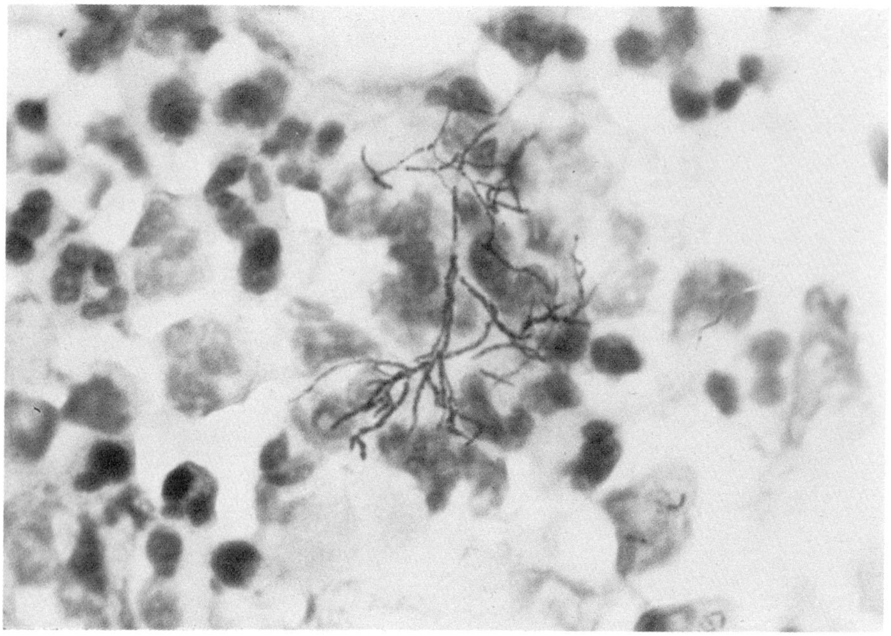

FIGURE 8-33 Gram stain of a corneal scraping showing multiple inflammatory cells and branching and beaded filaments. Cultures grew *Nocardia*.

The culture media recommended have the potential to support the growth of the bacteria and fungi responsible for most microbial keratitis (Table 8-6). Identification of other organisms may require special media. All refrigerated media should be warmed to room temperature before inoculation to prevent lethal cold shock to the organism.

Soybean casein digest broth (tryptic soy, trypticase soy) is used to saturate swabs for conjunctival and eyelid cultures and is a general nutrient that can be used for culture of aerobic and facultatively anaerobic bacteria without the addition of blood or serum.

Blood agar is the standard medium for the isolation of aerobic bacteria, and supports the growth of most saprophytic fungi at room temperature. Peptone agar is derived from seaweed and produces optimal surface moisture; the addition of 5 to 10 percent red blood cells provides nutrients and an index of hemolysis. Sheep blood is usually used; rabbit and horse sera are better for growth of *Haemophilus,* but are more expensive. Blood agar plates

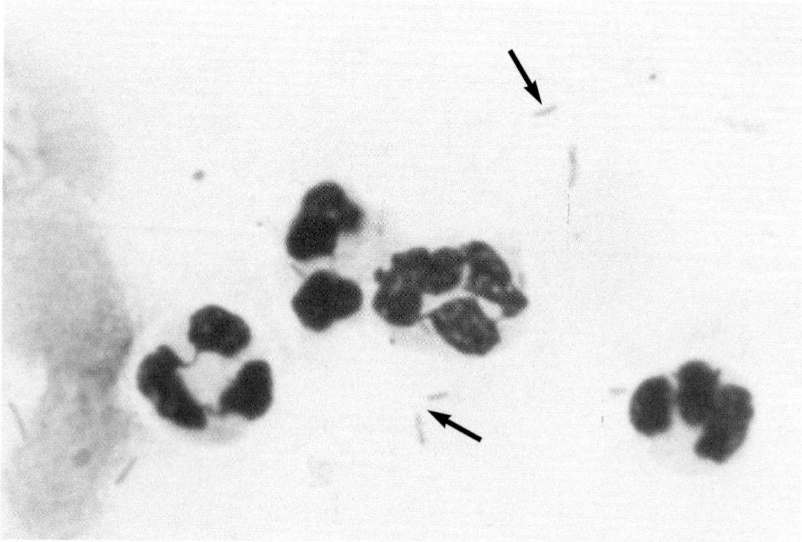

FIGURE 8-34 Giemsa stain of a corneal scraping demonstrating bacteria (arrows). Cultures grew *Pseudomonas aeruginosa,* an organism that is frequently difficult to see and can be missed on Gram stain.

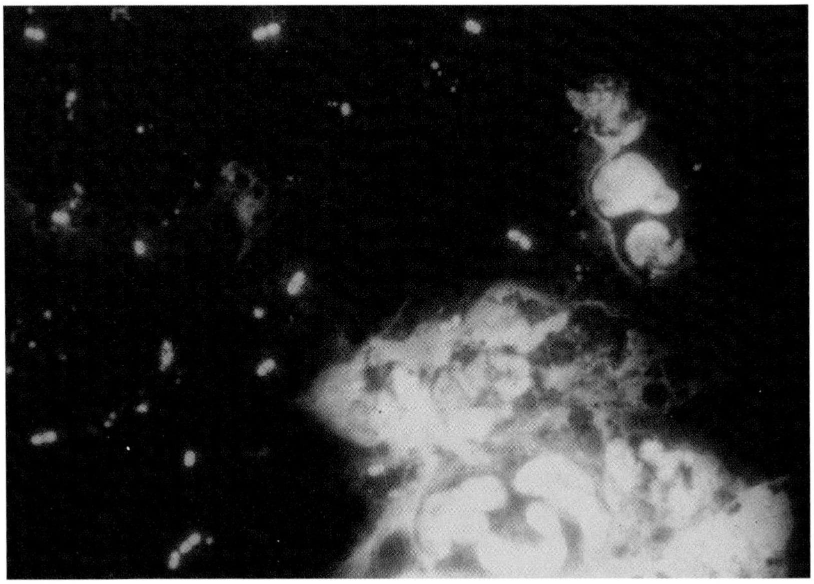

FIGURE 8-35 Acridine orange stain of a corneal scraping revealing yellow-orange boxcar-like diplobacilli. Cultures grew *Moraxella*. (Courtesy of Kirk Wilhelmus, M.D., Houston, TX.)

TABLE 8-6
Culture Media

Medium	*Purpose*	*Incubation Temperature*
Routine		
Soybean casein digest broth (tryptic or trypticase soy broth)	Saturation of swabs	
Blood agar	Aerobic and facultatively anaerobic bacteria, fungi	35°C with 3 to 10% CO_2
Chocolate agar	Aerobic and facultatively anaerobic bacteria, *Neisseria*, *Haemophilus*	35°C with 3 to 10% CO_2
Thioglycolate broth (enriched)	Aerobic and anaerobic bacteria	35°C
Sabouraud dextrose agar with antibiotic	Fungi	Room temperature
Brain-heart infusion (BHI) broth with antibiotic	Fungi	Room temperature (rotary shaker)
Special		
Cooked meat broth	Anaerobic bacteria	35°C
Schaedler agar	Anaerobic bacteria	35°C (anaerobic system)
Brucella blood agar	Anaerobic bacteria, nutritional variant streptococci	35°C (anaerobic system)
Thayer-Martin agar	*Neisseria*	35°C
Middlebrook-Cohn agar	*Mycobacterium, Nocardia*	35°C with 3 to 10% CO_2
Lowenstein-Jensen agar	*Mycobacterium*	35°C with 3 to 10% CO_2

are incubated at 35°C for bacteria, and at room temperature for fungi.

Chocolate agar is prepared by heat denaturation of blood, which releases hemoglobin and inactivates a diphosphopyridine nucleotide-hydrolytic enzyme. This medium provides hemin (X factor) and diphosphopyridine nucleotide (V factor) essential for growth of *Haemophilus*, and is also ideal for isolation of *Neisseria* and *Moraxella*. Chocolate agar plates are incubated at 35°C under 10 percent CO_2.

Thioglycolate broth contains basic nutrients for aerobic bacteria and also contains a sulfhydryl compound that acts as an oxygen-reducing agent to facilitate recovery of anaerobic bacteria. Thiol is a variation of thioglycolate broth and contains special complexes and 0.1 percent semisolid agar to prevent convection currents and promote the growth of aerobic bacteria as well as obligate and facultatively anaerobic organisms. It also supports a number of saprophytic fungi. The tubes should be stored and transported upright to preserve this division. The laboratory may modify the thioglycolate broth by adding polysorbate (Tween 80), vitamin K, and hemin to improve recovery of certain bacteria and to inactivate antimicrobial agents transferred with the inocula.[28]

The disadvantages of thioglycolate broth or thiol as the only anaerobic medium include the inability to monitor contamination, quantitate isolates, permit the growth of some anaerobes, and restrict aerobes from overgrowing the medium. However, thioglycolate broth is generally available, easy to store and inoculate, and does not require special equipment. Ideally, the tubes containing the medium are boiled for 10 minutes before use to drive out dissolved oxygen, then rapidly cooled in an ice bath. The medium is supplemented with sodium bicarbonate ($NaHCO_3$), Fildes' enrichment, or sterile animal serum.[180] Fresh chopped meat or egg is an effective inoculation and isolation medium but is not available in many laboratories.[37] Brain-heart infusion broth incubated in an anaerobic environment is another alternative for the culture of anaerobes. The preferred method for the collection and transport of clinical specimens for anaerobic cultures uses prereduced solid agar plates, gassed-out tubes or bottles, and special transport medium. Prereduced, enriched, anaerobic blood agar plates, such as the *Brucella* agar plate, may be used. The plates should not be exposed to the air any longer than necessary, and are incubated in an anaerobic system, such as an anaerobic jar, anaerobic bag system, or anaerobic chamber.[163] In the Gaspak system, an anaerobic environment is produced within the sealed jar by the generation of hydrogen and CO_2 from a packet containing sodium borohydride, sodium bicarbonate, and citric acid, to which water has been added. The *Brucella* agar plate or other anaerobic medium is also recommended for the isolation of nutritional variant streptococci, which can be causative agents in infectious crystalline keratopathy.[137] The further identification of anaerobes is based on staining characteristics, cell morphology, biochemical reactivity, and gas-liquid chromatographic analysis of free fatty acids.[36]

Sabouraud glucose and peptone agar is a readily available universal nonselective medium for primary isolation of opportunistic fungi.[181] Yeast extract is added to improve nutritional characteristics, and an antibiotic (gentamicin or chloramphenicol) is added to inhibit bacterial contamination. This medium must not contain any additives, such as cycloheximide, that inhibit the saprophytic fungi commonly responsible for ocular infections. After primary growth, the fungi are transferred to sporulating medium. Sabouraud agar plates are preferred over slants because of the ease of inoculation, observation of colony growth, transfer to secondary media, and the dilution of inhibitory substances for the fungi.[181] The agar medium must be thicker than usual to prevent desiccation during prolonged incubation, and the container should be taped closed during incubation and routine examination. Specimens in Sabouraud agar are incubated at room temperature.

Brain-heart infusion broth with neopeptone incubated in a gyrorotary platform shaker at room temperature enhances the recovery of filamentous fungi and yeasts. It gives the fungal elements more even exposure to essential nutrients and results in faster growth with a smaller inoculum. The broth is composed of calf brain and beef heart infusion with protease and dextrose; neopeptone is added to enhance fungal growth, and gentamicin is added to control bacterial contamination. Alternatively, brain-heart infusion agar is used in some laboratories. All fungal isolation media are incubated at room temperature.

Identification of other microorganisms requires the selection of special media. Selective media may contain a carbohydrate with an acid-base indicator or chemical substances that inhibit certain organisms while allowing specific organisms to grow. Examples include MacConkey agar (for isolating gram-negative bacilli), eosin-methylene blue agar, and mannitol agar slants (for isolating *Staphylococcus*). Thayer-Martin medium is a selective, chemically enriched, chocolate agar that suppresses the growth of inhibitory bacteria and fungi and allows the isolation of *Neisseria gonorrhoeae.* Atypical mycobacteria can grow on blood agar, but grow best on specific mycobacteria media, such as Löwenstein-Jensen or Middlebrook-Cohn medium. Growth is variable, both in appearance (rough or smooth colonies) and in time of development (days to weeks). *Actinomyces* can be isolated on anaerobic blood agar and *Nocardia* can be isolated on aerobic blood agar or in fungal media.

Culture Techniques Obtaining appropriate and adequate specimens from corneal ulcers is of paramount importance. Laboratory studies suggest that minimal antibiotic therapy may impair bacterial recovery without completely eradicating live organisms,[182] which emphasizes the need for culture prior to antibiotic therapy. The ophthalmologist should alert the microbiologist to have fresh media available and to be prepared for any special laboratory procedures. The media should be brought to room temperature before inoculation. A specialized tray carrying media, slides, and ancillary instruments is helpful. The materials should be inoculated directly onto the media by the ophthalmologist instead of adding the potential dilution factor of a transport medium for carrying these minute samples from the office to the laboratory.

Prior to corneal scraping, eyelid and conjunctival cultures from both eyes should be obtained and inoculated on blood agar plates and chocolate agar plates. Special circumstances may warrant inclusion of Sabouraud dextrose agar or an anaerobic medium. These cultures should be obtained before instillation of topical anesthetic because topical anesthetics

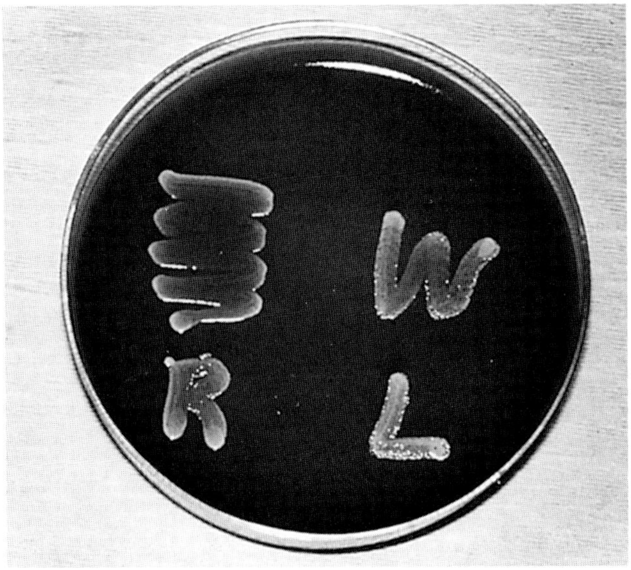

FIGURE 8-36 Conjunctival and eyelid cultures on an agar plate taken from a patient with microbial keratitis. Cultures of the right and left eyelids and conjunctiva can be distinguished by the streaking pattern.

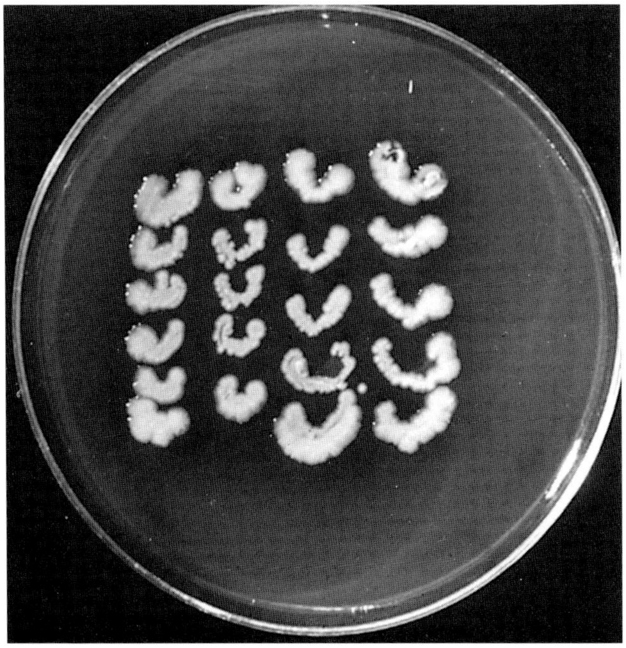

FIGURE 8-37 Exuberant mucoid growth of *Klebsiella* on a blood agar plate from all four rows of C streaks 36 hours after plating. There was no evidence of plate contamination.

contain preservatives that may interfere with recovery of certain organisms.[183] A cotton or calcium alginate applicator is immersed in trypticase soy broth (the saturated swab increases the recovery of organisms), and is swabbed across the anterior margin of the upper and lower eyelids. The applicator is gently rolled over the surface of the agar; the outside edge of the plate is avoided. The same procedure is repeated for the other eye. Conjunctival cultures are obtained by swabbing a saturated applicator over the surface of the conjunctiva and onto blood and chocolate agar plates. The same procedure is done for both eyes. It is convenient and economical to use one plate to culture the eyelids and conjunctiva from both eyes, with "R" and "L" designating the appropriate eyelids and a horizontal streak for the right conjunctiva and a vertical streak for the left conjunctiva (Figure 8-36). Eyelid and conjunctival cultures help to assess the possibility of contamination of the corneal culture by organisms in the tear film and may provide a clue to the source of the corneal pathogen.

Topical proparacaine is adequate for obtaining corneal cultures, although general anesthesia, sedation, or akinesia may be required in uncooperative adults, children, or mentally impaired patients. A Kimura platinum spatula is scraped over the base and edge of the ulcer with moderately firm strokes. The eyelids and eyelashes are avoided. Multiple areas of the ulcer are scraped. The use of multiple spatulas hastens the procedure. Each scraping should be used to inoculate only one medium or prepare one smear. The agar plates are inoculated by streaking the spatula lightly over the surface of the agar to produce a row of separate inoculation marks (C streaks). Each row of C streaks represents a separate scraping; this method of inoculation provides a means of distinguishing valid growth from plate contamination (Figure 8-37).

Thioglycolate broth is inoculated by transferring the corneal material from the spatula to a cotton-tipped applicator or calcium alginate swab, and inserting the swab into the bottom of the tube in the zone of reduced oxygen. Alternatively, a swab can be used to collect material directly from the ulcer and then inoculated into the broth.[165] Saturating the swab with trypticase soy broth reduces the amount of air delivered to the bottom of the tube and theoretically enhances the growth of anaerobic bacteria.

A blood agar plate, a chocolate agar plate, and thioglycolate broth are incubated at 35°C; another blood agar plate, a Sabouraud agar plate, and brain-heart infusion broth are incubated at room temperature. Incubation of the culture plates in a candle jar with 10 percent CO_2 enhances the initial growth of aerobic and microaerophilic organisms and provides an ideal method for recovering

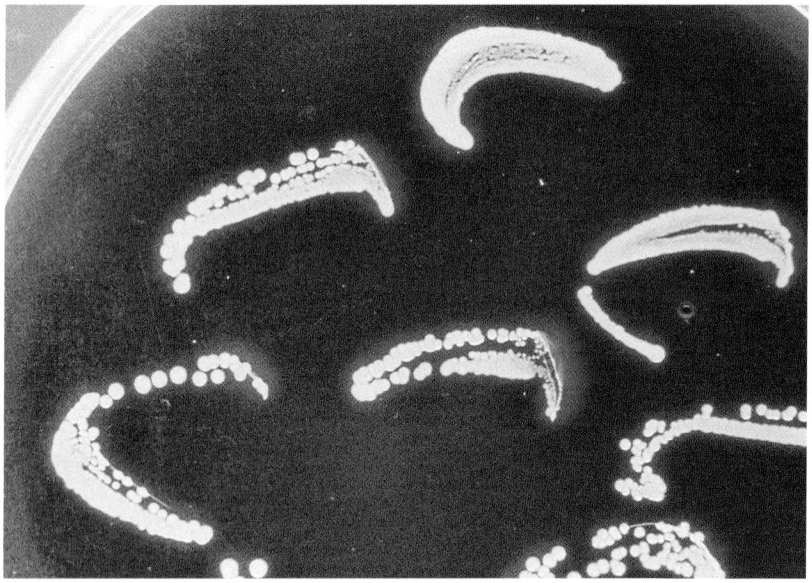

FIGURE 8-38 A blood agar plate demonstrating growth on the C streaks of glistening, smooth, white opaque colonies of *Staphylococcus aureus.*

Neisseria. Candle extinction in a tightly closed jar adequately provides this environment.

Culture Interpretation Most aerobic bacteria responsible for keratitis appear on standard culture media within 48 hours, and it is not unusual for the pathogen to be recognized within 12 to 15 hours. All plates should be examined daily with the magnification of a dissecting microscope, and liquid media should be observed for turbidity. In severe infections, the media should be examined 12 to 18 hours after inoculation. Growth outside the C streaks on solid media should be disregarded as a contaminant and circled with a wax pencil. Indigenous organisms in the tear film may appear on the inoculation marks, but can be distinguished by their sparse growth and the appearance of the same organism on the culture of the ipsilateral conjunctiva or eyelid. If growth is detected, an estimate of the number of colonies should be made, with a description of the colony morphology (Figures 8-37 to 8-39). As soon as growth is detected in either a solid plate or liquid medium (manifested as turbidity), a Gram stain should be done and the organism transferred to fresh media to encourage selection. Determination of antibiotic sensitivities can begin during the time identification is proceeding. Minimal inhibitory and bactericidal concentrations can be obtained within a few days and will thus be available when genus and species are fully identified.

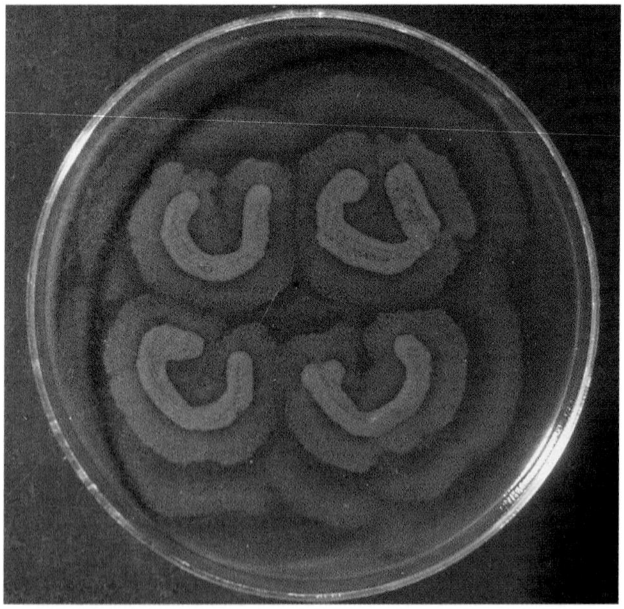

FIGURE 8-39 A chocolate agar plate demonstrating growth on the C streaks of gray colonies of *Proteus mirabilis* with a characteristic wave or swarm of growth.

Blood agar is the best medium for the isolation of aerobic bacteria, although other media will also isolate pathogenic organisms. Anaerobic bacteria are suspected when growth occurs on anaerobic plates or in the lower portion of the thiol tube. Because anaerobic bacteria are frequently slow growing, the cultures should be incubated for at least 10 days. Spherules are produced within the medium and over the surface of the swab before a noticeable turbidity.[28] Clues to a pathogenic anaerobe include the unique morphology seen on Gram stain of either the corneal smear or the culture (pleomorphic, slender, fusiform bacteria), growth in the anaerobic zone of the liquid medium or within the depth of the solid agar, production of gas in liquid media, and failure to grow organisms in aerobic media that were detected by Gram stain.[28]

The incidence of multiple organisms in corneal cultures varies from 6 to 32 percent, depending on the laboratory techniques and the criteria for infection or positive culture.[2,13,184] In one series of anaerobic corneal infections, one-third of the anaerobes isolated occurred in mixed infections.[37] The most frequent combination in polymicrobial keratitis has been an aerobic gram-positive coccus and a gram-negative rod[184]; the combination of fungi and bacteria has also been recorded.[2]

There are no established criteria that confirm a corneal process as infectious. Criteria for some authors have included the clinical signs of infection plus one of the following: (1) growth of an organism in two or more media; (2) confluent growth of a known ocular pathogen in one solid medium; or (3) growth in one medium of an organism identified on routine stain.[2] Jones[184] offered the following criteria: clinical signs of infection plus isolation of bacteria (10 or more colonies) on one solid medium and one additional medium, or isolation of fungi (any detectable growth) on any two media or one medium in the presence of a positive smear.

All these criteria have shortcomings. Some organisms may grow selectively in only one medium used in the schema for laboratory investigation (e.g., *Haemophilus* on chocolate agar or anaerobic bacteria in thiol broth). Small areas of corneal suppuration may yield only a few corneal samples that contain viable organisms. Additionally, antibiotics and other antimicrobial substances in the tear film may be transferred with the inoculum to solid media and inhibit growth, whereas these substances might be adequately diluted by liquid media.[184]

In the presence of incomplete criteria, a process may be judged as probable or suspicious for infection, and then clinical judgment becomes the deciding factor in therapy. The results of corneal cultures must be considered in view of the clinical situation, the confidence in the adequacy of sampling, and the likelihood of contamination by organisms present on the skin, eyelids, and conjunctiva. These concepts are important, especially when multiple organisms are isolated or when no organisms are isolated. Polymicrobial keratitis is a distinct entity whose frequency probably varies with the number of corneal scrapings and the diligence of the ocular microbiologist.[184] A negative culture is not uncommon; negative cultures were reported in 44 percent of 663 cases of suspected microbial keratitis.[2] Some negative cultures represent true sterile corneal ulcers, although other factors to consider are prior antibiotic treatment, inadequate sampling methods, improper selection of media, and improper interpretation of data. A device that removes antimicrobials has been used that permits the isolation of responsible organisms despite the presence of antibiotics.

Treatment

Most patients with bacterial keratitis are hospitalized because their families are unable to administer the antimicrobial drops with the necessary frequency, because the patient must be examined at regular intervals, and because it is never certain when the patient is first seen that compliance will be satisfactory, that the antimicrobial drops will be effective, and that rapid progression will not occur. Isolation is usually unnecessary, although contact should be avoided with patients anticipating intraocular surgery. With reliable patients or with milder disease, outpatient therapy is reasonable.[185]

The initial treatment of suspected microbial keratitis should be based on the clinical impression and the severity of the keratitis, predisposing factors, and the most likely responsible organisms and their antimicrobial susceptibility patterns.[13,170,186] The clinician is faced with the options of initiating specific or broad-spectrum antimicrobial treatment, initiating nonmicrobial treatment, or deferring treatment while following the clinical signs and awaiting the laboratory results. In general, the most rapidly destructive microbial keratitis is bacterial keratitis. Because of that fact, a suspected microbial ulcer should be treated as a bacterial ulcer until a definitive diagnosis is made. An ulcer that might be a fungal ulcer, for example, should be treated as a bacterial ulcer until the diagnosis of fungal keratitis is confirmed by laboratory studies.

The decision to base initial antibiotic therapy on the results of the Gram stain relies heavily on the technical proficiency of the microbiology laboratory, which under the best conditions, can identify the pathogen on Gram stain in 75 percent of cases of single-organism keratitis and 37 percent of cases of polymicrobial keratitis.[13] In view of the shortcomings of Gram and Giemsa stains, which may be inaccurate or nondiagnostic 30 percent of the time,[187] it is prudent to administer broad-spectrum antibiotic coverage in the initial treatment of all cases of serious suspected bacterial keratitis; the consequences of inadequate antibiotic coverage can be devastating.[188] Initial therapy may be modified by correlating the culture results with the results of Gram stain and the clinical response. This technique is less reliant on, but does not disregard the Gram stain findings. It takes into account the frequency of polymicrobial keratitis and the fact that gram-negative rods are frequently missed in the Gram stain.

The objective of treatment is to eliminate the organisms rapidly, reduce the inflammatory response, prevent structural damage, and promote re-epithelialization. Appropriate therapy implies an effective drug used efficaciously and quickly without causing severe toxicity. Close contact with the microbiology laboratory will allow maximum use of the initial stains and will direct more specific treatment as culture results and antibiotic sensitivities become available.

Antibiotics

Some factors that guide the choice of an appropriate antibiotic for systemic infection may not be applicable to the topical treatment of bacterial keratitis, for example, absorption characteristics, achievable serum levels, distribution space, mode of excretion, and influence of hepatic or renal function. Other factors remain important, such as efficacy, toxicity, and cost. The ideal antibiotic should be bactericidal at reasonable concentrations against the most common corneal pathogens, able to penetrate the cornea, and free of significant allergenicity and toxicity.[189] Other specific factors to consider are the route of administration, concentration and dosage, and frequency of administration. The past decade has witnessed the development of newer classes of antibiotics, including the fluoroquinolones, the carbapenems, and the monobactams. Older antibiotics, such as vancomycin, trimethoprim-sulfamethoxazole, and rifampin, are finding new applications.

Antibiotics used in ophthalmology have their effect on the cell wall, cytoplasmic membrane, protein synthesis, and cell DNA structure and synthesis (Tables 8-7 and 8-8). The mechanism of resistance to antibiotics includes the inability of the antibiotic to reach the organism, the inability to interact with the organism, and the production of enzymes by the organism, all of which inactivate the antibiotic. A detailed evaluation of antibiotics and the ocular pharmacology of antibiotics is available elsewhere.[190–197]

The penicillin family of antibiotics is ever expanding, with general properties of bactericidal activity, low toxicity, and good efficacy.[191] The action of the penicillins depends on the presence of a bacterial cell wall that contains mucopeptides. Natural penicillins (penicillin G and penicillin V) are effective against many gram-positive and a few gram-negative bacteria, as well as anaerobes. Penicillinase-resistant penicillins (methicillin, oxacillin, nafcillin, cloxacillin, and dicloxacillin) resist the action of penicillinase and are used mainly to treat infections caused by penicillinase-producing staphylococci. Their mechanism of resistance to the action of penicillinase is thought to be steric hinderance conveyed to the drug by the acyl side chain, which prevents opening of the β-lactam ring. Some strains of *S. aureus* in the United States are resistant to this group of drugs, as well as to similar antibiotics. If laboratory data indicate that a non-penicillinase-producing *Staphylococcus* is the causative infective agent, penicillin G is preferred because it is more active against such organisms, is less toxic, and is less expensive than the other penicillins. In vitro, oxacillin and cloxacillin are more effective than methicillin against penicillinase-producing *Staphylococcus,* although no clinical difference is evident.

The extended spectrum penicillins (ampicillin, amoxicillin, carbenicillin, ticarcillin, piperacillin, mezlocillin, and azolocillin) are effective against some gram-negative bacteria. They cannot resist the action of penicillinase and thus are ineffective against the staphylococci and gram-negative organisms that produce penicillinase. Ampicillin is active against *H. influenzae, E. coli, Proteus,* and *Listeria,* but is less active against most staphylococci and streptococci than is penicillin G. The emergence of ampicillin-resistant *H. influenzae* strains has necessitated treatment with chloramphenicol or a second- or third-generation cephalosporin. Carbenicillin has an antibiotic range similar to that of ampicillin, with additional activity against *P. aeruginosa,* indole-producing strains of *Proteus,* and anaerobes. Carbenicillin is less effective than penicillin G against gram-positive organisms and is ineffective against

TABLE 8-7
Mechanisms of Action of Antibiotics Used in Bacterial Keratitis

Inhibit bacterial cell wall synthesis
Penicillins, extended spectrum penicillins, semisynthetic penicillins
Cephalosporins
Carbapenems
Monobactams
Vancomycin
Bacitracin
Inhibit bacterial protein synthesis through ribosomal activity
Aminoglycosides/aminocyclitols
Erythromycin
Clindamycin
Tetracyclines
Chloramphenicol
Alter bacterial nucleic acid metabolism
Rifampin
Interfere with bacterial metabolism
Sulfonamides (inhibit modification of para-aminobenzoate into folic acid)
Trimethoprim (inhibits activity of bacterial dihydrofolate reductase)
Increase cell permeability
Polymyxins
Gramicidin
Inhibit supercoiling of DNA
Fluoroquinolones (inhibit DNA gyrase resulting in DNA entanglement)

TABLE 8-8
Antibiotics to Select for Use in Bacterial Keratitis

- Penicillins
  - Natural penicillins
    - Penicillin
  - Penicillinase-resistant penicillins
    - Methicillin
    - Oxacillin
    - Nafcillin
    - Cloxacillin
    - Dicloxacillin
  - Extended spectrum penicillins
    - Aminopenicillins
      - Ampicillin
      - Amoxicillin
      - Bacampicillin
      - Cyclacillin
    - Carboxypenicillins
      - Carbenicillin
      - Ticarcillin
    - Ureidopenicillins and piperazine penicillins
      - Mezlocillin
      - Azolocillin
      - Piperacillin
    - Combinations with β-lactamase inhibitors
      - Amoxicillin plus clavulanate
      - Ticarcillin plus clavulanate
      - Ampicillin plus sulbactam
- Cephalosporins
  - First-generation cephalosporins
    - Cephalothin
    - Cephapirin
    - Cephalexin
    - Cefaclor
    - Cephradine
    - Cefazolin
    - Cefadroxil
    - Cephaloridine
  - Second-generation cephalosporins
    - Cefamandole
    - Cefuroxime
    - Cefoxitin
    - Cefonicid
    - Cefotetan
    - Cefaclor
    - Cefmetazole
  - Third-generation cephalosporins
    - Cefotaxime
    - Ceftizoxime
    - Ceftriaxone
    - Cefoperazone
    - Ceftazidime
    - Cefsulodin
    - Cefixime
- Carbapenems
  - Imipenem plus cilastatin
- Monobactams
  - Aztreonam
- Aminoglycosides/aminocyclitols
  - Streptomycin
  - Kanamycin
  - Gentamicin
  - Netilmicin
  - Neomycin
  - Tobramycin
  - Amikacin
  - Spectinomycin
  - Paramycin
- Vancomycin
- Bacitracin
- Chloramphenicol
- Metronidazole
- Lincosamides
  - Lincomycin
  - Clindamycin
- Macrolides
  - Erythromycin
  - Azithromycin
  - Clarithromycin
- Tetracyclines
  - Tetracyline
  - Oxytetracycline
  - Chlortetracycline
  - Demeclocycline
  - Doxycycline
  - Methacycline
  - Minocycline
- Trimethoprim
- Trimethoprim-sulfamethoxazole
- Polymyxin
- Sulfonamides
- Rifampin
- Fluoroquinolones
  - Ciprofloxacin
  - Norfloxacin
  - Ofloxacin

penicillinase-producing streptococci. Ticarcillin has an antibiotic spectrum similar to that of carbenicillin, but is two to four times more active against *P. aeruginosa.* Carbenicillin or ticarcillin has been used with gentamicin in severe *Pseudomonas* infections because this combination is synergistic against many strains of *Pseudomonas* and because bacterial resistance may not develop as rapidly. Piperacillin has a wider spectrum of activity against both gram-positive and gram-negative bacteria, especially *Streptococcus, Enterococcus,* most Enterobacteriaceae, *Pseudomonas,* many anaerobes, and some β-lactamase-negative staphylococci. The major advantage of piperacillin is its increased activity against *P. aeruginosa* and *Klebsiella,* although studies have not confirmed clinical superiority. Piperacillin should be used in combination with an aminoglycoside because of the likelihood of development of resistance during treatment.

Allergic reactions are the chief side effects of the penicillins, and may be present in 3 to 5 percent of the general population and in as many as 10 percent of those who have previously received penicillin. Large doses or prolonged administration appears to be associated with a higher frequency of untoward reactions, with 10 percent mortality during anaphylaxis. Cross-allergenicity among the natural and semisynthetic penicillins reflects their common 6-aminopenicillinac acid nucleus and sensitizing derivatives.

The cephalosporin family of antibiotics are bactericidal agents of relatively low toxicity.[192] They are β-lactam antibiotics that act on the bacterial cell wall but also bind to proteins in the cellular membranes and initiate a complex chain of events that affect permeability and protein synthesis. In that the cephalosporins are generally active against many gram-positive, gram-negative, and anaerobic organisms, they are considered broad-spectrum antibiotics and are often used empirically. In general, first- and second-generation cephalosporins are most effective against *Staphylococcus* and *Streptococcus,* whereas third-generation cephalosporins are most effective against *P. aeruginosa* and Enterobacteriaceae. None of the currently available agents has adequate activity against methicillin-resistant *Staphylococcus,* penicillinase-resistant *S. pneumoniae,* or *Enterococcus.* Some Enterobacteriaceae *(Klebsiella, E. coli, P. mirabilis)* are sensitive to the cephalosporins, whereas other Enterobacteriaceae *(Enterobacter, Serratia)* are more resistant. *N. gonorrhoeae* is sensitive to the cephalosporins in general and to cefoxitin and ceftriaxone in particular. Second- and third-generation cephalosporins are effective against *H. influenzae. P. aeruginosa* is usually resistant to the cephalosporins except for some of the third-generation antibiotics. Because of their broad spectrum, good bactericidal activity, and low toxicity, cephalosporins are one of the first-line agents for the treatment of bacterial keratitis. Ceftazidime, a third-generation cephalosporin with potent activity against gram-negative bacilli, some gram-positive organisms, and anaerobes, may be effective as a topical treatment for suspected bacterial keratitis, either alone or in combination with an aminoglycoside.[191]

Cephalosporins are relatively lipid insoluble and do not penetrate ocular tissues well, although newer cephalosporins may penetrate better. If systemic administration is required, the majority of cephalosporins must be administered parenterally except for those resistant to hydrolysis by stomach acid, such as cephalexin, cefadroxil, cephradine, and cefaclor. The cephalosporins are excreted by the kidneys, but can be used with caution in patients with renal disease. Probenecid can block renal and ciliary body transport. Allergic reactions occur in up to 5 percent of individuals and are similar to penicillin reactions. There is cross-reactivity with penicillin allergy in about 8 percent of patients. Cephalosporins should not be used in patients who have a history of anaphylaxis or other severe or immediate reaction to any penicillin, or in those in whom skin testing shows reactivity to minor penicillin determinants. Milder delayed reactions to penicillin do not constitute a contraindication to the use of cephalosporins. Adverse reactions to cephalosporins may occur with or without a history of penicillin allergy.

In addition to the cephalosporins, other β-lactam antibiotics derived from the fungus *Cephalosporium* include the carbapenems and the monobactams. Carbapenems have a basic ring structure similar to that of penicillin. They are effective against gram-negative rods, gram-positive cocci, and anaerobes. Imipenem-cilastatin is a combination that combines a carbapenem (imipenem) with cilastatin, an inhibitor of renal dihydropeptide. This is an appropriate compound for some mixed infections.

Monobactams are a class of monocyclic antibiotics that have only the β-lactam ring as the core structure.[193] They have good activity against gram-negative bacilli, but little activity against either gram-positive cocci or anaerobes. Aztreonam is a monobactam that can be used as a substitute for an aminoglycoside.

Aminoglycosides (gentamicin, tobramycin, amikacin, streptomycin, kanamycin, neomycin) bind irreversibly to the 30-S bacterial ribosomal subunit, and thereby disrupt protein synthesis, and cause cell death by efflux of potassium, sodium, and other essential bacterial constituents.[194] They are bactericidal at high levels. Widespread antibiotic resistance among Enterobacteriaceae has restricted the use of streptomycin and kanamycin to a few clinical situations. Gentamicin, tobramycin, and amikacin are active against a wide range of Enterobacteriaceae and many *P. aeruginosa* strains, *H. influenzae,* and staphylococci (including penicillinase-producing strains). Gentamicin has been the mainstay of treatment of gram-negative corneal ulcers. It is not effective against streptococci at levels achievable in serum, but is effective topically at high concentrations. It may act synergistically with carbenicillin or ticarcillin against *P. aeruginosa* and *Proteus* species, but it is inactivated if mixed with carbenicillin in the same solution. Synergy has been reported between some cephalosporins and aminoglycosides.[198] *Pseudomonas* species other than *P. aeruginosa* are resistant to the aminoglycosides. Resistance to gentamicin appears to occur from acquired microbial enzymatic inactivation in the bacterial membrane or near the site of drug transport. Tobramycin closely resembles gentamicin in terms of antimicrobial spectrum and pharmacokinetics; it has comparable activity against *Klebsiella, Serratia,* and *Proteus,* and greater intrinsic activity against *P. aeruginosa.* Gentamicin-resistant strains of organisms are becoming increasingly frequent, and may be sensitive to tobramycin.[199] Systemic tobramycin may be less nephrotoxic than gentamicin.[200] Amikacin is similar in structure to kanamycin, but is resistant to aminoglycoside-modifying enzymes. Amikacin is active and more effective against a greater number of gram-negative bacilli than either gentamicin or tobramycin, although gentamicin and tobramycin are more effective if the organism is sensitive. *Nocardia* and nontuberculous mycobacteria may be sensitive to amikacin. Organisms resistant to gentamicin and tobramycin may be sensitive to amikacin and therefore, amikacin is used in hospitals where gentamicin resistance is prevalent. Neomycin is active against aerobic and facultatively anaerobic gram-positive and gram-negative bacteria. *Pseudomonas* is relatively resistant to neomycin. Because of its nephrotoxicity, neomycin is limited to topical administration and is usually formulated in combination with another antibiotic (e.g., polymyxin B, bacitracin, or gramicidin). Conjunctival and skin hypersensitivity reactions may occur with neomycin. Netilmicin is active against some strains of Enterobacteriaceae that are resistant to gentamicin and tobramycin, but has less intrinsic activity against *P. aeruginosa.* Systemic aminoglycosides have considerable vestibular, auditory, and renal toxicity; there is a narrow margin between efficacy and toxicity of these drugs. With topical use they can be associated with punctate epithelial keratitis and pseudomembranous conjunctivitis.[201] Chronic topical use should be avoided.

Vancomycin is a bactericidal glycopeptide antibiotic unrelated to other antibiotics.[195] It inhibits biosynthesis of peptidoglycan, the major structural cell wall polymer. It has a narrow spectrum against gram-positive bacteria, such as *Staphylococcus* (including penicillinase-producing strains), *Streptococcus,* and *Corynebacterium.* It is the antibiotic of choice for staphylococcal infections when penicillins, semisynthetic penicillins, or cephalosporins cannot be used or if the organism is resistant to these antibiotics.[202] It is extremely toxic systemically (ototoxicity and nephrotoxicity) and should be administered intravenously only under the supervision of an internist or infectious disease consultant. In ophthalmology, vancomycin is restricted to topical and intravitreal use. Vancomycin is acidic as dispensed and should be buffered before ophthalmic use, or tissue damage will occur. Subconjunctival injections can cause sloughing of the conjunctiva. Vancomycin used alone or with gentamicin for broad-spectrum coverage is more effective against some anaerobes, but has a narrower spectrum than cefazolin and gentamicin.

Bacitracin is bactericidal by binding to cell membranes. It is effective against most gram-positive cocci (including penicillinase-producing staphylococci) and is also effective against *Neisseria, Haemophilus,* and *Actinomyces.* Because of severe nephrotoxicity, it is not given systemically. It was once the preferred topical antibiotic for gram-positive bacterial keratitis, but the cephalosporins are now preferred because they are less toxic and more effective.

Chloramphenicol is a bacteriostatic drug that inhibits bacterial protein synthesis by binding irreversibly to the 50-S ribosomal subunit. Microbial resistance is caused by a specific plasmid. Chloramphenicol is active against *H. influenzae, Streptococcus, E. coli, Klebsiella,* and *Proteus,* and has moderate activity against *Staphylococcus.* It is not effective against *Pseudomonas.* Chloramphenicol has good penetration when administered by topical, subconjunctival, oral, or parenteral routes because of its lipid solubility. It is effective in serious ocular infections, but its use has declined as more effective antibiotics have been introduced and because of its potential for serious adverse reactions, including bone marrow suppression, which can occur as a dose-related or idiosyncratic reaction and can lead to aplastic anemia. Chloramphenicol can probably be administered topically with minimal risk of adverse systemic reactions, although bone marrow suppression after topical use has been reported.[203,204]

Macrolide antibiotics inhibit protein synthesis by binding to the 50-S subunit of bacterial ribosomes. Another unique property is the ability to penetrate polymorphonuclear leukocytes, macrophages, and lymphocytes. Erythromycin is the standard drug in this class and is used to treat mild bacterial conjunctivitis and blepharitis. Clarithromycin is a derivative of erythromycin that is more active against susceptible staphylococci, streptococci, chlamydia, *Borrelia,* and the nontuberculous mycobacteria. Azithromycin is a derivative of erythromycin with good potential for treatment of *Borrelia, Haemophilus influenzae,* chlamydia, and *Neisseria.*[196]

Clindamycin inhibits protein synthesis by binding to bacterial ribosomes. Plasmid-mediated resistance is possible. Clindamycin is active against *S. aureus, S. epidermidis, Streptococcus,* and anaerobes. It is most useful against gram-positive anaerobes (e.g., *Bacillus cereus*) as an alternative to penicillin or a cephalosporin. It can be administered orally or parenterally.

The antimicrobial combination of trimethoprim and sulfamethoxazole is active in vitro against a variety of gram-positive and gram-negative bacteria. Trimethoprim competitively inhibits the activity of bacterial dihydrofolate reductase; sulfamethoxazole competitively inhibits the modification of para-aminobenzoate into folic acid. Trimethoprim and sulfamethoxazole exert a synergistic bactericidal effect, with sequential inhibition of the synthesis of folinic acid in many gram-positive and gram-negative bacteria. The combination is the antimicrobial of choice in most *Nocardia* infections. Sulfamethoxazole is a broad-spectrum antibiotic with activity especially against Enterobacteriaceae and is useful in some bacteria resistant to the cephalosporins.

Polymyxins are surface-active agents that have a detergent-like bactericidal effect by changing the permeability and integrity of bacterial cytoplasmic cell membranes. Their effect is related to the phospholipid content of the bacterial cell wall, so that gram-negative bacteria are susceptible. The combination of trimethoprim and polymyxin B is available as a topical antibiotic drop, and is a useful addition in the treatment of conjunctivitis and blepharoconjunctivitis caused by susceptible strains of *Staphylococcus, Streptococcus,* and *Pseudomonas.* Its usefulness in deep corneal infections has not been adequately established.

Rifampin is an antituberculosis drug that also has antibiotic activity against other bacteria and chlamydia. It is a large, fat-soluble molecule that acts by inhibiting bacterial DNA-dependent RNA polymerase. Its main use in ophthalmology is against mycobacterial corneal ulcers. Other sensitive organisms include *S. aureus, S. epidermidis, Streptococcus, H. influenzae,* and *N. gonorrhoeae.*

Fluoroquinolones (ciprofloxacin, norfloxacin, ofloxacin, amifloxacin, perfloxacin, tosulfloxacin, and temafloxacin) are a group of antimicrobial agents structurally related to nalidixic acid.[205] They interfere with both the structure and function of bacterial DNA by blocking DNA gyrase, an essential enzyme that maintains the helical twist in DNA. In ophthalmology, the fluoroquinolones appear to have a broad spectrum with high potency and good pharmacokinetic and safety profiles. Acquired bacterial resistance to fluoroquinolones is uncommon. Plasmid-borne resistance is a common cause of failure of conventional antibiotics; the fluoroquinolones have not demonstrated plasmid-borne resistance, but resistance occurs through chromosomal mutations. Frequent use of fluoroquinolones is leading to the emergence of increasing resistance.[206,207]

Ciprofloxacin, norfloxacin, and ofloxacin have undergone evaluation in ophthalmology.[208–217] They offer a broad-spectrum monotherapy for corneal ulcers with a commercially available agent (rather than a fortified agent) and are effective against *Neisseria* and chlamydia.[218–220] Ciprofloxacin appears to be the most promising drug, with a broad spectrum of activity against both gram-positive and gram-negative bacteria, such as *Staphylococcus* (including methicillin-resistant *Staphylococcus*), *Pseudomonas,* and the Enterobacteriaceae. *Streptococcus* and anaerobes are mostly resistant. Some quinolones are effective against mycobacteria and mycoplasma. Ciprofloxacin is well absorbed orally and has a relatively long half-life. Optic nerve toxicity has been reported.[221] Because they may affect the development of cartilage, all fluoroquinolones are contraindicated in children, adolescents, pregnant women, and nursing mothers. Studies are accumulating that indicate the effectiveness of topical ciprofloxacin against *Staphylococcus* and *Pseudomonas* corneal ulcers in experimental animals and clinical situations.[222–225] Ciprofloxacin may precipitate within the corneal ulcer, but this usually resolves with time. A 0.3 percent ciprofloxacin ophthalmic ointment has been effective in one clinical trial.[226]

Route of Antibiotic Administration

Topical administration is the most efficient means of delivering antibiotics to the cornea (Table 8-9). In addition to providing therapeutically effective concentrations of the drug, topical drops wash away bacteria, bacterial antigens, and potentially destructive enzymes from the ocular surface. Penetration of topically applied drugs into the cornea is increased with higher concentrations of drug, greater frequency of application, more lipophilic antibiotics, and longer contact time, as provided by certain vehicles.[227–229] Absence of the epithelium also enhances penetration.

Some patients may respond to commercial strength topical antibiotics (e.g., ciprofloxacin) given at frequent intervals, but fortified topical antibiotics are usually more effective.[229,230,231] Fortified antibiotics are the primary form of therapy because when they are given with an initial loading dose, more drug is delivered to the cornea compared with subconjunctival injection, intra-

TABLE 8-9
Dosages of Principal Antibiotics Used in Bacterial Keratitis

Antibiotic	*Topical*	*Subconjunctival*[a]	*Intravenous*[a]
Cefazolin	50 mg/ml	100 mg	1 g/6 hr
Ceftazidime	50 mg/ml	100 mg	1 g/8 hr
Gentamicin or tobramycin	14 mg/ml	20 mg	3–7 mg/kg/day
Penicillin G	100,000 units/ml	500,000 units	2–6 million units/4 hr
Vancomycin	50 mg/ml	25 mg	[b]
Amikacin	20 mg/ml	20 mg	5 mg/kg/day
Trimethoprim-sulfamethoxazole	Trimethoprim (16 mg/ml)-sulfamethoxazole (80 mg/ml)	—	10–20 mg/kg/day
Ceftriaxone	50 mg/ml	—	1–2 g/day
Nafcillin	—	—	200 mg/kg/day
Chloramphenicol	5 mg/ml	100 mg	1 g/6 hr
Bacitracin	10,000 units/ml	—	—
Ampicillin	—	100 mg	2 g/4 hr
Clindamycin	—	40 mg	3 g/day
Piperacillin	20 mg/ml	100 mg	200 mg/kg/day
Ciprofloxacin	3 mg/ml	—	400 mg/12 hr
Norfloxacin	3 mg/ml	—	—
Ofloxacin	3 mg/ml	—	—
Clarithromycin	20 mg/ml	—	—

[a] Subconjunctival and intravenous therapy reserved for severe keratitis.
[b] Administered under the supervision of an internist.

venous, or intramuscular dosing, either alone or in combination.[232] Fortified topical antibiotics are prepared by adding the desired amount of parenteral agent to an artificial tear solution (Table 8-10). Two antibiotics should not be combined in one preparation. Fortified preparations can be kept at the bedside for 1 week without significant loss of antibiotic activity.[233-235] Although fortified antibiotics are generally prepared as solutions because of the ease of varying the concentration, laboratory data suggest that fortified topical antibiotic ointments may allow extended dose schedules[236]; however, the pharmacokinetics of such ointments need to be further defined.

Fortified topical antibiotics are given every 15 to 30 minutes (alternating drugs when multiple antibiotics are used) for the first 24 to 36 hours. One study indicates

TABLE 8-10
Preparation of Fortified Antibiotic Eye Drops

Antibiotic	*Method*	*Final Concentration*
Cefazolin	Add 5 ml of sterile water to 500 mg of cefazolin powder; mix, remove, and place into 5 ml of artificial tear solution	50 mg/ml
Gentamicin (tobramycin)	Add 2 ml of parenteral gentamicin (40 mg/ml) to 5-ml bottle of commercial ophthalmic gentamicin (3 mg/ml)	14 mg/ml
Penicillin G	Add 10 ml of artificial tears to 1 million-unit vial of penicillin G powder; mix, remove, and place into empty artificial tear bottle	100,000 units/ml
Vancomycin	Add 5 ml of sterile water to 500-mg vial of vancomycin powder; mix, remove, and place into 5 ml of artificial tear solution; buffer	50 mg/ml
Amikacin	Add 4 ml of parenteral amikacin (100 mg/2 ml) to 6-ml bottle of artificial tear solution	20 mg/ml
Bacitracin	Add 5 ml of artificial tears to 50,000-unit vial of bacitracin (lyophilized); mix, remove, and place into empty artificial tear bottle	10,000 units/ml
Trimethoprim-sulfamethoxazole	Use undiluted	Trimethoprim 16 mg/ml; sulfamethoxazole 80 mg/ml
Piperacillin	Add 10 ml sterile water to 2-g vial of piperacillin powder; mix, remove 1 ml, and place into 9-ml bottle of artificial tear solution	20 mg/ml

that fortified drops may be just as effective given every 30 minutes as every 15 minutes.[237] Commercial strength antibiotics should be used until the fortified antibiotics are prepared so that treatment is not delayed.

A collagen shield can be soaked in a commercially available concentration of antibiotic and placed on the cornea as soon as the patient is seen. This allows prompt and convenient antibiotic therapy while awaiting the formulation of fortified antibiotic eye drops. The presence of the shield on the cornea does not reduce the efficacy of subsequent topical antibiotic therapy. Topical antibiotic eye drops are rapidly diluted after they are instilled, and the concentration gradient encouraging their penetration into the eye is maintained for only a very short time. Collagen shields absorb antibiotics and present them to the eye over several hours, allowing high concentrations of antibiotics within the cornea and anterior chamber over a prolonged period. Although two studies[238,239] showed that collagen shields were not more effective than conventional fortified antibiotics, shields do provide a more convenient and less labor-intensive route of administration than frequent drops with equivalent efficacy in the treatment of bacterial ulcers.[240-244]

Subconjunctival antibiotic injections are painful and frightening for many patients, and may cause conjunctival inflammation, scarring, and possible necrosis. Penicillin G, vancomycin, and gentamicin are commonly used antibiotics with potential for conjunctival necrosis when given subconjunctivally.[201] Subconjunctival antibiotics also carry the risk of inadvertent intraocular penetration.

Antibiotics injected subconjunctivally reach the cornea through tissue diffusion and also by leakage through the conjunctival injection site and the intact conjunctiva.[93] Subconjunctival injections provide a higher drug level in the cornea than sub-Tenon's injections. Although subconjunctival antibiotic injections deliver therapeutic levels to the cornea and the anterior chamber,[245] a variety of studies indicate that fortified topical antibiotics are just as effective as subconjunctival antibiotics in microbial killing power and improving the clinical course in animal models.[93,237,246,247] Subconjunctival antibiotics add nothing to the microbial killing effect unless only commercially available antibiotic concentrations are being used[246,248-250] and collagen shields are not available.

Intravenous or intramuscular antibiotics do not appear to augment topical antibiotics in most situations.[251,252] Although pharmacologic and animal studies suggest that parenteral antibiotic therapy may enhance topical therapy, adequate clinical trials are lacking. Systemic antibiotics are poorly absorbed into the eye, and drug levels in the cornea can be achieved only with considerable risk of systemic toxicity. Ocular inflammation increases the ocular penetration of systemic antibiotics. Systemic antibiotics should be used concomitantly with local antibiotics in the presence of *N. gonorrhoeae* keratitis, or in *Pseudomonas* or *Haemophilus* keratitis in young children because of the risk of systemic spread.[253] Parenteral antibiotics are also indicated in scleral suppuration, in perforated ulcers, in severe keratitis with potential for intraocular spread, in association with perforating injuries to the cornea or sclera, or in situations where an ideal local regimen cannot be given.

Few clinical data are available to suggest the best parenteral agents. Cefazolin is the preferred cephalosporin for gram-positive cocci, although penetration is variable. Some prefer methicillin over other semisynthetic penicillins or cephalosporins because of greater familiarity with the drug, bacterial activity against *S. aureus,* low degree of protein binding, and knowledge of ocular penetration.[13] Gentamicin and tobramycin are the mainstays for susceptible organisms, but have significant renal and ototoxicity.

Antibiotic Therapy

Eighty-seven percent of bacterial corneal ulcers are caused by four groups of organisms.[13] Although no single antibiotic is effective against all organisms, it is possible to cover most organisms effectively with the use of two drugs (Table 8-11).

A cephalosporin is the drug of choice for unidentified gram-positive cocci. Penicillin has greater action against *S. pneumoniae* and other streptococci, but the frequency of penicillin-resistant *Staphylococcus* and *Micrococcus* substantiates the requirement that the primary agent be effective against penicillinase-producing organisms. Cephalosporins possess greater in vitro activity against *Staphylococcus* and *Streptococcus* than bacitracin, erythromycin, or lincomycin.[254] Cefazolin (50 mg/ml) is less toxic than bacitracin (10,000 units/ml) to the conjunctiva and cornea. Cefazolin can be used in selected patients who are allergic to penicillin. Recently, staphylococcal and streptococcal organisms that are resistant to penicillin and cefazolin have been recognized. Vancomycin is a useful alternative for these multiresistant staphylococcal organisms or in patients with a major penicillin allergy.[202] The fluoroquinolones appear to be useful alternatives.[214,218,219]

Tobramycin is the initial antibiotic of choice in suspected gram-negative rod keratitis because of its stability, corneal penetration, and bactericidal levels against *Pseudomonas, Enterobacter, Klebsiella,* and other gram-negative organisms. Tobramycin is preferred to gentamicin because of the increased number of gentamicin-resistant strains of *P. aeruginosa* and because tobramycin is more active by weight against *P. aeruginosa.*[255] Amikacin should be considered in gentamicin- and tobramycin-resistant infec-

TABLE 8-11
Initial Therapy for Bacterial Keratitis Based on Gram Stain

Smear Result	*Likely Organism*	*Initial Antibiotic Therapy*
Gram-positive cocci		Cefazolin
Aerobic	*Staphylococcus* *Streptococcus*	
Anaerobic	*Peptostreptococcus* *Streptococcus*	
Gram-positive rods		Cefazolin (tobramycin)
Aerobic	*Corynebacterium* *Bacillus* *Listeria*	
Anaerobic	*Clostridium* *Propionibacterium*	
Gram-positive filaments		Penicillin
Aerobic	*Mycobacterium* (acid fast) *Nocardia* (partially acid fast)	
Anaerobic	*Actinomyces*	
Gram-negative cocci		Systemic ceftriaxone
Aerobic	*Neisseria*	
Anaerobic	*Veillonella*	
Gram-negative rods		Tobramycin
Aerobic	*Pseudomonas* *Azotobacter* *Haemophilus* *Klebsiella* *Enterobacter* *Serratia* *Proteus* *Moraxella*	
Anaerobic	*Fusobacterium* *Bacteroides*	
No bacteria or multiple types of bacteria		Cefazolin and tobramycin
Acid-fast bacilli		Amikacin for *Mycobacterium*; trimethoprim-sulfamethoxazole for *Nocardia*

tions.[255] Gentamicin is effective against approximately 90 percent of *P. aeruginosa,* whereas tobramycin and amikacin are effective in approximately 95 percent. Unfortunately, these numbers are decreasing, especially in certain regions of the country. For multiresistant gram-negative rods, the addition of ticarcillin may give synergistic activity with other alternatives, including the extended spectrum cephalosporins, such as ceftazidime and cefoperazone; the ureidopenicillins, such as piperacillin; and the monobactams, such as aztreonam. There is limited clinical experience with most of these newer agents. Tobramycin is also an ideal choice for the initial treatment of gram-positive and gram-variable rods because *Azotobacter* and *Bacillus* species may be more susceptible to this agent than to penicillin.[31] Aminoglycosides are toxic when administered topically for a long time and therefore should not be used chronically. The availability of topical fluoroquinolones has expanded the armamentarium, especially against gram-negative organisms resistant to gentamicin.[256-258] Experimental and clinical studies suggest that ciprofloxacin may be an effective single drug because of increased potency, broad spectrum of antibacterial activity, and low frequency of organisms that are resistant.[218,259,260] There is evidence to suggest combined therapy may prevent the emergence of ciprofloxacin-resistant strains.[261]

Systemic ceftriaxone is the drug of choice for gram-negative cocci because of the likelihood of *N. gonorrhoeae* or *N. meningitidis* and because of a high prevalence of penicillin-resistant organisms.[262] *Neisseria* keratitis is rare. Cell wall damage by a variety of mechanisms may make gram-positive cocci appear to be gram-negative. If gram-negative coccobacilli are seen on the initial smears, chloramphenicol or ampicillin should be considered because of possible *Haemophilus* keratitis. Gram-positive filaments suggest Actinomycetes, and penicillin is appropriate pending final identification. Most gram-positive rods, both aerobic and anaerobic, remain sensitive to penicillin G or cefazolin, but clindamycin or carbenicillin may also be used.

The combination of cefazolin and tobramycin (or gentamicin) is indicated when two or more different types of bacteria are detected on the Gram stain, in the absence of an organism seen on Gram stain when the disease is judged to be a severe microbial process, or when antecedent antimicrobial therapy has been used.[170] This selection is effective against most organisms. Treatment with a topical aminoglycoside and piperacillin (or ticarcillin) is justified as initial therapy for severe keratitis caused by *P. aeruginosa* or an unidentified gram-negative bacillus. With increases in aminoglycoside-resistant *Pseudomonas* and other gram-positive organisms, fluoroquinolones, especially ciprofloxacin, have been investigated in vivo and in vitro for use against these organisms.[225,263,264]

Mycobacterium is usually sensitive to amikacin, although the emergence of clinical resistance to amikacin may occur during therapy.[46] *M. fortuitum* and *M. chelonae* specifically are more susceptible in vitro to amikacin than to streptomycin, kanamycin, or rifampin.[265] Erythromycin has shown a synergistic effect with amikacin in vitro,[266] and clarithromycin was effective in vivo in an animal model of *M. fortuitum* keratitis.[267] There is conflicting evidence of the in vitro and in vivo effectiveness of ciprofloxacin.[268–271] Surgical therapy with corneal transplantation may frequently be required.[268,272]

Therapy Modification

Modification of initial therapy may be indicated when the culture results become available. Virulent organisms (e.g., *Micrococcus, Staphylococcus, Streptococcus, Bacillus, Pseudomonas,* and *Enterobacter*) tend to be detected within 24 hours in culture. Slower growing organisms include *Haemophilus, Moraxella, Neisseria,* yeasts, some streptococci, and some anaerobes. The extremely slow-growing organisms may require 3 weeks for isolation; these include *Mycobacterium, Nocardia, Actinomyces,* some anaerobes, filamentous fungi, and *Acanthamoeba.* However, there can be considerable variation.[166] If the identified organism is substantially more susceptible to an antibiotic other than the one originally selected, the more effective antibiotic may be substituted. Table 8-12 indicates the preferred therapy for most bacterial organisms and also indicates acceptable alternatives. Variations from expected sensitivities do occur and require laboratory guidance. If broad coverage was initially selected and only one organism is isolated, the less effective drug is discontinued. If the culture is negative, the clinician must judge whether the initial impression of a microbial keratitis was correct.

All these decisions are tempered by the clinical response and tolerance to the initial therapy, the severity of the keratitis, and the anticipated or reported in vitro susceptibilities. If there is clinical improvement on the initiated course with a single antibiotic, there may be no advantage to switching to another agent. It must be remembered that up to 32 percent of cases of microbial keratitis may be characterized by two or more bacteria or fungi.[13]

If gram-positive cocci are confirmed by culture, cefazolin is continued. Alternatively, if the organism is anticipated or known to be sensitive to penicillin, treatment can be switched to the more effective therapy if there

TABLE 8-12
Therapy for Bacterial Keratitis Based on Culture Results

	Antibiotic		
Organism	*Topical (Alternative)*	*Subconjunctival*[a]	*Intravenous*[a]
Gram-positive			
Micrococcus, Staphylococcus (penicillin resistant)	Cefazolin (vancomycin, bacitracin, fluoroquinolone)	Cefazolin	Nafcillin
Micrococcus, Staphylococcus (methicillin resistant)	Vancomycin (bacitracin, fluoroquinolone)	Vancomycin	Vancomycin
Micrococcus, Staphylococcus (penicillin sensitive)	Penicillin (cefazolin, vancomycin, bacitracin, fluoroquinolone)	Penicillin G	Penicillin G
Streptococcus, S. pneumoniae	Penicillin G (cefazolin, vancomycin, bacitracin)	Penicillin G	Penicillin G
Enterococcus	Vancomycin (penicillin and tobramycin)	Vancomycin	Penicillin
Anaerobic gram-positive cocci	Penicillin G	Penicillin G	Penicillin
Corynebacterium	Vancomycin (erythromycin)	Vancomycin	Penicillin G
Propionibacterium	Penicillin	Penicillin	Penicillin
Bacillus cereus	Gentamicin and vancomycin	Gentamicin	Gentamicin
Listeria	Gentamicin and penicillin G	Gentamicin	Ampicillin
Gram-negative			
Pseudomonas species	Tobramycin and piperacillin (ceftazidime)	Tobramycin	Tobramycin
Enterobacteriaceae	Tobramycin (fluoroquinolone)	Tobramycin	Tobramycin
Moraxella	Tobramycin (fluoroquinolone)	Tobramycin	Tobramycin
Haemophilus	Chloramphenicol (ceftriaxone, fluoroquinolone)	Chloramphenicol	Chloramphenicol
Neisseria gonorrhoeae or *N. meningitidis*	Ceftriaxone (ceftazidime)	Ceftriaxone	Ceftriaxone[b]
Bacteroidaceae	Penicillin	Penicillin	Penicillin
Other			
Nocardia	Trimethoprim-sulfamethoxazole	—	Trimethoprim-sulfamethoxazole
Mycobacterium	Amikacin (rifampin, ciprofloxacin)	Amikacin	Amikacin

[a] Subconjunctival and intravenous therapy reserved for severe keratitis.
[b] Systemic therapy for associated conjunctivitis and systemic disease.

has not been adequate clinical improvement with cefazolin. Vancomycin should be considered in patients with a history of penicillin anaphylaxis or if the organism is resistant to multiple antistaphylococcal drugs.[273] The number of *S. epidermidis* and *S. aureus* organisms resistant to methicillin and other β-lactam antibiotics (including cephalosporin) and to the aminoglycosides is increasing. Treatment with vancomycin or ciprofloxacin is indicated for these organisms.

If an aerobic gram-negative rod is isolated, tobramycin or gentamicin is the drug of choice. Some experimental data suggest that an aminoglycoside combined with carbenicillin or ticarcillin or with a ureidopenicillin, such as piperacillin, is more effective against *P. aeruginosa* and other gram-negative organisms than single therapy; however, there was no synergism when a treatment regimen was evaluated in one model of experimental *Pseudomonas* keratitis.[274] If the organism is resistant to gentamicin or tobramycin, it may be sensitive to amikacin. Topical ceftazidime (a third-generation cephalosporin) and ciprofloxacin are potentially useful agents in *Pseudomonas* keratitis. *Pseudomonas* keratitis requires long-term, high-dose antibiotic therapy; it responds slowly and may persist for long periods within corneal tissue, only to recrudesce later. *Pseudomonas* keratitis also has a tendency to progress to perforation, scleral suppuration, and phthisis despite aggressive antibiotic therapy. *Moraxella* may progress, even with antibiotic treatment based on in vitro sensitivities, and may require surgical intervention; host factors may play a predominant role.[25] Mild *Haemophilus* keratitis is treated with topical chloramphenicol, but ceftriaxone (a third-generation cephalosporin) and ciprofloxacin are potential agents for severe keratitis.

For anaerobic organisms (either gram-positive cocci or gram-negative rods), penicillin is preferred; chloramphenicol or vancomycin is an alternative.[37] Aerobic and anaerobic gram-positive rods are infrequent causes of keratitis, and penicillin is recommended. *Bacillus* species should be treated with a combination of either clindamycin and amikacin, or gentamicin and vancomycin. For gram-positive filaments that suggest Actinomycetes, penicillin is effective. *Nocardia* responds to topical sulfonamides and tetracycline, but the present preferred treatment is a combination of trimethoprim (16 mg/ml) and sulfamethoxazole (80 mg/ml) eye drops.[275,276] If mixed organisms are cultured, effective drugs can be substituted if the initial selection of tobramycin and cefazolin is ineffective.

Although many bacteria have predictable antibiotic sensitivity patterns, sensitivity studies should be routinely performed on all corneal isolates. The laboratory should specifically perform antibiotic sensitivity testing with the aminoglycosides for all organisms because of the frequency of their primary use. Standardized, commercially available Kirby-Bauer disks impregnated with antibiotics are placed on Mueller-Hinton agar plates with a standardized bacterial inoculum. A zone of inhibition develops and the size determines sensitivity or resistance, correlating with clinically achievable levels in serum or body fluids. These in vitro sensitivities may guide antimicrobial therapy, although the determination of sensitivity and resistance by this method is arbitrary and does not reflect in vivo effectiveness of drugs in the tear film or cornea following standard routes of administration. Broth dilution methods to determine the minimal inhibitory or bactericidal concentration of antibiotics are a better guide and can be correlated with body fluid levels. A modification is the agar dilution technique, which allows use of a blood medium for more fastidious organisms and permits visualization of contaminants and mutants. This procedure may be available in a large laboratory, and has slightly more reproducible results than broth dilution, although it determines only the minimal inhibitory concentration.

Antibiotic sensitivity tests for anaerobes have been emphasized recently because of increasing recognition of anaerobes in corneal disease, the necessity for specific treatment, the introduction of new antibiotics, and the development of an agar dilution sensitivity test.

Bacterial β-lactamase production can be determined with filter paper by the chromogenic cephalosporin method (nitrocefin), the iodometric slide test, or the acidimetric test. On occasion, accurate determination of antibiotic serum concentrations may be necessary to ensure the adequacy of treatment and to prevent toxicity. Generally, these tests are performed when treatment involves antibiotics for which the margin between therapeutic and toxic levels is narrow, such as with the aminoglycosides or vancomycin. Several assay methods are available, including disk diffusion bioassay or chromatographic, immunologic, and radioenzymatic methods.

Signs of clinical improvement are based on frequent slit lamp microscopic examinations. The changes may be difficult to appreciate within the first few days because of the increased inflammation and edema related to corneal scrapings and the frequency of topical antibiotics. It is important to recognize that some bacteria, such as *Pseudomonas,* may continue to digest corneal collagen for up to 12 hours after the initiation of effective antibiotic therapy, so that there may be some degree of progression of the ulcer, although effective antibiotic therapy is being given. Within 2 or 3 days of effective therapy, the progression of the disease is halted; the size and density of the cellular infiltration and edema decrease, the periphery of the stromal suppuration is blunted, anterior chamber inflammation decreases, and epithelial and stromal healing begin.

Corneal vascularization is an indication of healing, although it heralds additional scarring. The improvement rate varies depending on the responsible organism, duration of infection, patient response, and other antecedent factors. Familiarity with the expected course of the infection, based on the virulence of the organism, will allow judgment of the effectiveness of antibiotic therapy. Keratitis caused by virulent gram-positive organisms, such as *S. aureus* and *S. pneumoniae,* may be relatively unchanged for 1 to 2 days and then may show rapid improvement with healing in 7 to 10 days. Keratitis caused by gram-negative bacilli, especially *Pseudomonas,* typically appears worse during the first 1 to 2 days of treatment because of rapid stromal destruction by enzymes; it may be difficult to distinguish areas of suppuration caused by replicating bacteria from the stromal inflammatory response. Bacteria persist for 10 to 14 days in the cornea and the time to healing may be prolonged. *Pseudomonas* keratitis requires prolonged antibiotic therapy. Keratitis caused by bacteria of relatively low virulence (e.g., *S. epidermidis, Moraxella*) generally improves rapidly within 1 to 2 days, with the organism eliminated in 5 to 7 days. Some organisms (e.g., *S. pneumoniae,* some strains of *Moraxella*) may cause rapid corneal perforation despite minimal suppuration and discharge. This melt may proceed despite appropriate topical antibiotics, especially in patients with rheumatoid arthritis and/or dry eyes.

After 36 hours, antibiotics can usually be tapered. Therapy may be converted to commercial strength antibiotic drops or ointments several days later. The end point of treatment is epithelial healing, but it must be recognized that toxic antibiotics may retard this process.[277] Repeat cultures are generally not reliable. Prolonged therapy is recommended for organisms known to persist in corneal tissue (i.e., *Pseudomonas*), and for bacteria that respond slowly to antibiotic therapy, such as *Mycobacterium, Nocardia,* anaerobic bacteria, and others.

Adjunctive Therapy

Local or systemic factors that might modify the patient's response should be investigated.[278] Structural eyelid deformities that cause or enhance keratitis, such as entropion or trichiasis, should be corrected (see Ch. 6). Lagophthalmos and dry eyes are particularly common antecedents of infected corneal ulcers. If they are not detected, the ulcers frequently will not heal even though appropriate antibiotic therapy has been given. Pain control with acetaminophen or other medication allows more effective delivery of the treatment regimen. Intraocular pressure should be monitored, and elevations treated with a topical β-blocker and an oral carbonic anhydrase inhibitor if necessary. Adequate cycloplegia and mydriasis are mandatory to help alleviate pain and inflammation and to prevent posterior synechiae formation.

Patching may be required to heal epithelial defects. However, patching should be avoided until the bacteria have been eliminated because of enhanced microbial growth, maceration of skin, and difficulty in delivering the treatment regimen. A bandage soft contact lens may be necessary for healing indolent epithelial defects, for severe stromal ulceration with or without active bacterial keratitis, and for small corneal perforations. Such a lens also provides comfort and may improve visual acuity.[279] Antibiotic therapy should be continued over the contact lens. Cholinergic agents (carbachol or echothiophate iodide) may stimulate epithelial growth through inhibition of adenosine 3′,5′-cyclic phosphate[280]; however, they are of little clinical benefit because they exacerbate iritis and pain.

If the keratitis progresses despite aggressive treatment, the clinician must consider other disease entities, such as atypical bacteria, fungi, protozoa, herpes, and nonmicrobial causes (Figures 8-40 and 8-41). Mixed infections or superinfections may also occur. Any abrupt worsening of clinical signs necessitates repeat corneal scrapings and laboratory evaluation. Suboptimal use of antibiotics or inactivation of the antibiotics in the delivery system or because of mixture with other drugs should be considered. Acquired antibiotic resistance is unlikely during a short period of treatment. Alternatively, the treatment may have been initiated at an advanced stage of the disease and may be ineffective in preventing progression and structural alterations.[281] Even in the absence of viable organisms, other mechanisms, such as necrotizing enzymes and toxins, may contribute to tissue destruction. Continued inflammation may produce severe structural alterations and lead to blindness by multiple pathways: corneal opacification, disorganization of the anterior segment, secondary glaucoma, scleral extension, and corneal perforation with endophthalmitis (Figures 8-42 and 8-43). Up to 24 percent of patients may go on to descemetocele formation, perforation, or endophthalmitis.[4,8]

A number of adjunctive modalities have been suggested to control corneal destruction in association with progressive bacterial keratitis: collagenase or proteoglycanase inhibitors,[282] heparin,[283] lysozyme,[284] corticosteroids,[122,285,286] and surgical procedures, including cryocurettage,[287,288] tissue adhesive,[289] argon, CO_2, and excimer lasers,[290–292] conjunctival flap, and penetrating keratoplasty.

The use of enzyme inhibitors in bacterial keratitis is controversial and probably not of much clinical value. Injured epithelial cells, polymorphonuclear leukocytes, and some bacteria elaborate various enzymes that contribute to corneal tissue destruction and melting. *Pseudomonas* produces a

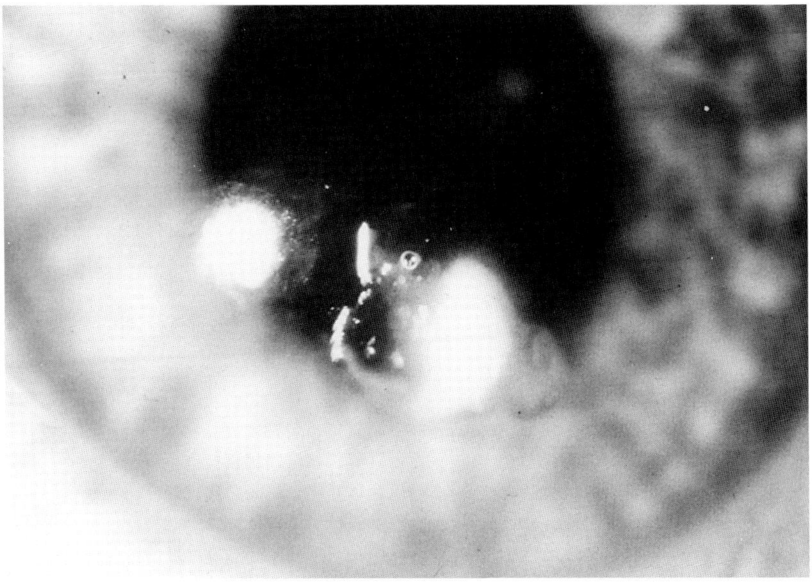

FIGURE 8-40 A corneal abscess in a soft contact lens wearer. There was no discharge or conjunctival reaction. Cultures and Gram stain were negative and the patient responded to discontinuing contact lens wear without the use of antibiotics.

variety of proteolytic enzymes. Collagenase is produced by the patient's corneal tissue. Inhibition of these enzymes with disodium edetate (0.05 M), acetylcysteine (20 percent), or heparin (2 percent) is effective experimentally, although there is no clear evidence of clinical efficacy in preventing stromal necrosis or ulceration. Disodium edetate binds calcium that is necessary for collagenase activity, but is toxic to the cornea. Acetylcysteine binds to enzymes and inhibits enzyme activity directly. Zinc sulfate (0.5 percent) may theoretically be helpful in *Moraxella* keratitis because it inhibits the action of proteolytic fermentation products of the organism. In an animal model of *Pseudomonas* keratitis, cyclo-oxygenase inhibitors caused worsening of the keratitis and a lipoxygenase inhibitor prevented this worsening.[293]

The goal of any treatment plan for bacterial keratitis is to prevent tissue necrosis and subsequent irreversible structural alterations. Corticosteroids impede host defenses by interfering with polymorphonuclear leukocyte activity at several levels (ingestion, degranulation, and lysozyme levels). Corticosteroids can effectively decrease the inflammatory component initiated by replicating organisms, bacterial endotoxins or exotoxins, host enzymes, and the release of hydrolytic enzymes from polymorphonuclear leukocytes. However, experimental

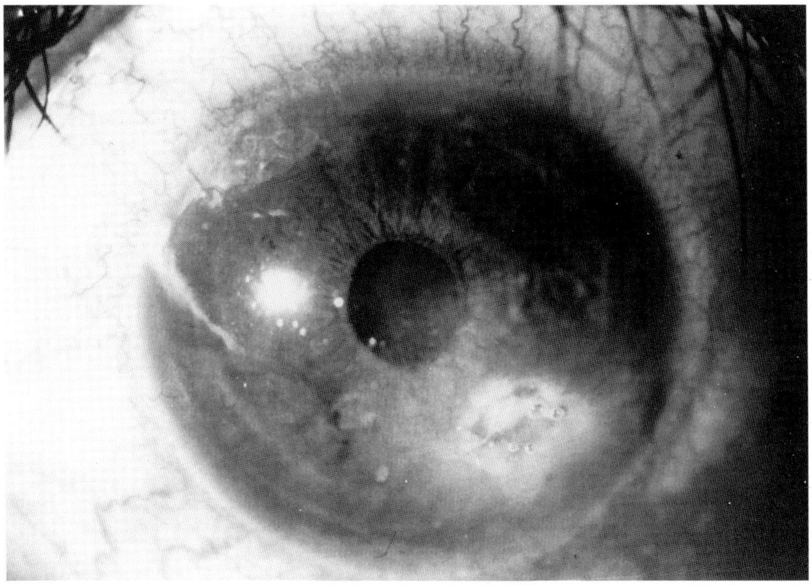

FIGURE 8-41 A patient with a 5th and 7th cranial nerve palsy after a neurosurgical procedure developed a dry corneal ulceration and edema without discharge or infiltrate. The patient responded to lubrication and patching.

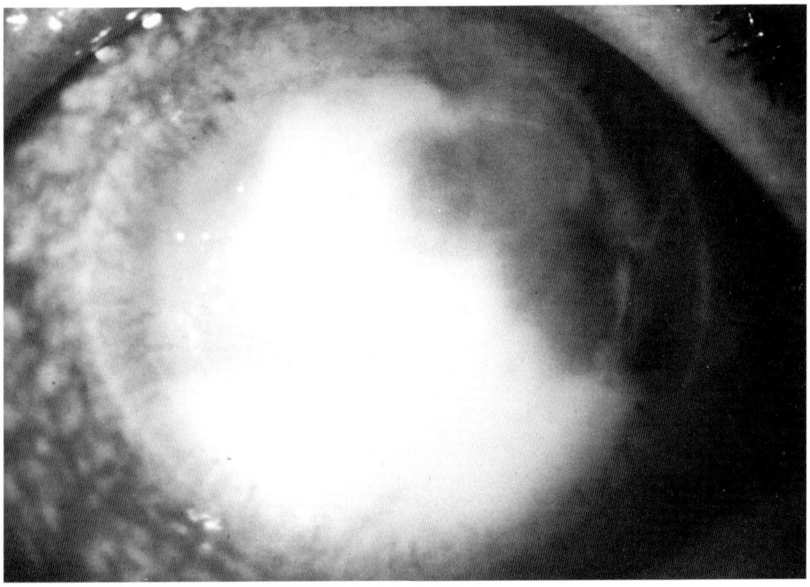

FIGURE 8-42 A corneal abscess caused by *Staphylococcus aureus* superimposed on herpes simplex stromal keratitis. Vascularization is beginning. The advanced stage of this infection may preclude satisfactory response to intensive antibiotics.

data on the efficacy of corticosteroids in bacterial keratitis are conflicting.[122] In experimental *Pseudomonas* keratitis, optimal topical fortified antibiotics and intensive corticosteroids did not adversely alter quantitative microbiological titers.[294] In experimental *S. aureus* keratitis and *Pseudomonas* keratitis, corticosteroids did not enhance replication if they were administered concurrently with an effective bactericidal antibiotic and if they were not instilled more frequently than the antibiotic.[285,286] In contrast, cultures from corneas after 3 days of gentamicin treatment had more bacteria in patients who received topical corticosteroids, and it took longer to eradicate the infection with this combined treatment.[285] In another study, combined corticosteroids and antibiotic did not improve the clinical course of the keratitis compared with antibiotic alone regardless of when the corticosteroids were started and in what strength.[295] Clinical experience with enhancement or recurrence of bacterial keratitis (especially *Pseudomonas*) with concomitant corticosteroids and antibiotics has been reported,[296,297] but severe inflammation alone may damage the eye. In patients with *Pseudomonas* keratitis that is effectively treated, there may be a sudden recrudescence of inflammation about 2 weeks after the initial inflammation. This

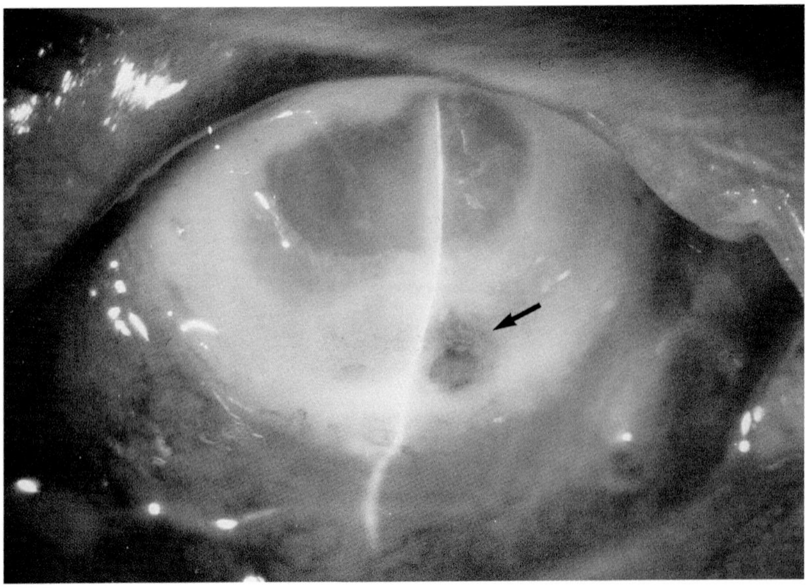

FIGURE 8-43 A corneal ring abscess caused by β-hemolytic *Streptococcus* in a patient with severe keratitis sicca. The flat anterior chamber and the brown pigment on the cornea (arrow) indicate a corneal perforation.

appears to be immunogenic and the addition of corticosteroids to antibiotics is valuable.

Antecedent use of corticosteroids may mask stromal and intraocular inflammation to the extent that bacterial invasion may not be recognized. Prior use also establishes the potential for resurgence of stromal inflammation and necrosis after withdrawal of corticosteroids during the initial management of the infection. If the infiltrate is deep or the cornea is thin, corticosteroids may also predispose to corneal perforation.

Corticosteroids may have a limited role in microbial keratitis, although their safety and efficacy in all forms of microbial keratitis have not been established.[4,122,129,298,299] Corticosteroids should not be used in the initial therapy for suspected microbial keratitis until there is adequate assurance of antimicrobial control of the responsible organism, except in patients who are already receiving corticosteroids. Topical corticosteroids should be considered in cases of stromal necrosis despite apparent control of replicating organisms; they may be helpful in reducing the harmful destructive components of the host inflammatory response, particularly in infections caused by gram-negative bacilli. Any corticosteroid use requires prior specific antibiotic coverage, knowledge of other immunologic abnormalities in the patient, ability to evaluate the patient, and adequate facilities to manage potential complications. Topical corticosteroids may be administered in low concentrations for 1 or 2 days on a trial basis to test for adverse effects, and then increased as necessary. Short-acting periocular corticosteroids may enhance the effect. Longer-acting periocular corticosteroids should be avoided; oral corticosteroids should also be avoided unless given preoperatively to reduce inflammation in cases requiring penetrating keratoplasty. Nonsteroidal anti-inflammatory drugs are probably not effective in bacterial keratitis.

Cryosurgery has shown bactericidal effects in an experimental animal model, but is too toxic for general use.[300] Nevertheless, it may have limited application in specific cases, such as localized peripheral corneal ulcers or uncontrolled *Pseudomonas* keratitis with scleral involvement.[288,301]

Medical grade cyanoacrylate tissue glue is useful for repair in progressive corneal necrosis, in thin descemetoceles, or perforated corneal ulcers. The glue may also have an inhibitory effect on bacteria.[289] It is toxic to the endothelium and lens, and should be used only in small perforations. It can quickly restore anterior segment integrity, thereby precluding the need for surgery altogether or at least until a later date, when the eye is less inflamed. Stromal ulcers must be debrided and dried before the glue is applied. Use of intracameral air or a viscoelastic substance facilitates adhesion of the glue in perforations. A bandage soft contact lens is placed over the glue to prevent irritation and to protect the glue from blinking of the eyelids.

A patch graft is an alternative to glue for a small perforation, but should be considered only after adequate antibiotic therapy has been given; otherwise the bacteria may invade and destroy the graft. Conjunctival flaps may be used in peripheral ulcers to promote healing, but are rarely indicated in central ulcers, except when associated factors prevent healing.[302] A conjunctival flap should not be placed over actively infected necrotic tissue because the flap will necrose; the corneal bed for the flap should be debrided until viable tissue is reached. If there is a large perforation, a small perforation with continued active microbial growth, an edematous necrotic cornea, or progressive suppuration despite optimal antibiotic therapy, penetrating keratoplasty may be indicated.[303,304] Penetrating keratoplasty is required in about 10 percent of patients with corneal ulcers, and is more frequently required with *S. pneumoniae,* staphylococcal species, *P. aeruginosa, Moraxella,* and β-hemolytic streptococci.[8] Penetrating keratoplasty may have a role in the more aggressive subacute treatment of *Pseudomonas* corneal ulcers or in the treatment of extensive scleral involvement.[305,306] The objectives of penetrating keratoplasty in bacterial keratitis are to eliminate infection, restore the integrity of the cornea, and preserve and/or restore vision. Decisions are based on the responsible organism (i.e., the potential for medical response) and also on the risk of subsequent endophthalmitis. Additional considerations are the previous status of the cornea (e.g., herpes simplex viral keratitis), the severity of the stromal inflammation and/or perforation (location and size of the required penetrating graft), and the status of intraocular structures. If penetrating keratoplasty is done for an infected corneal perforation, the graft has a better chance of remaining clear if temporary measures (such as glue, soft contact lens, or lamellar keratoplasty) are taken, and surgery is delayed until the eye is quiet.[303,307] In some ulcers, there is so much stromal necrosis that corneal vascularization is common. Some surgeons believe that penetrating keratoplasty should be done after the organisms are dead but before vascularization becomes severe.

When preparing for penetrating keratoplasty, it is ideal to try to sterilize the cornea and reduce inflammation to a minimum.[308] Intensive antibiotics should be used immediately before surgery. In general, even with a perforation, it is desirable to treat with antibiotics for 24 hours before surgery. Systemic corticosteroids (1 mg/kg) are given for at least 24 hours before surgery and for at least

1 week after surgery to reduce perioperative inflammation. A scleral support ring is essential. Care is taken during suturing of the ring to avoid pressure on the eye. It is desirable to re-form the anterior chamber with air or a viscoelastic substance before trephination. Viscoelastics are also useful for separating inflamed tissues and re-forming the eye at the end of the operation. An attempt can be made to close a small perforation with tissue adhesive at the beginning of the case in order to maintain the anterior chamber. The graft should encompass the entire area of visible infection. All necrotic tissue should be excised, even if it extends into the sclera. A healthy recipient tissue edge is essential to decrease the occurrence of postoperative suture erosion and wound dehiscence. A vacuum trephine, such as the Barron radial vacuum trephine, is helpful when the eye is soft.[309] If a large graft is required, adequate trephine sizes may not be available and a freehand cut may be necessary. If the cornea is perforated, the recipient cornea can be removed by inserting corneal scissors through the perforation, cutting radially to the trephine cut, and cutting circumferentially along the trephine cut. This method is safer than entering the anterior chamber with a blade through the trephine cut. It is desirable to try to retain the lens, if possible. Adequate iridectomies are mandatory, and an oversized graft helps to keep the anterior chamber angle open. Interrupted sutures are indicated because of the likelihood of differential healing of the wound. The sutures should be long enough to reach healthy recipient tissue; otherwise they will cheesewire through. The removed recipient cornea should be submitted for histopathologic examination to assess adequate surgical margins, and should be cultured to confirm the organism and to determine viability and sensitivity as guides to postoperative antimicrobial therapy. Intravenous antibiotics are indicated if there is suspicion of intraocular spread. Unfortunately, less than one-half of the patients who have corneal transplantation in the presence of a corneal infection gain improvement in visual acuity, compared with their presenting vision.[4]

BACTERIAL INTERSTITIAL KERATITIS

Interstitial keratitis is a nonsuppurative inflammation of the corneal stroma usually associated with a systemic disease. It may be diffuse or localized to various sectors of the central or peripheral cornea. On slit lamp examination, the cornea has a ground-glass appearance, with single or multiple areas of dense white stromal necrosis that may clear later, but leave stromal scars and corneal thinning. There is deep corneal vascularization from the anterior ciliary arteries, as well as superficial corneal vascularization from the conjunctival vessels. The inflammatory conditions may be caused by direct invasion of the cornea by organisms, but more often represent an immune response as an antigen-antibody-complement mediated disease or a delayed hypersensitivity reaction.

Interstitial keratitis may be caused by a number of conditions, including bacterial, viral, or protozoan infections as well as a number of systemic vasculitides and diseases of unknown etiology.[310] The bacterial causes considered here are those associated with *Treponema pallidum* (congenital and acquired syphilis), *Mycobacterium tuberculosis* (tuberculosis), *Mycobacterium leprae* (leprosy), and *Borrelia burgdorferi* (Lyme disease).

Syphilis

Treponema pallidum is a thin, delicate, helical-shaped spirochete with a unique motility that propels it quickly through tissues (e.g., placenta) and throughout the body. The cytoplasm is surrounded by a membrane, an inner micropeptide layer, and a mucoid slime layer. The organism is too small to be viewed by ordinary light microscopy, but can be observed by dark-field illumination, negative-staining, or phase-contrast microscopy.

There has been an increase in both acquired and congenital syphilis in the United States in recent years coinciding with the acquired immunodeficiency syndrome pandemic. Patients with acquired immunodeficiency syndrome have an increased risk of acquiring syphilis and vice versa. Syphilis is primarily a sexually transmitted disease but it can be spread by transfusion of fresh blood or accidental contact with an infected lesion.[311]

Congenital Syphilis

Congenital syphilis results from passage of *T. pallidum* to the fetus in utero. This may result in stillbirth. Children may be asymptomatic at birth but within a few months manifest infection with rhinitis, pneumonia, hepatosplenomegaly, osteochondritis, periostitis, nephritis, failure to thrive, and a vesicular or papulosquamous rash. Interstitial keratitis and other ocular manifestations of congenital syphilis usually appear after 2 years of age and are not a manifestation of active infection but rather an inflammatory response to previously present spirochetes.[312] In congenital interstitial keratitis, both corneas are usually involved within weeks of each other. The keratitis can be divided into three stages: progressive, florid, and retrogressive. In the progressive stage, there is photophobia, tearing, pain, blepharospasm, and perilimbal hyperemia. Nummular lesions appear in the anterior corneal stroma with keratic precipitates or sectorial interstitial stromal inflammation. Corneal edema, inflamma-

FIGURE 8-44 (A) Late syphilitic interstitial keratitis with corneal scarring, anterior corneal pigment, deep stromal vascularization (ghost vessels), and linear retrocorneal hyaline ridges from posterior collagen layers. (B) Slit beam demonstrates the marked stromal haze in the posterior cornea.

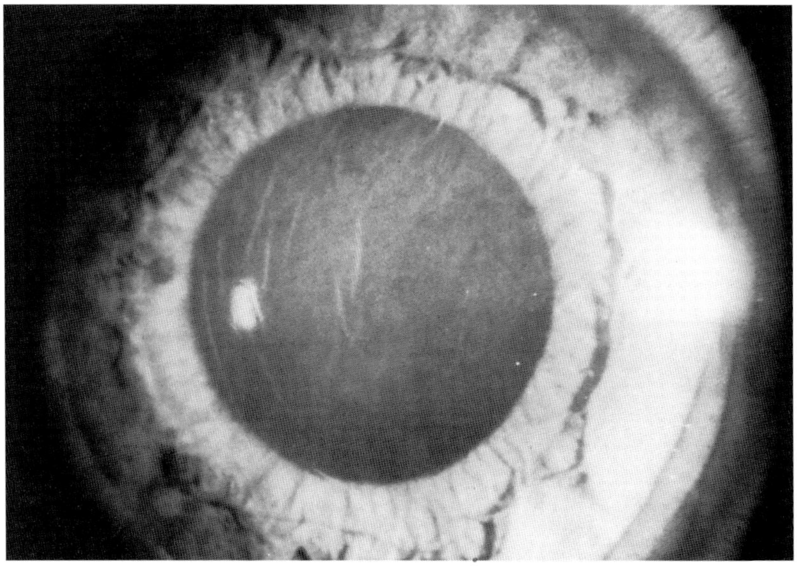

A

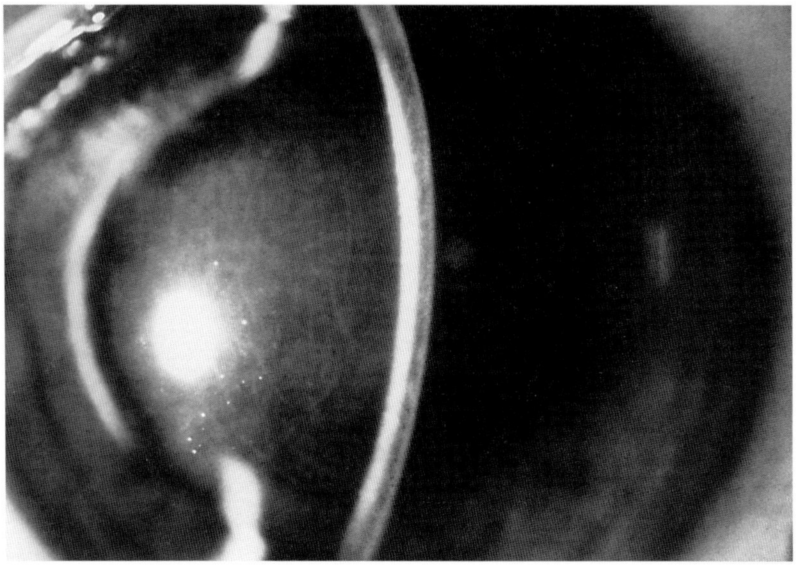

B

tion, vascularization, and iridocyclitis progress over months. In the florid stage, corneal vascularization flourishes and the cornea develops a pink color (salmon patch of Hutchinson). The retrogressive stage occurs over 1 to 2 years, with residual corneal scarring, thinning, and the appearance of ghost vessels (Figures 8-44 to 8-46). Later manifestations of congenital syphilis include osseous and dental abnormalities (saddle nose, palatal perforation, frontal bossing, sabre shins, mulberry molars, and Hutchinson teeth); 8th cranial nerve deafness; mental retardation and degenerative central nervous system disease (tabes dorsalis); and rhagades (circumoral radiating scars). Hutchinson's triad consists of interstitial keratitis, Hutchinson teeth, and deafness.

The histopathology of acute interstitial keratitis is a thinned edematous cornea that is diffusely infiltrated with lymphocytes in the middle and deeper layers. There is vascular inflammation and stromal necrosis, especially peripherally. With resolution, the edema and infiltration disappear, but ghost vessels persist. In chronic interstitial keratitis, there are changes in the deep corneal stroma, stromal thinning, and vascularization. There appears to be transformation of the endothelium by fibroblast-like cells that produce abnormal multilaminar base-

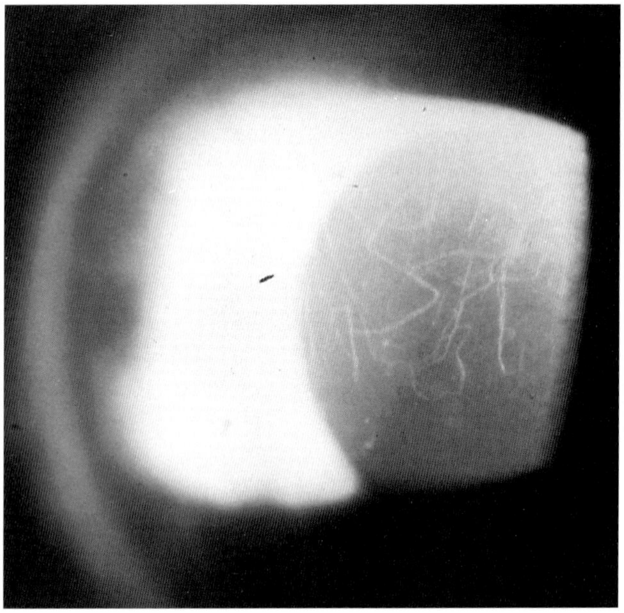

FIGURE 8-45 A patient with late syphilitic interstitial keratitis with corneal scarring and a myriad of ghost vessels coursing through the posterior corneal stroma.

ment membrane that is manifested by hyaline excrescences on Descemet's membrane with ridges that project into the anterior chamber.[313,314] Other anterior segment abnormalities include posterior synechiae, iris atrophy, iris papules, cataracts, glaucoma, episcleritis, and scleritis.

There is both a cellular and humoral response to *T. pallidum.* Cell-mediated immunity is the dominant mechanism in controlling treponemal infections. The humoral response consists of nonspecific antibodies (reagins) that react to cardiolipin (a substance that constitutes about 10 percent of treponemal lipids but is also present in mammalian tissues), and specific antibodies (immobilizing, agglutinating, or fluorescent treponemal) that react to specific components on treponemes (Table 8-13). Patients with congenital syphilis can become reinfected if exposed to *T. pallidum* during adulthood.

Patients with clinical signs of interstitial keratitis, especially in association with iris changes, chorioretinitis, optic atrophy, and central nervous system or cardiovascular disease, should have the fluorescent treponemal antibody absorption test (FTA-ABS) to confirm congenital syphilis. The Venereal Disease Research Laboratory test (VDRL) is positive only with active systemic disease.[315] The FTA-ABS, once positive, usually remains so for life, regardless

TABLE 8-13
Serologic Tests for Syphilis

Nonspecific
Venereal Disease Research Laboratory (VDRL) slide
Unheated serum reagin (USR)
Rapid plasma reagin (RPR) 18-mm Circle Card
Automated reagin test (ART)
Reagin screen test (RST)
Specific
Fluorescent treponemal antibody absorption (FTA-ABS)
Microhemmaglutination assay for antibodies to *T. pallidum* (MHA-TP)
Hemagglutination treponemal test for syphilis (HATTS)
Fluorescent treponemal antibody-absorption double-staining (FTA-ABS DS)

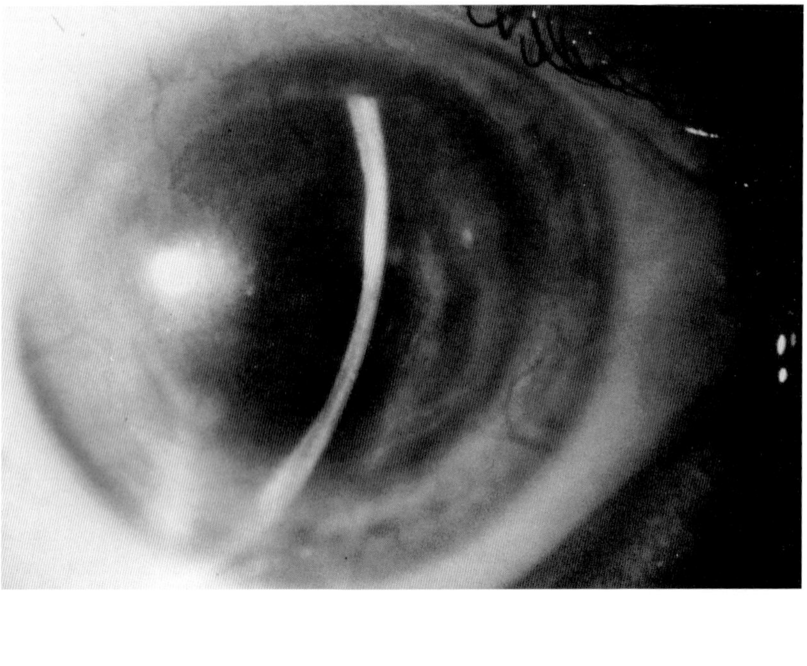

FIGURE 8-46 Slit beam illumination of a cornea with late syphilitic interstitial keratitis demonstrating the central corneal thinning along with the corneal scarring and extensive deep and superficial peripheral corneal vascularization.

of disease activity or treatment. With a positive FTA-ABS, cerebrospinal fluid examination is necessary to evaluate for central nervous system syphilis. Regardless of the results, these patients should be treated with penicillin, but the dose varies depending on whether the cerebrospinal fluid is normal or abnormal, and on the current guidelines from the Centers for Disease Control and Prevention.

Topical corticosteroids are the treatment for active interstitial keratitis; when given early, they are able to blunt the corneal damage. A topical cycloplegic agent is indicated in the presence of iritis. Systemic antisyphilitic treatment has no beneficial effect on the course of interstitial keratitis.[316] Residual corneal haze, scarring, thinning, astigmatism, and possible calcification can permanently reduce vision. The treatment of interstitial keratitis with penetrating keratoplasty has limitations because of the recurrence of iritis, potential wound problems related to thin recipient corneal tissue, the high prevalence of myopia, and associated retinopathy.[317] Systemic corticosteroids are routinely given preoperatively to patients with a history of syphilitic interstitial keratitis in an attempt to prevent exacerbation of iritis.

Acquired Syphilis

Acquired syphilis has three stages: primary, secondary, and tertiary. Primary syphilis manifests as a painless chancre that appears within 3 weeks of exposure on mucosal membranes at the site of inoculation and then resolves. Secondary syphilis can occur months to years later and has protean ocular manifestations, including iridocyclitis, retinochoroiditis, neuroretinitis, optic atrophy, and rarely, unilateral interstitial keratitis. Tertiary syphilis occurs when immune regulation falters and results in reactivation in certain targeted tissues. This stage may be divided into gummatous syphilis, cardiovascular syphilis, and neurosyphilis. Ocular findings include iridocyclitis, retinochoroiditis, optic atrophy, Argyll Robertson pupil (miotic pupil that reacts to accommodation, but poorly to light), and rarely, unilateral interstitial keratitis.

The clinical course of interstitial keratitis in acquired syphilis is usually seen approximately 10 years after the initial infection. It is similar to the keratitis associated with congenital syphilis except it is more commonly unilateral, has a female preponderance, is more likely to have a sectorial involvement, and is usually not accompanied by as much inflammation. Patients with concomitant human immunodeficiency virus infection have a high incidence of neurosyphilis, with a high relapse rate and frequent neurologic complications.[318] Patients should have cerebrospinal fluid evaluation for neurosyphilis and be treated depending on the results. Acquired syphilitic interstitial keratitis requires treatment with topical corticosteroids.

Tuberculosis

Interstitial keratitis associated with tuberculosis is uncommon. As in syphilitic interstitial keratitis, the keratitis appears to be an immune response to the tubercle bacillus rather than an active infection[311]; patients seldom have active pulmonary tuberculosis.[319,320] *Mycobacterium tuberculosis* has large quantities of waxes and lipids in the cell wall, which are probably responsible for sensitizing the patient and provoking the immune corneal reaction. The clinical presentation is an acute inflammation that is more frequently unilateral and involves peripheral sectorial portions of the cornea. The inflammation more frequently involves the superficial layers of the cornea rather than the deep layers characteristically involved in syphilis. The stromal reaction consists of edema, dense inflammatory infiltrates (like nodular abscesses), and sectorial vascularization of the peripheral anterior cornea. The clinical course can be prolonged, with residual dense corneal scarring (Figures 8-47 and 8-48). The vessels may be large on the surface and at midstroma. The diagnosis is made in the appropriate clinical setting of systemic tuberculosis with a positive tuberculin skin test and a negative FTA-ABS.

Treatment is with topical corticosteroids. Systemic treatment with antituberculous medications is indicated, although it has no effect on the interstitial keratitis.

Leprosy

Leprosy is caused by *Mycobacterium leprae,* an obligate intracellular parasite with an affinity for tissue macrophages associated with skin, nerves, and the lymphoreticular system.[321-324] Humans are the only significant infectious reservoir, with the portal of entry at the mucous membrane of the respiratory tract or the skin. Personal contact is important in spreading the disease, which has a high prevalence in certain areas of Africa, the Middle East, and southeast Asia. In the United States, however, the contact is usually not identified.

There are four basic forms of leprosy based on the patient's immune response: indeterminate, lepromatous, tuberculoid, and intermediate. If resistance is complete, the indeterminate short-lived form results, which either spontaneously resolves or evolves into one of the other three forms. The most severe form of the disease is the lepromatous form, which appears to result from a defect in cell-mediated immunity. The bacillus multiplies both extracellularly and intracellularly, especially within histiocytic cells. Patients with the lepromatous form have systemic involvement with multiple diffuse dermal lesions and neural lesions. In the tuberculoid form, a typical granulomatous reaction occurs in discrete areas of the dermis,

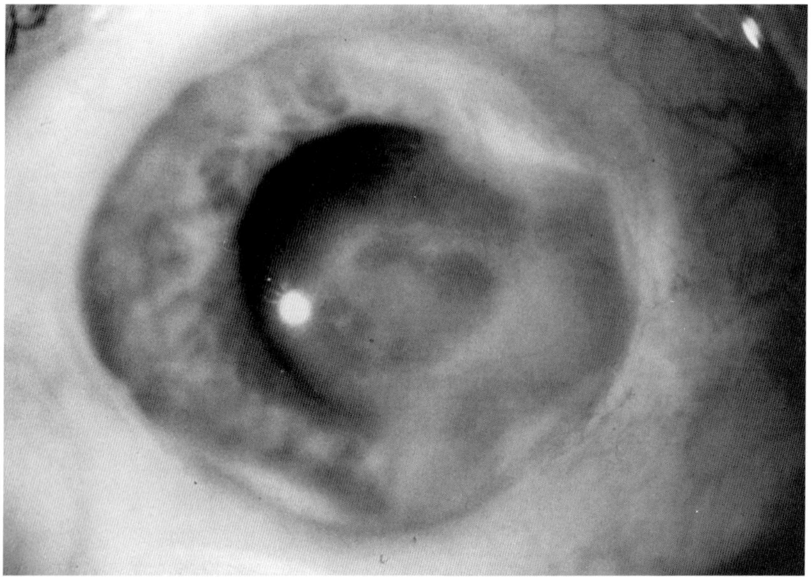

FIGURE 8-47 Late tuberculous interstitial keratitis with a peripheral sectorial scar involving the superficial and midstromal area of the cornea. Vascularization and linear lipid deposition are confined to the anterior cornea.

with sparse multiplication of the bacilli. Neural involvement is prominent, with sensory loss. Systemic or internal involvement is uncommon. The intermediate form has skin lesions of the tuberculoid form, but histologically, the disease is similar to the lepromatous form. Patients with the intermediate form have a more stable but variable expression of the infection, with numerous widespread dermal lesions.

The corneal findings in leprosy vary with the form of the disease. Exposure keratitis is associated with 7th cranial nerve involvement in tuberculoid leprosy. A concurrent neurotrophic keratitis from 5th cranial nerve involvement may aggravate this condition. Superficial punctate keratitis or avascular keratitis is predominantly seen in the superotemporal quadrant arising from miliary lepromas of lymphocytes and macrophages, and from invasion with *M. leprae.* A pannus may extend over the keratitis resulting in the classic corneal leproma. Thickened corneal nerves from *M. leprae* and the surrounding intraneural granulomatous reaction can produce beading of the corneal nerves.

The interstitial keratitis of leprosy is poorly understood and may take various forms. Superotemporal deep interstitial keratitis with ghost vessels may be a sequela to ciliary body involvement from either bacterial invasion or

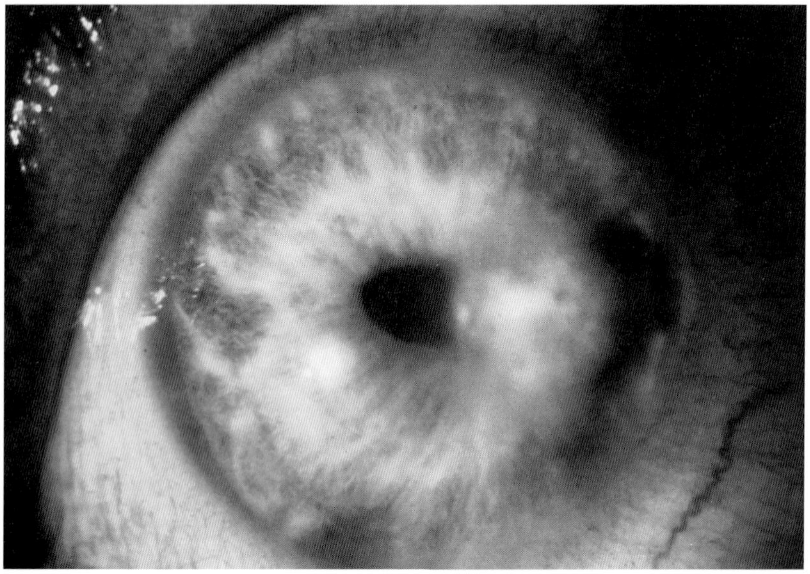

FIGURE 8-48 Late tuberculous interstitial keratitis with a peripheral sectorial stromal scar. There was a previous localized corneal perforation at the site of inflammation, leaving an irregular pupil and synechiae to the posterior aspect of the scar.

immunologic reaction. A more superficial stromal keratitis associated with vascular invasion and necrosis probably represents direct bacterial invasion and may obscure the visual axis.

Other ocular involvement includes scleritis, episcleritis, and uveal involvement, with iris pearls, acute granulomatous iridocyclitis, or chronic iridocyclitis with iris atrophy. Loss of eyebrows and eyelashes also occurs.

The diagnosis of leprosy will not be made unless it is entertained. Avascular keratitis in the superotemporal quadrant of the cornea is characteristic. The distinctive iris pearls and beaded corneal nerves are almost pathognomonic. Episcleritis, scleritis, and acute granulomatous uveitis are nonspecific except in the presence of skin or nerve lesions. The diagnosis is confirmed by skin biopsy revealing the granulomatous response and acid-fast bacilli. Smears from suspicious nasal or skin lesions can also confirm the diagnosis. *M. leprae* cannot be cultured on laboratory media.

Treatment of leprosy is with long-term systemic dapsone, rifampin, and clofazimine. The interstitial keratitis and uveitis are treated with topical corticosteroids and cycloplegic agents; rifampin ophthalmic ointment is used for the keratitis seen in the lepromatous form. Surgical therapy may be required for entropion, exposure keratitis, or to create an optical iridectomy.

Lyme Disease

Lyme disease (so named in 1975 because of an unusual clustering of children with inflammatory arthropathy in Lyme, CT) is a multisystemic disorder with prominent dermatologic, neurologic, cardiac, rheumatologic, and some ophthalmic manifestations.[325] The infectious agent, *Borrelia burgdorferi,* is a spirochete transmitted through the bite of its vector, the *Ixodes* tick. The pathognomonic criterion for the diagnosis of Lyme disease is the rash (erythema migrans), which occurs 4 to 20 days after the tick bite. The rash may not appear, however, in one-half of the patients. The incidence is increasing, especially in the Northeast, Midwest, and Northwest, corresponding to the distribution of the *Ixodes* tick.[326]

There are three stages of Lyme disease: infection, dissemination, and later immunologic reactions. There are wide variations in the signs during each stage. In the first stage, there may be flu-like symptoms, with fever, headache, stiff neck, malaise, nausea, and lymphadenopathy. In the second stage, the spirochete disseminates, causing multiple skin lesions, cardiac symptoms (arrhythmias, myocarditis), arthralgia, and neurologic symptoms (encephalitis, meningitis with papilledema, cranial neuritis, bilateral facial palsy, and painful radiculoneuritis). The third stage is characterized by immunologic symptoms, including dermatologic changes (acrodermatitis chronica atrophicans), arthralgia, and neurologic sequelae (encephalomyelitis, demyelination, dementia).

Ophthalmic manifestations can occur in all three stages. In the first stage, the only ocular manifestations are a nonspecific conjunctivitis and photophobia, which resolve. In the second stage, neuro-ophthalmic manifestations occur, including 7th cranial nerve and other cranial nerve palsies, causing diplopia, blurred vision, and headache. During the late second stage and third stage, more severe ocular manifestations occur, including keratitis, episcleritis, iritis, pars planitis, vitritis, choroiditis, panuveitis, retinal vasculitis, exudative retinal detachment, and branch retinal artery occlusion.[326] The main corneal involvement occurs in the third stage and consists of stromal keratitis and episcleritis related to an immune response.[327–330] The stromal keratitis is characterized by the appearance of multiple superficial and deep hazy corneal infiltrates (nummular or interstitial) that may respond to topical corticosteroids. Associated stromal vessels, keratic precipitates, and sectorial stromal edema have also been described.

B. burgdorferi has been isolated from blood, synovial fluid, spinal fluid, retina and vitreous, brain, and skin of experimental animals and patients with Lyme disease. The organism is notoriously difficult to culture from patients, and serologic tests are usually used in the diagnosis of the corneal disease. The enzyme-linked immunoabsorbent assay (ELISA) and indirect immunofluorescent antibody (IFA) are the most commonly used tests; both measure IgM and IgG in the patient's serum. Serologic testing is not well standardized and results vary. There are several other diagnostic procedures under investigation.[331]

When recognized during the first stage, Lyme disease is treated with oral tetracycline; erythromycin or penicillin is an alternative. For stage 2 disease with significant manifestations, ceftriaxone is recommended. The use of corticosteroids in Lyme disease is controversial, but certain stage 3 manifestations, such as keratitis, arthritis, and neurologic sequelae, may respond.[326,327,329,330] The ocular disease is probably mediated either by persistence of antigen with antigen-antibody and complement reaction, by a delayed hypersensitivity reaction, or by a vasculitis, all of which have been recognized in other components of this disease.

Note Added in Proof

Since this chapter was written, additional literature has been published in several controversial areas. This literature is important in advancing the clinical art and science, in providing better patient care, and in accomplishing cost containment, especially in this era of managed care.

The author recognizes that there remains a controversy about the need for culturing all corneal ulcers, about the use of fortified topical antibiotics versus monotherapy with the fluoroquinolones, and about the need to be vigilant for the changing resistance pattern of microbes. This chapter provides an overall approach to the management of patients with bacterial keratitis; newer data must be continually assimilated into our management protocols in order to offer the patient and the public the most appropriate and cost-effective evaluation and therapeutic alternatives. TJL/August 22, 1997

REFERENCES

1. Erie JC, Nevitt MP, Hodge DO, Ballard DJ: Incidence of ulcerative keratitis in a defined population from 1950 through 1988. Arch Ophthalmol 111:1665, 1993
2. Liesegang TJ, Forster RF: Spectrum of microbial keratitis in South Florida. Am J Ophthalmol 90:38, 1980
3. Koidou-Tsiligianni A, Alfonso E, Forster RK: Ulcerative keratitis associated with contact lens wear. Am J Ophthalmol 108:64, 1989
4. Gudmundsson OG, Ormerod LD, Kenyon KR, et al: Factors influencing predilection and outcome of bacterial keratitis. Cornea 8:115, 1989
5. Schein OD, Ormerod LD, Barraquer E, et al: Microbiology of contact-lens related keratitis. Cornea 8:281, 1989
6. Asbell P, Stenson LS: Ulcerative keratitis: survey of 30 years' laboratory experience. Arch Ophthalmol 100:77, 1982
7. Cohen EJ, Laibson PR, Arentsen JJ, et al: Corneal ulcers associated with cosmetic extended wear soft contact lenses. Ophthalmology 94:109, 1987
8. Ormerod LD, Hertzmark E, Gomez DS, et al: Epidemiology of microbial keratitis in southern California. Ophthalmology 94:1322, 1987
9. Upadhyay MP, Karmacharya PCD, Koirala S, et al: Epidemiologic characteristics, predisposing factors, and etiologic diagnosis of corneal ulceration in Nepal. Am J Ophthalmol 111:92, 1991
10. Ormerod LD: Causation and management of microbial keratitis in subtropical Africa. Ophthalmology 94:1662, 1987
11. Mahajan VM: Ulcerative keratitis: an analysis of laboratory data in 674 cases. J Ocul Ther Surg 4:138, 1985
12. Stein RM, Clinch TE, Cohen EJ, et al: Infected vs sterile corneal infiltrates in contact lens wearers. Am J Ophthalmol 105:632, 1988
13. Jones DB: Strategy for the initial management of suspected microbial keratitis. p. 86. In New Orleans Academy of Ophthalmology. Symposium on Medical and Surgical Diseases of the Cornea. CV Mosby, St. Louis, 1980
14. Coster DJ, Wilhelmus K, Peacock J, Jones BR: Suppurative keratitis in London. p. 395. In Trevor-Roper T (ed): European Society of Ophthalmology. The Cornea in Health and Disease. Academic Press, San Diego, 1981
15. Davis SD: *Pseudomonas*. p. II:54. In Tasman W, Jaeger EA (eds): Duane's Foundations of Clinical Ophthalmology. JB Lippincott, Philadelphia, 1990
16. Ostler HB, Okumoto M, Wilkey C: The changing pattern of the etiology of central bacterial corneal (hypopyon) ulcer. Trans Pac Coast Otoophthalmol Soc 57:235, 1976
17. Musch DC, Sugar A, Meyer RF: Demographic and predisposing factors in corneal ulceration. Arch Ophthalmol 101:1545,1983
18. Hassman G, Sugar J: Pseudomonas corneal ulcer with extended-wear soft contact lenses for myopia. Arch Ophthalmol 101:1549, 1983
19. Weissman BA, Mondino BJ, Pettit TH, Hofbauer JD: Corneal ulcers associated with extended-wear soft contact lenses. Am J Ophthalmol 97:476, 1984
20. Galentine PG, Cohen EJ, Laibson PR, et al: Corneal ulcers associated with contact lens wear. Arch Ophthamol 102:891,1984
21. Adams CP, Cohen EJ, Laibson PR, et al: Corneal ulcers in patients with cosmetic extended-wear contact lenses. Am J Ophthalmol 96:705, 1983
22. Lemp MA, Blackman HJ, Wilson LA, Leveille AS: Gram-negative corneal ulcers in elderly aphakic eyes with extended-wear lenses. Ophthalmology 90:60, 1984
23. Ormerod LD, Gomez DS, Murphree AL, et al: Microbial keratitis in children. Ophthalmology 93:449, 1986
24. Cruz DA, Sabir SM, Capo H, Alfonso EC: Microbial keratitis in childhood. Ophthalmology 100:192, 1993
25. Stern GA: Moraxella corneal ulcers: poor response to medical treatment. Ann Ophthalmol 14:295, 1982
26. Okumoto M: Other gram-negative aerobic rods. p. II:53. In Tasman W, Jaeger EA (eds): Duane's Foundations of Clinical Ophthalmology. JB Lippincott, Philadelphia, 1990
27. Cobo LM, Coster DJ, Peacock J: *Moraxella* keratitis. p. 409. In Trevor-Roper T (ed): European Society of Ophthalmology. The Cornea in Health and Disease. Academic Press, San Diego, 1981
28. Jones DB, Robinson NM: Anaerobic ocular infections. Trans Am Acad Ophthalmol Otolaryngol 83:390, 1977
29. Okumoto M: Enterobacteriaceae. p. II:52. In Tasman W, Jaeger EA (eds): Duane's Foundations of Clinical Ophthalmology. JB Lippincott, Philadelphia, 1990
30. Lass JF, Haaf J, Foster CS, Belcher C: Visual outcome in eight cases of *Serratia marcescens* keratitis. Am J Ophthalmol 92:384, 1981
31. Liesegang TJ, Jones DB, Robinson NM: *Azotobacter* keratitis. Arch Ophthalmol 99:1587, 1981
32. Chandler JW: Gram-negative cocci. p. II:50. In Tasman W, Jaeger EA (eds): Duane's Foundations of Clinical Ophthalmology. JB Lippincott, Philadelphia, 1990
33. Okumoto M: Gram-positive aerobic rods. p. II:51. In Tasman W, Jaeger EA (eds): Duane's Foundations of Clinical Ophthalmology. JB Lippincott, Philadelphia, 1990
34. O'Day DM, Ho PC, Andrews JS, et al: Mechanism of tissue destruction in ocular *Bacillus cereus* infections. p. 403.

In Trevor-Roper T (ed): European Society of Ophthalmology. The Cornea in Health and Disease. Academic Press, San Diego, 1981
35. Zaidman GW, Coudron P, Piros J: *Listeria monocytogenes* keratitis. Am J Ophthalmol 109:334, 1990
36. Osato MS, Jones DB: Anaerobic ocular infections. p. II:57. In Tasman W, Jaeger EA (eds): Duane's Foundations of Clinical Ophthalmology. JB Lippincott, Philadelphia, 1990
37. Perry LD, Brinser JF, Kolodner H: Anaerobic corneal ulcers. Ophthalmology 89:636, 1982
38. Liesegang TJ: Anaerobic corneal ulcers [discussion]. Ophthalmology 89:641, 1982
39. Stern GA, Hodes BL, Stock EL: *Clostridium perfringens* corneal ulcer. Arch Ophthalmol 97:661, 1979
40. Bullington RH, Lanier JD, Font RL: Nontuberculous mycobacterial keratitis: report of two cases and review of the literature. Arch Ophthalmol 110:519, 1992
41. Gangadharam PRJ, Lanier JD, Jones DB: Keratitis due to *Mycobacterium chelonei.* Tubercle 59:55, 1978
42. Turner L: Atypical mycobacterial infections in ophthalmology. Trans Am Ophthalmol Soc 68:667, 1970
43. Lazar M, Nemet P, Bracha R, Campus A: *Mycobacterium fortuitum* keratitis. Am J Ophthalmol 78:530, 1974
44. Newman PE, Goodman RA, Waring GO III, et al: A cluster of cases of *Mycobacterium chelonei* keratitis associated with outpatient office procedures. Am J Ophthalmol 97:344, 1984
45. Zimmerman LE, Turner L, McTigue JW: *Mycobacterium fortuitum* infection of the cornea. Arch Ophthalmol 82:596, 1969
46. Robin JB, Beatty RF, Dunn S, et al: *Mycobacterium chelonei* keratitis after radial keratotomy. Am J Ophthalmol 102:72, 1986
47. Hirst LW, Harrison GK, Merz WG, Stark WJ: *Nocardia asteroides* keratitis. Br J Ophthalmol 63:449, 1979
48. Perry HD, Nauheim JS, Donnenfeld ED: *Nocardia asteroides* keratitis presenting as a persistent epithelial defect. Cornea 8:41, 1989
49. Mondino BJ: Host defense against bacterial and fungal disease. p. II:45. In Tasman W, Jaeger EA (eds): Duane's Foundations of Clinical Ophthalmology. JB Lippincott, Philadelphia, 1990
50. Schein OD, Wasson PJ, Boruchoff SA, Kenyon KR: Microbial keratitis associated with contaminated ocular medications. Am J Ophthalmol 105:361, 1988
51. Aswad MI, Barza M, Baum J: Effect of lid closure on contact lens-associated *Pseudomonas* keratitis. Arch Ophthalmol 107:1667, 1989
52. Holden BA, Sweeney DR, Vannar A, et al: Effects of long-term extended contact lens wear on the human cornea. Invest Ophthalmol Vis Sci 26:1489, 1985
53. Duran JA, Refojo MF, Gipson IK, et al: *Pseudomonas* attachment to new hydrogel contact lenses. Arch Ophthalmol 105:106, 1987
54. Fowler SA, Allansmith MR: Evaluation of soft contact lens coatings. Arch Ophthalmol 98:95, 1980
55. Stern GA, Zam ZS: The pathogenesis of contact lens-associated *Pseudomonas aeruginosa* corneal ulceration I: the effect of contact lens coatings on adherence of *Pseudomonas aeruginosa* to soft contact lenses. Cornea 5:41, 1986
56. Klotz SA, Misra RP, Butrus SI: Contact lens wear enhances adherence of *Pseudomonas aeruginosa* and binding of lectins to the cornea. Cornea 9:266, 1990
57. Butrus SI, Klotz SA: Contact lens deposits increase the adhesion of *Pseudomonas aeruginosa.* Curr Eye Res 9:717, 1990
58. Fleiszig SMJ, Efron N, Pier GB: Extended contact lens wear enhances *Pseudomonas aeruginosa* adherence to human corneal epithelium. Invest Ophthalmol Vis Sci 33:2908, 1992
59. Miller MJ, Wilson LA, Ahearn DG: Adherence of *Pseudomonas aeruginosa* to rigid gas-permeable contact lenses. Arch Ophthalmol 109:1447, 1991
60. Chalupa E, Swarbrick HA, Holden BA, Sjöstrand J: Severe corneal infections associated with contact lens wear. Ophthalmology 94:17, 1987
61. Ormerod LD, Smith RE: Contact lens-associated microbial keratitis. Arch Ophthalmol 104:79, 1986
62. Poggio EC, Glynn RJ, Schein OD, et al: The incidence of ulcerative keratitis among users of daily-wear and extended wear soft contact lenses. N Engl J Med 321:779, 1989
63. Wilhelmus KR: Review of clinical experience with microbial keratitis associated with contact lenses. CLAO J 13:211, 1987
64. Palmer ML, Hyndiuk RA: Contact lens-related infectious keratitis. Int Ophthalmol Clin 33:23, 1993
65. Dart JKG: Predisposing factors in microbial keratitis: the significance of contact lens wear. Br J Ophthalmol 72:926, 1988
65. Dart JKG, Stapleton F, Minassian D: Contact lenses and other risk factors in microbial keratitis. Lancet 338:650, 1991
67. Buehler PO, Schein OD, Stamler JF, et al: The increased risk of ulcerative keratitis among disposable soft contact lens users. Arch Ophthalmol 110:1555, 1992
68. Matthews TD, Frazer DG, Minassian DC, et al: Risks of keratitis and patterns of use with disposable contact lenses. Arch Ophthalmol 110:1559, 1992
69. Laibson PR, Cohen EJ, Rajpal RK: Corneal ulcers related to contact lenses. CLAO J 19:73, 1993
70. Schein OD, Glynn RJ, Poggio EC, et al: The relative risk of ulcerative keratitis among users of daily wear and extended wear soft contact lenses. N Engl J Med 321:773, 1989
71. Glynn RJ, Schein OD, Seddon JM, et al: The incidence of ulcerative keratitis among aphakic contact lens wearers in New England. Arch Ophthalmol 109:104, 1991
72. Dunn JO, Mondino BJ, Weissman BA, et al: Corneal ulcers associated with disposable hydrogel contact lenses. Am J Ophthalmol 108:113, 1989
73. Donzis PB, Mondino BJ, Weissman BA, et al: Microbial contamination of contact lens care systems. Am J Ophthalmol 104:325, 1987
74. Kanpolat A, Kalayci D, Arman D, Duruk K: Contamination of contact lens care systems. CLAO J 18:105, 1992

75. Bowden FW, Cohen EJ, Arentsen JJ, Laibson PR: Patterns of lens care practices and lens product contamination in contact lens associated microbial keratitis. CLAO J 15:49, 1989
76. Maguen E, Tsai JC, Martinez M, et al: A retrospective study of disposable extended-wear lenses in 100 patients. Ophthalmology 98:1685, 1991
77. Tuberville AW, Wood TO: Corneal ulcers in corneal transplants. Curr Eye Res 8:479, 1981
78. Bates AK, Kirkness CM, Ficker A, et al: Microbial keratitis after penetrating keratoplasty. Eye 4:74, 1990
79. Varley GA, Meisler DM: Complications of penetrating keratoplasty: graft infections. Refract Corneal Surg 7:62, 1991
80. Leahey AB, Avery RL, Gottsch JD, et al: Suture abscesses after penetrating keratoplasty. Cornea 12:489, 1993
81. Tavakkoli H, Sugar J: Microbial keratitis following penetrating keratoplasty. Ophthalmic Surg 25:356, 1994
82. Badenoch PR, Aggarwal RK, Coster DJ: *Clostridium perfringens* keratitis after penetrating keratoplasty. Aust N Z J Ophthalmol 23:245, 1995
83. Al-Hazzaa SAF, Tabbara KF: Bacterial keratitis after penetrating keratoplasty. Ophthalmology 95:1504, 1988
84. Driebe WT, Stern GA: Microbial keratitis following corneal transplantation. Cornea 2:41, 1983
85. Harris DJ, Stulting RD, Waring GO, Wilson LA: Late bacterial and fungal keratitis after corneal transplantation. Ophthalmology 95:1450, 1988
86. Fong LP, Ormerod LD, Kenyon KR, Foster CS: Microbial keratitis complicating penetrating keratoplasty. Ophthalmology 95:1269, 1988
87. Snyder RW, Hyndiuk RA: Mechanisms of bacterial invasion of the cornea. p. II:44. In Tasman W, Jaeger EA (eds): Duane's Foundations of Clinical Ophthalmology. JB Lippincott, Philadelphia, 1990
88. Reichert R, Stern GA: Quantitative adherence of bacteria to human corneal epithelial cells. Arch Ophthalmol 102:1394, 1984
89. Panjwani N, Clark B, Cohen M, et al: Differential binding of *P. aeruginosa* and *S. aureus* to corneal epithelium in culture. Invest Ophthalmol Vis Sci 31:696, 1990
90. Stern GA: Bacterial adherence. p. II:42. In Tasman W, Jaeger EA (eds): Duane's Foundations of Clinical Ophthalmology. JB Lippincott, Philadelphia, 1990
91. Davis SD, Kushnaryov VM, Hyndiuk RA: Role of pili in virulence of *Pseudomonas aeruginosa* for scratched rabbit cornea. Presented at Ocular Microbiology and Immunology Group meeting, Chicago, 1983
92. Stern GA, Lubniewski A, Allen C: The interaction between *Pseudomonas aeruginosa* and the corneal epithelium. Arch Ophthalmol 103:1221, 1985
93. Hyndiuk RA: Experimental *Pseudomonas* keratitis. I. Sequential electron microscopy. II. Comparative therapy trials. Trans Am Ophthalmol Soc 79:541, 1981
94. John T, Refojo MF, Hanninen L, et al: Adherence of viable and nonviable bacteria to soft contact lenses. Cornea 8:21, 1989
95. Aswad MI, John T, Barza M, et al: Bacterial adherence to extended wear soft contact lenses. Ophthalmology 97:296, 1990
96. Klotz SA, An YK, Misra RP: A partial-thickness epithelial defect increases the adherence of *Pseudomonas aeruginosa* to the cornea. Invest Ophthalmol Vis Sci 30:1069, 1989
97. Spurr-Michaud SC, Barza M, Gipson IK: An organ culture system for study of adherence of *Pseudomonas aeruginosa* to normal and wounded corneas. Invest Ophthalmol Vis Sci 29:379, 1988
98. Butrus SM, Klotz SA, Misra RP: The adherence of *Pseudomonas aeruginosa* to soft contact lenses. Ophthalmology 94:1310, 1987
99. Ramphal R, McNiece MT, Polack FM: Adherence of *Pseudomonas aeruginosa* to the injured cornea: a step in the pathogenesis of corneal infections. Ann Ophthalmol 13:421, 1981
100. Slusher MM, Myrvik QN, Lewis JC, et al: Exended wear lenses, biofilm and bacterial adhesion. Arch Ophthalmol 105:110,1987
101. Stern GA, DiGaetano M, Zain S, Allen C: Pathogenesis of contact lens-associated *Pseudomonas* corneal ulcer. Presented at Ocular Microbiology and Immunology Group Meeting, San Francisco, 1985
102. Plant AG: Microbial IgA proteases. N Engl J Med 298:1459, 1978
103. Okumoto M: Infectious agents: bacteria. p. 105. In Smolin G, Thoft RA (eds): The Cornea: Scientific Foundations and Clinical Practice. Little, Brown, Boston, 1983
104. Johnson MK: Toxins and enzymes in ocular disease caused by gram-positive bacteria. p. II:43. In Tasman W, Jaeger EA (eds): Duane's Foundations of Clinical Ophthalmology. JB Lippincott, Philadelphia, 1990
105. Waldstrom T: Biological properties of extracellular proteins from *Staphylococcus.* Ann NY Acad Sci 236:343, 1974
106. Valenton MJ, Okumoto M: Toxin-producing strains of *Staphylococcus epidermidis.* Arch Ophthalmol 89:187, 1973
107. Jelyaszewicz J, Wadstrom T (eds): Bacterial Toxins and Cell Membranes. Academic Press, San Diego, 1978
108. Kamata R, Matsumoto K, Okamura R, et al: The serratial 56K protease as a major pathogenic factor in serratial keratitis. Ophthalmology 91:1452, 1985
109. Ohman DR, Burns RP, Iglewski BH: Corneal infections in mice with toxin A and elastase mutants of *Pseudomonas aeruginosa.* J Infect Dis 142:547, 1980
110. Brown SI, Bloomfield SE, Wai-fong IT: The cornea-destroying enzyme of *Pseudomonas aeruginosa.* Invest Ophthalmol 11:174, 1974
111. Kreger AS, Griffin OK: Physiochemical fractionation of extracellular cornea-damaging proteases of *Pseudomonas aeruginosa.* Infect Immun 9:829, 1974
112. Liu PV: Extracellular toxins of *Pseudomonas aeruginosa.* J Infect Dis 130(suppl):94, 1974
113. Johnson MK, Hobden JA, O'Callaghan RJ, Hill JM: Confirmation of the role of pneumolysin in ocular infections

with *Streptococcus pneumoniae.* Curr Eye Res 11:1221, 1992
114. Hsu C, Wiseman GM: Antibacterial substance from staphylococci. Can J Microbiol 13:947, 1967
115. Mondino BJ, Rabin BS, Kessler E, et al: Corneal rings with gram-negative bacteria. Arch Ophthalmol 95:2222, 1977
116. Belmont JB, Ostler HB, Chandler RD, Schwab I: Noninfectious ring-shaped keratitis associated with *Pseudomonas aeruginosa.* Am J Ophthalmol 93:338, 1982
117. Kessler E, Mondino B, Brown SI: The corneal response to *Pseudomonas aeruginosa:* histopathological and enzymatic characterization. Invest Ophthalmol Vis Sci 16:116, 1977
118. Twinning SS, Kirschner SE, Mahnke LA, Frank DW: Effect of *Pseudomonas aeruginosa* elastase, alkaline protease, and exotoxin A on corneal proteinases and proteins. Invest Ophthalmol Vis Sci 34:2699, 1993
119. Chusid MJ, Davis SD: Polymorphonuclear leukocyte kinetics in experimentally induced keratitis. Arch Ophthalmol 103:270, 1985
120. Babior BM: Oxygen-dependent microbial killing by phagocytes. N Engl J Med 298:721, 1978
121. Asbell PA, Gerson S, Friedman A: Effect of immunosuppression by cyclophosphamide on experimental *Pseudomonas* corneal ulceration in the rabbit model. Presented at Ocular Microbiology and Immunology Group Meeting, Chicago, 1983
122. Stern GA, Buttross M: Use of corticosteroids in combination with antimicrobial drugs in the treatment of infectious corneal disease. Ophthalmology 98:847, 1991
123. Epstein DL, Paton D: Keratitis from misuse of corneal anesthetics. N Engl J Med 279:396, 1968
124. Rosenwasser GOD, Holland S, Pflugfelder SC, et al: Topical anesthetic abuse. Ophthalmology 97:967, 1990
125. Abbott RL, Abrams MA: Bacterial corneal ulcers. p. IV:18. In Duane TD (ed): Clinical Ophthalmology. Harper & Row, Philadelphia, 1990
126. Harrison SM: Grading corneal ulcers. Ann Ophthalmol 7:537, 1975
127. Waring GO III, Laibson PR: A systematic method of drawing corneal pathologic conditions. Arch Ophthalmol 95:1540, 1977
128. Smolin G, Tabbara K, Whitcher J: Infectious Diseases of the Eye. Williams & Wilkins, Baltimore, 1984
129. Leibowitz HM: Bacterial keratitis. p. 353. In Leibowitz HM (ed): Corneal Disorders. WB Saunders, Philadelphia, 1984
130. Matoba AY, McCulley JP: Gram-positive cocci. p. II:49. In Tasman W, Jaeger EA (eds): Duane's Foundations of Clinical Ophthalmology. JB Lippincott, Philadelphia, 1990
131. Gorovoy MS, Stern GA, Hood I, Allen MS: Intrastromal noninflammatory bacterial colonization of a corneal graft. Arch Ophthalmol 101:1749, 1983
132. Meisler DM, Langston RHS, Naab TJ, et al: Infectious crystalline keratopathy. Am J Ophthalmol 97:337, 1984
133. Meisler DM, Langston RHS, Aaby AA, et al: Infectious corneal crystalline formation. ARVO abstract. Invest Ophthalmol Vis Sci 25(suppl):23, 1984
134. Samples JR, Baumgartner SD, Binder PS: Infectious crystalline keratopathy: an electron microscope analysis. Cornea 4:118, 1985
135. Reiss GR, Campbell RJ, Bourne WM: Infectious crystalline keratopathy. Surv Ophthalmol 31:69, 1986
136. James CB, McDonnell PJ, Falcon MG: Infectious crystalline keratopathy. Br J Ophthalmol 72:628, 1988
137. Ormerod LD, Ruoff KL, Meisler DM, et al: Infectious crystalline keratopathy. Role of nutritionally variant streptococci and other bacterial factors. Ophthalmology 98:159, 1991
138. Groden LR, Pascucci SE, Brinser JH: *Haemophilus aphrophilus* as a cause of crystalline keratopathy. Am J Ophthalmol 104:89, 1987
139. Lubniewski AJ, Houchin KW, Holland EJ, et al: Posterior infectious crystalline keratopathy with *Staphylococcus epidermidis.* Ophthalmology 97:1454, 1990
140. Stern GA: Infectious crystalline keratopathy. Int Ophthalmol Clin 33:1, 1993
141. Wilhelmus KR, Robinson NM: Infectious crystalline keratopathy caused by *Candida albicans.* Am J Ophthalmol 112:322, 1991
142. Hunts JH, Matoba AY, Osato Ms, Font RL: Infectious crystalline keratopathy. The role of bacterial exopolysaccharide. Arch Ophthalmol 111:528, 1993
143. Kincaid MC, Snip RC: Antibiotic resistance of crystalline bacterial ingrowth in a corneal graft. Ophthalmic Surg 18:268, 1987
144. Nanda M, Pflugfelder SC, Holland S: Fulminant pseudomonal keratitis and scleritis in human immunodeficiency virus infected patients. Arch Ophthalmol 109:503, 1991
145. Jones DB: Pathogenesis of bacterial and fungal keratitis. Trans Ophthalmol Soc UK 98:367, 1978
146. Rosenfeld ST, Mandelbaum S, Corrent GF, et al: Granular epithelial keratopathy as an unusual manifestation of *Pseudomonas* keratitis associated with extended-wear soft contact lenses. Am J Ophthalmol 109:17, 1990
147. Marioneaux SJ, Cohen EJ, Arentsen JJ, Laibson PR: *Moraxella* keratitis. Cornea 10:21, 1991
148. O'Day DM, Smith RS, Gregg CR, et al: The problem of *Bacillus* species infection with special emphasis on the virulence of *Bacillus cereus.* Ophthalmology 88:833, 1981
149. Liesegang TJ, Samples JR, Waller RW: Suppurative interstitial ring keratitis due to *Streptococcus.* Ann Ophthalmol 16:392, 1984
150. Holbach LM, Bialasiewicz AA, Boltze HJ: Necrotizing ring ulcer of the cornea caused by exogenous *Listeria monocytogenes* serotype IV 6 infection. Am J Ophthalmol 106:105, 1988
151. Paschal JF, Holland GN, Sison RF, et al: *Mycobacterium fortuitum* keratitis. Clinicopathologic correlates and cor-

ticosteroid effects in an animal model. Cornea 6:493, 1992
152. DiGaetano M, Ball SF, Straus JG: *Vibrio vulnificus* corneal ulcer. Arch Ophthalmol 107:323, 1989
153. Kiel RJ, Crane LR, Aguilar J, et al: Corneal perforation caused by dysgonic fermenter-2. JAMA 257:3269, 1987
154. deSmet MD, Chan CC, Nussenblatt RB, et al: *Capnocytophaga canimorsus* as the cause of chronic corneal infection. Am J Ophthalmol 109:240, 1990
155. Ticho BH, Urban RC, Safran MJ, et al: *Capnocytophaga* keratitis associated with poor dentition and human immunodeficiency virus. Am J Ophthalmol 109:352, 1990
156. Kelly L, Eliason J: *Eikenella corrodens* keratitis: case report. Br J Ophthalmol 73:22, 1989
157. Klein B, Couch J, Thompson J: Ocular infections associated with *Eikenella corrodens.* Am J Ophthalmol 109:127, 1990
158. Webb RM, Tabbara KF: Indolent bacterial corneal ulcers. Cornea 1:337, 1982
159. Rubinfeld RS, Cohen EJ, Arentsen JJ, Laibson PR: Diphtheroids as ocular pathogens. Am J Ophthalmol 108:251, 1989
160. Hyndiuk RA, Nassif KF, Burd EM: Bacterial disease. p. 147. In Smolin G, Thoft RA (eds): The Cornea: Scientific Foundations and Clinical Practice. Little, Brown, Boston, 1983
161. McDonnell PJ, Nobe J, Gauderman WJ, et al: Community care of corneal ulcers. Am J Ophthalmol 114:331, 1992
162. Pepose JS, Wilhelmus KR: Divergent approaches to the management of corneal ulcers. Am J Ophthalmol 114:630, 1992
163. Jones DB, Liesegang TJ, Robinson NM: Cumitech 13, Laboratory Diagnosis of Ocular Infections. Washington JA II (coord ed): American Society for Microbiology, Washington, DC, 1981
164. Brinser JH, Weiss A: Laboratory diagnosis in ocular disease. p. IV:1. In Tasman W, Jaeger EA (eds): Duane's Foundations of Clinical Ophthalmology. JB Lippincott, Philadelphia, 1990
165. Benson WH, Lanier JD: Comparison of techniques for culturing corneal ulcers. Ophthalmology 99:800, 1992
166. O'Day DM, Akrabawi PL, Head WS, Rather HB: Laboratory isolation techniques in human and experimental fungal infections. Am J Ophthalmol 87:688, 1979
167. Hwang DG: Lamellar flap corneal biopsy. Ophthalmic Surg 24:512, 1993
168. Jones BR, Jones DB, Richards AB: Surgery in the management of kerato-mycosis. Trans Ophthalmol Soc UK 89:887, 1969
169. Jones BR, Jones DB, Lim ASM, et al: Corneal and intraocular infection due to *Fusarium solani.* Trans Ophthalmol Soc UK 89:757, 1969
170. Jones DB: Initial therapy of suspected microbial corneal ulcers II: specific antibiotic therapy based on corneal smears. Surv Ophthalmol 24:97, 1979
171. Forster RK, Wirta MG, Solis M, Rebell G: Methenamine silver-stained corneal scrapings in keratomycosis. Am J Ophthalmol 82:261, 1976
172. Buttone EJ: The gram stain: the century-old quintessential rapid diagnostic test. Lab Med 19:288, 1988
173. Gomez JT, Robinson NM, Osato MS, et al: Comparison of acridine orange and gram stains in bacterial keratitis. Am J Ophthalmol 106:735, 1988
174. Groden LR, Rodnite J, Brinser JH, Genvert GI: Acridine orange and gram stains in infectious keratitis. Cornea 9:122, 1990
175. Wong IG: Diagnosis of ocular bacterial diseases. p. II:48. In Tasman W, Jaeger EA (eds): Duane's Foundations of Clinical Ophthalmology. JB Lippincott, Philadelphia, 1990
176. Rao NA: A laboratory approach to rapid diagnosis of ocular infections and prospects for the future. Am J Ophthalmol 107:283, 1989
177. McBeath J, Forster RK, Rebell G: Diagnostic limulus lysate assay for endophthalmitis and keratitis. Arch Ophthalmol 96:1265, 1978
178. Wolters RW, Jorgensen JH, Calyada E, Poirier RH: Limulus lysate assay for early detection of certain gram-negative corneal infections. Arch Ophthalmol 97:875, 1979
179. Alfonso EC, Miller D: Rapid detection of gram-negative endotoxin contamination of contact lens saline solutions. Arch Ophthalmol 110:1763, 1992
180. Finegold SM, Shepard WE, Spalding EH: Cumitech 5, Practical Anaerobic Bacteria. Shepard WE (coord ed): American Society for Microbiology, Washington, DC, 1977
181. Haley LD, Trandel J, Coyle MB: Cumitech 11, Practical Methods for Culture and Identification of Fungi in the Clinical Microbiology Laboratory. Sherris JC (coord ed): American Society for Microbiology, Washington, DC, 1980
182. Hodges EJ, Friedlaender MH, Lee A, Okumoto M: Effect of minimal antibiotic treatment on bacterial keratitis. Cornea 8:188, 1990
183. Badenoch PR, Coster DJ: Antimicrobial activity of topical anaesthetic preparations. Br J Ophthalmol 66:364, 1982
184. Jones DB: Polymicrobial keratitis. Trans Am Ophthalmol Soc 79:153, 1981
185. Groden LR, Brinser JH: Outpatient treatment of microbial corneal ulcers. Arch Ophthalmol 104:841, 1986
186. Wilhelmus KR: Bacterial corneal ulcers. Int Ophthalmol Clin 24:1, 1984
187. Jones DB: A plan for antimicrobial therapy in bacterial keratitis. Trans Am Acad Ophthalmol Otolaryngol 79:95, 1975
188. Baum JL: Initial therapy of suspected microbial corneal ulcers I: broad antibiotic therapy based on prevalence of organisms. Surv Ophthalmol 24:97, 1979
189. Steinert RF: Current therapy for bacterial keratitis and bacterial conjunctivitis. Am J Ophthalmol 112:105, 1991
190. Barza M, Baum J: Ocular pharmacology of antibiotics. p. II:61. In Duane TD, Jaeger EA (eds): Biomedical Foundations of Ophthalmology, Philadelphia, Harper & Row, 1987
191. Wright AJ, Wilkowske GJ: The penicillins. Mayo Clin Proc 66:1047, 1991
192. Gustaferro CA, Steckelberg JM: Cephalosporin antimicrobial agents and related compounds. Mayo Clin Proc 66:1064, 1991

193. Brewer NS, Hellinger WC: The monobactams. Mayo Clin Proc 66:1152, 1991
194. Edson RS, Terrell CL: The aminoglycosides. Mayo Clin Proc 66:1158, 1991
195. Wilhelm MP: Vancomycin. Mayo Clin Proc 66:1165, 1991
196. Smilack JD, Wilson WR, Cockerill FR III: Tetracyclines, chloramphenicol, erythromycin, clindamycin, and metronidazole. Mayo Clin Proc 66:1270, 1991
197. Jones DB: New horizons in antibacterial antibiotics. Int Ophthalmol Clin 33:179, 1993
198. Hooton TM, Blair AD, Turck M, Counts GW: Synergism at clinically attainable concentrations of aminoglycoside and beta-lactam antibiotics. Antimicrob Agents Chemother 26:535, 1984
199. Smolin G, Okumoto M, Wilson FM: The effect of tobramycin on gentamicin-resistant strains in *Pseudomonas* keratitis. Am J Ophthalmol 77:583, 1974
200. Smith CR, Lipsky JJ, Laskin OL, et al: Double-blind comparison of the nephrotoxicity and auditory toxicity of gentamicin and tobramycin. N Engl J Med 302:1106, 1980
201. Davison CR, Tuft SJ, Dart JKG: Conjunctival necrosis after administration of topical fortified aminoglycosides. Am J Ophthalmol 111:690, 1991
202. Wilhelmus KR: Vancomycin revived [editorial]. Cornea 1:103, 1982
203. Rosenthal RL, Blackman A: Bone marrow hypoplasia following use of chloramphenicol eyedrops. JAMA 191:136, 1965
204. Carpenter G: Chloramphenicol eyedrops and marrow aplasia [letter]. Lancet 2:236, 1975
205. Neu HC: Microbiologic aspects of fluoroquinolones. Am J Ophthalmol 112:155, 1991
206. Trucksis M, Hooper DC, Wolfson JS: Emerging resistance to fluoroquinolones in staphylococci: an alert. Ann Intern Med 114:424, 1991
207. Snyder ME, Katz HR: Ciprofloxacin-resistant bacterial keratitis. Am J Ophthalmol 114:336, 1992
208. Cokington CD, Hyndiuk RA: Insights from experimental data on ciprofloxacin in the treatment of bacterial keratitis and ocular infections. Am J Ophthalmol 112:255, 1991
209. Leibowitz HM: Clinical evaluation of ciprofloxacin 0.3% ophthalmic solution for treatment of bacterial keratitis. Am J Ophthalmol 112(4suppl):34S, 1991
210. Callegan MC, Hobden JA, Hill JM, et al: Topical antibiotic therapy for the treatment of experimental *Staphylococcus aureus* keratitis. Invest Ophthalmol Vis Sci 33:3017, 1992
211. Ophthalmic ciprofloxacin. Med Lett Drugs Ther 33:52, 1991
212. Cutarelli PE, Lass JH, Lazarus HM, et al: Topical fluoroquinolones: antimicrobial activity and in-vitro corneal epithelial toxicity. Curr Eye Res 10:557, 1991
213. Serdarevic ON: Role of fluoroquinolones in ophthalmology. Int Ophthalmol Clin 33:163, 1993
214. Parks DJ, Abrams DA, Sarfarazi FA, Katz HR: Comparison of topical ciprofloxacin to conventional antibiotic therapy in the treatment of ulcerative keratitis. Am J Ophthalmol 115:471, 1993
215. Veights SA, Dick JD, O'Brien TP, et al: Comparative in-vitro activities of fluoroquinolones vs aminoglycosides against ocular isolates. Invest Ophthalmol Vis Sci 33:936, 1992
216. Gritz DC, McDonnell PJ, Lee TY, et al: Topical ofloxacin in the treatment of *Pseudomonas* keratitis in a rabbit model. Cornea 11:143, 1992
217. Callegan MC, Hill JM, Insler MS, et al: Methicillin-resistant *Staphylococcus aureus* keratitis in the rabbit: therapy with ciprofloxacin, vancomycin and cefazolin. Curr Eye Res 11:1111, 1992
218. Reidy JJ, Hobden JA, Hill JM, et al: The efficacy of topical ciprofloxacin and norfloxacin in the treatment of experimental *Pseudomonas* keratitis. Cornea 10:25, 1991
219. Lauffenburger MD, Cohen KL: Topical ciprofloxacin versus topical fortified antibiotics in rabbit models of *Staphylococcus* and *Pseudomonas* keratitis. Cornea 12:517, 1993
220. McDermott ML, Tran TD, Cowden JW, Bugge CJ: Corneal stromal penetration of topical ciprofloxacin in humans. Ophthalmology 100:197, 1993
221. Vrabec TR, Sergott RC, Jaeger EA, et al: Reversible visual loss in a patient receiving high-dose ciprofloxacin hydrochloride. Ophthalmology 97:707, 1990
222. Pendleton KM, Hobden JA, Hill JM, et al: Antibacterial activity of ciprofloxacin against organisms isolated from patients with bacterial keratitis. ARVO abstract. Invest Ophthalmol Vis Sci 32 (suppl):1171, 1991
223. Abrams DA, Sarfarazi FA, Parks DJ, Katz HR: Topical ciprofloxacin versus conventional antibiotic therapy in the treatment of ulcerative keratitis. ARVO abstract. Invest Ophthalmol Vis Sci 32(suppl): 1171, 1991
224. Eiferman RA, Forgey DR, Snyder J: The successful treatment of bacterial corneal ulcers with ciprofloxacin. ARVO abstract. Invest Opthalmol Vis Sci 32(suppl):1171, 1991
225. Vajpayee RB, Gupta SK, Angra SK, Munjal A: Topical norfloxacin therapy in *Pseudomonas* corneal ulceration. Cornea 10:268, 1991
226. Wilhelmus KR, Hyndiuk RA, Caldwell DR, et al: 0.3% Ciprofloxacin ophthalmic ointment in the treatment of bacterial keratitis. Arch Ophthalmol 111:1210, 1993
227. Kupferman A, Leibowitz HM: Topical antibiotic therapy of *Pseudomonas aeruginosa* keratitis in guinea pigs. Arch Ophthalmol 97:1699, 1979
228. Davis SD, Sarff LD, Hyndiuk RA: Topical tobramycin therapy of experimental *Pseudomonas* keratitis: an evaluation of some factors that potentially enhance efficacy. Arch Ophthalmol 96:123, 1978
229. Baum J: Antibiotic mechanisms. p. 134. In Smolin G, Thoft RA (eds): The Cornea: Scientific Foundations and Clinical Practice. Little, Brown, Boston, 1983
230. Nassif KF, Davis SD, Hyndiuk RA, et al: Factors that influence the efficacy of topical gentamicin prophylaxis for experimental *Pseudomonas* keratitis. Am J Ophthalmol 94:216, 1982
231. Gilbert ML, Wilhelmus KR, Osato MS: Comparative bioavailability and efficacy of fortified topical tobramycin. Invest Ophthalmol Vis Sci 28:881, 1987

232. Glasser DB, Gardner S, Ellis JG, Pettit TH: Loading doses and extended dosing intervals in topical gentamicin therapy. Am J Ophthalmol 99:329, 1985
233. Osborn E, Baum JL, Ernst C, Koch P: The stability of 10 antibiotics in artificial tears. Am J Ophthalmol 82:775, 1976
234. Bowe BE, Snyder JW, Eiferman RA: An in vitro study of the potency and stability of fortified ophthalmic antibiotic preparations. Am J Ophthalmol 111:686, 1991
235. Charlton JF, Kniska A, Chao GM, et al: Stability of topical fortified antibiotic solutions. Invest Ophthalmol Vis Sci 33:937, 1992
236. Hyndiuk RA, Skorick DN, Davis SD, et al: Fortified antibiotic ointment in bacterial keratitis. Am J Ophthalmol 105:239,1988
237. Davis SD, Sarff LD, Hyndiuk RA: Antibiotic therapy of experimental *Pseudomonas* keratitis in guinea pigs. Arch Ophthalmol 95:1638, 1977
238. Assil KK, Zarnear SR, Fouraker BD, Schanzlin DJ: Efficacy of tobramycin-soaked collagen shields vs tobramycin eyedrops loading dose for sustained treatment of experimental *Pseudomonas aeruginosa*-induced keratitis in rabbits. Am J Ophthalmol 113:418, 1992
239. Finkelstein I, Trope GE, Menon IA, et al: Potential value of collagen shields as a subconjunctival depot release system. Curr Eye Res 9:653, 1990
240. Sawusch MR, O'Brien TP, Dick JD, Gottsch JD: Collagen corneal shields in the treatment of bacterial keratitis. Am J Ophthalmol 106:279, 1988
241. Hobden JA, Reidy JJ, O'Callaghan RJ, et al: Treatment of experimental *Pseudomonas* keratitis using collagen shields containing tobramycin. Arch Ophthalmol 106:1605, 1988
242. Phinney RB, Schwartz SD, Lee DA, et al: Collagen-shield delivery of gentamicin and vancomycin. Arch Ophthalmol 106:1599, 1988
245. Friedberg ML, Pleyer W, Mondino BJ: Device drug delivery to the eye. Ophthalmology 98:725, 1991
244. Hobden JA, Reidy JJ, O'Callaghan RJ, et al: Quinolones in collagen shields to treat aminoglycoside-resistant pseudomonal keratitis. Invest Ophthalmol Vis Sci 31:2241, 1990
245. Baum J, Barza M, Shushan D, Weinstein L: Concentration of gentamicin in experimental corneal ulcers. Arch Ophthalmol 92:315, 1974
246. Davis SD, Sarff LD, Hyndiuk RA: Comparison of therapeutic routes in experimental *Pseudomonas* keratitis. Am J Ophthalmol 87:710, 1979
247. Kupferman A, Leibowitz HM: Antibiotic therapy of bacterial keratitis: topical application or periocular injection? ARVO abstract. Invest Ophthalmol Vis Sci 19(suppl):112, 1980
248. Stern GA, Driebe WT: The effect of fortified antibiotic therapy on the visual outcome of severe bacterial corneal ulcers. Cornea 1:341, 1982
249. Leibowitz HM, Ryan WJ, Kupferman A: Route of antibiotic administration in bacterial keratitis. Arch Ophthalmol 99:1420, 1981
250. Baum J: Treatment of bacterial ulcers of the cornea in the rabbit: a comparison of administration by eyedrops and subconjunctival injections. Trans Am Ophthalmol Soc 80:369, 1982
251. Woo FL, Johnson AP, Insler MS, et al: Gentamicin, tobramycin, amikacin, and netilmicin levels in tears following intravenous administration. Arch Ophthalmol 103:216, 1985
252. Insler MS, Helm CJ, George WJ: Topical versus systemic gentamicin penetration into the human cornea and aqueous humor. Arch Ophthalmol 105:922, 1987
253. Burns RP, Rhodes DM: *Pseudomonas* eye infection as a cause of death in premature infants. Arch Ophthalmol 65:517, 1961
254. Finland M: Changing patterns of susceptibility of common bacterial pathogens to antimicrobial agents. Ann Intern Med 76:1006, 1972
255. Wilhelmus KR, Gilbert ML, Osato MS: Tobramycin in ophthalmology. Surv Ophthalmol 32:111, 1987
256. Wolfson JS, Hooper DC: The fluoroquinolones: structures, mechanisms of action and resistance, and spectra of activity in vitro. Antimicrob Agents Chemother 28:581, 1985
257. Barza M: Pharmacokinetics and efficacy of the new quinolones in infections of the eye, ear, nose, and throat. Rev Infect Dis 10:S241, 1988
258. Darrell RW, Modak SM, Fox CL Jr: Norfloxacin and silver norfloxacin in the treatment of *Pseudomonas* corneal ulcer in the rabbit. Trans Am Ophthalmol Soc 82:75, 1984
259. O'Brien TP, Sawusch MR, Dick JD, Gottsch JD: Topical ciprofloxacin treatment of *Pseudomonas* keratitis in rabbits. Arch Ophthalmol 106:1444, 1988
260. Hyndiuk RA, Eiferman RA, Caldwell DR, et al: Comparison of ciprofloxacin ophthalmic solution 0.3% to fortified tobramycin-cefazolin in treating bacterial corneal ulcers. Ophthalmology 103:1854, 1996
261. Kaatz GW, Seo SM: Mechanism of ciprofloxacin resistance in *Pseudomonas aeruginosa.* J Infect Dis 158:537, 1988
262. Jones RN: Disk diffusion antimicrobial susceptibility testing of *Neisseria gonorrhoeae.* MMWR 39:157, 1990
263. Borrmann LR, Leopold IH: The potential use of quinolones in future ocular antimicrobial therapy [editorial]. Am J Ophthalmol 106:227, 1988
264. Osato MS, Jensen HG, Trousdale MD, et al: The comparative in vitro activity of ofloxacin and selected ophthalmic antimicrobial agents against ocular bacterial isolates. Am J Ophthalmol 108:380, 1989
265. Sanders WE Jr, Hartwig EC, Schneider NJ, et al: Susceptibility of organisms in the *Mycobacterium fortuitum* complex to antituberculosis and other antimicrobial agents. Antimicrob Agents Chemother 12:295, 1972
266. Matoba AY, Lee BL, Robinson NM, et al: Combination drug testing of *Mycobacterium chelonae.* Invest Ophthalmol Vis Sci 34:2786, 1993
267. Helm CJ, Holland GN, Lin R, et al: Comparison of topical antibiotics for treating *Mycobacterium fortuitum* keratitis in an animal model. Am J Ophthalmol 116:700, 1993

268. Matoba A: *Mycobacterium chelonei* keratitis. Am J Ophthalmol 103:595, 1987
269. Dugel PU, Holland GN, Brown HH, et al: *Mycobacterium fortuitum* keratitis. Am J Ophthalmol 105:661, 1988
270. Young LS, Berlin OGW, Inderlied CB: Activity of ciprofloxacin and other fluorinated quinolones against mycobacteria. Am J Med 82:23, 1987
271. Stevens RK, Holland GN, Paschal JF, et al: *Mycobacterium fortuitum* keratitis: a comparison of topical ciprofloxacin and amikacin in an animal model. Cornea 11:500, 1992
272. Moore MB, Newton C, Kaufman HE: Chronic keratitis caused by *Mycobacterium gordonae.* Am J Ophthalmol 102:516, 1986
273. Goodman DF, Gottsch JD: Methicillin-resistant *Staphylococus epidermidis* keratitis treated with vancomycin. Arch Ophthalmol 106:1570, 1988
274. Bohigian G, Okumoto M, Valenton M: Experimental *Pseudomonas* keratitis. Arch Ophthalmol 86:432, 1971
275. Donnenfeld ED, Cohen EJ, Barza M, Baum J: Treatment of *Nocardia* keratitis with topical trimethoprim-sulfamethoxazole [letter]. Am J Ophthalmol 99:601, 1985
276. Enzenauer RW, Cornell FM, Brooke JD, Butler CE: *Nocardia asteroides* keratitis: a case associated with soft contact lens wear. CLAO J 15:72, 1989
277. Stern GA, Schemmer GB, Farber RD, et al: Effect of topical antibiotic solutions on corneal epithelial wound healing. Arch Ophthalmol 101:644, 1983
278. Coster DJ, Bodenoch PR: Host, microbial, and pharmacological factors affecting the outcome of suppurative keratitis. Br J Ophthalmol 71:96, 1987
279. Hurwitz JJ, Dixon NS, Sloan A: Therapeutic soft contact lenses: a survey. Can J Ophthalmol 9:72, 1974
280. Cavanagh HD, Pahlaja D, Thoft RA, Dohlman CH: The pathogenesis and treatment of persistent epithelial defects. Trans Am Acad Ophthalmol Otolaryngol 81:754, 1976
281. Reynolds MG, Alfonso E: Treatment of infectious scleritis and keratoscleritis. Am J Ophthalmol 112:543, 1991
282. Slansky HH, Dohlman CH, Berman MB: Prevention of corneal ulcers. Trans Am Acad Ophthalmol Otolaryngol 75:1208,1971
283. Ellison A, Poirier R: Therapeutic effects of heparin on *Pseudomonas*-induced corneal ulceration. Am J Ophthalmol 82:619, 1976
284. Mehra KS, Singh R, Bhatia RPS: Lysozyme in cornea ulcer. Ann Ophthalmol 7:1470, 1975
285. Smolin G, Okumoto M, Leong-Sit L: Combined gentamicin-tobramycin-corticosteroid treatment II: effect on gentamicin-resistant *Pseudomonas* keratitis. Arch Ophthalmol 98:473,1980
286. Leibowitz HM, Kupferman A: Topically administered corticosteroids: effect on antibiotic-treated bacterial keratitis. Arch Ophthalmol 98:1287, 1980
287. Velasquez O: Cryocurettage in the treatment of corneal ulcers. Ann Ophthalmol 6:733, 1974
288. Eiferman RA: Cryotherapy of *Pseudomonas* keratitis and scleritis. Arch Ophthalmol 97:1637, 1979
289. Eiferman RA, Snyder JW: Antibacterial effect of cyanoacrylate glue. Arch Ophthalmol 101:958, 1983
290. Sarno EM, Robin JB, Garabet A, Schanzlin DJ: Carbon dioxide laser therapy of *Pseudomonas aeruginosa* keratitis. Am J Ophthalmol 97:791, 1984
291. Serdarevic O, Darrell RW, Krueger RR, Trokel SL: Excimer laser therapy for experimental *Candida* keratitis. Am J Ophthalmol 99:534, 1985
292. Gottsch JD, Gilbert ML, Goodman DF, et al: Excimer laser ablative treatment of microbial keratitis. Ophthalmology 98:146, 1991
293. Moreira H, McDonnell PJ, Fasano AP, et al: Treatment of experimental *Pseudomonas* keratitis with cyclo-oxygenase and lipoxygenase inhibitors. Ophthalmology 98:1683, 1991
294. Davis SD, Sarff LD, Hyndiuk RA: Corticosteroid in experimentally induced *Pseudomonas* keratitis. Arch Ophthalmol 96:126, 1978
295. Bohigian GM, Foster CS: Treatment of *Pseudomonas* keratitis in rabbit with antibiotic-steroid combination. Invest Ophthalmol Vis Sci 16:553, 1977
296. Harbin T: Recurrence of a corneal *Pseudomonas* infection after topical steroid therapy: report of a case. Am J Ophthalmol 58:670, 1964
297. Burns RP: *Pseudomonas aeruginosa* keratitis: mixed infections of the eye. Am J Ophthalmol 67:257, 1969
298. Carmichael TR, Gelfand Y, Welsh NH: Topical steroids in the treatment of central and paracentral ulcers. Br J Ophthalmol 74:528, 1990
299. Hobden JA, O'Callaghan RJ, Hill JM, et al: Ciprofloxacin and prednisolone therapy for experimental *Pseudomonas* keratitis. Curr Eye Res 11:259, 1992
300. Alpren TVP, Hyndiuk RA, Davis SD, et al: Cryotherapy for experimental *Pseudomonas* keratitis. Arch Ophthalmol 97:711, 1979
301. Codere F, Brownstein S, Jackson B: *Pseudomonas aeruginosa* scleritis. Am J Ophthalmol 91:706, 1981
302. Buxton JN, Fox ML: Conjunctival flaps in the treatment of refractory pseudomonas corneal abscess. Ann Ophthalmol 18:315, 1986
303. Portnoy SL, Insler MS, Kaufman HE: Surgical management of corneal ulceration and perforation. Surv Ophthalmol 34:47, 1989
304. Killingsworth DW, Stern GA, Driebe WT, et al: Results of therapeutic penetrating keratoplasty. Ophthalmology 100:534,1993
305. Read JW: Penetating keratoplasty in the treatment of *Pseudomonas* corneal ulceration. Presented at the Castroviejo Society Meeting, Chicago, 1983
306. Malik SRK, Singh G: Therapeutic keratoplasty in *Pseudomonas pyocyaneus* corneal ulcers. Br J Ophthalmol 55:326, 1971
307. Nobe JR, Moura BT, Robin JB, Smith RE: Results of penetrating keratoplasty for the treatment of corneal perforations. Arch Ophthalmol 108:939, 1990
308. Mandelbaum S, Udell IJ: Corneal perforations associated with infectious agents. p. 87. In Abbott R (ed): Surgical

Intervention in Corneal and External Disease. Grune & Stratton, Orlando, FL, 1987
309. Phillips RL: Vacuum trephination of the hypotonous eye. Ophthalmic Surg 14:513, 1983
310. Yee RW, Hyndiuk RA: Interstitial keratitis. p. 601. In Tabbara KF, Hyndiuk RA (eds): Infections of the Eye. Little, Brown, Boston, 1986
311. Margo CE, Hamed LM: Ocular syphilis. Surv Ophthalmol 37:203, 1992
312. Wilhelmus KR: Syphilis. p. 73. In Insler MS (ed): AIDS and Other Sexually Transmitted Diseases and the Eye. Grune & Stratton, Orlando, FL, 1987
313. Scattergood KD, Green WR, Hirst LW: Scrolls of Descemet's membrane in healed syphilitic interstitial keratitis. Ophthalmology 90:1518, 1983
314. Waring GO, Font RL, Rodrigues MM, Mulberger RD: Alterations of Descemet's membrane in interstitial keratitis. Am J Ophthalmol 81:773, 1976
315. Tamesis RR, Foster S: Ocular syphilis. Ophthalmology 97:1281, 1990
316. Arffa RC: Grayson's Diseases of the Cornea. Chapter 11. Mosby-Year Book, St. Louis, MO, 1991
317. Rabb MF, Fine M: Penetrating keratoplasty in interstitial keratitis. Am J Ophthalmol 67:907, 1969
318. McLeish WM, Pulido JS, Holland S, et al: The ocular manifestations of syphilis in the human immunodeficiency virus type I-infected host. Ophthalmology 97:197, 1990
319. Helm CJ, Holland GN: Ocular tuberculosis. Surv Ophthalmol 38:229, 1993
320. Aclimandos WA, Kerr-Muir M: Tuberculous keratoconjunctivitis. Br J Ophthalmol 76:175, 1992
321. Schwab IR: Ocular leprosy. p. 613. In Tabbara KF, Hyndiuk RA (eds): Infections of the Eye. Little, Brown, Boston, 1986
322. Cameron AN: Leprosy and its ocular manifestations. Trans Ophthalmol Soc UK 81:637, 1961
323. Richards W: Ocular leprosy. Trans Pac Coast Otoophthalmol Soc 52:161, 1971
324. Schwab IR: Ocular leprosy. Infect Dis Clin North Am 6:953, 1992
325. Winterkorn JMS: Lyme disease. Neurologic and ophthalmic manifestations. Surv Ophthalmol 35:191, 1990
326. Zaidman GW: The ocular manifestations of Lyme disease. Int Ophthalmol Clin 33:8, 1993
327. Baum J, Barza M, Weinstein P, et al: Bilateral keratitis as a manifestation of Lyme disease. Am J Ophthalmol 105:75, 1988
328. Flack AJ, Lavoie PE: Episcleritis, conjunctivitis, and keratitis as ocular manifestations of Lyme disease. Ophthalmology 97:973, 1990
329. Kornmehl EW, Lesser RL, Jaros P, et al: Bilateral keratitis in Lyme disease. Ophthalmology 96:1194, 1989
330. Orlin SE, Lauffer JL: Lyme disease keratitis [letter]. Am J Ophthalmol 107:678, 1989
331. Steere AC: Lyme disease. N Engl J Med 321:586, 1989

9

Fungal Keratitis

THOMAS J. LIESEGANG

ORGANISMS

Fungi are primitive, nonmotile, plant-like structures that lack chlorophyll. They live as symbiotes, parasites, or saprophytes; when an organic compound supplies a carbon source, they can synthesize proteins and other essentials for growth. Fungi grow optimally between 20° and 30°C, but are capable of growth in the range of 0° to 35°C. They reproduce by fragmentation, fission, budding, and sexual or asexual spore formation. Unlike bacteria, fungi are eukaryotic. Their cell membranes are rich in sterols, which makes them susceptible to polyene antifungal agents, which have an affinity for these sterols. Fungi can also be distinguished from bacteria by the presence of a nucleolus, mitochondria, 80-S ribosomes and centrioles, and the preference for an acidic environment.

More than 70 genera of filamentous fungi and yeasts have been identified in fungal keratitis.[1-5] Fungi often are opportunistic invaders in compromised corneas as well as following trauma with plant or vegetable matter. The organisms implicated are ubiquitous as plant pathogens or exist in the soil, and are primarily saprophytic with regard to their disease potential elsewhere. The home environment is ideal for fungal growth.[6] Molds are easily isolated outdoors as far north as Canada,[7] and several of the organisms seen in fungal keratitis have been cultured on the beaches of Florida at different times of the year.[8] Fungi have the ability to grow at body temperature, to survive at the low redox potential of tissue, and to neutralize the humoral and cellular defenses of the host.[9] Frequently, fungi can be isolated from the flora of the normal eyelid and conjunctiva, especially in individuals who work outdoors. The increasing incidence of fungal keratitis is related to a greater recognition of the clinical features, improvement in laboratory techniques, better reporting, and increasingly widespread and indiscriminate use of corticosteroids, antibiotics, and immunosuppressive drugs.

The cell wall defines the fungus; 80 to 90 percent of the wall is polysaccharide, and the remainder is protein or lipid. The polysaccharide is either cellulose or chitin, and usually only one type is found in a given fungus.[10] The kingdom Fungi is divided into six classes: the Chytridiomycetes, the Zygomycetes, the Ascomycetes, the Basidiomycetes, the Fungi Imperfecti, and the lichens.[11] For purposes of discussing their role in ocular disease, it is easier to classify fungi into filamentous organisms (molds) and yeasts. This simple classification is helpful in discussing geographic distribution, predisposing and clinical features, laboratory diagnosis, and medical therapy. A dimorphic group, with both a filamentous phase (at 25° to 30°C) and yeast phase (at 37°C) is responsible for the deep mycoses. Included in this group are *Blastomyces, Coccidioides, Histoplasma,* and *Sporothrix.* These organisms rarely cause keratitis.

Filamentous fungi are multicellular organisms. They produce distinctive, long-branching hyphae that form a tangled feathery or powdery mass (mold or mycelium) above the culture medium. The hyphae are septate (divided by cross walls into definite cells, each containing one or more nuclei) or nonseptate (long tubes containing protoplasm with numerous nuclei scattered throughout). Fungi with nonseptate hyphae include *Mucor, Rhizopus,* and *Absidia.* They are responsible for lethal infections of the orbit and paranasal sinuses, but are rarely responsible for exogenous keratitis.[12] Most fungal keratitis is caused by fungi with septate hyphae. These septations may be either complete or incomplete; the incomplete septum allows the protoplasm to flow from one cell to another through a central pore. Fungi with septate hyphae are divided into nonpigmented fungi (Moniliaceae) and pigmented fungi (Dematiaceae), based on whether the hyphae are nonpigmented or pigmented on culture media (Table 9-1). Usually, the genus and species of a particular fungus cannot be identified from morphologic examination of tissue specimens, because conidia and their supporting structures, which are the principal identifying features in taxonomy, are absent. These features are produced after culture of the fungus on appropriate media.

Yeasts consist primarily of *Candida* species. These unicellular oval organisms reproduce by budding and form pseudohyphae under reduced oxygen tension or in tissue. The pseudohyphal phase is the most invasive and virulent phase.[13] The cell walls of pseudohyphae, unlike those of true hyphae, are not parallel to one another and have constrictions. *Candida* produces creamy, opaque, pasty colonies on culture media.

The predominant causes of fungal keratitis are *Fusarium solani* and other *Fusarium* species, *Aspergillus, Acremonium,* and *Penicillium,* which are all nonpigmented fungi.[1-5] Important pigmented fungi include *Curvularia, Alternaria, Bipolaris* (formerly *Drechslera*), *Exserohilum* (formerly *Drechslera*), *Phialophora,* and *Lasiodiplodia.*[14] Although *Fusarium* and *Aspergillus* clearly dominate the list, causative agents vary in different geographic areas.

In a series of 663 patients with suspected microbial keratitis in south Florida, 133 patients (35 percent of culture-positive ulcers) had fungi isolated from corneal scrapings.[1] Fifty-seven percent of these fungal isolates were *F. solani,* 21 percent were other nonpigmented fungi, 15 percent were pigmented fungi, and 7 percent were yeasts. Among the nonpigmented fungi were other *Fusarium* species, *Aspergillus fumigatus, Aspergillus flavus, Paecilomyces lilacinus,* and *Petriellidium boydii* (now called *Pseudallescheria boydii*). Among the pigmented fungi were *Curvularia, Drechslera* (now called *Bipolaris* or *Exserohilum*),[15] *Alternaria, Phialophora,* and the tropical fungi, *Lasiodiplodia* and *Colletrotrichum.* In a more recent review of 125 patients with culture-positive fungal keratitis in south Florida, the most common isolates were *F. oxysporum* (37 percent) and *F. solani* (23 percent).[5]

In a large series of microbial keratitis from New York City,[16] fungal keratitis represented only 1 percent of the cases and included five cases of *Candida,* two cases of *Fusarium,* and one of *Cryptococcus.* In a series of seven cases of fungal keratitis in Wisconsin, four were caused by *Candida,* and one each by *Penicillium, Aspergillus,* and *Alternaria.*[17] In 19 cases over a 10-year period in Minnesota, *Aspergillus* was isolated in six, *Candida* in six, *Alternaria* in four, and *Fusarium* in three.[18] Most fungal keratitis occurred in rural farmers and was associated with vegetable trauma. In studying fungal contamination within the media of organ-cultured corneas in Minnesota, the most common organism isolated was *Candida.*[19] The higher frequency of *Candida* in series outside the southern United States probably relates more to the universal distribution of *Candida* and lack of exposure to filamentous fungi in outdoor trauma than to any special factor promoting *Candida.*

F. solani is the most common fungal corneal pathogen in the southern United States and South America,[20] although it has been reported in all areas of the world. Although *Fusarium* species are primarily plant pathogens, they are ubiquitous in air, organic wastes, and soil. *F. solani* can replicate at 35°C and produces at least nine complex mycotoxins and destructive enzymes. Other *Fusarium* species, such as *F. oxysporum,* are being increasingly identified as causes of fungal keratitis.[5]

Aspergillus produces a variety of toxic metabolites, and causes many opportunistic and primary infections, such as infections of the lacrimal drainage system, orbital cellulitis, and endophthalmitis. *Aspergillus* was the most common cause of filamentous fungal keratitis in series from Minnesota,[18] India,[21,22] London,[23] Bangladesh,[24] Saudi Arabia,[25] and worldwide.[26] In Florida and all of the southern United States, however, *Aspergillus* is less common than other fungi as a cause of keratitis.[1,5,27,28]

Acremonium (formerly *Cephalosporium*) is a predominant genus in reported cases of postsurgical fungal endophthalmitis.[29] In addition to being associated with

TABLE 9-1
Fungi of Importance in Microbial Keratitis

Moniliaceae (nonpigmented filamentous fungi)
Fusarium (especially *F. solani*)
Aspergillus (especially *A. fumigatus, A. niger, A. flavus*)
Acremonium (formerly *Cephalosporium*)
Paecilomyces
Penicillium
Pseudallescheria (formerly *Allescheria, Petriellidium*)
Dematiaceae (pigmented filamentous fungi)
Curvularia
Alternaria
Phialophora
Bipolaris (formerly *Drechslera*)
Exserohilum (formerly *Drechslera*)
Cladosporium
Yeasts
Candida (especially *C. albicans, C. tropicalis, C. parapsilosis*)
Cryptococcus
Dimorphic fungi (rare in keratitis)
Blastomyces
Coccidioides
Histoplasma
Sporothrix

corneal ulceration by virtue of its proteolytic enzymes,[30] it can cause a suppurative abscess of the skin and subcutaneous tissues (mycetoma).

Candida is a ubiquitous yeast. Infection with *Candida* is not linked to environmental factors as is infection with filamentous fungi. *Candida* is an extreme example of an opportunistic organism, in that this infection may be the presenting feature in an immunocompromised individual.[31] It is the most common ocular fungal pathogen, because it is also implicated in diseases of the eyelids, conjunctiva, lacrimal drainage system, and retina.[32] *C. albicans* is the species most frequently identified, but *C. parapsilosis* and *C. tropicalis* are also seen. *C. albicans* can transform from a blastoconidial to a pseudohyphal phase under appropriate conditions. As with filamentous fungi, the large size of the pseudohyphae precludes complete ingestion by neutrophils.

PATHOGENESIS

Weather conditions, work habits, frequency of outdoor activity, and distribution of organisms in the environment in the warmer tropical climates are all factors that have led to a high incidence of keratitis with filamentous fungi. In the southern United States, fungal keratitis represents as much as 35 percent of all culture-positive cases of microbial keratitis.[1] A series of microbial keratitis in children from south Florida showed 18 percent of cultures positive for fungi.[33] Twenty-nine percent of children from New Orleans with microbial keratitis had fungi isolated on culture.[34] The principal risk factors for fungal keratitis in children were trauma, prior corneal surgery, systemic illness, and contact lens wear. In these endemic areas, filamentous fungi usually infect normal eyes of healthy young people who have had mild, abrasive corneal trauma with vegetable matter. Such trauma usually occurs in farmers or outdoor laborers. It is also seen occasionally in conjunction with the use of gardening tools (such as nylon line lawn trimmers[35]) without protective eye wear or in association with injury from an indoor plant. Filamentous fungi have frequently been isolated from the vegetable matter, and are implanted directly by the injuring material.[36] Filamentous fungal keratitis can occur after surgery such as penetrating keratoplasty[37] and radial keratotomy.[38] Rarely, there is no history of trauma, and an endogenous source may be responsible.[39] The incidence of fungal keratitis in south Florida peaks in the winter months (November to March), which are dry, cool, and windy.[1] In northern climates, fungal keratitis is more often the result of opportunistic infection, and occurs in compromised or immunosuppressed corneas. In the rural north, however, filamentous fungi may be associated with trauma from vegetable matter.[18]

Although predisposing ocular disease, systemic immunologic disease, or the use of corticosteroids or antibiotics are not prerequisites for filamentous fungal keratitis, the use of corticosteroids and antibiotics before a definitive diagnosis is made may worsen the disease process. Infection with human immunodeficiency virus (HIV) has been implicated as a risk factor in spontaneous or bilateral fungal keratitis.[40,41]

Candida and other yeasts are more frequently opportunistic than filamentous fungi and are seen in compromised corneas with multiple predisposing alterations in host defenses; many of these patients are immunocompromised. Any cornea with a chronic ulcer is prone to infection by this organism; exposure to vegetable matter and outdoor trauma are not inciting factors, as they are in filamentous fungal keratitis. *Candida* endophthalmitis can be seen as an endogenous infection in previously ill patients undergoing hyperalimentation, and the organism may secondarily infect the cornea.[42]

In fungal keratitis, the inflammatory reaction results from replicating and nonreplicating fungi, mycotoxins, proteolytic enzymes, and soluble fungal antigens.[43] Filamentous fungi proliferate within the corneal stroma without the release of the chemotactic substances that usually act to limit corneal damage.[28] The host response releases lysosomal substances from polymorphonuclear leukocytes, which contribute to the stromal destruction. The destructive potential of fungi ranges from the rapidly destructive *Fusarium* to the less virulent *Acremonium, Pseudallescheria, Aspergillus,* and *Penicillium,* and the more indolent *Bipolaris, Exserohilum,* and *Phialophora.* More than 200 mycotoxins from 50 genera of saprophytic filamentous fungi and yeasts have been isolated. These mycotoxins are primarily aflatoxins, trichothecenes, and zearalenones.[44] The pathogenicity of *C. albicans* may be the result of a proteolytic enzyme and lipase that cause lysis of host tissue[45] or the inhibitory substances in the cell wall that prevent the contact of neutrophils.[46] The virulence of yeasts also relates to their ability to transform from a blastoconidial to a pseudohyphal phase. *Aspergillus, F. solani, Acremonium,* and *Lasiodiplodia theobromae* produce enzymes that cause corneal destruction. The toxicity of *Fusarium* is related to its mycotoxin and its ability to replicate at 35°C. Hyphae tend to multiply extensively without inducing much cellular infiltration. The large size of the pseudohyphae of yeasts and the true hyphae of filamentous fungi precludes ingestion by neutrophils. Although Descemet's membrane is usually impermeable to bacteria, fungi can penetrate stromal lamellae, attack Descemet's membrane, and spread into the anterior chamber. *Fusarium* has a predilection for the posterior chamber, with accumulation around the

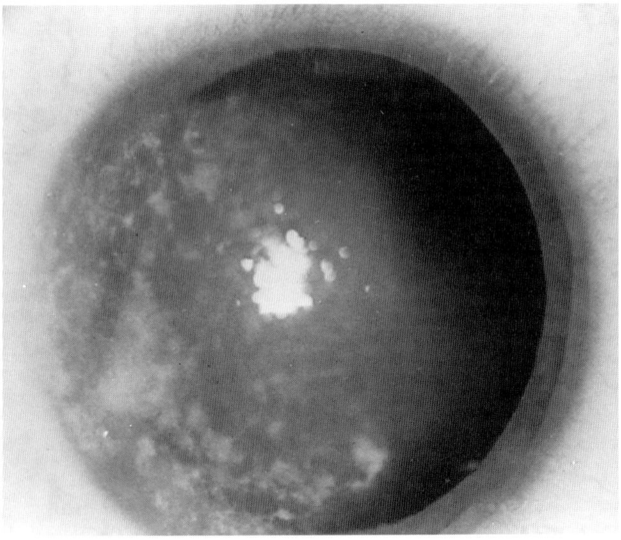

FIGURE 9-1 *Fusarium solani* keratitis in a young agricultural worker from south Florida. The epithelium is elevated and intact. There are coarse, granular infiltrates within the anterior stroma.

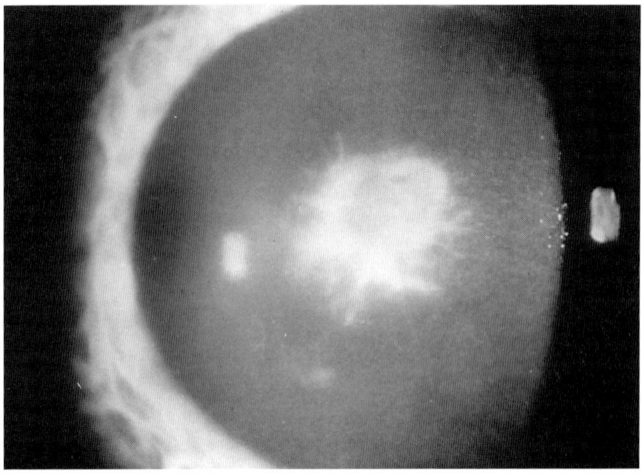

FIGURE 9-2 *Alternaria* keratitis in a farmer from rural Minnesota. Note the feathery branching hyphal infiltrates.

lens and seclusion of the pupil, which results in shallowing of the anterior chamber and severe fungal glaucoma.[47]

Under normal experimental conditions, saprophytic fungi are destroyed by humoral and cellular host defense mechanisms, and a large number of spores of *Aspergillus* and *Fusarium* generally produce only a mild keratitis.[44] However, when corticosteroids or immunosuppressive agents are given, the invasive ability of fungi is enhanced.[48] Nevertheless, corticosteroids are not a prerequisite in the pathogenesis of fungal keratitis.

Fungal keratitis is only occasionally associated with contact lens wear and represents 3 to 12 percent of infections associated with contact lenses.[28] Filamentous fungi are more likely associated with cosmetic or aphakic contact lenses, whereas yeasts are more frequently associated with bandage soft contact lenses.[49] Fungal growth is seen in about 14 percent of contact lens care systems,[50,51] and soft contact lenses themselves can be contaminated with fungi.[52,53] Neither heat nor chemical sterilization of contact lenses can completely protect against fungal or bacterial spoilage.

CLINICAL FEATURES

The salient clinical features of filamentous fungal keratitis were described in 1965.[54] The classic features may occur only in certain stages of keratitis caused by specific filamentous fungi. Although the disease process may be indolent, it frequently manifests within 24 to 36 hours following trauma, as in bacterial keratitis. The early biomicroscopic features consist of fine or coarse granular infiltrates within the epithelium and anterior stroma, with minimal cellular reaction. The epithelial surface has a dry, rough texture, and dirty, gray-white color (Figure 9-1). The epithelium may be elevated and intact, or occasionally, it may be ulcerated. The lack of marked stromal inflammation may permit direct visualization of pigment and delicate, feathery, branching hyphae with surrounding stromal infiltrates (Figure 9-2). Mild inflammation may contribute to the irregular edges of the feathery infiltrates. Concomitant use of corticosteroids may suppress the reaction and disclose the visible fungal elements. There may be multifocal suppurative microabscesses or satellite lesions (Figure 9-3). Occasionally, pigmentation in the ulcer bed is seen in dematiaceous fungal keratitis.[55]

A white ring in the cornea is frequently present, and presumably represents a toxic fungal diffusate or the junction and interaction of fungal antigen and host antibody (Figure 9-4). Other signs, such as conjunctival hyperemia, anterior chamber inflammation, hypopyon, and endothelial plaque, usually parallel the size and density of the lesion, but purulent discharge is generally absent. Mild iritis tends to occur early, but an endothelial plaque and hypopyon generally take several days to develop. Dense fibrinous material adheres to the endothelium and collects in the anterior chamber angle and over the surface of the iris. With advanced disease, the entire cornea becomes homogeneously yel-

FIGURE 9-3 Fungal keratitis with multiple satellite lesions.

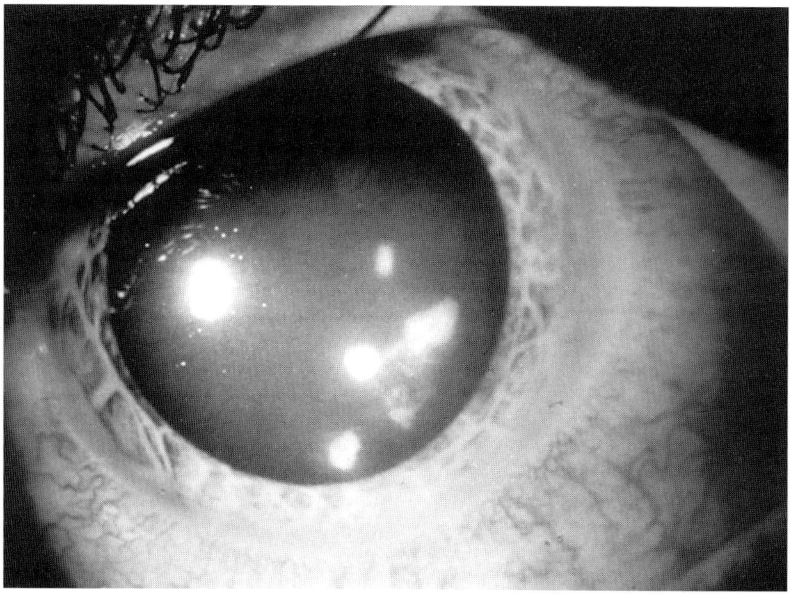

low-white, and can resemble any severe microbial keratitis. Stromal ulceration and necrosis can lead to perforation and endophthalmitis, particularly with *F. solani* keratitis associated with inappropriate use of topical corticosteroids. *Acremonium* can produce proteolytic enzymes and cause dense suppuration. The remainder of the filamentous fungi produce no distinctive features.

Satellite lesions, corneal rings, and endothelial plaques are less specific signs for fungal keratitis than the characteristic stromal infiltrates with feathery hyphate edges and the dry, gray, elevated epithelial surface. The condition most often mistaken for fungal keratitis is herpes simplex viral keratitis.[56] Conversely, fungal keratitis may mimic a number of other corneal diseases, which can lead to worsening of the infection with inappropriate corticosteroid therapy.

Yeast keratitis occurs in a different clinical setting. These patients have pre-existing ocular inflammatory disease or severe alterations in ocular structures. Trauma alone is rarely the initiating event. Yeast keratitis occurs in association with systemic diseases, such as Sjögren's syndrome, erythema multiforme, IgA deficiency, cell-mediated immune deficiency, human immunodeficiency virus infection, and endocrinopathies.[31] In contrast to filamentous fungal keratitis, yeast keratitis most often causes a small oval ulceration with an expanding, discrete, sharply demarcated, dense yellow-white stromal

FIGURE 9-4 Slit beam view of deep *Paecilomyces* keratitis with an adjacent white ring (arrows).

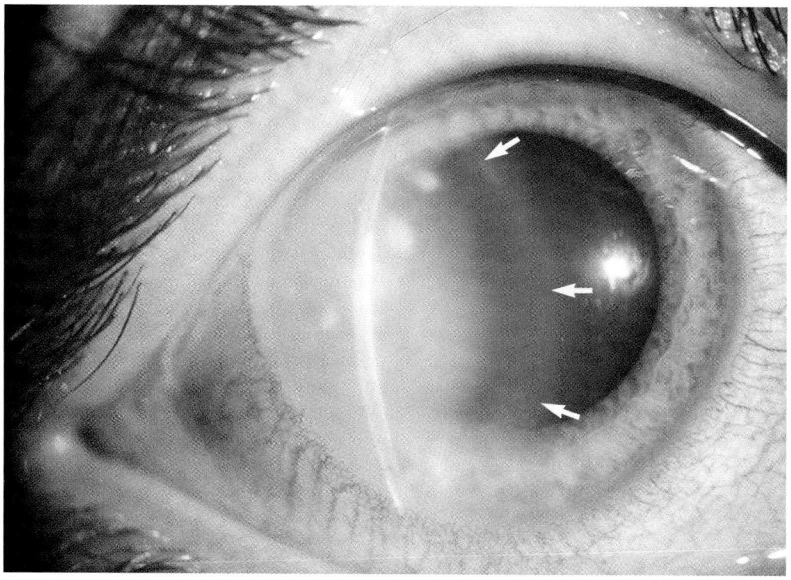

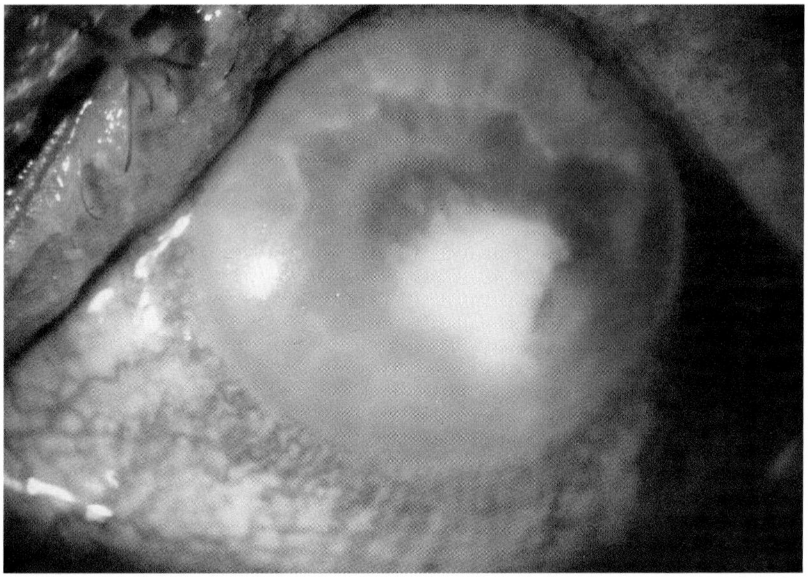

FIGURE 9-5 *Candida albicans* keratitis in a patient with immune suppression and thymoma. The dense yellow-white stromal infiltrate more closely resembles bacterial keratitis than fungal keratitis. There is a small hypopyon.

suppuration that lacks the delicate features of filamentous organisms (Figure 9-5). Frequently, there is a wide perimeter of stromal inflammation and edema, and fungal elements cannot be seen on slit lamp examination. Yeast keratitis resembles a gram-positive bacterial keratitis, such as *Staphylococcus aureus* or *Streptococcus pneumoniae* keratitis. Severe and chronic yeast keratitis may develop wet, necrotic stromal inflammation with features indistinguishable from those of other forms of microbial keratitis. Occasionally, the clinical picture can resemble that of infectious crystalline keratopathy.[57,58] The use of in vivo real time confocal microscopy for early detection of fungal keratitis is a novel investigatory procedure.[59-63] Confocal microscopy can differentiate fungal keratitis from other forms of microbial keratitis. In addition, it can differentiate filamentous keratitis from yeast keratitis.[60] Filamentous fungi appear to traverse the cornea in a plane that corresponds to the horizontal lamellae of the stroma, and can be observed within the cornea as multiple, linear, branching structures (Figure 9-6). Budding yeast grows in a plane perpendicular to the stromal lamellae and the surface of the cornea, and the confocal appearance is that of multiple, round, hyperreflective points scattered throughout the field.

HISTOPATHOLOGY

In filamentous fungal keratitis, the organism enters the corneal stroma at the time of the injury with vegetable matter. The fungi multiply by hyphal extension, with orientation parallel to the corneal lamellae[64,65] (Figure 9-7). They maintain this orientation as they extend deeper into the corneal stroma. The epithelium covers the defect, but is irregular. Often, fungi are absent from the superficial stroma of histopathologic specimens, which may explain the failure of scrapings to recover organisms and the failure of antifungal agents to effect a cure.

Limbal infiltration with round cells and plasma cells increases as the keratitis progresses, and a partial or complete ring abscess forms. Inflammatory cells migrate around the organisms and into the anterior chamber. A coagulative necrosis of the stroma develops, with loss of keratocytes and edema of the surrounding collagen fibrils. Satellite lesions, consisting of microabscesses, develop separately from the main lesion. Replicating or nonreplicating fungi, mycotoxins, proteolytic enzymes, and soluble fungal antigens contribute to stromal necrosis, inflammation, hypopyon formation, and corneal ring formation. Fungi can easily penetrate an intact Descemet's membrane,[64] and clinically can be seen waving in the anterior chamber from the back of Descemet's membrane (Figure 9-8). *F. solani* frequently invades the posterior chamber as well.

The histopathologic picture of fungal keratitis differs from that of bacterial keratitis in that the purulent inflammatory reaction is less marked, the periphery of the cornea is less likely to be involved, and a hypopyon is more often present.

If antifungal therapy has been successful in preventing further multiplication, the host defenses slowly aid in removing large fungal fragments from the corneal substance. The large size of these fragments precludes easy phagocytosis. There may be progressive inflammation,

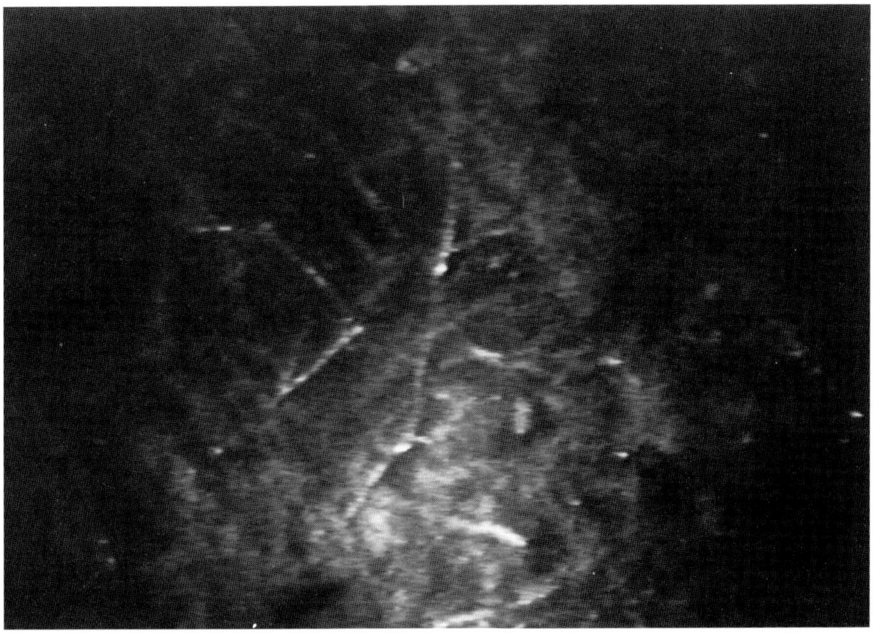

FIGURE 9-6 *Aspergillus fumigatus* fungal keratitis. Confocal micrograph shows multiple, fine, branching filaments within the disrupted corneal stroma. (Original magnification × 230.) (Courtesy of Stephen C. Kaufman, M.D., New Orleans, LA.)

necrosis, and ulceration in the absence of viable organisms, which is presumably secondary to immune mechanisms or persistent mycotoxins. A lamellar keratectomy, conjunctival flap, or penetrating keratoplasty may be required to terminate the process.[66]

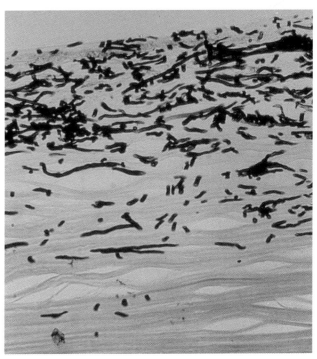

FIGURE 9-7 Gomori methenamine silver stain of fungal keratitis displaying the extensive hyphae in the anterior stroma lying parallel to the corneal lamellae.

LABORATORY TECHNIQUES

Stains

Cytologic or histologic confirmation of fungal keratitis is extremely important.[67] Because fungal infections are usually within the stroma, the use of calcium alginate swabs with trypticase soy broth is probably not adequate for obtaining specimens.[68] A vigorous scraping combined with special stains is generally necessary, but if these are not positive, a corneal biopsy should be done to confirm the diagnosis before therapy is begun.[69] If fungal keratitis is suspected, corneal smears are examined for yeasts, pseudohyphae, and hyphae. (Techniques for obtaining material for smears are discussed in Ch. 8.) Gram and Giemsa stains do not stain the cell wall or septa of fungal hyphae, but are absorbed by the protoplasm of filamentous fungi (Figure 9-9). However, the staining characteristics of the hyphae are inconsistent and nonspecific. High dry magnification is sufficient to detect fungal organisms; oil immersion is not necessary. The elements that allow specific classification of fungi are rarely present in corneal smears. Small hyphae branching at 45 degrees with distinct cross septa are characteristic of *Aspergillus* species. These need to be distinguished from the

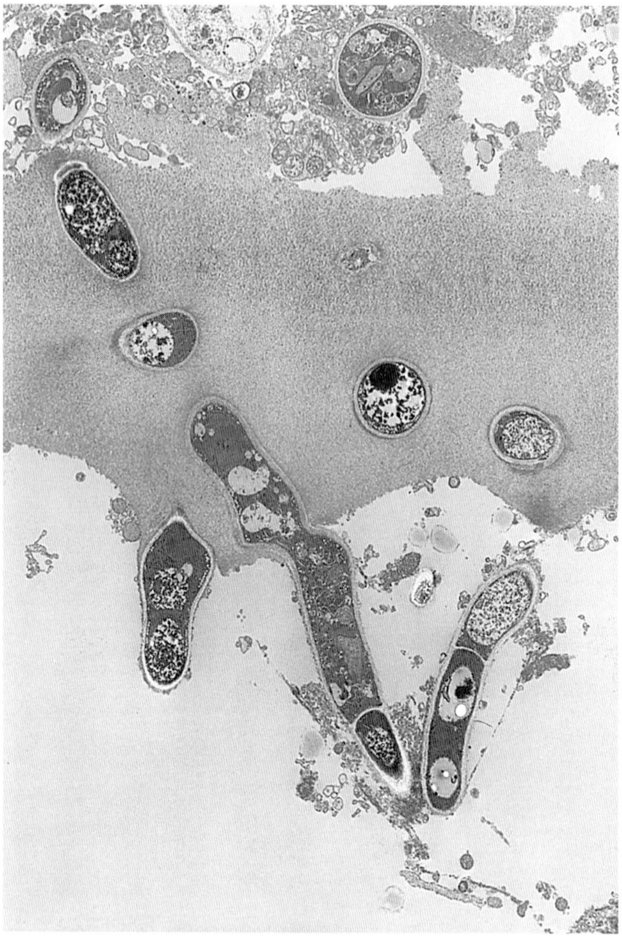

FIGURE 9-8 Transmission electron micrograph of fungi penetrating Descemet's membrane into the anterior chamber in a case of *Paecilomyces* keratitis unresponsive to medical therapy. (Courtesy of Bruce Barron, M.D., New Orleans, LA.)

delicate branching filaments of the bacterium *Nocardia,* which is gram-positive and partially acid fast. Yeasts typically stain dark blue and may have forms that allow specific identification. *Candida* shows yeast forms, with budding characteristically off the main axis of the parent cell, and also pseudohyphal forms, with elongated buds strung together in chains that resemble septate hyphae.

In one series, the hyphal fragments of filamentous fungi or the blastoconidia and pseudohyphae of yeast were detected by Gram or Giemsa stain in 75 percent of cases of fungal keratitis.[70] In another series of 133 fungal ulcers, fungal elements were seen by Giemsa stain 66 percent of the time and by Gram stain 55 percent of the time.[1] A more recent series reported fungal elements seen by Giemsa stain 27 percent of the time and by Gram stain 33 percent of the time in patients with culture-positive fungal keratitis.[5] There is probably no difference in the accuracy between Gram and Giemsa stains for the detection of fungi; multiple sampling is the most important factor in the detection of fungal elements. Yeasts can grow in neglected gentian violet used in Gram stain, which can lead to false-positive identification of yeasts in corneal smears and a misdiagnosis.

The wet mount potassium hydroxide (KOH) procedure has been largely abandoned, although it proved to be more effective than fungal cultures in identifying fungal elements in one study from India.[71] Lactophenol cotton blue mounts have also been accurate in another study from India.[72] An ink-potassium hydroxide preparation (nine parts 10 percent potassium hydroxide and one part ink) is effective in distinguishing fungal elements[73] (Figure 9-10). Calcofluor white, a fluorescent dye used to enhance the brightness of fabrics, has an affinity for several β-linked polysaccharide polymers, such as cellu-

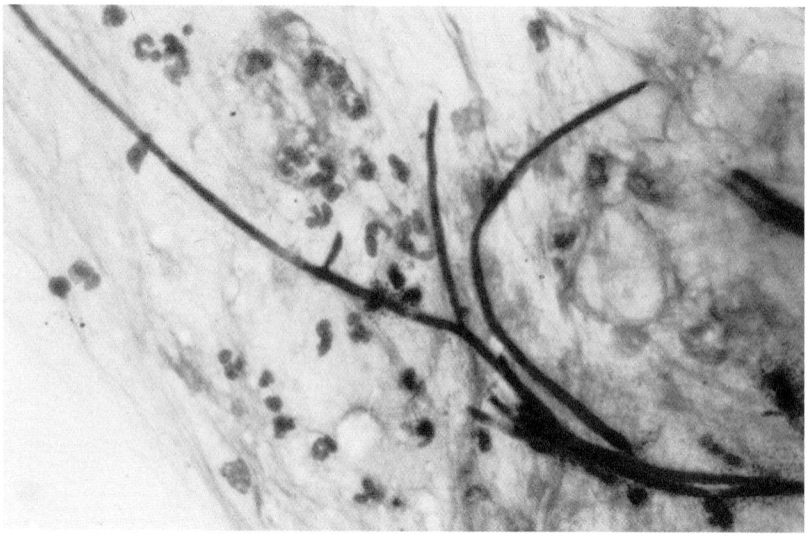

FIGURE 9-9 Gram stain of a corneal smear from a patient with *Fusarium solani* keratitis. Large, branching, septate hyphal fragments are easily identified with high dry magnification.

FIGURE 9-10 Ink-potassium hydroxide stain demonstrating hyphal elements of *Aspergillus*. (Courtesy of Robert Arffa, M.D., Pittsburgh, PA.)

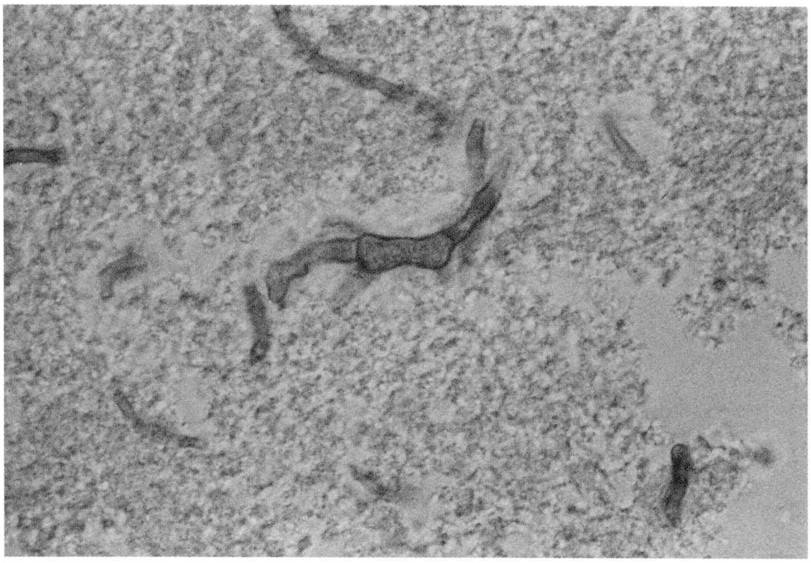

lose and chitin, both present in fungal cell walls. Calcofluor white is used to detect filamentous fungi, yeasts, and *Acanthamoeba* cysts in corneal smears and tissue sections. When Evans blue is used as a counterstain and the specimen is viewed with a fluorescence microscope, these organisms appear as bright apple-green against an orange background[74] (Figure 9-11). Some fungal organisms, such as *Candida* and *Aspergillus,* exhibit autofluorescence when examined with ultraviolet light. This property usually persists even if the specimen has undergone fixation, paraffin embedding, and staining with hematoxylin and eosin.[75]

Lectins, ubiquitous proteins found predominantly in plant seeds, have the unique property of binding specifically to carbohydrate groups. When conjugated with fluorescein, they can be seen with a fluorescence microscope. Lectins bind to the cell walls of filamentous fungi, yeasts, and atypical mycobacteria, and also to the cysts and trophozoites of *Acanthamoeba.*[76-78] Selective staining with different fluorescein-conjugated lectins permits a more specific diagnosis.[76] *Fusarium* and *Aspergillus* are preferentially stained with wheat germ agglutinin, *Candida, Aspergillus,* and *Fusarium* with concanavalin-A, and *Candida* with lens cutinaris agglutinin.

A modification of the Gomori methenamine silver (GMS) stain is the most specific tissue stain for the identification of fungal elements.[79] The test is run with controls and requires 2 to 3 hours for processing. Chromic acid oxidizes polysaccharides in the cell walls of fungi to aldehydes, which reduce methenamine silver to metallic silver, and appear black. The black cell walls and septa of fungi are easily recognized against the light green counterstain (Figure 9-12). Ideally, corneal scrapings should be smeared on gelatin-coated slides for this technique. In one series of fungal keratitis, the Gomori methenamine silver stain was more accurate than Gram or Giemsa stain in detection of fungal elements.[1] Equivocal Gram- or Giemsa-stained specimens can be restained by the Gomori methenamine silver technique.

Periodic acid-Schiff (PAS) stain is similarly helpful for the identification of fungal elements. Periodic acid oxidizes fungal cell wall polysaccharides to aldehydes, which are subsequently colored red by the Schiff reagent. Fungal hyphae stain bright red (Figure 9-13). The genus or species is difficult to identify in histopathologic tissue, although *Candida* can frequently be distinguished by the simultaneous presence of yeast cells and pseudohyphae (Figure 9-14).

The acridine fluorescence technique has been effective in detecting filamentous fungi.[80,81] Acridine orange dye binds to the DNA of fungi and is more sensitive than Gram stain in detecting microorganisms in clinical specimens.[28,82] With a fluorescence microscope, the fungi appear brilliant yellow-orange against a dark background.

Cultures

The appropriate culture media for suspected fungal keratitis are addressed in Chapter 8. The majority of fungi that infect the cornea grow within 3 days,[1,5,83] but it is not unusual for them to take 5 to 7 days to grow, and up to one-fourth of all fungi may not grow until after more than 14 days.[84] Therefore, cultures should be kept for 3 weeks. Sabouraud agar with gentamicin and without cyclohex-

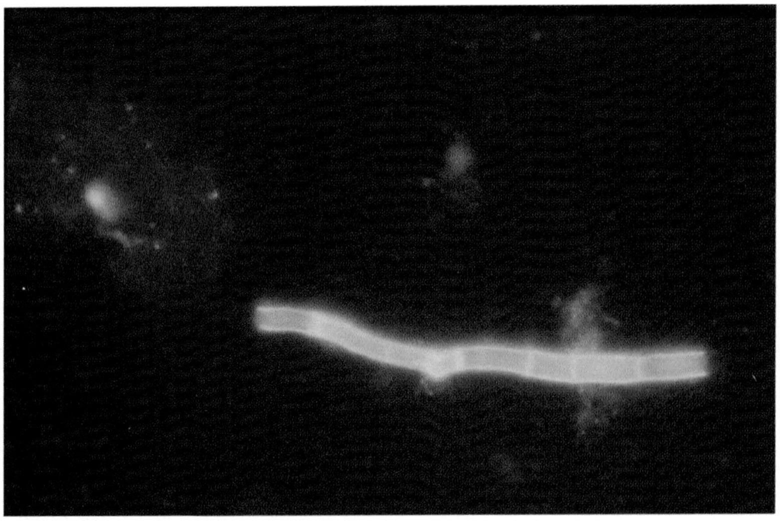

FIGURE 9-11 A calcofluor white-stained hyphal fragment confirming a septate filamentous fungal keratitis.

imide incubated at room temperature is the most sensitive medium for the isolation of ocular fungi. Most filamentous fungal pathogens and virtually all *Candida* species grow on blood agar at 35°C, but Sabouraud agar at room temperature enhances the isolation of less thermophilic organisms. In one series, sheep or rabbit blood agar and Sabouraud agar at room temperature produced comparable frequencies of isolation of filamentous fungi and yeasts; blood agar supported growth 71 percent of the time and Sabouraud agar 79 percent of the time.[1] In the same series, brain-heart infusion (BHI) broth demonstrated growth 55 percent of the time. Others report that this broth is the most reliable medium for the isolation of ocular fungi.[85] A slower growth of fungi from eye cultures was reported from a Tennessee study,[84] in contrast to a series from south Florida.[1] The reason for these regional differences is not clear.

C. albicans grows readily as smooth flat colonies that are pasty and milky white, and resemble bacterial colonies, especially at 35°C (Figure 9-15). The colonies of other *Candida* species appear beige, but all have a yeast-like odor. Several methods are used to identify *C.*

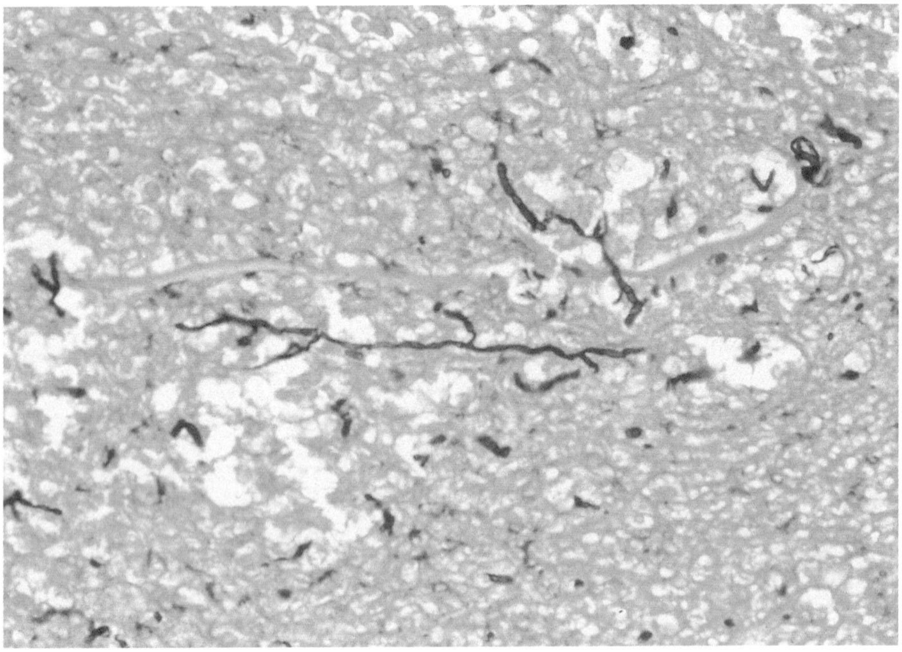

FIGURE 9-12 Gomori methenamine silver stain of a corneal transplant specimen from a patient with *Paecilomyces* keratitis. Fungal hyphae appear black.

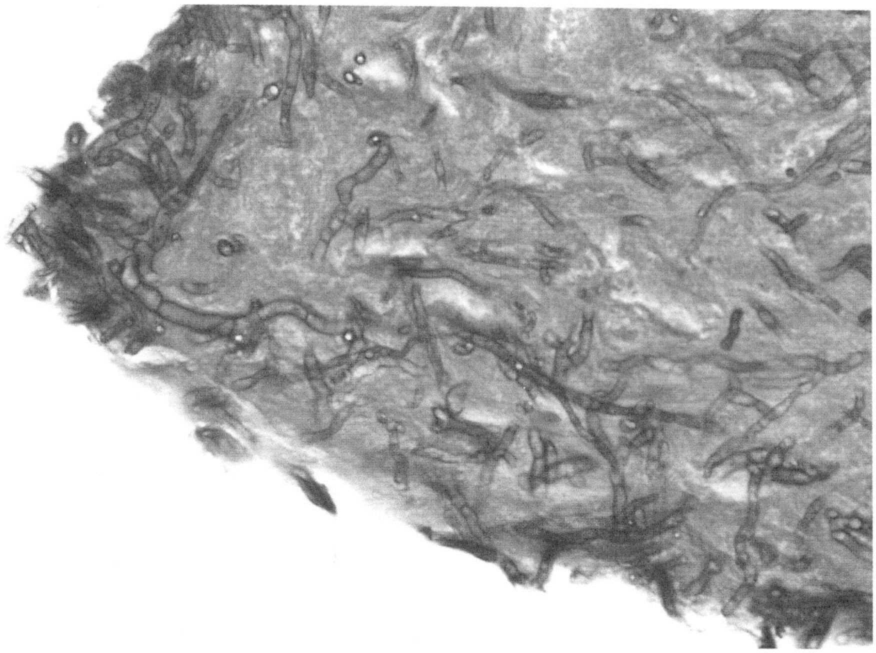

FIGURE 9-13 Periodic acid–Schiff stain of a corneal biopsy specimen from a patient with *Curvularia* keratitis. The septate hyphae are easily seen.

albicans: the germ tube test, the production of chlamydospores on cornmeal agar, the demonstration of spider-like colonies of organisms on eosin-methylene blue agar, or the use of packaged tests with basic biochemical procedures.[9]

Filamentous fungi appear as aerial fluffy colonies on solid media and as a feathery mycelium in liquid media (Figures 9-16 and 9-17). Some colonies are pigmented, especially on the undersurface of the colony (reverse pigmentation), which helps in identification. *Fusarium* is white in its early stages but acquires a buff color as the colony matures. *Aspergillus fumigatus* is white initially but later turns velvety green. *Aspergillus niger* is white but turns black as sporulation begins (Figure 9-18). *Acremonium* is compact early, but later develops a typical woolly appearance.

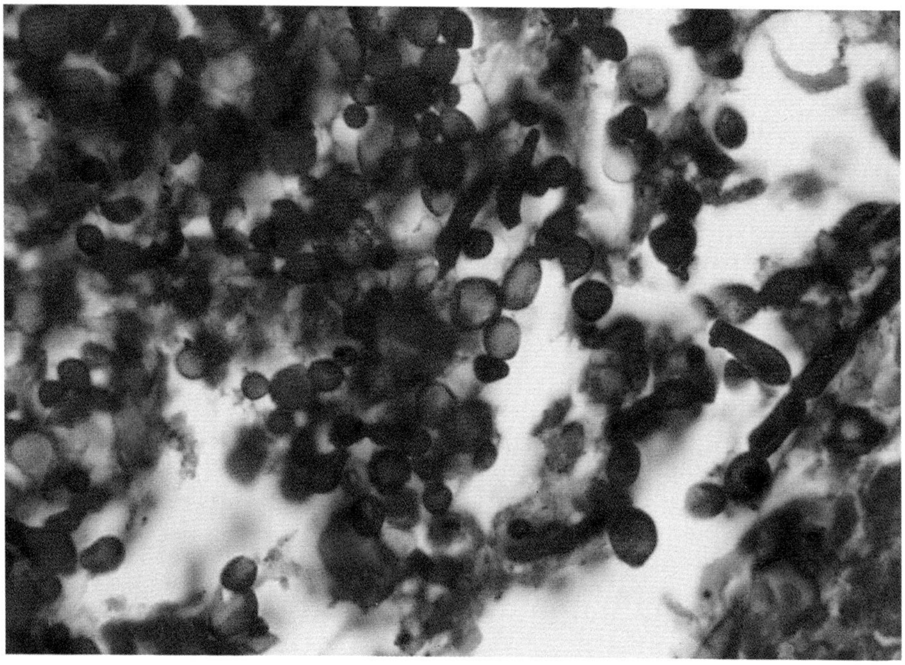

FIGURE 9-14 Periodic acid–Schiff stain of a smear of a corneal abscess caused by *Candida albicans* demonstrating budding yeasts.

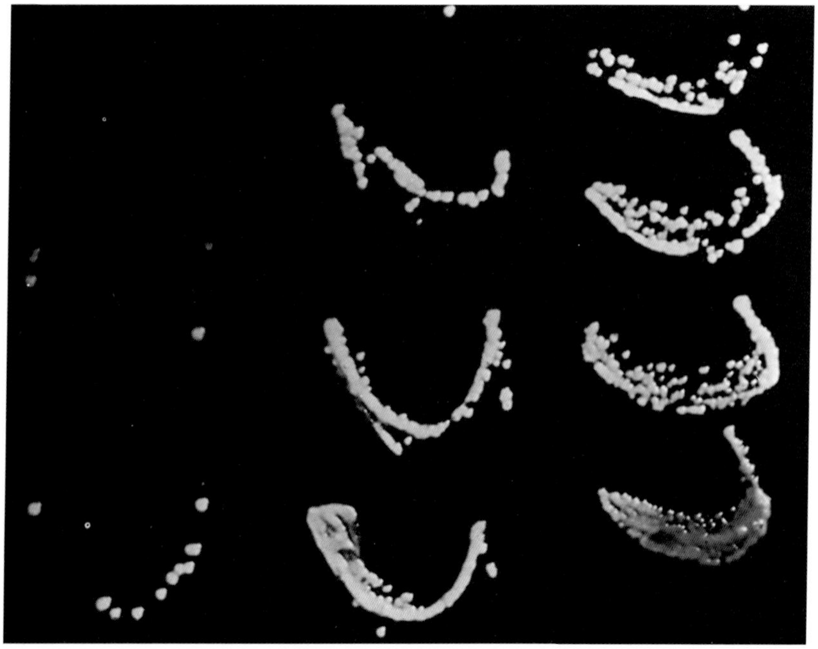

FIGURE 9-15 Blood agar plate incubated at 35°C. *Candida albicans* was isolated from each of three rows of C streaks within 48 hours after plating from a corneal scraping. Colonies are white, smooth, domed, shiny, and moist.

The microscopic morphology, surface texture, color, growth rate, and pigmentation on the reverse side are the initial identifying features for fungi (Figure 9-19). Once fungal growth has appeared on the primary isolation medium, colonies should be subcultured promptly to fresh medium for isolation and identification in pure culture and for preservation as a stock culture before mutation occurs. For specific identification it is necessary to induce a fungus to display characteristic conidia, sporangiospores, or other elements by the use of a special medium or growth conditions.[86-88] Potato dextrose agar, cornmeal agar, Czapek-Dox agar, and other special media are used.[89] A cellophane tape slide mount made directly from the sporulating culture, stained with a drop of lactophenol cotton blue and examined under the microscope, can show identifying fungal elements, especially conidia morphology.[9] *Fusarium* species are characterized by distinctive, large, banana-shaped conidia, which are produced on short lateral hyphae or conidiophores (Figure 9-20). *Aspergillus* has a conidiophore with a swollen terminal end (vesicle) surrounded by flask-shaped phialids; it also has dichotomous branching (Figure 9-21). *Acremonium* produces only conidiophores. *Penicillium* has brush-like (penicillate) conidiophores (Figure 9-22). Similar laboratory findings are found with *Paecilomyces*. *Curvularia* has multiseptate conidia that are characteristically curved (Figure 9-23). *Bipolaris* has cylindrical multiseptate conidia (Figure 9-24). Incubation of yeast cells permits observation of germ tube production *(C. albicans)* or detection of a pseudomycelium, a true mycelium, chlamydospores, or ascospores characteristic of various species. Reserve cultures (consisting of conidia suspended in skim milk) may be maintained by lyophilization or storage at −70°C to prevent mutation.[87]

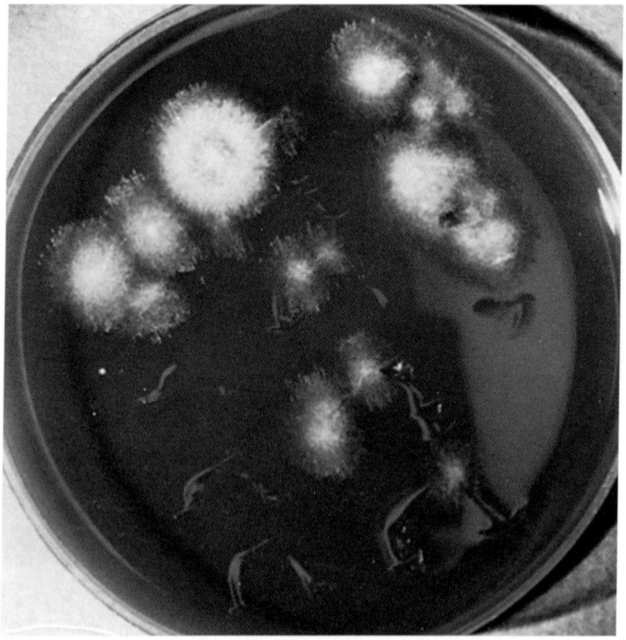

FIGURE 9-16 Fluffy mycelial colonies of *Fusarium solani* isolated from several C streaks on a blood agar plate incubated at 25°C (room temperature) for 2 days.

Fungi can also be identified by biochemical tests, immunodiffusion, counterimmunoelectrophoresis, latex

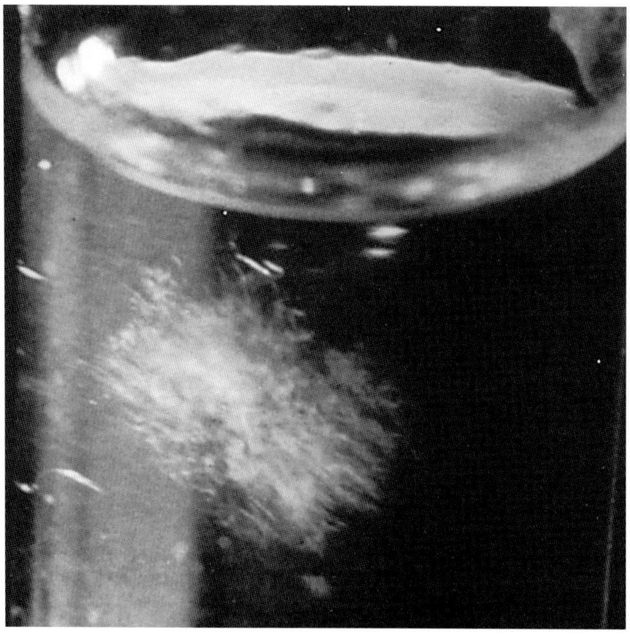

FIGURE 9-17 Feathery mycelium within thioglycolate broth after 3 days incubation at 35°C from a corneal scraping of a patient with *Fusarium solani* keratitis.

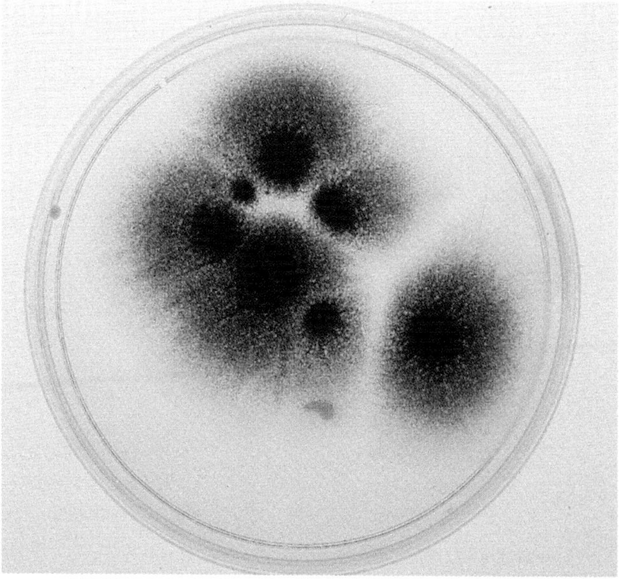

FIGURE 9-18 Fluffy mycelial colonies of *Aspergillus niger* that were originally white and turned black, which is characteristic of aged colonies.

agglutination, crossed electrophoresis, and enzyme-linked immunosorbent assays (ELISA).[89]

TREATMENT

Antifungal Agents

In corneal tissue, yeasts and filamentous fungi are present only in filamentous (hyphal) form. The fungal cell membrane acts as a barrier, modulates electrolyte and solute exchange, controls homeostasis of the fungal cell, and is the site of antifungal therapy. The ergosterol in the cell membrane is unique to fungi and is the site of action of most antifungal agents. Although many antifungal agents have been isolated or synthesized, none of the presently available agents has the features of an ideal drug, which are broad spectrum of action, minimal propensity to cause development of resistant organisms, high solubility in effective vehicles of delivery, stability in solution, effective penetration into the eye, and lack of local or systemic toxicity.[90,91] Present antifungals generally have poor solubility, low potency, restrictive pharmacokinetic properties, noticeable variability between the in vitro sensitivity pattern and the in vivo effect, marked potential for the development of resistant organisms, and a tendency to be toxic at therapeutic concentrations. The development of oral antifungal agents has aided the therapy of fungal keratitis; nevertheless, the best that can be accomplished with the present agents is the inhibition of fungal growth by long-term administration of effective nontoxic agents to allow host defense mechanisms to eradicate the infection. Invariably, prolonged treatment (6 weeks to 3 months) is needed for fungal keratitis.

The most important antifungal agents are the polyene and azole compounds, which affect the cell membrane of fungi, and the pyrimidines, which interfere with fungal protein synthesis[92] (Table 9-2). Most clinical experience has been with the polyene antifungals; the evidence for efficacy of the azole compounds is based on in vitro sensitivity determinations[23] and is now accumulating in case reports and series. Combinations of polyenes, azoles, and pyrimidines have been additive when tested in vitro, except for the polyenes and azoles, which appear to be antagonistic.[23] Clinical reports and in vitro studies substantiate the concept that fungi resemble bacteria in their varied sensitivity to agents within the genus and species, but the relationship is more complex.[93,94] Antifungal sensitivity testing has not been standardized and remains clinically unreliable. Results of in vitro data on minimal inhibitory concentrations should be interpreted with caution because these values vary with the type and the pH of the medium and the size of the inoculum. Animal models of fungal keratitis have been difficult to establish and to reproduce

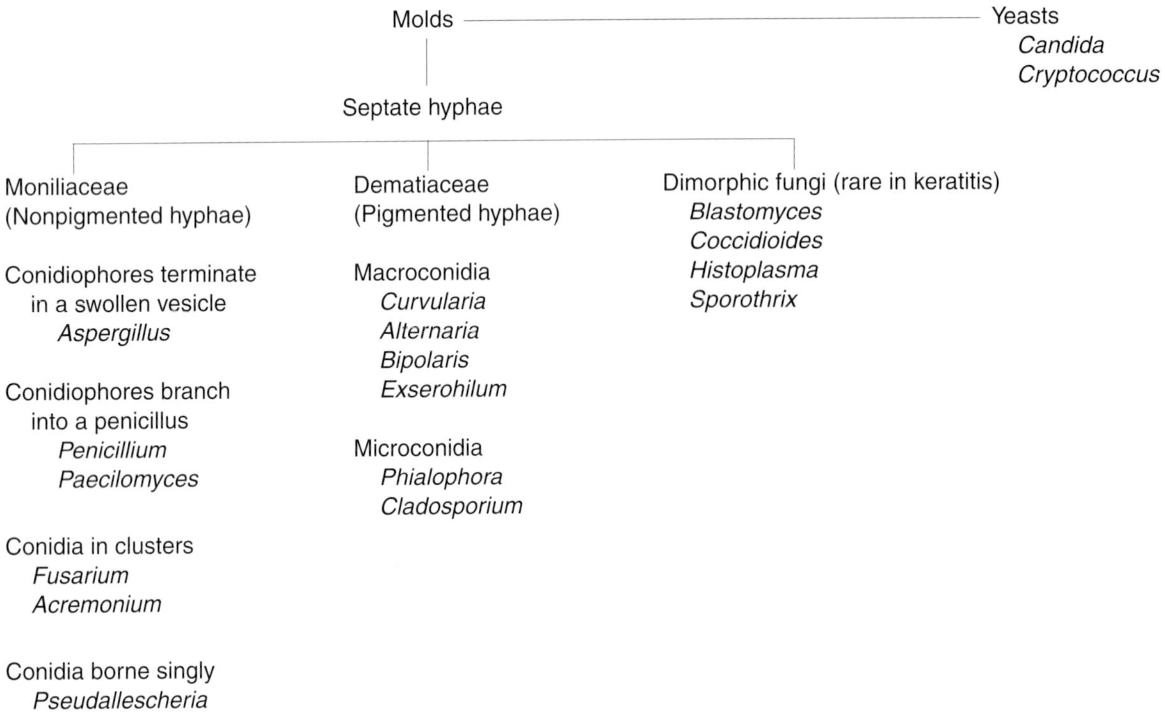

FIGURE 9-19 Flow chart for the identification of fungi important in keratitis.

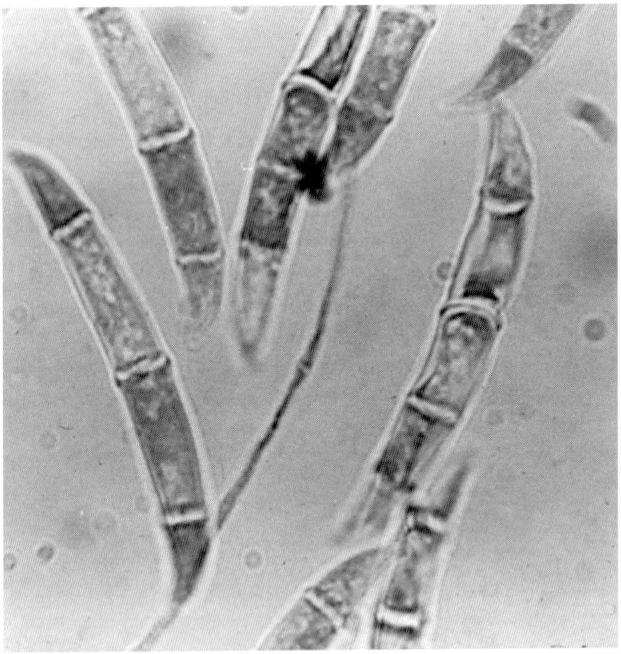

FIGURE 9-20 Lactophenol cotton blue stain of a cellophane mount demonstrating the banana-like conidia of *Fusarium solani.*

reliably, which has hampered the investigation of effective agents.[95] Ideally, decisions would be made based on drug properties, in vitro sensitivity testing, findings in animal models of fungal keratitis, and the results of clinical trials, but firm data are lacking. Except for natamycin, topical ophthalmic antifungal agents are not yet available commercially, so the physician must prepare topical preparations from systemic compounds. The topical drugs are generally administered every hour over the first 2 days. Collagen shields soaked in amphotericin B have been an effective treatment for *Candida* keratitis in rabbits.[96]

Polyenes

The polyenes were isolated from various species of *Streptomyces* and demonstrate the greatest antifungal activity against filamentous fungi and yeasts in vitro. They have a complex molecular structure consisting of a large conjugated system in a lactose ring linked to mycosamine, an amino acid sugar. They are classified according to the number of double bonds. The major drugs in this group are the large polyenes (nystatin and amphotericin B) and the small polyenes (natamycin). Polyenes bind to the ergosterol moiety in the cell membranes of sensitive fungi and produce an osmotic pressure change and electrolyte imbalance (reversible or irreversible) in the cell.[97] They have no effect on cell membranes that lack sterols. The large polyenes form narrow circular channels in the cell membrane that allow the passage of ions, which ultimately leads to a reversible electrolyte imbalance. The small polyenes accumulate in the cell membrane and irreversibly disrupt the membrane.[83] In general, these agents are highly insoluble in water, some are unstable, and many irritate the eye. They penetrate poorly into ocular tissues. Systemic toxicity is related to the sterol moiety binding to renal tubular cells and erythrocytes. Clinically tested polyenes are nystatin, amphotericin A and B, natamycin, candicidin, hamycin, trichomycin, dermostatin, endomycin, and lucimycin.

Nystatin was one of the first antifungal drugs, but has only superficial activity in vivo and is no longer used. It is less effective than amphotericin B against *Candida* and other filamentous fungi.

Amphotericin B is a haptene polyene that is insoluble in water, unstable at 37°C, and degrades rapidly when exposed to light. It was first isolated from a soil actinomycete, *Streptomyces nodosus,* and became available as a colloidal suspension with deoxycholate added as a stabilizing agent. It is active against *Candida, Cryptococcus,* and *Aspergillus,* and has variable activity against *Fusarium* and other filamentous fungi. Studies of experimental *C. albicans* keratitis have shown that topical amphotericin B in concentrations of 0.5 to 0.75 percent is superior in efficacy to 5 percent natamycin, 1 percent flucytosine, 1 percent miconazole, and 1 percent ketoconazole.[98] The development of resistance to amphotericin B is uncommon, but sensitivity to amphotericin B may vary.[99] Topical application causes punctate epithelial erosions and a greenish discoloration of the cornea. Subconjunctival

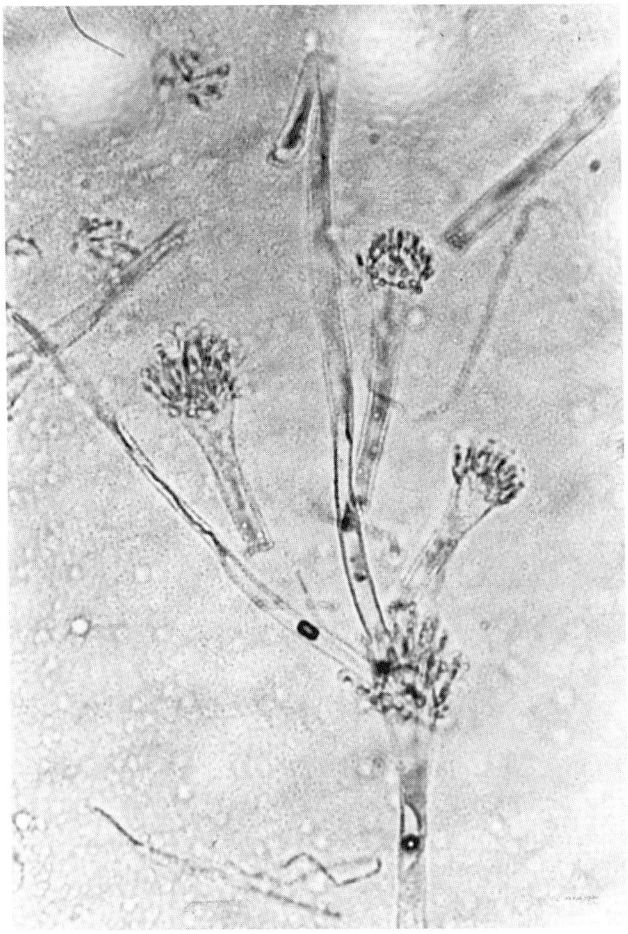

FIGURE 9-21 Lactophenol cotton blue stain of the conidiophores and conidia of *Aspergillus fumigatus.*

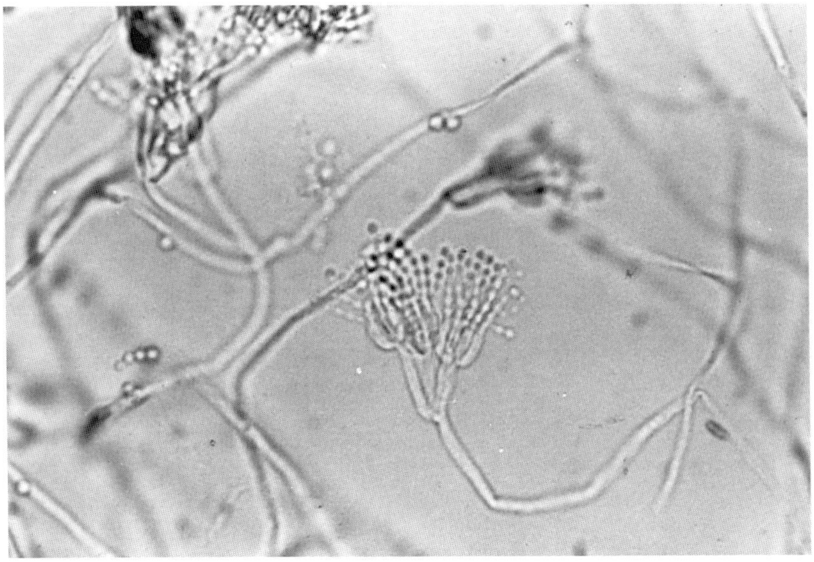

FIGURE 9-22 Lactophenol cotton blue stain of *Penicillium* demonstrating septate hyphae and conidiophores forming a characteristic brush-like flask.

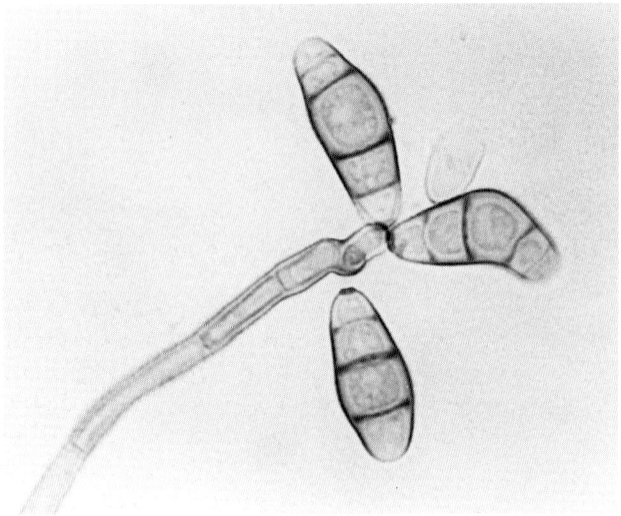

FIGURE 9-23 Lactophenol cotton blue stain of the characteristically curved multiseptate conidia of *Curvularia.*

TABLE 9-2
Antifungal Agents for Fungal Keratitis

Polyenes
Large polyenes
Nystatin
Amphotericin B
Amphotericin B methylester
Small polyenes
Natamycin
Azoles
Imidazoles
Miconazole
Ketoconazole
Clotrimazole
Econazole
Thiabendazole
Triazoles
Fluconazole
Itraconazole
Saperconazole
Pyrimidines
Flucytosine

amphotericin B in dosages as small as 0.1 mg causes transient conjunctival nodules, and permanent yellow discoloration of the conjunctiva may occur.[100] Topical 1 percent amphotericin B is more toxic than other antifungal agents,[101] although experience with 0.05 to 0.15 percent amphotericin B suggests that it is a well tolerated and effective antifungal agent.[94,98,102] There is some evidence that topical amphotericin B at a concentration of 0.15 percent can penetrate the deep cornea and aqueous of inflamed animal eyes and that epithelial debridement substantially improves corneal penetration. Although the optimal rate of administration is not known, animal experiments suggest that with very rapid administration (every 5 minutes for 1 hour), drug levels within the therapeutic range can be achieved rapidly in the cornea[103]; less frequent administration can then be used to maintain that level. Amphotericin B is available as a parenteral drug that also contains sodium deoxycholate and sodium buffer. The topical preparation is prepared by diluting the parenteral formulation with distilled water without a bacteriostatic agent; topical toxicity is partially related to the deoxycholate, which keeps the amphotericin B in colloidal suspension. There is

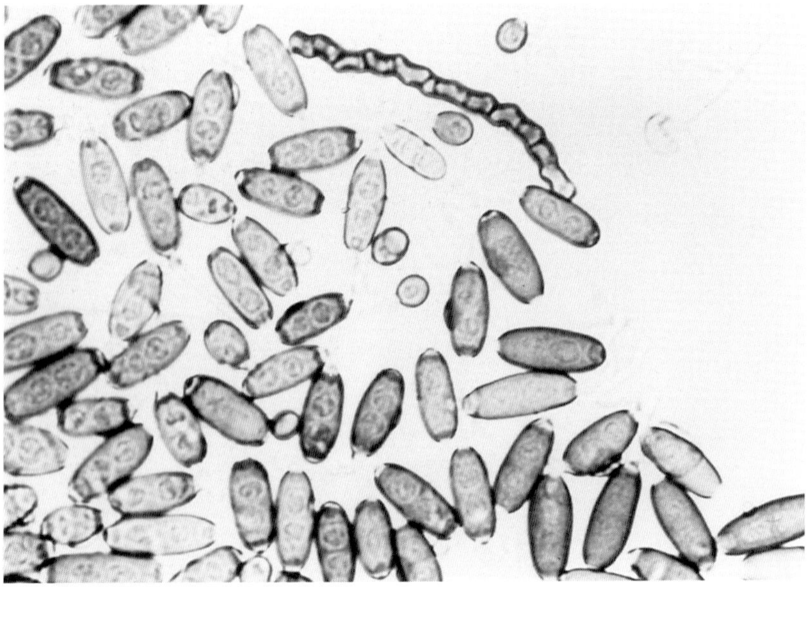

FIGURE 9-24 Cylindrical multiseptate conidia of *Bipolaris* with thickened cell walls after growth on potato dextrose agar.

a dose-related parenteral nephrotoxicity with amphotericin B, which may not be reversible. This toxicity is reduced by alternate-day intravenous administration. Intravenous amphotericin B for keratitis is generally not justified because of toxicity, limited intraocular penetration, and lack of in vivo effectiveness. If intravenous administration is used, however, the patient should be carefully monitored and the dosage increased slowly over the first few days according to a specific protocol.[104]

Although amphotericin B is highly effective in vitro, in an animal model of *Candida* keratitis,[98] and in some clinical infections,[102] these findings must be interpreted against the background of its previously poor clinical record against filamentous fungal keratitis, compared with natamycin.[105,106] Amphotericin B methylester may be as effective as amphotericin B, and may also be effective in deep stromal disease, once the epithelium is removed.[107] However, amphotericin B methylester has been withdrawn by the Food and Drug Administration because of central nervous system leukoencephalopathy that occurred with parenteral use.

Natamycin is a small tetraene polyene antibiotic that was isolated from a South African strain of *Streptomyces* in 1955. It is active in vitro against a variety of filamentous fungi (especially *Fusarium*) and yeasts. Natamycin irreversibly alters cell membranes. When introduced in the United States in 1968, it reversed the previously disastrous experience with *Fusarium* keratitis in south Florida,[105] and it has continued to be an effective preparation. It was successful as the initial treatment of 85 percent of cases caused by *F. solani,* 20 percent of cases caused by other nonpigmented fungi, 90 percent of cases caused by brown pigmented fungi, and 75 percent of cases caused by yeasts.[108] A 5 percent microfine suspension of natamycin is stable. It adheres to the surface of the ulcer and forms a rope-like strand in the inferior fornix, perhaps prolonging the contact time of the drug. It is relatively nonirritating and nontoxic to the cornea, but moderately severe conjunctival hyperemia, follicle formation, and persistent epithelial ulceration have been noted with prolonged use.[109] Although it has been considered to penetrate the cornea poorly, clinical effectiveness in extensive fungal keratitis suggests otherwise.[91] Tissue toxicity and the lack of absorption preclude its periocular or intravenous use.

On the basis of its broad spectrum of activity, lack of toxicity, and established efficacy against a variety of superficial corneal pathogens, natamycin is the preferred initial agent for the treatment of filamentous fungal keratitis.[27,56,105] It was approved by the Food and Drug Administration in 1979. Although the optimal dosing schedule is unknown, treatment is usually begun with application every 30 minutes followed by a tapering schedule after 3 to 4 days.[91] Treatment failures occur in filamentous fungal keratitis, even in some infections caused by *Fusarium* and *Aspergillus.* Yeasts are less sensitive to natamycin than are filamentous fungi.

Azoles

The azole compounds consist of the imidazoles and the triazoles. They contain a five-member azole ring that is attached by a carbon-nitrogen bond to the aromatic rings. The imidazoles affect the fungal cell membrane by inhibiting cytochrome enzymes and interfering with the synthesis of ergosterol and by binding to fatty acids,[110] which alter cell-membrane permeability. The imidazoles have a low solubility. Included in this group are thiabendazole, miconazole, clotrimazole, econazole, and ketoconazole.

Although thiabendazole is effective against *Fusarium, Aspergillus,* and other filamentous fungi, it is no longer used because it has been replaced by more effective agents.

Miconazole has a broad spectrum of activity against yeast and filamentous fungi. It is more effective than clotrimazole against *Fusarium,* although neither is very effective against this fungus. Topical application (10 mg/ml in arachis oil) or subconjunctival injection (5 to 10 mg) of the undiluted parenteral preparation is relatively well tolerated by the conjunctiva and cornea. Miconazole was approved by the Food and Drug Administration in 1978 as a parenteral agent for systemic candidiasis and other infections caused by susceptible fungi. Miconazole is used topically and subconjunctivally in superficial and deep keratitis caused by *C. albicans, Aspergillus,* and other fungal species that fail to respond to other therapy.[111] Definitive proof of its efficacy is not substantial, although laboratory data are accumulating.[112] Intravenous administration (30 mg/kg/day), although potentially toxic, produces inhibitory concentrations of the drug in the aqueous humor of inflamed eyes and may aid in treating fungal endophthalmitis that develops sequential to deep keratitis.[29,113] Oral ketoconazole and fluconazole offer just as effective in vitro activity as intravenous miconazole, and are preferred because of fewer serious adverse reactions.[28] In vitro data concerning potential enhanced therapeutic effectiveness of combined polyene (natamycin) and imidazole (e.g., miconazole) treatment are conflicting. Adverse reactions to intravenous miconazole include fever, chills, nausea, anorexia, anemia, altered sensorium, transient increase in serum lipids, and possibly, cardiac arrest.

Topical or oral clotrimazole has a broad antifungal action. It has a greater tendency to bind to fatty acids than miconazole or ketoconazole, but is too toxic to be given systemically. It was used successfully as 1 percent arachis oil drops and ointment in a series of 13 cases of fungal keratitis caused by *Aspergillus, Candida, Fusarium moniliforme,* and *Drechslera rostrata* (now called *Exserohilum rostratum*).[114] Clotrimazole drops have been somewhat effective in a rabbit model of *Candida* keratitis,[115] and Foster[116] has reported the use of the 1 percent cream originally approved for vaginal fungal infections topically in patients with fungal keratitis, especially keratitis caused by yeast.

Econazole may be the most widely acting imidazole compound, but its clinical efficacy has been disappointing.

Ketoconazole has in vitro activity comparable to that of other imidazoles, and clinical trials suggest efficacy in a large variety of chronic fungal infections. It is available orally as a 200-mg capsule, and the recommended dosage is 400 to 800 mg/day. Both topical and oral ketoconazole are effective in the treatment of keratitis caused by filamentous fungi,[117] especially *Aspergillus, Fusarium, Curvularia,* and *Candida.* Studies have confirmed intraocular penetration of ketoconazole after topical administration.[118] Although its efficacy in laboratory studies is not convincing,[119] oral ketoconazole has also been used clinically alone and in conjunction with topical and subconjunctival miconazole in filamentous fungal keratitis.[91,120] Studies are also beginning to accumulate on the effectiveness of systemic imidazoles (miconazole and ketoconazole) as single agents for the treatment of fungal keratitis.[113,119,121] Systemic ketoconazole has been associated with impotence, decreased libido, and gynecomastia.

The triazoles are water soluble with good oral absorption, have good first-order pharmacokinetics, have few side effects, and achieve corneal levels sufficient to treat keratitis caused by filamentous fungi (especially *Aspergillus*) and yeasts. The triazoles, including itraconazole, fluconazole, and saperconazole, show promise in the treatment of ocular fungal infections with oral medication.[91] Oral itraconazole is effective against *Aspergillus, Cryptococcus,* and *Candida* in various experimental and clinical studies.[122–124] Elegant laboratory studies have been designed, but the effectiveness of the triazoles in experimental keratitis has been difficult to establish. A combination of topical and oral itraconazole was effective in the treatment of 69 percent of 110 patients with fungal keratitis from India.[125]

Oral fluconazole is well tolerated; it is preferentially taken up by the cornea and may allow treatment of fungal keratitis with systemic therapy.[126,127] The drug has a broad spectrum and also inhibits ergosterol biosynthesis. It is water soluble and has a low molecular weight and a reduced affinity for plasma proteins, compared with other azoles. Laboratory studies with oral fluconazole have demonstrated an excellent ocular pharmacokinetic profile.[95,128] Topical fluconazole is effective in *C. albicans* keratitis in rabbits.[129] Oral fluconazole may be valuable in the treatment of fungal keratitis caused by a variety of fungi.[130] Oral fluconazole should probably be substituted for ketoconazole because of its pharmacokinetic properties, penetration into ocular tissues, lack of adverse reactions, and proven efficacy in certain nonocular fungal infections.[28]

Pyrimidines

Unlike polyene or azole compounds, which act on cell membranes, the pyrimidine flucytosine is incorporated into fungal RNA and interferes with protein synthesis. Fungi have a permease that allows entry of the drug, and a deaminase that converts flucytosine to fluorouracil, which is incorporated into fungal RNA and inhibits synthesis of both DNA and RNA.[131] Flucytosine is effective mainly against *Candida, Cryptococcus,* and certain strains of *Aspergillus, Penicillium,* and *Cladosporium.*[26] It is not effective against *Acremonium* or *Fusarium.* There is a high incidence of acquired resistance, so combined treatment (usually with amphotericin B) is indicated when it is used for prolonged periods. Tube dilution sensitivity studies, animal model studies, and limited clinical trials suggest that the combination of flucytosine and amphotericin B is more effective than single drug therapy against a variety of fungi.[26] Flucytosine is best used in combination with amphotericin B, because the resultant altered permeability of fungal cell membranes by amphotericin B allows enhanced uptake of flucytosine by strains that are usually resistant.[130]

Effective aqueous and cerebrospinal fluid levels are obtained using oral flucytosine, which may contribute to the control of deep stromal suppuration or endophthalmitis caused by susceptible fungi. Adverse reactions include gastrointestinal upset, hepatic dysfunction, leukopenia, and thrombocytopenia. A 1 percent topical solution can be prepared by dissolving capsules in distilled water and removing insoluble filler substances by filtration. The topical solution is stable at room temperature and is well tolerated. Flucytosine has mostly been replaced by the polyenes and imidazoles in the treatment of fungal keratitis.

Antifungal Therapy

A simple classification of fungi into filamentous fungi or yeasts based on clinical features and the results of corneal smears permits organization of therapy (Tables 9-3 and 9-4). It is preferable to withhold antifungal therapy until there is laboratory confirmation that the infection is fungal, especially in view of the potential toxicity of antifungal drugs.[101] Fungal elements can be detected in the initial smears 75 to 80 percent of the time.[1] In general, fungal keratitis progresses more slowly than bacterial keratitis, and the clinician should not institute therapy without a definitive diagnosis; too many misdiagnoses will be made if the history and clinical appearance alone are used to make a diagnosis of fungal keratitis. Sometimes the infection is deep in the cornea and a corneal biopsy may be necessary for diagnosis. In the presence of indolent keratitis, unusual organisms such as *Mycobacterium*, anaerobes, and protozoa should be suspected, and then special stains or more technical microbiologic investigations of the smear are indicated.

Despite prompt identification of the causative agent, management of fungal keratitis is a challenge because of the paucity of effective antifungal agents.[132] Most of the recommendations for treatment are derived largely from uncontrolled clinical studies or laboratory models. The lack of good reproducible models of the disease, as well as a means of quantifying the response, makes recommendations difficult.

Natamycin as a 5 percent suspension, topically applied, is the initial drug of choice when hyphal fragments are seen in the corneal smear. It has a broad spectrum of action against filamentous fungi, established efficacy against a variety of corneal pathogens, and lack of toxicity. Most *Fusarium, Candida, Acremonium, Aspergillus,* and *Curvularia* species are susceptible in vitro and do not acquire resistance. Animal models and clinical trials suggest that topical amphotericin B (0.15 percent) is the treatment of choice for yeast or pseudohyphal keratitis and is a good second agent for filamentous fungal keratitis.[94,98,102,133] In a rabbit model of invasive *Candida* keratitis, 0.15 percent amphotericin B was more effective than 5 percent natamycin both in vitro and in vivo.[134] Prior clinical experience with more concentrated amphotericin B showed that it was poorly tolerated and probably ineffective in the treatment of *Fusarium* keratitis,[106] but effective against *Aspergillus*.

Topical natamycin or amphotericin B is given at 60-minute intervals for the first 48 hours. A loading pattern for amphotericin may be considered. Subconjunctival

TABLE 9-3
Initial Therapy for Fungal Keratitis

	Antifungal		
	Topical	*Subconjunctival*[a]	*Oral*[a]
Hyphal fragments	Natamycin	Miconazole	Fluconazole
Yeasts or pseudohyphae	Amphotericin B	Miconazole	Flucytosine

[a] Subconjunctival and oral therapy reserved for severe keratitis.

miconazole or subconjunctival fluconazole may be indicated for deep suppuration or impending perforation, although this route of administration has largely been replaced by oral therapy. Natamycin and amphotericin B are too toxic to be given subconjunctivally.[100] Systemic amphotericin B is seldom indicated for corneal disease; it is quite toxic by this route and does not penetrate ocular tissues well. Because poor penetration of topical antifungals is the rule, the routine use of oral systemic antifungal agents seems justified, especially the azole agents. Oral fluconazole or oral ketoconazole is given daily depending on the clinical severity, the clinical response, and the identification of the organism. Atropine or scopolamine is given for cycloplegia, and a topical β-blocker or oral carbonic anhydrase inhibitor is given to control the intraocular pressure, which is frequently elevated in these cases.

Modification of Therapy

When the fungus is identified, more selective antifungal treatment may be indicated (Table 9-5). Treatment may be further altered after sensitivity testing.[91] If a *Fusarium* species is identified, topical natamycin is the drug of choice. Addition of oral fluconazole or ketoconazole should be considered for severe or deep keratitis. Topical miconazole, fluconazole, or amphotericin B along with

TABLE 9-4
Dosages of Principal Antifungal Agents Used in Fungal Keratitis

Agent	*Topical*	*Subconjunctival*[a]	*Systemic*[a]
Natamycin	50 mg/ml (5%)	—	—
Amphotericin B	0.5–2.5 mg/ml (0.05 to 0.25%)	—	—
Miconazole	10 mg/ml (1%)	5 mg	30 mg/kg/day (IV)
Fluconazole	2 mg/ml (0.2%)	1 mg	200–400 mg/day (oral)
Ketoconazole	10 mg/ml (1%)	—	400–600 mg/day (oral)

[a] Subconjunctival and systemic therapy reserved for severe keratitis.

subconjunctival miconazole or fluconazole should be considered if the keratitis is unresponsive.[111] In vitro data on the potential enhancing therapeutic effectiveness of combined antifungal agents are conflicting.[114] Combining two polyenes, such as amphotericin B and natamycin, enhances drug toxicity without enhancing clinical effectiveness. Combining a polyene with an azole agent might have an additive effect.

If a filamentous fungus other than *Fusarium* is isolated, the same guidelines are suggested, although natamycin has more variable activity against these organisms. The addition or substitution of amphotericin B or miconazole should be considered. Topical and subconjunctival miconazole along with oral ketoconazole have been effective in selected cases of filamentous fungal keratitis.[121] Miconazole is especially effective against *Aspergillus.* Some strains of *Aspergillus, Penicillium,* and *Cladosporium* may be sensitive to flucytosine. Topical ketoconazole has been reported to be effective against *Aspergillus.*[117]

If *Candida* or an unidentified yeast is isolated, topical amphotericin B should be continued. Addition of oral flucytosine should be considered for severe or deep keratitis. Alternative therapy with topical fluconazole or miconazole could be considered for advancing keratitis. Subconjunctival miconazole or fluconazole combined with oral ketoconazole or fluconazole may be indicated in selected circumstances. Combined treatment is indicated more often in yeast keratitis because yeasts replicate more rapidly than filamentous fungi. Oral rifampin with topical amphotericin B may enhance the killing of *Candida.*[135] Patients with yeast keratitis may be more difficult to treat than those with filamentous fungal keratitis because of the underlying local corneal abnormalities that are usually present. It should be emphasized that the efficacy of the azoles and pyrimidines in fungal keratitis is based on in vitro determination and on a few clinical cases.

Generally, fungal keratitis improves slowly, despite proper selection of agents, and prolonged therapy should be anticipated. Debridement is valuable and should accompany drug therapy. Clinical signs of improvement include rounding of the perimeter of the lesions, loss of the irregular feathery linear borders, resolution of satellite lesions, reduction in the density of stromal suppuration, and improvement in epithelial and stromal edema. Persistence of an epithelial defect may indicate excessive topical medication. Repeated smears may not be helpful because the organisms are frequently deep within the stroma and a positive smear may identify only nonreplicating hyphal forms. If there is a change in the clinical picture, cultures should be repeated because secondary bacterial infection may occur.

Sensitivity testing of fungi has not been standardized and the value in directing therapy for ocular fungal infections is not established.[136,137] There is no uniform agreement among laboratories concerning specific media and methods, inoculation phase or size, incubation conditions, solubilization of the antifungal agent, or endpoint determinations.[138] There is little correlation between susceptibility testing results and the clinical response to the use of an antifungal agent. Therefore, sole dependence on these studies is not recommended. Nevertheless, performing tube dilution sensitivity studies on a variety of fungal isolates allows one to tabulate the likely sensitivity pattern for a large number of isolates from ocular infections. Several reference laboratories are now performing these functions.

Disk diffusion tests are more variable, and the broth dilution method is the preferred technique for sensitivity testing of ocular yeasts and filamentous fungi.[139] Determination should include the antifungal agents of potential value in the treatment of ocular infections. A modification of the standard tube dilution method that uses saturated paper disks and multiwell tissue culture plates has been used.[140]

Results from some laboratories have shown that *F. solani* is uniformly sensitive to natamycin. *F. solani* and most other *Fusarium* species are relatively resistant to the imidazoles in vitro, but almost all other isolates of fila-

TABLE 9-5
Modified Therapy for Fungal Keratitis Based on Culture Results

Organism	*Topical (Alternatives)*	*Subconjunctival[a] (Alternatives)*	*Oral[a] (Alternatives)*
Filamentous fungi	Natamycin (amphotericin B, miconazole, fluconazole)	Miconazole (fluconazole)	Fluconazole (ketoconazole)
Yeast	Amphotericin B (fluconazole, miconazole)	Miconazole (fluconazole)	Flucytosine (ketoconazole, fluconazole)

[a] Subconjunctival and oral therapy reserved for severe keratitis.

mentous fungi are sensitive to the imidazoles in vitro.[83] Clotrimazole has been the most effective in vitro, but is also the most toxic because of its binding properties.

Adjunctive Therapy

Interactions between the organism and the host in fungal keratitis are complex. There may be progressive corneal inflammation stimulated by replicating and nonreplicating fungi, their mycotoxins and enzymes, drugs, and the immune response. The presence of *Candida* keratitis suggests the need for an immunologic work-up. Strains of *F. solani* produce at least nine mycotoxins, and there are more than 200 mycotoxins among opportunistic fungi, with evidence supporting their role in tissue destruction.[141] The inflammatory response may persist long after effective antifungal therapy; reduction in this inflammation may minimize or eliminate structural alterations. A mydriatic-cycloplegic agent is indicated to reduce intraocular inflammation, relieve ciliary spasm, and prevent or break posterior synechiae.

In some situations, prostaglandin synthetase inhibitors or corticosteroids can be beneficial in combination with effective specific antifungal therapy.[26] Corticosteroids are contraindicated in the early treatment of fungal keratitis because they enhance the growth of both yeasts and filamentous fungi. The efficacy of antifungal agents is marginal and is easily negated by the adverse effects of corticosteroids.[48,142] In the cornea, treatment with topical corticosteroids may further inhibit the ability of neutrophils to ingest and destroy the hyphae.[143] Patients on antecedent topical corticosteroids should have these tapered, although abrupt cessation should be avoided because a rebound response is possible. Effective antifungal therapy must be established before any topical corticosteroids are started. Treatment should begin cautiously in immunologically competent patients, with monitoring of the clinical response; the clinician must be prepared to supervene surgically if necessary. Systemic corticosteroids have no role except to decrease intraocular inflammation prior to penetrating keratoplasty.

Aside from corneal biopsy for diagnostic purposes, surgery has been proposed for a number of conditions when optimal antifungal therapy has failed.[144] Debridement may be used to remove a concentrated abscess and to facilitate topical antifungal therapy. Initially, as treatment is begun, it may be necessary to debride the ulcer daily to eliminate all of the easily removable superficial necrotic material and fungal elements. Scraping the ulcer with a spatula or scalpel blade can facilitate treatment. More extensive surgery with a superficial or lamellar keratectomy may be effective in small, localized, superficial peripheral infections.[145] The excimer laser has been tested experimentally in this regard.[146,147] The results of excimer laser phototherapeutic keratectomy in rabbit eyes 24 and 72 hours after experimental infection with *Fusarium* suggested that this modality might be useful for the treatment of early, localized, superficial infections.[147] Treatment of deeper infections, however, carries a marked risk of perforation that would make careful patient selection critical.

In the presence of a large necrotic ulcer, advancing disease, or corneal perforation, more aggressive treatment is indicated. A deep keratectomy that excises most of the visibly necrotic tissue followed by placement of a thin inlay conjunctival flap in the keratectomy bed may control superficial infections by providing vascularization and additional host factors (Figure 9-25). This procedure is generally indicated for structural alterations when there is control of replicating organisms but a contraindication to penetrating keratoplasty exists. In peripheral ulcers, this procedure may, in fact, be preferable to prolonged medical therapy, especially in poorly compliant patients or in patients who do not respond to medical therapy.

Penetrating keratoplasty is an effective way to remove the fungus-laden cornea along with the dense polymorphonuclear leukocytic infiltrate, the antigen or immune complex precipitates, and the further stimulus for inflammation and vascularization. Penetrating keratoplasty is indicated for progressive ulceration or abscess formation, uncontrolled inflammation, corneal thinning or perforation, and extensive drug toxicity. Corneal transplantation is more commonly required in fungal keratitis than in bacterial keratitis (Figure 9-26).

The graft must be full thickness and larger than the visibly infected area. The addition of topical or systemic corticosteroids, or both, preoperatively, may facilitate penetrating keratoplasty in eyes that fail to respond to optimal medical therapy as directed by sensitivity determination. Use of general anesthesia, generous peripheral iridectomies, lysis of anterior and posterior synechiae, multiple interrupted 10-0 nylon sutures, viscoelastic substances, and intraoperative re-formation of the anterior chamber are important concepts in the surgical treatment of fungal keratitis. Examination of the keratoplasty specimen may reveal fungal elements at the edge, implicating corneal involvement beyond the clinically apparent ulcer. Even when hyphae penetrate Descemet's membrane into the anterior chamber, endophthalmitis is rare and the infection does not usually become intraocular. Cultures from the keratoplasty specimen are usually negative, but organisms in the specimen may stain with periodic acid–Schiff or Gomori methenamine silver.

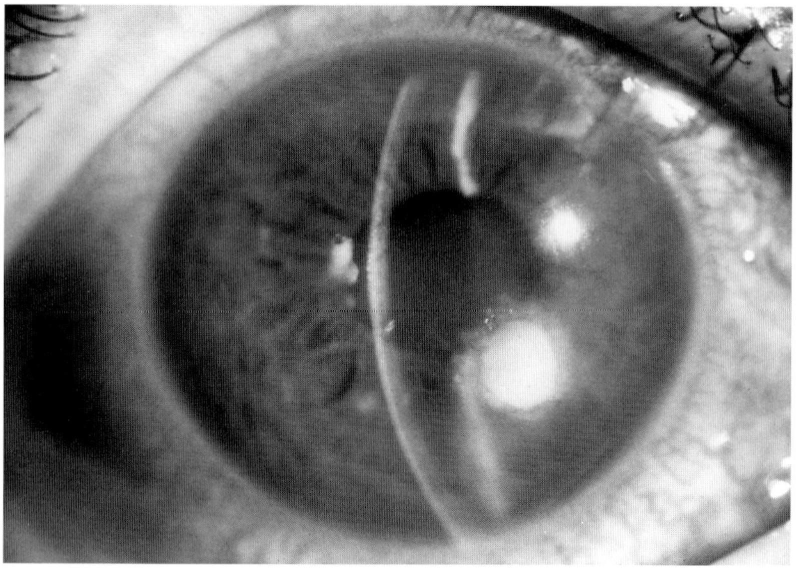

A

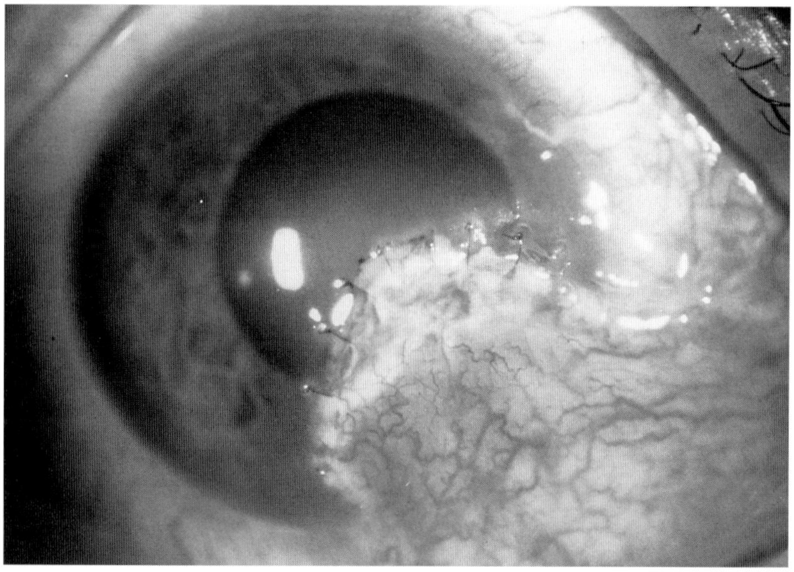

B

FIGURE 9-25 **(A)** Patient with *Curvularia* keratitis. **(B)** A lamellar keratectomy and inlay conjunctival flap were done because the keratitis progressed despite medical therapy. Visual acuity was 20/30 after the flap healed.

Lamellar keratoplasty is contraindicated in fungal keratitis because of the tendency for the fungi to exist deep in the stroma with danger of recurrence in the bed and frequent sloughing of the tissue.[27,148] Topical and oral antifungal agents should be continued postoperatively. Corticosteroids are not used in the early postoperative period unless there is marked inflammation, but may be used cautiously later to avoid vascularization or graft rejection. Recurrences at the graft edge may occur early or late.

Penetrating keratoplasty and conjunctival flaps were the main therapeutic options for fungal infection before the advent of antifungal agents.[66,149] Penetrating keratoplasty, however, carries the risk, although low, of conversion of fungal keratitis to fungal endophthalmitis.[150] The management of glaucoma induced by the accumulation of *Fusarium* species around the lens in the posterior chamber[47] requires removal of the lens and establishment of a flow of aqueous humor from the posterior to the anterior chamber.

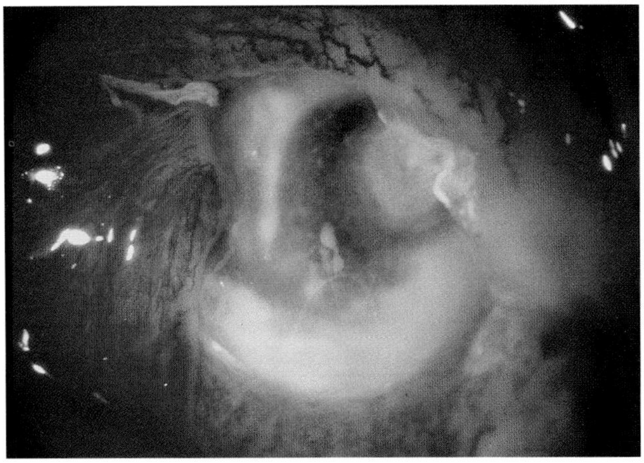

A

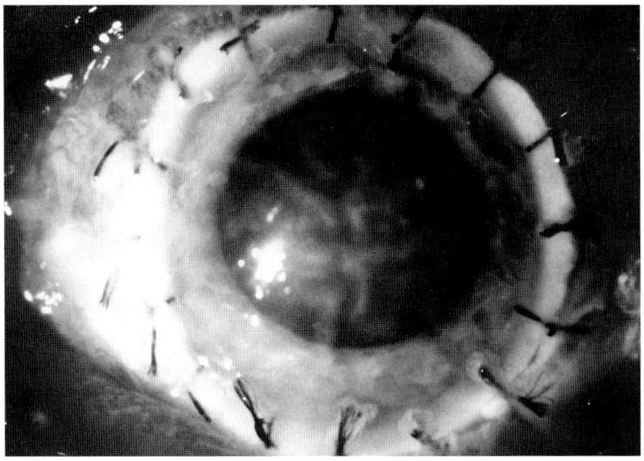

B

FIGURE 9-26 **(A)** A 45-year-old farmer from Minnesota with advanced *Aspergillus fumigatus* keratitis. Subconjunctival injections of amphotericin B caused marked conjunctival swelling and yellow nodules. **(B)** A large tectonic penetrating keratoplasty was required to control the infection. **(C)** After a second penetrating keratoplasty, visual acuity was 20/25.

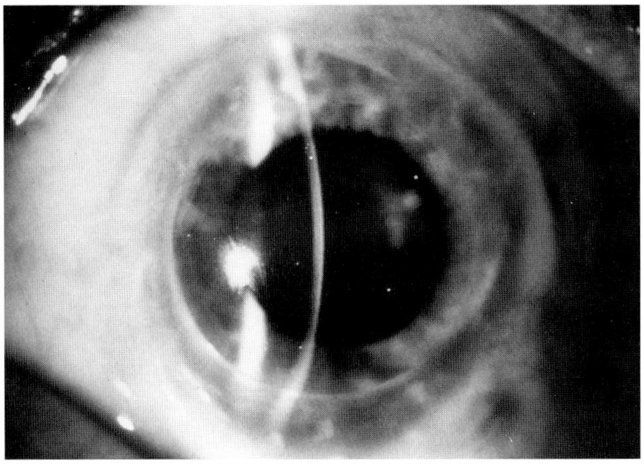

C

Note Added in Proof

Since this chapter was written, additional literature has been published describing other fungal species involved in corneal infection and describing the effective use of other/newer antifungal agents in therapy. This literature is important in advancing the clinical art and science, in providing better patient care, and in accomplishing cost containment. This chapter provides an overall approach to the management of patients with fungal keratitis; newer data must be assimilated continually into our management protocols in order to offer the patient and the public the most appropriate and cost-effective evaluation and therapeutic alternatives. TJL/August 22, 1997

REFERENCES

1. Liesegang TJ, Forster RF: Spectrum of microbial keratitis in South Florida. Am J Ophthalmol 90:38, 1980
2. Jones BR, Richards AB, Morgan G: Direct fungal infection of the eye in Britain. Trans Ophthalmol Soc UK 89:727, 1969
3. Jones DB: Opportunistic fungal infections in ophthalmology: fungal keratitis. p. 103. In Chic ED, Balows A, Furcolow ML (eds): Opportunistic Fungal Infections. Charles C Thomas, Springfield, IL, 1975
4. DeVoe AG, Silva-Hutner M: Fungal infections in the eye. p. 208. In Locatcher-Khorazo D, Seegal BC (eds): Microbiology of the Eye. CV Mosby, St. Louis, 1972
5. Rosa RH Jr, Miller D, Alfonso EC: The changing spectrum of fungal keratitis in South Florida. Ophthalmology 101:1005, 1994
6. Levitin E, Hurewitz D: A one-year survey of the airborne molds of Tulsa, Oklahoma II: indoor survey. Ann Allergy 41:25,1978
7. Thachyk SJ, Khan RS: Airborne mold survey—Edmonton. J Asthma Res 14:103, 1977
8. Bergen L, Wagner-Merner DT: Comparative survey of fungi and potential pathogenic fungi from selected beaches in the Tampa Bay area. Mycologia 69:299, 1977

9. Margo CE, Brinser JH: Microbiologic diagnosis: mycology. p. 171. In Karcioglu ZA (ed): Laboratory Diagnosis in Ophthalmology. Macmillan, New York, 1987
10. Bartnicki-Garcia S: Cell wall chemistry, morphogenesis, and taxonomy of fungi. Annu Rev Microbiol 22:87, 1968
11. Rippon JW: Medical Mycology: The Pathogenic Fungi and the Pathogenic Actinomycetes. 3rd Ed. WB Saunders, Philadelphia, 1988
12. Schwartz LK, Loignon LM, Webster RG, Jr: Post-traumatic phycomycosis of the anterior segment. Arch Ophthalmol 96:860, 1978
13. Manning M, Mitchell TG: Morphogenesis of *Candida albicans* and cytoplasmic proteins associated with differences in morphology, strain, or temperature. J Bacteriol 144:258, 1980
14. Forster RK, Rebell G, Wilson LA: Dematiaceous fungal keratitis. Br J Ophthalmol 59:372, 1975
15. Adam RD, Paquin ML, Petersen EA, et al: Phaeohyphomycosis caused by the fungal genera *Bipolaris* and *Exserohilum.* Medicine 65:203, 1986
16. Asbell P, Stenson LS: Ulcerative keratitis: survey of 30 years' laboratory experience. Arch Ophthalmol 100:77, 1982
17. Chin GN, Hyndiuk RA, Kwasny GP, Schultz RO: Keratomycosis in Wisconsin. Am J Ophthalmol 79:121, 1975
18. Doughman DJ, Leavenworth NM, Campbell RC, Lindstrom RL: Fungal keratitis at the University of Minnesota: 1971–1981. Trans Am Ophthalmol Soc 80:235, 1982
19. Nelson JD, Mindrup EA, Chung CK, et al: Fungal contamination in organ culture. Arch Ophthalmol 101:280, 1983
20. Mino de Kaspar H, Zoulek G, Paredes ME, et al: Mycotic keratitis in Paraguay. Mycoses 34:251, 1991
21. Venugopal PL, Venugopal TL, Gomathi A, et al: Mycotic keratitis in Madras. Indian J Pathol Microbiol 32:190, 1989
22. Sundaram BM, Badrinath S, Subramanian S: Studies on mycotic keratitis. Mycoses 32:568, 1989
23. Jones BR, Clayton YM, Oji EO: Recognition and chemotherapy of oculomycosis. Postgrad Med J 55:625, 1979
24. Williams G, McClellan K, Billson F: Suppurative keratitis in rural Bangladesh: the value of gram stain in planning management. Int Ophthalmol (Netherlands) 15:131, 1991
25. Khairallah SH, Byrne KA, Tabbara KF: Fungal keratitis in Saudi Arabia. Doc Ophthalmol 79:269, 1992
26. Jones BR: Principles in the management of oculomycosis. Am J Ophthalmol 79:719, 1975
27. Polack FM, Kaufman HE, Newmark E: Keratomycosis, medical and surgical treatment. Arch Ophthalmol 85:410, 1971
28. Jones DB: Fungal keratitis. p. IV:21. In Duane TD (ed): Clinical Ophthalmology. Harper & Row, Philadelphia, 1978
29. Jones DB: Therapy of postsurgical fungal endophthalmitis. Trans Am Acad Ophthalmol Otolaryngol 95:357, 1978
30. Burda CD, Fisher E Jr: Corneal destruction by extracts of *Cephalosporium* mycelium. Am J Ophthalmol 50:926, 1960
31. Liesegang TJ, Palestine RF, Su WPD: Chronic mucocutaneous candidiasis and keratitis associated with malignant thymoma. Ann Ophthalmol 15:174, 1983
32. Thygeson P, Okumoto M: Keratomycoses: a preventable disease. Trans Am Acad Ophthalmol Otolaryngol 78:433, 1974
33. Cruz OA, Sabis SM, Capo H, Alfonso EC: Microbial keratitis in childhood. Ophthalmology 100:192, 1993
34. Clinch TE, Palmon FE, Robinson MJ, et al: Microbial keratitis in children. Am J Ophthalmol 117:65, 1994
35. Clinch TE, Robinson MJ, Barron BA, et al: Fungal keratitis from nylon line lawn trimmers. Am J Ophthalmol 114:437,1992
36. Lim G: Distribution of *Fusarium* in some British soils. Mycopathol Mycologia Appl 52:231, 1974
37. Harris DJ Jr, Stulting RD, Waring GO, Wilson LA: Late bacterial and fungal keratitis after corneal transplantation. Ophthalmology 95:1450, 1988
38. Maskin SL, Alfonso E: Fungal keratitis after radial keratotomy. Am J Ophthalmol 114:369, 1992
39. Hirst LW, Sebban A, Whitby RM, et al: Non-traumatic mycotic keratitis. Eye 6:391, 1992
40. Parrish CM, O'Day DM, Hoyle TC: Spontaneous fungal corneal ulcer as an ocular manifestation of AIDS. Am J Ophthalmol 104:302, 1987
41. Santos C, Parker J, Dawson C, et al: Bilateral fungal corneal ulcers in a patient with AIDS-related complex. Am J Ophthalmol 102:118, 1986
42. Michelson PE, Rupp R, Efthimiadis B: Endogenous *Candida* endophthalmitis leading to bilateral corneal perforation. Am J Ophthalmol 80:800, 1975
43. Zhu WS, Wojdyla K, Donlan K, et al: Extracellular protease of *Aspergillus flavus:* fungal keratitis, proteases, and pathogenesis. Diagn Microbiol Infect Dis 13:491, 1990
44. Wogan GN: Mycotoxins. Annu Rev Pharmacol 15:437, 1975
45. Howlett JA, Squier CA: *Candida albicans* ultrastructure: colonization and invasion of oral epithelium. Infect Immun 29:252, 1980
46. Diamond RD, Oppenheim F, Nakagawa Y, et al: Properties of a product of *Candida albicans* hyphae and pseudohyphae that inhibits contact between the fungi and human neutrophils in vitro. J Immunol 125:2797, 1980
47. Jones BR, Jones DB, Lim ASM, et al: Corneal and intraocular infection due to *Fusarium solani.* Trans Ophthalmol Soc UK 89:757, 1969
48. Stern GA, Buttross M: Use of corticosteroids in combination with antimicrobial drugs in the treatment of infectious corneal disease. Ophthalmology 98:847, 1991
49. Wilhelmus KR, Robinson NM, Font RA, et al: Fungal keratitis in contact lens wearers. Am J Ophthalmol 106:708, 1988
50. Pitts RD, Krachmer JH: Evaluation of soft contact lens disinfection in the home environment. Arch Ophthalmol 97:470,1979
51. Donzis PB, Mondino BJ, Weissman BA, Bruckner DA: Microbial contamination of contact lens care systems. Am J Ophthalmol 104:325, 1987
52. Wilson LA, Ahearn DG: Association of fungi with extended-wear soft contact lenses. Am J Ophthalmol 101:434, 1986

53. Simmons RB, Buffington JR, Ward M, et al: Morphology and ultrastructure of fungi in extended-wear soft contact lenses. J Clin Microbiol 24:21, 1986
54. Kaufman HE, Wood RM: Mycotic keratitis. Am J Ophthalmol 59:993, 1965
55. Berger ST, Katsev DA, Mondino BJ, Pettit TH: Macroscopic pigmentation in a dematiacious fungal keratitis. Cornea 10:272, 1991
56. Forster RK, Rebell G: The diagnosis and management of keratomycoses I: cause and diagnosis. Ophthalmology 93:975,1975
57. Wilhelmus KR, Robinson NM: Infectious crystalline keratopathy caused by *Candida albicans.* Am J Ophthalmol 112:322,1991
58. Sassani JU, Rosenwasser GO: Fungal contact lens infiltration simulating crystalline deposits. CLAO J 17:205, 1991
59. Chew SJ, Beuerman RW, Assouline M, et al: Early diagnosis of infectious keratitis with in vivo real time confocal microscopy. CLAO J 18:197, 1992
60. Kaufman SC, Beuerman RW, Greer DL: In vivo identification of morphologically different fungi with the tandem scanning confocal microscope. ARVO abstract. Invest Ophthalmol Vis Sci 34(suppl):851, 1993
61. Kaufman SC, Laird J, Beuerman RW: In vivo, real-time confocal mcroscopy of fungal, bacterial, and acanthamoeba keratitis. ARVO abstract. Invest Ophthalmol Vis Sci 36(suppl):S1022, 1995
62. Auran JD, Florakis GJ, Siegal S, et al: Scanning slit confocal microscopy of fungal keratitis. ARVO abstract. Invest Ophthalmol Vis Sci 36(suppl):S1022, 1995
63. Winchester K, Elgin RG, Mathers WD, Sutphin JE: Confocal microscopy of fungal keratitis. ARVO abstract. Invest Ophthalmol Vis Sci 36(suppl):S1022, 1995
64. Naumann G, Green WR, Zimmerman LE: Mycotic keratitis. Am J Ophthalmol 64:668, 1969
65. Fons A, Garcia de Lomas J, Nogueira JM, et al: Histopathology of experimental *Aspergillus fumigatus* keratitis. Mycopathologia 101:129, 1988
66. Forster RK, Rebell G: Therapeutic surgery in failures of medical treatment for fungal keratitis. Br J Ophthalmol 59:366, 1975
67. Pincus DH, Salkin IF, McGinnis MR: Rapid methods in medical mycology. Lab Med 19:310, 1988
68. Benson WH, Lanier JD: Comparison of techniques for culturing corneal ulcers. Ophthalmology 99:800, 1992
69. Ishibashi Y, Hommura S, Matsumoto Y: Direct examination vs. culture of biopsy specimens for the diagnosis of keratomycosis. Am J Ophthalmol 103:636, 1987
70. Jones DB: Strategy for the initial management of suspected microbial keratitis. p. 86. In New Orleans Academy of Ophthalmology. Symposium on Medical and Surgical Diseases of the Cornea. CV Mosby, St. Louis, 1980
71. Vajpayee RB, Angra SK, Sandramouli S, et al: Laboratory diagnoses of keratomycoses: comparative evaluation of direct microscopy and culture results. Ann Ophthalmol 25:68, 1993
72. Thomas PA, Kuriakose T, Kirupashankes MP, Maharajan VS: Use of lactophenol cotton blue mounts of corneal scrapings as an aid to the diagnosis of mycotic keratitis. Diagn Microbiol Infect Dis 14:219, 1991
73. Arffa RC, Avni I, Ishibashi Y, et al: Calcofluor and ink-potassium hydroxide preparations for identifying fungi. Am J Ophthalmol 100:719, 1985
74. Marines HM, Osato MS, Font RL: The value of calcofluor white in the diagnosis of mycotic and acanthamoeba infections of the eye and ocular adnexa. Ophthalmology 94:23, 1987
75. Margo CE, Bombardier T: The diagnostic value of fungal autofluorescence. Surv Ophthalmol 29:374, 1985
76. Robin JB, Arffa RC, Avni I, et al: Rapid visualization of three common fungi using fluorescein-conjugated lectins. Invest Ophthalmol Vis Sci 27:500, 1986
77. Jackson M, Chan R, Matoba AY, et al: The use of fluorescein conjugated lectins for visualizing atypical mycobacteria. Arch Ophthalmol 107:1206, 1989
78. Robin JB, Chan R, Rao NA, et al: Fluorescein-conjugated lectin visualization of fungi and acanthamoeba in infectious keratitis. Ophthalmology 96:1198, 1989
79. Forster RK, Wirta MG, Solis M, Rebell G: Methenamine silver-stained corneal scrapings in keratomycosis. Am J Ophthalmol 82:261, 1976
80. Kanungo R, Svinivasan R, Rao RS: Acridine orange staining in early diagnosis of mycotic keratitis. Acta Ophthalmol (Copenh) 69:750, 1991
81. Groden LR, Rodnite J, Brinser JH, Genvert GI: Acridine orange and Gram stains in infectious keratitis. Cornea 9:122, 1990
82. Torres-Gomez J, Robinson NM, Wilhelmus KR, et al: Comparison of acridine orange and Gram stain in bacterial keratitis. Am J Ophthalmol 106:735, 1988
83. Forster RK: Fungal keratitis and conjunctivitis. p. 239. In Smolin G, Thoft RA (eds): The Cornea: Scientific Foundations and Clinical Practice. Little, Brown, Boston, 1994
84. O'Day DM, Akrabawi PL, Head WS, Rather HB: Laboratory isolation techniques in human and experimental fungal infections. Am J Ophthalmol 87:688, 1979
85. Hyndiuk RA, Nassif KF, Burd EM: Bacterial disease. p. 147. In Smolin G, Thoft RA (eds): The Cornea: Scientific Foundations and Clinical Practice. Little, Brown, Boston, 1983
86. Haley LD, Trandel J, Coyle MB: Cumitech 11, Practical Methods for Culture and Identification of Fungi in the Clinical Microbiology Laboratory. Sherris JC (coord ed): American Society for Microbiology, Washington, DC, 1980
87. Rebell GC, Forster RK: Fungi of keratomycosis. p. 553. In Lennette EH, Balows A, Hausler WJ Jr, Truant JP (eds): Manual of Clinical Mycology. 3rd Ed. American Society for Microbiology, Washington, DC, 1980
88. Roberts GD: Laboratory methods in basic mycology. p. 678. In Finegold SM, Baron EJ (eds): Bailey and Scott's Diagnostic Microbiology. CV Mosby, St. Louis, 1986
89. Okumoto M: Infectious agents: fungi. p. 127. In Smolin G, Thoft RA (eds): The Cornea: Scientific Foundations and Clinical Practice. Little, Brown, Boston, 1983

90. Jones BR: Antifungal drugs for oculomycoses I: selection of possible useful substances. Trans Ophthalmol Soc UK 89:819, 1969
91. Johns KJ, O'Day DM: Pharmacologic management of keratomycoses. Surv Ophthalmol 33:178, 1988
92. O'Day DM: Antifungal agents. p. 345. In Leibowitz HM (ed): Corneal Disorders. WB Saunders, Philadelphia, 1984
93. O'Day DM, Ray WA, Robinson RD, Head WS: Correlation of in vitro and in vivo susceptibility of *Candida albicans* to amphotericin B and natamycin. Invest Ophthalmol Vis Sci 28:596, 1987
94. Wood TO, Williford W: Treatment of keratomycosis with amphotericin B 0.15%. Am J Ophthalmol 81:847, 1976
95. O'Day DM, Head WS, Robinson RD, et al: The evaluation of therapeutic responses in experimental keratomycosis. Curr Eye Res 11:35, 1992
96. Pleyer V, Legmann A, Mondino BJ, Lee DA: Use of collagen shields containing amphotericin B in the treatment of experimental *Candida albicans*-induced keratomycosis in rabbits. Am J Ophthalmol 113:303, 1992
97. Kotler-Brajtburg J, Medoff G, Kobayashi GS, et al: Classification of polyene antibiotics according to chemical structure and biological effects. Antimicrob Agents Chemother 15:716, 1979
98. O'Day DM, Robinson R, Head WS: Efficacy of antifungal agents in the cornea. Invest Ophthalmol Vis Sci 24:1098, 1983
99. O'Day DM, Ray WA, Robinson RD, et al: Differences in response in vivo to amphotericin B among *Candida albicans* strains. Invest Ophthalmol Vis Sci 32:1569, 1991
100. O'Day DM, Smith R, Stevens JB, et al: Toxicity and pharmacokinetics of subconjunctival amphotericin B. Cornea 10:411, 1991
101. Foster CS, Lass JH, Moran-Wallace K, Giovanoni R: Ocular toxicity of topical antifungal agents. Arch Ophthalmol 99:1081, 1981
102. Wood TO, Tuberville AW, Monnett R: Keratomycosis and amphotericin B. Trans Am Ophthalmol Soc 83:397, 1985
103. O'Day DM, Head WS, Robinson RD, Clanton JA: Bioavailability and penetration of topical amphotericin B in the anterior segment of the rabbit eye. J Ocul Pharmacol 2:371, 1986
104. Drutz DJ, Spickard A, Rogers DE, Koenig MG: Treatment of disseminated mycotic infections—a new approach to amphotericin B therapy. Am J Med 45:405, 1968
105. Jones DB, Forster RK, Rebell G: *Fusarium solani* keratitis treated with natamycin (pimaricin): 18 consecutive cases. Arch Ophthalmol 88:147, 1972
106. Jones DB, Sexton RR, Rebell G: Mycotic keratitis in South Florida: a review of 39 cases. Trans Ophthalmol Soc UK 89:781, 1969
107. O'Day DM, Ray WA, Head WS, Robinson RD: Efficacy of antifungal agents in the cornea IV: amphotericin B methylester. Invest Ophthalmol Vis Sci 25:851, 1984
108. Forster RK, Rebell G: The diagnosis and management of keratomycoses II: medical and surgical management. Arch Ophthalmol 93:1134, 1975
109. Jones DB: Decision-making in the management of microbial keratitis. Ophthalmology 88:814, 1982
110. Sud IT, Feingold DS: Heterogeneity of action mechanisms among antimycotic imidazoles. Antimicrob Agents Chemother 20:71, 1981
111. Foster CS: Miconazole therapy for keratomycosis. Am J Ophthalmol 91:622, 1981
112. Ishibashi Y, Kaufman HE: The effects of subconjunctival miconazole in the treatment of experimental *Candida* keratitis in rabbits. Arch Ophthalmol 103:1570, 1985
113. Ishibashi Y, Matsumoto Y: Intravenous miconazole in the treatment of keratomycosis. Am J Ophthalmol 97:646, 1984
114. Jones DB, Jones BR, Robinson NM: Clotrimazole (Canesten) therapy of fungal keratitis. Chemotherapy 6:189, 1975
115. Behrens-Baumann W, Klinge B, Uter W: Clotrimazole and bifonazole in the topical treatment of *Candida* keratitis in rabbits. Mycoses 33:567, 1990
116. Foster CS: Fungal keratitis. Infect Dis Clin North Am 6:851, 1992
117. Torres MA, Mohamed J, Cavazos-Adame H, Martinez LA: Topical ketoconazole for fungal keratitis. Am J Ophthalmol 100:293, 1985
118. Hemady RK, Foster CS: Intraocular penetration of ketoconazole in rabbits. Cornea 11:329, 1992
119. Komadina RG, Wilkes TDI, Shock JP, et al: Treatment of *Aspergillus fumigatus* keratitis in rabbits with oral and topical ketoconazole. Am J Ophthalmol 99:476, 1985
120. Ishibashi Y: Oral ketoconazole therapy for keratomycosis. Am J Ophthalmol 95:342, 1983
121. Fitzsimons R, Peter AL: Miconazole and ketoconazole as a satisfactory first-line treatment for keratomycoses. Am J Ophthalmol 101:605, 1986
122. Thomas PA, Abraham BJ, Kalavathy CM, et al: Oral itraconazole therapy for mycotic keratitis. Mycoses 31:271, 1988
123. Saag MS, Dismukes WE: Azole antifungal agents: emphasis on new triazoles. Antimicrob Agents Chemother 32:1, 1988
124. Hay RJ: First international symposium on itraconazole: a summary. Rev Infect Dis 9:51, 1987
125. Rajasekarau J, Thomas PA, Kalavathy CM, et al: Itraconazole therapy for fungal keratitis. Indian J Ophthalmol 35:157, 1987
126. Savani DV, Perfect JR, Cobo LM, Durack DT: Penetration of new azole compounds into the eye and efficacy in experimental *Candida* endophthalmitis. Antimicrob Agents Chemother 31:6, 1987
127. O'Day DM: Orally administered antifungal therapy for experimental keratomycosis. Trans Am Ophthalmol Soc 88:685, 1990
128. O'Day DM, Foulds G, Williams TE, et al: Ocular uptake of fluconazole following oral administration. Arch Ophthalmol 108:1006, 1990
129. Behrens-Baumann W, Klinge B, Ruchel T: Topical fluconazole for experimental *Candida* keratitis in rabbits. Br J Ophthalmol 74:40, 1990

130. Terrell CL, Hughes CE: Antifungal agents used in deep-seated mycotic infections. Mayo Clin Proc 67:69, 1992
131. Wagner GE, Shadomy S: Studies on the mode of action of 5-flucytosine in *Aspergillus* species. Chemotherapy 25:61, 1979
132. O'Day DM: Fungal keratitis. p. 420. In Leibowitz HM (ed): Corneal Disorders. WB Saunders, Philadelphia, 1984
133. O'Day DM: Selection of appropriate antifungal therapy. Cornea 6:238, 1987
134. O'Day DM, Ray WA, Robinson RD, et al: In vitro and in vivo susceptibility of *Candida* keratitis to topical polyenes. Invest Ophthalmol Vis Sci 28:874, 1987
135. Stern GA, Okumoto M, Smolin G: Combined amphotericin B and rifampin treatment of experimental *Candida albicans* keratitis. Arch Ophthalmol 97:721, 1979
136. Stevens DA: Antifungal susceptibility testing: a critical review. Mycopathologia 87:135, 1984
137. Galgiani JN: Antifungal susceptibility tests. Antimicrob Agents Chemother 31:1867, 1987
138. Roberts GD: Fungi. p. 473. In Washington JA (ed): Laboratory Procedures in Clinical Microbiology. Springer-Verlag, New York, 1981
139. Shadomy S, Espinel-Ingroff A: Susceptibility testing with antifungal drugs. p. 647. In Lennette EH, Balows A, Hausler WJ Jr, Truant JP (eds): Manual of Clinical Microbiology. 3rd Ed. American Society for Microbiology, Washington, DC, 1980
140. Jones DB, Liesegang TJ, Robinson NM: Cumitech 13, Laboratory Diagnosis of Ocular Infections. Washington JA II (coord ed): American Society for Microbiology, Washington, DC, 1981
141. Chick EW: Opportunistic fungi as producers of mycotoxins. p. 235. In Chick EW, Balows A, Furcolow ML (eds): Opportunistic Fungal Infections. Charles C Thomas, Springfield, IL, 1975
142. O'Day DM, Ray WA, Head WS, et al: Influence of corticosteroid on experimentally induced keratomycosis. Arch Ophthalmol 109:1601, 1991
143. Kiryu H, Yoshida S, Suenaga Y, Asahi M: Invasion and survival of *Fusaria solani* in the dexamethasone treated cornea of rabbits. J Med Vet Mycol 29:395, 1991
144. Jones BR, Jones DB, Richards AB: Surgery in the management of keratomycosis. Trans Ophthalmol Soc UK 89:887, 1969
145. Sanitato JJ, Kelley CG, Kaufman HE: Surgical management of peripheral fungal keratitis. Arch Ophthalmol 102:1507, 1984
146. Serdarevic O, Darrell RW, Krueger RR, Trokel SL: Excimer laser therapy for experimental *Candida* keratitis. Am J Ophthalmol 99:534, 1985
147. Gottsch JD, Gilbert ML, Goodman DF, et al: Excimer laser ablative treatment of microbial keratitis. Ophthalmology 98:146, 1991
148. Singh G, Malik SR: Therapeutic keratoplasty in fungal corneal ulcers. Br J Ophthalmol 56:41, 1972
149. Sanders N: Penetrating keratoplasty in treatment of fungal keratitis. Am J Ophthalmol 70:24, 1970
150. Wilson LA, Cavanagh HD: Penetrating keratoplasty for exogenous *Paecilomyces* keratitis followed by postoperative endophthalmitis. Am J Ophthalmol 98:552, 1984

10

Herpes Simplex Viral Infections

HERBERT E. KAUFMAN, MARK A. RAYFIELD, AND BRYAN M. GEBHARDT

VIRAL STRUCTURE AND CLASSIFICATION

Herpes simplex virus (HSV) is a member of the family Herpesviridae, which also includes varicella-zoster virus, Epstein-Barr virus, and cytomegalovirus. The virus has a rather complex structure[1] (Figure 10-1). A 100-nm icosahedral-shaped (20-sided) capsid encloses a core of double-stranded DNA and various phosphoproteins of the viral chromatin. The capsid is encompassed by an envelope of glycoproteins, carbohydrates, and lipids. All known proteins associated with the envelope arise from either virus-specified de novo synthesis or by modification of host cell proteins. The lipid portion of the envelope appears to be derived principally from the phospholipids of the nuclear membrane of the host cell. The enveloped viral particle has a diameter of approximately 180 nm. Quantitatively, the mature viral particle is composed of approximately 70 percent protein, 22 percent lipid, 7 percent nucleic acid, and 2 percent carbohydrate.

During replication, the elaborate demands of viral propagation gradually blur the distinction between the components of the host cell and the virus. The virus progressively cannibalizes the synthetic pathways of the host cell, shuttling nascent proteins from the cytoplasm to the nucleus and inserting its own glycoproteins into the cell membrane of the host cell.

Virus-specific antigens differentiate HSV into two types: type 1 (HSV-1) and type 2 (HSV-2).[2,3] Although an oversimplification, it has been stated that HSV-1 causes infections above the waist and HSV-2 causes infections below the waist. This is usually the case; however, either type is capable of causing infection in either location.[4]

Within each type, no specific subgroups have been identified. The term *viral strain,* which is used frequently in descriptions and explanations of both clinical and experimental viral behavior, simply denotes a single viral isolate obtained from an infected individual and propagated in the laboratory. For example, the classic McKrae strain was isolated from a patient named McKrae and is the laboratory strain used to produce spontaneous recurrences of herpetic keratitis in rabbits that resemble those occurring in humans. One viral strain can be differentiated from another by various means, including DNA mapping. More information about the theories associated with specific strain behavior is provided in the section on clinical behavior.

EPIDEMIOLOGY

Available evidence indicates that HSV is ubiquitous and that contact with the virus occurs frequently and generally at an early age. Primary infection usually occurs between 6 months and 5 years of age. Some studies indicate that more than 80 percent of adults have been infected with and have antibodies to HSV.

HSV first infects a peripheral end organ and then travels to the ganglia, where it may become latent. Early studies that examined cadavers at random demonstrated that more than 50 percent had HSV latent in the trigeminal or cervical ganglia.[5,6] Considering that the methods used in these studies for detecting latent virus were not very sensitive, the true percentage was probably higher. More recent studies using molecular biologic techniques have found percentages ranging from 55 to 94.[7-11]

Although most adults have been infected with HSV-1, only about 20 to 25 percent give any history of clinical manifestations of ocular or cutaneous herpetic disease. Most primary herpetic infections, therefore, are

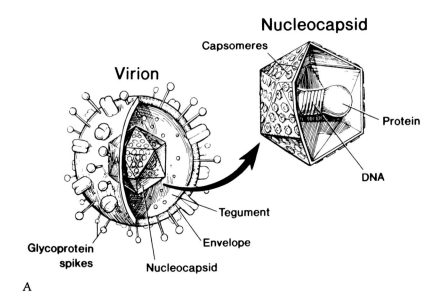

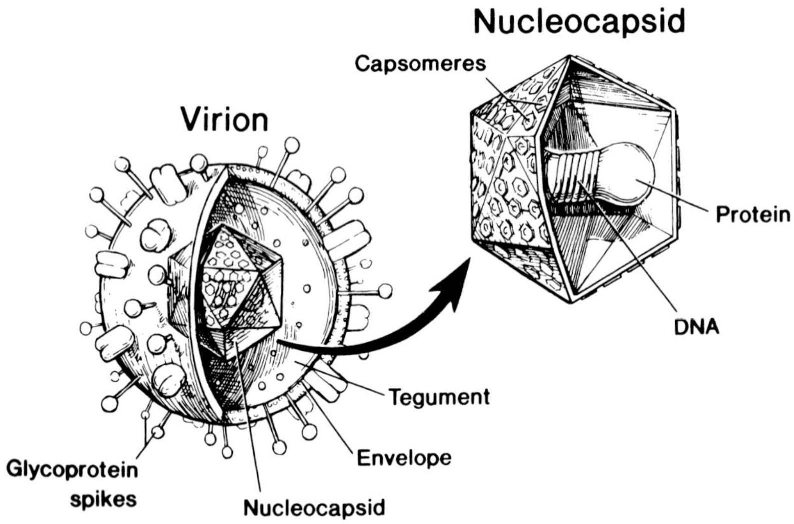

A

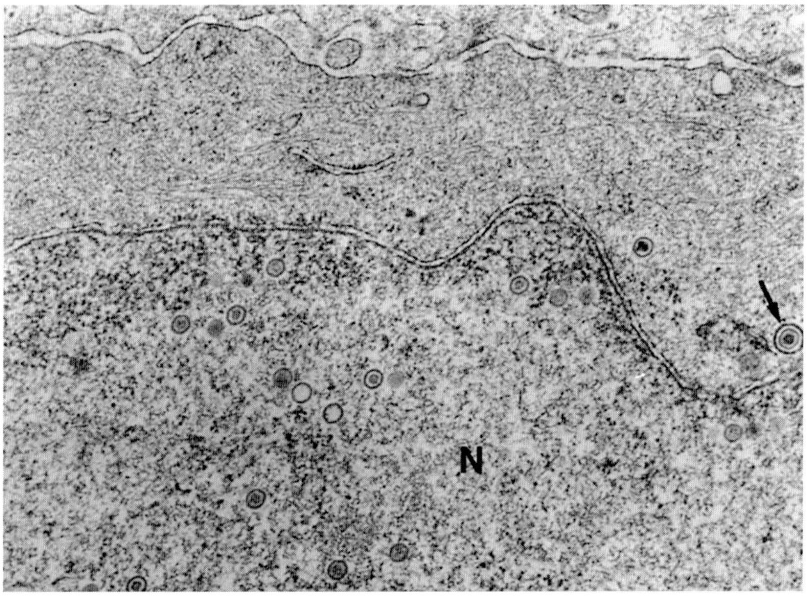

B

FIGURE 10-1 **(A)** Schematic drawing of a herpesvirus. (Reprinted with permission from TJ Liesegang: Biology and molecular aspects of herpes simplex and varicella-zoster virus infections. Ophthalmology 99:781, 1992. Courtesy of Ophthalmology.) **(B)** Transmission electron micrograph depicting herpes simplex virions within the nucleus *(N)* of a basal epithelial cell. The nucleocapsids become enveloped with nuclear membrane (arrow) on passing into the cytoplasm of the cell (× 42,000). (Courtesy of Roger W. Beuerman, Ph.D., New Orleans, LA.)

subclinical, and more than 95 percent of the clinical disease seen is a recurrence that develops long after a possibly asymptomatic primary infection. In an epidemiologic study of the population of Rochester, Minnesota, over a 33-year period,[12,13] the annual incidence of new cases of ocular herpes simplex was 8.4 per 100,000, and the overall annual incidence (new and recurrent cases combined) was 20.7 cases per 100,000. For patients with one episode of disease, the cumulative rate of recurrence, assessed by life table methods, was about 10 percent at 1 year, 23 percent at 2 years, and 63 percent at 20 years. Approximately 12 percent of the patients had bilateral disease.

Because of the ubiquitous nature of HSV, there has been some question whether to treat it as a potentially transmissible infectious agent or to ignore it as something to which a potential contact has almost certainly already been exposed. We do not treat herpes as a highly transmissible disease and do not isolate patients with herpetic infections. Exceptions include parents with young children and patients with a potential contact who is immunocompromised or in whom a herpetic infection might prove fatal.

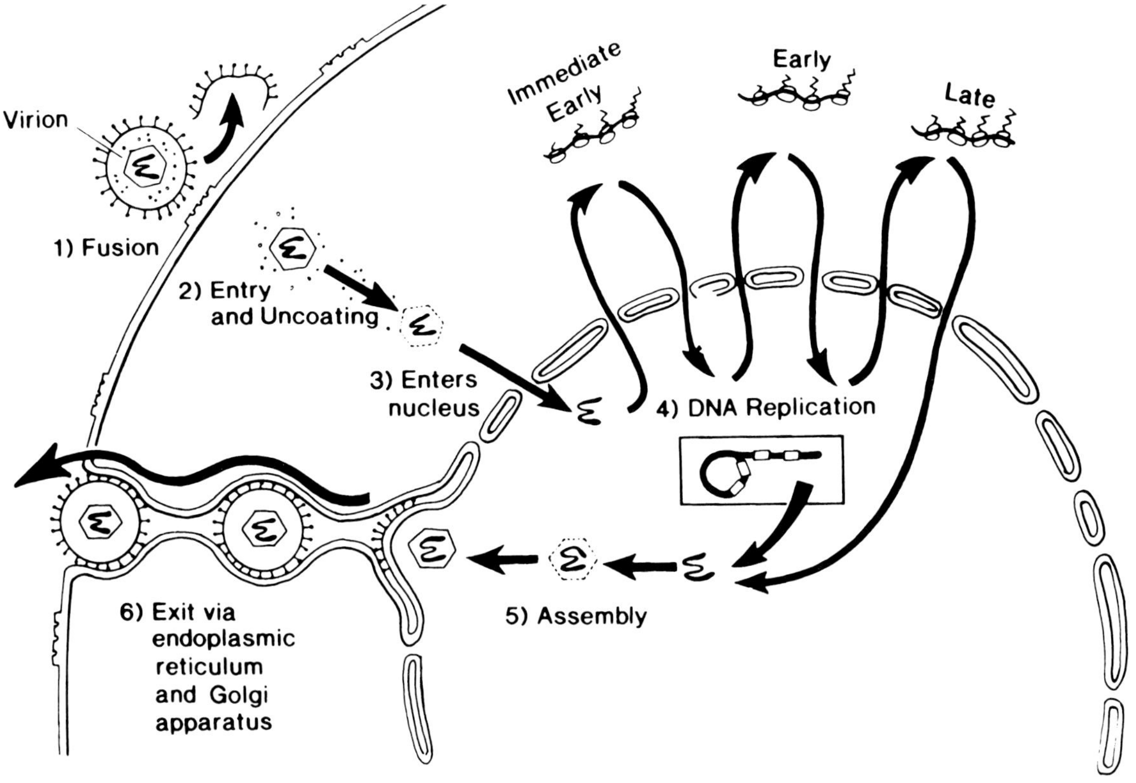

FIGURE 10-2 Schematic replication of herpes simplex virus in a susceptible cell. (Reprinted with permission from TJ Liesegang: Biology and molecular aspects of herpes simplex and varicella-zoster virus infections. Ophthalmology 99:781, 1992. Courtesy of Ophthalmology.)

CLINICAL BEHAVIOR

After entering through a peripheral nerve, HSV travels by axonal transport to neuronal cell bodies and then into the nucleus of neurons of the superior cervical and trigeminal ganglia.[14,15] The virus persists in the ganglia in a latent state and, from time to time, is reactivated and travels via the axons to the cornea, where it is shed and may produce recurrent disease.

During the lytic or infectious phase, which, for ocular herpes, takes place largely in the corneal epithelial cells, the virus loses its envelope on passage through the cell membrane and the capsid is stripped away before the virus enters the nucleus[1] (Figure 10-2). In the nucleus, the uncoated DNA takes on a circular shape (episome). The activation of a cascade of immediate early (α), early (β), and late (γ) genes leads to production of viral structural proteins in the cytoplasm and replication of viral DNA in the nucleus. The proteins are transported to the nucleus, where they and the viral DNA are assembled into nucleocapsids that are released through the nuclear membrane to the cytoplasm. The nucleocapsids are enveloped before leaving the cell and are then capable of infecting nearby cells. One of the nonstructural proteins produced during this cycle, infected cell protein zero (ICP0), is an immediate early regulatory protein, and its presence is a marker for actively replicating virus.

During the establishment of latency, the virus enters the neural cells and travels to the nucleus, where the viral DNA takes on the episomal form, but the cascade of genetic activity seen in the epithelial cells during the lytic phase does not occur, transcription is limited, and infectious particles are not made. The only transcription of DNA to RNA during latency appears to be the generation of latency-associated transcripts (LATs), which are considered a marker for latently infected cells.[1,16] LATs are transcribed from portions of the DNA strand complementary to and overlapping the region that codes for ICP0. These LATs do not exit the host nucleus to the cytoplasm and apparently do not take part in the usual function of messenger RNA, in that, to date, no LAT-associated protein has been identified.

When LATs were discovered, many thought that a "controlling" factor for latency had been found. Since then, researchers have shown that HSV strains bioengineered without LAT regions in their DNA are also capable of becoming latent and remaining latent, although the in vivo reactivation rates for LAT-negative strains are low.[1,16] It is now believed that LATs are not essential for the establishment or maintenance of latency but that they do play an as yet unidentified role in viral reactivation.

The molecular biology of viral replication, latency, and reactivation is under intense investigation in the hope of identifying one or more fundamental mechanisms that can be disrupted or inhibited to prevent disease. However, despite a considerable increase in our knowledge, our understanding of the events underlying the shift of HSV from the latent to the active state and back again is incomplete, and so far no practical applications have resulted.

Molecular biologic techniques have also been applied to the investigation of extraneuronal latency.[17,18] A variety of studies have used techniques such as in situ hybridization, immunofluorescence assays, and the polymerase chain reaction (PCR) to demonstrate the presence of putatively latent HSV in corneal tissue; the site of corneal latency is generally thought to be within the nuclei of stromal keratocytes. The criteria that must be met to fulfill the definition of latency in the cornea, to discriminate between "true" latency and low-level chronic infection or viral replication, are sufficiently rigorous that no study has yet conclusively demonstrated this type of latency. Although the controversy continues, it seems likely that the frequency of latency in the cornea, if any, is low and that this phenomenon, therefore, may have little or no clinical significance. To date, no patient has been shown to develop herpetic keratitis from transplanted corneal tissue. In ocular disease, the trigeminal and superior cervical ganglia are the major sources of latent virus and the corneal innervation is the main conduit for the transport of reactivated virus to the cornea.

HSV colonizes not only the superior cervical and trigeminal ganglia but possibly also the brain stem, especially in animals, and has been found in the brain stem in humans.[19] The role of the brain stem in providing a source of latent virus is unclear, and the viral function in the brain stem is uncertain. True encephalitis caused by HSV-1 is extremely rare, although it does occur.

The evidence is now great that the initial infecting viral strain colonizes all the ganglia in most cases and that for each individual there is a single strain of virus present in all of the ganglia. Studies involving mapping of the viral DNA confirm this.[20] Experiments in rabbits have shown that when, for example, the eye is infected with a particular HSV strain, this strain usually colonizes the superior cervical and trigeminal ganglia on both sides. More important, once a ganglion is infected, it seems to be impossible to superinfect it with a different HSV strain.[21] It is the initial infecting strain that colonizes the ganglion, and although a second strain can infect the peripheral end organ and may remain for as long as 2 weeks, it does not take up residence in the ganglion.

In animals, infection with a strain that causes mild superficial disease results in that strain occupying the ganglia, and later superinfection, even with a highly neurovirulent strain that could produce spontaneous recurrent herpetic disease, does not displace the original strain. The superinfecting strain may cause end organ disease, but it does not become latent in the ganglia. Only the initial infecting strain is found in the ganglia and only the initial strain is shed in the tears.[21,22] Strains used for superinfection have been looked for in the ganglia by very sensitive methods, including DNA hybridization and DNA mapping techniques. Superinfection has also been performed with a viral strain that does not produce glycoprotein C. Antiglycoprotein C neutralizing antibody inhibits normal viral replication but permits glycoprotein C-deficient strains to grow. In the presence of neutralizing antibody, no growth could be detected in the ganglia, even with sophisticated cocultivation techniques.

In the laboratory, it is possible to make exceptions to this general rule of a single strain of virus for a single individual. For example, if both eyes of a rabbit are simultaneously infected with different viral strains, each homolateral trigeminal ganglion may become infected with the homolateral infecting strain.[23] Similarly, if primary infection is produced with a defective laboratory viral strain that causes poor and partial infection because of manipulation of the viral DNA, it is possible to superinfect a ganglion. In humans, occasional examples of ganglionic colonization by more than one viral strain have been documented, but these are the exception and not the rule.

The history of the understanding of strain differences in HSV is, in a way, a history of fads in science. It has been known for several years that total-body radiation or total immunosuppression could disseminate the virus and make herpetic disease worse. Similarly, it was known that corticosteroids could worsen herpetic disease. From these observations, it was assumed that differences in manifestations and severity of herpetic disease among different individuals must be caused by differences in immunologic resistance and that severe disease must in some way be the result of a relative immunodeficiency. The assumption was made that HSV was a simple virus with no variation in virulence, that variations in disease were host related, and that somehow a particular host could have lowered immunologic resistance to this one virus but be resistant to other organisms and be otherwise healthy.

Recurrences, too, were thought to be lapses in immunocompetence. It was known that in humans, sudden fevers, exposure to sunlight, and stress could cause herpetic recurrences, that preganglionic neurectomy for trigeminal pain could cause herpetic disease along the distribution of the nerve, and that, in animals, iontophoresis of various substances[24] or even the stripping of adhesive tape from a mouse ear[25] could cause herpetic recurrences, all without obvious change in immune status. Nevertheless, all this information was ignored and the assumption was made that, in humans, immunodeficiency for only one agent must somehow be responsible for herpetic recurrences and that immunocompetence, if sufficient, could somehow prevent recurrences.

Although it is clear that severe immunodeficiency can make herpetic disease worse, there is no evidence that variations in immunologic status and differences in host susceptibility are related to the severity of herpetic disease in otherwise healthy people. Similarly, there is no evidence that variations in immunologic status make possible or prevent recurrences in otherwise healthy people. Logically, it is difficult to credit the idea that somehow people could have an immunodeficiency to this one virus but otherwise be well and immunocompetent in all other respects.

An alternative approach to the recognition and explanation of differences in herpetic disease patterns is the understanding that the viral genome contains large amounts of genetic material that can determine the manifestations and severity of herpetic infection. Based on the epidemiology of HSV and the fact that so many people have been infected but so few actually express clinical disease, it seems likely that most HSV-1 strains produce subclinical disease or such mild disease that it is not recognized. Most strains of the virus, therefore, are virulent in the sense of invading the body and colonizing the ganglia but are not disease producing under normal circumstances. Some strains of virus, however, do produce eye disease or labial disease of varying degrees of severity.

In the laboratory, strains of HSV have been obtained that produce different kinds of dendritic ulcers in rabbits and in mice.[26-28] Each strain always produces dendritic ulcers typical of that particular strain, and the different strains can be differentiated simply by the appearance of the ulcer. In other words, the extent, length, and shape of the ulcer are determined by the genetic material contained in the virus.

We looked at two different strains of HSV in rabbits, all of which were equally immunocompetent. One strain produced small dendrites and a high incidence of stromal disease, and another produced long, filamentous dendrites and virtually no stromal disease.[27] The DNA from these two viral strains was broken up with digestive enzymes and recombined to make "daughter virus." Patterns of dendrites and patterns of stromal disease varied in the five daughter strains. It was clear that dendritic disease was an inherent property of the viral genome and peculiar to the specific strain. It was also clear that stromal disease was determined by the viral genome and was not connected with or determined by the epithelial disease but rather segregated separately from it. It appears that strains that produce a high incidence of stromal disease also produce large amounts of highly antigenic glycoproteins,[29,30] so that the occurrence of stromal disease, although immunogenic, may be determined by the virus in terms of how much and what kind of antigen it produces, rather than being a primary function of immunoreactivity of the host. Others[28] have suggested that genetically determined, nonimmunologic differences in the ability of the host cell to restrict virus replication may play a role in susceptibility to stromal disease.

Recurrence rates also appear to be determined in part by the viral genome. For example, a study was performed in rabbits in which one eye was infected with McKrae strain, which has a high recurrence rate, and the other eye was infected simultaneously with MacIntyre strain, which has a low recurrence rate.[23] Each homolateral trigeminal ganglion became infected with the viral strain used to infect the corresponding eye. The rabbits had a higher recurrence rate in the eye infected with McKrae strain than in the eye infected with MacIntyre strain. This occurred in the same animal with the same immunologic status but with a different viral strain infecting each eye, indicating that immunologic status alone cannot explain differences in recurrence rates, just as it cannot explain patterns of disease.

This work has been carried further. For example, some viral strains cause an epithelial keratitis that is made worse with corticosteroids. Other strains, however, do not.[31] How can this be explained if the effect of corticosteroids is based on local immunosuppression? The answer is that it cannot. The ability of corticosteroids to make herpetic infection worse has been documented in tissue culture[32] where no immunologic elements are present. The explanation for the corticosteroid effect on HSV growth remains unclear at this time.

The site of an eruption of herpetic disease may also be determined by the viral genome. Different strains of HSV grow preferentially at different temperatures; some grow better at warmer temperatures (near core body temperature) and others grow better at lower temperatures (nearer corneal temperature).[33,34] Although both kinds of strains can infect the cornea, evidence suggests that strains that prefer cooler temperatures are more likely to cause corneal reinfection, whereas strains that prefer higher temperatures are more likely to produce mucocutaneous infection. Similarly, it seems likely that strains that cause encephalitis might prefer still higher temperatures. This is now a hypothesis with some evidence, and although unproven, might explain why, although virus may colonize the whole trigeminal ganglion, some people get labial infections and others get corneal infections. It may also explain the tendency of the virus to cause lesions in some individuals when fever develops and body temperature rises.

Our hypothesis of the mechanism of HSV infection is that most of us are infected early in life. The ganglia are colonized by virus, in most people a "good virus" that is incapable of producing disease except under extreme conditions. Others, however, in a "virologic roulette," are colonized by a more virulent virus that produces more severe clinical disease and frequent recurrences. Once a ganglion is infected, it appears impossible to superinfect that ganglion under normal circumstances, and the initial infecting viral strain probably stays with the individual for life. This accounts for the fact that in herpetic infections, recurrences in a given individual seem to be caused by virus with the same DNA composition (i.e., the same virus from the same ganglion).[35] Both the severity of the disease and the frequency of recurrences are determined to a large extent by the viral genome and its inherent patterns of virulence.

Although the precise role of the immune system is not clear, it is not our intent to imply that it has no role.[36] Stromal disease is almost certainly, in part, an immune reaction to viral antigen. The differences in the occurrence of stromal disease, however, appear likely to be not differences in immunoreactivity from one person to another, but rather differences in the amounts and types of individual glycoproteins produced by the different viral strains that stimulate this immunoreactive process.

If these findings and the consequent hypothesis are true, several things follow. First, recurrences are probably triggered by factors other than immunologic factors when they occur at times of fever, trauma, stress, or other stimuli that are poorly understood. There are, therefore, specific neuronal triggers that may be important in determining recurrences, in addition to the inherent genetic material of the virus. Second, immunization after infection has occurred is unlikely to play a major role in controlling herpetic disease. In fact, immunization and vaccination after ganglionic colonization has occurred could make herpetic disease worse. Finally, it seems likely that the most effective type of vaccination may be an inoculation early in life with a non-disease-producing virus that colonizes the ganglia and blocks later colonization by virulent virus. In this case, the colonizing virus must be known to be safe not only in terms of not producing disease but also in terms of being unlikely to be associated with tumorigenesis (HSV-1 has been associated with nasopharyngeal tumors and HSV-2 with cervical carcinoma and other malignancies). Similarly, there must be sufficient experimental evidence to indicate that this virus, which in nature can be genetically unstable, will remain stable in the vaccinated host and, if secreted, will not change enough to endanger others.

CLINICAL MANIFESTATIONS

The clinical manifestations of HSV infection are varied. The virus may produce a primary infection of the skin or mucous membranes, which can spread over the face, but tends to recur, if at all, at the mucocutaneous junctions of the lip and nose. In the mouth, the virus can cause recurrent intraoral herpetic disease and a diffuse vesicular eruption in the mouth and throat. Aphthous stomatitis (the ordinary canker sore) does not appear to be caused by herpes simplex virus. Cutaneous infections can occur, especially in wrestlers (herpes gladiatorum) and dentists (herpetic whitlow), in which there is direct inoculation of the virus. In immunocompromised or atopic individuals, the virus may spread all over the body, causing a herpes varicelliform eruption that has a mortality of approximately 50 percent (Figure 10-3).

Ocular manifestations of HSV infection are equally varied and include blepharitis, canalicular obstruction, conjunctivitis, keratitis, uveitis, and retinitis. Herpetic eye disease is a leading cause of corneal blindness caused by infectious disease in the United States. The social and economic impact of this disease is, therefore, substantial.

Blepharitis

Herpetic blepharitis is most likely to occur at the time of a primary infection, with virus present on the skin around the eyelids, on the eyelid margins, and on the eye. Vesicular lesions on an erythematous base occur on the eyelids and surrounding skin and go through the typical stages of ulceration and crusting (Figures 10-4 and 10-5). The lesions do not cause scarring unless they become secondarily infected. Scrapings of the base of a lesion stained with

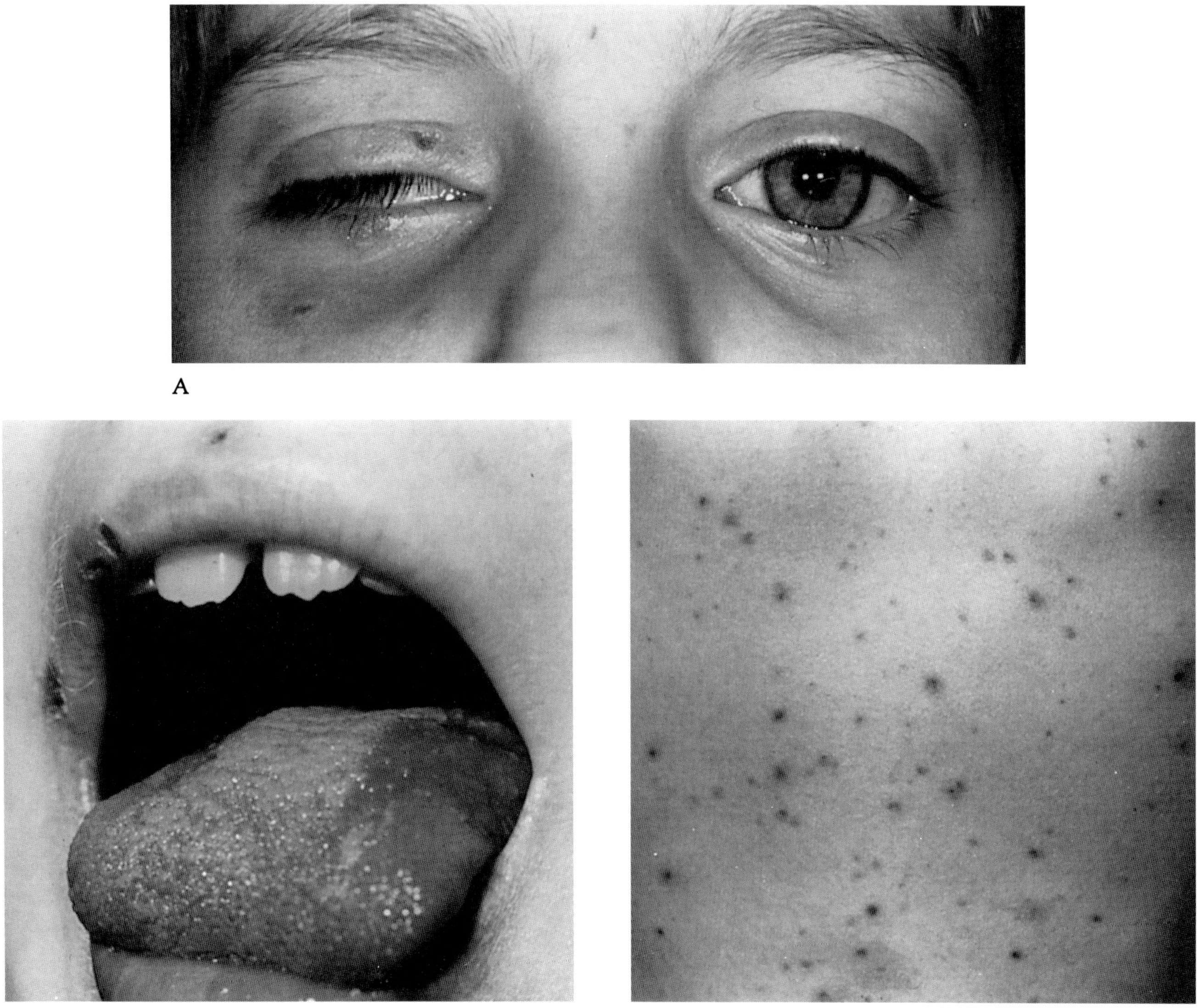

A

B

C

FIGURE 10-3 Disseminated herpes simplex viral infection, involving **(A)** the eye, **(B)** oral mucous membranes, and **(C)** skin of the extremities.

FIGURE 10-4 Blepharoconjunctivitis caused by herpes simplex virus. Note the ulcerated vesicles.

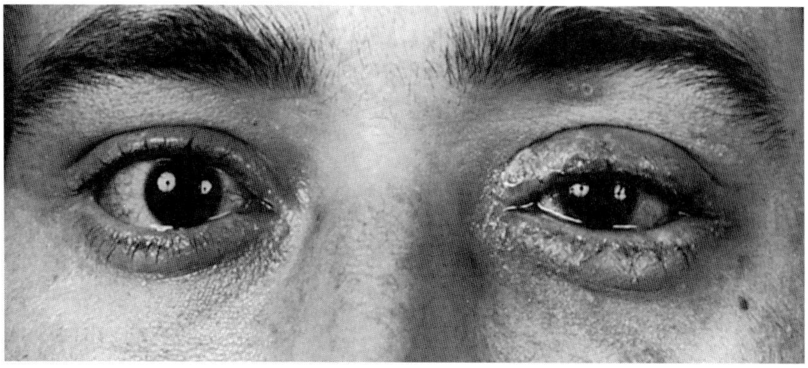

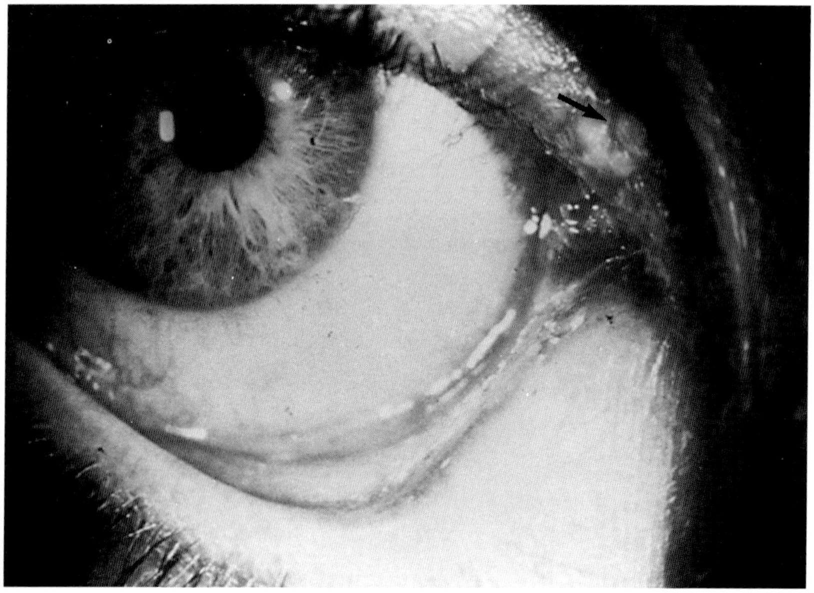

FIGURE 10-5 Group of herpes simplex virus vesicles on the eyelid (arrow).

Giemsa stain (Tzanck preparation) may demonstrate the characteristic multinucleated giant cells or intranuclear inclusions. The random distribution of the lesions helps to differentiate them from lesions of herpes zoster ophthalmicus; however, sometimes the distinction is difficult. Definitive diagnosis may be made by characteristic ocular findings, if present, or by viral culture of the lesions.

Herpetic blepharitis, either primary or recurrent, may occur in the absence of other herpetic eye disease. One of the questions often raised is whether the eye of a patient with herpetic blepharitis should be protected with an antiviral agent, since most of these patients will not develop corneal disease. Our custom is to use an antiviral agent because herpetic infection of the eye itself, although rare, occurs often enough that prophylaxis is justified in patients who do not react adversely to the antiviral agent.

Conjunctivitis

During primary infection with HSV, follicular conjunctivitis may occur and may precede corneal infection (Figure 10-6). HSV may also produce recurrent follicular

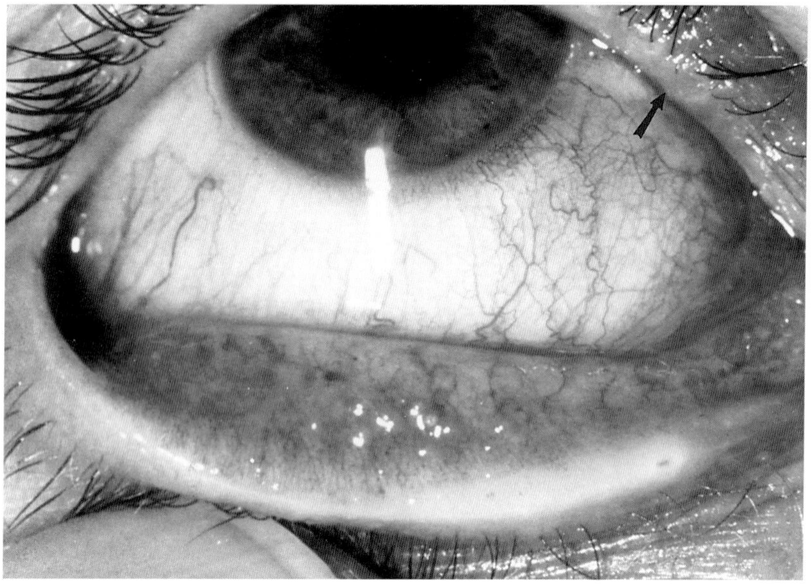

FIGURE 10-6 Follicular conjunctivitis caused by herpes simplex virus. Note the accompanying ulcerated lesion on the eyelid (arrow). The eyelids should be examined carefully for the presence of vesicles in any patient with follicular conjunctivitis. (Courtesy of Chandler R. Dawson, M.D., San Francisco, CA.)

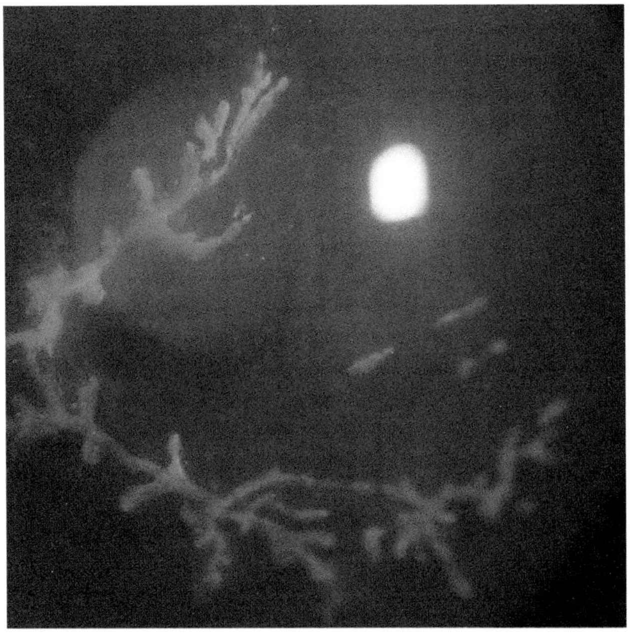

FIGURE 10-7 Pathognomonic fluorescein-stained dendrite caused by herpes simplex virus. Note the linear branching pattern and the "terminal bulbs" at the end of each branch.

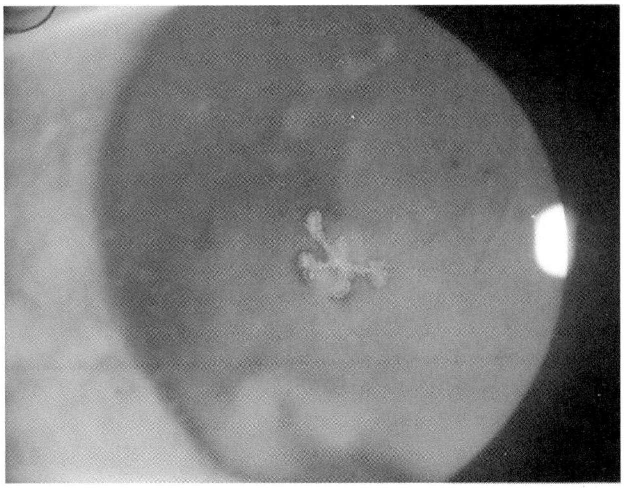

FIGURE 10-8 Small herpes simplex viral dendrite (fluorescein stain).

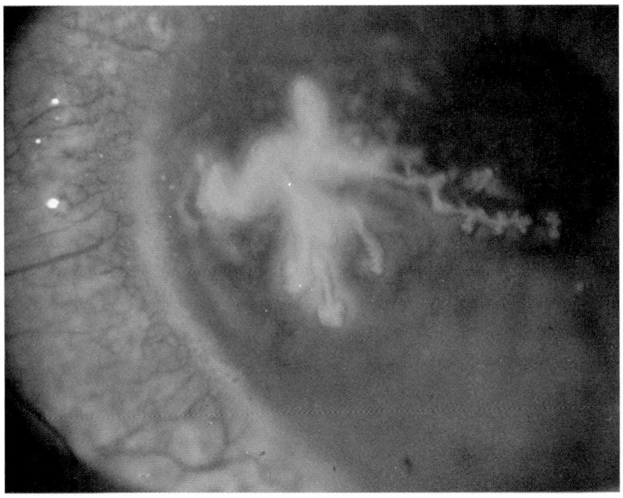

FIGURE 10-9 Herpes simplex viral dendrite nearly large enough to be considered a geographic ulcer (fluorescein stain).

conjunctivitis, and even conjunctival scarring, in the absence of corneal disease. This phenomenon is often unrecognized because conjunctival ulcers are rarely seen, and the diagnosis cannot be made without viral cultures, which are not generally available outside of large institutional laboratories. Many of these patients give a history of having had previously diagnosed herpetic disease; however, some do not. Therefore, any patient with recurrent follicular conjunctivitis of unknown origin should be suspected of having recurrent herpetic conjunctivitis. It is important to include herpetic conjunctivitis in the differential diagnosis because the result of using topical corticosteroids for the treatment of follicular conjunctivitis caused by HSV can be devastating.

Epithelial Keratitis

In the cornea, HSV infection may present as punctate keratitis, small bullous epithelial lesions, a dendritic ulcer, or a geographic ulcer. Most cases of herpetic epithelial keratitis present initially as a pathognomonic dendrite, which is a branching linear lesion (Figure 10-7). The base of the dendrite is devoid of epithelium and stains with fluorescein; the edges contain actively replicating virus in epithelial cells and stain with rose bengal. The reason for the dendritic pattern is not clear.

Dendrites occur in many shapes and sizes (Figures 10-8 to 10-10). Some may be extremely small and can sometimes be confused with the coarse superficial punctate keratitis described by Thygeson.[37] In coarse superficial punctate keratitis, the history is one of chronicity, with many remissions and exacerbations. The disease is usually bilateral, symptoms are minimal, and the eye is relatively quiet. Herpetic epithelial keratitis may transiently resemble this disorder for a day or so, but its morphology changes rapidly; herpetic disease is not chronic in this form and should never be mistaken for coarse superficial punctate keratitis. Whereas

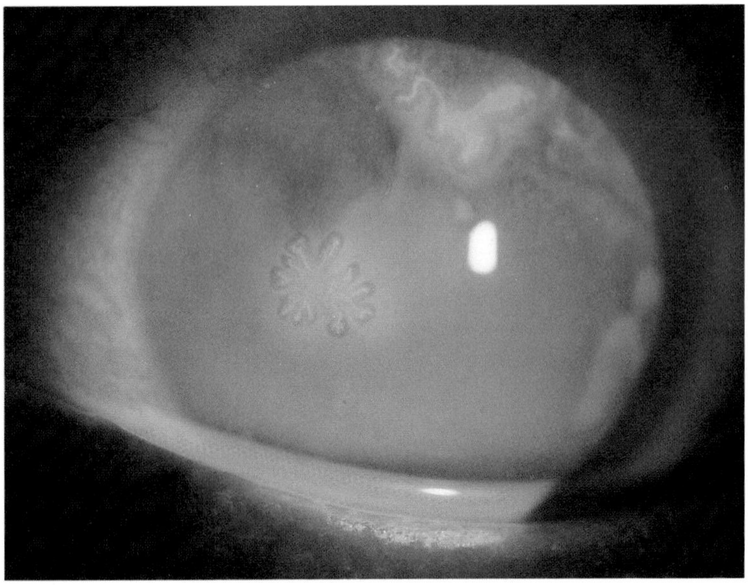

FIGURE 10-10 Two herpes simplex viral dendrites in the same eye that have different shapes (fluorescein stain).

coarse superficial punctate keratitis responds to corticosteroids, herpetic epithelial keratitis is made worse. The distinction is also important because antivirals may make coarse superficial punctate keratitis worse.

If the area of active herpetic ulceration is large, it is referred to as a geographic ulcer (Figure 10-11). Geographic ulcers may have dendritic edges, which are useful in differentiating them from corneal ulcers not caused by HSV. Geographic ulcers respond more slowly than dendritic ulcers to antiviral agents, and re-epithelialization of the bed of the ulcer is difficult. An ulcer that persists after active herpetic infection is referred to as a *postinfectious ulcer,* although other terms, such as *metaherpetic* or *trophic ulcer,* have been used.

One of the potentially confusing manifestations of herpetic epithelial keratitis is the limbal ulcer, which may appear at first glance to resemble marginal keratitis caused by *Staphylococcus aureus,* although the herpetic lesions are always ulcerated (Figures 10-12 and 10-13). Sometimes there are dendritic edges to the ulcer, which confirms the viral cause, but the diagnosis must often be made in the laboratory, either with fluorescent antibody studies or viral culture. Peripheral herpetic epithelial keratitis is difficult to treat and responds more slowly

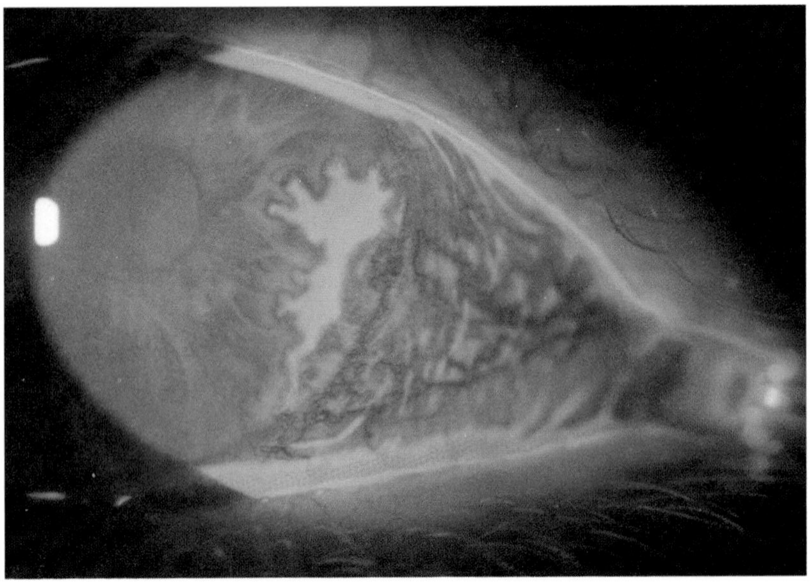

FIGURE 10-11 Geographic ulcer caused by herpes simplex virus (fluorescein stain).

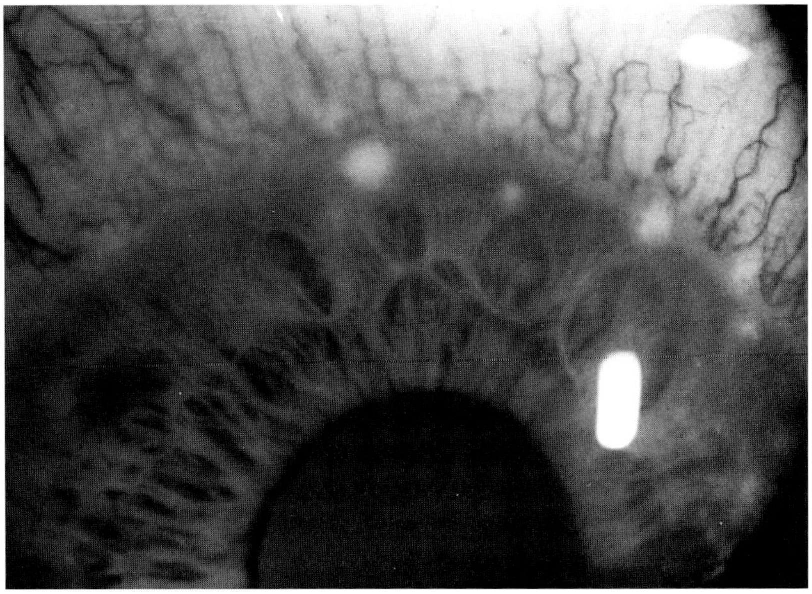

FIGURE 10-12 Peripheral corneal infiltrates caused by herpes simplex virus. Unlike marginal keratitis from *Staphylococcus aureus* blepharoconjunctivitis, these lesions usually begin as ulcerations, followed by infiltration.

to antiviral agents than its centrally located counterpart.[38]

Herpetic epithelial infections occasionally present with a clinically atypical appearance that delays or confounds diagnosis in patients who have no history of herpetic disease. Among the circumstances that may stimulate these masquerade infections are corneal surgery and trauma. Prompted by experimental studies in which previously infected rabbits demonstrated recurrent herpes after penetrating keratoplasty followed by corticosteroid treatment,[39,40] we looked more closely at patients without a history of herpes who, after surgery, developed persistent epithelial defects with none of the typical characteristics of herpes. Despite the lack of pathognomonic signs, herpesvirus was found in several of these lesions. We[41] and others[42] have described cases of early- and late-onset postkeratoplasty epithelial defects that have had cultures positive for HSV and have responded to antiviral treatment. Similarly, a Japanese study[43] used immunofluorescence techniques to demonstrate that about one-quarter of patients with recurrent erosions, superficial punctate keratitis, marginal ulcer, or follicular conjunctivitis had herpes antigen, although there was no overt evidence or history of herpes. In that most adults probably carry latent herpesvirus whether or not

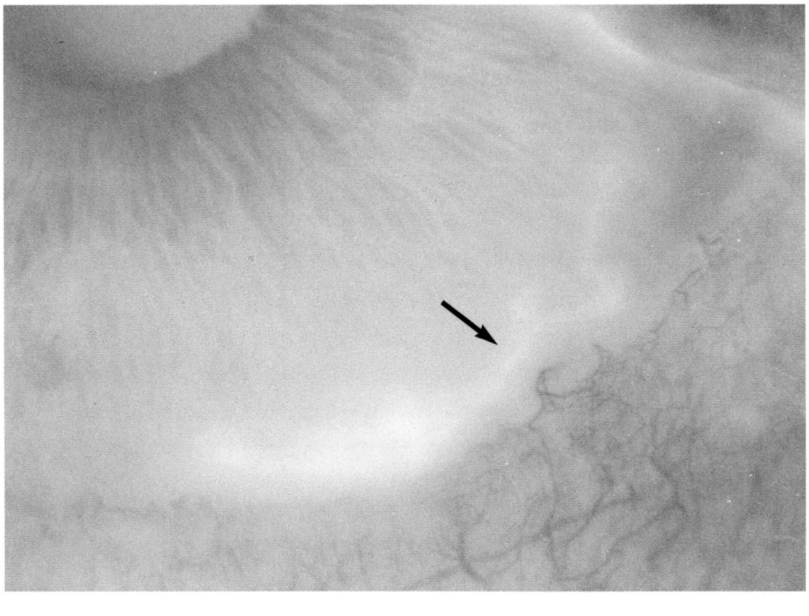

FIGURE 10-13 Peripheral dendrite (arrow) caused by herpes simplex virus (fluorescein stain).

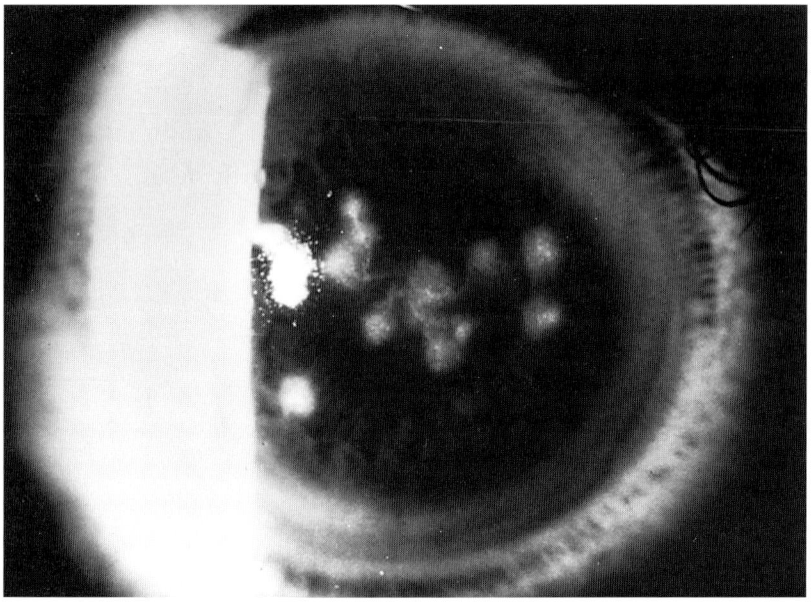

FIGURE 10-14 Superficial stromal scarring beneath a resolving herpes simplex viral dendrite. The dendritic shape of the scarring is characteristic.

they are aware of previous disease, this phenomenon may be more common than has been recognized. HSV should be considered as a possible cause of epithelial keratitis after any intraocular surgery when postoperative corticosteroids are used. In particular, when the patient has no history of ocular herpetic disease, a high index of suspicion on the part of the ophthalmologist is necessary for accurate diagnosis, as well as timely and effective therapy.

Stromal Keratitis

There are several types of herpetic stromal disease that must be differentiated from one another for clinical management to be effective: superficial stromal scarring, necrotizing stromal keratitis, and disciform edema.

Superficial Stromal Scarring

Faint superficial scars can develop under an epithelial dendrite or ulcer, especially if it is chronic and treatment has been inadequate or delayed (Figure 10-14). These scars are simply an extension of damage from the superficial ulcer and are not an indication for corticosteroids. Treatment should be directed toward healing the epithelium.

Necrotizing Stromal Keratitis

In necrotizing stromal keratitis, the lesion appears white, necrotic, and heavily infiltrated (Figure 10-15). It may extend deep into the stroma, resulting in marked corneal thinning or perforation.

The exact pathogenesis of necrotizing stromal keratitis is not known. We believe that it is caused by direct viral invasion of the stroma and that the visible disease is largely the immune reaction to this process. It is clear that when a herpetic epithelial ulcer is treated extensively with corticosteroids without antiviral coverage, viral particles can be found within the stroma[44,45] (Figure 10-16). In addition to these viral particles, viral antigens may be present in the cell membranes of keratocytes. We believe that virus often persists in the cornea in these deep necrotic scars and that in patients who need corneal transplantation, stromal invasion of the transplant by the virus is a significant hazard if the visible stromal scar cannot be completely excised.

In a rabbit model, it is possible to destroy host defenses and to show that direct viral invasion results in stromal necrosis and severe corneal damage. Similarly, in both rabbits and humans, there is evidence that the virus can insert viral glycoproteins into the host cell membrane,[46,47] rendering the membrane antigenically different and recognizable by host immune mechanisms, creating, in effect, an "autoimmune" mechanism for chronic disease.

Some HSV strains produce stromal disease and others do not. If a rabbit eye is inoculated with one of the stromal disease-producing strains, it appears that the virus must multiply within the stroma for about 1 week before significant stromal disease appears.[48] At the end of the period of viral multiplication, when the amount of virus decreases rapidly, the host reaction against the virus and viral antigens produces severe necrotizing keratitis. This is, for all practical purposes, a pure antigen-induced stromal disease secondary to HSV infection and is highly strain specific. In animal models, if the eye is treated with an antiviral agent during the first day or two after infection, stromal disease can be prevented.[49] If antiviral treat-

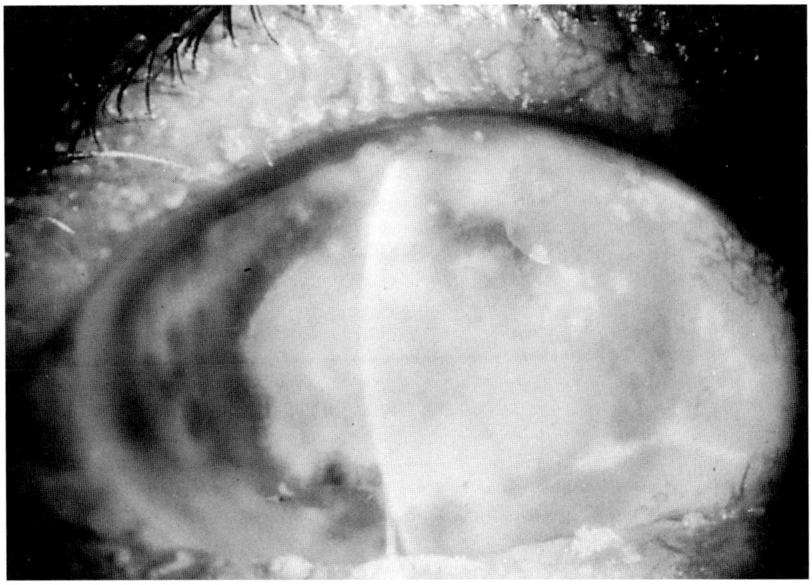

FIGURE 10-15 Necrotizing stromal keratitis caused by herpes simplex virus.

ment is delayed beyond this initial period so that the stroma has been colonized with virus and viral antigens have been produced, antiviral agents are of no use. At this point, however, corticosteroids seem to be of benefit and appear to carry little or no additional risk of worsening the disease.

An understanding of the pathogenesis of the human form of this disease would be important for successful treatment. If necrotizing stromal keratitis is caused by multiplying virus, antiviral treatment should be highly effective. If it is largely an antigenic disease, with only a modest component of viral multiplication occurring before the obvious manifestations of the disease, antiviral therapy may have little effect by the time the disease becomes evident. Unfortunately, the precise pathogenesis is not known.

Therapeutic or preventative approaches to necrotizing stromal keratitis must be considered with caution. For example, if an immune reaction is responsible for stromal necrosis, an increase in immunity by vaccination or the administration of antibodies may worsen the disease. A parallel situation occurred several years ago, when it was

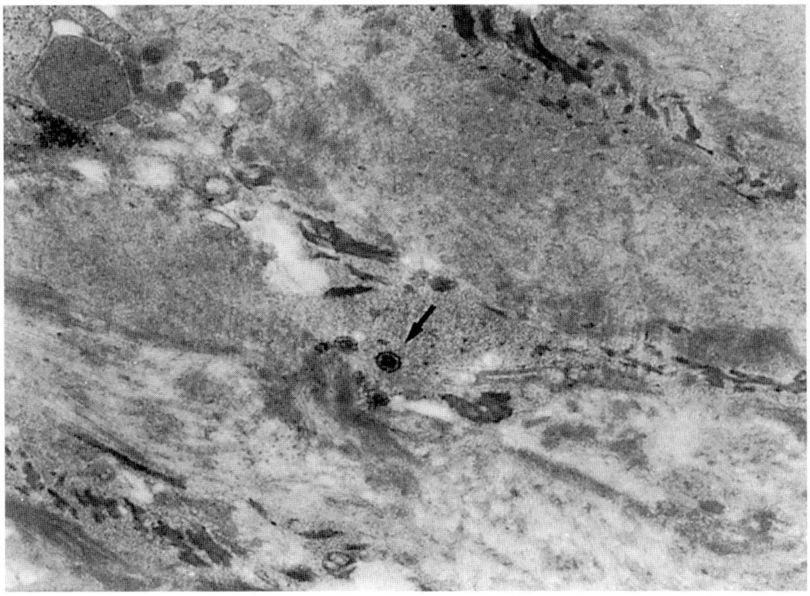

FIGURE 10-16 Herpesvirus particles (arrow) in a degenerated keratocyte in the stroma of a patient who had necrotizing stromal keratitis. (Reprinted with permission from JJ Sanitato, PA Asbell, ED Varnell, et al: Acyclovir in the treatment of herpetic stromal disease. Am J Ophthalmol 98:537, 1984. Copyright by The Ophthalmic Publishing Company.)

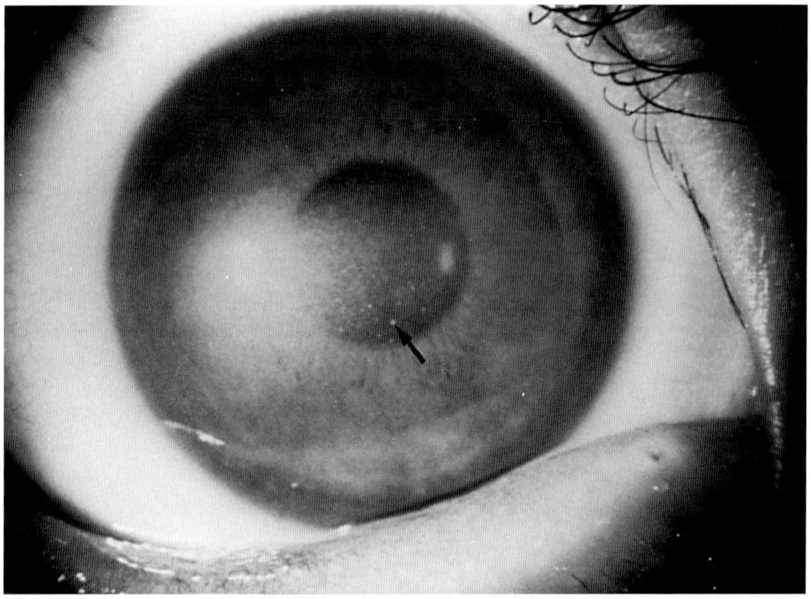

FIGURE 10-17 Disciform edema caused by herpes simplex virus. Note the keratic precipitates (arrow).

proposed that human vaccinial keratitis (which is similar to herpes simplex keratitis in many ways) be treated with vaccinial immune globulin. The immune globulin made the ocular disease significantly worse. Vaccination and immunization might well have the same result in cases of herpes simplex keratitis.

Disciform Edema

Disciform edema is clinically quite different from necrotizing stromal keratitis. It generally occurs centrally as a disk of corneal edema similar to that caused by Fuchs' dystrophy, hydrops, or a traumatic tear in Descemet's membrane (Figure 10-17). Although the differentiation of herpetic disciform edema from these diseases is usually simple, sometimes it is not. Two signs are present in herpetic disciform edema that aid in this differentiation. First, herpetic disciform edema is generally associated with keratic precipitates. These are difficult to see through the edema but are often most visible at the lower edge of the lesion, where they settle by gravity. They do not generally extend onto normal cornea. Second, herpetic disciform edema virtually always responds to corticosteroids, and as the corneal edema clears (usually within 7 to 10 days), the keratic precipitates may be seen. None of the other diseases is associated with keratic precipitates or responds to corticosteroids. Herpetic disciform edema may occasionally be eccentric, occurring near the limbus, or it may be diffuse, in the form of bullous keratopathy, in which case it is likely to be more severe and more difficult to treat (Figure 10-18). Disciform edema frequently results in corneal scarring and thinning and may stimulate the growth of blood vessels into the stroma (Figure 10-19).

Disciform edema is always accompanied by iritis, but the iritis is usually not clinically diagnosable because cells and flare cannot be seen through the edematous cornea. They are visible only around the lesion after the edema begins to clear.

The exact pathogenesis of herpetic disciform edema is not known. In our experience, specimens of aqueous humor obtained by paracentesis from patients with disciform edema have yielded a low incidence of positive viral cultures even though viral antigens have been found.[50] This finding, along with the almost uniform response of disciform edema to corticosteroids and the relatively minor destruction of endothelial cells documented by specular microscopy, suggests that disciform edema may be a reversible toxic reaction caused, perhaps, by the presence of antigen-antibody complexes. Sundmacher and Neumann-Haefelin[51] obtained a higher incidence of positive viral cultures than we did and believe that herpetic disciform edema is a true endotheliitis caused by direct invasion of the endothelium by the virus. This seems to us to be incompatible with the rapid response to corticosteroids. It may be that, although clinically the populations in the two studies[50,51] appeared to be similar, there were significant differences between them. The conflict between these observations is not trivial when one considers the possible therapeutic options, such as antiviral therapy.

It is assumed in the literature that stromal keratitis always follows superficial epithelial keratitis and that

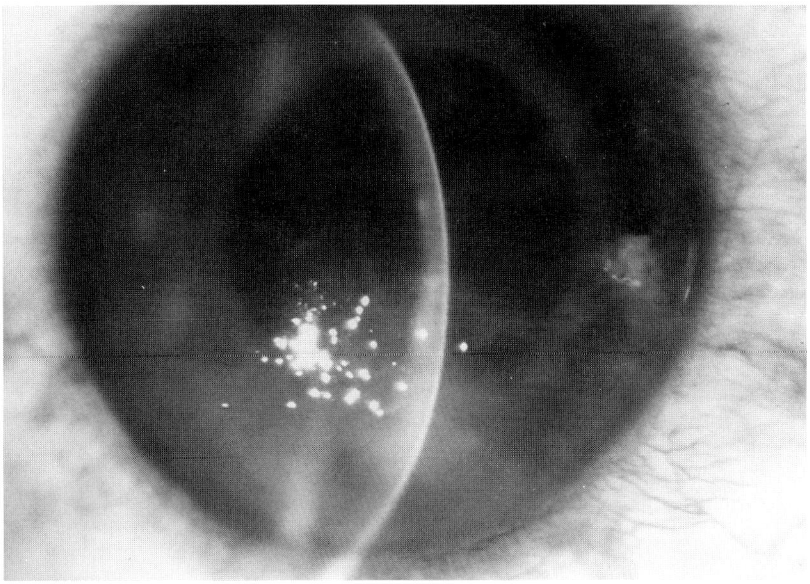

FIGURE 10-18 Bullous keratopathy caused by herpes simplex virus.

there is some cause-and-effect relationship between them. Although this may be so, we have seen several patients with epithelial keratitis who had healed rapidly several months before and later developed stromal keratitis in the absence of recent epithelial keratitis. Similarly, we have seen patients with stromal keratitis who deny ever having had epithelial keratitis and yet who, when treated with corticosteroids without antiviral coverage, develop dendritic ulcers. In animal studies, we have shown that stromal virulence is determined in the virus genome, and is independent of the presence of epithelial disease.[27]

Endotheliitis

Herpetic endotheliitis is rare. It is usually associated with anterior uveitis and is nonprogressive. However, we reported a case in which the endotheliitis was progressive and had the clinical appearance of an endothelial rejection line, with advancing keratic precipitates and corneal edema[52] (Figure 10-20). Aspirated samples of aqueous humor and keratic precipitates were positive for herpes simplex antigens and viral growth. Since that time, other cases have been reported.[53,54]

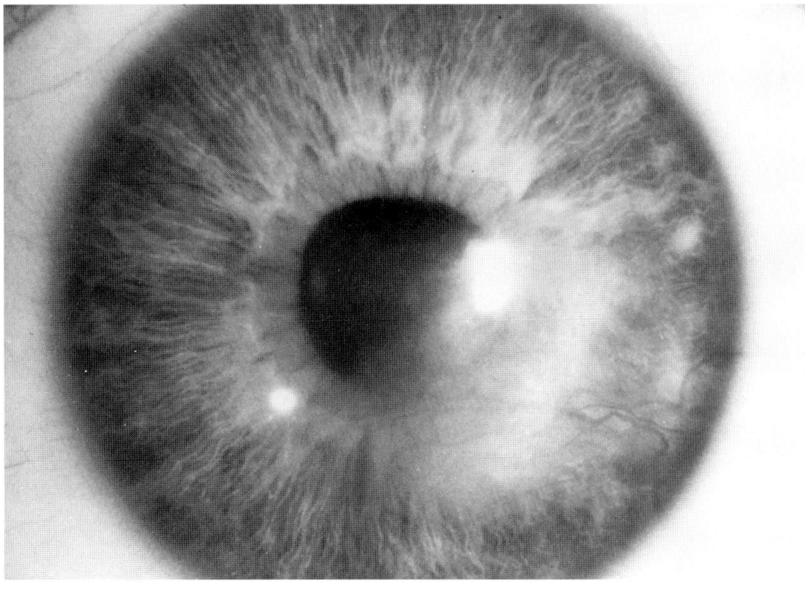

FIGURE 10-19 Scarring and vascularization resulting from herpes simplex viral stromal keratitis.

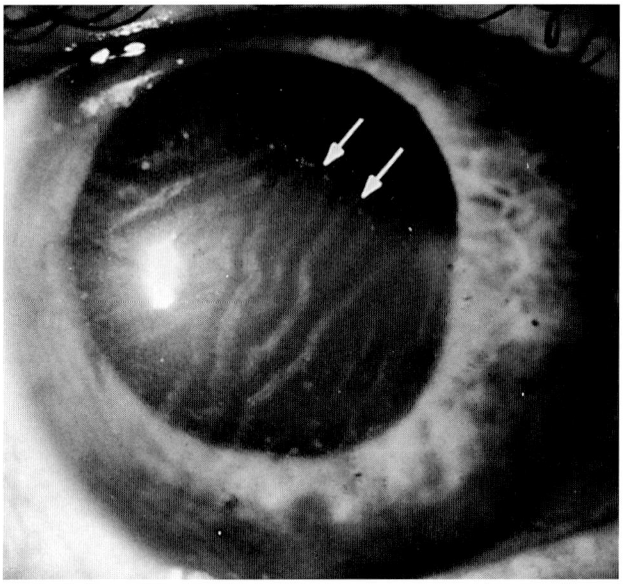

FIGURE 10-20 Herpetic endotheliitis demonstrating stromal edema and a line of pigmented keratic precipitates (arrows) at the junction of edematous and nonedematous cornea. (Reprinted with permission from JB Robin, JB Steigner, HE Kaufman: Progressive corneal endotheliitis. Am J Ophthalmol 100:336, 1985. Copyright by The Ophthalmic Publishing Company.)

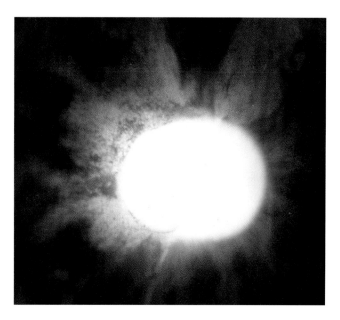

FIGURE 10-21 Several areas of focal iris necrosis caused by herpetic uveitis. (Courtesy of Chandler R. Dawson, M.D., San Francisco, CA.)

Uveitis

HSV can produce uveitis, although severe herpetic uveitis is rare. In some patients, the iris may develop segmental necrosis (Figure 10-21); in others the entire iris may develop intravascular thromboses and become ischemic and necrotic. The ciliary body may even develop areas of necrosis. With severe iritis, membranes sometimes grow into the anterior chamber angle, producing not only secondary glaucoma from inflammatory debris but also angle closure glaucoma from the membranes themselves. Hyphema from severe herpetic iritis, although uncommon, is not atypical.

Herpetic uveitis with no other signs of herpetic disease is difficult to diagnose. We have had several patients with a vague history of herpetic ocular disease who presented with severe iritis of undiagnosed etiology. Anterior chamber paracentesis and fluorescent antibody staining were done. Two drops of aqueous humor were allowed to air dry on a slide; one was treated with nonimmune rabbit serum and the other with fluorescein-labeled rabbit anti-HSV, followed by examination with an immunofluorescence microscope. This procedure revealed viral antigens within white cells. Occasional viral particles were seen by electron microscopic examination.[50]

Retinitis

Herpes simplex viral retinitis has been diagnosed primarily in association with herpetic encephalitis. It may occur suddenly, is typically bilateral, and is devastating. There are large exudative retinal detachments, which lead to blindness. HSV can cause the acute retinal necrosis (ARN) syndrome,[55-60] but other herpesviruses, such as varicella-zoster virus, have also been implicated.[60-63] HSV and varicella-zoster virus account for most, if not all, cases of the acute retinal necrosis syndrome. Intravenous acyclovir is the current medical treatment of choice.[60]

LABORATORY DIAGNOSIS

A typical herpetic epithelial dendrite is pathognomonic of HSV infection of the cornea, and clinical observation of such a dendrite by an experienced physician provides an accurate diagnosis. For patients who do not present with a typical corneal lesion, however, one or more laboratory tests can be done to confirm the presence of the virus. Among these are tissue culture, which assays for live virus; various generic and commercial immunoassays, which confirm the presence of viral antigen; and molecular biologic techniques such as the polymerase chain reaction, which amplifies and identifies viral DNA.

Tissue Culture

The gold standard of laboratory tests for HSV is tissue culture. Specificity is 100 percent (all patients with positive cultures have herpes), but sensitivity may range from 85 to 100 percent (occasionally, a patient with a negative culture may be infected, but sampling error or culture conditions may produce a false-negative result). An advantage of tissue culture for HSV is that further studies of the isolated virus are possible. The major disadvantages are the need for laboratory facilities and the length of time required to obtain the results (days to weeks).

To culture for ocular herpes, one drop of a topical anesthetic eye drop (0.5 percent proparacaine) is applied to the patient's cornea. A sterile cotton- or dacron-tipped swab is dipped into a test tube containing tissue culture medium (Medium 199, Eagle's Minimal Essential Medium, or any other widely available tissue culture medium containing antibiotics) and pressed against the side of the tube to remove excess medium. The wet swab is gently touched to the lesion, then swept through the upper and lower fornices of the eye, and returned to the test tube. The tube containing the swab can be stored in a refrigerator for up to 8 hours before it is transferred to the laboratory for further processing.

In the laboratory, the tube is vortexed on a mechanical laboratory vortexing instrument. Then the tube is opened and the swab is pressed against the side of the tube to remove the absorbed tissue culture medium. Aliquots (0.1 ml) of the tissue culture medium from the tube are added to previously prepared monolayer cultures of susceptible cells. Some laboratories use African green monkey kidney cells, such as CV-1, whereas others prefer to use the human cell line designated A549. The inoculated cell cultures are incubated at 37°C and observed daily, by means of an inverted tissue culture microscope, for the appearance of cytopathic effect.

Cytopathic effect, which denotes the presence of growing virus, is evidenced as a focal destruction of the monolayer of cells in the culture dish (Figure 10-22). The effect may be seen as early as 48 hours or as late as 10 to 14 days after inoculation. That the cytopathic effect is caused by herpes simplex virus can be confirmed immunohistochemically.

Immunoassays

Some physicians prefer to confirm a diagnosis of ocular herpes using an immunoassay to detect viral antigen in the presumably HSV-infected cornea. In particular, a patient who has already been treated with an antiviral agent may have a negative viral culture, but the presence of HSV antigen would still provide confirmation of the diagnosis.

In cases in which a clinical diagnosis of superficial corneal herpetic infection based purely on clinical grounds is not possible, immunofluorescent staining of the cells obtained from the corneal lesion may aid in the identification of the causative agent. The advantage of immunofluorescent staining is that the results are available more rapidly than are the results of viral culture. The major disadvantage is the need for a well-equipped laboratory and an experienced technician to perform the assay. The results are reasonably reliable; one study reported a sensitivity of 90 percent and a specificity of 100 percent,[64] although these parameters may vary depending on the type of test and the controls involved.

To obtain a specimen for immunofluorescent staining, the cornea is first anesthetized with topical proparacaine. A sterile spatula or less ideally, a sterile cotton- or dacron-tipped swab, is gently applied to the cornea. Particular effort is made to collect material from the lesion on the spatula. The specimen is then gently smeared on a microscope slide and allowed to air dry.

When the collected material has dried, the slide is immersed in acetone for 1 minute and then in saline for 1 minute. An aliquot (0.1 ml) of diluted (1:1,000) fluorescein-labeled, anti-HSV antibody is applied directly onto the cells collected from the patient's lesion. The slide is incubated for 30 minutes at room temperature, after which it is washed in physiologic saline for three successive 5-minute periods. The slide is then coverslipped and observed with a fluorescence microscope fitted with the appropriate excitation and barrier filters for visualizing fluorescein isothiocyanate-labeled molecules. The corneal cells that contain herpesvirus display a bright apple green fluorescence; if no fluorescence is seen, the cells may not be infected or the amount of virus may be too small to be detected by this test.

One of the chief drawbacks of the immunofluorescence test is that false-negative results may occur because of sampling errors and false-positive results may occur due to nonspecific sticking of the antibody to cellular components. If two or more specimen slides are available, one is incubated first in a 1:100 dilution of unlabeled anti-HSV antibody and then both are incubated in the fluorescein-labeled antibody. The unlabeled antibody blocks binding of the labeled antibody, providing a specificity control.

In recent years, a number of assays that use immunologic principles and techniques, such as the enzyme-linked immunosorbent assay (ELISA), have been developed and marketed.[65-72] At the present time, however, most of these assays are expensive and require a skilled and experienced technician with a fully equipped laboratory to carry them

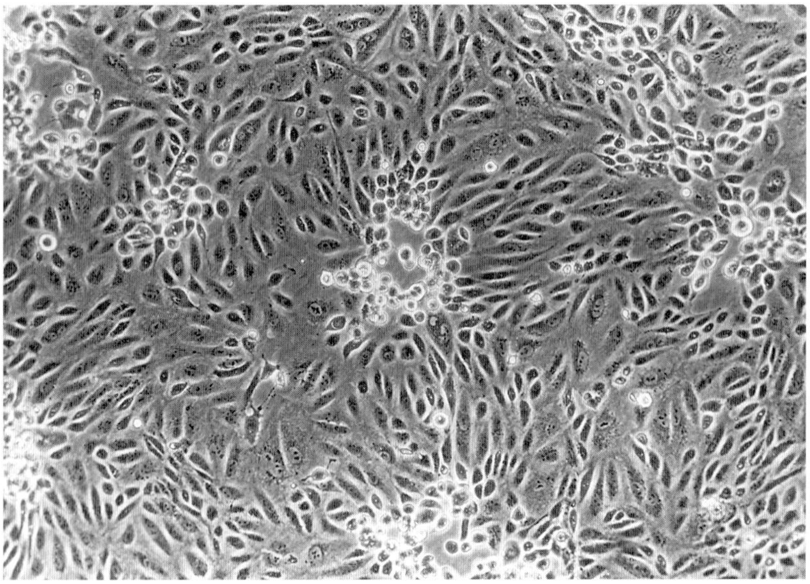

FIGURE 10-22 Tissue culture for herpes simplex virus. A monolayer of CV-1 cells inoculated with a specimen obtained from a cornea by debridement shows several areas of focal destruction of cells by multiplying virus, known as *cytopathic effect.*

out and to interpret the results, which generally precludes their use in an office practice setting.

For one such test, HERPCHEK, the sample is obtained by swabbing the inferior and superior fornices with a cotton- or dacron-tipped swab. Then the swab is stored and/or transported in a special medium until processing begins. Laboratory processing involves preparation of a multiwell plate and addition of the specimen-containing medium, followed by a series of incubations, washings, and additions of solutions. In the final step, the optical density of the wells is read in an ELISA plate reader (spectrophotometer). The entire procedure takes about 5 hours. When the appropriate equipment and trained personnel are available, the results are good; clinical evaluation of ocular specimens showed a sensitivity of 65 percent and a specificity of 100 percent for the original version[65] and both sensitivity and specificity of 100 percent for the latest version.[71] This is a rapid test, and we use it frequently.

One kit, Kodak Surecell, which was developed to test for genital herpes in the physician's office, took only 15 minutes. In this test, the swab was placed in extraction buffer, which was then dropped into three wells; wash solution, peroxide, monoclonal antibody, and dye were added and the results were read visually as the presence or absence of color in each well. Evaluation using clinical ocular samples, however, showed a sensitivity of 27 percent and a specificity of 80 percent.[72] The authors concluded that although the test was rapid and simple, it was not useful for routine diagnosis of ocular herpes because of its low efficiency. This kit is no longer available commercially.

A small cottage industry has developed around the use of membrane immunoassays for the diagnosis of epithelial herpetic infections[73-76]; none of these assays is currently commercially available. Variously referred to as impression debridement,[73,74] corneal impression cytology,[76] or the affinity membrane test,[75] the assays are based on the attachment of virus-infected cells to cellulose acetate or nylon protein-binding membranes and visualization with dye-labeled (e.g., fluorescein) or enzyme-labeled (e.g., peroxidase) antiherpes antibodies. In the simplest and most direct form of this kind of test,[75] the membrane is touched directly to the corneal lesion, incubated in a high protein/antibody mixture, and developed in a substrate solution. The results, which are available in less than 30 minutes, are seen as a colorful (in this case, blue) image of the original lesion (Figure 10-23). To our knowledge, however, most of these tests have not been widely evaluated in patients with ocular herpetic disease; one study showed a sensitivity of 100 percent and a specificity of 92 percent for corneal impression cytology.[76]

Polymerase Chain Reaction

The polymerase chain reaction (PCR) can be used to amplify small amounts of nucleic acid sequences in body fluids and extracts of cells and tissues. This method has been applied to the search for HSV DNA in the cerebrospinal fluid of patients with herpes encephalitis,[77-79] in oral and genital lesions,[80,81] in ocular fluids from patients with cytomegalovirus retinitis,[82] and in corneal epithelium from HSV-infected and uninfected eyes.[70,83,84] In ocu-

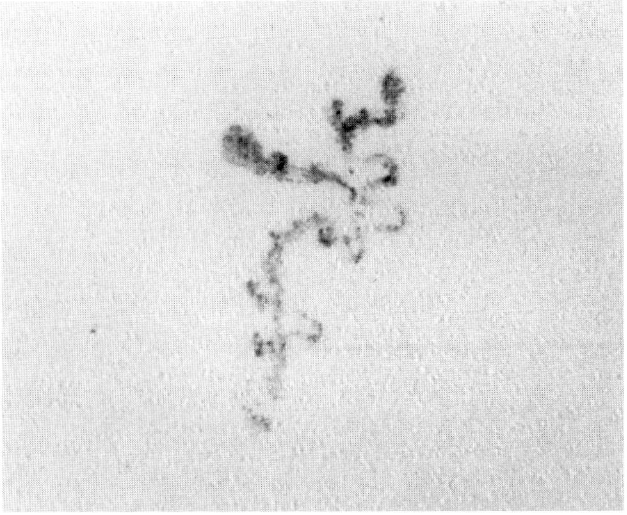

FIGURE 10-23 Positive affinity membrane test for herpes simplex virus. The image corresponds to the shape of the dendrite.

lar specimens, sensitivity ranged from 86 percent to 100 percent and specificity from 65 percent to 87 percent.[71,84] In one study, four specimens from patients who responded to antiviral treatment were positive for HSV by PCR but were culture negative.[84] Small numbers of uninfected control corneas also were PCR positive, possibly as a result of contamination or asymptomatic viral shedding.[83,84]

The PCR technique requires a well-equipped laboratory, a skilled technician, and 1 day or more to complete. Thus, PCR is neither generally useful nor available to most clinicians at the present time.

In summary, the best and most reliable approach to the diagnosis of superficial corneal infection with HSV is the observation of a dendrite. The time-tested technique of tissue culture for the isolation and identification of the virus remains an important adjunct to clinical diagnosis. Newer tests are constantly being improved, and new techniques are being adapted, but a rapid, simple, and accurate diagnostic assay that can be used in the physician's office is not yet available.

TREATMENT

Antiviral Agents

Idoxuridine

Idoxuridine (5-iodo-2′-deoxyuridine) (Figure 10-24) was synthesized as an anticancer agent in the early 1950s by William Prusoff at Yale University. Prusoff found that idoxuridine was an effective inhibitor of DNA polymerase in Ehrlich ascites tumor cells,[85] but it proved not to be a good anticancer agent and was generally abandoned. Hermann[86] found that idoxuridine had some activity against HSV in tissue culture, but at that time, there were hundreds of drugs that had been shown to be active against HSV in tissue culture, and it was not clear that idoxuridine was different from any of the other drugs.

In a review of the literature on the treatment of viral disease, it appeared that many antimetabolites had been tried as potential antiviral agents. Most of these compounds could reduce the yield of virus in virus-infected tissue cultures, but none was effective in animals, and none had been shown to be effective in humans. After discussing the matter with Igor Tamm at the Rockefeller Institute, I (H.E.K.) was encouraged about the prospects for the treatment of viral disease. David Cogan and Edwin B. Dunphy encouraged me in this work, and in 1959, I developed a hypothesis through which an effective antiviral drug might be found.

Previously investigated antimetabolites and antivirals depended on the inhibition of normal cellular synthetic processes that either provided energy or made nucleotides that were used in the synthesis of the genetic material of both the host cell and the virus. It appeared from perusal of the literature that there might be a viral DNA polymerase, distinct from cellular DNA polymerase, that assembled nucleotides into viral DNA, and that this viral DNA polymerase would have a higher affinity for nucleotides than would cellular DNA polymerase. If this were true, there would be little chance of inhibiting viral replication with a drug that simply inhibited the production of energy or nucleotides without killing the host cells. My hypothesis was that if an antiviral drug were to be effective, its site of action would have to be at the final step: the actual polymerization of nucleotides into DNA. At that time, the only drug known to inhibit DNA polymerase was idoxuridine.

Idoxuridine was commercially available, although it was expensive. Because the solubility of idoxuridine was low, and only a 0.1 percent solution could be formulated, it would have to be administered frequently. It was hypothesized that, for maximal effect, it should be given every hour during the day and every 2 hours at night. With no other evidence, animal experiments were begun.

Idoxuridine was proved effective in rabbits[87,88] and subsequently, in 1962, was shown to be effective in humans as well.[89] Shortly thereafter, it became clear that there were multiple phases of herpetic eye disease and that any antiviral drug, including idoxuridine, could treat only those phases associated with viral replication. Idoxuridine was unquestionably effective in the treatment of dendritic ulcers. In the laboratory,[90] and clinically in humans,[91] it

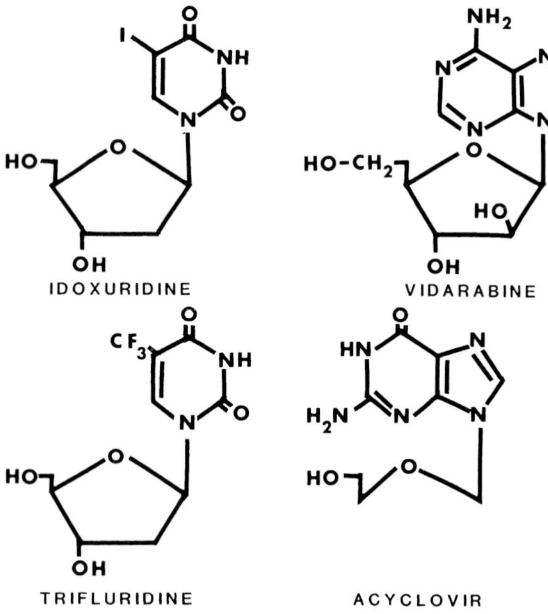

FIGURE 10-24 Antiviral agents used in the treatment of herpes simplex virus. Idoxuridine and trifluridine consist of a halogenated pyrimidine coupled to a deoxyribose sugar. Vidarabine and acyclovir consist of a purine coupled to a sugar incapable of 3′ to 5′ linkage.

seemed able to antagonize the effect that corticosteroids have in worsening herpetic disease caused by replicating virus. It was then that it was hypothesized that dendritic ulcers were caused by replicating virus, that necrotizing stromal keratitis was caused primarily by replicating virus and a significant immunologic component, and that disciform edema was caused primarily by an immunologic phenomenon suppressible by corticosteroids. It was also suggested that the potential danger of corticosteroids worsening infectious herpetic disease could be counteracted by the simultaneous administration of an antiviral agent. It was also at that time that I suggested that disciform edema could be treated safely and effectively with a corticosteroid-antiviral combination.[91,92]

Although idoxuridine was the first effective antiviral drug, it is now obsolete because of the requirement for frequent application and its relatively low potency, compared with more recently developed antiviral drugs.

Vidarabine

The second antiviral agent developed for human use was vidarabine (1-β-D-arabinofuranosyladenine).[93] Its insolubility requires that it be given in ointment form, and its acute toxicity appears to be at least as great as that of idoxuridine, although some have hypothesized, without evidence, that its long-term toxicity may be less. Its relative lack of potency and lack of clear superiority to idoxuridine make it, too, an obsolete drug, except for treatment of disease caused by occasional viral strains resistant to other antiviral agents. In test systems, it is less active than topical trifluridine or acyclovir, and it is rarely used.

Vidarabine is not a completely selective antiviral agent. Although it is an inhibitor of DNA synthesis and presumably causes DNA damage in normal cells, it is sufficiently safe to be used systemically. Because of its insolubility, however, approximately 2 L/day of fluid are required to administer a therapeutic intravenous dose to the average patient. The ester, although more soluble, appears to be more toxic. Vidarabine was the first drug shown to be effective systemically against herpetic encephalitis and other herpetic diseases.[94] It has been given systemically to patients with herpetic uveitis,[95] but the effect is slight, the treatment difficult, and the net long-term value uncertain.

Trifluridine

Trifluridine (5-trifluoromethyl-2′-deoxyuridine), the drug of choice for the topical treatment of herpetic epithelial keratitis in the United States, was developed by Heidelberger for the treatment of cancer.[96] Although it was not terribly effective as an anticancer drug, our group showed its efficacy as a topical antiviral agent.[97] Topical administration of a 1 percent solution of trifluridine 5 to 10 times a day cures at least 97 percent of dendritic ulcers within about 2 weeks.[98] Published studies indicate that it is superior to idoxuridine or vidarabine.[99] Resistance to trifluridine is rare. Because trifluridine is not selective enough in sparing host DNA and inhibiting viral DNA synthesis and is rapidly degraded in the bloodstream, the drug is neither effective nor useful as a systemic antiviral agent. Given topically, it appears to be more effective than idoxuridine or vidarabine in antagonizing the corticosteroid effect, and if corticosteroids are used, trifluridine is the drug of choice for antiviral coverage. Trifluridine is approximately as effective as acyclovir.[100,101] The potential for developing resistance to a systemic antiviral is minimized by the use of the topical medication, and eye drops blur vision less than ointment.

Acyclovir

Acyclovir [9-(2-hydroxyethoxymethyl)guanine] is a highly potent antiviral agent[102] and is active against HSV types 1 and 2, varicella-zoster virus, Epstein-Barr virus, and, to a limited extent, cytomegalovirus. Topical acyclovir penetrates the cornea well and provides therapeutic levels of the drug in the aqueous humor.[103] Theoretically, it is therefore superior to other topical antiviral agents in terms of corneal penetration. Topical 3 percent acyclovir ointment is an effective treatment for HSV epithelial keratitis[104–109] and has been shown to be better than idoxuridine[110–113] or vidarabine[114–118] and as good as trifluridine.[100,101] (The ointment is not available in the United States.) Oral acyclovir provides therapeutic levels of the drug in the tear film, as well as the aqueous humor, and has also been shown to be an effective treatment for HSV epithelial keratitis.[109,119–122]

Conflicting reports have appeared in the literature regarding the efficacy of acyclovir in the treatment of HSV stromal keratitis.[115,122–129] It is difficult to interpret these reports because they contain many anecdotal cases and open, uncontrolled trials. Interpretation is further confounded by the fact that many patients had concomitant HSV epithelial keratitis, and it is not clear to what extent clinical improvement was due to the antiviral effect of acyclovir in the stroma and to what extent it was due, secondarily, to resolution of the HSV infection in the epithelium. In addition, when topical corticosteroids were used, the dosage was not always standardized, making it difficult to separate the effects of acyclovir from those of the corticosteroids. In the Herpetic Eye Disease Study (HEDS), a group of multicenter clinical trials supported by the National Eye Institute, there was no significant benefit derived from adding oral acyclovir (400 mg five times a day) to a standardized regimen of topical corticosteroids and topical trifluridine in the treatment of patients with HSV stromal keratitis.[130] A similar trial evaluating oral acyclovir for herpetic iritis suggested some benefit from oral acyclovir, although the findings were not statistically significant.[131] A recent report of another trial of the Herpetic Eye Disease Study showed that oral acyclovir was not effective in preventing stromal keratits in patients with herpetic epithelial keratitis who were treated concomitantly with topical trifluridine.[132]

There are three situations in which we have found oral acyclovir to be useful in patients with ocular herpes, although there have been no proper controlled trials of these therapies. First, we give acyclovir to children younger than 10 years of age who have herpetic epithelial keratitis; these young patients appear to respond less well to topical trifluridine alone, compared with adults. Second, oral acyclovir in doses of 400 mg five times a day is useful for handicapped patients or those who cannot use eye drops; this regimen may also be tried when compliance with topical application is uncertain. Third, patients with herpes who undergo corneal transplantation tend to have an exacerbated, severe iritis immediately after surgery. If there are no systemic contraindications, oral acyclovir (400 mg five times a day) is given, along with oral prednisone and topical corticosteroids and trifluridine.

Valacyclovir is the valyl ester of acyclovir and is better absorbed after oral administration.[133] It is hydrolyzed to acyclovir, which is active in the blood stream. The therapeutic dose is 1,000 mg three times a day, and the maintenance prophylactic dose is 500 mg twice a day. It should probably replace oral acyclovir for clinical use.

Mechanisms of Antiviral Action

The DNA double helix contains a core of nitrogenous bases linked to each other through a backbone of sugar molecules formed in two intertwined spiral chains. As an analogy, the two strands of the DNA helix may be envisioned as the two arms of a zipper: the purine and pyrimidine bases that form the core of the helix are the teeth, and the sugar backbone is the fabric that holds all the elements together. Like the teeth of a zipper, the purine and pyrimidine bases complement each other so that in the native state the two strands are tightly intermeshed and the helix is closed. Events such as replication and protein synthesis are initiated by enzyme complexes that move up and down the helix, opening and closing it like a zipper.

Drugs that have a normal sugar but an abnormal substituent on the base, such as idoxuridine and trifluridine, appear to act primarily by being incorporated into RNA as a mismatch that codes for abnormal proteins, which in turn impair viral replication, or by binding to DNA polymerase and inhibiting DNA polymerization. Other drugs, such as vidarabine and acyclovir, have normal bases but abnormal substituents for the sugar moiety. Although all the antivirals have multiple sites of activity, those with abnormal sugars probably do not permit normal 3′-5′ linkage at the sugar during polymerization of the DNA backbone and, therefore, act as chain terminators, generating short pieces of DNA that cannot elongate into normal chains.

For any of these antiviral agents to be effective, they must be phosphorylated. The first phosphorylation is by the enzyme thymidine kinase. After this initial activation, the other two phosphates are rapidly attached, and the drug can inhibit viral DNA polymerase. Although thymidine kinase is present in the host cell, the virus encodes for a different thymidine kinase with affinities for phosphorylation that are different from those of cellular thymidine kinase. Cellular thymidine kinase may be thought of as more discriminating and less in demand for rapid synthesis, and viral thymidine kinase as less discriminating and more rapid in its synthetic potential for virus growth. Certain drugs are selectively phosphorylated largely by viral thymidine kinase and very little by cellular thymidine kinase. This means that there is a potential for a truly selective antiviral agent that is not activated by phosphorylation in normal cells but is activated by phosphorylation only in virus-infected cells that contain viral thymidine kinase.

Acyclovir, valacyclovir, and famciclovir (a prodrug of penciclovir) are currently the most important and useful of the thymidine kinase-selective antiviral drugs. There are also a number of extremely effective experimental antivirals, such as bromovinyldeoxyuridine (BVDU), that are selectively activated by viral thymidine kinase. The activation of BVDU is so selective that it is very effective against HSV-1 but relatively ineffective against HSV-2.[134]

Do the thymidine kinase-selective drugs have any advantage when used as topical antivirals? Theoretically, when administered topically, they should be less toxic than the other antivirals, but double-masked studies do not support this.[113] These drugs also have potential disadvantages. In the test tube, HSV easily becomes resistant to these agents. Any large virus stock has a proportion of mutants that are thymidine kinase deficient; these mutants do not require viral thymidine kinase to multiply and can use the thymidine kinase of the host cell to grow. They are, therefore, not affected by these drugs. This kind of resistance occurs even with pools of virus that have never been exposed to the drug. Similarly, viruses have been isolated that alter their thymidine kinase so that it is more like cellular thymidine kinase and does not phosphorylate these drugs. Viruses can even alter their DNA polymerase so that the fully phosphorylated drug is no longer effective. The importance of this resistance in clinical terms is unclear because most resistant mutants appear to be less virulent, but some virulent mutants have been isolated from treated patients.[135–141] If the virus is continually reactivated from the ganglion and returned to the ganglion to resume latency, even if peripheral virus becomes resistant, the host ganglion may not be reinfected with this mutant, but the mutant could be spread to others, creating a pool of resistant virus in the general population.

For antiviral agents to be systemically active, they must not only inhibit viral replication but also spare the host immune system. Vidarabine and all the newer thymidine kinase-selective drugs appear to meet these qualifications.

Foscarnet represents a different kind of antiviral (Figure 10-25). It is an extremely potent drug that does not require cellular activation to inhibit virus multiplication. Rather, the phosphonates bind selectively to viral DNA polymerase and thus directly inhibit the synthesis of viral DNA. For years, the phosphonates were viewed suspiciously because they tend to accumulate in bone, and the long-term effects of this accumulation, if any, are not clear. Foscarnet is presently approved for intravenous use against cytomegalovirus retinitis in acquired immunodeficiency syndrome (AIDS) patients, with a number of cautions, including renal toxicity and mineral and electrolyte imbalances. Phosphonylmethoxyethyl adenine (PMEA) and hydroxyphosphonylmethoxypropyl cytosine (HPMPC; cidofovir) are similarly selective and are potent against clinical strains of herpes, including thymidine kinase-negative strains that are resistant to acyclovir and BVDU.[134] HPMPC is effective against HSV epithelial keratitis,[142] but there is no evidence that it is more effective or can be administered less frequently than trifluridine. HPMPC is currently approved for intravenous use against cytomegalovirus retinitis in patients with acquired immunodeficiency syndrome.

Corticosteroids

Although trifluridine can inhibit herpetic stromal keratitis in rabbits when given early, it cannot do so when given late in the course of the disease.[49] Some have suggested that trifluridine, given frequently, may be of some benefit in occasional patients with stromal keratitis. However, it is our clinical impression that trifluridine does not help except that it heals an epithelial defect, which has some secondary benefit to the stroma. It also permits the use of corticosteroids. Although antiviral agents alone are effective in the treatment of herpetic eye diseases caused by actively replicating virus (dendritic and geographic ulcers), they do not appear to be effective in the treatment of herpetic eye diseases in which immunologic components play a major role (disciform edema).

Corticosteroids appear to be indicated for the treatment of stromal keratitis. Support for this long-standing but generally empiric practice has recently been supplied by the results of the Herpetic Eye Disease Study. This study showed earlier resolution of stromal keratitis in patients with herpes simplex stromal keratitis who received topical corticosteroids in conjunction with topical trifluridine, compared with those receiving trifluridine and a placebo, and no adverse effects over the 6-month period of follow-up.[143]

It is important to remember that corticosteroids do not cure anything; they only suppress inflammation, which minimizes stromal necrosis, scarring, and vascularization until the disease has run its course. In general, when a patient with disciform edema has eccentric edema or minimal central edema without much discomfort or decreased vision, corticosteroids are not necessary. If the patient is symptomatic or vision is reduced, corticosteroids should be used, and they appear to reduce scarring and vascularization, relieve pain, and restore vision. The exception to this is in children younger than 5 years of age, in whom corticosteroid treatment is sometimes associated with more complications. In this age group, it may be better

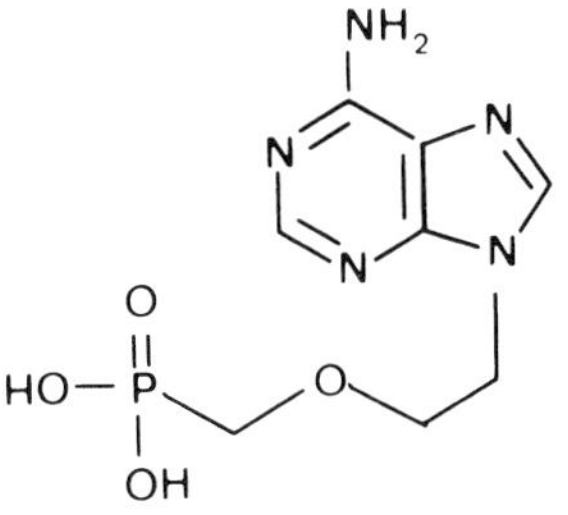

PMEA

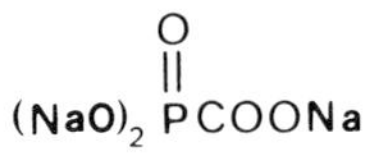

Foscarnet

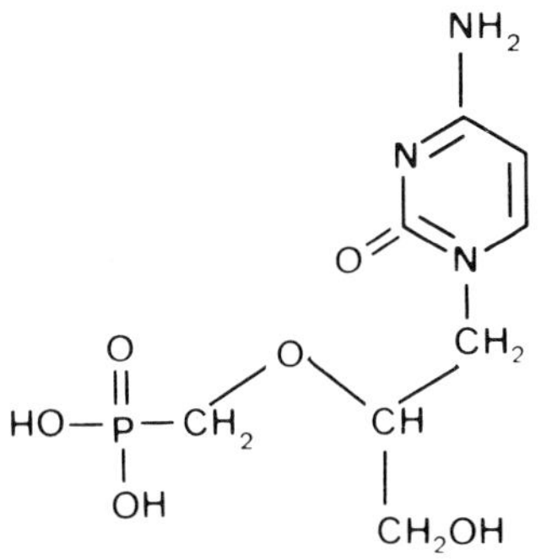

HPMPC

FIGURE 10-25 Three antiviral drugs that act by binding phosphonates to viral DNA polymerase and inhibiting the synthesis of viral DNA. These drugs do not require activation by viral thymidine kinase and are generally potent against viral strains resistant to acyclovir or bromovinyldeoxyuridine. Foscarnet and HPMPC have been approved for clinical use in patients with acquired immunodeficiency syndrome and cytomegalovirus retinitis.

to let the disease run its course or to give oral acyclovir along with the topical corticosteroids.

Although there are many effective corticosteroid regimens for the treatment of active stromal disease, our preference is to begin with dexamethasone sodium phosphate 1 percent, five times a day, and trifluridine given with equal frequency. After 4 or 5 days, the stromal edema begins to clear; this is the primary indicator of therapeutic efficacy. As the edema clears, the corticosteroids can generally be tapered to once or twice a day; again, trifluridine is given with equal frequency. The question is often raised, when the corticosteroids are tapered to once or twice a day, whether the risk of reactivation of herpetic epithelial keratitis is sufficiently high to warrant antiviral coverage. In our experience, most patients receiving low doses of topical corticosteroids do not develop herpetic epithelial keratitis, but some certainly will. For this reason, an antiviral agent is given as long as corticosteroids are used, provided there is no allergic reaction to or other untoward complications from the antiviral agent. If the patient is allergic or reacts adversely to the antiviral agent, it is worth the small risk of doing without it.

In our experience, about 85 percent of patients can be weaned from corticosteroids after approximately 3 months. Continuing corticosteroids once or twice a day for 3 months appears to represent both minimal nuisance and minimal risk. Discontinuing corticosteroids prematurely causes reinflammation of the eye, and the reentrance of inflammatory cells, whose pepsins and digestive enzymes can cause increased stromal necrosis, which is clinically like turning back the clock. Although some patients may be able to discontinue corticosteroids before 3 months, it does not seem worthwhile to try it. After 3 months, corticosteroids are tapered and stopped; if the disease flares up, they are resumed. For the small proportion of patients who are refractory to treatment, it may be necessary to continue corticosteroids for longer periods with a drop or two a day, but this is no different from treating chronic uveitis. At present, there is no evidence that any of the antiviral agents alone can treat herpetic disciform edema.

Occasionally, the use of topical corticosteroids is undesirable because of persistent epithelial defects or complications associated with topical corticosteroids. When this occurs, systemic corticosteroids can be given, beginning with 60 to 80 mg/day of prednisone and tapering to 20 mg after 4 or 5 days. It is interesting to speculate that if the primary problem with disciform edema is caused by antigen-antibody complexes at the endothelial surface or perhaps within the anterior chamber, topical application of drugs may be a relatively inefficient means of delivering the drug. Achieving therapeutic levels of corticosteroids in the anterior chamber by topical application requires enormous concentrations at the corneal surface, causing an increased risk of epithelial complications. In contrast, the administration of systemic corticosteroids causes a high concentration in the anterior chamber and a relatively low concentration in the epithelium, and as a consequence there should be fewer epithelial complications. Nevertheless, because of the other side effects of systemic corticosteroids, only rarely is systemic administration preferable to topical administration.

The response of necrotizing stromal keratitis to topical corticosteroids and antivirals is more erratic and less predictable, compared with the response of disciform edema, which is almost uniformly good. As stated above, a rational approach to the treatment of necrotizing stromal keratitis requires an understanding of what causes it, but the pathogenesis of this disease remains uncertain. If viral multiplication is minimal or very slow, antiviral agents probably will not be very effective; they certainly will not be effective in stopping necrosis if it is primarily an immunologic reaction. If more potent antiviral agents can be administered safely and effectively, stromal necrosis may be treatable. However, experience with present antiviral agents does not yet suggest that this is the case.

Interferons

Although interferon has some antiviral effect against HSV,[144–150] at this time the effect seems too slight for it to be considered as a therapeutic drug or adjunct to therapy.

Prevention of Recurrences

It is not the single acute infection that makes herpetic eye disease one of the leading infectious causes of corneal blindness but rather the recurrent infections. The likelihood of a recurrence of herpetic eye disease has been reported to vary from 10 percent in the first year to 50 percent in 10 years.[13] If a patient has had one recurrence, the chance for future recurrences increases; reported rates range from about 25 percent in 1 year to 72 percent in 10 years for a third episode,[13,147] and 27 percent in 1 year to 89 percent in 10 years for a fifth episode.[13] Increasing numbers of recurrences are characterized by shorter intervals between bouts of disease.[13,143] Because each recurrence usually causes irreversible structural damage to the eye and increases the likelihood of further recurrences, an important therapeutic goal is to prevent recurrences.

At the present time, there is no known method to prevent recurrences of herpetic eye disease. No currently available antiviral drug eliminates the virus from the ganglia. The chronic administration of antiviral eye drops does not prevent recurrences in animals or humans, but the drops may be useful for brief periods in patients who have clear-cut inciting factors. For example, if a child has recurrences with a high fever, the administration of trifluridine during such an episode seems sensible. Similar use at times of stress in selected individuals may be worthwhile. However, chronic administration at other times is not indicated.

In patients with genital[151,152] and nongenital cutaneous[153] herpetic disease, the administration of oral acyclovir prevents recurrent episodes of the disease as long as the drug is administered. As soon as it is stopped, however, recurrences occur. The possibility of preventing ocular recurrences with acyclovir has been studied in rabbits.[154,155] We were not able to prevent recurrences of viral shedding or overt disease experimentally with acyclovir or BVDU,[154] although the concentration of drug used was similar to that achieved in human studies in which suppression of recurrent genital disease was observed. It may be that for genital and cutaneous lesions to occur, there must be not only ganglionic reactivation but also significant end organ viral multiplication. Acyclovir may prevent the end organ multiplication and therefore suppress the mucocutaneous lesions, whereas ocular lesions may result from virus liberated directly by the activated neuron and may not require the same degree of end organ multiplication. Studies in mice[156] have shown that acyclovir does not prevent the replication of viral DNA in the ganglion during recurrences, although it reduces virus in the cornea. Some experimental drugs such as β-blockers[157] and specific viral thymidine kinase inhibitors[158] prevent ganglionic viral DNA emergence. A trial of the Herpetic Eye Disease Study is presently evaluating the efficacy of oral acyclovir in preventing recurrent HSV eye disease in patients with one or more previous episodes of HSV eye disease.

Treatment of Postinfectious Ulcers

The longer a herpetic ulcer has been present, the more difficult it is to treat and the more slowly it heals. It is clear that persistent epithelial defects and persistent viral infection can damage the hemidesmosomes, basement membrane, and superficial stroma of the cornea, resulting in slower healing of corneal ulcers. Whereas active herpetic ulcers usually have dendritic edges, postinfectious ulcers (also called metaherpetic ulcers or trophic ulcers) are likely to be ovoid (Figure 10-26), with smooth heaped-up gray edges, so that an active geographic ulcer can usually be differentiated from a postinfectious ulcer.[159] Sometimes, however, fluorescent antibody or culture studies must be performed to differentiate the two.

The importance of differentiating a geographic ulcer from a postinfectious ulcer is that an ulcer caused by rapidly multiplying virus can be treated effectively with an antiviral agent, whereas an ulcer caused by fragile epithelium that does not adhere to its basement membrane responds poorly to frequent opening and closing of the eyelids and frequent administration of topical antiviral medication. A postinfectious ulcer can be treated either by patching, a bandage soft contact lens that protects the epithelium, or a temporary tarsorrhaphy. When there is doubt about whether active virus is present, a bandage lens may be used so that a topical antiviral agent can be given concomitantly.

In patients with herpetic eye disease, tear flow is frequently deficient, lagophthalmos is common, and corneal sensation is often decreased. Because of this, compound disease, (i.e., a herpetic ulcer complicated by dryness and exposure) is common, and the ulcer will not heal unless the drying and exposure are treated. Ulcers that are unresponsive to the above measures can be treated with a conjunctival flap.

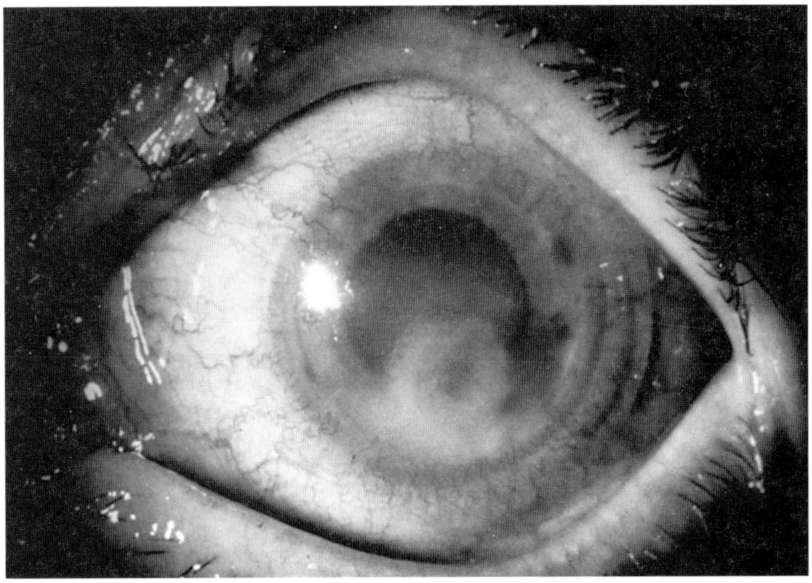

FIGURE 10-26 Postinfectious herpetic ulcer. Healing is impeded by the abnormal bed of the ulcer rather than by active infection.

Surgical Treatment

Conjunctival Flap

In chronic ulcers that are peripheral and off the visual axis, a peripheral inlay conjunctival flap is extremely effective, aborting what would otherwise be a prolonged course of therapy, rapidly quieting the eye, and giving the patient instant comfort (Figure 10-27). Patients with chronic central ulcers who have good vision in the unaffected eye and for whom vision-restoring surgery, such as penetrating keratoplasty, is not indicated are often better off with a total conjunctival flap than with months or years of chronic corticosteroids, antiviral therapy, and bandage lenses. The complex chronic medical treatment of a blind eye for which visual rehabilitation is not contemplated in the near future may be more trouble than it is worth to the patient, and a conjunctival flap may be the best way to give the patient a lasting solution to a miserable problem. Even in eyes that have visual potential, a total conjunctival flap can provide a temporary respite, until the eye is quiet, when penetrating keratoplasty can be performed.

We do inlay flaps and total flaps more often than many groups, because we think it is often easier for the patient to have surgery to quiet the eye rather than go through many months of repeated office visits and complex medical regimens that may not achieve as good a result. Penetrating keratoplasty can be performed in the future at a time when the eye is no longer inflamed. The techniques of conjunctival flaps are described in Chapter 29.

Lamellar Keratoplasty

Except for sealing small perforations with lamellar patches, lamellar keratoplasty is not recommended for patients with herpetic keratitis because the infection may reactivate at the interface.

Penetrating Keratoplasty

There are, in general, two reasons for penetrating keratoplasty in herpetic keratitis. The first is acute perforation and the second is a stromal scar that precludes good vision. In cases with acute perforation, the eye is likely to be inflamed. In general, frequent topical antiviral treatment and oral corticosteroids (usually 80 mg/day of prednisone for an adult) are begun before surgery if possible, or at the time of surgery, along with oral acyclovir. Surgical techniques are described in Chapter 34. A viscoelastic substance is placed in the anterior chamber angle to prevent anterior synechiae and synechiae to the graft. One or two peripheral iridectomies are performed in case pupillary block occurs postoperatively. High-dose oral corticosteroids and oral acyclovir are continued for 1 or 2 weeks after surgery; otherwise severe inflammation may destroy the graft and sometimes cause synechiae that destroy the eye.

In a patient with a stromal scar in a quiet eye, a similar dose of oral corticosteroids is given beginning 1 or 2 days before surgery and continuing for 1 or 2 weeks afterward because these patients frequently develop severe iritis at the time of surgery. In all cases, topical corticosteroids are begun along with the systemic corticosteroids. Oral acyclovir (400 mg five times a day) is used, and topical trifluridine is given

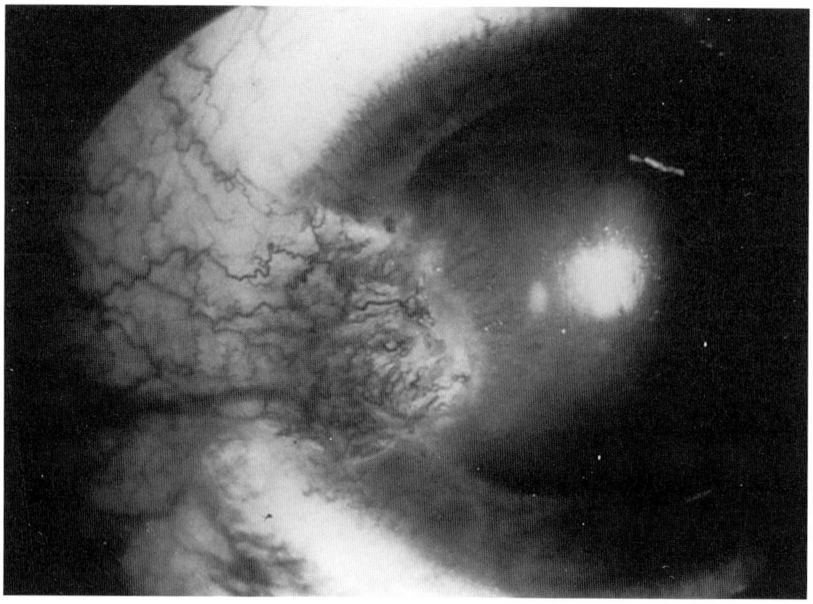

FIGURE 10-27 Peripheral inlay conjunctival flap for persistent herpetic keratitis.

with a frequency at least equal to that of the topical corticosteroids. This regimen does not appear to be toxic to the epithelium or to affect the graft in any adverse way; no clinically obvious effects on wound healing have been observed. By the end of 1 to 2 weeks, the oral corticosteroids and acyclovir are discontinued, but high-dose topical corticosteroids and trifluridine are continued usually for 2 or 3 weeks and then gradually tapered, depending on the amount of inflammation. It is our clinical impression that if the stromal scar can be completely excised and all visible stromal disease removed, the patients do significantly better than if stromal scarring or necrotic stroma is left behind. It may be that multiplying virus or virus that can be potentially activated remains in the white necrotic stroma. Many surgeons believe that the rate of recurrence seems to be reduced after a herpetic scar has been totally removed, and this is our clinical impression, although there are no objective substantiating data. We do not remove the scar totally if this would result in an unacceptably large or eccentric graft, however, because of the increased incidence of graft rejection. Recent reports suggest that prolonged acyclovir therapy after penetrating keratoplasty may improve graft prognosis,[160,161] and some surgeons give small doses of acyclovir for up to 1 year after surgery, although the efficacy of this has not been established definitively.

Acknowledgment

This work was supported in part by U.S. Public Health Service grants EY02672, EY08701, and EY02377 from the National Eye Institute, National Institutes of Health, Bethesda, MD.

REFERENCES

1. Liesegang TJ: Biology and molecular aspects of herpes simplex and varicella-zoster virus infections. Ophthalmology 99:781, 1992
2. Nahmias AJ, Josey WE, Naib ZM: Neonatal herpes simplex infection: role of genital infection in mother as the source of virus in the newborn. JAMA 199:164, 1967
3. Dowdle WR, Nahmias AJ, Harwell RW, Pauls FP: Association of antigenic type of herpesvirus hominis with site of viral recovery. J Immunol 99:974, 1967
4. Lafferty WE, Coombs RW, Benedetti J, et al: Recurrences after oral and genital herpes simplex virus infection. Influence of site of infection and viral type. N Engl J Med 316:1444, 1987
5. Baringer JR, Swoveland P: Recovery of herpes-simplex virus from human trigeminal ganglions. N Engl J Med 288:648, 1973
6. Warren KG, Moira Brown S, Wroblewska Z, et al: Isolation of latent herpes simplex virus from the superior cervical and vagus ganglions of human beings. N Engl J Med 298:1068, 1978
7. Stevens JG, Haarr L, Porter DD, et al: Prominence of the herpes simplex virus latency-associated transcript in trigeminal ganglia from seropositive humans. J Infect Dis 158:117, 1988
8. Croen KD, Ostrove JM, Dragovic LJ, Straus SE: Patterns of gene expression and sites of latency in human nerve ganglia are different for varicella-zoster and herpes simplex viruses. Proc Natl Acad Sci USA 85:9773, 1988

9. Takasu T, Furuta Y, Sato KC, et al: Detection of latent herpes simplex virus DNA and RNA in human geniculate ganglia by the polymerase chain reaction. Acta Otolaryngol (Stockh)112:1004, 1992
10. Furuta Y, Takasu Y, Sato KC, et al: Latent herpes simplex virus type 1 in human geniculate ganglia. Acta Neuropathol 84:39, 1992
11. Mahalingam R, Wellish MC, Dueland AN, et al: Localization of herpes simplex virus and varicella zoster virus DNA in human ganglia. Ann Neurol 31:444, 1992
12. Liesegang TJ, Melton LJ, Daly PJ, Ilstrup DM: Epidemiology of ocular herpes simplex: incidence in Rochester, Minnesota, 1950 through 1982. Arch Ophthalmol 107:1155, 1989
13. Liesegang TJ: Epidemiology of ocular herpes simplex: natural history in Rochester, Minnesota, 1950 through 1982. Arch Ophthalmol 107:1160, 1989
14. Stevens JG, Nesburn AB, Cook ML: Latent herpes simplex virus from trigeminal ganglia of rabbits with recurrent eye infection. Nature 235:216, 1972
15. Stevens JG, Cook ML: Latent herpes simplex virus in spinal ganglia of mice. Science 173:843, 1971
16. McGill J: Herpes simplex latency and the eye [editorial]. Br J Ophthalmol 75:641, 1991
17. Cook SD, Hill JM: Herpes simplex virus: molecular biology and the possibility of corneal latency. Surv Ophthalmol 36:140,1991
18. Petrash JM: Applications of molecular biological techniques to the understanding of visual system disorders. Am J Ophthalmol 113:573, 1992
19. Fraser N, Lawrence W, Wroblewska Z, et al: Herpes simplex type I DNA in human brain tissue. Proc Natl Acad Sci USA 78:6461, 1981
20. Lonsdale DM, Moira Brown S, Subak-Sharpe JH, et al: The polypeptide and the DNA restriction enzyme profiles of spontaneous isolates of herpes simplex virus type I from explants of human trigeminal, superior cervical, and vagus ganglia. J Gen Virol 43:151, 1979
21. Centifanto-Fitzgerald YM, Varnell ED, Kaufman HE: Initial herpes simplex virus type 1 infection prevents ganglionic superinfection by other strains. Infect Immunol 35:1125, 1982
22. Centifanto-Fitzgerald YM, Rayfield M, Tian PY, Kaufman HE: Herpes simplex virus latency in the rabbit trigeminal ganglia: ganglionic superinfection. Proc Soc Exp Biol Med 179:55, 1985
23. Gerdes JC, Smith DS: Recurrence phenotypes and establishment of latency following rabbit keratitis produced by multiple herpes simplex virus strains. J Gen Virol 64:2441, 1983
24. Hill JM, Haruta Y, Rootman DS: Adrenergically induced recurrent HSV-1 corneal epithelial lesions. Curr Eye Res 6:1065,1987
25. Hill TJ, Blyth WA, Harbour DA: Trauma to the skin causes recurrence of herpes simplex in the mouse. J Gen Virol 39:21, 1978
26. Wander AH, Centifanto YM, Kaufman HE: Strain specificity of clinical isolates of herpes simplex virus. Arch Ophthalmol 98:1458, 1980.
27. Centifanto-Fitzgerald YM, Yamaguchi T, Kaufman HE, et al: Ocular disease pattern induced by herpes simplex virus is genetically determined by a specific region of viral DNA. J Exp Med 155:475, 1982
28. Stulting RD, Kindle JC, Nahmias AJ: Pattern of herpes simplex keratitis in inbred mice. Invest Ophthalmol Vis Sci 25:1360, 1985
29. Centifanto-Fitzgerald YM, Fenger T, Kaufman HE: Virus proteins in herpetic keratitis. Exp Eye Res 35:425, 1982
30. Smeraglia R, Hochadel J, Varnell ED, et al: The role of herpes simplex virus secreted glycoproteins in herpetic keratitis. Exp Eye Res 35:443, 1982
31. Kaufman HE, Varnell ED, Centifanto YM, Kissling GE: Effect of the herpes simplex virus genome on the response of infection to corticosteroids. Am J Ophthalmol 100:114, 1985
32. Nishiyama Y, Rapp F: Regulation of persistent infection with herpes simplex virus in vitro by hydrocortisone. J Virol 31:841, 1979
33. Centifanto-Fitzgerald Y: Recurrent and non-recurrent HSV-1 strains: effect of temperature. p. 27. In Maudgal PC, Missotten L (eds): Herpetic Eye Diseases. Dr. W. Junk, Dordrecht, 1985
34. Centifanto-Fitzgerald YM: Pathogenicity of recurrent and non-recurrent herpes simplex virus strains. p. 3. In Kono R (ed): Herpes Viruses and Virus Chemotherapy. Elsevier Science Publishers, Amsterdam, 1985
35. Asbell PA, Centifanto-Fitzgerald YM, Chandler JW, Kaufman HE: Analysis of viral DNA in isolates from patients with recurrent herpetic keratitis. Invest Ophthalmol Vis Sci 25:951, 1984
36. Chandler JW: Herpes keratitis and the immune system. Ophthalmic Forum 2:189, 1984
37. Thygeson P: Superficial punctate keratitis. JAMA 144:1544, 1950
38. Thygeson P: Marginal herpes simplex keratitis simulating catarrhal ulcer. Invest Ophthalmol 10:1006, 1971
39. Beyer CF, Arens MQ, Hill JM, et al: Penetrating keratoplasty in rabbits induces latent HSV-1 reactivation when corticosteroids are used. Curr Eye Res 8:1323, 1989
40. Portnoy SL, Beyer CF, Hill JM, Kaufman HE: The coincidence of HSV-1 ocular cultures with HSV-1 corneal epithelial defects in rabbits after experimental penetrating keratoplasty. Cornea 10:17, 1991
41. Beyer CF, Byrd TJ, Hill JM, Kaufman HE: Herpes simplex virus and persistent epithelial defects after penetrating keratoplasty. Am J Ophthalmol 109:95, 1990
42. Mannis MJ, Plotnik RD, Schwab IR, Newton RD: Herpes simplex dendritic keratitis after keratoplasty. Am J Ophthalmol 111:480, 1991
43. Kodama T, Hayasaka S, Setogawa T: Immunofluorescent staining and corneal sensitivity in patients suspected of having herpes simplex keratitis. Am J Ophthalmol 113:187, 1992

44. Shimeld C, Tullo AB, Easty DL, Thomsitt J: Isolation of herpes simplex virus from the cornea in chronic stromal keratitis. Br J Ophthalmol 66:643, 1982
45. Sanitato JJ, Asbell PA, Varnell ED, et al: Acyclovir in the treatment of herpetic stromal disease. Am J Ophthalmol 98:537, 1984
46. Spear PG: Membrane proteins specified by herpes simplex viruses I: identification of four glyoprotein precursors and their products in type-1 infected cells. J Virol 17:991, 1976
47. Baucke RB, Spear PG: Membrane proteins specified by herpes simplex viruses V: identification of an Fc-binding glycoprotein. J Virol 32:779, 1979
48. Metcalf JF, McNeill JI, Kaufman HE: Experimental disciform edema and necrotizing keratitis in the rabbit. Invest Ophthalmol 15:979, 1976
49. McNeill JI, Kaufman HE: Local antivirals in a herpes simplex stromal keratitis model. Arch Ophthalmol 97:727, 1979
50. Kaufman HE, Kanai A, Ellison ED: Herpetic iritis: demonstration of virus in the anterior chamber by fluorescent antibody techniques and electron microscopy. Am J Ophthalmol 71:465, 1971
51. Sundmacher R, Neumann-Haefelin D: Herpes simplex Virus Isolierung aus dem Kammerwasser bei fokaler Iritis, Endotheliitis und langdauernder Keratitis disciformis mit Sekundarglaukom. Klin Monatsbl Augenheilkd 175:488, 1979
52. Robin JB, Steigner JB, Kaufman HE: Progressive corneal endotheliitis. Am J Ophthalmol 100:336, 1985
53. Ohashi Y, Yamamoto S, Nishida K, et al: Demonstration of herpes simplex virus DNA in idiopathic corneal endotheliopathy. Am J Ophthalmol 112:419, 1991
54. Cheng C-K, Chang S-W, Hu F-R: Acyclovir treatment for linear endotheliitis on grafted corneas. Cornea 14:311, 1995
55. Ludwig IH, Zegarra H, Zakov ZN: The acute retinal necrosis syndrome: possible herpes simplex retinitis. Ophthalmology 91:1659, 1981
56. Peyman GA, Goldberg MF, Uninsky E, et al: Vitrectomy and intravitreal antiviral drug therapy in acute retinal necrosis syndrome. Arch Ophthalmol 102:1618, 1984
57. Freeman WR, Thomas EL, Rao NA, et al: Demonstration of herpes group virus in acute retinal necrosis syndrome. Am J Ophthalmol 102:701, 1986
58. Lewis ML, Culbertson WW, Post JD, et al: Herpes simplex virus type 1: a cause of the acute retinal necrosis syndrome. Ophthalmology 96:875, 1989
59. Duker JS, Nielsen J, Eagle RC, et al: Rapidly progressive, acute retinal necrosis (ARN) secondary to herpes simplex virus, type 1. Ophthalmology 97:1638, 1990
60. Duker JS, Blumenkranz MS: Diagnosis and management of the acute retinal necrosis (ARN) syndrome. Surv Ophthalmol 35:327, 1991
61. Culbertson WW, Blumenkranz MS, Pepose JS, et al: Varicella zoster virus is a cause of the acute retinal necrosis syndrome. Ophthalmology 93:559, 1986
62. Yeo JH, Pepose JS, Stewart JA, et al: Acute retinal necrosis syndrome following herpes zoster dermatitis. Ophthalmology 93:1418, 1986
63. Browning DJ, Blumenkranz MS, Culbertson WW, et al: Association of varicella zoster dermatitis with acute retinal necrosis syndrome. Ophthalmology 94:602, 1987
64. Bordin P, Merlin U, Pugina P, et al: Reliability of the herpes simplex virus immunofluorescent test in corneal disease. Eur J Ophthalmol 2:175, 1992
65. Kowalski RP, Gordon YJ: Evaluation of immunologic tests for the detection of ocular herpes simplex virus. Ophthalmology 96:1583, 1989
66. Wu TC, Zaza S, Callaway J: Evaluation of the Du Pont HERPCHEK herpes simplex virus antigen test with clinical specimens. J Clin Microbiol 27:1903, 1989
67. Pavan-Langston D, Dunkel EC: A rapid diagnostic test for herpes simplex infectious keratitis. Am J Ophthalmol 107:675, 1989
68. Lee SF, Pepose JS: Sandwich enzyme immunoassay and latex agglutination test for herpes simplex virus keratitis. J Clin Microbiol 28:785, 1990
69. Lipson SM, Salo RJ, Leonard GP: Evaluation of five monoclonal antibody-based kits or reagents for the identification and culture confirmation of herpes simplex virus. J Clin Microbiol 29:466, 1991
70. Needham CA, Hurlbert P: Evaluation of an enzyme-linked immunoassay employing a covalently bound capture antibody for direct detection of herpes simplex virus. J Clin Microbiol 30:531, 1992
71. Kowalski RP, Gordon YJ, Romanowski EG, et al: A comparison of enzyme immunoassay and polymerase chain reaction with the clinical examination for diagnosing ocular herpetic disease. Ophthalmology 100:530, 1993
72. Kowalski RP, Portnoy SL, Karenchak LM, Arffa RC: The evaluation of the Kodak Surecell test for the detection of ocular herpes simplex virus. Am J Ophthalmol 112:214, 1991
73. Wittpenn JR, Pepose JS: Impression debridement of herpes simplex dendritic keratitis. Cornea 5:245, 1987
74. Pepose JS: Applications of immunologic technology to the diagnosis of viral infections of the ocular surface. Cornea 7:36, 1988
75. Gebhardt BM, Reidy J, Kaufman HE: An affinity membrane test for superficial corneal herpes. Am J Ophthalmol 105:686, 1988
76. Simon MW, Miller D, Pflugfelder SC, et al: Comparison of immunocytology to tissue culture for diagnosis of presumed herpesvirus dendritic keratitis. Ophthalmology 99:1408, 1992
77. Rowley AH, Whitley RJ, Lakeman FD, Wolinsky SM: Rapid detection of herpes-simplex-virus DNA in cerebrospinal fluid of patients with herpes simplex encephalitis. Lancet 335:440, 1990
78. Yamamoto LJ, Tedder DG, Ashley R, Levin MJ: Herpes simplex virus type 1 DNA in cerebrospinal fluid of a patient with Mollaret's meningitis. N Engl J Med 325:1082, 1991

79. Dennett C, Klapper PE, Cleator GM, Lewis AG: Short communication: CSF pretreatment and the diagnosis of herpes encephalitis using the polymerase chain reaction. J Virol Methods 34:101, 1991
80. Kimura H, Shibata M, Kuzushima K, et al: Detection and direct typing of herpes simplex virus by polymerase chain reaction. Med Microbiol Immunol 179:17, 1990
81. Cone RW, Hobson AC, Palmer J, et al: Extended duration of herpes simplex virus DNA in genital lesions detected by the polymerase chain reaction. J Infect Dis 164:757, 1991
82. Fox GM, Crouse CA, Chuang EL, et al: Detection of herpesvirus DNA in vitreous and aqueous specimens by the polymerase chain reaction. Arch Ophthalmol 109:266, 1991
83. Crouse CA, Pflugfelder SC, Pereira I, et al: Detection of herpes viral genomes in normal and diseased corneal epithelium. Curr Eye Res 9:569, 1990
84. Dumas LA, de Ancos E, Herbort CP: Evaluation de la methode d'amplification de L'ADN (PCR, polymerase chain reaction) pour le diagnostic de l'herpes oculaire superficiel. Klin Monatsbl Augenheilkd 200:472, 1992
85. Welch AD, Prusoff WH: Synopsis of recent investigations of 5-iodo-2'-deoxyuridine. Cancer Chemother (Rep. 6):29, 1960
86. Hermann EC Jr: Plaque inhibition test for detection of specific inhibitions of DNA containing viruses. Proc Soc Exp Biol Med 107:142, 1961
87. Kaufman HE: Clinical cure of herpes simplex keratitis by 5-iodo-2'-deoxyuridine. Proc Soc Exp Biol Med 109:251, 1962
88. Kaufman HE, Nesburn AB, Maloney ED: IDU therapy of herpes simplex. Arch Ophthalmol 67:583, 1962
89. Kaufman HE, Martola E-L, Dohlman CH: The use of 5-iodo-2'-deoxyuridine (IDU) in the treatment of herpes simplex keratitis. Arch Ophthalmol 68:235, 1962
90. Kaufman HE, Maloney ED: IDU and hydrocortisone in experimental herpes simplex keratitis. Arch Ophthalmol 68:396, 1962
91. Kaufman HE, Martola E-L, Dohlman CH: Herpes simplex treatment with IDU and corticosteroids. Arch Ophthalmol 69:468, 1963
92. Kaufman HE: Treatment of deep herpetic keratitis with IDU and corticosteroids. EENT Digest 25:37, 1963
93. Pavan-Langston D, Dohlman CH: A double-blind clinical study of adenine arabinoside therapy of viral keratoconjunctivitis. Am J Ophthalmol 74:81, 1972
94. Whitley RJ, Soong SJ, Dolin R, et al: Adenine arabinoside therapy of biopsy-proved herpes simplex encephalitis. N Engl J Med 297:289, 1977
95. Abel R, Kaufman HE, Sugar J: Intravenous adenine arabinoside against herpes simplex keratouveitis in humans. Am J Ophthalmol 79:659, 1975
96. Heidelberger C, Parsons DG, Remy DC: Syntheses of 5-trifluoromethyluracil and 5-trifluoromethyl-2'-deoxyuridine. J Med Chem 7:1, 1964
97. Kaufman HE, Heidelberger C: Therapeutic anti-viral action of 5-trifluoromethyl-2'-deoxyuridine. Science 145:585, 1964
98. Wellings PC, Awdry PN, Bors FH, et al: Clinical evaluation of trifluorothymidine in the treatment of herpes simplex corneal ulcers. Am J Ophthalmol 73:932, 1972
99. Heidelberger C, King DH: Trifluorothymidine. Pharmacol Ther 6:427, 1979
100. La Lau C, Oosterhuis JA, Versteeg G, et al: Acyclovir and trifluorothymidine in herpetic keratitis: preliminary report of a multicentered trial. Doc Ophthalmol 50:287, 1981
101. Høvding G: A comparison between acyclovir and trifluorothymidine ophthalmic ointment in the treatment of epithelial dendritic keratitis: a double blind, randomized parallel group trial. Acta Ophthalmol (Copenh) 67:51, 1989
102. Schaeffer HJ, Beauchamp L, deMiranda P, Elion GB: 9-(2-Hydroxyethoxymethyl)guanine activity against viruses of the herpes group. Nature 272:583, 1978
103. Poirier RH, Kingham JD, deMiranda P, Annel M: Intraocular antiviral penetration. Arch Ophthalmol 100:1964, 1982
104. Jones BR, Fison PN, Cobo LM, et al: Efficacy of acycloguanosine (Wellcome 248U) against herpes-simplex cornea ulcers. Lancet 1:243, 1979
105. Wilhelmus KR, Coster DJ, Jones BR: Acyclovir and debridement in the treatment of ulcerative herpetic keratitis. Am J Ophthalmol 91:323, 1981
106. Tormey P, McGill J, Walker C: Use of acyclovir in herpes simplex corneal ulcers. Trans Ophthalmol Soc UK 101:6, 1981
107. Colin J, Chastel C, Renard G, Cantell K: Combination therapy for dendritic keratitis with human leukocytic interferon and acyclovir. Am J Ophthalmol 95:346, 1983
108. de Koning EWJ, van Bijsterveld OP, Cantell K: Combination therapy for dendritic keratitis with acyclovir and alpha-interferon. Arch Ophthalmol 101:1866, 1983
109. Porter SM, Patterson A, Kho P: A comparison of local and systemic acyclovir in the management of herpetic disciform keratitis. Br J Ophthalmol 74:283, 1990
110. Coster DJ, Wilhelmus KR, Michaud R, Jones BR: A comparison of acyclovir and idoxuridine as treatment for ulcerative herpetic keratitis. Br J Ophthalmol 64:763, 1980
111. Collum LMT, Benedict-Smith A, Hillary IB: Randomised double-blind trial of acyclovir and idoxuridine in dendritic corneal ulceration. Br J Ophthalmol 64:766, 1980
112. Klauber A, Ottovay E: Acyclovir and idoxuridine treatment of herpes simplex keratitis—a double-blind clinical study. Acta Ophthalmol (Copenh) 838:60, 1982
113. McCulley JP, Binder PS, Kaufman HE, et al: A double-blind, multicenter clinical trial of acyclovir vs idoxuridine for treatment of epithelial herpes simplex keratitis. Ophthalmology 89:1195, 1982
114. Pavan-Langston D, Lass J, Hettinger M, Udell I: Acyclovir and vidarabine in the treatment of ulcerative herpes simplex keratitis. Am J Ophthalmol 92:829, 1981
115. McGill J, Tormey P, Walker CB: Comparative trial of acyclovir and adenine arabinoside in the treatment of herpes simplex corneal ulcers. Br J Ophthalmol 65:610, 1981

116. Laibson PR, Pavan-Langston D, Yeakley WR, Lass J: Acyclovir and vidarabine for the treatment of herpes simplex keratitis. Am J Med 73:281, 1982
117. Young BJ, Patterson A, Ravenscroft T: A randomised double-blind clinical trial of acyclovir (Zovirax) and adenine arabinoside in herpes simplex corneal ulceration. Br J Ophthalmol 66:361, 1982
118. Jackson WB, Breslin CW, Lorenzetti DWC, Michaud R: Treatment of herpes simplex keratitis: comparison of acyclovir and vidarabine. Can J Ophthalmol 19:107, 1984
119. Hung SO, Patterson A, Clark DI, Rees PJ: Oral acyclovir in the management of dendritic herpetic corneal ulceration. Br J Ophthalmol 68:398, 1984
120. Collum LMT, Akhtar J, McGettrick P: Oral acyclovir in herpetic keratitis. Trans Ophthalmol Soc UK 104:629, 1985
121. Collum LMT, McGettrick P, Akhtar J, et al: Oral acyclovir (Zovirax) in herpes simplex dendritic corneal ulceration. Br J Ophthalmol 70:435, 1986
122. Schwab IR: Oral acyclovir in the management of herpes simplex ocular infections. Ophthalmology 95:423, 1988
123. Van der Meer JWM, Versteeg J: Acyclovir in severe herpes virus infections. Am J Med 73:271, 1982
124. Van Ganswijk R, Oosterhuis JA, Swart-Van Den Berg M, Versteeg J: Acyclovir treatment in stromal herpetic keratitis. Doc Ophthalmol 55:57, 1983
125. Collum LMT, O'Connor M, Logan P: Comparison of the efficacy and toxicity of acyclovir and of adenine arabinoside when combined with dilute betamethasone in herpetic disciform keratitis: preliminary results of a double-blind trial. Trans Ophthalmol Soc UK 103:597, 1983
126. Sundmacher R: Orale Acyclovir-Therapie virologish nachgewiesener intraokularer Herpes simplex Virus Infectionen. Klin Monatsbl Augenheilkd 183:246, 1983
127. Collum LMT, Logan P, Ravenscroft T: Acyclovir (Zovirax) in herpetic disciform keratitis. Br J Ophthalmol 67:115, 1983
128. Bialasiewicz AA, Jahn GJ: Systemische Acyclovir-Therapie bei rezi divierender durch Herpes simplex Virus bedingter Keratouveitis. Klin Monatsbl Augenheilkd 185:539, 1984
129. Colin J, Mazet D, Chastel C: Treatment of herpes keratouveitis: comparative action of vidarabine, trifluorothymidine and acyclovir in combination with corticoids. p. 227. In Maudgal PC, Missotten L (eds): Herpetic Eye Diseases. Dr. W. Junk, Dordrecht, 1985
130. Barron BA, Gee L, Hauck WW, et al: Herpetic Eye Disease Study: a controlled trial of oral acyclovir for herpes simplex stromal keratitis. Ophthalmology 101:1871, 1994
131. The Herpetic Eye Disease Study Group: A controlled trial of oral acyclovir for iridocyclitis caused by herpes simplex virus. Arch Ophthalmol 114:1065, 1996
132. The Herpetic Eye Disease Study Group: A controlled trial of oral acyclovir for the prevention of stromal keratitis or iritis in patients with herpes simplex virus epithelial keratitis. The epithelial keratitis trial. Arch Ophthalmol 115:703, 1997
133. Rolan P: Pharmacokinetics of new antiherpetic agents. Clin Pharmacokinet 29:333, 1995
134. Andrei G, Snoeck R, Goubau P, et al: Comparative activity of various compounds against clinical strains of herpes simplex virus. Eur J Clin Microbiol Infect Dis 11:143, 1992
135. Crumpacker CS, Schnipper LE, Marlowe SI, et al: Resistance to antiviral drugs of herpes simplex virus isolated from a patient treated with acyclovir. N Engl J Med 306:343, 1982
136. Burns WH, Saral R, Santos GW, et al: Isolation and characterization of resistant herpes simplex virus after acyclovir therapy. Lancet 1:421, 1982
137. Sibrack CD, Gutman LT, Wilfert CM, et al: Pathogenicity of acyclovir-resistant herpes simplex virus type 1 from an immunodeficient child. J Infect Dis 146:673, 1982
138. Erlich KS, Mills J, Chatis P, et al: Acyclovir-resistant herpes simplex virus infections in patients with the acquired immunodeficiency syndrome. N Engl J Med 320:293, 1989
139. Charles SJ, Gray JJ: Ocular herpes simplex virus infection: reduced sensitivity to acyclovir in primary disease. Br J Ophthalmol 74:286, 1990
140. McLeish W, Pflugfelder SC, Crouse C, et al: Interferon treatment of herpetic keratitis in a patient with acquired immunodeficiency syndrome [letter]. Am J Ophthalmol 109:93, 1990
141. Sonkin PL, Baratz KH, Frothingham R, Cobo LM: Acyclovir-resistant herpes simplex keratouveitis after penetrating keratoplasty. Ophthalmology 99:1805, 1992
142. Maudgal PC, De Clercq E:(S)-1-(3-hydroxy-2-phosphonyl-methoxypropyl)cytosine in the therapy of thymidine kinase-positive and -deficient herpes simplex virus experimental keratitis. Invest Ophthalmol Vis Sci 32:1816, 1991
143. Wilhelmus KR, Gee L, Hauck WW, et al: Herpetic Eye Disease Study (HEDS): a controlled trial of topical corticosteroids for herpes simplex stromal keratitis. Ophthalmology 101:1883, 1994
144. Pestka S (ed): Methods in Enzymology. Vol. 78. Interferons. Part A. Academic Press, San Diego, 1981
145. Jones BR, Coster DJ, Falcon MG, Cantell K: Topical therapy of ulcerative herpetic keratitis with human interferon. Lancet 2:128, 1976
146. Kaufman HE, Meyer RF, Laibson PR, et al: Human leukocyte interferon for the prevention of recurrences of herpetic keratitis. J Infect Dis 133:A165, 1976
147. Shuster JJ, Kaufman HE, Nesburn AB: Statistical analysis of the rate of recurrence of herpesvirus ocular epithelial disease. Am J Ophthalmol 91:328, 1981
148. Sundmacher R, Cantell K, Neumann-Haefelin D: Combination therapy of dendritic keratitis with trifluorothymidine and interferon. Lancet 2:687, 1978
149. de Koning EWJ, van Bijsterveld OP, Cantell K: Combination therapy for dendritic keratitis with human leucocyte interferon and trifluorothymidine. Br J Ophthalmol 66:509, 1982
150. Sundmacher R, Mattes A, Neumann-Haefelin D, et al: The potency of interferon-alpha-2 and interferon-gamma in a combination therapy of dendritic keratitis. A controlled clinical study. Curr Eye Res 6:273, 1987

151. Straus SE, Takiff HE, Seidlin M, et al: Suppression of frequently recurring genital herpes: a placebo-controlled double-blind trial of oral acyclovir. N Engl J Med 310:1543, 1984
152. Douglas JM, Critchlow C, Benedetti J, et al: A double-blind study of oral acyclovir for suppression of recurrences of genital herpes simplex virus infection. N Engl J Med 310:1551, 1984
153. Meyrick Thomas RH, Dodd HJ, Yeo JM, et al: Oral acyclovir in the suppression of recurrent non-genital herpes simplex virus infection. Br J Dermatol 113:731, 1985
154. Kaufman HE, Varnell ED, Centifanto-Fitzgerald YM, et al: Oral antiviral drugs in experimental herpes simplex keratitis. Antimicrob Agents Chemother 24:888, 1983
155. Nesburn AB, Willey DE, Trousdale MD: Effect of intensive acyclovir therapy during artificial reactivation of latent herpes simplex virus (41563). Proc Soc Exp Biol Med 172:316, 1983
156. Gebhardt BM, Kaufman HE, Hill JM: Effect of acyclovir on thermal stress-induced viral reactivation. Antiviral Res, submitted
157. Gebhardt BM, Kaufman HE: Propranolol suppresses reactivation of herpes virus. Antiviral Res 27:255, 1995
158. Gebhardt BM, Wright GE, Xu H, et al.: 9-(4-Hydroxybutyl)-N^2-phenylguanine, HBPG, a thymidine kinase inhibitor, suppresses herpes virus reactivation in mice. Antiviral Res 30:87, 1996
159. Kaufman HE: Epithelial erosion syndrome: metaherpetic keratitis. Am J Ophthalmol 57:983, 1964
160. Barney NP, Foster CS: A prospective randomized trial of oral acyclovir after penetrating keratoplasty for herpes simplex keratitis. Cornea 13:232, 1994
161. Moyes AL, Sugar A, Musch DC, Barnes RD: Antiviral therapy after penetrating keratoplasty for herpes simplex keratitis. Arch Ophthalmol 112:601, 1994

11

Varicella-Zoster Viral Infections

KEITH H. BARATZ, KENNETH GOINS, AND MICHAEL COBO

The term *herpes zoster* is derived from the Greek words *herpein,* "to creep and spread," and *zoster,* "a girdle, belt, or zone," which refers to the belt-like dermatomal distribution of the disease. Herpes zoster, commonly known as *shingles,* is caused by reactivation of latent varicella-zoster virus present in sensory ganglia after varicella (chickenpox). Varicella is caused by primary infection with the virus, usually during childhood.[1]

Herpes zoster ophthalmicus involves the tissues innervated by the ophthalmic division of the trigeminal nerve and accounts for 10 to 25 percent of all cases of herpes zoster.[2] Herpes zoster ophthalmicus differs from herpes zoster involvement of other dermatomes inasmuch as the ocular counterpart of visceral involvement (i.e., involvement of the eye itself) occurs in a significant proportion of patients. Herpes zoster involvement of other dermatomes is typically limited to localized cutaneous disease, and metastasis of the virus to the viscera is uncommon. The sequelae of herpes zoster ophthalmicus can be devastating and include chronic ocular inflammation, visual loss, and debilitating pain. Until recently, only corticosteroids and palliative therapy were used to manage the ocular complications and chronic pain.[3–5] Now, however, specific antiviral therapies are available.

VIRUS STRUCTURE AND BEHAVIOR

Varicella-zoster virus (VZV) is a double-stranded DNA virus and is classified in the same family (Herpesviridae) as herpes simplex virus (HSV), Epstein-Barr virus (EBV), and cytomegalovirus (CMV). Varicella zoster virus is more closely related to herpes simplex virus than it is to other herpesviruses.[6]

Replication of varicella-zoster occurs in the host cell nucleus and produces an intranuclear inclusion body. After transcription of viral DNA to messenger RNA, viral proteins are synthesized in the host cell cytoplasm. These proteins are then transported to the host cell nucleus, where they are assembled with replicated viral DNA into nucleocapsids. The virus acquires an outer envelope as it passes through the cytoplasm and is then released from the cell.[7]

After transmission from a contagious individual, varicella-zoster virus initially infects the upper respiratory mucosa or conjunctiva. During the prodrome of varicella, local viral replication results in a primary viremia, with subsequent systemic dissemination of the virus and later, a secondary viremia that coincides with the clinical signs and symptoms of the infection.[8] In varicella, the virus infects the capillary endothelium and then spreads locally to the epidermis, where it causes skin lesions. Vesicles form by the accumulation of fluid between the infected basal layer and the superficial layers of the epidermis. The fluid contains inflammatory cells, fibrin, and many viable virions. The histologic appearance of the skin lesions is that of balloon degeneration (intracellular edema), intercellular edema, and multinucleated giant cells. The intranuclear inclusion bodies are eosinophilic, proteinaceous collections that are separated from the nuclear membrane by a wide clear zone. These findings are present in almost all infected tissues.[9]

After the primary infection, varicella-zoster virus, like herpes simplex virus, remains latent in sensory ganglia, where it produces no clinical signs or symptoms. Studies that use radiolabeled nucleic acid probes for varicella-zoster viral genes have found viral genetic material in the trigeminal and spinal sensory ganglia of asymptomatic individuals.[10–12] Originally, the specific cell type that harbors latent varicella-zoster virus was thought to be the neuron,[10,11] as it is for herpes simplex virus. Varicella-zoster virus, however, is probably also latent in the satellite cells, as well as the neuron, and it is not unlikely that the satellite cells are the major site of latency for this virus.[12]

Latency implies that the virus exists in a noninfectious state.[13] To become latent, the virus must limit its cytotoxicity and prevent recognition by or activation of the host immune system. The viral genetic material must also remain stored in infected host cells, awaiting transcription and assembly of complete virions when the virus is reactivated.[14] Cytotoxicity is limited by halting the production of complete virions, although portions of viral DNA continue to be transcribed in infected cells. Limitation of viral DNA transcription also aids the latent virus in its evasion of immune surveillance. Specifically, reduction of viral glycoproteins on cell membranes makes the virus "invisible" to the host cellular and humoral immune systems.

Knowledge of the molecular biology of varicella-zoster virus latency is incomplete. Studies of herpes simplex virus have identified a specific portion of the viral genome that is transcribed during latency, while the rest of the genome is quiescent; the RNA products of this transcription are termed *latency-associated transcripts* (LATs).[15-17] Latency-associated transcripts are markers of, but are not essential for, establishment or maintenance of latency, although they appear to play a role in reactivation. In contrast, at least three widely separated areas of the varicella-zoster viral genome are transcribed during latency, including some of the immediate early and early genes involved in the production of infectious virus, which implies a more complex, multifactorial process underlying varicella-zoster viral latency compared with herpes simplex viral latency.[18]

To cause recurrent disease, latent varicella-zoster virus must be induced to reactivate, at which time it replicates within the ganglion and spreads to the area of skin (dermis) innervated by a nerve of that ganglion. Differences in the mechanisms of latency and the preferred cell type within the ganglia for latent virus help to explain the different manifestations of varicella-zoster virus and herpes simplex virus reactivation. The larger dermatomal area involved in the infrequent, yet explosive, recurrences of varicella-zoster virus compared with the more localized, frequent recurrences of herpes simplex virus may be related to the pattern of latent infection within the sensory ganglia and the genetic mechanisms and expressivity of the latent virus.[17]

Although the inciting factors are unclear, the reactivation of varicella-zoster virus may be the result of an inability of the host immune system to check an episode of renewed viral replication. Specific cell-mediated immunity to varicella-zoster virus, as measured by skin testing to varicella-zoster viral antigens as well as more sensitive in vitro methods, is disproportionately deficient in elderly populations, compared with the normal age-related decline in immune functions. Humoral immunity to varicella-zoster virus is also affected, although less so, by age.[19-21] These points help to explain the increased frequency of herpes zoster with advancing age and its recurrence in the presence of detectable serum antibodies to varicella-zoster virus.[22] Subclinical, episodic reactivation of varicella-zoster virus can occur, as evidenced by transient elevations in virus-specific antibodies.[23] Exogenous reinfection with varicella-zoster virus can also occur and has been detected by elevations in antibodies to varicella-zoster virus in household contacts of patients with varicella.[24] Such episodes of reactivated virus may cause no clinical disease or may be associated with mild disease, as in zoster sine herpete, in which dermatomal neurologic symptoms occur without the accompanying skin lesions.[3,25]

EPIDEMIOLOGY

The incidence of herpes zoster, as derived from a population-based study of 590 cases in Rochester, Minnesota, is approximately 131 cases per 100,000 persons per year.[2] The incidence is lowest in childhood and rises steadily with age. The correlation with age is even more pronounced in herpes zoster ophthalmicus.

An attack of herpes zoster does not impart subsequent immunity, and recurrence in the same dermatome is not unusual.[26] The chance for a recurrent bout in a previously affected individual is at least as great as the chance for an initial attack in an individual without a prior history of herpes zoster.

Thoracic dermatomes are most commonly affected in herpes zoster and account for more than half the cases. The ophthalmic division of the trigeminal nerve is involved in 10 to 25 percent of all cases. These high frequencies of sensory nerve involvement in herpes zoster coincide with the greatest density of involvement of the dermatomes in varicella.[20,26] Isolated infection of the maxillary or mandibular branches of the trigeminal nerve accounts for 2 percent of cases.[2] Simultaneous infection of the ophthalmic division and other divisions of the trigeminal nerve is atypical, and bilateral disease is even less common (about 1 percent).[3,27]

The incidence of reported ocular involvement in herpes zoster ophthalmicus ranges from 20 to 72 percent, depending on the particular study and whether eyelid involvement is included in the statistics. The more recent reviews in the ophthalmic literature tend to give percentages toward the upper end of this range.[2,3,28]

In addition to age, several immunodeficient conditions predispose individuals to the development of herpes zoster, including malignancy (especially hematologic), radiation therapy, systemic lupus erythematosus, acquired immunodeficiency syndrome (AIDS), and therapeutic immunosuppression.[29-32] Patients with such conditions may be prone to more severe disease and to a greater than average risk of dissemination of the virus.[29,33] Within the group of immunosuppressed patients, it has long been recognized that patients with hematologic malignancies, especially Hodgkin's disease, have a particular tendency to develop herpes zoster.[30,34] The occurrence rate for herpes zoster in all patients with hematologic malignancies is 3 to 10 percent; in Hodgkin's disease, the occurrence rate may be as high as 22 percent.[29,30,35] By contrast, patients with nonhematologic malignancies have a risk that is only moderately higher than or even approaches the rate in the general population.[30,31] The unusual susceptibility of patients with Hodgkin's disease may be linked to a specific impairment in cell-mediated immunity to varicella-zoster virus, a situation analogous to that in the elderly.[36,37]

The presentation of herpes zoster in patients with AIDS is not unexpected in view of the altered cell-mediated immunity in these patients. In a study population of patients with herpes zoster ophthalmicus in New York City, most patients younger than 45 years of age were in a high-risk group for the development of AIDS.[38] Indeed, at the time of diagnosis of herpes zoster ophthalmicus, many of these patients did not have a previous diagnosis of AIDS but had laboratory evidence of infection with human immunodeficiency virus (HIV). Older patients with herpes zoster ophthalmicus in the same population were rarely in a high-risk group for AIDS. The incidence of herpes zoster ophthalmicus was greatest for patients in their fourth decade, an unexpected finding for a normally geriatric disease. This finding may reflect the changing epidemiology of herpes zoster that parallels the age-related prevalence of AIDS. Other studies have confirmed that herpes zoster may be a marker for AIDS in high-risk groups and may be a harbinger of a rapidly waning immune status.[39-41] In a young, otherwise healthy person, herpes zoster should alert the clinician to the possible presence of AIDS, and the appropriate medical history, physical examination, and laboratory work-up should be undertaken.

Although herpes zoster has been associated with immune suppression, most individuals with herpes zoster have no underlying illness, nor are they at an increased risk of subsequently developing cancer. Ragozzino and associates[42] described a large cohort of patients with herpes zoster in which they found no increase in the incidence of subsequent cancer. These results suggest that in the absence of clinical signs or symptoms of malignancy, an elaborate search for occult malignancy at the time of diagnosis of herpes zoster, as well as repeated probing thereafter, is unnecessary.

Although herpes zoster per se is not transmitted directly, the shedding of varicella-zoster virus during an episode of herpes zoster can result in transmission of the virus and subsequent primary infection (i.e., varicella) in previously uninfected individuals. Pregnant women and immunosuppressed patients with no history of varicella are at high risk of complications of varicella.[43-45] Maternal infection with varicella-zoster virus is associated with spontaneous abortion, major fetal malformations, maternal death from pneumonitis, and when the disease occurs near delivery, a high rate of infant mortality.[44] Although most adults with no clinical history of varicella have been exposed to the virus, had subclinical disease, and are not susceptible to infection, about 25 percent have never been exposed to the virus and are at risk from exposure to infected individuals. Because of the danger to both mother and child, patients with herpes zoster should limit contact with pregnant women who have not had varicella.[46] Should such contact occur, the women should be tested for serologic evidence of prior exposure to the virus and counseled appropriately.

CLINICAL MANIFESTATIONS

Sixty percent of patients with herpes zoster ophthalmicus experience dermatomal pain before the typical vesicular skin lesions.[47-49] The lesions first appear as nummular or geographic areas of erythematous papules that worsen and evolve over several days into vesicles that contain clear serous fluid (Figure 11-1A) and, later, into pustules (Figure 11-1B). As these rupture or are resorbed, they typically become covered with crusts (Figure 11-1C) that take one to several weeks to heal completely.[50] In severe cases, a large proportion of the skin within a dermatome may be affected, but the lesions do not cross the midline of the face. In mild cases, the papular rash can resolve without vesiculation. Shedding of varicella-zoster virus from the skin lesions persists for an average of 3 days but can continue for as long as 14 days in some patients.[48] The course of the acute dermatologic features of herpes zoster ophthalmicus is self limited. The duration and severity of the skin lesions vary greatly and are not predictors of subsequent eye involvement.

Constitutional symptoms include fatigue, malaise, and a low-grade fever. The erythrocyte sedimentation rate may be elevated, although leukocytosis is not typical. In fact,

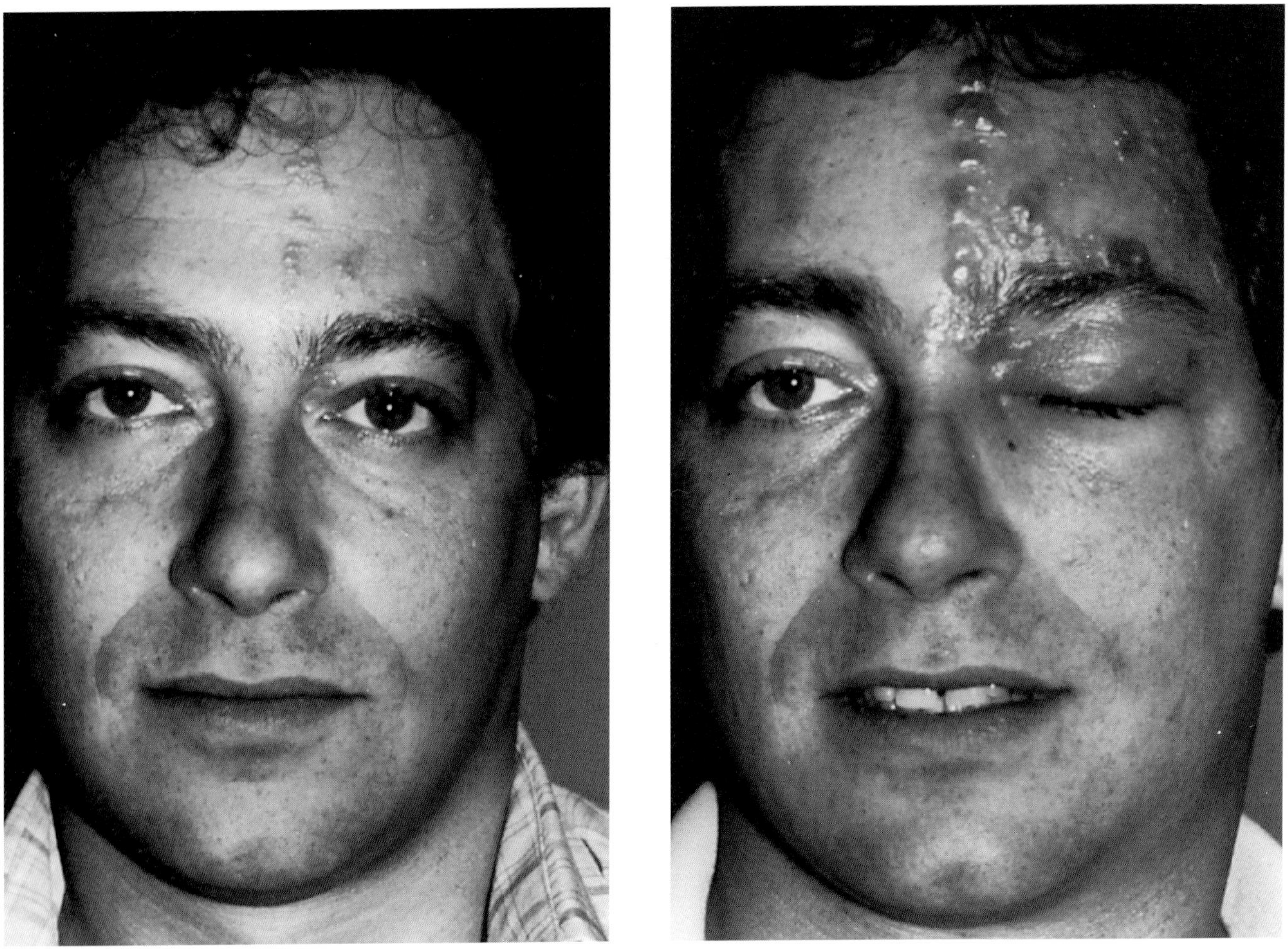

A B

FIGURE 11-1 Herpes zoster ophthalmicus, with progression of the lesions from **(A)** vesicles to **(B)** pustules to *(continues)*

a large study of patients with herpes zoster revealed a significant depression in absolute neutrophil and lymphocyte counts compared with the counts in healthy controls.[51]

OCULAR MANIFESTATIONS OF HERPES ZOSTER

The ocular manifestations of herpes zoster ophthalmicus may be varied, prolonged, and recurrent. The anterior segment and ocular adnexa are commonly involved in clinically significant disease. Hutchinson sign, or involvement of the tip of the nose, has classically been quoted as a clinical predictor of ocular involvement. The nasociliary nerve is the main sensory nerve to the eye and sends posterior ciliary nerves to the eye and sensory branches to the tip of the nose. The assumption is that involvement of one portion of a particular nerve with the virus will be associated with involvement of all end organs supplied by that nerve. However, caution should be exercised in applying this to clinical practice, because it is unreliable.[28] Although patients with a positive Hutchinson sign may have twice the incidence of ocular involvement (76 percent versus 34 percent), about one-third of patients without the sign develop ocular manifestations.[52]

Conjunctiva

Mucopurulent conjunctivitis is common in herpes zoster ophthalmicus. It is self limited and is not an indication that more serious ocular complications are developing. Conjunctival vesicles may develop. These are typically unroofed by eyelid movement, which results in a focal area of con-

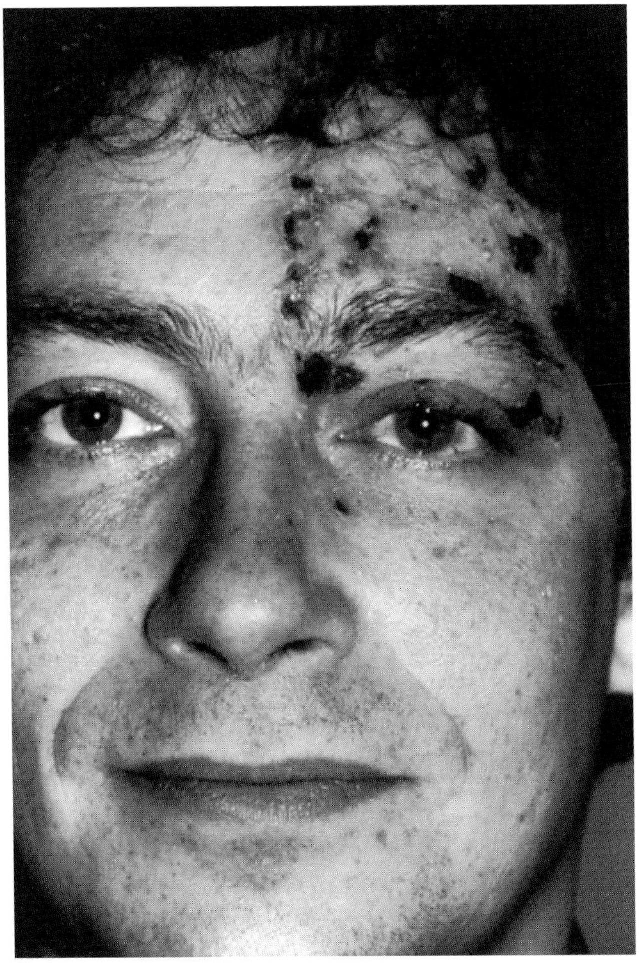

C

FIGURE 11-1 *(continued)* (C) crusts.

junctival inflammation and an erosion that stains with rose bengal (Figure 11-2). Although these lesions are of interest, they typically resolve and do not appear to be directly correlated with specific long-term ocular complications.

Cornea and Sclera

The cornea becomes involved in herpes zoster ophthalmicus in about 65 percent of patients. The clinical features of corneal disease represent a spectrum of virus-induced pathology, including direct viral infection, antigen-antibody reactions or delayed cell-mediated hypersensitivity reactions, vasculitis, and neurotrophic keratitis. Through clinical observation and laboratory studies, the diverse corneal findings have been classified in an attempt to aid ophthalmologists in the diagnosis, treatment, and basic understanding of the pathologic processes of the disease.

Keratitis associated with herpes zoster ophthalmicus can be divided into two stages: early and late. Liesegang[27] noted that the earliest corneal finding is punctate epithelial keratitis (PEK), which consists of multiple focal areas of swollen epithelial cells that stain with rose bengal. These lesions may be present as early as 1 or 2 days after the initial skin rash. Resolution may be spontaneous. In many patients, however, punctate epithelial keratitis progresses during the first week to dendritic keratitis (Figure 11-3), which, in turn, may be followed by anterior stromal inflammation.[27]

The occurrence rate of dendritic keratitis varies from 13 to 60 percent of all cases of herpes zoster ophthalmicus.[49,53] The appearance of dendrites was first thought to be caused by the coexistence of herpes simplex virus and varicella-

FIGURE 11-2 Conjunctival and eyelid margin erosions in a patient with acute herpes zoster ophthalmicus (rose bengal stain).

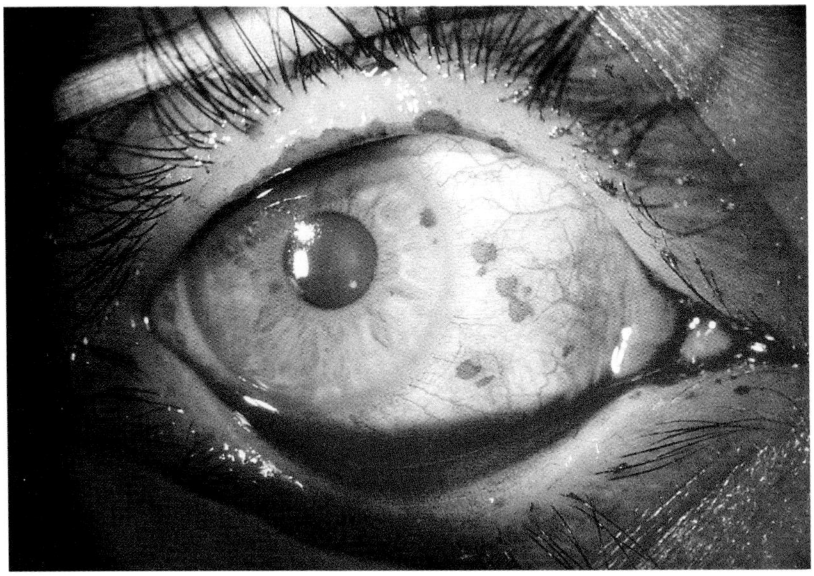

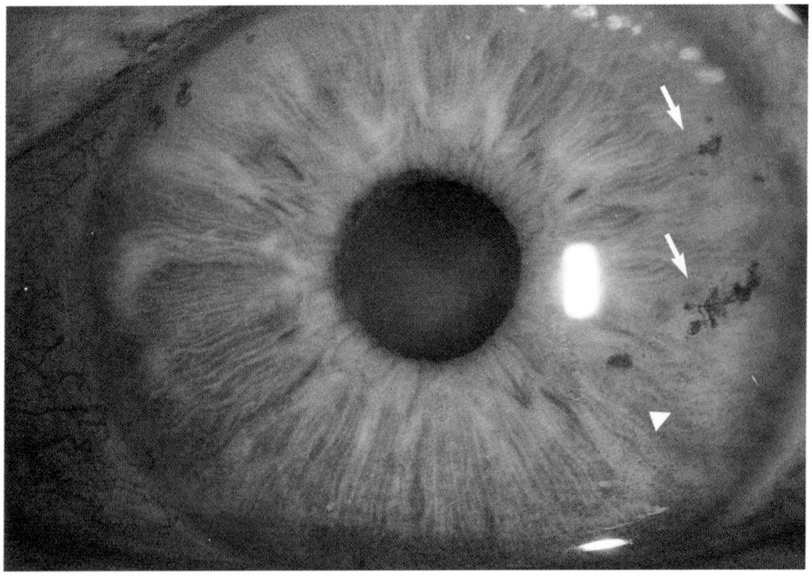

FIGURE 11-3 Early viral punctate epithelial keratitis (arrowhead) and small dendrites (arrows) in a patient with acute herpes zoster ophthalmicus (rose bengal stain).

zoster virus.[54-56] Although the two infections can coexist, they usually do not, and herpes zoster virus produces dendrites that are generally quite different from those produced by herpes simplex virus. In three patients reported by Kaufman et al[54] and one patient reported by Giles,[55] prior treatment of herpes zoster-related uveitis with corticosteroids was thought to predispose the cornea to secondary infection with herpes simplex virus. The theory was reinforced by the apparent responsiveness of the dendrites to topical idoxuridine. In 1973, however, Pavan-Langston and McCulley[57] offered evidence that the typical herpes zoster dendrites are a manifestation of direct infection of the corneal epithelium with varicella-zoster virus. The authors described three patients whose corneal scrapings grew varicella-zoster virus but not herpes simplex virus. Further support was provided by a later case of a child with varicella-related dendritic keratitis. Epithelial cells from the cornea examined by direct immunofluorescence were positive for varicella-zoster viral antigens but were negative for herpes simplex viral antigens.[58]

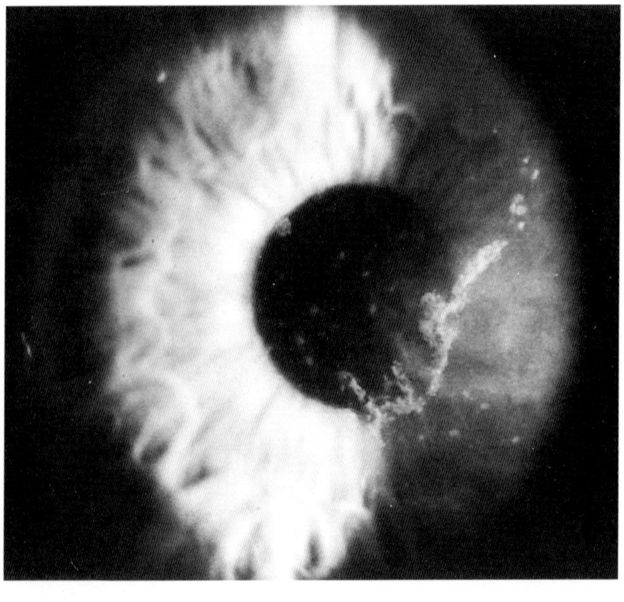

FIGURE 11-4 Dendrite in a patient with concurrent herpes zoster disciform keratitis and uveitis. The dendrite is plaque-like and nonulcerated. Several keratic precipitates can be seen.

Early herpes zoster dendrites are morphologically distinct from herpes simplex dendrites. Herpes zoster dendrites are whitish, elevated, and plaque-like and consist of swollen epithelial cells without ulceration (Figure 11-4). They are coarse and form branching or "medusa-like" patterns. The branches may be broken or coalescent. The dendrites stain with rose bengal but minimally with fluorescein. In contrast, herpes simplex dendrites are ulcerated and characteristically appear as fine, branching epithelial defects that stain brightly with fluorescein. Terminal bulbs are typical of herpes simplex dendrites but are absent in herpes zoster dendrites.[59,60] Like the initial punctate epithelial keratitis but unlike herpes simplex virus epithelial disease, zoster dendrites do not appear to respond to topical antivirals nor are they worsened by corticosteroids.[27,53]

Marsh et al[4] distinguished between the acute and late varieties of herpes zoster epithelial keratitis, and this distinction has been continued in later clinical studies. Of 238

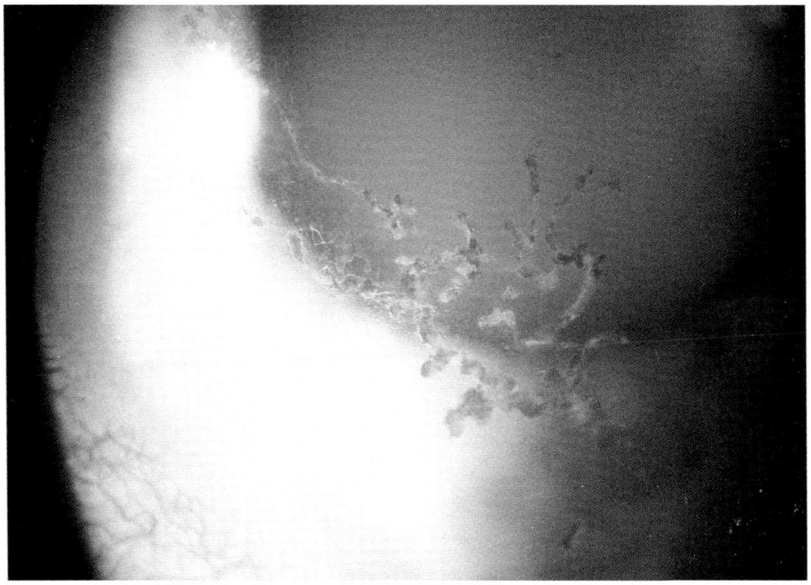

FIGURE 11-5 Late dendriform epithelial lesion secondary to herpes zoster. Rose bengal staining reveals staining of a mucous plaque adherent to nonulcerated corneal epithelium.

patients with herpes zoster ophthalmicus, 13 percent had epithelial dendrites in the acute phase of the disease. Another 7 percent developed mucous plaque keratitis, usually several months after the initial onset of the disease. These plaques were of various shapes and sizes and varied in dimension from day to day (Figure 11-5). They were seen in conjunction with an unstable tear film, epithelial bedewing, stromal haze, and anterior chamber inflammation. Scrapings from mucous plaques stained positively with Alcian blue, in contrast to specimens from corneas with acute epithelial keratitis, which did not stain. Unlike dendrites, mucous plaques could be debrided without removing the underlying epithelium. Interestingly, examination of scrapings from both dendrites and plaques revealed large multinucleated epithelial cells,[60] whereas similar-appearing mucous plaques in patients with keratoconjunctivitis sicca showed no multinucleated cells.[61]

The early stage of stromal keratitis presents during the second week of the disease and consists of superficial stromal inflammation. There are patches of granular, grayish stromal infiltrates immediately beneath Bowman's layer in 20 to 35 percent of patients with herpes zoster ophthalmicus[28] (Figure 11-6). The patches may arise in a setting in which pre-existing epithelial disease was not evi-

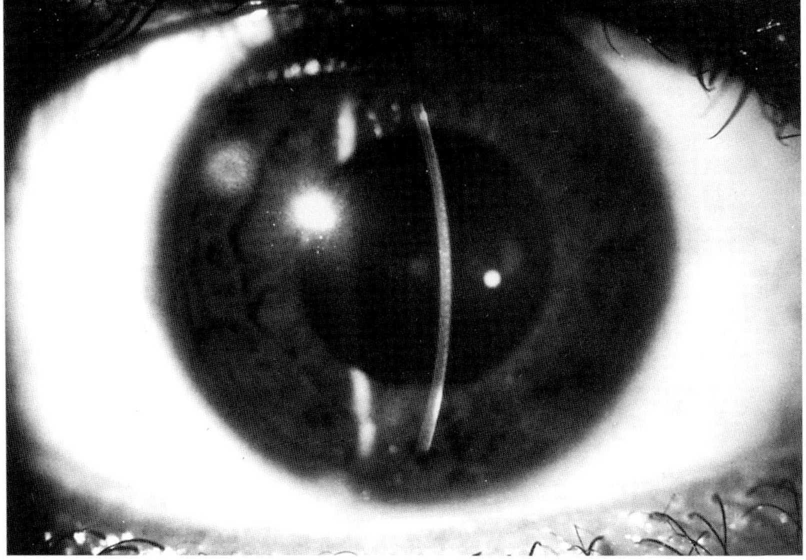

FIGURE 11-6 Multiple subepithelial infiltrates revealed in the anterior portion of the slit beam in a patient with herpes zoster ophthalmicus.

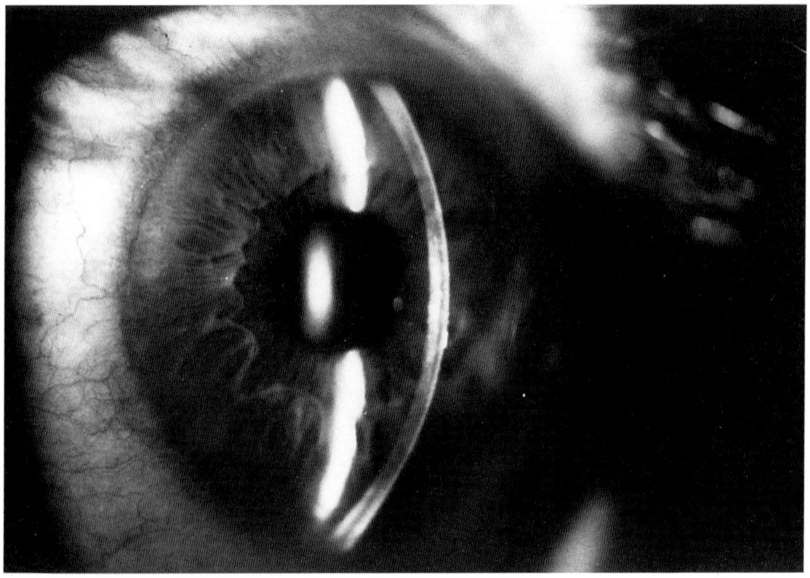

FIGURE 11-7 Late disciform stromal keratitis after herpes zoster ophthalmicus. Note the central anterior and posterior opacification in the slit beam.

dent, but most are preceded by dendrites and lie directly beneath them. The inflammatory nature of such infiltrates is evidenced by their responsiveness to topical corticosteroids and their propensity for scarring. Possible etiologies for these lesions have been suggested. They have been noted to occur along the course of corneal nerves, which may implicate a perineuritis from viral destruction of the sensory nerves. Another possible cause is an antigen-antibody reaction resulting from viral proliferation in the overlying epithelium.[27,53] Anterior stromal keratitis may be prolonged and recurrent.[49,53]

The late stage of stromal keratitis is characterized by deep stromal inflammation with edema and can occur one or more months after the onset of herpes zoster ophthalmicus. The keratitis may present as a typical disciform lesion, consisting of a localized area of inflammation affecting all levels of the stroma (Figure 11-7), or as peripheral infiltrates that may have a surrounding immune ring or may be contiguous with an area of scleritis. Corneal edema may be a prominent feature at this stage, and anterior chamber inflammation is common. Deep stromal keratitis is less common than superficial keratitis. A chronic or relapsing course is not unusual. Without corticosteroid therapy, continued inflammation leads to vascularization, scarring, or ulceration (Figure 11-8). Lipid deposition in the stroma is prominent in chronically affected

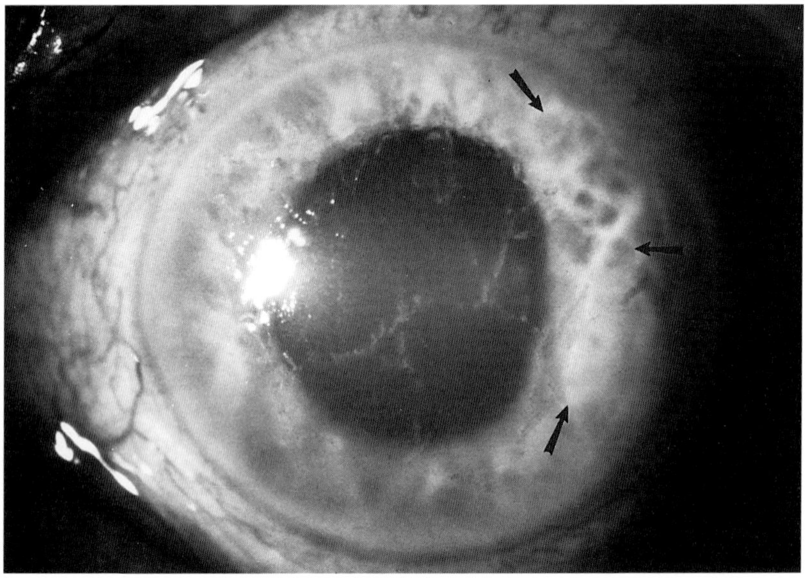

FIGURE 11-8 Severe keratouveitis in a patient with herpes zoster ophthalmicus. Several dendrites are present, the cornea is hazy, and the iris is atrophic (arrows).

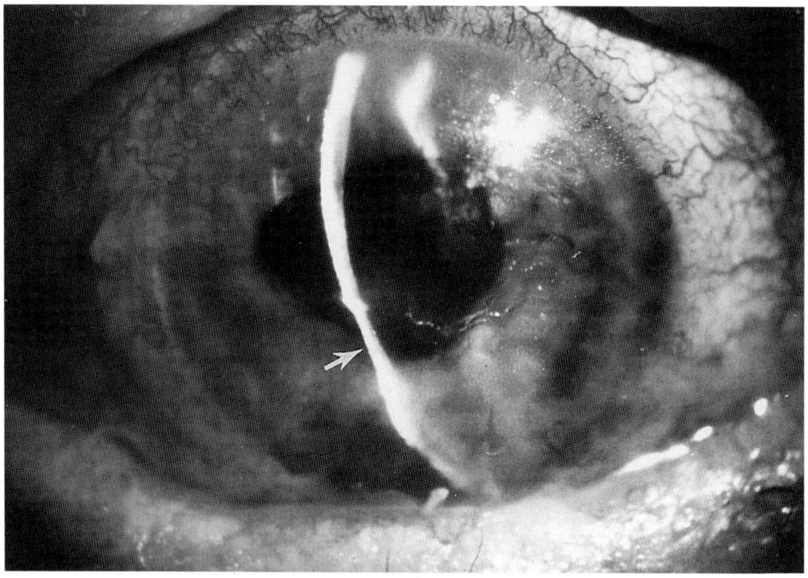

FIGURE 11-9 Neurotrophic keratitis secondary to herpes zoster in a patient with profoundly reduced corneal sensation, eyelid margin scarring, and lagophthalmos. Note corneal thinning (arrow) in the interpalpebral fissure.

corneas. The mechanism involved in disciform keratitis is probably a delayed cell-mediated hypersensitivity reaction; chronic active infection is unlikely.

Endothelial involvement in herpes zoster ophthalmicus has received little attention in the literature. Endotheliitis has been reported to be a not-infrequent occurrence in the course of the keratitis; however, the presence of stromal inflammation with resulting corneal swelling can be difficult to differentiate from isolated endothelial dysfunction. Several studies have evaluated specular microscopic imaging in patients in whom the eye with prior herpes zoster keratouveitis had decreased endothelial cell density compared with the normal contralateral eye. These changes were described as patchy areas of endothelial cell loss.[62,63] Another report found herpes-like viral particles in an endothelial biopsy of an inflamed eye; however, the diagnosis of varicella-zoster viral infection and not herpes simplex viral infection in this atypical case was questionable.[64]

During the acute phase of herpes zoster ophthalmicus, the inflamed eyelids often do not close, although they may appear almost swollen shut. Lagophthalmos is common and is critical to recognize because, if untreated, it can lead to corneal ulceration and stromal scarring. Treatment with ointments and occlusive dressings can reduce these complications.

Neurotrophic keratitis is a potentially severe complication of herpes zoster ophthalmicus. Neurotrophic disease is the end result of multiple factors affecting an insensate cornea, including susceptibility to mechanical trauma, decreased lacrimation, and delayed epithelial healing. Animal models of neurotrophic corneal disease have shown thinning of the epithelium and decreased mitotic rates, even in the presence of a complete tarsorrhaphy.[65-67] There is evidence for an epithelial trophic function of cholinergic neurotransmitters, present as acetylcholine in high concentration in normal corneal epithelium.[68] Because varicella-zoster viral infection originates in the sensory nerve and destroys the neuron, it would seem logical that lack of sensation would be evident early in the course of the disease. Cobo et al[49] found that the mean presentation time of central corneal hypesthesia, as measured with an esthesiometer, was approximately 3 days after the onset of the rash. Roughly one-half of cases of herpes zoster ophthalmicus have decreased corneal sensation, but in most, sensation is not completely lost and is often recovered. The more worrisome patient is the one in whom corneal hypesthesia is profound, especially if there is any eyelid malposition or dysfunction caused by the skin lesions. The clinical appearance of neurotrophic keratitis begins as a lack of corneal luster and the presence of punctate epithelial erosions. If sensation remains absent, the condition can progress to an epithelial defect and indolent ulceration, with edematous grayish stroma and a cellular infiltrate. At this stage, the cornea is prone to secondary infection but may have progressive stromal thinning, leading to perforation even in a sterile environment[27,53] (Figure 11-9). One study of herpes zoster ophthalmicus in 86 patients found neurotrophic keratitis as a cause of visual loss in 8 (9 percent), second only to stromal scarring.[28]

An unusual sequela of herpes zoster keratitis is peripheral corneal ulceration, which consists of crescent-shaped furrowing accompanied by edema and cellular infiltra-

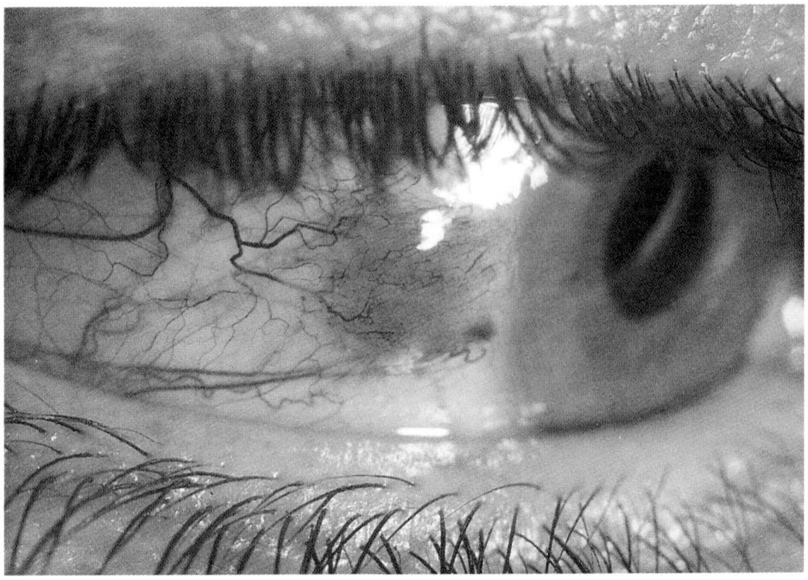

FIGURE 11-10 Episcleritis associated with herpes zoster ophthalmicus.

tion, as well as decreased corneal and conjunctival sensation. The central border of the ulcer is steep, and the ulcer can lead to vascularization and pannus formation or to stromal melting and perforation.[69] The ulceration is not caused solely by neurotrophic disease but may be a manifestation of a concurrent immune or inflammatory reaction.[27,69]

Scleritis or episcleritis as an isolated finding without corneal inflammation has been reported in herpes zoster ophthalmicus[70] (Figure 11-10). Vasculitis and ischemia are important factors to be considered in the pathogenesis of scleritis. Evidence for anterior segment ischemia is atrophy of the iris pigment epithelium, which is most easily observed at the slit lamp by retroillumination (see next section). These retroillumination defects may occur in the same sector as the concomitant scleritis.[27,53]

Uvea

Uveitis is a common occurrence in the setting of herpes zoster stromal keratitis or corneal edema, although it may be difficult to grade because of poor visibility due to corneal opacification. The incidence varies from 43 to 60 percent.[28,49,71] Uveitis typically appears within the first 1 to 2 weeks of the onset of herpes zoster ophthalmicus. It is successfully treated with topical corticosteroids, but the course, like that of stromal keratitis, may be prolonged over months to years, with more severe cases developing posterior synechiae, glaucoma, and cataracts. In Womack and Liesegang's retrospective review of 86 patients with herpes zoster ophthalmicus,[28] 7 of the 37 patients with uveitis developed cataracts. Six of the seven had been on topical corticosteroids for longer than 3 months. The presence of uveitis may be difficult to diagnose in a patient with corneal scars, yet persistence of uveitis makes the prognosis for penetrating keratoplasty poor.

Increased intraocular pressure is a complication in at least one-third of herpes zoster uveitis cases.[28,49] This form of glaucoma is usually transient and, in most cases, resolves with corticosteroid treatment of the causative uveitic inflammation, but prolonged intraocular pressure elevation and glaucomatous optic nerve damage can develop. The treatment of glaucoma may be complicated if intraocular pressure elevation is further exacerbated by chronic corticosteroid use.

Iris atrophy is an interesting aspect of herpes zoster ophthalmicus, and there is evidence for multiplication of virus in the iris. Slit lamp findings of iris transillumination defects in a sectorial pattern or in the peripupillary area corresponding to the iris sphincter muscle are typical (Figure 11-11). There may be poor pupillary motility in the involved sector. A few patients have massive iris atrophy. Iris transillumination defects are not clinically apparent immediately but develop and progress over weeks to months, even after the uveitis subsides.[71] Fluorescein angiography of the iris has provided insight into the pathogenesis of anterior segment disease. On fluorescein angiography, there is diffuse leakage of iris vessels early in the course of the uveitis. Shortly thereafter, delayed filling or complete closure of sectorial radial vessels and some of the basal arcades occurs. In cases affecting the iris sphincter muscle, there are additional filling defects in the circumferential arterial arcade.

A variety of other rare complications have been reported in herpes zoster ophthalmicus. Most of these complications are severe forms of the basic ischemic and inflammatory processes present in more typical cases. Some of these cases include irreversible corneal decompensation and anterior segment ischemic syndrome. Phthisis bulbi may occur, probably a result of generalized ischemia with extensive ciliary body necrosis.

Ocular Adnexa

Unlike the vesicular rash of varicella, which usually does not cause scarring, the skin lesions of herpes zoster tend to cicatrize. Crusted lesions may leave pits, scars, or areas of altered pigmentation (Figure 11-12); these sequelae are more likely to be prominent on the forehead and eyelids than on other parts of the body.[72] Initially, the eyelids are edematous with a degree of swelling that causes a mechanical type of ptosis. Lagophthalmos is common with acute eyelid involvement and must be treated to prevent corneal scarring. If scarring of eyelid lesions occurs, a variety of eyelid malformations, such as eyelid retraction, ectropion or entropion of either the upper or lower eyelid, trichiasis, and punctal occlusion, can result. The extent of cicatricial changes or sloughing of tissue may be great and is compounded by necrosis secondary to ischemic vasculitis.[5,28,33,72–75] Many of these eyelid sequelae result in impaired eyelid function and exposure of an ocular surface that may already be compromised. Nasr et al[74] found herpes zoster-related eyelid deformities to be amenable to surgical correction for functional rehabilitation.

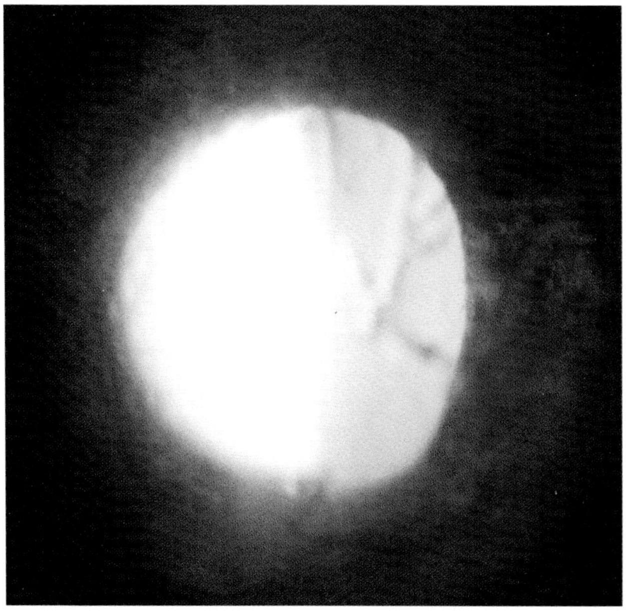

FIGURE 11-11 Peripupillary iris atrophy (seen with transillumination) associated with herpes zoster ophthalmicus.

Ophthalmic Innervation, Posterior Segment, and Central Nervous System

Neuro-ophthalmic and posterior segment sequelae of herpes zoster ophthalmicus are highly varied and generally rare. Oculomotor nerve palsy reportedly occurs in 4 to 50 percent of patients and is generally transient. Retinitis is a rare, although devastating complication, as is optic

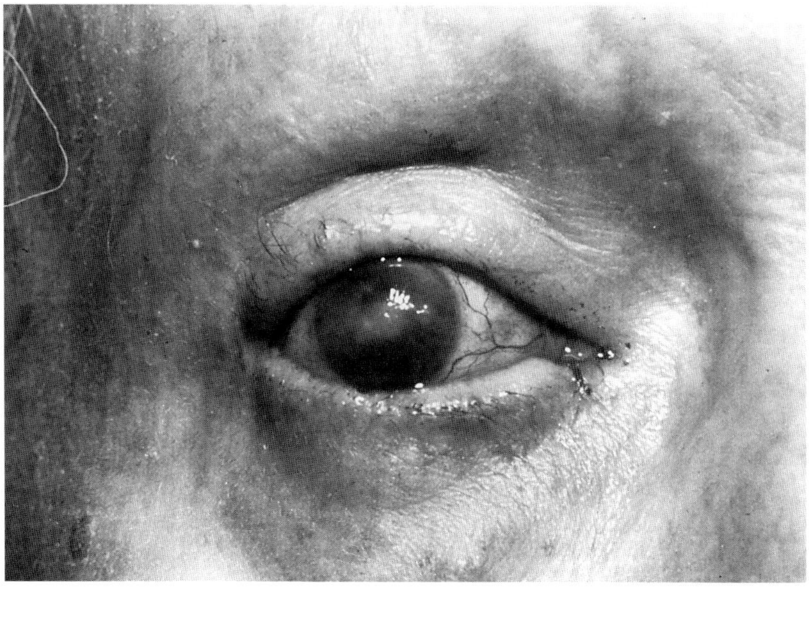

FIGURE 11-12 Scarring of the eyebrow and eyelids in a patient after acute herpes zoster ophthalmicus. The cornea is also scarred.

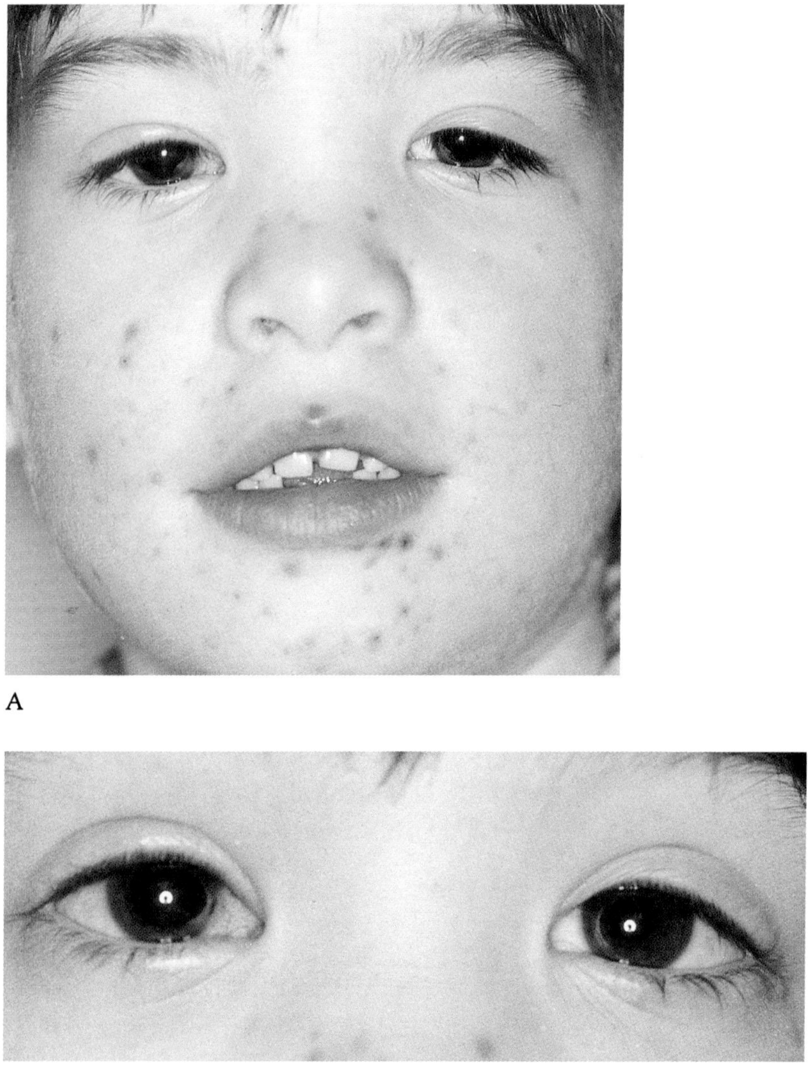

A

B

FIGURE 11-13 (A) Typical appearance of chickenpox. (B) There is mild conjunctivitis and iritis in the right eye.

neuritis. Considering the threat to vision from a possibly virus-productive process, it may be appropriate to treat these complications of herpes zoster ophthalmicus with intravenous antiviral therapy. Cerebral vasculitis is an uncommon but catastrophic complication of herpes zoster ophthalmicus and is associated with a vasculitis and virus production within the intima of blood vessels.[76] The classic manifestation is late-onset contralateral hemiplegia as a consequence of a middle cerebral arteritis. This illness is life threatening and must be recognized as distinct from other cerebrovascular entities of the elderly. In this setting, the ophthalmologist can be instrumental in providing the correct diagnosis, thereby facilitating prompt therapy.

OCULAR MANIFESTATIONS OF VARICELLA

Primary varicella infection has been shown to cause ocular disease that mimics the sequelae of herpes zoster ophthalmicus. Eyelid vesiculation and conjunctivitis are fairly common in the acute stage of the illness (Figure 11-13). Conjunctivitis may be accompanied by phlyctenular nodules or perilimbal infiltrates, punctate epithelial keratitis, or dendrites. Less common are uveitis and stromal keratitis that present shortly after the infection, but these manifestations can be severe and vision threatening. Like herpes zoster keratouveitis, varicella keratouveitis may become chronic and require prolonged therapy.[77] Because varicella is extremely common in children and could occur coincidentally in association with other eye diseases, it is wise to consider other causes of keratouveitis, such as herpes simplex virus, Epstein-Barr virus, mumps, syphilis, Lyme disease, or tuberculosis, in the differential diagnosis.

HISTOPATHOLOGY

Retrospective studies of histologic specimens from more than 30 eyes affected by herpes zoster ophthalmicus have reported inflammation in almost all ocular tissues.[78,79] The trigeminal ganglion is infiltrated with lymphocytes and plasma cells, and there is necrosis and demyelination of the sensory nerves, as well as the sensory nucleus of the 5th cranial nerve in the brain stem. There is also local spread of inflammation, which may include an arteritis marked by giant cells and granulomatous involvement of the vessels that supply the intracranial structures.[79]

Naumann et al[78] reviewed the pathology of 21 eyes obtained 1 week to 8 years after the first clinical signs of herpes zoster ophthalmicus. The most notable feature shared by almost all eyes was perineural or intraneural lymphocytic infiltration of the long posterior ciliary nerves. The anterior segment findings included episcleritis and scleritis, thickening and inflammation of the perilimbal tissues, corneal ulceration and perforation, pseudoepitheliomatous hyperplasia of the corneal epithelium, band keratopathy, stromal inflammation and vascularization, granulomatous reaction to Descemet's membrane, and loss of endothelial cells. These were severely affected eyes; most were enucleated because of perforated corneal ulcers or because they had become blind and painful from glaucoma. Other characteristic anterior segment changes included patchy ciliary body necrosis and disruption of areas of iris pigment epithelium.[78,79]

DIAGNOSIS

The diagnosis of herpes zoster ophthalmicus can usually be made on clinical presentation alone. Prodromal dysesthesia followed by a painful papulovesicular rash in a unilateral dermatomal distribution is sufficient evidence for the diagnosis. Atypical cases may require the help of adjunctive laboratory tests. Patients may present with a mild rash or a rash that involves only one or several small branches of the ophthalmic division of the trigeminal nerve.[3] If the area of skin involvement is small or displaced away from the midline of the face, the clinically useful sign of a vertical demarcation may be absent. Another diagnostic dilemma may be the new patient with ocular inflammation or surface disease who does not have a definite history of previous herpes zoster ophthalmicus. Included in the differential diagnosis of ocular disease are herpes simplex, syphilis, tuberculosis, atopic keratoconjunctivitis, neurotrophic keratitis, keratoconjunctivitis sicca, and autoimmune causes of ocular inflammation. Also to be considered in the differential diagnosis of dermatologic or neurologic conditions are impetigo, facial cellulitis, chemical or thermal burns, trigeminal neuralgia, contact dermatitis, and other noninfectious dermatitides.

A quick and easy laboratory test for herpes zoster is the Tzanck smear, which is prepared by scraping the base of a fresh vesicle. After staining with Giemsa, hematoxylin-eosin, Papanicolaou, or Paragon Multiple stain, multinucleated giant cells and intranuclear inclusions are seen in about 50 percent of specimens. A major limitation of the Tzanck smear is that herpes simplex yields the same findings.[80,81]

Immunofluorescence staining or counterimmunoelectrophoresis can be used on vesicular fluid or swabs of vesicular fluid or crusted lesions. Direct and indirect immunofluorescence allow application of monoclonal antibodies against varicella-zoster viral glycoproteins or hyperimmune serum to smears of infected tissue. Direct immunofluorescence uses fluorescein conjugated to varicella-zoster viral antibodies, whereas indirect immunofluorescence uses unconjugated varicella-zoster virus antibodies followed by fluorescein-conjugated immunoglobulin to anti–varicella-zoster virus antibodies. These tests are specific for varicella-zoster virus and do not crossreact with other herpesviruses.[82-84] Another advantage is that these tests require only viral antigen and may remain positive after viable virus can no longer be isolated from the skin lesions.[82]

A variety of serologic tests for varicella-zoster virus-specific antibodies are available, including a fluorescent antibody to virus membrane antigen (FAMA), enzyme-linked immunosorbent assay (ELISA), and others.[85] A negative FAMA correlates with susceptibility to primary varicella. A fourfold or greater increase in convalescent serum IgG titer compared with the acute serum IgG titer is evidence of disease activation.[86] The presence of varicella-zoster virus-specific IgM also is indicative of recent or active disease and may be useful in the case of a patient with ocular inflammation without a definite history of herpes zoster dermatitis. Increases in antibody titer are seen in household contacts of acutely infected individuals, suggesting subclinical reinfection. Elevated antibody levels, however, do not correlate with reduced susceptibility to herpes zoster.[22,87]

Culture of varicella-zoster virus yields a definitive diagnosis. However, the cultivation of the virus may be difficult, making it one of the few viruses for which culture is less sensitive than other diagnostic methods. If culture is to be attempted, the suggested method is to aspirate the fluid from a fresh vesicle with a tuberculin syringe and immediately add it to a viral transport medium that is on ice. The specimen should be inoculated onto viral culture medium as soon as possible. The virus may be grown on a variety of human cell lines as well as a few simian cell types.[88] Crusted lesions do not usually yield positive culture results, although scraping the base of an unroofed lesion will provide material for culture if no vesicle fluid is obtainable.[9]

TREATMENT

Dermatitis

There has been great progress in antiviral therapy in the past several decades, and several antiviral agents have been investigated with possible applications for varicella-zoster viral infection. Idoxuridine has been tried clinically, but its toxicity, when used systemically, has limited its use. Topical idoxuridine reportedly has benefits when applied to the skin lesions of herpes zoster.[89] Beneficial effects in the healing of the dermatomal rash and decreased systemic spread of the virus have been reported with intravenous vidarabine and human leukocyte interferon. In the past, these drugs were particularly useful in immunosuppressed patients, but with the recent development of newer antiviral agents, acyclovir has become the drug of choice for the treatment of herpes zoster in this high-risk group.[90–92]

The use of systemic acyclovir has become widespread in recent years as an effective treatment for a variety of herpes simplex virus-related and varicella-zoster virus-related conditions. Acyclovir is specific for herpesviruses. It is selectively phosphorylated by viral thymidine kinase, which is produced only in virus-infected cells. The active compound, acyclovir triphosphate, inhibits DNA polymerase and is incorporated into growing chains of DNA, where it causes the chains to terminate.

Early clinical trials of intravenous acyclovir in the treatment of herpes zoster revealed a beneficial effect in preventing new vesicle formation and decreasing the duration of viral shedding.[93–95] These studies found that intravenous acyclovir was of questionable use in otherwise healthy adults, considering the need for intravenous administration and lack of proof of a reduction in postherpetic neuralgia, which is the most common complication of non-ophthalmic herpes zoster in this population.[43,96] Subsequent clinical reports on oral acyclovir found a reduction in the time course of the rash, although its effect on postherpetic neuralgia is still debated. Current data show alleviation of pain with oral acyclovir during the acute stages of the disease, especially if the drug is given within the first 3 days, and tend to favor a positive effect on postherpetic neuralgia.[97–99] The data supporting the effect on postherpetic neuralgia, however, do not approach statistical significance in most studies.[93,95,96,100–102] The unresolved discrepancies found in the literature may be related to the need for high-dose medication, 800 mg orally five times a day for 7 days as opposed to 400 mg on the same schedule used in some studies.[99] Realizing that the benefits of acyclovir may be minimal in immunocompetent patients, some clinicians still recommend treatment of non-ophthalmic herpes zoster in adults, except pregnant women, with high-dose acyclovir within 3 days of the onset of the rash. If the patient presents later than 3 or 4 days after onset, the decision to treat may be based on the severity of symptoms and the inflammation.[97]

The indications for acyclovir in immunocompromised patients are more readily agreed on. Such patients have a relatively high rate of viral dissemination to the viscera and other areas of the skin. Of 94 patients studied by Balfour et al,[43] six had life-threatening visceral involvement; two of these patients died. Intravenous acyclovir prevents and halts widespread dissemination of virus to the skin and the progression of visceral disease. Intravenous acyclovir is indicated in herpes zoster patients with malignancy (particularly hematologic malignancy), patients on cytotoxic drugs, AIDS patients, and transplant recipients.[43,103,104] Balfour[103] also recommends intravenous acyclovir in patients with systemic lupus erythematosus or immunosuppression resulting from other autoimmune diseases. He advocates only observation in corticosteroid-dependent patients, such as asthmatics.

Topical 1 percent silver sulfadiazine applied to the affected skin four times a day results in complete drying of vesicles, marked reduction of erythema and edema, and elimination of pain and burning sensation within 24 to 72 hours, without evidence of local or systemic toxicity.[105] Also, topical 5 to 40 percent idoxuridine in dimethyl sulfoxide (DMSO) relieves pain and accelerates healing. At this time, idoxuridine is unavailable in this formulation in the United States.[89] Some authors have appropriately warned that application of drying preparations, such as powder, should be avoided, because these preparations may increase permanent scarring of the skin, which could promote immobilization of the eyelids and exposure keratopathy.[4] Some patients may develop bacterial superinfection of skin lesions that requires topical and/or systemic antibiotics.

A variety of drugs have been developed with the aims of improving the antiviral activity and the pharmacokinetic characteristics as compared with acyclovir. Valacyclovir, a prodrug of acyclovir, is converted to acyclovir after absorption from the intestinal tract. Oral valacyclovir is more readily absorbed than acyclovir, so the prodrug has greater bioavailability, which allows a more convenient dosing schedule.[106] In 1995, valacyclovir (Valtrex) was approved by the U.S. Food and Drug Administration (FDA) for the treatment of herpes zoster. The recommended dose is 1 g orally every 8 hours for 7 days. Dosage reduction is recommended in patients with reduced renal function.

Another prodrug, famciclovir, has a high rate of systemic absorption after oral administration and is converted to penciclovir in the intestinal wall and the liver.[107] Penciclovir is phosphorylated in virus-infected cells, where the active triphosphate is more stable than its acyclovir counterpart.[108] These pharmacologic properties allow the use of a lower effective dose at less frequent intervals. One study comparing famciclovir to placebo in immunocompetent patients found that herpes zoster lesions healed more quickly, the duration of viral shedding was reduced, and the resolution of postherpetic neuralgia was more rapid in famciclovir recipients than in placebo recipients.[109] In 1994, famciclovir (Famvir) was approved by the FDA for the treatment of herpes zoster. The recommended dose is 500 mg every 8 hours for 7 days, beginning within 72 hours of the diagnosis of herpes zoster. Dosage reduction is recommended in patients with reduced renal function. Whether famciclovir offers therapeutic advantages over acyclovir or valacyclovir remains to be established. Degreef[110] reported similar times to crusting of herpes zoster lesions and resolution of acute pain in famciclovir recipients and acyclovir recipients.

Another antiviral, unavailable in the United States, is bromovinyldeoxyuridine (BVDU), which has potential both as an oral agent for the treatment of herpes zoster dermatitis and as a topical agent for the treatment of herpes zoster and herpes simplex keratouveitis.[111-113] Like acyclovir and penciclovir, BVDU is selectively phosphorylated by viral thymidine kinase and inhibits viral DNA polymerase. In cell culture, BVDU is more potent than acyclovir, trifluridine, or idoxuridine against herpesviruses.

Pain

Intractable pain is one of the most difficult therapeutic problems encountered in patients with herpes zoster. No established regimen eliminates this severe pain, which often leads to psychological problems and social withdrawal. The management of pain-related problems may require a multispecialty approach, including consultation with an internist, psychiatrist, and anesthesiologist or other pain management specialist.

Acute Pain

The acute pain of herpes zoster may be severe, requiring analgesics, and occasionally, the short-term use of narcotics. Cimetidine is a histamine H_2-receptor antagonist that has received transient advocacy in the treatment of the acute pain and itching of herpes zoster.[114,115] Many anecdotal reports have indicated a dramatic improvement in signs and symptoms with a dose of 300 mg orally four times a day. Conclusive evidence of the efficacy of cimetidine is lacking, however, and a double-masked study of cimetidine versus placebo showed no benefit with respect to pain.[116] Additionally, cimetidine increases the blood level of many drugs through an effect on certain microsomal enzymes, which makes the use of this otherwise well-tolerated drug potentially problematic. Topical percutaneous local anesthesia with 9 percent lidocaine ointment has been reported for control of cutaneous pain of acute herpes zoster.[117]

In addition to pain, patients with acute herpes zoster are generally plagued by pruritus, nausea, insomnia, malaise, and agitation. Empiric therapy with an oral antihistamine, such as hydroxyzine, can produce a palliative effect on these signs and symptoms; a daytime dose of 25 mg three times a day is used for the treatment of pruritus and nausea, and a bedtime dose of 50 to 100 mg is used for sedation.

Chronic Pain (Postherpetic Neuralgia)

The incidence of postherpetic neuralgia (defined as dermatomal pain lasting more than 1 month after disease onset) for all types of herpes zoster is between 9 and 14 percent.[118] Corresponding rates in herpes zoster ophthalmicus are similar or even higher. It is acknowledged that older patients are more prone to the development of postherpetic neuralgia, but there are no other obvious manifestations of herpes zoster that serve as predictors.[52] The pain can have a variety of characteristics, from a constant burning or ache to a pruritic sensation to a fleeting lancinating pain. In approximately 20 percent of patients with postherpetic neuralgia, the pain lasts longer than 1 year.[2]

Many nontraditional analgesics have been used in the management of postherpetic neuralgia, including tricyclic antidepressants, phenothiazine, corticosteroids, anticonvulsants, levodopa, and amantadine.[119] Amitriptyline, a tricyclic antidepressant, has been used extensively in the treatment of postherpetic neuralgia to ameliorate pain and to alleviate the depression that often accompanies it. Because the dosage can be problematic in elderly patients, the ophthalmologist may wish to defer to an internist or psychiatrist. Alternatively, one may initiate therapy with a low bedtime dose of 25 mg, gradually increasing to 75 mg as tolerance develops. Once a full bedtime dose is established, a dose of 25 mg three times a day may be added to obtain the recommended therapeutic dose. However, the full antidepressant dose of amitriptyline is not always required to achieve pain reduction; some patients may benefit from relatively low doses of the drug.

Oral prednisone administered during the acute phase of herpes zoster dermatitis has been reported to reduce the incidence and duration of postherpetic neuralgia.[120] Controversy about its use persists, however, because studies of prednisone and acute herpes zoster dermatitis vary greatly with respect to definition of postherpetic neuralgia, dose administered, and study design. The point of controversy is the short-term use of an immunosuppressive drug in a disease caused by a virus that is prone to dissemination. Of nonimmunocompromised patients with herpes zoster ophthalmicus who are not treated with prednisone, 6 to 14 percent develop vesicular lesions involving other dermatomes (microdissemination); the percentages are higher in immunocompromised patients, in whom possible further dissemination of the virus to the viscera carries a high rate of morbidity and mortality.[47,48,103] A placebo-controlled study of prednisone combined with acyclovir in the treatment of acute herpes zoster showed no difference in the development or duration of postherpetic neuralgia, although the corticosteroid-treated group apparently obtained added relief of pain during the first 3 days of drug therapy.[121] Based on lack of evidence for long-term benefits from corticosteroids, coupled with their potential drawbacks, other analgesics should probably be used in the early stages of herpes zoster in most cases.

Drugs that deplete chemomediators of pain impulses have been evaluated for the treatment of postherpetic neuralgia. Capsaicin is a natural chemical that, when applied topically, depletes and prevents the accumulation of substance P, which is involved in the transmission of pain impulses. High levels of substance P have been demonstrated in sensory nerves at sites of chronic inflammation. Preliminary clinical trials indicate that topical capsaicin may reduce or eliminate the chronic pain associated with herpes zoster.[122] Capsaicin is available as a topical cream and can be applied to affected skin three to four times a day. The drug is extremely irritating to the eye, and under no circumstances should it be applied to a site adjacent to the eye. The most common side effect of cutaneous application is transient burning of the skin.

Ocular Disease

Treatment of the ocular complications of herpes zoster ophthalmicus requires a thorough understanding of the variety of problems that may occur during the course of the disease and the potential side effects of therapy. A treatment regimen must be individualized, depending on the stage of the disease, the severity of symptoms and inflammation, the patient's tendency toward adverse reactions to therapy (such as corticosteroid-induced intraocular pressure elevation), and the integrity of the ocular surface as affected by neural and mechanical factors.

The mainstay of treatment of ocular inflammation caused by herpes zoster has been topical corticosteroids. Topical corticosteroids carry the risks of intraocular pressure elevation, cataract formation, and secondary infection in patients with corneal epithelial instability. Another theoretical disadvantage is the potential for prolonging the course of the disease or increasing the frequency of recurrences due to uninhibited viral replication in the presence of corticosteroids.[123]

Cobo et al[47] studied 71 patients presenting within 1 week of onset of herpes zoster ophthalmicus in a randomized, placebo-controlled trial to determine the efficacy of oral acyclovir on ocular complications. At a dose of 600 mg, five times a day for 10 days, acyclovir had a significant clinical effect, especially on anterior segment inflammation. There was also a marginally significant effect on the incidence of dendritic keratitis but no significant effect on episcleritis. The rate of development and severity of stromal keratitis were notably decreased in the acyclovir-treated group. Similarly, the incidence and severity of uveitis were markedly decreased by acyclovir.[47,48]

Topical 3 percent acyclovir ointment has been used in Great Britain but is not available in the United States. Topical acyclovir appears to be as effective as topical corticosteroids in the treatment of most cases of acute herpes zoster ocular disease and more effective in eliminating the early dendrites. However, severe cases still need additional topical corticosteroids to quiet the inflammation. The theoretical advantage of topical acyclovir is that it may eradicate the virus rather than mask the inflammatory reaction to continued viral replication. This phenomenon was evident in one study that compared topical acyclovir to topical corticosteroids, in which the duration of treatment was shorter for the acyclovir group. Recurrences were common in the corticosteroid group, which necessitated reinstitution of prolonged treatment, but were absent in the acyclovir group.[124,125]

General Recommendations

Our recommendation for the treatment of acute herpes zoster ophthalmicus in otherwise healthy patients who present in the first week of disease is either valacyclovir 1 g every 8 hours or famciclovir 500 mg every 8 hours for 7 to 10 days. There is evidence that these drugs, especially famciclovir, shorten the duration of postherpetic neuralgia. In patients with chronic renal failure or who are on dialysis, adjustments in dosage may be necessary. In immunocompromised patients or patients with particularly severe signs and symptoms, hospitalization, administration of intravenous acyclovir, and observation by a consulting internist may be needed. Currently, we do not recommend systemic corticosteroids for most patients. The early ocular manifestations, which usually consist of conjunctivitis and dendritic keratitis, require only the palliative measures of topical lubricants or mucolytics, such as 10 percent acetylcysteine.[126] There is no evidence that the topical antivirals currently available in the United States (vidarabine and trifluridine) are effective in eradicating epithelial disease. At the earliest sign of stromal inflammation, corneal edema, or uveitis, frequent topical corticosteroids should be administered. Doses of 1 percent prednisolone every hour may be needed for the initial treatment of moderate or severe inflammation. Acutely increased intraocular pressure should respond to corticosteroids as well, in addition to aqueous suppressants and cycloplegics. The indications for topical corticosteroids as the primary therapeutic agent in the treatment of the inflammatory ocular sequelae of herpes zoster ophthalmicus may change as new topical antivirals are introduced. Until that time, we must accept the potential for a prolonged clinical course and frequent recrudescences inherent with corticosteroid therapy.

During initial eyelid involvement and neurotrophic keratitis, it is important to recognize the presence of corneal exposure, which requires a different approach and complicates therapeutic decisions in the setting of corticosteroid-responsive inflammation. Topical lubricants, patching, or a bandage soft contact lens can be used, although these are temporizing measures. A generous tarsorrhaphy is curative and is recommended if epithelial defects are slow to heal or if corticosteroids are concurrently needed in an eye with poor sensation and epithelial abnormalities. More aggressive therapies, such as systemic corticosteroids and a total conjunctival flap, are reserved for cases of unrelenting inflammation or stromal melting with impending perforation.[127,128] In progressive corneal stromal ulceration, it may be necessary to rule out a secondary infection, such as bacterial keratitis.

Another important consideration in the care of the herpes zoster ophthalmicus patient is the safety and efficacy of surgical procedures that are necessary to visually rehabilitate the eye or control glaucoma. Marsh and Cooper[129] reported their experience with cataract extraction, trabeculectomy, and penetrating keratoplasty in patients with herpes zoster ophthalmicus. In general, the results were optimistic, although there was a reluctance to perform penetrating keratoplasty in patients with neurotrophic keratitis. Another study specifically addressed this question; the authors found that the absence of corneal sensation need not doom the graft to failure.[130] If penetrating keratoplasty in an insensate eye is being considered, a temporary complete tarsorrhaphy or a permanent lateral tarsorrhaphy at the time of surgery should be considered strongly. Other factors that should be taken into account are intraocular pressure control, tear film integrity, eyelid function, and the presence of active inflammation, which may be difficult to assess preoperatively.

REFERENCES

1. Bastian FO, Rabson AS, Yee CL, Tralka TS: Herpes virus varicellae isolated from human dorsal root ganglia. Arch Pathol 97:331, 1974
2. Ragozzino MW, Melton LJ III, Kurland LT, et al: Population-based study on herpes zoster and its sequelae. Medicine 61:310, 1982
3. Edgerton AE: Herpes zoster ophthalmicus: report of cases and review of literature. Arch Ophthalmol 34:40, 1945
4. Marsh RJ, Fraunfelder FT, McGill JL: Herpetic corneal epithelial disease. Arch Ophthalmol 94:1899, 1976
5. Liesegang TJ: The varicella-zoster virus: systemic and ocular features. J Am Acad Dermatol 11:165, 1984
6. Murphy FA, Kingsbury DW: Virus taxonomy. p. 29. In Fields BN, Knipe DM (eds): Virology. Raven Press, New York, 1990
7. Ben-Porat T, Kaplan AS: Replication—biochemical aspects. p. 163. In Kaplan AS (ed): The Herpesviruses. Academic Press, San Diego, 1973
8. Feldman S, Epp E: Detection of viremia during incubation of varicella. J Pediatr 94:746, 1979
9. Gelb LD: Varicella-zoster virus. p. 2011. In Fields BN, Knipe DM (eds): Virology. Raven Press, New York, 1990
10. Hyman RW, Ecker JR, Tenser RB: Varicella-zoster virus RNA in human trigeminal ganglia. Lancet 2:814, 1983
11. Gilden DH, Rozenman Y, Murray R, et al: Detection of varicella-zoster virus nucleic acid in neurons of normal human thoracic ganglia. Ann Neurol 22:377, 1987
12. Croen KD, Ostrove JM, Dragovic LJ, Straus S: Patterns of gene expression and sites of latency in human nerve ganglia are different for varicella-zoster and herpes simplex viruses. Proc Natl Acad Sci USA 85:9773, 1988
13. Roizman B, Sears AE: An inquiry into the mechanism of herpes simplex virus latency. Annu Rev Microbiol 41:543, 1987
14. Oldstone MB: Viral persistence. Cell 56:517, 1989
15. Stevens JG, Haarr L, Porter DD, et al: Prominence of the herpes simplex virus latency-associated transcript in trigeminal ganglia from seropositive humans. J Infect Dis 158:117, 1988
16. Stevens JG, Wagner EK, Devi-Rao GB, et al: RNA complementary to a herpesvirus alpha gene mRNA is prominent in latently infected neurons. Science 235:1056, 1987

17. Straus SE: Clinical and biological differences between recurrent herpes simplex virus and varicella-zoster virus infections. JAMA 262:3455, 1989
18. Meier JL, Straus SE: Comparative biology of latent varicella-zoster virus and herpes simplex virus infections. J Infect Dis 166(suppl):S13, 1992
19. Burke BL, Steele RW, Beard OW, et al: Immune responses to varicella-zoster in the aged. Arch Intern Med 142:291, 1982
20. Miller AE: Selective decline in cellular immune response to varicella zoster in the elderly. Neurology 30:582, 1980
21. Berger R, Florent G, Just M: Decrease of the lymphoproliferative response to varicella-zoster virus antigen in the aged. Infect Immunol 32:24, 1981
22. Brunell PA, Gershon AA, Uduman SA, Steinberg S: Varicella-zoster immunoglobulins during varicella, latency, and zoster. J Infect Dis 132:49, 1975
23. Luby JP, Ramirez-Ronda C, Rinner S, et al: A longitudinal study of varicella-zoster virus infections in renal transplant recipients. J Infect Dis 135:659, 1977
24. Arvin AM, Koropchak CM, Wittek AE: Immunologic evidence of reinfection with varicella-zoster virus. J Infect Dis 148:200, 1983
25. Lewis GW: Zoster sine herpete. Br Med J 2:418, 1958
26. Hope-Simpson RE: The nature of herpes zoster: a long-term study and a new hypothesis. Proc R Soc Med 58:9, 1965
27. Liesegang TJ: Corneal complications from herpes zoster ophthalmicus. Ophthalmology 92:316, 1985
28. Womack LW, Leisegang TJ: Complications of herpes zoster ophthalmicus. Arch Ophthalmol 101:42, 1983
29. Mazur MH, Dolin R: Herpes zoster at the NIH: a 20 year experience. Am J Med 65:738, 1978
30. Wright ET, Winer LH: Herpes zoster and malignancy. Arch Dermatol 84:110, 1961
31. Dolin R, Reichman RC, Mazur MH, Whitley RJ: Herpes zoster-varicella infections in immunosuppressed patients. Ann Intern Med 89:375, 1978
32. Rifkind D: The activation of varicella-zoster virus by immunosuppressive therapy. J Lab Clin Med 68:463, 1966
33. Blodi FC: Ophthalmic zoster in malignant disease. Am J Ophthalmol 65:686, 1968
34. Pancoast HK, Pendergrass EP: The occurrence of herpes zoster in Hodgkin's disease. Am J Med Sci 168:326, 1924
35. Feldman S, Hughes WT, Kim HY: Herpes zoster in children with cancer. Am J Dis Child 126:178, 1973
36. Ruckdeschel JC, Schimpff SC, Smyth AC, Mardiney MR: Herpes zoster and impaired cell-associated immunity to the varicella-zoster virus in patients with Hodgkin's disease. Am J Med 62:77, 1977
37. Gershon AA, Steinberg SP: Cellular and humoral immune responses to varicella-zoster virus in immunocompromised patients during and after varicella-zoster infections. Infect Immun 25:170, 1979
38. Sandor EV, Millman A, Croxson TS, Mildvan D: Herpes zoster ophthalmicus in patients at risk for the acquired immune deficiency syndrome (AIDS). Am J Ophthalmol 101:153, 1986
39. Friedman-Kien AE, Lafleur FL, Gendler E, et al: Herpes zoster: a possible early clinical sign for development of acquired immunodeficiency syndrome in high-risk individuals. J Am Acad Dermatol 14:1023, 1986
40. Cole EL, Meisler DM, Calabrese LH, et al: Herpes zoster ophthalmicus and acquired immune deficiency syndrome. Arch Ophthalmol 102:1027, 1984
41. Melbye M, Grossman RJ, Goedert JJ, et al: Risk of AIDS after herpes zoster. Lancet 1:728, 1987
42. Ragozzino MW, Melton LJ, Kurland LT, et al: Risk of cancer after herpes zoster. N Engl J Med 307:393, 1982
43. Balfour HH, Bean B, Laskin OL, et al: Acyclovir halts progression of herpes zoster in immunocompromised patients. N Engl J Med 308:1448, 1983
44. Paryani SG, Arvin AM: Intrauterine infection with varicella-zoster virus after maternal varicella. N Engl J Med 314:1542, 1986
45. Stagno S, Whitley RJ: Herpesvirus infections of pregnancy. Part II. Herpes simplex virus and varicella-zoster infections. N Engl J Med 313:1327, 1985
46. Steele RW, Coleman MA, Fiser M, Bradsher RW: Varicella zoster in hospital personnel: skin test reactivity to monitor susceptibility. Pediatrics 70:604, 1982
47. Cobo LM, Foulks GN, Leisegang T, et al: Oral acyclovir in the therapy of acute herpes zoster ophthalmicus: an interim report. Ophthalmology 92:1574, 1985
48. Cobo LM, Foulks GN, Liesegang T, et al: Oral acyclovir in the treatment of acute herpes zoster ophthalmicus. Ophthalmology 93:763, 1986
49. Cobo LM, Foulks GN, Leisegang T, et al: Observations on the natural history of herpes zoster ophthalmicus. Curr Eye Res 6:195, 1987
50. Burgoon CF, Burgoon JS, Baldridge GD: The natural history of herpes zoster. JAMA 164:265, 1957
51. Hellgren L, Hersle K: A statistical and clinical study of herpes zoster. Gerontol Clin 8:70, 1966
52. Harding SP, Lipton JR, Wells JCD: Natural history of herpes zoster ophthalmicus—predictors of postherpetic neuralgia and ocular involvement. Br J Ophthalmol 71:353, 1987
53. Marsh RJ: Herpes zoster keratitis. Trans Ophthalmol Soc UK 93:181, 1973
54. Kaufman H, Dohlman CH, Martola EL: Herpes simplex treatment with IDU and corticosteroids. Arch Ophthalmol 69:468, 1963
55. Giles C: Coexisting herpes zoster and herpes simplex: ocular involvement. Eye Ear Nose Throat Mon 48:216, 1969
56. Acers TE, Vaile V: Coexisting herpes zoster and herpes simplex. Am J Ophthalmol 63:992, 1967
57. Pavan-Langston D, McCulley JP: Herpes zoster dendritic keratitis. Arch Ophthalmol 89:25, 1973
58. Uchida Y, Kaneko M, Hayashi K: Varicella dendritic keratitis. Am J Ophthalmol 89:259, 1980
59. Piebanga LW, Laibson PR: Dendritic lesions in herpes zoster ophthalmicus. Arch Ophthalmol 90:268, 1973
60. Marsh RJ: Ophthalmic herpes zoster. Br J Hosp Med 15:609, 1976

61. Fraunfelder FT, Wright P, Tripathi RC: Corneal mucus plaques. Am J Ophthalmol 83:191, 1977
62. Reijo A, Antti V, Jukka M: Endothelial cell loss in herpes zoster keratouveitis. Br J Ophthalmol 67:751, 1983
63. Sundmacher R, Mutter O: Das Hornhautendothel bei Zoster Ophthalmicus. Klin Monatsbl Augenheilkd 180:271, 1982
64. Maudgal PC, Missotten L, DeClerq E, Descamps J: Varicella-zoster virus in the human corneal endothelium: a case report. Bull Soc Belge Ophtalmol 190:71, 1980
65. Alper MG: The anesthetic eye: an investigation of changes in the anterior ocular segment of the monkey caused by interrupting the trigeminal nerve at various levels along its course. Trans Am Ophthalmol Soc 73:323, 1975
66. Mishima S: The effects of the denervation and the stimulation of the sympathetic and the trigeminal nerve on the mitotic rate of the corneal epithelium in the rabbit. Jpn J Ophthalmol 1:65, 1957
67. Sigelman S, Friedenwald JS: Mitotic and wound-healing activities of the corneal epithelium. Arch Ophthalmol 52:46, 1954
68. Cavanagh HD, Colley A, Pihlaja DJ: Persistent corneal epithelial defects. Int Ophthalmol Clin 19:197, 1979
69. Mondino BJ, Brown SI, Mondzelewski JP: Peripheral corneal ulcers with herpes zoster ophthalmicus. Am J Ophthalmol 86:611, 1978
70. Penman GG: Scleritis as a sequel of herpes ophthalmicus. Br J Ophthalmol 15:585, 1931
71. Marsh RJ, Easty DL, Jones BR: Iritis and iris atrophy in herpes zoster ophthalmicus. Am J Ophthalmol 78:255, 1974
72. Scheie HG: Herpes zoster ophthalmicus. Trans Ophthalmol Soc UK 90:899, 1970
73. Bouzas A: Canalicular inflammation in ophthalmic cases of herpes zoster and herpes simplex. Am J Ophthalmol 60:713, 1965
74. Nasr AM, Beyer-Machule CK, Yeatts RP: Cicatricial ectropion secondary to herpes zoster. Ophthalmic Surg 14:763, 1983
75. Smith JP, Lavine DM: Cicatricial ectropion of the upper lid secondary to herpes zoster ophthalmicus. Ann Ophthalmol 13:579, 1981
76. Linnemann CC Jr, Alvira MM: Pathogenesis of varicella-zoster angiitis in the CNS. Arch Neurol 37:239, 1980
77. Wilhelmus KR, Hamill MB, Jones DB: Varicella disciform stromal keratitis. Am J Ophthalmol 111:575, 1991
78. Naumann G, Gass JDM, Font RL: Histopathology of herpes zoster ophthalmicus. Am J Ophthalmol 65:533, 1968
79. Hedges TR III, Albert DM: The progression of the ocular abnormalities of herpes zoster. Ophthalmology 89:165, 1982
80. Blank H, Burgoon CF, Baldridge GD, et al: Cytologic smears in diagnosis of herpes simplex, herpes zoster, and varicella. JAMA 146:1410, 1951
81. Barr RJ, Herten RJ, Graham JH: Rapid method for Tzanck preparations. JAMA 237:1119, 1977
82. Schmidt NJ, Gallo D, Devlin V, et al: Direct immunofluorescence staining for detection of herpes simplex and varicella-zoster virus antigens in vesicular lesions and certain tissue specimens. J Clin Microbiol 12:651, 1980
83. Schmidt NJ, Lennette EH, Woodie JD, Ho HH: Immunofluorescent staining in the laboratory diagnosis of varicella-zoster virus infections. J Lab Clin Med 66:403, 1965
84. Weigle KA, Grose C: Common expression of varicella-zoster viral glycoprotein antigens in vitro and in chickenpox and zoster vesicles. J Infect Dis 148:630, 1983
85. Landry ML, Cohen SD, Mayo DR, et al: Comparison of fluorescent-antibody-to-membrane-antigen test, indirect immunofluorescence assay, and a commercial enzyme-linked immunosorbent assay for determination of antibody to varicella-zoster virus. J Clin Microbiol 25:832, 1987
86. Gershon AA, Krugman S: Seroepidemiologic survey of varicella: value of specific fluorescent antibody test. Pediatrics 56:1005, 1975
87. Weigle KA, Grose C: Molecular dissection of the humoral immune response to individual varicella-zoster viral proteins during chickenpox, quiescence, reinfection, and reactivation. J Infect Dis 149:741, 1984
88. Weller TH, Witton HM, Bell EJ: The etiologic agents of varicella and herpes zoster. J Exp Med 108:843, 1958
89. Juel-Jensen BE, MacCallum FO, Mackenzie AMR, Pike MC: Treatment of zoster with idoxuridine in dimethyl sulphoxide—results of two double-blind controlled trials. Br Med J 4:776, 1970
90. Merigan TC, Rand KH, Pollard RB, et al: Human leukocyte interferon for the treatment of herpes zoster in patients with cancer. N Engl J Med 298:981, 1978
91. Whitley RC, Soong SJ, Dolin R, et al: Early vidarabine therapy to control the complications of herpes zoster in immunosuppressed patients. N Engl J Med 307:971, 1982
92. Whitley RC, Ch'ien LT, Dolin R, et al: Adenine arabinoside therapy of herpes zoster in the immunosuppressed. NIAID Collaborative antiviral study. N Engl J Med 294:1193, 1976
93. McGill J, MacDonald DR, Fall C, et al: Intravenous acyclovir in acute herpes zoster infection. J Infect 6:157, 1983
94. Peterslund NA, Seyer-Hansen K, Ipsen J, et al: Acyclovir in herpes zoster. Lancet 2:827, 1981
95. Bean B, Braun C, Balfour HH: Acyclovir therapy for acute herpes zoster. Lancet 2:118, 1982
96. Juel-Jensen BE, Khan JA, Pasvol G: High-dose intravenous acyclovir in the treatment of zoster: a double-blind placebo-controlled trial. J Infect 6(suppl):31, 1983
97. Peterslund NA: Management of varicella zoster infections in immunocompetent hosts. Am J Med 85(suppl):74, 1988
98. Morton P, Thomson AN: Oral acyclovir in the treatment of herpes zoster in general practice. N Z Med J 102:93, 1989
99. Huff JC, Bean B, Balfour HH, et al: Therapy of herpes zoster with oral acyclovir. Am J Med 85(suppl):84, 1988
100. McKendrick MW, McGill JI, White JE, Wood MJ: Oral acyclovir in acute herpes zoster. Br Med J 293:1529, 1986

101. McKendrick MW, McGill JI, Wood MJ: Lack of effect of acyclovir on postherpetic neuralgia. Br Med J 298:431, 1989
102. Wood MJ, Ogan PH, McKendrick MW, et al: Efficacy of oral acyclovir treatment of acute herpes zoster. Am J Med 85(suppl):79, 1985
103. Balfour HH: Varicella zoster virus infections in immunocompromised hosts. Am J Med 85(suppl):68, 1985
104. Shepp DH, Dandliker PS, Meyers JD: Current therapy of varicella zoster virus infection in immunocompromised patients. A comparison of acyclovir and vidarabine. Am J Med 85(suppl):96, 1985
105. Montes LF, Muchinik G, Fox CL: Response of varicella zoster virus to silver sulfadiazine. Cutis 38:363, 1986
106. Burnette TC, deMiranda P: Purification and characterization of an enzyme from rat liver that hydrolyzes 256487, the L-valyl ester prodrug of acyclovir. Antiviral Res 20(suppl):S144, 1993
107. Vere Hodge RA, Sutton D, Boyd MR, et al: Selection of an oral prodrug (BRL 42810; famciclovir) for the antiherpes agent BRL 39123 [9-(4-hydroxy-3-hydroxymethylbut-1-yl) guanine; penciclovir]. Antimicrob Agents Chemother 33:1765, 1989
108. Earnshaw DL, Bacon TH, Darlison SJ, et al: Mode of antiviral action of penciclovir in MRC-5 cells infected with herpes simplex virus type 1 (HSV-1), HSV-2 and varicella zoster virus. Antimicrob Agents Chemother 36:2747, 1992
109. Tyring S, Barbarash RA, Nahlik JE, et al: Famciclovir for the treatment of acute herpes zoster: effects on acute disease and postherpetic neuralgia. A randomized, double-blind, placebo-controlled trial. Collaborative Famciclovir Herpes Zoster Study Group. Ann Intern Med 123(2):89, 1995
110. Degreef H: Famciclovir, a new oral antiherpes drug: results of the first controlled clinical study demonstrating its efficacy and safety in the treatment of uncomplicated herpes zoster in immunocompetent patients. Int J Antimicrob Agents 4:241, 1994
111. DeClerq E, Degreef H, Wildiers J, et al: Oral (E)-5-(2-bromovinyl)-2'-deoxyuridine in severe herpes zoster. Br Med J 282:1178, 1980
112. Maudgal PC, DeClerq E, Missotten L: Efficacy of bromovinyldeoxyuridine in the treatment of herpes simplex virus and varicella zoster virus eye infections. Antiviral Res 4:281, 1984
113. Ameye C, Sundmacher R, DeClerq E: Topical BVDU plus low-dosage steroids in the treatment of chronic relapsing zoster keratouveitis. Graefes Arch Clin Exp Ophthalmol 227:118, 1989
114. Van der Spuy S, Levy D, Levin W: Cimetidine in the treatment of herpes virus infection. S Afr Med J 58:112, 1980
115. Mavligit GM, Talpaz M: Cimetidine for herpes zoster [letter]. N Engl J Med 310:318, 1984
116. Levy DW, Banerjee AK, Glenny HP: Cimetidine in the treatment of herpes zoster. J R Coll Physicians Lond 19:96, 1985
117. Riopelle J, Lopez-Anaya A, Cork RC, et al: Treatment of the cutaneous pain of acute herpes zoster with 9% lidocaine (base) in petrolatum/paraffin ointment. J Am Acad Dermatol 30:757, 1994
118. Watson PN, Evans RJ: Postherpetic neuralgia. Arch Neurol 43:836, 1986
119. Thompson M, Bones M: Nontraditional analgesics for the management of post-herpetic neuralgia. Clin Pharm 4:170, 1985
120. Keczkes K, Basheer AM: Do corticosteroids prevent post-herpetic neuralgia? Br J Dermatol 102:551, 1980
121. Esmann V, Geil JP, Kroon S, et al: Prednisolone does not prevent post-herpetic neuralgia. Lancet 2:126, 1987
122. Bernstein JE, Bickers DR, Dahl MV, Roshal JY: Treatment of chronic post-herpetic neuralgia with topical capsaicin. A preliminary study. J Am Acad Dermatol 17:93, 1987
123. McGill J, Chapman C, Mahakasingam M: Acyclovir therapy in herpes zoster infection—a practical guide. Trans Ophthalmol Soc UK 103:111, 1983
124. McGill J: Topical acyclovir in herpes zoster ocular involvement. Br J Ophthalmol 65:542, 1981
125. McGill J, Chapman C: A comparison of topical acyclovir with steroids in the treatment of herpes zoster keratouveitis. Br J Ophthalmol 67:746, 1983
126. Cobo LM: Corneal complications from herpes zoster ophthalmicus. Cornea 7:50, 1988
127. Gundersen T: Conjunctival flaps in the treatment of corneal disease with reference to a new technique of application. Arch Ophthalmol 60:880, 1958
128. Lugo M, Arentsen JJ: Treatment of neurotrophic ulcers with conjunctival flap. Am J Ophthalmol 103:711, 1987
129. Marsh RJ, Cooper M: Ocular surgery in ophthalmic zoster. Eye 3:313, 1989
130. Soong HK, Schartz AE, Meyer RF, Sugar A: Penetrating keratoplasty for corneal scarring due to herpes zoster ophthalmicus. Br J Ophthalmol 73:19, 1989

12

Epstein-Barr Viral Infections

ALICE Y. MATOBA

Epstein-Barr virus (EBV) is a member of the herpes group of viruses. It was first detected in 1964 in cultured lymphoblasts from Burkitt's lymphoma.[1] The virus has a worldwide distribution, and more than 95 percent of the adult population is seropositive.[2] Epstein-Barr virus is the most common cause of infectious mononucleosis syndrome, which is the clinical manifestation of primary infection with the virus. Epstein-Barr virus has been strongly linked to endemic Burkitt's lymphoma[3] and nasopharyngeal carcinoma[4] and has also been implicated in the pathogenesis of thymic carcinoma,[5] lymphoproliferative disorders in immunocompromised patients,[6] and oral hairy leukoplakia in patients with acquired immunodeficiency syndrome (AIDS).[7] Recently, an association of the virus with rheumatoid arthritis[8] and Sjögren syndrome[9,10] has been suggested.

Epstein-Barr virus predominantly infects oropharyngeal epithelial cells[11] and resting B cells.[12] Epstein-Barr viral DNA has also been detected in periocular tissues, including the lacrimal gland[9] and cornea.[13] Infection with Epstein-Barr virus leads to a life-long carrier state. Infection of oropharyngeal epithelial cells leads to viral replication, with intermittent shedding of live virus throughout life.[14] Infection of B cells leads for the most part to viral latency, but the virus can be reactivated from B cells by certain chemicals or antibodies,[12] and the virus has the capacity to transform these lymphocytes into lymphoblasts that can proliferate indefinitely.[15] Control of Epstein-Barr viral infection depends on T-cell activity.[16,17] Most reported cases of Epstein-Barr virus–related ocular disease are noted in patients with apparently normal systemic immunologic reactions to the virus.

CLINICAL MANIFESTATIONS

Anterior segment disorders associated with Epstein-Barr viral infection include Parinaud oculoglandular syndrome,[18] conjunctival inflammation ranging from hyperemia to follicular conjunctivitis,[19,20] Sjögren syndrome,[9,10] keratitis,[19-24] and uveitis.[24]

Epstein-Barr viral epithelial keratitis may manifest as multifocal microdendrites in association with acute infectious mononucleosis.[22] Multifocal dendritic keratitis has also been reported after a chemical facial peel.[23] In this case, Epstein-Barr viral antigens were detected by monoclonal antibody testing in corneal epithelial specimens obtained by impression cytology. It was hypothesized that the phorbol esters in the chemical used for the facial peel may have been instrumental in activating latent virus.

Epstein-Barr viral stromal keratitis may involve all depths of the stroma. Subepithelial infiltrates that resemble those of adenoviral keratitis have been described in two patients[20,25] (Figure 12-1). Persistent follicular conjunctivitis was associated with one of these cases. The diagnosis was based on serologic tests that documented recent infection with Epstein-Barr virus and ruled out adenoviral infection. Anterior and deep stromal keratitis associated with Epstein-Barr viral infection have been described by several authors.[19,21,24,25] The most distinctive form of stromal keratitis consists of multifocal, discrete, granular, circular or ring-shaped opacities 0.1 to 2 mm in size that are scattered throughout the anterior and mid stroma[25] (Figure 12-2). The overlying epithelium is usually intact, and the intervening stroma is clear.[19] A less distinctive form of stromal keratitis is the dense, peripheral, full-thickness or deep stromal infiltration associated with vary-

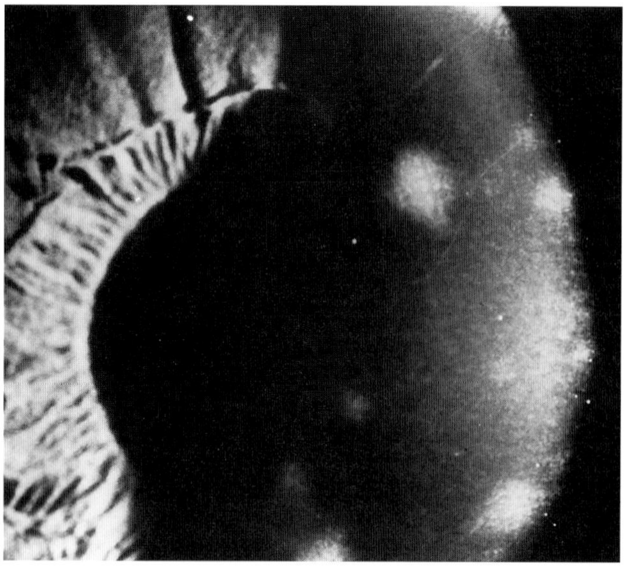

FIGURE 12-1 Subepithelial infiltrates in Epstein-Barr viral keratitis. (Reprinted with permission from AY Matoba: Ocular disease associated with Epstein-Barr virus infection. Surv Ophthalmol 35:145, 1990.)

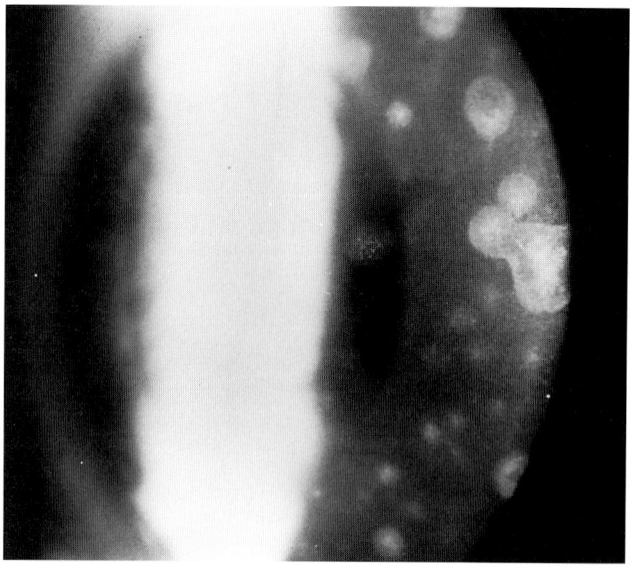

FIGURE 12-2 Multifocal, discrete, granular, anterior and midstromal opacities in Epstein-Barr viral keratitis. (Reprinted with permission from AY Matoba: Ocular disease associated with Epstein-Barr virus infection. Surv Ophthalmol 35:145, 1990.)

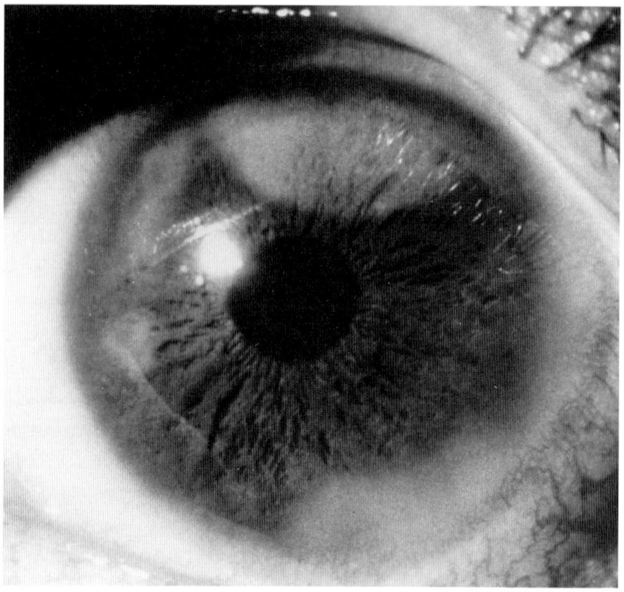

FIGURE 12-3 Multifocal peripheral mid- and deep stromal infiltrates in Epstein-Barr viral keratitis. (Reprinted with permission from AY Matoba, KR Wilhelmus, DB Jones: Epstein-Barr viral stromal keratitis. Ophthalmology 93:746, 1986. Courtesy of Ophthalmology.)

ing degrees of vascularization (Figure 12-3). This form of keratitis is usually associated with significant conjunctival and episcleral inflammation. Peripheral stromal edema overlying confluent, geographic patches of white endothelial precipitates has also been described.[24] In all reported cases of stromal keratitis associated with Epstein-Barr virus, the diagnosis was based on a serologic profile consistent with systemic Epstein-Barr viral infection and negative serologic tests for other potential etiologic agents, or a serologic profile and systemic symptoms compatible with recent primary Epstein-Barr viral infection. Although Epstein-Barr virus has been cultured from the conjunctiva and tears in a case of epithelial keratitis,[22] it has not been cultured from stromal lesions, nor have viral antigens been detected in corneal stromal tissue.

DIAGNOSIS

The clinical diagnosis of primary Epstein-Barr viral infection (infectious mononucleosis) depends on identification of the classic triad of fever, sore throat, and lymphadenopathy. Enlargement of the liver and spleen is also frequently noted. In some patients, however, primary infection with Epstein-Barr virus may be subclinical.

The laboratory diagnosis of systemic Epstein-Barr viral infection is based on hematologic and serologic tests.

Hematologic abnormalities include a relative and absolute lymphocytosis in 70 percent of patients, a mild relative and absolute neutropenia in 60 to 90 percent of patients, and mild thrombocytopenia in 50 percent of patients.[26] Usually 30 percent of lymphocytes are atypical.[26] The serologic profile of acute primary Epstein-Barr viral infection includes an early rise in the titer of antibodies (both IgM and IgG) against viral capsid antigen (VCA), followed within several weeks by a rise in the titer of antibodies against early antigen (EA)[2,26] (Table 12-1). Antibodies against nuclear antigen (EBNA or NA) become detectable several weeks to months after the acute infection.[2,26] IgG, but not IgM, antibodies against viral capsid antigen and antibodies against nuclear antigen persist for life, but in patients with appropriate immunologic control of viral replication, antibodies against early antigen usually become undetectable within 6 to 9 months.[2] In a small percentage of healthy individuals, a significant titer of antibodies against early antigen may persist.[27,28]

Epstein-Barr viral keratitis is uncommon, and the diagnosis usually depends on clinical and/or serologic evidence of systemic infection with the virus. Epithelial dendrites can be caused by herpes simplex virus, varicella-zoster virus, and Epstein-Barr virus. Epstein-Barr viral dendrites are rare and have occurred only in association with acute infectious mononucleosis or after a chemical facial peel. Subepithelial infiltrates caused by Epstein-Barr virus closely mimic those caused by adenovirus but have an atypical and prolonged course and are more resistant to treatment with topical corticosteroids. The granular, circular or ring-shaped anterior and midstromal opacities are almost pathognomonic of Epstein-Barr viral infection.

TABLE 12-1
EBV-Specific Antibodies: Laboratory Diagnosis

	Mean Titer	
Antibody	*Acute Infection*	*Long Past Primary Infection*
Viral capsid antigen (VCA)		
IgM	160	Undetectable
IgG	>160	>40
Nuclear antigen (EBNA or NA)	<1:2[a]	>40
Early antigen (EA)		
Diffuse (EA-D)	>40[b]	<10
Restricted (EA-R)	<10	<10

[a] Rises weeks to several months after acute infection.
[b] Observed in 80% of patients.
Source: Reprinted with permission from AY Matoba: Ocular disease associated with Epstein-Barr virus infection. Surv Ophthalmol 35:145, 1990.

Deep stromal keratitis caused by Epstein-Barr virus is not sufficiently distinctive to be diagnosed on the basis of clinical examination. Herpes simplex virus and syphilis are much more common causes of deep stromal keratitis than is Epstein-Barr virus.

TREATMENT

There are no strict guidelines for the treatment of keratitis associated with Epstein-Barr virus because it is uncommon and only a few cases have been described in the literature. Epstein-Barr virus is resistant to available ocular antiviral medications, although several antiviral agents, including acyclovir, ganciclovir, foscarnet, zidovudine, and bromovinyldeoxyuridine, effectively inhibit viral replication or B-cell transformation in vitro.[12] Epithelial keratitis may be treated with oral acyclovir, but the natural history of epithelial keratitis associated with infectious mononucleosis is unknown. The pauci-inflammatory, granular, multifocal stromal keratitis generally requires no specific therapy. However, the peripheral deep stromal infiltrative keratitis is usually associated with significant inflammation. This form of keratitis responds well to topical corticosteroids; in rare instances, recurrent or chronic inflammation may occur. Concomitant antiviral therapy is not necessary if herpes simplex viral infection has been excluded as the cause of the keratitis.

REFERENCES

1. Epstein MA, Achong BG, Barr YM: Virus particle in cultured lymphoblasts from Burkitt's lymphoma. Lancet 1:702, 1964
2. Ooka T, de Turenne-Tessier M, Stolzenburg MC: Relationship between antibody production to Epstein-Barr Virus (EBV) early antigens and various EBV-related disorders. Springer Semin Immunopathol 13:233, 1991
3. Lenoir GM: Role of the virus, chromosomal translocations and cellular oncogenes in the etiology of Burkitt's lymphoma. p. 184. In Epstein MA, Achong BG (eds): The Epstein-Barr Virus: Recent Advances. John Wiley & Sons, New York, 1986
4. Klein G: The relationship of the virus to nasopharyngeal carcinoma. p. 340. In Epstein MA, Achong BG (eds): The Epstein-Barr Virus. Springer, New York, 1979
5. Leyvraz S, Henle W, Chahinian AP, et al: Association of Epstein-Barr virus with thymic carcinoma. N Engl J Med 312:1296, 1985
6. Saemundsen AK, Purtilo DT, Sakamoto K, et al: Documentation of Epstein-Barr virus infection in immunodeficient patients with life-threatening lymphoproliferative diseases by Epstein-Barr virus complementary RNA/DNA

and viral DNA/RNA hybridization. Cancer Res 41:4237, 1981
7. Greenspan JS, Greenspan D, Lennette ET: Replication of Epstein-Barr virus within the epithelial cells of oral hairy leukoplakia, an AIDS-associated lesion. N Engl J Med 985:1564, 1985
8. Alspaugh MA, Jensen PC, Rabio H, et al: Lymphocytes transformed by Epstein-Barr virus: induction of nuclear antigen reactive with antibody in rheumatoid arthritis. J Exp Med 147:1018, 1987
9. Pflugfelder SC, Crouse C, Pereira I, Atherton S: Amplification of Epstein-Barr virus genomic sequences in blood cells, lacrimal glands, and tears from primary Sjögren's syndrome patients. Ophthalmology 97:976, 1990
10. Pflugfelder SC, Tseng SCG, Pepose JS, et al: Epstein-Barr virus infection and immunologic dysfunction in patients with aqueous tear deficiency. Ophthalmology 97:313, 1990
11. Sixby JM, Nedrud JG, Raab-Traub N, et al: Epstein-Barr virus replication in oropharyngeal epithelial cells. N Engl J Med 310:1225, 1984
12. Strauss SE, Cohen JI, Tosato G, et al: Epstein-Barr virus: biology, pathogenesis, and management. Ann Intern Med 118:45, 1993
13. Crouse CA, Pflugfelder SC, Pereira I, et al: Detection of herpes viral genomes in normal and diseased corneal epithelium. Curr Eye Res 9:569, 1990
14. Gerber P, Nonoyama M, Lucas S, et al: Oral secretion of Epstein-Barr virus by healthy subjects and patients with infectious mononucleosis. Lancet 11:988, 1972
15. Nilsson K, Klein G, Henle W, Henle G: The establishment of lymphoblastoid cell lines from adult and from foetal human lymphoid tissue and its dependence on EBV. Int J Cancer 8:443, 1971
16. Tosato G: The Epstein-Barr virus and the immune system. p. 49. In Klein G, Weinhouse S (eds): Advances in Cancer Research. Academic Press, San Diego, 1987
17. Rickinson AB: Cellular immunological responses to the virus infection. p. 75. In Epstein MA, Achong BG (eds): The Epstein-Barr Virus: Recent Advances. Wiley Medical Publications, New York, 1990
18. Meisler DM, Bosworth DE, Krachmer JH: Ocular infectious mononucleosis manifested as Parinaud's oculoglandular syndrome. Am J Ophthalmol 92:722, 1981
19. Matoba AY, Wilhelmus KR, Jones DB: Epstein-Barr viral stromal keratitis. Ophthalmology 93:746, 1986
20. Matoba AY, Jones DB: Corneal subepithelial infiltrates associated with systemic Epstein-Barr viral infection. Ophthalmology 94:1669, 1987
21. Pinnolis M, McCulley JP, Urman JD: Nummular keratitis associated with infectious mononucleosis. Am J Ophthalmol 89:791, 1980
22. Wilhelmus KR: Ocular involvement in infectious mononucleosis. Am J Ophthalmol 91:117, 1981
23. Pflugfelder SC, Huang A, Crouse C: Epstein-Barr virus keratitis after a chemical facial peel. Am J Ophthalmol 110:571, 1990
24. Wong KW, D'Amico DJ, Hedges TR, et al: Ocular involvement associated with chronic Epstein-Barr virus disease. Arch Ophthalmol 105:788, 1987
25. Matoba AY: Ocular disease associated with Epstein-Barr virus infection. Surv Ophthalmol 35:145, 1990
26. Benson CA, Kessler HA: Update: Epstein-Barr virus-related disease. Compr Ther 14(3):58, 1988
27. Henle W, Henle G, Zajac BA, et al: Differential reactivity of human serums with early antigens induced by Epstein-Barr virus. Science 169:188, 1970
28. Horwitz CA, Henle W, Henle G, et al: Long-term serological follow-up of patients for Epstein-Barr virus after recovery from infectious mononucleosis. J Infect Dis 151:1150, 1985

13

Nonherpetic Viral Infections

H. Bruce Ostler and John R. Bierly

Several nonherpetic viruses cause external ocular infections (Table 13-1). These infections are covered in this chapter; infections caused by herpesviruses are covered in Chapters 10, 11, and 12.

ADENOVIRAL INFECTIONS

Adenoviruses are small, nonenveloped, double-stranded DNA viruses 70 to 90 nm in diameter. They are stable in the environment and are resistant to lipid solvents, which permits their transmission through fomites, unwashed hands, and swimming pools. Six subgenera (A through F) and at least 47 serotypes of adenoviruses have been identified.[1]

Adenoviral infections appear to be unique to humans and cause several clinical syndromes. In the eye, these syndromes include an acute follicular conjunctivitis, epidemic keratoconjunctivitis, pharyngoconjunctival fever, and rarely, chronic keratoconjunctivitis.

Epidemic Keratoconjunctivitis

Epidemic keratoconjunctivitis (EKC) is caused most commonly by adenovirus types 8 and 19, and less commonly by types 2, 3, 4, 5, 7, 9, 10, 11, 14, 16, 21, 29, and 37. The disease is highly contagious and occurs worldwide. Epidemics are common; however, sporadic cases do occur. Subclinical infections are also possible.

Iatrogenic epidemics can be caused by hands, instruments (especially applanation tonometers), and solutions contaminated with the virus.[2–5] Therefore, handwashing and proper disinfection of instruments after contact with any patient suspected of having adenoviral infection are mandatory. Adenovirus can survive on a variety of surfaces in optometrists' and ophthalmologists' offices and can remain potentially infectious for up to 35 days.[6] This survivability permits transmission of the virus through fomites in waiting areas. Adenovirus type 19 has been isolated from the genital tract, which suggests that the virus can be transmitted sexually as well.[7] Patients with epidemic keratoconjunctivitis remain infectious for 14 days from the onset of symptoms.[8]

Clinical Features

The interval from exposure to adenovirus to onset of symptoms ranges from 5 to 12 days. Systemic symptoms of fever, sore throat, and gastrointestinal disturbances are unusual in adults with epidemic keratoconjunctivitis but may be seen in children. Ocular symptoms may be mild or severe and include foreign body sensation, tearing, and photophobia. Ocular involvement is usually bilateral but can be unilateral in as many as 25 percent of cases. Often, symptoms develop in one eye and the infection then spreads to the other eye. Manifestations of the infection in the second eye may take several days to evolve and are frequently less severe.

The onset of epidemic keratoconjunctivitis is usually acute, with follicular conjunctivitis and commonly a tender, enlarged preauricular lymph node. Eyelid edema, blepharoptosis,[9] and occasionally, ecchymosis may occur. During the first 2 days, the conjunctiva becomes hyperemic, chemotic, and infiltrated (Figure 13-1). Petechiae and subconjunctival hemorrhage may also occur. Usually, there is a watery to fibrinous discharge. By the third day, follicles develop in the fornix and on the tarsal conjunctiva (Figure 13-2). The follicles may persist for 2 to 3 weeks. Pseudomembrane formation can occur and can lead to scarring and symblepharon formation.[10]

TABLE 13-1
Nonherpetic Viruses That Cause External Ocular Infections

	Family	*Virus*
DNA Viruses		
	Adenoviridae	Adenoviruses
	Poxviridae	Variola virus
		Vaccinia virus
		Molluscum contagiosum virus
	Papovaviridae	Papillomaviruses
RNA Viruses		
	Picornaviridae	Enteroviruses
		Coxsackieviruses
	Paramyxoviridae	Measles virus
		Mumps virus
		Newcastle disease virus
	Togaviridae	Rubella virus

Punctate epithelial keratitis develops diffusely over the central cornea between days 7 and 14 and is caused by direct infection and multiplication of adenovirus in corneal epithelial cells. The keratitis evolves over the next 7 to 10 days into a combined epithelial and subepithelial keratitis, then later into discrete, round subepithelial infiltrates (Figure 13-3). The subepithelial infiltrates consist of mononuclear cells, a few polymorphonuclear leukocytes, and degenerated epithelium and stroma. The infiltrates probably represent a delayed hypersensitivity reaction to viral antigen. Rarely, marked stromal edema accompanied by keratic precipitates occurs.

Photophobia is often intense at the peak of the epithelial keratitis. Visual acuity is frequently reduced during the acute infection, and vision may be impaired for weeks to months because of persistent subepithelial infiltrates. Visual debility may be exacerbated by recurrent breakdown of corneal epithelium over the infiltrates.

Occasionally, a mild nongranulomatous iritis can occur in association with the keratitis.[11] Uncommon associated

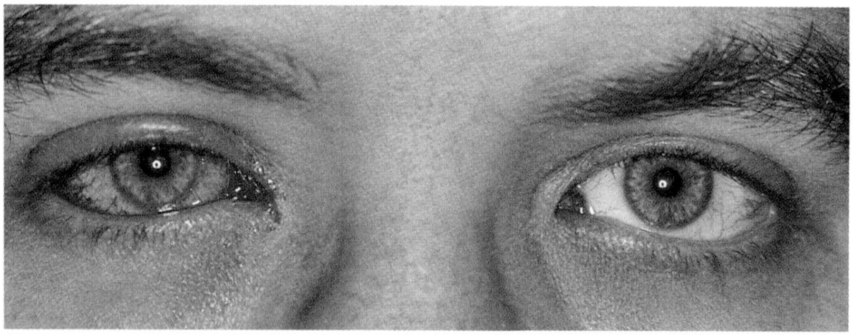

FIGURE 13-1 Epidemic keratoconjunctivitis. The eyelids are swollen, the conjunctiva is hyperemic, and there is profuse tearing. (Courtesy of Steven A. Dingeldein, M.D., Burlington, NC.)

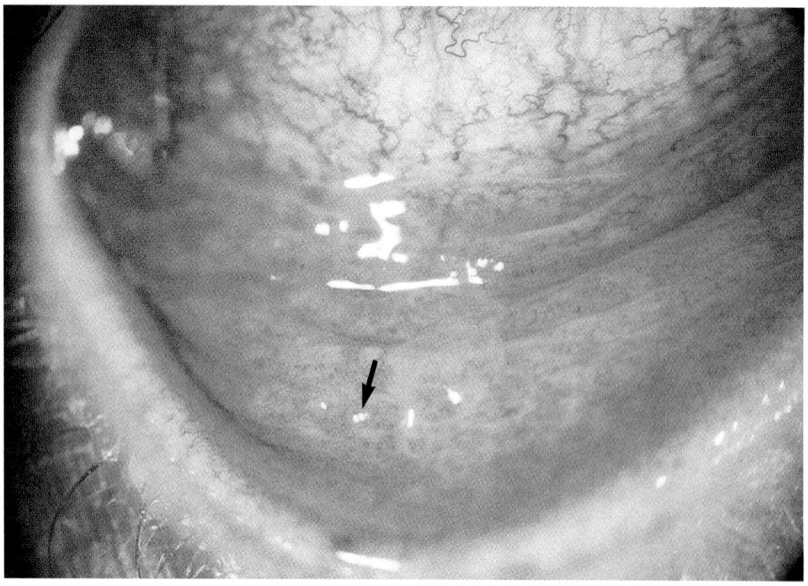

FIGURE 13-2 Conjunctival follicles (arrow) in epidemic keratoconjunctivitis. (Courtesy of Steven A. Dingeldein, M.D., Burlington, N.C.)

findings include a diffuse anterior scleritis and an acute optic neuritis.[12]

Epidemic keratoconjunctivitis may be confused with Thygeson's superficial punctate keratitis.[13] However, several features distinguish Thygeson's superficial punctate keratitis: conjunctivitis is absent; subepithelial infiltrates are small and uncommon; and the disorder is either chronic or recurrent, in contrast to the acute nature of epidemic keratoconjunctivitis. Also, the eye is relatively quiet and symptoms are minimal. Coarse, punctate, gray epithelial opacities are slightly raised above the corneal surface (Figure 13-4). These opacities may occur anywhere in the cornea but are more common centrally. The disorder is usually bilateral, although one eye may be affected and then clear before the other eye is affected. Thygeson's superficial punctate keratitis improves rapidly with low-dose topical corticosteroids but recurs when corticosteroids are discontinued. It typically lasts many months or even years. Removal of the corneal epithelium is not helpful.

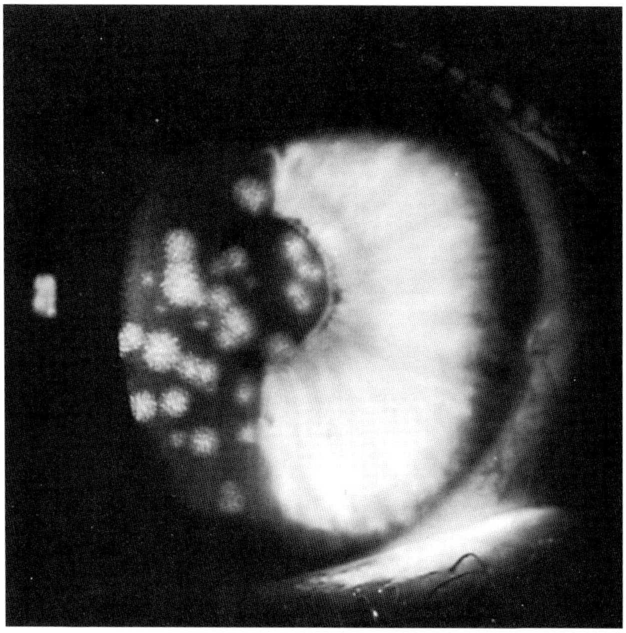

FIGURE 13-3 Subepithelial infiltrates in epidemic keratoconjunctivitis.

Diagnosis

A definitive diagnosis of epidemic keratoconjunctivitis can be made by isolation of adenovirus from the conjunctiva. The virus can be cultured in primary human embryonic kidney cells, continuous human cell lines, such as HeLa or Hep-2, or diploid cell cultures. Viral isolation is most likely during the first week of infection; it is unreliable after the second week.

Conjunctival scrapings reveal predominantly lymphocytes with a few polymorphonuclear leukocytes. If there is pseudomembrane formation, polymorphonuclear leukocytes predominate. Direct and indirect immunofluorescence staining of conjunctival scrapings have been used to diagnose epidemic keratoconjunctivitis, but a fluorescence microscope is required. A direct enzyme immunoassay test for the detection of adenoviral antigen in conjunctival swabs is available (Adenoclone). When com-

FIGURE 13-4 Superficial punctate keratitis of Thygeson. Several lesions are demonstrated by the slit beam and by retroillumination. The reflexes to the left of the slit beam are artifacts.

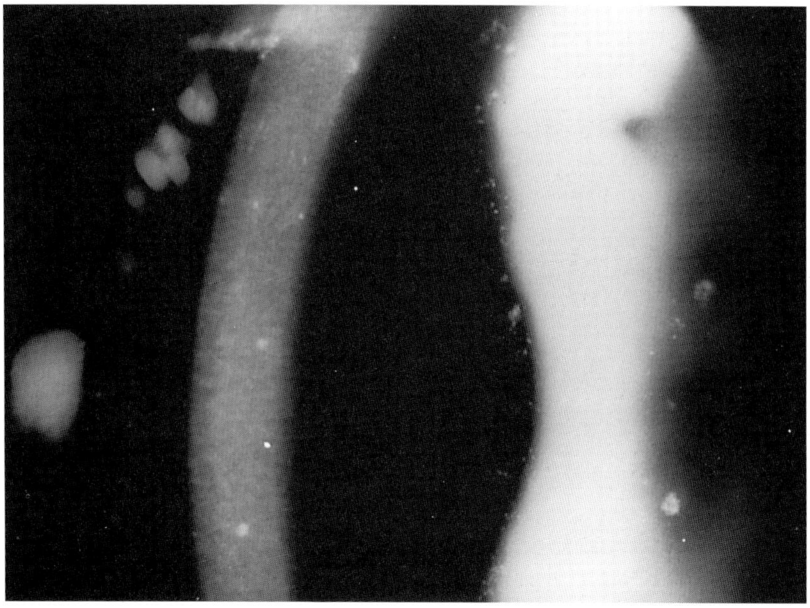

pared with conventional cultures, this test is 100 percent specific and 77 to 81 percent sensitive in patients tested within 1 week of onset of symptoms.[14,15]

Serology has also been used to diagnose adenoviral ocular infections. Paired blood samples drawn several weeks apart may establish the diagnosis by revealing a fourfold or greater increase in serum antibody titers to adenovirus.[16]

Treatment

In general, acute epidemic keratoconjunctivitis is a self-limited infection. Supportive therapy, such as cold compresses, artificial tears, topical vasoconstrictors, and systemic analgesics, is often helpful. In cases of symblepharon formation, the inferior fornix can be swept with a blunt instrument or the tip of an ointment tube on a daily basis. Low-dose topical corticosteroids may help when corneal subepithelial infiltrates are in the visual axis and are causing decreased visual acuity. Before corticosteroids are instituted, herpes simplex virus must be excluded as the cause of the keratoconjunctivitis. The subepithelial infiltrates may reappear when the corticosteroids are tapered. Corticosteroids may limit the lymphocytic response to viral antigen in the superficial stroma, but they do not remove the antigen. With or without corticosteroids, the infiltrates may last for several years.

Pharyngoconjunctival Fever

Pharyngoconjunctival fever is usually caused by adenovirus types 3, 4, and 7 and rarely by types 1, 5, and 14. It often occurs in small epidemics, especially in children and young adults; however, sporadic cases can occur. Unlike epidemic keratoconjunctivitis, pharyngoconjunctival fever is transmitted by aerosolized droplets and occasionally in swimming pools.[17] The incubation period ranges from 2 to 14 days. After the onset of symptoms, the patient remains infectious for 7 to 10 days.

Pharyngoconjunctival fever typically consists of an acute follicular conjunctivitis with an associated pharyngitis. The pharyngitis may be accompanied by tender cervical lymph nodes. Headache, malaise, myalgia, abdominal discomfort, diarrhea, and low-grade fever can occur. The pharyngitis and fever are typically short lived and resolve before the conjunctivitis disappears.

The conjunctivitis begins acutely and is associated with irritation, foreign body sensation, tearing, and watery discharge. A small- to medium-size preauricular lymph node is common. The eyelids are erythematous and often edematous. Typically, conjunctival hyperemia and chemosis precede the development of follicles. The inferior forniceal and tarsal conjunctiva are involved more than the superior forniceal and tarsal conjunctiva. The conjunctivitis lasts 7 to 10 days. In general, patients with pharyngoconjunctival fever do not develop the severe keratitis seen in epidemic keratoconjunctivitis. However, a diffuse epithelial keratitis may occur 3 to 5 days after the onset of the conjunctivitis and may occasionally lead to subepithelial infiltrates.

Diagnosis can be established by culture or by demonstration of a rise in serum antibody titers. Conjunctival scrapings reveal a predominantly lymphocytic response.

Pharyngoconjunctival fever is self limited and therapy should be directed to relief of symptoms.

Chronic Adenoviral Conjunctivitis

Chronic infections of the eye with adenovirus are rare.[18-20] The patient develops an acute follicular conjunctivitis that is followed by intermittent and prolonged symptoms of photophobia, tearing, and conjunctival hyperemia. The chronic conjunctivitis is papillary in type and may be associated with focal superficial keratitis. Subepithelial infiltrates may occur. Adenoviruses thought to be associated with the chronic form of infection include type 2 (chronic keratitis) and types 3, 4, 5, and 19 (chronic keratoconjunctivitis).

The diagnosis can be established by isolating adenovirus from the conjunctiva and cornea, demonstrating serotype-specific serum antibodies to the adenovirus recovered, and excluding other causes of chronic papillary conjunctivitis.

ACUTE HEMORRHAGIC CONJUNCTIVITIS

Acute hemorrhagic conjunctivitis is caused by coxsackievirus type A-24 and enterovirus type 70. Both are members of the picornavirus family and are single-stranded, nonenveloped RNA viruses with an icosahedral (20-sided) structure. Two pandemics have occurred since the infection was first described in 1969.[21] Smaller epidemics and sporadic cases have also been observed.[22] The relatively few cases that have occurred in the United States have been located in Florida and Minnesota.[23,24] Transmission is usually from person to person by hand-to-eye contact or through fomites. The incubation period varies from 12 to 48 hours. Hand washing, sterilization of instruments, and patient quarantine may prevent the spread of the virus.

Ocular irritation, foreign body sensation, periocular pain, photophobia, tearing, and a mucoid discharge develop acutely. Headache, malaise, myalgia, and sore

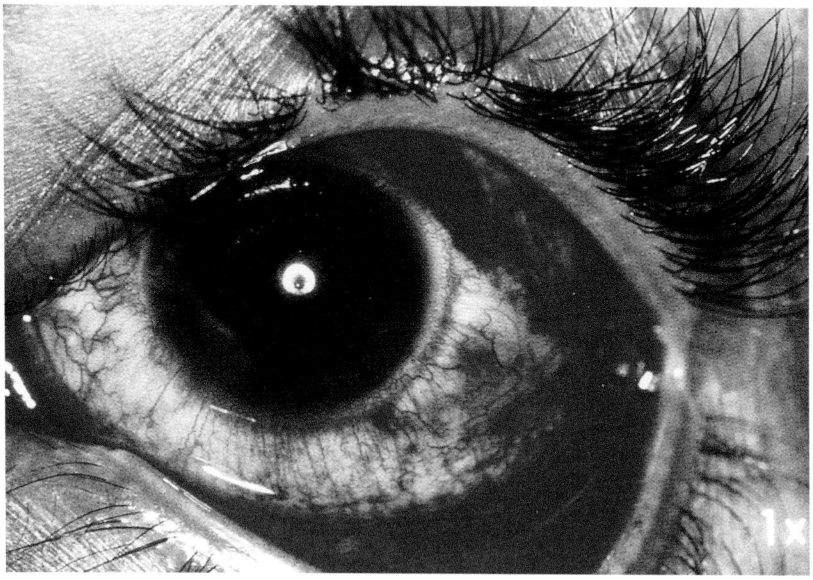

FIGURE 13-5 Conjunctival hemorrhage in acute hemorrhagic conjunctivitis.

throat often develop during the course of infection and subside by the third or fourth day.

The conjunctivitis is an acute follicular type, with chemosis and subconjunctival hemorrhage (Figure 13-5). The hemorrhage affects both the bulbar and tarsal conjunctiva and is more prominent superiorly. The conjunctivitis usually begins in one eye but quickly becomes bilateral. It persists for 3 to 5 days. Eyelid edema and tender preauricular lymphadenopathy are common. Transient, diffuse, superficial punctate keratitis usually becomes apparent at the height of the disease and persists for 1 to 2 weeks. It may be accompanied by mild iritis. Flaccid radiculomyelitis and transient facial nerve palsy may occur.[25] Uncommon complications include gonococcal ocular infection when urine is used as a folk-remedy eyewash.[26]

The diagnosis of hemorrhagic conjunctivitis can be confirmed by viral cultures, which reveal either enterovirus type 70 or an antigenic variant of coxsackievirus type A-24. The virus can be isolated from the conjunctiva, throat, or stool. Serologic diagnosis depends on the demonstration of virus-specific antibodies. Conjunctival scrapings reveal a predominantly lymphocytic reaction.

Therapy is directed toward the relief of symptoms with cold compresses, topical vasoconstrictors, and systemic analgesics. In general, the infection is self limited, with complete recovery occurring within 4 to 12 days.[27] There is evidence that topical interferon-α eye drops can prevent and halt the spread of infection in contacts, but they are not beneficial in an established infection and do not prevent infection in the second clinically uninvolved eye.[28]

MEASLES, MUMPS, AND NEWCASTLE DISEASE

Measles, mumps, and Newcastle disease are all caused by members of the paramyxovirus family. They are roughly spherical single-stranded RNA viruses with a lipid envelope.

Measles (Rubeola)

Measles (rubeola) is a highly infectious disease that occurs worldwide. More than 90 percent of susceptible contacts develop the disease when exposed to the virus. Measles can be devastating in crowded living conditions, where the disease occurs in young infants and has a high mortality rate. Measles vaccine has markedly decreased the incidence of the disease in industrialized countries. Humans are the major reservoir of measles virus. Infection occurs through aerosolized droplets that reach the conjunctiva or mucous membrane of the upper respiratory tract.[29] The patient is infectious from several days before to 5 days after the skin rash appears.

The manifestations of measles become evident 9 to 11 days after exposure to the virus and consist of malaise, fever, cough, coryza, periorbital edema, conjunctivitis, and photophobia. Koplik spots may appear at this time and are considered pathognomonic of the disease. These spots are small bluish-white dots with an erythematous base and are found on the buccal mucosa opposite the lower molars. Similar lesions may also be found on the conjunctiva or caruncle. Within the next

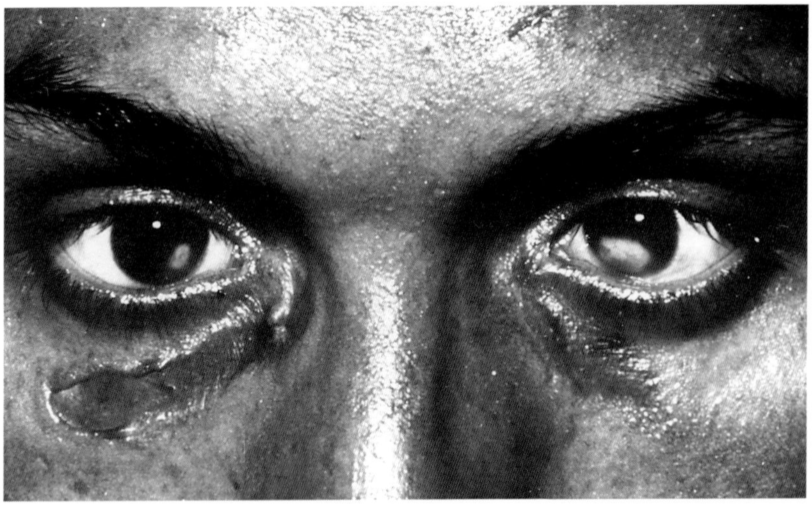

FIGURE 13-6 Bilateral corneal scars caused by measles.

few days, a rash appears, usually on the forehead, then gradually spreads downward to involve the face, trunk, and extremities.

An acute catarrhal conjunctivitis with associated eyelid edema is often seen before the rash and may persist for the duration of the illness. Epithelial keratitis is most prominent with the appearance of the rash and consists of superficial, fine, gray or white dots grouped into larger lesions.[30] The keratitis usually clears spontaneously and leaves no permanent loss of vision. However, the keratitis can be severe, especially in protein malnourished and vitamin A–deficient patients, in whom keratomalacia, perforation, and blindness can occur (Figure 13-6). The exact role of the measles infection in the pathogenesis of postmeasles blindness is unclear.[31,32]

Diagnosis of measles is confirmed by recovery of measles virus from mucous membranes or blood or by demonstration of a serum antibody response.

In general, the prognosis is good except in immunocompromised patients. Uncommon complications, such as interstitial giant cell pneumonia, encephalitis, and subacute sclerosing panencephalitis, can occur. Vaccination with live attenuated measles virus provides adequate protection against the infection.

Mumps

Mumps is an acute generalized infection that typically affects children and young adults. Transmission occurs by infected droplets, saliva, contaminated fomites, and direct contact. The incubation period is 14 to 25 days after exposure. Patients are probably contagious from at least 7 days before to 9 days after the onset of symptoms.

Prodromal symptoms include myalgia, anorexia, malaise, headache, and fever. The major clinical manifestation is parotitis, which classically appears in one parotid gland 1 to 2 days after the onset of symptoms and, in most cases, involves the other parotid gland within a few days. The swelling increases over several days and then gradually subsides over 1 to 2 weeks.

A bilateral dacryoadenitis frequently accompanies the parotitis and usually resolves within 1 week. An acute catarrhal conjunctivitis is common.[33] Diffuse episcleritis or scleritis and, rarely, sclerokeratitis can occur. Acute unilateral interstitial keratitis occasionally occurs approximately 5 days after the onset of the parotitis.[34,35] Photophobia and tearing are common, and there may be an associated iritis. The interstitial keratitis is avascular, with prominent stromal infiltrates and edema. Folds in Descemet's membrane are evident, as is microcystic epithelial edema, but the intraocular pressure is normal. The keratitis resolves spontaneously in 2 to 3 weeks but may leave nebulous opacities that can interfere with vision.

The diagnosis of mumps is made by the constellation of clinical findings and is confirmed by isolation of the virus or by demonstration of a serum antibody response.

Therapy includes cold compresses for the conjunctivitis and cycloplegics for the keratitis and iritis. Topical corticosteroids may shorten the duration of the keratitis, scleritis, and iritis. Live attenuated mumps vaccine is effective in preventing infections.

Newcastle Disease

Newcastle disease virus primarily affects fowl, such as chickens and turkeys; humans are infected secondarily.

Poultry handlers, laboratory technicians, and veterinarians are, therefore, at highest risk of acquiring the disease. The usual portal of entry is the conjunctiva, and the incubation period is 18 to 48 hours.

Systemic symptoms are uncommon but can develop within hours of exposure. They include headache, malaise, a mild fever, and arthralgia.[36] The virus usually causes an acute unilateral follicular conjunctivitis. The follicles are more prominent in the inferior fornix and persist for 7 to 10 days. Irritation, burning, pain, and blurred vision are common, as are preauricular lymphadenopathy and eyelid edema. Superficial punctate keratitis is also common; rarely, round subepithelial infiltrates are found.[37]

Conjunctival scrapings show a predominantly lymphocytic response. The diagnosis can be confirmed by recovery of the virus from the hen's eggs or by demonstration of a serum antibody response in the patient.

Therapy is supportive and the disease is self limited without sequelae. Immunity is short lived and reinfection is possible in the same individual.

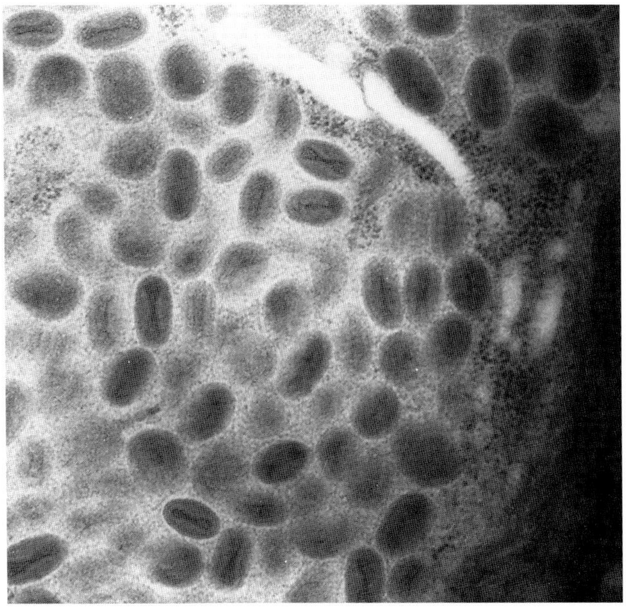

FIGURE 13-7 Molluscum contagiosum virus.

RUBELLA (GERMAN MEASLES)

Rubella (German measles) is caused by a single-stranded RNA virus that is a member of the togavirus family. Children and young adults are most frequently affected. Typically, the virus causes a self-limited, acute viral syndrome characterized by malaise, fever, headache, and sometimes polyarthritis. Lymphadenopathy and skin rash are common; rarely, meningoencephalitis or thrombocytopenia may occur.

A mild acute follicular conjunctivitis may occur, usually appearing 2 to 3 days before the rash and lasting only a few days. Superficial punctate keratitis can occur with the conjunctivitis.

Congenital rubella is the result of maternal infection with the virus, especially in the first trimester of pregnancy. Affected offspring demonstrate a variety of birth defects; the classic triad consists of congenital heart defects, deafness, and cataracts.[38] Microphthalmos, anterior chamber angle abnormalities and glaucoma, and a pigmentary retinopathy are observed. The cornea is often edematous and cloudy centrally at birth, which is caused either by an absence of or ruptures in Descemet's membrane or by congenital glaucoma. The cornea may gradually clear with time.

A suspected diagnosis of rubella is based on the constellation of clinical findings. In pregnant women, viral isolation or serologic study should be undertaken. Live attenuated virus is effective in preventing the disease but should not be given to pregnant women.

VARIOLA AND VACCINIA

Variola virus (smallpox virus) and vaccinia virus (the vaccine strain) are members of the poxviruses, which are large double-stranded DNA viruses and are among the largest viruses known. With the probable eradication of smallpox by the World Health Organization in 1977, ocular infections with variola virus have virtually disappeared. Routine vaccination is no longer considered necessary in much of the world. Ocular infections with vaccinia virus are attributed to autoinoculation after vaccination and are, therefore, rare.

Vaccinia virus can cause typical "kissing lesions" of the eyelids. Viral conjunctivitis caused by variola or vaccinia virus is similar to that caused by herpes simplex virus. Punctate epithelial keratitis, ulcerative keratitis, disciform edema, and necrotizing pustular keratitis can occur with either virus. The keratitis can be treated with topical trifluridine.

MOLLUSCUM CONTAGIOSUM

Molluscum contagiosum is caused by a member of the poxvirus family (Figure 13-7). The virus causes an epidermal infection manifested by the appearance of round, waxy, pearly white, umbilicated lesions 2 to 5 mm in diameter (Figure 13-8). The lesions can occur anywhere on the skin except the palms and soles. The infection is autoinoc-

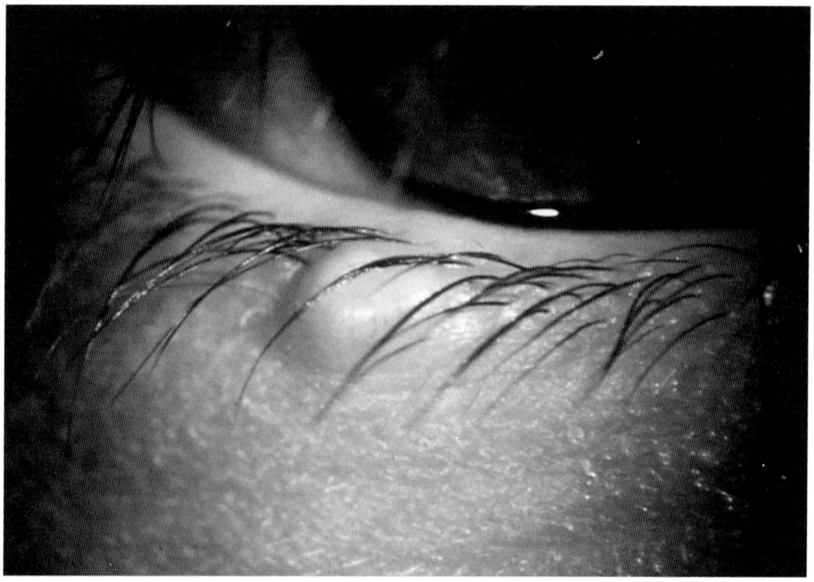

FIGURE 13-8 Umbilicated eyelid lesion of molluscum contagiosum.

ulable, is often transmitted by direct contact, and is occasionally transmitted sexually. The incubation time varies from days to several months.

Skin lesions are common on the face and eyelids. Primary involvement of the conjunctiva or cornea by molluscum lesions is rare.[39] Eyelid lesions can cause a chronic follicular conjunctivitis (Figure 13-9). Superficial keratitis can occur and can cause photophobia and blurred vision. The keratitis is composed of fine grouped epithelial erosions and intraepithelial and subepithelial infiltrates that stain slightly with fluorescein.[40] The keratitis frequently involves the entire cornea but is more pronounced superiorly and may evolve into a superficial pannus that mimics trachoma.[41]

Typically, molluscum contagiosum is a self-limited disease but may persist for up to 4 years. The course of the disease can be particularly aggressive in immunocompromised patients[42,43] (Figure 13-10). Removal or expression of the lesion, electrocautery, cryotherapy, or incision of the lesion so that blood permeates it are all satisfactory forms of therapy in nonimmunocompromised patients. Pathologic examination of excised lesions reveals acanthotic epithelium surrounding lobules of keratinized debris and epithelial cells that contain intracy-

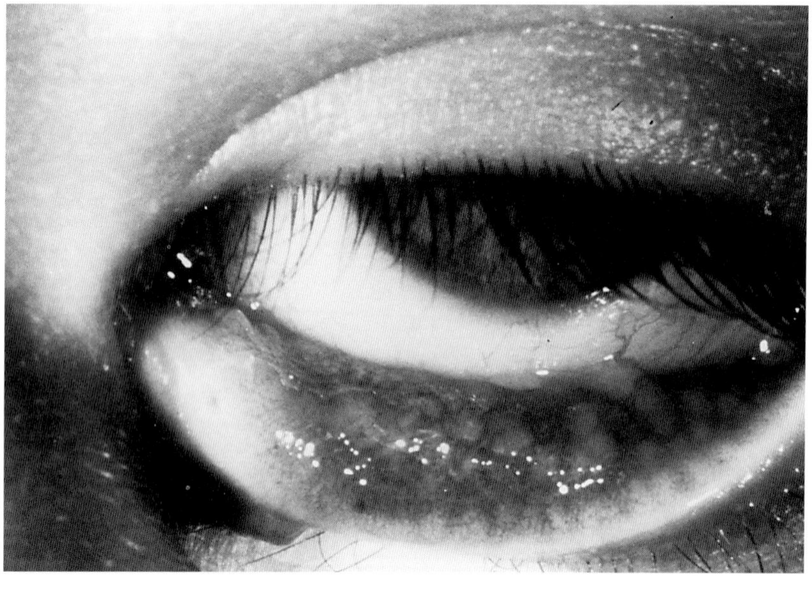

FIGURE 13-9 Chronic follicular conjunctivitis associated with molluscum contagiosum.

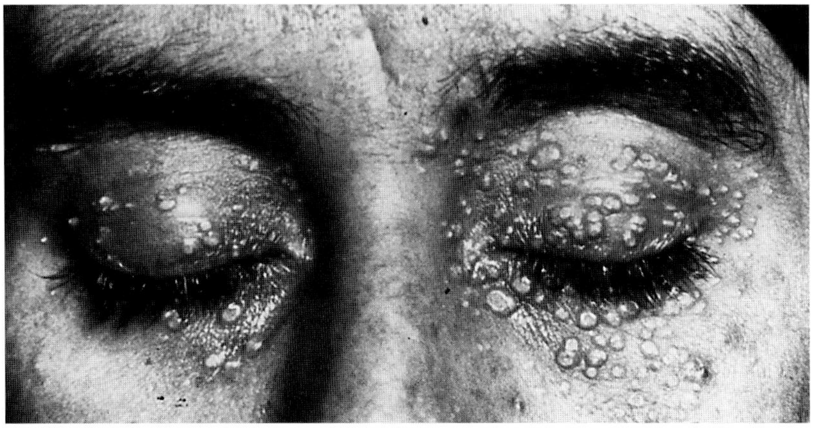

FIGURE 13-10 Multiple lesions of molluscum contagiosum in a patient with acquired immunodeficiency syndrome. (Reprinted with permission from SR Kohn: Molluscum contagiosum in patients with acquired immune deficiency syndrome. Arch Ophthalmol 105:458, 1987. Copyright 1987, American Medical Association.)

toplasmic inclusions known as molluscum bodies (Figure 13-11).

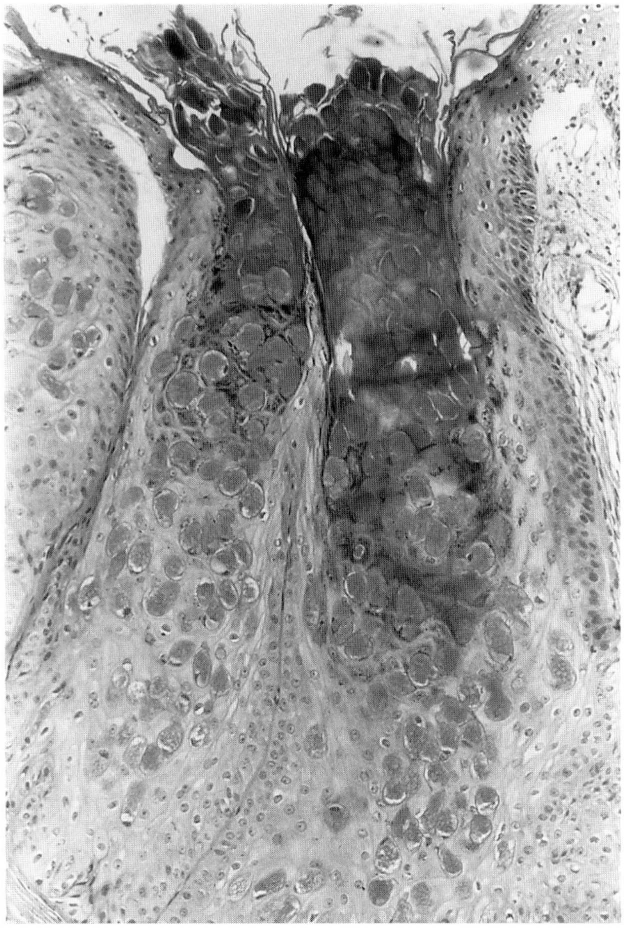

FIGURE 13-11 Pathognomonic histopathologic appearance of molluscum contagiosum, demonstrating many molluscum bodies.

PAPILLOMAVIRAL INFECTIONS

Papillomaviruses are small, nonenveloped, double-stranded DNA viruses that are members of the papovavirus family. They infect surface epithelia and produce a variety of lesions of the skin and mucous membranes. With regard to the eye, papillomaviruses are most commonly found in verrucous lesions of the eyelids (verruca vulgaris) and papillomas of the conjunctiva. Papillomaviruses are oncogenic viruses and have also been found in a variety of epithelial neoplasms of the eye, including squamous cell carcinoma of the eyelid,[44] conjunctival dysplasia,[45] conjunctival intraepithelial neoplasia,[46] conjunctival squamous cell carcinoma,[45] and corneal epithelial dysplasia.[45]

Papillomaviruses are divided into types based on homologous characteristics of their DNA sequences. At least 50 types have been identified in humans. Each type is associated with a particular lesion. Types 6 and 11 are found in benign and premalignant lesions and have been identified in conjunctival papillomas.[47,48] Types 16 and 18 are more common in carcinomas and have been identified in squamous cell carcinoma of the eyelid[44] and conjunctival and corneal epithelial neoplasms.[45,46]

Papillomaviral infections are transmitted through abrasions of the skin or mucous membrane, by sexual contact, and during passage through an infected birth canal.

Verruca Vulgaris

Verrucae are common warty elevations that often occur on the eyelid margin between the eyelashes or on the skin

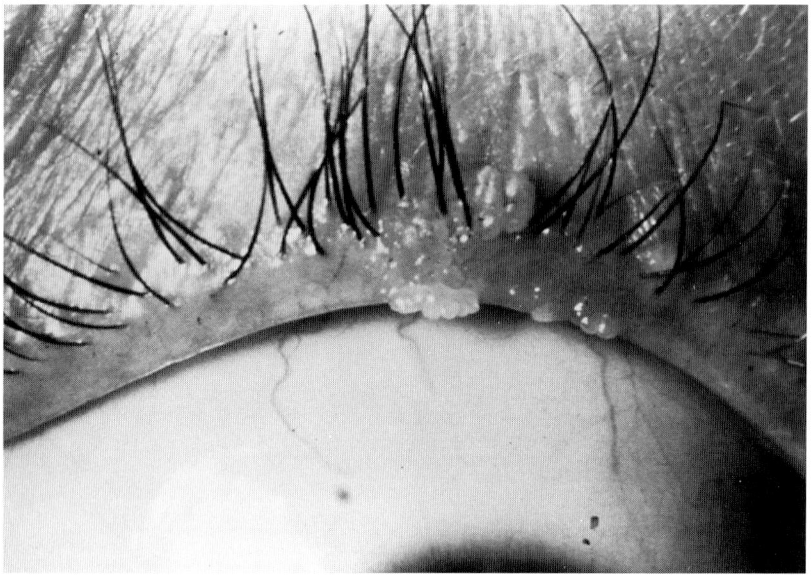

FIGURE 13-12 Verrucae on the upper eyelid margin.

of the eyelid (Figure 13-12). They are flat, digitate, or filiform in shape and can produce a low-grade, chronic papillary conjunctivitis. There may be an associated punctate epithelial keratitis, often in the area of the cornea closest to the eyelid lesion. In severe, long-standing cases, superficial wedge-shaped vascularization of the cornea can develop. Histologically, verrucae exhibit papillomatosis with acanthosis, hyperkeratosis, and parakeratosis. The upper malpighian and granular layers contain vacuolated cells with deeply basophilic nuclei that contain numerous viral particles[49] (Figure 13-13).

Verrucae often disappear spontaneously after 1 to 2 years. Surgical excision and cautery or cryotherapy can be used to treat the lesions.

Conjunctival Papillomas

Conjunctival papillomas (squamous papillomas of the conjunctiva) frequently occur in children and young adults. They are sessile or pedunculated lesions usually found in the inferior fornix, although they can occur anywhere on the conjunctiva, semilunar fold, caruncle, or limbus (Fig-

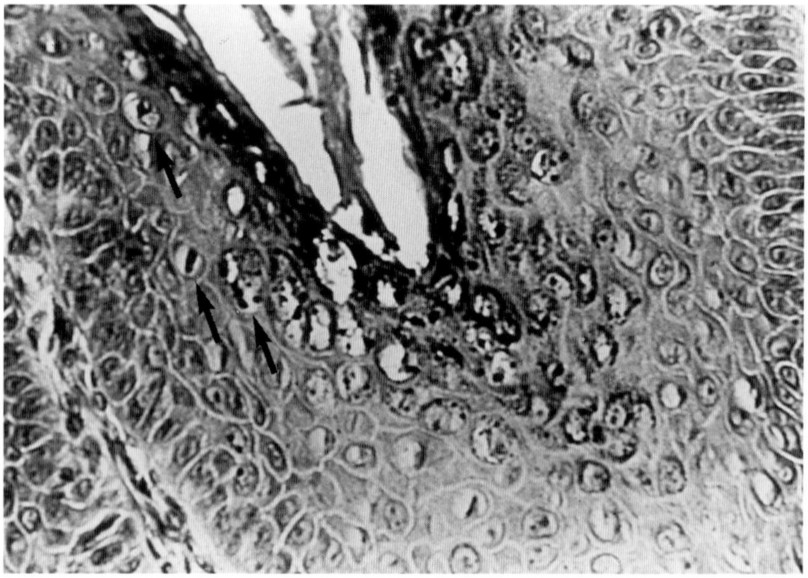

FIGURE 13-13 Histopathologic appearance of verruca vulgaris, demonstrating vacuolated cells with basophilic intranuclear viral inclusions (arrows). (Reprinted with permission from Lancaster Course in Ophthalmology. FA Davis, Philadelphia, 1981.)

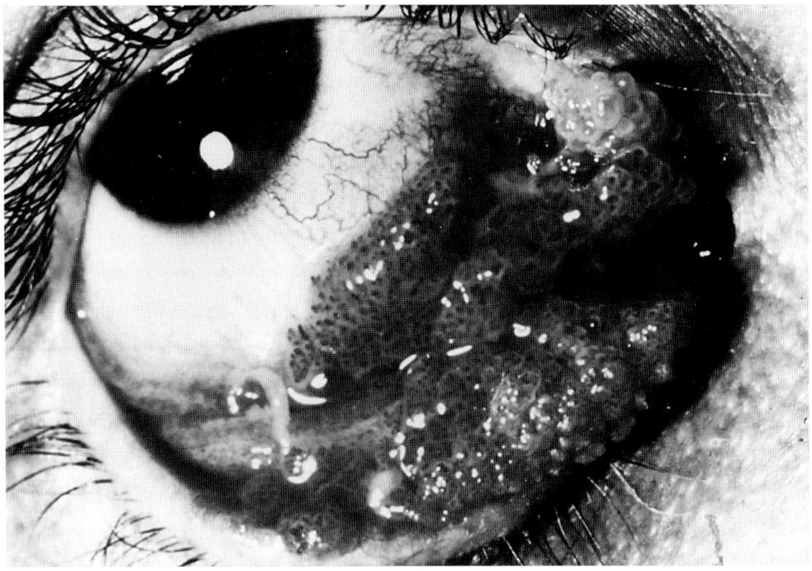

FIGURE 13-14 Massive conjunctival papilloma caused by papillomavirus. (Courtesy of the Armed Forces Institute of Pathology, Washington, DC)

ure 13-14). The lesions have a raspberry- or cauliflower-like appearance, with multiple delicate fronds of semitransparent tissue containing central red dots, which represent the central fibrovascular cores of the fronds. The histopathology of conjunctival papillomas is described further in Chapter 24.

If possible, conjunctival papillomas should probably be allowed to involute spontaneously, because multiple recurrent lesions are common after excision. Other than excision, treatment modalities described for conjunctival papillomas include cautery, liquid nitrogen cryotherapy,[50] CO_2 laser therapy,[51] immunotherapy with topical dinitrochlorobenzene,[52,53] and systemic interferon-α therapy.[54]

REFERENCES

1. Wadell G: Adenoviruses. p. 267. In Zuckerman AJ, Banatvala JE, Parrison JR (eds): Principles and Practice of Clinical Virology. 2nd Ed. John Wiley & Sons, New York, 1990
2. Colon LE: Keratoconjunctivitis due to adenovirus type 8: report on a large outbreak. Ann Ophthalmol 23:63, 1991
3. Warren D, Nelson KE, Farrar JA, et al: A large outbreak of epidemic keratoconjunctivitis: problems in controlling nosocomial spread. J Infect Dis 160:938, 1989
4. Koo D, Bauvier B, Wesley M, et al: Epidemic keratoconjunctivitis in a university medical center ophthalmology clinic; need for re-evaluation of the design and disinfection of instruments. Infect Control Hosp Epidemiol 10:547, 1989
5. Ford E, Nelson KE, Warren D: Epidemiology of epidemic keratoconjunctivitis. Epidemiol Rev 9:244, 1987
6. Nauheim RC, Romanowski EG, Araullo-Cruz T, et al: Prolonged recoverability of desiccated adenovirus type 19 from various surfaces. Ophthalmology 97:1450, 1990
7. Harnett GB, Newnham WA: Isolation of adenovirus type 19 from the male and female genital tracts. Br J Vener Dis 57:55, 1981
8. Dawson CR, Hanna L, Wood RT, et al: Adenovirus type 8 keratoconjunctivitis in the United States. III. Epidemiologic, clinical, and microbiologic features. Am J Ophthalmol 69:473, 1970
9. Corin S, Harvey J: Epidemic keratoconjunctivitis associated with blepharoptosis. Am J Ophthalmol 106:360, 1988
10. Hammer LH, Perry HD, Donnenfeld ED, Rahn EK: Symblepharon formation in epidemic keratoconjunctivitis. Cornea 9:338, 1990
11. Duke-Elder S, Perkins ES: Viral uveitis. p. 332. In Duke-Elder S (ed): System of Ophthalmology. Vol. IX. Diseases of the Uveal Tract. CV Mosby, St. Louis, 1966
12. Walsh FB, Hoyt WF: Infections and parasitic invasions of the nervous system. p. 1312. In: Clinical Neuro-ophthalmology. 3rd Ed. Williams & Wilkins, Baltimore, 1969
13. Thygeson P: Superficial punctate keratitis. JAMA 144:1544, 1950
14. Wiley L, Springer D, Kowalski RP, et al: Rapid diagnostic test for ocular adenovirus. Ophthalmology 95:431, 1988
15. Kowalski RP, Gordon YJ: Comparison of direct rapid tests for the detection of adenovirus antigen in routine conjunctival specimens. Ophthalmology 96:1106, 1989
16. Knopf HL, Hierholzer JC: Clinical and immunologic responses in patients with viral keratoconjunctivitis. Am J Ophthalmol 80:661, 1975
17. D'Angelo LJ: Pharyngoconjunctival fever caused by adenovirus type 4: report of a swimming pool-related outbreak with recovery of virus from pool water. J Infect Dis 140:42, 1979

18. Boniuk M, Phillips CA, Friedman JB: Chronic adenovirus type 2 keratitis in man. N Engl J Med 273:924, 1965
19. Pettit TH, Holland GM: Chronic keratoconjunctivitis associated with ocular adenovirus infection. Am J Ophthalmol 88:748, 1979
20. Darougar S, Quinlan MP, Gibson JA, et al: Epidemic keratoconjunctivitis and chronic papillary conjunctivitis in London due to adenovirus type 19. Br J Ophthalmol 61:76, 1977
21. Chatterjee S, Quarcoopome CO, Apenteng A: Unusual type of epidemic conjunctivitis in Ghana. Br J Ophthalmol 54:628, 1970
22. Ghendon Y: Ocular enterovirus infections of the world. p. 3. In Ishii K, Uchida Y, Miyamura K, Yamazaki S (eds): Acute Hemorrhagic Conjunctivitis: Etiology, Epidemiology and Clinical Manifestations. University of Tokyo Press, Tokyo, 1989
23. Patriarca PA, Onorato IM, Sklar VE, et al: Acute hemorrhagic conjunctivitis. Investigation of a large-scale community outbreak in Dade County, Florida. JAMA 249:1283, 1983
24. Kuritsky JN, Weaver JH, Bernard KW, et al: An outbreak of acute hemorrhagic conjunctivitis in central Minnesota. Am J Ophthalmol 96:449, 1983
25. Chopra JS, Sawhney IMS, Dhand UK, et al: Neurological complications of acute hemorrhagic conjunctivitis. J Neurol Sci 73:177, 1986
26. Sklar VEF: Clinical findings and results of treatment in an outbreak of acute hemorrhagic conjunctivitis in southern Florida. Am J Ophthalmol 95:45, 1983
27. Christopher S, Theogaraj S, Godbole S, John TJ: An epidemic of acute hemorrhagic conjunctivitis due to coxsackie virus A24. J Infect Dis 146:16, 1982
28. Stansfield SK, de la Pena W, Koenig S, et al: Human leukocyte interferon in the treatment and prophylaxis of acute hemorrhagic conjunctivitis. J Infect Dis 149:822, 1984
29. Banks HS: Infection across the intact conjunctiva. Lancet 2:518, 1958
30. Deckard PS, Bergstrom TJ: Rubeola keratitis. Ophthalmology 88:812, 1981
31. Foster A, Sommer A: Corneal ulceration, measles, and childhood blindness in Tanzania. Br J Ophthalmol 71:331, 1987
32. James HO, Wester CE, Duggan MB, Magwa M: A controlled study on the effect of injected water-miscible retinyl palmitate on plasma concentrations of retinol and retinol-binding protein in children with measles in northern Nigeria. Acta Paediatr Scand 73:22, 1984
33. Meyer RF, Sullivan JH, Oh J: Mumps conjunctivitis. Am J Ophthalmol 78:1022, 1974
34. Fields J: Ocular manifestations of mumps. Am J Ophthalmol 30:591, 1947
35. Riffenburg R: Ocular manifestations of mumps. Arch Ophthalmol 66:739, 1961
36. Keeney AH, Hunter MC: Human infection with Newcastle virus of fowls. Arch Ophthalmol 44:573, 1950
37. Hales RH, Ostler BH: Newcastle disease conjunctivitis with subepithelial infiltrates. Br J Ophthalmol 57:694, 1973
38. Wolff SM: Ocular manifestations of congenital rubella. A prospective study of 328 cases of congenital rubella. J Pediatr Ophthalmol 10:101, 1973
39. Charles NC, Friedberg DN: Epibulbar molluscum contagiosum in acquired immune deficiency syndrome. Ophthalmology 99:1123, 1992
40. Lee OS Jr: Keratitis with molluscum contagiosum. Arch Ophthalmol 31:64, 1944
41. Julianelle LA, James WM: Molluscum contagiosum of the eye, its clinical course and transmissibility and the cultivability of the virus. Am J Ophthalmol 26:565, 1943
42. Robinson MR, Udell IJ, Perry FG, et al: Molluscum contagiosum of the eyelids in patients with acquired immune deficiency syndrome. Ophthalmology 99:1745, 1992
43. Kohn SR: Molluscum contagiosum in patients with acquired immunodeficiency syndrome. Arch Ophthalmol 105:458, 1987
44. McDonnell JM, McDonnell PJ, Stout WC, Martin J: Human papillomavirus DNA in a recurrent squamous carcinoma of the eyelid. Arch Ophthalmol 107:1631, 1989
45. McDonnell JM, Mayr AJ, Martin WJ: DNA of human papillomavirus type 16 in dysplastic and malignant lesions of the conjunctiva and cornea. N Engl J Med 320:1442, 1989
46. Lauer SA, Malter JS, Meier JR: Human papillomavirus type 18 in conjunctival intraepithelial neoplasia. Am J Ophthalmol 110:23, 1990
47. Lass JH, Grove AS, Papale JJ, et al: Detection of human papillomavirus DNA sequences in conjunctival papilloma. Am J Ophthalmol 96:670, 1983
48. McDonnell PJ, McDonnell JM, Kessis T, et al: Detection of human papillomavirus type 6/11 DNA in conjunctival papillomas by in situ hybridization with radioactive probes. Hum Pathol 18:1115, 1987
49. Lancaster Course in Ophthalmology. FA Davis, Philadelphia, 1981
50. Harkey ME, Metz HS: Cryotherapy of conjunctival papillomata. Am J Ophthalmol 66:872, 1968
51. Schachat A, Iliff WJ, Kashima HK: Carbon dioxide laser therapy of recurrent squamous papilloma of the conjunctiva. Ophthalmic Surg 13:916, 1982
52. Petrelli R, Cotlier E, Robins S, Stoessel K: Dini trochlorobenzene immunotherapy of recurrent squamous papilloma of the conjunctiva. Ophthalmology 88:1221, 1981
53. Burns RP, Wankum G, Giangiacomo J, Anderson PC: Dinitrochlorobenzene and debulking therapy of conjunctival papilloma. J Pediatr Ophthalmol Strabismus 20:221, 1983
54. Lass JH, Foster CS, Grove AS, et al: Interferon-alpha therapy of recurrent conjunctival papillomas. Am J Ophthalmol 103:294, 1987

14

Chlamydial Infections

CHANDLER DAWSON

Chlamydial infections cause a variety of clinical diseases. Although many of these have only recently been recognized, the clinical and microbiologic features of chlamydial eye infections (trachoma, adult inclusion conjunctivitis, and neonatal inclusion conjunctivitis) have been well understood since the first decade of this century.[1,2] Trachoma is highly endemic in some developing countries, where it affects 300 to 400 million people and has blinded at least 6 million.[3] Sexually transmitted chlamydial infections are common in the urban populations of both industrialized and developing countries. Although sexually transmitted chlamydial infections infrequently involve the eye in adults, they are common causes of conjunctivitis and pneumonia in neonates.[4]

Although there have been rapid advances in the microbiology, immunology, and laboratory diagnosis of chlamydial infections, the pathogenesis of these infections is not well understood. Chlamydial eye infections are often chronic, and new episodes of disease occur with re-exposure to the organism.

ORGANISM

Classification

Chlamydiae are eubacteria that were originally grouped together as the psittacosis-lymphogranuloma venereum-trachoma agents because they have several common characteristics: (1) an obligate intracellular life cycle, (2) a common complement-fixing antigen, and (3) sensitivity to certain antibiotics.[5] Gordon and Quan[6] divided the chlamydiae into two groups based on the morphology of the inclusion (the intracytoplasmic vacuole in the host cell that contains the organism) and the presence or absence of glycogen in the inclusion. Subsequent taxonomic classification added sensitivity to sulfonamides as a criterion. Chlamydiae are now classified as a single order (Chlamydiales), a single family (Chlamydiaceae), one genus *(Chlamydia)*, and three species: *C. trachomatis* (glycogen positive and sulfonamide sensitive), *C. psittaci* (glycogen negative and sulfonamide resistant), and *C. pneumoniae* (glycogen negative and sulfonamide resistant).[5]

Three biovariants (biovars) of *C. trachomatis* are recognized: the trachoma, lymphogranuloma venereum (LGV), and mouse pneumonitis biovars. With the exception of the mouse pneumonitis biovar, *C. trachomatis* has a single host: humans. The trachoma biovar, once referred to as TRIC (trachoma-inclusion conjunctivitis) agents, replicates in the epithelial cells of mucosal surfaces and can infect the conjunctiva, respiratory tract, lower gastrointestinal tract, and genital tract (including the urethra), as well as the cervix, endometrium, and fallopian tubes. The trachoma biovar consists of several serovariants (serovars), which are distinguished by the microimmunofluorescence (micro-IF) test.[7] Serovars A, B, Ba, and C are usually associated with classic endemic trachoma; serovars D, Da, E, F, G, H, I, Ia, J, and K are usually associated with sexually transmitted infections. The lymphogranuloma venereum biovar consists of four serovars: L1, L2, L2a, and L3.

C. psittaci strains that are pathogenic for human eyes include the agents of feline pneumonitis and psittacosis, an acute infectious disease transmitted to humans by parrots and other fowl.[8–10] Another *C. psittaci* strain causes guinea pig inclusion conjunctivitis, which has been extensively studied as a model of human chlamydial eye disease.[11–13]

The most recently described chlamydial species, *C. pneumoniae,* was first isolated from children with trachoma in Taiwan and Iran.[14] Originally identified as the

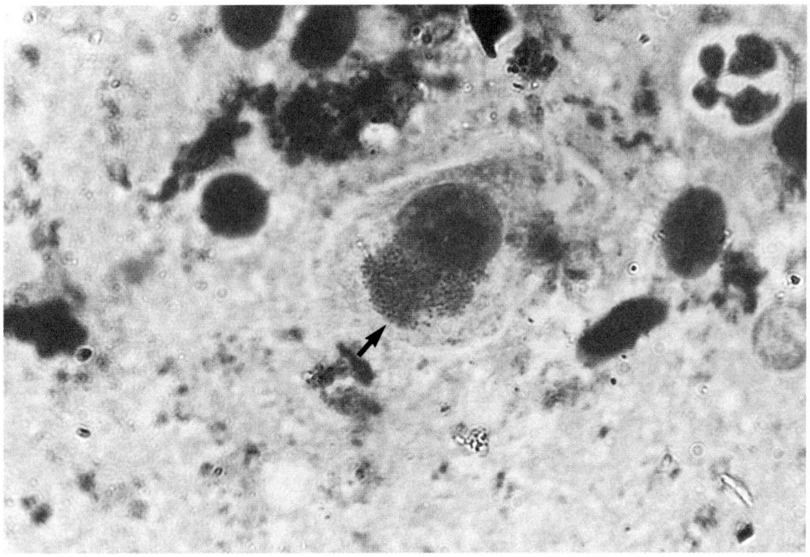

FIGURE 14-1 Chlamydial inclusion (arrow) next to the nucleus in a conjunctival epithelial cell. In this conjunctival scraping, the inclusion consists of individual blue particles in the cytoplasm of the epithelial cell (Giemsa stain).

TWAR (Taiwan acute respiratory) agent, it is now designated *C. pneumoniae.* This human pathogen appears to be immunologically distinct from *C. trachomatis* and *C. psittaci.*

Growth and Structure

Chlamydiae have a growth cycle within a membrane-bound vacuole (inclusion) in the cytoplasm of the host cell (Figure 14-1). The organism has two distinct forms: (1) the elementary body and (2) the initial, or reticulate, body. The elementary body is the extracellular infectious form and is responsible for cell-to-cell and host-to-host transmission. It contains a dense central core of DNA and has a rigid cell wall, which, on electron microscopy, sometimes appears to have many infoldings. The initial body is the noninfectious replicative form. It is found within the inclusion and cannot survive outside the host cell. On light microscopy, the initial body stains blue with Giemsa stain. On electron microscopy, it has a trilaminar cell wall and the appearance of a small bacterium. Similarly to bacteria, the initial body appears to divide by cross-wall formation.

The first step in the growth cycle is the attachment of the elementary body to the surface of a susceptible host cell[15] (Figure 14-2). The elementary body enters the cell in a cytoplasmic vacuole and is, therefore, protected from attack by the host's lysosomal enzymes.[16,17] It then reorganizes and within 6 to 8 hours becomes an initial body. The metabolically active initial body uses host cell substrates to synthesize RNA, DNA, and protein and divides by binary fission for 18 to 24 hours after infection. Some initial bodies then reorganize to become elementary bodies, which are released from the cell.

More than 60 percent of the total protein of the chlamydial cell wall consists of major outer membrane protein (MOMP), which has a molecular weight of about 40,000. The major outer membrane protein provides the structural integrity of the elementary body. The shift in the highly cross-linked, impermeable, major outer membrane protein of the elementary body to the permeable major outer membrane protein of the initial body is mediated by the reduction of disulfide bonds and the formation of pore-like structures (porins).[18]

The antigens responsible for genus specificity, species specificity, and subspecies (serovar) specificity appear to be located on the major outer membrane protein,[19] which suggests both constant and variable domains.[20–22] The identification of these antigenic determinants may provide the basis for developing recombinant or synthetic vaccines to chlamydiae.

CLINICAL MANIFESTATIONS

Ocular Infections with *C. trachomatis*

The clinical diseases associated with *C. trachomatis* ocular infections appear to occur in two distinct epidemiologic patterns. One pattern is the classic blinding endemic trachoma of developing countries, which is spread by eye-to-eye transmission of the organism. Trachoma is usually caused by *C. trachomatis* serovars A, B, Ba, or C.

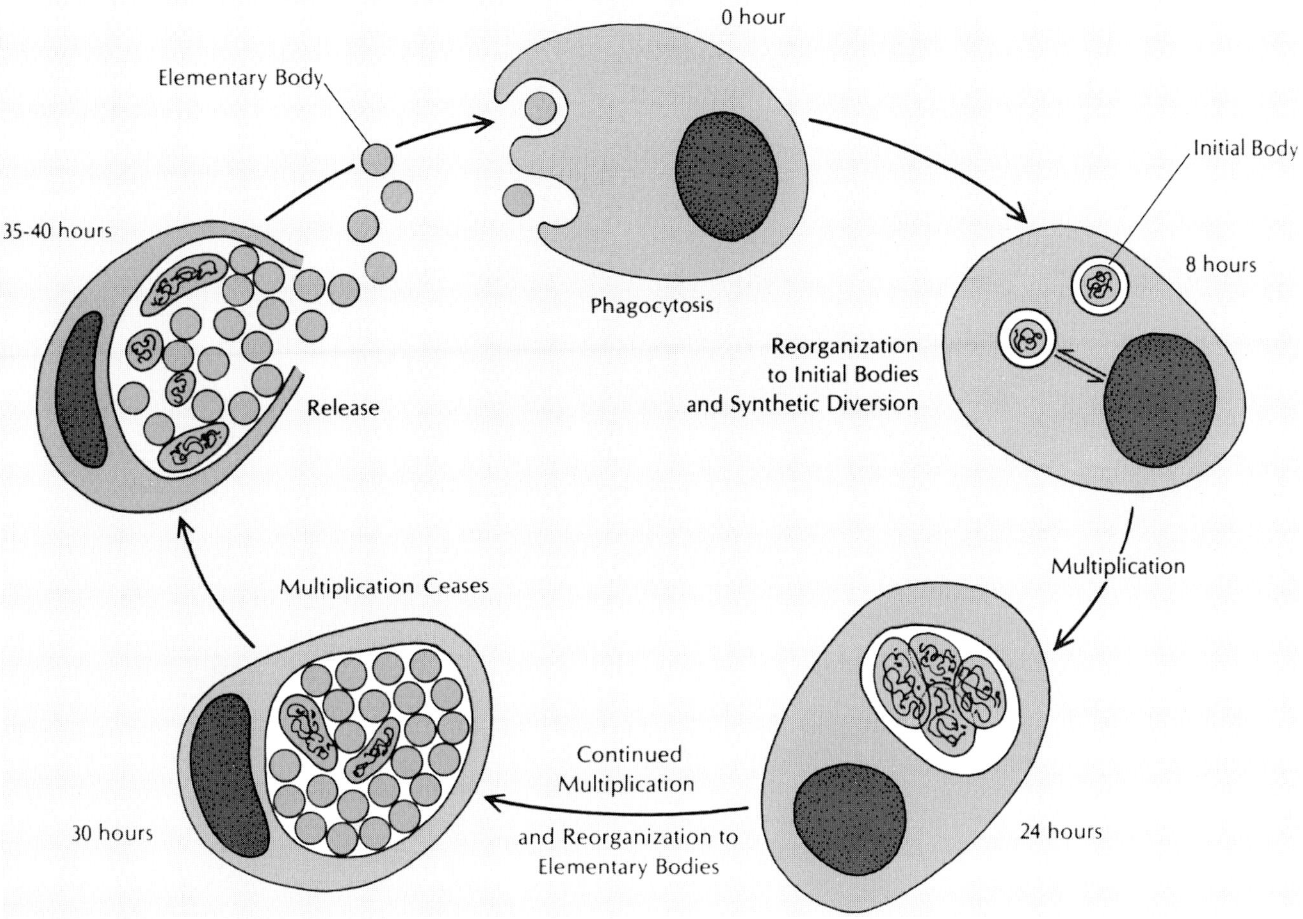

FIGURE 14-2 Schematic representation of the life cycle of chlamydial organisms. (Reprinted with permission from ER Alexander: *Chlamydia:* the organism and neonatal infection. Hosp Prac 14:63, 1979. © 1979, The McGraw-Hill Companies. Illustration by Nancy Lou Makris.)

The second pattern of ocular infections is inclusion conjunctivitis and is usually caused by the sexually transmitted *C. trachomatis* serovars D through K, although occasionally serovar B is isolated. These infections may be difficult to distinguish from the early inflammatory phases of endemic trachoma, hence the name *paratrachoma*. Although these sporadic chlamydial infections of the eye rarely cause permanent visual loss, the involvement of other sites (genital and respiratory tracts) produces other significant diseases in both adults and neonates. In adults, sexually transmitted chlamydiae are an important cause of diseases of the genital tract, including nongonococcal urethritis, in both men and women. In women, endometritis and salpingitis may be followed by fallopian tube scarring and sterility. Women can also develop perihepatitis by an ascending infection into the peritoneum (Fitzhugh-Curtis syndrome). In neonates, sexually transmitted chlamydiae can cause pneumonia and gastrointestinal infection in addition to inclusion conjunctivitis.

Trachoma

In communities with endemic trachoma, the onset of disease, frequently in the first year of life, often is not apparent or is so gradual that it goes unnoticed by the parents. In the early stages, trachoma manifests as conjunctivitis characterized by the formation of lymphoid follicles in the subconjunctival tissue and a papillary reaction with inflammatory infiltration and thickening of the conjunctiva (Figure 14-3). In children younger than 2 years of age, follicles may not be visible, so that the papillary reaction and conjunctival inflammation become the predominant signs. Trachoma involves the entire conjunctiva, but its effects are most noticeable on the superior tarsus, which has been selected as a convenient area of examination to represent the degree of

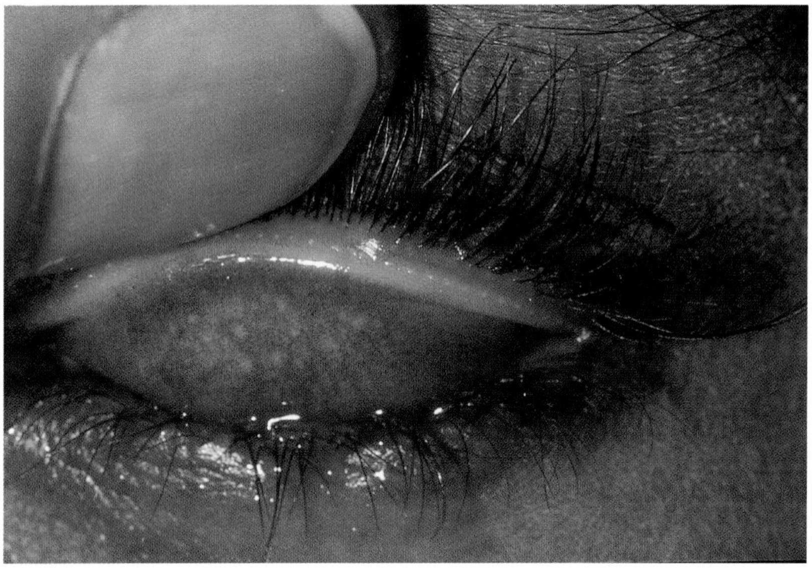

FIGURE 14-3 Active trachoma inflammation. The tarsal conjunctiva is used as a diagnostic area in evaluating trachoma. In this patient, there are individual lymphoid follicles seen as white or avascular spots surrounded by diffuse inflammation and infiltration of the conjunctiva (papillary hypertrophy), which partially obscure the normal deep conjunctival vessels.

trachomatous inflammation and scarring for the eye as a whole.[23]

Corneal lesions in the inflammatory phase include epithelial keratitis (usually in the superior portion of the cornea), anterior stromal infiltrates, and superficial neovascularization (vascular pannus)[24] (Figure 14-4). Neovascularization is usually twice as extensive at the superior limbus as it is at the inferior limbus. A unique characteristic of trachoma is the formation of lymphoid follicles in the limbal conjunctiva, which on resolution leave characteristic depressions of the limbus called *Herbert's pits*[25] (Figure 14-5).

Trachoma is a chronic disease. As it progresses, it causes scarring of the conjunctiva, with small stellate or fine linear scars in mild cases and broad confluent or synechial scars in severe cases (Figure 14-6). Blindness in trachoma is caused mainly by this scarring, which produces distortion of the eyelids, particularly of the superior tarsus, with resultant entropion and trichiasis[26] (Figure 14-7). The disease also destroys goblet cells and injures lacrimal glands and tear ducts. Deficient tear secretion and constant corneal abrasion by the trichiatic eyelashes often lead to corneal ulceration, followed by opacification and visual loss. In addition, the deep trachomatous scarring

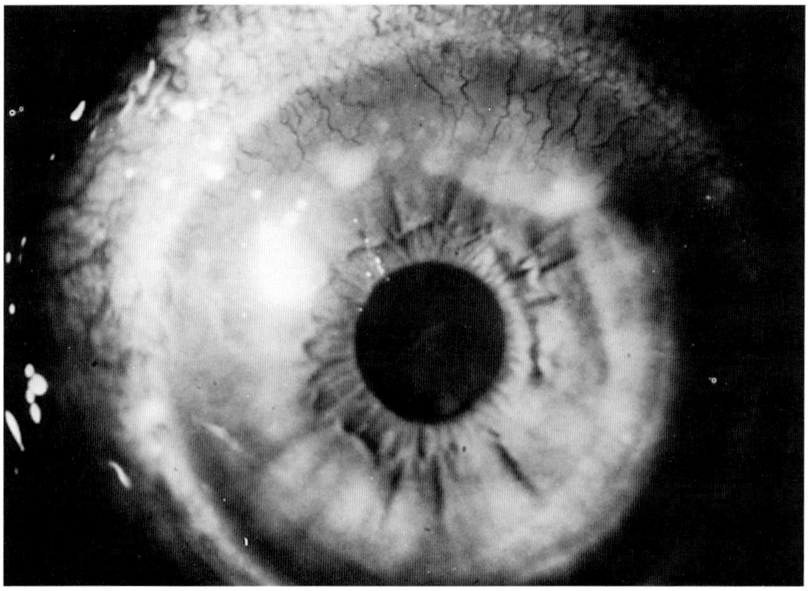

FIGURE 14-4 Superior pannus caused by trachoma.

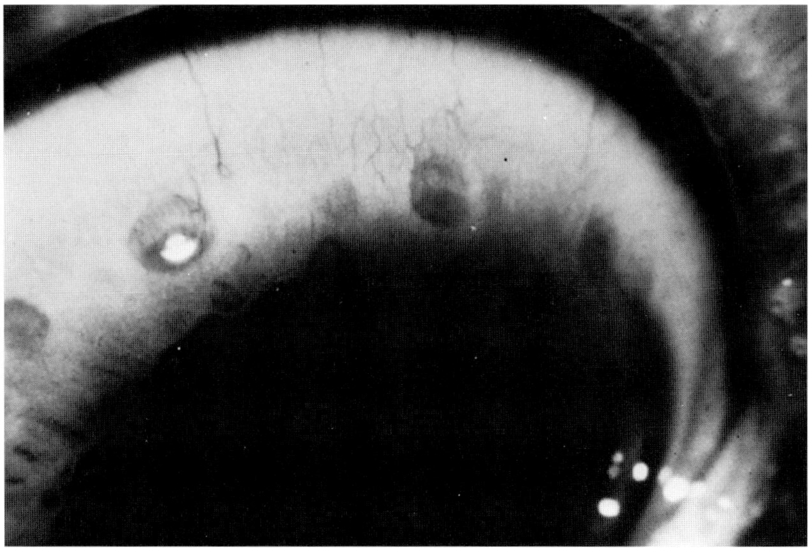

FIGURE 14-5 Herbert's pits.

in the superior tarsus and fornix may produce defects in eyelid closure that predispose the cornea to traumatic and infectious damage.

The degree of conjunctival scarring is thought to be directly proportional to the intensity and duration of inflammation. Severe scarring may occur in children as young as 4 or 5 years of age. However, entropion is uncommon at this age and tends not to occur until late adolescence and early adulthood, long after the active inflammatory disease has subsided.[27] This late onset of entropion is the result of gradual contraction of the scars, particularly the deeper scars close to the eyelid margin.

The presence of trachoma in a community can be confirmed if suspected cases have at least two of the following signs[23]: (1) superior tarsal conjunctival follicles; (2) limbal follicles or their sequelae (Herbert's pits); (3) typical conjunctival scarring; and (4) vascular pannus that is marked at the superior limbus.

Adult Inclusion Conjunctivitis

Adult inclusion conjunctivitis presents as acute follicular conjunctivitis with a palpable preauricular lymph node on the side of the involved eye[28] (Figure 14-8). The follicles are most prominent in the inferior conjunctiva but may be present in the superior tarsal conjunctiva. There is a small amount of mucopurulent discharge. Corneal involvement includes epithelial keratitis, marginal and central infiltrates, and the formation of subepithelial opacities similar to those of epidemic keratoconjunctivitis (Figure 14-9). There may also be corneal neovascularization (micropannus) in some cases. Conjunctival scarring has been reported in chronic cases.[28] The presence of tarsal follicles, corneal neovascularization, and rarely, conjunctival scarring can lead to confusion in the clinical diagnosis; some acute cases have been misdiagnosed as acute trachoma, although the infections were clearly caused by sexually transmitted strains of *C. trachomatis*.[28] In naturally occurring and experimentally induced disease, anterior uveitis is an uncommon complication, but otitis media is a typical feature of the infection.[28-32]

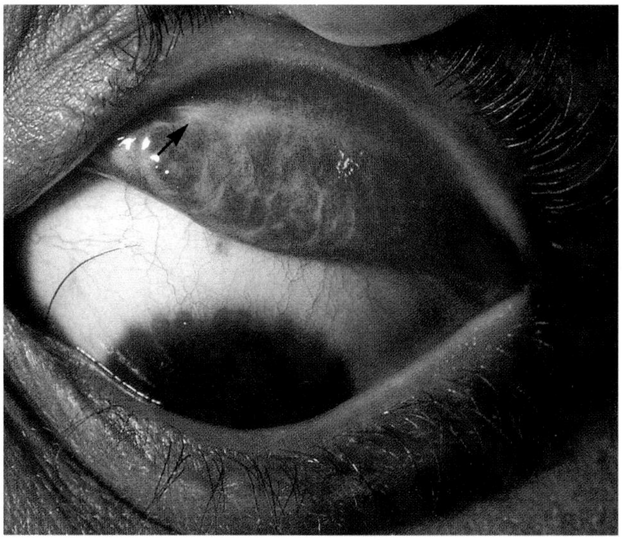

FIGURE 14-6 Conjunctival scarring from trachoma. In this Tunisian child, there is marked scarring of the tarsal conjunctiva. The solid white band of fibrosis (arrow) is called an *Arlt's line*. Between the scars, the conjunctiva appears to be inflamed; follicles may be present. The crenulated appearance at the limbus is caused by Herbert's pits, which are depressions left by trachoma follicles that formed at this site.

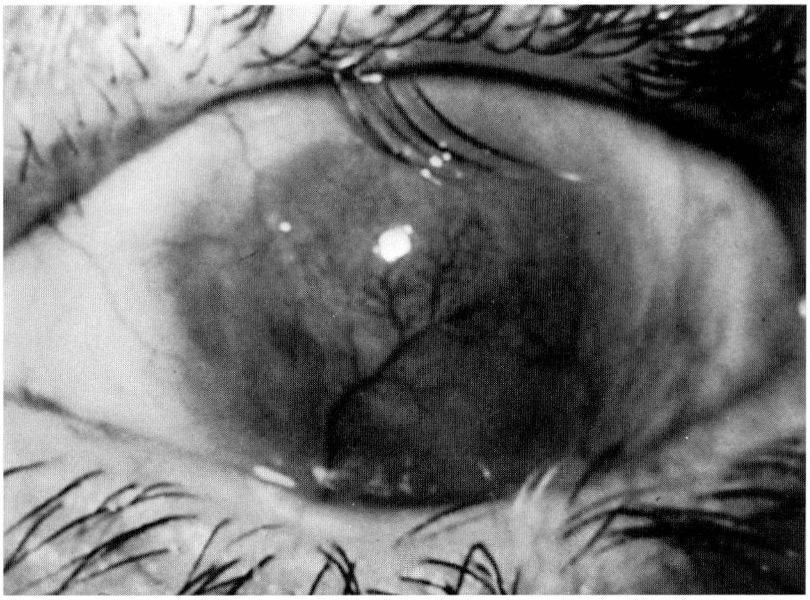

FIGURE 14-7 Trichiasis and corneal scarring caused by trachoma. (Reprinted with permission from the World Health Organization. ML Tarizzo: Field Methods for the Control of Trachoma. WHO, Geneva, 1973.)

In adult inclusion conjunctivitis, the clinical appearance of the disease evolves during the course of the infection, which if untreated, may last from 3 to 12 months, unlike follicular conjunctivitis caused by adenoviruses, which resolves within a few weeks. During the first 2 weeks, conjunctival hyperemia, infiltration, and discharge dominate the clinical picture. After 2 weeks, conjunctival follicles and superficial keratitis become more prominent. The follicles may be less prominent in cases that have persisted for several months.

Adult inclusion conjunctivitis is relatively uncommon. It is estimated to occur in about 1 in 300 cases of chlamydial genital infection in the United Kingdom.[33] Ocular infection appears to occur by autoinoculation from an infected genital tract to the eye by the fingers or by genital-to-eye inoculation from an infected sexual partner. The highest rates of sexually transmitted chlamydial eye infections are among patients 15 to 30 years old.[29]

Sexually transmitted strains of *C. trachomatis* were once a common cause of swimming pool conjunctivi-

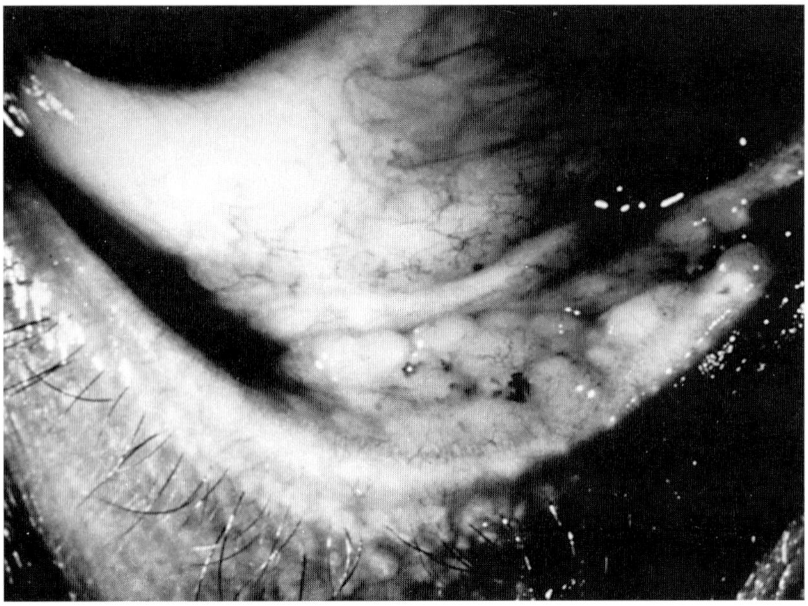

FIGURE 14-8 Follicles in the inferior fornix in adult inclusion conjunctivitis. (Courtesy of John W. Chandler, M.D., Bellingham, WA.)

tis, presumably because the pools were not chlorinated adequately.[34] There has been some spread of the infection in families of infected newborns.[35] Several gynecologists have been reported to have acquired the infection by accidental ocular inoculation with genital material.[35]

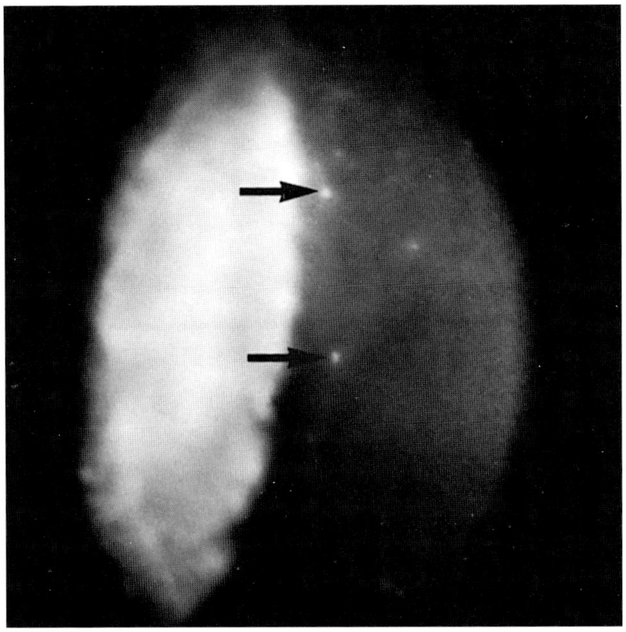

FIGURE 14-9 Superficial keratitis in a patient with adult inclusion conjunctivitis. Note the punctate lesions (arrows). (Courtesy of Jay H. Krachmer, M.D., Minneapolis, MN.)

Neonatal Inclusion Conjunctivitis

Neonatal inclusion conjunctivitis (inclusion blennorrhea) usually appears 5 to 19 days after birth; however, infection can occur earlier if the placental membranes rupture before delivery.[36,37]

Neonatal inclusion conjunctivitis is characterized by swelling of the eyelids, hyperemia and infiltration of the conjunctiva, and a purulent discharge (Figure 14-10). Keratitis has been reported in some cases. Newborns who are treated late or not at all develop conjunctival scarring and superficial corneal vascularization.[38-40] Systemic infection with respiratory tract involvement is well documented.[4,36] As in all cases of ophthalmia neonatorum, gonococcal infection must be excluded by the use of appropriate cultures and smears.

Lymphogranuloma Venereum

Ocular infection with the lymphogranuloma venereum biovar of *C. trachomatis* can present as Parinaud's oculoglandular conjunctivitis, which manifests as conjunctival inflammation associated with massive preauricular, submandibular, and cervical lymphadenopathy[41,42] (Figure 14-11).

The lymphogranuloma venereum biovar is a less common cause of genital tract infection than are *C. trachomatis* serovars D through K. However, lymphogranuloma venereum infection of the rectum and lower bowel is common in male homosexuals,[43] although the exact prevalence is not known. Infection with the lymphogranuloma venereum biovar appears to be highly associated with clinically manifest disease, in contrast to the milder dis-

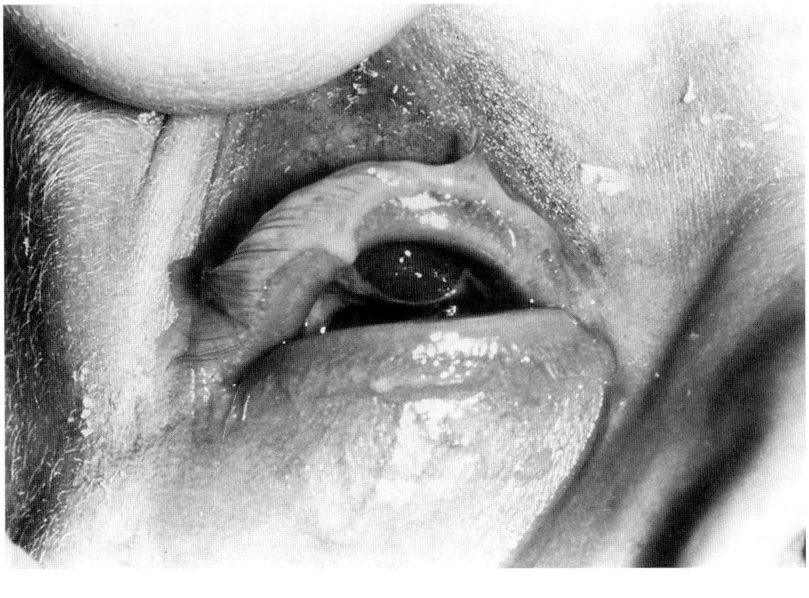

FIGURE 14-10 Neonatal inclusion conjunctivitis. (Courtesy of Mark J. Mannis, M.D., Sacramento, CA.)

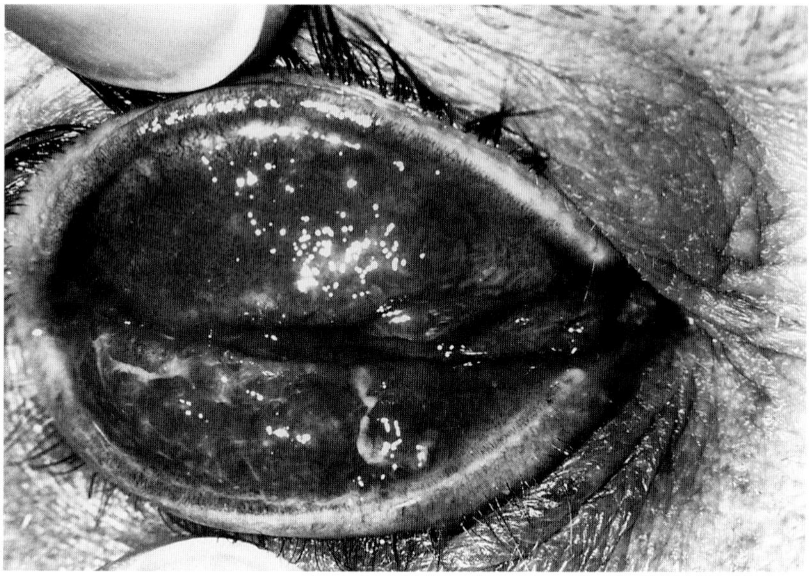

FIGURE 14-11 Papillary conjunctivitis caused by lymphogranuloma venereum. In this patient, the primary site of inoculation was probably the eye. The patient developed Parinaud's oculoglandular conjunctivitis.

ease caused by rectal infection with *C. trachomatis* serovars D through K.

Ocular Infections with *C. psittaci*

Conjunctivitis has been reported in association with infection with *C. psittaci,* the cause of feline pneumonitis and psittacosis.[8-10] Feline pneumonitis is a naturally occurring disease of cats that manifests as conjunctivitis and pneumonia in kittens. Human ocular infection results in a subacute follicular conjunctivitis with minimal mucopurulent discharge.[8-10] There can be a diffuse epithelial keratitis; corneal pannus does not occur. Without treatment, the disease can persist for months.

Unilateral subacute conjunctivitis with minimal mucopurulent discharge and a small preauricular lymph node has been reported in one patient with laboratory-acquired infection with the psittacosis strain of *C. psittaci.*[9] There was a diffuse superficial keratitis with subepithelial infiltrates but no corneal neovascularization. The infection responded slowly to treatment with oral tetracycline for 6 weeks. *C. psittaci* was isolated from the eye before treatment and after 2 weeks of oral tetracycline.

Ocular Infection with *C. pneumoniae*

C. pneumoniae appears to be a common cause of respiratory disease in adults and children,[14] but naturally occurring ocular infections have not been demonstrated since the original isolations in Taiwan and Iran. A single laboratory ocular infection has been reported with *C. pneumoniae.*[44] Papillary and follicular conjunctivitis occurred without keratitis, but with mild rhinitis. The disease resolved after treatment with systemic doxycycline and topical chlortetracycline.

HISTOPATHOLOGY

The host response of the conjunctiva infected with *C. trachomatis* is characterized both clinically and histologically by the presence of lymphoid follicles with germinal centers. In the early stages of trachoma, the epithelial and subepithelial tissues are infiltrated with lymphocytes and polymorphonuclear leukocytes. The tarsal conjunctiva is thrown into villous processes to form papillae with a central vascular tuft and folds of epithelium between the elevations.[45-47]

Early in the disease, collections of lymphocytes are seen just beneath the epithelium or deeper within the connective tissue. These early follicles do not have germinal centers and appear to consist mostly of small lymphocytes. As the disease progresses, the collections of lymphocytes develop a structure like that of lymph nodes, with an outer layer of small, dense lymphocytes and an inner center of lighter-staining lymphocytes with more cytoplasm. Unlike in central lymph nodes, the germinal center in these follicles is displaced toward the surface. The lymphocytes of the follicle appear to infiltrate the conjunctival epithelium, which is relatively flattened and loosened over the follicle itself, allowing foreign material ready access to the follicle. This structure may be analogous to Peyer's patches in the intestinal tract. Follicles can also occur deeper in the conjunctival connective tissue.

In the more advanced stages of trachoma, the follicles themselves or the germinal centers of the follicles become necrotic, and connective tissue forms around the follicle, a reaction that produces scarring.[45,46] Follicles at the limbus form Herbert's pits.

Macrophages are frequently found in the epithelium and in the follicles themselves. Plasma cells appear to be distributed throughout the conjunctiva. There is marked lymphocytic infiltration between the follicles. In addition, the capillaries are dilated, and the whole conjunctiva can be considerably thickened by the cellular infiltration, with the formation of papillary villi or fronds. As scarring takes place, the islands of epithelium between the elevated papillae may become trapped and form epithelium-lined cysts that are identified clinically as post-trachomatous degeneration.

Despite increased knowledge of the immunology of *C. trachomatis* infections, the pathologic processes in the diseased tissue itself are still poorly understood. In sporadic infection of the eye with the sexually transmitted *C. trachomatis* serovars in industrialized countries, the disease may be prolonged but self limited. However, with endemic trachoma in developing countries, children with the greatest degree of conjunctival inflammation (severe intensity trachoma) have the highest rates of chlamydial infection and the highest titers of antibodies in the serum and tears.[48,49] Moreover, the intensity in individual cases tends to remain the same for many months or years. Thus, some individuals appear to be permissive of infection despite clear evidence of a good immune response. It is these patients who develop the greatest degree of scarring and who are at the highest risk of becoming blind as adults. The inflammation and damage to the eye are proportional to the number of organisms present, and the inflammatory response is driven by replicating organisms.

It is not clear what events that occur in the conjunctival tissue lead to destruction of tissue with scar formation in trachoma. The cicatricial pathways in trachoma have been associated with a hypersensitivity or a T-cell-mediated immune response. In trachoma, the T cells and other lymphocytes (perhaps natural killer cells) are the predominant cells in the inflamed conjunctiva. This cell-mediated immune response, then, may not only be ineffective in controlling the infection but may also lead to tissue destruction.

IMMUNOLOGY

Immunity to chlamydial infections is not well understood. In nonhuman primate models and the early human vaccine trials, immunity was serovar specific, secretory antibody mediated, T-cell dependent, dose dependent, and relatively short lived.[50-52] More severe eye disease resulted from reinfection when vaccines failed to protect due to either inadequate potency or the use of a heterologous serovar.[53] It is now thought that the damaging conjunctival scarring in trachoma is caused by the immunologic response and prolonged inflammation caused by repeated or persistent infection.

Antibody Response

Much of the earlier work on the antibody response in chlamydial infections was done with the complement fixation test, which measures antibodies to *Chlamydia* group antigen (i.e., the antigen common to all three chlamydial species). In lymphogranuloma venereum, the complement fixation test usually reveals a serum antibody titer of at least 1:16; in many cases, the titer can be extremely elevated, often far greater than 1:128.[54,55] Although this test has been widely available in public health laboratories, it has limited usefulness for the diagnosis of superficial chlamydial infections such as trachoma and oculogenital chlamydial infections.

As detected with the microimmunofluorescence test, ocular infection with *C. trachomatis* serovars A, B, Ba, and C or serovars D through K can produce an antibody response narrowly limited to the infecting serovar and its closely related serovars or broadly reactive to all serovars.[7,48,55] After initial infection with *C. trachomatis,* serum IgM antibodies appear in 2 to 3 weeks and persist for 4 to 8 weeks. IgG antibodies appear about the same time or slightly later but continue to persist after the IgM antibodies disappear. During recurrent disease episodes, serum IgM antibodies may reappear.

Serum antibodies have been found in about 80 percent of children with severe endemic trachoma in North Africa.[56] In American Indian children with mild trachoma, only 1 child in 46 was found to have serum antibodies, but in American Indian adolescents with trachoma, antibodies were present in almost 50 percent.[49] About 90 percent of adult patients in the general population with oculogenital chlamydial infections have serum antibodies.[49]

Antibodies in tears appear to occur less frequently than serum antibodies, even in the presence of active infection of the conjunctiva. Tear antibodies are found infrequently (about 5 percent) in the absence of serum antibodies.[49] However, in endemic trachoma, about half the patients have antibodies in both the serum and tears. The prevalence of antibodies in the serum and tears appears to be directly related to the intensity of disease. In one study of children in southern Tunisia, the titer of tear antibodies declined with decreasing intensity of disease.[56] Tear antibodies were present in 80 percent of those with severe endemic trachoma, in 31 percent with moderate trachoma, and in only 17 percent with mild trachoma. Tear antibodies also occur more frequently and in a higher titer in patients with trachoma who have *Chlamydia* isolated from the conjunctiva compared with those who do not.[56] Tear antibodies to *Chlamydia* are predominantly IgG, not IgA. The titer of tear antibodies is usually lower than the titer of serum antibodies in the same patient.[49]

Cell-Mediated Immunity

The intradermal skin test for delayed hypersensitivity to *Chlamydia* was described by Frei,[57] who used pus from the buboes of lymphogranuloma venereum patients. With the isolation of the causative agent of lymphogranuloma venereum, antigen for the Frei intradermal skin test was obtained from infected mouse brain, and in 1940, a purified skin test antigen, Lygranum, was obtained from organisms grown in yolk sacs of developing chicken embryos.[58] The Frei skin test is positive in some patients with lymphogranuloma venereum but rarely in patients with other chlamydial infections. Even in proven cases of lymphogranuloma venereum, the Frei test may be positive in only one-third of patients, and a negative Frei test has occurred even when *C. trachomatis* has been isolated from the patient.[49]

LABORATORY DIAGNOSIS

Available techniques to identify infection with chlamydia are summarized in Table 14-1 and include (1) morphologic identification of chlamydial inclusions by Giemsa or iodine staining of smears; (2) identification of chlamydial antigen by direct fluorescent antibodies to species-specific or group-specific antigen or by enzyme immunoassay (EIA); (3) isolation of the organism in cell culture; (4) DNA probes for chlamydial DNA or its plasmid; (5) identification of chlamydial DNA by polymerase chain reaction (PCR) or ligase chain reaction (LCR); and (6) detection of antibodies to *C. trachomatis* in serum, tears, or other secretions.

Cytology

In Giemsa-stained smears, chlamydial organisms are seen as clusters of distinct particles (inclusions) in the cytoplasm of conjunctival epithelial cells. With an oil immersion lens (× 400 to × 1,000), the elementary bodies stain reddish purple and the larger initial bodies stain deep blue.[59,60] The common sources of misdiagnosis in Giemsa-stained smears include pigment granules, keratin, nuclear extrusions, goblet cells, eosinophilic granules, and bacteria.[59] In trachoma, the accompanying conjunctival cytology can be used as a guide to screen smears. Inclusions are usually found only when polymorphonuclear leukocytes and epithelial cells are present; the prevalence of inclusions increases progressively with the presence of other inflammatory cells (lymphocytes, plasma cells, macrophages, and multinucleated giant cells).

Staining with Lugol's iodine demonstrates the presence of glycogen matrix in the inclusions by staining the glycogen brown.[61] Iodine staining of conjunctival smears is insensitive, but the technique has been used to identify inclusions in cell culture.

TABLE 14-1
Sensitivity of Tests to Detect Chlamydial Eye Infections

		Inclusion Conjunctivitis (%)	
	Trachoma (%)	*Adult*	*Neonatal*
Cytology			
Giemsa stain	30	60	95
Detection of antigen			
Direct fluorescent antibody stain	50–80	+[a]	100
Enzyme immunoassay	80	+	+[a]
Isolation			
Cell culture	85	+	90
Serology			
Complement fixation	–[b]	–[b]	–[b]
Microimmunofluorescence	±[c]	±[c]	+[a] (IgM)

[a] Useful test but no data on sensitivity and specificity.
[b] Not useful in this situation.
[c] A negative test cannot rule out a chlamydial infection.

Detection of Chlamydial Antigen

Staining of conjunctival smears with fluorescein-conjugated polyclonal antibodies produced in rabbits was conducted in several research laboratories in the 1960s and 1970s.[32] Direct fluorescein-conjugated monoclonal antibody preparations (direct fluorescent antibodies) to *C. trachomatis* are now widely available for the detection of the organism in smears.[19,62] With this stain, individual elementary bodies are identified as brightly fluorescing extracellular particles, but intracellular inclusions are not well identified. With fluorescent antibodies to species-specific antigen (Syva MicroTrak *Chlamydial trachomatis* Direct Specimen Test), the manufacturer recommends that, for a positive test, at least 10 elementary bodies should be identified in cervical or urethral smears, but only 5 or more are required for conjunctival smears. For trachoma, the direct fluorescent antibody stain is 80 percent as sensitive as culture and is highly specific. The technique requires a fluorescence microscope and an experienced microscopist who can recognize the typical morphology of free elementary bodies. Other stains use antibodies to chlamydial lipopolysaccharide to identify all three chlamydial species.

Enzyme immunoassay techniques (Chlamydiazyme Diagnostic Kit, Syva MicroTrak *Chlamydia* EIA) detect chlamydial antigen in clinical specimens with about the same sensitivity and specificity as fluorescent antibody techniques.[63] A somewhat less sensitive test kit (Kodak Surecell Chlamydia Test Kit) was marketed for office and small hospital laboratories,[64] but is no longer commercially available.

Culture

Isolation of *C. trachomatis* in cell culture is the definitive way to identify the organism. Although chlamydial culture is the standard by which other methods for the detection of *C. trachomatis* are judged, few laboratories are prepared to perform this procedure.

Serologic Diagnosis

In individual patients, the detection of antibodies to *Chlamydia* in the serum or tears is usually not useful for the diagnosis of chlamydial eye infections, because in most populations, the infections are chronic and endemic. Because patients are rarely tested during the early phases of infection, serologic testing is usually performed with a single serum or tear specimen rather than paired specimens. However, testing for antibodies has been applied in epidemiologic studies.

The microimmunofluorescence (micro-IF) test is of use for diagnosing active chlamydial infections in newborns but not in older children and adults. Microimmunofluorescence testing is limited to a few laboratories with research interests. It measures the serovar-specific antibodies produced against chlamydiae. Newborns who develop inclusion conjunctivitis usually carry serum IgG antibodies transferred from the mother during pregnancy. If the chlamydial infection of the newborn is limited to the eye, there is little if any rise in serum IgM antibodies, particularly during the first 4 weeks of life. In newborns who develop pneumonia due to *C. trachomatis,* there is a rise in serum IgG antibodies, and IgM antibodies appear.

The older complement fixation (CF) test measures antibody levels to chlamydial group-specific antigen. It is a genus-specific test and detects antibodies against a lipopolysaccharide antigen common to all chlamydiae.

Detection of Chlamydial DNA

A polymerase chain reaction (PCR) test (Amplicor) was developed to detect chlamydial DNA. Evaluation of this test in adult conjunctival specimens revealed a sensitivity of 88 percent and a specificity of 100 percent.[65]

Comparison of Diagnostic Techniques

In endemic trachoma, direct fluorescent antibody staining and enzyme immunoassay are more sensitive than Giemsa staining in detecting chlamydiae. Isolation of the organism in cell culture is less widely available but has greater sensitivity and specificity. Microimmunofluorescence testing for serovar-specific antibodies may be useful for epidemiologic studies but is not as sensitive for individual cases.[66]

In adult inclusion conjunctivitis, Giemsa staining is less sensitive than direct fluorescent antibody staining, enzyme immunoassay techniques, or cell culture; microimmunofluorescence serology has only limited usefulness.

Giemsa staining, direct fluorescent antibody staining, and cell culture are all highly sensitive and specific for the diagnosis of neonatal inclusion conjunctivitis. Testing for serum IgM antibodies is useful for the detection of chlamydial pneumonia after the second or third month of life. Giemsa-stained conjunctival smears from infected neonates often contain large numbers of inclusions. In a study comparing cell culture, Giemsa staining, and direct fluorescent antibody staining in neonatal conjunctivitis, 43 of 100 cultures yielded *C. trachomatis;* Giemsa staining was positive in 42 percent, and direct fluorescent antibody staining was positive in 100 percent of the culture-positive cases.[37]

TREATMENT

Trachoma

In regions where trachoma is endemic, treatment is based on public health efforts to prevent blindness. These efforts include medical therapy, surgical correction of eyelid deformities, and preventive measures. The objectives of medical therapy are to reduce the intensity of disease (and thus the risk of blindness) in the individual and to reduce the transmission rate in the population.

Sulfonamides, tetracyclines, erythromycin and its derivatives, and rifampin are all effective in the treatment of active trachoma. Topical tetracyclines (eye ointments or suspensions) are recommended for large-scale treatment of trachoma,[23] and current trachoma control programs are based on the mass application of topical antibiotics. In theory, initial, intensive, large-scale medical therapy is intended to reduce the ocular reservoir of chlamydia in the population and is to be followed by intermittent, family-based topical treatment to control further eye-to-eye transmission. However, this strategy has not been effective in endemic areas except when accompanied by economic development.

In communities with severe endemic trachoma, face washing of young children and use of latrines by adults in their households appear to protect these children from potentially blinding inflammatory trachoma.[67,68] Thus, health education to encourage these two health-related behaviors should accompany community-wide antibiotic treatment programs.

In children older than 8 years of age with severe-intensity infectious trachoma, systemic antibiotic treatment with a tetracycline or erythromycin derivative is more effective than topical treatment and should eliminate the extraocular reservoirs of *C. trachomatis*. Currently, the World Health Organization recommends systemic antibiotics for individuals with moderate-to-severe trachoma. This selective therapy involves screening the affected population for disease and assumes the monitoring of treated children for side effects.

In Tunisia, oral doxycycline (50 mg/day) given to school-age children with trachoma once daily on an intermittent schedule (5 days/mo for 6 months) significantly reduced the intensity of trachoma.[69] The tetracyclines, however, should not be used in children younger than 8 years of age, the group with the highest rates of active infectious trachoma. Although oral erythromycin can be used to treat these younger children, the pediatric suspensions (in doses of 30 to 50 mg/kg/day) are impractical for use in remote rural areas of developing countries.[70] Oral sulfonamides were once used for community-wide treatment of trachoma, but they had an unacceptably high rate of untoward reactions, some of which were very serious. Studies with the new long-acting azalide, azithromycin, have shown that a single dose (20 mg/kg) is as effective for active trachoma as 30 doses of topical tetracycline.[71,72] This erythromycin-like drug could well be the drug of choice for childhood trachoma. Azithromycin also has the advantage that it can be administered to children as young as 4 months of age.

Because trachoma is still a worldwide problem that is difficult to control by the present means of mass antibiotic therapy, possible specific vaccines are being developed in several laboratories.

The surgical correction of trichiasis and/or entropion has an immediate effect on preventing blindness. These simple procedures can be carried out in affected communities by mobile teams. Where ophthalmologists are not available, general physicians or auxiliary personnel can be trained to do these eyelid operations. In general, eyelid margin rotation procedures have been most successful[73] (see Ch. 6).

Excimer laser photoablation of superficial corneal opacities from trachoma has been reported, with improvement in visual acuity in two of three cases.[74] When appropriate, optical iridectomy may be useful and safe in restoring vision in patients with central corneal scarring. Penetrating keratoplasty has a poor prognosis in patients with trachoma. Reduced flow of aqueous tears, loss of mucin caused by goblet cell destruction, and poor mechanical surfacing as a result of eyelid deformities contribute to postoperative complications and graft opacification. Prosthokeratoplasty may be considered in patients with severe scarring in whom penetrating keratoplasty has no chance of success (see Ch. 36).

Adult Inclusion Conjunctivitis

Current recommendations for the treatment of genital *C. trachomatis* infections in adults are oral doxycycline, 100 mg twice a day for 7 days; ofloxacin, 300 mg twice a day for 7 days; erythromycin, 500 mg four times a day for 7 days; or azithromycin, 1.0 g as a single dose.[75] The duration of treatment for patients with the adult eye infection has not been determined but probably should be 10 to 14 days as a minimum. Adult inclusion conjunctivitis usually responds promptly to treatment for 3 weeks with full doses of systemic tetracycline (1.0 to 1.5 g daily) or erythromycin derivatives. Tetracycline should be administered 30 minutes before or 2 hours after meals and should not be given with milk, antacids, or other agents that inhibit gastric absorption. Tetracycline should not be used by pregnant women, nursing mothers, or children younger than the age of 8 years. In such patients, erythromycin or azithromycin are alternatives. Because adult inclusion conjunctivitis is a sexually transmitted disease, it is recommended that sexual partners be treated at the same time.

Topical tetracycline or erythromycin may temporarily suppress the ocular symptoms, but they do not affect the genital reservoir of the disease, and neither is satisfactory as the sole therapeutic agent. In addition, they do not improve outcome when given with systemic antibiotics.

Neonatal Inclusion Conjunctivitis

Untreated cases of neonatal inclusion conjunctivitis run a course of 3 to 12 months. The eye disease clears slowly with topical antibiotic treatment alone; however, topical treatment is insufficient to cure the frequently accompanying systemic infection. Oral erythromycin (40 mg/kg/day in four divided doses) for 2 weeks is indicated to treat not only the ocular infection but also the extraocular infection and to prevent pneumonia.[75] Parents should also be treated with systemic tetracycline, erythromycin, or azithromycin for their genital tract infections.

REFERENCES

1. Halberstaedter L, von Prowazek S: Zur Atiologie des Trachomas. Dtsch Med Wochenschr 33:1285, 1907
2. Linder K: Gonoblennorrhoe, Einschlussblennorrhoe und Trachom. Albrecht von Graefe's Arch Ophthalmol 78:380, 1911
3. World Health Organization: Strategies for the Prevention of Blindness. WHO, Geneva, 1984
4. Beem MO, Saxon EM: Respiratory tract colonization and a distinctive pneumonia syndrome in infants infected with *Chlamydia trachomatis.* N Engl J Med 293:306, 1977
5. Stephens RS: Challenge of *Chlamydia* research. Infect Agents Dis 1:279, 1992
6. Gordon FB, Quan AL: Occurrence of glycogen inclusions of psittacosis-lymphogranuloma venereum-trachoma agents. J Infect Dis 115:186, 1965
7. Wang SP, Grayston JT: Microimmunofluorescence antibody responses in *Chlamydia trachomatis* infection: a review. p. 301. In Mardh PA, Holmes KK, Oriel JD, et al (eds): Chlamydial Infections. Elsevier Biomedical Press, Amsterdam, 1982
8. Ostler HB, Schachter J, Dawson CR: Acute follicular conjunctivitis of epizootic origin. Arch Ophthalmol 82:587, 1969
9. Schachter J, Arnstein P, Dawson CR, et al: Human follicular conjunctivitis caused by infection with psittacosis agent. Proc Soc Exp Biol Med 127:292, 1968
10. Schachter J, Ostler HB, Meyer KF: Human infection with the agent of feline pneumonitis. Lancet 1:1063, 1969
11. Murray ES: Guinea pig inclusion conjunctivitis virus. I. Isolation and identification as a member of the psittacosis-lymphogranuloma-trachoma group of organisms. J Infect Dis 114:1, 1964
12. Kazdan JJ, Schachter J, Okumoto M: Inclusion conjunctivitis in the guinea pig. Am J Ophthalmol 64:116, 1967
13. Malaty M, Dawson CR, Wong I, et al: Serum and tear antibodies to *Chlamydia* after reinfection with guinea pig inclusion conjunctivitis agent. Invest Ophthalmol Vis Sci 21:833, 1981
14. Grayston JT, Kuo CC, Wang SP, Altman J: A new *Chlamydia psittaci* strain, TWAR, isolated in acute respiratory tract infections. N Engl J Med 315:161, 1987
15. Alexander ER: *Chlamydia:* the organism and neonatal infection. Hosp Prac 14:63, 1979
16. Friis RR: Interaction of L cells and *Chlamydia psittaci:* entry of the parasite and host responses to its development. J Bacteriol 110:706, 1972
17. Wyrick PB, Brownridge EM: Growth of *Chlamydia psittaci* in macrophages. Infect Immun 19:1054, 1978
18. Bavoil P, Ohlin A, Schachter JS: The role of disulfide bonding in outer membrane structure and permeability in *Chlamydia trachomatis.* Infect Immun 44:479, 1984
19. Caldwell H, Kromhout J, Schachter J: Purification and partial characterization of the major outer membrane protein of *Chlamydia trachomatis.* Infect Immun 31:1161, 1981
20. Stephens RS, Tam MI, Kuo CC, Nowinski RC: Monoclonal antibodies to *C. trachomatis:* antibody specificities and antigen characterization. J Immunol 128:1083, 1982
21. Stephens RS, Mullenbach G, Sanchez-Pescador R, Agabian N: Sequence analysis of the major outer membrane protein gene from *Chlamydia trachomatis* serovar L2. J Bacteriol 168:1277, 1986
22. Stephens RS, Sanchez-Pescador R, Wagar EA, et al: Diversity of *Chlamydia trachomatis* major outer membrane protein genes. J Bacteriol 169:3879, 1987
23. Dawson CR, Jones BR, Tarizzo M: Guide to the Control of Trachoma. World Health Organization, Geneva, 1981
24. Dawson CR, Juster JP, Lyon C, Schachter J: Response to treatment in ocular chlamydial infections (trachoma inclusion conjunctivitis): analogies with nongonococcal urethritis. p. 135. In Hobson D, Holmes KK (eds): Nongonococcal Urethritis and Related Infections. American Society for Microbiology, Washington, DC, 1977
25. Dawson CR, Juster R, Marx R, et al: Limbal disease in trachoma and other ocular chlamydial infections: risk factor for corneal vascularization. Eye 3:204, 1989
26. World Health Organization: Diagnosis of Trachoma. WHO, Geneva, 1973
27. Kupka K, Nizetic B, Reinhards J: Sampling studies of epidemiology and control of trachoma in southern Morocco. WHO Bull 39:547, 1968
28. Dawson CR, Schachter J, Ostler HB, et al: Inclusion conjunctivitis and Reiter's syndrome in a married couple. Arch Ophthalmol 83:300, 1970
29. Dawson CR, Schachter J: TRIC agent infections of the eye and genital tract. Am J Ophthalmol 63:1288, 1967
30. Gow JA, Ostler HB, Schachter J: Inclusion conjunctivitis with hearing loss. JAMA 229:519, 1974

31. Dawson CR, Jawetz E, Hanna L, et al: Experimental inclusion conjunctivitis in man. II. Partial resistance to infection. Am J Epidemiol 84:411, 1966
32. Dawson CR, Wood TR, Rose L, Hanna L: Experimental inclusion conjunctivitis. III. Keratitis and other complications. Arch Ophthalmol 78:341, 1967
33. Tullo AB, Richmond SJ, Easty DL: The presentation and incidence of paratrachoma in adults. J Hyg (Lond) 87:63, 1981
34. Morax V: Les Conjonctivities Folliculaires. Masson et Cie, Paris, 1933
35. Thygeson P, Stone W: Epidemiology of inclusion conjunctivitis. Arch Ophthalmol 27:91, 1942
36. Schachter J, Holt J, Goodner E, et al: Prospective study of chlamydial infection in neonates. Lancet 2:377, 1979
37. Rapoza PA, Quinn TC, Kiessling LA, et al: Assessment of neonatal conjunctivitis with a direct immunofluorescent monoclonal antibody stain for *Chlamydia*. JAMA 255:3369, 1986
38. Mordhorst C, Dawson CR: Sequelae of neonatal inclusion conjunctivitis and associated disease in parents. Am J Ophthalmol 71:861, 1971
39. Forster R, Dawson CR, Schachter J: Late follow-up of patients with neonatal inclusion conjunctivitis. Am J Ophthalmol 69:467, 1970
40. Goscienski PJ, Sexton RR: Follow-up studies in neonatal inclusion conjunctivitis. Am J Dis Child 124:180, 1972
41. Curth W, Curth HO, Sanders M: Chronic conjunctivitis due to the virus of venereal lymphogranuloma. JAMA 115:445, 1941
42. Applemans M: Conjonctivite infectious de Parinaud. Ophthalmologica 96:321, 1939
43. Klotz SA, Durtz JN, Milton RT, Reed HR: Hemorrhagic proctitis due to lymphogranuloma venereum serogroup L2. Diagnosis by fluorescent monoclonal antibody. N Engl J Med 308:1563, 1983
44. Forsey T, Darougar S: Acute conjunctivitis caused by an atypical *Chlamydia* strain IOL 207. Br J Ophthalmol 68:409, 1984
45. Badir G, Wilson RP, Maxwell-Lyons F: The histopathology of trachoma. Bull Egypt Ophthalmol Soc 46:129, 1953
46. Dhermy P, Coscas G, Nataf R, Levaditi JC: Histopathologie des follicules au cours du trachome et des conjonctivites folliculaires. Rev Int Trach 4:295, 1968
47. Duke-Elder S, Leigh AG: System of Ophthalmology. Vol. VIII. Diseases of the Outer Eye. Part I. Henry Kimpton, London, 1965
48. Treharne JD, Dines RJ, Darougar S: Serological responses to chlamydial ocular and genital infections in the United Kingdom and the Middle East. p. 249. In Hobson K, Holmes KK (eds): Nongonococcal Urethritis and Related Infections. American Society of Microbiology, Washington, DC, 1977
49. Hanna L, Jawetz E, Briones OC, et al: Antibodies to TRIC agents in tears and serum of naturally infected humans. J Infect Dis 127:95, 1973
50. Nichols RL, Oertley RE, Fraser CEO, et al: Immunity to chlamydial infections of the eye. VI. Homologous neutralization of trachoma infectivity for the owl monkey conjunctivae by eye secretions from humans with trachoma. J Infect Dis 127:429, 1973
51. Wang SP, Grayston JT: Pannus with experimental trachoma and inclusion conjunctivitis infection of Taiwan monkeys. Am J Ophthalmol 63:1133, 1967
52. Grayston JT, Kim KSW, Alexander ER, Wang SP: Protective studies in monkeys with trivalent and monovalent trachoma vaccines. p. 357. In Nichols RL (ed): Trachoma and Related Disorders Caused by Chlamydial Agents. Excerpta Med Int Congr Ser, Amsterdam, 1971
53. Wang SP, Grayston JT, Alexander ER: Trachoma vaccine studies in monkeys. Am J Ophthalmol 63:1615, 1962
54. Schachter J, Osoba AO: Lymphogranuloma venereum. Br Med Bull 39:151, 1983
55. Wang SP, Grayston JT, Kuo CC, et al: Serodiagnosis of *Chlamydia trachomatis* infections with the microimmunofluorescence test. p. 237. In Hobson K, Holmes KK (eds): Nongonococcal Urethritis and Related Infections. American Society of Microbiology, Washington, DC, 1977
56. Treharne JD, Dwyer STC, Darougar S, et al: Antichlamydial antibody in tears and sera and serotypes of *Chlamydia trachomatis* isolated from school children in southern Tunisia. Br J Ophthalmol 62:509, 1978
57. Frei W: Eine neue Hautreaktion bei Lymphogranuloma inguinale. Klin Wochenschr 4:2148, 1925
58. Grace AW, Rake G, Schaffer MF: A new material (Lygranum) for the performance of the Frei test for lymphogranuloma venereum. Proc Soc Biol Med 45:259, 1940
59. Yoneda C, Dawson CR, Daghfous T, et al: Cytology as a guide to the presence of chlamydial inclusions in Giemsa-stained conjunctival smears. Br J Ophthalmol 59:116, 1975
60. World Health Organization: Guide to the Laboratory Diagnosis of Trachoma. WHO, Geneva, 1975
61. Rice CE: Carbohydrate matrix of epithelial-cell inclusion in trachoma. Am J Ophthalmol 19:1, 1936
62. Tam MR, Stamm WE, Handsfield HH, et al: Culture independent diagnosis of *Chlamydia trachomatis* using monoclonal antibody. N Engl J Med 310:1146, 1984
63. Shepard JD, Kowalski RP, Meyer MP, et al: Immunodiagnosis of adult chlamydial conjunctivitis. Ophthalmology 95:434, 1988
64. Tantisira JG, Kowalski RP, Gordon YJ: Evaluation of the Kodak Surecell *Chlamydia* test for the laboratory diagnosis of adult inclusion conjunctivitis. Ophthalmology 102:1035, 1995
65. Kowalski RP, Uhrin M, Karenchak LM, et al: Evaluation of the polymerase chain reaction test for detecting chlamydial DNA in adult chlamydial conjunctivitis. Ophthalmology 102:1016, 1995
66. Schacter J, Moncada J, Dawson CR, et al: Nonculture methods for diagnosing chlamydial infection in patients with trachoma: a clue to the pathogenesis of the disease. J Infect Dis 158:1347, 1988
67. West SK, Congdon N, Katala S, Mele L: Facial cleanliness and risk of trachoma in families. Arch Ophthalmol 109:855, 1991

68. Courtright P, Sheppard J, Lane S: Latrine ownership as a protective factor in inflammatory trachoma in Egypt. Br J Ophthalmol 75:322, 1991
69. Dawson CR, Schachter J: Strategies for treatment and control of blinding trachoma. Cost-effectiveness of topical or systemic antibiotics. J Infect Dis 7:768, 1985
70. Dawson CR, Daghfous T, Hoshiwara I, et al: Trachoma therapy with topical tetracycline and oral erythromycin: a comparative trial. Bull WHO 60:347, 1982
71. Dawson CR, Sallam S, Sheta A, et al: Trachoma treatment with oral azithromycin or topical tetracycline. Invest Ophthalmol Vis Sci 34:851, 1993
72. Bailey RL, Arullendran P, Whittle HC, Mabey DE: Randomization controlled trial of single dose azithromycin in treatment of trachoma. Lancet 342:453, 1993
73. Bog H, David Y, Foster A: Results of community based eyelid surgery for trichiasis due to trachoma. Br J Ophthalmol 77:81, 1993
74. Goldstein M, Loewenstein A, Rosner M, et al: Phototherapeutic keratectomy in the treatment of corneal scarring from trachoma. J Corneal Refract Surg 10(suppl):S290, 1994
75. Centers for Disease Control and Prevention: 1993 Sexually Transmitted Diseases. Treatment Guidelines. MMWR 42(No. RR-14):51, 1993

15

Parasitic Infections

ALLAN RICHARD RUTZEN AND MARY BETH MOORE

A variety of organisms ranging from unicellular protozoa to insects can be grouped together as parasites. Parasites live on or in a host organism to obtain nutrition. Some, such as *Acanthamoeba,* are facultative parasites, capable of living apart from the host organism, whereas others are obligate parasites, incapable of living without the host. This chapter is concerned with the following parasitic diseases that affect the cornea: *Acanthamoeba* keratitis; infections caused by other unicellular protozoa; infections caused by worms, including a variety of roundworms, tapeworms, and flukes; and ocular disorders caused by arthropods.

ACANTHAMOEBA KERATITIS

Organism

In 1930, Sir Aldo Castellani[1] described an ameba with morphologic features now considered characteristic of the genus *Acanthamoeba.* Early in the study of amebae, confusion existed regarding the taxonomy and nomenclature because there was no agreement on categorization based on features such as morphology, nutritional requirements, and serology.[2] According to current nomenclature, only two genera of free-living amebae cause human disease: *Acanthamoeba* and *Naegleria.*[3] The species responsible for *Acanthamoeba* keratitis include *A. castellani, A. polyphaga, A. culbertsoni, A. rhysodes,* and *A. hatchetti.* However, differentiation of *Acanthamoeba* at the species level is difficult and unreliable and is of limited clinical importance.[2,4] Even within a particular species, various isolates have different degrees of virulence and sensitivity to antiamebic therapy. In addition to keratitis, *Acanthamoeba* can cause other rare diseases, such as granulomatous amebic encephalitis, pneumonitis, and subacute granulomatous dermatitis. Inoculation with *Naegleria*-contaminated water can result in primary amebic encephalitis, an uncommon and rapidly fatal infection of the central nervous system.

Acanthamoeba is widely distributed in the environment and has been isolated from air, soil, swimming pools, hot tubs, ponds, municipal water supplies, bottled drinking water, contact lenses, and contact lens solutions.[5-7] *Acanthamoeba* has also been isolated from the nasal and oral mucosa of asymptomatic individuals.[8] Recent evidence indicates, however, that only a fraction of *Acanthamoeba* isolates from environmental sources or asymptomatic individuals are pathogenic.[5]

Acanthamoeba may be found in two forms: trophozoites and cysts (Figure 15-1). The metabolically active and motile trophozoites are the infective and invasive form of the organism. They reproduce by binary fission. Trophozoites usually feed on bacteria or fungi in their environment and may rarely infect human corneal or brain tissue. When trophozoites are exposed to unfavorable environmental conditions or exhaust their supply of nutrients, they encyst. Encystation renders the organism resistant to heat, cold, desiccation, changes in pH, and medical therapy.[5,9] Cysts are truly dormant, with no detectable metabolic activity. Because they are relatively resistant to attack by the host immune system, cysts may persist in host tissues for many months.[10,11] Under favorable environmental conditions, cysts excyst to the trophozoite form.

Epidemiology

Acanthamoeba keratitis was first reported in 1973.[12] Since then, many cases have been reported. Although exposure to *Acanthamoeba* is common, infection is relatively rare.

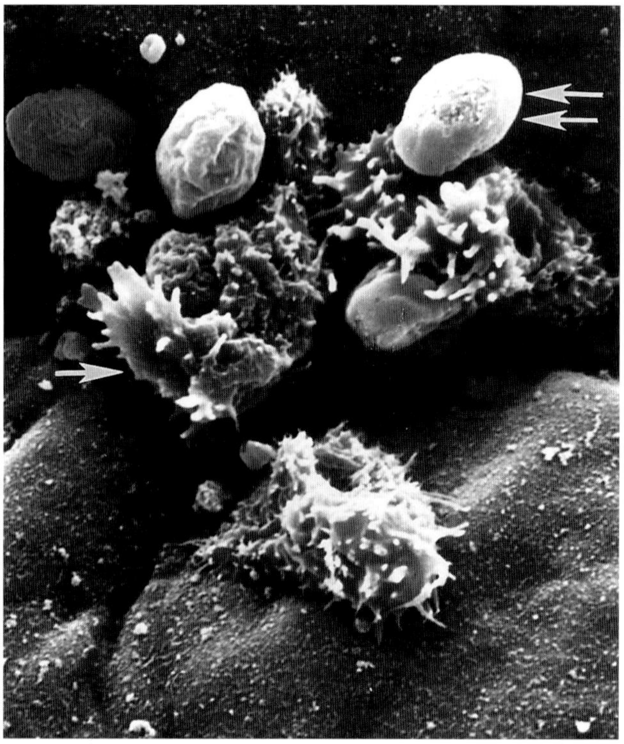

FIGURE 15-1 Scanning electron micrograph of *Acanthamoeba castellani* trophozoites (single arrow) and cysts (double arrow). Note acanthopodia on the trophozoites. Trophozoites measure 16 to 47 μm in length and cysts are 10 to 25 μm in diameter (× 5,000). (Courtesy of Mel Trousdale, Ph.D., Los Angeles, CA.)

Acanthamoeba keratitis comprises fewer than 1 percent of cases of infectious keratitis.[13]

Risk factors include contact lens wear, corneal trauma, and exposure to contaminated water. The predominant risk factor is contact lens wear; approximately 85 percent of patients with *Acanthamoeba* keratitis have worn contact lenses.[14] All types of contact lenses have been implicated, including daily-wear soft, extended-wear soft, disposable soft, rigid gas-permeable, and polymethyl methacrylate contact lenses. Homemade saline solutions, infrequent lens disinfection, and exposure to contaminated water while wearing contact lenses are factors that play a role in contact lens–associated *Acanthamoeba* keratitis.[10,14–17]

Risk factors for patients who do not wear contact lenses include corneal trauma, exposure to contaminated water, and exposure to vegetable matter or insects.[18–20] In some patients, however, no identifiable predisposing factor can be identified. *Acanthamoeba* keratitis usually occurs in immunologically normal individuals.[20]

Pathogenesis

The pathogenesis of *Acanthamoeba* keratitis is poorly understood. Corneal infection depends on inoculation with a virulent isolate of *Acanthamoeba*, the presence of a suitable environment for its growth, and the host response. As noted above, the virulence of *Acanthamoeba* isolates is variable.[4] It is not known whether the inoculum must contain trophozoites to initiate a corneal infection or whether cysts can excyst on the ocular surface and cause an active infection.

The association between contact lens wear and *Acanthamoeba* keratitis has prompted studies of contact lens systems. The potential for contamination of contact lenses with *Acanthamoeba* is great because of the widespread distribution of the organism in the environment. *Acanthamoeba* has been demonstrated in contact lens cases and contact lens solutions of patients with *Acanthamoeba* keratitis.[15,16,21–23] Lens care systems contaminated with *Acanthamoeba* are also frequently contaminated with bacteria or fungi, which may be a food source for *Acanthamoeba*.[15,24] Some studies have shown that as many as 7 percent of lens storage cases used by asymptomatic lens wearers are contaminated with *Acanthamoeba*.[25]

Acanthamoeba trophozoites and cysts are capable of adhering to soft and hard contact lenses,[26–31] and cysts have been found on the surface of a contact lens from a patient with *Acanthamoeba* keratitis.[32] In vitro studies have shown that *Acanthamoeba* binds to contact lenses exposed to the organism for as little as 10 seconds.[28,31] Although *Acanthamoeba* is capable of adhering to new contact lenses, the biofilm and particulate debris on used lenses may increase the adherence and viability of the organism.[26,29] Heat disinfection kills *Acanthamoeba* trophozoites and cysts, but the lenses may become contaminated if nonsterile solutions, such as homemade saline solution or tap water, are used to rinse, store, or lubricate the lenses. In addition, some methods of chemical contact lens disinfection are ineffective in eradicating *Acanthamoeba*, as described below in the section on prevention.

It is not known whether *Acanthamoeba* is capable of invading healthy corneal epithelium or whether a break in the surface is required. In vitro morphologic studies show that *Acanthamoeba* can adhere to intact corneal epithelium and burrow between epithelial cells.[4,26,33] Although epithelial damage may not be a prerequisite for amebic infection, breaks in the epithelium or damage from contact lens–related hypoxia probably facilitate the development of amebic keratitis. In a hamster model, greater numbers of *Acanthamoeba* bound to de-epithelialized corneas, compared with corneas with intact epithelium.[34,35] Similarly, application of *Acanthamoeba*-laden contact lenses to de-epithelialized corneas resulted in keratitis, whereas an intact epithelium appeared to prevent the development of infection.[35]

Acanthamoeba initially invades the superficial stroma. Histopathologic specimens from the initial stages of the infection are rare, but early cases show trophozoites and cysts in the anterior stroma, with little inflammatory cell infiltration.[36] As the infection progresses, decreased numbers of keratocytes are observed histologically, especially in the anterior stroma. The inflammatory response is predominantly composed of polymorphonuclear leukocytes and rare macrophages.[11,36] Lymphocytes are notably absent, and leukocytic infiltration is found more in the anterior stroma than in the posterior stroma. In established infections, it is common to observe full-thickness invasion of trophozoites and cysts, but the leukocytic infiltration is found mainly in the anterior stroma.[36] Various degrees of stromal necrosis and necrotic inflammatory cells are seen on histopathologic examination. The stromal necrosis and thinning may be attributable to enzymes released by the inflammatory cells or to enzymes released by *Acanthamoeba*.[36] In almost all cases, there is a striking lack of corneal neovascularization, even in cases with severe and chronic inflammation.[11,36]

Bacterial coinfection may play a role in the development of *Acanthamoeba* keratitis. Corneal cultures from patients with suspected *Acanthamoeba* keratitis reveal a variable rate of bacterial coinfection, with some studies reporting a coinfection rate as high as 58 percent.[23,37] It has been suggested that bacteria may enhance the pathogenicity of *Acanthamoeba* by serving as a source of nutrition for the amebae until the nutrients liberated by stromal necrosis become available. When *Acanthamoeba* was injected into the stroma of immunologically normal rats, corneal manifestations were mild and self limited; infection resolved over several weeks without treatment.[38,39] When avirulent bacteria were added to the *Acanthamoeba* inoculum, however, a severe suppurative keratitis rapidly ensued.[39]

The host response to *Acanthamoeba* is poorly understood. Humoral immunity, cellular immunity, and complement activation may each play a role in the prevention of infection and in the eradication of an established infection. Probably as the result of environmental exposure, human serum contains antibodies to *Acanthamoeba*.[40] These antibodies may be important in opsonization of *Acanthamoeba*, in fixation of complement on the amebic plasma membrane, and in the neutralization of amebic toxins.[40] Studies using an animal model have suggested that local mucosal immune mechanisms are important in immunity to *Acanthamoeba* keratitis.[41] Animals were protected against challenges with *Acanthamoeba* after oral and topical immunization with *Acanthamoeba* antigen but not after intramuscular or subconjunctival immunization, despite high levels of serum antibody titers. It has been hypothesized that secretory IgA antibodies may account for this immunity.

As stated above, the cellular response to *Acanthamoeba* keratitis consists mainly of polymorphonuclear leukocytes; macrophages and lymphocytes are rarely seen.[11,20,36,42–44] The cell-mediated response is important in the eradication of both trophozoites and cysts from the cornea, but *Acanthamoeba* cysts appear to be capable of evading the host response for extended periods of time and reactivating to cause recurrence late in the course of the infection.

In vitro studies have shown that *Acanthamoeba* is capable of activating complement by the alternative pathway.[40] Activation of complement may generate opsonic factors used for the phagocytosis of the organism and may lead to the production of inflammatory mediators important in the pathogenesis of *Acanthamoeba* keratitis.

Clinical Features

The early signs and symptoms of *Acanthamoeba* keratitis are usually nonspecific, with the hallmark features developing only as the infection progresses into the later stages. A review of the literature reveals a remarkably high frequency of misdiagnosis early in the course of *Acanthamoeba* keratitis.[20,23] *Acanthamoeba* keratitis can mimic keratitis caused by herpesvirus, bacteria, mycobacteria, and fungi. Table 15-1 lists the principal clinical features of this infection.

Acanthamoeba keratitis begins with an insidious onset of symptoms. The rate of development is variable, however, and symptoms may emerge slowly over weeks to months or may rapidly worsen within several days after the

TABLE 15-1
Clinical Features of Acanthamoeba Keratitis

Young, healthy, immunocompetent individuals
History of corneal contact with
Contact lens
Contaminated fluids (distilled water, tap water, well water, hot-tub water, saliva, saline)
Foreign body, minor trauma
Usually unilateral (rarely bilateral)
Severe eye pain
Epithelial irregularities
Patchy stromal infiltrates, ring infiltrates, perineural infiltrates, satellite lesions
Absence of corneal neovascularization
Mild anterior chamber inflammation, rare hypopyon
Scleritis

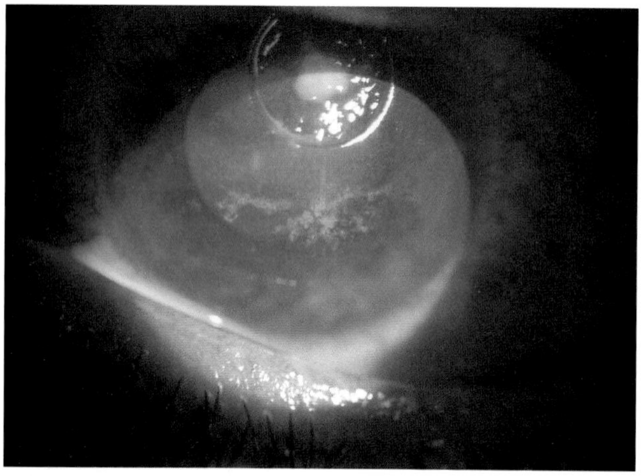

FIGURE 15-2 Dendritiform epithelial lesions demonstrated by fluorescein staining in a patient with *Acanthamoeba* keratitis. A circular biopsy site is seen superior to the lesions.

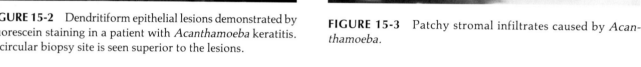

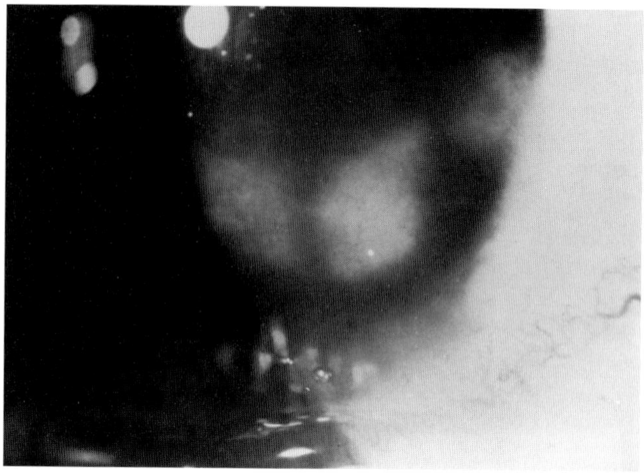

FIGURE 15-3 Patchy stromal infiltrates caused by *Acanthamoeba.*

presumed inciting event.[20] Overall, the course of the infection is usually chronic and gradually progressive and may, in some patients, have periods of temporary remission.[20,42]

As with other forms of keratitis, patients may report a foreign body sensation, ocular pain, tearing, photophobia, and/or blurred vision. The pain from *Acanthamoeba* keratitis is relatively severe and helps to distinguish this infection from other infections. The pain is usually out of proportion to the objective clinical findings and may require strong analgesics, narcotics, or a modified retrobulbar alcohol injection for alleviation.

Because the portal of entry of *Acanthamoeba* is presumably through the corneal epithelium, the superficial layers of the cornea are the first to be affected. In most cases, the epithelium is abnormal; in some patients, however, the epithelium appears relatively unaffected. Nonspecific epitheliopathy may be one of the first clinical manifestations of *Acanthamoeba* infection and may be characterized by punctate keratitis, elevated epithelial lines, or dendritiform irregularities[45] (Figure 15-2). These dendritiform lesions are frequently white or gray, plaque-like, and slightly raised and stain variably with fluorescein. As the lesions progress, epithelial ulceration may occur.

As the infection progresses over a period of weeks, stromal involvement generally increases. Stromal infiltrates occur centrally or paracentrally and may appear patchy or confluent (Figure 15-3). Early stromal infiltrates may be subepithelial or located within the anterior stroma. They frequently develop into a partial or complete ring configuration that is highly indicative of *Acanthamoeba* keratitis (Figure 15-4). The stroma central to the ring may appear normal or have a granular whitish infiltrate. In rare cases, a concentric double-ring infiltrate may occur. The presence of a partial or complete ring infiltrate may be rare in the early stages of the infection but is common in advanced stages.[23] The percentage of patients demonstrating a ring infiltrate varies from 19 to 93 percent, depending on the stage of infection, whether and when antiamebic treatment was initiated, and whether topical corticosteroids have been used.[23,44] The epithelium overlying the stromal infiltrates may be intact or ulcerated. A distinctive feature of *Acanthamoeba* keratitis is the absence of stromal neovascularization, even in relatively severe and long-standing cases.[11] As the infection progresses, the full thickness of the stroma may become involved, with extensive necrosis, thinning, and eventual corneal perforation.

Linear infiltrates may be observed along the corneal nerves (Figure 15-5), resulting in radial keratoneuritis.[46] This finding is nearly pathognomonic of *Acanthamoeba* keratitis; only one case of radial keratoneuritis has been reported in a patient who did not have *Acanthamoeba* keratitis but rather *Pseudomonas* keratitis.[47] The perineural infiltrates arise relatively early in the course of *Acanthamoeba* keratitis and may be present in as many as 71 percent of patients. These infiltrates are found in the mid stroma and may extend from the paracentral cornea to the limbus. The propensity of *Acanthamoeba* to cause perineural infiltrates may explain the unusually severe pain and corneal hypesthesia found in many patients with *Acanthamoeba* keratitis.[48]

Scleritis may be observed in advanced cases and is characterized by severe ocular pain, deep scleral vascular engorgement, and scleral nodules.[49-51] The frequency of scleritis ranges from 11 to 42 percent, depending on the

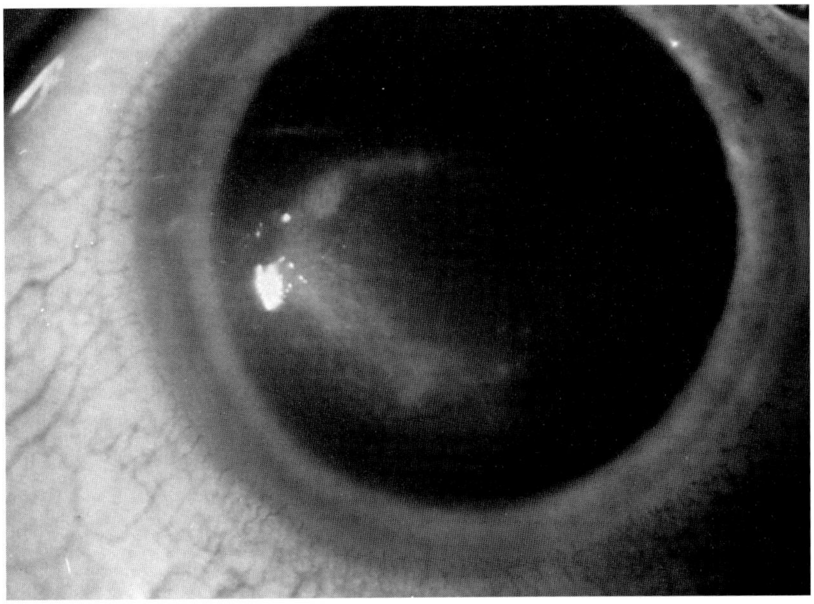

FIGURE 15-4 Ring infiltrate caused by *Acanthamoeba*. (Courtesy of Wayne Bowman, M.D., Dallas, TX.)

stage of the infection.[23,50] Most patients have sectorial areas of anterior scleritis contiguous with areas of keratitis. In one advanced case, posterior scleritis and optic neuritis were observed.[50] In most cases, the scleritis is probably a secondary immunologic response, rather than a true scleral infection with *Acanthamoeba*. After resolution of inflammation, scleral ectasia may occur.[50,51] *Acanthamoeba* has not been detected in scleral tissue in the vast majority of reported biopsy and enucleation specimens; only one case of scleral infection has been described—in an enucleation specimen from a patient who developed an overwhelming *Acanthamoeba* infection despite treatment with antiamebic medications, topical corticosteroids, penetrating keratoplasty, and scleral cryotherapy.[36,49]

Anterior chamber inflammation in cases of early *Acanthamoeba* keratitis is usually mild but increases as the infection progresses.[23] In late stages, uveitis is present in most patients, and a hypopyon is observed in as many as 46 percent of patients.[23] Occasionally, elevated intraocular pressure and cataracts are observed, most often in patients with severe and prolonged intraocular inflammation.[20,23]

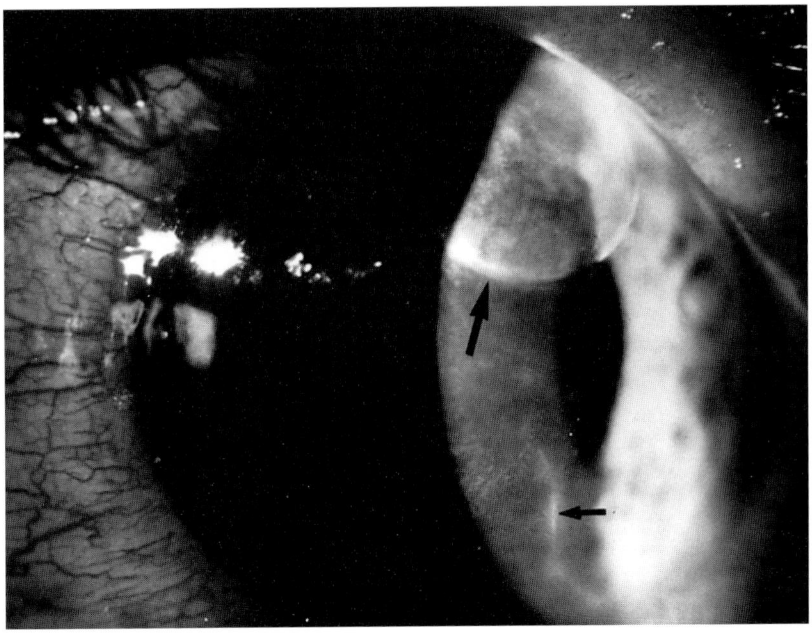

FIGURE 15-5 Radial corneal nerve infiltrate (small arrow) that is nearly pathognomonic of *Acanthamoeba* keratitis. (Large arrow, biopsy site.) (Reprinted with permission from MB Moore, JP McCulley, HE Kaufman, JB Robin: Radial keratoneuritis as a presenting sign in *Acanthamoeba* keratitis. Ophthalmology 93:1310, 1986. Courtesy of Ophthalmology.)

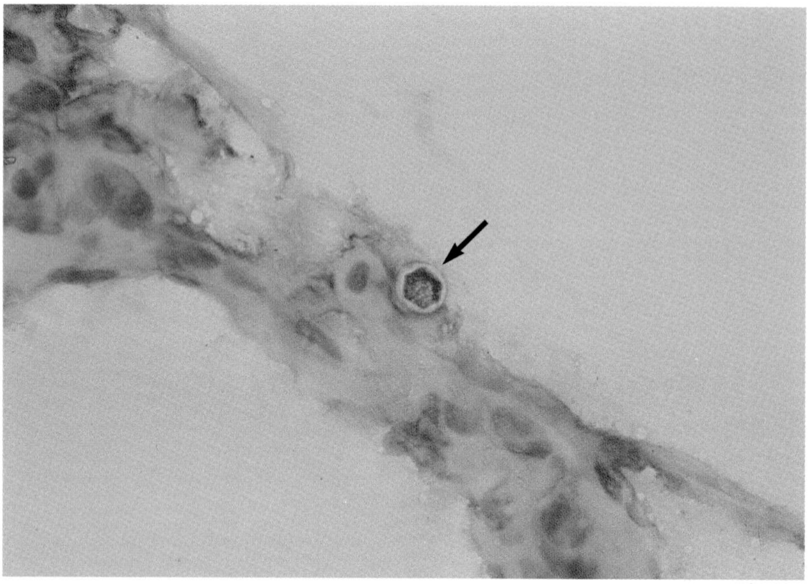

FIGURE 15-6 Corneal scraping stained with Masson trichrome stain demonstrating a polygonal cyst of *Acanthamoeba* (arrow). (Courtesy of Catherine Newton, M.D., Louisville, KY.)

Late in the course of the infection, after other clinical signs of inflammation have resolved, patients may develop subepithelial corneal infiltrates.[52] Many small, round subepithelial infiltrates may be found widely distributed in the cornea, including areas distant from the previous focus of infection. One report described clinical improvement with topical corticosteroids after antiamebic therapy had been discontinued, suggesting an immunologic rather than an actively infectious basis for this clinical finding. Caution must be exercised in the interpretation of late corneal infiltrates because recurrent or persistent infection may be present.

Laboratory Diagnosis

In cases of suspected *Acanthamoeba* keratitis, even when the index of suspicion is high, it is essential to confirm the diagnosis with laboratory techniques before instituting antiamebic therapy. Because of its varied clinical presentation, *Acanthamoeba* keratitis may be mistaken for other clinical disorders, such as herpetic, fungal, bacterial, or sterile contact lens-related keratitis. Corneal scrapings and cultures, as well as examination and culture of contact lenses and contact lens solutions, are usually sufficient to identify the causative organism (Figure 15-6). In some cases, however, a corneal biopsy is required. If available, confocal microscopy may be a useful noninvasive method to detect *Acanthamoeba* in vivo.

Corneal scrapings may be taken from areas of abnormal epithelium or ulceration but may fail to reveal the presence of *Acanthamoeba* in early cases when the epithelium is intact or in cases in which the superficial cornea is relatively unaffected. To maximize the diagnostic yield of corneal scrapings, the affected cornea should be scraped aggressively with a spatula or a # 15 Bard-Parker blade. The scraping is then touched to a glass slide and is immediately fixed with methyl alcohol for 3 to 5 minutes to prevent air drying, which may rupture trophozoites.

Various stains may be used to demonstate *Acanthamoeba,* including calcofluor white, Gram, Giemsa, Wright, trichrome, Hemacolor, methylene blue, Congo red, Janus green, lugol solution, periodic acid–Schiff, Gomori's methenamine silver, and immunofluorescent antibody stains.[53,54] With some stains, *Acanthamoeba* may be confused with macrophages or other mononuclear cells. For this reason, calcofluor white stain is recommended because of the ease of identification of *Acanthamoeba.*

Calcofluor white stain is a relatively simple and reliable method for the detection of *Acanthamoeba,* even in cases in which Gram and Giemsa stains fail to reveal organisms.[53] Calcofluor white is a fabric brightener that has an affinity for chitin and cellulose, which are components of the cell walls of *Acanthamoeba* cysts and fungi but not of *Acanthamoeba* trophozoites. A solution containing 0.1 percent calcofluor white and 0.1 percent Evans blue counterstain is applied to the specimen for 5 minutes. The excess solution is removed, a coverslip is placed, and the specimen is examined with a fluorescence microscope. *Acanthamoeba* cysts appear as apple-green structures 10 to 25 μm in diameter[53,55,56] (Figure 15-7). Trophozoites are considerably more difficult to detect with this method because they do not absorb calcofluor white. However,

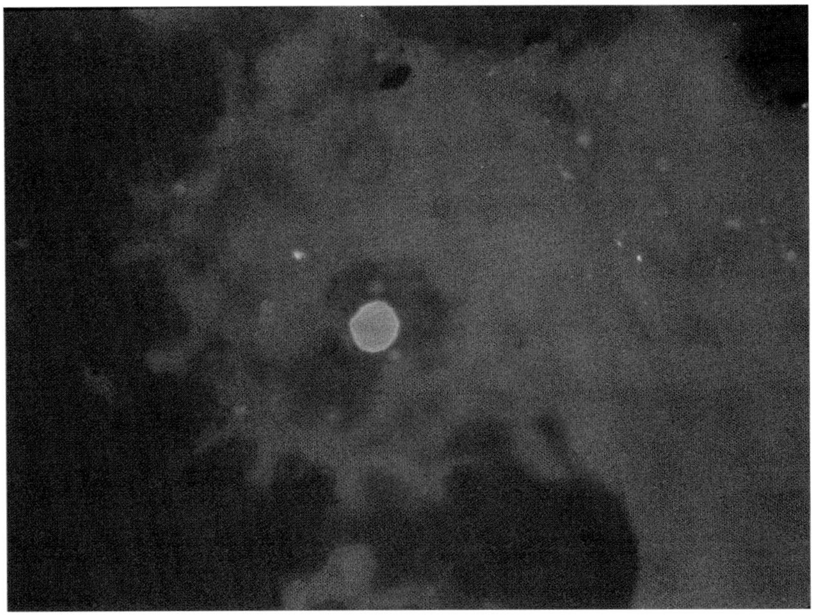

FIGURE 15-7 Calcofluor white-stained cyst in a corneal scraping from a patient with culture-proven *Acanthamoeba* keratitis. (Courtesy of Kirk R. Wilhelmus, M.D., Houston, TX.)

the Evans blue counterstain shows the trophozoites as red-brown, irregularly shaped structures 15 to 20 μm in length. Enzymatic digestion of the background stroma may enhance visualization of *Acanthamoeba* trophozoites and cysts in tissue sections stained with calcofluor white, but this additional step is not ordinarily necessary.[56]

Although *Acanthamoeba* may grow on blood or chocolate agar, cultures of *Acanthamoeba* should include inoculation onto non-nutrient agar with an *Escherichia coli* overlay. This may be accomplished by inoculating the scraping onto non-nutrient agar with a pre-existing *E. coli* overlay or by inoculating the scraping onto non-nutrient agar, which is then coated with a suspension of *E. coli.* Immediate inoculation of the scraping onto the culture plate prevents evaporation and maximizes the likelihood of recovering *Acanthamoeba.* If immediate inoculation is not possible, the scraping may be placed in ameba transport medium. Two cultures on non-nutrient agar and *E. coli* should be inoculated; one should be incubated at 22°C and the other at 37°C. The culture plates should be sealed with adhesive tape to prevent evaporation and loss of *Acanthamoeba* organisms from drying. When these plates are examined under a microscope, one may see wavy tracts created by the trophozoites as they traverse the culture plate consuming *E. coli* in their path (Figure 15-8). Under high magnification, irregularly shaped trophozoites may be observed directly. Large numbers of trophozoites are usually evident by 3 days of incubation but may appear as early as 1 day.[45] *Acanthamoeba* encyst when the *E. coli* food source is consumed. If no organisms are initially detected, the culture plates should be incubated for 2 weeks before a negative culture result is reported. Occasionally, fine wavy tracts of *Acanthamoeba* trophozoites may be detected on blood or chocolate agar cultures without an *E. coli* overlay.

If a patient with suspected *Acanthamoeba* keratitis is a contact lens wearer, the lenses and lens care solutions should be cultured for *Acanthamoeba.* A positive culture from the lenses or solutions is helpful when corneal scrapings and cultures are negative. A fragment of the contact lens may be placed directly onto non-nutrient agar with an *E. coli* overlay. If *Acanthamoeba* is present, the trophozoites will migrate onto the culture plate. Large volumes of contact lens solutions can be filtered through a 5-μm polycarbonate membrane filter, which is then placed upside down on the culture plate.

Contact lenses can be examined directly with light microscopy to provide rapid confirmation of *Acanthamoeba* keratitis.[32] An excised fragment of the contact lens is placed on a microscope slide with a coverslip and examined unstained or after staining with several drops of 0.1 percent calcofluor white. Evans blue counterstain should not be used because it stains the contact lens intensely. The anterior and posterior surfaces of the contact lens are examined with ×200 to ×400 magnification for the presence of *Acanthamoeba.*

Confocal microscopy can be used for the noninvasive detection of *Acanthamoeba* in vivo.[57–59] *Acanthamoeba* cysts appear as highly refractile, spherical structures 10 to 20 μm in diameter (Figure 15-9). Other ovoid objects may be observed during confocal microscopy of patients with *Acanthamoeba* keratitis and may represent inflammatory cells, trophozoites, or altered keratocytes.

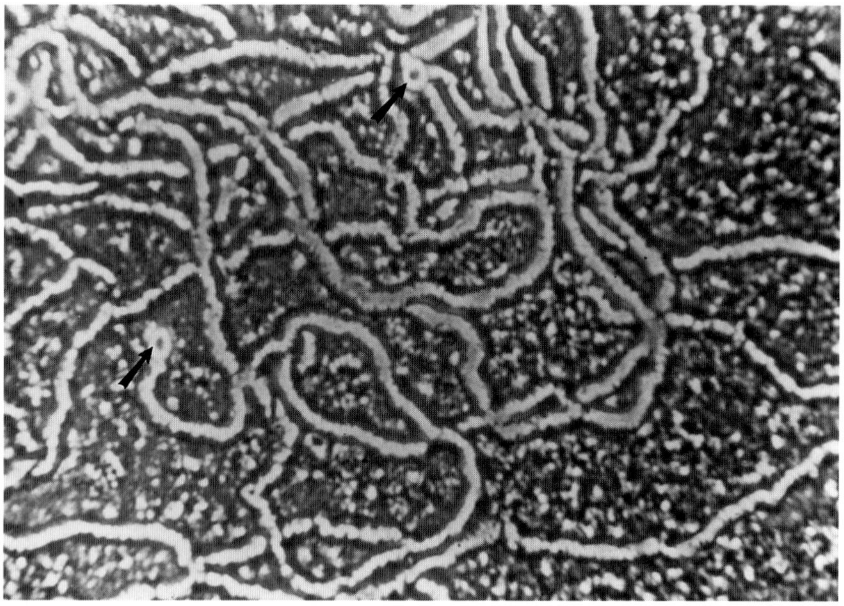

FIGURE 15-8 Maze of paths on a culture plate created by the consumption of *E. coli* by *Acanthamoeba* trophozoites (arrows).

If the initial laboratory evaluation is negative for *Acanthamoeba*, a corneal biopsy may be required to confirm the diagnosis (Figure 15-10). A corneal biopsy is particularly valuable in cases in which the infiltrate is deep in the cornea. A 1.5- or 2-mm corneal trephine may be used to obtain a biopsy specimen from an area of infiltration peripheral to the visual axis. The specimen should be cultured and processed for histopathologic examination and electron microscopy, if available (Figure 15-11). Scrapings from the base of the biopsy site can be stained as described above and may provide a rapid diagnosis in some cases.

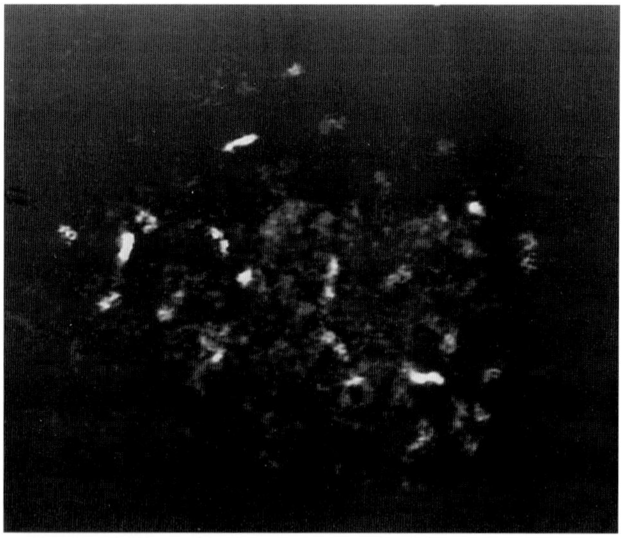

FIGURE 15-9 Confocal micrograph of *Acanthamoeba*. The circular bright structures are cysts; the elongated irregularly shaped structures are trophozoites. (Courtesy of Stephen C. Kaufman, M.D., New Orleans, LA.)

Treatment

Medical treatment of *Acanthamoeba* keratitis is difficult, partly because the cysts are not as sensitive to antiamebic agents as are the trophozoites. It is therefore important to consider the efficacy of various agents against cysts, and not only trophozoites, because cysts represent the most difficult obstacle to the eradication of *Acanthamoeba* from infected tissues. The optimal medical regimen for the treatment of *Acanthamoeba* keratitis is not well defined. Current clinical practices have been based on studies of in vitro efficacy of medications and retrospective reports of the results of treatment with various medical regimens. Confusion exists about the in vitro efficacy of antiamebic medications because of a lack of standardized methodology in various reports, including differences in the phase of the cultures during antiamebic challenge, methods of culture preparation, size of the inoculum, duration of exposure to the agents tested, and criteria for determination of antiamebic efficacy.[60]

Although in vitro susceptibility data have been used as a basis for the selection of certain antiamebic agents for clinical use, the results of clinical studies have not shown a strong correlation between in vitro susceptibility and in vivo clinical efficacy.[9,61] The lack of correlation may be

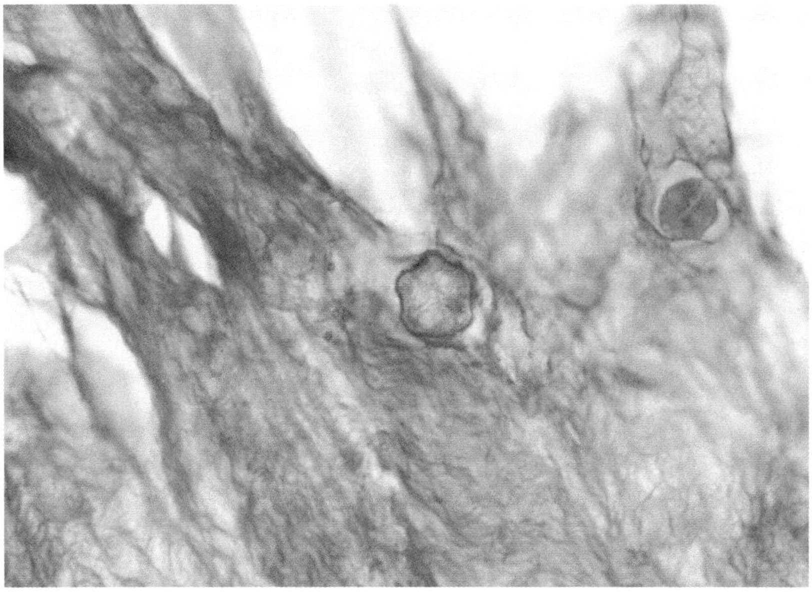

FIGURE 15-10 *Acanthamoeba* cysts in a corneal biopsy specimen (periodic acid–Schiff stain).

due, in part, to differences in the susceptibility of different *Acanthamoeba* isolates to various antiamebic compounds. Interpretation of clinical reports of *Acanthamoeba* treatment is problematic because of differences in the severity of infection, the duration of infection at the onset of therapy, the frequent misdiagnosis and use of topical corticosteroids before the initiation of antiamebic therapy, the combined use of medical therapy and penetrating keratoplasty at various stages of the infection, and variation in the duration and intensity of treatment.[60] In addition, it is difficult to compare treatment regimens when various combinations of as many as five agents (both topical and oral) are studied.

Several agents have been studied to assess their in vitro antiamebic effect. These agents include the cationic antiseptics (polyhexamethylene biguanide, chlorhexidine), the aromatic diamidines (propamidine isethionate, dibromopropamidine, stilbamidine isethionate, hydroxystilbamidine, pentamidine), the aminoglycosides (neomycin, paromomycin), the imidazoles (miconazole, ketocona-

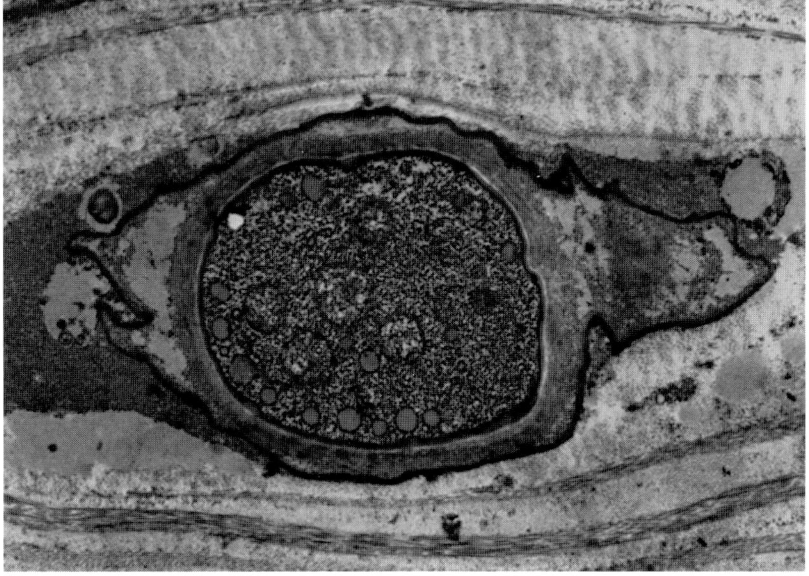

FIGURE 15-11 Electron micrograph of an encysted amebic organism. (Courtesy of Lia Pedroza, New Orleans, LA.)

zole, clotrimazole, itraconazole), and others (pimaricin, ciclopirox olamine).[60,62-66] Only a few agents from this extensive list have demonstrated the ability to destroy cysts in concentrations that might be achievable in the cornea. Although susceptibility of various *Acanthamoeba* isolates varies widely, in vitro studies generally demonstrate cysticidal activity of polyhexamethylene biguanide, propamidine, neomycin, paromomycin, miconazole, ketoconazole, pimaricin, and ciclopirox olamine. Clinical experience with many of these agents is limited, however.

Polyhexamethylene biguanide is perhaps the most promising antiamebic agent under investigation. Although the number of clinical cases reported is relatively small, favorable clinical results have been reported when topical polyhexamethylene biguanide is used in combination with other agents.[9,23,61,65,67,68] This compound is the active ingredient in a pool cleaning product (Baquacil) but is not commercially available as an ophthalmic medication and has not been approved for ophthalmic use by the Food and Drug Administration. When used in experimental protocols, polyhexamethylene biguanide is diluted in an unpreserved artificial tear vehicle from a 20 percent stock solution to a final 0.02 percent solution. In vitro studies generally report that polyhexamethylene biguanide is both trophocidal and cysticidal at relatively low concentrations and is effective against many species of gram-positive and gram-negative bacteria. When sensitivity testing is performed using various *Acanthamoeba* isolates, polyhexamethylene biguanide is consistently effective against these isolates, in contrast to other agents, which show wide variation in their effectiveness against various *Acanthamoeba* isolates.[61,68] This compound appears to be well tolerated by patients and has low levels of epithelial toxicity, unlike propamidine, neomycin, and other agents.[9,23,61,68]

Topical propamidine isethionate, in combination with other medications, is the most commonly used drug to treat *Acanthamoeba* keratitis.[23,69] In 1985, the first medical cure of *Acanthamoeba* keratitis was reported; the medical regimen included a combination of topical propamidine isethionate, dibromopropamidine, and neomycin.[70] Subsequently, other reports of treatment with propamidine isethionate described only fair results, with a small proportion of patients showing progression despite a variety of intensive combination regimens that included propamidine isethionate.[71,72] More recent reports of treatment with this drug have shown excellent cure rates and improved prognoses.[9,23,68,69,73] This may be due to several factors, including early diagnosis. Propamidine isethionate (0.1 percent) is not commercially available in the United States and has not been approved by the Food and Drug Administration but is available as a nonprescription medication (Brolene eye drops) in the United Kingdom and many European countries. Dibromopropamidine (0.15 percent Brolene ointment) is a closely related form of this agent and has been used in conjunction with propamidine isethionate to treat *Acanthamoeba* keratitis. In vitro sensitivity testing has shown that propamidine isethionate has excellent trophocidal activity. Although propamidine isethionate is usually cysticidal against most *Acanthamoeba* isolates, the sensitivity of various *Acanthamoeba* isolates to propamidine isethionate is variable.[9,60,61,65] A slightly additive effect in cysticidal activity is found when propamidine isethionate is combined with neomycin or paromomycin.[60] Propamidine isethionate has low levels of toxicity, but reversible epithelial toxicity may occur during prolonged treatment.[74]

Almost all reports on the treatment of *Acanthamoeba* keratitis have described combination therapy that included either neomycin or paromomycin. Neomycin is readily available as a topical ophthalmic solution. Paromomycin is available in 250-mg capsules that must be dissolved in an artificial tear vehicle to a final concentration of 2.5 percent (25 mg/ml). In vitro sensitivity studies have shown excellent trophocidal activity of these two agents but variable cysticidal activity.[9,60,65,70] Because of their strong trophocidal activity, it has been postulated that their therapeutic effect is due to their ability to reduce the trophozoite population and possibly to eliminate bacterial coinfection.[9] Adverse reactions to prolonged use of these agents are common and may include corneal epithelial toxicity, slow epithelial healing, conjunctival hyperemia, and other signs and symptoms of local toxicity.[68,70]

The role of oral medications in the treatment of *Acanthamoeba* keratitis is not clear. Oral itraconazole and ketoconazole have been used successfully in combination with topical medications in several reports, but in vitro sensitivity studies show that most *Acanthamoeba* isolates are not sensitive to these agents.[9,10,63,67] These oral medications may cause serious side effects such as headache, gastritis, and liver dysfunction.

Because no single agent has been shown to be exceedingly effective in the treatment of *Acanthamoeba* keratitis, it is generally agreed that a multiple-drug regimen is required. If possible, the initial treatment of *Acanthamoeba* keratitis should begin with a combination of topical polyhexamethylene biguanide, propamidine isethionate, and neomycin. These drops are given every 15 to 60 minutes for the first week. If epithelial toxicity is observed, the neomycin should be discontinued. If the patient shows clinical improvement, the drops may be tapered to four times a day and should be continued for several months. Long-term maintenance therapy to prevent recurrence should be continued using polyhexamethylene biguanide

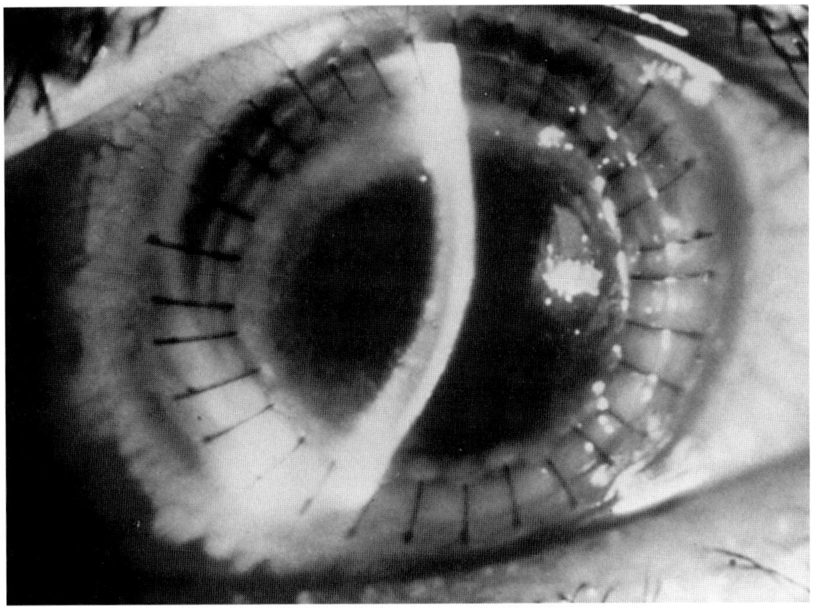

FIGURE 15-12 Recurrent *Acanthamoeba* keratitis in a corneal graft. (Courtesy of Henry Gelender, M.D., Dallas, TX.)

once or twice a day for 1 year or longer after the signs of active infection have resolved. Some clinicians have advocated the use of epithelial debridement at the time of diagnosis because it may reduce the number of infectious organisms and may facilitate the corneal penetration of some antiamebic medications.[63,72,75]

Corticosteroids should not be used in the treatment of *Acanthamoeba* keratitis. Some authors have advocated their use because of their ability to suppress corneal inflammation, to decrease pain, and to treat associated scleritis.[69,73] However, suppression of the host immune response by corticosteroids may have a detrimental effect on the eradication of *Acanthamoeba* and may facilitate further corneal invasion by the organism.[48,64,76] The host response to *Acanthamoeba* consists primarily of polymorphonuclear leukocytes, which may be inhibited by corticosteroids.[43] Additionally, because treatment of *Acanthamoeba* keratitis usually continues for months, it is advisable to avoid the long-term complications of corticosteroid administration, such as cataract formation and glaucoma. Although many patients are given corticosteroids before the establishment of the correct diagnosis of *Acanthamoeba* keratitis, corticosteroids should be quickly tapered and stopped once the infection is diagnosed.[64]

Penetrating keratoplasty is indicated for the treatment of *Acanthamoeba* keratitis only in patients with impending or actual corneal perforation and in patients who have visually significant corneal scarring after the infection has resolved with medical treatment. Penetrating keratoplasty should not be performed in the setting of active *Acanthamoeba* infection, except for impending or actual corneal perforation, and it is not recommended as a method of decreasing the infectious load of the organism. The success rate of penetrating keratoplasty during active *Acanthamoeba* infection is poor because the infection frequently recurs in the graft, and the graft fails. Recurrence of the infection is caused by residual organisms peripheral to the clinically apparent infiltrate that were not excised during keratoplasty. Cryotherapy of the cornea has been attempted to eradicate residual *Acanthamoeba* organisms, but results have been unsatisfactory.[18,77-79] When *Acanthamoeba* recurs in a graft, an arcuate infiltrate central to the keratoplasty wound is usually apparent (Figure 15-12). Recurrent *Acanthamoeba* keratitis after penetrating keratoplasty is difficult to treat and typically results in graft failure. When penetrating keratoplasty is performed after signs of active infection have disappeared, graft survival and visual results are good.[73,80]

Although conjunctival flaps have been attempted to cure the infection and alleviate symptoms, they should not be performed in patients with active infection because the infection progresses beneath the flap and erodes through the flap in 1 to 3 weeks.[20]

The importance of early diagnosis and treatment of *Acanthamoeba* keratitis cannot be overemphasized. There is a clear association between early diagnosis and successful medical treatment.[10,20,23,68,69,72] In patients treated within 1 month of initial symptoms, the prognosis for medical

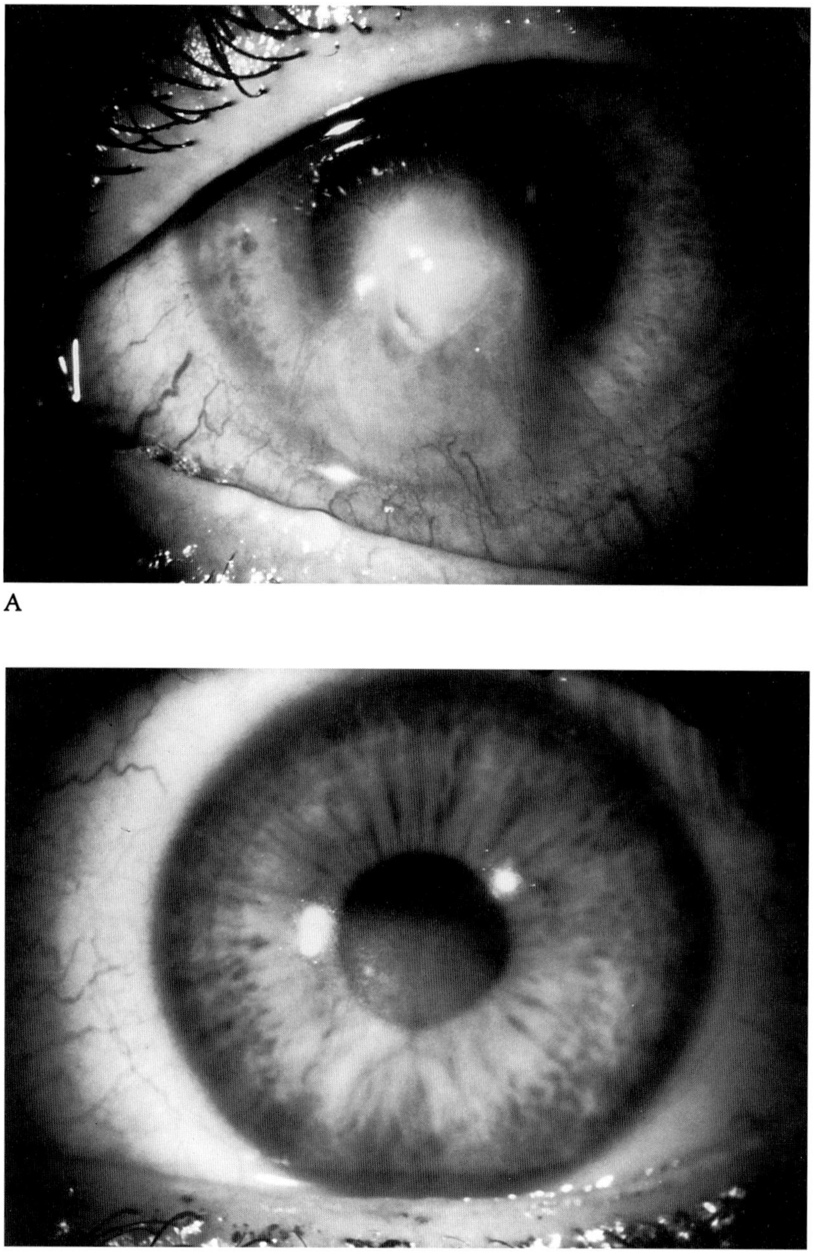

A

B

FIGURE 15-13 **(A)** Active *Acanthamoeba* keratitis diagnosed in a contact lens wearer in 1984. **(B)** After treatment with topical Brolene, Neosporin, and miconazole, the keratitis resolved, leaving a faint scar.

cure and preservation of vision is excellent[23,68,69,72] (Figure 15-13). In patients with a delay in diagnosis, the prognosis is poor. One report described a final visual acuity of at least 20/40 in all 15 eyes of patients who were treated within 1 month of initial symptoms, whereas only 17 (53 percent) of 32 eyes of patients who presented late in the course of the infection achieved a final visual acuity of 20/40 or better.[69] A correspondingly higher percentage of patients treated late in the course of the infection require penetrating keratoplasty to restore good vision. In addition to corneal scarring, other causes of poor visual outcome include uncontrollable *Acanthamoeba* infection, failed penetrating keratoplasty, glaucoma, and cataract.[20,23,69,70,80,81]

Prevention

Because 85 percent of cases of *Acanthamoeba* keratitis occur in contact lens wearers, preventive measures have focused on this subgroup of individuals. It may be possible to minimize the risk of *Acanthamoeba* keratitis through the education of eye care practitioners and ultimately contact lens wearers. Contact lens wearers must be informed of appropriate lens care and wearing practices to effectively eradicate viable *Acanthamoeba* organisms and to reduce the likelihood of subsequent contamination. Conscientious contact lens care should involve meticulous hand washing, thorough lens cleaning, effective lens disinfection, and suitable lens rinsing and storage practices.

The cleaning step using commercially prepared contact lens cleaners is an important measure to decrease *Acanthamoeba* and bacterial contamination. In vitro studies have shown that *Acanthamoeba* trophozoites and cysts readily adhere to soft contact lenses,[26,29,30] but the number of adherent *Acanthamoeba* organisms is decreased after washing.[29-31] In addition, particulate debris on contact lenses probably facilitates *Acanthamoeba* adhesion.[29] It is, therefore, advantageous to thoroughly clean lenses to decrease the number of adherent *Acanthamoeba* organisms as well as to remove particulate debris and to decrease the population of viable bacteria.

Effective disinfection to eradicate *Acanthamoeba* from contact lenses may be accomplished by heat disinfection or by several commercially available chemical disinfection systems. Heat disinfection is suitable only for certain types of lenses and is not advisable for high-water-content soft lenses or rigid gas-permeable lenses. This method is effective in eradicating *Acanthamoeba* trophozoites and cysts only when adequate temperatures are achieved.[21,82,83] In vitro studies have shown that 15 minutes at 65°C or 2 minutes at 70°C is adequate to kill *Acanthamoeba* cysts.[82] In practice, some heat disinfection units may fail to kill *Acanthamoeba* if they do not attain suitable temperatures.[82]

Many chemical disinfection solutions are commercially available. However, the ability to kill *Acanthamoeba* is not required by the Food and Drug Administration, and as a result, only a few are capable of eradicating *Acanthamoeba*. Solutions containing hydrogen peroxide, benzalkonium chloride, chlorhexidine, and thimerosal in combination with ethylenediaminetetraacetic acid (EDTA) are generally effective, given the appropriate concentration and exposure times.

Disinfection solutions containing hydrogen peroxide are effective in killing *Acanthamoeba* cysts and trophozoites but require adequate exposure times. In vitro studies have shown that 3 percent hydrogen peroxide requires at least 2 to 4 hours to kill *Acanthamoeba* cysts.[21,84-86] Hydrogen peroxide can be used in a two-step process in which the lenses are disinfected in 3 percent hydrogen peroxide for at least 4 hours, followed by neutralization with a catalytic neutralizing agent. Other hydrogen peroxide disinfection systems use a metal catalyst that is present from the beginning of the disinfection step. In these systems, however, the hydrogen peroxide concentration decreases relatively rapidly, and therefore the exposure to hydrogen peroxide is not sufficient to kill *Acanthamoeba*.[85]

There is wide variation in the effectiveness of other agents. Some studies have shown that solutions containing 0.005 percent chlorhexidine are effective against *Acanthamoeba*, with exposure times as short as 30 minutes.[84,85] Other studies have variable results but show generally that chlorhexidine is amebicidal within 4 hours of exposure.[21,86,87] Solutions containing 0.004 percent benzalkonium chloride are effective in killing *Acanthamoeba* after 1 hour of exposure.[84,85] Thimerosal alone is not effective, but commercially available solutions containing 0.002 or 0.004 percent thimerosal combined with 0.1 percent edetate disodium are effective after 4 to 8 hours.[84-86] Polyaminopropyl biguanide (0.00005 percent) and 0.001 percent polyquaternium-1 are not effective, even with long exposure times.[84,85]

It is important to avoid lens contamination subsequent to disinfection. Lenses may become contaminated from irrigation or storage in contaminated solutions or when the contact lens wearer is exposed to water while swimming, bathing, or using a hot tub. Contact lens wearers should not use homemade saline solution. Preserved saline solution or nonpreserved solution in an aerosol container is preferable to nonpreserved saline solution in a squirt bottle. Saline solution should be purchased in relatively small quantities and discarded 1 or 2 weeks after it is opened; after the expiration date, even unopened containers should be thrown away. The use of contact lens cases with two separate wells may be preferable to single-well cases because it decreases the risk of cross contamination. After prolonged storage, contact lenses should be disinfected before use. Through conscientious contact lens care and wear, it should be possible to decrease the risk of *Acanthamoeba* keratitis. Contact lenses that are worn for 1 day and then thrown away are now available commercially. Because these lenses are not disinfected by patients, the risk of *Acanthamoeba* keratitis from improper disinfection is nil.

UNICELLULAR PROTOZOA

Leishmaniasis

Leishmania spp. are obligate intracellular protozoa transmitted by the bites of infected sandflies. Leishmaniasis is classified as a zoonosis because it is a disease of animals that is capable of afflicting humans. Rodents and dogs are the usual reservoir hosts for *Leishmania*. When

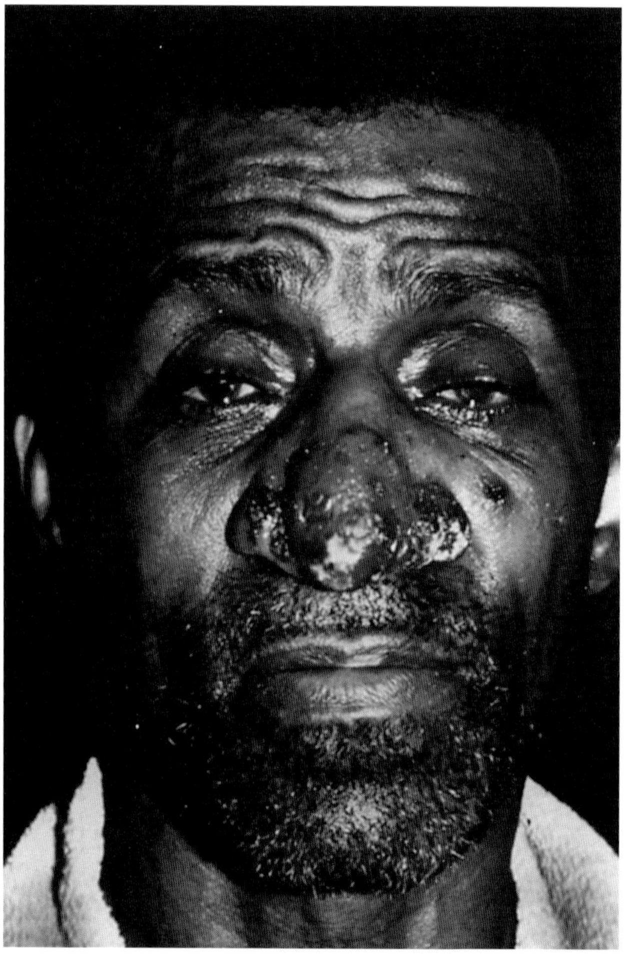

A

sandflies suck the blood from infected animals, they become infected and are capable of transmitting the parasite to humans. The sandfly vectors are found throughout the Middle East, India, Africa, Central America, and South America. Depending on the parasite species, *Leishmania* can cause cutaneous, mucocutaneous, or visceral disease.

The cutaneous form, the so-called oriental sore, develops as a single nodule at the site of a sandfly bite. On injection into human skin, the organisms are ingested by local macrophages and multiply intracellularly. Parasite-laden macrophages eventually lyse, releasing organisms that infect new macrophages. The lesion enlarges centrifugally, ulcerates, and scars. Flies biting active lesions become infected and are capable of transmitting the disease. Mucocutaneous leishmaniasis is characterized by cutaneous lesions as well as destructive lesions involving the mucous membranes and cartilage of the oral cavity, nasal septum, and larynx. Visceral leishmaniasis, also known as kala-azar or black fever, causes splenomegaly and liver and bone marrow involvement, but the eyes are usually not affected.

Infection of the eyelids and conjunctiva results in inflammation, ulceration, and scarring. When the eyelids are affected, cicatricial ectropion may occur. Nodular granulomas of the conjunctiva[88] and interstitial keratitis[89] have been reported (Figure 15-14). Corneal involvement begins with superficial phlyctenules that quickly become deep infiltrates. Corneal abscess formation can lead to corneal perforation. Ocular infection is presumed to be the result of direct inoculation of the

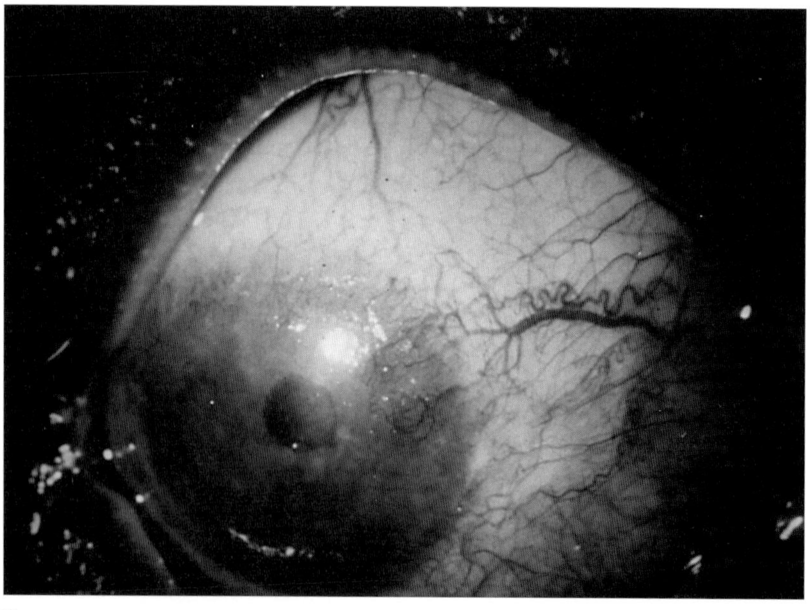

B

FIGURE 15-14 **(A)** A 58-year-old man with mucocutaneous leishmaniasis. **(B)** Diffuse leukoma, superficial vascularization, and cellular infiltration of the cornea. (Reprinted with permission from J Roizenblatt: Interstitial keratitis caused by American [mucocutaneous] leishmaniasis. Am J Ophthalmol 87:175, 1979. Copyright by The Ophthalmic Publishing Company.)

conjunctiva, contiguous spread from skin lesions near the eye, or hematogenous spread.

In endemic areas, the diagnosis of leishmaniasis is usually made on clinical grounds. The diagnosis can be confirmed with scrapings from the leading edge of an ulcer or with aspiration of fluid from beneath the ulcer. When stained with Wright or Giemsa stain, intracellular *Leishmania* organisms may be detected. Scrapings or aspirated fluid can be cultured for *Leishmania* if the stains are nondiagnostic. Skin tests using *Leishmania* antigen may be helpful in some cases.

Depending on the species of *Leishmania,* some cutaneous lesions may heal spontaneously, whereas others require systemic therapy. When ocular involvement is present, a combination of systemic and topical therapy is advisable. Meglumine antimoniate or sodium stibogluconate is given either intravenously or intramuscularly and is capable of eradicating the intracellular parasites. Topical therapy with stilbamidine hydrochloride drops may be beneficial. Secondary infections, such as bacterial cellulitis or myiasis (infection with fly maggots), may occur in some settings and should be treated accordingly.

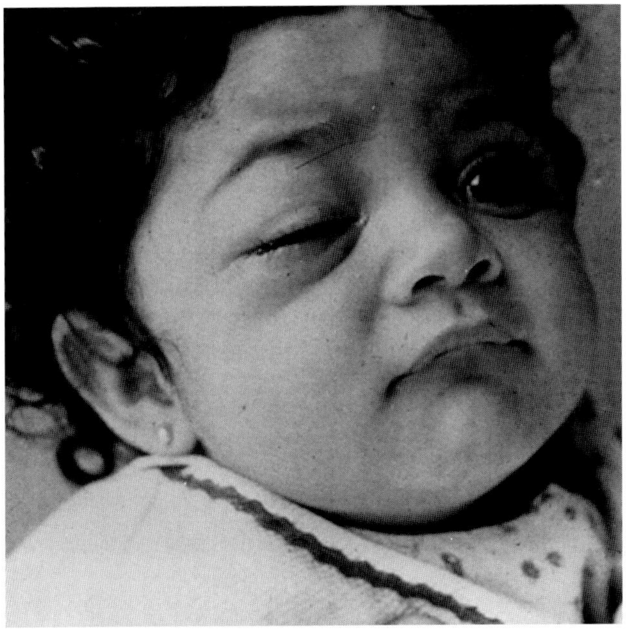

FIGURE 15-15 Child with Romaña sign caused by trypanosomiasis. (Reprinted with permission from CH Binford, DH Connor [eds]: Pathology of Tropical and Extraordinary Diseases. Armed Forces Institute of Pathology, Washington, DC, 1976. Courtesy of the Armed Forces Institute of Pathology, AFIP 62-3934-6.)

Trypanosomiasis

Trypanosoma spp. are capable of producing two distinct diseases commonly referred to as African trypanosomiasis and American trypanosomiasis. Only American trypanosomiasis is associated with ocular involvement. American trypanosomiasis, also known as Chagas' disease, is caused by the organism *Trypanosoma cruzii* and is found in South America, Central America, and rarely, North America.

This disease is classified as a zoonosis. A variety of animals are reservoir hosts, and the parasite is transmitted to humans by reduviid bugs. The infectious form of *Trypanosoma* is found in the feces of the reduviid bug. At the time of taking a blood meal, the reduviid bug usually defecates, depositing infectious organisms on the skin near the bite. The organisms enter the human host either through the bite or through mucous membranes that are rubbed with contaminated fingers. The organisms proliferate within the subcutaneous tissues or mucous membranes and spread to the regional lymph nodes. The erythematous nodule that develops on the skin or conjunctiva is known as a chagoma. When the trypanosomes enter through the conjunctiva, the constellation of eyelid edema, conjunctivitis, and preauricular lymphadenopathy is known as *Romaña sign*[90] (Figure 15-15). Interstitial keratitis (similar to syphilitic keratitis), iritis, and conjunctival hyperemia have been described in experimental studies in dogs and in humans.[91-93] Histology of corneal sections reveals trypanosomes between corneal lamellae. Symptoms of disseminated infection usually appear weeks after the initial bite. Fever, malaise, lymphadenopathy, hepatosplenomegaly, meningoencephalitis, and cardiac arrhythmias may develop. The severity of the disease is variable; it is most severe in young children.

The diagnosis is usually made by detection of trypanosomes in the blood or through serologic testing. Treatment is problematic because the reproductive form of the organism is intracellular in host tissues and is difficult to eradicate. Nifurtimox or benznidazole is recommended as initial therapy.

Microsporidiosis

Microsporidiosis is caused by organisms of the phylum Microspora. Three genera have been associated with ophthalmic disease: *Microsporidium, Nosema,* and *Encephalitozoon.* These organisms are minute, obligate intracellular parasites that multiply within the cytoplasm of infected host cells, followed by the formation of spores. Ocular microsporidiosis is an uncommon disease in immuno-

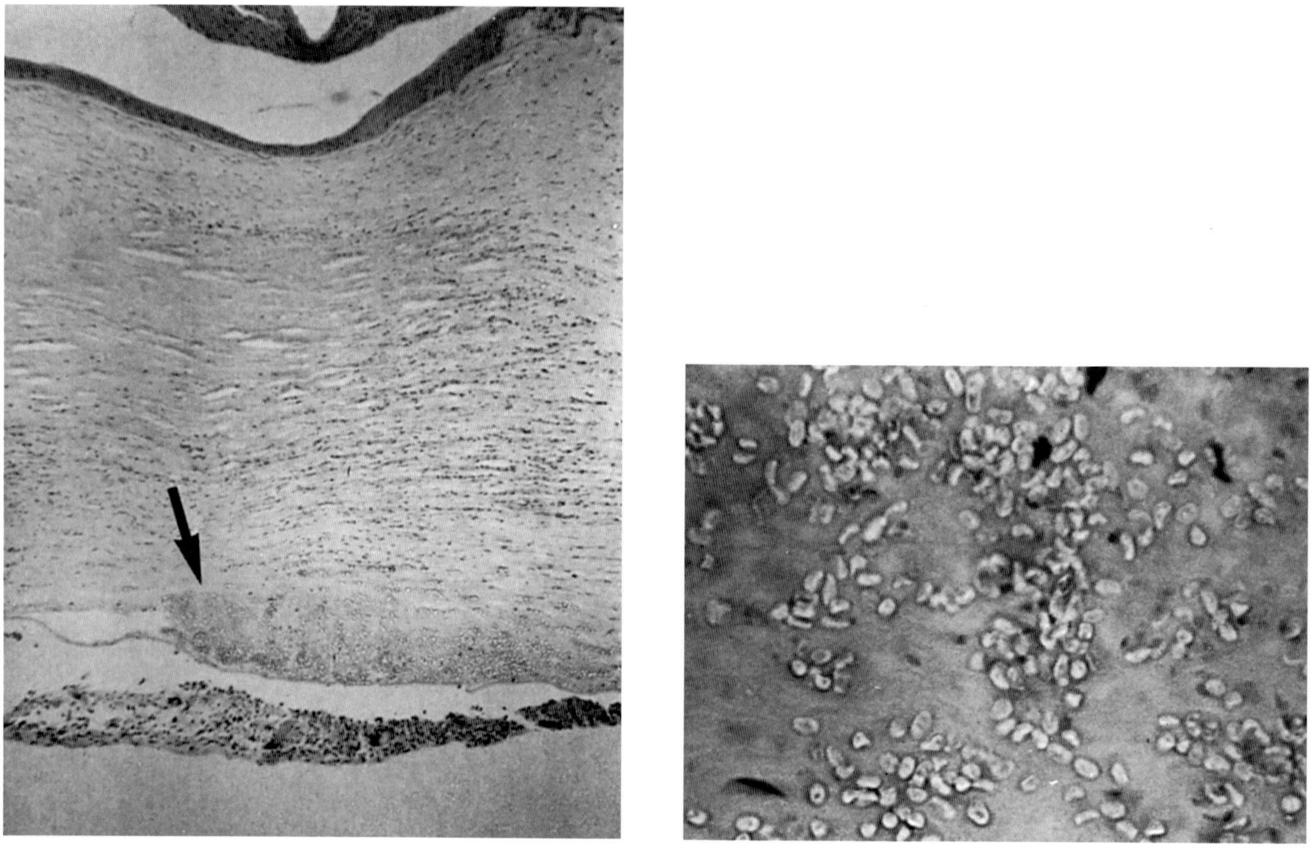

A B

FIGURE 15-16 **(A)** Corneal button from an 11-year-old boy with nosematosis demonstrating refractile spores anterior to Descemet's membrane (arrow). Note the inflammatory exudate on the posterior surface of the cornea. **(B)** Higher magnification of the area near the arrow in Fig. A showing many refractile spores. (Reprinted with permission from CH Binford, DH Connor [eds]: Pathology of Tropical and Extraordinary Diseases. Armed Forces Institute of Pathology, Washington, DC, 1976. Courtesy of the Armed Forces Institute of Pathology, AFIP 73-10783 and 73-10784.)

competent individuals but has been recognized with increasing frequency in patients with acquired immunodeficiency syndrome.

Corneal microsporidiosis exhibits characteristic clinical features depending on the genus involved. *Microsporidium* and *Nosema* usually infect immunocompetent individuals after direct ocular inoculation of the organisms from a contaminated source or by trauma.[94–97] The organisms penetrate the deep stroma, where they may cause corneal ulceration, disciform keratitis, necrotizing keratitis, and corneal perforation (Figure 15-16). The infection generally remains localized to the eye.

Encephalitozoon usually infects individuals with acquired immunodeficiency syndrome who have a CD4 (T-helper cell) count less than 100 cells/μl.[97–107] Infection is limited to the superficial cornea and conjunctiva, causing ocular irritation, photophobia, and decreased vision. Infected individuals have bilateral epithelial keratitis characterized by diffuse, fine punctate epithelial opacities that may be worse in the interpalpebral area (Figure 15-17). These lesions stain variably with fluorescein, and the conjunctiva usually shows little or no hyperemia. Deep corneal involvement has not been observed in these patients. Individuals with ocular encephalitozoon infection usually show systemic infection with the parasite and frequently shed parasites in the urine.[107]

The diagnosis of ocular microsporidiosis is established through scraping or biopsy of the conjunctiva or cornea. Microsporidial organisms may be observed with Giemsa, Gram, hematoxylin-eosin, or calcofluor white stains. Specimens stained with Giemsa stain show spores with blue cytoplasm and a red-purple nucleus. Gram stain

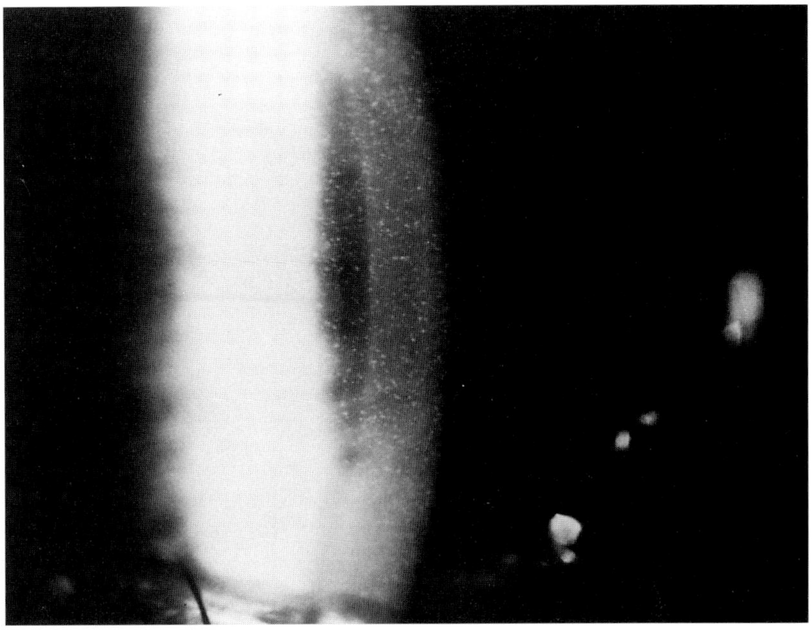

FIGURE 15-17 Microsporidial keratitis in a patient with acquired immunodeficiency syndrome. (Reprinted with permission from DN Friedberg, SM Stenson, JM Orenstein, et al: Microsporidial keratoconjunctivitis in acquired immunodeficiency syndrome. Arch Ophthalmol 108:504, 1990. Copyright 1990, American Medical Association.)

reveals gram-positive intracellular spores (Figure 15-18). Electron microscopy is useful to confirm the diagnosis and to determine the species of the organism[108] (Figure 15-19).

Treatment of ocular microsporidiosis is problematic because the organism is resistant to antimicrobial agents.[109] Treatment with topical fumagillin, topical propamidine isethionate, or oral itraconazole may be effective in controlling the symptoms of this infection.[100,110,111] Treatment must be continued indefinitely because symptoms usually recur if the medications are discontinued.

NEMATODES (ROUNDWORMS)

Onchocerciasis

Onchocerciasis is caused by *Onchocerca volvulus* and involves mainly the skin, subcutaneous tissue, and eyes. Onchocerciasis is a leading cause of blindness worldwide.[112-117] Humans are the principal host of this nematode; there are no animal reservoirs. The intermediate host and vector of *Onchocerca* is the blackfly *(Simulium)*. Blackflies live only near fast-flowing rivers and streams

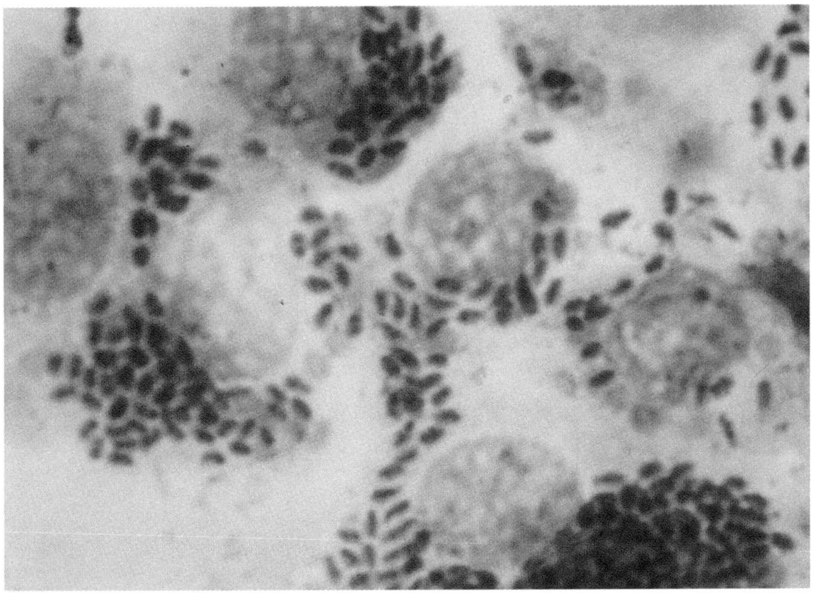

FIGURE 15-18 Gram stain of a conjunctival scraping from a patient with microsporidial keratoconjunctivitis showing many large gram-positive ovoid organisms within conjunctival epithelial cells. (Reprinted with permission from DN Friedberg, SM Stenson, JM Orenstein, et al: Microsporidial keratoconjunctivitis in acquired immunodeficiency syndrome. Arch Ophthalmol 108:504, 1990. Copyright 1990, American Medical Association.)

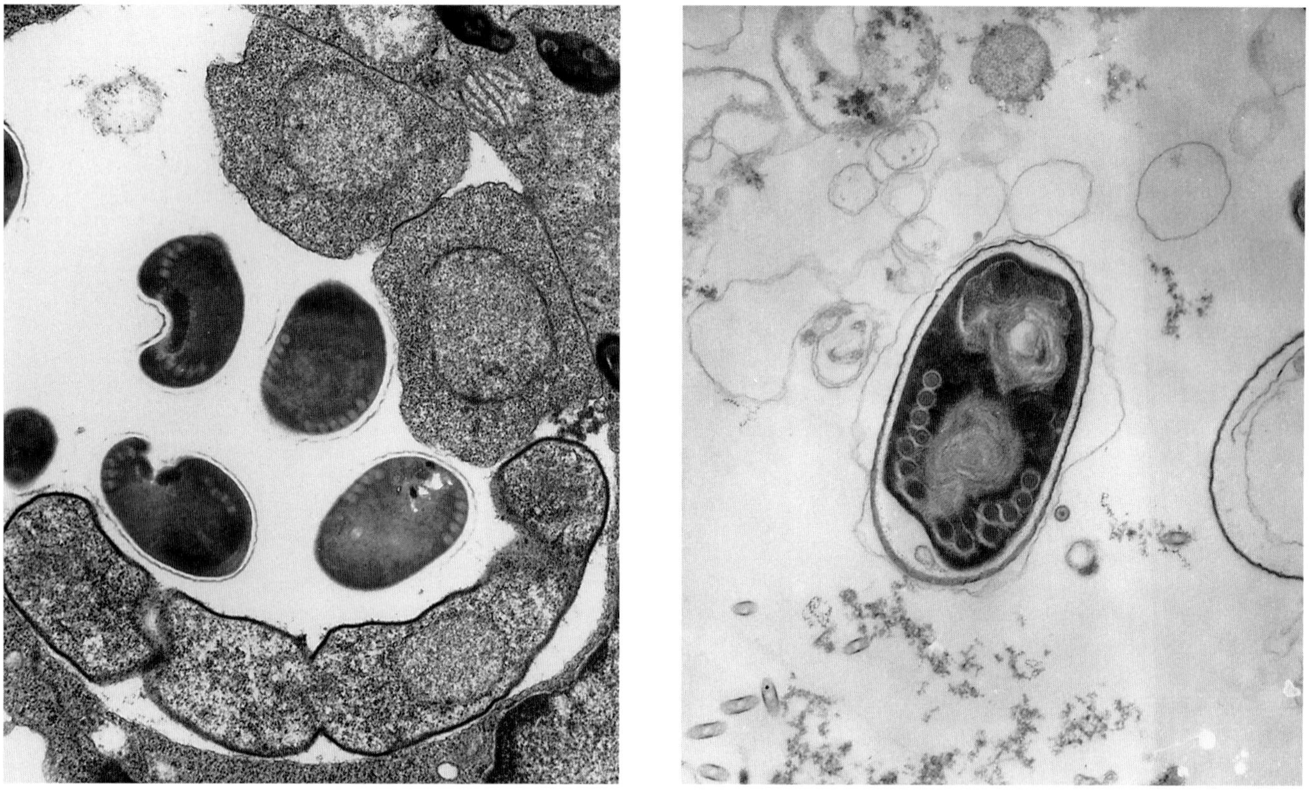

A B

FIGURE 15-19 **(A)** Electron micrograph demonstrating several stages of microsporidial development. Spores are located centrally and contain a polar tubule with several coils. **(B)** Electron micrograph of *Encephalitozoon* spore. (Reprinted with permission from PJ Didier, ES Didier, JM Orenstein, JA Shadduck: Fine structure of a new human microsporidian, *Encephalitozoon hellem*, in culture. J Protozool 38:502, 1991.)

because they rely on the humidity and vegetation, hence the common term for the disease, *river blindness*. Black fly vectors are found in Africa, Mexico, Central America, and South America. Blackflies become infected by ingesting microfilariae during a blood meal from an infected individual. The microfilariae penetrate the fly's gut, enter the flight muscles, and grow through several molts to become infective larvae. Infected blackflies introduce larvae to new individuals during subsequent blood meals. In the human host, the larvae develop into adult worms that migrate through the subcutaneous tissues before settling in small groups to form encapsulated nodules. These nodules are most commonly found beneath the skin but are occasionally observed in deeper tissues. Gravid female worms release microfilariae that migrate out of the nodule and throughout host tissues, concentrating in the dermis.[118] Disseminated microfilariae cause severe dermatitis characterized by itching, depigmentation, and thickening of the skin.

Ocular involvement is the result of microfilarial invasion and is the most serious complication of this infection.[119,120] Ocular manifestations may take years to develop as increasing numbers of microfilariae populate the ocular tissues. Living microfilariae are apparently well tolerated; with slit lamp microscopy, they may be seen floating in the anterior chamber or moving slowly in the cornea at the level of Bowman's layer.[121] Histology of the cornea and conjunctival nodules reveals microfilariae[122–125] (Figure 15-20). Photophobia, lacrimation, and conjunctival hyperemia are seen in early infection. With the death of intracorneal microfilariae, a severe inflammatory reaction ensues.[124] Corneal lesions begin as fluffy longitudinal infiltrates around dead organisms and progress to disk-shaped opacities approximately 0.5 mm in diameter.[126] These infiltrates have also been described as "nummular" or like "snowflakes melting on the window." They are usually located in the anterior stroma, are moderate in number, and are found near the limbus in the interpalpebral area (Figure 15-21). Early

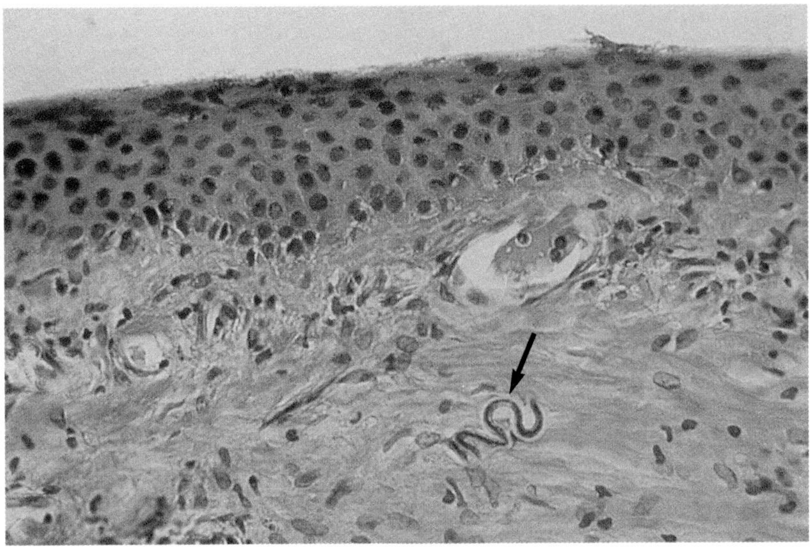

FIGURE 15-20 Microfilaria of *Onchocerca volvulus* (arrow) in the superficial corneal stroma (hematoxylin and eosin). (Reprinted with permission from CH Binford, DH Connor [eds]: Pathology of Tropical and Extraordinary Diseases. Armed Forces Institute of Pathology, Washington, DC, 1976. Courtesy of the Armed Forces Institute of Pathology, AFIP 65-2023.)

in the course of the infection, the infiltrates are reversible and represent the manifestations of relatively mild disease. On the severe end of the clinical spectrum, sclerosing keratitis may develop in response to a high-intensity infection of several years duration.[117] Many microfilariae are observed advancing across the cornea. The advancing microfilariae are usually most dense at the 3- and 9-o'clock positions (Figure 15-22). The area behind the advancing border of microfilariae becomes edematous and opacified and eventually results in a confluent opacification of the cornea (Figure 15-23). In other individuals, onchocerciasis causes blindness as the result of severe exudative iridocyclitis with pupillary membrane formation.

In patients with ocular involvement, the identification of microfilariae in the cornea or anterior chamber is sufficient to diagnose onchocerciasis. In other patients with conjunctival or cutaneous disease, the diagnosis can be made through the identification of microfilariae in a skin biopsy. A small specimen of excised skin may be placed in saline and observed over a period of several hours for the emergence of microfilariae. A skin

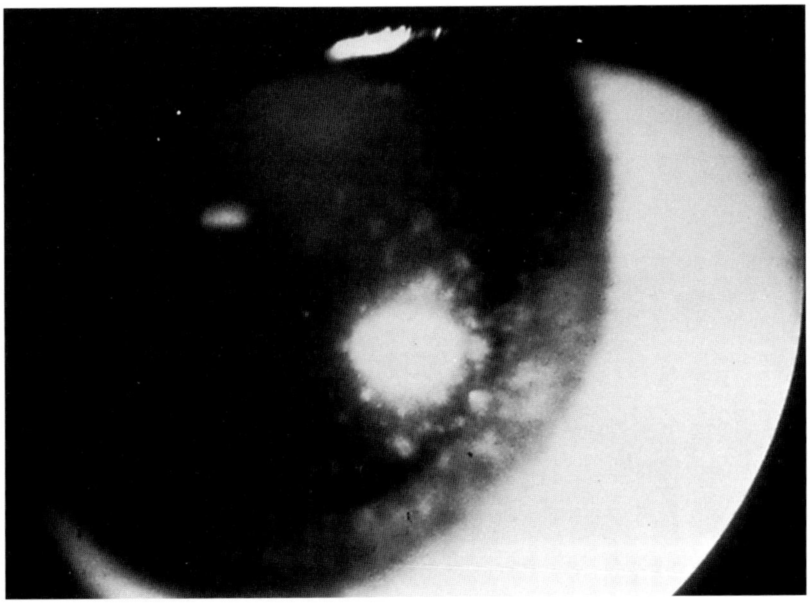

FIGURE 15-21 Many corneal opacities caused by an inflammatory reaction to *Onchocerca volvulus.* (Reprinted with permission from CH Binford, DH Connor [eds]: Pathology of Tropical and Extraordinary Diseases. Armed Forces Institute of Pathology, Washington, DC, 1976. Courtesy of the Armed Forces Institute of Pathology, AFIP 75-1622.)

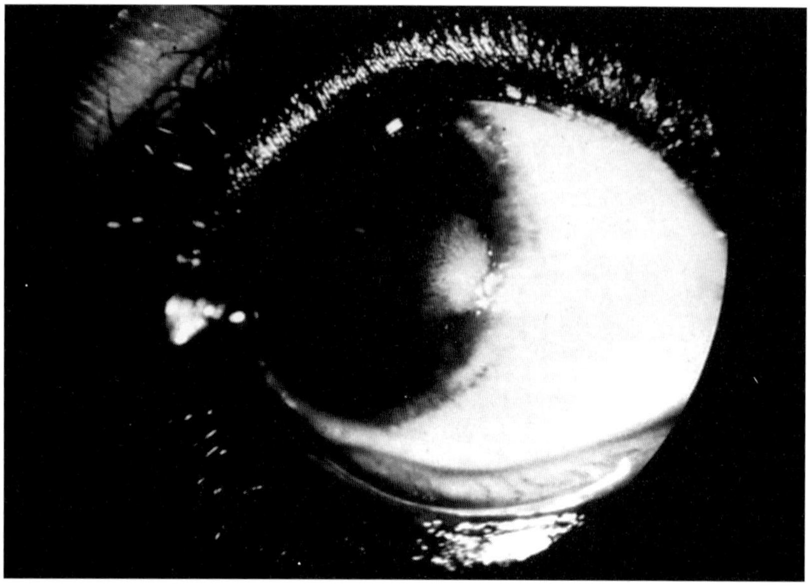

FIGURE 15-22 Early sclerosing keratitis involving the peripheral cornea caused by onchocerciasis. (Reprinted with permission from CH Binford, DH Connor [eds]: Pathology of Tropical and Extraordinary Diseases. Armed Forces Institute of Pathology, Washington, DC, 1976. Courtesy of the Armed Forces Institute of Pathology, AFIP 75-1623.)

antigen test is available but is of limited use in areas where *Onchocerca* is endemic and exposure to the organism is common.

The treatment of choice for onchocerciasis is oral ivermectin. This medication is effective in reducing the numbers of microfilariae but does not kill the adult worms. Oral diethylcarbamazine has been used to treat onchocerciasis but results in rapid death of microfilariae. In response to the sudden death of large numbers of microfilariae, severe inflammatory reactions in the skin and eye may result which may require the use of antihistamines and corticosteroids. Ivermectin is effective, is better tolerated by the patient, and appears to have fewer ocular complications than diethylcarbamazine.[127] Suramin kills both microfilariae and adult worms, but its use has decreased because of severe toxicity.[128] Ocular therapy is directed toward symptoms, and some patients may benefit from topical corticosteroids to reduce the inflammatory response to dead organisms. Topical treatment with diethylcarbamazine, levamisole, and mebendazole has been reported but is of uncertain efficacy.[129,130] Surgical excision of skin nodules, especially those located on the scalp, may pro-

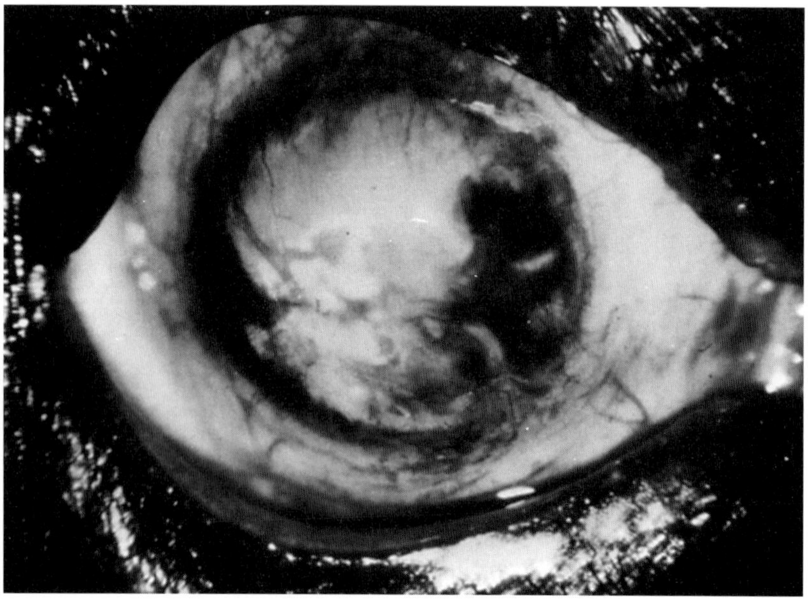

FIGURE 15-23 Advanced sclerosing keratitis caused by onchocerciasis. (Reprinted with permission from CH Binford, DH Connor [eds]: Pathology of Tropical and Extraordinary Diseases. Armed Forces Institute of Pathology, Washington, DC, 1976. Courtesy of the Armed Forces Institute of Pathology, AFIP 75-1626.)

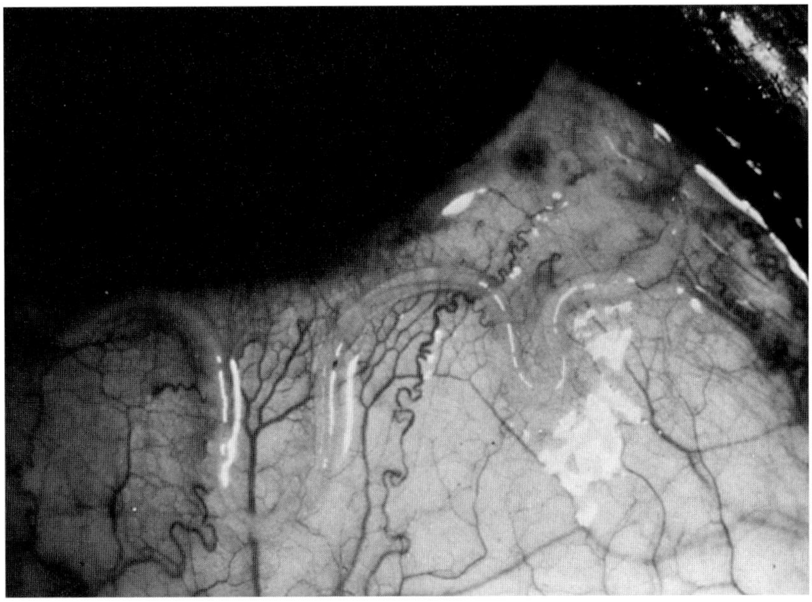

FIGURE 15-24 *Loa loa* beneath the conjunctiva. (Reprinted with permission from CH Binford, DH Connor [eds]: Pathology of Tropical and Extraordinary Diseases. Armed Forces Institute of Pathology, Washington, DC, 1976. Courtesy of the Armed Forces Institute of Pathology, AFIP 73-6654.)

vide some benefit by reducing the number of microfilariae and reducing ocular complications.[131]

Ascariasis

Ascariasis is caused by *Ascaris lumbricoides* and, rarely, *A. suum*. These large roundworms resemble earthworms and live in the small intestine, where they may grow to lengths of 30 cm or more. *Ascaris* is distributed worldwide and is found in large numbers in areas with poor sanitation.

Infection is acquired by ingesting the eggs in food, vegetables, water, and soil. When the eggs reach the small intestine, the larvae hatch and penetrate the intestinal wall and are carried to the liver and lungs. From there, the larvae migrate up the respiratory passages and are swallowed, eventually returning to the small intestine as adult worms. The adult worm matures in the small intestine and passes eggs into the host feces.

Heavy infections may be associated with aberrant migration of larvae which may settle in various tissues, including intraocular or periocular locations. Ocular manifestations of ascariasis include eyelid edema and urticaria, subconjunctival nodules containing parasites, conjunctivitis, larvae in the lacrimal puncta, uveitis, glaucoma, lens subluxation, recurrent vitreous hemorrhage, chorioretinitis, papilledema, and pseudotumor.[132,133] The diagnosis of ascariasis is made by detecting characteristic eggs or worms in a fecal smear. Pyrantel pamoate or mebendazole is effective against *Ascaris*. Alternative drugs include piperazine and thiabendazole.

Loiasis

Loiasis is caused by *Loa loa*, a nematode transmitted to humans by the bite of the mango fly *(Chrysops)*. The infection is confined to Africa, and there are no reservoir hosts. Larvae are inoculated into the skin of the host during the bite of the mango fly and attain sexual maturity in the subcutaneous tissues. Adult worms continuously migrate throughout the subcutaneous tissues and can live as long as 15 years. Microfilariae are released into the peripheral blood and do not generally cause significant morbidity to the host.

As the adult worms migrate through subcutaneous tissues, they provoke a mild inflammatory response known as Calabar swellings. Ocular involvement becomes apparent when adult worms meander through the conjunctival tissues (Figure 15-24). Adult worms, which may grow as long as 5 cm in length, have also been found in the eyelids, orbit, and anterior chamber.[134–136]

The diagnosis of loiasis is clear when the organism is observed in the conjunctiva. Surgical removal of the worm is simple and effective (Figure 15-25), but other adult worms may be undetectable in other locations. Treatment with ivermectin or diethylcarbamazine may be used, but patients with large numbers of microfilariae in the blood must be monitored carefully for adverse reactions to large

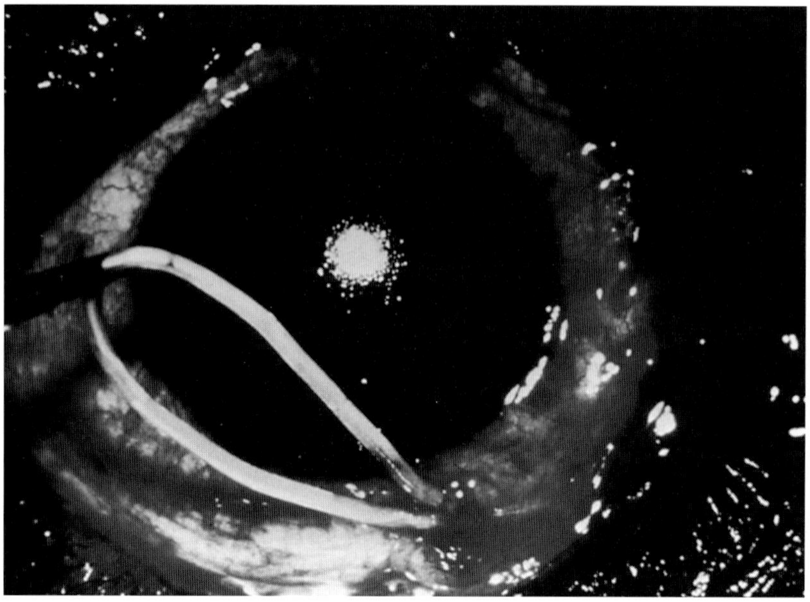

FIGURE 15-25 Extraction of *Loa loa* from the conjunctiva. (Reprinted with permission from CH Binford, DH Connor [eds]: Pathology of Tropical and Extraordinary Diseases. Armed Forces Institute of Pathology, Washington, DC, 1976. Courtesy of the Armed Forces Institute of Pathology, AFIP 75-1789-4.)

numbers of dead microfilariae, such as fever, purpura, and encephalitis.

Thelaziasis

Thelaziasis may be caused by *Thelazia callipaeda* or *T. californiensis. T. callipaeda* is normally found on the conjunctiva of dogs, cats, and other mammals in China, Korea, and southeast Asia. *T. californiensis* is normally found on the conjunctiva of deer, jackrabbits, and coyotes in North America. These nematodes are transmitted by flies belonging to the genera *Musca* and *Fannia.*

Clinical manifestations include ocular irritation and conjunctival hyperemia due to the presence of adult worms that attach to the conjunctival surface. The worms are white and thread-like and can be seen moving in the conjunctival fornix. Rarely, the worms invade the conjunctiva, cornea, and eyelid. Ectropion and cicatricial changes in the eyelids are occasionally observed. Filariform larvae may penetrate human skin and wander aimlessly, producing serpiginous tunnels and indurated pruritic papules. Adult worms can be easily removed, and systemic treatment with diethylcarbamazine is rarely necessary.

Trichinosis

Trichinosis is an infection caused by the nematode *Trichinella spiralis* and is found worldwide. It is acquired in carnivores, including humans, by ingesting the encysted larvae found in undercooked pork, horse, walrus, or bear meat. The cysts are digested and release larvae that develop into adult worms in the intestine. Female worms release eggs, which hatch into larvae that penetrate the gut wall and migrate into the bloodstream, where they are disseminated to various organs. They have a predilection to invade and become encysted in skeletal muscles.

Most cases of trichinosis go undetected because symptoms may be nonspecific or relatively mild. Systemic symptoms such as fever, malaise and generalized myalgias are common. During the stage of muscle invasion, the extraocular muscles are frequently involved, resulting in the classic symptoms of trichinosis: edema and pain of the periorbital area and face (Figure 15-26). The conjunctiva may become edematous and hyperemic, with occasional subconjunctival hemorrhages.

The diagnosis is confirmed through biopsy of skeletal muscle, most often the deltoid muscle. A skin test using *Trichinella* antigen is also available. Mebendazole and thiabendazole may be used in the early stages of the active infection. Systemic corticosteroids may be used in the late stages of the infection to treat the inflammation that occurs when organisms die in the tissues.

Dirofilariasis

Nematodes of the genus *Dirofilaria* ordinarily infect cats, dogs, and other mammals. Rarely, these worms are found in humans. *Dirofilaria* is worldwide in distribution, with most patients living in the United States. Transmission to humans occurs through the bite of an infected mosquito.

The parasites either remain in the subcutaneous tissues or migrate into the bloodstream, which carries them into the lungs, where they may form small nodules.

The eyelid and conjunctiva are occasionally infected[137-139] (Figure 15-27), and intraocular involvement has been reported.[140] Other reported ocular manifestations include pseudotumor, proptosis, and scleral nodules. Treatment consists of surgical excision if the worms are accessible.

Dracunculiasis

Dracunculus medinensis is a nematode found in the Middle East, Africa, India, and South America. The infection is contracted through the ingestion of infected water fleas, which are commonly found in water in endemic areas. The fleas degenerate and liberate larvae, which penetrate the intestinal mucosa and migrate to the retroperitoneal tissues, where they mature and mate. The gravid female worm migrates to the skin, where it causes a blister, usually on the lower leg. The worm contains many larvae that are released when the skin comes in contact with water. The larvae are swallowed by water fleas to complete the life cycle.

Lesions containing a single gravid female worm usually occur on the extremities but may occasionally appear on the face, thorax, and abdomen. Conjunctival, eyelid, and orbital lesions have been reported. Secondary bacterial infection can occur, leading to cellulitis and gangrene.

The diagnosis is usually clear when the characteristic cutaneous lesion is present. If the diagnosis is in question, larvae from the lesion may be examined microscopically. Treatment is usually accomplished by surgical removal of the adult worm from the skin lesion. In primitive areas, cold water may be applied to the worm, which stimulates expulsion of larvae and facilitates removal of the worm. A common practice is to pull a small length of the worm from the lesion each day to avoid inadvertently breaking

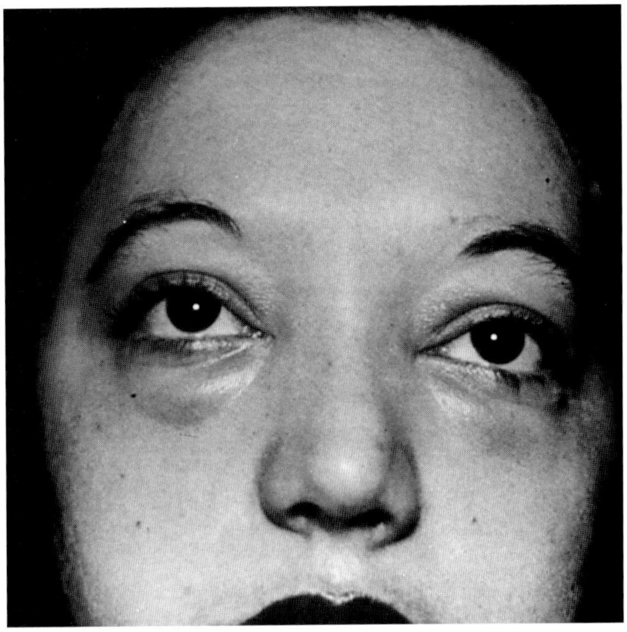

FIGURE 15-26 Woman with periorbital edema caused by *Trichinella spiralis.* (Reprinted with permission from CH Binford, DH Connor [eds]: Pathology of Tropical and Extraordinary Diseases. Armed Forces Institute of Pathology, Washington, DC, 1976. Courtesy of the Armed Forces Institute of Pathology, AFIP 52-8038.)

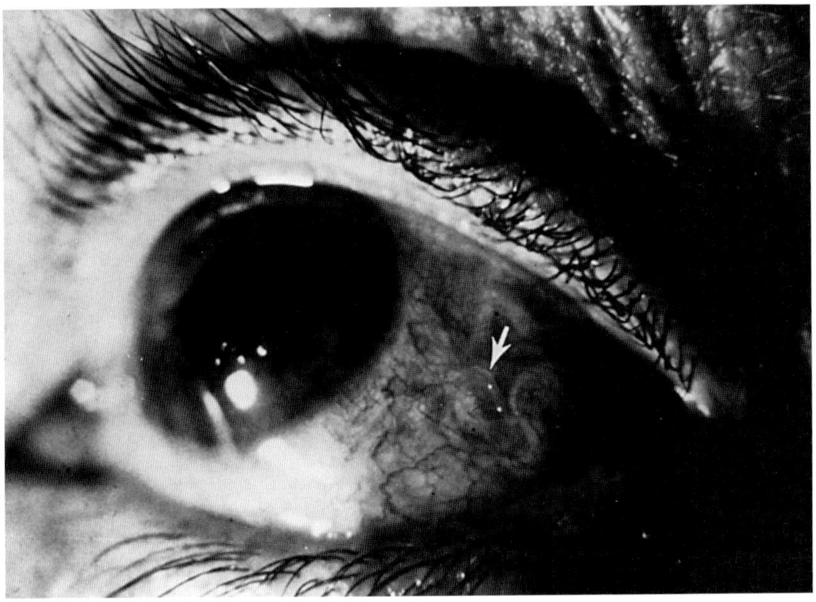

FIGURE 15-27 *Dirofilaria tenuis* (arrow) beneath the conjunctiva. (Reprinted with permission from CH Binford, DH Connor [eds]: Pathology of Tropical and Extraordinary Diseases. Armed Forces Institute of Pathology, Washington, DC, 1976. Courtesy of the Armed Forces Institute of Pathology, AFIP 74-6351-2.)

the worm. In cases in which the worm remains in deep tissues, several oral medications may be useful, including niridazole, thiabendazole, or metronidazole.

CESTODES (TAPEWORMS)

Cysticercosis

Cysticercosis is caused by the pork tapeworm, *Taenia solium,* which is found worldwide. Humans become infected by ingesting raw or undercooked pork containing cysticerci (encysted larvae). Once ingested, the larva attaches to the intestinal mucosa, where it develops into an adult tapeworm. The adult worm releases eggs into the feces, which may be ingested by the infected person or others. Ingestion of eggs results in the migration of hatched larvae through the intestinal mucosa and into the bloodstream, then to the subcutaneous tissues, eyes, brain, muscles, heart, and lungs. In these tissues, the larvae form cysticerci which are usually well tolerated. When a cysticercus dies, a severe inflammatory response ensues. Symptoms are variable, depending on the location of the cysticercus, and the infection can be fatal.

Reported sites of ocular involvement include the eyelid, conjunctiva, lacrimal gland, and vitreous.[141–145] Uveitis, retinal detachment, chorioretinal scar formation, papilledema, and optic atrophy have been described. The most dramatic ocular finding is the intravitreal cysticercus. Treatment is accomplished through the surgical removal of conjunctival and intravitreal cysticerci. Niclosamide or praziquantel can be used to eradicate the intestinal worm.

Echinococcosis (Hydatid Disease)

Echinococcosis is caused by larval tapeworms of *Echinococcus granulosus* or *E. multilocularis.* It is found worldwide and parallels sheep husbandry in distribution. Only the larval form of the parasite is found in the human host, where it causes space-occupying lesions known as hydatid cysts. The adult worm lives in the small intestine of the dog and sheds eggs into the feces. When an egg is ingested by humans or sheep, the embryo is released from its surrounding membranes through the action of gastrointestinal enzymes. The embryo migrates through the intestinal wall and is carried in the bloodstream to tissues, most commonly the liver and lungs. The embryo develops into a hydatid cyst, which contains thousands of infectious organisms (protoscolices). Cysts can grow and rupture, causing anaphylactic reactions and seeding of new tissues that results in the formation of second-generation cysts. The life cycle is completed when infected sheep are fed to sheepdogs.

Symptoms are those of space-occupying lesions in the liver, lungs, spleen, kidney, brain, bone, and heart. Many asymptomatic cysts of the lungs or liver are discovered incidentally from radiologic or ultrasound studies. Cysts have been found in the eyelid, lacrimal gland, vitreous, and retina. Cysts can erode the orbital roof and become intracranial.[146]

A skin test and serologic tests are available to assist the diagnosis of echinococcosis. Treatment involves surgical excision if the cysts are accessible. Inoperable cysts may be treated with albendazole.

Coenurosis

Coenurosis is a rare infection caused by *Multiceps multiceps,* a tapeworm usually found in dogs and wolves but occasionally in humans, cattle, horses, and sheep. Most cases occur in Africa, but sporadic cases have been reported in the United States, Great Britain, and France. The eggs of *M. multiceps* are found in the feces of infected dogs or wolves. After the eggs are ingested by humans or other intermediate hosts, the embryo form of the organism hatches in the small intestine, penetrates the intestinal wall, migrates to various organs via the bloodstream, and develops into a cyst. When cysts are eaten by carnivores they develop into adult worms, completing the life cycle.

Coenurus cysts are typically present in the central nervous system but may be found in other tissues. Ocular manifestations include conjunctival cysts, intraocular inflammation, retinal detachment, chorioretinitis, proptosis, and intravitreal cysts.[147,148] When possible, the cyst should be surgically excised. Systemic corticosteroids may be used to control inflammation.

Sparganosis

Sparganosis is caused by the larvae of various tapeworms of the genus *Diphyllobothrium.* The larvae are commonly referred to as *sparganum,* a term that arose when these larvae were thought to represent a distinct genus. The adult worm usually infects the intestines of cats and dogs. Eggs are passed in the stool and hatch in fresh water. The larvae are ingested by microscopic crustaceans. When the microscopic crustaceans are swallowed by snakes, frogs, birds, or other animals, the larvae pierce the intestinal wall and migrate to the skin or muscle. Humans can be infected by drinking water containing these microscopic crustaceans or by eating raw or uncooked frogs, snakes, birds, or other infected animals. In the Orient, especially China and Vietnam, the flesh of frogs or snakes is occasionally applied to skin or eye wounds as a traditional healing practice.[149] If the flesh is infected, larvae may enter the wound and infect the individual.

When the worm matures in a tissue, it elicits an inflammatory reaction. Ocular sparganosis results in marked swelling of the eyelids, with intense pain, irritation, and lacrimation. If the worm is superficial, it can occasionally be expressed from the conjunctiva. If the worm migrates to a retrobulbar location, it may cause proptosis, lagophthalmos, and corneal ulceration. Treatment is surgical excision. Medical therapy with praziquantel may be effective.

TREMATODES (FLUKES)

Paragonimiasis

Paragonimiasis is a disease caused by trematodes of the genus *Paragonimus. P. westermani, P. heterotrema, P. skrjabini, P. siamensis, P. africanus,* and *P. uterobilateralis* produce infections in humans. They are found in the Far East, Africa, and South America. Humans acquire the infection by eating raw or undercooked crustacea or undercooked or raw flesh of intermediate hosts containing the encysted stage of the worm (metacercaria). The cysts excyst in the small intestine, and the worms migrate to the lungs, where they mature into adult worms. The worms live in a fibrotic capsule in the lung periphery, releasing fertilized eggs, which are coughed up in sputum or swallowed and passed in the stool. The eggs hatch in fresh water into miracidia (first-stage larvae), which penetrate snail hosts. Cercariae (last-stage larvae) develop in the snail and exit, later to encyst in the freshwater crab.

Ophthalmic manifestations include invasion of the subconjunctival space, eyelid, and intraocular or orbital tissue by the worm.[150–152] Treatment is surgical excision.

Schistosomiasis (Bilharziasis)

Schistosomiasis is caused by the trematodes *Schistosoma japonicum, S. mansoni,* and *S. haematobium.* It is endemic in the Orient, the Middle East, Africa, and South America. The parasite is transmitted through the snail, which serves as an intermediate host. In humans, cercariae (last-stage larvae) penetrate through the skin and enter the bloodstream, where they are carried to the liver and intestine. Mature worms migrate against the flow of blood in the portal vein to settle in the mesenteric veins. Eggs are released by the adult worms and may be found in the urine, stool, and blood. Eggs form emboli in the liver and lungs, causing cirrhosis and pulmonary fibrosis. Emboli to the postpulmonary circulation are uncommon but may involve the eyes, orbits, and central nervous system.[153–155] Eggs escaping in the urine and feces are deposited in fresh water, hatch into miracidia (first-stage larvae), penetrate the snail, develop into cercariae, leave the snail, and penetrate the skin of humans, thus completing the cycle.

Schistosoma eggs have been found in the conjunctiva, in caruncle granulomas, and in the lacrimal gland.[156–159] Niridazole, metrifonate, praziquantel, and oxamniquine are used systemically to treat schistosomiasis. Corticosteroids and surgical excision are also used.

ARTHROPODS

Demodicosis

Hair follicle mites *(Demodex folliculorum)* and sebaceous gland mites *(Demodex brevis)* are permanent ectoparasites of humans and are found predominantly on the skin of the nose, nasolabial folds, and eyelids.[160] The mites are 0.4 mm long, spindle shaped, and colorless. The female mite deposits eggs in the hair follicle or sebaceous gland. The life cycle is approximately 15 days. Both adults and larvae eat follicular and sebaceous cells. Adults "transfer" from one gland or follicle to another and may serve as potential vectors of other disease organisms.

Microscopic examination of an eyelash after epilation may demonstrate infestation with *Demodex;* however, the organism's role in the pathogenesis of blepharitis is unclear.[161–163] Histology shows dilation and destruction of hair follicles and sebaceous glands. In heavy infestations, the signs and symptoms include itching, burning, blepharitis, madarosis (loss of eyelashes), and conjunctival hyperemia. Treatment includes lid scrubs and the application of antibiotic ointment to the eyelid margins.

Ophthalmomyiasis

Infestation of host tissues with fly larvae (maggots) is called myiasis. Certain species of flies are obligate parasites requiring living tissue for development, whereas others develop facultatively in either living or dead tissue. A third group may cause accidental myiasis. Damage to the skin or ocular surface by trauma, infection, surgery, or malignancy can increase the risk of myiasis.

Most larvae identified in the ocular adnexa are *Oestrus ovis* (sheep or goat botfly). These larvae are usually deposited in the nostrils of sheep and goats but may also be deposited in the nasal passages of humans, causing severe frontal headaches. In patients with ophthalmomyiasis, fly larvae are most commonly detected in the

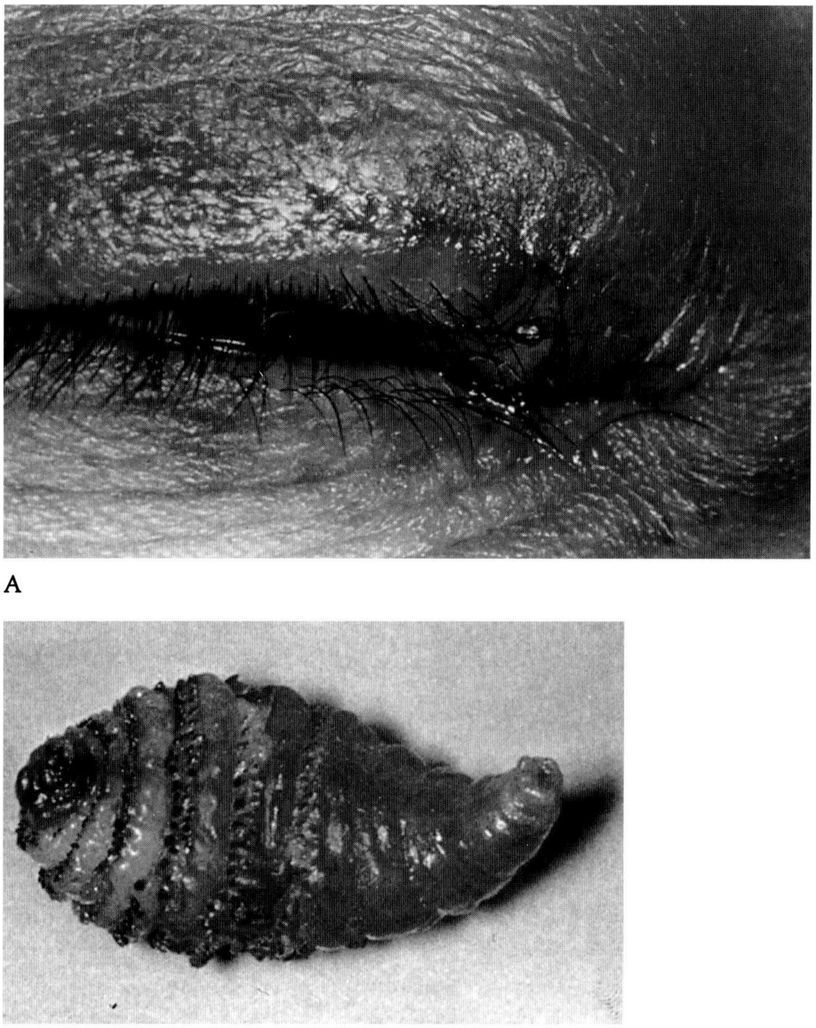

FIGURE 15-28 (A) Eyelid cellulitis caused by *Dermatobia hominis.* (B) *Dermatobia hominis* extracted from the eyelid. (Reprinted with permission from KR Wilhelmus: Myiasis palpebrarum. Am J Ophthalmol 101:496, 1986. Copyright by The Ophthalmic Publishing Company.)

conjunctiva[164–166] but have also been observed in the vitreous, subretinal space, and periorbital tissues.[167–169] When the larvae migrate through the subretinal space, characteristic tracks may be observed by ophthalmoscopy. Other reported causes of ophthalmomyiasis include *Dermatobia hominis* (human botfly)[170] (Figure 15-28), *Chrysomya bezziana* (Old World screwworm), *Wohlfahrtia magnifica* (screwworm), *Cochliomyia hominivorax* (screwworm), *Cochliomyia macellaria* (screwworm), *Hypoderma bovis* (cattle grub), *Calliphora vomitoria* (bluebottle fly), *Oedemagena tarandi* (caribou or reindeer warble fly), and *Cuterebra* (rodent and rabbit botfly).

Eyelid lesions may be covered with petrolatum, forcing maggots to the surface for air, followed by gentle manual or surgical removal.

Phthiriasis Palpebrarum

Phthiriasis is caused by the pubic louse, *Phthirus pubis,* which is usually found on the hairs in the pubic region but may occasionally be found on the eyelashes, eyebrows, beard, and hairs of the axilla.[171] Neither the human body louse *(Pediculus humanus corporis)* nor the human head louse *(Pediculus humanus capitis)* normally infest the ocular area.

P. pubis is approximately 2 mm long, has stout claw-like legs for grasping hair shafts, and tends to remain in one location (Figures 15-29 and 15-30). The louse is found at the base of the hair with the mouth parts inserted in the skin to suck blood from the host. Adult females lay eggs (nits), which are firmly glued to the eyelashes (Figure 15-31). Transmission is through close contact, sexual contact, bedding, and clothing.

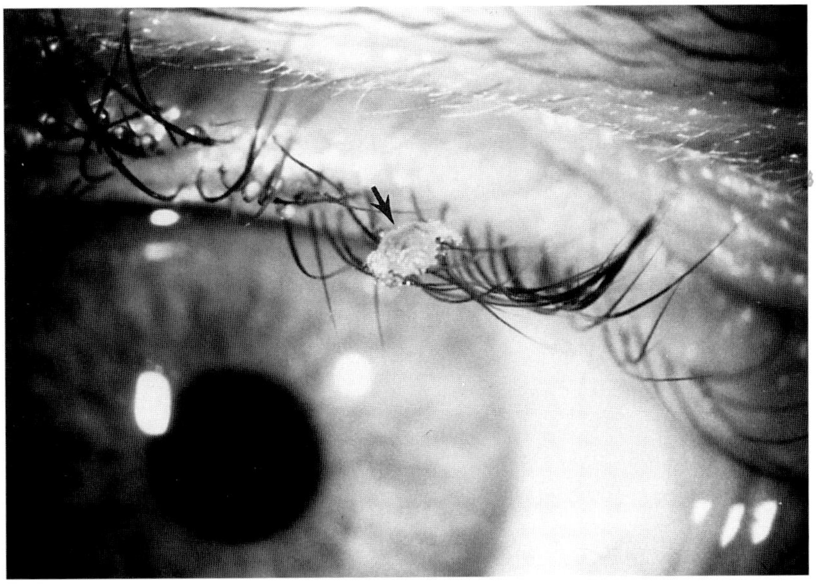

FIGURE 15-29 *Phthirus pubis* (arrow) grasping eyelashes. Several nits are seen on the eyelashes in the upper left-hand corner.

The presence of *P. pubis* on the eyelids causes irritation and itching of the eyelids and conjunctiva. Superficial punctate keratitis, marginal keratitis, secondary infection at bite sites, and madarosis have been reported. Reddish brown granular material or blood-tinged deposits may form on the eyelid margins. The diagnosis is often made by the observation of nits on eyelashes, which are usually easier to detect than the lice themselves.

Treatment of *P. pubis* palpebrarum consists of chemical treatment or mechanical removal of lice and nits with forceps. In cases of heavy infestation, the eyelashes can be trimmed. The use of pediculocides around the eye is not recommended. The simplest and safest chemical treatment for *P. pubis* palpebrarum, and the one recommended by the Centers for Disease Control and Prevention, is ophthalmic ointment applied twice a day for 10 days.[172] The ointment kills lice by mechanically obstructing their respiratory apparatus and smothering them. It is ineffective against nits, however, and must be used long enough to cover the entire life cycle of lice. Anticholinesterase agents, such as physostigmine, have been reported as an effective chemical treatment because of their adverse effect on nerve transmission in lice.[173] The side effects of these agents limit

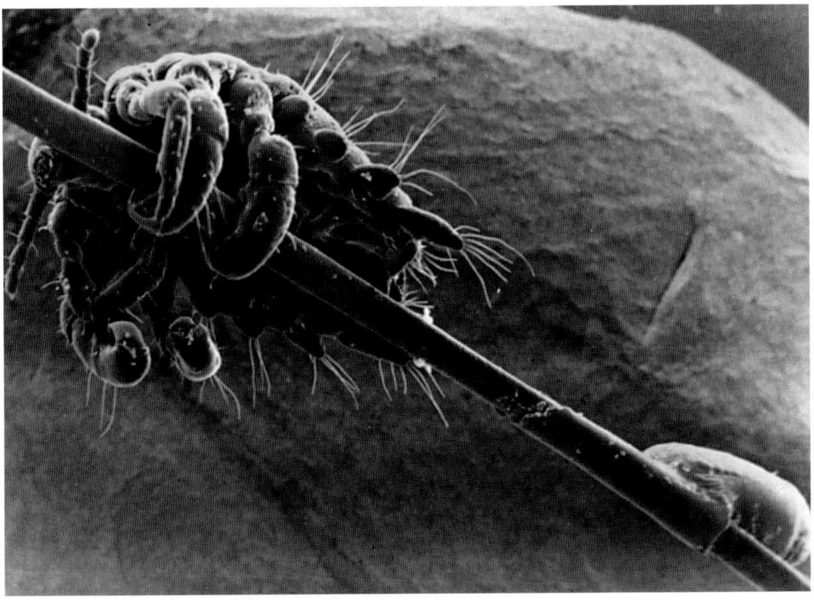

FIGURE 15-30 Scanning electron micrograph of a nit and a louse grasping an eyelash. (Reprinted with permission from JM Couch, WR Green, LW Hirst, ZC De La Cruz: Diagnosing and treating *Phthirus pubis* palbebrarum. Surv Ophthalmol 26:219, 1982.)

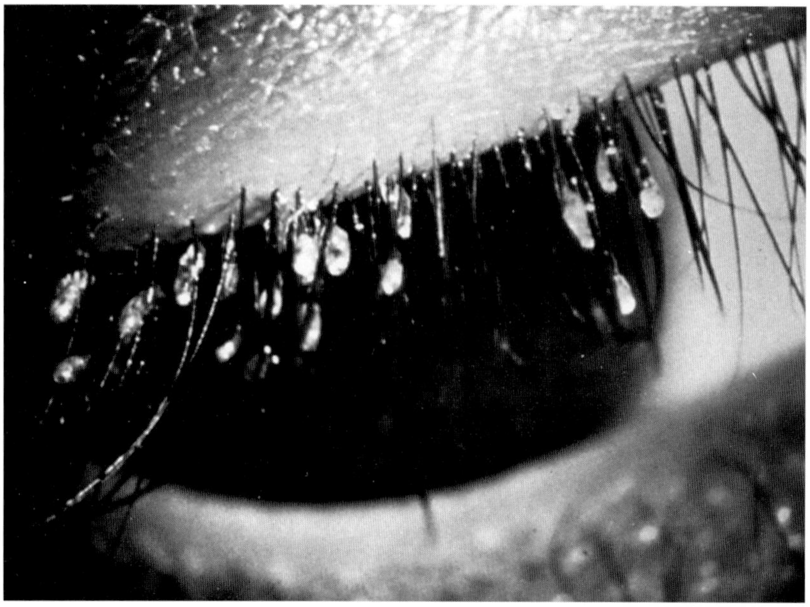

FIGURE 15-31 Many *Phthirus pubis* eggs (nits) on the eyelashes.

their usefulness, however. A 20 percent solution of fluorescein has also been shown to be pediculicidal.[174]

Infestation of other areas of the body should be treated with a 1 percent permethrin creme rinse (Nix Creme Rinse), which is applied to affected areas for 10 minutes and washed off.[172] Alternatives include pyrethrins and piperonyl butoxide, which are applied for 10 minutes, and 1 percent lindane shampoo (Kwell Shampoo), which is applied for 4 minutes. Lindane is not recommended for pregnant or lactating women. Clothing and fomites that have been contaminated should be washed in hot water (125°F) or dry cleaned, which kills the adults, nymphs, and nits. Nonwashable items should be treated with a disinfectant that contains pyrethrins and piperonyl butoxide (e.g., Raid, Black Flag).

Ticks

Ticks are bloodsucking arthropods that attach to hosts by glue-like salivary secretions and mouth parts that penetrate the skin. Ticks act as vectors for bacterial diseases such as Rocky Mountain spotted fever and Lyme disease (see Ch. 8). Ticks may be found anywhere on the human body, most often at the base of the scalp or in the scalp.

Eyelid involvement with the dog tick was reported in a 34-year-old man who had slept in a tent, and conjunctival infestation with a seed tick was reported in a 28-year-old man who had been chopping wood.[175,176] No adverse reactions were reported, and the ticks were successfully removed. Removal is performed manually, with care taken not to leave the head or mouth parts in the epidermis. Application of kerosene, camphorated phenol, iodine, or ether has been recommended to facilitate the removal of ticks in the skin but is not advisable around the eye.

Acariasis

The term *acariasis* is derived from the order Acari, which contains the human scabies mite, *Sarcoptes sabiei.* This mite is ubiquitous and is capable of infesting humans as well as a variety of other animals. The infestation is usually transmitted through close personal contact. The mites are approximately 0.5 mm long and mate on the skin of the host. Male mites remain on the surface, whereas female mites burrow into the skin. As the female mite digs tortuous, thread-like channels in the skin, she deposits eggs, cuticles, and excrement, causing a pruritic rash. The eggs hatch into larvae after 3 to 7 days, and the larvae migrate to the surface of the skin.

The skin between the fingers, the flexor surfaces of the elbows and knees, and the skin of the groin are preferentially affected. Mites may burrow into the skin of the eyelids and cause itching, burning, and crusting. Treatment with 1 percent lindane lotion or 5 percent permethrin cream is recommended for skin lesions, but care must be taken to keep these compounds away from the eyes.

Ophthalmia Nodosa

Ophthalmia nodosa is the descriptive term for inflammatory reactions in the eye in response to insect hairs

FIGURE 15-32 Corneal infiltrate surrounding a tarantula hair (arrow).

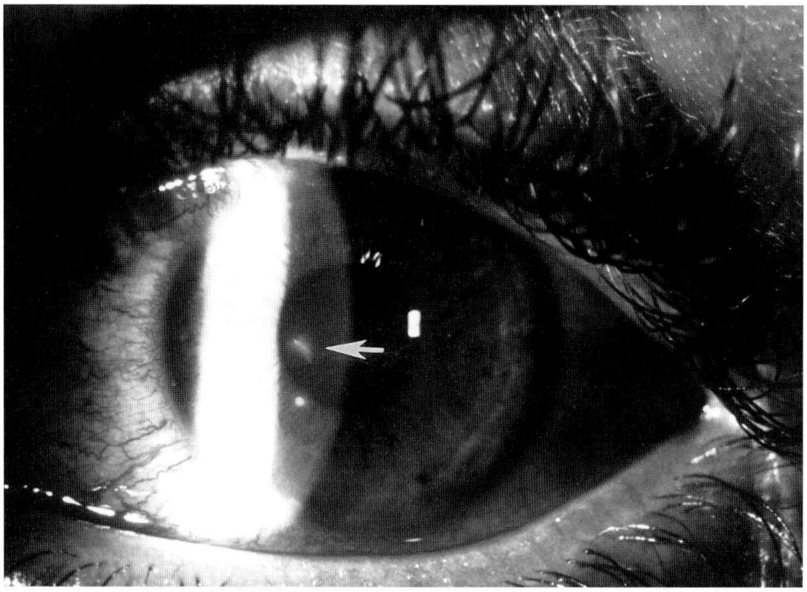

or vegetable matter. This syndrome derives its name from the nodular inflammatory reaction observed in the conjunctiva of affected individuals. Various insects possess hairs capable of causing irritation if they become embedded in the ocular surface. Caterpillar and tarantula hairs may be blown into the eye, may become lodged in the eye as the result of direct contact, or may be transferred to the eye after hand contact with these insects.[177–182] These hairs have a pointed tip as well as many barbs along the shaft and have been observed to migrate into deeper ocular tissues.

On examination, fine, white insect hairs may occasionally be observed in the cornea. These hairs are frequently surrounded by a small nummular corneal infiltrate[182] (Figure 15-32). In patients with a large number of hairs in the cornea, the anterior chamber may show moderately severe inflammation. Rarely, hairs can be observed to migrate through the cornea into the anterior chamber and may be seen on gonioscopy in the anterior chamber angle. Although the hairs are difficult to detect in the conjunctiva, erythematous nodules in the conjunctiva are often present.

Initial treatment begins with an attempt to remove as many of the exposed hairs as possible. This task is difficult because the hairs are extremely delicate and tend to break easily, leaving a portion embedded in the tissue. The inflammatory reaction in the cornea and conjunctiva usually responds well to topical corticosteroids.[182] After several months, the topical corticosteroids can usually be discontinued without recurrence of inflammation. Occasionally, it is necessary to surgically remove an inflammatory nodule from the conjunctiva.

REFERENCES

1. Castellani A: An amoeba found in cultures of yeast: preliminary note. J Trop Med Hyg 33:160, 1930
2. Visvesvara GS: Classification of *Acanthamoeba*. Rev Infect Dis 13(suppl): S369, 1991
3. Martinez AJ: Infection of the central nervous system due to *Acanthamoeba*. Rev Infect Dis 13(suppl):S399, 1991
4. Badenoch PR: The pathogenesis of *Acanthamoeba* keratitis. Aust N Z J Ophthalmol 19:9, 1991
5. De Jonckheere JF: Ecology of *Acanthamoeba*. Rev Infect Dis 13(suppl):S385, 1991
6. Mergeryan H: The prevalence of *Acanthamoeba* in the human environment. Rev Infect Dis 13(suppl):S390, 1991
7. Rivera F, Lares F, Ramirez E, et al: Pathogenic *Acanthamoeba* isolated during an atmospheric survey in Mexico City. Rev Infect Dis 13(suppl):S388, 1991
8. Rivera F, Medina F, Ramirez P, et al: Pathogenic and free-living protozoa cultured from the nasopharyngeal and oral regions of dental patients. Environ Res 33:428, 1984
9. Elder MJ, Kilvington S, Dart JKG: A clinicopathologic study of in vitro sensitivity testing and *Acanthamoeba* keratitis. Invest Ophthalmol Vis Sci 35:1059, 1994
10. Cohen EJ, Parlato CJ, Arentsen JJ, et al: Medical and surgical treatment of *Acanthamoeba* keratitis. Am J Ophthalmol 103:615, 1987
11. Kremer I, Cohen EJ, Eagle RC Jr, et al: Histopathologic evaluation of stromal inflammation in *Acanthamoeba* keratitis. CLAO J 20:45, 1994
12. Jones DB, Visvesvara GS, Robinson NM: *Acanthamoeba polyphaga* keratitis and *Acanthamoeba* uveitis associated with fatal meningoencephalitis. Trans Ophthalmol Soc UK 95:221, 1975

13. Wilhelmus KR: Microbial keratitis associated with contact lens wear. p. 41.1. In Contact Lenses: Update 3. Little, Brown, Boston, 1988
14. Stehr-Green JK, Bailey TM, Visvesvara GS: The epidemiology of *Acanthamoeba* keratitis in the United States. Am J Ophthalmol 107:331, 1989
15. Stehr-Green JK, Bailey TM, Brandt FH, et al: *Acanthamoeba* keratitis in soft contact lens wearers. JAMA 258:57, 1987
16. Moore MB, McCulley JP, Newton C, et al: *Acanthamoeba* keratitis: a growing problem in soft and hard contact lens wearers. Ophthalmology 94:1654, 1987
17. Heideman DG, Verdier DD, Dunn SP, Stamler JF: *Acanthamoeba* keratitis associated with disposable contact lenses. Am J Ophthalmol 110:630, 1990
18. Samples JR, Binder PS, Luibel FJ, et al: *Acanthamoeba* keratitis possibly acquired from a hot tub. Arch Ophthalmol 102:707, 1984
19. Sharma S, Srinivasan M, George C: *Acanthamoeba* keratitis in non-contact lens wearers. Arch Ophthalmol 108:676, 1990
20. Auran JD, Starr MB, Jakobiec FA: *Acanthamoeba* keratitis: a review of the literature. Cornea 6:2, 1987
21. Ludwig IH, Meisler DM, Rutherford I, et al: Susceptibility of *Acanthamoeba* to soft contact lens disinfection systems. Invest Ophthalmol Vis Sci 27:626, 1986
22. Moore MB, McCulley JP, Luckenbach M, et al: *Acanthamoeba* keratitis associated with soft contact lenses. Am J Ophthalmol 100:396, 1985
23. Bacon AS, Frazer G, Dart JKG, et al: A review of 72 consecutive cases of *Acanthamoeba* keratitis, 1984–1992. Eye 7:719, 1993
24. Donzis PB, Mondino BJ, Weissman BA, Bruckner DA: Microbial analysis of contact lens care systems contaminated with *Acanthamoeba*. Am J Ophthalmol 108:53, 1989
25. Devonshire P, Munro FA, Abernethy C, Clark BJ: Microbial contamination of contact lens cases in the west of Scotland. Br J Ophthalmol 77:41, 1993
26. Moore MB, Ubelaker J, Silvany R, et al: Scanning electron microscopy of *Acanthamoeba castellanii*: adherence to surfaces of new and used contact lenses and to human corneal button epithelium. Rev Infect Dis 13(suppl 5):S423, 1991
27. Kelly LD, Xu L: The effect of *Acanthamoeba* concentration on adherence to four types of unworn soft contact lenses. CLAO J 21:27, 1995
28. Kelly LD, Long D, Mitra D: Quantitative comparison of *Acanthamoeba castellanii* adherence to rigid versus soft contact lenses. CLAO J 21:111, 1995
29. Perkovitch BT, Meisler DM, McMahon JT, Rutherford I: *Acanthamoeba* adherence to soft contact lenses. ARVO abstract. Invest Ophthalmol Vis Sci 30(suppl):198, 1988
30. John T, Desai D, Sahm D: Adherence of *Acanthamoeba castellanii* cysts and trophozoites to extended wear soft contact lenses. Rev Infect Dis 13(suppl):S419, 1991
31. John T, Desai D, Sahm D: Adherence of *Acanthamoeba castellanii* cysts and trophozoites to unworn soft contact lenses. Am J Ophthalmol 108:658, 1989
32. Johns KJ, Head WS, Parrish CM, et al: Examination of hydrophilic contact lenses with light microscopy to aid in the diagnosis of *Acanthamoeba* keratitis [letter]. Am J Ophthalmol 108:329, 1989
33. Morton LD, McLaughlin GL, Whitely HE: Adherence characteristics of three strains of *Acanthamoeba*. Rev Infect Dis 13(suppl):S424, 1991
34. Alizadeh H, Stewart GL, Silvany RE, et al: Chemotactic activity and adherence of pathogenic and nonpathogenic strains of *Acanthamoeba* to different layers of pig cornea. ARVO abstract. Invest Ophthalmol Vis Sci 33(suppl):1320, 1992
35. van Klink F, Alizadeh H, He Y, et al: The role of contact lenses, trauma, and Langerhans cells in a Chinese hamster model of *Acanthamoeba* keratitis. Invest Ophthalmol Vis Sci 34:1937, 1993
36. Garner A: Pathogenesis of acanthamoebic keratitis: hypothesis based on a histological analysis of 30 cases. Br J Ophthalmol 77:366, 1993
37. Osato M, Pyron M, Penland R, Robinson N: Epidemiology of *Acanthamoeba* keratitis: an update. ARVO abstract. Invest Ophthalmol Vis Sci 33(suppl):1318, 1992
38. Larkin DFP, Easty DL: Experimental *Acanthamoeba* keratitis. I. Preliminary findings. Br J Ophthalmol 74:551, 1990
39. Badenoch PR, Johnson AM, Christy PE, Coster DJ: Pathogenicity of *Acanthamoeba* and a *Corynebacterium* in the rat cornea. Arch Ophthalmol 108:107, 1990
40. Ferrante A: Immunity to *Acanthamoeba*. Rev Infect Dis 13(suppl):S403, 1991
41. McCulley JP, Alizadeh H, Niederkorn JY: *Acanthamoeba* keratitis. CLAO J 21:73, 1995
42. Blackman HJ, Rao NA, Lemp MA, Visvesvara GS: *Acanthamoeba* keratitis successfully treated with penetrating keratoplasty: suggested immunogenic mechanisms of action. Cornea 3:125, 1984
43. Mathers W, Stevens G, Rodrigues M, et al: Immunopathology and electron microscopy of *Acanthamoeba* keratitis. Am J Ophthalmol 103:626, 1987
44. Theodore FH, Jakobiec FA, Juechter KB, et al: The diagnostic value of a ring infiltrate in acanthamoebic keratitis. Ophthalmology 92:1471, 1985
45. Florakis GJ, Folberg R, Krachmer JH, et al: Elevated corneal epithelial lines in *Acanthamoeba* keratitis. Arch Ophthalmol 106:1202, 1988
46. Moore MB, McCulley JP, Kaufman HE, Robin JB: Radial keratoneuritis as a presenting sign in *Acanthamoeba* keratitis. Ophthalmology 93:1310, 1986
47. Feist RM, Sugar J, Tessler H: Radial keratoneuritis in *Pseudomonas* keratitis. Arch Ophthalmol 109:774, 1991
48. Rabinovitch T, Weissman SS, Ostler HB, et al: *Acanthamoeba* keratitis: clinical signs and analysis of outcome. Rev Infect Dis 13(suppl):427, 1991
49. Dougherty PJ, Binder PS, Mondino BJ, Glasgow BJ: *Acanthamoeba* sclerokeratitis. Am J Ophthalmol 117:475, 1994
50. Mannis MJ, Tamaru R, Roth AM, et al: *Acanthamoeba* sclerokeratitis. Determining diagnostic criteria. Arch Ophthalmol 104:1313, 1986

51. Lindquist TD, Fritsche TR, Grutzmacher RD: Scleral ectasia secondary to *Acanthamoeba* keratitis. Cornea 9:74, 1990
52. Holland EJ, Alul IH, Meisler DM, et al: Subepithelial infiltrates in *Acanthamoeba* keratitis. Am J Ophthalmol 112:414, 1991
53. Wilhelmus KR, Osato MS, Font RL, et al: Rapid diagnosis of *Acanthamoeba* keratitis using calcofluor white. Arch Ophthalmol 104:1309, 1986
54. Epstein RJ, Wilson LA, Visvesvara GS, Plourde EG Jr: Rapid diagnosis of *Acanthamoeba* keratitis from corneal scrapings using indirect fluorescent antibody staining. Arch Ophthalmol 104:1318, 1986
55. Marines HM, Osato MS, Font RL: The value of calcofluor white in the diagnosis of mycotic and *Acanthamoeba* infections of the eye and ocular adnexa. Ophthalmology 94:23, 1987
56. Silvany RE, Luckenbach MW, Moore MB: The rapid detection of *Acanthamoeba* in paraffin-embedded sections of corneal tissue with calcofluor white. Arch Ophthalmol 105:1366, 1987
57. Chew SJ, Beuerman RW, Assouline M, et al: Early diagnosis of infectious keratitis with in vivo real time confocal microscopy. CLAO J 18:197, 1992
58. Auran JD, Starr MB, Koester CJ, LaBombardi VJ: In vivo scanning slit confocal microscopy of *Acanthamoeba* keratitis. Cornea 13:183, 1994.
59. Winchester K, Mathers WD, Sutphin JE, Daley TE: Diagnosis of *Acanthamoeba* keratitis in vivo with confocal microscopy. Cornea 14:10, 1995
60. Osato MS, Robinson NM, Wilhelmus KR, Jones DB: In vitro evaluation of antimicrobial compounds for cysticidal activity against *Acanthamoeba*. Rev Infect Dis 13(suppl):431, 1991
61. Larkin DFP, Kilvington S, Dart JKG: Treatment of *Acanthamoeba* keratitis with polyhexamethylene biguanide. Ophthalmology 99:185, 1992
62. Hay J, Kirkness CM, Seal DV, Wright P: Drug resistance and *Acanthamoeba* keratitis: the quest for alternative antiprotozoal chemotherapy. Eye 8:555, 1994
63. Ishibashi Y, Matsumoto Y, Kabata T, et al: Oral itraconazole and topical miconazole with debridement for *Acanthamoeba* keratitis. Am J Ophthalmol 109:121, 1990
64. Driebe WT Jr, Stern GA, Epstein RJ, et al: *Acanthamoeba* keratitis. Potential role for topical clotrimazole in combination chemotherapy. Arch Ophthalmol 106:1196, 1988
65. Mills RA, Wilhelmus KR, Osato MS, Pyron M: Polyhexamethylene biguanide in the treatment of *Acanthamoeba* keratitis [letter]. Aust N Z J Ophthalmol 21:277, 1993
66. Seal D, Hay J, Wright P, Kirkness C: In vitro drug sensitivity testing for alternate therapy in resistant strains of *Acanthamoebae*. ARVO abstract. Invest Ophthalmol Vis Sci 34(suppl):979, 1993
67. Gray TB, Gross KA, Cursons RT, Shewan JF: *Acanthamoeba* keratitis: a sobering case and a promising new treatment. Aust NZ J Ophthalmol 22:73, 1994
68. Varga JH, Wolf TC, Jensen HG, et al: Combined treatment of *Acanthamoeba* keratitis with propamidine, neomycin, and polyhexamethylene biguanide. Am J Ophthalmol 115:466, 1993
69. Bacon AS, Dart JKG, Ficker LA, et al: *Acanthamoeba* keratitis. The value of early diagnosis. Ophthalmology 100:1238, 1238
70. Wright P, Warhurst D, Jones BR: *Acanthamoeba* keratitis successful treated medically. Br J Ophthalmol 69:778, 1985
71. Cohen EJ, Buchanan HW, Laughrea PA, et al: Diagnosis and management of *Acanthamoeba* keratitis. Am J Ophthalmol 100:389, 1985
72. Lindquist TD, Sher NA, Doughman DJ: Clinical signs and medical therapy of early *Acanthamoeba* keratitis. Arch Ophthalmol 106:73, 1988
73. Berger ST, Mondino BJ, Hoft RH, et al: Successful medical management of *Acanthamoeba* keratitis. Am J Ophthalmol 110:395 1990
74. Johns KJ, Head WS, O'Day DM: Corneal toxicity of propamidine. Arch Ophthalmol 106:68, 1988
75. Holland GN, Donzis PB: Rapid resolution of early *Acanthamoeba* keratitis after epithelial debridement [letter]. Am J Ophthalmol 104:87, 1987
76. Stern GA, Buttross M: Use of corticosteroids in combination with antimicrobial drugs in the treatment of infectious corneal disease. Ophthalmology 98:847, 1991
77. Meisler DM, Rutherford I: Freezing and *Acanthamoeba* [letter]. Arch Ophthalmol 107:1420, 1989
78. Hirst L, Green WR, Merz W, et al: Management of *Acanthamoeba* keratitis. A case report and review of the literature. Ophthalmology 91:1105, 1984
79. Meisler DM, Ludwig IH, Rutherford I, et al: Susceptibility of *Acanthamoeba* to cryotherapeutic method. Arch Ophthalmol 104:130, 1985
80. Ficker L, Kirkness C, Wright P: Prognosis for keratoplasty in *Acanthamoeba* keratitis. Ophthalmology 100:105, 1993
81. Cohen EJ, Higgins SE, Arentsen JJ, et al: *Acanthamoeba* keratitis: extended abstracts. Rev Infect Dis 13(suppl):426, 1991
82. Kilvington S: Moist-heat disinfection of *Acanthamoeba* cysts. Rev Infect Dis 13(suppl):418, 1991
83. Lindquist TD, Doughman DJ, Rubenstein JB, Moore JW: *Acanthamoeba*-infected hydrogel contact lenses: susceptibility to disinfection. ARVO abstract. Invest Ophthalmol Vis Sci 28(suppl):371, 1987
84. Silvany RE, Dougherty JM, McCulley JP: Effect of contact lens preservatives on *Acanthamoeba*. Ophthalmology 98:854, 1993.
85. Silvany R, Dougherty JM, McCulley JP, et al: The effect of currently available contact lens disinfection systems on *Acanthamoeba castellanii* and *Acanthamoeba polyphaga*. Ophthalmology 97:286, 1990
86. Kilvington S, Anthony Y, Davies DJG, Meakin BJ: Effect of contact lens disinfectants against *Acanthamoeba* cysts. Rev Infect Dis 13(suppl):414, 1991
87. Rutherford I, Katanik MT, Meisler DM: Efficacy of a chlorhexidine tablet system for disinfection of soft contact

lenses against *Acanthamoeba* species. Rev Infect Dis 13(suppl):S416, 1991
88. Tomkins A, Bryceson A: Cutaneous leishmaniasis and pentamidine diabetes. Trans R Soc Ther Med Hyg 66:948, 1972
89. Roizenblatt J: Interstitial keratitis caused by American (mucocutaneous) leishmaniasis. Am J Ophthalmol 87:175, 1979
90. Binford CH, Connor DH (eds): Pathology of Tropical and Extraordinary Diseases. Armed Forces Institute of Pathology, Washington, DC, 1976
91. de Schweinitz GE, Woods AC: Experimental trypanosomiasis of the eye. Br J Ophthalmol 1:774, 1917
92. de Schweinitz GE, Woods AC: Trypanosome keratitis: an experimental study. Trans Am Ophthalmol Soc 5:106, 1917
93. Neame H: Parenchymatous keratitis in trypanosomiasis in cattle and in dogs and in man. Br J Ophthalmol 11:209, 1927
94. Ashton N, Wirasinha P: Encephalitozoonosis (nosematosis) of the cornea. Br J Ophthalmol 57:669, 1973
95. Pinnolis M, Egbert PR, Font RL, Winter FC: Nosematosis of the cornea. Arch Ophthalmol 99:1044, 1981
96. Davis RM, Font RL, Keisler MS, Shadduck JA: Corneal microsporidiosis: a case report including ultrastructural observations. Ophthalmology 97:953, 1990
97. Cali A, Meisler DM, Lowder CY, et al: Corneal microsporidioses: characterization and identification. J Protozool 39:215, 1991
98. Friedberg DN, Stenson SM, Orenstein JM, et al: Microsporidial keratoconjunctivitis in acquired immunodeficiency syndrome. Arch Ophthalmol 108:504, 1990
99. Didier ES, Didier PJ, Friedberg DN, et al: Isolation and characterization of a new human microsporidian, *Encephalitozoon hellem* (n.sp.), from three AIDS patients with keratoconjunctivitis. J Infect Dis 163:617, 1991
100. Yee RW, Tio FO, Martinez A, et al: Resolution of microsporidial epithelial keratopathy in a patient with AIDS. Ophthalmology 98:196, 1991
101. Lowder CY, Meisler DM, McMahon JT, et al: Microsporidial infection of the cornea in a man seropositive for human immunodeficiency virus. Am J Ophthalmol 109:242, 1990
102. Metcalf TW, Doran RML, Rowlands PL, et al: Microsporidial keratoconjunctivitis in a patient with AIDS. Br J Ophthalmol 76:177, 1992
103. Lacey CJ, Clard AM Fraser P, et al: Chronic microsporidian infection of the nasal mucosae sinuses and conjunctivae in HIV disease. Genitourin Med 68:179, 1992
104. Canning EU, Hollister WS: Human infections with microsporidia. Rev Med Microbiol 3:35, 1992
105. Margileth A, Strano A, Chandra R, et al: Disseminated nosematosis in an immunologically compromised infant. Arch Pathol 95:145, 1973
106. Weber R, Kuster H, Visvesvara GS, et al: Disseminated microsporidiosis due to *Encephalitozoon hellem*: pulmonary colonization, microhematuria, and mild conjunctivitis in a patient with AIDS. Clin Infect Dis 17:415, 1993
107. Schwartz DA, Visvesvara GS, Diesenhouse MC, et al: Pathologic features and immunofluorescent antibody demonstration of ocular microsporidiosis (*Encephalitozoon hellem*) in seven patients with AIDS. Am J Ophthalmol 115:285, 1993
108. Didier PJ, Didier ES, Orenstein JM, Shadduck JA: Fine structure of a new human microsporidian, *Encephalitozoon hellem*, in culture. J Protozool 38:502, 1991
109. Rastrelli PD, Didier E, Yee RW: Microsporidial keratitis. Ophthalmol Clin North Am 7:617, 1994
110. Diesenhouse MC, Wilson LA, Corrent GF, et al: Treatment of microsporidial keratoconjunctivitis with topical fumagillin. Am J Ophthalmol 115:293, 1993
111. Rosberger DF, Serdarevic ON, Erlandson RA, et al: Successful treatment of microsporidial keratoconjunctivitis with topical fumagillin in a patient with AIDS. Cornea 12:261, 1993
112. Choyce DP: Some observations on the ocular complications of onchocerciasis and their relationship to blindness. Trans R Soc Trop Med Hyg 52:112, 1958
113. Rodger FC: Living larvae of *Onchocerca volvulus*. Br J Ophthalmol 64:223, 1980
114. Solanes MP, Noble BR, Fonte A: Ocular onchocerciasis. Am J Ophthalmol 32:1207, 1949
115. Budden FH: Natural history of onchocerciasis. Br J Ophthalmol 41:214, 1957
116. Anderson J, Fuglsang H: Ocular onchocerciasis. Trop Disease Bull 74:257, 1977
117. Thylefors B: Ocular onchocerciasis. Bull WHO 56:63:1978
118. Semba R, Day S, Spencer W: Conjunctival nodules associated with onchocerciasis. Arch Ophthalmol 103:823, 1985
119. Duke B: Route of entry of *Onchocerca volvulus* microfilariae into the eye. Trans R Soc Trop Med Hyg 70:90, 1976
120. Sakla AA, Donnelly JJ, Lok JB, et al: Punctate keratitis induced by subconjunctivally injected microfilariae of *Onchocerca lienalis*. Arch Ophthalmol 104:894, 1986
121. Fuglsang JA: Living microfilariae of *Onchocerca volvulus* in the cornea. Br J Ophthalmol 57:712, 1983
122. Paul EV, Zimmerman LE: Some observations on the ocular pathology of onchocerciasis. Hum Pathol 1:581, 1970
123. Rodger FC, Chir M: The pathogenesis and pathology of ocular onchocerciasis. Am J Ophthalmol 49:560, 1960
124. Rodger FC, Chir M: The pathogenesis and pathology of ocular onchocerciasis. Am J Ophthalmol 49:104, 1960
125. Donnelly JJ, Rockey JH, Bianco AE, Soulsby EJ: Ocular immunopathologic findings of experimental onchocerciasis. Arch Ophthalmol 102:628, 1984
126. Jones BR, Anderson J, Fuglsang H: Evaluation of microfilaricidal effects in the cornea from topically applied drugs in ocular onchocerciasis: trials with levamisole and mebendazole. Br J Ophthalmol 62:440, 1978
127. Taylor HR, Murphy RP, Newland HS, et al: Treatment of onchocerciasis. The ocular effects of ivermectin and diethylcarbamazine. Arch Ophthalmol 104:863, 1986
128. Anderson J, Fuglsang H: Further studies on the treatment of ocular onchocerciasis with diethylcarbamazine and suramin. Br J Ophthalmol 62:450, 1978
129. Tonjum AM, Thylefors B: Aspects of corneal changes in onchocerciasis. Br J Ophthalmol 62:458, 1978

130. Jones BR, Anderson J, Fuglsang H: Effects of various concentrations of diethylcarbamazine citrate applied as eyedrops in ocular onchocerciasis and the possibilities of improved therapy from continuous non-pulsed delivery. Br J Ophthalmol 62:428, 1978
131. Fuglsang H, Anderson J: Further observations on the relationship between ocular onchocerciasis and the head nodule and on the possible benefit of nodulectomy. Br J Ophthalmol 62:445, 1978
132. Rockey JH, Donnelly JJ, Stromberg BE, et al: Immunopathology of ascarid infection of the eye. Arch Ophthalmol 99:1831, 1981
133. Ashton N, Cook C: Allergic granulomatous nodules of eyelid and conjunctiva. Am J Ophthalmol 87:1, 1979
134. Stein MF, Finkelstein WE: Loiasis in Westchester County. NY State J Med 79:1882, 1979
135. Osuntokun O, Olurin O: Filarial worm (*Loa loa*) in the anterior chamber. Report of two cases. Br J Ophthalmol 59:166, 1975
136. Farrer WE, Wittner M, Tanowitz HB: African eye worm (*Loa loa*) in a tourist. Ann Ophthalmol 13:1177, 1981
137. Font RL, Neafie RC, Perry HD: Subcutaneous dirofilariasis of the eyelid and ocular adnexa. Report of six cases. Arch Ophthalmol 98:1079, 1980
138. Jariva P, Sucharit S: *Dirofilaria repens* from the eyelid of a woman in Thailand. Am J Trop Med Hyg 32:1456, 1983
139. Orsoni JG, Coggiola G, Minazzi P: Filaria conjunctivae. Ophthalmologica 190:243, 1985
140. Moorhouse DE: *Dirofilaria immitis*: a cause of human intraocular infection. Infection 6:192, 1978
141. Sen DK: Acute suppurative dacryodenitis caused by a *Cysticercus cellulosae*. J Pediatr Ophthalmol Strabismus 19:100, 1982
142. Singh E, Kaur J: Cysticercosis of the eyelid. Ann Ophthalmol 14:947, 1982
143. Perry HD, Font RL: Cysticercosis of the eyelid. Arch Ophthalmol 96:1255, 1978
144. Sen DK, Thomas A: Incidence of subconjunctival cysticercosis. Acta Ophthalmol (Copenh) 47:395, 1969
145. Singh I, Phogat AC, Chohan BS, Malik KPS: Conjunctival cysticercosis. J Indian Med Assoc 70:136, 1978
146. Apple DJ, Fajoni ML, Garland PE, et al: Orbital hydatid cyst. J Pediatr Ophthalmol Strabismus 17:380, 1980
147. Boase AJ: *Coenurus* cyst of the eye. Br J Ophthalmol 40:183, 1956
148. Williams PH, Templeton AC: Infection of the eye by tapeworm *Coenurus*. Br J Ophthalmol 55:766, 1971
149. Hui-lan Z, Lan S, De Run L, et al: Ocular sparganosis caused blindness. Chin Med J 96:73, 1983
150. Wang WJ, Xin YJ, Robinson NL, et al: Intraocular paragonimiasis. Br J Ophthalmol 68:85, 1984
151. Luo WB: Paragonimiasis of the eye. Report of 20 cases. Chin Med J 83:453, 1964
152. Jiang MF, Wang HF, Huang SY: Anterior chamber and eyelid paragonimiasis. Report of 7 cases. Chin J Ophthalmol 18:245, 1982
153. Newton JC, Kanchanaranya C, Previte LR: Intraocular *Schistosoma mansoni*. Am J Ophthalmol 65:774, 1968
154. Abboud IA, Hanna LS, Ragab HAA: Experimental ocular schistosomiasis. Br J Ophthalmol 55:106, 1971
155. Lester RJG, Freeman RS: Eye penetration by cercariae of *Schistosoma mansoni*. J Parasitol 61:970, 1975
156. Badir G: Schistosomiasis of the conjunctiva. Br J Ophthalmol 30:215, 1946
157. Fatt-Hi A, Kamel I: Ectopic bilharziasis. J Laryngol Otol 94:1179, 1980
158. Welsh NH: Bilharzial conjunctivitis. Am J Ophthalmol 66:933, 1968
159. Jakobiec FA, Gess L, Zimmerman LE: Granulomatous dacryoadenitis caused by *Schistosoma haematobium*. Arch Ophthalmol 95:278, 1977
160. Rufli T, Mumcuoglu Y: The hair follicle mites *Demodex folliculorum* and *Demodex brevis*: biology and medical importance. Dermatologica 162:1, 1981
161. English FP, Nutting WB: Demodicosis of ophthalmic concern. Am J Ophthalmol 92:362, 1981
162. Norn MS: *Demodex folliculorum*. Incidence and possible pathogenic role in the human eyelid. Acta Ophthalmol (Copenh) 108(suppl): 85, 1970
163. Gutgesell VJ, Stern GA, Hood CI: Histopathology of meibomian gland dysfunction. Am J Ophthalmol 94:383, 1982
164. de Vries LAM, van Bijsterveld OP: Ophthalmooestriasis conjunctivae. Ophthalmologica 192:193, 1986
165. Romanes GJ: Ocular myiasis. Br J Ophthalmol 67:332, 1983
166. Wong D: External ophthalmomyiasis caused by the sheep bot *Oestrus ovis*. Br J Ophthalmol 66:786, 1982
167. Ziemianski MC, Lee KY, Sabates FN: Ophthalmomyiasis interna. Arch Ophthalmol 98:1588, 1980
168. Slusher MM, Holland WD, Weaver RG, Tyler ME: Ophthalmomyiasis interna posterior. Arch Ophthalmol 97:885, 1979
169. Syrdalen P, Nitter T, Mehl R: Ophthalmomyiasis interna posterior: report of a case caused by the reindeer warble fly larvae and review of previously reported cases. Br J Ophthalmol 66:589, 1982
170. Wilhelmus KR: Myiasis palpebrarum. Am J Ophthalmol 101:496, 1986
171. Couch JM, Green WR, Hirst LW, De La Cruz ZC: Diagnosing and treating *Phthirus pubis* palbebrarum. Surv Ophthalmol 26:219, 1982
172. Centers for Disease Control: 1989 Sexually transmitted diseases treatment guidelines. MMWR 38:i, 1989
173. Cogan DG, Grant WM: Treatment of pediculosis ciliaris with anticholinesterase agents. Arch Ophthalmol 41:627, 1949
174. Mathew M, D'Souza P, Mehta DK: A new treatment of *Phthiriasis palpebrarum*. Ann Ophthalmol 14:439, 1982
175. Terry JE, Williams RE: *Dermacentor variabilis*. Uncomplicated lid involvement. Arch Ophthalmol 98:514, 1980
176. Bode D Speicher P, Harlan H: A seed tick infestation of the conjunctiva: *Amblyomma americanum* larva. Ann Ophthalmol 19:63, 1987

177. Knapp G: Ophthalmia nodosa. Am J Ophthalmol 24:247, 1897
178. Watson PG, Sevel D: Ophthalmia nodosa. Br J Ophthalmol 50:209, 1966
179. Gundersen T, Heath P, Garron LK: Ophthalmia nodosa. Trans Am Ophthalmol Soc 48:151, 1950
180. Stulting RD, Hooper RJ, Cavanagh ND: Ocular injury caused by tarantula hairs. Am J Ophthalmol 96:118, 1983
181. Hered RW, Spaulding AG, Sanitato JJ, Wander AH: Ophthalmia nodosa caused by tarantula hairs. Ophthalmology 95:166, 1988
182. Rutzen AR, Weiss JS, Kachadoorian H: Tarantula hair ophthalmia nodosa. Am J Ophthalmol 116:381, 1993

16

Congenital Anomalies of the Cornea

William M. Townsend

Describing a corneal anomaly as congenital implies that the anomaly is discovered at birth. Such a definition, however, excludes conditions that are determined at the moment of conception but do not manifest themselves until adulthood, such as many corneal dystrophies. Similarly, acquired conditions, such as those caused by intrauterine trauma or infection, may be classified as congenital merely because they are recognized at birth. The term *congenital* has no connotation with regard to the genetic versus acquired status of an anomaly, and assumptions about the cause of a lesion noted at birth are unwarranted until a diagnosis has been made.

ETIOLOGY OF CONGENITAL ANOMALIES

The time-honored concept that divided developmental anomalies into genetically and environmentally determined processes has been replaced by the understanding that these two processes often coexist. To be sure, approximately 1,500 systemic diseases have a genetic basis,[1] and chromosomal mapping has pinpointed the defective gene in at least 68 ocular and 338 systemic diseases.[2] New cases arising from gene mutation add to the group of genetically determined disorders.[3] Teratogenic agents acting on parental germ cells not only induce gene mutations (which may become hereditary) but also induce chromosomal aberrations (which are usually not hereditary). These same teratogenic agents may also affect the zygote, embryo, or fetus, producing anomalies of varying severity. Fetal alcohol syndrome[4] is a good example of the effects of a teratogenic agent; severe ocular and systemic malformations may result from maternal alcohol abuse during the first trimester of pregnancy. Separating gene-determined disease from nonhereditary, teratogen-induced disease is important in genetic counseling. Nevertheless, anomalies are often too similar to permit the differentiation of genetic versus nongenetic causes on the basis of appearance alone. The only reliable method is a thorough pedigree analysis.

Table 16-1 lists some of the causative factors implicated in congenital anomalies.[5]

NATURE OF CONGENITAL ANOMALIES

Congenital anomalies usually represent the end stage of pathologic intrauterine events. The clinician can only conjecture or deduce the true nature of such events. There are three major types of developmental anomalies: developmental arrest, aberration, and a combination of the two.[6] In developmental arrest, the differentiation of a particular ocular structure appears to be normal but stops at an early stage, while the rest of the eye continues to develop. The fetal anterior chamber angle in patients with congenital glaucoma is an example. In aberration, abnormal development changes the normal pattern of differentiation. Myelinated nerve fibers are an example. In developmental arrest plus aberration, aberrant development is superimposed on developmental arrest at a certain stage. An example of this is persistent hyperplastic primary vitreous, in which there is an arrest in the development of the hyaloid system, with persistence of the hyaloid vessels, and aberrant retrolental fibrous tissue formation.

An important determinant of a corneal anomaly caused by an intrauterine insult is the time at which the insult occurs. If it occurs early in embryogenesis, the entire organ may be absent or disorganized. As fetal age progresses, the impact of the insult becomes more limited in severity and extent. Most anomalies affecting the cornea, as well as the eye in general, are caused by insults that occur dur-

TABLE 16-1
Causes of Congenital Anomalies

- Hereditary disorders
  - Transmitted from past generations: gene induced
    - Inborn errors of metabolism
    - Dystrophies
    - Hereditary syndromes
      - Mesodermal
      - Craniofacial
      - Osseous
      - Neurologic
      - Ectodermal
  - Spontaneous, "random" mutations
  - Induced in parental germ cells by exposure to teratogenic agents
- Nonhereditary disorders
  - Acting on parental germ cells: chromosomal aberrations
    - Numerical abnormalities: aneuploidy
    - Structural abnormalities
      - Deletions and duplications
      - Translocations
      - Inversions
      - Fragmentation
      - Ring formation
  - Acting on zygote, embryo, or fetus: specific tissue anomalies
    - Physical agents: radiation, hypothermia, hyperthermia
    - Chemical agents: drugs, dyes, metals, antimetabolites
    - Trauma
    - Maternal disturbance: malnutrition, hormonal imbalance
    - Rh incompatibility
    - Placental dysfunction
    - Anoxia
    - Infection
    - Maternal alcohol abuse

TABLE 16-2
Classification of Congenital Anomalies of the Cornea

- Absence of the cornea and related anomalies
- Anomalies of size
  - Megalocornea
  - Microcornea
- Anomalies of shape
  - Oval cornea
  - Astigmatism
  - Keratoconus
  - Keratoglobus
  - Cornea plana
- Anomalies of transparency
  - Developmental congenital corneal opacities
    - Diffuse corneal opacities
      - Sclerocornea
    - Central corneal opacities
      - Peters' anomaly type I
      - Peters' anomaly type II
      - Posterior keratoconus
      - Congenital anterior staphyloma
    - Peripheral corneal opacities
      - Posterior embryotoxon
      - Axenfeld's and Rieger's anomalies
  - Dystrophic congenital corneal opacities
    - Congenital hereditary endothelial dystrophy
    - Congenital cornea guttata
    - Posterior polymorphous dystrophy
    - Posterior amorphous dystrophy
    - Congenital hereditary stromal dystrophy
  - Congenital opacities caused by inborn errors of metabolism
    - Amino acid abnormalities
    - Mucopolysaccharidoses
    - Sphingolipidoses
    - Mucolipidoses
    - Miscellaneous metabolic disorders
  - Congenital opacities in hereditary syndromes
    - Mesodermal: Marfan, Weill-Marchesani
    - Craniofacial: craniofacial dysostosis, cleft lip and palate, hemifacial hypoplasia, brachycephaly, Aarskog, Neuhauser, Peters' plus
    - Osseous: osteogenesis imperfecta, onycho-osteodysplasia, Mietens, Conradi, Léri, dermochondrodystrophy, Rosenthal-Kloepfer, Robinow, SHORT, Krause-Kivlin
    - Neurologic: Smith-Lemli-Opitz, lissencephaly, Cockayne, Norrie
    - Ectodermal: ichthyosis, anhydrotic ectodermal dysplasia, epidermolysis bullosa, keratoses, Melkersson-Rosenthal, acrodermatitis, Kyrle's disease, palmoplantar keratosis, Richner-Hanhart, Rothmund-Thomson
  - Congenital opacities in chromosomal aberrations
  - Congenital opacities caused by infection
  - Congenital opacities caused by glaucoma
  - Congenital opacities caused by trauma
- Congenital mass lesions of the cornea
  - Dermoid
  - Keloid
  - Dyskeratosis

ing the period of organogenesis (between the fourth and sixth weeks of gestation). Anomalies limited to the cornea and anterior chamber develop later, during the period of differentiation (between the sixth week and fourth month). Beyond this stage, corneal anomalies resemble those occurring after birth. This gradient of severity provides the clinician with a clue as to when the noxious insult occurred. At the same time, it accounts for variations in anomalies that share a common pathologic nature.

Table 16-2 presents a classification of congenital corneal anomalies, combining causative factors with elements of differential diagnosis.

ABSENCE OF THE CORNEA

True absence of the cornea is extremely rare. The case reported by Manschot[7] was accompanied by primary aphakia, which illustrates the inducing function of the lens in corneogenesis. The induction of the lens, in turn,

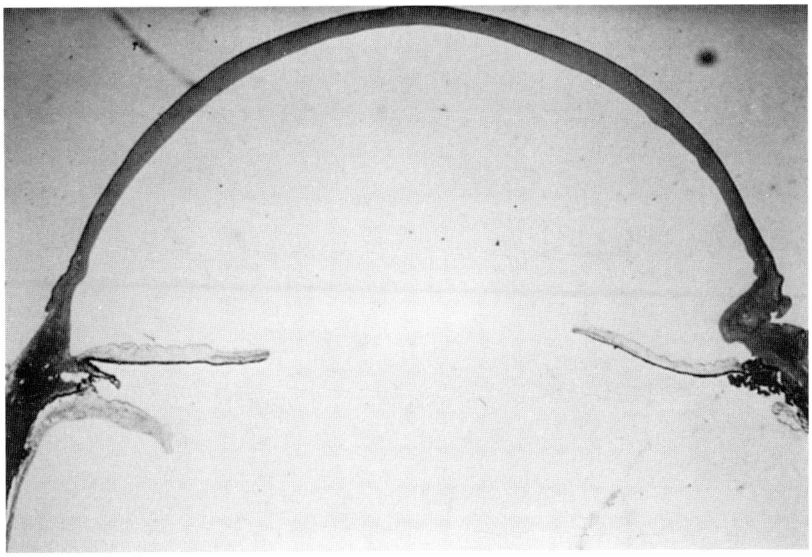

FIGURE 16-1 Megalocornea. Note that the entire anterior segment and ciliary girdle are grossly enlarged. The lens dislocated spontaneously (hematoxylin and eosin).

depends on the anatomic proximity of the optic cup to the surface ectoderm. In cryptophthalmos, the cornea is not truly absent; failure of eyelid formation results in metaplasia of the corneal epithelium into skin.

ANOMALIES OF SIZE

Megalocornea

Normally, the horizontal (largest) corneal diameter is 10.0 to 12.8 mm in the newborn infant.[8] In megalocornea, this diameter is exceeded, often considerably. The entire anterior segment is disproportionately larger than the rest of the eye[9] (Figure 16-1). Megalocornea is usually bilateral. It is nonprogressive, and the cornea remains clear except over sites of tears in Descemet's membrane. The limbal region is sharply delimited, in contrast to buphthalmos, the main condition from which megalocornea must be differentiated. Megalocornea presents most frequently as an isolated finding in healthy males; it is most frequently transmitted as an X-linked recessive trait.[5] The gene locus has been located in the region Xq12q26, near the locus for Aarskog syndrome.[10] Autosomal transmission has been found in families also presenting with congenital glaucoma.[11]

In addition to frequent myopia and astigmatism, complications of megalocornea include cataract formation and lens dislocation, presumably caused by stretching of the zonules in the presence of a widened ciliary girdle. Even in the absence of these complications, iridodonesis and phakodonesis from zonular instability are common. In some instances, other anomalies are present, especially iris and pupillary anomalies (Figure 16-2). Less commonly associated ocular anomalies include posterior embryotoxon, mosaic corneal dystrophy,[12] infantile or juvenile glaucoma,[13] and pigmentary dispersion with Krukenberg spindle.[14]

Systemic syndromes associated with megalocornea include Marfan syndrome,[15] Apert syndrome,[16] osteogenesis imperfecta, mucolipidosis type II,[17] and Neuhauser syndrome, which is a recessively inherited syndrome that includes mental retardation, seizures, short stature, and dyscephaly.[18]

The size of the anterior segment is determined largely by the location of the optic cup margins.[6] A slowing of forward growth of the optic cup between the 12- and 40-mm stage, together with failure to bend axially during the third month, leaves an excessively large, broad ciliary girdle and anterior segment. The frequent finding of borderline large corneas in Marfan syndrome[19] and the occurrence of megalocornea in connective tissue diseases raise the possibility that some collagen abnormality may be involved. Perhaps then, the fault lies not only with the optic cup but also with the keratocytes, which are derived from neural ectoderm.[20]

Microcornea

In true microcornea, the globe is normal in size; only the cornea and anterior segment are abnormally small. The corneal diameter is 10 mm or less. Occurring as frequently bilaterally as unilaterally, microcornea shows no sex predilection. When microcornea occurs as an isolated condition, visual acuity is excellent despite a tendency

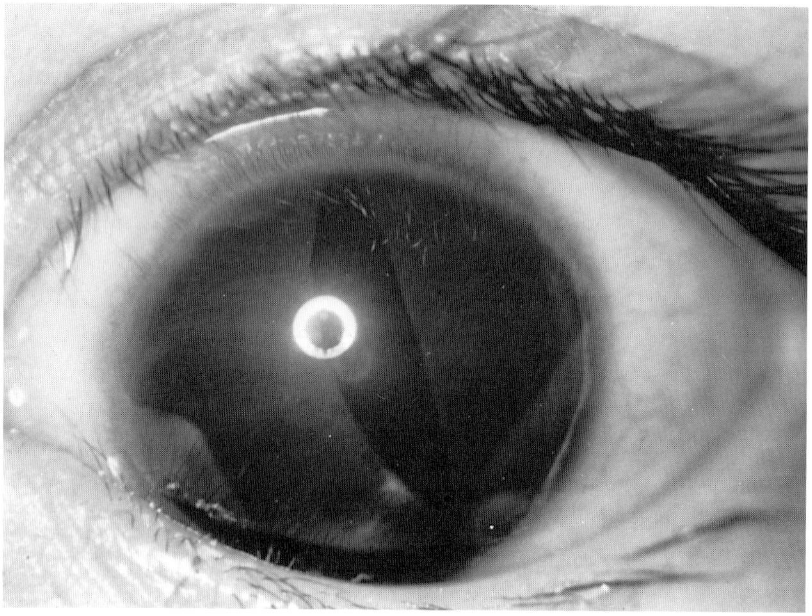

FIGURE 16-2 Megalocornea. The corneal diameter is 13.8 mm. There are associated anomalies, including posterior embryotoxon, dyscoria, and iris hypoplasia.

toward a steepened corneal curvature. In these cases, hereditary transmission is the rule and follows an autosomal dominant pattern.[21] Unlike megalocornea, microcornea is a frequent companion to several anterior segment anomalies (Figure 16-3). The degree of corneal differentiation is often affected. Systemic associations are also frequent[22-40] (Table 16-3). Patients with microcornea are subject to angle closure glaucoma in adult life because the growing lens crowds the small anterior segment[41] (Figure 16-4). A variant of microcornea is seen with a vertically oval cornea in the syndrome of microphthalmos with coloboma[32] (Figure 16-5). The cause of microcornea remains obscure. There appears to be an arrest in the growth of the cornea, a process that begins after the fifth month of gestation, when differentiation is complete.[6]

ANOMALIES OF CORNEAL SHAPE

Oval Cornea

A vertically oval cornea of fairly normal size has been described in Rieger's anomaly[42] and Turner syndrome.[36] It also occurs with microcornea, as noted above (see Figure 16-5).

A horizontally oval cornea is almost always caused by sclerocornea, in which the sclera is more prominent than normal along the superior and inferior limbus.

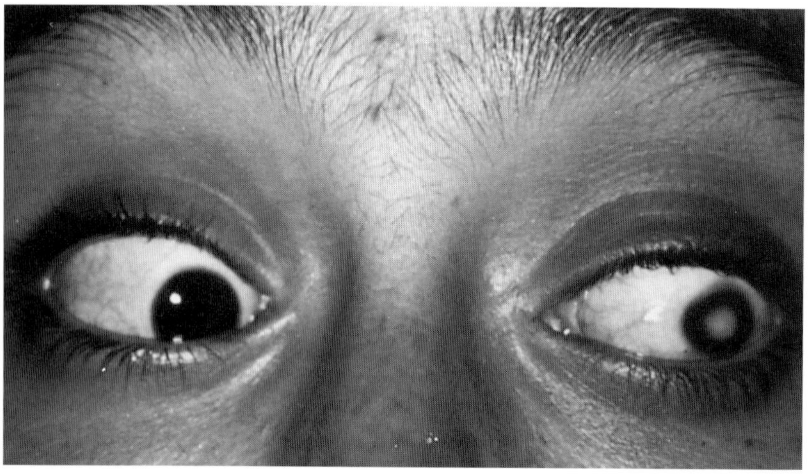

FIGURE 16-3 Microcornea, left eye. The horizontal diameter of the cornea is 10.0 mm. There is also a congenital cataract.

TABLE 16-3
Systemic Associations of Microcornea

Mesodermal syndromes	
	Ehlers-Danlos[22]
	Weill-Marchesani[23]
	Rieger[24]
Craniofacial syndromes	
	Hallerman-Streiff[25]
	Waardenburg[26]
	Meyer-Schwickerath[27]
	Greig's hypertelorism[28]
Osseous syndromes	
	Onycho-osteo-dysplasia (Hood)[29]
	Kohn-Romano[30]
	Nance-Horan[31]
Neurologic syndromes	
	Norrie[32]
	Meckel[33]
	Progeria[34]
	Smith-Lemli-Opitz[35]
	Sjögren-Larsson[32]
	Cornelia de Lange[32]
	Goltz[32]
Chromosomal syndromes	
	Turner[36]
	de Grouchy[37]
	Trisomy 13-15[38]
	Duplication of 2p[39]
Infections	
	Rubella[40]

Corneal Astigmatism

In most instances, corneal astigmatism falls within the definition of a variation or "a departure from the theoretical normal."[6] The normal pattern of postnatal development tends toward with-the-rule astigmatism (steep vertical meridian) in the first decades of life and against-the-rule astigmatism (steep horizontal meridian) in later years.[43] Significant amounts of astigmatism may follow a hereditary pattern, usually that of an autosomal dominant trait.[34] Large, frequent changes in astigmatism and increasing axis obliquity should raise the suspicion of keratoconus.

Keratoconus

Keratoconus is a progressive, noninflammatory ectasia of the central and paracentral cornea, which assumes a conical configuration (Figure 16-6). The classification of keratoconus as a degeneration by some and as a dystrophy by others emphasizes the uncertainty about its causes and pathogenesis. Keratoconus usually occurs in a sporadic, isolated fashion, although autosomal dominant transmission has been documented in some cases.[44] It is usually bilateral, and females are more frequently affected than males.[45] The rare patient who presents with keratoconus at birth usually has other congenital anomalies. Typically, keratoconus is not evident until puberty, when relentless, progressive oblique astigmatism suddenly occurs. Franceschetti documented progression of the ectasia until age 32, after which most cases showed slowing of the process.[46] Occasionally, progression becomes arrested very early (forme fruste) or there is only slight slow progression throughout life. Several disorders have been associated with keratoconus[28,47-58] (Table 16-4). Keratoconus is discussed in further detail in Chapter 22.

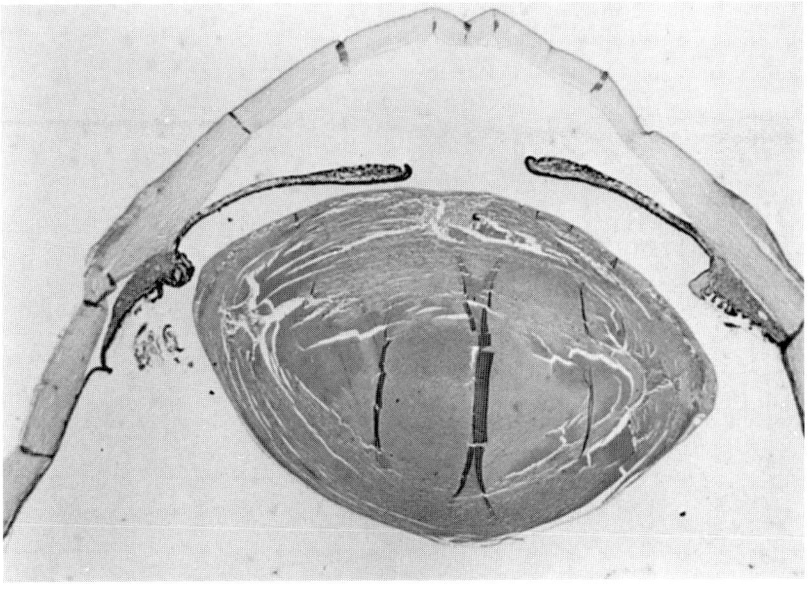

FIGURE 16-4 Microcornea. Note that the entire anterior segment and ciliary girdle are smaller than normal. The cataractous lens has induced a pupillary block, with the apposition of iris root against the anterior chamber angle (hematoxylin and eosin).

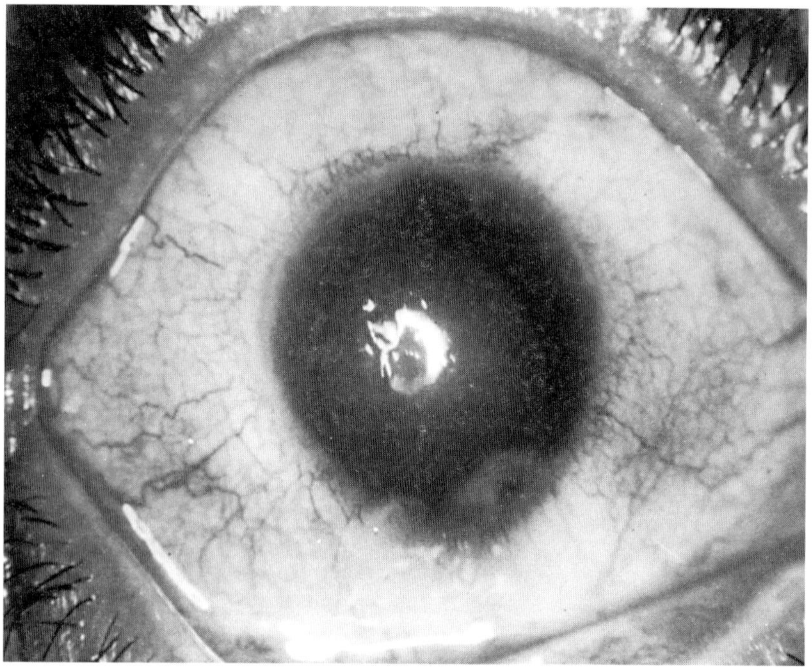

FIGURE 16-5 Vertically oval cornea and microcornea. The lens is cataractous, and pupillary block is present. Intraocular pressure is 46 mmHg. Note the typical iris coloboma, later found to include the choroid.

Keratoglobus

In keratoglobus, the entire cornea, not just the apical portion, is thin and ectatic (Figure 16-7). The condition is rare compared with keratoconus, from which it is said to differ qualitatively.[59] Nevertheless, the occurrence of keratoconus and keratoglobus in the same family[59] and the similar ectatic nature of both processes suggest that the two conditions are related. The histopathologic features are similar in both.[60] Keratoglobus is discussed further in Chapter 22, as is pellucid marginal degeneration,[61] which is another corneal ectasia.

Cornea Plana

In cornea plana, the cornea is extremely flat; keratometry readings may be as low as 20 to 30 diopters. The cornea

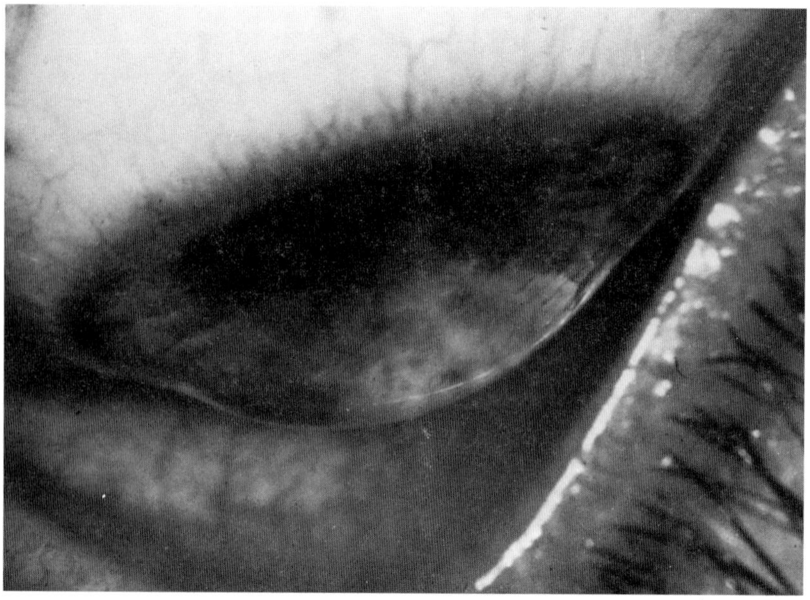

FIGURE 16-6 Keratoconus. The central cornea is thin and ectatic.

TABLE 16-4
Disorders Associated with Keratoconus

Van der Hoeve's fragilitas ossium[47]
Apert syndrome[48]
Marfan syndrome[49]
Ehlers-Danlos syndrome[50]
Down syndrome[51]
Crouzon syndrome[52]
Tapetoretinal degenerations[53]
Atopy[54]
Vernal conjunctivitis[55]
Hypothyroidism[56]
Noonan syndrome[57a]
Chandler syndrome[58]
Greig's hypertelorism[28]

[a] This case may have represented an example of posterior keratoconus.

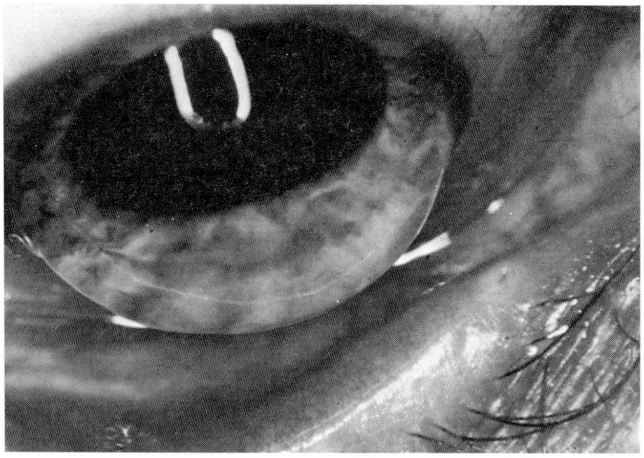

FIGURE 16-7 Keratoglobus. The entire cornea is thin and ectatic except for a small limbal rim.

is opaque peripherally and frequently centrally as well. All reported cases of cornea plana[62] have shown peripheral scleralization. In fact, the condition is indistinguishable clinically from peripheral sclerocornea. The term *cornea plana* is used mostly in Europe,[63-65] whereas in the United States the term *sclerocornea* is used. The associated ocular and systemic abnormalities are similar for both conditions[29,33,65-71] (Table 16-5). In the absence of histologic differentiation, distinguishing them as two separate entities should be viewed with skepticism.

ANOMALIES OF TRANSPARENCY

The various causes of congenital corneal opacities are outlined in Table 16-2.

Developmental Congenital Corneal Opacities

The term *anterior chamber cleavage syndrome* was introduced by Reese and Ellsworth[72] in 1966 and includes all the lesions described below; others[73,74] have emphasized the usefulness of this unifying concept. However, the term *anterior chamber cleavage* is based on a theory of embryology that no longer appears to be fully accurate.[75] Additionally, it is clear that each of the lesions included in the "syndrome" has a separate origin, identity, and destiny. A true syndrome may present isolated lesions as partial manifestations of a polymorphic or multifaceted whole, but the full range of signs must appear together to constitute a clearly defined syndrome. The anterior chamber cleavage syndrome has never met this criterion for the

TABLE 16-5
Comparison of Ocular Findings and Systemic Associations of Cornea Plana and Sclerocornea

Ocular Findings		*Systemic Associations*	
Cornea Plana	*Sclerocornea*	*Cornea Plana*	*Sclerocornea*
Congenital anterior synechiae	Congenital anterior synechiae	Osteogenesis imperfecta	Osteogenesis imperfecta[65]
Iris coloboma	Iris coloboma, dyscoria	Epidermolysis bullosa[66]	Epidermolysis bullosa[66]
Cataract	Cataract		Polydactyly[67]
Glaucoma	Glaucoma		Cranial dystrophies[67]
Ectopia lentis	Ectopia lentis		Ear deformities[67]
Blue sclera	Blue sclera		Cerebellar anomalies[67]
Microphthalmos	Microphthalmos		Hereditary onycho-osteo-dysplasia syndrome[29]
Choroidal coloboma	Choroidal coloboma		Cryptorchidism[67]
Retinal aplasia			Trisomy 18[68]
			Mietens syndrome[69]
			Smith-Lemli-Opitz syndrome[70]
			Meckel syndrome[33]
			Unbalanced translocation (17p,10q)[71]

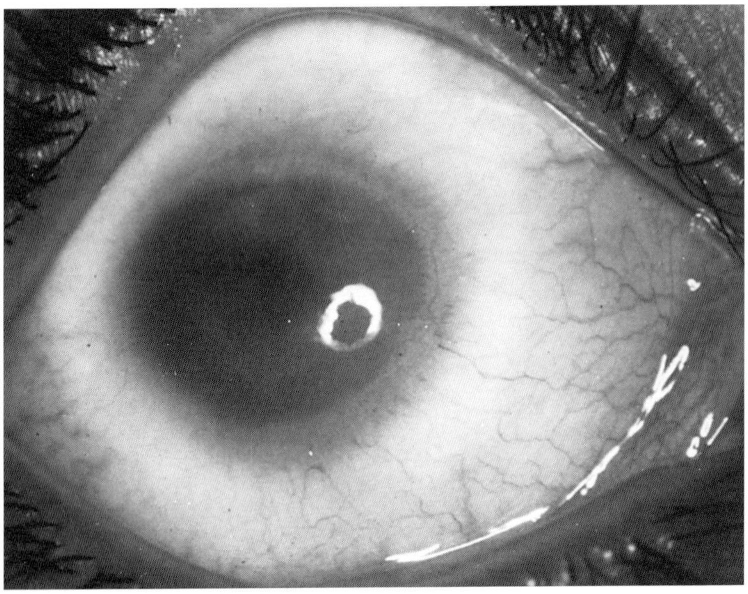

FIGURE 16-8 Peripheral sclerocornea. The central cornea is nebulous, but only the peripheral cornea shows the characteristic dense opacification. Microcornea also is present, and the corneal curvature is flat.

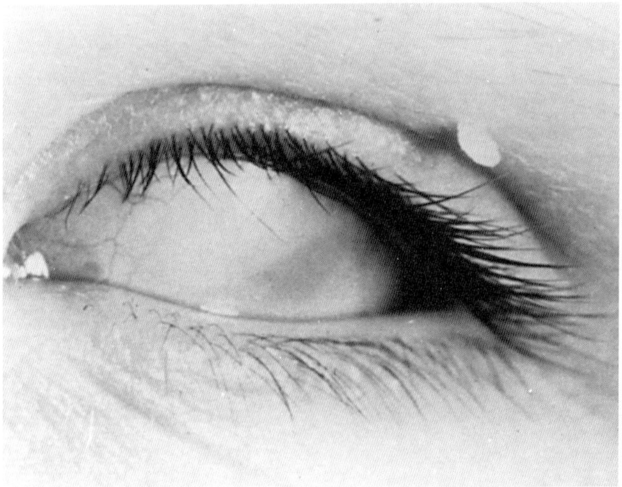

FIGURE 16-9 Diffuse sclerocornea. There is marble-like opacification of the entire cornea, and the corneal curvature is flat.

simple reason that it does not exist. The lumping together of qualitatively different lesions serves no useful purpose.

Diffuse Corneal Opacities

Sclerocornea In sclerocornea, a diffuse, marble-like, white opacification of the entire corneal thickness blends imperceptibly with the sclera circumferentially, obliterating the limbal region. In some cases, only the corneal periphery is involved (Figure 16-8), whereas in others, most or all of the cornea is opacified (Figure 16-9). Most reported cases have flattening of the corneal curvature,[76] as already mentioned. Sclerocornea is frequently bilateral; it shows no sex predilection. Most cases appear sporadically, although pedigrees showing autosomal dominant and recessive patterns of inheritance have been described.[77]

In sclerocornea, Bowman's layer is usually absent. The diameter of the collagen fibrils is greater in the superficial stroma than in the deeper stroma,[78] which is the opposite of the situation in normal cornea (where the fibril diameter is greater in the deeper stroma), and similar to normal sclera. Orderly lamellar orientation is absent at all levels, and scattered blood vessels are intermingled with the abnormal fibrils. The endothelium and Descemet's membrane appear normal in some patients,[71] whereas in others they are either abnormal[69] or entirely absent.[79] Of importance to the surgeon is the frequent finding of anterior chamber angle abnormalities, varying from congenital anterior synechiae to total lack of differentiation.[67,79] Because of angle abnormalities, glaucoma may present initially or, more commonly, after penetrating keratoplasty.

The mesenchymal cells of neural crest origin, which normally would develop into corneal and scleral stroma, remain as a single continuous homogeneous sheet until the limbal anlage becomes interposed between the two at the 24-mm stage (seventh week). By the 40-mm stage (tenth week), the limbal anlage becomes defined as a clearly visible, well-demarcated condensation. This limbal condensation, by virtue of being denser than the adjacent tissue, is thought to provide a ring of rigid stability that allows for the subsequent development of increased corneal curvature, relative to the curvature of the sclera.[80] Thus,

FIGURE 16-10 Peters' anomaly type I. Note the central location of the nebular opacity and the adherent iris strands from the collarette.

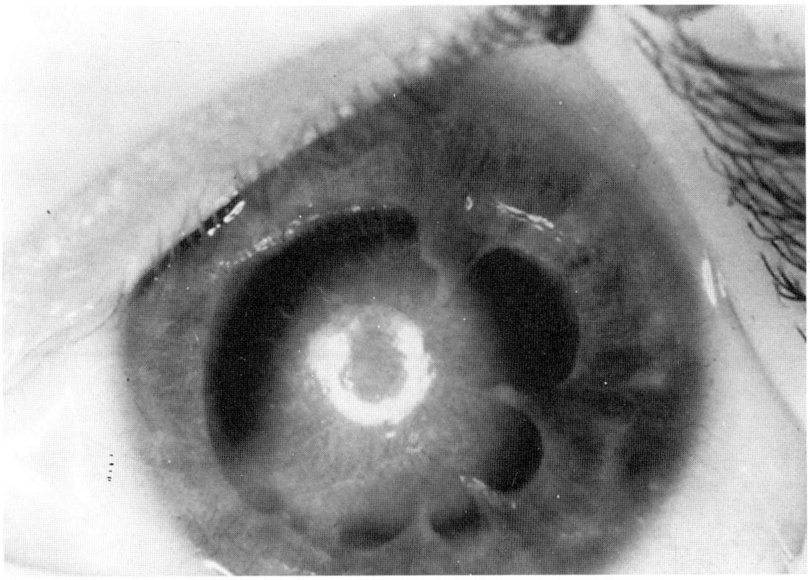

absence of the limbal anlage results in a flat cornea with a curvature approximating that of the sclera, a condition normally present in the fetal eye until the 40-mm stage. The simultaneous presence of a flat cornea and an undefined limbus in sclerocornea bears testimony to the close relationship between corneal curvature and limbal differentiation. Although a developmental arrest at the 24-mm stage can explain these two features of sclerocornea,[78] the frequent finding of total endothelial undifferentiation or absence suggests an earlier arrest. The fault may lie with the undifferentiated corneogenic mesenchyme that is adjacent to the optic cup at the 16-mm stage.[81]

Central Corneal Opacities

In contrast to the diffuse, full-thickness, marble-like opacity of sclerocornea is a group of developmental anomalies characterized by opacities limited to a portion of the cornea and localized to the deeper layers of the stroma. Most, if not all, of these conditions result from focal defects in the endothelium and Descemet's membrane. Unless these opacities are dense, they are compatible with good vision and rarely require corneal transplantation.

Peters' Anomaly Type I Peters' anomaly has acquired a long list of names through the years: primary mesodermal dysgenesis of the cornea, congenital anterior synechiae, posterior keratoconus, and anterior chamber cleavage syndrome. Additionally, different authors have used the same term to label different lesions, further confusing the subject.

The clinical appearance of Peters' anomaly type I is a nebular opacity in the pupillary axis bordered (but not covered) by one or more iris strands that cross the anterior chamber from the iris collarette (Figure 16-10). In some cases, the iris adhesions have broken off, and only microscopic examination shows their presence as uveal fragments attached to the posterior surface of the cornea. The lens is positioned normally and remains clear, although a discrete anterior pyramidal cataract is occasionally present. Associated anomalies include microcornea, sclerocornea, and infantile glaucoma. For the most part, however, the lesion is an isolated one, and there are no other ocular or systemic abnormalities. A familial pattern has been recorded in some instances, but extensive pedigree studies are lacking. Both sexes are affected, and unilateral involvement appears to predominate. Histologic examination[82] confirms an absence of Descemet's membrane and endothelium limited to the area of the opacity. On light microscopy, the overlying stroma, Bowman's layer, and epithelium are uninvolved.

The pathogenesis of Peters' anomaly type I is the subject of speculation. In the absence of lenticular changes, it is impossible to invoke a lenticular role, as proposed by Peters.[83] Furthermore, the focal nature of the defect and the normal differentiation of adjacent structures militate against the idea of an arrest early in development, as proposed by Collins[84] and Seefelder.[85] Even Ballantyne,[86] as far back as 1905, noted this and maintained that the lesion must develop after full differentiation of the anterior segment (40-mm stage, tenth week). The lesion must occur, however, before Descemet's membrane is well formed (70- to 90-mm stage, fourth month). During development, the volume of the anterior segment

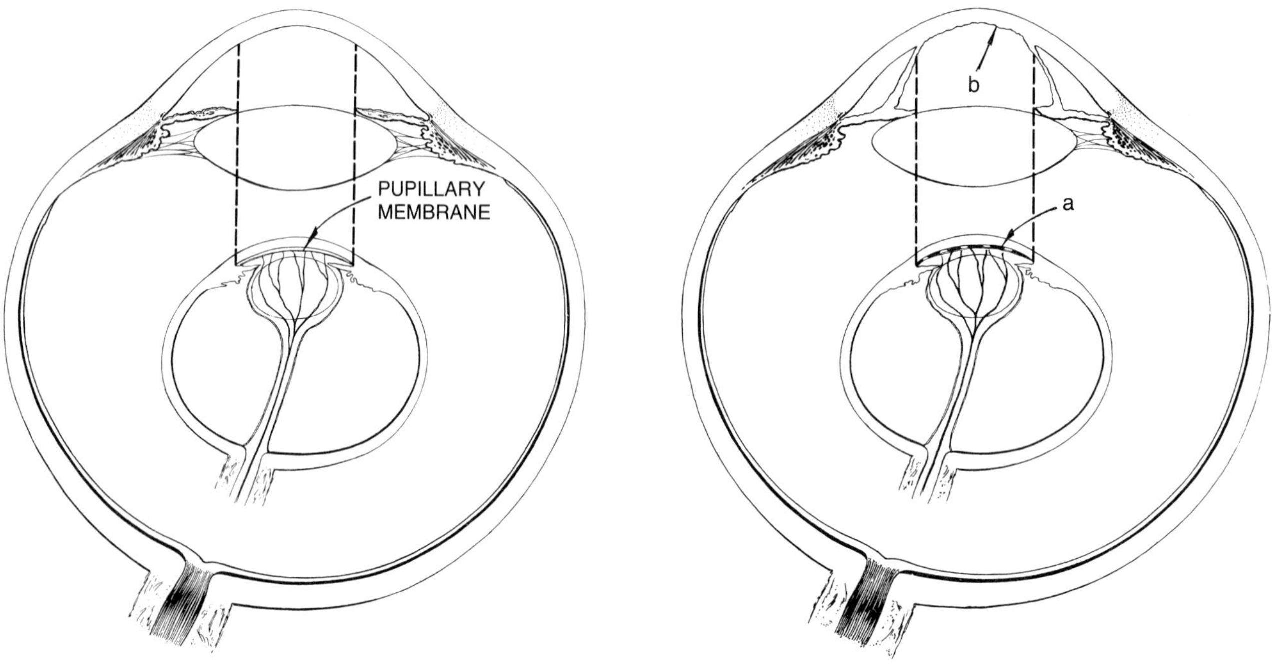

A B

FIGURE 16-11 Presumed pathogenesis of Peters' anomaly type I. **(A)** The size of the pupillary membrane in the fetal eye corresponds to the size of a Peters' type I lesion in the adult eye. **(B)** Apposition of the pupillary membrane to the cornea (a) may cause the posterior corneal defect in Peters' anomaly (b).

is such that the entire fetal anterior chamber would fit into the normal adult pupillary diameter[87] (Figure 16-11A). This area in the fetal anterior segment is occupied by a well-defined vascular membrane that constitutes the anterior hyaloid vascular plexus. The membrane remains prominent until the 40-mm stage, when it begins slowly to involute. Anoxia and other insults may induce increased vascular permeability, with serum transudation and displacement of the membrane against the cornea, damaging the endothelium and Descemet's membrane (Figure 16-11B). Although this type of accidental pathophysiologic event may explain the sporadic cases, it is less reasonable to rely on this explanation for genetically determined, primary lesions; the pathogenesis of the adhesion of the pupillary membrane anlage to the developing endothelium remains obscure.

Peters' Anomaly Type II In Peters' anomaly type II, in addition to the central corneal opacity and iridocorneal synechiae, the lens is abnormal. The most characteristic pattern of involvement presents the lens adherent to the posterior corneal surface or at least firmly pressed against it. In other cases, only lens fragments adhere to the cornea. In still others, the lens is in normal position but is cataractous. The corneal opacity (and corresponding defect in Descemet's membrane and endothelium) shows consistent alignment along the extent of the corneolenticular contact. Usually central in position, the opaque area may be slightly eccentric if the pupil and related area of lenticular apposition are eccentric as well. In contrast to Peters' anomaly type I, the opacity is denser, is most frequently bilateral, and usually is accompanied by many ocular or systemic abnormalities.[82]

It appears that multiple mechanisms may produce corneolenticular adhesion or contact (Figure 16-12). Faulty separation of the lens vesicle from the surface ectoderm was proposed by Peters[83] in 1906. In many cases, however, the lens assumes the abnormal position by being pushed forward instead of failing to separate.[82] Thus, in aniridia, the microspherophakic lens commonly spontaneously dislocates anteriorly (Figure 16-12A). A similar mechanism may play a role in cases associated with microphthalmos and choroidal coloboma. Another group of cases in which corneolenticular contact is common is characterized by microphthalmos and persistent hyperplastic primary vitreous. Here, the lens may be pushed anteriorly into a shallow anterior chamber by the retrolental tissue (Figure 16-12B). In patients with trisomy 13-15, the entire globe suffers gross arrest and aberration so

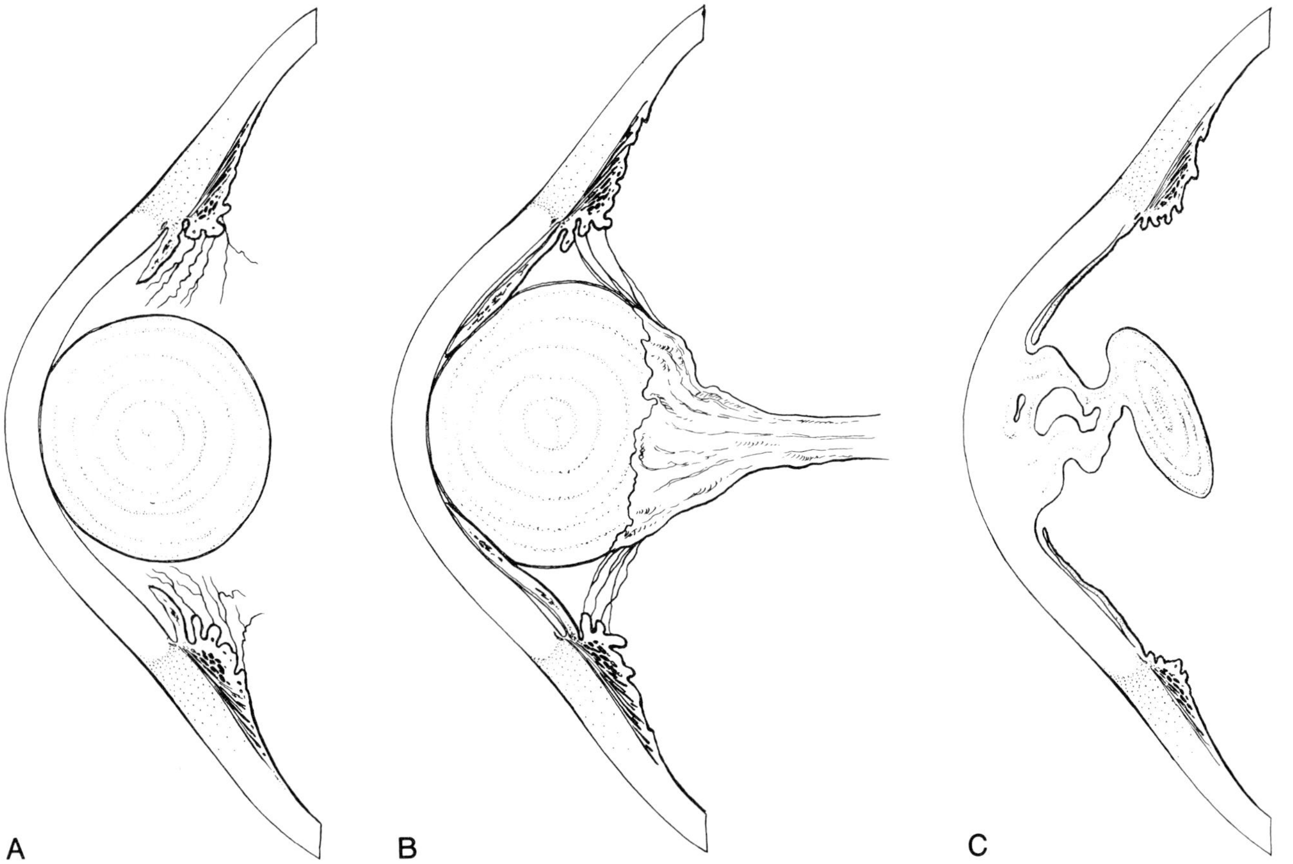

FIGURE 16-12 Derivation of Peters' anomaly type II by different pathogenetic mechanisms. **(A)** Microspherophakic lens dislocated anteriorly. **(B)** Retrolenticular tissue pushing the lens anteriorly. **(C)** Faulty separation of the lens vesicle from the surface ectoderm.

that dysgenesis may play an additional role (Figure 16-12C).

Kupfer and Kayser-Kupfer[88] suggested abnormal mesenchymal wave migration and Kenyon[81] coined the term *mesenchymal dysgenesis* to explain the anomaly. Bahn et al[89] proposed abnormal neural crest cell migration to explain the occurrence of sclerocornea, as well as Peters', Axenfeld's, and Rieger's anomalies. Certain hereditary cases of Peters' anomaly type II have indeed revealed other members of the family presenting with Rieger's anomaly in Robinow syndrome[90] and displaying all four anomalies in the pedigree described by Holmstrom et al.[91]

Hereditary syndromes featuring Peters' anomaly type II as the only anterior segment disturbance include Krause-Kivlin syndrome[92,93] and Peters' plus syndrome (Peters' anomaly plus short stature, brachymorphy, mental retardation, abnormal ears, and, in some patients, cleft lip and palate).[94] Familial transmission of the lesion as a primary isolated anomaly has been rarely documented as an autosomal recessive trait.[95]

In summary, Peters' anomaly type II must be seen as occurring both as the incidental result of mechanical events precipitated by anomalies in adjacent tissues and as a primary lesion. Either of these modes of derivation can, in turn, result from nongenetic and genetic influences.

Posterior Keratoconus The term *posterior keratoconus* has been applied to two different lesions. Hagedoorn and Belzeboer,[96] Forsius and Metsala,[97] Reese and Ellsworth,[72] and others used the term synonymously with the term *Von Hippel's internal ulcer.* This lesion has not been reported since 1902, and in all likelihood, it represented a Peters' anomaly type I modified by the absence of anterior synechiae (probably broken off) and showing only the concave central defect of Descemet's membrane and endothelium. Independently, in 1930, Butler[98] used the term to describe a different disorder:

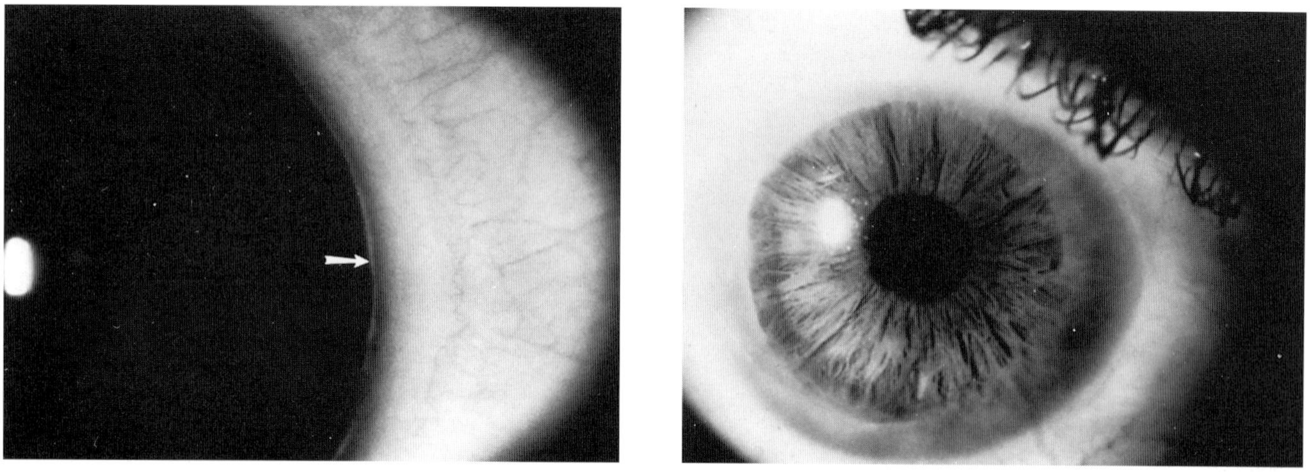

A B

FIGURE 16-13 **(A)** Posterior embryotoxon demonstrating an anteriorly displaced Schwalbe's ring (arrow). **(B)** Marked anterior displacement of Schwalbe's ring.

circumscribed, crater-like, round lesions occurring centrally or eccentrically, singly or multiply, wherever the posterior corneal surface showed an anterior concavity. A nebular opacity usually coincided with the area of concavity. The condition also occurred in a generalized form,[99] the concavity then involving the entire posterior surface of the cornea. Often bilateral, it has been "discovered" mostly in adults, who cannot recall any incident to explain the lesion, suggesting a congenital onset. Most reported cases have been sporadic, although there are exceptions.[100,101] Histopathologic studies have shown that Descemet's membrane and endothelium are present but altered.[102] The pathogenesis and causes of this condition are unclear.

Congenital Anterior Staphyloma Congenital staphylomas are corneal ectasias characterized by a disproportionately large and disorganized anterior segment. The cornea itself is usually thin and lined posteriorly by the remaining pigment epithelium of a markedly atrophic iris. The enlarged cornea usually protrudes beyond the plane of the eyelids, and secondary epithelial metaplasia into keratinized, stratified, squamous epithelium occurs in all cases. Prognosis for vision is usually nil, and only cosmetic considerations are pertinent.

A varied pathogenesis is evident from reports in the literature. Intrauterine maternal and fetal infection with corneal perforation have been noted.[103] In several cases, one eye showed a frank staphyloma while the other eye demonstrated a Peters' anomaly type II.[104] The suggestion that many staphylomas are caused by pathophysiologic intrauterine events is strengthened by the frequent finding of a microphakic lens adherent to the posterior corneal surface.[104] Peters' concept of a defective separation of the lens vesicle is consistent with the severe aberrations observed in the anterior segment of these eyes.

Peripheral Corneal Opacities

Posterior Embryotoxon Posterior embryotoxon (Figure 16-13) is an anomaly of Schwalbe's ring, which is the anterior boundary of the trabecular meshwork and the posterior boundary of Descemet's membrane. Normally, Schwalbe's ring is visible only gonioscopically unless it is exposed by a partial limbal coloboma of Ascher[105] (Figure 16-14). In posterior embryotoxon, Schwalbe's ring is thickened or hypertrophied and is located more anteriorly than normal, so that it is visible behind clear cornea. It appears as a glass-like hyaline membrane, sharply defined and concentric with the limbus. It occurs in approximately 15 percent of normal eyes[106]; the high prevalence suggests that the condition, when solitary, is merely an anatomic variation. Autosomal dominant transmission has been described frequently. Posterior embryotoxon has been described in association with megalocornea, aniridia, and corectopia. Systemic associations include Noonan,[57] Alagille,[107] and Aarskog (facial-digital-genital)[108] syndromes.

Axenfeld's Anomaly and Rieger's Anomaly In 1920, Axenfeld[109] described the anomaly that came to bear his name: a prominent, anteriorly displaced Schwalbe's ring to which multiple peripheral iris strands adhere (Figures 16-15 and 16-16). Axenfeld himself chose the name *posterior embryotoxon* to label this anomaly, which is applied

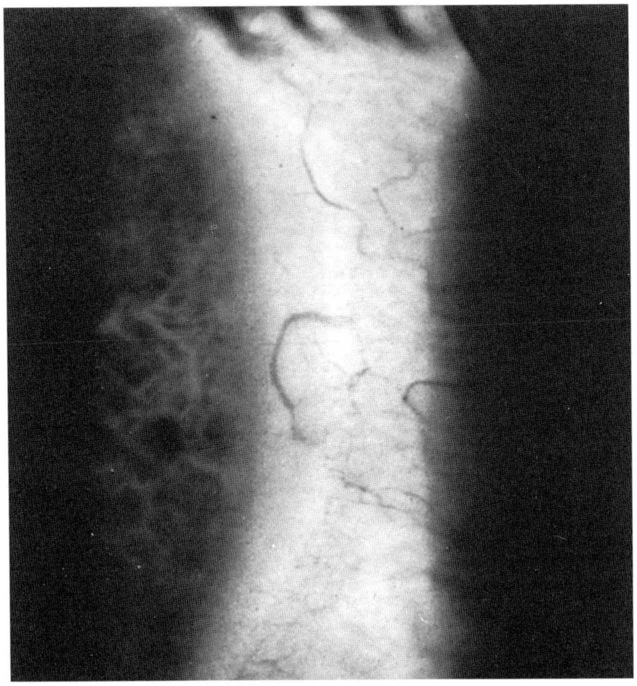

FIGURE 16-14 Limbal coloboma of Ascher. Absence of the anterior scleral lamellae of the limbal region bares Schwalbe's ring.

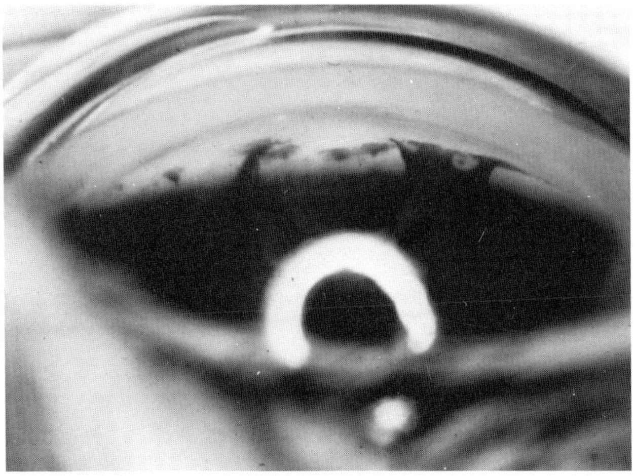

FIGURE 16-15 Axenfeld's anomaly. Gonioscopic view showing iris processes bridging the anterior chamber and adhering to a centrally displaced Schwalbe's ring.

today to a different lesion, as described above. Axenfeld's anomaly may occur alone or in association with glaucoma, in which case it is called Axenfeld syndrome.[110]

The three cardinal features of Rieger's anomaly are posterior embryotoxon with iris adhesions, hypoplasia of the iris stroma, and bilateral involvement (Figure 16-17). There may be associated findings, both ocular (dyscoria, glaucoma, congenital anterior synechiae) and systemic (osteogenesis imperfecta, Marfan syndrome, Ehlers-Danlos syndrome, Down syndrome, oculodentodigital dysplasia, and Franceschetti syndrome).[42] Rieger's anomaly has also been described as a feature of the Robinow syndrome[90] and SHORT (short stature, hernia and/or hyperextensibility of joints, ocular abnormalities, Rieger's anomaly, and tooth eruption delay) syndrome.[111] Less frequently associated ocular findings include megalocornea, microcornea, aniridia, and Peters' anomaly type I.

The occurrence of Peters' anomaly type I in Rieger's anomaly is purely a secondary event.[42] The secondary nature of this central leukoma is better appreciated when the entire spectrum of corneal opacities that occur in Rieger's anomaly is viewed. Congenital anterior synechiae are common in Rieger's anomaly. Most are located eccentrically. They usually produce opacities where the iris tents up and attaches to the posterior corneal surface (Figure 16-18). The area lacking Descemet's membrane and endothelium corresponds to the area of synechiae.[112] As part of this same tendency to form anterior synechiae, when the pupillary membrane itself adheres at some point between the tenth week and fifth month, the "secondary" Peters' anomaly type I appears as part of Rieger's anomaly. The importance of this concept cannot be overemphasized. Several authors have mistakenly described a hereditary pattern to the corneal lesion as if the pedigree were that of Peters', while in reality, it represented a Rieger's pedigree.[113,114] However, Peters' anomaly type II has been observed in pedigrees also featuring Rieger's anomaly.[90,91]

In the presence of developmental defects of the teeth and facial bones, Rieger's anomaly becomes Rieger syndrome. Transmission follows an autosomal dominant pattern. Iridogoniodysgenesis with glaucoma is a variation of Rieger syndrome that lacks the element of posterior embryotoxon. In some instances, a juvenile cataract is present.[115]

Although Axenfeld's anomaly and syndrome and Rieger's anomaly and syndrome have been described as distinct entities here, it is sometimes difficult to sort a particular case into one of these traditional categories. The occurrence of the anomaly described by Axenfeld in pedigrees that include patients with Rieger's anomaly[113,116] suggests that Axenfeld's anomaly is, in most instances, a mild expression of Rieger's anomaly.[115] Axenfeld's anomaly and syndrome and Rieger's anomaly and syndrome probably represent a spectrum of developmental disorders; therefore, a single diagnostic category of Axenfeld-Reiger syndrome has been proposed.[75]

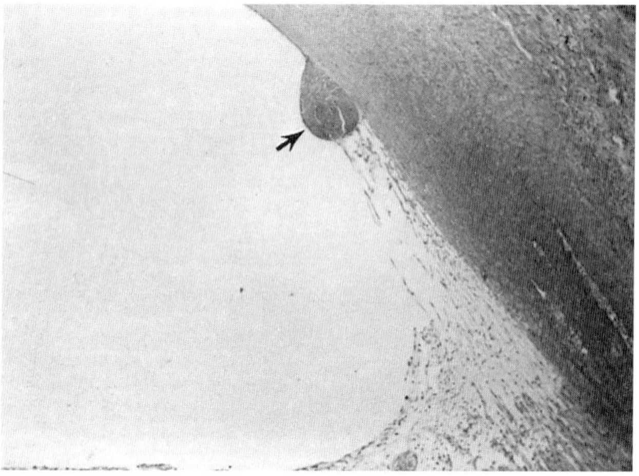

FIGURE 16-16 Axenfeld's anomaly. Hypertrophied Schwalbe's ring (arrow) with iris processes attached to it. Abnormal trabecular meshwork is partly covered by the anterior insertion of the iris root (hematoxylin and eosin).

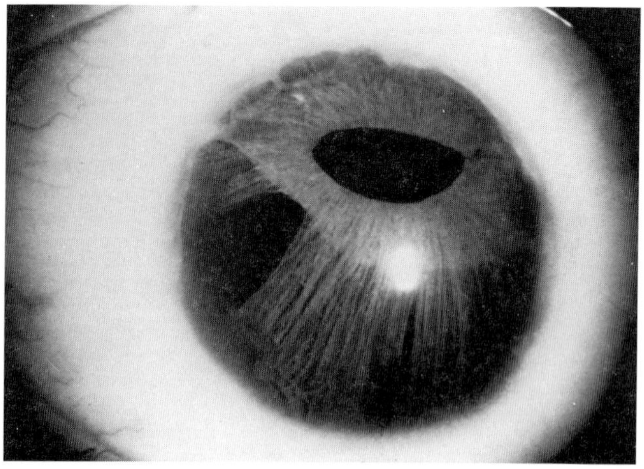

FIGURE 16-17 Rieger's anomaly. Note the posterior embryotoxon, iris synechiae, iris hypoplasia, and corectopia.

Dystrophic Congenital Corneal Opacities

Congenital Hereditary Endothelial Dystrophy

Congenital hereditary endothelial dystrophy is the most commonly encountered congenital dystrophy. It occurs in both dominant and recessive forms. The latter is more severe and is usually present at birth.[117] The entire stroma is markedly edematous, giving the cornea a uniformly diffuse, milky appearance (Figure 16-19). Little if any variation is observed throughout life, and epithelial edema does not usually develop to a significant degree. A spectrum of severity varying from minimal to severe involvement may be observed in the families of those affected with the dominant form.[118] The parents often have posterior polymorphous changes in the cornea.

Histologic surveys have consistently shown increased collagen fibril diameter, an irregular Descemet's membrane, and severe endothelial abnormalities.[119,120] The anterior banded portion of Descemet's membrane forms before the fifth month of gestation and appears intact. The posterior nonbanded portion forms after the fifth month of gestation and is abnormal, suggesting that the

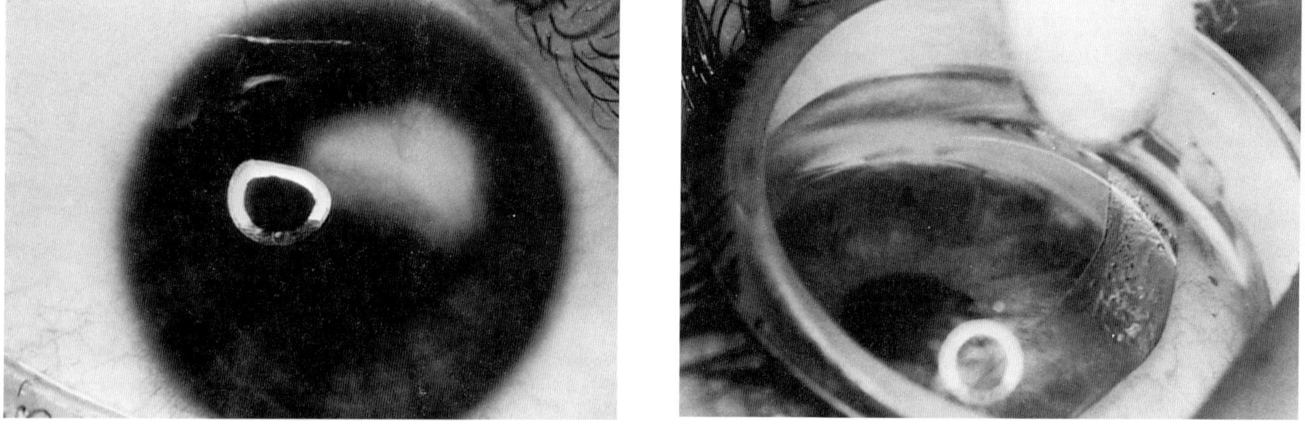

A B

FIGURE 16-18 **(A)** Noncentral congenital opacity in Rieger's anomaly. **(B)** The opacity corresponds to an area of iris attachment to the cornea.

endothelial dysfunction does not begin until that period in fetal development.[119,120]

Congenital Cornea Guttata

In congenital cornea guttata,[121] the deeper stromal layers may show some degree of opacification, but unlike the typical adult form of Fuchs' dystrophy, which tends to progress relentlessly, the congenital form remains stationary and epithelial edema is not significant.

Posterior Polymorphous Dystrophy

Posterior polymorphous dystrophy is often present at birth, but opacification of the cornea is not present in this age group. The condition is described in Chapter 19.

Posterior Amorphous Dystrophy

Dunn et al[122] documented the congenital nature of this rare dystrophy. Of autosomal dominant inheritance, it is bilateral, symmetrical, and seemingly stationary. Vision is unaffected despite the presence of sheet-like, diffuse, posterior stromal opacification.

Congenital Hereditary Stromal Dystrophy

Congenital hereditary stromal dystrophy is an extremely rare disorder with autosomal dominant transmission. It is present at birth and appears as a nebular opacification of the central cornea, especially over the more superficial layers. Corneal thickness appears normal. The condition is not progressive. Tightly packed, normally oriented collagen fibrils alternate in layers with loosely and haphazardly arranged collagen fibrils.[123]

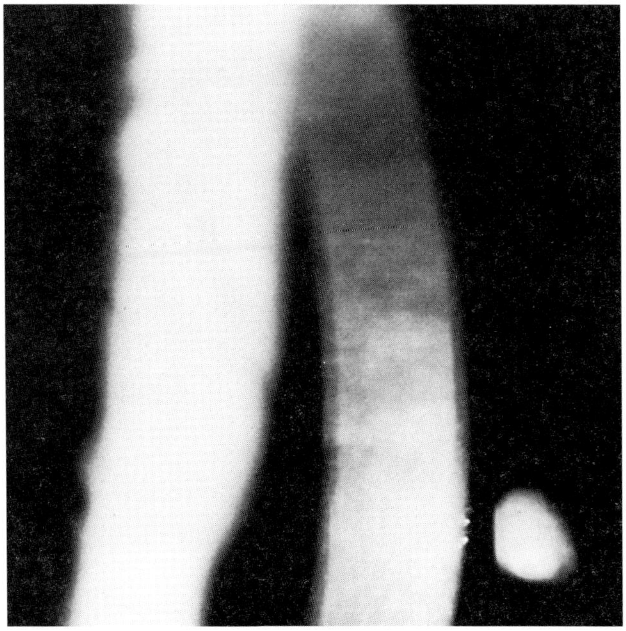

FIGURE 16-19 Congenital hereditary endothelial dystrophy. There is a diffuse increase in stromal thickness.

Congenital Corneal Opacities Caused by Inborn Errors of Metabolism

Metabolic disorders of the cornea are reviewed in Chapter 17. Some of the disorders that cause corneal abnormalities observable at birth are summarized here.

Amino Acid Abnormalities

In cystinosis, iridescent corneal crystals may be present at birth or appear soon thereafter. The stromal deposition of needle-like cystine crystals progresses until the entire thickness of the cornea becomes affected. The most severe form, which is infantile, is usually associated with death from renal failure in early childhood.[124] More benign adolescent and adult forms also occur.[125]

Mucopolysaccharidoses

Gross clouding of the cornea, which often has a ground-glass appearance, is a feature of several mucopolysaccharidoses (MPS), including Hurler (MPS I-H), Scheie (MPS I-S), and Morquio (MPS IV) syndromes. In Hurler and Scheie syndromes, the clouding is present at birth or develops during the first 6 months of life. Although the pattern is diffuse in Hurler syndrome, it tends to be more pronounced in the corneal periphery in Scheie syndrome.[126] In patients with Morquio syndrome, the clouding is usually not apparent until after the age of 10 years.[127]

Clinically detectable clouding of the cornea does not occur in Sanfilippo syndrome (MPS III). Faint opacities, usually not discernible macroscopically, may occur in the severe form of Hunter syndrome (MPS II).[128] Similarly, in the Maroteaux-Lamy syndrome (MPS VI), the punctate opacities often cannot be seen without a slit lamp microscope although they are always present.[129]

Histologic examination has shown similar findings in most reports: the basal epithelial cells appear swollen, their cytoplasm distended with mucopolysaccharide-containing vacuoles. Similar changes are evident in the stromal keratocytes, accounting for the punctate opacities visible clinically. Often a row of prominent vacuolated histiocytes is present under the basal lamina of the epithelium.[130]

Penetrating keratoplasty has a reasonable chance of therapeutic success, but retinal degeneration is a common concomitant and preoperative electroretinography (ERG) is mandatory to assess retinal function.

Sphingolipidoses
Corneal opacities have been noted occasionally in G_{M1} gangliosidosis type I (generalized gangliosidosis),[131] G_{M2} gangliosidosis type II (Sandhoff's disease),[132] Nieman-Pick disease,[133] and infantile metachromatic leukodystrophy. In Fabry's disease, a characteristic form of subepithelial opacity has been observed in infants as young as 6 months of age.[134] The whorl-like lines, tenuous and gold-colored, are produced by ridge-like elevations of the epithelial basement membrane. The overlying basal epithelial cells contain sphingolipid deposits in the apical portion of their cytoplasm.[135] This sign is so typical that, although not pathognomonic, it may be of great importance in diagnosing the systemic disease.

Mucolipidoses
Corneal opacities may occur in these disorders of both mucopolysaccharide and glycolipid metabolism. They have been described in mucolipidoses (MLS) I through IV and in the Goldberg-Cotlier syndrome.[136] However, the opacities are commonly present at birth only in MLS II and MLS IV.[16,137] Other lysosomal storage diseases such as mannosidosis and fucosidosis have faint corneal opacities that usually do not occur until later in childhood.[138]

Miscellaneous Metabolic Disorders
In Lowe syndrome, corneal clouding is usually a result of the glaucoma that is frequently present.[139] However, a case has been described in which the opacity was produced by a Peters' anomaly type II. In Alport syndrome, posterior polymorphous dystrophy without actual corneal opacification has been described.[140]

Refsum's disease is a disease of phytanic acid storage and produces predominantly posterior segment changes. Baum et al[141] reported epithelial changes and pannus formation in an affected male.

Congenital Corneal Opacities in Hereditary Syndromes and Chromosomal Aberrations

Congenital corneal opacities are associated with several hereditary syndromes and chromosomal aberrations[5,18,29,57,65,68–71,82,89,90,91,108,111,142–163] (Table 16-6).

Congenital Infections

Corneal opacities may follow congenital infections. With rubella, the opacification may result from several mechanisms: parenchymal inflammation and scarring, corneal edema caused by glaucoma and ruptures of Descemet's membrane, and Peters' anomaly type II.[164] Congenital syphilis may occasionally produce deep parenchymatous inflammation, vascularization, and scarring.[165] At least two cases of congenital herpes simplex keratitis have been reported.[166,167]

Glaucoma

Primary glaucoma and the multiple secondary forms[168] may result in corneal enlargement and opacification due to edema and tears in Descemet's membrane.

Trauma

Corneal perforation, and more commonly, tears in Descemet's membrane may result from trauma in utero or at birth. Persistent corneal edema caused by ocular injury from obstetric forceps at birth is uncommon; however, corneal edema and bullous keratopathy may develop several years later, and tears in Descemet's membrane may not be visible after the cornea becomes edematous. A patient with unexplained corneal edema should be questioned about forceps injury at birth and should be examined for periorbital forceps depressions and posterior skull depressions 180 degrees from the affected cornea (which correlates with the opposite blade of the forceps).[169]

CONGENITAL MASS LESIONS OF THE CORNEA

Dermoids

Dermoids of the limbus and cornea are solid tumors. They are classified as choristomas[170] because they contain cellular elements not normally present in that location: ectodermal derivatives, such as hair follicles, as well as sebaceous and sweat glands embedded in connective tissue and covered by squamous epithelium. Dermolipomas are also choristomas, but are usually localized to the temporal conjunctiva near the lateral canthus. Choristomas contrast with teratomas in that only the latter are true neoplasms, which in addition contain cellular derivatives from all three basic layers: ectoderm, mesoderm, and endoderm.

The solid dermoids occurring on the limbus and cornea appear grossly as fleshy white masses with a smooth domed surface that often bears hair shafts (Figure 16-20). There are three types of dermoids, characterized by the extent of involvement.[6] The small limbal dermoid is typically seen straddling the limbus and usually measures 5 mm in diameter. The second type is much larger, often covering the entire corneal surface, but with variable posterior extension, stopping short of Descemet's membrane;

TABLE 16-6
Congenital Corneal Opacities in Hereditary Syndromes and Chromosomal Aberrations

Syndrome	*Corneal Opacity*
Mesodermal syndromes	
Marfan[142]	Rieger's anomaly
Weill-Marchesani[143]	Congenital anterior synechiae; Rieger's anomaly
Craniofacial syndromes	
Craniofacial dysostosis[144]	Congenital anterior synechiae with corresponding corneal opacities
Aarskog[108]	Posterior embryotoxon
Neuhauser[18]	Megalocornea
Cleft lip and palate[145]	Peters' anomaly type II
Hemifacial hypoplasia[146]	Peters' anomaly type II
Osseous syndromes	
Osteogenesis imperfecta[65]	Sclerocornea
Onycho-osteo-dysplasia[29]	Sclerocornea
Mietens[69]	Sclerocornea
Conradi[144]	Diffuse corneal clouding
Léri[144]	Diffuse corneal clouding
Dermochondrocorneal dystrophy	Subepithelial opacities in late childhood
Rosenthal-Kloepfer[147]	Dense corneal opacities in young adults
Krause-Kivlin[89]	Peters' anomaly type II
Robinow[90]	Peters' anomaly type II
Peters' plus[91]	Peters' anomaly type II
SHORT[111]	Rieger's anomaly
Neurologic syndromes	
Smith-Lemli-Opitz[70]	Sclerocornea
Lissencephaly[5]	Diffuse opacification of the corneal periphery
Cockayne[148]	Diffuse opacification of the corneal periphery
Norrie[149]	Peters' anomaly type II; band keratopathy
Ectodermal syndromes	
Sex-linked congenital ichthyosis[150]	Salzmann's-like nodules; pre-Descemet's filiform opacities; band keratopathy; exposure keratopathy
Anhidrotic ectodermal dysplasia[151]	Inferior punctiform epithelial dystrophy
Epidermolysis bullosa[152]	Congenital corneal clouding; recurrent erosions
Darier	Punctiform epithelial opacities; sinuous lines
Melkersson-Rosenthal[153]	Linear epithelial opacities
Acrodermatitis enteropathica[154]	Linear epithelial opacities
Kyrle's disease[155]	Superficial punctiform opacities
Palmoplantar keratosis[152,156]	Inferior punctiform lesions; herpetiform lesions
Richner-Hanhart[157]	Pseudodendrites
Rothmund-Thomson	Band keratopathy
Chromosomal aberrations	
17p,10q translocation[71]	Sclerocornea
Trisomy 18[68]	Sclerocornea
Trisomy 13-15[82]	Peters' anomaly type II
Mosaic trisomy 9	Peters' anomaly type II
Partial deletion of 11q[158]	Peters' anomaly type II
Duplication of 6q	Congenital anterior synechiae
Deletion of 18p	Posterior keratoconus
Trisomy 21	Keratoconus; Axenfeld syndrome
Noonan syndrome[57]	Keratoconus; Rieger's anomaly with secondary corneal changes
Deletion or translocation of Xp22[159]	Sclerocornea
Deletion of 2q14q21[160]	Peters' anomaly type II
Deletion of 4p[161]	Peters' anomaly type II; Rieger's anomaly
Deletion of 13[162]	Rieger syndrome
Inversion of 6[163]	Rieger syndrome

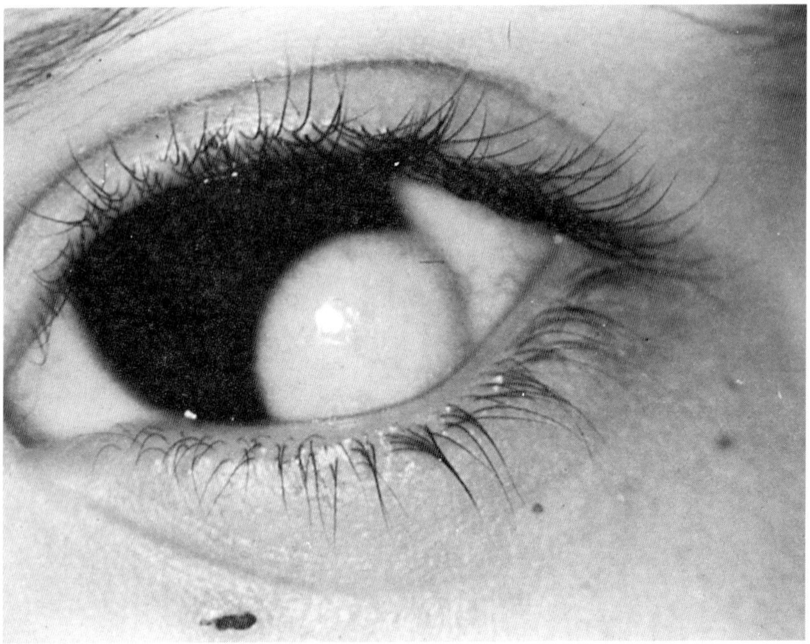

A

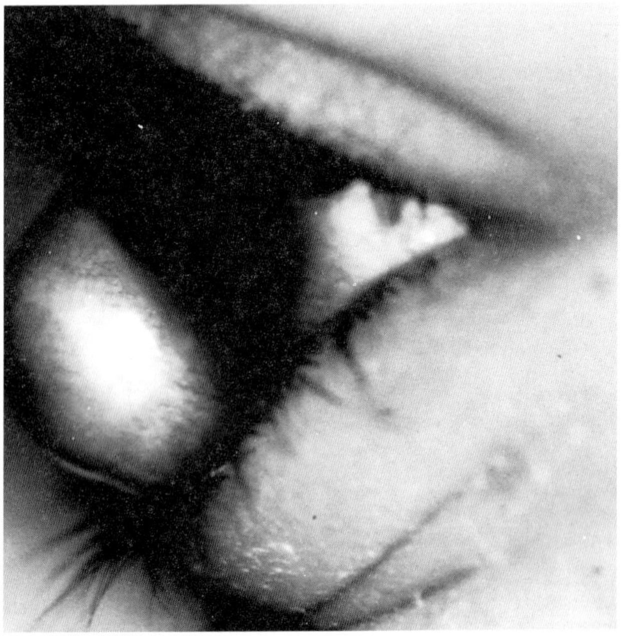

B

FIGURE 16-20 **(A)** Dermoid in characteristic limbal position in a 5-year-old patient with Goldenhar syndrome. **(B)** Large dermoid involving more than half the corneal surface.

intermediate forms are common. The third and most severe type is also the most rare. In this type, the tumor replaces the cornea, anterior chamber, and iris stroma and is lined posteriorly by the pigment epithelium of the iris. These variations are attributed to the different times during fetal development that the teratogenic event becomes operative. The earlier the onset, the more severe the malformation. These tumors usually occur in sporadic fashion, although their occurrence in cousins has been described.[171]

The small limbal tumor is the most common dermoid. Already present at birth, it may enlarge, especially at puberty. Vision may be impaired if there is encroachment on the pupillary area by either the tumor or the often present lipid infiltration around its periphery. In some instances, irregular astigmatism appears. Limbal dermoids are common in Goldenhar syndrome, affecting as many as 30 percent of patients.[172] Dermoids occur with many ocular and systemic abnormalities: Duane syndrome, coloboma of the upper eyelid, neuroparalytic keratitis, lacrimal stenosis, anophthalmos, and many others.[172]

Approaches to treatment for cosmetic improvement or chronic irritation should take into account the high potential for unsightly scarring in these patients.[173] The tumor should be cut flush with the corneal surface. No effort should be made to excise the entire tumor, as the deeply located segment of clear cornea may be too thin and perforation may occur. If the dermoid covers the corneal surface and visual improvement is the goal, lamellar or, more commonly, penetrating keratoplasty is indicated.

Keloids

Keloids[174] are reactive fibrous tissue proliferations that represent the exuberant response of embryonic connective tissue to injury. They often assume tumoral proportions and bear a superficial resemblance to dermoids. Like dermoids, keloids show variable degrees of extension and may replace the cornea or the entire anterior segment.[175] Grossly, they appear as chalky white masses that are solid but have a glistening gelatinous texture, which distinguishes them from dermoids.

Hereditary Benign Intraepithelial Dyskeratosis

Hereditary benign intraepithelial dyskeratosis[176] is a bilateral, horseshoe-shaped limbal plaque associated with similar lesions in the buccal mucosa. It is inherited as an autosomal dominant trait and is benign in character.

MANAGEMENT OF CONGENITAL ANOMALIES OF THE CORNEA

Management of congenital anomalies of the cornea depends on the causes, nature, and extent of the anomaly, the time at which the anomaly is discovered, the presence of associated ocular or systemic abnormalities, and the degree of parental cooperation available. Based on the results of the ophthalmologic examination (including ultrasonography, electroretinography, and visual evoked response testing), physical examination, and family history, a diagnosis can usually be made, the prognosis given, and treatment planned.

Corneal opacifications that interfere with vision may be treated with penetrating keratoplasty. Penetrating keratoplasty in infants is technically more difficult than in adults because of the frequently associated anterior segment abnormalities, elasticity of the recipient cornea, scleral collapse, and anterior movement of the lens-iris diaphragm despite the use of a scleral support ring. In addition to preoperative ocular massage, hyperventilation and the avoidance of depolarizing relaxants lessen the risk of extrusion of intraocular contents.

Postoperative management of penetrating keratoplasty in infants is difficult because of lack of patient cooperation, inability of the patient to communicate effectively, dependence on the parents for compliance, and the threat of amblyopia. A surgically successful graft is doomed if postoperative compliance is poor. The rapid healing rate in infants requires that sutures be removed 4 to 6 weeks postoperatively; otherwise, the sutures will loosen, collect mucus, and stimulate vascularization, all of which increase the incidence of graft failure. Correction of refractive errors and initiation of amblyopia therapy as soon as possible after surgery are of paramount importance for a graft to be visually successful.

Several authors have reported the results of penetrating keratoplasty in infants and children with congenital corneal anomalies[164,177–187] (Table 16-7). In the series by Stulting et al,[183] survival analysis showed that the probability of obtaining a clear graft 1 year after surgery was 60 ± 8 percent (45 eyes); however, only 1 of 34 eyes in which visual acuity could be measured saw better than 20/40. They found that preoperative corneal vascularization, persistent epithelial defects, and lensectomy-vitrectomy performed at the time of penetrating keratoplasty correlated significantly with poor graft survival, whereas amblyopia, strabismus, nystagmus, and glaucoma limited visual rehabilitation. Dana et al[187] reported that the probability of obtaining a clear graft 1 year after surgery was 80 percent. Vitrectomy and postoperative complications were associated with loss of graft clarity. Vitrectomy, postoperative complications, and lack of optical refractive or amblyopia management were significantly associated with poor visual outcome.

Penetrating keratoplasty in infants with congenital corneal anomalies appears to be most successful in cases with isolated central corneal opacification. These cases have a sufficiently high success rate to warrant penetrating keratoplasty not only in patients with bilateral disease but also in patients with unilateral disease if postoperative compliance can be ensured. If other anterior segment abnormalities are present, such as anterior chamber angle abnormalities or cataract, the success rate is low. In bilateral cases, surgery is justified in an attempt to obtain vision in at least one eye; in unilateral cases, it is questionable whether surgery is warranted.

TABLE 16-7
Penetrating Keratoplasty in Infants and Children with Congenital Corneal Anomalies

		No. of				
Authors	*Disorder*	*Patients*	*Eyes*	*Grafts*	*No. of Clear Grafts*	*Length of Follow-up*
Picetti and Fine, 1966[177]	Keratoconus	1	1	1	1	>1 yr
	Lipoidal dystrophy	1	2	2	2	>1 yr
Wood and Kaufman, 1970[178]	Bilateral sclerocornea	1	1	1	1	3 mo
Brown, 1970[179]	Peters' anomaly	1	1	1	1	10 mo
Brown, 1974[180]	Peters' anomaly	1	2	2	2	34–42 mo
	Bilateral opacity (rubella)	1	2	2	1 partially clear	16 mo
	Corneal keloid	1	1	2	1 partially clear	14 mo
Stone et al, 1976[181]	Peters' anomaly	3	3	3	2	6 wk–15 mo
Waring and Laibson, 1977[182]	Vascularized corneal opacity	7	8	10	1	2 wk–3 yr
	Sclerocornea	1	1	1	0	2 mo
Schanzlin et al, 1980[164]	Peters' anomaly	5	8	8	6 clear, 1 semitransparent	1–10 yr
	Bilateral opacity (rubella)	1	2	2	0	
	Corneal keloid	1	1	2	0	18 mo
	Epithelialization of anterior chamber	1	1	1	Semitransparent	5.5 yr
	Sclerocornea	3	4	4	1 clear, 1 partially clear	5–17 mo
Stulting et al, 1984[183]	Peters' anomaly	Total of 33 patients	27	Total of 72 grafts	Total of 31 eyes with clear grafts	2–75 mo
	Congenital glaucoma		6			
	Posterior polymorphous dystrophy		5			
	Multiple anterior segment anomalies		4			
	Sclerocornea		3			
Feldman et al, 1987[184]	Microphthalmos	5	9	9	7	About 2 yr
Frucht-Pery et al, 1989[185]	Buphthalmos	3	4	4	3	5 mo–6 yr
Cowden, 1990[186]	Peters' anomaly	Total of 20 patients	Total of 25 eyes	8	3	1 yr
	Congenital glaucoma			7	7	
	Sclerocornea			4	1	
	Congenital anterior staphyloma			2	0	
	Dermoid (Goldenhar syndrome)			1	1	
	Mucopolysaccharidosis			1	1	
	Rubella			2	1	
Dana, 1995[187]	Anterior segment dysgenesis	Total of 63 patients	Total of 84 eyes	48	Total eyes with clear grafts approximately 62%	6 mo
	Congenital hereditary endothelial dystrophy			21		
	Sclerocornea			12		
	Congenital glaucoma			12		
	Posterior polymorphous dystrophy			3		
	Dermoid			2		
	In utero perforation			2		
	Neurofibromatosis			1		
	Unknown			8		

REFERENCES

1. McKusick VA: Heritable Disorders of Connective Tissue. 4th Ed. CV Mosby, St. Louis, 1972
2. Mets MB, Maumenee IH: The eye and the chromosome. Surv Ophthalmol 28:20, 1983
3. Neel JV: Mutation in the human population. p. 203. In Bordette WJ (ed): Methodology in Mammalian Genetics. Holden Day, San Francisco, 1962
4. Chan T, Bowell R, O'Keefe M, Lanigan B: Ocular manifestations in fetal alcohol syndrome. Br J Ophthalmol 75:524, 1991
5. Duke-Elder S: System of Ophthalmology. Vol. III. Normal and Abnormal Development. Part 2, Congenital Deformities. CV Mosby, St. Louis, 1963
6. Mann I: Developmental Abnormalities of the Eye. 2nd Ed. JB Lippincott, Philadelphia, 1957
7. Manschot WA: Primary congenital aphakia. Arch Ophthalmol 69:571, 1963
8. Friede R: Surface area of cornea and sclera in embryos and in newborn infants and its relation to megalocornea in adults. Z Augenheilkd 81:213, 1933
9. Vail DT: Adult hereditary anterior megalophthalmos sine glaucoma: a definite disease entity. Arch Ophthalmol 6:39, 1931
10. Mackey DA, Buttery RG, Wise GM, Denton MJ: Description of X-linked megalocornea with identification of the gene locus. Arch Ophthalmol 109:829, 1991
11. Pearce WG: Autosomal dominant megalocornea with congenital glaucoma: evidence for germ-line mosaicism. Can J Ophthalmol 26:21, 1991
12. Malbran EP: Megalocornea with mosaic-like dystrophy. Arch Ophthalmol 74:130, 1965
13. Malbran E, Dodds R: Megalocornea and its relation to congenital glaucoma. Am J Ophthalmol 49:908, 1960
14. Friede R: Megalocornea congenita, a phylogenetic anomaly. Arch Ophthalmol 148:716, 1948
15. Allen RA, Straatsma BR, Apt L, Hall MO: Manifestations of the Marfan syndrome. Trans Am Acad Ophthalmol Otolaryngol 71:18, 1967
16. Calamandrei D: Megalocornea in due pazienti con syndrome craniosinostocia. Q Ital Ophthalmol 3:278, 1950
17. Libert J, Vanhoof F, Farreaux JP, Tousseant D: Ocular findings in I cell disease (mucolipidosis type II). Am J Ophthalmol 83:617, 1977
18. Frydman M, Berkenstadt M, Raas-Rothschild A, Goodman RM: Megalocornea, macrocephaly, mental and motor retardation (MMMM). Clin Genet 38:149, 1990
19. Maumenee IM: The cornea in connective tissue diseases. Trans Am Acad Ophthalmol Otolaryngol 85:1014, 1978
20. Johnston MC, Noden DM, Hazelton RD, et al: Origins of avian ocular and periocular tissues. Exp Eye Res 29:27, 1979
21. François J, Neetens A: Microcornea. Acta Genet Med Gemellol (Roma) 4:217, 1955
22. Durham DG: Cutis hyperelastica (Ehlers-Danlos syndrome) with blue scleras, microcornea, and glaucoma. Arch Ophthalmol 49:220, 1953
23. Feiler-Ofry V, Stein R, Godel V: Marchesani syndrome and chamber angle anomalies. Am J Ophthalmol 65:862, 1968
24. Henkind P, Siegel IM, Carr RE: Mesodermal dysgenesis of the anterior segment: Rieger's anomaly. Arch Ophthalmol 73:810, 1965
25. Sugar A, Bigger JF, Podos SM: Hallerman-Streiff-François syndrome. J Pediatr Ophthalmol 8:234, 1971
26. Goldberg G: Waardenburg's syndrome with fundus and other anomalies. Arch Ophthalmol 76:797, 1966
27. Meyer-Schwickerath G, Gruterich E, Weyers H: Mikrophthalmussyndrome. Klin Monatsbl Augenheilkd 131:18, 1957
28. Friede R: Uber physiologische Euryopie und pathologischen Hypertelorismus Ocularis. Albrecht von Graefes Arch Ophthalmol 155:359, 1954
29. Fenske HD, Spitalny LA: Hereditary onycho-osteodysplasia. Am J Ophthalmol 70:604, 1970
30. Kohn R, Romano R: Ptosis, blepharophimosis, epicanthus inversus and telecanthus—the syndrome with no name. Am J Ophthalmol 72:625, 1971
31. Lewis RA, Nussbaum RL, Stambolian D: Mapping X-linked ophthalmic diseases. IV. Provisional assignment of the locus for X-linked congenital cataracts and microcornea (the Nance-Horan syndrome) to Xp22.2-p22.3. Ophthalmology 97:110, 1990
32. Warburg M: The heterogeneity of microphthalmia in the mentally retarded. p. 146. In Bergsma D (ed): The Eye. Vol. 7. Williams & Wilkins, Baltimore, 1971
33. McRae DW, Howard RO, Albert DM, Hsia YE: Ocular manifestations of the Meckel syndrome. Arch Ophthalmol 88:106, 1972
34. François J: Heredity in Ophthalmology. CV Mosby, St. Louis, 1961
35. Gold JD, Pfaffenbach DD: Ocular abnormalities in the Smith-Lemli-Opitz syndrome. J Pediatr Ophthalmol 12:228, 1975
36. Lessel S, Forbes AP: Eye signs in Turner's syndrome. Arch Ophthalmol 76:211, 1966
37. Levenson JE, Crandall BF, Sparkes RS: Partial deletion syndromes of chromosomes 18. Ann Ophthalmol 3:756, 1971
38. Ginsberg J, Bove KE: Ocular pathology of trisomy 13. Ann Ophthalmol 6:113, 1974
39. Heathcote JG, Sholdice J, Walton JC, et al: Anterior segment mesenchymal dysgenesis associated with partial duplication of the short arm of chromosome 2. Can J Ophthalmol 26:35, 1991
40. Boniuk V, Boniuk M: Congenital rubella syndrome. Int Ophthalmol Clin 8:487, 1968
41. Sugar HS: Oculodentodigital dysplasia syndrome with angle closure glaucoma. Am J Ophthalmol 86:36, 1978
42. Alkemade PPH: Dysgenesis Mesodermalis of the Iris and the Cornea. Charles C Thomas, Springfield, IL, 1961
43. Strenström S: Variations and correlations of the optical components of the eye. In Sorsby A (ed): Modern Trends in Ophthalmology. Paul Hoeber, New York, 1948

44. Stähli J: Weitere Mitteilunger uber die Vererbung des Keratoconus. Klin Monatsbl Augenheilkd 75:465, 1925
45. Thomas CI: The Cornea. Charles C Thomas, Springfield, IL, 1955
46. Franceschetti A: Keratoconus. In King JH, McTigue JW (eds): The Cornea. World Congress. Butterworths, Washington, DC, 1965
47. Greenfield G, Romano A, Stein R, et al: Blue sclera and keratoconus. Clin Genet 4:8, 1973
48. Seelenfreund M, Gartner S: Acrocephalosyndactyly (Apert's syndrome). Arch Ophthalmol 78:8, 1967
49. Storck H: Ein Fall von Arachnodaktylie (Dystrophia mesodermalis congenita). Dermatologica 104:321, 1952
50. Robertson I: Keratoconus and the Ehlers-Danlos syndrome. Med J Aust 1:571, 1975
51. Slusher MM, Laibson PR, Mullberger KD: Acute keratoconus in Down's syndrome. Am J Ophthalmol 63:1137, 1968
52. Walter JR: Bilateral keratoconus in Crouzon's syndrome with unilateral hydrops. Ann Ophthalmol 14:141, 1976
53. Strieff EB: Kératocone et rétinite pigmentaire. Bull Mem Soc Fr Ophtalmol 63:323, 1952
54. Spencer WH, Fischer JJ: The association of keratoconus with atopic dermatitis. Am J Ophthalmol 43:331, 1959
55. Gomez A, Eggers C: On the secondary nature of keratoconus to vernal conjunctivitis. Colombian Society of Ophthalmology, 15th National Congress, Medellin, Colombia, 1969
56. King EF: Keratoconus following thyroidectomy. Trans Ophthalmol Soc UK 73:31, 1953
57. Schwartz DE: Noonan's syndrome associated with ocular abnormalities. Am J Ophthalmol 75:955, 1972
58. Gasset AR, Worthen DM: Keratoconus and Chandler's syndrome. Ann Ophthalmol 6:819, 1974
59. Cavara V: Keratoconus and keratoglobus: a contribution to the nosological interpretation of keratoglobus. Br J Ophthalmol 34:621, 1950
60. Jacobs DS, Green RW, Maumenee AE: Acquired keratoglobus. Am J Ophthalmol 77:393, 1974
61. François J, Hanssens M, Stockmans L: Dégénérescence marginale pellucide de la cornea. Ophthalmologica 155:337, 1968
62. Forsius H: Studien über Cornea Plana Congenita. Bei 19 Kranken in 9 Familien. Acta Ophthalmol (Copenh) 39:203, 1961
63. Felix CH: Kongenitale familiäre Cornea Plana. Klin Monatsbl Augenheilkd 74:710, 1925
64. Eriksson AW, Lahmann W, Forsius H: Congenital cornea plana in Finland. Clin Genet 4:301, 1973
65. Desvignes P, Pouliquen Y, Legras M, Guyot JD: Aspect iconographique d'une cornea plana dans une maladie de Lobstein. Arch Ophtalmol (Paris) 27:43, 1967
66. Sharkey JA, Kervick GN, Jackson AJ, Johnston PB: Cornea plana and sclerocornea in association with recessive epidermolysis bullosa dystrophica. Case report. Cornea 11:83, 1992
67. Goldstein TE, Cogan DG: Sclerocornea and associated congenital anomalies. Arch Ophthalmol 67:761, 1962
68. Kolbert GS, Seelenfreund M: Sclerocornea, anterior cleavage syndrome, and trisomy 18. Ann Ophthalmol 2:26, 1970
69. Waring GO, Rodrigues MM: Ultrastructure and successful keratoplasty of sclerocornea in Mietens' syndrome. Am J Ophthalmol 90:469, 1980
70. Harbin RL, Katz JI, Frias JL, et al: Sclerocornea associated with the Smith-Lemli-Opitz syndrome. Am J Ophthalmol 84:72, 1977
71. Rodrigues MM, Calhoun J, Weinreb S: Sclerocornea with an unbalanced translocation (17p, 10q). Am J Ophthalmol 78:49, 1974
72. Reese AB, Ellsworth RM: The anterior chamber cleavage syndrome. Arch Ophthalmol 75:307, 1966
73. Waring GO, Rodrigues MM, Laibson PR: Anterior chamber cleavage syndrome: a stepladder classification. Surv Ophthalmol 20:3, 1975
74. Wilson FM: Congenital anomalies. In Smolin G, Thoft RA (eds): The Cornea. Scientific Foundations and Clinical Practice. Little, Brown, Boston, 1983
75. Shields MB, Buckley E, Klintworth GK, Thresher R: Axenfeld-Rieger syndrome. A spectrum of developmental disorders. Surv Ophthalmol 29:387, 1985
76. Howard RO, Abrahams IW: Sclerocornea. Am J Ophthalmol 71:1254, 1971
77. Block N: Les differents types de sclerocornée, leurs modes d'heredité et les malformations congénitales concomitantes. J Génét Hum 15:133, 1965
78. Kanai A, Wood TC, Polack FM, Kaufman HE: The fine structure of sclerocornea. Invest Ophthalmol 9:687, 1971
79. Friedman AH, Weingeist S, Brackup A, Marinoff G: Sclerocornea and defective mesodermal migration. Br J Ophthalmol 59:683, 1975
80. Coulombre AJ, Coulombre JL: The development of the structural and optical properties of the cornea. p. 405. In Smelser GK (ed): The Structure of the Eye. Academic Press, San Diego, 1961
81. Kenyon KR: Mesenchymal dysgenesis in Peters' anomaly, sclerocornea and congenital endothelial dystrophy. Exp Eye Res 21:125, 1975
82. Townsend WM, Font RL, Zimmerman LE: Congenital corneal leukomas. II. Histopathologic findings in 19 eyes with central defect in Descemet's membrane. Am J Ophthalmol 77:192, 1974
83. Peters A: Ueber angeborene Defektbildung der Descemetschen Membran. Klin Monatsbl Augenheilkd 44:27, 1906
84. Collins ET: Adhesion of a persistent pupillary membrane to the cornea in the eye of a cat. Trans Ophthalmol Soc UK 27:203, 1907
85. Seefelder R: Patologish-anatomische Beitrage sur Frage der angeborenen zentralen Defektbildung der Hornhauthinterflache. Klin Monatsbl Augenheilkd 65:539, 1920
86. Ballantyne AJ: Synechiae of the iris and pupillary membrane. Trans Ophthalmol Soc UK 23:319, 1905
87. Duke-Elder S: System of Ophthalmology. Vol. III. Normal and Abnormal Development. Part 1, Embryology. CV Mosby, St. Louis, 1963

88. Kupfer CM, Kayser-Kupfer M: New hypothesis of developmental anomalies of the anterior chamber associated with glaucoma. Trans Ophthalmol Soc UK 98:213, 1978
89. Bahn C, Falls H, Varley G, et al: Classification of corneal endothelial disorders based on neural crest origin. Ophthalmology 91:558, 1984
90. Saal HM, Greenstein RM, Weinbaum PJ, Poole AE: Autosomal recessive Robinow-like syndrome with anterior chamber cleavage anomalies. Am J Med Genet 30:709, 1988
91. Holmstrom GE, Reardon WP, Baraitser M, et al: Heterogeneity in dominant anterior segment malformations. Br J Ophthalmol 75:591, 1991
92. Kivlin J, Fineman RM, Crandall AS, Olson RA: Peters' anomaly as a consequence of genetic and nongenetic syndromes. Arch Ophthalmol 104:61, 1986
93. Frydman M, Weinstock AL, Cohen HA, et al: Autosomal recessive Peters' anomaly, typical facies appearance, failure to thrive, hydrocephalus, and other anomalies: further delineation of the Krause-Kivlin syndrome. Am J Genet 40:34, 1991
94. Van Schooneveld MS, Dellerman JW, Beemer FA, Bleeker-Wagemakers EM: Peters' plus: a new syndrome. Ophthalmol Paediatr Genet 4:141, 1984
95. Boel M, Timmermans J, Emmery L, et al: Primary mesodermal dysgenesis of the cornea (Peters' anomaly) in two brothers. Hum Genet 51:237, 1979
96. Hagedoorn A, Belzeboer CMT: Postnatal partial spontaneous correction of a severe anomaly of the anterior segment of the eye. Arch Ophthalmol 62:685, 1959
97. Forsius M, Metsala P: Keratoconus posticus. Acta Ophthalmol (Copenh) 41:768, 1963
98. Butler TM: Keratoconus posticus. Trans Ophthalmol Soc UK 50:551, 1930
99. Ingram HU: Keratoconus posticus. Trans Ophthalmol Soc UK 56:563, 1963
100. Jacobs HB: Posterior conical cornea. Br J Ophthalmol 41:31, 1957
101. Haney WP, Falls HF: The occurrence of congenital keratoconus posticus circumscriptus in two siblings presenting a previously unrecognized syndrome. Am J Ophthalmol 52:53, 1961
102. Walter JR, Haney WP: Histopathology of keratoconus posticus circumscriptus. Arch Ophthalmol 19:357, 1963
103. Pratt JC, Richards RD: Bilateral secondary congenital aphakia. Arch Ophthalmol 80:420, 1968
104. Peters A: Weiterer Beitrage zur Kenntnis der angeborenen Defektbildung der Descemetschen Membran. Klin Monatsbl Augenheilkd 46:241, 1908
105. Ascher KW: Partial coloboma of the scleral limbus zone with visible Schlemm's canal. Am J Ophthalmol 24:615, 1941
106. Forsius H, Eriksson A, Fellman J: Embryotoxon corneae posterius in an isolated population. Acta Ophthalmol (Copenh) 42:42, 1964
107. Ricci B, Lepore D, Iossa M, et al: Ocular anomalies in Alagille's syndrome. J Fr Ophtalmol 14:481, 1991
108. Brodsky MC, Keppen LD, Rice CD, Ranells JD: Ocular and systemic findings in the Aarskog (facial-digital-genital) syndrome. Am J Ophthalmol 109:450, 1990
109. Axenfeld TH: Embryotoxon corneae posterius. Klin Monatsbl Augenheilkd 65:381, 1920
110. Sugar HS: Juvenile glaucoma with Axenfeld syndrome. Am J Ophthalmol 59:1012, 1965
111. Gorlin RJ: A selected miscellany. p. 39. In Bergsma D (ed): Malformation Syndromes. Excerpta Medica, Amsterdam, 1975
112. Kupfer C, Kuwabara J, Stark WJ: Ocular manifestations of trisomy 18. Am J Ophthalmol 80:653, 1975
113. Falls JF: A gene producing various defects of the anterior segment of the eye. Am J Ophthalmol 32:41, 1949
114. Jaeger W: Angeborene scheibenförmige Hornhauttrübung mit recessiven Erbgang. Klin Monatsbl Augenheilkd 134:124, 1959
115. Henkind P, Friedman AH: Iridogoniodysgenesis with cataract. Am J Ophthalmol 72:949, 1971
116. Pearce WG, Kerr CB: Inherited variations in Rieger's malformation. Br J Ophthalmol 49:530, 1969
117. Maumenee AE: Congenital hereditary corneal dystrophy. Am J Ophthalmol 50:1114, 1960
118. Levenson JE, Chandler JW, Kaufman HE: Affected asymptomatic relatives in congenital hereditary endothelial dystrophy. Am J Ophthalmol 76:967, 1973
119. Kenyon KR, Maumenee AE: The histological and ultrastructural pathology of congenital hereditary corneal dystrophy: a case report. Invest Ophthalmol 7:475, 1968
120. Kanai A, Waltman S, Polack FM, Kaufman HE: Electron microscopic study of hereditary corneal edema. Invest Ophthalmol 10:89, 1971
121. Dohlman CH: Familial congenital corneal guttata in association with anterior polar cataract. Acta Ophthalmol (Copenh) 29:445, 1951
122. Dunn SP, Drachner JN, Ching SST: New findings in posterior amorphous corneal dystrophy. Arch Ophthalmol 102:236, 1984
123. Witschel H, Fine BS, Grutzner P, McTique JW: Congenital hereditary stromal dystrophy of the cornea. Arch Ophthalmol 96:1043, 1978
124. Cogan DG, Kuwabara T, Kinoshita J, et al: Ocular manifestations of systematic cystinosis. Arch Ophthalmol 55:36, 1962
125. Cogan DG, Kuwabara T, Kinoshita HJ, et al: Cystinosis in an adult. JAMA 164:394, 1957
126. Scheie HG, Hambrick GW, Barness LA: A newly recognized forme fruste of Hurler's disease (gargoylism). Am J Ophthalmol 53:753, 1952
127. Von Noorden GK, Zellweger H, Ponsetti I: Ocular findings in Morquio-Ullrich's disease. Arch Ophthalmol 64:585, 1960
128. Topping TM, Kenyon KR, Goldberg MF, Maumenee AE: Ultrastructural ocular pathology of Hunter's syndrome. Arch Ophthalmol 86:164, 1971
129. Goldberg MF, Scott CI, McKusick VA: Hydrocephalus and papilledema in Maroteaux-Lamy syndrome. Am J Ophthalmol 69:969, 1970

130. Kenyon KH: Ocular ultrastructure of inherited metabolic disease. p. 139. In Goldberg MF (ed): Genetic and Metabolic Eye Diseases. Little, Brown, Boston, 1974
131. Emery JM, Greene WR, Wyllie RG, Howell RR: GM-1 gangliosidosis. Ocular and pathological manifestations. Arch Ophthalmol 85:177, 1971
132. Tremblay M, Szots F: GM2 Type 2 gangliosidosis (Sandhoff's disease)—ocular and pathological manifestations. Can J Ophthalmol 9:338, 1974
133. Hibert T, Toussaint D, Guiselings R: Ocular findings in Niemann-Pick disease. Am J Ophthalmol 80:991, 1975
134. Spaeth GL, Frost P: Fabry's disease. Arch Ophthalmol 74:760, 1965
135. Weingeist TA, Blodi FC: Fabry's disease: ocular findings in a carrier female. Arch Ophthalmol 85:169, 1971
136. Goldberg MF, Cotlier E, Fichenscher LG, et al: Macular cherry-red spot, corneal clouding and beta-galactosidase deficiency. Clinical, biochemical and electron microscope study of a new autosomal recessive storage disease. Arch Intern Med 128:387, 1971
137. Berman ER, Livni N, Shapira E, et al: Congenital corneal clouding with abnormal systemic storage bodies: a new variant of mucolipidosis. J Pediatr 84:519, 1974
138. Snyder RD, Carlow TJ, Ledman J, Wenger DA: Ocular findings in fucosidosis. Birth Defects 12:241, 1976
139. Ginsberg J, Bove KE, Bogelson MH: Pathological features of the eye in the oculocerebrorenal (Lowe) syndrome. J Pediatr Ophthalmol Strabismus 18:16, 1981
140. Sabates R, Krachmer JM, Weingeist TA: Ocular findings in Alport's syndrome. Ophthalmologica 186:204, 1983
141. Baum JL, Tannenbaum M, Kolodny EH: Refsum's syndrome with corneal involvement. Am J Ophthalmol 60:699, 1965
142. Schocket SS: Anterior cleavage syndrome in a patient with Marfan's syndrome. Am J Ophthalmol 66:272, 1968
143. Harcourt B: Anterior chamber cleavage syndrome associated with Weill-Marchesani syndrome and craniofacial dysostosis. J Pediatr Ophthalmol Strabismus 7:24, 1970
144. Franceschetti A, Klein D, Forni D, et al: Heredity in ophthalmology. p. 226. In Clinical and Social Aspects of Heredity in Ophthalmology. Stapes, Herts, England, 1958
145. Ide CH, Matta C, Holt JE, et al: Dysgenesis mesodermalis of the cornea (Peters' anomaly) associated with cleft lip and palate. Ann Ophthalmol 7:841, 1975
146. Riise D: Congenital leucoma of the cornea (Peters' anomaly). Acta Ophthalmol (Copenh) 42:1063, 1964
147. McKusick VA: Mendelian Inheritance in Man. Heinemann, London, 1966
148. Broderick J, Dark AJ: Corneal dystrophy in Cockayne's syndrome. Br J Ophthalmol 57:391, 1973
149. Warburg M: Norrie's disease. p. 117. In Bergsma D (ed): Birth Defects. Part VIII. Williams & Wilkins, Baltimore, 1971
150. Franceschetti A, Maeder G: Dystrophie profonde de la cornée dans un cas d'ichtyose congenitale. Bull Mem Soc Fr Ophtalmol 67:146, 1954
151. Franceschetti A: Les dysplasies ectodermiques et les syndromes héréditaires apparentes. Dermatologica 106:129, 1953
152. Franceschetti AL: Hereditary skin diseases (genodermatoses) and corneal affections. In: Symposium on Surgical and Medical Management of Congenital Anomalies of the Eye. Transactions of the New Orleans Academy of Ophthalmology. CV Mosby, St. Louis, 1968
153. Mulvihill JJ, Echman WW, Fraumeni JF, et al: Melkersson-Rosenthal syndrome, Hodgkin disease, and corneal keratopathy. Arch Intern Med 132:116, 1972
154. Warshawsky RS, Hill CW, Doughman DJ, Harris JE: Acrodermatitis enteropathica. Arch Ophthalmol 93:194, 1975
155. Tessler HH, Apple DJ, Goldberg MF: Ocular findings in a kindred with Kyrle disease. Arch Ophthalmol 90:278, 1973
156. Grayson M: Corneal manifestations of keratosis plantaris and palmaris. Am J Ophthalmol 59:483, 1965
157. Burns RP: Soluble tyrosine aminotransferase deficiency. An unusual cause of corneal ulcers. Am J Ophthalmol 73:400, 1972
158. Bateman TB, Maumenee IH, Sparkes RS: Peters' anomaly associated with partial deletion of the long arm of chromosome 11. Am J Ophthalmol 97:11, 1984
159. Temple IK, Hurst JA, Hing S, et al: De novo deletion of Xp22.2-pter in a female with linear skin lesions of the face and neck, microphthalmia and anterior chamber eye anomalies. J Med Genet 27:56, 1990
160. Frydman M, Steinberger J, Shabtai F, et al: Interstitial deletion 2q14q21. Am J Genet 34:476, 1989
161. Bialasiewicz AA: Ocular findings in 4 p-deletion syndrome (Wolf-Hirshhorn). Ophthalmol Paediatr Genet 10:69, 1989
162. Stathacopoulus R, Bateman B, Sparkes R, Hepler R: The Rieger syndrome and a chromosome 13 deletion. J Pediatr Ophthalmol Strabismus 24:198, 1987
163. Heinemann M, Breg R, Cotlier E: Rieger's syndrome with pericentric inversion of chromosome 6. Br J Ophthalmol 63:40, 1979
164. Schanzlin DJ, Goldberg DB, Brown SI: Transplantation of congenitally opaque corneas. Ophthalmology 87:1253, 1980
165. Spicer WTH: Parenchymatous Keratitis. Interstitial Keratitis-Uveitis Anterior. George Pulman, London, 1924
166. Nahmias AJ, Visintine AM, Caldwell DR, Wilson LA: Eye infections with herpes simplex viruses in neonates. Surv Ophthalmol 21:100, 1976
167. Hutchison DS, Smith RE, Haughton PB: Congenital herpetic keratitis. Arch Ophthalmol 93:70, 1975
168. Townsend WM: The pathogenesis of secondary congenital glaucoma. In Halberg GP (ed): Glaucoma Update. Paul Hoeber, New York, 1974
169. McDonald MB, Burgess SK: Contralateral occipital depression related to obstetric forceps injury to the eye. Am J Ophthalmol 114:318, 1992
170. Hogan M, Zimmerman LE (eds): Ophthalmic Pathology. 2nd Ed. WB Saunders, Philadelphia, 1962
171. Henkind P, Marinsoff G, Manas A, Friedman A: Bilateral corneal dermoids. Am J Ophthalmol 76:972, 1973

172. Baum JL, Feingold M: Ocular aspects of Goldenhar's syndrome. Am J Ophthalmol 75:250, 1953
173. Dailey EG, Lubowitz RM: Dermoids of the limbus and cornea. Am J Ophthalmol 53:661, 1962
174. O'Grady RB, Kirk HQ: Corneal keloids. Am J Ophthalmol 73:206, 1972
175. Weizenblatt S: Congenital malformations of cornea associated with embryonic arrest of ectodermal and mesodermal structures. Arch Ophthalmol 52:415, 1954
176. Von Sallman L, Paton D: Hereditary benign intraepithelial dyskeratosis. Arch Ophthalmol 63:421, 1960
177. Picetti B, Fine M: Keratoplasty in children. Am J Ophthalmol 61:782, 1966
178. Wood TO, Kaufman HE: Penetrating keratoplasty in an infant with sclerocornea. Am J Ophthalmol 70:609, 1970
179. Brown SI: Corneal transplantation in the anterior chamber cleavage syndrome. Am J Ophthalmol 70:942, 1970
180. Brown SI: Corneal transplantation of the infant cornea. Trans Am Acad Ophthalmol Otolaryngol 78:OP461, 1974
181. Stone DL, Kenyon KR, Green WR, Ryan SJ: Congenital central corneal leukoma (Peters' anomaly). Am J Ophthalmol 81:173, 1976
182. Waring GO, Laibson PR: Keratoplasty in infants and children. Trans Am Acad Ophthalmol Otolaryngol 83:OP283, 1977
183. Stulting RD, Sumers KD, Cavanagh HD, et al: Penetrating keratoplasty in children. Ophthalmology 91:1222, 1984
184. Feldman ST, Frucht-Pery J, Brown SI: Corneal transplantation in microphthalmic eyes. Am J Ophthalmol 104:164, 1987
185. Frucht-Pery J, Feldman ST, Brown SI: Transplantation of congenitally opaque corneas from eyes with exaggerated buphthalmos. Am J Ophthalmol 107:655, 1989
186. Cowden JW: Penetrating keratoplasty in infants and children. Ophthalmology 97:324, 1990
187. Dana MR, Moyes AL, Gomes JAP, et al: The indications for and outcome in pediatric keratoplasty: a multicenter study. Ophthalmology 102:1129, 1995

17

Metabolic Disorders of the Cornea

JOEL SUGAR

Metabolic disorders of the cornea are those in which a systemic metabolic abnormality leads to an accumulation of an abnormal substance in the cornea. In contrast to the corneal dystrophies, these disorders often are inherited in an autosomal recessive fashion and involve more than one layer of the cornea; they involve the peripheral as well as the central cornea, are progressive, and are associated with systemic abnormalities. For organizational purposes, these disorders are discussed in groups based on the biochemical substance accumulated or the abnormal metabolic pathway.

DISORDERS OF PROTEIN AND AMINO ACID METABOLISM

This is a diverse group of disorders from both the biochemical and the clinical standpoint (Table 17-1). They are grouped together more for convenience of discussion than on the basis of biochemical similarities.

Cystinosis

Cystinosis is an autosomal recessive disorder of cystine storage and occurs in three forms: infantile, adolescent, and adult. The infantile or nephropathic form has severe renal involvement, with Fanconi syndrome and rickets. Cystine is deposited in multiple organs, and death from renal failure often occurs in the first decade of life. The adolescent or intermediate form has less severe renal involvement, with death usually occurring in the second or third decade. The adult form has no renal involvement and a normal life expectancy.[1] In all these forms, cystine is found in the involved organs in intracytoplasmic, membrane-bound vacuoles.

Ocular manifestations of cystinosis depend on the form of the disease, but all forms have conjunctival and corneal involvement. The infantile and adolescent forms also have retinal involvement, with patchy pigmentary abnormalities and, occasionally, macular changes.[2] Ocular symptoms are limited to photophobia.

Corneal involvement consists of the presence of needle-shaped, refractile, polychromatic crystals that are most dense in the peripheral cornea, where the full thickness of the stroma is typically involved (Figure 17-1). The crystals may also occur in the central cornea, where only the anterior stroma is typically involved.[3] This pattern is seen even late in life in patients with the adult form.[4] Deposits accumulate progressively throughout the cornea, even centrally, in patients with the infantile form whose survival has been prolonged by renal transplantation.[5] Band keratopathy may also develop. Patients with cystinosis and corneal involvement have decreased corneal sensation.[6]

The corneal crystals have been observed by means of clinical specular[7] and electron[3] microscopy and are presumed to be cystine, although they are more needle shaped than the rectangular and hexagonal crystals that are present in the conjunctiva, which have been demonstrated to be L-cystine.[2]

The differential diagnosis of the corneal changes in cystinosis includes those seen in monoclonal gammopathies, Schnyder's crystalline dystrophy, Bietti's crystalline dystrophy, gout, and chrysiasis (Table 17-2). The corneal changes, however, are sufficiently characteristic to suggest the diagnosis of cystinosis in most cases.

Treatment is that of the systemic disease. No treatment is necessary for the adult form. Unfortunately, renal trans-

TABLE 17-1
Ocular Manifestations of Disorders of Protein and Amino Acid Metabolism

Disorder	*Enzyme Deficiency*	*Metabolite Accumulated*	*Mode of Inheritance*	*Ocular Manifestations*
Cystinosis	Probably an abnormality in lysosomal transport of cysteine or cystine	Cystine	Autosomal recessive	All forms: conjunctival and corneal cystine crystal deposition (needle-shaped, refractile polychromatic crystals in full thickness of peripheral stroma and in anterior central stroma), band keratopathy, photophobia. Infantile and adolescent forms: patchy retinal pigment abnormalities, occasional macular changes
Tyrosinemia type II (tyrosinosis; Richner-Hanhart syndrome)	Tyrosine aminotransferase	Tyrosine	Autosomal recessive	Dendritiform corneal epithelial changes (branched or snowflake opacities); red eye; photophobia
Alkaptonuria	Homogentisic acid oxidase	Homogentisic acid	Autosomal recessive	Triangular patches of intrascleral pigmentation near insertion of horizontal rectus muscles; "oil-droplet" opacities in limbal corneal epithelium and Bowman's layer; pigmented pingueculae; irregular pigmented granules in episclera; no functional changes
Wilson's disease	Unknown	Copper (due to reduced ceruloplasmin)	Autosomal recessive	Kayser-Fleischer ring; "sunflower" cataract
Amyloidosis				
Lattice dystrophy type I	Gene defect on chromosome 5q	Amyloid	Autosomal dominant	Classic lattice dystrophy
Lattice dystrophy type II (Meretoja syndrome)	Gelsolin gene defect on chromosome 9	Amyloid	Autosomal dominant	Lattice lines
Lattice dystrophy type III	Unknown	Amyloid	Autosomal recessive	Lattice lines
Lattice dystrophy type IIIA	Unknown	Amyloid	Autosomal dominant	Lattice lines
Granular-lattice dystrophy (Avellino dystrophy)	Gene defect on chromosome 5q	Amyloid; phospholipids and microfibrillar protein	Autosomal dominant	Granular deposits; lattice lines
Gelatinous drop-like dystrophy	Unknown	Amyloid	Autosomal recessive	Mulberry-like subepithelial deposits
Ehlers-Danlos syndrome (type VI)	Lysyl hydroxylase	Abnormal collagen	Autosomal recessive	Keratoconus

plantation does not halt progressive tissue accumulation of cystine.[5] Oral cysteamine appears to reduce cystine levels in leukocytes and prolongs renal function. Topical cysteamine eye drops, when used for prolonged periods, appear to both prevent and reverse corneal accumulation of crystals.[8,9] Recurrent crystal deposition has been reported after penetrating keratoplasty.[10,11]

Tyrosinemia

Genetic disorders of tyrosine metabolism are rare. Type I tyrosinemia is a severe disorder associated with hepatic and renal disease, but not ocular disease. Type II tyrosinemia, also known as tyrosinosis, or Richner-Hanhart syndrome, is an autosomal recessive disorder characterized by corneal abnormalities, painful palmar and plantar hyperkeratosis (Figure 17-2A), and often, mental retardation. The enzyme defect is in hepatic tyrosine aminotransferase and leads to excess tyrosine in the blood and urine.[12]

The ocular manifestations of tyrosinosis consist of dendritiform epithelial changes in the cornea, with ocular redness and photophobia. The epithelial changes appear as fine, branched or snowflake opacities and do not stain with fluorescein (Figure 17-2B). Corneal vascularization and scarring have been reported but may be related to therapies for presumed herpes simplex viral keratitis before proper diagnosis. Conjunctival translucency has also been described.[13]

Histopathologic examination of the conjunctiva reveals membrane-bound intraepithelial inclusions, with thickening of the subepithelial connective tissue and infiltration with plasma cells.[13] Excess dietary tyrosine in rats produces a disease that mimics the clinical disorder in humans, with snowflake corneal opacities and the development of paw erythema.[14] The opacities are followed by stromal thickening, vascular ingrowth, and eventual regression of the lesions. Histopathologic study reveals cytoplasmic inclusions.[15]

Clinical suspicion of tyrosinosis may lead to effective therapy, because dietary restriction of tyrosine and phenylalanine can reduce both corneal and skin changes.[16,17]

Alkaptonuria (Ochronosis)

Another defect in the metabolic pathway of tyrosine is the absence of homogentisic acid oxidase in alkaptonuria. In this autosomal recessive disorder, homogentisic acid accumulates, oxidizes, and polymerizes to cause darkening of the urine and pigmentation of connective tissues (ochronosis). Clinically, patients have arthropathy, with joint pain and ankylosis, as well as pigmentation of cartilaginous structures, renal calculi, and darkening of the urine in the presence of strong alkali.

Ocular findings include triangular patches of intrascleral pigmentation near the insertion of the horizontal rectus muscles (Figure 17-3), darkly pigmented, round, "oil-droplet" opacities in the limbal corneal epithelium and Bowman's layer, pigmented pingueculae, and irregular pigmented granules in the episclera.[18] Histologically, the pigment granules are extracellular[19] and stain differently from melanin. The ocular changes are of no functional significance but may be important in establishing the diagnosis. Differential diagnosis includes senile scleral plaques, melanoma, and drug-induced pigmentation as seen with quinacrine. No specific therapy is available.

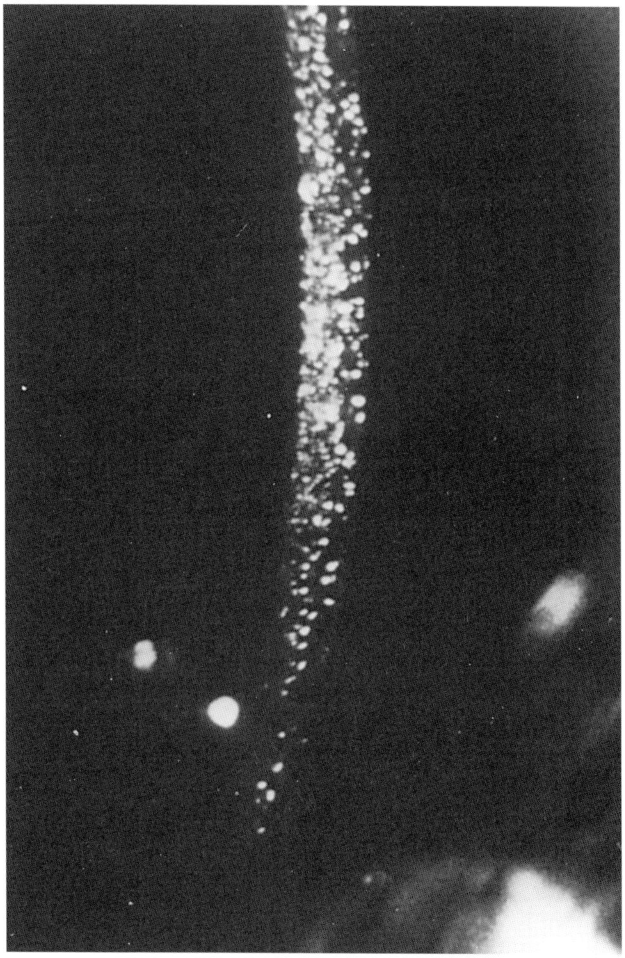

FIGURE 17-1 Crystals in the cornea in cystinosis.

Wilson's Disease

This recessively inherited disorder typically presents in the first two decades of life with liver dysfunction, often with jaundice and hemolysis. Later, neurologic symptoms develop, including dysarthria, loss of coordination, involuntary movements, and abnormal muscle tone. Loss of intellect and behavioral disturbances ensue, and bulbar palsies may lead to death. Joint changes and renal dysfunction are common.

Ocular findings are important in Wilson's disease, not because of any functional ophthalmic significance but because of their usefulness in making or confirming the diagnosis. The Kayser-Fleischer ring consists of copper deposits in Descemet's membrane, which give an orange, brown, green-brown, or gray appearance to the

TABLE 17-2
Differential Diagnosis of Corneal Crystals

Disorder	*Metabolite Accumulated*	*Clinical Appearance*
Cystinosis	Cystine	Needle-shaped, refractile polychromatic crystals in full thickness of peripheral stroma and in anterior central stroma
Monoclonal gammopathies	Immunoglobulin aggregates	White, yellow, gray, or polychromatic crystals at varying levels of the stroma
Schnyder's crystalline dystrophy	Cholesterol and neutral fats	White, red-green, or polychromatic needle-shaped crystals in a central ring-shaped pattern in the anterior stroma and Bowman's layer; may extend deeper and cause a milky opalescence of the cornea
Bietti's crystalline dystrophy	Lipid	Yellow-white needle-like crystals in the anterior stroma of the peripheral cornea
Other lipid keratopathies (LCAT deficiency, Tangier disease, fish-eye disease)	Cholesterol, lipid	Arcus-like changes, fine stromal dots
Gout	Monosodium urate	Fine refractile yellow epithelial and subepithelial crystals, most dense in the interpalpebral area
Chrysiasis	Gold[a]	Irregular yellowish brown to violet glistening deposits most commonly in the superficial cornea; may extend deeper
Clofazimine keratopathy	Clofazimine	Purple-brown small crystals in the epithelium and anterior stroma
Infectious crystalline keratopathy	None[b]	Noninflammatory-appearing white stromal infiltrate with crystalline edges
Dieffenbachia (plant) keratopathy	Calcium oxalate	Clear needle-shaped stromal crystals
Corneal stromal fibrosis	None	White stromal crystal-like opacities

Abbreviation: LCAT, Lecithin:cholesterol acyltransferase.
[a] From intramuscular gold therapy.
[b] Various microorganisms can cause infectious crystalline keratopathy.

deep corneal periphery (Figure 17-4). These deposits initially appear as a thin crescent superiorly, then inferiorly, and ultimately circumferentially. With an anterior Schwalbe's ring, a clear space may separate the Kayser-Fleischer ring from the limbus. The reason for the pattern of copper deposition is unknown but may be related to the pattern of aqueous circulation in the anterior chamber.[20]

Histopathologic study demonstrates copper deposition in Descemet's membrane in the form of granules that are smallest near the corneal endothelium, suggesting a possible active role of endothelial cells in this phenomenon.[21] X-ray and atomic absorption spectroscopy demonstrate copper deposition in the central as well as the peripheral cornea, with the copper bound to sulfur.[22] Corneal copper deposition can also be seen with copper intraocular foreign bodies, and pigmented corneal rings indistinguishable from Kayser-Fleischer rings have been reported with non-Wilsonian liver diseases.[23] Copper may also be deposited in the lens as a sunflower cataract, which appears as green or brown circular and petaloid pigmentation of the anterior and posterior lens capsules.

The pathogenetic biochemical defect in Wilson's disease is unknown. Slowed hepatic production of ceruloplasmin (the protein that carries copper in the blood) and poor biliary excretion of copper appear to be basic defects. Involvement of nonhepatic organs, including the eye and brain, appears to be the result of overflow of excess copper from the liver.[24] Diagnostic laboratory test results include decreased serum ceruloplasmin and serum copper levels, increased urinary excretion of copper, and increased hepatic copper levels in biopsy specimens.

Treatment with D-penicillamine is effective in preventing the long-term complications of Wilson's disease and reducing complications already present. Corneal examination may be helpful in following therapy, because the Kayser-Fleischer ring regresses and may ultimately disappear in a pattern that is the reverse of the progression of deposition: the nasal-temporal portions of the ring disappear first, followed by the inferior and then the superior portions of the ring.

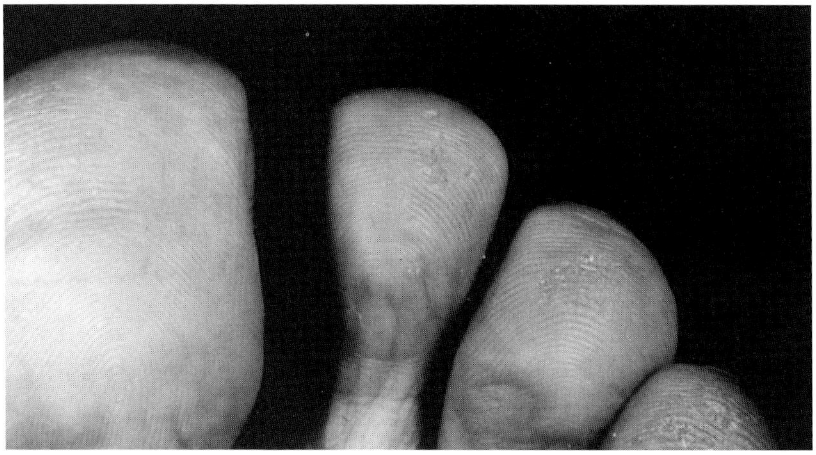
A

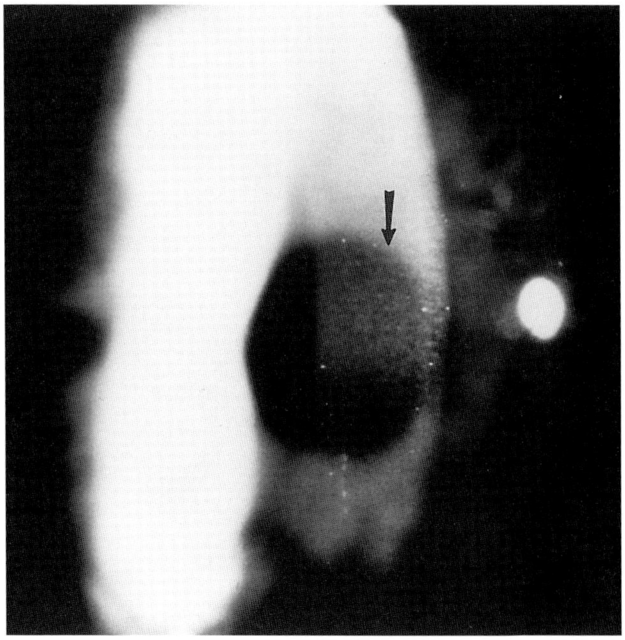
B

FIGURE 17-2 (A) Hyperkeratotic plaques on the toes of a 56-year-old man with tyrosinemia type II. (B) Cornea demonstrating snowflake epithelial opacities (arrow). (Courtesy of Marian Macsai, M.D., Morgantown, WV.)

Amyloidosis

Amyloid is a β-pleated fibrillar group of substances that accumulate in tissues in several disorders. In the cornea, inherited forms of amyloidosis include classic lattice dystrophy (lattice dystrophy type I), Meretoja syndrome of neuropathic amyloidosis and corneal changes (lattice dystrophy type II), lattice dystrophy types III and IIIA, granular-lattice (Avellino) dystrophy, and primary familial corneal amyloidosis (gelatinous drop-like dystrophy). Recently, lattice dystrophy type I has been mapped to chromosome 5q, along with granular and granular-lattice dystrophies.[25] A specific genetic mutation involving the gene on chromosome 9 for the actin-binding protein gelsolin has been identified in lattice dystrophy type II patients.[26] These disorders are discussed in Chapters 18 and 20.

Ehlers-Danlos Syndrome

Ehlers-Danlos syndrome type VI is an autosomal recessive disorder and is associated with keratoconus. It is discussed in Chapter 22.

DISORDERS OF PURINE AND PYRIMIDINE METABOLISM

Disorders of purine and pyrimidine metabolism are infrequently encountered as ophthalmic problems but nonetheless deserve mention (Table 17-3).

Gout

Gout is a form of arthritis caused by the deposition of monosodium urate crystals in and around joints. Classically, this occurs in the great toe (podagra). Accumulation of urate crystals in tissues occurs as tophi. Renal calculi may occur as well.

The cause of gout appears to be related to identified defects in purine metabolic pathways in only a minority of patients, and the clinical disorder appears to result from a combination of genetic and environmental factors.

The ocular changes of gout include conjunctival, scleral, and corneal deposition of monosodium urate crystals, which can cause conjunctivitis, episcleritis, and scleritis. The corneal deposits may appear as fine, refractile, yellow crystals, most dense in the interpalpebral fissure,[27] or in a form indistinguishable from that of calcific

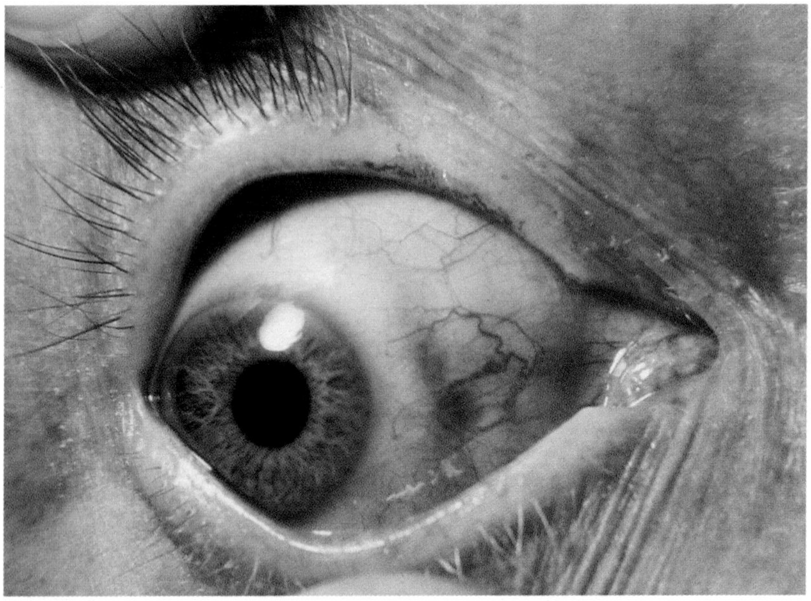

FIGURE 17-3 Intrascleral pigmentation in alkaptonuria.

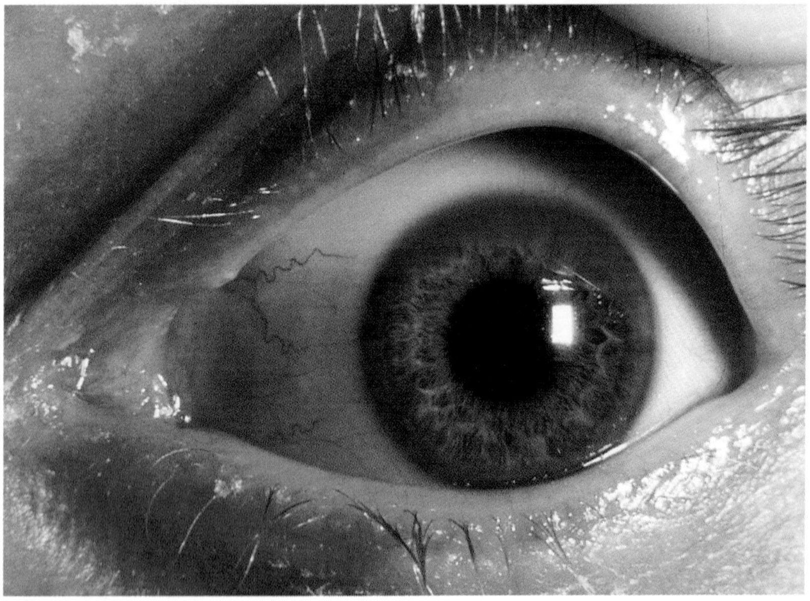

FIGURE 17-4 Kayser-Fleischer ring in Wilson's disease.

TABLE 17-3
Ocular Manifestations of Disorders of Purine and Pyrimidine Metabolism

Disorder	*Enzyme Deficiency*	*Metabolite Accumulated*	*Mode of Inheritance*	*Ocular Manifestations*
Gout	Environmental, physiologic, and genetic abnormalities, including excessive synthesis of purine precursors of uric acid	Monosodium urate	—	Corneal deposition of monosodium urate crystals (as fine refractile yellow crystals); conjunctivitis; episcleritis; scleritis
Xeroderma pigmentosum	Defect in DNA repair (endonuclease)	—	Autosomal recessive	Eyelid and conjunctival tumors (basal and squamous cell); juvenile cataract

band keratopathy.[28] The corneal manifestations of gout must be distinguished from urate keratopathy, a disorder in which there is localized corneal urate deposition without systemic hyperuricemia.

Treatment includes the use of nonsteroidal anti-inflammatory drugs, colchicine, and occasionally, corticosteroids during acute episodes. Chronic use of allopurinol prevents hyperuricemia. Corneal deposits may occasionally require scraping or superficial keratectomy.

Xeroderma Pigmentosum

This autosomal recessive disorder is caused by a defect in the ability of cells to repair DNA damaged by ultraviolet light. While a specific enzyme defect has not been identified, tissue cell culture fusion studies demonstrate eight different complementation groups. Fusion of cells from two patients in different groups overcomes the DNA repair defect present in the unfused cells from either individual.[29] Clinically, these patients develop skin hyper- and hypopigmentation, dryness, scaling, and many skin tumors, both benign and malignant, in sun-exposed areas (Figure 17-5A).

Ocular findings include eyelid tumors, especially basal and squamous cell carcinomas, with eyelid deformities developing subsequent to these lesions and their excision (Figure 17-5B). Recurrent conjunctival inflammation and infection occur, and conjunctival membranes develop.[30] Corneal involvement includes scarring and vascularization, as well as development of squamous cell carcinoma (Figure 17-6).

Treatment includes prevention of tumors by the use of sunscreening agents and avoiding exposure to sunlight, as well as local excision of tumors. Penetrating keratoplasty has a poor prognosis in this disorder.[29]

DISORDERS OF CARBOHYDRATE METABOLISM

Mucopolysaccharidoses

The mucopolysaccharidoses are a group of inherited disorders characterized by the accumulation of excess mucopolysaccharides, or glycosaminoglycans (GAGs), in lysosomes (Table 17-4). Glycosaminoglycans are long-chain carbohydrates made up of uronic acids, amino sugars, and neutral sugars; glycosaminoglycans linked to proteins form proteoglycans, the ground substance of connective tissue.

The normal cornea contains 4 to 4.5 percent glycosaminoglycans. Three major glycosaminoglycans are found in the corneal stroma. Keratan sulfate I is found exclusively in the corneal stroma and accounts for 50 percent

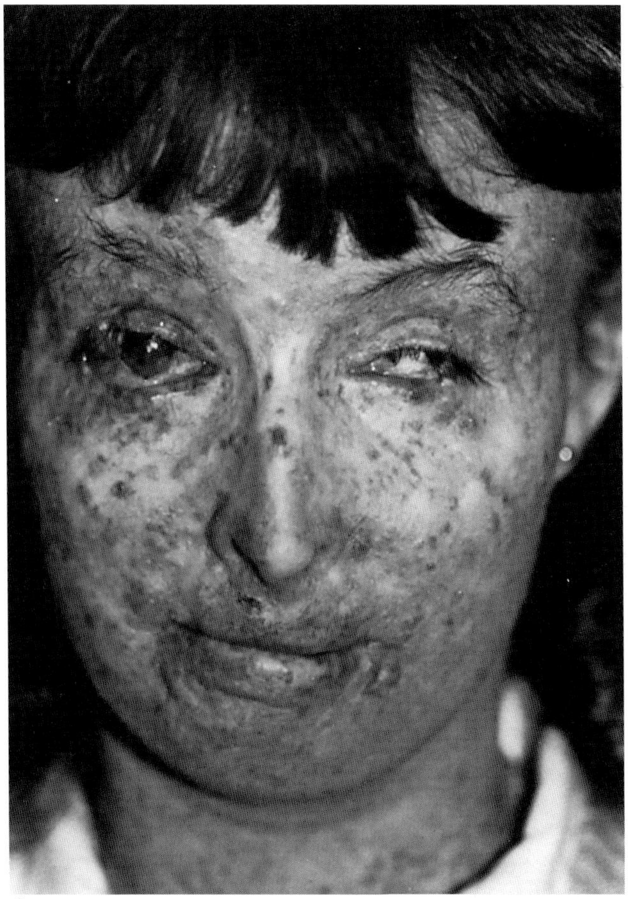

A

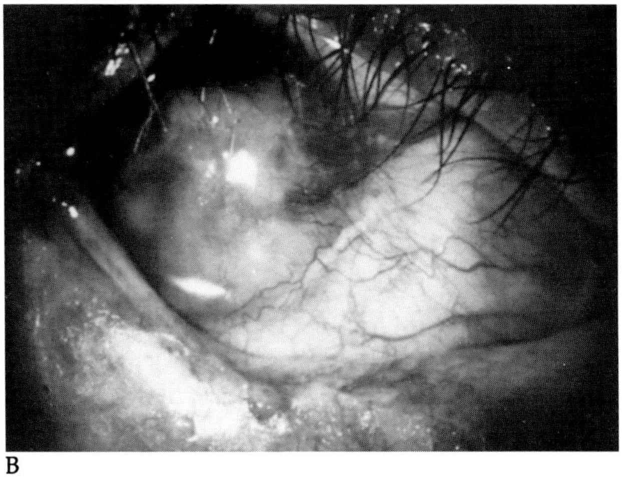

B

FIGURE 17-5 **(A)** Patient with xeroderma pigmentosum demonstrating many skin tumors. **(B)** The right eyelids are severely deformed. Corneal damage has been caused by trichiasis and exposure.

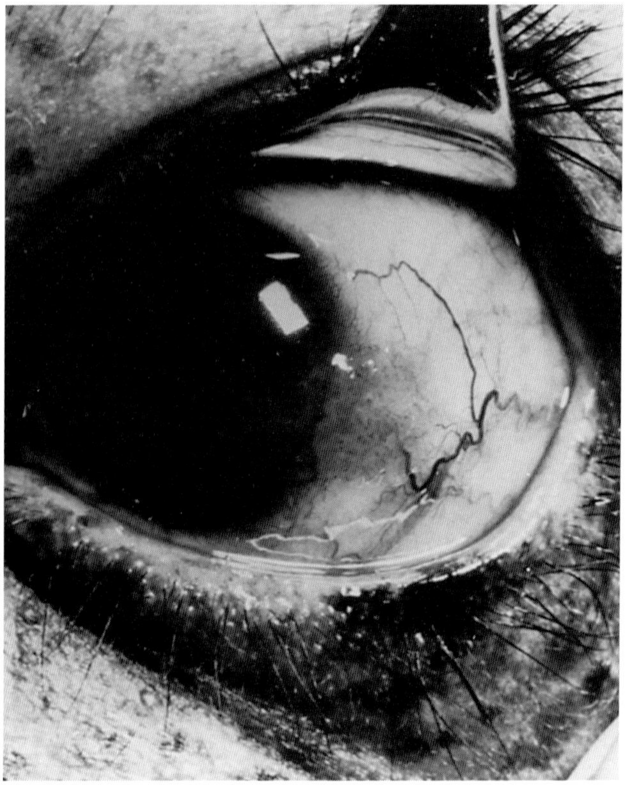

FIGURE 17-6 Limbal carcinoma in situ in a patient with xeroderma pigmentosum.

of the glycosaminoglycans, whereas chondroitin and chondroitin-4-sulfate each account for 25 percent.[31] Dermatan sulfate is not present in the normal cornea but is present in corneal scars.

Normally, glycosaminoglycans are catabolized by lysosomal acid hydrolases, but in the mucopolysaccharidoses, deficiencies of these enzymes lead to glycosaminoglycan accumulation. Dermatan sulfate and keratan sulfate accumulate in the cornea and cause corneal clouding, whereas heparan sulfate affects the function of the retina and central nervous system. The specific enzyme deficiency determines the substance that accumulates and the clinical manifestations of the disorder. Histopathologically, however, all the mucopolysaccharidoses show characteristic pathologic changes in the cornea, consisting of intracytoplasmic vacuolation of epithelium, subepithelial histiocytes, stromal keratocytes, and endothelium. Granular material surrounds the stromal keratocytes and accumulates in these cells and in the cytoplasm of epithelial cells. The degree of accumulation of such material determines the degree of corneal clouding.

Hurler (MPS I-H) and Scheie (MPS I-S) syndromes are allelic, in that they are both caused by abnormalities in the function of the same enzyme, α-L-iduronidase, but presumably the specific abnormalities are different. The Hurler-Scheie compound disorder (MPS I-H/S) is the result of a heterozygous combination of the two allelic defects.

MPS I-H (Hurler Syndrome)

Hurler syndrome is characterized by gargoyle-like facial dysmorphism, progressive mental degeneration, dwarfism, and skeletal dysplasia (dysostosis multiplex). These features become more evident with age, and the typical appearance is usually seen by 1 year of age. Death usually occurs by mid-adolescence from cardiac or pulmonary disease. Diffuse corneal clouding develops after birth as a ground-glass haze (Figure 17-7). Retinal pigmentary changes and optic atrophy occur as well. Trabecular involvement can lead to glaucoma.[32]

MPS I-S (Scheie Syndrome)

Scheie syndrome is the result of the same enzyme defect as Hurler syndrome but is less severe. Facial features are coarse, there is claw-like deformity of the hands, and there may be aortic valve disease. Intelligence, however, is not impaired. Progressive corneal clouding occurs, as do pigmentary retinopathy, optic atrophy, and glaucoma.[33] Penetrating keratoplasty may be successful in clearing the visual axis, but vision may be limited by retinal and optic nerve disease.

MPS I-H/S (Hurler-Scheie Compound)

Patients with Hurler-Scheie compound have disease that is phenotypically more severe than patients with Scheie syndrome but less severe than those with Hurler syndrome. Corneal clouding, abnormal facies, and aortic valve disease occur. Bone deformities and mental retardation are less severe. Retinitis-pigmentosa-like changes are present in the retina.[34]

MPS II (Hunter Syndrome)

Hunter syndrome is the only X-linked recessive mucopolysaccharidosis and is caused by a deficiency of iduronate sulfate sulfatase. The severe form (MPS II-A) is similar to Hurler syndrome, but skeletal changes are less severe and corneal clouding is rare. A milder form (MPS II-B) exists without mental retardation but with coarse features and heart disease. These patients have hearing deficits and poor vision because of retinal and optic nerve changes. Corneal clouding may be evident on slit lamp examination of older patients, and mucopolysaccharide can be seen on histopathologic examination of the cornea. Presumably, the less evident corneal clouding is related to decreased production and accumulation of dermatan sulfate.

TABLE 17-4
Ocular Manifestations of Disorders of Carbohydrate Metabolism

Disorder	Enzyme Deficiency	Metabolite Accumulated	Mode of Inheritance	Ocular Manifestations
MPS I-H (Hurler syndrome)	α-L-iduronidase	Heparan sulfate Dermatan sulfate	Autosomal recessive	Corneal clouding; pigmentary retinopathy; optic atrophy; glaucoma
MPS I-S (Scheie syndrome)	α-L-iduronidase	Heparan sulfate Dermatan sulfate	Autosomal recessive	Corneal clouding; pigmentary retinopathy; optic atrophy; glaucoma
MPS I-H/S (Hurler-Scheie)	α-L-iduronidase	Heparan sulfate Dermatan sulfate	Autosomal recessive	Corneal clouding; pigmentary retinopathy; optic atrophy
MPS II (Hunter syndrome)	Iduronate sulfate sulfatase (iduronate sulfatase)	Heparan sulfate Dermatan sulfate	X-linked recessive	Rare corneal clouding; pigmentary retinopathy; optic atrophy
MPS III (Sanfilippo syndrome)	A: heparan-*S*-sulfaminidase (heparan sulfate *N*-sulfatase)	Heparan sulfate	Autosomal recessive	All forms: clinically clear cornea; occasional slit lamp corneal opacities (mucopolysaccharide accumulation in intracytoplasmic vacuoles in keratocytes, endothelium, and epithelium); pigmentary retinopathy; optic atrophy
	B: α-*N*-acetyl-glucosaminidase (*N*-acetyl-α-D-glucosaminidase)	Heparan sulfate	Autosomal recessive	
	C: acetyl-CoA-α-glucosaminide-*N*-*N*-acetyl-transferase	Heparan sulfate	Autosomal recessive	
	D: *N*-acetyl-glucosamine-6-sulfate sulfatase	Heparan sulfate	Autosomal recessive	
MPS IV (Morquio syndrome)	A: *N*-acetyl-galactosamine-6-sulfate sulfatase	Keratan sulfate	Autosomal recessive	Corneal clouding; optic atrophy
	B: β-galactosidase	Keratan sulfate	Autosomal recessive	
MPS V (reclassified as MPS I-S)	—	—	—	—
MPS VI (Maroteaux-Lamy syndrome)	*N*-acetyl-galactosamine-4-sulfate sulfatase (arylsulfatase B)	Dermatan sulfate	Autosomal recessive	Corneal clouding; optic atrophy
MPS VII	β-Glucuronidase	Dermatan sulfate Heparan sulfate	Autosomal recessive	Corneal clouding

Abbreviation: MPS, mucopolysaccharidosis.

MPS III (Sanfilippo Syndrome)

Sanfilippo syndrome is actually the phenotypic expression of any of four possible enzyme defects involved in the degradation of heparan sulfate. MPS III-A is due to deficiency in heparan sulfate *N*-sulfatase, MPS III-B to a deficiency in α-*N*-acetyl-glucosaminidase, MPS III-C to a deficiency in acetyl-CoA-α-glucosaminide-*N*-*N*-acetyl-transferase, and MPS III-D to a deficiency in *N*-acetylglucosamine-6-sulfate sulfatase.[35]

Clinically, Sanfilippo syndrome is characterized by mild dysmorphism and progressive dementia. The cornea appears grossly clear (Figure 17-8), but slit lamp examination occasionally reveals opacities.[36] Histopathologic examination shows mucopolysaccharide accumulation in membrane-bound intracytoplasmic vacuoles in corneal epithelium, keratocytes, and endothelium.[37,38] Accumulation in the retinal pigment epithelium is associated with retinitis-pigmentosa–like photoreceptor damage.

MPS IV (Morquio Syndrome)

In Morquio syndrome, facial appearance and intelligence are normal, but bone deformities are severe (Figure 17-9). Slit lamp examination shows evidence of corneal clouding, and optic atrophy is common. The corneal changes are insufficient to warrant penetrating keratoplasty.[39] Spinal cord compression from vertebral deformities and aortic valve disease occur. MPS IV-A, the more severe type, is caused by *N*-acetyl-galactosamine-6-sulfate sulfatase deficiency, whereas the milder IV-B is the result of a specific β-galactosidase deficiency.

MPS V

MPS V is vacant, having previously been filled by Scheie syndrome, now known to be a form of MPS I.

MPS VI (Maroteaux-Lamy Syndrome)

Maroteaux-Lamy syndrome is characterized by deformities similar to those of Hurler syndrome, but intelligence

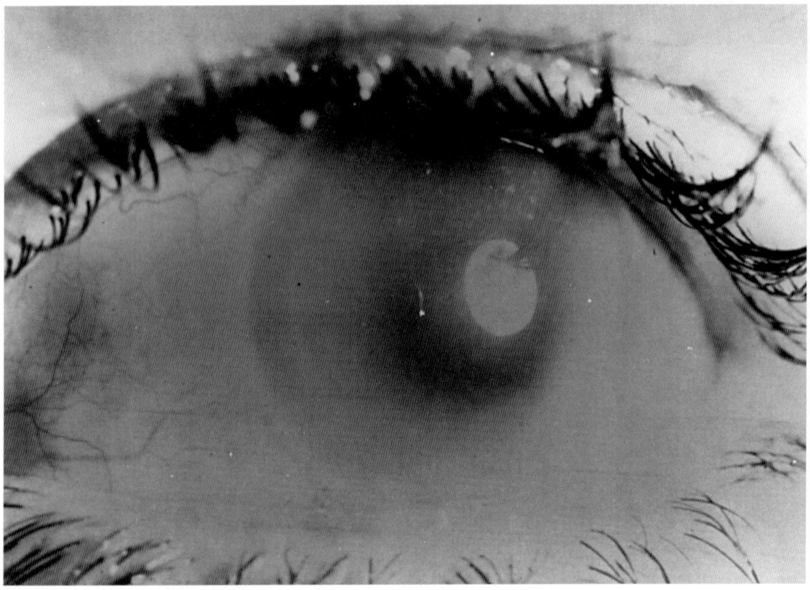

FIGURE 17-7 Corneal clouding in Hurler syndrome.

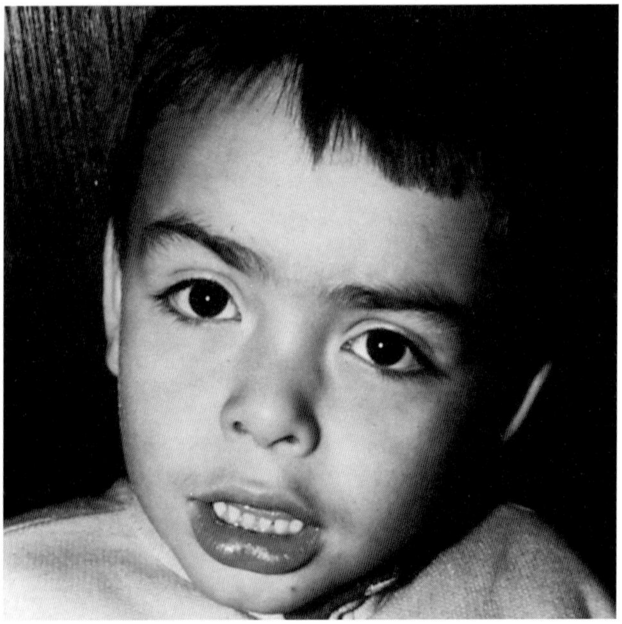

FIGURE 17-8 Patient with Sanfilippo syndrome. The corneas are grossly clear. (Courtesy of Yves Lacassie, M.D., New Orleans, LA.)

is normal. Hydrocephalus with optic atrophy can occur. Corneal clouding is marked and may necessitate penetrating keratoplasty.[40] The retina is normal. There are two allelic forms, one severe (MPS VI-A) and one mild (MPS VI-B); the deficient enzyme is *N*-acetyl-galactosamine-4-sulfate sulfatase (arylsulfatase B). An analogous disorder with the same enzyme defect and corneal clouding occurs as a recessively inherited disorder in cats.[41]

MPS VII

This disorder is caused by β-glucuronidase deficiency and results in facial and bone abnormalities similar to those listed above, in addition to mental retardation, hepatosplenomegaly, and frequent respiratory infections. Corneal clouding is present in approximately 75 percent of cases.[42]

Treatments for all the mucopolysaccharidoses are likely to change dramatically with the advent of molecular genetic approaches to the treatment of inherited metabolic diseases. Other approaches have included transplantation of healthy donor tissues. In the mucopolysaccharidoses, bone marrow transplantation in infancy has led to improvements in corneal clouding in some patients with MPS types I-H, II, IIIA, and IIIB.[43]

DISORDERS OF LIPID METABOLISM AND STORAGE

Sphingolipidoses

The sphingolipidoses are disorders of lipid storage, and except for Fabry's disease, are inherited in an autosomal recessive manner. They are caused by deficient activity of specific catabolic enzymes, which leads to intracellular accumulation of lipid (Table 17-5). Functional deficits occur in those tissues in which the involved sphingolipid is an important constituent. Neural sphingolipids are involved in G_{M2} gangliosidosis and metachromatic leukodystrophy, and accumulation leads to central nervous system dysfunction. Visceral sphingolipids are involved in Fabry's disease, and accumulation leads to renal failure without central nervous system involvement. Clinical disorders have been correlated with defects in metabolism of each of the major sphingolipids. Only those disorders with corneal involvement, however, are discussed here.

G_{M2} Gangliosidosis Type II (Sandhoff's Disease)

Sandhoff's disease is similar to Tay-Sachs disease (G_{M2} gangliosidosis type I) but differs in its enzyme defect. In Sandhoff's disease, hexosaminidase A and B are deficient, whereas in Tay-Sachs disease only hexosaminidase A is deficient. Patients with Sandhoff's disease have severe psychomotor retardation, hepatosplenomegaly, and cherry-red maculas with blindness. Corneas are clear, even on slit lamp evaluation, but pathologic examination reveals single membrane-bound vacuoles within keratocytes.[44]

Metachromatic Leukodystrophy (Austin's Juvenile Form)

Metachromatic leukodystrophy is caused by a deficiency in arylsulfatases A, B, and C, as well as other sulfatases. This disorder manifests in the first few years of life as slow development, psychomotor retardation, seizures, and features resembling Hurler syndrome. Corneal clouding may occur.[42]

Fabry's Disease

Fabry's disease is the only sphingolipidosis that is inherited as an X-linked recessive disorder. It is characterized by renal failure, peripheral neuropathy with painful dysesthesias in the lower extremities, and skin lesions. The skin lesions, called angiokeratoma corporis diffusum, are symmetrical, small, and round (Figure 17-10). They are caused by accumulation of sphingolipid in vascular endothelium.

Ocular findings include conjunctival and retinal vascular tortuosity; whitish, granular, anterior subcapsular lens opacities; oculomotor abnormalities; and corneal changes. The corneal changes consist of whorl-like lines (cornea verticillata) that appear to flow together in the inferocentral corneal epithelium (Figure 17-11A). The lines appear to be made up of many powdery, white, yellow, or brown dots in the corneal epithelium or subepithelium.[45] These corneal changes are present in affected patients as well as in the female carriers. The corneal changes are evident only on slit lamp examination and are of no visual significance. Their presence, however, can be important in making or confirming the diagnosis. The corneal changes of Fabry's disease appear to be the result of intracellular lipid inclusions in the basal epithelium,[46] although Weingeist and Blodi[47] suggested that the whorl-like lines may represent reduplications of epithelial basement membrane, as well as material accumulated between the basement membrane and Bowman's layer. Differential diagnosis includes the corneal opacities seen with chloroquine, phenothiazine, and amiodarone (Figure 17-11B) and striate melanokeratosis (Figure 17-11C).

Treatment of the renal failure of Fabry's disease with renal transplantation provides only temporary relief of renal symptoms and fails to alter the systemic enzyme deficiency of α-galactosidase.

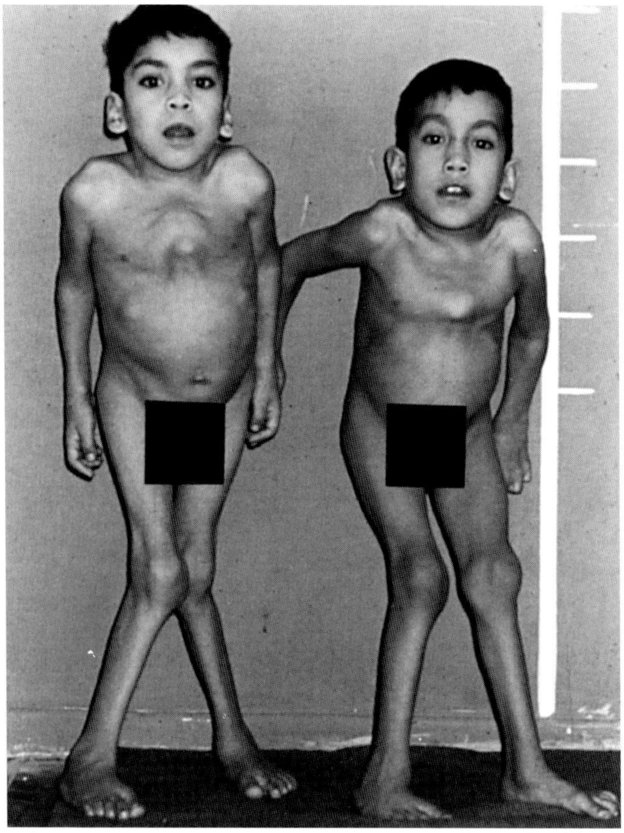

FIGURE 17-9 Severe bone deformities in two patients with Morquio syndrome. (Courtesy of Yves Lacassie, M.D., New Orleans, LA.)

TABLE 17-5
Ocular Manifestations of Disorders of Lipid Metabolism and Storage

Disorder	*Enzyme Deficiency*	*Metabolite Accumulated*	*Mode of Inheritance*	*Ocular Manifestations*
G_{M2} gangliosidosis II (Sandhoff's disease)	Hexosaminidase A and B	G_{M2}-ganglioside	Autosomal recessive	Membrane-bound vacuoles within corneal keratocytes; cherry-red macula
Metachromatic leukodystrophy (Austin's juvenile form)	Arylsulfatases A, B, and C and other sulfatases	Sulfatide	Autosomal recessive	Corneal clouding
Fabry's disease	α-Galactosidase	Ceramide trihexoside	X-linked recessive	Conjunctival and retinal vascular tortuosity; white granular anterior subcapsular lens opacities; oculomotor abnormalities; whorl-like corneal epithelial changes (cornea verticillata)
LCAT deficiency	Lecithin:cholesterol acyltransferase	Free cholesterol	Autosomal recessive	Dense peripheral arcus; diffuse grayish dots in central stroma; no visual changes
Tangier disease	Unknown	Triglycerides (low HDL, cholesterol, and phospholipids)	Autosomal recessive	Fine dot corneal clouding; no visual changes; no arcus
Fish-eye disease	α-Lecithin:cholesterol acyltransferase	Triglycerides, VLDL	Unknown (rare)	Progressive gray-white-yellow dot corneal clouding; increased corneal thickness
Hyperlipoproteinemia I (hyperchylomicronemia)	Lipoprotein lipase	Triglycerides; chylomicrons	Autosomal recessive	Lipemia retinalis; palpebral eruptive xanthomas
Hyperlipoproteinemia II				
IIa. Hyper-β-lipoproteinemia	Thought to be defective or absent LDL receptors	LDL; cholesterol	Autosomal dominant	Both forms: corneal arcus; conjunctival xanthomas; xanthelasma
IIb. Hyper-β- and hyperpre-β-lipoproteinemia	Unknown	LDL; VLDL; cholesterol, triglycerides	Autosomal dominant	
Hyperlipoproteinemia III (dys-β-lipoproteinemia) (Broad beta disease)	Defective remnant metabolism in the liver caused by an abnormality in apo-E	VLDL remnants; cholesterol; triglycerides	Autosomal recessive	Arcus; xanthelasma; lipemia retinalis
Hyperlipoproteinemia IV (hyperpre-β-lipoproteinemia)	Unknown	Triglycerides; VLDL; cholesterol	Autosomal dominant	Arcus; xanthelasma; lipemia retinalis
Hyperlipoproteinemia V (hyperpre-β-lipoproteinemia and hyperchylomicronemia)	Unknown	VLDL; cholesterol; triglycerides; chylomicrons	Unknown	Lipemia retinalis; no arcus

Abbreviations: HDL, high-density lipoprotein; VLDL, very-low-density lipoprotein; LDL, low-density lipoprotein.

Dyslipoproteinemias

The dyslipoproteinemias include several lipid metabolic abnormalities with corneal manifestations.

LCAT Deficiency

In this autosomal recessive disorder located on chromosome 16q22,[48] lack of the enzyme lecithin:cholesterol acyltransferase (LCAT) leads to the inability to esterify free cholesterol. Free cholesterol then accumulates in vessels and causes atherosclerosis and renal insufficiency. Abnormal lipids in the red blood cells result in anemia. Phagocytosis of lipids leads to "sea-blue" histiocytes in the bone marrow and spleen. In the cornea, changes are present from early childhood. Homozygous enzyme-deficient patients have stromal deposition of fine gray dots centrally with peripheral arcus-like changes (Figure 17-12). Symptoms of

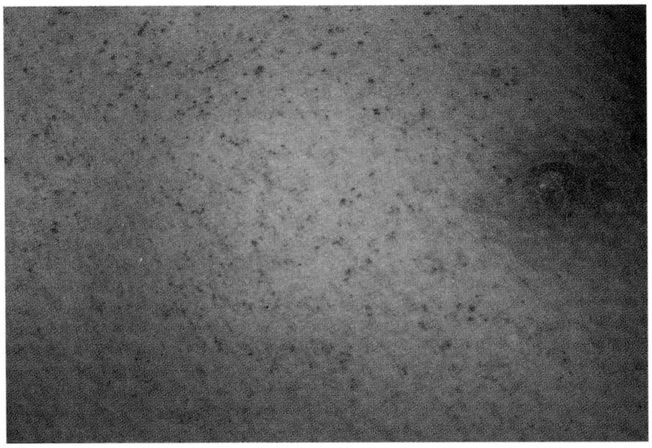

FIGURE 17-10 Skin lesions on the torso of a patient with Fabry's disease.

photophobia and mild blurring of vision may occur. Heterozygotes have peripheral arcus-like changes only.[49]

Tangier Disease (Familial High-Density Lipoprotein Deficiency)

Tangier disease is an autosomal recessive disorder characterized by low plasma levels of cholesterol and high-density lipoproteins, in which the precursors of high-density lipoproteins are abnormally catabolized. Clinically, these patients have orange tonsils, lymphadenopathy, hepatosplenomegaly, peripheral neuropathy, and coronary artery disease. Corneal clouding, consisting of many fine dots, occurs and is most dense centrally and posteriorly in the stroma. Arcus is not seen. Vision is not affected. Lipid particles have been demonstrated in degenerating pericytes of conjunctival vessels.[50]

Fish-Eye Disease

Fish-eye disease is a rare disorder characterized genetically by an abnormality in the LCAT gene that causes a loss of α-LCAT activity.[51] Patients have abnormal serum lipoproteins and corneal clouding with no other evidence of systemic disease. Triglycerides are elevated, as are very-low-density lipoproteins (VLDL). The disorder is named for the corneal opacification that eventually resembles a boiled fish eye. Corneal clouding first becomes evident late in the second decade of life and slowly progresses. Visual acuity and color discrimination slowly decline. The corneal opacities are gray-white-yellow dots distributed in a mosaic pattern throughout the corneal stroma, most densely in the periphery. Corneal thickness is increased. The clouding can become sufficient to require penetrating keratoplasty. Histopathologic examination reveals many extracellular vacuoles made up of a cholesterol-containing lipid sandwiched between the collagen fibrils throughout the corneal stroma.[52]

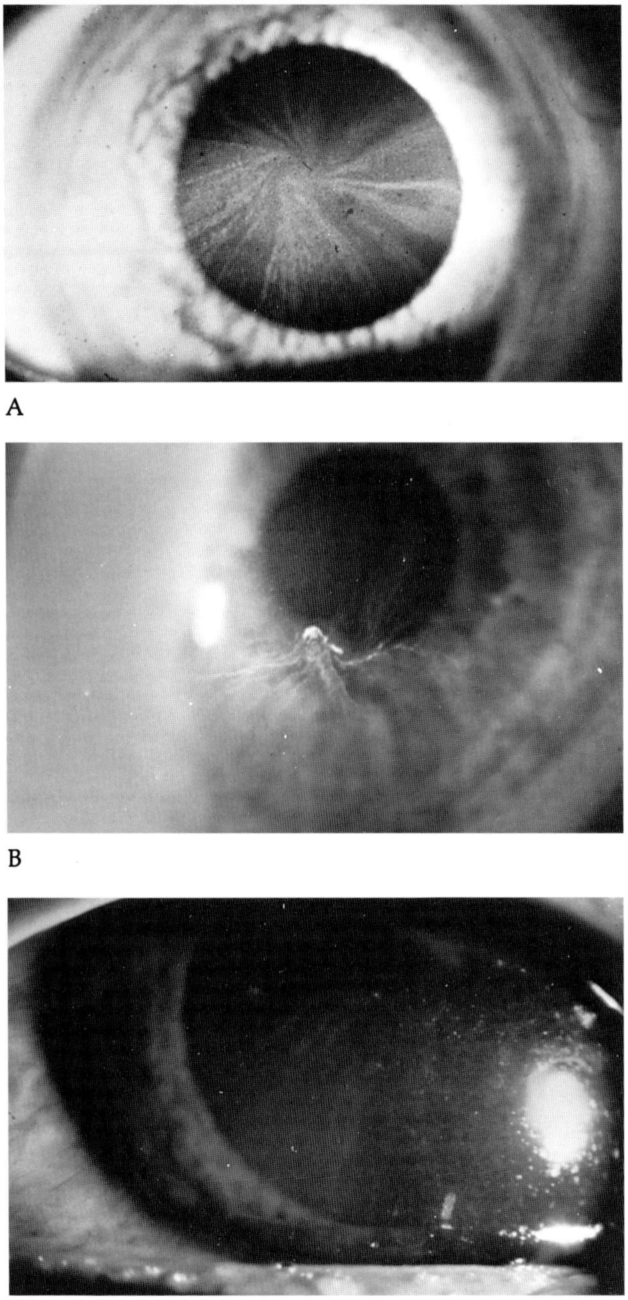

A

B

C

FIGURE 17-11 **(A)** Cornea verticillata in Fabry's disease. **(B)** Cornea verticillata caused by amiodarone. **(C)** Striate melanokeratosis.

Hyperlipoproteinemias

Fredrickson and co-workers[53] described five major phenotypes of hyperlipoproteinemia, characterized by lipoprotein electrophoresis patterns. Subsequently, the lipoproteinemias have been separated by other physical and chemical techniques. The normal fasting lipoproteins are very low-den-

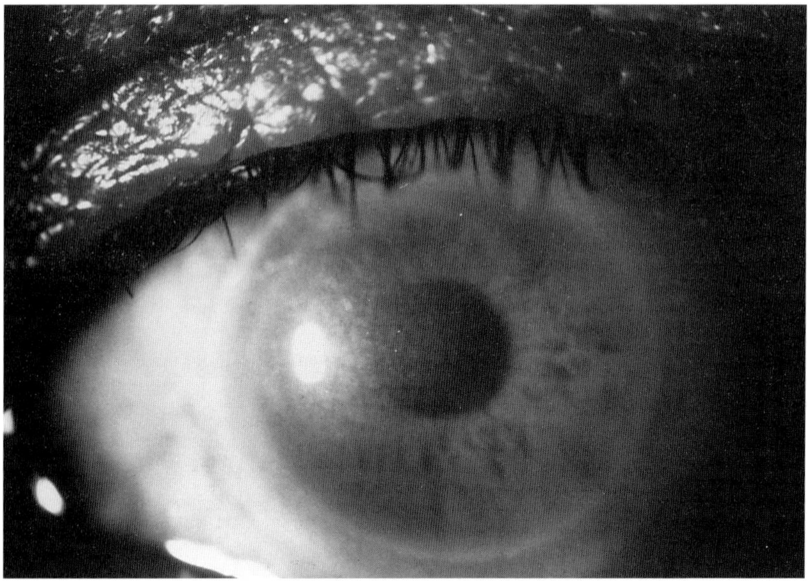

FIGURE 17-12 A 42-year-old man with LCAT deficiency. Note the arcus-like changes and stromal haze. (Courtesy of Michael B. Shapiro, M.D., Madison, WI.)

sity lipoproteins (VLDL) or pre-β-lipoproteins, low-density lipoproteins (LDL) or β-lipoproteins, and high-density lipoproteins (HDL) or α-1-lipoproteins. In various disorders, these and/or chylomicrons and intermediate-density lipoproteins (IDL) may be elevated. Corneal changes, particularly corneal arcus, may occur in many of these disorders.

Arcus is the result of deposition of lipids in the corneal stroma, Bowman's layer, and Descemet's membrane. It occurs in the peripheral cornea, and there is a clear space between it and the limbus (Figure 17-13). The central cornea is not affected. Arcus appears to develop first in the superior and then the inferior cornea and then becomes confluent. Descemet's membrane, then Bowman's layer, and eventually the deeper stroma become involved. In a study of patients with hyperlipoproteinemias, arcus was strongly correlated with age but not with the pattern of hyperlipoproteinemia.[54] An Israeli study showed a positive correlation between arcus and levels of cholesterol and LDL.[55] Treatment of hyperlipoproteinemias is not associated with reduction in arcus.

Type I hyperlipoproteinemia (hyperchylomicronemia) is an autosomal recessive disorder. It is not associated with arcus, but is associated with lipemia retinalis and palpebral eruptive xanthomas. These patients also have hepatosplenomegaly and diffuse eruptive xanthomas.

Type II hyperlipoproteinemia (hyper-β; hyper-β and hyperpre-β-lipoproteinemia) is inherited as an autosomal dominant disorder. Patients have xanthelasma, corneal arcus, and conjunctival xanthomas, in addition to tendinous xanthomas and coronary artery disease.

Type III hyperlipoproteinemia (dys-β-lipoproteinemia) is an autosomal recessive disorder. Xanthelasma, corneal arcus, and lipemia retinalis occur. These patients have peripheral vascular disease, coronary artery disease, and diabetes mellitus.

Type IV hyperlipoproteinemia (hyperpre-β-lipoproteinemia) is inherited as an autosomal dominant disorder. Arcus, xanthelasma, and lipemia retinalis are present, in addition to vascular disease and diabetes.

Type V hyperlipoproteinemia (hyperpre-β-lipoproteinemia plus hyperchylomicronemia) is associated with lipemia retinalis without corneal arcus. Xanthomas and hepatosplenomegaly occur without significant vascular disease.

As mentioned previously, this classification of hyperlipoproteinemia was established before the recognition of additional lipoprotein disorders, and newer pathophysiologic approaches may help in future classification of these disorders.[56]

DISORDERS OF COMBINED CARBOHYDRATE AND LIPID METABOLISM

Mucolipidoses (Oligosaccharidoses)

A group of disorders with changes similar to those seen in the mucopolysaccharidoses as well as the visceral changes seen in the sphingolipidoses has been described; the definition and classification of these disorders have evolved as biochemical understanding has improved. The common characteristic of these disorders appears to be abnormal metabolism of the carbohydrate in glycoproteins and glycolipids,[57] leading to accumulation and excess excretion of oligosaccharides (Table 17-6). Corneal clouding is seen in

FIGURE 17-13 Corneal arcus.

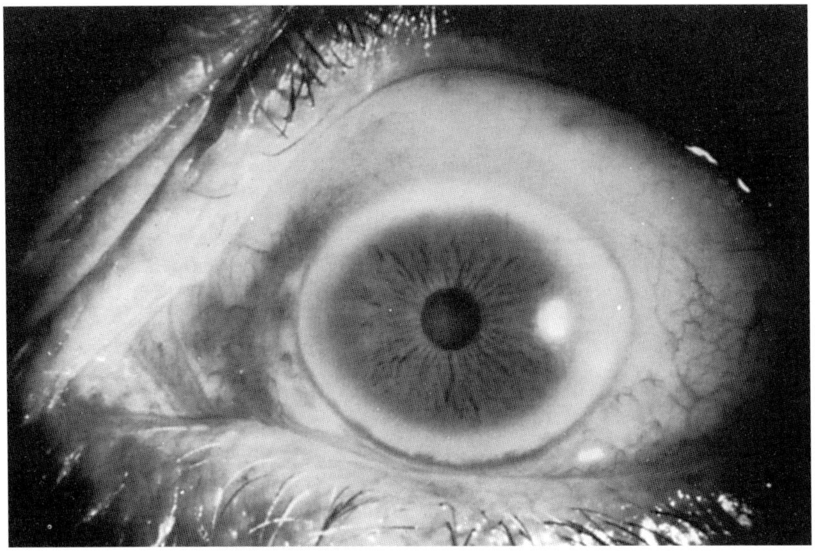

several of these disorders. All are inherited in an autosomal recessive manner, and all are caused by defects in lysosomal acid hydrolase enzymes.

MLS I (Dysmorphic Sialidosis, Spranger Syndrome)

Spranger syndrome is characterized by coarse facies, kyphosis, slow psychomotor development, and hearing loss. With advancing age, increasing neurologic deficits occur, with ataxia, muscle weakness, tremors, and muscle twitching. Mobility becomes limited because of the neurologic difficulties, and death occurs in adolescence or early adulthood.

Ocular findings include macular cherry-red spot, tortuous retinal and conjunctival vessels, and spoke-like lens opacities. Progressive stromal and epithelial corneal clouding similar to that seen in the mucopolysaccharidoses is seen in some patients.[58] Histopathologic appearance is similar to that of the mucopolysaccharidoses, with single membrane-bound inclusions in corneal epithelial cells and keratocytes. Rare lamellar bodies, as seen in the sphingolipidoses, are seen in this disorder as well.

MLS II (I-Cell Disease)

MLS II is a disorder with facies resembling that seen in Hurler syndrome, orthopedic deformities, mental retardation, severe growth retardation, thickened skin, and death in childhood. The orbits are small, with hypoplastic supraorbital ridges and prominent eyes. Corneal haze, which can be seen on slit lamp examination, develops gradually. Glaucoma and megalocornea with normal intraocular pressure have been reported.[59] Granular inclusions are seen on phase-contrast examination of keratocytes and fibroblasts, leading to the name *I-cell (inclusion-cell) disease.* Conjunctival biopsy reveals these cells in the substantia propria.[59]

MLS III (Pseudo-Hurler Polydystrophy)

MLS III is similar to MLS II but is less severe, with milder growth and mental retardation and greater life expectancy. Corneal clouding is visible with the slit lamp. The I-cell phenomenon, as seen in MLS II, is also present in these patients.[57]

MLS IV (Berman Syndrome)

MLS IV is a disorder seen most frequently in Ashkenazic Jews. Slowed psychomotor development becomes evident in the first year of life. Facial and joint changes are not present. Corneal clouding is prominent from birth or early infancy, and retinal degeneration occurs.[60] Histologically, membrane-bound intracytoplasmic vacuoles show a predilection for the corneal and conjunctival epithelium, with much less involvement of keratocytes and conjunctival substantia propria.[61,62] Corneal grafting in one patient improved visual acuity, but recurrence of opacification was noted 9 months later.[63] Epithelial debridement in another patient improved corneal clarity, but the improvement lasted only until corneal re-epithelialization occurred. Conjunctival transplantation from a normal sibling led to marked improvement in corneal clarity.[64]

Goldberg Syndrome (Goldberg-Cotlier Syndrome, Goldberg-Wenger Syndrome)

Goldberg syndrome appears to combine sialidase deficiency, as in MLS I, with β-D-galactosidase deficiency. These patients have seizures, mental retardation, coarse

TABLE 17-6
Ocular Manifestations of Disorders of Combined Carbohydrate and Lipid Metabolism

Disorder	*Enzyme Deficiency*	*Metabolite Accumulated*	*Mode of Inheritance*	*Ocular Manifestations*
MLS I (Dysmorphic sialidosis; Spranger syndrome)	Glycoprotein sialidase (neuroaminidase)	Unknown	Autosomal recessive	Macular cherry-red spot; tortuous retinal and conjunctival vessels; spoke-like lens opacities; progressive corneal clouding
MLS II (I-cell disease)	GluNac-1-phosphotransferase	Unknown	Autosomal recessive	Small orbits; hypoplastic supraorbital ridges and prominent eyes; glaucoma; megalocornea; corneal clouding
MLS III (pseudo-Hurler polydystrophy)	GluNac-1-phosphotransferase	Unknown	Autosomal recessive	Corneal clouding; hyperopic astigmatism; retinal tortuosity and surface maculopathy; optic nerve head swelling
MLS IV (Berman syndrome)	Ganglioside sialidase	Sialogangliosides; mucopolysaccharides	Autosomal recessive	Corneal clouding; retinal degeneration
Goldberg syndrome	Sialidase; β-D-galactosidase	Unknown	Autosomal recessive	Macular cherry-red spot; diffuse mild corneal clouding
Mannosidosis and fucosidosis	α-D-Mannosidase, α-D-fucosidase	Unknown	Autosomal recessive	No corneal abnormalities

Abbreviation: MLS, mucolipidosis (oligosaccharidosis).

facies, skeletal abnormalities, macular cherry-red spot, and mild, diffuse corneal clouding.[65,66]

Mannosidosis and Fucosidosis

Mannosidosis and fucosidosis also fit into this group of disorders, but no corneal abnormalities are present. A variant of fucosidosis with angiokeratoma corporis diffusum and corneal clouding has been described.[67] A patient with fucosidosis who died at the age of 25 years with clinically clear corneas was found to have inclusions of fibrillogranular and multilaminar material in the cytoplasm of the cells of all corneal layers.[68]

MISCELLANEOUS METABOLIC DISORDERS

Familial Dysautonomia (Riley-Day Syndrome)

Although not associated with the accumulation of an abnormal metabolite in the cornea, familial dysautonomia (hereditary sensory neuropathy type III) is an autosomal recessive disorder and, therefore, presumably a metabolic disorder in which corneal changes can be significant.

Familial dysautonomia is characterized by both sensory and autonomic dysfunction. Infants experience feeding difficulty, recurrent aspiration, vomiting crises, and dehydration. Development is delayed and growth is poor, although intelligence is normal. Sensory deficits include poor temperature discrimination and insensitivity to bone and skin pain despite normal sensitivity to visceral pain. Fungiform papillae on the tongue are absent (Figure 17-14), and taste perception is decreased. Autonomic dysfunction is characterized by postural hypotension, skin blotching, and hyperhidrosis.[69]

Ocular findings (Table 17-7) include absent corneal sensation and absent reflex tearing. Ptosis, exotropia, myopia, anisometropia, anisocoria, and retinal vascular tortuosity are commonly seen.[70] Methacholine (2.5 percent) induces miosis in affected patients but not in normals, suggesting cholinergic supersensitivity or perhaps increased corneal penetration because of epithelial damage from decreased tearing and absent corneal sensation. Decreased tearing and corneal sensation may lead to significant problems, such as punctate staining, ulceration, perforation, scarring, and vascularization.

The cause of familial dysautonomia is not known. Axelrod[69] considers it a developmental arrest of the sensory and autonomic systems. Abnormalities occur in sympa-

FIGURE 17-14 Absent fungiform papillae in a patient with Riley-Day syndrome.

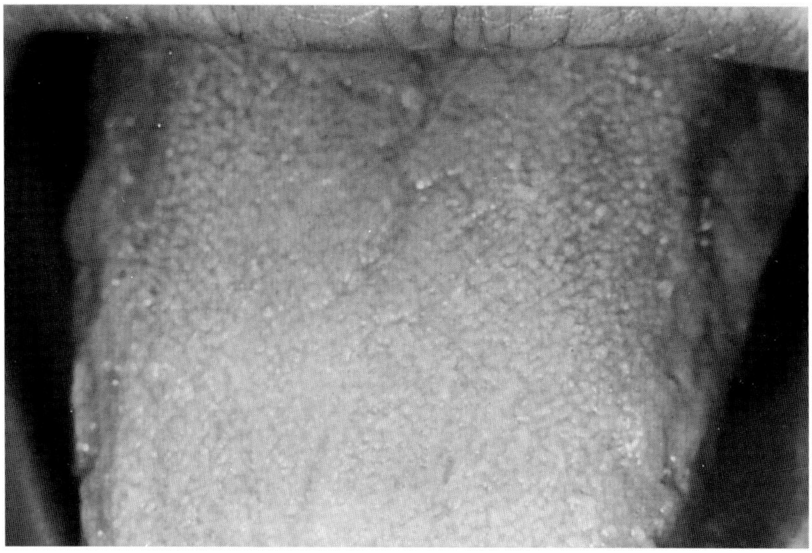

thetic ganglia, with decreased size and numbers of neurons. Excretion of epinephrine and norepinephrine breakdown products is decreased, and dopamine-β-hydroxylase levels have been suggested to be decreased, although this has not been confirmed in comparison with age-matched controls.[69] One in 50 Ashkenazic Jews carries the gene associated with the disorder; non-Jewish patients are rare.[71]

Systemic treatment consists of support during vomiting crises, special feeding of infants, and attention to chronically poor hydration. Ocular therapy consists of tear replacement and frequent use of ointments. Punctal occlusion is helpful, and at times, a bandage soft contact lens or tarsorrhaphy may be necessary, especially in the presence of decreased blink frequency and corneal exposure during sleep. Prevention of systemic dehydration may also be helpful. Long-term follow-up data on corneal grafting for these patients are lacking.[72]

Lowe Syndrome (Oculocerebrorenal Syndrome)

Lowe syndrome is an X-linked recessive disorder consisting of mental and psychomotor retardation, renal abnormalities with aminoaciduria, proteinuria, renal tubular acidosis, and rickets, as well as ocular changes. The specific biochemical defect is unknown.

Many ocular anomalies are found, including cataracts in all patients, congenital glaucoma in 60 percent of patients, and occasional iris and retinal abnormalities[73] (see Table 17-7). Corneal abnormalities have usually been

TABLE 17-7
Ocular Manifestations of Miscellaneous Metabolic Disorders

Disorder	*Enzyme Deficiency*	*Metabolite Accumulated*	*Mode of Inheritance*	*Ocular Manifestations*
Familial dysautonomia (Riley-Day syndrome)	Unknown	—	Autosomal recessive	Absent corneal sensation; absent reflex tearing; ptosis; exotropia; myopia; anisometropia; anisocoria; retinal vascular tortuosity
Lowe syndrome (oculocerebrorenal syndrome)	Unknown	—	X-linked recessive	Cataract (100%); congenital glaucoma (60%); iris and retinal abnormalities; buphthalmos; stromal vascularization and scarring

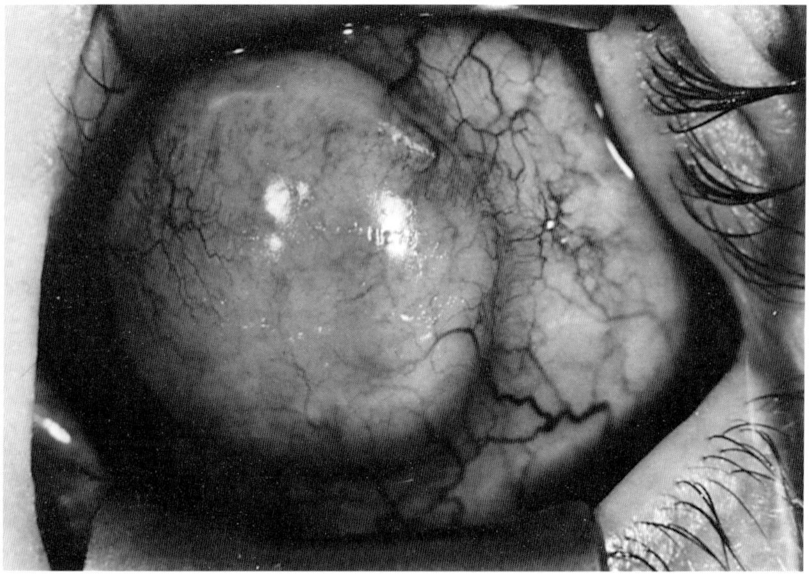

FIGURE 17-15 Large corneal keloid in Lowe syndrome.

described as those typical of buphthalmos. Stromal vascularization and scarring have been described as well. Exuberant corneal scarring has been examined histopathologically and diagnosed as corneal keloid formation.[74] The cause of this is unknown and may be related to glaucoma, multiple surgical procedures, or self-traumatization through oculodigital manipulation, which is often exhibited by these patients. Alternatively, the metabolic disorder itself may in some way be causative.

Specific treatment of the corneal problems is usually unnecessary. One patient in my care, however, had discomfort from marked protuberance of his corneal keloid (Figure 17-15). Three surgical excisions of the keloid were followed by recurrences of the lesion. A conjunctival flap over the involved cornea following a fourth excision of the keloid halted further proliferation.

REFERENCES

1. Kroll W, Lichte K: Cystinosis: a review of the different forms and of recent advances. Humangenetik 20:75, 1973
2. Wong V: Ocular manifestations in cystinosis. Birth Defects 12:181, 1976
3. Melles RB, Schneider JA, Rao NA, Katz B: Spatial and temporal sequence of corneal crystal deposition in nephropathic cystinosis. Am J Ophthalmol 104:598, 1987
4. Dodd MJ, Pusin SM, Green WR: Adult cystinosis: a case report. Arch Ophthalmol 96:1054, 1978
5. Yamamoto GK, Schulman JD, Schneider JA, Wong VG: Long-term ocular changes in cystinosis: observation in renal transplant recipients. J Pediatr Ophthalmol Strabismus 16:21, 1979
6. Katz B, Melles RB, Schneider JA: Corneal sensitivity in nephropathic cystinosis. Am J Ophthalmol 104:413, 1987
7. Dale RT, Rao GN, Aquavella JV, Metz HS: Adolescent cystinosis: a clinical and specular microscopic study of an unusual sibship. Br J Ophthalmol 65:828, 1981
8. Gahl WA, Thoene JG, Scheider JA, et al: NIH Conference. Cystinosis: progress in a prototypic disease. Ann Intern Med 109:557, 1988
9. Kaiser-Kupfer MI, Gazzo MA, Datiles MB, et al: A randomized placebo-controlled trial of cysteamine eye drops in nephropathic cystinosis. Arch Ophthalmol 108:689, 1990
10. Katz B, Melles RB, Schneider JA: Recurrent crystal deposition after keratoplasty in nephropathic cystinosis. Am J Ophthalmol 104:190, 1987
11. Katz B, Melles RB, Schneider JA: Crystal deposition following keratoplasty in nephropathic cystinosis. Arch Ophthalmol 107:1727, 1989
12. Goldsmith LA, Kang E, Bienfang DC, et al: Tyrosinemia with plantar and palmar keratosis and keratitis. J Pediatr 83:798, 1973
13. Bienfang DC, Kuwabara T, Pueschel SM: The Richner-Hanhart syndrome. Arch Ophthalmol 94:1133, 1976
14. Rich LF, Beard ME, Burns RP: Excess dietary tyrosine and corneal lesions. Exp Eye Res 17:87, 1973
15. Burns RP, Gipson IK, Murray MJ: Keratopathy in tyrosinemia. Birth Defects 12:169, 1976
16. Bardeli AM, Borgogni P, Farnetani MA, et al: Familial tyrosinemia with eye and skin lesions. Ophthalmologica 175:5, 1977
17. Heidemann DJ, Dunne SP, Bawle EV, Shepherd DM: Early diagnosis of tyrosinemia type II. Am J Ophthalmol 197:559, 1989
18. Wirtschafter JD: The eye in alkaptonuria. Birth Defects 12:279, 1976

19. Kampik A, Sani JN, Green WR: Ocular ochronosis: clinicopathological, histochemical, and ultrastructural studies. Arch Ophthalmol 98:1441, 1980
20. Walshe JM: The eye in Wilson disease. Birth Defects 12:187, 1976
21. Tso MOM, Fine BS, Thorpe HE: Kayser-Fleischer ring and associated cataract in Wilson's disease. Am J Ophthalmol 79:479, 1975
22. Johnson RE, Campbell RJ: Wilson's disease: electron microscopic, X-ray energy spectroscopic, and atomic absorption spectroscopic studies of corneal copper deposition and distribution. Lab Invest 46:564, 1982
23. Fleming CR, Dickson ER, Waner HW, et al: Pigmented corneal rings in non-Wilsonian liver disease. Ann Intern Med 86:285, 1977
24. Panks PM: Disorders of copper metabolism. p. 1319. In Emery AEH, Rimoin DL (eds): Principles and Practice of Medical Genetics. Churchill Livingstone, New York, 1983
25. Stone EN, Mathers WD, Rosenwasser GOD, et al: Three autosomal dominant corneal dystrophies map to chromosome 5q. Nature Genet 6:47, 1994
26. Gorevic PD, Munoz PC, Gorgone G, et al: Amyloidosis due to a mutation of the gelsolin gene in an American family with lattice corneal dystrophy type II. N Engl J Med 325:1780, 1991
27. Slansky HH, Kuwabara T: Intranuclear urate crystals in corneal epithelium. Arch Ophthalmol 80:338, 1968
28. Fishman RA, Sunderman FW: Band keratopathy in gout. Arch Ophthalmol 75:367, 1966
29. Gaasterland DE, Rodrigues MM, Moshell AN: Ocular involvement in xeroderma pigmentosum. Ophthalmology 89:980, 1982
30. Stenson S: Ocular findings in xeroderma pigmentosum: report of two cases. Ann Ophthalmol 14:580, 1982
31. Cotlier E: The cornea. p. 38. In Moses RA (ed): Adler's Physiology of the Eye. CV Mosby, St. Louis, 1975
32. Spellacy E, Bankes KJL, Crow J, et al: Glaucoma in a case of Hurler disease. Br J Ophthalmol 64:773, 1980
33. Kenyon KR: Ocular manifestations and pathology of systemic mucopolysaccharidoses. Birth Defects 12:133, 1976
34. Chijiiwa T, Inomata H, Yamana Y, Kaibara N: Ocular manifestations of Hurler/Scheie phenotype in two sibs. Jpn J Ophthalmol 27:54, 1983
35. Spranger J: The mucopolysaccharidoses. p. 1339. In Emery AEH, Rimoin DL (eds): Principles and Practice of Medical Genetics. Churchill Livingstone, New York, 1983
36. Sanfilippo SJ, Podosin R, Langer L, et al: Mental retardation associated with acid mucopolysacchariduria (heparitin sulfate type). J Pediatr 63:837, 1963
37. DelMonte MA, Maumenee IH, Green WR, Kenyon KR: Histopathology of Sanfilippo's syndrome. Arch Ophthalmol 101:1255, 1983
38. Lavery MA, Green WR, Jabs EW, et al: Ocular histopathology and ultrastructure of Sanfilippo's syndrome: type III-B. Arch Ophthalmol 101:1263, 1983
39. Ghosh M, McCulloch C: The Morquio syndrome: light and electron microscopic findings from two corneas. Can J Ophthalmol 9:445, 1974
40. Suveges I: Histological and ultrastructural studies of the cornea in Maroteaux-Lamy syndrome. Albrecht von Graefes Arch Klin Exp Ophthalmol 212:29, 1979
41. Aguirre G, Stramm L, Haskins M: Feline mucopolysaccharidosis VI: general ocular and pigment epithelial pathology. Invest Ophthalmol Vis Sci 24:991, 1983
42. François J: Metabolic disorders and corneal changes. Dev Ophthalmol 4:1, 1981
43. Summers CJ, Purple RL, Kribic W, et al: Ocular changes in the mucopolysaccharidoses after bone marrow transplantation. Ophthalmology 96:977, 1989
44. Brownstein S, Carpenter S, Polomeno RD, Little JM: Sandhoff's disease (G_{M2} gangliosidosis type 2), histopathology and ultrastructure of the eye. Arch Ophthalmol 98:1089, 1980
45. Franceschetti AT: Fabry's disease: ocular manifestations. Birth Defects 12:195, 1976
46. François J, Hanssens M, Teuchy H: Corneal ultrastructural changes in Fabry's disease. Ophthalmologica 176:313, 1978
47. Weingeist TA, Blodi FC: Fabry's disease: ocular findings in a female carrier. A light and electron microscopic study. Arch Ophthalmol 85:169, 1971
48. Gjone E: Familial lecithin:cholesterol acyltransferase (LCAT) deficiency. Ophthalmic Paediatr Genet 9:167, 1988
49. Vrabec MP, Shapiro MB, Koller E, et al: Ophthalmic observation in lecithin cholesterol acyltransferase deficiency. Arch Ophthalmol 106:225, 1988
50. Chu FC, Kuwabara T, Cogan DG, et al: Ocular manifestations of familial high-density lipoprotein deficiency (Tangier disease). Arch Ophthalmol 97:1926, 1979
51. Funke H, von Eckardstein A, Pritchard PH, et al: A molecular defect causing fish-eye disease: an amino acid exchange in lecithin-cholesterol acyltransferase (LCAT) leads to the selective loss of α-LCAT activity. Proc Natl Acad Sci USA 88:4855, 1991
52. Philipson BT: Fish eye disease. Birth Defects 18:441, 1979
53. Fredrickson DS, Levy RJ, Lees R: Fat transport in lipoproteins: an integrated approach to mechanisms and disorders. N Engl J Med 276:34, 1967
54. Winder AF: Relationship between corneal arcus and hyperlipidaemia is clarified by studies in familial hypercholesterolaemia. Br J Ophthalmol 67:789, 1983
55. Pe'er J, Vidaurri J, Siman-Tov H, et al: Association between corneal arcus and some of the risk factors for coronary artery disease. Br J Ophthalmol 67:795, 1983
56. Barchiesi BJ, Eckel RH, Ellis PP: The cornea and disorders of lipid metabolism. Surv Ophthalmol 36:1, 1991
57. Leroy JG: The oligosaccharidoses (formerly mucolipidoses). p. 1348. In Emery AEH, Rimoin DL (eds): Principles and Practice of Medical Genetics. Churchill Livingstone, New York, 1983
58. Cibis GW, Harris DJ, Chapman AL, Tripathi RC: Mucolipidosis I. Arch Ophthalmol 101:933, 1983

59. Libert J, Van Hoof F, Farriaux J, Toussaint D: Ocular findings in I-cell disease (mucolipidosis type II). Am J Ophthalmol 83:617, 1977
60. Merin S, Livni N, Berman ER, Yatsiv S: Mucolipidosis IV: ocular, systemic, and ultrastructural findings. Invest Ophthalmol 14:437, 1975
61. Kenyon KR, Maumenee IH, Green WR, et al: Mucolipidosis IV: histopathology of conjunctiva, cornea, and skin. Arch Ophthalmol 97:1106, 1979
62. Zwann J, Kenyon KR: Two brothers with presumed mucolipidosis IV. Birth Defects 18:381, 1982
63. Lake BD, Milla PJ, Taylor DSI, Young EP: A mild variant of mucolipidosis type 4 (ML_4). Birth Defects 18:391, 1982
64. Dangel ME, Bremer DL, Rogers GL: Treatment of corneal opacification in mucolipidosis IV with conjunctival transplantation. Am J Ophthalmol 99:137, 1985
65. Goldberg MF, Cotlier E, Fichenscher LG, et al: Macular cherry-red spot, corneal clouding, and β-galactosidase deficiency. Arch Intern Med 128:387, 1971
66. Emery JM, Green WR, Wyllie RG, Howell RR: G_{MI}-gangliosidosis, ocular and pathological manifestations. Arch Ophthalmol 85:177, 1971
67. Snyder RD, Carlow TJ, Ledman J, Wenger DA: Ocular findings in fucosidosis. Birth Defects 12:241, 1976
68. Hoshino M, O'Brien TP, McDonell JM, et al: Fucosidosis: ultrastructural studies of the eye in an adult. Graefes Arch Clin Exp Ophthalmol 227:162, 1989
69. Axelrod F: Autonomic and sensory disorders. p. 248. In Emery AEH, Rimoin DL (eds): Principles and Practice of Medical Genetics. Churchill Livingstone, New York, 1983
70. Goldberg MF, Payne JW, Brunt PW: Ophthalmological studies of familial dysautonomia. The Riley-Day syndrome. Arch Ophthalmol 80:732, 1968
71. Mensher JH: Familial dysautonomia: report of a case in a non-Jewish child. J Pediatr Ophthalmol 12:40, 1975
72. Karpik AG, Streeten BW, Spitzer KH, McGraw JL: Corneal transplantation in familial dysautonomia. Am J Ophthalmol 88:993, 1979
73. Ginsberg J, Bore KE, Fogelson MH: Pathological features of the eye in the oculocerebrorenal (Lowe) syndrome. J Pediatr Ophthalmol Strabismus 18:16, 1981
74. Cibis GW, Tripathi RC, Tripathi BJ, Harris DJ: Corneal keloid in Lowe's syndrome. Arch Ophthalmol 100:1795, 1982

18

Epithelial and Stromal Dystrophies

COREY A. MILLER AND JAY H. KRACHMER

Corneal dystrophies are inherited, bilateral, primary alterations of the cornea that are not associated with prior inflammation or systemic disease.[1-6] Although corneal dystrophies are rare, the relative frequency of a single dystrophy varies greatly depending on the population studied.[7] Most corneal dystrophies show an autosomal dominant inheritance pattern and present in the first few decades of life. They may be stationary or slowly progressive in their appearance. Corneal dystrophies are distinguished from corneal degenerations, which are usually age-related changes often accompanied by other ocular or systemic diseases (see Ch. 20). Characteristically, the age of onset, symptoms, clinical presentation, and progression of the dystrophy are similar among affected members of the same pedigree. Nevertheless, like other disorders with autosomal dominant inheritance, altered expressivity of the genetic defect may result in striking variations in the natural history of the dystrophy within the same family. Therefore, all available family members should be examined. The diagnosis of a case with an unusual appearance or atypical presentation may become easier when family members with more typical changes are examined. This is especially true of the early clinical stages of the dystrophy, as well as late stages in which secondary vascularization and scarring may obscure the primary dystrophic process.

Some conditions commonly labeled as dystrophies, such as pre-Descemet's dystrophy, are probably not inherited and may represent degenerations. Others, such as epithelial basement membrane dystrophy and Fuchs' dystrophy, may be familial but in most instances do not display a regular genetic pattern. The corneal changes associated with systemic metabolic disorders may mimic changes seen in corneal dystrophies[6,8] (see Ch. 17). The term *dystrophy* should, however, be reserved for primary changes unassociated with systemic manifestations. Because patients with corneal dystrophies are rare and are therefore often studied extensively, associated ocular and systemic diseases have been encountered.

Characteristic histopathologic findings, especially those observed on electron microscopy, are known for many of the dystrophies.[9-12] However, the reported findings are often skewed toward the later or more severe stages of the dystrophy, when surgical intervention becomes necessary. Immunohistochemical and electron microscopic methods have greatly increased our knowledge of the accumulated products in the dystrophies, but our understanding of their pathogenesis is relatively limited. The study of patterns of recurrence of some of the dystrophies in corneal grafts has given rise to theories regarding their initial onset. Further understanding may be provided by tissue culture techniques, which permit study of involved tissue in more than just the static state.

The visual impact varies with the individual dystrophy, the age of the patient, the occurrence of secondary complications, and the phenotypic expression within the individual and family. The ophthalmologist's first responsibility is proper diagnosis and patient and family education regarding the disorder. In addition to decreased vision, complications often involve loss of the epithelial layer with recurrent erosions, which require appropriate therapy.[13] In more severe cases, debridement and lamellar or penetrating keratoplasty may be indicated. Recurrences following these procedures have been reported in many of the dystrophies.

Corneal dystrophies have been classified in many different ways.[2,4,14,15] Because the initial clinical findings usually appear in a single corneal layer, anatomic classifications have been most accepted. Embryologic or causative classifications may become more appropriate

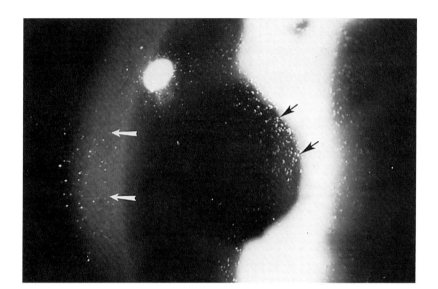

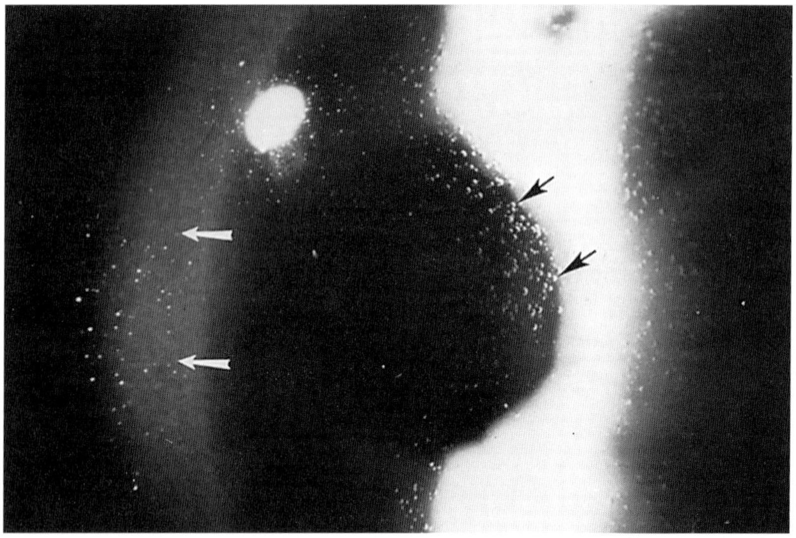

FIGURE 18-1 Meesmann's dystrophy. The intraepithelial cysts appear as gray dots with focal illumination (white arrows) and as refractile vesicles with indirect illumination (black arrows).

when more is known about the pathogenesis of the dystrophies.

Dystrophies that primarily involve the epithelium, epithelial basement membrane, Bowman's layer, and stroma are described in this chapter. Endothelial dystrophies are covered in Chapter 19.

DYSTROPHIES OF THE EPITHELIUM, EPITHELIAL BASEMENT MEMBRANE, AND BOWMAN'S LAYER

Meesmann's Dystrophy

Meesmann's dystrophy, or juvenile hereditary epithelial dystrophy, is a rare, bilaterally symmetrical, autosomal dominant disorder of the corneal epithelium.[16-19] It may present in the first year of life as epithelial microcysts visible only by slit lamp magnification.[20] The number and density of these epithelial cysts increase throughout life. Usually, the cysts are first noted during routine examination for other ocular conditions. Symptoms rarely occur until early adulthood or middle age when the cysts begin to rupture onto the ocular surface, causing intermittent erosive symptoms. Vision may be temporarily diminished during erosive episodes or permanently decreased if there is resultant subepithelial scarring. In most patients, treatment is rarely required and usually involves only symptomatic management of the corneal surface problems.

In adults with Meesmann's dystrophy, myriads of fine round cysts are present in the epithelium, most prominently in the interpalpebral zone. However, slit lamp microscopy demonstrates that the cysts involve the entire cornea. With retroillumination, the cysts appear as fine droplets or vesicles that are regular in size and shape (Figure 18-1). Direct focal illumination shows the cysts as focal, discrete, gray dots or partially filled cyst-like structures. As the cysts coalesce, they may form refractile clusters or lines (Figure 18-2). Fluorescein staining of the ocular surface brilliantly highlights cysts that have ruptured onto the ocular surface; however, the deeper cysts do not stain with fluorescein or rose bengal. The microcysts are usually dispersed diffusely, although whorl, crescentic, wedge, and cluster distributions have been reported.[18] These patterns may change with time as the cysts rise and rupture onto the ocular surface. In advanced stages, serpiginous gray lines and small amorphous subepithelial opacities, in addition to the characteristic uniform microcysts, may be found.[21] Central corneal thickness may be reduced, especially in younger patients.[22]

Although the appearance of Meesmann's dystrophy is characteristic, epithelial cysts are seen in a variety of other disorders, particularly epithelial basement membrane dystrophy. The microcysts in Meesmann's dystrophy differ from those in epithelial basement membrane dystrophy in that they are not white, and are more vesicular, more uniform in size and shape, and more diffusely distributed. A similar pattern may be seen in mild diffuse epithelial edema, contact lens wear, or toxicity from topical medications.

By light microscopy, the epithelial layer in Meesmann's dystrophy is usually thickened but may be flattened or thin.[19,23,24] Typically, there is cytoplasmic vacuolation, as well as diffuse disorganization of the epithelium, with a lack of normal transition from the deeper epithelial cells to the more superficial, mature epithelial cells. Small, usually round, debris-filled intraepithelial cysts are found

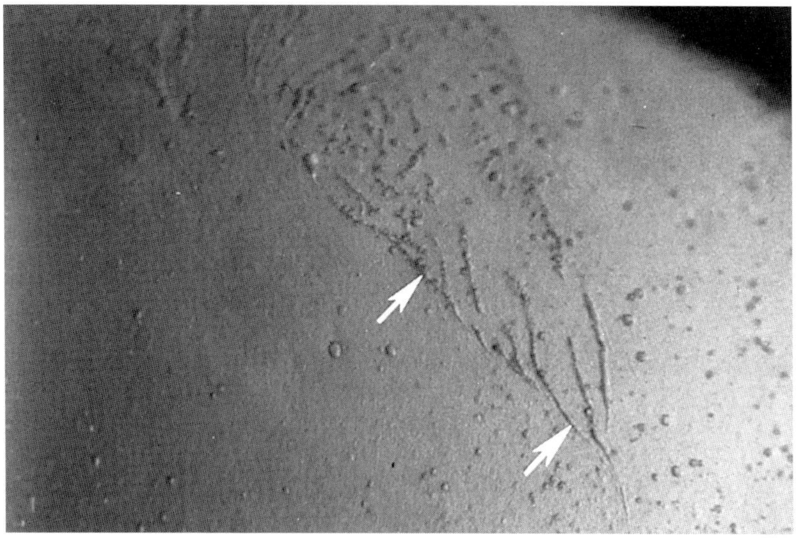

FIGURE 18-2 Retroillumination of the intraepithelial cysts in Meesmann's dystrophy shows clusters and refractile lines (arrows).

throughout the epithelium but occur most characteristically in the anterior third. Some of these cysts may open onto the corneal surface. Often, basal cell mitoses are present. Increased amounts of glycogen have been reported in the more superficial epithelial cells, presumably on the basis of increased epithelial cell turnover.[18,25] The intracystic debris stains for acid mucopolysaccharides (glycosaminoglycans) with Alcian blue and colloidal iron stains, and is also periodic acid–Schiff (PAS)-positive and diastase- and neuraminidase-resistant. An abnormally thickened, often multilaminar epithelial basement membrane may be present with pedunculated excrescences extending into the epithelium. Like the intracystic debris, the anterior portion of this membrane stains for glycosaminoglycans.

The characteristic ultrastructural finding of Meesmann's dystrophy is a focal collection of electron-dense, fibrillogranular material described as "peculiar" substance within the cytoplasm of the epithelial cells[19,23,24,26] (Figure 18-3). These unusual accumulations occur most prominently in the basal epithelial cell layer and are often surrounded by aggregates of tonofilaments and desmosomes. The walls of the intraepithelial cysts are formed by the cell membranes of adjacent epithelial cells and have a corrugated, microvillous appearance. The intracystic debris comprises a spectrum of degenerated cell products from recognizable cell organelles to a vacuolated homogeneous substance. However, little "peculiar" substance is found among this debris. Electron-dense bodies similar to lysosomes have also been described.[27] The thickened basement membrane

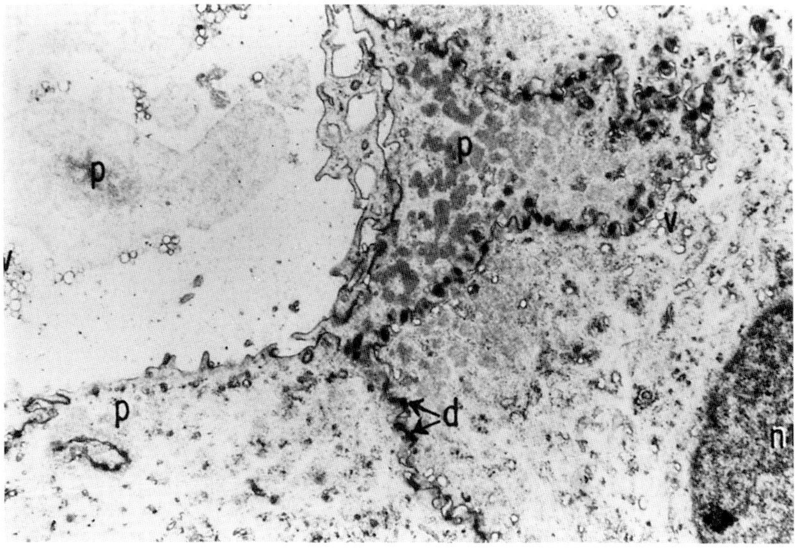

FIGURE 18-3 Electron micrograph of corneal epithelium in Meesmann's dystrophy. There are several cells in different stages of degeneration with "peculiar" substance *(p)* in dense accumulation, numerous vacuoles *(v)*, and a degenerated cell showing huge ballooning of "peculiar substance." (× 8,420.) *n*, nucleus; *d*, desmosomes. (Reprinted with permission from RP Burns: Meesmann's corneal dystrophy. Trans Am Ophthalmol Soc 66:530, 1968.)

is formed by an anterior, often multilaminar, accumulation of basement membrane and a more diffuse, posterior, homogeneous, filamentous material. In most cases, the remainder of the cornea, including Bowman's layer, stroma, and endothelium, is normal.

The cause and specific nature of the "peculiar" substance in Meesmann's dystrophy remains unknown. The accumulation of this material in the cytoplasm of the epithelial cells may be the primary manifestation of this dystrophy. The increased cell turnover and thickening of the basement membrane are probably secondary changes. Most affected individuals retain normal visual acuity and are only intermittently symptomatic. However, repeated episodes of erosion and inflammation may result in subepithelial scarring and irregular corneal astigmatism. Epithelial debridement is usually followed by a recurrence of the intraepithelial cysts. Nevertheless, these cysts may be slow to form and are not always as severe as the original involvement. Superficial keratectomy has been reported with normal re-epithelialization,[25] but epithelial involvement has recurred following this and other lamellar and penetrating keratoplasty procedures for Meesmann's dystrophy.[21]

Another unusual epithelial dystrophy, with band-shaped or whorled opacities composed of tightly packed fine microcysts, has been described in five family members in one pedigree and in three unrelated patients.[28] Histopathology in three patients showed vacuolation of the epithelial cells in the involved areas with sharp demarcations between the involved areas and the surrounding uninvolved corneal epithelium.[28]

Epithelial Basement Membrane Dystrophy (Map-Dot-Fingerprint Dystrophy)

Epithelial basement membrane dystrophy is the most common anterior dystrophy encountered in clinical practice. A variety of previously described anterior corneal disorders fall into this group, including Cogan's microcystic epithelial dystrophy, map-dot-fingerprint dystrophy, anterior basement membrane dystrophy, fingerprint dystrophy, and certain net- and bleb-like patterns that occur separately or in conjunction with the above morphologies. This category may also include some of the cases previously reported as dystrophic recurrent erosion. Although the term *epithelial basement membrane dystrophy* is used for this group of disorders, each may have a different clinical presentation and representative histopathologic appearance. Part of the confusion in terminology in this dystrophy is due to the historical sequence of recognition of its individual clinical components.

Microcystic dystrophy of the corneal epithelium was first described by Cogan et al,[29] who noted bilateral, grayish white spheres of varying sizes in the superficial corneas of five unrelated women. The spheres were centrally located and irregularly shaped, and they did not significantly decrease visual acuity. The location and morphologies of the individual lesions changed with time. Histopathologic studies from two patients showed intraepithelial cysts containing pyknotic nuclei and cytoplasmic debris. An anomalous basement membrane was found insinuated within the epithelial layer.

Guerry[30] described additional patients with subtle, geographic configurations sometimes found in association with putty-gray dots. This map-like epithelial dystrophy of the cornea was usually asymptomatic and nonprogressive, but the map figures themselves were noted to change location, contour, and size over time. Fingerprint lines of the cornea had been previously elucidated by Guerry,[31] although similar, but more marked changes had been described decades previously by Vogt.[32] The fingerprint lines had a whorl-like contour and no familial predisposition. Histopathologic examination demonstrated folding and reduplication of the epithelial basement membrane.[33] Other studies[34–36] demonstrated the concomitant appearance of map, dot, and fingerprint changes of the cornea in characteristic configurations. Related bleb- and net-like patterns with a distinctive histopathologic character have also been reported.[35]

The terms *map-dot-fingerprint dystrophy* and *epithelial basement membrane dystrophy* have been used to refer to this group of associated presentations. The pattern of familial occurrence suggests autosomal dominant inheritance.[37] Subsequent studies have shown similar but milder clinical findings in a large percentage of the asymptomatic general population.[38] Some of the clinical features of epithelial basement membrane dystrophy may appear in the relatively common syndrome of post-traumatic recurrent erosion. There appears to be a spectrum of similar epithelial changes occurring in normal individuals, following trauma, and in the genetically determined dystrophic state. The similarities in these epithelial changes may be due to the limited ways the anterior cornea can respond to a variety of insults.

The most common and probably earliest clinical change in epithelial basement membrane dystrophy is the map-like pattern. Maps are circumscribed areas with a central ground-glass appearance often punctuated with clear oval lacunae (Figure 18-4). They are best seen with broad, oblique-beam, focal illumination with an undilated pupil and are highlighted by retroillumination with a dilated pupil. The margins of the maps may be sharply demarcated, with a rolled or elevated edge around part of the circumference of the pattern. Other portions of the map may blend into the surrounding clear stroma. Fluorescein applied to the corneal surface overlying the map figures shows negative staining over elevated areas. The patches range in size from several hundred microns in diameter to several square millimeters or more.

Dots are fine, gray-white, round, oblong, or comma-shaped opacities often seen beneath or near the map-like patches (see Figure 18-4). They are easily visible on direct illumination, are of various sizes, and may be confluent with lobulated, smooth margins. Smaller dots are often closely clustered and take on a refractile cyst-like appearance with retroillumination. Fluorescein may stain the superficial microcysts or show negative staining over elevated areas where the cysts have not ruptured onto the ocular surface.

Fingerprint lines are the least frequently encountered of the triad of characteristic changes in epithelial basement membrane dystrophy. They are concentric, often curvilinear, parallel lines clustered in the central or midperipheral cornea, frequently surrounding the maps (Figure 18-5). They are seen best by indirect illumination from the iris or by retroillumination, where they take on a refractile quality. Some fingerprint lines appear as cylindrical processes that may branch, while others have club-shaped terminations. Topical fluorescein may highlight the presence of the fingerprint lines although they are usually not seen by focal illumination. Similar superficial corneal lines are found in a variety of other conditions.[39] Fibrillary lines[40] are often seen in normal corneas; shift lines may be present with epithelial edema of any cause and are especially characteristic in Fuchs' dystrophy. Mares' tails and tram lines are also variants of fingerprints with characteristic aggregate morphologies.

Blebs are clustered, fine, clear, bubble-like structures that are best seen by indirect illumination or retroillumination.[39] They are uniform in size and shape and may form a refractile-appearing layer with an irregular border in the central cornea. Nets are refractile lines or rows of blebs that seem to follow the normal anterior corneal mosaic. Neither blebs nor nets alone disrupt the corneal surface.

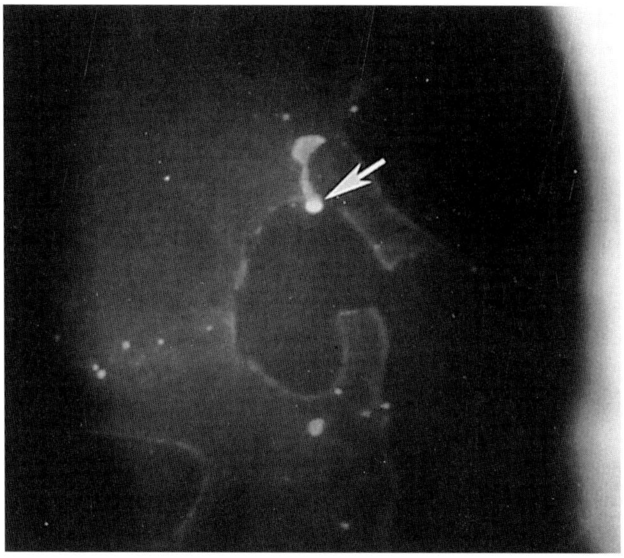

FIGURE 18-4 Epithelial basement membrane dystrophy with large, putty-like dots (arrow) extending from beneath the intraepithelial gray map opacification.

Most patients with epithelial basement membrane dystrophy remain asymptomatic; however, painful recurrent epithelial erosions or transient decreases in visual acuity may occur, usually after the third decade of life. The ero-

FIGURE 18-5 Fingerprint lines in epithelial basement membrane dystrophy.

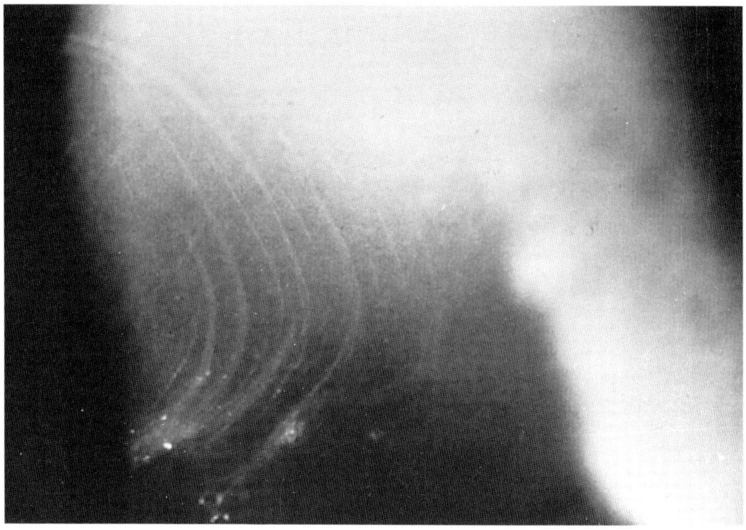

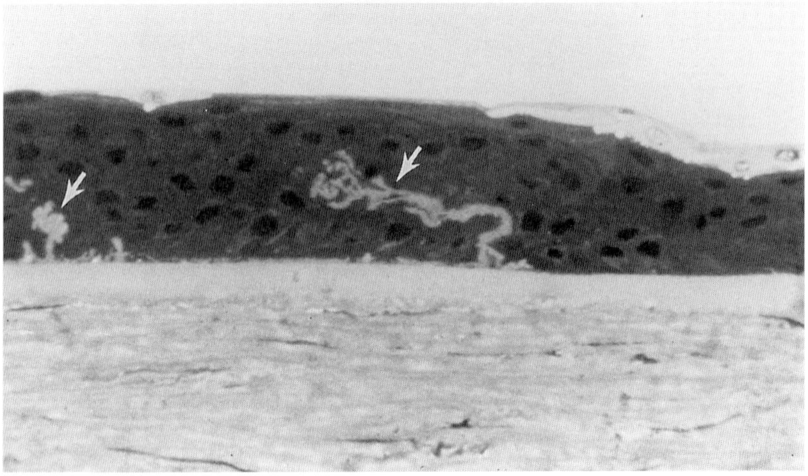

FIGURE 18-6 Projections (arrows) of basement membrane into the epithelium in epithelial basement membrane dystrophy (carbol fuchsin stain).

sions characteristically recur over a period of up to a few years, with spontaneous improvement and no significant residual effect on visual acuity.[41] Stromal keratitis may complicate the erosive episodes associated with epithelial basement membrane dystrophy.[42]

Histopathologic studies in epithelial basement membrane dystrophy[43–45] demonstrate that the map-like changes are formed by aberrant multilaminar projections of a thickened basement membrane into the overlying epithelium (Figure 18-6). The projections are composed of a fine fibrillogranular material and may be fragmented or discontinuous, with rolled or club-shaped terminations. The 2- to 6-μm wide layer of intraepithelial basement membrane separates the epithelium into anterior and posterior lamellae. The epithelial cells surrounding this layer show normal intercellular junctions but do not develop good hemidesmosomal connections to the aberrant basement membrane.

Dots are pseudocysts that contain nuclear and cytoplasmic debris. Pseudocysts usually abut the posterior surface of the abnormal intraepithelial basement membrane, imparting a wavy appearance to the posterior margin of the material (Figure 18-7). The pseudocysts are occasionally surrounded by multinucleated cells. Villous processes of the surrounding epithelial cells may give a corrugated appearance to the borders of the pseudocysts on electron microscopy (Figure 18-8). Similar, although usually smaller pseudocysts may appear at the edges of the map changes and occasionally are seen opening onto the anterior epithelial surface.

Fingerprint lines are formed by an insinuation of basement-membrane-enclosed material into the overlying epithelium (Figure 18-9). The core of these projections is made up of closely packed granules with a diameter of approximately 80 Å. Larger fibrils with diameters of 125 to 170 Å are located near the free ends of the intraepithelial projections. A similar fibrillogranular substance may form a thickened basement membrane layer (Figure 18-10). Subepithelial plaques, sometimes with mushroom-shaped

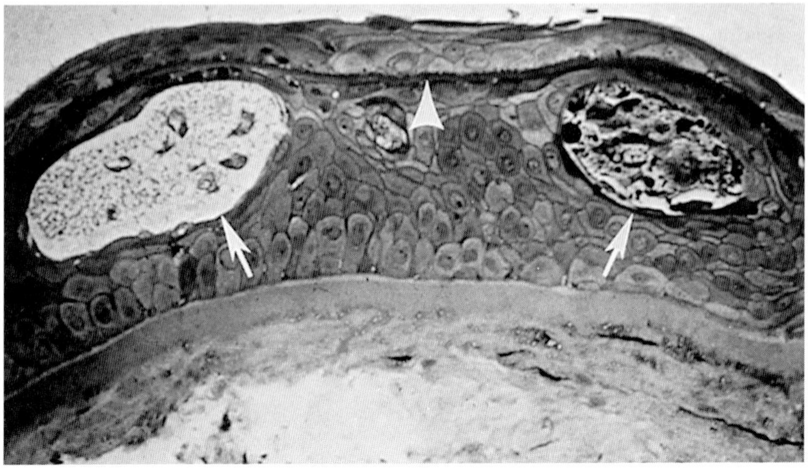

FIGURE 18-7 Epithelial basement membrane dystrophy. Light photomicrograph demonstrates intraepithelial microcysts (arrows) just posterior to the abnormal intraepithelial basement membrane (arrowhead). (Paraphenylenediamine, $\times$ 165.) (Reprinted with permission from MM Rodrigues, BS Fine, PR Laibson, LE Zimmerman: Disorders of the corneal epithelium: a clinicopathologic study of dot, geographic, and fingerprint patterns. Arch Ophthalmol 92:475, 1974.)

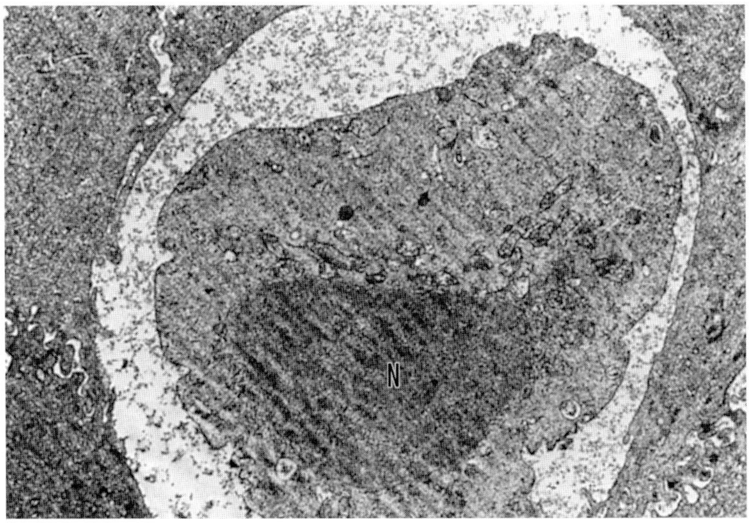

FIGURE 18-8 Transmission electron micrograph of an intraepithelial cyst in epithelial basement membrane dystrophy. Located within the cyst are the pyknotic nucleus *(N)* and cytoplasmic debris. (× 12,880.) (Reprinted with permission from GO Waring, MM Rodrigues, PR Laibson: Corneal dystrophies. I. Dystrophies of the epithelium, Bowman's layer and stroma. Surv Ophthalmol 23:71, 1978.)

configurations, have also been noted. Usually, Bowman's layer and the stroma are not involved.

Bleb-like figures are formed by deposition of a fibrillogranular protein between Bowman's layer and the epithelial basement membrane in a mound configuration. Where isolated blebs occur, the overlying epithelium is usually relatively normal.[46]

The pathogenesis of epithelial basement membrane dystrophy probably involves the primary synthesis of an abnormal basement membrane with intraepithelial extensions. Once present, these midepithelial layers block the normal maturation and desquamation of the underlying epithelial cells, resulting in aberrancy and degeneration of the cells and focal collections of cellular debris.[43] The cause of the fine fibrillogranular material remains unclear. Recurrent epithelial erosions in the disorder probably result from poor epithelial adhesion to the abnormal basement membrane or mechanical shearing of the membrane.

Treatment of acute erosive episodes in map-dot-fingerprint dystrophy is directed toward re-establishment of the epithelial layer. Patching with cycloplegia and prophylactic antibiotic coverage is the usual initial treatment. The use of topical 5 percent sodium chloride ointment or any bland ophthalmic ointment at night is thought to decrease the recurrence of erosions by providing a lubricating layer between the eyelids and the epithelium. Topical mucolytic agents and osmotic colloidal solutions at bedtime have also been successful.[47] Recalcitrant cases may require a bandage soft contact lens worn continuously for an extended period with the concomitant use of sodium chloride drops.[4] Vigorous mechanical debridement of the involved epithelium and basement membrane

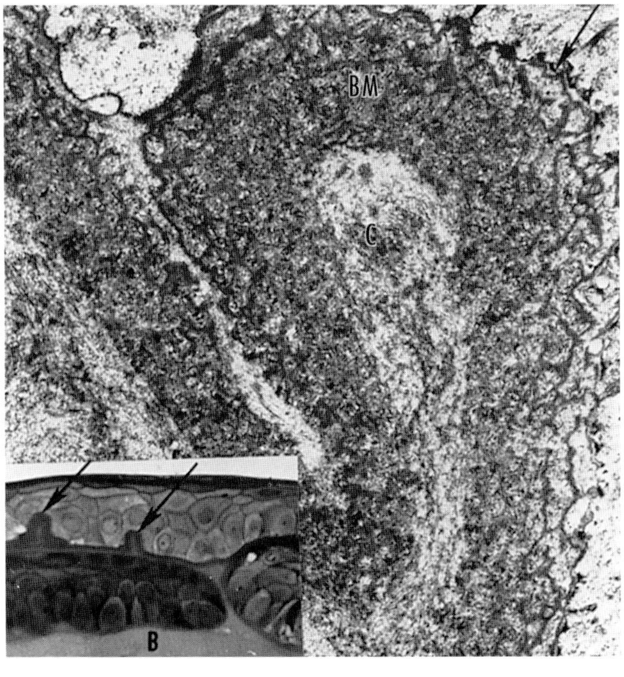

FIGURE 18-9 Histopathologic specimen of fingerprint lines in epithelial basement membrane dystrophy. Inset: Ridges (arrows) project anteriorly from the abnormal mid-epithelial layer. Bowman's layer *(B)* is intact. (Toluidine blue, × 55.) Transmission electron micrograph shows a fibrillogranular core *(C)*, which is enclosed in basement membrane *(BM)*. The overlying epithelial cells show hemidesmosomal attachments (arrow) to the basement membrane. (× 1,250.) (Reprinted with permission from GO Waring, MM Rodrigues, PR Laibson: Corneal dystrophies. I. Dystrophies of the epithelium, Bowman's layer and stroma. Surv Ophthalmol 23:71, 1978.)

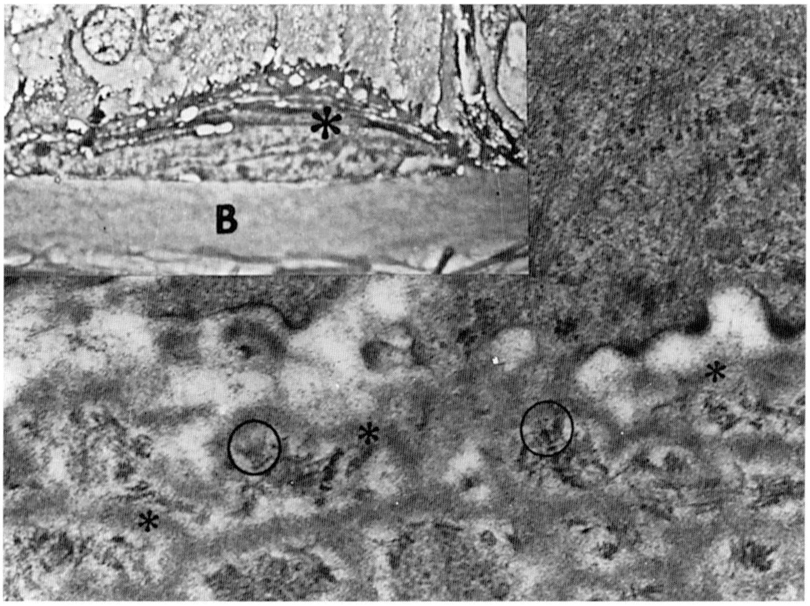

FIGURE 18-10 Transmission electron micrograph of the abnormal subepithelial layer in epithelial basement membrane dystrophy. Multiple fine laminations of basement membrane material (asterisks) are present with associated increased numbers of anchoring fibrils (circles). The number of hemidesmosomes is decreased. *B,* Bowman's layer. (× 40,000.) (Courtesy of Kenneth R. Kenyon, M.D., Boston, MA.)

often results in re-epithelialization with a more normal epithelium, relief of symptoms, and a long-lasting therapeutic effect.[48,49] Micropuncture of the epithelial basement membrane and anterior stroma has been advocated by some to reduce recurrent erosions.[50,51] Excimer laser photoablation of the anterior corneal surface has also been used to treat refractory cases.

Dystrophic Recurrent Erosion

Noninherited recurrent corneal erosion is a common clinical disorder that can usually be linked to previous trauma but may occur spontaneously.[42,52] Pedigrees with a dominant family history of recurrent erosions spanning several generations have been reported,[53] following the initial description by Franceschetti.[54] In most of these families, the onset of symptoms occurred in the first decade of life and erosions were often bilateral. The recurrences in these patients appeared at multiple sites in the cornea, in contrast to the typical course of acquired post-traumatic erosion, where recurrences are usually limited to the site of previous trauma.

Epithelial slippage, microcyst formation, epithelial edema, bullae, filaments, and frank epithelial loss may be apparent during an acute erosive episode, which characteristically awakens the individual from sleep in the early morning hours. Pain, photophobia, tearing, and blepharospasm are prominent. Although vision is usually reduced during an acute episode and early convalescence, recovery is usually complete. Subtle changes may persist between erosive episodes, including epithelial irregularity and edema, intraepithelial microcysts, and mild subepithelial haze. As the patient grows older, the severity and frequency of these episodes decrease. Significant subepithelial scarring, which results in diminished visual acuity, is unusual in the absence of secondary complications and may suggest the presence of other underlying dystrophies or systemic diseases.

Although no specific pathologic basis has been reported in cases of known, inherited, recurrent corneal erosion, cases of spontaneous erosion have demonstrated intraepithelial cysts, epithelial edema, and deficiency or lack of normal basement membrane connections (hemidesmosomes).[55] Similar changes have also been demonstrated in post-traumatic corneal erosions.[56]

Recurrent erosions may occur secondarily as a result of other primary corneal dystrophies.[13] These erosions occur most frequently in epithelial basement membrane dystrophy. In fact, some of the previously reported cases of dystrophic recurrent erosion may have been examples of epithelial basement membrane dystrophy. Reis-Bücklers', macular, and lattice dystrophies may also present with frequent and prominent recurrent corneal erosions at certain stages. Erosions are less frequently encountered in Meesmann's dystrophy and the variants of Reis-Bücklers' dystrophy, including anterior membrane dystrophy and honeycomb dystrophy. Fuchs' dystrophy may present with epithelial breakdown, presumably on the basis of epithelial edema, although congenital hereditary endothelial dystrophy, which is associated with marked corneal edema, usually does not manifest as corneal erosion.

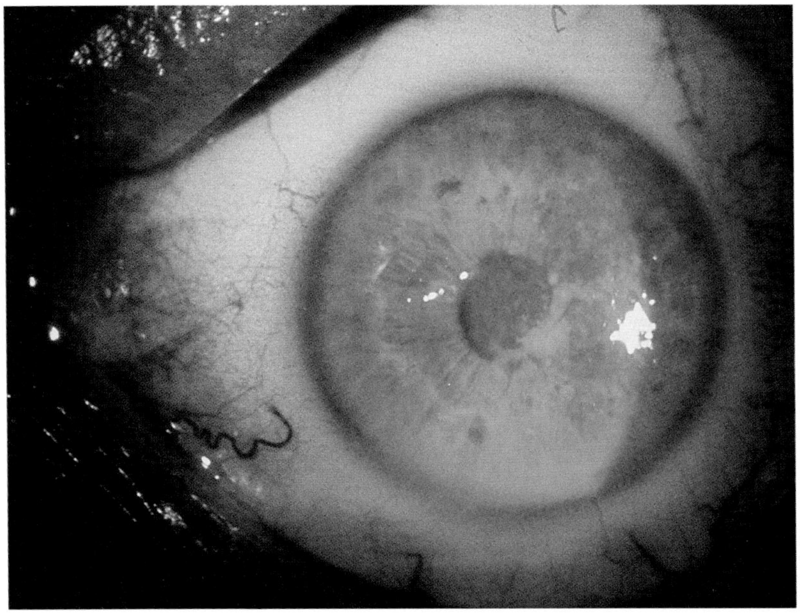

FIGURE 18-11 Fluorescein staining in a patient with Reis-Bücklers' dystrophy demonstrating surface irregularity and an erosion.

There is general agreement that recurrent erosions, whether inherited or post-traumatic, are a result of poor epithelial attachment. One of the pathogenetic mechanisms appears to be that the tear flow at night is minimal and what few tears there are flow around the limbal gutter rather than over the corneal surface, so that the epithelium partially adheres to the eyelid. When the epithelium is poorly attached to the underlying cornea, rapid eye movements during the early morning hours or opening of the eyelids on arising tears off the epithelium. Long-lasting ophthalmic ointment at bedtime provides a lubricating layer between the epithelium and the eyelids, and can reduce the risk of recurrent erosions. After an erosion has healed, the use of ointment at bedtime for at least 3 weeks can reduce the risk of later recurrences. Similarly, a bandage soft contact lens can protect the epithelium and reduce the risk of recurrences. Stromal puncture apparently causes a fine fibroblastic layer to grow through Bowman's layer, to which the epithelium preferentially adheres. Excimer laser photoablation of abnormal basement membrane also permits epithelial reattachment and is a treatment for recurrent erosions.

Reis-Bücklers' Dystrophy

Reis-Bücklers' dystrophy was first clearly described by Reis[57] and subsequently detailed by Bücklers,[58] who documented the dominant inheritance and strong penetrance. This bilaterally symmetrical central corneal dystrophy presents in childhood with recurrent attacks of photophobia and irritation. Subsequent progressive visual loss is the result of anterior corneal opacification and irregular astigmatism.[59] Most patients experience erosive episodes three or four times a year, with gradual progression of the slit lamp findings and diminished corneal sensation. Acute erosive episodes generally diminish in frequency over 5 to 20 years and usually stabilize after the third decade of life. The pattern of erosions, rate of progression, and extent of visual impairment have been variable even within the same pedigree.

The earliest slit lamp findings in affected children include a fine reticular opacification at the level of Bowman's layer. Clinical examination of the more advanced stages shows an irregular corneal surface or epithelium of various thicknesses. Usually, epithelial edema is not present. Fluorescein staining is apparent only in patients with erosions (Figure 18-11). Characteristic discrete, gray-white opacities in the subepithelial area assume a variety of forms (Figure 18-12); some opacities are linear, while others have a geographic, ring-like, honeycomb, fishnet, or alveolar pattern.[60] All of these patterns are created by ridges or blunt spokes that project anteriorly from the level of Bowman's layer into the overlying epithelium. The overall patterns are seen best with broad oblique illumination, while the depth and individual peak-like projections are seen best with a narrow slit beam (Figure 18-13). The opacities are most dense in the central or midperipheral cornea, often creating an annular appearance. The peripheral cornea is grossly spared; however, on closer examination, a fine diffuse haze usually extends to the limbus and is best seen with retroillumination. The central anterior stroma may contain discrete refractile opacities or show a similar

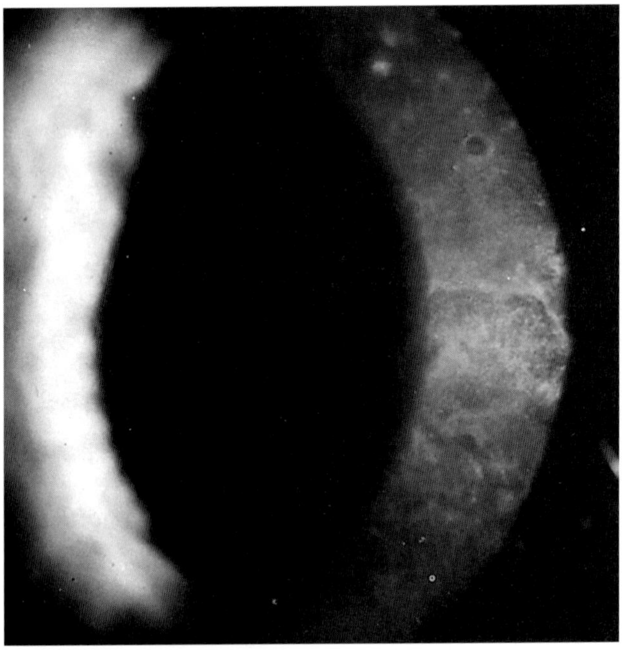

FIGURE 18-12 Slit lamp photograph of Reis-Bücklers' dystrophy shows diffuse superficial corneal haze with superimposed localized opacities of various morphologies.

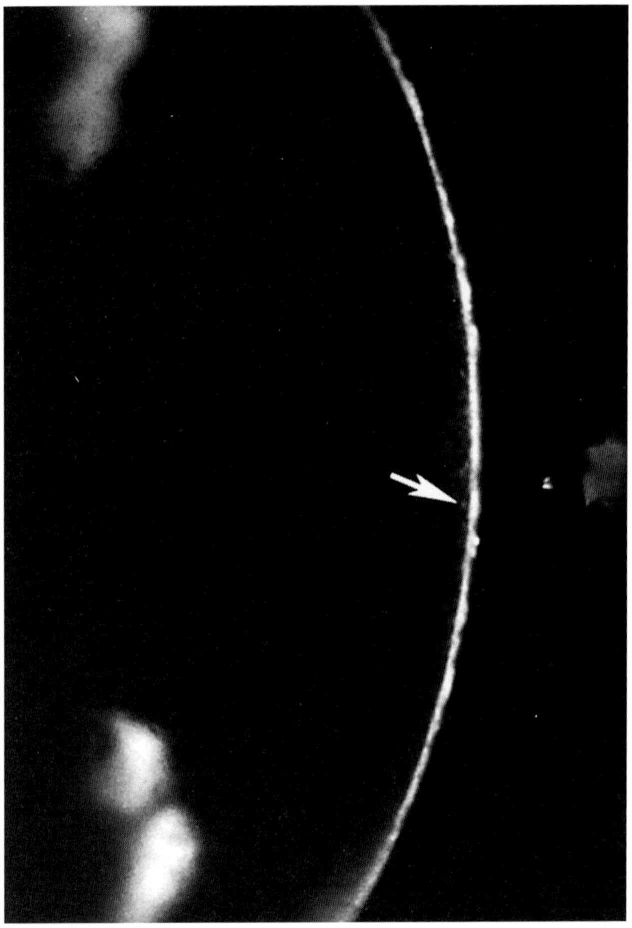

FIGURE 18-13 The anterior location of opacification and the irregular corneal surface are demonstrated in this slit lamp photograph of Reis-Bücklers' dystrophy. Smaller punctate opacities (arrow) are seen in the underlying stroma.

ground-glass appearance. Iron lines, which may be dense or fragmented, and prominent corneal nerves are often present.[61] Irregular astigmatism, distorted keratoscopic mires, negative fluorescein staining, and increased central corneal thickness may be found in all stages. Vascularization is unusual even in erosive cases.

Light microscopy[62–64] often demonstrates a sawtooth configuration of the epithelial layer in late cases. The epithelial cells show degenerative changes with intracellular and intercellular edema. A prominent subepithelial layer is present and contains fragments of Bowman's layer, fibroblasts, and fibrous tissue (Figure 18-14). Projections of this subepithelial layer extend into the epithelium, and a similar material may also be present in the anterior stroma. Inflammatory changes are conspicuously absent.

The ultrastructure[62–65] of the fibrocellular layer that replaces Bowman's layer (Figure 18-15) demonstrates closely packed, larger collagen fibrils with a diameter of 250 to 400 Å and normal periodicity interspersed with clumps and sheets of short, dense, half-moon–shaped tubular microfibrils with diameters of approximately 100 Å. These curly fibrils have tapering ends and may show cross striations. Their appearance is probably caused by histologic sectioning of longer wavy or corkscrew-like fibers. Loss of hemidesmosomes and disordered basement membrane complexes may be demonstrated overlying the areas of accumulation of these fibrils and also in areas where the basement membrane is absent.[65] In areas where Bowman's layer remains intact, an accumulation of collagen and microfibrils occurs between Bowman's layer and the overlying epithelium. The posterior stroma, Descemet's membrane, and endothelium are usually normal. In one case of recurrent Reis-Bücklers' dystrophy following a superficial keratectomy, biopsy of the bulbar conjunctiva showed duplication of the epithelial basement membrane.[66]

The cause and specific nature of the characteristic microfibrils in Reis-Bücklers' dystrophy remain unclear. Some investigators believe there is a primary degeneration of Bowman's layer with resultant basement membrane and epithelial changes.[62,63] In the late stages, Bowman's layer is replaced with collagen and microfibrils, which seem to be produced by the fibroblast-like cells in the ante-

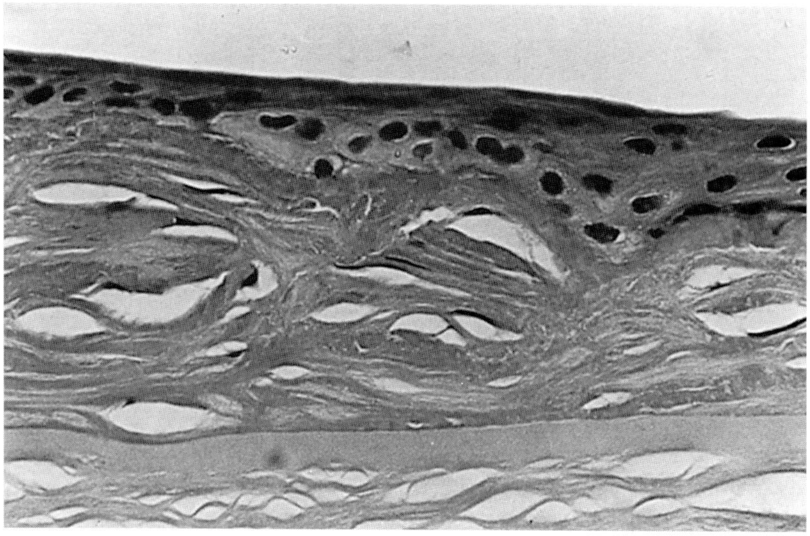

FIGURE 18-14 Light microscopy of Reis-Bücklers' dystrophy demonstrates the saw-tooth configuration of the epithelial layer and prominent subepithelial fibrous tissue. In this area, Bowman's layer is intact. (Hematoxylin and eosin, × 500.)

rior stroma. Other theories include primary epithelial, epithelial basement membrane, and neurotrophic causes.[66]

Treatment includes medical management of the erosive episodes. Persistent epithelial defects may be troublesome in advanced cases. The superficial opacification may be treated by curettage and superficial keratectomy.[67] More advanced cases have been treated with lamellar or penetrating keratoplasty. Delayed recurrence of this dystrophy in successful grafts has been documented[66]; earlier superficial recurrence of the annular pattern may occur in some patients (Figure 18-16). Although experience is not extensive, it seems likely that excimer laser photoablation may be the method of choice for the treatment of Reis-Bücklers' dystrophy.

Anterior Membrane Dystrophy (Grayson-Wilbrandt Dystrophy)

Anterior membrane dystrophy, a disorder with a clinical appearance similar to that of Reis-Bücklers' dystrophy, was initially described as an autosomal dominant trait in two generations of a single pedigree.[68] The disorder did not become clinically apparent in these patients until they were 10 years of age; erosive symptoms were infrequent and

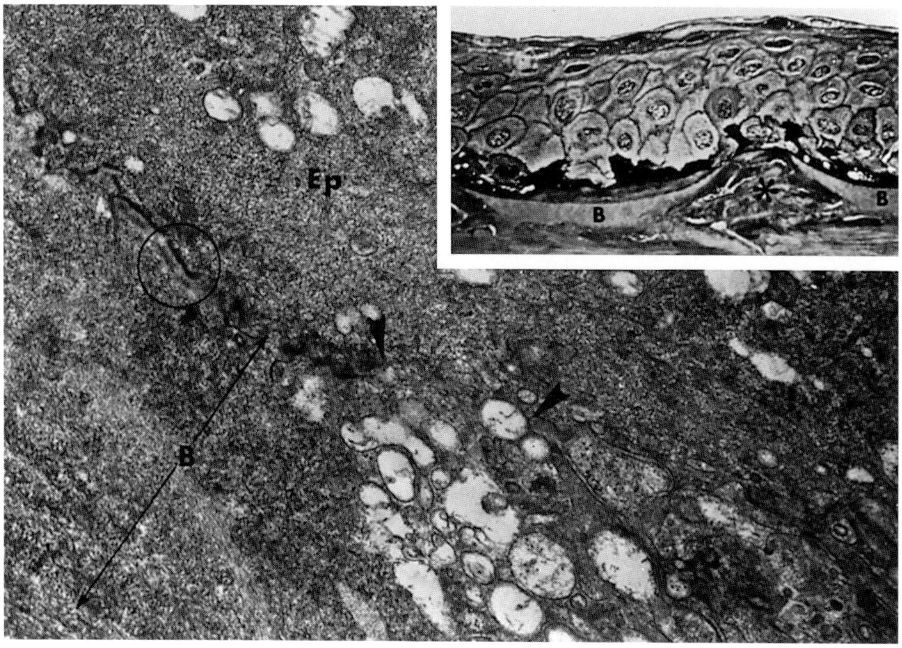

FIGURE 18-15 Reis-Bücklers' dystrophy. Inset: Phase contrast photomicrograph demonstrates focal disruption of Bowman's layer *(B)* by a fibrous appearing material (asterisk). (Paraphenylenediamine, × 800.) Transmission electron micrograph shows remnants of Bowman's layer *(B)* and masses of small-diameter fibrils. Hemidesmosomes (circle) are discontinuous and there is apparent continuity (arrowheads) between the basal cell cytoplasm *(Ep)* and underlying cellular debris. (× 30,000.) (Reprinted with permission from JA Fogle, KR Kenyon, WJ Stark, WR Green: Defective epithelial adhesion in anterior corneal dystrophies. Am J Ophthalmol 79:925, 1975. Copyright by The Ophthalmic Publishing Company.)

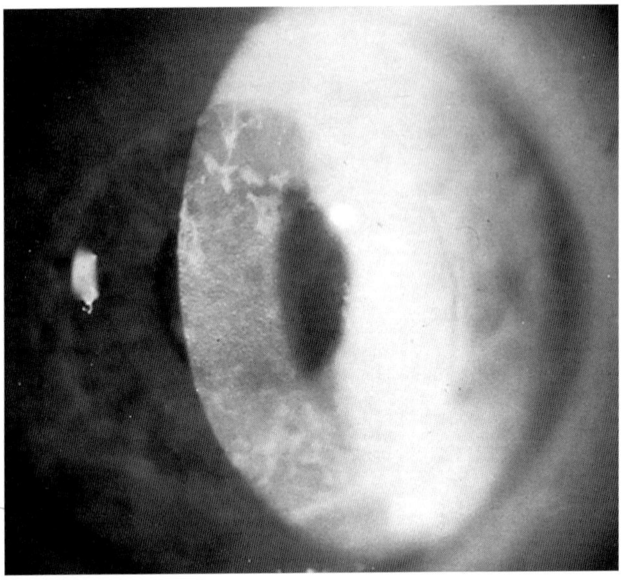

FIGURE 18-16 Recurrent Reis-Bücklers' dystrophy in a graft. There is a fine granular appearance of the central graft and a more typical superficial opacification in the periphery.

lacked a specific pattern. Vision was variably affected, ranging from 20/20 to 20/200. Anterior membrane dystrophy differs from Reis-Bücklers' dystrophy in several ways, including a less severe effect on visual acuity, sparing of the peripheral cornea, normal corneal sensation, and characteristic epithelial basement membrane and subepithelial changes.

Slit lamp examination demonstrated gray-white, amorphous opacities of various sizes over the central cornea, consisting of mounds extending into the epithelium from a thickened Bowman's layer. The intervening cornea remained relatively clear, and small refractile figures were present in the stroma. Corneal sensation was normal, and the corneal nerves were usually prominent.

Light microscopy performed on a lamellar specimen from the most severely involved family member showed a regular periodic acid-Schiff-positive subepithelial layer extending into the basal epithelial layer. In some locations, Bowman's layer was absent or replaced by this material. There were no stromal changes that corresponded to the clinically detected refractile bodies.

Honeycomb Dystrophy (Thiel and Behnke Dystrophy)

Honeycomb dystrophy is an unusual subepithelial dystrophy transmitted as an autosomal dominant trait.[69] Honeycomb dystrophy presents in childhood and runs a progressive course, with painful erosive episodes and gradually deteriorating vision. A characteristic honeycomb-like opacity develops in the subepithelial region of the cornea in the second decade of life. The fully developed clinical appearance affects the central cornea at the level of Bowman's layer and fades toward the periphery, leaving a clear margin 1 to 2 mm wide. Despite projections from the underlying opacity into the epithelium, the corneal surface is described as smooth and mirror-like. Corneal sensation is not significantly decreased and vision varies from 20/25 in younger patients to approximately 20/100 at 40 to 60 years of age.

Histopathologic findings were reported in one case of clinical honeycomb dystrophy in which there was also a positive family history of Reis-Bücklers' dystrophy.[60] Light and electron microscopy demonstrated a thickened, split, or duplicated epithelial basement membrane and a fibrillogranular subepithelial layer with nodular protrusions into the overlying epithelium.

Epithelial basement membrane changes, especially thickening of this layer, are present in most of the anterior dystrophies and may also be found in chronic corneal edema. Thickening of the epithelial basement membrane is a prominent feature of both honeycomb dystrophy and anterior membrane dystrophy. However, it is not typically a feature of Reis-Bücklers' dystrophy. Despite these differences, the wide spectrum of clinical findings in patients with Reis-Bücklers' dystrophy and the concurrent appearance of Reis-Bücklers' dystrophy and honeycomb dystrophy in a single pedigree favor the classification of this latter disorder, along with anterior membrane dystrophy, as a variant of Reis-Bücklers' dystrophy.[70] Honeycomb dystrophy is differentiated by later onset, normal corneal sensation, typical honeycomb morphology, and a smooth corneal surface.

Inherited Band Keratopathy

Although band keratopathy is usually seen in degenerative ocular conditions and systemic diseases, it can also be inherited and considered a dystrophy. Inherited band keratopathy has been described in both childhood and senile forms.[1] The childhood form was seen in an 11-year-old boy and his 16-year-old sister,[71] and was also seen in three of nine children in a consanguineous pedigree.[72] The involvement was congenital in one of these siblings and developed at puberty in the other two. Clinically, the opacity was denser in the central cornea and consisted of small gray opacities having the appearance of tapioca grains. The senile form was documented in a report of two brothers, 66 and 71 years of age, who demonstrated band keratopathy.[73] Vertical transmission in pedigrees has been described in other cases,[74] but the inheritance of this disorder remains unclear.

A pedigree with yellow- to amber-colored globules with a central band configuration has been reported.[75] A younger family member manifested only geographic subepithelial hazy lesions. Electron microscopy in this familial disorder showed homogeneous electron-dense material in globules in the anterior cornea.[75]

Anterior Mosaic Dystrophy

Anterior mosaic dystrophy is rare, bilaterally symmetrical, and manifests as gray-white polygonal opacities separated by clear spaces, imparting a crocodile-skin appearance to Bowman's layer. The axial pattern usually appears as a sporadic senile change (anterior crocodile shagreen), but familial juvenile and adult-onset forms have been described.[76] Dominant inheritance was documented over two generations in one family.[77] The corneal changes occurred later in life and there was no significant effect on visual acuity or corneal sensation. A similar pattern may be seen in early band keratopathy and in association with X-linked recessive megalocornea.[78,79] Secondary forms have been described following trauma and in phthisical globes.[80]

The dystrophy is thought to take its morphology from the anterior corneal mosaic.[81] The pattern can be demonstrated in the normal cornea by flattening the corneal surface, and is most frequently seen clinically in the fluorescein pattern with applanation tonometry or following ocular massage. Anterior mosaic dystrophy should be differentiated from posterior crocodile shagreen, which is an aging change that is most dense in the posterior stroma, but sometimes extends anteriorly to Bowman's layer.

STROMAL DYSTROPHIES

In 1890, Groenouw[82] described a form of corneal degeneration termed *noduli corneae*. He later traced the disease through four generations of the original pedigree family. In 1938, Bücklers[83] concluded that the cases initially described by Groenouw represented two different dystrophies. The nodular type (Groenouw type I), with a dominant transmission, is now known as *granular dystrophy*, and the other type (Groenouw type II), with recessive inheritance, is termed *macular dystrophy*. In the same year as Groenouw's original description, Biber[84] described a reticular dystrophy that subsequently was shown to have a dominant mode of inheritance.[85,86] This dystrophy completes the triad of the classic stromal dystrophies and is termed *lattice dystrophy* (Table 18-1).

Since these classic observations, other dystrophies that principally involve the stroma have been described. Those discussed in the following section include central crystalline dystrophy of Schnyder, fleck dystrophy, central cloudy corneal dystrophy of François, posterior amorphous corneal dystrophy, congenital hereditary stromal dystrophy, and a group of disorders collected under the appellation of pre-Descemet's dystrophy. Polymorphic stromal dystrophy is also discussed, although like most of the conditions similar to pre-Descemet's dystrophy, it is probably a degenerative process and not a dystrophy. Gelatinous drop-like dystrophy is covered in this section because of its similarity to lattice dystrophy, although its primary manifestations are at the level of Bowman's layer.

Granular Dystrophy

Granular dystrophy (Groenouw type I) is an autosomal dominant condition that usually becomes apparent in the first or second decade of life.[87] Fine, discrete, gray-white dots or radial lines are seen in the anterior central stroma (Figure 18-17). The intervening stroma remains clear, and vision is usually not affected early in the course. Slowly and insidiously, the opacities enlarge, coalesce, and multiply; often they spread to involve the deeper and more peripheral stroma. The peripheral 2 to 3 mm of the stroma, however, remain uninvolved. Although the lesions may involve Bowman's layer and result in surface irregularity, epithelial erosions occur infrequently. In most cases, visual impairment is rarely severe until after the fifth decade and usually occurs secondary to intervening stromal opacification. Corneal sensation is variably affected. Isolated cases have been reported, although in most cases, familial occurrence with a dominant mode of inheritance is well documented.[1,88,89] The features of the dystrophy, especially the presence of erosions and the morphology of the individual lesions, tend to be uniform within families. Granular dystrophy has been mapped to a single locus on the long arm of chromosome 5, along with granular-lattice (Avellino) and lattice type I corneal dystrophies.[90]

Slit lamp examination of early cases shows fine dots and radial lines in the superficial stroma, usually in the first decade of life. Later, focal white opacities in the anterior stroma may take on a variety of shapes. The dots are opaque on focal illumination and may be partially translucent on retroillumination (Figure 18-18). More homogeneous opacities resemble bread crumbs or snowflakes and have sharp, irregular margins. Other lesions show sinuous geographic margins and relatively clear centers. There may be any number of these opacities. They usually occur

TABLE 18-1
Characteristics of the Three Major Stromal Dystrophies

Feature	*Granular Dystrophy*	*Macular Dystrophy*	*Lattice Dystrophy (Type I)*
Age of onset			
Deposits	1st decade	1st decade	1st decade
Symptoms	3rd decade or asymptomatic	1st decade	2nd decade
Heredity	Autosomal dominant	Autosomal recessive	Autosomal dominant
Reduced vision	By 4th–5th decade	By 1st–2nd decade	By 2nd–3rd decade
Erosions	Uncommon	Common	Frequent
Opacities	Discrete with sharp borders Intervening stroma clear early but becomes hazy Not to limbus	Indistinct margins Hazy intervening stroma early Extends to limbus Endothelium affected Central lesions more anterior, peripheral lesions more posterior	Early Refractile tiny lines and dots Subepithelial spots Diffuse central haze Becomes Lattice lines with knobs Amorphous various-sized deposits Stromal haze Limbal zone clear except in extreme cases
Corneal thickness	Normal	Thinned	Normal
Characteristic histochemical stains	Masson's trichrome Luxol fast blue Antibodies to microfibrillar protein	Periodic acid-Schiff Colloidal iron Alcian blue Metachromatic dyes	Periodic acid–Schiff Congo red Thioflavine-T (fluorescence) Crystal violet (metachromasia) Positive birefringence and dichroism
Material accumulated	Phospholipids and microfibrillar protein	Glycosaminoglycans	Amyloid
Ultrastructure	Electron-dense, rod-shaped structures surrounded by 8- to 10-nm microfibrils	Intracytoplasmic membrane-limited vacuoles filled with fibrillogranular material or lamellar bodies Similar vacuoles in endothelium	Characteristic 8- to 10-nm electron-dense, nonbranching amyloid fibrils
Distinguishing clinical characteristics	Clear limbal zone	Opacities reach limbus Cornea thinned unless decompensated	Lattice lines

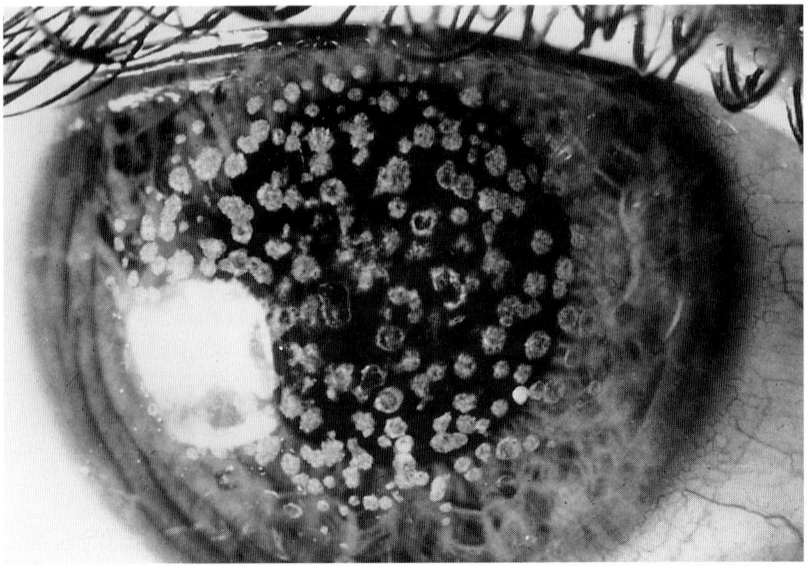

FIGURE 18-17 Granular dystrophy. Discrete stromal opacities with clear intervening stroma and peripheral cornea. (Courtesy of the Armed Forces Institute of Pathology, Washington, DC, AFIP 63-5288.)

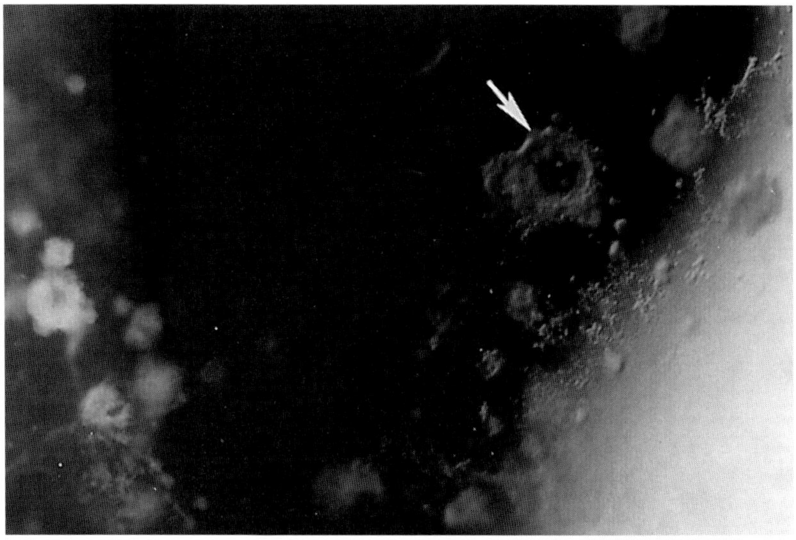

FIGURE 18-18 Individual lesions in granular dystrophy are opaque with focal illumination and partially translucent, sometimes with clear centers, on retroillumination (arrow).

in a random distribution; however, aggregates of the lesions may take on many forms, including chains, rings, or branching patterns.

Initially, the intervening cornea is clear, but with progression, the stroma develops a diffuse, ground-glass appearance, which can best be seen as a slight haze with broad oblique illumination and as a fine granularity on retroillumination. Indirect illumination may demonstrate a myriad of fine punctate opacities. Fluorescein staining of the corneal surface highlights areas of tear film breakup or negative staining over the more superficial lesions.

Most patients with granular dystrophy require no treatment and do not require penetrating keratoplasty. Mild photophobia may be present due to scattering of incident light by the opacities. Erosive episodes are unusual. When erosions do occur, they tend to be a common feature among affected family members.

Variants of granular dystrophy with an earlier onset, atypical appearance, higher frequency of erosive episodes, and more severe eventual visual impairment have been described.[88,89,91,92] In these exceptional cases, snowflake-like opacities form a diffuse superficial stromal haze with progressive opacification and erosion resembling Reis-Bücklers' dystrophy.

The morphology and nature of the staining of the lesions in typical granular dystrophy are characteristic. Light microscopy demonstrates deeply staining, eosinophilic, rod- or trapezoidal-shaped deposits in the stroma or subepithelial areas. The individual opacities stain bright red with Masson's trichrome stain (Figure 18-19) and are argyrophilic

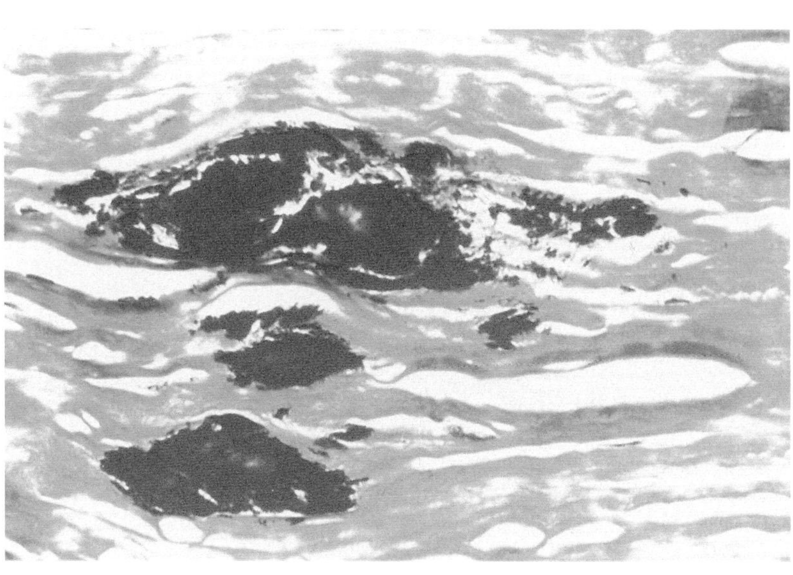

FIGURE 18-19 Granular dystrophy. Red stromal deposits with Masson's trichrome stain. (× 500.)

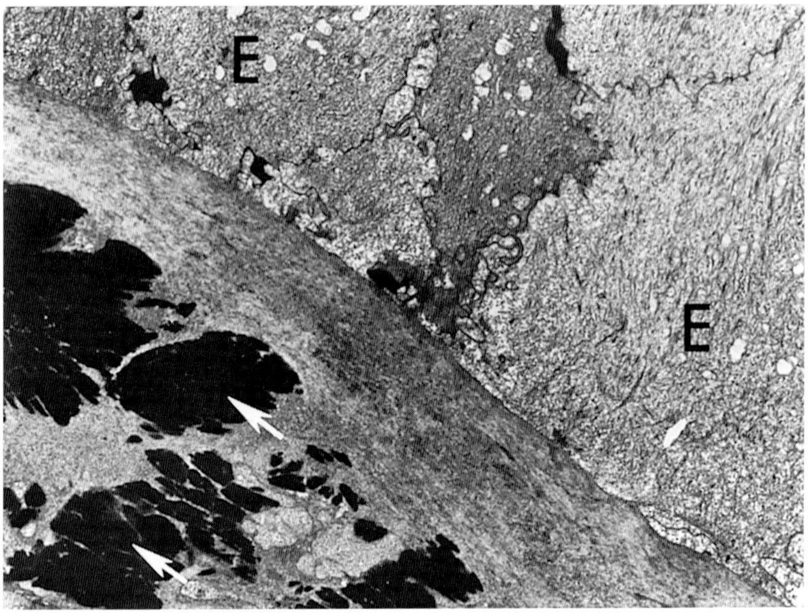

FIGURE 18-20 Transmission electron micrograph of granular dystrophy. Dense deposits (arrows) are seen in the superficial stroma and between basal epithelial cells *(E)*. (× 12,900.) (Reprinted with permission from MM Rodrigues, BW Streeten, JH Krachmer: Microfibrillar protein and phospholipid in granular corneal dystrophy. Arch Ophthalmol 101:802, 1983.)

with reticulin stains. The deposits stain with Luxol fast blue and protein stains. Frozen sections of the lesions reveal a positive reaction with antibodies to microfibrillar proteins.[93] Filipin staining has demonstrated secondary accumulation of unesterified cholesterol.[94] Biochemical analysis of corneas with granular dystrophy has shown excess phospholipids in addition to microfibrillar protein. Analytical microscopy has not revealed further significant information regarding the specific character of the lesions.

Transmission electron microscopy demonstrates irregular, electron-dense, rod-shaped structures 100 to 500 μm wide in the extracellular spaces.[4,95,96] These structures are found most commonly in the superficial stroma, but on occasion have been identified in the epithelial intercellular spaces or within degenerated basal epithelial cells (Figure 18-20). Higher magnification of the individual lesions demonstrates variable inner structural organization. Some lesions seem to be composed of closely packed filaments oriented along the long axis of the rod-shaped structures. Others show a "moth-eaten" pattern or a diffuse, fine, homogeneous morphology. Surrounding these lesions may be 8- to 10-nm tubular microfibrils (Figure 18-21). Although originally thought to be amyloid on the basis of Congo red stain, these fibrils usually lack the typical spatial orientation of amyloid.[93] Stromal keratocytes may be normal in appearance or show various stages of degeneration, with dilation of the endoplasmic reticulum and Golgi apparatus and vacuolation of the cytoplasm.[97]

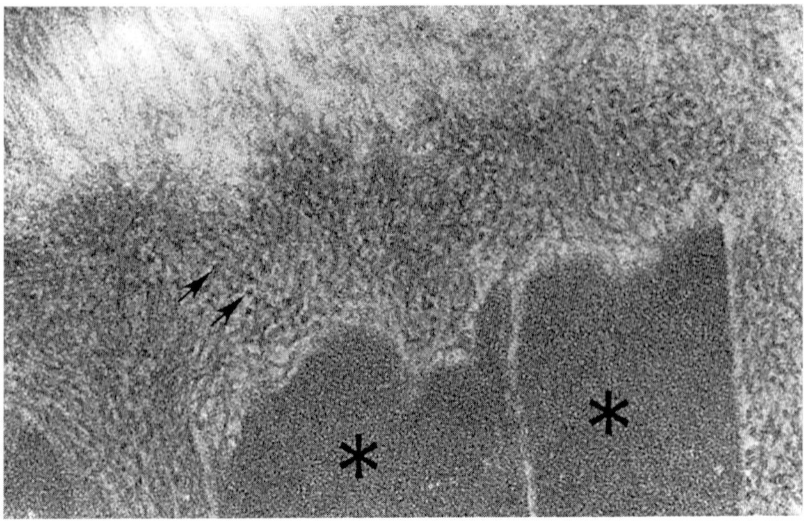

FIGURE 18-21 Higher magnification of the rod-shaped deposits (asterisks) with surrounding 8- to 10-nm microfibrils (arrows). (× 165,000.) (Reprinted with permission from MM Rodrigues, BW Streeten, JH Krachmer: Microfibrillar protein and phospholipid in granular corneal dystrophy. Arch Ophthalmol 101:802, 1983.)

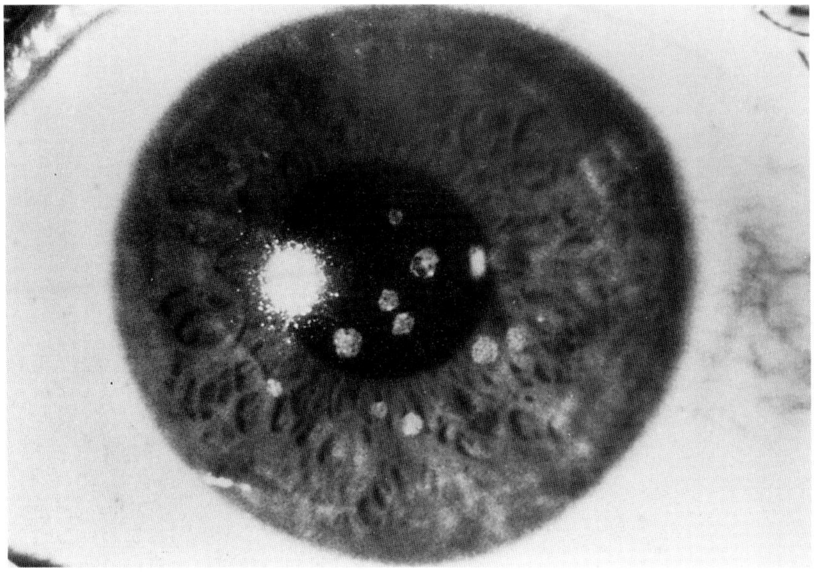

FIGURE 18-22 Slit lamp photograph of well-circumscribed anterior stromal and subepithelial lesions in a patient with granular-lattice (Avellino) dystrophy. (Courtesy of Edward J. Holland, M.D., Minneapolis, MN.)

The exact nature of the stromal deposits in granular dystrophy remains unclear. Hyaline is a descriptive, light microscopy term that does not indicate the chemical nature of the deposits. The dystrophy probably is the result of abnormal synthesis or handling of protein or phospholipids, which are the principal components of biologic cell membranes. The predominance of epithelial findings in recurrent granular dystrophy is cited by some as evidence for an epithelial genesis of this disorder, while other investigators think the stromal keratocyte is the primary source of the material.[95,98–100]

Most patients with granular dystrophy do not require therapy. Recurrent epithelial erosions should be appropriately managed as previously described. Lamellar keratectomy, either manually or with the excimer laser, has been used successfully to treat some of the superficial forms of the dystrophy.[101] Penetrating keratoplasty is indicated in cases of significant visual loss with more typical stromal involvement. However, recurrences may occur soon after keratoplasty, and consist clinically of a diffuse, subepithelial, fibrovascular invasion of the graft from the periphery, or recurrence of typical granular lesions in the middle and posterior portions of the donor stroma.[102] Sometimes the superficial recurrence can be removed by debridement or superficial keratectomy.[103]

An unusual variant of granular dystrophy has been described in families who trace their ancestry to the Italian province of Avellino.[101,104–106] The clinical and pathologic findings of both granular and lattice dystrophies are found in granular-lattice (Avellino) corneal dystrophy, which seems to be a highly penetrant autosomal dominant trait in the reported pedigrees.[105] All three dystrophies have been linked independently to markers on the long arm of chromosome 5, suggesting that these dystrophies are caused by mutations in the same gene.[90,107]

Although the phenotypic variation within families with granular-lattice dystrophy is substantial,[106] discrete subepithelial or anterior stromal granular deposits are seen in younger family members (Figure 18-22). Mid- to posterior stromal refractile lattice lines develop in the second or third decade as the granular lesions progress, especially in the inferior cornea (Figure 18-23). By the sixth decade of life, an anterior stromal haze appears in addition to the progressive granular- and lattice-like lesions, and functional vision is impaired (Figure 18-24). Recurrent erosions are more common than in typical granular dystrophy.

The histopathology of Avellino dystrophy shows typical superficial granular lesions with trichrome stain. Numerous fusiform amyloid deposits are seen in the deeper stromal layers.[101,104,105] Lectin binding characteristics of the granular deposits in these cases differ from those of typical granular dystrophy.[104]

In this dystrophy, recurrent granular deposits have been seen clinically in grafts.

Macular Dystrophy

Macular dystrophy is the least common of the classic stromal dystrophies. Unlike granular and lattice dystrophies, macular dystrophy is inherited as an autosomal recessive trait. Like other recessive disorders, it is clinically more severe and occurs often in pedigrees with consanguinity. The dystrophy may appear to occur as sporadic cases because the heterozygous carriers do not manifest corneal

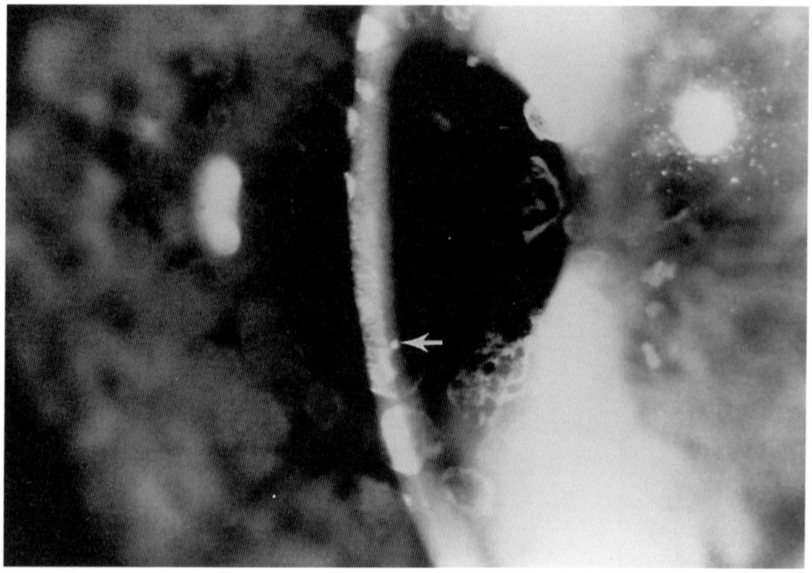

FIGURE 18-23 More advanced gray-white opacities of the anterior stroma in granular-lattice dystrophy. The slit beam shows a deep fusiform lesion (arrow) in the stroma characteristic of the lattice-like opacities seen in the later stages of granular-lattice dystrophy. (Courtesy of Edward J. Holland, M.D., Minneapolis, MN.)

changes. Extensive genealogical investigation of involved families with macular dystrophy has linked some of the families together by common ancestry.[11,108] The gene frequency in the population is small, but the frequency of homozygous individuals has been amplified by inbreeding within pedigrees.

Macular dystrophy usually shows symmetrical changes that begin in the first decade of life, starting with a fine superficial stromal haze. This opacification begins centrally, extends to the periphery, and usually involves the entire thickness of the cornea by the second decade (Figure 18-25). Multiple, irregular, gray-white nodules develop within the haze and may project into the anterior chamber posteriorly or protrude anteriorly, causing surface irregularity.[2] However, recurrent erosion occurs much less frequently in macular dystrophy than in lattice dystrophy.

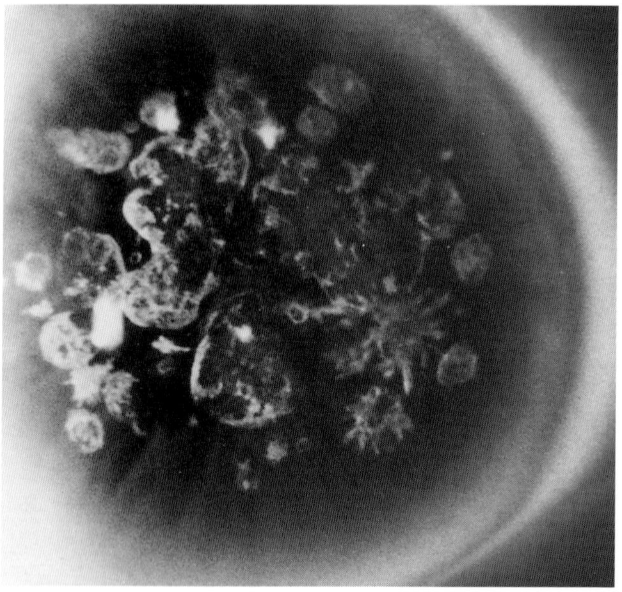

FIGURE 18-24 Larger anterior stromal and fusiform deeper lesions are seen in the later stages of granular-lattice dystrophy. (Courtesy of Edward J. Holland, M.D., Minneapolis, MN.)

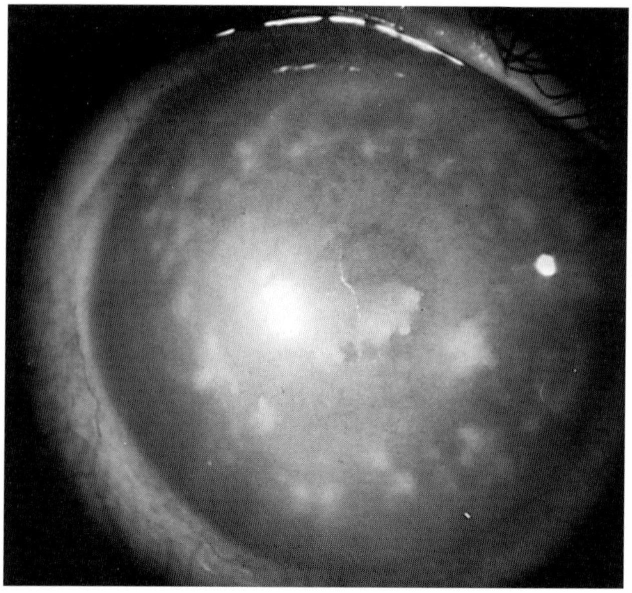

FIGURE 18-25 Macular dystrophy extending to the limbus in a 20-year-old man.

Photophobia is a prominent feature of macular dystrophy and often seems out of proportion to the clinical corneal involvement. Usually by 20 to 30 years of age, the patient has lost useful vision and requires penetrating keratoplasty.

Slit lamp examination in the early stages of macular dystrophy shows a central, faint, ground-glass–like haze in the superficial stroma, which is best seen by broad oblique illumination. Developing within this hazy matrix are multiple, small, pleomorphic, gray-white opacities with irregular borders. These opacities are more prominent and superficial in the central cornea and deeper and more discrete in the peripheral cornea (Figure 18-26). They are opaque to focal illumination; with indirect illumination, they are highlighted against the background haze. The opacities may enlarge, taking on a nodular appearance and becoming more confluent centrally and superficially, with overlying surface irregularity. As the dystrophy progresses, Descemet's membrane takes on a slate-gray appearance and multiple corneal guttae are seen. In the later stages, the stroma is diffusely involved, there are opaque nodules, and surface irregularity may become prominent. However, unlike the other classic stromal dystrophies, which show normal corneal thickness, macular dystrophy shows significantly reduced central corneal thickness by pachymetry and generally manifests with-the-rule astigmatism.[109,110]

Clinical distinction between the early stages of macular and granular dystrophies may be difficult. Focal, rather discrete opacities in the superficial stroma appear early in both conditions. However, the very early intervening stromal haze, involvement of the peripheral and deep stroma, decreased corneal thickness, with-the-rule astigmatism, and recessive family history help to distinguish macular dystrophy. The autosomal dominant inheritance and sparing of the peripheral 2 to 3 mm of the cornea help to distinguish the late changes of granular dystrophy. Similarly, late opacification in lattice dystrophy may occur, but typical filaments are usually seen peripheral to the opacification, and the peripheral stroma is spared except in the most severe cases.

Histologically, macular dystrophy is characterized by the accumulation of glycosaminoglycans within stromal keratocytes, as well as in the surrounding stroma, subepithelial area, Bowman's layer, histiocytes, Descemet's membrane, and endothelium.[111-114] These accumulations show positive staining for glycosaminoglycans with several histochemical stains, including periodic acid-Schiff, Alcian blue, metachromatic dyes, and colloidal iron (Figures 18-27 and 18-28). Light microscopy shows nonspecific epithelial changes with degeneration of the basal epithelial cells. Mononuclear cells and collections of glycosaminoglycans have been noted in the subepithelial area.[113,114] Bowman's

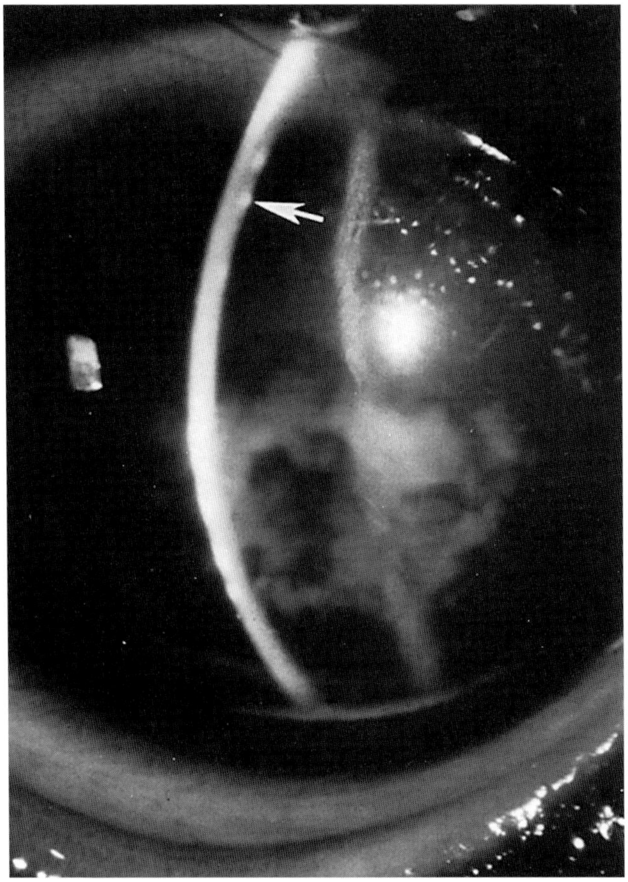

FIGURE 18-26 Slit lamp photograph of macular dystrophy demonstrates mottled central superficial opacification and deep discrete peripheral opacities (arrow).

layer may be irregular and either partially or totally destroyed. Portions of Bowman's layer may be replaced by a basement-membrane–like material or a hyaline-like membrane, often with embedded histiocytes.[114,115] The stroma contains distended, vacuolated keratocytes with pyknotic nuclei. The keratocytes are normal in number, with the most involved cells usually concentrated in the superficial or deep layers of the stroma and the least involved keratocytes in the mid- and peripheral stroma.[116]

Electron microscopy shows abundant endoplasmic reticulum and prominent Golgi systems in the epithelial cells.[113] The keratocytes contain membrane-limited intracytoplasmic vacuoles of various sizes (Figure 18-29). Smaller vacuoles are often found in conjunction with the rough endoplasmic reticulum.[115] The vacuoles may appear clear or may contain a granular or fibrillar material of moderate electron density, as well as lamellar bodies. Keratocytes may be distended up to three times their normal size by the large

FIGURE 18-27 Alcian blue stain of macular dystrophy. (× 500.)

intracytoplasmic vacuoles.[115-117] Similar vacuoles may be seen extracellularly in the collagen lamellae. These membrane-limited vesicles may also contain osmiophilic granular deposits (Figure 18-30). Degenerated keratocyte components and patches of fibrillogranular substance have also been found. Both the intracellular and extracellular accumulations of glycosaminoglycans can be localized by means of silver stains used in conjunction with electron microscopy.[11]

The anterior banded portion of Descemet's membrane is normal.[113,115] However, the posterior portion is usually filled with small, electron-lucent vacuoles and osmiophilic membrane-like structures, creating a honeycomb pattern.[115,118] This posterior layer also contains numerous focal thickenings that resemble corneal guttae. The endothelium has sometimes been reported to contain small vesicles filled with a fibrillogranular substance, similar to those found in the keratocytes.[115,119]

In normal corneas, the extracellular matrix consists of mainly type I collagen and two proteoglycans, one of which is a keratan sulfate proteoglycan.[120] Organ culture studies show that little or no keratan sulfate proteoglycan is synthesized by corneas in macular dystrophy.[121] Instead, an unusual glycoprotein with large unsulfated oligosaccharide side chains accumulates and reacts positively with antibodies to the protein core of the normal keratan sulfate proteoglycan. Enzyme-linked immunosorbent assay (ELISA) studies using monoclonal antibodies to sulfated keratan sulfate have shown no reactivity in either the cornea or the serum of most studied patients with macular dystrophy (type I).[122] A smaller subgroup

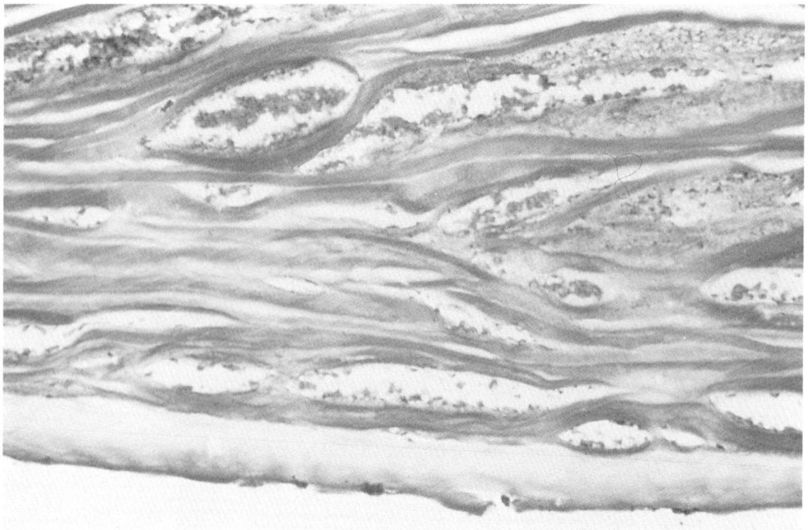

FIGURE 18-28 Colloidal iron stain of macular dystrophy. (× 250.)

(type II) shows antigenic keratan sulfate in both the serum and cornea. This assay may become useful in diagnosing type I macular dystrophy early in life before the appearance of corneal changes. Studies of families, bilateral pathologic specimens, and extraocular tissues have shown significant heterogeneity in this proposed classification.[123–125]

Macular dystrophy can be distinguished from other disorders involving glycosaminoglycans, including the systemic mucopolysaccharidoses.[126] In these latter disorders, there is a deficiency in the breakdown of the glycosaminoglycan portion of different proteoglycans, resulting in their accumulation and deposition in a variety of tissues. In the cornea this material initially accumulates within Golgi-derived lysosomes, in contrast to the vesicles associated with endoplasmic reticulum seen in macular dystrophy. In the systemic mucopolysaccharidoses, histopathologic evidence of epithelial involvement is prominent, while Descemet's membrane is usually normal, which is also in contrast to the findings in macular dystrophy. However, the systemic mucopolysaccharidoses are most easily differentiated from macular corneal dystrophy by the associated clinical features and extracorneal tissue and urine studies (see Ch. 17).

Treatment of macular dystrophy involves the use of tinted lenses to reduce photophobia, medical management of occasional erosions, and ultimately, penetrating keratoplasty, which has a favorable prognosis. However, the disease may recur in both lamellar[127–129] and penetrating keratoplasty grafts.[128,129] The pattern of recurrence usually involves the peripheral donor stroma, most prominently in the superficial and deep stromal layers. Later, spread of the involvement tends to blur the area of the graft-host junction and may simulate the primary dystrophy, with opacification of Descemet's membrane and the appearance of corneal guttae. Although donor keratocytes may sur-

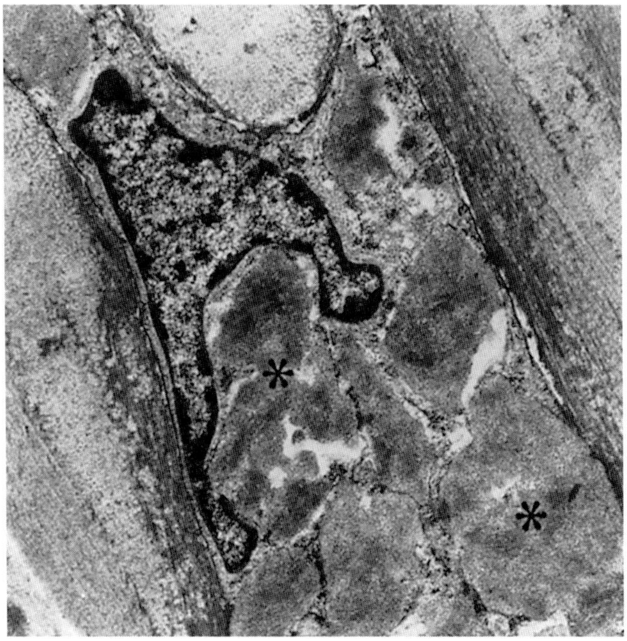

FIGURE 18-29 Stromal keratocyte in macular dystrophy is distended by membrane-limited cytoplasmic vacuoles containing a fine fibrillogranular material (asterisks). (× 16,545.) (Reprinted with permission from GO Waring, MM Rodrigues, PR Laibson: Corneal dystrophies. I. Dystrophies of the epithelium, Bowman's layer and stroma. Surv Ophthalmol 23:71, 1978.)

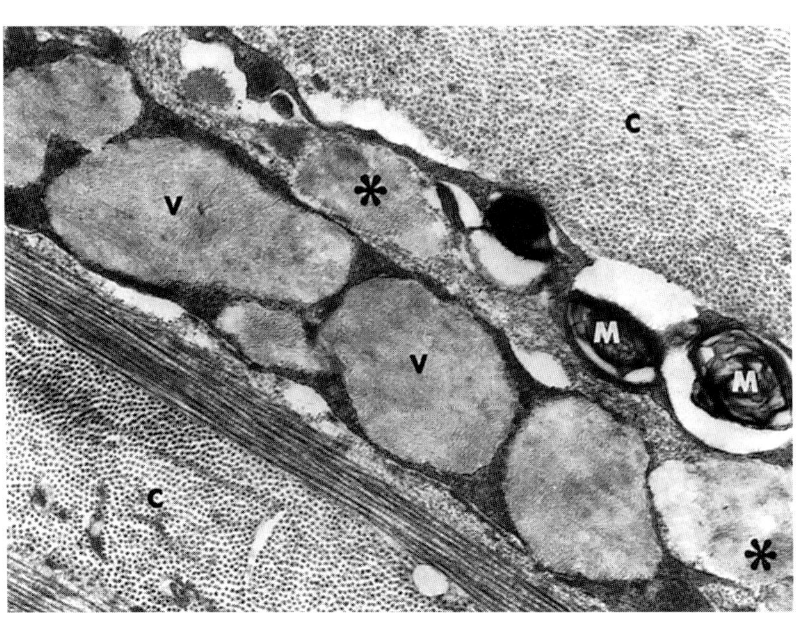

FIGURE 18-30 Electron micrograph of macular dystrophy. A stromal keratocyte is distended by vacuoles *(V)* filled with a fibrillogranular material. Similar fibrillogranular deposits (asterisks), in addition to membranous osmiophilic whorls *(M)*, are present adjacent to the keratocyte in the extracellular space. The stromal collagen fibrils *(C)* appear normal. (× 22,700.) (Reprinted with permission from RC Snip, KR Kenyon, WR Green: Macular corneal dystrophy: ultrastructural pathology of corneal endothelium and Descemet's membrane. Invest Ophthalmol 12:88, 1973.)

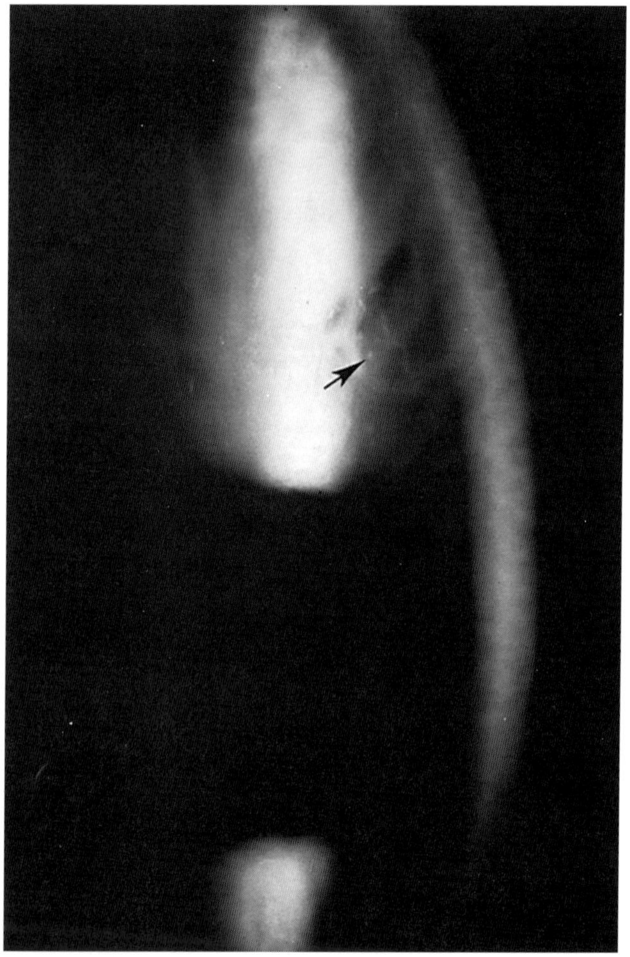

FIGURE 18-31 Refractile stromal dots (arrow) without accompanying lattice lines in a 13-year-old patient with early lattice dystrophy.

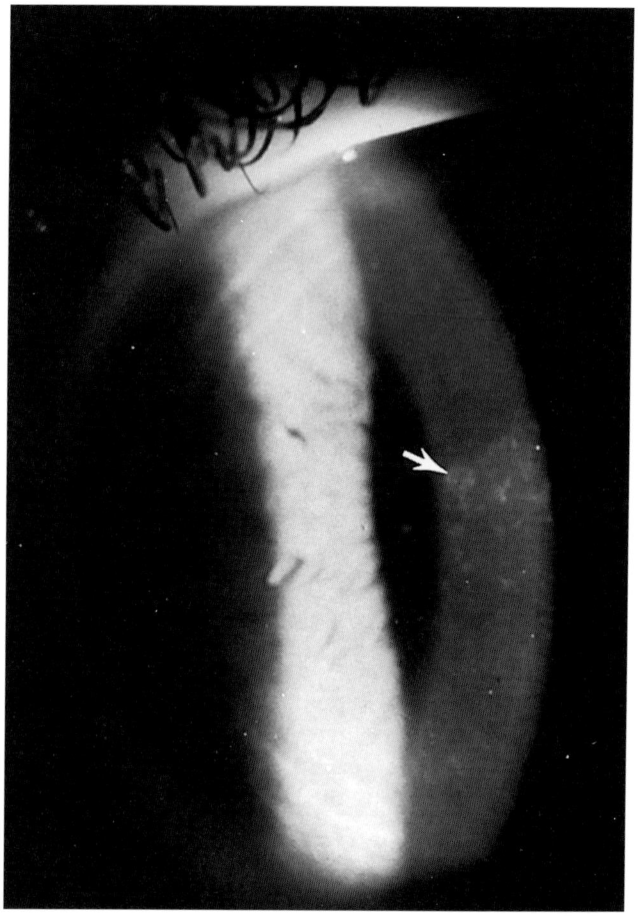

FIGURE 18-32 Subepithelial opacities (arrow) are seen in the central cornea of a 10-year-old patient with early lattice dystrophy.

vive for prolonged periods with normal production of keratan sulfate proteoglycan,[128,130] the host keratocytes continue to produce abnormal glycoproteins and do not synthesize normal keratan sulfate proteoglycan. The accumulation of abnormal glycoproteins produced by the host keratocytes is thought to be the cause of recurrent dystrophy in the donor tissue; this mechanism would also explain the initial peripheral localization of such recurrences.

Lattice Dystrophy

Lattice dystrophy type I is an autosomal dominant disorder that usually presents in the first decade of life with symptoms of recurrent erosion or visual disturbance.[131] As is common in disorders with autosomal dominant inheritance, the penetrance and expression of the trait vary, as do clinical onset and presentation. Although the dystrophy is usually bilateral and symmetrical, asymmetrical and unilateral cases of lattice dystrophy have been reported.[132–134] These unusual presentations tend to have a later onset and a more benign clinical course than typical lattice dystrophy. Lattice dystrophy type I has been mapped to chromosome 5q, as have granular and granular-lattice (Avellino) dystrophies.[90]

Careful examination of family members may reveal typical findings of lattice dystrophy in asymptomatic individuals.[135] Young patients may show characteristic early findings, including anterior refractile stromal dots (Figure 18-31), filamentary lines, subepithelial white spots (Figure 18-32), and central stromal haze (Figure 18-33). Other members of involved pedigrees may show only recurrent erosions with minimal stromal involvement or opacification.[136] These findings may often be confused with herpetic keratitis.

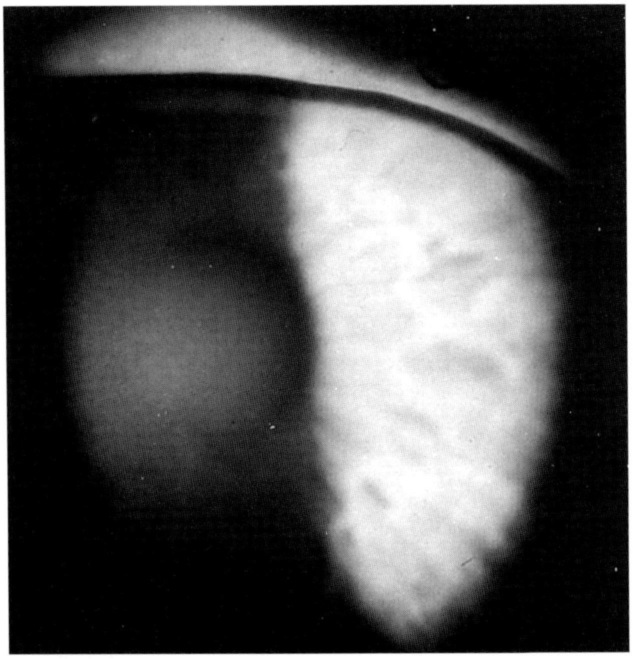

FIGURE 18-33 Diffuse anterior stromal haze in a young asymptomatic patient with lattice dystrophy.

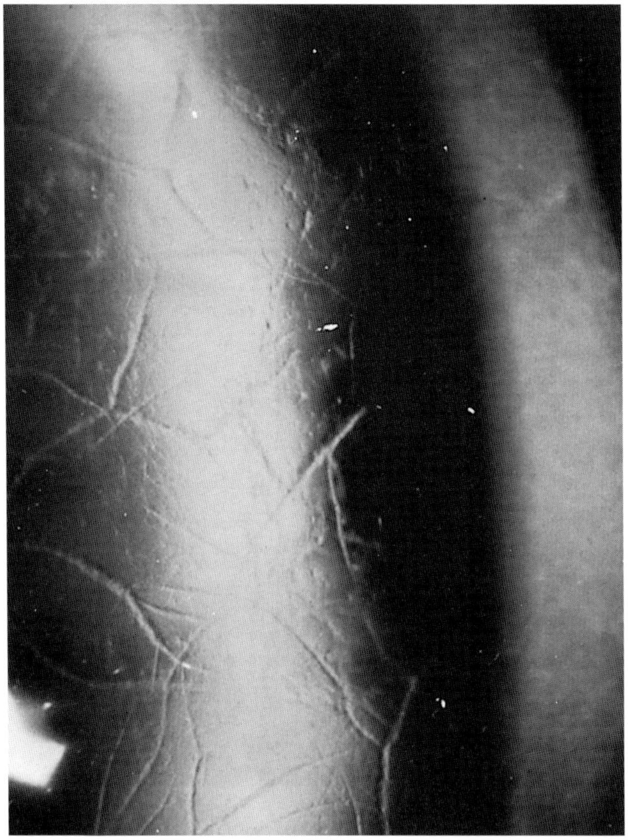

FIGURE 18-34 Lattice dystrophy. Small refractile dots and delicate, branching, refractile filaments are seen on indirect illumination.

Clinical involvement typically begins in the superficial and middle portions of the central stroma. With age, the fine refractile lines spread to involve the deeper and more peripheral layers of the stroma. Recurrent erosions result in irregularity of the epithelial surface with accompanying decreased visual acuity. Patients with typical stromal involvement without erosions may be asymptomatic and retain good visual acuity. Progressive clouding of the intervening stroma and scarring from recurrent erosions may result in dense, subepithelial opacities and in extreme cases, vascularization. Opacification may obscure the underlying lattice pattern. At this stage, the disorder may resemble the later stages of macular and granular dystrophies; however, with careful examination, typical branching lattice lines are usually seen and the peripheral cornea appears to be relatively uninvolved. Concomitant decreased central corneal sensation occurs in the later stages and may result in symptomatic improvement.

Slit lamp examination shows fine, refractile filamentary lines, refractile and nonrefractile dots, and less frequently, a diffuse stromal haze. The typical lattice filaments vary in appearance from delicate fine lines (Figure 18-34) to broad coarse bands with nodular dilations (Figure 18-35). In focal slit lamp illumination, the filaments are opaque with finely irregular margins. They are radially oriented with dichotomous branching near their central terminations. The lines overlap one another in various stromal levels, creating a latticework pattern. Indirect or retroillumination shows the lattice lines as rodlike, with a double contour and an optically clear core. They look like glassy rods with smooth refractile edges, often resembling icicles. In advanced cases, the lines fluoresce with cobalt-blue slit lamp illumination.

Refractile, glassy, homogeneous, discrete dots or more irregular opacities are seen with the filaments. They may also occur in a linear configuration, creating the appearance of a pseudofilament. Minute gray nebulae in the superficial stroma may be early findings in lattice, granular, and macular dystrophies. However, on retroillumination the opacities in lattice dystrophy take on a refractile quality that differs from the more homogeneous-appearing opacities in the other classic stromal dystrophies.

In lattice dystrophy, a fine, central, anterior stromal haze may be present and is best seen with a broad oblique beam. As the dystrophy progresses, this haze may intensify and spread to involve the deeper stromal layers. Gradually, the dot-like opacities coalesce, the lattice lines

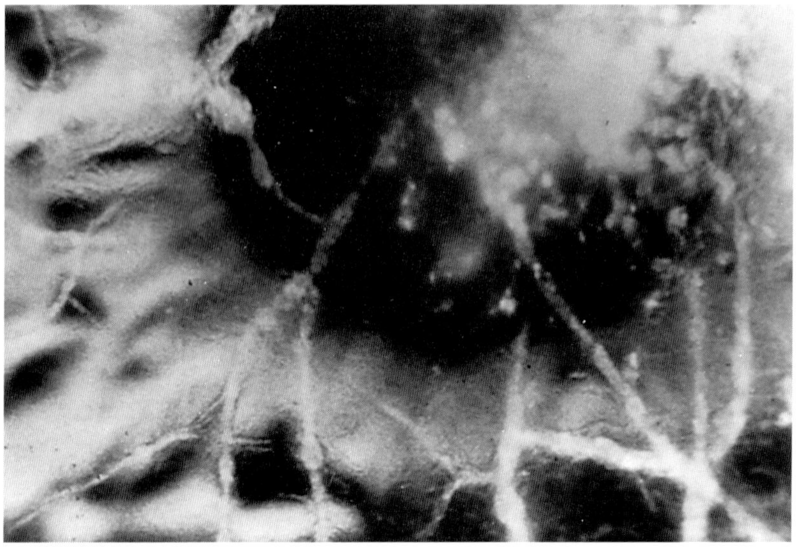

FIGURE 18-35 Coarse bands with nodular dilations in lattice dystrophy.

become thicker and more opaque, and opacification of the intervening stroma progresses. Yellow or amber refractile material has been seen in the subepithelial areas in some cases and has been identified histopathologically as elastotic degeneration.[136,137]

Histopathologic study in lattice dystrophy type I reveals an irregular epithelium, with degeneration of the basal epithelial cells.[120,138] The epithelial basement membrane is usually thickened and lacks normal hemidesmosomal structures.[13] Bowman's layer may be thicker or thinner than normal and is frequently fragmented in its periphery. A variably thick, eosinophilic layer separating the epithelial basement membrane from Bowman's layer is present and is composed of amyloid and collagen.[139] The stroma contains a myriad of large, irregular, eosinophilic deposits, which distort the normal configuration of the corneal lamellae (Figure 18-36).

The histochemical staining and polarization microscopy of the deposits in lattice dystrophy are characteristic.[138] Deposits stain orange-red with Congo red and manifest green birefringence when viewed with a microscope that polarizes light. There is no loss of Congo red stain when the tissue is pretreated with dilute potassium permanganate. Fluorescence of the material is present with thioflavine-T stain and ultraviolet light. With crystal violet stain, metachromasia is usually apparent. Some lesions have shown elastotic material by Verhoeff-van Gieson stain. Polarization microscopy may demonstrate epithe-

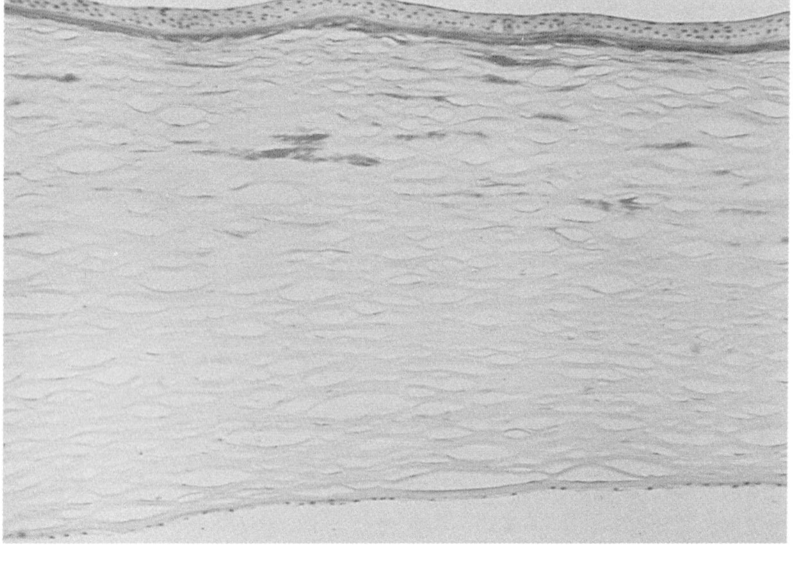

FIGURE 18-36 Fusiform lesions and a similar Congo-red–staining material forming a subepithelial layer in lattice dystrophy. (× 125.)

lial or Bowman's layer involvement that is not apparent on initial histologic examination.

Ultrastructural examination shows the lesions to be amyloid, consisting of extracellular masses of fine, electron-dense fibrils with diameters of 8 to 10 nm[140,141] (Figure 18-37). Most of the fibrils are highly aligned, which explains the birefringence and dichroism; however, most do not show periodicity. Normal or electron-dense collagen fibrils may admix with finer amyloid fibrils near the edges of the lesions. Associated amorphous electron-dense elastoid material has been noted in some cases. Keratocytes in the involved areas are decreased in number and may show cytoplasmic vacuolation and degeneration, while others appear metabolically active, with prominent dilated endoplasmic reticulum and Golgi apparatus.[140,142,143] Descemet's membrane is usually normal but sometimes contains amyloid deposits. The endothelium in lattice dystrophy is usually normal.[139,142]

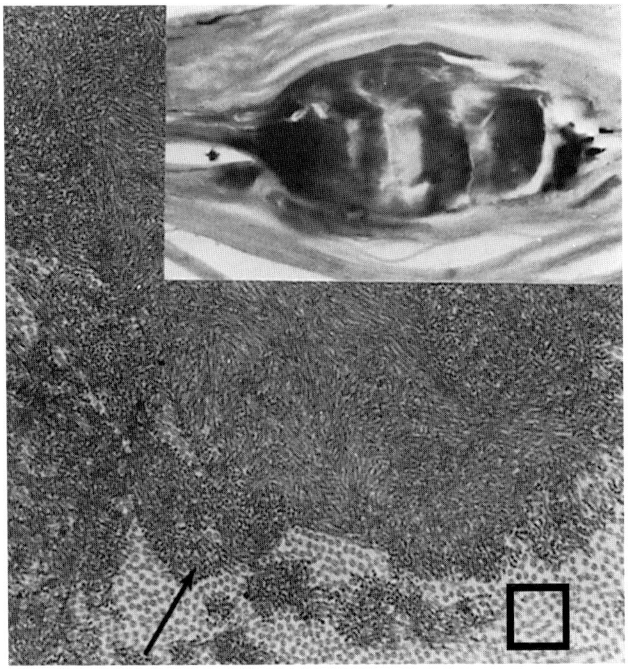

FIGURE 18-37 Lattice dystrophy. Inset: Fusiform lesion that distorts the normal stromal lamellar architecture. (Congo red, × 500.) Transmission electron micrograph shows masses of 10-nm-diameter amyloid filaments (arrow) with adjacent normal stromal collagen fibrils (box). (× 45,000.) (Reprinted with permission from GO Waring, MM Rodrigues, PR Laibson: Corneal dystrophies. I. Dystrophies of the epithelium, Bowman's layer and stroma. Surv Ophthalmol 23:71, 1978.)

Amyloid is a glycoprotein with a fibrous component that differs from collagen in amino acid content and fibril character. Amyloidosis is classified into two basic groups: systemic and localized. Each group is subdivided into primary and secondary amyloidosis.[144] In primary systemic amyloidosis, the amyloid contains fragments of immunoglobulin light chains. A similar component (M-component) is found in the serum or urine. In secondary amyloidosis, the main amyloid component is a nonimmunoglobulin protein (protein AA) usually found in association with an elevated serum amyloid A-related protein (SAA). All types of systemic amyloidosis, as well as several localized forms of amyloidosis, are associated with a structural protein (protein AP), which is also present in normal serum.

Evaluation of corneas with lattice dystrophy type I has not demonstrated the presence of the immunoglobulin light chains. The presence of the structural protein (protein AP) has been documented. Staining with antibodies to protein AA was initially reported as positive.[145,146] However, more detailed studies were unable to corroborate the presence of protein AA in lattice dystrophy.[147] Amyloid deposits have not been found in other excised tissues from patients with lattice dystrophy type I.[142,148] Lectin binding studies of corneal specimens from lattice dystrophy have shown that the amyloid in the stromal lesions is at least in part glycoconjugated.[147,149] Immunospecific binding has identified some of the sugar residues involved.[150] Concurrent deposition of extracellular glycoprotein is more widespread in the stroma.[149] The source of this material has yet to be elucidated.

Lattice dystrophy type II (Meretoja syndrome) is associated with type IV familial neuropathic syndrome, a form of systemic amyloidosis.[148,151] It has rarely been described other than in patients of Finnish origin.[152] The onset of clinical corneal changes in this generalized amyloidosis is later, erosive symptoms are less frequent, and the visual outcome is more favorable than in lattice dystrophy type I.[11] Other systemic manifestations, including cranial and peripheral neuropathies and dermatologic involvement, become prominent with age. Histopathologic examination demonstrates amyloid deposits in the arteries, basement membranes, skin, peripheral nerves, sclera, and other tissues. Open-angle glaucoma and pseudoexfoliation with or without glaucoma are frequently found.[153]

In lattice dystrophy type II, clinical examination shows lattice lines that are fewer and more radially oriented than those seen in lattice dystrophy type I; type II lattice lines mainly involve the peripheral cornea, with relative central sparing. The amorphic dots are fewer in number and more confined in distribution than in lattice dystrophy type I. Histopathologic study demonstrates a regular amyloid layer formed beneath a normal-appearing Bowman's layer, in contrast to the disrupted Bowman's layer encountered in lattice dystrophy type I. Fewer, but similar stromal lesions with typical amyloid-staining characteristics are found.[148] A variant gelsolin molecule, caused by mutations in the gelsolin gene on chromosome 9, has been identified as the major constituent of amyloid deposits in lattice dystrophy type II.[154]

Clinical variants of lattice dystrophy have been reported in five Asian patients (lattice dystrophy type III) and two families of Italian descent (lattice dystrophy type IIIA).[155,156] These patients presented with decreased vision late in life. Deep, large lattice lines were seen to nearly traverse the cornea with relative central sparing. Diffuse subepithelial opacities, nodular deposits, and stromal haze were less prominent findings. Systemic amyloidosis was absent. Histopathology showed significantly larger stromal amyloid deposits and a discontinuous band of amyloid between Bowman's layer and the stroma.[156,157] Unlike in the other types of lattice corneal dystrophy, no significant subepithelial deposits were found. Immunohistochemical studies showed mild staining of the deposits with antibodies to amyloid protein AA.[157] The differences between lattice dystrophies types I, II, III, and IIIA are summarized in Table 18-2.

Amyloid deposits may occur in the cornea in other disorders, including primary familial amyloidosis of the cornea[158,159] (gelatinous drop-like dystrophy[160,161]), the Avellino variant of granular corneal dystrophy,[101,104,105] and polymorphic amyloid degeneration.[162] Amyloid may also be found in association with local ocular diseases and trauma.[163]

The treatment of lattice dystrophy includes management of recurrent epithelial erosions in the early course and excimer laser phototherapeutic keratectomy or penetrating keratoplasty in the later stages if visual acuity is poor. Penetrating keratoplasty carries a good prognosis. However, recurrence in the graft occurs more commonly than in granular or macular dystrophy.[164] In these recurrences, elevated subepithelial opacities, fine lattice lines, or diffuse haze in the anterior stroma are usually seen in the periphery but may also appear centrally. These findings must be differentiated from signs of graft rejection or disciform edema. Electron microscopy has confirmed the amyloid nature of these deposits even when typical staining characteristics have not been demonstrated on light microscopy.[143]

TABLE 18-2
Differentiation of the Lattice Dystrophies

Feature	*Lattice Dystrophy Type I (Classic Lattice Dystrophy)*	*Lattice Dystrophy Type II (Meretoja Syndrome)*	*Lattice Dystrophy Type III*	*Lattice Dystrophy Type IIIA*
Age of onset	1st decade	3rd decade or later	5th decade or later	4th–5th decade
Inheritance	Autosomal dominant	Autosomal dominant	Autosomal recessive	Autosomal dominant
Systemic involvement	None	Cranial and peripheral neuropathies Skin masses including eyelids Lacrimal gland Arteries throughout body Kidneys and other organs	None	None
Reduced vision	By 2nd–3rd decade	Not present except in extreme cases	By 7th decade	By 5th decade
Erosions	Frequent	Unusual	None	Frequent
Slit lamp findings	Early Refractile tiny lines and dots Subepithelial spots Diffuse central haze Becomes Lattice lines with knobs Various-sized amorphous deposits Stromal haze Limbal zone clear except in extreme cases	Lattice lines Fewer in number Tendency toward radial orientation Most reach limbus Densest in corneal midperiphery Relative axial sparing Coarser than type I Cornea between lines Clearer than type I Fewer amorphous deposits	Lattice lines Much thicker More numerous More opaque Limbus to limbus Ribbon-like Cornea between lines Diffuse subepithelial opacities	Lattice lines Ropy, branching Nearly limbus to limbus Deep lines thicker Superficial lines shorter and thinner Cornea between lines Small dots Nodular opacities Haze
Material accumulated	Amyloid	Amyloid	Amyloid	Amyloid

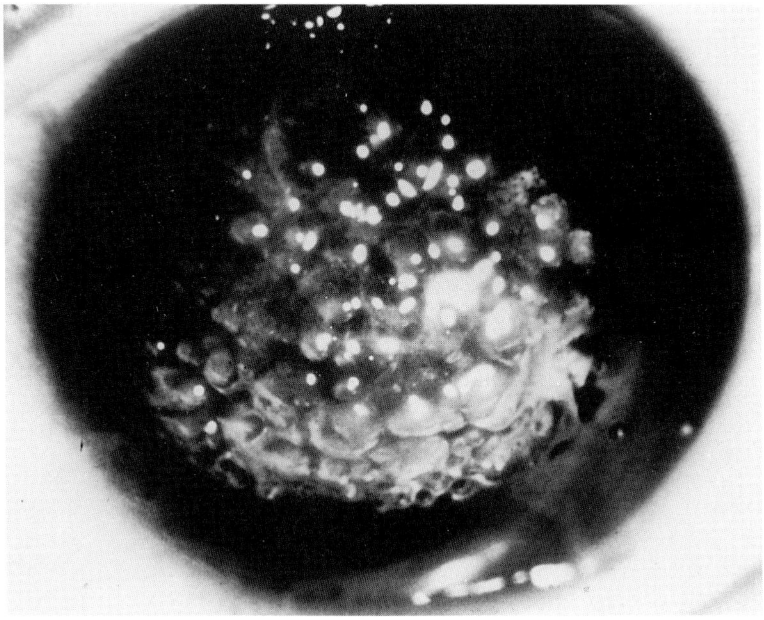

FIGURE 18-38 Gelatinous drop-like dystrophy. Deposition of amyloid has a mulberry-like appearance. (Courtesy of the Armed Forces Institute of Pathology, Washington, DC, AFIP 22-1590.)

Gelatinous Drop-Like Dystrophy

Gelatinous drop-like dystrophy is a rare, familial disorder that has been well documented in the Japanese literature since it was first reported by Nakaizumi in 1914.[165] A similar condition was described in the European literature in 1930.[166] Later, investigators in the United States termed the dystrophy *primary familial amyloidosis of the cornea*.[158,159] The inheritance of the dystrophy appears to be autosomal recessive with low penetrance. A significant number of the reported cases have shown ancestral consanguinity. There are no known associated systemic findings in this inherited form of corneal amyloidosis.

This bilateral dystrophy usually presents in the first decade of life with photophobia, lacrimation, and decreased visual acuity. Early in the dystrophy, the changes may resemble those of primary band keratopathy.[167] Examination shows a central mulberry-like opacity with protuberant subepithelial mounds that appear white on focal illumination and semitransparent on retroillumination (Figure 18-38). With age, the opacities increase in number and depth. Surrounding the mound-like excrescences, flat, often dense subepithelial opacities are seen. Vascularization, if present, is usually minimal, and anterior and posterior cortical lens changes have been reported.[158]

Multiple subepithelial deposits with typical staining and polarization findings of amyloid are present[158-161,168-171] (Figure 18-39). Bowman's layer is usually absent. A flat, more uniform layer of a similar material may surround the nodular masses. Ultrastructural examination demonstrates the amyloid nature of these deposits. Fusiform stromal amyloid deposits that resemble those found in lattice dystrophy have also been seen. The origin of the amyloid deposits has been attributed to the basal epithelial cells.[170,171] Rapid superficial recurrence of this dystrophy following lamellar keratoplasty has been reported.[172,173]

Central Crystalline Dystrophy (Schnyder's Dystrophy)

Central crystalline dystrophy is one of the most rare and least severe types of stromal corneal dystrophy. Characteristic findings were first described by Van Went and Wibaut in three generations of a single pedigree.[174] Schnyder clarified the entity and documented its stable and asymptomatic initial clinical course and autosomal dominant inheritance.[175,176] Typically, a ring-shaped, yellow-white opacity develops in the central cornea or is noted early in life[177-179] (Figure 18-40). Involvement is usually bilateral and symmetrical. Reported unilateral cases usually have shown eventual bilaterality. The opacity has a regular border and consists of numerous fine polychromatic crystals located in the anterior stroma and Bowman's layer. A variety of overall morphologies of the crystalline aggregates have been described, in addition to a disciform central opacification of the cornea without crystals.[180] A single pedigree may have any combination of the various morphologies, and there may be great variability in the extent of the involvement within a single family.[181]

Although the crystals are probably present early in life, the pattern of a central stromal opacity usually has devel-

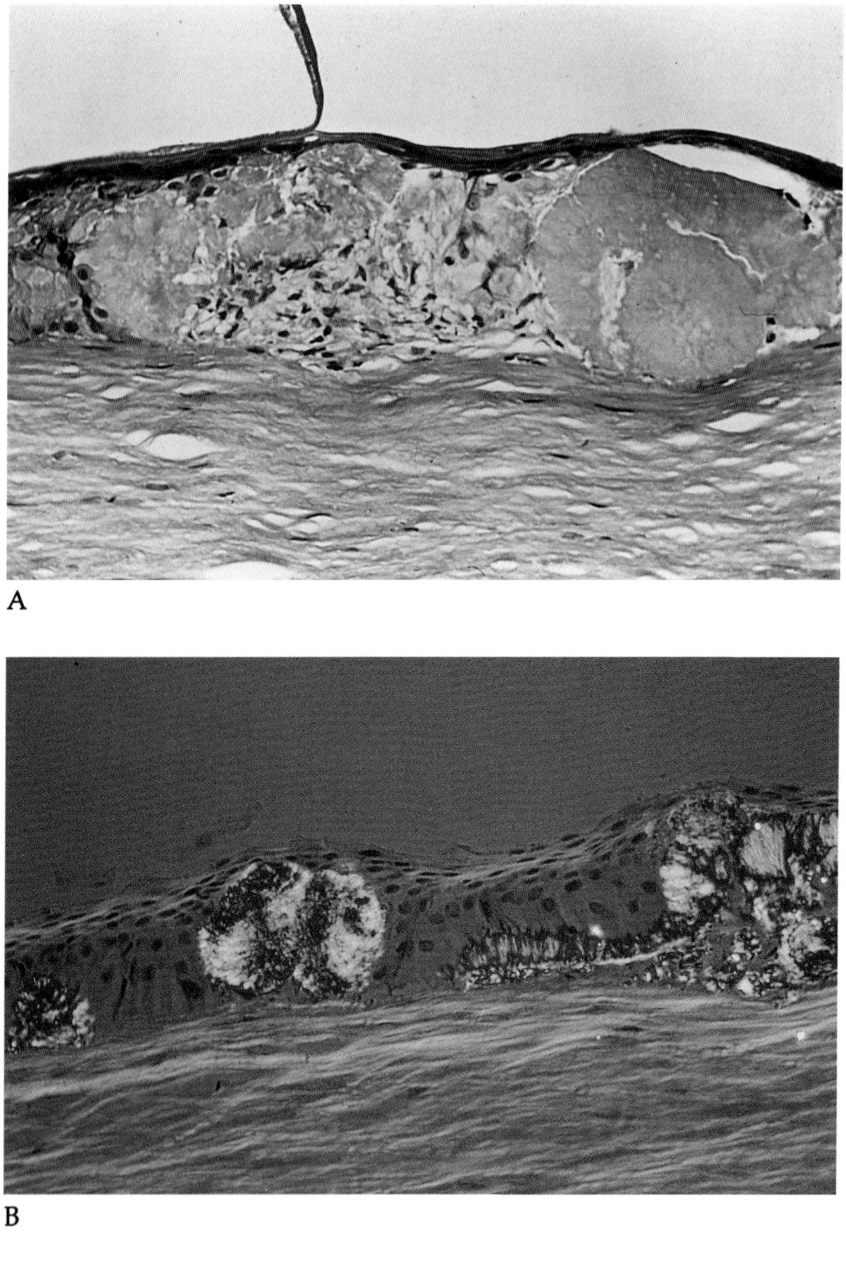

A

B

FIGURE 18-39 Subepithelial deposits of amyloid in gelatinous drop-like dystrophy. **(A)** Hematoxylin and eosin. **(B)** Congo red stain and polarized light. (Courtesy of the Armed Forces Institute of Pathology, Washington, DC, AFIP 11-15874.)

oped by the second or third decade.[180,182] From this point on, a prominent arcus lipoides is usually seen as an opacification of the peripheral cornea with relative central sparing. The progression of the corneal changes may slow in later life and significant visual loss, when present, is related to the development of central corneal opacification, often with decreased corneal sensation.[182]

Chondrodystrophy and genu valgum have appeared in certain pedigrees.[180,183–186] Hyperlipidemia has been reported in a significant percentage of patients with central crystalline dystrophy, although no correlation between the presence or extent of the dystrophy and the type of lipid elevation exists.[184,185,187,188] In a single family, individuals may have crystalline dystrophy, the dystrophy and hyperlipidemia, or only hyperlipidemia.

Slit lamp examination shows a myriad of minute, needle-like crystals that usually appear polychromatic on focal and indirect illumination. Palisades, aggregates, or meshwork clumps of these crystals in the anterior stroma often take on a geographic, annular, or disciform appearance. Although the crystals are usually most prevalent in the anterior third of the cornea, they may extend to the deeper

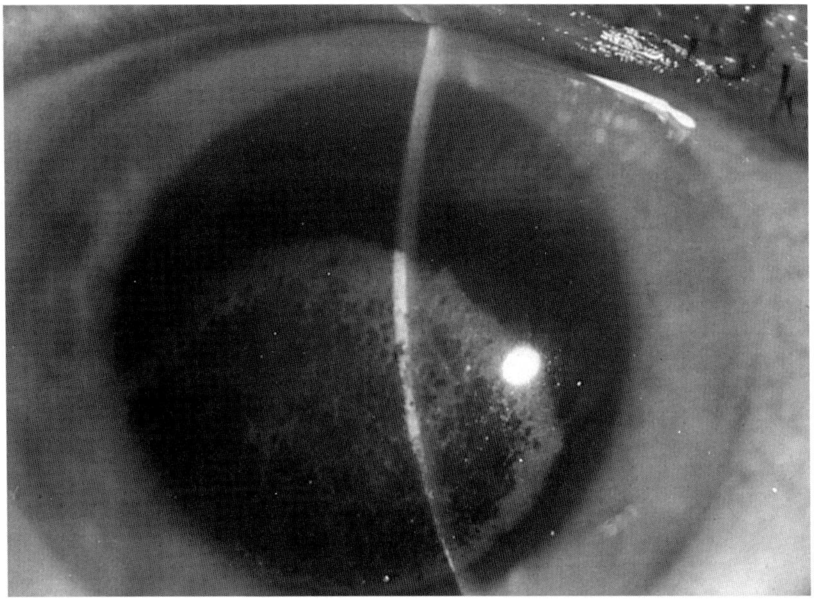

FIGURE 18-40 Characteristic anterior corneal opacity in central crystalline dystrophy.

stromal layers and cause a milky opalescence of the cornea.[185] The intervening stroma is usually clear but may be hazy due to smaller punctate stromal opacities.[178,181,184] Descemet's membrane and the endothelium usually appear uninvolved. The associated arcus may be very dense and involves all stromal layers. The stroma on either side of the arcus usually remains clear but may become diffusely involved with an atypical appearance in some cases.[185] Corneal sensation is usually normal but may be diminished diffusely or locally over the axial lesions.

Frozen light microscopy specimens show birefringent cholesterol crystals and globular neutral fats that correspond to the needle-like crystals and finer stromal opacities seen clinically.[181,189-193] The epithelium varies in thickness, and Bowman's layer and the overlying epithelial basement membrane may be replaced in places with fibrous tissue. Oil red O staining for cholesterol esters and triglycerides shows deposits primarily in Bowman's layer, the anterior stroma, and just anterior to Descemet's membrane. Studies have shown deposits that stain with filipin, a marker for unesterified cholesterol, and that can also be seen by electron microscopy.[91,193] These unesterified cholesterol deposits are localized primarily to the extracellular stromal matrix.[181]

Ultrastructural examination[181,190-192,194-197] shows focal degeneration of the basal epithelial layers and partial replacement of Bowman's layer with abnormal collagen and fibroblasts. Characteristic larger trapezoidal or smaller oblong-shaped spaces disrupt the normal stromal architecture and are seen primarily in the superficial to middle stroma. The clear spaces result from extraction of the cholesterol and lipids by the embedding solvents (Figure 18-41). A fine granular or fibrillar electron-dense material may be found at the edges of the larger cholesterol clefts. Although most cases have shown relatively normal posterior layers, a pathologic specimen in an advanced clinical case showed extensive vesicular spaces anterior to Descemet's membrane.[192] The presence of progressive corneal lipid deposition in central crystalline dystrophy, without vascularization or consistent serum lipid abnormalities, suggests localization of the metabolic abnormality to the cornea. Although the composition of the deposits has been clarified, their pathogenesis remains unknown.[181,193]

All patients with crystalline dystrophy should be investigated for systemic hyperlipidemia with the appropriate fasting blood studies. In those individuals with normal serum cholesterol and triglyceride levels, lipoprotein electrophoresis should also be performed. Excimer laser phototherapeutic keratectomy may be used to treat central crystalline dystrophy. Lamellar or penetrating keratoplasty has been required in a minority of patients. Recurrences of the crystals have occurred in both penetrating[180] and lamellar grafts.[180,189]

Corneal conditions other than central crystalline dystrophy clinically manifest similar polychromatic crystals. Bietti's crystalline dystrophy shows tiny anterior stromal and subepithelial crystals in the peripheral cornea with similar refractile bodies within the retina.[198,199] The pathologic findings are similar to those of central crystalline dystrophy with the exception that in Bietti's, crystals are also found in circulating lymphocytes.[199]

Corneal crystals may also be seen in the various types of monoclonal gammopathies,[200,201] although the per-

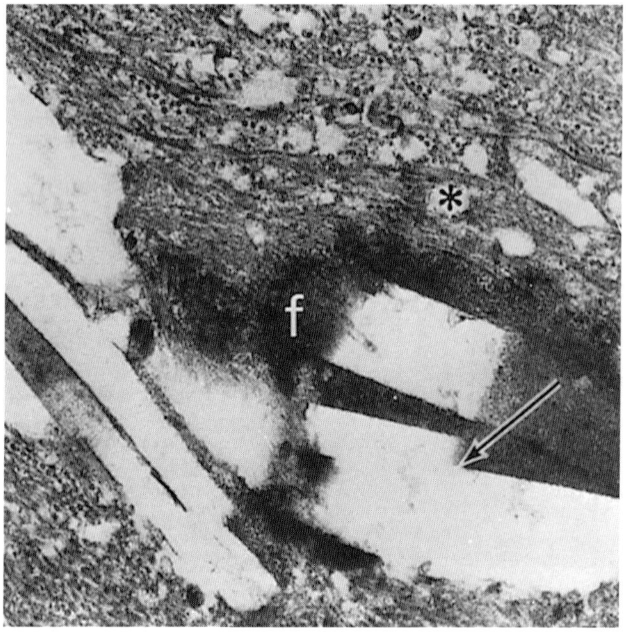

FIGURE 18-41 Central crystalline dystrophy. Transmission electron micrograph demonstrates geometric-shaped crystal spaces (arrow) surrounded by fine electron-dense fibrillogranular deposits *(f)*. Small round empty spaces (asterisk) are seen in the surrounding stroma. (× 45,000.) (Reprinted with permission from GO Waring, MM Rodrigues, PR Laibson: Corneal dystrophies. I. Dystrophies of the epithelium, Bowman's layer and stroma. Surv Ophthalmol 23:71, 1978.)

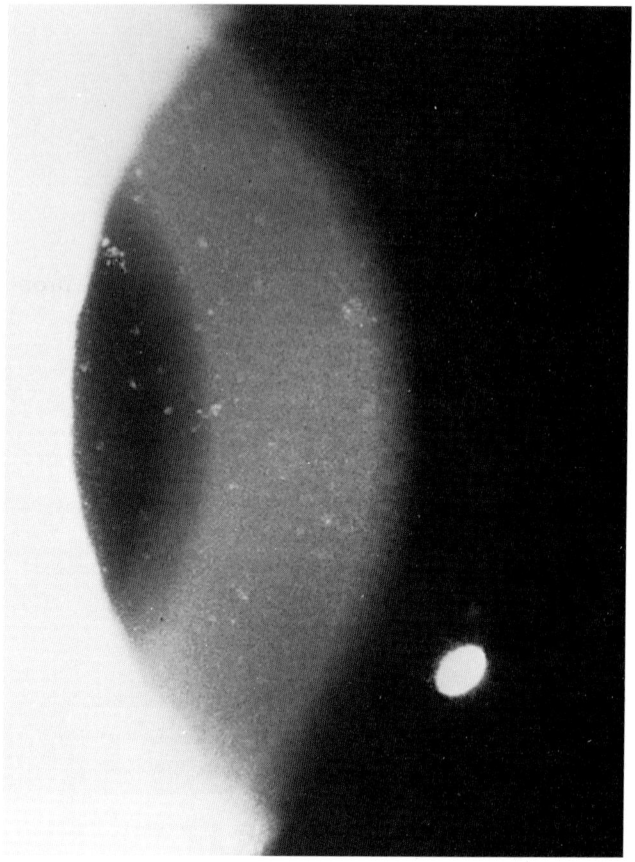

FIGURE 18-42 Slit lamp photograph of fleck dystrophy with diffuse, irregularly shaped opacities.

centage of these patients with clinically visible crystals is low.[202] Cystine corneal crystals may be seen in all three forms (infantile, adolescent, and adult) of cystinosis[203–205] (see Ch. 17).

Other causes of corneal crystals include lipid keratopathy, primary lipoidal degeneration of the cornea, climatic droplet keratopathy,[206] gout, chronic renal failure, hypercalcemia, chronic drug therapy,[207] graft rejection, and familial lecithin:cholesterol acyltransferase (LCAT) deficiency.[208]

Fleck Dystrophy

François and Neetens[209] first described fleck dystrophy in 31 members of a single pedigree. This rare, autosomal dominant dystrophy may be congenital and is usually noted as an incidental finding on routine examination. Although generally bilateral, it may be asymmetrical, and strictly unilateral cases have been reported.[210–212] An occasional patient may have mild photophobia, but no symptoms or erosions are present, and vision is unaffected. Once documented, fleck dystrophy is stable or slowly progressive and is characterized by small, gray-white, discrete opacities that extend to the limbus in all stromal levels. The corneal changes are subtle and are seen only with careful slit lamp examination. The opacities vary in size, configuration, depth, and number (Figure 18-42). With focal illumination, homogeneous dots and flecks are present, as are comma-shaped, stellate, circular, and wreath-like opacities. Individual opacities often show a doughnut-like peripheral opacity with sharp borders and a relatively clear center. On optical section, the individual opacities appear flat or disk-shaped, with very little anteroposterior thickness (Figure 18-43). The intervening stroma, epithelium, and endothelium are normal. The opacities are usually widely dispersed but occasionally form aggregations in the more anterior stromal levels. Corneal sensation is normal, although cases of familial decreased corneal sensation have appeared.[213]

There are no regularly associated ocular or systemic disorders. A variety of ocular conditions, including esotropia,[209] central cloudy corneal dystrophy,[209,214,215] granular corneal dystrophy,[216] keratoconus,[217] limbal dermoid,[217] papillitis,[217] angioid streaks,[217] and punctate cortical lens opacities[218] have been reported in patients with fleck dystrophy. However, these combinations are probably random coincidences. Extensive systemic evaluation has failed to demonstrate any generalized mucopolysaccharide abnormality.[211]

Light microscopic findings are limited to occasional abnormally distended keratocytes, which are found at all stromal levels. The remainder of the stroma, as well as the epithelium, Bowman's layer, Descemet's membrane, and endothelium, is histopathologically normal. The presence of lipid in these involved keratocytes is readily demonstrated by staining with Sudan black B and oil red O stains. Alcian blue and colloidal iron stains for glycosaminoglycans are also positive; staining corresponds to the distended keratocytes.[219,220] Congo red stain for amyloid is negative.[219] As with macular dystrophy, no significant staining for glycosaminoglycans is present in the conjunctival cells.

Electron microscopy demonstrates extensive membrane-limited cytoplasmic vacuolations within the keratocytes (Figure 18-44). The majority of the vacuoles contain a fibrillogranular material, while other vacuoles contain smaller vesicles.[220] Both of these types of vacuoles contain occasional membranous inclusions and pleomorphic electron-dense deposits.[219,220] In the less involved keratocytes,

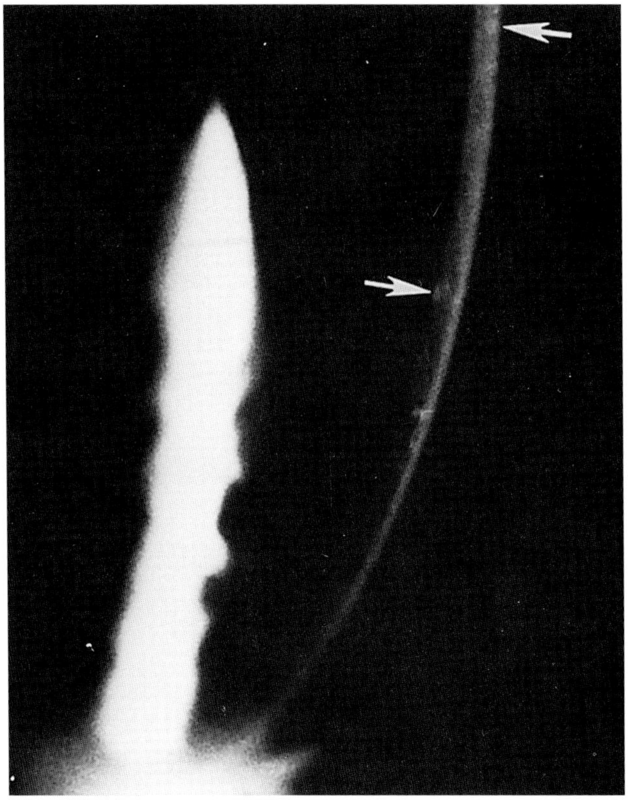

FIGURE 18-43 Individual stromal opacities (arrows) in fleck dystrophy are located at various stromal levels as demonstrated by slit lamp examination with a narrow beam.

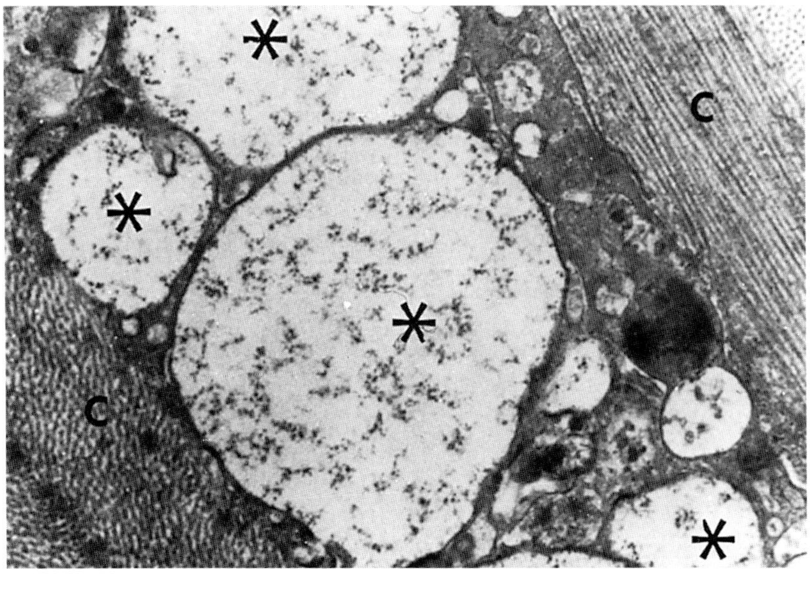

FIGURE 18-44 Fleck dystrophy. Transmission electron micrograph shows large, membrane-limited intracytoplasmic vacuoles (asterisks) that contain a fine fibrillogranular material. The surrounding collagen fibrils *(C)* are normal.

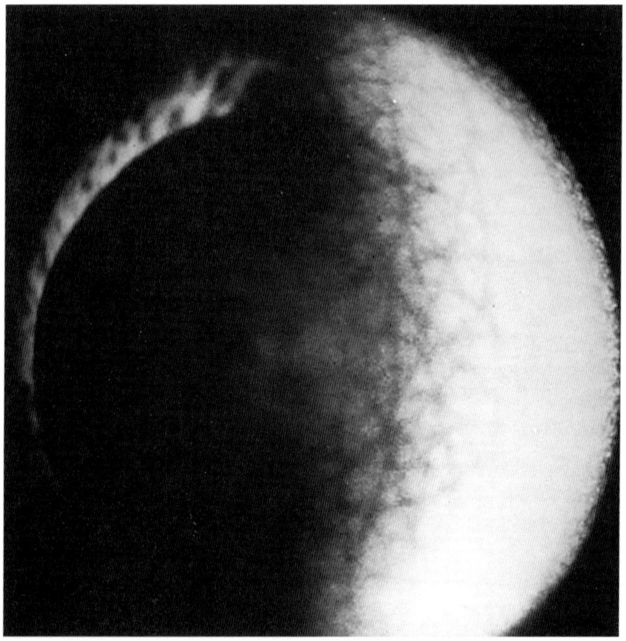

FIGURE 18-45 Slit lamp photograph of diffuse posterior crocodile shagreen.

the vacuoles appear to be associated principally with prominent Golgi complexes. Nonspecific electron microscopic changes can be seen in the surrounding stroma, but no specific extracellular material is identifiable. This finding differs from the histopathologic appearance in macular dystrophy in that only isolated keratocytes are involved, with no extracellular glycosaminoglycan accumulation.

Based on the histologic findings, fleck dystrophy appears to be a storage disorder that involves glycosaminoglycans and complex lipids; it is limited to the cornea. Fleck dystrophy is inherited as an autosomal dominant trait, which is unique genetically, because metabolic disorders typically show recessive inheritance. No associated systemic abnormalities or ocular disorders are uniformly present, progression is minimal, and treatment is not required.

Polymorphic Stromal "Dystrophy" (Polymorphic Amyloid Degeneration)

In this bilaterally symmetrical disorder, polymorphic gray opacities are seen in the middle and deep layers of the stroma, usually after the fifth decade of life.[162] Patients are asymptomatic, and no associated systemic or ocular diseases are usually present. The heritability of this condition has not been demonstrated in family studies.[162,221] It is considered a degeneration associated with aging and is appropriately termed *polymorphic amyloid degeneration*.

Examination reveals heterogeneous stromal opacities of the central cornea. These opacities may resemble the individual lesions found in lattice dystrophy.[222] Deep stromal opacities indent Descemet's membrane and can alter the red reflex. The individual lesions are gray-white on focal illumination, refractile or glass-like with indirect lighting, and transparent on retroillumination. In contrast to lattice dystrophy, in this disorder the intervening stroma is clear, corneal sensation is intact, the corneal surface remains smooth, and vision is not affected. Histochemical and electron microscopic studies have confirmed the amyloid nature of the deposits.[162,223] The surrounding keratocytes show increased rough endoplasmic reticulum.[162]

Central Cloudy Dystrophy

Central cloudy dystrophy is a bilaterally symmetrical, nonprogressive dystrophy that was first described as a faint, deep opacification in the central stroma occurring in two siblings and six additional unrelated patients.[224] Subsequent reports documented the familial nature of this entity, and an autosomal dominant inheritance was observed.[225,226] Central cloudy dystrophy has been reported as early as the first decade of life, and unilateral cases have appeared.[224,227,228] Some patients have presented with other ocular disorders, including fleck and pre-Descemet's dystrophies, spherophakia, and glaucoma. Corneal thickness and sensation are normal, vision is not affected, and treatment is not required in central cloudy dystrophy.

The lesions are not macroscopically visible and rarely progress. Slit lamp examination shows involvement of the central two-thirds of the cornea, with multiple grayish opacities in the deep stroma that are separated by narrow lines of relatively clear stroma. The opacities have been described as snowflake-like and are best seen with broad oblique illumination or sclerotic scatter. They are most dense posteriorly but can extend into the anterior third of the stroma. The margins of the lesions are fluffy and indistinct, but the intervening crack-like areas of clear stroma impart a polygonal structure to the opacities. This mosaic pattern is similar to that seen in anterior mosaic dystrophy and is also seen in a significant percentage of the aging population.[228] Descemet's membrane and the endothelium are clinically normal. This disorder seems clinically identical to posterior crocodile shagreen[229] (Figure 18-45). Unless multiple family members, preferably in more than one generation and over a wide range of ages, have the findings, it is probably more appropriate to diagnose the condition as posterior crocodile shagreen.[223,230]

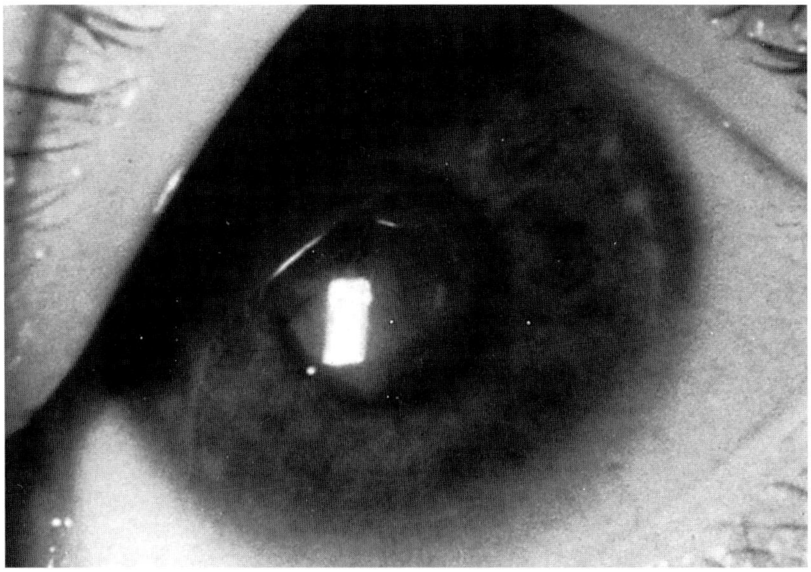

FIGURE 18-46 Posterior amorphous corneal dystrophy in a 6-month-old infant.

Ultrastructural examination in one case of clinical posterior crocodile shagreen demonstrated a unique configuration of the collagen lamellae.[223] Some of the lamellae were oriented at right angles to others and interspersed in these areas were patches of abnormal collagen with 100-nm banding. The uninvolved peripheral and anterior stromal architecture was normal.

The absence of increased corneal thickness or Descemet's folds makes central corneal dystrophy easily distinguishable from central corneal edema. Although located in the same stromal layers, the more diffuse nature of the opacities in central corneal dystrophy should be readily differentiated from the discrete lesions of pre-Descemet's dystrophy and cornea farinata. Unlike posterior amorphous stromal dystrophy, which manifests as anterior and peripheral stromal involvement and significant corneal thinning, central cloudy dystrophy shows normal corneal thickness and does not extend to the periphery.

Posterior Amorphous Corneal Dystrophy

Posterior amorphous corneal dystrophy is an extremely rare autosomal dominant condition that was first described in three generations of a single pedigree in 1977.[231] A study of eight affected members spanning five generations in a second pedigree confirmed the autosomal dominant inheritance.[232] Posterior amorphous corneal dystrophy is characterized by deep stromal opacification and corneal thinning in the absence of vascularization or inflammation.[231] Additional features include extension to the limbus, flattened corneal topography, hypermetropia, and anterior iris abnormalities.[232] The presence of the dystrophy in a 6-month-old infant (Figure 18-46) who was noted to have corneal clouding at the age of 16 weeks suggests that the changes may be congenital.

Slit lamp examination reveals layers of gray, sheet-like opacities in the posterior stroma. These amorphous opacities occur in central, central-peripheral, diffuse, and peripheral forms. Although they are most prominent in the deeper stromal layers, all stromal layers have been reported to be involved in some cases (Figure 18-47). Clear stromal breaks in the sheets of the opacification can be seen with focal or retroillumination. Descemet's membrane may be involved with posterior bowing and distortion of the endothelial pattern. Central, often uniform corneal thinning, with flattened keratometry readings, is present in patients who have central involvement. Specular microscopy may show nonspecific findings in the underlying endothelial mosaic.[232]

Gonioscopy may demonstrate a prominent Schwalbe's ring with numerous fine iris processes. Various iris anomalies including prominent pupillary membrane remnants,[232] anterior stromal tags,[232] corectopia,[231] iridocorneal adhesions,[231] and a generalized sponginess of the iris stroma have been described. There are no reported nonocular associated conditions.

The clinical appearance of posterior amorphous corneal dystrophy can be differentiated from other forms of corneal clouding seen in early life. Thinning of the central cornea may also be found in macular dystrophy and interstitial keratitis. The stromal pathology is similar to that of the mesenchymal dysgeneses, including Peters' anomaly, sclerocornea, and congenital endothelial corneal dystrophy. The documented involvement at a young age,

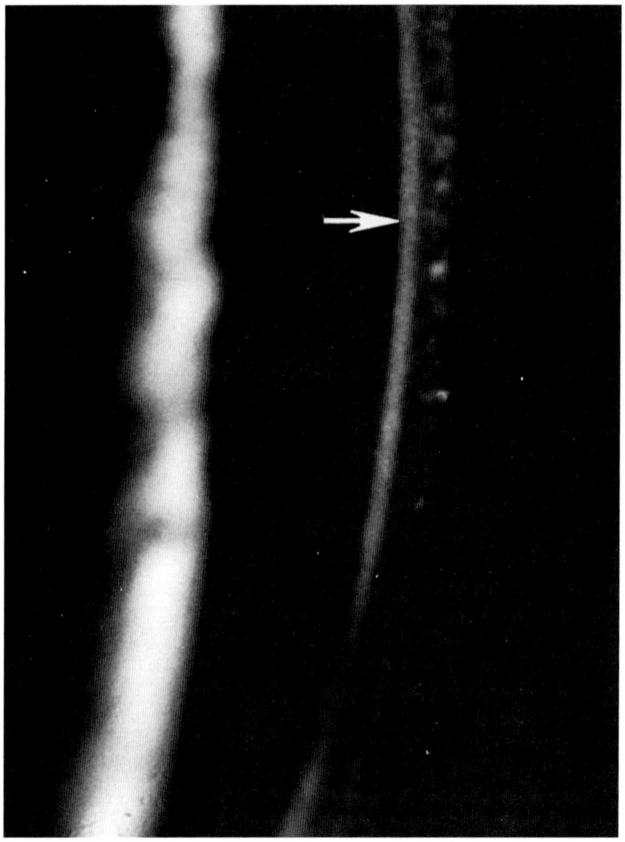

FIGURE 18-47 Posterior amorphous corneal dystrophy. A gray sheet of opacification (arrow) is demonstrated deep in the posterior cornea on slit beam section. Less dense opacities are located more anteriorly.

the lack of evidence of significant progression, and the disorganized pathologic appearance suggest a congenital origin. The variability in the reported pathology of the fetal portion of Descemet's membrane leaves the embryonic development of this dystrophy unclear.[233,234]

Congenital Hereditary Stromal Dystrophy

Primary, inherited, bilateral congenital opacification of the cornea has been classified in a number of different ways.[3,14] Most congenital corneal clouding has been linked to endothelial dysfunction and fits into the categories of congenital hereditary endothelial dystrophy or posterior polymorphous dystrophy. One nonprogressive corneal dystrophy has been separated from other causes of congenital corneal opacification on the basis of unique clinical corneal findings and a characteristic electron microscopic appearance.[235] This disorder, termed *congenital hereditary stromal dystrophy,* appears to be the result of disordered stromal fibrogenesis. Two pedigrees with typical electron microscopic findings have been studied, although there may be other reports in the literature with similar clinical and light microscopic presentations.[235,236] In both of the families documented by electron microscopy, the dystrophy appeared to be inherited in an autosomal dominant fashion.

Clinical examination shows a diffuse, flaky or feathery haze most evident in the central anterior stroma and less obvious in the deep peripheral stroma. The opacification is present at birth and appears stationary with periodic observations over a period as long as 11 years. In contrast to congenital hereditary endothelial dystrophy, the stromal disorder is characterized by the normal appearance of the anterior and posterior layers of the cornea, as well as normal central corneal thickness. Corneal sensation is also normal, and epithelial edema and recurrent erosions do not occur. Early visual deprivation may result in nystagmus and strabismus, which are often present at an early age.[235]

The epithelium and Bowman's layer are normal by both light and electron microscopy. The stromal lamellae show clefting or fine layering without significant stromal edema. The distinctive ultrastructural picture consists of alternating layers of small-diameter collagen fibrils of approximately one-half the normal fibril diameter. The layers consist of tightly packed, aligned fibrils in a lamella sandwiched by layers of smaller fibrils arranged in a more random fashion. Although collagen fibrils of similar diameter may be found in granular and lattice dystrophies, the alternating lamellar pattern is distinctive for congenital hereditary stromal dystrophy. The anterior banded portion of Descemet's membrane is poorly developed, although the posterior portion of Descemet's membrane and its overall thickness are normal. Unlike congenital hereditary endothelial dystrophy, which demonstrates a markedly abnormal endothelium and disorganization of the posterior portion of Descemet's membrane, the endothelium in congenital hereditary stromal dystrophy is normal.[235]

The pathogenesis of congenital hereditary stromal dystrophy remains unclear, but probably involves disordered fibrogenesis of stromal collagen. The endothelium may play an early role in the production of this disorder as evidenced by the abnormal anterior portion of Descemet's membrane. However, later endothelial function and morphology appear to be normal.[235]

Penetrating keratoplasty has been performed with no known clinical recurrence of the stromal pattern. However, as in other congenital anomalies of the visual axis, the resultant visual acuity following penetrating keratoplasty is determined by the extent of the deprivation amblyopia. Earlier and more aggressive intervention with penetrating keratoplasty, although technically difficult, may result in improved rehabilitation.

Pre-Descemet's Dystrophies

A number of disorders involving fine opacities limited to the extreme posterior stroma have been reported. Although more than one case has been seen in some families, inheritance of these conditions has been questioned. They may represent a spectrum of sporadically appearing or degenerative changes.[4] The opacities usually appear between the fourth and seventh decades of life and may show a variety of morphologies. Previous descriptions of this group of heterogeneous disorders have included cornea farinata, deep filiform dystrophy,[237,238] posterior punctiform dystrophy,[239] punctate pre-Descemet's dystrophy,[240] and pre-Descemet's dystrophy.[241]

Cornea farinata is the most frequently encountered of these disorders. Myriads of fine dust or flour-like opacities are found diffusely in the deep stroma. The opacities are more prominent in the central cornea and are best seen with broad oblique or retroillumination. Familial occurrence of cornea farinata has been described,[242,243] but it is generally thought to be a degenerative process associated with aging.

Pre-Descemet's dystrophy exhibits opacities at the same level, but they are larger and more polymorphous in appearance than those present in cornea farinata (Figure 18-48). However, these two entities have been reported to occur concomitantly in the same eye or as separate lesions in opposite eyes of the same patient.[241] Differing morphologies of the discrete deposits, including dendritic, boomerang, circular, dot-like, comma-shaped, linear, filiform, and semicircular shapes, have been described.[241,244] The distribution of these homogeneous deposits may be central or diffuse, or they may form an annular pattern with sparing of the central and far peripheral cornea. Inheritance over two generations was described in three pedigrees, and the disorder occurred in siblings in another family.[241] Similar opacities have been seen in patients with other ocular and systemic conditions, including keratoconus,[237,241,245] epithelial basement membrane dystrophy,[241] posterior polymorphous dystrophy,[241] central cloudy corneal dystrophy,[246] pseudoxanthoma elasticum,[247] and juvenile asteroid hyalosis.[248] Identical lesions can also be found in affected males and carriers of X-linked recessive ichthyosis.[249]

Histopathologic studies obtained in one case with the clinical diagnosis of pre-Descemet's dystrophy showed the pathologic involvement to be limited to the posterior stromal keratocytes, with striking vacuolation and enlargement of the affected cells and histochemical staining of lipid-like material.[244] Transmission electron microscopy showed cytoplasmic membrane-bound vacuoles containing a fibrillogranular material and electron-dense lamellar inclusions. No extracellular deposition of a similar material was noted. These pathologic findings suggest the accumulation of a lipofuscin-like material, which supports the hypothesis that pre-Descemet's dystrophy is actually a degeneration associated with aging. Recent histopathologic and immunochemical studies of a patient presenting with more optically dense opacities just anterior to Descemet's membrane showed immunoglobulin deposits.[250] Serum studies failed to reveal any detectable dysproteinemia in this case. Consideration should be given to serum study for evaluation of dysproteinemia in patients with unusual deposits in the posterior stroma.[250,251]

A clinically distinct disorder termed *punctiform and polychromatic pre-Descemet's dominant corneal dystrophy* has been described in four generations of a single pedigree.[252]

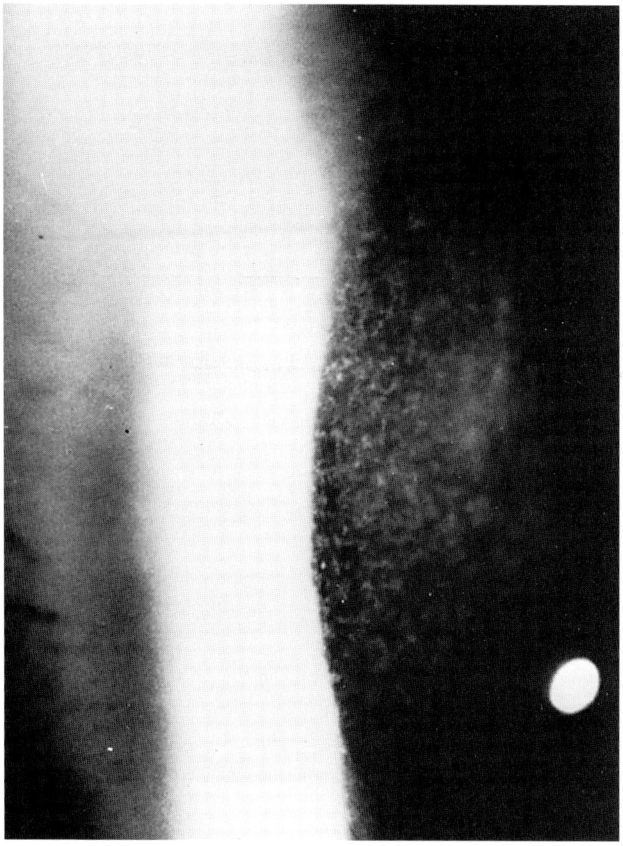

FIGURE 18-48 Slit lamp photograph of pre-Descemet's dystrophy demonstrates numerous, irregular, deep stromal opacities that are highlighted by indirect illumination.

This disorder differed from pre-Descemet's dystrophy by exhibiting more uniform, polychromatic, deep stromal filaments extending to the limbus. No particular aggregations or annular patterns were observed, and Descemet's membrane and the endothelium were not clinically affected. An autosomal dominant inheritance was suggested in a study of 46 family members. No histopathologic specimens from this clinical variant have been described.

REFERENCES

1. Duke-Elder SS: System of Ophthalmology. Vol. VIII, Part 2. Diseases of the Outer Eye. CV Mosby, St. Louis, 1965
2. François J: Heredo-familial corneal dystrophies. Trans Ophthalmol Soc UK 86:367, 1966
3. Malbran ES: Corneal dystrophies: a clinical, pathological and surgical approach. Trans Am Acad Ophthalmol Otolaryngol 76:573, 1972
4. Waring GO, Rodrigues MM, Laibson PR: Corneal dystrophies. I. Dystrophies of the epithelium, Bowman's layer and stroma. Surv Ophthalmol 23:71, 1978
5. Waring GO, Rodrigues MM, Laibson PR: Corneal dystrophies. II. Endothelial dystrophies. Surv Ophthalmol 23:147, 1978
6. Miller CA, Krachmer JH: Corneal diseases. In Renie WA (ed): Goldberg's Genetic and Metabolic Eye Disease. Little, Brown, Boston, 1986
7. Lang GK, Naumann GO: The frequency of corneal dystrophies requiring keratoplasty in Europe and the USA. Cornea 6:209, 1987
8. François J: Metabolic disorders and corneal changes. Dev Ophthalmol 4:1, 1981
9. McTigue JW: The human cornea: a light and electron microscopic study of the normal cornea and its alterations in various dystrophies. Trans Am Ophthalmol Soc 65:591, 1967
10. Polack FM: Contributions of electron microscopy to the study of corneal pathology. Surv Ophthalmol 20:375, 1976
11. Klintworth GK: Corneal dystrophies. p. 23. In Nicholson DH (ed): Ocular Pathology Upate. Masson, New York, 1980
12. Rodrigues MM, Krachmer JH: Recent advances in corneal stromal dystrophies. Cornea 7:19, 1988
13. Fogle JA, Kenyon KR, Stark WJ, Green WR: Defective epithelial adhesion in anterior corneal dystrophies. Am J Ophthalmol 79:925, 1975
14. Franceschetti A: Classification and treatment of hereditary corneal dystrophies. Arch Ophthalmol 52:1, 1954
15. François J: Heredofamilial corneal dystrophies. p. 114. In Symposium on Surgical and Medical Management of Congenital Anomalies of the Eye, Transactions of the New Orleans Academy of Ophthalmology. CV Mosby, St. Louis, 1968
16. Pameijer JK: Uber eine fremdartige familiäre oberflächliche Hornhautveranderung. Klin Monatsbl Augenheilkd 95:516, 1935
17. Meesmann A: Uber eine bisher nicht beschriebene dominant vererbte Dystrophia epithelialis corneae. Ber Zusammenkunft Dtsch Ophthalmol Ges 52:154, 1938
18. Meesmann A, Wilke F: Klinische und anatomische Untersuchungen über eine bisher unbekannte, dominant vererbte Epitheldystrophie der Hornaut. Klin Monatsbl Augenheilkd 103:361, 1939
19. Burns RP: Meesmann's corneal dystrophy. Trans Am Ophthalmol Soc 66:530, 1968
20. Snyder WB: Hereditary epithelial corneal dystrophy. Am J Ophthalmol 55:56, 1963
21. Stocker FW, Holt LB: Rare form of hereditary epithelial dystrophy. Arch Ophthalmol 53:536, 1955
22. Wittebol-Post D, van Bijsterveld OP, Delleman JW: Meesmann's epithelial dystrophy of the cornea: biometrics and a hypothesis. Ophthalmologica 194:44, 1987
23. Kuwabara T, Ciccarelli EC: Meesmann's corneal dystrophy. Arch Ophthalmol 71:676, 1964
24. Fine BS, Yanoff M, Pitts E, Slaughter FD: Meesmann's epithelial dystrophy of the cornea. Am J Ophthalmol 83:633, 1977
25. Cogan DG, Kuwabara T, Donaldson DD, Collins E: Microscopic dystrophy of the cornea: a partial explanation for its pathogenesis. Arch Ophthalmol 92:470, 1974
26. Tremblay M, Dubé I: Meesmann's corneal dystrophy: ultrastructural features. Can J Ophthalmol 17:24, 1982
27. Nakanishi I, Brown SI: Ultrastructure of the epithelial dystrophy of Meesmann. Arch Ophthalmol 93:259, 1975
28. Lisch W, Steuhl KP, Lisch C, et al: A new, band-shaped and whorled microcystic dystrophy of the corneal epithelium. Am J Ophthalmol 114:35, 1992
29. Cogan DG, Donaldson DD, Kuwabara T, Marshall D: Microcystic dystrophy of the corneal epithelium. Trans Am Ophthalmol Soc 63:213, 1964
30. Guerry D: Observations on Cogan's microcystic dystrophy of the corneal epithelium. Trans Am Ophthalmol Soc 63:320, 1965
31. Guerry D: Fingerprint lines in the cornea. Am J Ophthalmol 33:724, 1950
32. Vogt A: Lehrbuch und Atlas der Spaltlampenmikroskopie des Lebenden Auges. Vol. I. Julius Springer, Berlin, 1930
33. DeVoe AG: Certain abnormalities of Bowman's membrane with particular reference to fingerprint lines in the cornea. Trans Am Ophthalmol Soc 60:195, 1962
34. Wolter JR, Fralick FB: Microcystic dystrophy of corneal epithelium. Arch Ophthalmol 75:380, 1966
35. Trobe JD, Laibson PR: Dystrophic changes in the anterior cornea. Arch Ophthalmol 87:378, 1972
36. Laibson PR: Microcystic corneal dystrophy. Trans Am Ophthalmol Soc 74:488, 1976
37. Laibson PR, Krachmer JH: Familial occurrence of dot (microcystic), map, fingerprint dystrophy of the cornea. Invest Ophthalmol 14:397, 1975
38. Werblin TP, Hirst LW, Stark WJ, Maumenee IH: Prevalence of map-dot-fingerprint change in the cornea. Br J Ophthalmol 65:401, 1981

39. Bron AJ, Brown NA: Some superficial corneal disorders. Trans Ophthalmol Soc UK 91:13, 1971
40. Bron AJ: Superficial fibrillary lines: a feature of the normal cornea. Br J Ophthalmol 59:133, 1975
41. Brown NA, Bron AJ: Recurrent erosion of the cornea. Br J Ophthalmol 60:84, 1976
42. Schoch DE, Stock EL, Schwartz AE: Stromal keratitis complicating anterior membrane dystrophy. Am J Ophthalmol 100:199, 1985
43. Rodrigues MM, Fine BS, Laibson PR, Zimmerman LE: Disorders of the corneal epithelium: a clinicopathologic study of dot, geographic, and fingerprint patterns. Arch Ophthalmol 92:475, 1974
44. Brodrick JD, Dark AJ, Peace GW: Fingerprint dystrophy of the cornea: a histological study. Arch Ophthalmol 92:483, 1974
45. Dark AJ: Cogan's microcystic dystrophy of the cornea: ultrastructure and photomicroscopy. Br J Ophthalmol 62:821, 1978
46. Dark AJ: Bleb dystrophy of the cornea: histochemistry and ultrastructure. Br J Ophthalmol 61:65, 1977
47. Foulks GN: Treatment of recurrent corneal erosion and corneal edema with topical osmotic colloidal solution. Ophthalmology 88:801, 1981
48. Buxton JN, Constad WH: Superficial epithelial keratectomy in the treatment of epithelial basement membrane dystrophy. Ann Ophthalmol 19:92, 1987
49. Wood TO, Griffith ME: Surgery for corneal epithelial basement membrane dystrophy. Ophthalmic Surg 19:20, 1988
50. Rubinfeld RS, Laibson PR, Cohen EJ, et al: Anterior stromal puncture for recurrent erosion: further experience and new instrumentation. Ophthalmic Surg 21:318, 1990
51. Geggel HS: Successful treatment of recurrent corneal erosion with Nd:YAG anterior stromal puncture. Am J Ophthalmol 110:404, 1990
52. Cavanagh HD, Pihlaja D, Thoft R, Dohlman CH: Pathogenesis and treatment of persistent epithelial defects. Trans Am Acad Ophthalmol Otolaryngol 81:754, 1976
53. Wales HJ: A family history of corneal erosions. Trans Ophthalmol Soc NZ 8:77, 1955
54. Franceschetti A: Hereditäre rezidivierende Erosion der Hornhaut. Z Augenheilkd 66:309, 1928
55. Goldman JN, Dohlman CH, Kravitt BW: The basement membrane of the human cornea in recurrent epithelial erosion syndrome. Trans Am Acad Ophthalmol Otolaryngol 73:471, 1969
56. François J: Erosion dystrophique récidivante de l'epithélium cornéen. Ophthalmologica (Basel) 177:121, 1978
57. Reis W: Familiäre fleckige Hornhautentartung. Dtsch Med Wochenschr 43:575, 1917
58. Bücklers M: Über eine weitere familiäre Hornhautdystrophie (Reis). Klin Monatsbl Augenheilkd 114:386, 1949
59. Hall P: Reis-Bücklers' dystrophy. Arch Ophthalmol 91:170, 1974
60. Yamaguchi T, Polack FM, Rowsey JJ: Honeycomb-shaped corneal dystrophy: a variation of Reis-Bücklers' dystrophy. Cornea 1:71, 1982
61. Jones ST, Stauffer LH: Reis-Bücklers' corneal dystrophy. Trans Am Acad Ophthalmol Otolaryngol 74:417, 1970
62. Griffith DG, Fine BS: Light and electron microscopic observations in a superficial corneal dystrophy. Am J Ophthalmol 63:1659, 1967
63. Hogan MJ, Wood I: Reis-Bücklers' corneal dystrophy. Trans Ophthalmol Soc UK 91:41, 1971
64. Perry HD, Fine BS, Caldwell DR: Reis-Bücklers' dystrophy. Arch Ophthalmol 97:664, 1979
65. Akiya S, Brown SI: The ultrastructure of Reis-Bücklers' dystrophy. Am J Ophthalmol 72:549, 1973
66. Yamaguchi T, Polack FM, Valenti J: Electron microscopic study of recurrent Reis-Bücklers' corneal dystrophy. Am J Ophthalmol 90:95, 1980
67. Wood TO, Fleming JC, Dotson RS, Cotten MS: Treatment of Reis-Bücklers' corneal dystrophy by removal of subepithelial fibrous tissue. Am J Ophthalmol 85:360, 1978
68. Grayson M, Wilbrandt H: Dystrophy of the anterior limiting membrane of the cornea (Reis-Bückler type). Am J Ophthalmol 61:345, 1966
69. Thiel H-J, Behnke H: Eine bisher unbekannte subepitheliale hereditäre Hornhautdystrophie. Klin Monatsbl Augenheilkd 150:862, 1967
70. Weidle EG: Differentialdiagnose der hornhautdystrophien vom typ Groenouw I, Reis-Bücklers, und Thiel-Behnke. Fortschr Ophthalmol 86:265, 1989
71. Fuchs A: Über primäre qeurtelfoermige Hornhauttrübung. Klin Monatsbl Augenheilkd 103:300, 1939
72. Streiff EB, Zwahlen P: Une famille avec dégénérescence en bandelette de la cornée. Ophthalmologica 111:129, 1946
73. Velhagen CH: Über die primäre bandförmige Hornhauttrübung. Klin Monatsbl Augenheilkd 42:428, 1904
74. Glees M: Über familiäres Auftreten der primären, bandfoermigen Hornhautdegeneration. Klin Monatsbl Augenheilkd 116:185, 1950
75. Meisler DM, Tabbara KF, Wood IS, et al: Familial band-shaped nodular keratopathy. Ophthalmology 92:217, 1985
76. Pouliquen Y, Dhermy P, Presles D, Tollard MF: Dégénérescence en Chagrin de crocodile de Vogt ou dégénérescence en mosaique de Valerio. Arch Ophtalmol (Paris) 36:395, 1976
77. Kopsa M, Marusic K: Contribution à l'étude de la dégénérescence en mosaïque de la membrane de Bowman de la cornée. Ophthalmologica 136:83, 1958
78. Boles-Carenini B: Juvenile familial mosaic degeneration of the cornea associated with megalocornea. Br J Ophthalmol 45:64, 1961
79. Malbran E, D'Alessandro C, Valenzuela J: Megalocornea and mosaic dystrophy of the cornea. Ophthalmologica 149:161, 1965
80. Tripathi RC, Bron AJ: Secondary anterior crocodile shagreen of Vogt. Br J Ophthalmol 59:59, 1975
81. Bron AJ: Anterior corneal mosaic. Br J Ophthalmol 52:659, 1968

82. Groenouw A: Knötchenförmige Hornhauttrübungen (noduli corneae). Arch Augenheilkd 21:281, 1890
83. Bücklers M: Die erblichen Hornhautdystrophie: Dystrophiae corneae hereditariae. Ferdinand Enke Verlag, Stuttgart, 1938
84. Biber H: Ueber einige seltene Hornhauterkrankungen. (Diss). Zurich, 1890
85. Haab O: Die gittrige Keratitis. Z Augenheilkd 2:235, 1899
86. Dimmer F: Über oberflächliche gittrige Hornhauttrübung. Z Augenheilkd 2:354, 1899
87. Bourquin JB, Babel J, Klein D: Nouvel arbre généalogique de dystrophie cornéene granuleuse (Groenouw I). J Genet Hum 3:137, 1954
88. Waardenburg PJ, Jonkers GH: A specific type of dominant progressive dystrophy of the cornea, developing after birth. Acta Ophthalmol (Copenh) 39:919, 1961
89. Haddad R, Font RL, Fine BS: Unusual superficial variant of granular dystrophy of the cornea. Am J Ophthalmol 83:213, 1977
90. Stone EN, Mathers WD, Rosenwasser GOD, et al: Three autosomal dominant corneal dystrophies map to chromosome 5q. Nature Genet 6:47, 1994
91. Rodrigues MM Gaster RN, Pratt MV: Unusual superficial confluent form of granular corneal dystrophy. Ophthalmology 90:1507, 1983
92. Sajjidi SH, Javadu MA: Superficial juvenile granular dystrophy. Ophthalmology 99:95, 1992
93. Rodrigues MM, Streeten BW, Krachmer JH: Microfibrillar protein and phospholipid in granular corneal dystrophy. Arch Ophthalmol 101:802, 1983
94. Rodrigues MM, Kruth HS, Rajagopalan S, Jones K: Unesterified cholesterol in granular, lattice, and macular dystrophies. Am J Ophthalmol 115:112, 1993
95. Akiya S, Brown SI: Granular dystrophy of the cornea. Arch Ophthalmol 84:179, 1970
96. Iwamoto T, Stuart JC, Srinivasan BD, et al: Ultrastructural variations in granular dystrophy of the cornea. Albrecht von Graefes Arch Klin Exp Ophthalmol 194:1, 1975
97. Sornson ET: Granular dystrophy of the cornea: an electron microscopic study. Am J Ophthalmol 59:1001, 1965
98. Garner A: Histochemistry of corneal granular dystrophy. Br J Ophthalmol 8:475, 1969
99. Johnson BL, Brown SI, Zaidman GW: A light and electron microscopic study of recurrent granular dystrophy of the cornea. Am J Ophthalmol 92:49, 1981
100. Klintworth GK: Proteins in ocular disease. In Garner A, Klintworth GK (eds): Pathology of Ocular Disease: A Dynamic Approach, Part B. Marcel Dekker, New York, 1982
101. Sassani JW, Smith SG, Rabinowitz YS: Keratoconus and bilateral lattice-granular corneal dystrophies. Cornea 11:343, 1992
102. Witschel H, Sundmacher R: Bilateral recurrence of granular corneal dystrophy in the grafts. Albrecht von Graefes Arch Klin Exp Ophthalmol 209:179, 1979
103. Lempert SL, Jenkins MS, Johnson BL, Brown SI: A simple technique for removal of recurring granular dystrophy in corneal grafts. Am J Ophthalmol 86:89, 1978
104. Folberg R, Alfonso E, Croxatto JO, et al: Clinically atypical granular corneal dystrophy with pathologic features of lattice-like amyloid deposits: a study of three families. Ophthalmology 95:46, 1988
105. Holland EJ, Daya SM, Stone EM, et al: Avellino corneal dystrophy: clinical manifestations and natural history. Ophthalmology 99:1564, 1992
106. Rosenwasser GOD, Sucheski BM, Rosa N, et al: Phenotypic variation in combined granular-lattice (Avellino) corneal dystrophy. Arch Ophthalmol 111:1546, 1993
107. Folberg R, Stone EM, Sheffield VC, Mathers WD: The relationship between granular, lattice type 1, and Avellino corneal dystrophies—a histopathologic study. Arch Ophthalmol 112:1080, 1994
108. Jonasson F, Johannsson JH, Garner A, Rice NSC: Macular corneal dystrophy in Iceland. Eye 3:446, 1989
109. Donnenfeld ED, Cohen EJ, Ingraham HJ, et al: Corneal thinning in macular corneal dystrophy. Am J Ophthalmol 101:112, 1986
110. Ehlers N, Bramsen T: Central thickness in corneal disorders. Acta Ophthalmol (Copenh) 56:412, 1978
111. Jones ST, Zimmerman LE: Histopathologic differentiation of granular, macular, and lattice dystrophies of the cornea. Am J Ophthalmol 51:394, 1961
112. Garner A: Histochemistry of corneal macular dystrophy. Invest Ophthalmol 8:473, 1969
113. Snip RC, Kenyon KR, Green WR: Macular corneal dystrophy: ultrastructural pathology of corneal endothelium and Descemet's membrane. Invest Ophthalmol 12:88, 1973
114. Teng CC: Macular dystrophy of the cornea: a histochemical and electron microscopic study. Am J Ophthalmol 62:436, 1966
115. François J, Hanssens M, Teuchy H, Sebruyns M: Ultrastructural findings in corneal macular dystrophy (Groenouw II type). Ophthalmic Res 7:80, 1975
116. Klintworth GK, Vogel FS: Macular corneal dystrophy: an inherited acid mucopolysaccharide storage disease of the corneal fibroblast. Am J Pathol 45:565, 1964
117. Tremblay M, Dubé I: Macular dystrophy of the cornea: ultrastructure of two cases. Can J Ophthalmol 8:47, 1973
118. Ghosh M, McCulloch C: Macular corneal dystrophy. Can J Ophthalmol 8:515, 1973
119. Livni N, Abraham FA, Zauberman H: Groenouw's macular dystrophy: histochemistry and ultrastructure of the cornea. Doc Ophthalmol 37:327, 1974
120. Hassell JR, Newsome DA, Hascall VC: Characterization and biosynthesis of proteoglycans of corneal stroma from rhesus monkey. J Biol Chem 254:12346, 1979
121. Klintworth GK, Smith CF: Abnormal product of corneal explants from patients with macular corneal dystrophy. Am J Pathol 101:143, 1980
122. Thonar EJ, Meyer RF, Dennis RF, et al: Absence of normal keratan sulfate in the blood of patients with macular corneal dystrophy. Am J Ophthalmol 102:561, 1986
123. Yang CJ, SundarRaj N, Thonar EJ, Klintworth GK: Immunohistochemical evidence of heterogeneity in

macular corneal dystrophy. Am J Ophthalmol 106:65, 1988
124. Edward DP, Yue BY, Sugar J, et al: Heterogeneity in macular corneal dystrophy. Arch Ophthalmol 106:1579, 1988
125. Edward DP, Thonar EJ, Srinivasan M, et al: Macular dystrophy of the cornea: a systemic disorder of keratan sulfate metabolism. Ophthalmology 97:1194, 1990
126. Quigley HA, Goldberg MF: Scheie syndrome and macular corneal dystrophy. Arch Ophthalmol 85:553, 1971
127. Robin AL, Green WR, Lapsa TP, et al: Recurrence of macular corneal dystrophy after lamellar keratoplasty. Am J Ophthalmol 85:457, 1977
128. Klintworth GK, Reed J, Stainer GA, Binder PS: Recurrence of macular corneal dystrophy within grafts. Am J Ophthalmol 95:60, 1983
129. Akova YA, Kirkness CM, McCartney AC, et al: Recurrent macular corneal dystrophy following penetrating keratoplasty. Eye 4:698, 1990
130. Newsome DA, Hassell JR, Rodrigues MM, et al: Biochemical and histological analysis of "recurrent" macular corneal dystrophy. Arch Ophthalmol 100:1125, 1982
131. Stansbury FC: Lattice type of hereditary corneal degeneration: report of five cases, including one of a child of two years. Arch Ophthalmol 40:189, 1948
132. Raab MF, Blodi F, Boniuk M: Unilateral lattice dystrophy of the cornea. Trans Am Acad Ophthalmol Otolaryngol 78:440, 1974
133. Lanier JD, Fine M, Togni B: Lattice corneal dystrophy. Arch Ophthalmol 94:921, 1976
134. Mehta RF: Unilateral lattice dystrophy of the cornea. Br J Ophthalmol 64:53, 1980
135. Dubord PJ, Krachmer JH: Diagnosis of early lattice corneal dystrophy. Arch Ophthalmol 100:788, 1982
136. Dark AJ, Thompson DS: Lattice dystrophy of the cornea: a clinical and microscopic study. Br J Ophthalmol 44:275, 1960
137. Dubord PJ, Rodrigues MM, Krachmer JH: Corneal elastosis in lattice corneal dystrophy. Ophthalmology 88:1239, 1981
138. Yanoff M, Fine BS, Colosi NJ, Katowitz JA: Lattice corneal dystrophy: report of an unusual case. Arch Ophthalmol 95:651, 1977
139. François J, Feher J: Light microscopy and polarization optical study of the lattice dystrophy of the cornea. Ophthalmologica 164:1, 1972
140. McTigue JW, Fine BS: The stromal lesion in lattice dystrophy of the cornea: a light and electron microscopic study. Invest Ophthalmol 3:355, 1964
141. François J, Hanssens M, Teuchy H: Ultrastructural changes in lattice dystrophy of the cornea. Ophthalmic Res 7:321, 1975
142. Klintworth GK: Lattice corneal dystrophy: an inherited variety of amyloidosis restricted to the cornea. Am J Pathol 50:371, 1967
143. Hogan MJ, Alvarado J: Ultrastructure of lattice dystrophy of the cornea: a case report. Am J Ophthalmol 64:656, 1967
144. Brownstein MH, Elliott R, Helwig EB: Ophthalmologic aspects of amyloidosis. Am J Ophthalmol 69:423, 1970
145. Mondino BJ, Raj CVS, Skinner M, et al: Protein AA and lattice corneal dystrophy. Am J Ophthalmol 89:377, 1980
146. Wheeler GE, Eiferman RA: Immunohistochemical identifications of the AA protein in lattice dystrophy. Exp Eye Res 36:181, 1983
147. Gorevic PE, Rodrigues MM, Krachmer JH, et al: Lack of evidence for protein AA reactivity in amyloid deposits of lattice corneal dystrophy and amyloid corneal degeneration. Am J Ophthalmol 98:216, 1984
148. Meretoja J: Comparative histopathological and clinical findings in eyes with lattice corneal dystrophy of two different types. Ophthalmologica 165:15, 1972
149. Bishop PN, Bonshek RE, Jones CJ, et al: Lectin binding sites in normal, scarred, and lattice dystrophy corneas. Br J Ophthalmol 75:22, 1991
150. Panjwani N, Rodrigues MM, Free K, et al: Lectin receptors of amyloid in corneas with lattice dystrophy. Arch Ophthalmol 105:688, 1987
151. Purcell JJ Jr, Rodrigues MM, Chishti MI, et al: Lattice corneal dystrophy associated with familial systemic amyloidosis (Meretoja's syndrome). Ophthalmology 90:1512, 1983
152. Starck T, Kenyon KR, Hanninen LA, et al: Clinical and histopathologic studies of two families with lattice corneal dystrophy and familial systemic amyloidosis (Meretoja syndrome). Ophthalmology 98:1197, 1991
153. Meretoja J, Tarkkanen A: Pseudoexfoliation syndrome in familial systemic amyloidosis with lattice corneal dystrophy. Ophthalmic Res 7:194, 1975
154. Rodrigues MM, Rajagopalan S, Jones K, et al: Gelsolin immunoreactivity in corneal amyloid, wound healing, and macular and granular dystrophies. Am J Ophthalmol 115:664, 1993
155. Hida T, Tsubota K, Kigasawa K, et al: Clinical features of a newly recognized type of lattice corneal dystrophy. Am J Ophthalmol 104:241, 1987
156. Stock EL, Feder RS, O'Grady RB, et al: Lattice corneal dystrophy type IIIA: clinical and histopathologic correlations. Arch Ophthalmol 109:354, 1991
157. Hida T, Proia AD, Kigasawa K, et al: Histopathologic and immunochemical features of lattice corneal dystrophy type III. Am J Ophthalmol 104:249, 1987
158. Kirk HG, Rabb H, Hattenhauer J, Smith R: Primary familial amyloidosis of the cornea. Trans Am Acad Ophthalmol Otolaryngol 77:411, 1973
159. Stock EL, Kielar RA: Primary familial amyloidosis of the cornea. Am J Ophthalmol 82:266, 1976
160. Akiya S, Ito I, Matsui M: Gelatinous drop-like dystrophy of the cornea: light and electron microscopic study of superficial stromal lesion. Jpn J Clin Ophthalmol 26:815, 1972
161. Weber FL, Babel J: Gelatinous drop-like dystrophy. Arch Ophthalmol 98:144, 1980
162. Mannis MJ, Krachmer JH, Rodrigues MM, Pardos GJ: Polymorphic amyloid degeneration of the cornea. Arch Ophthalmol 99:1217, 1981

163. Garner A: Amyloidosis of the cornea. Arch Ophthalmol 53:73, 1969
164. Meisler DM, Fine M: Recurrence of the clinical signs of lattice corneal dystrophy (type I) in corneal transplants. Am J Ophthalmol 97:210, 1984
165. Nakaizumi K: A rare case of corneal dystrophy. Nippon Ganka Gakkai Zasshi 18:949, 1914
166. Lewkojewa EF: Über einen Fall primärer Degenerationamyloidose der Kornea. Klin Monatsbl Augenheilkd 85:117, 1930
167. Kanai A, Kaufman HE: Electron microscopic studies of primary band-shaped keratopathy and gelatinous, drop-like corneal dystrophy in two brothers. Ann Ophthalmol 14:535, 1982
168. Akiya S, Furukawa H, Sakamoto H, et al: Histopathologic and immunohistochemical findings in gelatinous drop-like corneal dystrophy. Ophthalmic Res 22:371, 1990
169. Gartry DS, Falcon MG, Cox RW: Primary gelatinous drop-like keratopathy. Br J Ophthalmol 73:661, 1989
170. Takahashi M, Yokota T, Yamashita Y, et al: Unusual inclusions in stromal macrophages in a case of gelatinous drop-like corneal dystrophy. Am J Ophthalmol 99:312, 1985
171. Ohnishi Y, Shinoda Y, Ishibashi T, Taniguchi Y: The origin of amyloid in gelatinous drop-like corneal dystrophy. Curr Eye Res 2:225, 1982
172. Nagataki S, Tanishima T, Sakamoto T: A case of primary gelatinous drop-like corneal dystrophy. Jpn J Ophthalmol 16:107, 1972
173. Matsui M, Ito K, Akiya S: Histochemical and electron microscopic examinations on so-called gelatinous drop-like dystrophy of the cornea. Nippon Ganka Kiyo 23:466, 1972
174. Van Went JM, Wibaut F: Een zeldzame erfelijke hoornvliesaandoening. Ned Tijdschr Geneeskd 68:2996, 1924
175. Schnyder WF: Mitteilung über einen neuen Typus von familiärer Hornhauterkrankung. Schweiz Med Wochenschr 59:559, 1929
176. Schnyder WF: Scheibenförmige Kristalleinlagerungen in der Hornhautmitte als Erbleiden. Klin Monatsbl Augenheilkd 103:494, 1939
177. Karseras A, Price A: Central crystalline corneal dystrophy. Br J Ophthalmol 54:659, 1970
178. Ehlers N, Matthiessen M: Hereditary crystalline corneal dystrophy of Schnyder. Acta Ophthalmol (Copenh) 51:316, 1973
179. Grop K: Clinical and histological findings in crystalline corneal dystrophy. Acta Ophthalmol (Copenh) 120:52, 1973
180. Delleman JW, Winkelman JE: Degeneratio corneae cristallinea hereditaria: a clinical, genetical, and histological study. Ophthalmologica 155:409, 1968
181. Weiss JS, Rodrigues MM, Kruth HS, et al: Panstromal Schnyder's corneal dystrophy: ultrastructural and histochemical studies. Ophthalmology 99:1072, 1992
182. Weiss JS: Schnyder's dystrophy of the cornea: a Swede-Finn connection. Cornea 11:93, 1992
183. Fry WE, Pickett WE: Crystalline dystrophy of the cornea. Trans Am Ophthalmol Soc 48:220, 1950
184. Luxenberg M: Hereditary crystalline dystrophy of the cornea. Am J Ophthalmol 63:507, 1967
185. Bron AJ, Williams HP, Carruthers ME: Hereditary crystalline stromal dystrophy of Schnyder. I. Clinical features of a family with hyperlipoproteinaemia. Br J Ophthalmol 56:383, 1972
186. Hoang-Xuan T, Pouliquen Y, Gastau J: Dystrophie cristalline de Schnyder. II. Association a un genu valgum. J Fr Ophtalmol 8:743, 1985
187. Kaden R, Feurle G: Schnydersche Hornhautdystrophie und Hyperlipidämie. Albrecht von Graefes Arch Klin Exp Ophthalmol 198:129, 1976
188. Lisch W, Weidle EG, Lisch C, et al: Schnyder's dystrophy: progression and metabolism. Ophthalmic Paediatr Genet 7:45, 1986
189. Garner A, Tripathi RC: Hereditary crystalline stromal dystrophy of Schnyder. II. Histopathology and ultrastructure. Br J Ophthalmol 56:400, 1972
190. Weller RO, Rodger FC: Crystalline stromal dystrophy: histochemistry and ultrastructure of the cornea. Br J Ophthalmol 64:46, 1980
191. Rodrigues MM, Kruth HS, Krachmer JH, Willis R: Unesterified cholesterol in Schnyder's corneal crystalline dystrophy. Am J Ophthalmol 104:157, 1987
192. Freddo TF, Polack FM, Leibowitz HM: Ultrastructural changes in the posterior layers of the cornea in Schnyder's crystalline dystrophy. Cornea 8:170, 1989
193. Rodrigues MM, Kruth HS, Krachmer JH, et al: Cholesterol localization in ultrathin frozen sections in Schnyder's corneal crystalline dystrophy. Am J Ophthalmol 110:513 1990
194. Hoang-Xuan T, Pouliquen Y, Savoldelli M, Gasteau J: Dystrophie cristalline de Schnyder. I. Étude d'un cas en microscopie optique et en ultrastructure. J Fr Ophtalmol 8:735, 1985
195. Babel J, Englert U, Ricci A: La dystrophie cristalline de la cornée; étude histologique et ultrastructurale. Arch Ophtalmol (Paris) 33:721, 1973
196. Ghosh M, McCulloch C: Crystalline dystrophy of the cornea: a light and electron microscopic study. Can J Ophthalmol 12:321, 1977
197. Eiferman RA, Rodrigues MM, Laibson PR, Arentsen J: Schnyder's crystalline dystrophy associated with amyloid deposition. Metab Pediatr Ophthalmol 3:15, 1979
198. Bagolini B, Ioli-Spada G: Bietti's tapetoretinal degeneration with marginal corneal dystrophy. Am J Ophthalmol 65:53, 1968
199. Wilson DJ, Weleber RG, Klein ML, et al: Bietti's crystalline dystrophy: a clinicopathologic correlative study. Arch Ophthalmol 107:213, 1989
200. Barr CC, Gelender H, Font RL: Corneal crystalline deposits associated with dysproteinemia. Arch Ophthalmol 98:884, 1980
201. Orellana J, Friedman AH: Ocular manifestations of multiple myeloma, Waldenström's macroglobulinemia and

benign monoclonal gammopathy. Surv Ophthalmol 25:157, 1981
202. Bourne WM, Kyle RA, Brubaker RF, Greipp PR: Incidence of corneal crystals in the monoclonal gammopathies. Am J Ophthalmol 107:192, 1989
203. Sanderson P, Kuwabara T, Stark W, et al: Cystinosis, a clinical, histological and ultrastructural study. Arch Ophthalmol 91:270, 1974
204. Dodd MJ, Pusin SM, Green WR: Adult cystinosis: a case report. Arch Ophthalmol 96:1054, 1978
205. Melles RB, Schneider JA, Rao NA, Katz B: Spatial and temporal sequence of corneal crystal deposition in nephropathic cystinosis. Am J Ophthalmol 104:598, 1987
206. Gray RH, Johnson GJ, Freedman A: Climatic droplet keratopathy. Surv Ophthalmol 36:241, 1992
207. Font RL, Sobol W, Matoba A: Polychromatic corneal and conjunctival crystals secondary to clofazimine therapy in a leper. Ophthalmology 96:311, 1989
208. Gjone E: Familial lecithin:cholesterol acyltransferase (LCAT) deficiency: an updated review Spring 1988. Ophthalmic Paediatr Genet (Netherlands) 9:167, 1988
209. François J, Neetens A: Nouvelle dystrophie hérédo-familiale du parenchyme cornéen (hérédodystrophie Mouchetée). Bull Soc Belge Ophtalmol 114:641, 1957
210. Streeten BW, Falls HF: Hereditary fleck dystrophy of the cornea. Am J Ophthalmol 51:275, 1961
211. Patten JT, Hyndiuk RA, Donaldson DD, et al: Fleck (mouchetée) dystrophy of the cornea. Ann Ophthalmol 8:25, 1976
212. Goldberg MF, Krimmer B, Sugar J, et al: Variable expression in flecked (speckled) dystrophy of the cornea. Ann Ophthalmol 9:889, 1977
213. Birndorf LA, Ginsberg SP: Hereditary fleck dystrophy associated with decreased corneal sensitivity. Am J Ophthalmol 73:670, 1972
214. Gillespie F, Covelli B: Fleck (mouchetée) dystrophy of the cornea: report of a family. South Med J 56:1265, 1963
215. Collier M: Dystrophie mouchetée parenchyme cornéen avec dystrophie muageuse centrale. Bull Soc Ophtalmol Fr 64:608, 1964
216. Forsius H, Eriksson AW, Karna J, et al: Granular corneal dystrophy with late manifestation. Acta Ophthalmol (Copenh) 61:514, 1983
217. Purcell JJ Jr, Krachmer JH, Weingeist TA: Fleck corneal dystrophy. Arch Ophthalmol 95:440, 1977
218. Stankovic I, Stojanovic D: L'hérédodystrophie mouchetée du parenchyme cornéen. Ann Oculist (Paris) 197:52, 1964
219. Nicholson DH, Green WR, Cross HE, et al: A clinical and histopathological study of François-Neetens speckled corneal dystrophy. Am J Ophthalmol 83:554, 1977
220. Kiskaddon BM, Campbell RJ, Waller RR, Bourne W: Fleck dystrophy of the cornea: case report. Ann Ophthalmol 12:700, 1980
221. Strachan IM: Pre-Descemetic corneal dystrophy. Br J Ophthalmol 52:716, 1968
222. Thomsitt J, Bron AJ: Polymorphic stromal dystrophy. Br J Ophthalmol 59:125, 1975
223. Krachmer JH, Dubord PJ, Rodrigues MM, Mannis MJ: Corneal posterior crocodile shagreen and polymorphic amyloid degeneration. Arch Ophthalmol 101:54, 1983
224. François J: Une nouvelle dystrophie hérédo-familiale de la cornée. J Genet Hum 5:189, 1956
225. Strachan IM: Cloudy central dystrophy of François. Br J Ophthalmol 53:192, 1969
226. Bramsen T, Ehlers N, Baggesen LH: Central cloudy corneal dystrophy of François. Acta Ophthalmol (Copenh) 54:221, 1976
227. Bietti GB: Contribution à la connoissance des dégénérescences cornéennes seniles. Arch Ophtalmol (Paris) 25:37, 1965
228. Ansons AM, Atkinson PL: Corneal mosaic patterns—morphology and epidemiology. Eye 3:811, 1989
229. Vogt A: Corneal degenerations of various etiology. p. 120. In Blodi FC (trans): Textbook and Atlas of Slit Lamp Microscopy of the Living Eye. Vol. I. JP Wayenborgh, Bonn, 1981
230. Goodside V: Posterior crocodile shagreen. Am J Ophthalmol 46:748, 1958
231. Carpel EF, Sigelman RJ, Doughman DJ: Posterior amorphous corneal dystrophy. Am J Ophthalmol 83:629, 1977
232. Dunn SP, Krachmer JH, Ching SS: New findings in posterior amorphous dystrophy. Arch Ophthalmol 102:236, 1984
233. Johnson AT, Folberg R, Vrabec MP, et al: The pathology of posterior amorphous corneal dystrophy. Ophthalmology 97:104, 1990
234. Roth SI, Mittelman D, Stock EL: Posterior amorphous corneal dystrophy: an ultrastructural study of a variant with histopathological features of an endothelial dystrophy. Cornea 11:165, 1992
235. Witschel H, Fine BS, Grutzner P, McTigue JW: Congenital hereditary stromal dystrophy of the cornea. Arch Ophthalmol 96:1043, 1978
236. Desvignes P, Vigo A: À propos d'un cas de dystrophie cornéenne parenchymateuse familiale a heredite dominate. Bull Soc Ophtalmol Fr 55:220, 1955
237. Maeder G, Danis P: Sur une nouvelle forme de dystrophie cornéenne (dystrophia filiformis profunda corneae) associée à un keratôcone. Ophthalmologica 114:246, 1947
238. Franceschetti A, Chodos J, Dierterle P, Forni S: Severe filiforme dystrophy of the cornea. Bull Mem Soc Fr Ophtalmol 70:175, 1957
239. Franceschetti A, Maeder G: Dystrophic profonde de la cornée dans un cas d'ichtyose congénitale. Bull Mem Soc Fr Ophtalmol 64:146, 1954
240. Collier MM: Caractère hérédo-familial de la dystrophie ponciforme prédéscemetique. Bull Mem Soc Fr Ophtalmol 64:731, 1964
241. Grayson M, Wilbrandt H: Pre-Descemet dystrophy. Am J Ophthalmol 64:276, 1967
242. Pippow G: Zur Erbbedingtheit der Cornea Farinata. (Mehlstaubartige Hornhautdegeneration). Albrecht von Graefes Arch Ophthalmol 144:276, 1941
243. Paufigue L, Etienne R: La "cornea farinata." Bull Soc Ophtalmol Fr 50:522, 1950

244. Curran RE, Kenyon KR, Green WR: Pre-Descemet's membrane corneal dystrophy. Am J Ophthalmol 77:711, 1974
245. Collier M: Dystrophie filiforme profonde de la cornée. Bull Soc Ophtalmol Fr 64:1034, 1964
246. Collier M: Dystrophie nuageuse centrale et dystrophie pontiforme prédéscemtique dans une même famille. Bull Soc Ophtalmol Fr 66:575, 1966
247. Collier M: Elastorrhexie systématisée et dystrophies cornéennes chez deux soeur. Bull Soc Ophtalmol Fr 65:301, 1965
248. Dodwell DG, Freeman K, Shoch D: Juvenile asteroid hyalosis and pre-Descemet's dystrophy. Am J Ophthalmol 106:504, 1988
249. Sever RJ, Frost P, Weinstein G: Eye changes in ichthyosis. JAMA 206:2283, 1968
250. Yassa NH, Font RL, Fine BS, Koffler BH: Corneal immunoglobulin deposit in the posterior stroma: a case report including immunohistochemical and ultrastructural observations. Arch Ophthalmol 105:99, 1987
251. Rodrigues MM, Krachmer JH, Miller SD, et al: Posterior corneal crystalline deposits in benign monoclonal gammopathy: a clinicopathologic case report. Arch Ophthalmol 97:124, 1979
252. Fernandez-Sasso D, Acosta JEP, Malbran E: Punctiform and polychromatic pre-Descemet's dominant corneal dystrophy. Br J Ophthalmol 63:336, 1979

19

Endothelial Dystrophies

COREY A. MILLER AND JAY H. KRACHMER

Corneal transparency is maintained by the barrier and pump functions of the corneal endothelium (see Ch. 1). The structure and function of the endothelial cells can be affected by aging; by a variety of insults, such as trauma, medications, contact lens wear, and surgery; and by ocular disorders, such as glaucoma, interstitial keratitis, uveitis, and congenital anterior segment anomalies. Dystrophies that involve primarily the endothelium are not associated with ocular inflammation or systemic disease. Corneal endothelial dystrophies are important because they can reduce vision markedly as a result of endothelial cell dysfunction and the subsequent loss of corneal clarity. Two major endothelial dystrophies, Fuchs' dystrophy and posterior polymorphous dystrophy, are discussed in this chapter. Congenital hereditary endothelial dystrophy is discussed in Chapter 16. Although not considered a dystrophy, iridocorneal endothelial syndrome is included in this chapter to differentiate it from posterior polymorphous dystrophy and because it is thought to be a primary corneal endothelial disorder.

FUCHS' DYSTROPHY

In 1910, Ernst Fuchs described a condition that he termed *dystrophia epithelialis corneae*.[1] The disorder occurred in patients with corneal epithelial edema, stromal clouding, and decreased corneal sensation. At that time, the slit lamp microscope had not been invented, so Fuchs was unaware of the concomitant pathologic changes in the corneal endothelium. Longitudinal slit lamp microscopy later documented that endothelial changes precede the edematous epithelial changes by many years. Vogt was the first to use the Latin term *cornea guttata* to describe the slit lamp appearance of small excrescences on the posterior corneal surface.[2] Some confusion has occurred in the literature about this term, because the word *guttata* is often used to denote the individual lesions, more properly termed *guttae.*

Fuchs' dystrophy is a bilateral condition; however, it is often asymmetrical.[3] It may be associated with hypermetropia, short axial length, and a shallow anterior chamber.[4] Women are affected more severely and two and one-half times more frequently than men.[5,6] The earliest findings, the corneal guttae, are not specific for this disease in that most patients with guttae never develop the classic signs of Fuchs' dystrophy. In some patients, however, the guttae progress and the corneal endothelial cell layer loses its ability to maintain corneal clarity, resulting in stromal and epithelial edema and corneal scarring.

Clinical Features

Corneal Guttae

Corneal guttae are excrescences of Descemet's membrane produced by abnormal endothelial cells. Multiple central guttae associated with a fine stippling of pigment on the posterior corneal surface are seen by slit lamp microscopy. With direct illumination, the guttae appear as golden refractile mounds on the posterior corneal surface (Figure 19-1). With specular reflection, they appear as black holes in the endothelial cell mosaic (Figure 19-2). As the guttae become more extensive, dark areas appear throughout, and endothelial cells can no longer be seen (Figure 19-3). Guttae can involve the entire posterior corneal surface. Descemet's membrane has a beaten metal appearance, is thickened, and has faint gray irregular opacities, which are best seen on tangential focal illumination (Figure 19-4). The red reflex of retinoscopy reveals the diffuse mottled appearance of Descemet's membrane.

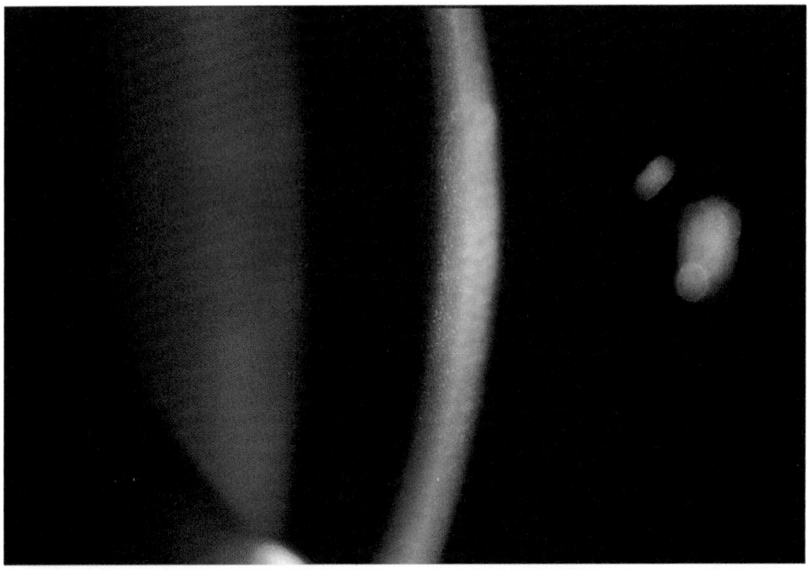

FIGURE 19-1 Pigmented guttae in a patient with Fuchs' dystrophy.

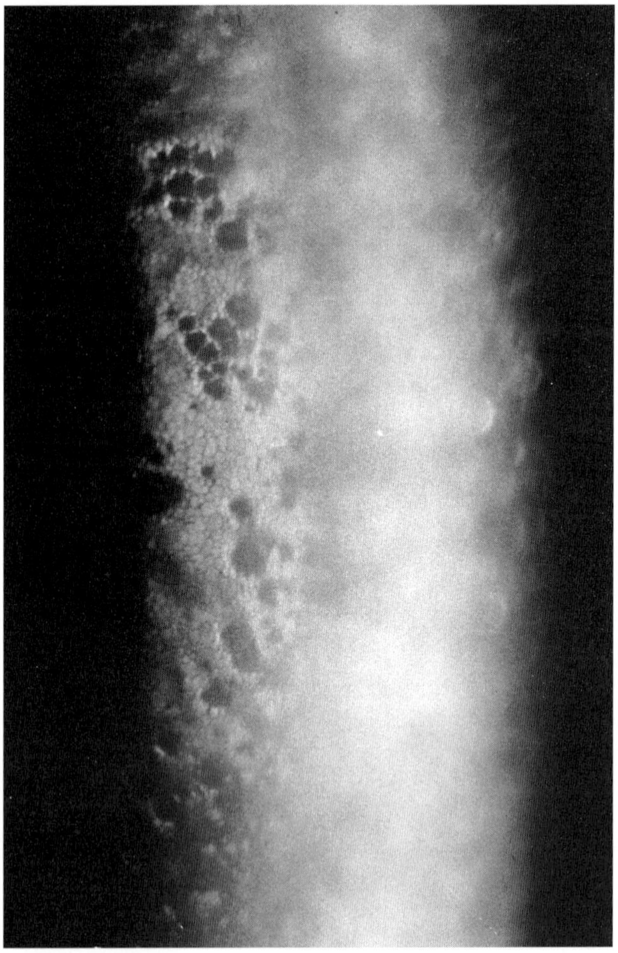

FIGURE 19-2 Specular photomicrograph of a patient with corneal guttae. Dark holes in the endothelial mosaic represent the guttae.

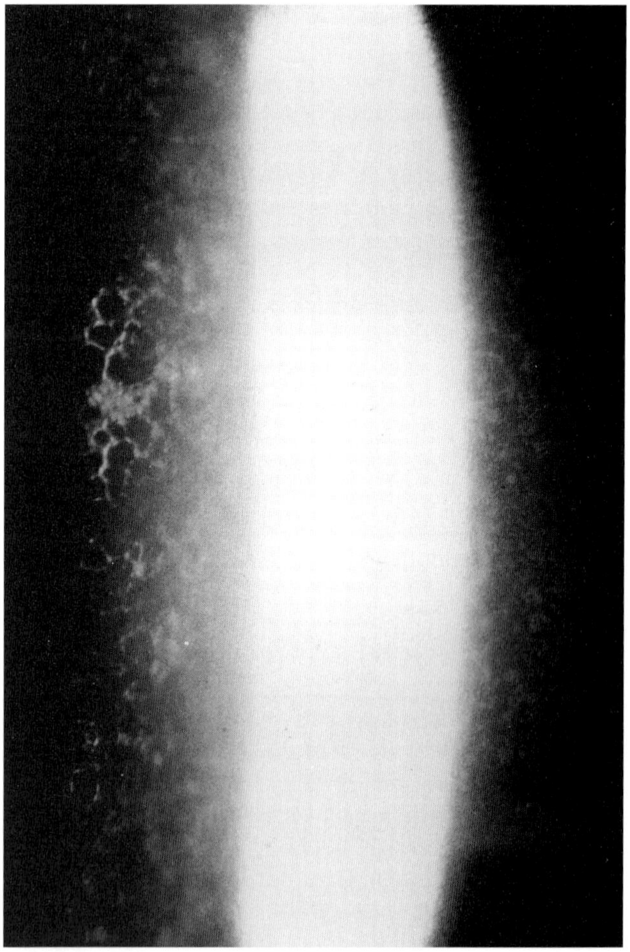

FIGURE 19-3 Specular photomicrograph of a patient with extensive corneal guttae. There is almost complete loss of the endothelial mosaic.

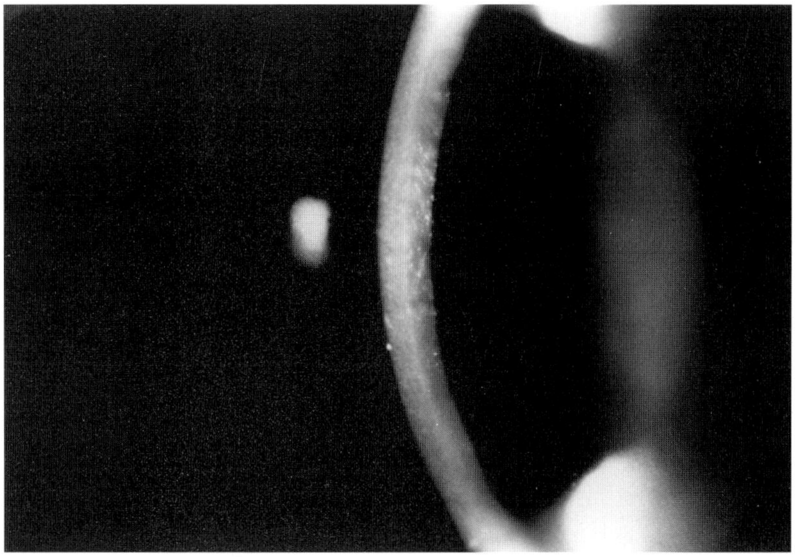

FIGURE 19-4 Beaten metal appearance of Descemet's membrane in a patient with Fuchs' dystrophy.

It is common to see a few central guttae in middle-aged and older individuals. Up to 70 percent of people older than 40 years have one or more guttae[7,8]; 3.9 percent of individuals older than 40 years have confluent guttae that may be associated with increased corneal thickness.[9,10]

The influence of heredity on the presence of guttae is not clear. In a study of 64 families in which 228 relatives were examined, guttae did not appear in a strictly autosomal dominant inheritance pattern. However, it is thought that heredity does play a role, and some form of dominant inheritance is suspected.[5,11] Both men and women, as well as successive generations, are affected. In the families of patients with relatively extensive guttae, approximately 40 percent of blood relatives older than 40 years have confluent guttae.[5]

Guttae are not pathognomonic of Fuchs' dystrophy. They are produced by abnormal endothelial cells resulting from a variety of conditions, including aging and inflammation.[12] Guttae can be seen in interstitial keratitis, other postuveitic conditions, and macular corneal dystrophy, and after trauma. Pseudoguttae may appear in a transient form in cases of trauma, contact lens wear, or iritis.[13] Specular microscopy of pseudoguttae reveals small dark spots localized to individual endothelial cells or very small groups of endothelial cells. Histologically, pseudoguttae are the result of endothelial cell edema.

Stromal Edema with or without Epithelial Edema

If the pump function of the endothelial cells is sufficiently compromised or discontinuities in the endothelial cell layer permit excessive leakage of aqueous humor into the cornea, aqueous humor accumulates in the corneal stroma and epithelium, which produces stromal and epithelial edema. Thickening of the stroma alone generally causes only minimal reduction in vision, and a significant increase in corneal thickness can be demonstrated in some asymptomatic individuals with confluent guttae.[10] As greater numbers of endothelial cells decompensate, the epithelium becomes edematous and vision decreases. The superficial epithelial cells have intercellular tight junctions through which fluid cannot pass. As a result, the fluid from the aqueous humor accumulates beneath this barrier and forms microcysts and bullae.

In the earliest stages of stromal edema, a faint sheen appears just anterior to Descemet's membrane, and minor folds in the membrane are seen (Figure 19-5). Because Descemet's membrane is inelastic, the excess length is thrown into folds as stromal swelling flattens the posterior corneal curvature. A diffuse ground glass-like stromal haze may develop as the stroma thickens. Typically, the central cornea is the most edematous region. However, it is not unusual for the edema to be eccentric, and significant variability in corneal thickness may be demonstrated across the cornea by ultrasonic pachymetry.[14]

Early epithelial edema can be difficult to diagnose. Indirect illumination reveals a slight clouding of the anterior cornea and sometimes microcysts. Sclerotic scatter (placement of the slit beam at the limbus) helps demonstrate the haze caused by epithelial edema. It is usually easier to see the haze by looking from the side of the slit lamp rather than through the oculars. Topical fluorescein is helpful in demonstrating microcysts. Although the microcysts do not stain with fluorescein, they cause disruptions in the fluorescein-laden tear film and appear as dark areas (Fig-

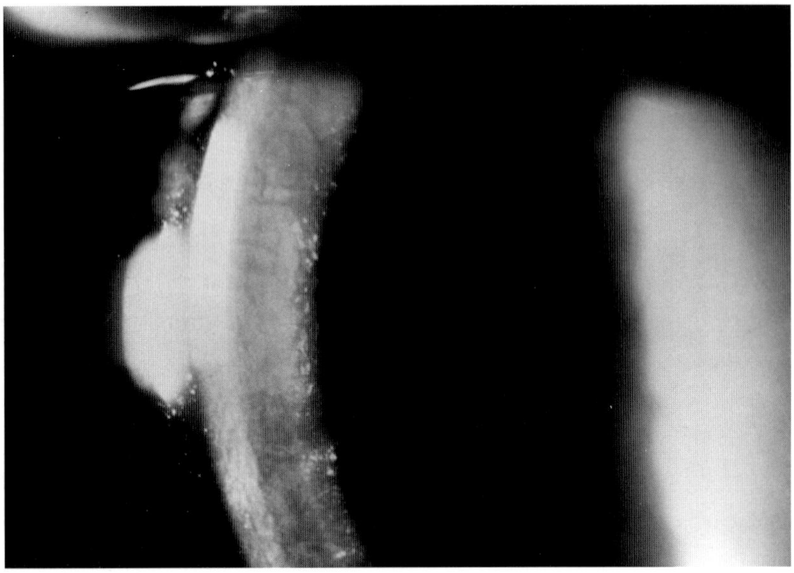

FIGURE 19-5 Stromal edema and folds in Descemet's membrane in a patient with Fuchs' dystrophy. Note the beaten metal appearance of Descemet's membrane.

ure 19-6). As the edema progresses, the epithelium can shift, resulting in fingerprint-like lines (Figure 19-7). With progression of epithelial edema, retroillumination reveals a fine beaten metal or pigskin-like texture to the anterior corneal surface. Microcysts coalesce to form intra-epithelial or subepithelial bullae (Figure 19-8). Bullous keratopathy with subsequent epithelial breakdown can cause photophobia, scarring, vascularization, and irritation ranging from mild discomfort to severe pain. Not uncommonly, a bulla may rupture, creating an epithelial erosion that can become infected.

Even the mild surface irregularity accompanying the earliest stages of epithelial edema can significantly impair vision, and increasing epithelial edema can cause a marked reduction in visual acuity (Figure 19-9). Irregularities in Descemet's membrane also produce reductions in vision, which is why smoothing of surface irregularities from epithelial edema with a contact lens provides only minimal improvement in vision once stromal edema is sufficient to cause folds in Descemet's membrane.

At first, edema occurs only in the morning as a consequence of decreased transcellular fluid evaporation and tear osmolarity during the night when the eyelids are closed. During the waking hours, increased tear evaporation and tear osmolarity draw fluid out of the edematous epithelium. The result is glare and decreased vision in the morning, followed by improvement later in the day. Deturgescence of the swollen epithelium during the

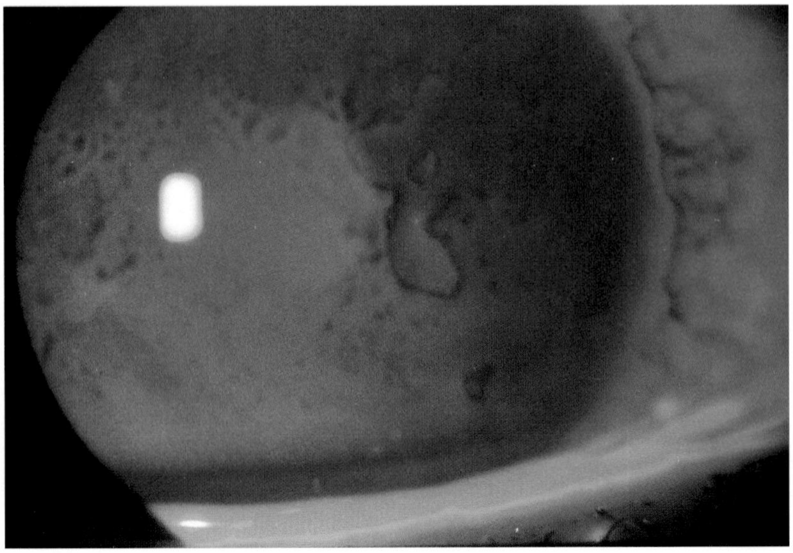

FIGURE 19-6 Corneal epithelial edema demonstrated with fluorescein. Edematous areas cause disruptions in the fluorescein and appear as dark areas. Note the numerous microcysts and the area of early bulla formation.

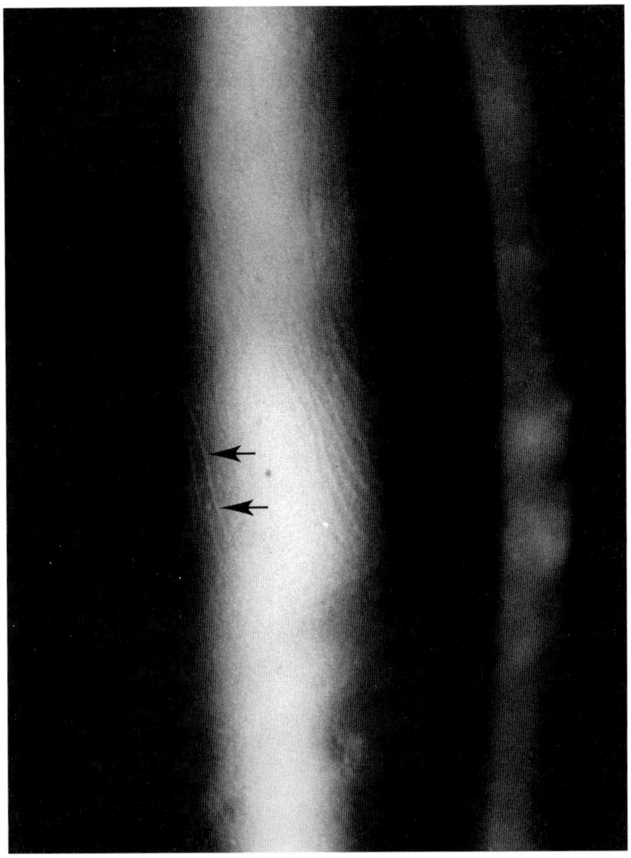

FIGURE 19-7 Epithelial edema in a patient with Fuchs' dystrophy. Shift lines (arrows) produce a fingerprint-like pattern.

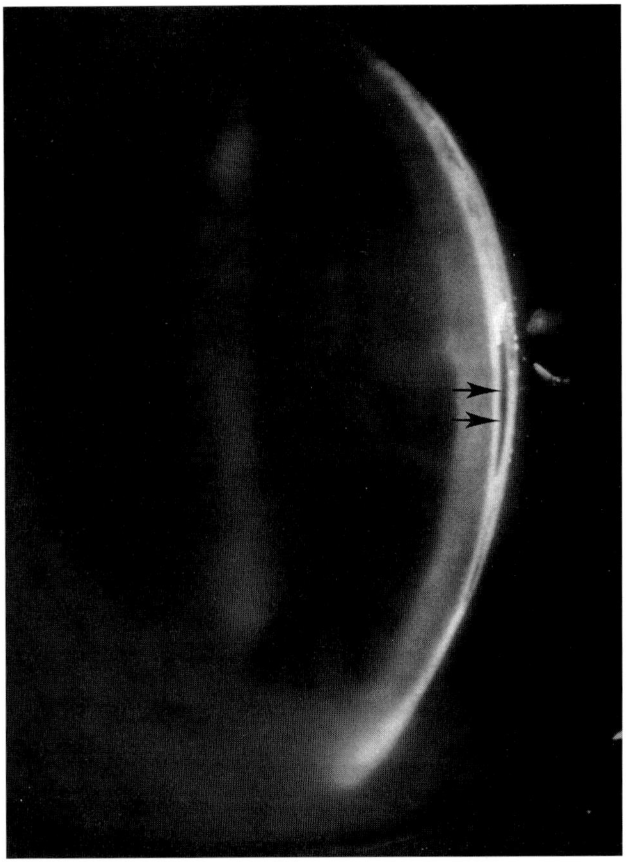

FIGURE 19-8 Patient with Fuchs' dystrophy in whom coalescent epithelial edema has produced bullae (arrows).

FIGURE 19-9 Patient with Fuchs' dystrophy in whom surface irregularity from epithelial edema is demonstrated by the irregular light reflex.

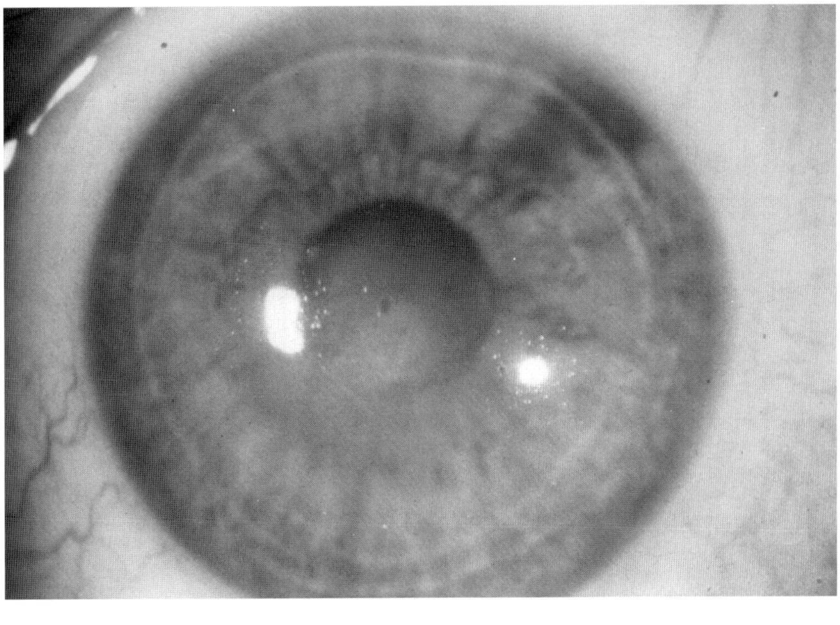

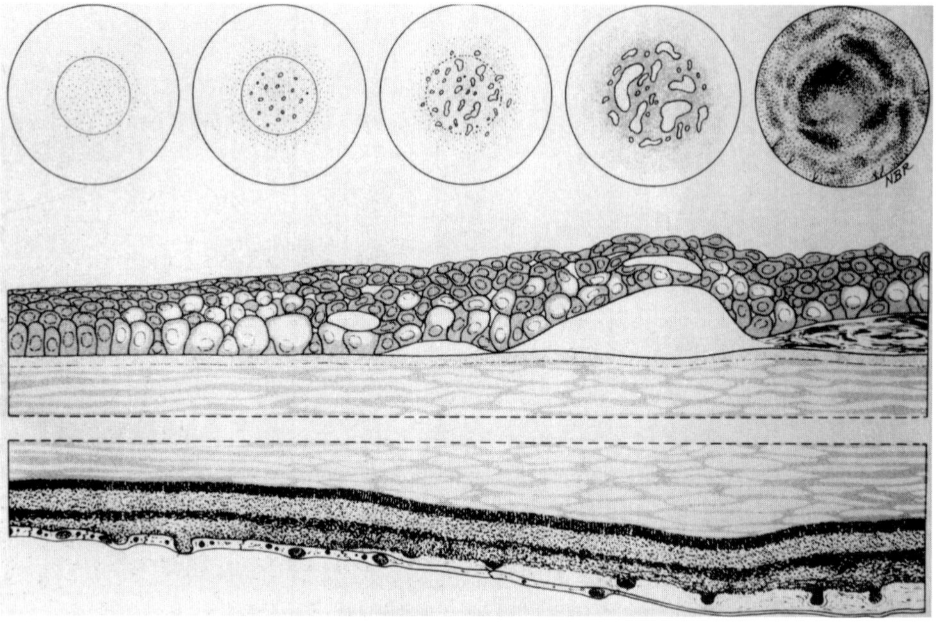

FIGURE 19-10 Composite drawing of the progressive clinical and histopathologic changes in Fuchs' dystrophy. At the left, corneal guttae are present posterior to Descemet's membrane. If the endothelium decompensates, fluid accumulates in the basal epithelial cells and stroma. Abnormal endothelial cells produce a posterior collagenous layer. The endothelium phagocytizes pigment and becomes progressively atrophic. Epithelial edema coalesces into bullae. A collagenous layer forms beneath the epithelium. Less edema is present if cicatrization is severe. (Reprinted with permission from GO Waring, MM Rodrigues, PR Laibson: Corneal dystrophies. II. Endothelial dystrophies. Surv Ophthalmol 23:147, 1978.)

day is impeded by high humidity, contact lens wear, and eyelid closure. Patients with Fuchs' dystrophy tend to become more symptomatic during the humid summer months. Also, patients with bilateral Fuchs' dystrophy who undergo penetrating keratoplasty in one eye may notice decreased vision in the unoperated eye because of a tendency to keep the unoperated eye closed more than usual. This results in decreased tear evaporation and persistence of corneal edema.[15] Patients should be warned preoperatively of this possibility.

Subepithelial Scarring

As corneal edema progresses and becomes chronic, a diffuse subepithelial sheet of scar tissue may form, separating the epithelium from the stroma and leading to end-stage cicatrization. Corneal sensation is usually diminished. Epithelial edema usually decreases at this stage, and overall corneal thickness may become more normal or remain increased. Erosions, ulcers, vascularization, calcific degeneration, chronic macular edema, glaucoma, and cataract formation can be secondary complications of Fuchs' dystrophy.

Histopathology

Figure 19-10 is a composite drawing of the progressive clinical and histopathologic features of Fuchs' dystrophy.[16] Because histopathology specimens are obtained from patients undergoing penetrating keratoplasty, histopathologic descriptions of corneas with Fuchs' dystrophy are skewed to the more advanced stages in which secondary complications have already begun. Clinical and histopathologic correlation of varying stages of edema in different portions of the cornea in patients with Fuchs' dystrophy shows that areas of attenuation of corneal endothelial cells and marked thickening of Descemet's membrane with multiple guttae correspond to areas of severe clinical edema.[14] Edema is not present clinically in the absence of these histopathologic changes.

Light microscopy of more involved areas shows multilaminar thickening of Descemet's membrane up to nearly three times the normal thickness. Periodic acid–Schiff positive excrescences protrude into the anterior chamber or are buried within a thickened posterior collagenous layer[14] (Figure 19-11). The endothelial cells are attenuated, with widely spaced nuclei, especially in the areas of the excrescences.[17] Widening of the interfibrillar spaces of the stromal collagen is noted in more edematous corneas. In some cases, Bowman's layer contains focal disruptions that are sealed with connective tissue. In advanced cases, a thick fibrocellular layer is found between Bowman's layer and the epithelial basement membrane. Both intracellular and intercellular edema of the epithelial cells are seen, along with large clear spaces under the basement membrane corresponding to bullae (Figure 19-12).

Transmission electron microscopy provides evidence of degeneration of the endothelial cells, including vacuolization and cell membrane disruption.[14,17] Some

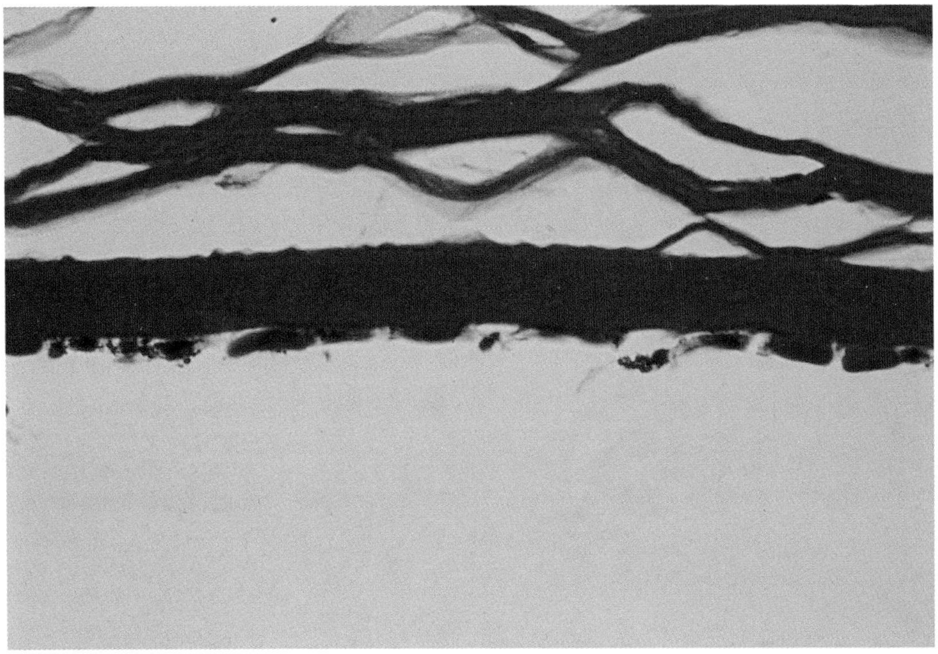

FIGURE 19-11 Typical wart-like configuration of Descemet's membrane in Fuchs' dystrophy (periodic acid–Schiff stain).

endothelial cells have increased cytoplasmic filaments, ribosomes, and rough endoplasmic reticulum, similar to fibroblasts.[17,18] Endothelial cells have a more normal ultrastructure in clinically nonedematous areas.[14]

The most striking electron microscopic finding in Fuchs' dystrophy is the profound alteration in Descemet's membrane.[14,18,19] In the normal cornea, Descemet's membrane consists of two layers. The anterior banded layer, which averages 3 μm in width, is produced during fetal development and contains characteristic 110-nm banded collagen. The posterior nonbanded layer is produced by the endothelium throughout life at an average rate of 1 to 2 μm per decade. In Fuchs' dystrophy, the anterior banded layer appears normal; however, the posterior nonbanded layer is attenuated or absent. The increase in the overall thickness of Descemet's membrane is caused by the presence of a prominent posterior collagenous layer. This layer contains 110-nm banded fibrils similar to those in the anterior banded layer but in a more patchy distribution and in association with amorphous ground substance[19] (Figure 19-13). Also found are more randomly oriented spindle-shaped bundles of collagen with 64-nm periodicity and microfibrils with diameters of 10 to 20 nm.[14,19,20] The organization of the posterior collagenous layer becomes more random and distorted toward its more posterior extent.[18] Guttae, if present, are located in this area. Larger guttae have a laminar configuration with areas of pigment granules.[14] Small oxytalan microfibrils, which belong to the elastic family of fibers, are most prominent around guttae.[14,20]

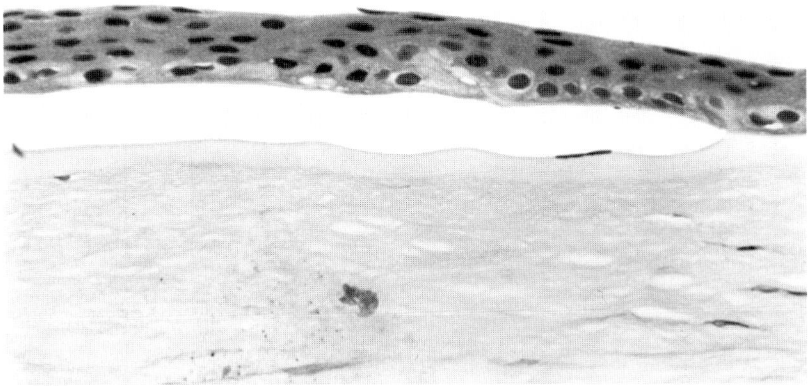

FIGURE 19-12 Corneal bulla in a patient with Fuchs' dystrophy. The corneal epithelium is separated from Bowman's layer (hematoxylin and eosin stain).

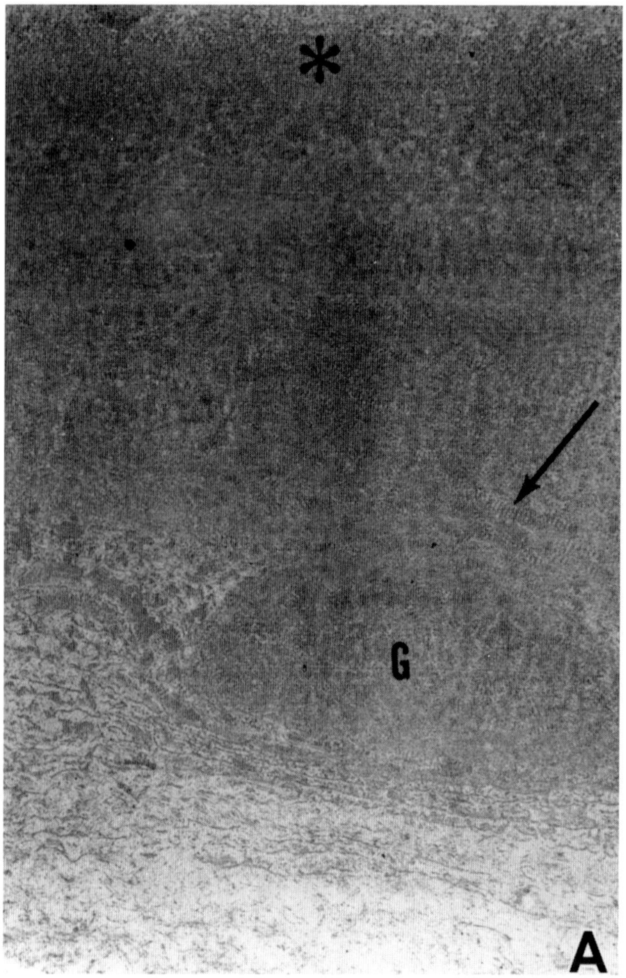

FIGURE 19-13 Transmission electron micrograph from a case of advanced Fuchs' dystrophy. The anterior portion of Descemet's membrane (asterisk) appears normal. Abnormal 110-nm banded collagen fibrils (arrow) are seen within a background of amorphous material in the posterior portion of Descemet's membrane. Loose fibrillar material (*A*) is seen posterior to a focal guttate excrescence (*G*). (Reprinted with permission from GO Waring, MM Rodrigues, PR Laibson: Corneal dystrophies. II. Endothelial dystrophies. Surv Ophthalmol 23:147, 1978.)

Scanning electron microscopy demonstrates the irregular contour of the posterior corneal surface caused by the guttae and the partial loss of endothelial cells[21] (Figure 19-14).

Generally, ultrastructural studies show Bowman's layer to be intact except for occasional focal defects. A subepithelial avascular layer, consisting of active fibroblasts, collagen fibrils 10 to 20 nm in diameter, and amorphous material, may be as thick as 350 nm.[18] Stromal and epithelial edema are apparent. Granular or filamentous material is found around stromal keratocytes and within collagen lamellae.[18]

The primary pathologic change in Fuchs' dystrophy is thought to be in the corneal endothelium, manifested by its production of a thickened, abnormal basement membrane. The elaboration of this material, which begins early in life, predates the onset of clinical symptoms by many decades. Electrophoretic studies comparing the dystrophic posterior collagenous layer in diseased corneas with age-matched normal corneas show no consistent differences in amino acid composition or collagen types.[22,23] However, levels of amino acids in aqueous humor from patients with Fuchs' dystrophy are altered compared with normal controls and age-matched patients with senile cataracts, probably as a result of abnormal endothelial function.[24] It has been suggested that the disordered appearance of the posterior collagenous layer in Fuchs' dystrophy is the result of alterations in the assembly of collagen molecules rather than deposition of new types of collagen.[22]

The endothelial barrier function in Fuchs' dystrophy has been evaluated by fluorophotometric techniques that monitor fluorescein movement into the aqueous humor.[10,25] The original studies showed increased permeability in Fuchs' dystrophy.[25] A later evaluation[10] demonstrated no significant differences in endothelial permeability between patients with mild guttae, patients with confluent guttae and increased corneal thickness, and individuals with normal corneas. Because corneal transparency is maintained by both barrier and active metabolic pump mechanisms, changes in the pump function are implied. Radioactive labeling of endothelial Na^+/K^+ ATPase pump sites has shown an increase in pump site density and, presumably, pump function in corneas with guttae.[26] This interaction of barrier function and pump capacity may explain the variability of measurements of stromal edema in the early stages of Fuchs' dystrophy.[10,26]

Disorders that should be differentiated from the edematous stages of Fuchs' dystrophy include aphakic or pseudophakic bullous keratopathy, congenital hereditary endothelial dystrophy,[27] and unilateral nonguttate corneal endothelial degeneration.[24] Fuchs' dystrophy has been implicated as a causative factor in many cases of postsurgical bullous keratopathy. The posterior collagenous layer in nondystrophic aphakic or pseudophakic bullous keratopathy differs in structure and collagen content from that found in Fuchs' dystrophy.[28-30] In one tissue culture study, Descemet's membrane from patients with pseudophakic bullous keratopathy did not support growth of endothelial cells, whereas the cells could be grown to

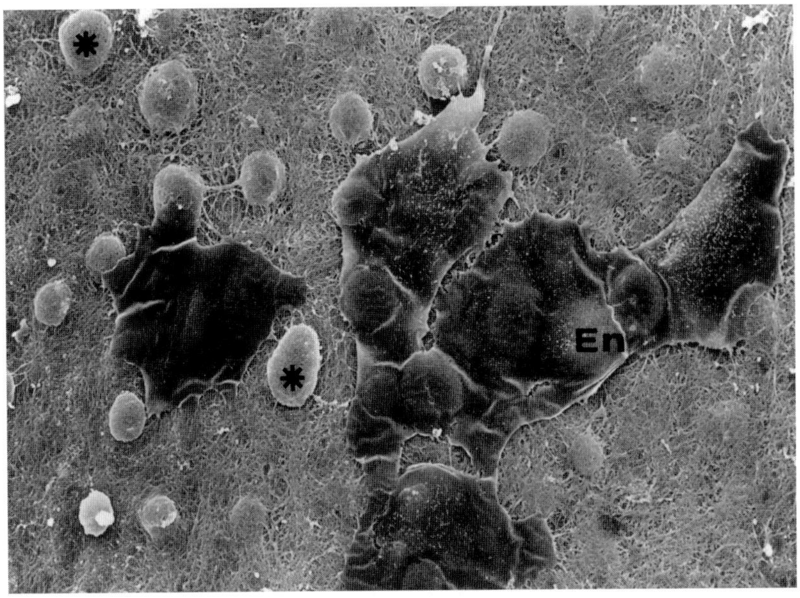

FIGURE 19-14 Scanning electron micrograph from a patient with advanced Fuchs' dystrophy. Numerous guttae (asterisks) and severely degenerated endothelial cells (*En*) are seen. The exposed surface beneath missing endothelial cells appears as a fibrous network of collagen tissue. (Courtesy of Kenneth R. Kenyon, M.D., Boston, MA.)

confluence on Descemet's membrane from patients with Fuchs' dystrophy.[31]

Treatment

Corneal guttae need not be treated if the cornea has not decompensated and stromal and epithelial edema are absent. Topical hyperosmotic agents, such as 5 percent sodium chloride drops or ointment, used frequently in the morning may be beneficial in the treatment of morning edema. Five percent sodium chloride ointment applied at bedtime reduces edema the following morning. Five percent sodium chloride drops used throughout the day may also be helpful. Some patients use a hair dryer set at low heat or air only and held at arm's length to create air currents across the cornea, which helps reduce edema by increasing evaporation. The use of hyperosmotic agents and a hair dryer may improve morning visual acuity to what it would be later in the day without these aids.

Treatment with topical glaucoma medications or oral carbonic anhydrase inhibitors may decrease corneal edema in patients with elevated intraocular pressure. A cornea with endothelium that is beginning to decompensate is especially sensitive to even minimal increases in intraocular pressure and becomes edematous more quickly than a cornea with normal endothelium. Topical corticosteroids probably have no direct effect on the dystrophic process and should be used only for the management of secondary complications.[32] Conditions that increase occlusion and decrease tear evaporation, such as ptosis, should be corrected.

Contact lenses have varying effects on corneal edema. A hard lens reduces irregular astigmatism but may worsen the edema and decrease visual acuity because it reduces evaporation from the corneal surface. A high-water-content soft contact lens permits evaporation from the surface of the lens and may improve visual acuity by reducing irregular astigmatism. If there are folds in Descemet's membrane, however, a contact lens is of little or no benefit in improving visual acuity.

A bandage soft contact lens can help reduce discomfort in a patient with advanced corneal edema and bullae. It should not be worn on a long-term basis, however, because of the risk of infection. When visual rehabilitation is desired, penetrating keratoplasty is indicated and has an excellent prognosis. For a patient with limited visual potential from a cause other than corneal edema, such as age-related macular degeneration, a total conjunctival flap carries fewer risks than long-term bandage soft contact lens wear.

Cataracts are common in patients with Fuchs' dystrophy. Whether to graft the cornea at the time of cataract extraction depends on the stage of the dystrophy. If the patient's cornea is not thickened or edematous, no matter how low the endothelial cell density or how large the amount of pigment in the guttae, cataract extraction alone, either by an extracapsular technique or by phacoemulsification, with posterior chamber intraocular lens implantation, is indicated. If the cornea is slightly thickened but the central corneal thickness is less than 600 μm and the patient has no epithelial edema at any time of the day, cataract extraction alone, with posterior chamber intraocular lens implantation, is usually

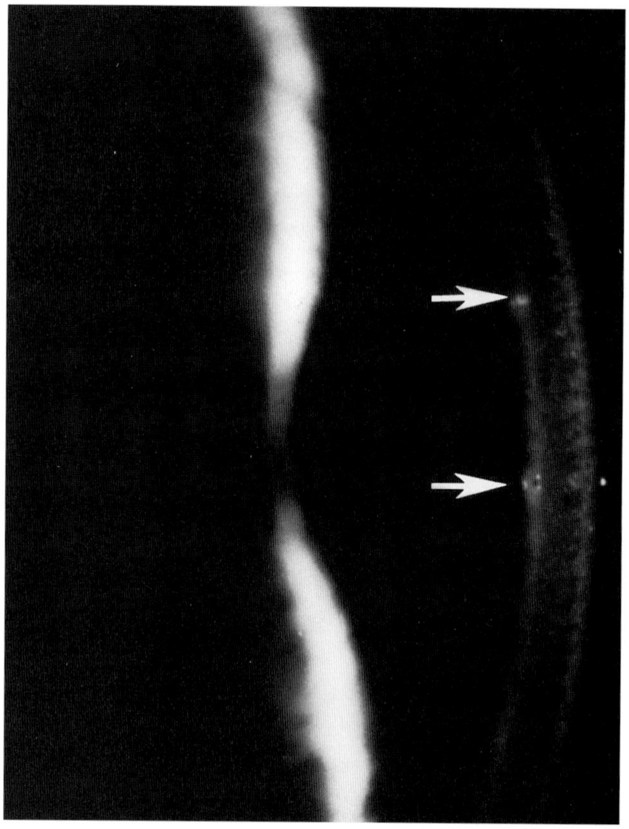

FIGURE 19-15 Small scattered posterior corneal vesicles (arrows) in the father of a patient with severe posterior polymorphous dystrophy.

successful. If, on the other hand, the central corneal thickness is 600 μm or greater or if the patient has any epithelial edema or reports that vision is cloudy in the morning and clears later in the day, the potential for taking out the cataract and not having the cornea decompensate is so low that combined penetrating keratoplasty and cataract extraction are indicated.

In general, if penetrating keratoplasty is indicated and a cataract exists, most surgeons prefer to combine penetrating keratoplasty with extracapsular cataract extraction and posterior chamber intraocular lens implantation.[33-35] Even if the cataract is relatively immature (around 20/40), it will progress after penetrating keratoplasty, especially in patients older than 50 years.[36] Therefore, cataract extraction is recommended at the time of penetrating keratoplasty rather than later,[6] because cataract extraction in an eye with a successful corneal graft causes the graft to fail in a significant percentage of cases.[3,6]

The cataract should be extracted through the recipient corneal opening as described in Chapter 34.

POSTERIOR POLYMORPHOUS DYSTROPHY

Posterior polymorphous dystrophy was first reported by Koeppe in 1916.[37] It is a bilateral, dominantly inherited (rarely recessively inherited) disorder of the corneal endothelium, characterized by a spectrum of changes in the posterior cornea and, less commonly, in the iris and anterior chamber angle structures.[38-40]

As is typical of dominantly inherited diseases, there is wide variation in expression among affected members of a family.[39,40] In some cases, a child can have much more severe involvement than the parent (Figures 19-15 and 19-16). The same gene that causes corneal edema in an offspring can cause a nonprogressive polymorphous dystrophy in the parent or other family members. The disorder may even be unilateral within a family demonstrating bilateral disease. Sometimes changes in the fellow eye are so minimal that the case may be falsely diagnosed as unilateral. The pathologic changes can be sectorial or even peripheral.[39]

Posterior polymorphous dystrophy usually does not progress to corneal edema, and most affected individuals are asymptomatic. Some cases of posterior polymorphous dystrophy are congenital, exhibiting corneal edema at birth.[41] Because the age of onset of the dystrophy in asymptomatic individuals is not known, it is possible that they, too, may have had pathologic changes at birth. This theory is supported by ultrastructural studies of Descemet's membrane that show focal areas of attenuation of the anterior layer (which develops before birth) and abnormal banding in the posterior layer.[42,43]

Some patients, especially those with no family history of posterior polymorphous dystrophy, have polymorphous excrescences of Descemet's membrane and progressive endothelial decompensation. This syndrome is clinically similar to a variant of Fuchs' dystrophy.

Chance associations have occurred with posterior polymorphous dystrophy, other dystrophies, and ocular disorders.[40] A significant number of cases associated with keratoconus have been reported.[44-47] Clinical changes of posterior polymorphous dystrophy have been described in a small number of patients with Alport syndrome.[48-50]

Linkage of posterior polymorphous dystrophy to the long arm of chromosome 20 (20q11) was reported in a family that had 21 members with this disorder.[51]

Clinical Features

Slit lamp examination of patients with posterior polymorphous dystrophy reveals a spectrum of findings, including isolated or coalescent posterior corneal vesicles

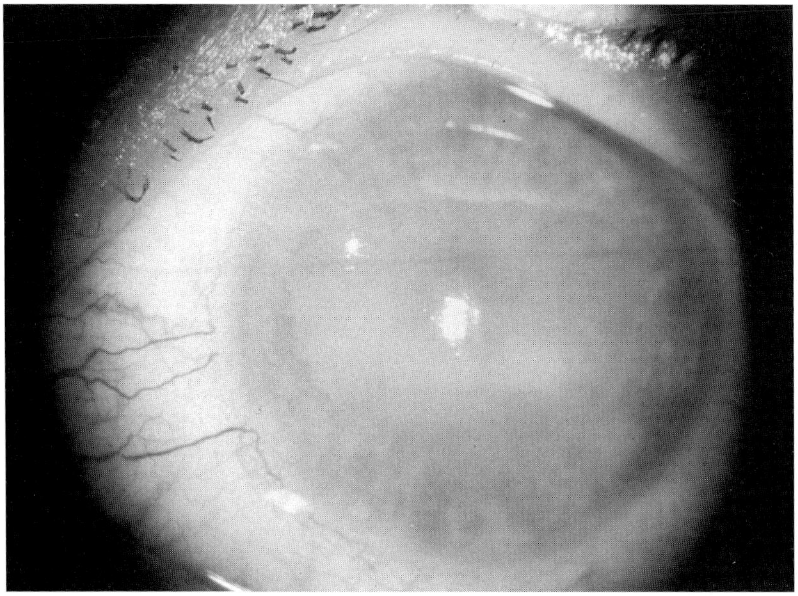

FIGURE 19-16 Severe posterior polymorphous dystrophy in the 12-year-old daughter of the patient in Figure 19-15.

(usually without corneal edema), thickening of Descemet's membrane, band-like figures on the posterior corneal surface, diffuse stromal and epithelial edema, and fine peripheral anterior synechiae or broad-based iridocorneal adhesions, sometimes with ectropion uveae and corectopia. Calcific and lipid corneal degeneration are seen in severe cases.[38,40]

Vesicles can range from one lesion in the posterior cornea to total coalescence (Figures 19-17 and 19-18). The lesions appear as small excavations or blisters on Descemet's membrane with sharp scalloped margins, surrounded by halos of gray-white haze. Cluster, linear, geographic, or arborizing configurations are created by groups of vesicles. The presence of vesicles in the posterior cornea is the most distinctive clinical characteristic of posterior polymorphous dystrophy. Similar vesicular lesions have been reported unilaterally in asymptomatic patients without a family history of this disorder.[52]

Descemet's membrane may show diffuse, geographic, or band-like thickening, and opacification (Figure 19-19). Focal white patches and projections into the anterior chamber have been described. With retroillumination, the thickened Descemet's membrane takes on a *peau d'orange* appearance. Band-like lesions similar to Haab's striae may be seen at the level of Descemet's membrane (Figure 19-20).

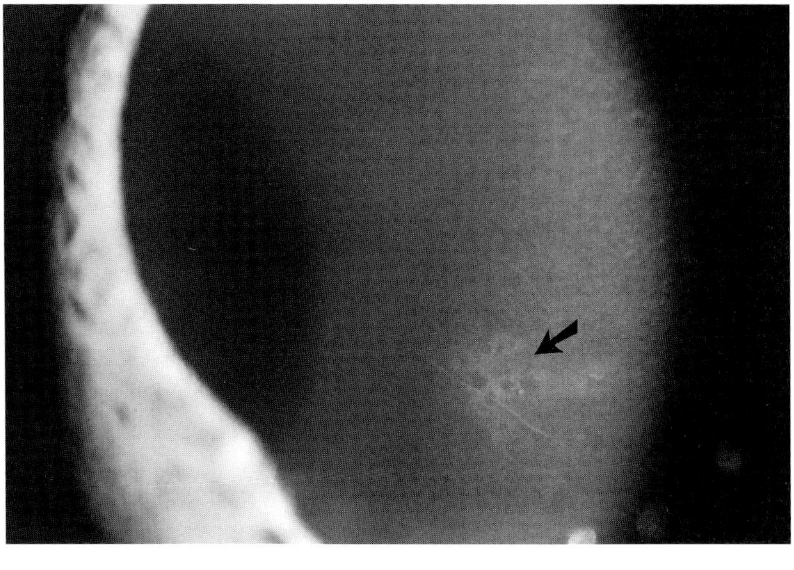

FIGURE 19-17 Several posterior corneal vesicles (arrow) in a patient with posterior polymorphous dystrophy.

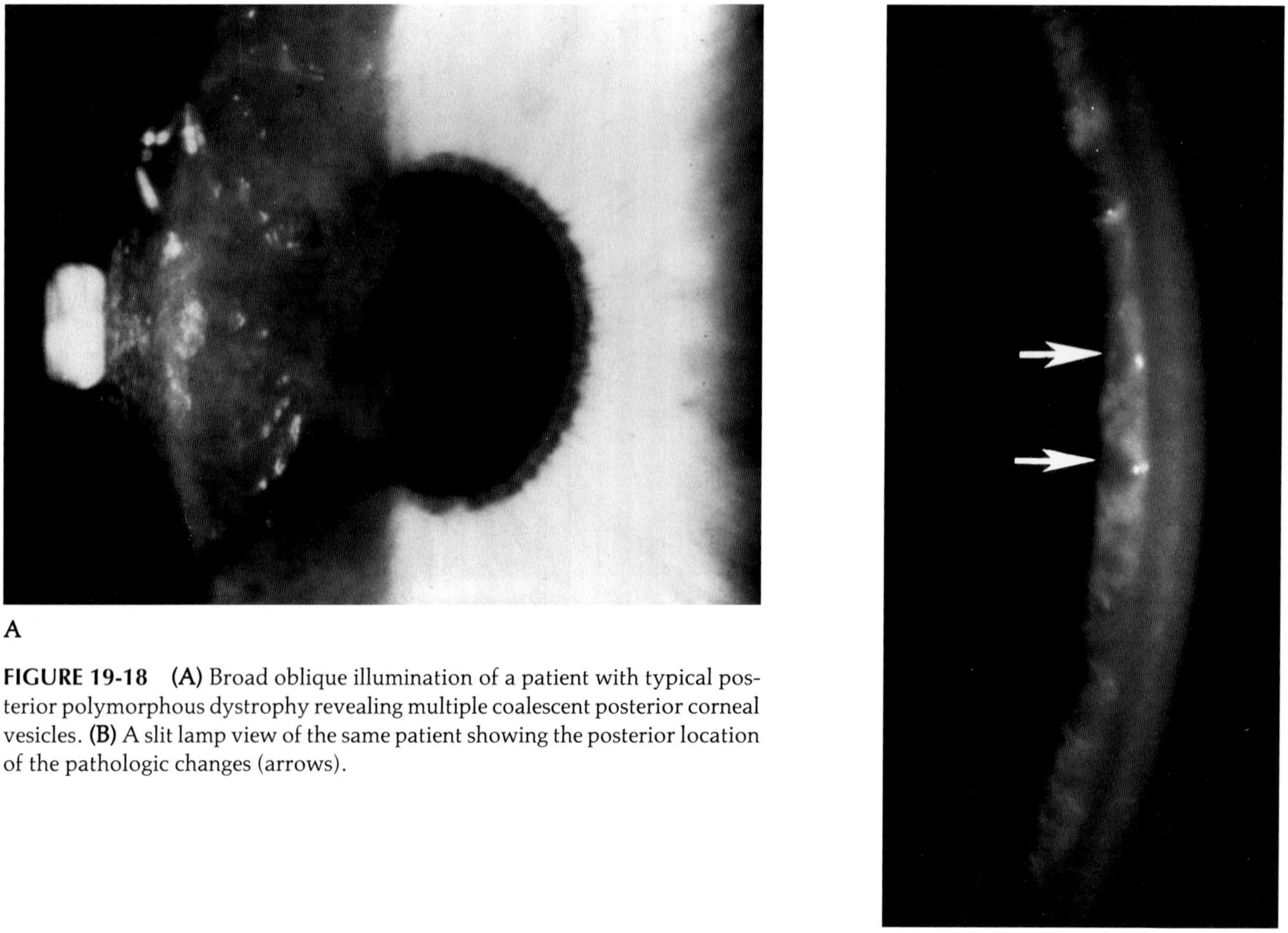

A

B

FIGURE 19-18 **(A)** Broad oblique illumination of a patient with typical posterior polymorphous dystrophy revealing multiple coalescent posterior corneal vesicles. **(B)** A slit lamp view of the same patient showing the posterior location of the pathologic changes (arrows).

These lesions can be differentiated from tears in Descemet's membrane by their scalloped, irregular, white margins and nontapering terminations.[53]

Specular microscopy shows that vesicles and bands are composed of abnormal pleomorphic cells with indistinct borders and reflective septa that may create black areas in the endothelial mosaic (Figure 19-21). The surrounding endothelial cells may be enlarged, with bright intracellular structures.[54–56] Interface cells are more pleomorphic and circumferentially aligned. Geographic lesions are often surrounded by a more normal appearing endothelial mosaic.[54]

Small basal iridocorneal adhesions, visible only with gonioscopy and not necessarily associated with glaucoma, may be seen in up to 25 percent of patients with posterior polymorphous dystrophy.[40] Corneal findings are usually most prominent in the area or sector of the adhesions.[40,57] Other patients show broad-based iris synechiae attached to the cornea by a glassy membrane. These adhesions may cause ectropion uveae and corectopia (Figures 19-22 and 19-23). The complete spectrum of iridocorneal adhesions and total corneal opacification can be seen in families in which some members have only minor vesicular lesions.[53,58]

Approximately 15 percent of patients with posterior polymorphous dystrophy have elevated intraocular pressure. Most patients with extensive iris involvement have glaucoma that is difficult to manage. Filtering procedures are complicated by an overgrowth of the abnormal endothelium, which blocks the passage of aqueous humor.

Because some cases of posterior polymorphous dystrophy involve both the cornea and iris and are associated with a displaced pupil and glaucoma, the differential diagnosis of posterior polymorphous dystrophy must include iridocorneal endothelial syndrome (see Iridocorneal Endothelial Syndrome below).[43,47,57,59] The major difference between posterior polymorphous dystrophy and iridocorneal endothelial syndrome is that posterior polymorphous dystrophy is bilateral, dominantly inherited, and slowly progressive or nonprogressive, whereas iridocorneal endothelial syndrome is usually unilateral, not inherited, and rapidly progressive.

Histopathology

The histopathology of posterior polymorphous dystrophy has been limited to more severely affected corneas obtained at the time of penetrating keratoplasty. Light microscopic findings include irregular thickening of the epithelial layer, basal epithelial cell edema, subepithelial calcific deposits, focal disruptions in Bowman's layer, and stromal edema. Descemet's membrane is variably thickened, with multiple laminations and usually with associated guttate excrescences.[43,60-63] Attenuation of the endothelium is seen in some specimens, and areas of multilayered endothelium are seen in others. Occasional pits caused by infolding of Descemet's membrane are seen on the posterior corneal surface.[63]

Scanning electron microscopy of the posterior corneal surface shows two types of endothelial cells.[42,61,63,64] The first cell type consists of pleomorphic hexagonal cells with scant microvilli, prominent nuclei, collapsed cytoplasm, and junctional complexes that appear normal. The second type of cell is larger, more squamous, and has numerous microvilli. Tissue culture of posterior corneal specimens has shown that these cells have some of the characteristics of epithelial cells, including rapid growth, squamous morphology, microvilli, desmosomal attachments, and indirect immunofluorescent staining for keratin.[65] Actin and keratin staining have been localized to the areas of epithelial-like cells.[64,66] A sharp

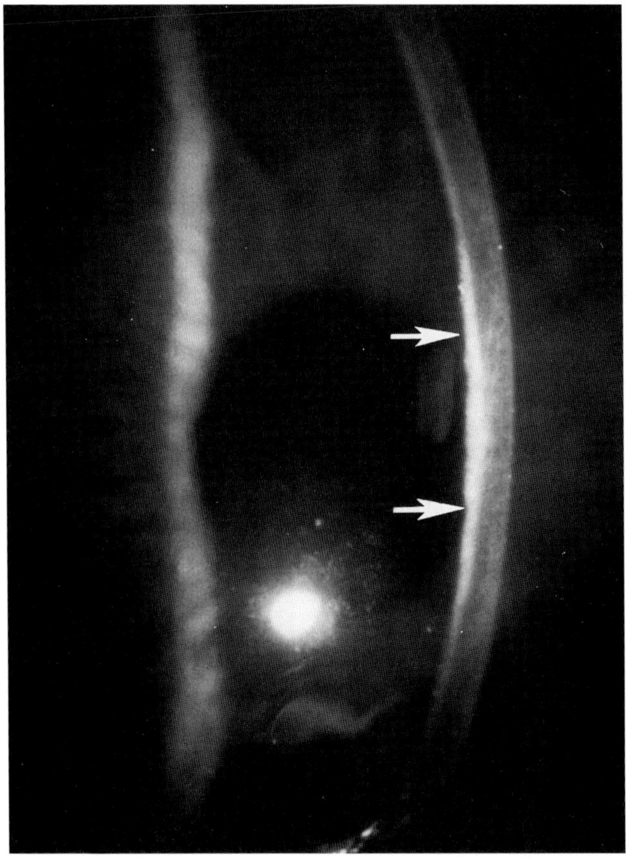

FIGURE 19-19 Thickening of Descemet's membrane (arrows) in a patient with posterior polymorphous dystrophy.

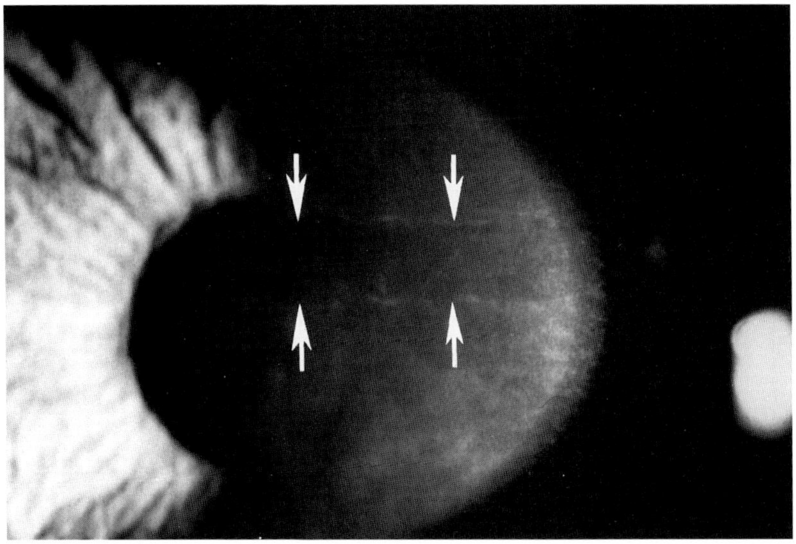

FIGURE 19-20 Broad oblique illumination revealing band-like configuration of the posterior cornea (arrows) in a patient with posterior polymorphous dystrophy. It is important to differentiate this condition from a break in Descemet's membrane.

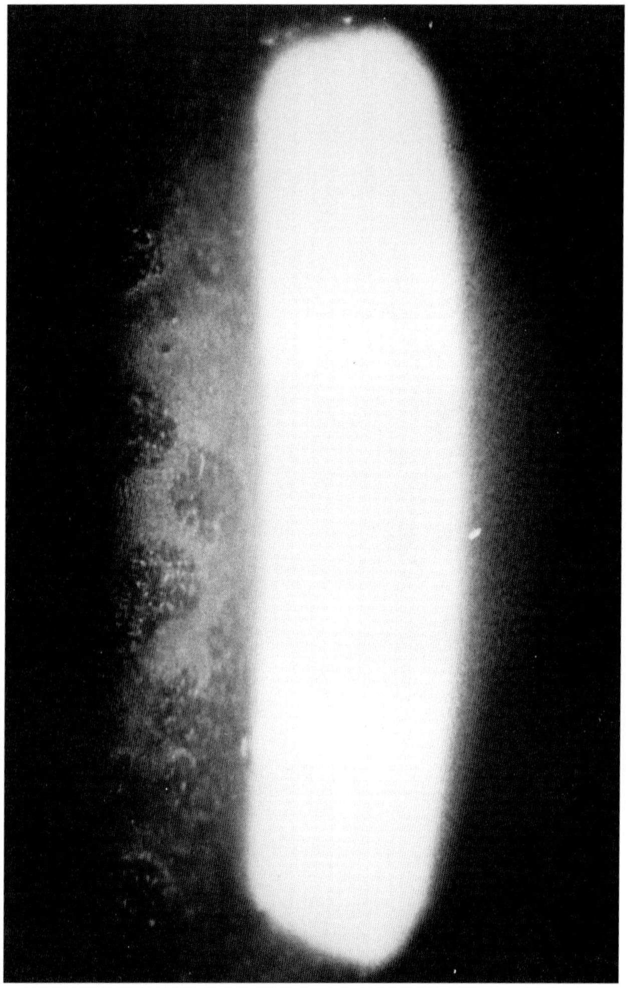

FIGURE 19-21 Specular photomicrograph of a patient with moderate posterior polymorphous dystrophy showing islands of abnormal endothelial cells.

transition border between the two cell types may be present. There may be areas of advanced cellular degeneration and cell loss, revealing bare areas of Descemet's membrane.

Transmission electron microscopy shows abnormal lamination of Descemet's membrane, with irregular deposition of collagen and basement membrane material in the posterior layer.[42,43,57,60,63,67–69] A few congenital cases have demonstrated more profound alterations in Descemet's membrane.[42,70] Ultrastructural examination of the endothelial layer generally shows degenerated endothelial cells with phagosomal inclusions, disorganized organelles, and disordered cell membranes.[63,68,70] Scattered fibroblastic cells with prominent endoplasmic reticulum have been noted around guttae and filling excavations in Descemet's membrane.[61] The epithelial-like cells usually are arranged in layers, with prominent desmosomal junctions, cytoplasmic filaments, sparse mitochondria, and microvillous projections facing the anterior chamber [42,57,60,63,64,67,68] (Figure 19-24). Small clear spaces may separate the otherwise tightly adherent cells.[60]

Epithelial-like cells have been demonstrated on the trabecular meshwork and iris in patients with posterior polymorphous dystrophy and glaucoma.[57,64] Trabeculectomy and iridectomy specimens reveal an abnormal insertion of the iris into the trabecular meshwork or epithelial-like cells extending across the inner trabecular meshwork and onto the anterior surface of the iris.[57,71] These cells have all the characteristics of the epithelial-like endothelial cells found on the posterior surface of the cornea.

Posterior polymorphous dystrophy involves the presence of four different cell types on the posterior cornea: normal endothelial cells, attenuated and degenerated cells, fibroblast-like cells, and the characteristic epithelial-like cells. The changes in Descemet's membrane, including lamination, deposition of abnormal collagen, guttae, and pits, are thought to be secondary to the primary alterations in the endothelium.[38,72] The exact pathogenesis of the different lines of endothelial cells remains unclear. The presence of findings at a young age, the relatively stable appearance in most cases, and the structure of Descemet's membrane suggest a congenital onset. Theories of development from cell nests, altered differentiation from neural crest cells, and transformation from endothelial to more epithelial-like cells have been proposed.[39,40,61,63,73]

Treatment

Most cases of posterior polymorphous dystrophy are asymptomatic and do not require treatment. If endothelial decompensation occurs and results in stromal and epithelial edema, the treatment is similar to that of Fuchs' dystrophy. Early edema can be treated with hyperosmotic agents, whereas more advanced edema requires penetrating keratoplasty for visual rehabilitation. Penetrating keratoplasty is most successful in patients who do not have iridocorneal adhesions or glaucoma.[40,57,71] Some cases in which abnormal endothelium has grown over the anterior chamber angle are successful, but many fail because of postoperative glaucoma, which is difficult to manage.[40] Recurrences of posterior polymorphous dystrophy in a corneal graft presenting as diffuse graft edema or as a retrocorneal membrane have shown histopathologic changes of posterior polymorphous dystrophy.[40,74]

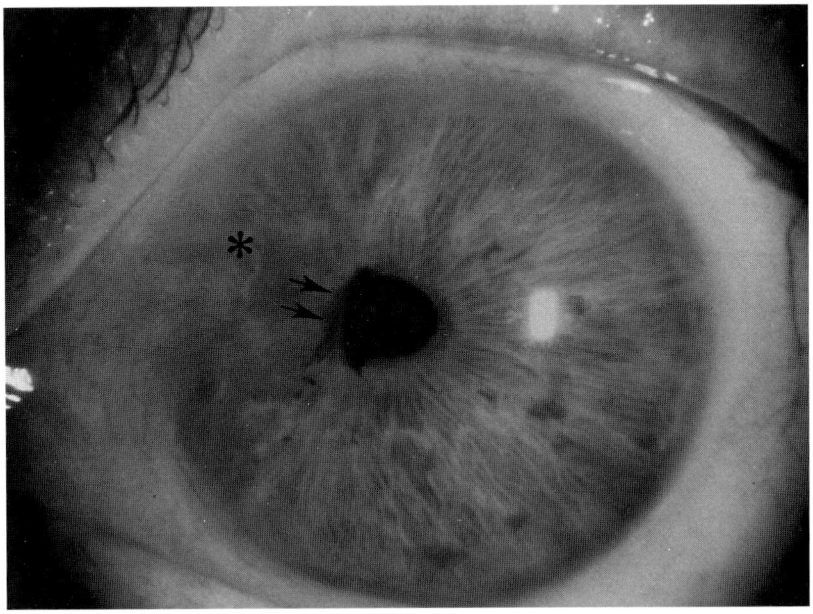

FIGURE 19-22 Area of broad-based iris adhesion to the cornea (asterisk) resulting in uveal ectropion (arrows) in a patient with posterior polymorphous dystrophy.

IRIDOCORNEAL ENDOTHELIAL SYNDROME

The term *iridocorneal endothelial syndrome* was proposed by Yanoff[75] in 1979 to group essential iris atrophy, Chandler syndrome, and iris nevus syndrome as varying clinical manifestations of a single disease entity involving a primary abnormality of the corneal endothelium. Although not considered an endothelial dystrophy, iridocorneal endothelial syndrome is included here to differentiate it from posterior polymorphous dystrophy. In contrast to the corneal endothelial dystrophies, which are bilateral, familial, and slowly progressive, iridocorneal endothelial syndrome is usually unilateral, nonfamilial, and more rapidly progressive.

In the late 19th century, several reports appeared in the literature describing isolated cases of unilateral glaucoma with progressive atrophy of the iris and occasional corneal edema. Harms[76] is generally given credit for the first precise description of this condition, which became known as essential iris atrophy. In the mid-1950s, Chandler[77,78] described a form of essential iris atrophy in four women and two men. The syndrome was characterized by slight atrophy of the iris stroma without hole formation, peripheral anterior synechiae, normal or slightly elevated intraocular pressure, corneal endothelial abnormalities similar to those seen in Fuchs' dystrophy, and corneal edema. This condition, in which the predominant clinical findings are corneal edema (even at a near normal intraocular pressure) and minimal iris abnormalities, became known as *Chandler syndrome*. In 1969, Cogan and Reese[79]

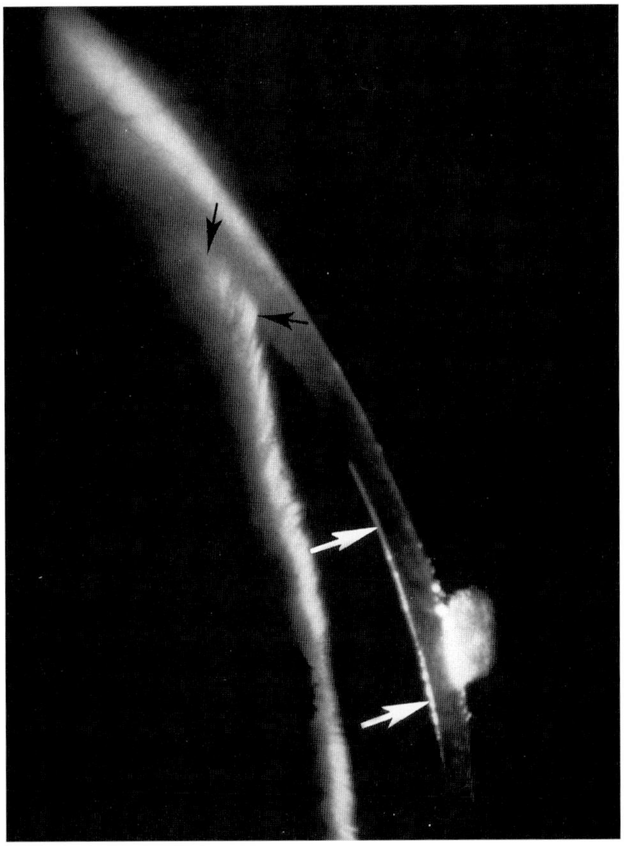

FIGURE 19-23 Slit lamp view of a patient with posterior polymorphous corneal dystrophy showing a large iris adhesion to the cornea (black arrows) and thickening of Descemet's membrane (white arrows).

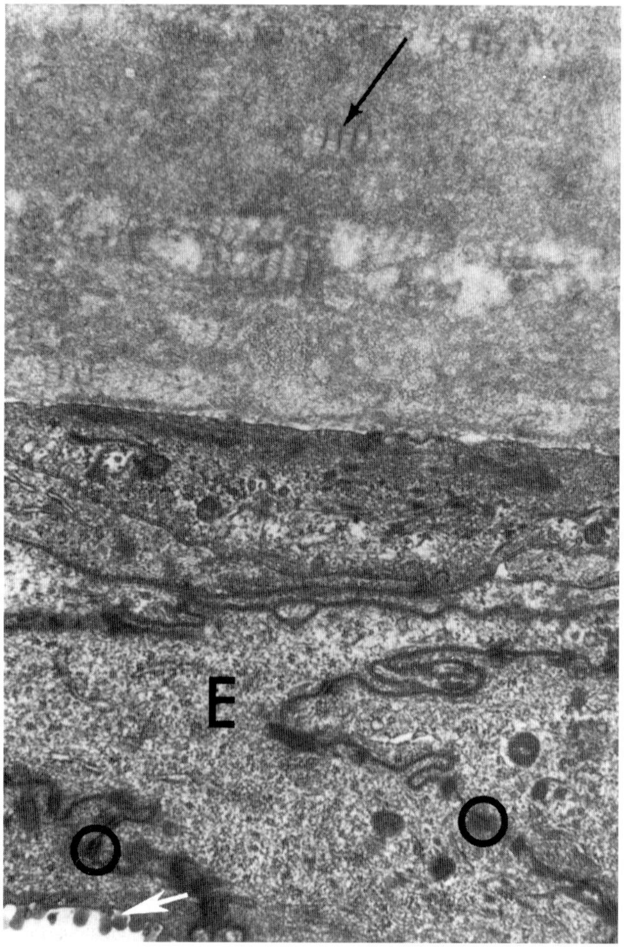

FIGURE 19-24 Transmission electron micrograph of a cornea with posterior polymorphous dystrophy showing abnormal posterior Descemet's banding (black arrow), a multilaminar endothelium (*E*), desmosomal junctions between endothelial cells (circles), and microvillous projections from the endothelial surface into the anterior chamber (white arrow).

described clinical and histologic abnormalities in two women with unilateral glaucoma, focal iris stromal atrophy without hole formation, distortion of the pupil, ectropion uveae, and sectorial pigmented pedunculated iris nodules thought to be melanomas. Pathologically, both eyes showed nevus-like clusters of cells on the iris that were covered by ectopic Descemet's membrane and endothelium extending from the posterior surface of the cornea. The name *Cogan-Reese syndrome* was given to this disorder. Scheie and Yanoff[80] reviewed ten women and four men with findings similar to those described by Cogan and Reese,[79] and coined the term *iris nevus syndrome* for this disorder.

As it became apparent that the originally distinct disorders of essential iris atrophy, Chandler syndrome, and iris nevus syndrome shared the same spectrum of clinical and histopathologic findings, the term *iridocorneal endothelial syndrome* (ICE) was proposed to unify them.[75,81] These disorders have a common pathogenic mechanism in which abnormal corneal endothelium produces an abnormal basement membrane, resulting in a spectrum of clinical presentations. Iridocorneal endothelial syndrome classically affects young to middle-aged women, although men can also be affected. The male/female ratio varies from 1:2 to 1:5.

Clinical Features

The diagnosis of iridocorneal endothelial syndrome is made when two of three main clinical features are present in one eye: abnormal corneal endothelium, peripheral anterior synechiae, and iris changes.

Clinically, corneal endothelial changes are generally diffuse and the posterior corneal surface is described as having the appearance of beaten metal or hammered silver [77,78] (Figure 19-25). Corneal guttae have also been described. The focal endothelial changes characteristic of posterior polymorphous dystrophy, such as vesicles, ridges, and bands, are not seen in iridocorneal endothelial syndrome. Specular microscopy may show iridocorneal endothelial cells, which are typically enlarged pleomorphic cells with a large, dark, central area that has a central highlight and contrasts with a light peripheral surround. The dark cell borders are usually visible [82-86] (Figure 19-26). Partial or geographic endothelial changes, with sharp demarcations between the normal endothelial mosaic and the iridocorneal endothelial cells, have been seen.[82,87,88] Progression and regression of the specular microscopic endothelial changes have been described.[88] Specular microscopy may be useful in establishing the diagnosis of iridocorneal endothelial syndrome in cases in which there is diffuse endotheliopathy and the typical beaten silver appearance is absent.[89] Although endothelial pleomorphism and polymegethism, iris transillumination, and decreased outflow facility have been described in contralateral eyes,[90-92] the clinical and specular microscopic changes are most often unilateral. Some early cases of bilateral corneal involvement reported as iridocorneal endothelial syndrome were most likely variants of posterior polymorphous dystrophy, because cases of posterior polymorphous dystrophy were identified when additional family members were examined.[43,93]

Peripheral anterior synechiae, the second component in the clinical triad, are most commonly broad based, located anterior to Schwalbe's line, and result in corectopia toward the synechiae and iris hole formation on the

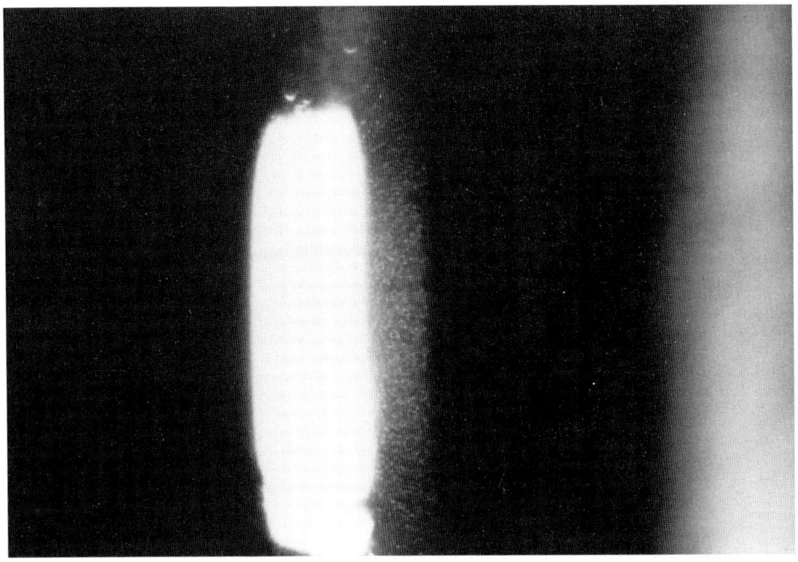

FIGURE 19-25 Hammered silver appearance of the posterior corneal surface in iridocorneal endothelial syndrome.

opposite side (Figure 19-27). Basal synechiae, endothelialization of the anterior chamber angle, and small peripheral iris holes are best seen with gonioscopy. Blunting of the normal anatomic landmarks of the angle occurs due to the presence of a clear or slightly opaque membrane over all or part of the angle. Progressive angle closure occurs in cases studied longitudinally and is often associated with glaucoma and visual loss.[84,88]

The clinical iris changes are the major determinant of the subtype classification of iridocorneal endothelial syndrome.[94] When iris atrophy, iris holes, and corectopia predominate, the diagnosis of essential (progressive) iris atrophy is given, as illustrated in Figure 19-27. Chandler syndrome is characterized by minimal iris changes and prominent corneal changes (Figure 19-28). The least frequent presentation is iris nevus syndrome, in which there is flattening of the normal iris architecture punctuated by elevated areas of protruding light or dark colored iris stromal nodules[79,80] (Figure 19-29). Other iris changes include heterochromia and ectropion uveae.

The clinical presentation of iridocorneal endothelial syndrome varies depending on the predominant features, the duration of the disorder, and any secondary complications.[94] Intermittent blurred vision and a noticeable change in the pupil are the most common presenting symptoms.[84] Halos around lights and photophobia are often mentioned by patients with corneal edema. Iris changes have been noted at the time of routine eye examinations in asymptomatic individuals. Conjunctival hyperemia and ocular pain have been reported less frequently. Pain is usually confined to patients with high intraocular pressure and corneal edema.[95,96] Varying degrees of iridocyclitis with keratic precipitates have been reported occasionally. Visual acuity decreases with the development of corneal edema but remains remarkably good when iris changes alone predominate, despite rather dramatic changes in iris architecture.

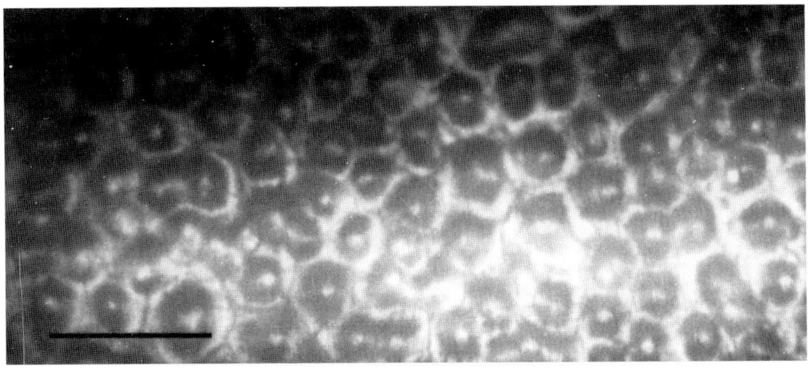

FIGURE 19-26 Specular photomicrograph of a patient with iridocorneal endothelial syndrome showing pleomorphic endothelial cells with darkened centers, central light points, and light peripheries. (Bar, 100 μm.) (Reprinted with permission from WM Bourne, RF Brubaker: Progression and regression of partial corneal involvement in the iridocorneal endothelial syndrome. Am J Ophthalmol 114:171, 1992. Copyright by The Ophthalmic Publishing Company.) (Courtesy of Ophthalmic Publishing Company, Chicago, and William M. Bourne, M.D., Rochester, MN.)

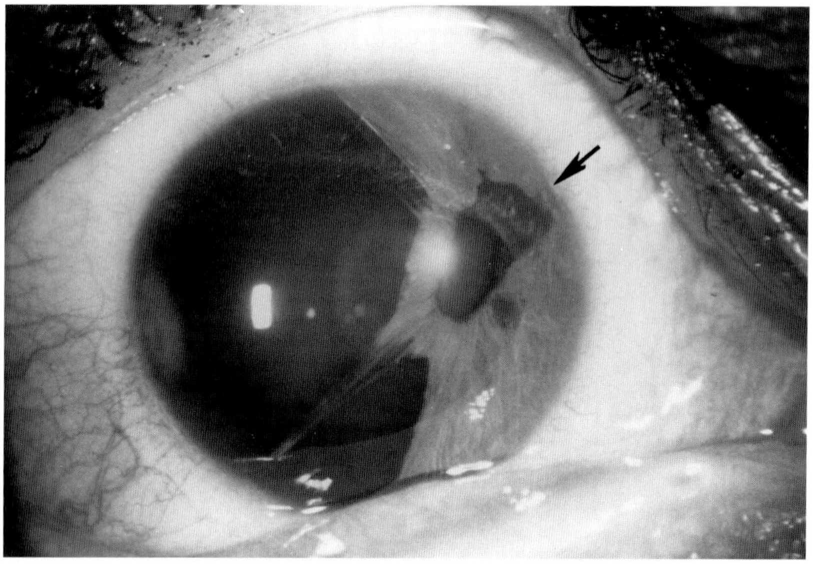

FIGURE 19-27 Large peripheral anterior synechia (arrow) with corectopia, iris holes, and ectropion uveae in a patient with essential iris atrophy.

Histopathology

Light microscopic corneal findings in iridocorneal endothelial syndrome have generally been described in edematous corneas removed at the time of penetrating keratoplasty.[82,97] Aside from edema and secondary inflammatory changes, the anterior cornea is usually normal. The endothelium is generally attenuated, with an underlying fibrous layer and a thickened Descemet's membrane. The endothelial layer may be seen in the anterior chamber angle overlying a hypoplastic trabecular meshwork[58] and on the surface of the iris, with a periodic acid–Schiff positive basement membrane and extracellular matrix.[98]

In addition to pleomorphism and attenuation of the endothelial cells, scanning electron microscopy has generally demonstrated relatively normal endothelial cells with filopodial cytoplasmic projections.[97] A second population of cells with epithelial characteristics, such as surface microvilli, cell membrane blebs, and abnormal intercellular borders, has been reported in some cases.[99,100] A few of the previous reports of epithelial-like endothelial cells in iridocorneal endothelial syn-

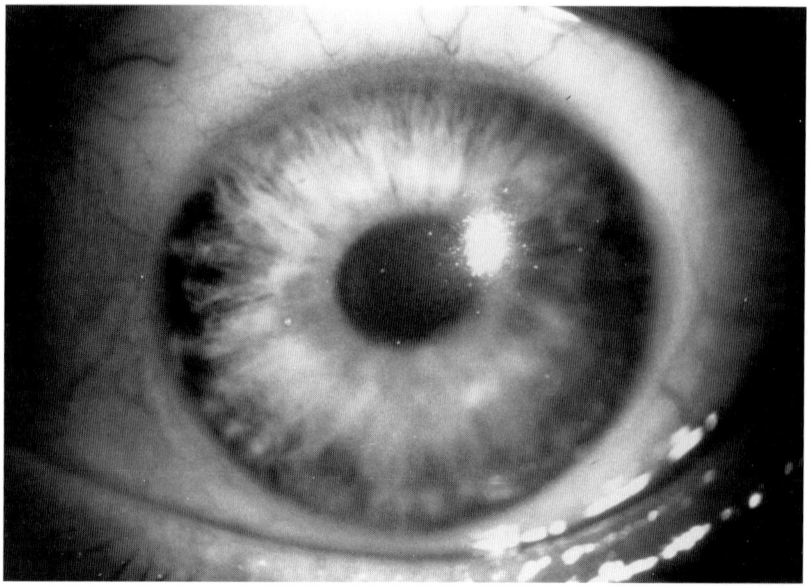

FIGURE 19-28 Corneal edema in a patient with Chandler syndrome.

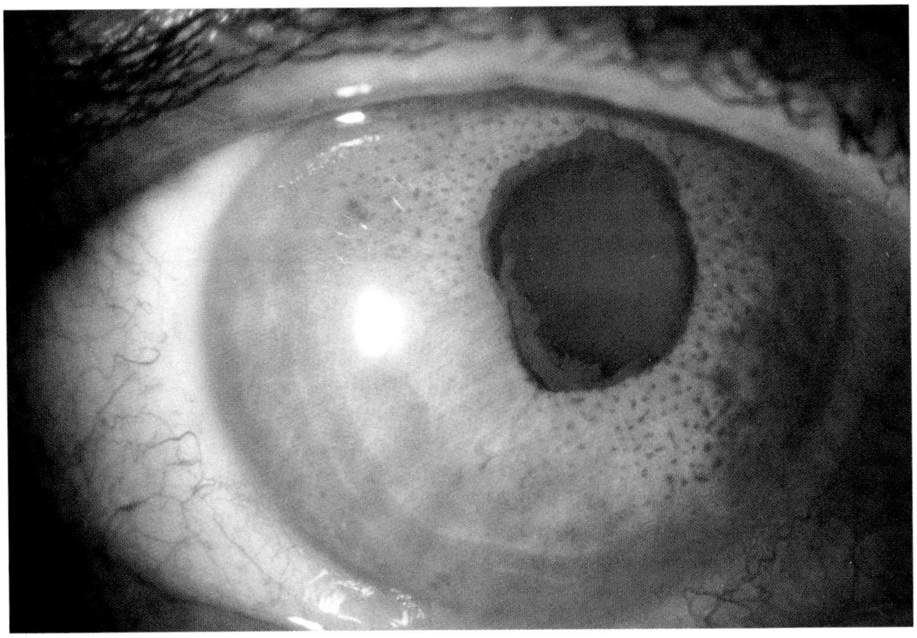

FIGURE 19-29 Numerous dark brown iris nodules, ectropion uveae, and corectopia in a patient with iris nevus syndrome.

drome actually were examples of posterior polymorphous dystrophy.[97]

Transmission electron microscopy in suspected cases of iridocorneal endothelial syndrome has shown that Descemet's membrane has a normal anterior fetal layer and a homogeneous posterior layer, as well as an abnormal banded or fibrillar layer anterior to the endothelium, indicating that the syndrome is an acquired disorder.[82,97,98,101] The endothelial cells have generally shown increased intracytoplasmic filaments, filopodial cytoplasmic projections, and ruptured or distended cytoplasmic blebs in addition to areas of apoptosis and cellular pleomorphism.[82,97] Moderate increases in surface microvilli, fibroblast-like cells, and lymphocytes have occasionally been seen, although mitotic figures and viral particles are absent.[101] Study of trabeculectomy and iridectomy specimens and post mortem globes has demonstrated that the abnormal endothelium and basement membrane extend over the trabecular meshwork, bridge the cornea and iris in areas of synechial closure, and extend onto the iris surface[58,82,98,101] (Figure 19-30). This "endothelialization" of the anterior chamber from loss of the normal contact inhibition is not unique to iridocorneal endothelial syndrome or posterior polymorphous dystrophy and is also seen rarely

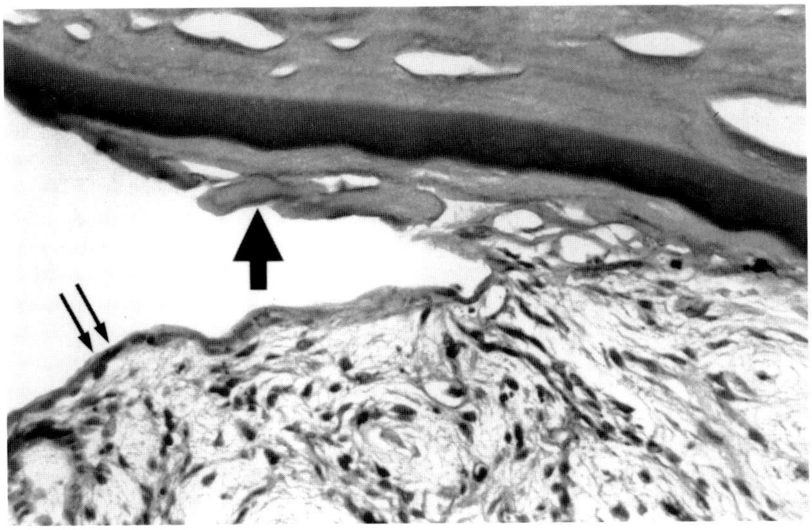

FIGURE 19-30 Sheets and rodlets of extracellular matrix material (large arrow) are interposed between cornea and iris in the pseudoangle formed by the synechial closure in a patient with essential iris atrophy. Newly formed Descemet's membrane is present on the anterior surface of the iris (small arrows). (Periodic acid–Schiff and hematoxylin stains; original magnification × 160). (Reprinted with permission from RC Eagle, JA Shields: Iridocorneal endothelial syndrome with contralateral guttate endothelial dystrophy. A light and electron microscopic study. Ophthalmology 94:862, 1987. Courtesy of Ophthalmology.) (Photograph courtesy of Ophthalmology and Ralph C. Eagle, Jr., M.D., Philadelphia, PA.)

in traumatic, inflammatory, or vascular conditions involving the anterior segment of the eye.[58,102,103]

Although a variety of possible causes for the acquisition of iridocorneal endothelial syndrome have been proposed, no clear-cut etiology has been defined.[104] The fact that most cases are acquired, unilateral, rapidly progressive, and occasionally associated with signs of inflammation, lymphocytic infiltration, and spontaneous resolution has led some to propose a viral etiology.[101,105] An elevation in serum antibody levels to Epstein-Barr viral capsid antigen has been reported in patients with this disorder.[106] More recently, herpes simplex viral DNA was demonstrated by polymerase chain reaction in a significant percentage (64 percent) of corneas from patients with iridocorneal endothelial syndrome[105]; the possibility of an underlying genetic susceptibility to postnatal infection or transformation by herpes simplex virus has been proposed.[92]

Treatment

Clinical intervention in iridocorneal endothelial syndrome varies with the dominant features of the various subtypes and the duration of the disorder. Corneal edema, even at a normal intraocular pressure, predominates in Chandler syndrome. Glaucoma, as manifested by optic nerve cupping and visual field loss, and varying degrees of corneal edema are seen at the essential iris atrophy end of the spectrum.[93] Early corneal edema may respond to topical hyperosmotic solutions or ointment. Lowering intraocular pressure initially with aqueous suppressants and eventually with a surgical filtering procedure improves corneal clarity and visual acuity in some patients.[84,107,108]

Penetrating keratoplasty is indicated in cases in which corneal edema significantly reduces vision, precludes visualization of the posterior pole to monitor concurrent glaucoma therapy, or causes pain from bullous keratopathy, recurrent corneal erosions, or secondary infectious keratitis.[96,109,110] The success rate for penetrating keratoplasty in iridocorneal endothelial syndrome has generally been favorable despite the poor overall clinical prognosis for the disorder.[96,109,111] The role of concomitant surgical pupilloplasty and lysis of peripheral anterior synechiae at the time of keratoplasty has not been clarified.[109]

Prevention of glaucomatous optic nerve damage in iridocorneal endothelial syndrome is the major therapeutic challenge in determining final visual outcome. Most patients require some intervention to lower intraocular pressure in the course of their disease. Medical management has generally been found to be ineffective over the long term,[84] although newer topical medications may extend the period of successful presurgical topical therapy. Laser trabeculoplasty has not been effective in iridocorneal endothelial syndrome. The success rates of functioning filtering blebs following trabeculectomy have varied from poor to nearly comparable to those of age-matched patients with primary open-angle glaucoma.[84,108] Progressive endothelialization of the blebs and the young age of patients with iridocorneal endothelial syndrome are the common explanations for bleb failure.[84] The use of concurrent antimetabolites and setons may improve the results of secondary filtering procedures in recalcitrant cases.[112] Vigorous control of inflammation following filtering procedures is recommended. If the suggested viral etiology is confirmed,[92,105] topical and systemic antiviral treatment may be therapeutic.

REFERENCES

1. Fuchs E: Dystrophia epithelialis corneae. Albrecht von Graefes Arch Ophthalmol 76:478, 1910
2. Vogt A: Textbook and atlas of slit-lamp. In: Microscopy of the Living Eye. Vol. 1. Springer-Verlag, Bonn, 1981 [reprint].
3. Wilson SE, Bourne WM: Fuchs' dystrophy. Cornea 7:2, 1988
4. Pitts JF, Jay JL: The association of Fuchs' corneal endothelial dystrophy with axial hypermetropia, shallow anterior chamber, and angle closure glaucoma. Br J Ophthalmol 74:601, 1990
5. Krachmer JH, Purcell JJ, Young CW, Bucher KD: Corneal endothelial dystrophy. A study of 64 families. Arch Ophthalmol 96:2036, 1978
6. Payant JA, Gordon LW, VanderZwaag R, Wood TO: Cataract formation following corneal transplantation in eyes with Fuchs' endothelial dystrophy. Cornea 9:286, 1990
7. Moeschler H: Untersuchungen über Pigmentierung der Hornhautrueckflaeche bei 395 am Spaltlampenmikroskop untersuchten Augen gesunder Personen. Z Augenheilkd 48:195, 1922
8. Goar EL: Dystrophy of the cornea endothelium (cornea guttata), with a report of a histological examination. Am J Ophthalmol 17:215, 1934
9. Lorenzetti DWC, Uotila MH, Parikh N, Kaufman HE: Central cornea guttata. Incidence in the general population. Am J Ophthalmol 64:1155, 1967
10. Wilson SE, Bourne WM, O'Brien PC, Brubaker RF: Endothelial function and aqueous humor flow rate in patients with Fuchs' dystrophy. Am J Ophthalmol 106:270, 1988
11. Krachmer JH, Bucher KD, Purcell JJ, Young CW: Inheritance of endothelial dystrophy of the cornea. Ophthalmologica 181:301, 1980
12. Waring GO, Font RL, Rodrigues MM, Mulberger RD: Alterations of Descemet's membrane in interstitial keratitis. Am J Ophthalmol 81:773, 1976
13. Krachmer JH, Schnitzer JI, Fratkin J: Cornea pseudoguttata. A clinical and histopathologic description of endothelial cell edema. Arch Ophthalmol 99:1377, 1981

14. Rodrigues MM, Krachmer JH, Hackett J, et al: Fuchs' corneal dystrophy. A clinicopathologic study of the variation in corneal edema. Ophthalmology 93:789, 1986
15. Mosteller MW, Goosey JD, Kaufman HE: Nosocomial exacerbation of Fuchs' endothelial dystrophy. Am J Ophthalmol 98:513, 1984
16. Waring GO, Rodrigues MM, Laibson PR: Corneal dystrophies. II. Endothelial dystrophies. Surv Ophthalmol 23:147, 1978
17. Hogan MJ, Wood I, Fine M: Fuchs' endothelial dystrophy of the cornea. Am J Ophthalmol 10:9, 1971
18. Iwamoto T, DeVoe A: Electron microscopic studies on Fuchs' combined dystrophy: II. Anterior portion of the cornea. Invest Ophthalmol 10:29, 1971
19. Bourne WM, Johnson DH, Campbell RJ: The ultrastructure of Descemet's membrane. III. Fuchs' dystrophy. Arch Ophthalmol 100:1952, 1982
20. Alexander RA, Grierson I, Garner A: Oxytalan fibers in Fuchs' endothelial dystrophy. Arch Ophthalmol 99:1622, 1981
21. Polack FM: The posterior corneal surface in Fuchs' dystrophy. Scanning electron microscope study. Invest Ophthalmol 13:913, 1974
22. Kenney MC, Labermeier U, Hinds D, Waring GO III: Characterization of the Descemet's membrane/posterior collagenous layer isolated from Fuchs' endothelial dystrophy corneas. Exp Eye Res 39:267, 1984
23. Wilson SE, Lloyd SA, Lloyd WC III: Two-dimensional gel electrophoretic comparison of endothelial cell-Descemet's membrane proteins in Fuchs' dystrophy and normal corneas. Cornea 11:315, 1992
24. Rosenthal WN, Blitzer M, Insler MS: Aqueous amino acid levels in Fuchs' corneal dystrophy. Am J Ophthalmol 102:570, 1986
25. Burns RR, Bourne WM, Brubaker RF: Endothelial function in patients with cornea guttata. Invest Ophthalmol Vis Sci 20:77, 1981
26. Geroski DH, Matsuda M, Yee RW, Edelhauser HF: Pump function of the human corneal endothelium. Effects of age and cornea guttata. Ophthalmology 92:759, 1985
27. Kirkness CM, McCartney A, Rice NS, et al: Congenital hereditary corneal edema of Maumenee: its clinical features, management, and pathology. Br J Ophthalmol 71:130, 1987
28. Johnson DH, Bourne WM, Campbell JC: The ultrastructure of Descemet's membrane. II. Aphakic bullous keratopathy. Arch Ophthalmol 100:1948, 1982
29. Tuberville A, Wood TO, Hasty K: The posterior collagenous layer does contain collagen. Invest Ophthalmol Vis Sci 30:336, 1989
30. Kenney MC, Chwa M: Abnormal extracellular matrix in corneas with pseudophakic bullous keratopathy. Cornea 9:115, 1990
31. Raphael B, Lange T, Wood TO, McLaughlin BJ: Growth of human corneal endothelium on altered Descemet's membrane. Cornea 11:242, 1992
32. Wilson SE, Bourne WM: Effect of dexamethasone on corneal endothelial function in Fuchs' dystrophy. Invest Ophthalmol Vis Sci 29:357, 1988
33. Arentsen JJ, Laibson PR: Penetrating keratoplasty and cataract extraction. Combined vs. nonsimultaneous surgery. Arch Ophthalmol 96:75, 1978
34. Binder PS: Intraocular lens powers used in the triple procedure. Effect on visual acuity and refractive error. Ophthalmology 92:1561, 1985
35. Pineros OE, Cohen EJ, Rapuano CJ, Laibson PR: Triple vs nonsimultaneous procedures in Fuchs' dystrophy and cataract. Arch Ophthalmol 114:525, 1996
36. Pineros OE, Cohen EJ, Rapuano CJ, Laibson PR: Long-term results after penetrating keratoplasty for Fuchs' endothelial dystrophy. Arch Ophthalmol 114:15, 1996
37. Koeppe L: Klinische Beobachtungen mit der Nernstspaltlampe und dem Hornhautmikroskop. I. Mitteilung. Fruhjahrskatarrh. Streifentrubung ohne Faltenbildung. Keratitis bullosa interna. Angeborene Dellen-bildung der Hornhauthinterflache. Albrecht von Graefes Arch Ophthalmol 91:363, 1916
38. Grayson M: The nature of hereditary deep polymorphous dystrophy of the cornea: its association with iris and anterior chamber dysgenesis. Trans Am Ophthalmol Soc 72:516, 1974
39. Cibis JW, Krachmer JH, Phelps CD, Weingeist TA: The clinical spectrum of posterior polymorphous dystrophy. Arch Ophthalmol 95:1529, 1977
40. Krachmer JH: Posterior polymorphous corneal dystrophy: a disease characterized by epithelial-like endothelial cells which influence management and prognosis. Trans Am Ophthalmol Soc 83:413, 1985
41. Levy SG, Moss J, Noble BA, McCartney AC: Early-onset posterior polymorphous dystrophy. Arch Ophthalmol 114:1265, 1996
42. Richardson WP, Hettinger ME: Endothelial and epithelial-like cell formations in a case of posterior polymorphous dystrophy. Arch Ophthalmol 103:1520, 1985
43. Presberg SE, Quigley HA, Forster RK, Green WR: Posterior polymorphous corneal dystrophy. Cornea 4:239, 1986
44. Gassett AR, Zimmerman TJ: Posterior polymorphous dystrophy associated with keratoconus. Am J Ophthalmol 78:535, 1974
45. Weissman BA, Ehrlich M, Levenson JE, Pettit TH: Four cases of keratoconus and posterior polymorphous corneal dystrophy. Optom Vis Sci 66:243, 1989
46. Bechara SJ, Grossniklaus NE, Waring GO, Well JA: Keratoconus associated with posterior polymorphous dystrophy. Am J Ophthalmol 112:729, 1991
47. Blair SD, Seabrooks D, Shields WJ, et al: Bilateral progressive essential iris atrophy and keratoconus with coincident features of posterior polymorphous dystrophy: a case report and proposed pathogenesis. Cornea 11:255, 1992
48. Sabates R, Krachmer JH, Weingeist TA: Ocular findings in Alport's syndrome. Ophthalmologica 186:204, 1983
49. Thompson SM, Deady JP, Wilshaw HE, White RHR: Ocular signs in Alport's syndrome. Eye 1:146, 1987
50. Teekhasaenee C, Nimmanit S, Wutthiphan S, et al: Posterior polymorphous dystrophy and Alport syndrome. Ophthalmology 98:1207, 1991

51. Heon E, Mathers WD, Alward WL, et al: Linkage of posterior polymorphous corneal dystrophy to 20q11. Hum Mol Genet 4:485, 1995
52. Pardos GJ, Krachmer JH, Mannis MJ: Posterior corneal vesicles. Arch Ophthalmol 99:1573, 1981
53. Cibis GW, Tripathi RC: The differential diagnosis of Descemet's tears (Haab's striae) and posterior polymorphous dystrophy bands. Ophthalmology 89:614, 1982
54. Hirst LW, Waring GO III: Clinical specular microscopy of posterior polymorphous endothelial dystrophy. Am J Ophthalmol 95:143, 1983
55. Mashima Y, Hida T, Akiya S, Uemura Y: Specular microscopy of posterior polymorphous endothelial dystrophy. Ophthalmic Paediatr Genet 7:101, 1986
56. Laganowski HC, Sherrard HS, Muir MG: The posterior corneal surface in posterior polymorphous dystrophy: a specular microscopical study. Cornea 10:224, 1991
57. Rodrigues MM, Phelps CD, Krachmer JH, et al: Glaucoma due to endothelialization of the anterior chamber angle. A comparison of posterior polymorphous dystrophy of the cornea and Chandler's syndrome. Arch Ophthalmol 98:688, 1980
58. Cibis GW, Krachmer JH, Phelps CD, Weingeist TA: Iridocorneal adhesions in posterior polymorphous dystrophy. Trans Am Acad Ophthalmol Otolaryngol 81:770, 1976
59. Eagle RC, Ront RL, Yanoff M, Fine BS: Proliferative endotheliopathy with iris abnormalities. The iridocorneal endothelial syndrome. Arch Ophthalmol 97:2104, 1979
60. Chan CC, Green WR, Barraquer J, et al: Similarities between posterior polymorphous and congenital hereditary endothelial dystrophies: a study of 14 buttons of 11 cases. Cornea 1:155, 1982
61. Polack FM, Bourne WM, Forstot SL, Yamaguchi T: Scanning electron microscopy of posterior polymorphous corneal dystrophy. Am J Ophthalmol 89:575, 1980
62. Rodrigues MM, Waring GO, Laibson PR, Weinreb S: Endothelial alterations in congenital corneal dystrophies. Am J Ophthalmol 80:678, 1975
63. Henriquez AS, Kenyon KR, Dohlman CH, et al: Morphologic characteristics of posterior polymorphous dystrophy: a study of nine corneas and review of the literature. Surv Ophthalmol 29:139, 1984
64. Rodrigues MM, Sun T, Krachmer JH, Newsome D: Epithelialization of the corneal endothelium in posterior polymorphous dystrophy. Invest Ophthalmol Vis Sci 19:832, 1980
65. Rodrigues MM, Sun T, Krachmer JH, Newsome D: Posterior polymorphous corneal dystrophy. Birth Defects 18:479, 1982
66. Rodrigues MM, Krachmer JH, Rajogopalan S, Ben-Zvi A: Actin filament localization in developing and pathologic human corneas. Cornea 6:190, 1987
67. Boruchoff SA, Kuwabara T: Electron microscopy of posterior polymorphous degeneration. Am J Ophthalmol 73:879, 1971
68. Tripathi RC, Casey TA, Wise EG: Hereditary posterior polymorphous dystrophy. An ultrastructural and clinical report. Trans Ophthalmol Soc UK 94:211, 1974
69. McCartney AC, Kirkness CM: Comparison between posterior polymorphous dystrophy and congenital hereditary endothelial dystrophy of the cornea. Eye 2:63, 1988
70. de Felice GP, Braidotti P, Viale G, et al: Posterior polymorphous dystrophy of the cornea. An ultrastructural study. Graefes Arch Clin Exp Ophthalmol 223:265, 1985
71. Bourgeois J, Shields B, Thresher R: Open-angle glaucoma associated with posterior polymorphous dystrophy: a clinicopathologic study. Ophthalmology 91:420, 1984
72. Waring GO: Posterior collagenous layer (PCL) of the cornea. Arch Ophthalmol 100:122, 1982
73. Johnston MC, Noden DM, Hazelton RD, et al: Origins of avian ocular and periocular tissues. Exp Eye Res 29:27, 1979
74. Boruchoff SA, Weiner MJ, Albert DM: Recurrence of posterior polymorphous corneal dystrophy after penetrating keratoplasty. Am J Ophthalmol 109:323, 1990
75. Yanoff M: Iridocorneal endothelial syndrome: unification of a disease spectrum. Surv Ophthalmol 24:1, 1979
76. Harms C: Einseitige spontane Luckenbildung der Iris durch Atrophie ohne mechanische Zerrung. Klin Monatsbl Augenheilkd 41:522, 1903
77. Chandler PA: Atrophy of the stroma of the iris, endothelial dystrophy, corneal edema, and glaucoma. Trans Am Ophthalmol Soc 53:75, 1955
78. Chandler PA: Atrophy of the stroma of the iris. Am J Ophthalmol 41:607, 1956
79. Cogan DG, Reese AB: A syndrome of the iris nodules, ectopic Descemet's membrane, and unilateral glaucoma. Doc Ophthalmol 26:424, 1969
80. Scheie HG, Yanoff M: Iris nevus (Cogan-Reese) syndrome. Arch Ophthalmol 93:963, 1975
81. Yanoff M: Discussion of Shields MB, McCracken JS, Klintworth GK, Campbell DG: Corneal edema in essential iris atrophy. Ophthalmology 86:1533, 1979
82. Patel A, Kenyon KR, Hirst LW, et al: Clinicopathologic features of Chandler's syndrome. Surv Ophthalmol 27:327, 1983
83. Sherrard ES, Frangoulis MA, Muir MG, Buckley RJ: The posterior surface of the cornea in the irido-corneal endothelial syndrome: a specular microscopical study. Trans Ophthalmol Soc UK 104:766, 1985
84. Laganowski HC, Kerr-Muir MG, Hitchings RA: Glaucoma and the iridocorneal endothelial syndrome. Arch Ophthalmol 110:346, 1992
85. Sherrard ES, Frangoulis MA, Kerr-Muir MG: On the morphology of cells of posterior cornea in the iridocorneal endothelial syndrome. Cornea 10:233, 1991
86. Neubauer L, Lund O, Leibowitz HM: Specular microscopic appearance of the corneal endothelium in iridocorneal endothelial syndrome. Arch Ophthalmol 101:916, 1983
87. Bourne WM: Partial corneal involvement in the iridocorneal endothelial syndrome. Am J Ophthalmol 94:774, 1982
88. Bourne WM, Brubaker RF: Progression and regression of partial corneal involvement in the iridocorneal endothelial syndrome. Am J Ophthalmol 114:171, 1992

89. Shields MB: Axenfeld Rieger syndrome: a theory of mechanism and distinctions from the iridocorneal endothelial syndrome. Trans Am Ophthalmol Soc 81:736, 1983
90. Kupfer C, Kaiser-Kupfer MI, Datiles M, McCain L: The contralateral eye in the iridocorneal endothelial (ICE) syndrome. Ophthalmology 90:1343, 1983
91. Hemady RK, Patel A, Blum S, Nirankari VS: Bilateral iridocorneal endothelial syndrome: case report and review of the literature. Cornea 13:368, 1994
92. Lucas-Glass TC, Baratz KH, Nelson LR, et al: The contralateral corneal endothelium in the iridocorneal endothelial syndrome. Arch Ophthalmol 115:40, 1997
93. Quigley HA, Forster RF: Histopathology of cornea and iris in Chandler's syndrome. Arch Ophthalmol 96:1878, 1978
94. Wilson MC, Shields MB: A comparison of the clinical variations of the iridocorneal endothelial syndrome. Arch Ophthalmol 107:1465, 1989
95. Shields MB, Campbell DG, Simmons RJ: The essential iris atrophies. Am J Ophthalmol 85:749, 1978
96. Buxton JN, Lash RS: Results of penetrating keratoplasty in the iridocorneal endothelial syndrome. Am J Ophthalmol 98:297, 1984
97. Rodrigues MM, Stulting RD, Waring GO: Clinical, electron microscopic, and immunohistochemical study of the corneal endothelium and Descemet's membrane in the iridocorneal endothelial syndrome. Am J Ophthalmol 101:16, 1986
98. Eagle RC, Shields JA: Iridocorneal endothelial syndrome with contralateral guttate endothelial dystrophy. A light and electron microscopic study. Ophthalmology 94:862, 1987
99. Alvarado JA, Murphy CG, Maglio M, Hetherington J: Pathogenesis of Chandler's syndrome, essential iris atrophy and the Cogan-Reese syndrome. I. Alterations of the corneal endothelium. Invest Ophthalmol Vis Sci 27:853, 1986
100. Levy SG, Kirkness CM, Ficker L, McCartney ACE: The histopathology of the iridocorneal-endothelial syndrome. Cornea 15:46, 1996
101. Alvarado JA, Murphy CG, Juster RP, Hetherington J: Pathogenesis of Chandler's syndrome, essential iris atrophy and Cogan-Reese syndrome: II. Estimated age at disease onset. Invest Ophthalmol Vis Sci 27:873, 1986
102. Gartner S, Taffet S, Friedman AH: The association of rubeosis iridis with endothelialization of the anterior chamber: report of a clinical case with histopathological review of 16 additional cases. Br J Ophthalmol 61:267, 1977
103. Colosi NJ, Yanoff M: Reactive corneal endothelialization. Am J Ophthalmol 83:219, 1977
104. Carpet EF: Iridocorneal endothelial syndrome. p. 1107. In Krachmer JH, Mannis MJ, Holland EJ (eds): Cornea. Vol II. CV Mosby, New York, 1997
105. Alvarado JA, Underwood JL, Green WR, et al: Detection of herpes simplex viral DNA in the iridocorneal endothelial syndrome. Arch Ophthalmol 112:1601, 1994
106. Tsai CS, Ritch R, Straus SE, et al: Antibodies to Epstein-Barr virus in iridocorneal endothelial syndrome. Arch Ophthalmol 108:1572, 1990
107. Shields MB, McCracken JS, Klintworth GK, Campbell DG: Corneal edema in essential iris atrophy. Ophthalmology 86:1533, 1979
108. Kidd M, Hetherington J, Magee S: Surgical results in iridocorneal endothelial syndrome. Arch Ophthalmol 106:199, 1988
109. Crawford GJ, Stulting RD, Cavanagh HD, Waring GO III: Penetrating keratoplasty in the management of iridocorneal endothelial syndrome. Cornea 8:34, 1989
110. DeBroff BM, Thoft RA: Surgical results of penetrating keratoplasty in essential iris atrophy. J Refract Corneal Surg 10:428, 1994
111. Chang PCT, Soong HK, Couto MF, et al: Prognosis for penetrating keratoplasty in iridocorneal endothelial syndrome. Refract Corneal Surg 9:129, 1993
112. Wright MM, Grajewski AL, Cristol SM, Parrish RK: 5-Fluorouracil after trabeculectomy and the iridocorneal endothelial syndrome. Ophthalmology 98:314, 1991

20

Corneal and Conjunctival Degenerations

ALAN SUGAR

A degeneration is a deterioration or change in a tissue that makes it less functional. Because this definition is not often rigidly applied in the classification of corneal and conjunctival disorders, there is frequent confusion about the categorization of degenerations, dystrophies, deposition of abnormal materials, and other pathologic processes. Some conditions that have been described as dystrophies, such as Salzmann's dystrophy, are actually degenerations. Conversely, some conditions classified as degenerations have familial forms, a feature that usually qualifies a disorder as a dystrophy.

Because the cause of most degenerative conditions is unknown, classification is descriptive rather than causal. Some degenerative corneal lesions may be normal aging processes, such as cornea farinata or corneal arcus, while others may be pathologic, such as band keratopathy or amyloidosis. An association with prior ocular or systemic disease is present in many cases. Unlike dystrophies, degenerations may be characterized by vascularization, unilateral occurrence, rapid progression, or late onset. However, there are many exceptions to these categorizing features.

The clinical importance of degenerative conditions varies. Many degenerations are subtle incidental findings, usually on slit lamp examination, of interest only from a descriptive standpoint; others are vision threatening. Some degenerations require therapy, but most either require no treatment, or an effective treatment is not available. However, recognition of and accurate diagnosis of these degenerations allow appropriate prognostication and therapeutic planning.

In this chapter, conjunctival degenerations are discussed briefly. These conditions overlap with corneal degenerations, which are considered in greater detail. Superficial corneal degenerations are considered first, followed by a discussion of the deeper corneal degenerations.

CONJUNCTIVAL DEGENERATIONS

Pinguecula

A pinguecula is a horizontal, triangular or oval, elevated, gray-to-yellow area of bulbar conjunctival thickening in the palpebral fissure adjacent to the limbus (Figure 20-1). It occurs nasally more often and earlier than temporally, and is usually bilateral. The elevated tissue is usually more opaque than the normal conjunctiva, and often appears as if lipid has infiltrated the subepithelial tissues, obscuring the vessels. A pinguecula may encroach on the limbus, but when the cornea is reached, it becomes, by definition, a pterygium, although the progression from one condition to the other is disputed.

The cause of pingueculae is uncertain. There is a definite relationship with increasing age; most people older than 70 years, and virtually all people older than 80 years, have pingueculae.[1,2] Repeated trauma to the interpalpebral bulbar conjunctiva from eyelid closure has also been considered a factor.[3] It is likely that a more important factor is chronic exposure to ultraviolet irradiation from sunlight.[4] The predominantly nasal location of pingueculae has been attributed to reflection of sunlight from the nose. Pingueculae occur in the same populations as pterygia, which are also thought to have an actinic basis. Both occur more often in outdoor workers and in people who live close to the equator.[5] The relationship of pingueculae to ultraviolet light exposure is weak, however, while the relationship of pterygia to ultraviolet light exposure is strong, suggesting that these conditions may have different causes.[5] Other consequences of exposure, such as drying and trauma from wind and dust, may also play a role. Another condition thought to have an actinic basis, spheroidal degeneration, is almost always associated with pingueculae.[4]

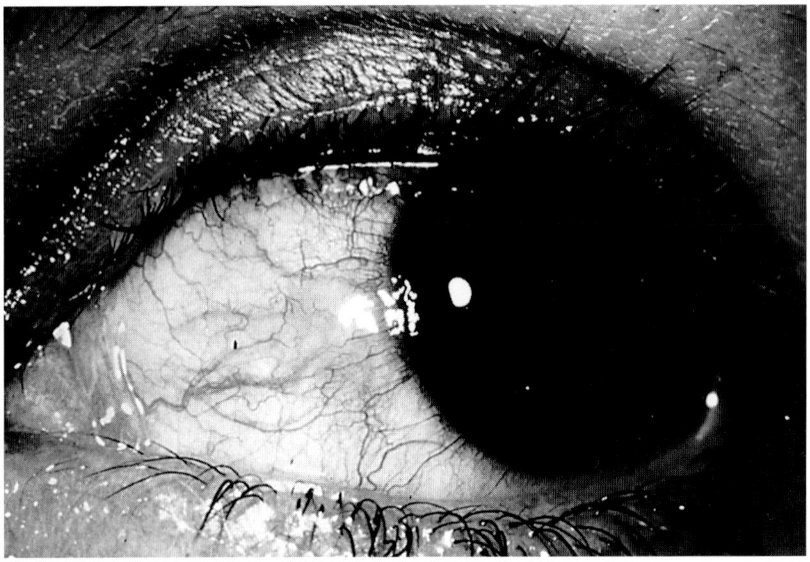

FIGURE 20-1 Nasal pinguecula with an associated corneal delle.

Although pingueculae may increase in size and elevation, they rarely spread beyond the interpalpebral area. Pingueculae are usually asymptomatic, presenting, at most, a cosmetic problem. Occasionally pingueculae may become reddened and irritated, and a white, roughened, leukoplakic surface may develop. The term *pingueculitis* refers to an inflamed pinguecula.[5] Such lesions may be treated with short-term use of topical corticosteroids or by excision. In general, however, pingueculae do not require treatment.

Pingueculae are rarely confused with other lesions. Epithelial neoplasms are distinguished by their epithelial location, compared with the subepithelial location of pingueculae. Brown, pinguecula-like lesions can occur in adults with Gaucher's disease, a sphingolipid metabolic disorder.[6]

The pathologic appearance of pingueculae was described in detail by Fuchs[7] in 1891. He reported hyalinization of the subepithelial connective tissue, increased basophilic elastotic fibers (elastotic degeneration), increased granular material, and concretions (Figure 20-2). The elastotic fibers are resistant to elastase, and have been thought to be the result of ultraviolet-light–induced degeneration of collagen.[8] One study suggests that the fibers are the product of damaged fibroblasts, which produce abnormal elastic fibers that subsequently degenerate.[9] Epithelial thinning and thickening have been described. Usually

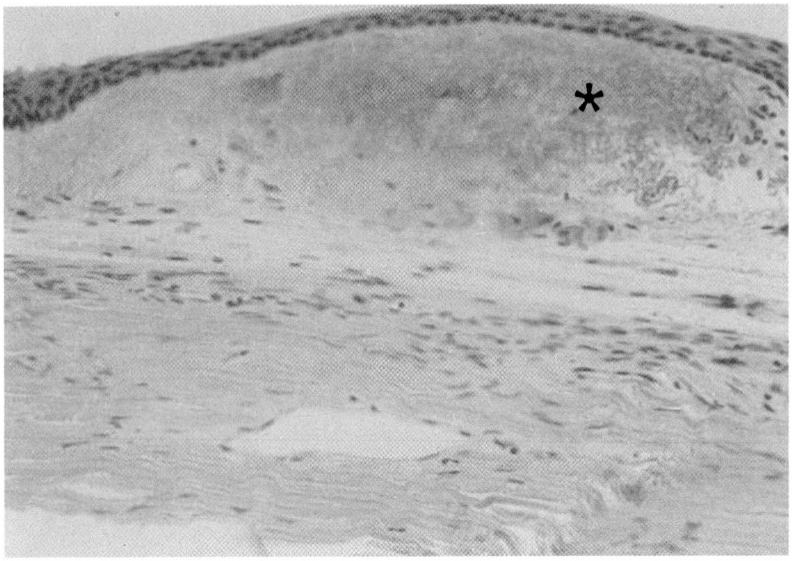

FIGURE 20-2 Pinguecula demonstrating subepithelial elastotic degeneration (asterisk). (Courtesy of the Armed Forces Institute of Pathology, Washington, DC, AFIP 61823.)

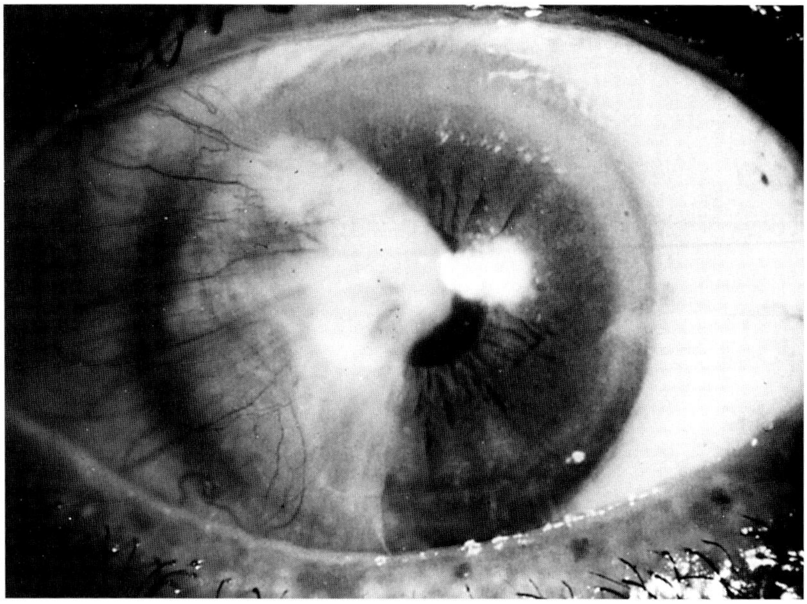

FIGURE 20-3 Extensive nasal pterygium.

there are no inflammatory cells, although they may appear within the epithelium during pingueculitis.[5]

Pterygium

A pterygium is a triangular growth of fibrovascular tissue onto the cornea. Like a pinguecula, with which it is associated, and from which it may originate, a pterygium is more frequently located nasally than temporally. Pterygia always occur in the interpalpebral fissure. A true pterygium is a degenerative lesion, whereas a pseudopterygium is a conjunctival adherence to the cornea caused by limbal or corneal inflammation or trauma. A pseudopterygium can be distinguished by its lack of adherence at the limbus (a probe can be passed beneath it at some point), and often by its atypical position.[10] As a pterygium progresses, it approaches the visual axis and may interfere with vision (Figure 20-3). It may cross the center of the cornea. The progression may be extremely slow, over many years, or rapid, over several months. Signs of activity, besides measured growth, are vascular injection, a gray, leading edge in the cornea central to the pterygium head, and punctate staining at the leading edge. Iron may be deposited in the corneal epithelium central to the leading edge of a stable pterygium (Stocker's line).[11] Symptoms are often absent or only cosmetic. A pterygium should be removed if the leading edge threatens to encroach on the visual axis, if it causes local irritation, or if there is restriction of lateral gaze.

Many causes have been proposed for pterygia, but the most likely relate to exposure to ultraviolet light. Pterygia are most prevalent in outdoor workers in equatorial regions, and are less common and less aggressive in temperate climates. The incidence of pterygium has been correlated with ultraviolet and visible blue light exposure in Chesapeake Bay watermen.[5,12] They occur only in areas not protected by the eyelids. Pterygia also occur in association with other disorders thought to have an actinic origin, such as pingueculae and spheroidal degeneration.[13] It has been suggested that a pinguecula disturbs the distribution of the tear film, leading to localized drying and delle formation, and that the advancement of a pterygium is a protective response of the conjunctiva to this damage.[14]

The histologic appearance of a pterygium is similar to that of a pinguecula, except that a pterygium involves the cornea and there is destruction of Bowman's layer.[8,9,15,16]

Chapter 21 presents a more in-depth discussion of pterygia, including medical and surgical treatment.

Other Conjunctival Degenerations

Other conjunctival degenerations, such as conjunctival amyloidosis, spheroidal degeneration, and calcium deposition, are discussed below in conjunction with the corresponding corneal degenerations.

CORNEAL DEGENERATIONS

The classification of corneal degenerations defies any single system of categorization. Many lesions involve either the superficial or deep cornea, or both. In this chap-

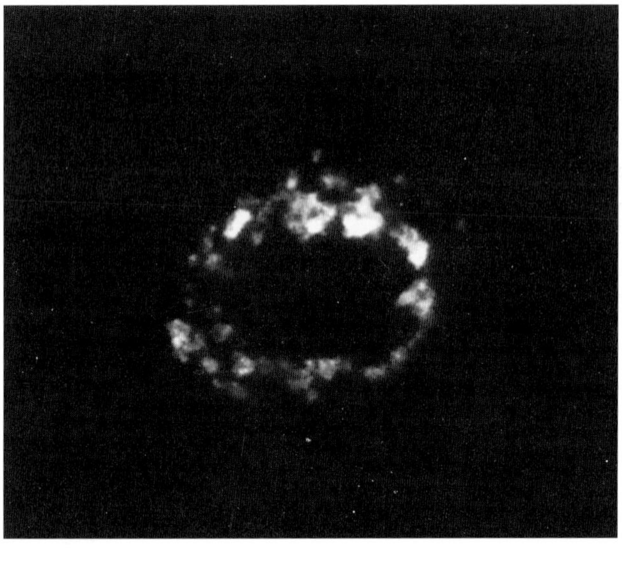

FIGURE 20-4 Coats' white ring, high magnification.

ter, superficial lesions are discussed first, followed by deeper lesions.

Iron Deposition

Iron deposition in the corneal epithelium occurs in many situations. The most common is the Hudson-Stähli line, termed by Vogt[17] the "spontaneous senile corneal line." This line may be green, brown, yellow, or rarely, white. It is located in the deep epithelium at the line of eyelid closure (the juncture of the middle and inferior third of the cornea), is approximately 0.5 mm wide, extends horizontally with a downward arc in its center, and does not usually reach the limbus. The line may be single, double, or split at the ends, and deviates around anterior corneal scars[17-19]; it is most visible against the black pupil. The line averages 1.5 mm in length, increases with age,[18] and is longer in brown eyes than in blue eyes.[20]

Rose and Lavin[20] detected Hudson-Stähli lines in 69 percent of 550 patients. Gass[18] estimated that Hudson-Stähli lines occur in more than 75 percent of patients over 50 years of age. Norn[19] examined 700 patients and found Hudson-Stähli lines in 29 percent. There was no sex predominance. The prevalence increased with age up to the 60- to 69-year age group (44 percent), then decreased to 31 percent in the 80- to 89-year age group. The intensity of the lines followed a similar age course, decreasing after age 70, despite increasing intensity of corneal arcus, another age-related degenerative phenomenon, in the same population.[19]

Histologic study shows intracellular deposition of iron in basal corneal epithelial cells. The deposits are thought to be hemosiderin. Vogt[17] described a relationship with breaks in Bowman's layer, but this relationship has not been confirmed by others.[19,21] When clinically normal corneas were stained for iron, almost all, including a cornea from a 2 year old, showed deposition in the paracentral epithelium.[18,21] This frequency led Gass[18] to conclude that the process is physiologic rather than pathologic.

The cause of the Hudson-Stähli line is unknown, although the tear film is the most likely source of the iron.[22] Other possible sources are limbal or corneal vessels, aqueous humor, or breakdown of iron-containing enzymes in the corneal tissues.[18] Histologically identical iron deposition occurs around elevations in the cornea, most notably as the Fleischer ring at the base of the cone in keratoconus,[18] the Ferry line around a filtering bleb,[23] and the Stocker line at the head of a pterygium.[11] Iron may also be deposited in the epithelium over or around corneal scars and around the nodules in Salzmann's degeneration.[17,24] Iron deposition inside the rim of corneal grafts and around refractive corneal procedures has been demonstrated, suggesting that alteration of the shape of the cornea and the resultant disturbance of tear flow are causative factors.[25,26] It is likely that migration patterns of corneal epithelium play a role in iron line position and morphology.[27] These iron lines cause no symptoms and require no therapy.

Coats' White Ring

Coats' white ring is another form of iron deposition, occurring at the level of Bowman's layer (Figure 20-4). A small oval ring made up of discrete white dots, it is asymptomatic, usually found in the inferior cornea,[28] and is associated with previous corneal foreign bodies. In the past it was thought that Coats' white ring contained lipid or calcium.[29] However, it actually contains iron, probably from the foreign body.[30]

White Limbal Girdle of Vogt

In 1930, Vogt[17] described two types of white, crescentic opacities of the peripheral cornea inside the limbus in the interpalpebral area. Type I opacity is separated from the limbus by a clear zone, and has irregular, clear holes similar to those seen in band keratopathy. Type I is rare, and probably is not a distinct entity, but rather an early manifestation of calcific band keratopathy.[31] Type II opacity is also semilunar, but has no clear zone between it and the limbus. Type II is made of fine white lines that run radially and are best seen in combined retroillumination and sclerotic scatter (Figure 20-5). The nasal limbus is involved 1.7 times more often than the temporal limbus;

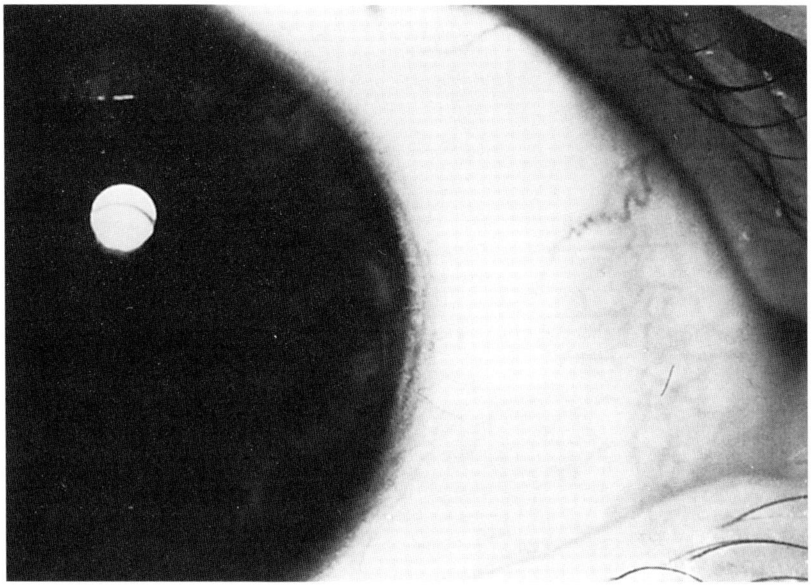

FIGURE 20-5 White limbal girdle of Vogt.

the inferior limbus may be involved if the resting interpalpebral fissure exposes that area.

Vogt's limbal girdle is directly associated with age. The opacities occur in 55 percent of normal eyes of patients 40 to 60 years of age, 67 percent of those 60 to 69 years of age, 93 percent of those 70 to 79 years of age, and 100 percent of those over age 80.[31]

Histologically, the lesion is subepithelial, with hyperelastosis and mild hyaline degeneration, similar to the findings in pingueculae.[7,8] It is peripheral to Bowman's layer. Reports of calcification in Bowman's layer probably represent type I opacity or calcific band keratopathy.[32] Type II opacity causes no symptoms and requires no therapy, but should be distinguished from band keratopathy.

Degenerative Calcific Band Keratopathy

Calcific band keratopathy can result from several inflammatory and degenerative conditions, and in most cases, is not itself a specific entity.[33] It can appear following chronic ocular disease, repeated ocular trauma, or systemic disease with elevated calcium or phosphate, and rarely occurs in a primary form. In children, calcific band keratopathy is most common after chronic uveitis, particularly when associated with juvenile rheumatoid arthritis. In adults, band keratopathy has been seen in eyes with long-standing glaucoma, corneal edema, and old interstitial keratitis. Associations with repeated trauma from chemical exposure, particularly mercury, and climatic exposure have been noted.[34] Band keratopathy has also been associated with prolonged use of pilocarpine that contains a mercurial preservative.[35,36] Associated systemic diseases are primarily those with elevated serum calcium, such as hyperparathyroidism, milk-alkali syndrome, sarcoidosis, and metastatic neoplastic disease.[37] Elevated serum phosphate caused by chronic renal failure or secondary hyperparathyroidism in patients on hemodialysis can also lead to band keratopathy.[38] Primary band keratopathy rarely occurs in patients with no history of ocular or systemic disease. Hereditary forms occur in Norrie's disease, hypophosphatasia, autosomal recessive congenital band keratopathy, and a syndrome of band keratopathy, deafness, and abnormal calcium turnover.[34] Intraocular substances, including emulsified silicone oil for retinal detachment repair[39] and viscoelastic substances with elevated phosphate concentration,[40] have been shown to cause band keratopathy.

Band keratopathy usually begins near the limbus as a grayish haze at the level of Bowman's layer. It has a sharp peripheral border separated from the limbus by a clear zone and a tapering central border. Clear circular areas within the band give it a "Swiss cheese" appearance. These areas are thought to occur at sites where nerve endings perforate Bowman's layer. As the condition progresses, the band extends centrally from both sides, affecting the central cornea last. The deposits of calcium salts eventually become white and chalky and can elevate the overlying epithelium (Figure 20-6). Only the area within the interpalpebral fissure is involved, with the center of the band slightly inferior to the center of the cornea. Although the calcium deposits normally take several years to develop in eyes with long-standing inflammation, they may develop rapidly in dry eyes.[41] Advanced band keratopathy may decrease visual

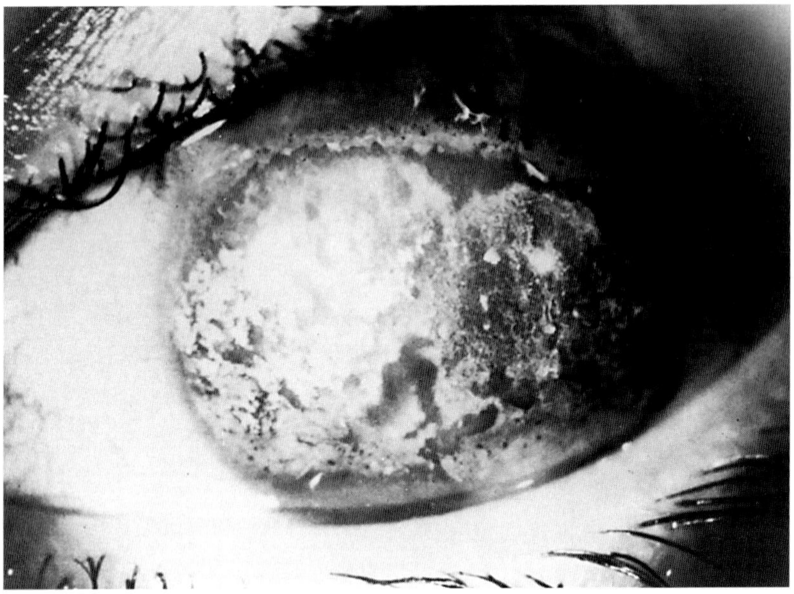

FIGURE 20-6 Extensive calcific band keratopathy in a blind eye with long-standing uveitis.

acuity, and when heavy deposits are present, may also cause irritative symptoms and epithelial erosions.

The reasons for the deposition of calcium salts in the typical band shape are not known. In an experimental animal model involving induced ocular inflammation and overdoses of vitamin D, band keratopathy did not develop if the eyelids were kept closed. However, when the eyelids were open but the animals were kept in total darkness, the band developed as it did in the light. Evaporation of tears, which causes calcium salt precipitation, was thought to be the cause.[42] Exposure of the corneal surface and tear film also allows release of carbon dioxide, which makes the surface more alkaline. Calcium phosphate can then precipitate in the more alkaline medium. O'Connor[33] suggested that the limbal blood supply provides a buffering capacity not available centrally in the cornea, which explains the clear limbal zone.

Histologically, the first sign of band keratopathy is basophilic staining of the corneal epithelial basement membrane. In band keratopathy associated with hypercalcemia, there may be intracellular calcium deposition in the basal epithelial cells, whereas in other forms the deposits are extracellular. Later, Bowman's layer calcifies and may become disrupted (Figure 20-7). The anterior

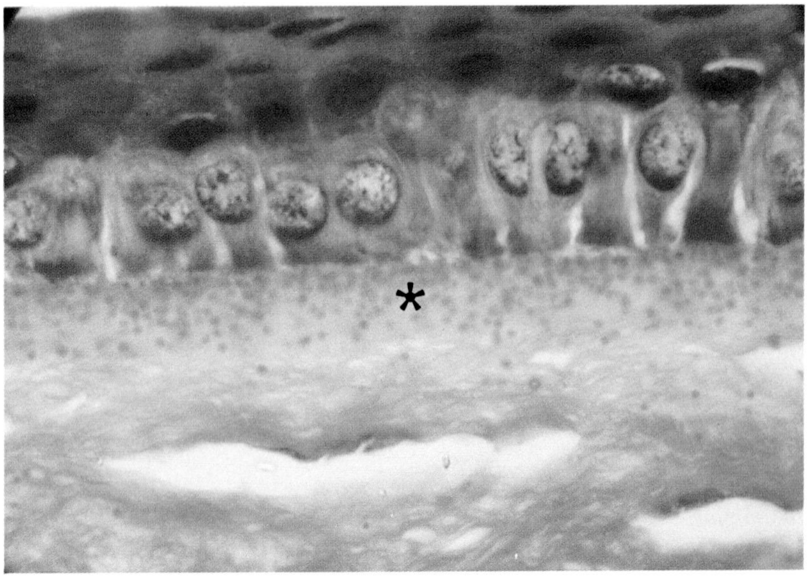

FIGURE 20-7 Calcific band keratopathy. Bowman's layer (asterisk) is stippled with basophilic-staining dots (hematoxylin and eosin stain).

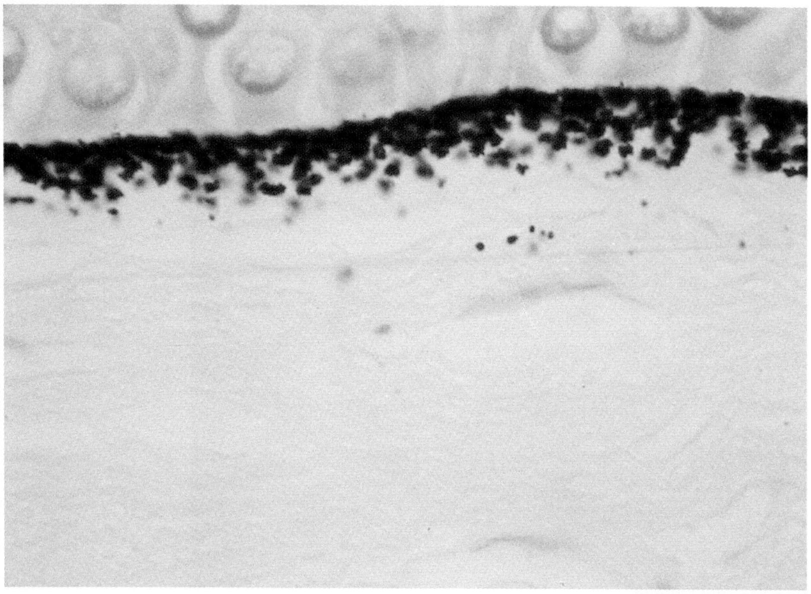

FIGURE 20-8 Von Kossa stain of calcific band keratopathy.

stroma can also be involved. Hyaline material deposited beneath the epithelium gives the appearance of duplication of Bowman's layer.[33,43] The calcium is deposited in the hydroxyapatite form, which is a phosphate salt. Calcium stains black with von Kossa stain and red with alizarin red stain (Figure 20-8).

Treatment of band keratopathy is necessary only if vision is decreased or if the calcific deposits mechanically irritate the eyelids. The usual treatment is chelation with ethylenediaminetetraacetic acid (EDTA). The epithelium must first be removed. The EDTA is then applied repeatedly as a 0.05 M solution on a saturated cellulose sponge. Because EDTA irritates the cornea, its application should be limited to the area of pathologic change. After several minutes, the corneal surface is rubbed with sponges, scraped with a blade, or polished with a diamond burr. The process is repeated as necessary.[44,45] Scraping alone with a blade can also be done.[46] Phototherapeutic keratectomy with the excimer laser effectively removes band keratopathy.[47] Although excimer laser photoablation is associated with a hyperopic shift in refractive error, continued improvements in methods are likely to make this an increasingly useful treatment modality for band keratopathy.

Calcareous Degeneration

Calcareous degeneration is a term used for what may be merely an advanced form of calcific band keratopathy. Unlike band keratopathy, however, calcareous degeneration involves the deep cornea as well as Bowman's layer. It is seen in grossly distorted globes, and may be associated with intraocular bone formation.[33]

Salzmann's Nodular Degeneration

Although originally described by Salzmann[48] in 1925 as a dystrophy, Salzmann's nodular degeneration is a gradually developing process that appears in corneas that have been inflamed many years earlier. Past phlyctenular keratitis is the most common association, followed by trachoma, vernal keratitis, keratitis sicca, exposure keratopathy, interstitial keratitis, Thygeson's superficial punctate keratitis, and other forms of chronic keratitis.[49-51] Occasionally patients have lesions typical of Salzmann's degeneration with no history of keratitis.[24] Most patients with Salzmann's degeneration are female (65 percent). Some reports state that 80 percent of cases are unilateral[51]; other reports state that 80 percent of cases are bilateral[50]; the latter conforms with my experience. The age range varies from late childhood to old age, with most patients in the older group.

The lesions of Salzmann's degeneration appear as elevated, gray to blue-gray, fibrous nodules in the superficial stroma, just beneath the epithelium. There are usually one to several discrete lesions, often in a circular array, with clear intervening cornea, unless the past keratitis has left residual scarring in these areas (Figure 20-9). The nodules tend to occur within the area of scarring or at the junction of scarred and clear cornea, often at the central edge of pannus. The nodules themselves are not vascularized, although the underlying stroma may be.[50] Iron

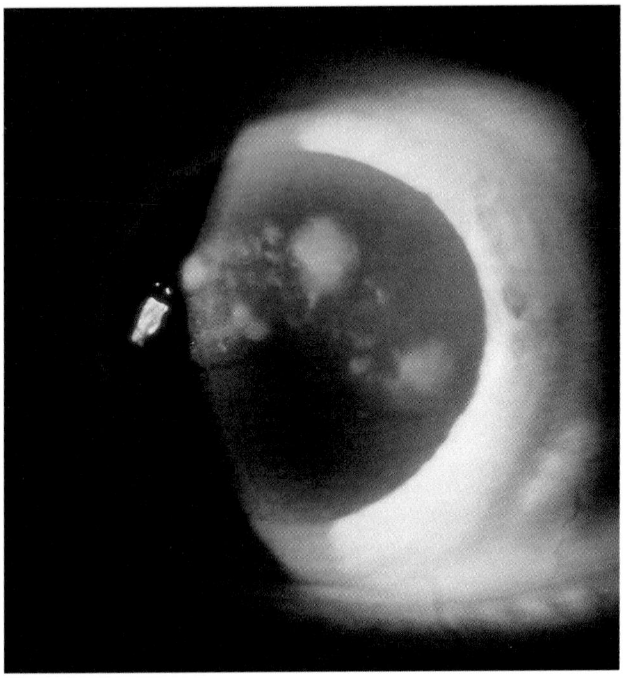

FIGURE 20-9 Salzmann's nodular degeneration of the cornea.

rings may be seen at the base of the nodules.[24] The nodules may increase in size, elevation, and number, and demonstrate no tendency to regress. They are often asymptomatic, but when central, may cause decreased vision. Some patients may also complain of irritation resulting from the elevated nodules as well as epithelial erosions overlying the elevations.

Histologically, there is evidence of old corneal inflammation with scarring and vascularization, although there are no vessels or inflammatory cells in the nodules. The epithelium is thinned and flattened, with degeneration of basal epithelial cells. The nodule consists of a mound of dense collagenous tissue (Figure 20-10). In most cases, Bowman's layer is replaced by eosinophilic material that does not stain for reticulin, amyloid, or elastic fibers,[50] and the underlying stromal collagen is disorganized.

Treatment is often unnecessary, but is indicated when vision is decreased, when recurrent erosions occur, and when contact lens wear is hampered. Nodules can usually be removed by superficial keratectomy or direct peeling of the fibrous plaques from the corneal surface.[52] The excimer laser has been used to remove similar nodules.[53]

Spheroidal Degeneration

Spheroidal degeneration has been described under a variety of names, including hyaline degeneration, Labrador keratopathy, Bietti's band-shaped nodular dystrophy, climatic droplet keratopathy, keratinoid corneal degeneration, degeneration sphaerularis elaiodes, and chronic actinic keratopathy.[54,55] Because of confusion as to nomenclature and cause, this degeneration is difficult to classify. Currently, spheroidal degeneration is the most widely used term.

There are three types of spheroidal degeneration. Type 1 is considered a primary corneal degeneration, type 2 is a corneal degeneration secondary to other ocular disease, and type 3 is a conjunctival degeneration.[55-57] In practice, however, these classifications are not always easy to apply.

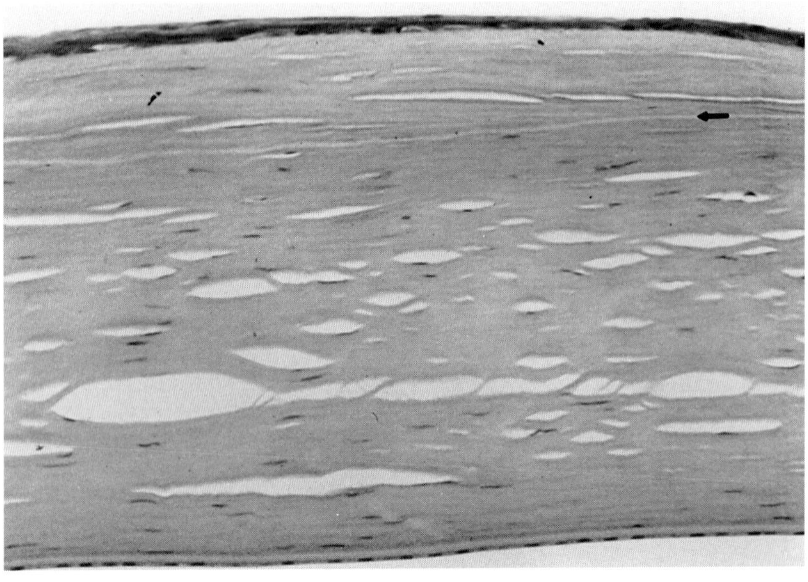

FIGURE 20-10 Nodule of dense collagenous tissue between the epithelium and Bowman's layer (arrow) in Salzmann's nodular degeneration. (Courtesy of the Armed Forces Institute of Pathology, Washington, DC, AFIP 94-1176.)

The forms of the disease ascribed to climatic exposure can be considered type 2 because they are probably secondary to actinic exposure, dry eyes, and other trauma. However, the lesions classified as type 1 and related to aging may be related to length of actinic exposure and trauma from dry eyes as well. Taylor[13] prefers to distinguish "climatic droplet keratopathy" from "spheroidal degeneration" to avoid this problem with nomenclature, whereas others prefer to combine them on the basis of similarities in clinical and pathologic features.[4]

Clinically, spheroidal degeneration is seen as clusters of fine, yellow, gray, or gold droplets beneath the epithelium of the cornea or conjunctiva (Figure 20-11). They may initially be clear, and later become opalescent or opaque. They begin peripherally and advance centrally. When advanced, they may be grossly nodular and elevate the epithelium in a band-shaped distribution[58] (Figure 20-12). Only exposed areas are involved. A clear zone may be left between the deposits and the limbus in early cases, but this zone is later lost.[59] Gray et al[54] distinguish three grades of spheroidal degeneration. In grade 1, opacities are limited to the medial and lateral corneal periphery, and are visible only in retroillumination as fine, glistening droplets; no symptoms are present. In grade 2, the central cornea is involved, with larger deposits in the anterior stroma, and vision is reduced to 20/100. In grade 3, large yellow nodules elevate the epithelium, and visual acuity is 20/200 or worse. This pattern of progression and distribution does not necessarily apply to the forms that occur secondary to corneal disease, in which the deposits may be present only over scarred areas.

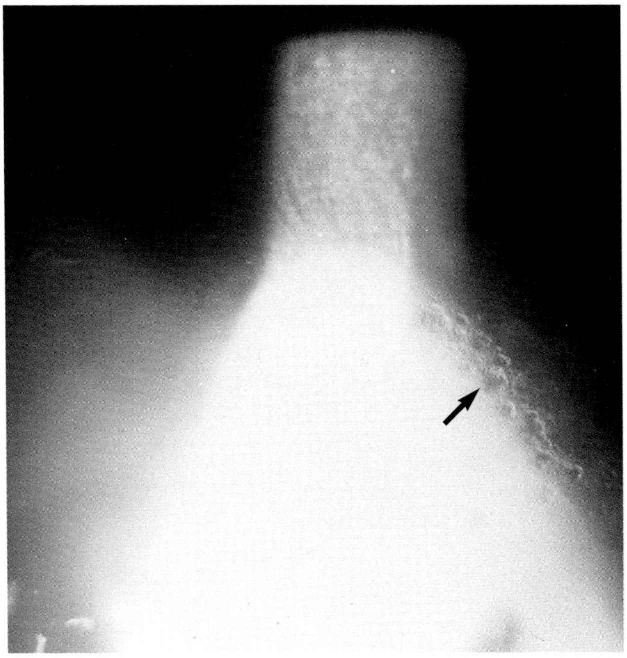

FIGURE 20-11 Deposits of spheroidal degeneration (arrow) at the limbus in a cornea with scarring from trauma.

When the lesions are subtle, they can be distinguished by autofluorescence in ultraviolet light.[56] Spheroidal degeneration is bilateral, except when it is associated with previous unilateral disease.

The frequency of spheroidal degeneration varies in different geographic regions[60] and increases with age. Actinic

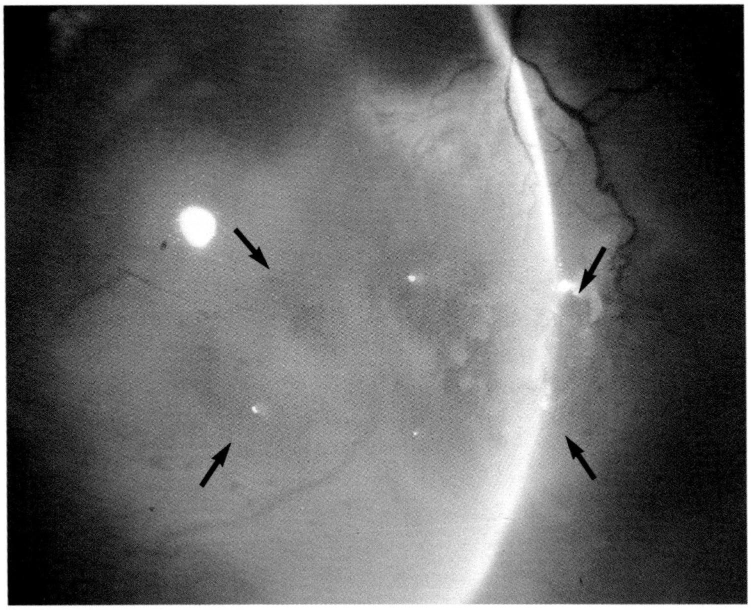

FIGURE 20-12 Advanced band-shaped spheroidal degeneration (arrows) in a scarred cornea.

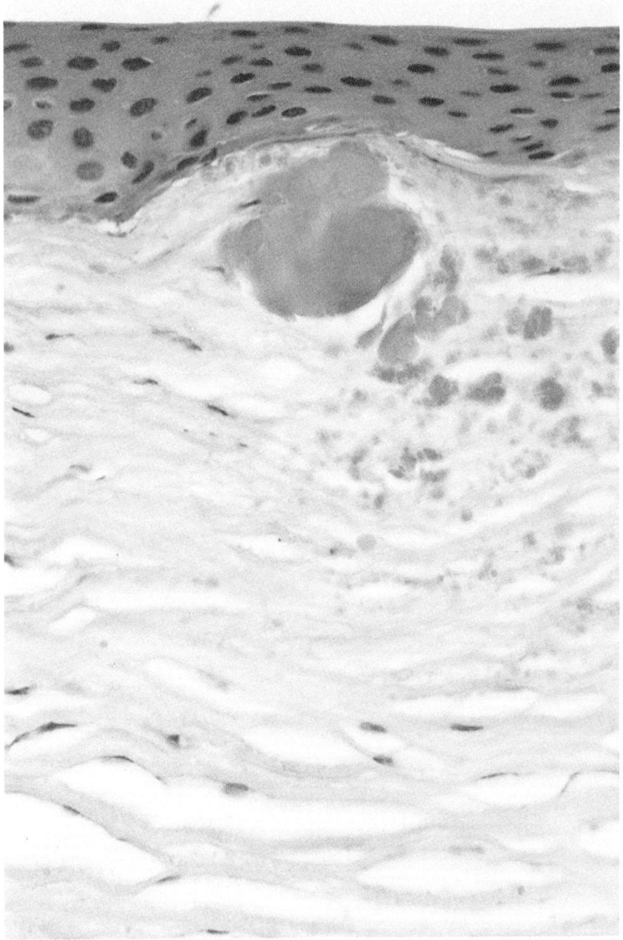

FIGURE 20-13 Homogeneous globular deposits in Bowman's layer and anterior stroma in spheroidal degeneration (hematoxylin and eosin stain).

exposure is the most likely basis for the varying geographic distribution. For example, the incidence is lower in England than in Arkansas, in a relationship best accounted for by the length of exposure to sunlight.[60] In a southern United States population, spheroidal degeneration was reported to occur in 43 percent of people over 50 years of age, and in at least 50 percent of people over 70 years of age. Studies of welders[2] and watermen[5,12] confirm a relationship between both prevalence and severity of deposits and ultraviolet and visible light exposure.

The cause of spheroidal degeneration is unknown. The climatic forms have been attributed to corneal drying, exposure to ice and sand in the wind, and ultraviolet light. The forms occurring secondary to pre-existing ocular disease have been seen in eyes with traumatic corneal scars, chronic corneal edema, herpetic keratitis, lattice corneal dystrophy, and glaucoma. A high incidence of open-angle glaucoma (21 percent) has been reported in the primary form.[56] The conjunctival form is frequently (86 percent) associated with pingueculae.

Histologically, the corneal droplets appear as hyaline spheres in the anterior corneal stroma and Bowman's layer (Figure 20-13). They are extracellular, and are composed of a proteinaceous material. This material was originally considered by Garner et al[60,61] to have features of keratin and later to be of collagenous origin. Others have stressed the presence of elastoid material, as seen in pingueculae.[62,63] The material may originate from proteins generated in the limbal conjunctiva that diffuse into the corneal stroma and precipitate.[4]

The lesions are asymptomatic in most cases. Treatment, therefore, either is not necessary or is directed toward the underlying corneal disease. In some patients, particularly those with advanced lesions, lamellar keratectomy or keratoplasty is indicated.

Corneal Arcus (Arcus Senilis)

Classification of corneal arcus as a degenerative change recognizes its frequent association with aging. It is not associated with tissue breakdown but rather with deposition of material not normally present in the healthy young cornea.[64,65]

Corneal arcus occurs initially in the inferior, then in the superior, peripheral cornea as a band of gray, white, or yellow deposits, made up of fine dots, separated from the limbus by a clear interval (Figure 20-14). This clear interval was described by Vogt[17,66] as being 0.2 to 0.3 mm wide. The arcus has a sharp peripheral border and a diffuse central border. As the deposits increase, the arcus spreads to involve the entire corneal circumference, although the density and width are greatest superiorly and often remain less in the horizontal meridian.[67] Deposition begins first in the deep cornea just anterior to Descemet's membrane, then in the area of Bowman's layer, forming two triangles, apex to apex. With time, the two triangles join, giving an hourglass configuration in cross section.[64] Dark crossing lines may occasionally be seen within the central hazy region of the arcus.[17] When abnormal vessels are present at the limbus and extend into the cornea, the arcus deviates centrally, maintaining a clear area of separation from the vessels.[17] Arcus may also form most densely, or earliest, at an area of corneal or limbal vascularization.

In the normal population, the frequency of corneal arcus increases with age. Arcus appears in 60 percent of men between the ages of 40 and 60 years, and 90 percent of men between 70 and 80 years of age. It is ubiquitous in men over the age of 80 years.[66] It tends to occur about

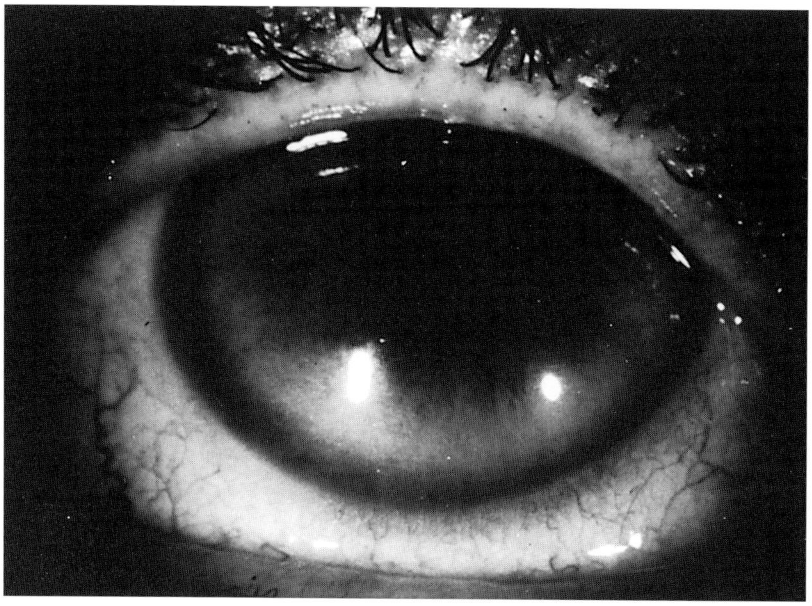

FIGURE 20-14 Corneal arcus.

10 years later in women than in men, and blacks are affected at an earlier age than whites.[34] Corneal arcus is almost nonexistent in some populations, such as Canadian Eskimos.[68] It is almost always bilateral. Unilateral occurrence may indicate vascular occlusive disease on the side without arcus.[69]

The association of corneal arcus with systemic vascular disease has been debated for decades. The presence of corneal arcus in persons under 50 years of age is a significant risk factor for coronary artery disease.[70] The relative risk of death from coronary artery disease or cardiovascular disease is increased four times in men 30 to 49 years of age with corneal arcus. This relationship is independent of the association with hyperlipidemia, and does not exist after the age of 50.[71] The most definite association is with types II and III hyperlipoproteinemias.[68] Levels of low-density lipoproteins are elevated in both. The presence of corneal arcus prior to age 40 is an indication for evaluation for systemic lipid abnormalities to detect these treatable conditions. Two very rare lipid abnormalities may also be associated with arcus. Lecithin:cholesterol acyltransferase (LCAT) deficiency is a recessive condition with anemia and renal disease associated with arcus and fine, central, stromal corneal haze.[72] Tangier disease, a deficiency of high-density lipoproteins, can also cause lipid deposits in the cornea[73] (see Ch. 17).

Histological and histochemical studies of arcus have demonstrated lipid deposits in the peripheral cornea and sclera.[64] These deposits are made up of sterol esters, mostly low-density lipoproteins.[65,74] Animal models and observations in humans suggest that both increased vascular permeability and elevated serum low-density lipoproteins are factors in arcus formation.[75]

Lipid Keratopathy

Lipid keratopathy[76] or degeneration, also known as fatty degeneration of the cornea, occurs in two forms, primary and secondary; the secondary form is more common than the primary form.

The secondary form of lipid keratopathy is related to the presence of corneal blood vessels. Typically, a dense, yellow-white infiltrate develops in the corneal stroma around an area of vessels. Occasionally the infiltrate develops gradually, but generally it appears suddenly around vessels that have been present for a long time. This sudden appearance is frequently alarming to the patient. Lipid keratopathy may seem to be similar to corneal arcus, with feathery edges, but more often occurs as a single mass and looks quite different from the circumferential arcus; it may also be made up of discrete crystals. It may take the form of a circular or oval disk, or may occur as a fan-like arc around the ends of the vessels (Figure 20-15). Although lipid keratopathy may be seen in any condition with corneal neovascularization, it typically occurs after corneal trauma, ulceration, interstitial keratitis, and herpetic keratitis.[77] A case has been reported following corneal hydrops of uncertain cause, and corneal edema has been considered to be a possible factor.[78] Both intra- and extracellular lipid deposition occur around abnormal blood vessels.[79] The lipids are the same as those seen in corneal arcus, suggesting vascular leakage as a factor in both.[74] Attempts

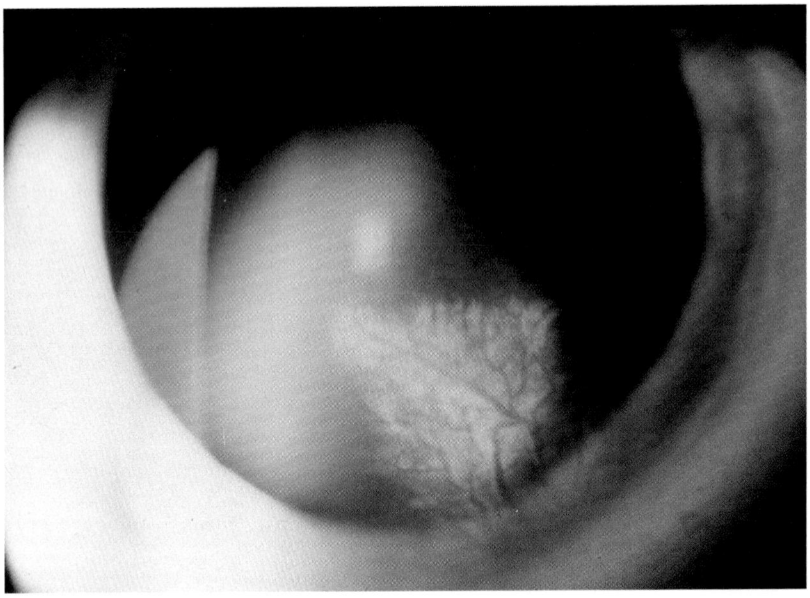

FIGURE 20-15 Lipid deposits central to corneal vascularization.

to permanently close vessels associated with lipid deposition are usually unsuccessful.

The primary form of lipid keratopathy occurs in a cornea that has not been previously altered by vascularization or inflammation, and in the absence of serum lipid elevation.[80,81] It is usually bilateral and may decrease vision. In some cases, it may represent an exaggeration of corneal arcus, extending into the central cornea.[80] Cholesterol crystals are present within the stroma. This condition has been treated by penetrating keratoplasty, although the lipid deposits may recur in the graft.[77,78]

Anterior and Posterior Crocodile Shagreen

Vogt[17] first described a gray shagreen in a circular area of Bowman's layer, including the central third of the cornea, in a 90-year-old woman. The shagreen was composed of "angular or round gray dots separated by dark lines." These areas were larger in the center and became gradually smaller as the opacity faded peripherally. A small tear or crack in Bowman's layer was visible in this patient. The condition was given the name *anterior crocodile shagreen.* A similar mosaic-like or cobblestone pattern was seen in the deep stroma or Descemet's membrane in other patients, and was termed *posterior crocodile shagreen.*

Anterior crocodile shagreen (Figure 20-16) is usually bilateral and is seen in the elderly. This involutional form usually causes minimal, if any, visual loss but may rarely cause significantly decreased visual acuity. Similar mosaic changes may be seen following trauma or in association with band keratopathy. Familial types may occur with X-linked megalocornea, or in a dominant juvenile form. Histologically, ridges with calcium deposition are seen in Bowman's layer.[82] Bron and Tripathi[82,83] relate the mosaic pattern to the normal anterior corneal mosaic, a pattern seen when the fluorescein-stained cornea is examined after pressure is applied through the eyelid. This pattern is thought to be related to the collagen structure of the anterior cornea, with areas of oblique insertion of collagen fibers into Bowman's layer. The pattern also manifests when tension on the cornea is decreased, as in hypotony, and in keratoconus patients who wear hard contact lenses.[84]

Generally, posterior crocodile shagreen is considered to be a result of aging. It is characterized by polygonal gray opacities, similar to those seen in anterior shagreen, but occurring in the central deep cornea (Figure 20-17). Occasionally, they also occur in the periphery, where they may be indistinguishable from corneal arcus. A dystrophic form of the same disorder has been described as central cloudy dystrophy by François[85] (see Ch. 18). It is dominantly inherited and can occur at any age. Vision is usually not impaired in either the dystrophic or senile form.[86] Histologically, there is irregularity of stromal collagen lamellae, with an irregular sawtooth pattern on electron microscopy.[87]

In most cases, neither anterior nor posterior crocodile shagreen requires therapy. However, in the senile form it is often difficult to determine whether a concurrent cataract accounts for the visual loss. Lamellar or penetrating keratoplasty is rarely indicated.

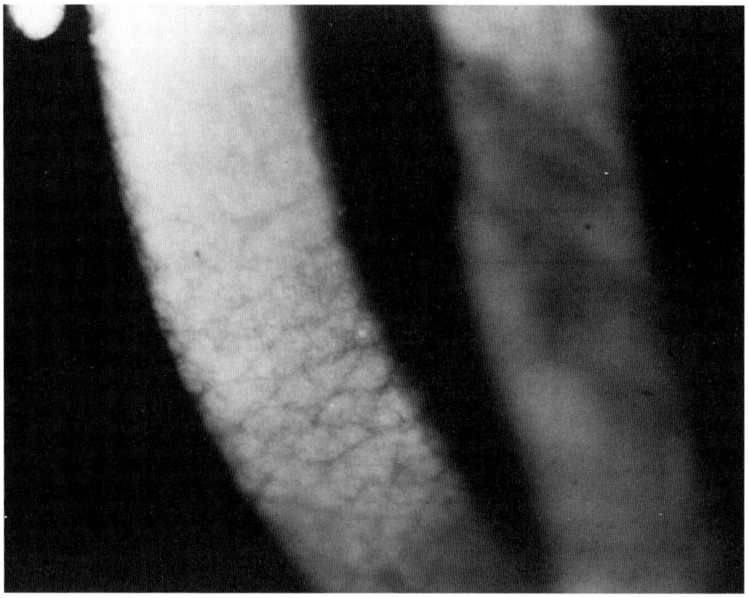

FIGURE 20-16 Anterior crocodile shagreen.

Cornea Farinata

Cornea farinata was first described by Vogt[17] in 1930. This condition is commonly seen in aging corneas and is asymptomatic. Discrete tiny, gray-to-white opacities are scattered throughout the deep corneal stroma, giving the appearance of flour dust (Figure 20-18). The manifestations are often subtle, and can be seen only on retroillumination. They are most prominent axially, and occur bilaterally. Their appearance is similar to that of the pre-Descemet's dystrophies, with which they have been classified by some,[88] although they are smaller and are usually seen at a later age. Familial cases have been reported.[89] The cause is unknown. Histologic studies of similar pre-Descemet's lesions have shown vacuoles in posterior keratocytes that contain lipofuscin-like material.[90] Lipofuscin is thought to be a pigment resulting from aging and wear and tear on cells; the presence of this material is consistent with a degenerative origin.

Amyloid of the Cornea and Conjunctiva

Amyloidosis is a group of disorders characterized by deposition of a particular group of hyaline proteins in tissues.

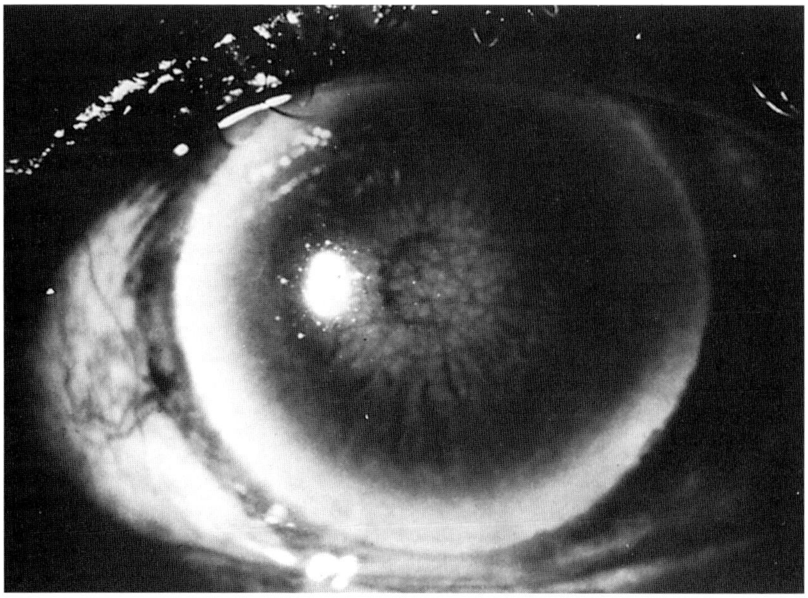

FIGURE 20-17 Posterior crocodile shagreen and dense corneal arcus.

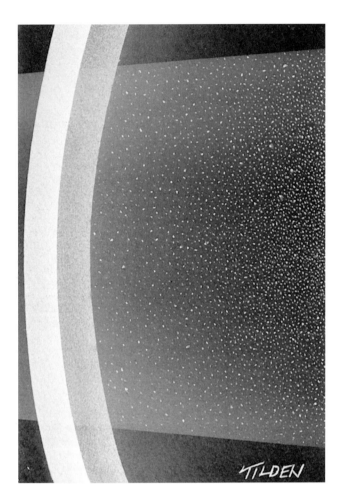

FIGURE 20-18 Fine deep corneal dusting of cornea farinata (artist's impression).

The various forms of amyloidosis may be localized or systemic, primary or secondary. The primary forms may be familial or nonfamilial. The proteins of amyloid may be derived from immunoglobulin λ- or κ-light chains (primary systemic amyloidosis); protein AA, a protein of unknown origin found in secondary amyloidosis; specific proteins of prealbumin origin found in some forms of familial amyloidosis; and protein AP, which is found in all types of amyloid.[91,92]

Primary systemic amyloidosis is usually nonfamilial. In this form, generalized organ involvement leads to nephrotic syndrome, congestive heart failure, tongue enlargement, and neuropathies.[91] Ocular involvement is unusual, although ophthalmoplegias and ptosis may occur. Eyelid skin is frequently involved. In the familial form of primary systemic amyloidosis, which is much rarer than the nonfamilial form, veil-like vitreous opacities and glaucoma may occur.[93] This is a dominantly inherited condition. Meretoja syndrome, which is a separate form of dominantly inherited, primary, familial amyloidosis, has been reported in Finland.[94] These patients have cranial nerve palsies beginning in middle age, with paresis of the upper face and blepharochalasis. They have corneal involvement (lattice dystrophy type II) similar to classic lattice corneal dystrophy (lattice dystrophy type I), but with fewer lattice lines and less central deposition. Visual loss occurs in patients in their seventh decade, much later than in lattice dystrophy type I. Glaucoma may also occur (see Ch. 18).

Secondary systemic amyloidosis is the most common systemic form of amyloidosis and follows long-standing rheumatoid arthritis, tuberculosis, leprosy, syphilis, and other chronic inflammatory conditions. Ocular involvement is rare, although histologic involvement of choroidal blood vessels and Bruch's membrane is reported.[95–97]

Localized amyloidosis may also be primary or secondary, familial or nonfamilial. Primary localized amyloidosis can involve the conjunctiva, eyelids, and orbit.[97–99] This presents as a soft, yellow, nodular thickening or mass in the eyelid or conjunctiva. Although evaluation for systemic disease is advised for such patients in the literature, the results of the work-up are almost always negative. Treatment is by local excision.

Lattice dystrophy type I may be considered a familial form of primary localized amyloidosis, and is discussed in Chapter 18. A recessive form of corneal amyloidosis has been reported, mostly in Japanese patients, as gelatinous drop-like corneal dystrophy, and is also discussed in Chapter 18. It occurs as bilateral, subepithelial opacities that cause irritation, photophobia, and visual loss. As the lesions progress, they become mulberry-like, yellow, white, or milky translucent nodular masses in the anterior cornea. Amyloid is deposited initially beneath the corneal epithelium and later in the anterior stroma. The material may be derived from the basal epithelial cells. Treatment with lamellar or penetrating keratoplasty has been successful in the short term, but deposits of amyloid may recur in the graft.[100–103]

Secondary localized corneal amyloidosis has been reported to occur following ocular trauma, phlyctenular keratitis, trachoma, chronic uveitis, and keratoconus.[104–106] The diagnosis is usually made histologically rather than clinically. The deposits occur as perivascular gray opacities, pannus, or nonspecific stromal opacities. In a review of 200 corneal specimens by an ophthalmic pathology laboratory, 3.5 percent were found to have amyloid deposits.[104] Amyloid deposits in the corneal stroma were found in about one-third of corneal buttons removed at keratoplasty for old syphilitic interstitial keratitis.[107] The histologic diagnosis of amyloidosis in ocular tissue is made on

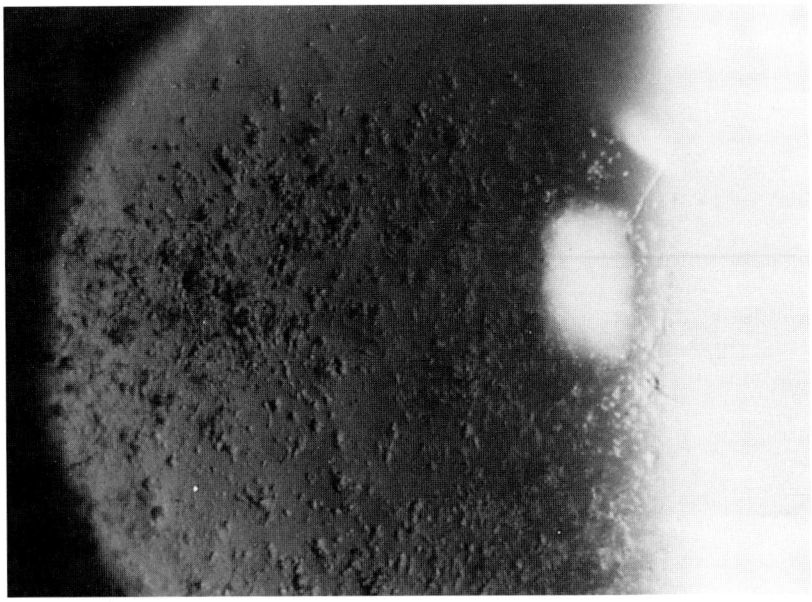

FIGURE 20-19 Polymorphic amyloid degeneration of the cornea as seen on retroillumination.

the basis of Congo red stain of the hyaline, amorphous, extracellular material, and dichroism in polarized light. Thioflavine T stain is also helpful.[98] Recent studies have used immunofluorescence techniques to characterize the proteins.[92] On electron microscopy, a characteristic fibrillar pattern is seen.

Another form of corneal amyloid deposition, polymorphic amyloid degeneration, will be considered as a separate entity, although it may be classified as a form of primary, localized amyloidosis of the cornea. Unlike gelatinous drop-like dystrophy and lattice corneal dystrophy, polymorphic amyloid degeneration of the cornea is probably more appropriately classified as a degeneration than a dystrophy.[108-110] It is usually asymptomatic, but may account for a decrease of no more than one line in visual acuity.[108] The lesions are seen as punctate and filamentous opacities in the corneal stroma, which appear gray on direct examination and transparent and glassy on retroillumination (Figure 20-19). They may be punctiform or branching, with clear intervening stroma, identical in appearance to the lesions of lattice dystrophy. However, they tend to be axial and more posteriorly located. Frequently, the deposits displace Descemet's membrane toward the anterior chamber. The longer lattice-like lesions may have a beaded appearance. The anterior and peripheral stroma are usually not involved. The lesions are bilateral, avascular, and usually not associated with other ocular or corneal disease. Cases have been reported in patients from the late fifth to the ninth decade, with an average age of 64.5 years.[108,110] Family studies have found no definite evidence of hereditary transmission.[110] Histologic studies have confirmed the amyloid nature of the deposits.[87,110] No cause has been determined, although mild elevation of serum globulins was found in five of eight cases.[108]

Unlike lattice corneal dystrophy, polymorphic amyloid degeneration is characterized by late onset, lack of inheritance, good visual acuity, central and posterior distribution, and the absence of epithelial erosions.

Terrien's Marginal Corneal Degeneration

Terrien[111] described a symmetrical, ectatic, marginal corneal dystrophy in 1900. Since that time, this condition has been reported in men more often than women, and can occur at any age. Although most series suggest a predominance of middle-aged and older men,[66] I have seen more cases in adolescent girls. Because the disease may take 20 or more years to develop, the cases noted in older adults may often have had a much earlier onset. The disease is usually bilateral (86 percent), although the development may be asymmetrical.[112]

Terrien's degeneration usually begins in the superior cornea but may occur anywhere around the limbus; it begins as a fine, punctate, stromal opacity similar to corneal arcus, with a lucid zone. This area becomes superficially vascularized by radial extension of vessels from the limbal arcades. An indentation develops parallel to the limbus, followed by slowly progressive thinning. The thin area has a sloping peripheral edge and fairly

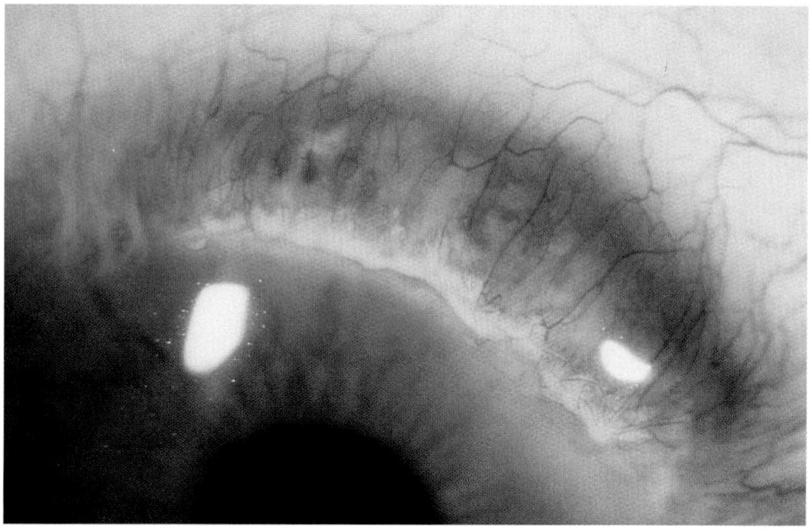

FIGURE 20-20 Superior corneal thinning and vascularization with lipid deposition at the central edge in Terrien's marginal corneal degeneration.

sharp central edge highlighted by a central white line of arcus-like material (Figure 20-20). During this stage, flattening in the involved area leads to a high degree of astigmatism that is often irregular.[113] Although the epithelium remains intact, the thinned area may bulge ectatically. Perforation or hydrops may occur spontaneously or after minor trauma.[114] The involved area slowly spreads circumferentially and rarely, centrally.[115,116] An oblique pseudopterygium, not in the usual axis for a true pterygium, is present in about 20 percent of cases and may be the presenting sign.[10,112] The process of corneal thinning is usually noninflammatory and painless. The patient may note only the visual change caused by the astigmatism. Some patients, however, may have recurrent episodes of painful inflammation, as well as coexistent episcleritis or superficial scleritis.[112]

The differential diagnosis of Terrien's degeneration includes Mooren's ulcer (see Ch. 23), which is an inflammatory autoimmune process. The epithelium is not intact in Mooren's ulcer, the central edge is undermined, and the process is generally much more rapid and destructive, although in the elderly, a relatively quiet, unilateral form may be difficult to distinguish from Terrien's degeneration.[117] Pellucid marginal corneal degeneration (see Ch. 22) does not have lipid infiltrates and usually occurs inferiorly. Marginal ulcerations related to systemic disease usually have a more rapid course.

Histologic study of Terrien's degeneration shows subepithelial connective tissue and vessels with fibrillar degeneration of collagen. Electron microscopy shows stromal material in phagocytic cells.[115,116,118,119]

No medical treatments have been effective in Terrien's degeneration. Peripheral inlay lamellar keratoplasty is necessary in cases of extreme thinning or perforation[114] (see Ch. 31).

Senile Furrow Degeneration

Senile furrow degeneration is rarely discussed in the literature, but it occurs occasionally and is usually noted as an incidental finding. Vogt[17] pointed out the false appearance of a furrow that may occur in the lucid interval between an arcus and the limbus. True thinning, however, may occur in the same region in the elderly. The "false" furrow is usually shallow, 0.5 mm or less in width, and not vascularized. The central and peripheral edges slope. The epithelium is intact, and there is no inflammation or change in vision. If these furrows progress, they do so slowly, and perforation does not occur.

Peripheral Corneal Guttae: Hassall-Henle Bodies

Peripheral guttate changes in Descemet's membrane occur with normal aging. Descemet's membrane has an anterior banded layer and a posterior nonbanded layer. The posterior layer thickens progressively with increasing age.[120] Localized areas of nodular thickening are visible in the peripheral cornea from early adulthood in the specular reflection of the slit lamp microscope. They are called Hassall-Henle bodies or warts, but are identical in structure to guttae occurring centrally in the cornea. The incidence of central guttae (cornea guttata) increases with age.[121] This condition is discussed with the endothelial dystrophies in Chapter 19.

PREVALENCE OF DEGENERATIONS IN A CORNEA CLINIC POPULATION

One hundred consecutive adult patients seen in my corneal practice were examined specifically for the corneal degenerations described in this chapter. All were examined with the Haag-Streit slit lamp microscope at high magnification. Patient ages ranged from 23 to 94 years, with a mean of 62.7 years (SD 16.5), and median of 65 years. Fifty-six percent of the patients were women. Most patients were referred for some pathologic change other than the corneal degeneration. Examinations were conducted specifically for each degeneration, and the most subtle findings were considered positive. Patients had from one to seven degenerations; the mean was 2.97 degenerations (SD 1.6, median 3). The most common degenerations were corneal arcus (67 percent); iron line (57 percent), mostly Hudson-Stähli, but some associated with Salzmann's nodular degeneration, pterygia, and keratoconus; guttae (56 percent), many as part of Fuchs' dystrophy; Vogt's limbal girdle (50 percent); and pinguecula (32 percent). Spheroidal degeneration, mostly of the conjunctiva, was seen in eight patients; lipid keratopathy in seven; and pterygium and Salzmann's degeneration in four each. The other degenerations were seen in three or fewer patients. No cases of Coats' white ring or known amyloid were seen (Table 20-1).

Although the bias of this small survey is obvious because of the source of patients referred for anterior segment disease, it is also obvious that these conditions occur with great frequency, making their recognition an important part of the corneal and conjunctival examination.

TABLE 20-1
Prevalence of Corneal Degenerations in 100 Consecutive Adult Cornea Clinic Patients (%)

Corneal arcus	67
Iron line	57
Guttae	56
Vogt's limbal girdle	50
Pinguecula	32
Spheroidal degeneration	8
Lipid keratopathy	7
Pterygium	4
Salzmann's degeneration	4
Band keratopathy	3
Cornea farinata	3
Crocodile shagreen	2
Senile furrow	2
Terrien's degeneration	1
Coats' white ring	0
Amyloid	0

REFERENCES

1. Hinnen E: Die Altersveranderungen des vorderen Bulbusabschnittes. Z Augenheilkd 45:129, 1921
2. Norn M, Franck C: Long-term changes in the outer part of the eye in welders. Acta Ophthalmol (Copenh) 69:382, 1991
3. Sugar S, Kobernick S: The pinguecula. Am J Ophthalmol 47:341, 1959
4. Klintworth GK: Chronic actinic keratopathy—a condition associated with conjunctival elastosis (pingueculae) and typified by characteristic extracellular concretions. Am J Pathol 67:327, 1972
5. Taylor HR, West SK, Rosenthal FS, et al: Corneal changes associated with chronic UV irradiation. Arch Ophthalmol 107:1481, 1989
6. Petrohelos M, Tricoulis D, Kotsiras I, Vouzoukos A: Ocular manifestations of Gaucher's disease. Am J Ophthalmol 80:1006, 1975
7. Fuchs E: Zur Anatomie der Pinguecula. Albrecht von Graefes Arch Ophthalmol 37:143, 1891
8. Hogan MJ, Alvarado J: Pterygium and pinguecula: electron microscopic study. Arch Ophthalmol 78:74, 1967
9. Austin P, Jakobiec FA, Iwamoto T: Elastodysplasia and elastodystrophy as pathologic bases of ocular pterygium and pinguecula. Ophthalmology 90:96, 1983
10. Goldman KN, Kaufman HE: Atypical pterygium, a clinical feature of Terrien's marginal degeneration. Arch Ophthalmol 96:1027, 1978
11. Stocker FW: Demonstrationen: eine pigmentierte Hornhautlinie bei Pterygium. Schweiz Med Wochenschr 20:19, 1939
12. Taylor HR, West S, Munoz B, et al: The long-term effects of visible light on the eye. Arch Ophthalmol 110:99, 1992
13. Taylor HR: Aetiology of climatic droplet keratopathy and pterygium. Br J Ophthalmol 64:154, 1980
14. Paton D: Pterygium management based upon a theory of pathogenesis. Trans Am Acad Ophthalmol Otolaryngol 79:603, 1975
15. Ansari MW, Rahi HS, Sukla BR: Pseudoelastic nature of pterygium. Br J Ophthalmol 54:473, 1970
16. Cameron MF: Histology of pterygium, an electron microscopic study. Br J Ophthalmol 67:604, 1983
17. Vogt A: Textbook and Atlas of Slit Lamp Microscopy of the Living Eye. Wayenborgh Editions, Bonn, 1981
18. Gass JD: The iron lines of the superficial cornea. Arch Ophthalmol 71:348, 1964
19. Norn MS: Hudson-Stähli's line of cornea. I. Incidence and morphology. Acta Ophthalmol (Copenh) 46:106, 1968
20. Rose GE, Lavin MJ: The Hudson-Stähli line. I. An epidemiologic study. Eye 1:466, 1987
21. Barraquer-Somers E, Chan CC, Green WR: Corneal epithelial iron deposition. Ophthalmology 90:729, 1983
22. Norn MS: Hudson-Stähli's line of cornea. II. Aetiological studies. Acta Ophthalmol (Copenh) 46:119, 1968
23. Ferry AP: A "new" line of the superficial cornea: occurrence in patients with filtering blebs. Arch Ophthalmol 79:142 1968

24. Reinach NW, Baum J: A corneal pigmented line associated with Salzmann's nodular degeneration. Am J Ophthalmol 91:677, 1981
25. Mannis MJ: Iron deposition in the corneal graft. Arch Ophthalmol 101:1858, 1983
26. Koenig SB, McDonald MB, Yamaguchi T, et al: Corneal iron lines after refractive keratoplasty. Arch Ophthalmol 101:1862, 1983
27. Rose GE, Lavin MJ: The Hudson-Stähli line. III. Observations on morphology, a critical review of aetiology and a unified theory for the formation of iron lines of the corneal epithelium. Eye 1:475, 1987
28. Coats G: Small superficial opaque white rings in the cornea. Trans Ophthalmol Soc UK 32:53, 1912
29. Miller EM: Genesis of white rings of the cornea. Am J Ophthalmol 61:904, 1966
30. Nevins RC, Davis WH, Elliott JH: Coats' white ring of the cornea—unsettled metal fettle. Arch Ophthalmol 80:145, 1968
31. Sugar HS, Kobernick S: The white limbus girdle of Vogt. Am J Ophthalmol 50:101, 1960
32. Franceschetti A, Forgács J: Aspect histologique de la dégéneresence limbique en ceinture ("Weisser limbusgürtel" de Vogt) et son analogie avec la dégénerescence primitive en bandelette de la cornée. Ophthalmologica 138:393, 1959
33. O'Connor GR: Calcific band keratopathy. Trans Am Ophthalmol Soc 70:58, 1972
34. Klintworth G: Degenerations, depositions, and miscellaneous reactions of the cornea, conjunctiva, and sclera. p. 1431. In Garner A, Klintworth G (eds): Pathobiology of Ocular Disease. Marcel Dekker, New York, 1982
35. Kennedy RE, Roca PD, Landers PH: Atypical band keratopathy in glaucomatous patients. Am J Ophthalmol 72:917, 1971
36. Brazier DJ, Hitchings RA: Atypial band keratopathy following long-term pilocarpine treatment. Br J Ophthalmol 73:294, 1989
37. Cogan DG, Albright F, Bartter FC: Hypercalcemia and band keratopathy. Arch Ophthalmol 40:624, 1948
38. Porter R, Crombie AL: Corneal and conjunctival calcification in chronic renal failure. Br J Ophthalmol 57:339, 1973
39. Bennett SR, Abrams GW: Band keratopathy from emulsified silicone oil. Arch Ophthalmol 108:1387, 1990
40. Nevyas AS, Raber IM, Eagle RC, et al: Acute band keratopathy following intracameral Viscoat. Arch Ophthalmol 105:958, 1987
41. Lemp MA, Ralph RA: Rapid development of band keratopathy in dry eyes. Am J Ophthalmol 83:657, 1977
42. Doughman DJ, Olson GA, Nolan S, Hajny RG: Experimental band keratopathy. Arch Ophthalmol 81:264, 1969
43. Cursino JW, Fine BS: A histologic study of calcific and noncalcific band keratopathy. Am J Ophthalmol 82:395, 1976
44. Breinin GM, DeVoe AG: Chelation of calcium with EDTA in band keratopathy and corneal calcium affections. Arch Ophthalmol 52:846, 1954
45. Bokosky JE, Meyer RF, Sugar A: Surgical treatment of calcific band keratopathy. Ophthalmic Surg 16:645, 1985
46. Wood TO, Walker GG: Treatment of band keratopathy. Am J Ophthalmol 80:553, 1975
47. Gartry D, Kerr Muir M, Marshall J: Excimer laser treatment of corneal surface pathology: a laboratory and clinical study. Br J Ophthalmol 75:258, 1991
48. Salzmann M: Über eine Abart der knotchenformigen Hornhautdystrophie. Z Augenheilkd 57:92, 1925
49. Abbott RL, Forster RK: Superficial punctate keratitis of Thygeson associated with scarring and Salzmann's nodular degeneration. Am J Ophthalmol 87:296, 1979
50. Vannas A, Hogan MJ, Wood I: Salzmann's nodular degeneration of the cornea. Am J Ophthalmol 79:211, 1975
51. Katz D: Salzmann's nodular corneal dystrophy. Acta Ophthalmol (Copenh) 31:377, 1953
52. Wood TO: Salzmann's nodular degeneration. Cornea 9:17, 1990
53. Steinert RF, Puliafito CA: Excimer laser phototherapeutic keratectomy for a corneal nodule. Refract Corneal Surg 6:352, 1990
54. Gray RH, Johnson GJ, Freedman A: Climatic droplet keratopathy. Surv Ophthalmol 36:241, 1992
55. Fraunfelder FT, Hanna C: Spheroidal degeneration of the cornea and conjunctiva. 3. Incidence, classification, and etiology. Am J Ophthalmol 76:41, 1973
56. Fraunfelder FT, Hanna C, Parker JM: Spheroidal degeneration of the cornea and conjunctiva. 1. Clinical course and characteristics. Am J Ophthalmol 74:821, 1972
57. Hanna C, Fraunfelder FT: Spheroidal degeneration of the cornea and conjunctiva. 2. Pathology. Am J Ophthalmol 74:829, 1972
58. Etzine S, Kaufmann JCE: Band-shaped nodular dystrophy of the cornea. Am J Ophthalmol 57:760, 1964
59. Young JDH, Finlay RD: Primary spheroidal degeneration of the cornea in Labrador and northern Newfoundland. Am J Ophthalmol 79:129, 1975
60. Garner A, Fraunfelder FT, Barras TC, Hinspeter EN: Spheroidal degeneration of cornea and conjunctiva. Br J Ophthalmol 60:473, 1976
61. Garner A, Morgan G, Tripathi RC: Climatic droplet keratopathy. II. Pathologic findings. Arch Ophthalmol 89:198, 1973
62. Brownstein S, Rodrigues MM, Fine BS, Albert EN: The elastotic nature of hyaline corneal deposits. Am J Ophthalmol 75:799, 1973
63. Rodrigues MM, Laibson PR, Weinreb S: Corneal elastosis, appearance of band-like keratopathy and spheroidal degeneration. Arch Ophthalmol 93:111, 1975
64. Cogan DG, Kuwabara T: Arcus senilis, its pathology and histochemistry. Arch Ophthalmol 61:353, 1959
65. Walton KW: Studies on the pathogenesis of corneal arcus formation. 1. The human corneal arcus and its relation to atherosclerosis as studied by immunofluorescence. J Pathol 111:263, 1973
66. Duke-Elder S, Leigh AG: System of Ophthalmology. Vol. 8. Diseases of the Outer Eye. Kimpton, London, 1965

67. Phillips CI, Tsukahara S, Gore SM: Corneal arcus: some morphology and applied pathophysiology. Jpn J Ophthalmol 34:442, 1990
68. Rifkind BM: Corneal arcus and hyperlipoproteinaemia. Surv Ophthalmol 16:295, 1972
69. Smith JL, Susac JO: Unilateral arcus senilis: sign of occlusive disease of the carotid artery. JAMA 225:676, 1973
70. Rosenman RH, Brand RJ, Sholtz BJ, Jenkins CD: Relation of corneal arcus to cardiovascular risk factors and incidence of coronary disease. N Engl J Med 29:1322, 1974
71. Chambless LE, Fuchs FD, Linn S, et al: The association of corneal arcus with coronary heart disease and cardiovascular disease mortality in the Lipid Research Clinics mortality follow-up study. Am J Public Health 80:1200, 1990
72. Horven I, Egge K, Gjone E: Corneal and fundus changes in familial LCAT deficiency. Acta Ophthalmol (Copenh) 52:201, 1974
73. Fredrickson DS, Gotto AM, Levy RI: Familial lipoprotein deficiency. p. 493. In Stanbury JB, Wyngaarden JB, Fredrickson DS (eds): The Metabolic Basis of Inherited Disease. 3rd Ed. McGraw-Hill, New York, 1972
74. Andrews JS: The lipids of arcus senilis. Arch Ophthalmol 68:264, 1962
75. Walton KW, Dunkerley DJ: Studies on the pathogenesis of corneal arcus formation. II. Immunofluorescent studies on lipid deposition in the eye of the lipid-fed rabbit. J Pathol 114:217, 1974
76. Cogan DG, Kuwabara T: Lipid keratopathy and atheromas. Circulation 18:519, 1958
77. Friedlaender MH, Cavanagh HD, Sullivan WR, et al: Bilateral central lipid infiltrates of the cornea. Am J Ophthalmol 84:781, 1977
78. Shapiro LA, Farkas TG: Lipid keratopathy following cornea hydrops. Arch Ophthalmol 95:456, 1977
79. Jack RL, Lase SA: Lipid keratopathy, an electron microscopic study. Arch Ophthalmol 83:678, 1970
80. Fine BS, Townsend WM, Zimmerman LE, Lashkari MH: Primary lipoidal degeneration of the cornea. Am J Ophthalmol 78:12, 1974
81. Baum JL: Cholesterol keratopathy. Am J Ophthalmol 67:372, 1969
82. Tripathi RC, Bron AJ: Secondary anterior crocodile shagreen of Vogt. Br J Ophthalmol 59:59, 1975
83. Bron AJ, Tripathi RC: Anterior corneal mosaic, further observations. Br J Ophthalmol 53:760, 1969
84. Dangel ME, Kracher GP, Stark WJ: Anterior corneal mosaic in eyes with keratoconus wearing hard contact lenses. Arch Ophthalmol 102:888, 1984
85. François J: Une nouvelle dystrophie hérédo-familiale de la cornée. J Génét Hum 5:189, 1956
86. Goodside V: Posterior crocodile shagreen. Am J Ophthalmol 46:748, 1958
87. Krachmer JH, Dubord PJ, Rodrigues MM, Mannis MJ: Corneal posterior crocodile shagreen and polymorphic amyloid degeneration. Arch Ophthalmol 101:54, 1983
88. Grayson M, Wilbrandt H: Pre-Descemet dystrophy. Am J Ophthalmol 64:276 1967
89. Paufique L, Etienne R: La cornea farinata. Bull Soc Ophtalmol Fr 50:522, 1950
90. Curran RE, Kenyon KR, Green WR: Pre-Descemet's membrane corneal dystrophy. Am J Ophthalmol 77:711, 1974
91. Kyle RA, Grapp RP: Amyloidosis (A2), clinical and laboratory features in 229 cases. Mayo Clin Proc 58:665, 1983
92. Mondino BJ, Raj CV, Skinner M, et al: Protein AA and lattice corneal dystrophy. Am J Ophthalmol 89:377, 1980
93. Kaufman HE: Primary familial amyloidosis. Arch Ophthalmol 60:1036, 1958
94. Starck T, Kenyon KR, Hanninen LA, et al: Clinical and histopathologic studies of two families with lattice corneal dystrophy and familial systemic amyloidosis (Meretoja syndrome). Ophthalmology 98:1197, 1991
95. Rodriques M, Zimmerman LE: Secondary amyloidosis in ocular leprosy. Arch Ophthalmol 85:277, 1971
96. Doughman DJ: Ocular amyloidosis. Surv Ophthalmol 13:133, 1968
97. Brownstein MH, Elliott R, Helwig EB: Ophthalmologic aspects of amyloidosis. Am J Ophthalmol 69:423, 1970
98. Smith ME, Zimmerman LE: Amyloidosis of the eyelid and conjunctiva. Arch Ophthalmol 88:346, 1979
99. Blodi FC, Apple DJ: Localized conjunctival amyloidosis. Am J Ophthalmol 88:346, 1979
100. Ramsey MS, Fine BS, Cohen SW: Localized corneal amyloidosis. Am J Ophthalmol 73:560, 1972
101. Stock EL, Keilar RA: Primary familial amyloidosis of the cornea. Am J Ophthalmol 82:266, 1976
102. Weber FL, Babel J: Gelatinous drop-like dystrophy, a form of primary corneal amyloidosis. Arch Ophthalmol 98:144, 1980
103. Ohnishi Y, Shinoda Y, Ishibashi T, Taniguchi Y: The origin of amyloid in gelatinous drop-like corneal dystrophy. Curr Eye Res 2:225, 1982/1983
104. McPherson SD, Kiffney GT, Freed CC: Corneal amyloidosis. Am J Ophthalmol 62:1025, 1966
105. Stafford WR, Fine BS: Amyloidosis of the cornea, report of a case without conjunctival involvement. Arch Ophthalmol 75:53, 1966
106. Collyer RT: Amyloidosis of the cornea. Can J Ophthalmol 3:35, 1968
107. Dutt S, Elner VM, Soong HK, et al: Secondary localized amyloidosis in interstitial keratitis (IK): clinicopathologic findings. Ophthalmology 99:817, 1992
108. Thomsitt J, Bron AJ: Polymorphic stromal dystrophy. Br J Ophthalmol 59:125, 1975
109. Drobec P: Senile Gitterstrukturen im Parenchym der Kornea. Klin Monatsbl Augenheilkd 171:636, 1977
110. Mannis MJ, Krachmer JH, Rodrigues MM, Pardos GJ: Polymorphic amyloid degeneration of the cornea. Arch Ophthalmol 99:1217, 1981
111. Terrien F: Dystrophie marginale symetrique des deux cornées. Arch Ophtalmol (Paris) 20:12, 1900
112. Etzine S, Friedmann A: Marginal dystrophy of the cornea with total ectasia. Am J Ophthalmol 55:150, 1963

113. Wilson SE, Lin DTC, Klyce SD, Insler MS: Terrien's marginal degeneration: corneal topography. Refract Corneal Surg 6:15, 1990
114. Soong HK, Fitzgerald J, Boruchoff SA, et al: Corneal hydrops in Terrien's marginal degeneration. Ophthalmology 93:340, 1986
115. Suveges I, Levai G, Alberth B: Pathology of Terrien's disease. Am J Ophthalmol 74:1191, 1972
116. Lopez JS, Price FW, Whitcup SM, et al: Immunohistochemistry of Terrien's and Mooren's corneal degeneration. Arch Ophthalmol 109:988, 1991
117. Wood TO, Kaufman HE: Mooren's ulcer. Am J Ophthalmol 71:417, 1971
118. Iwamoto T, DeVoe AG, Farris RL: Electron microscopy in cases of marginal degeneration of the cornea. Invest Ophthalmol 11:241, 1972
119. Austin P, Brown SI: Inflammatory Terrien's marginal corneal disease. Am J Ophthalmol 92:189, 1981
120. Johnson DH, Bourne WM, Campbell RJ: The ultrastructure of Descemet's membrane. I. Changes with age in normal corneas. Arch Ophthalmol 100:1942, 1982
121. Lorenzetti DW, Uotila MH, Parikh N, Kaufman HE: Central cornea guttata, incidence in the general population. Am J Ophthalmol 64:1155, 1967

21

Pterygium

BRADLEY P. GARDNER AND WILLIAM M. TOWNSEND

Most textbooks evade the question of what a pterygium really is and merely describe the lesion instead of truly defining it. A pterygium, to borrow from Amsler's comment about keratoconus, is a condition that resembles only itself. Since the days of Susruta, the world's first ophthalmic surgeon who lived more than a thousand years before the birth of Christ, pterygia have been recognized as triangular sheets of fibrovascular tissue that appear on the epibulbar conjunctiva and cornea, disturbing both the patient because of their unsightly appearance and the surgeon because of their tendency to recur.[1] A definitive classification of the lesion continues to elude us, and its cause and pathogenesis remain uncertain. In our present state of knowledge, we can only characterize the lesion as accurately as possible and point out the best available methods for successful medical management and surgical removal.

INCIDENCE AND PREVALENCE

Cameron's map of world prevalence rates of pterygia (Figure 21-1) establishes a direct relationship between prevalence and proximity to the equator: the nearer to the equator, the greater the prevalence.[2] Thus, on an island such as Aruba, situated only 12 degrees of latitude from the equator, the prevalence may be as high as 22.5 percent.[3] In Puerto Rico (latitude 18 degrees), it is approximately 18 percent. Within the continental United States, higher rates prevail in the South. Texas, Louisiana, New Mexico, southern California, and Florida, which occupy latitudes between 28 and 36 degrees, have rates between 5 and 15 percent.[4] Beyond the 40th parallel, the prevalence of pterygia is negligible (2 percent or less).

Factors other than geographic location also affect the prevalence of pterygia. Pterygia are seen nearly twice as often in men as in women. They are also more common in farmers than in city dwellers, and in those who do not wear eyeglasses.[2] Prevalence and incidence rates differ with respect to age. Although the elderly have the highest prevalence rate, a much younger (20- to 40-year-old) group has the highest incidence rate. Pterygia rarely occur in patients under the age of 20 years. Curiously, the discrepancy between incidence and prevalence rates is not seen with pingueculae, which are widely held to be the precursors of pterygia.[5] Both the incidence and prevalence of pingueculae increase with age. Another difference between pingueculae and pterygia is that pingueculae occur with similar frequency in both sexes. Also, pingueculae are common even in regions where pterygia rarely occur.

CLINICAL FEATURES

A pterygium appears as a fleshy triangular band of fibrovascular tissue. It has a broad base on the nasal or temporal epibulbar surface, and a blunted apex on the cornea (Figure 21-2). The axis of the triangle is not exactly horizontal; instead, it gently slopes superiorly on the corneal side.

A pterygium has several components. A gray zone, or cap, precedes the apex, or head. The cap is a flat, grayish white avascular zone of variable size located in the subepithelial corneal tissue, surrounding the head of the pterygium like a halo. Sometimes, round, gray, coin-like extensions of the cap precede it ("lots of Fuchs").[6] In some cases, a golden-yellow iron line (Stocker's line)[7] is evident in the corneal epithelium, bordering the corneal side of the head. Between the head and the cap are small capillaries that often anastomose with the limbal plexus. The head itself is slightly elevated and white. It is the one site of firm adhesion of the

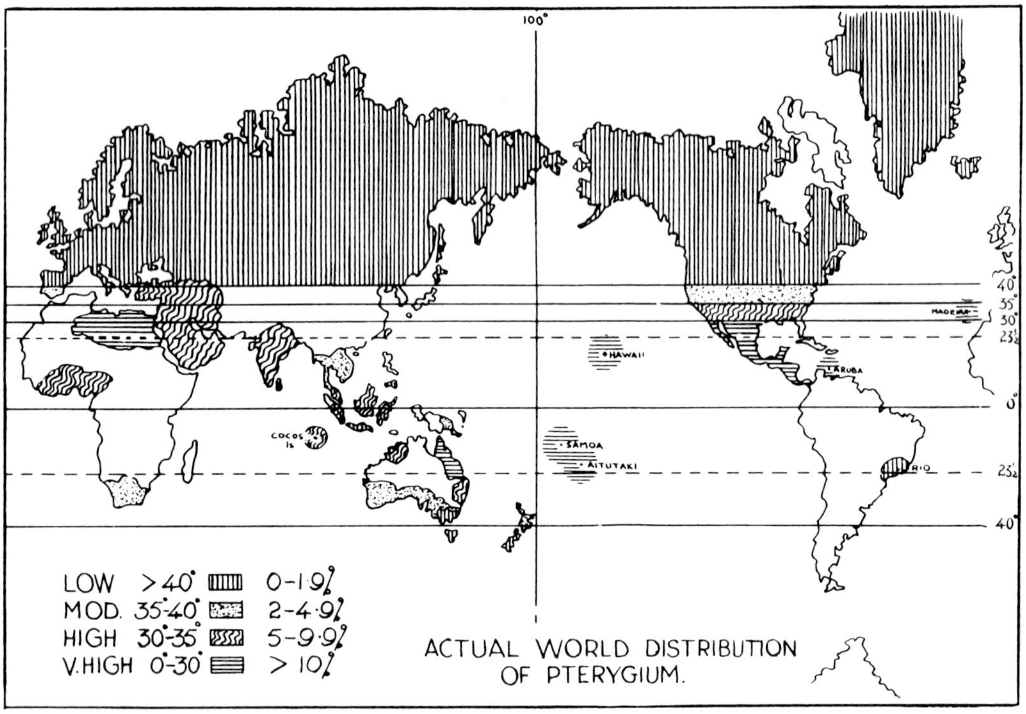

FIGURE 21-1 Cameron's map of world prevalence rates of pterygia. (Reprinted with permission from ME Cameron: Pterygium throughout the World. Charles C Thomas, Springfield, IL, 1965. Courtesy of Charles C. Thomas, Publisher, Springfield, IL.)

pterygium to the globe; the body of the pterygium can be readily lifted from the epibulbar surface. The body is a fleshy sheet of pink, highly vascularized tissue that is delineated from the normal conjunctiva superiorly and inferiorly by sharp folds and attaches on a broad base. The body is under horizontal tension, as evidenced by the vessels, which appear stretched and straight. Application of fluorescein frequently reveals punctate staining over the epithelial surface of the body and occasionally on the cornea immediately in front of the head. Corneal dellen may occur, but are rare, although central dry spots are common.

More often than not, a pterygium is already fully developed when the patient first seeks help. Usually, the history reveals that the lesion grew rapidly over a period not exceeding 2 or 3 months. In some cases, the patient acknowledges that prior to the onset of rapid growth, the

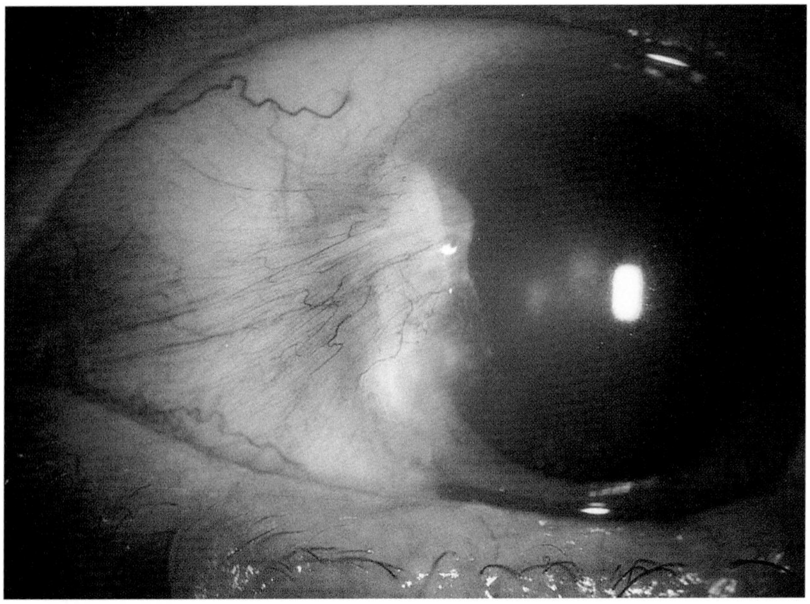

FIGURE 21-2 Nasal pterygium. Note the various components described in the text.

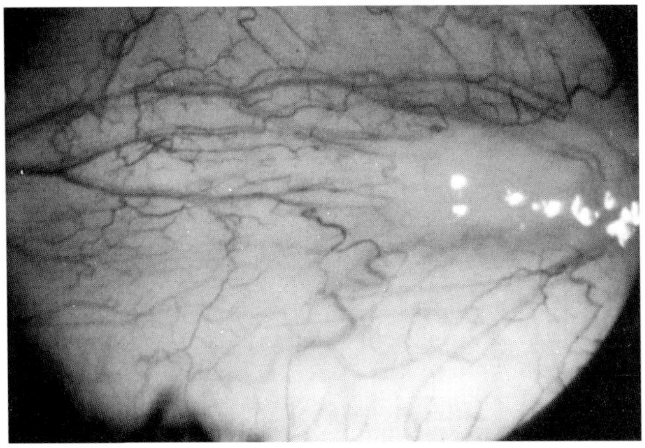

FIGURE 21-3 Beginning pterygium. The appearance is similar to that of a pinguecula.

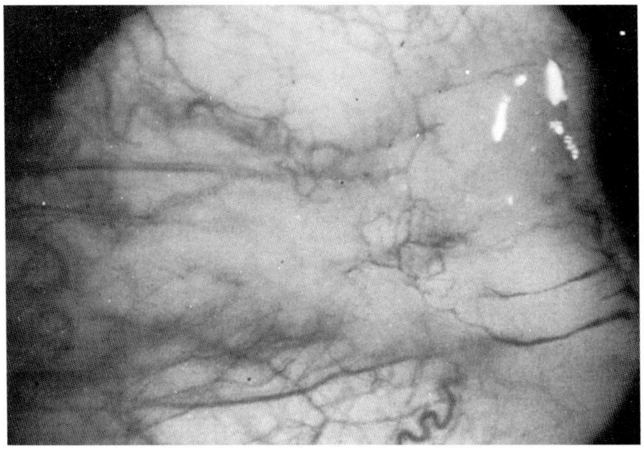

FIGURE 21-4 As a pterygium evolves, the tissue elongates and neovascularization appears on its conjunctival side and its corneal side. Also, there is congestion of the limbal plexus.

lesion had been a small mound present for many months or even years.

Rarely, the full evolution of a pterygium can be witnessed. In these cases, the initial lesion is indistinguishable from a pinguecula (Figure 21-3), which suddenly has attracted vessels from both the conjunctiva and underlying tissue. The yellow mound elongates and assumes the shape of an hourglass (Figure 21-4). In the weeks or months following, prominent new vessels continue to appear on the conjunctival side of the mound, while on the corneal side many delicate vascular twigs project toward segmentally engorged limbal vessels. With the appearance of superior and inferior folds, the body of the pterygium is defined. The entire lesion becomes a true pterygium when the yellow mound, now the head, encroaches on the cornea (Figure 21-5). Actual encroachment is heralded by the appearance of a halo-like subepithelial cap in the cornea.

In contrast to the relatively rapid formation, growth across the cornea is slow, and the pterygium usually takes several years to reach the entrance pupil. Often, however, growth abruptly ceases. This inactivation is characterized by the absence of episodic congestion, disappearance of punctate staining over the body, and shrinkage of the halo-like cap. The lesion may remain stationary for several years. Eventually, involutional changes occur. The head progressively thins and flattens, leaving a scar that blends imperceptibly with the adjacent cornea, and the body withers into a veil-like membrane traversed by only a few delicate blood vessels.

Actively growing pterygia typically occur in the young age group (20- to 30-year-old patients), the group with the highest incidence of pterygium. The most exuberant

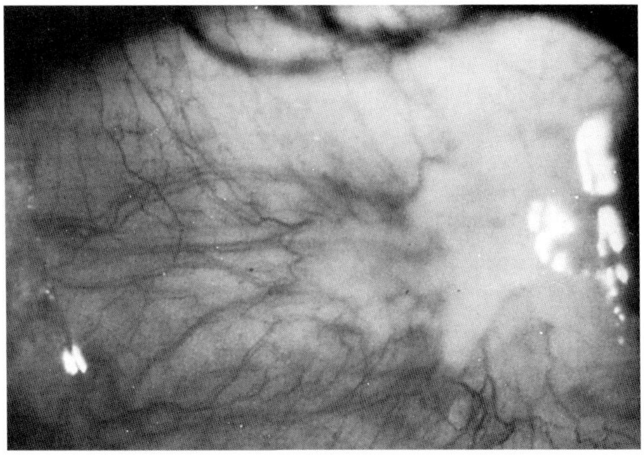

FIGURE 21-5 With further evolution of a pterygium, there is consolidation of the tissue into a head and body.

pterygia, that is, extremely fleshy masses with marked corneal extension, are seen in people who are exposed to the elements, such as farmers and construction workers.

Pterygia can be classified into five groups: (1) actively growing pterygia, (2) slowly growing pterygia, (3) stationary pterygia, (4) fleshy pterygia, and (5) atrophic pterygia.

Symptoms result from decreased visual acuity and intermittent episodes of inflammation, during which the pterygium becomes hyperemic and causes photophobia, tearing, and foreign body sensation. The cosmetic blemish is always present. Visual acuity may decrease as a result of astigmatism, increased glare and decreased contrast sensitivity, or encroachment of the pterygium on the

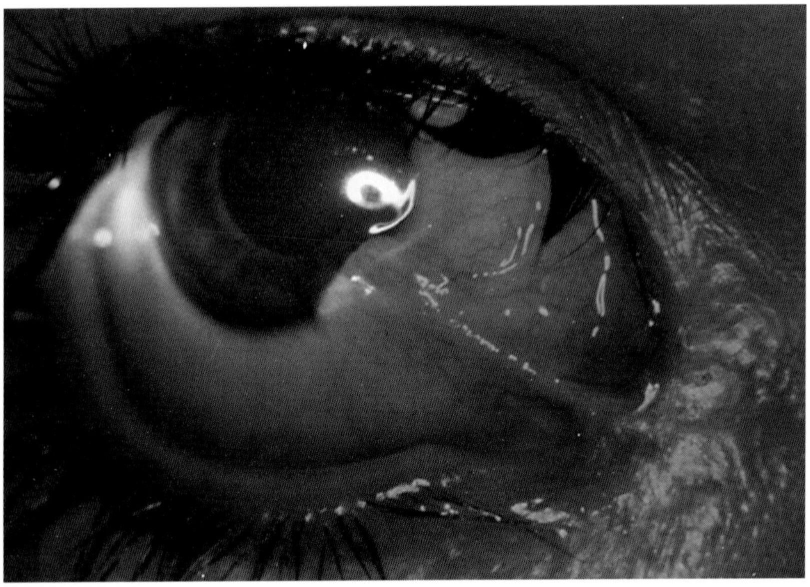

FIGURE 21-6 Symblepharon caused by a pterygium.

visual axis.[8,9] In severe cases, diplopia may be caused by symblepharon formation and limitation of ocular motility (Figure 21-6). Astigmatism induced by a pterygium is most commonly with-the-rule (steep vertical axis), but can be against-the-rule, oblique, or irregular.[8,10] As much as 9 diopters of astigmatism can occur.[10] Regular astigmatism induced by a pterygium occurs long before the pterygium encroaches on the entrance pupil and certainly before it reaches the visual axis.[10] One possible explanation for the astigmatism is the exertion of tractional forces by contractile elements within the pterygium that mechanically distort and flatten the cornea.[11] However, corneal topography has shown that the distortion of the precorneal tear film by the leading edge of a pterygium alters the topographic mires, thereby effectively flattening the horizontal meridian and creating with-the-rule astigmatism[12] (Figure 21-7). The absence of myofibroblasts within a pterygium, coupled with evidence of distortion of the tear

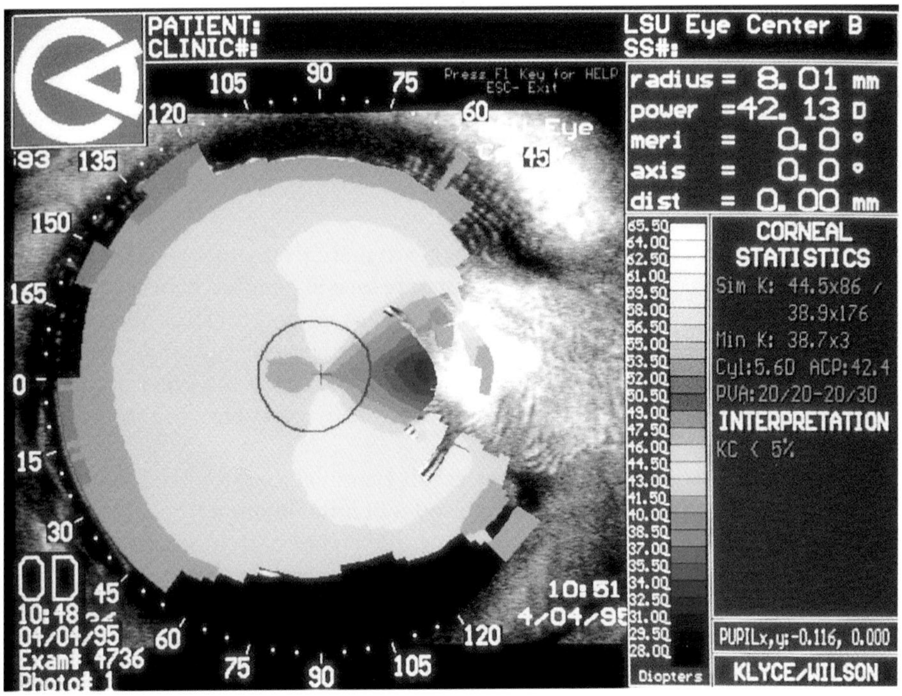

FIGURE 21-7 Videokeratograph of a cornea with a pterygium. There is flattening immediately central to the head of the pterygium, and with-the-rule astigmatism.

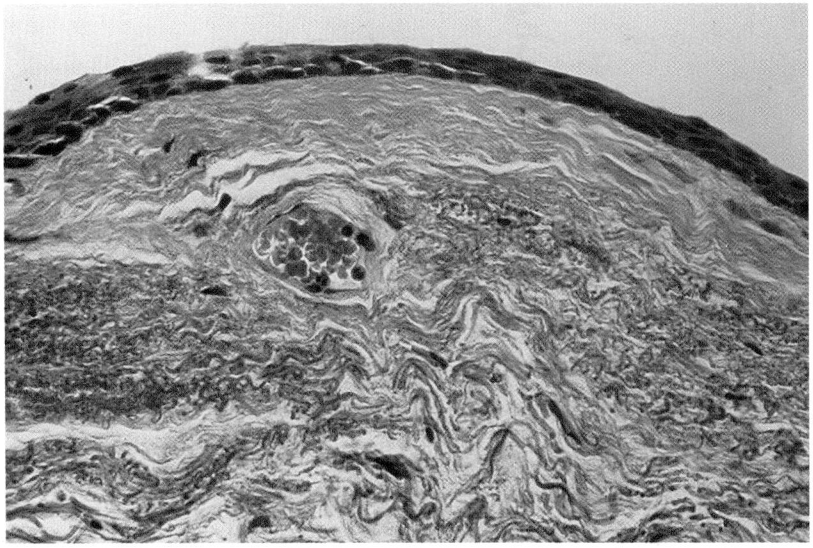

FIGURE 21-8 Histologic appearance of a pterygium. Note the corkscrew appearance of the elastotic degeneration (hematoxylin and eosin).

film, suggests that tear film distortion is a more likely cause of the induced astigmatism.[12]

HISTOPATHOLOGY

Three basic elements characterize the histologic appearance of a pterygium. The first element is an epithelial covering of atrophic conjunctiva that extends beyond its normal anatomic confines onto the cornea. It overlies the second element: a bulky mass of thickened, hypertrophied, and degenerated connective tissue, the collagen component of which assumes a coiled, fibrillated pattern reminiscent of elastic tissue (Figure 21-8). The abnormal collagen shows basophilia and an affinity for elastic tissue stains, but is not digested by elastase.[13] Hence, it is not elastic tissue, but falls into a category of elastotic degeneration. The third element is vascular. New blood vessels, usually congested, are dispersed among the hypertrophied collagen fibers. Additionally, the episcleral bed beneath the pterygium is hyperemic.

Because Tenon's capsule is absent at the limbus, the subepithelial connective tissue at this site lies directly over the episclera (Figure 21-9A). A short distance posterior to

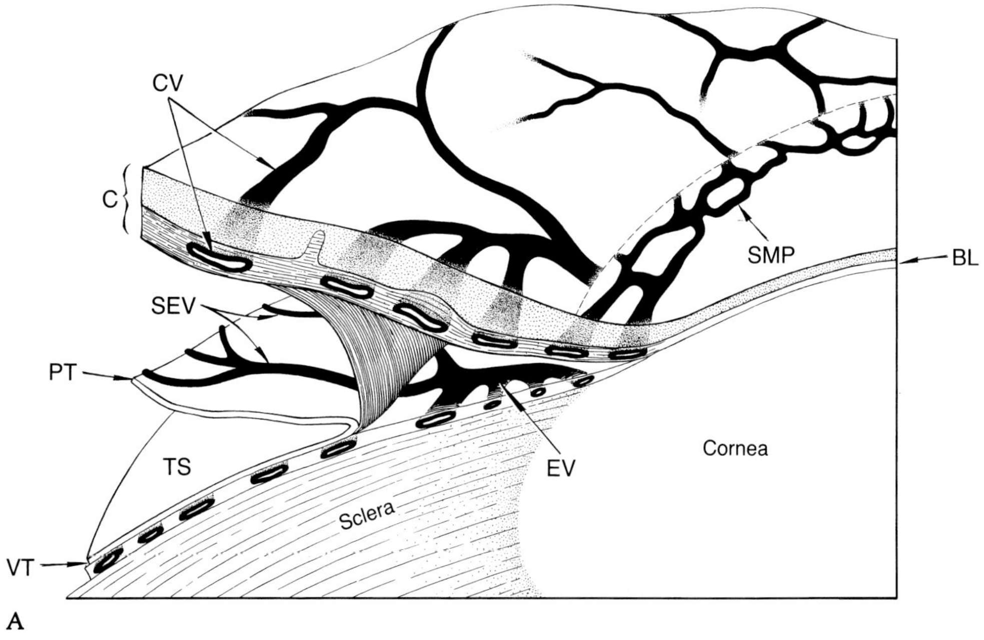

FIGURE 21-9 (A) Limbal anatomy. The conjunctival subepithelial tissue is in the same plane as Bowman's layer *(BL)*. The episcleral vessels lie directly under the conjunctival subepithelial tissue for only 2 mm because Tenon's capsule is interposed distally. *C,* conjunctiva; *PT,* parietal Tenon's capsule; *TS,* Tenon's space; *VT,* visceral Tenon's capsule; *SMP,* superficial marginal plexus; *SEV,* superficial episcleral vessels; *CV,* conjunctival vessels; *EV,* episcleral vessels. *(continues)*

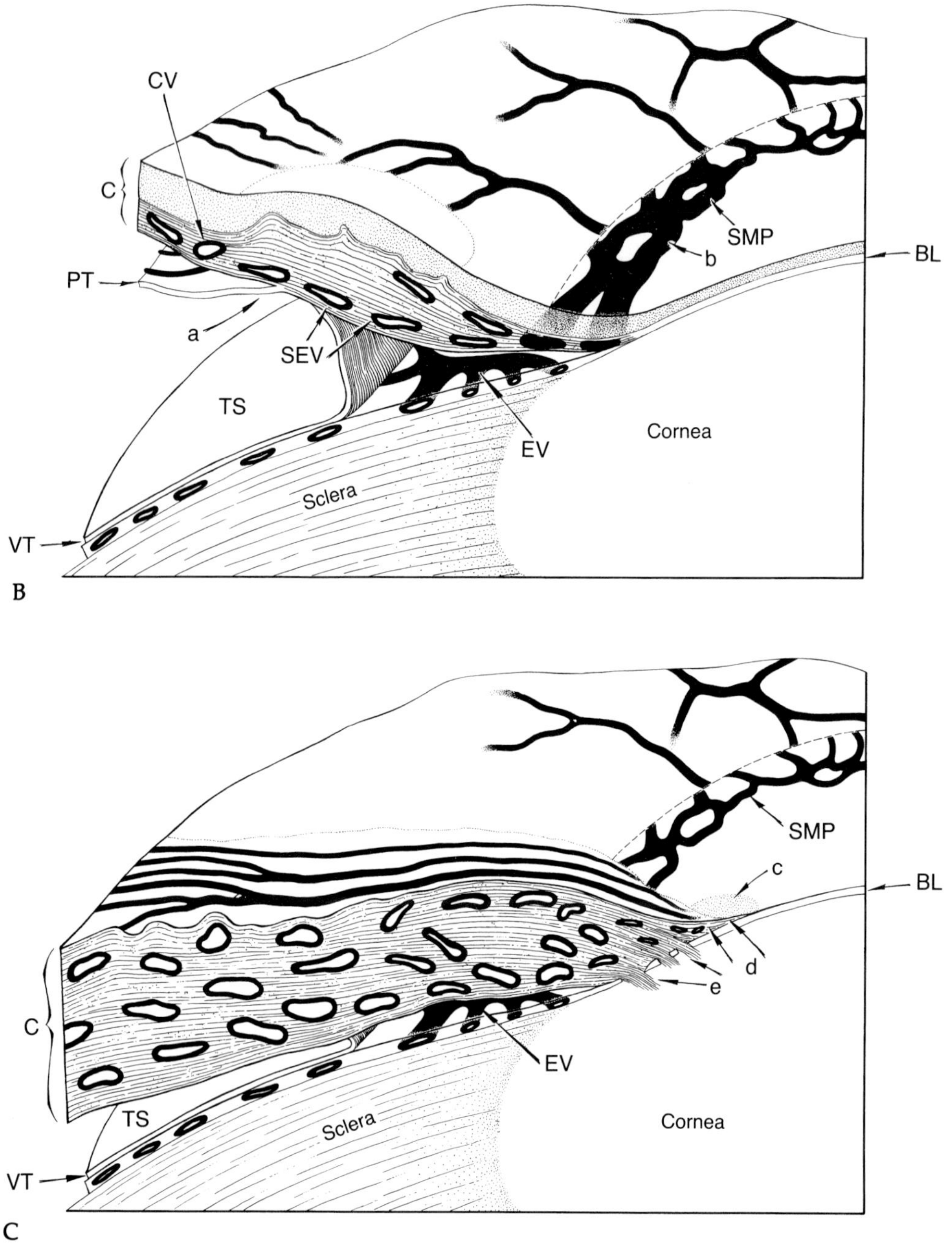

FIGURE 21-9 *(continued)* **(B)** Evolving pterygium. Abnormal connective tissue mound incorporates parietal Tenon's capsule *(PT)* and superficial episcleral vessels *(SEV)* at *a*. The superficial marginal plexus *(SMP)* is engorged at *b*. The abnormal connective tissue is encroaching upon the cornea. **(C)** Formed pterygium. The pterygium head is preceded by fibroblasts that lie between Bowman's layer (*BL*) and the epithelium, giving rise to the clinically apparent gray zone (*c*). Vascularized connective tissue is seen detaching the corneal epithelial basement membrane from Bowman's layer at *d*, while at *e*, it is penetrating the stroma through dehiscences in Bowman's layer. These are the only sites of adhesion of a pterygium to the globe because the bare episclera and Tenon's space (*TS*) are not invaded.

the limbus, Tenon's capsule is present, so that in this location the same connective tissue does not lie over episclera but rather over Tenon's capsule. Tenon's capsule is incorporated into the body of the pterygium and contributes to its vasculature and bulk (Figure 21-9B). Because Tenon's capsule is interposed between the pterygium and the episclera, the body of the pterygium is loose and is not adherent to the sclera.

On the corneal side immediately in front of the head of the pterygium, an advancing row of fibroblasts penetrates the cornea between Bowman's layer and the basement membrane of the overlying epithelium (Figure 21-9C). This plane of invasion corresponds anatomically to that of the subconjunctival connective tissue. These fibroblasts account for the gray zone, or cap, and are thought to prepare a path for fibrovascular tissue to enter the cornea.

As this tissue enters the cornea, Bowman's layer is pushed posteriorly and eventually becomes fragmented. The head of the pterygium becomes firmly adherent to the superficial stroma over these sites of focal interruptions in Bowman's layer.

PATHOGENESIS

Many theories have been proposed to explain the cause of pterygia. However, most of these theories cannot be reconciled with known facts. Scarpa,[14] Friede,[15] and Kamel[16] believed that chronic inflammation in the form of conjunctivitis or episcleritis initiates the process. Yet inflammatory cells are rarely prominent in a pterygium, and clinical observation fails to reveal this element in the evolution of the lesion. Redslob,[17] and more recently, Austin et al[18] argued in favor of dysplasia of the subepithelial fibroblasts. However, the histologic appearance is consistently one of hyperplasia, not dysplasia.

Aside from corneal invasiveness, the most impressive characteristic of a pterygium is the exuberant fibrous tissue proliferation that is observed clinically as a thick head and a bulky body. This feature has been likened to keloid formation,[2] and is reminiscent of the subepithelial scar tissue prominent in alkali burns. Indeed, many of the findings suggest that a pterygium is a type of burn that is produced over several years by the cumulative absorption of infrared and ultraviolet radiation from sunlight.[19]

All the risk factors previously cited point to sunlight as a causative factor. In addition, the anatomic location in the interpalpebral region also implicates sunlight as an etiologic agent. The conjunctiva and cornea absorb most of the infrared and ultraviolet radiation from sunlight, which can damage epibulbar tissue. Although the proportion of infrared radiation greatly exceeds that of ultraviolet radiation (40 percent vs. 2 percent), the latter is much more biologically active.

Experimental studies in rats have shown that ultraviolet radiation can induce proliferative changes ranging from hyperplasia to neoplasia in both epithelial and connective tissues.[20] Cameron[2] pinpoints the 290- to 320-nm wavelengths (ultraviolet-B radiation) as directly involved in the production of pterygia, emphasizing that the greater absorption of these wavelengths at the subepithelial level may explain the subepithelial tissue proliferation. Pico[21] places greater importance on the role of infrared radiation in producing thermal effects and the consequent tissue response. Diponegoro and Houwer,[22] Talbot,[19] Kerkenesov,[23] Elliot,[24] and others have argued in favor of the theory that sunlight causes pterygia, whereas others have stressed additional factors to account for the progression of a pterygium onto the cornea. Hilgers[25] believed that ultraviolet radiation denatures corneal proteins, provoking an antigen-antibody reaction that stimulates fibrovascular proliferation.

To further support the theory of ultraviolet radiation as a causative factor in pterygium formation, Mackenzie et al[26] found an increased risk of pterygium among persons who, in their third decade of life, worked outdoors in an environment with high surface reflectance of ultraviolet light compared with those who worked indoors. Those who worked outdoors mainly in a sandy environment had an increased risk of several hundredfold; those who worked in a concrete environment had an increased risk of 20-fold. Persons who spent their first 5 years of life at latitudes less than 30 degrees had almost 40 times the risk of pterygium formation compared with those who spent their first 5 years of life at latitudes greater than 40 degrees. Persons who spent the majority of their time outdoors in these early years had a 20-fold risk of developing pterygia compared with those who spent the majority of their time indoors. Mackenzie et al[26] concluded that there is a strong causal relationship between the development of pterygia and ultraviolet light exposure during the early years of life combined with cumulative exposure over the next two to three decades in occupations in which there is a high component of reflected ultraviolet light. Eyeglasses, sunglasses, and headgear with brims, all of which shield the eyes from ultraviolet-A and -B radiation, were found to provide a strong protective effect.

Barraquer[27] proposed that the limbal elevation produced by a pinguecula leads to poor apposition of the eyelids to the globe, which causes tear film discontinuity and leads to micro-ulcerations of the epithelium and dellen formation, which initiate fibrovascular invasion. Caldwell[28] also supported this theory. He proposed that the iron line seen at the head of an advanced pterygium is evidence of drying and exposure from the stagnation of tears and failure of the tear film to spread over the area. He hypothesized that loss of moisture from the tear interface may induce an anoxic condition, stimulating the release of an angiogenic factor, which in turn leads to fibrovascular ingrowth into the cornea. Postoperative recurrences of pterygia are thought to occur secondary to an angiogenic factor released by polymorphonuclear leukocytes that are stimulated by the surgical insult. Opponents of this theory argue that neither dellen nor micro-ulcerations of the corneal epithelium are consistent findings in active pterygia. In addition, they believe that the presence of an iron line at the head of a pterygium suggests pooling of tears in this area, quite the opposite of a proposed mechanism based on corneal desiccation.

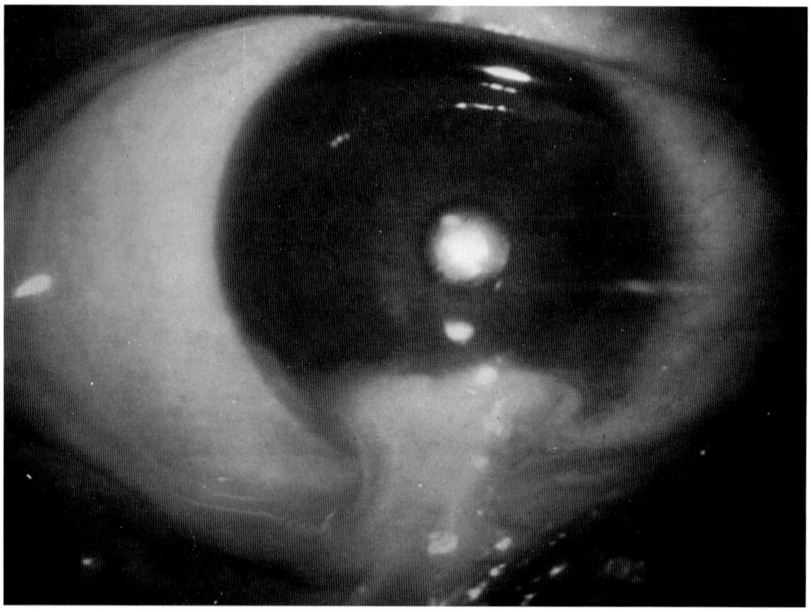

FIGURE 21-10 Pseudopterygium caused by an alkali burn. Note the inferior location.

DIAGNOSIS

The differential diagnosis of pterygium includes pseudopterygium and neoplasia. A pseudopterygium is fibrovascular tissue that may occur on any quadrant of the cornea. Like pterygia, the majority of these lesions develop at the 3 o'clock and 9 o'clock positions because these areas are constantly exposed to dryness and irritation. In contrast to a pterygium, a pseudopterygium lacks organization into different regions (cap, head, and body). A pseudopterygium also lacks firm adhesion at the limbus. Pseudopterygia may be evoked by peripheral corneal disease, such as marginal ulceration. They may also be seen after chemical burns and cicatricial conjunctivitis (Figure 21-10). Pseudopterygia may also occur secondary to hard contact lens wear,[29,30] especially with a lens that rocks on a steep vertical axis in a cornea with significant with-the-rule astigmatism. Chronic mechanical irritation from contact lens movement and abnormal tear wetting may induce a punctate keratopathy that can stimulate peripheral corneal vascular ingrowth. A pseudopterygium caused by contact lens wear differs from a true pterygium in that a pseudopterygium has a broad, ill-defined leading edge on the corneal surface, unlike the well-defined head of a true pterygium. Furthermore, a pseudopterygium caused by hard contact lens wear may regress after removal of the lens.

A conjunctival malignancy, such as squamous cell carcinoma, must be differentiated from a pterygium.[31] Rarely, the epithelium overlying a pterygium may undergo malignant degeneration. Therefore, all surgical specimens should be submitted for pathologic examination to rule out neoplasia.

TREATMENT

Medical Treatment

Surgical manipulation of a pterygium should not be undertaken casually. The possibility of a recurrent pterygium is high, and the recurrence is often worse than the primary lesion. In addition, complications may be associated with any surgical technique. Therefore, medical management should be attempted first, when possible.

A small pterygium that does not involve the visual axis may be amenable to medical management. Such a pterygium can cause signs and symptoms suggestive of local inflammation, including hyperemia, foreign body sensation, and tearing. These signs and symptoms may be alleviated with artificial tears, lubricants, and even brief courses of topical corticosteroids. Any associated blepharitis should be treated. The eye should be protected from a hostile environment, including exposure to ultraviolet light, dust, and dry hot wind. Sunglasses that filter ultraviolet light are also recommended.

Surgical Treatment

Many of the signs and symptoms of pterygium are not amenable to medical management and require surgical intervention. These include a significant cosmetic blemish, decreased visual acuity from encroachment of the pterygium on the visual axis, regular or irregular astigmatism, restriction of ocular motility, formation of a delle, or recurrent inflammation unresponsive to medical therapy.

Pterygia would certainly arouse less interest were it not for their tendency to recur despite various surgical therapies designed to avoid just that. Rich et al[32] stated that "to manage pterygia, we can incise, excise, bury, transplant, graft, freeze, burn, cauterize, diathermize, divulse, avulse, chemically assault, irradiate or simply leave them to fate." The many therapeutic options available for the treatment of pterygia imply that no single method is universally successful.[33]

Avulsion, the earliest technique used to treat pterygia, was practiced by the ancient Greeks, and still has its proponents.[34] The method that followed, simple excision, has the same high recurrence rate as avulsion (23 to 75 percent).[35] This complication spurred the development of alternative and adjunctive surgical procedures.

Desmarres[36] first suggested that a pterygium would atrophy if the pterygium head was dissected and transposed to a new position away from the cornea. Many variations of this technique have been described[37]: Knapp favored dissecting the pterygium, splitting it in half, and suturing the halves to the conjunctiva; McReynolds[38] buried the head of the pterygium under the conjunctiva; Blaskovics folded the head under the body; and Wilson and Bourne[39] modified Stocker's technique[40] by using a conjunctival Z-plasty to divert the head of the pterygium away from the cornea.

Concurrent with the establishment of techniques for transposing the pterygium head, newer excision techniques were evolving. Some thought it was crucial to cover the entire exposed epibulbar defect with normal conjunctiva. Arlt, Terson, Campodonico, Arruga, and Bangerter designed various rotating conjunctival flaps to accomplish this.[1] Others recommended the use of a free graft to cover the defect, and introduced the barrier concept, wherein the grafted tissue forms a barrier against the passage of new vessels into the cornea, thus helping to avoid recurrence.[1] Various tissues have been suggested as grafts. Elschnig,[1] Majoros, Gomez-Marquez, and others favored the use of bulbar conjunctiva obtained from the same or opposite eye (conjunctival autograft). Svoboda favored buccal mucous membrane, Gifford advocated the use of skin, and Castroviejo recommended cornea.

The barrier effect of conjunctiva is limited because the plane followed by new vessels that foster recurrence is deep, over the episclera itself. D'Ombain,[1] McGavic, Sugar, and King were proponents of leaving an area of bare sclera adjacent to the limbus to give the raw corneal surface time to heal before the conjunctiva grew up to the limbus again. The authors that introduced the bare-sclera concept emphasized the importance of excising subconjunctival connective tissue present under the body of a pterygium in deterring recurrence. Pico[21] agreed with Alger[41] that the source of recurrence is the formation of granulation tissue on the raw corneal and scleral surfaces.

Proponents of conjunctival flaps think that the precise placement of the flap ensures proper wound healing, decreases recurrences, and provides a smooth surface at the limbus to encourage proper tear film distribution. Rapid epithelialization of the epibulbar surface provided by the conjunctival flap also helps to diminish the formation of new capillary endothelium and granulation tissue that may lead to recurrences. Probably the first to suture the conjunctiva to cover the exposed epibulbar surface was Coccius.[1] Several types of sliding conjunctival flaps have been designed to cover the epibulbar defect created by the excision of a pterygium. Czermack's technique involved approximating the superior and inferior edges of the conjunctiva with sutures that also passed through superficial sclera for added stabilization.[42] The design advocated by Bangerter consisted of a rotating conjunctival flap from the superior or inferior bulbar conjunctiva to cover the defect.[1] In one study, Tomas[43] constructed sliding conjunctival flaps from the superior and inferior bulbar conjunctiva using incisions parallel to the limbus. He reported a recurrence rate of 5 percent with this technique.

Conjunctival autografts were popularized by Kenyon et al.[44] Conjunctival autografts allow coverage of large defects that occur from large excisions, which are often encountered in advanced and recurrent pterygia. The grafts can cover large areas of sclera and exposed extraocular muscle and provide tissue for reconstruction of the fornix. A recurrence rate of 5 percent was reported when this technique was used on advanced and recurrent pterygia[44]; two of the three recurrences were successfully treated with repeat conjunctival autografts. However, a recurrence rate of 21 percent after conjunctival autografting was found in a study in the Caribbean, where the risk of pterygium recurrence is high.[45]

In tropical countries, where many patients have trachomatous scarring and xerosis, sufficient conjunctiva for a graft cannot always be obtained. To overcome this obstacle, labial or buccal mucous membrane may be used. Trivedi et al[46] reported no recurrences with oral mucous membrane harvested from the lower lip. However, 6 percent of the patients complained of a cosmetically unsatisfactory result because of the color differences between the graft and ocular tissues.

The successful removal of a pterygium depends not only on the surgical technique used, but also on the type of lesion encountered. Slow-growing, stationary, and atrophic

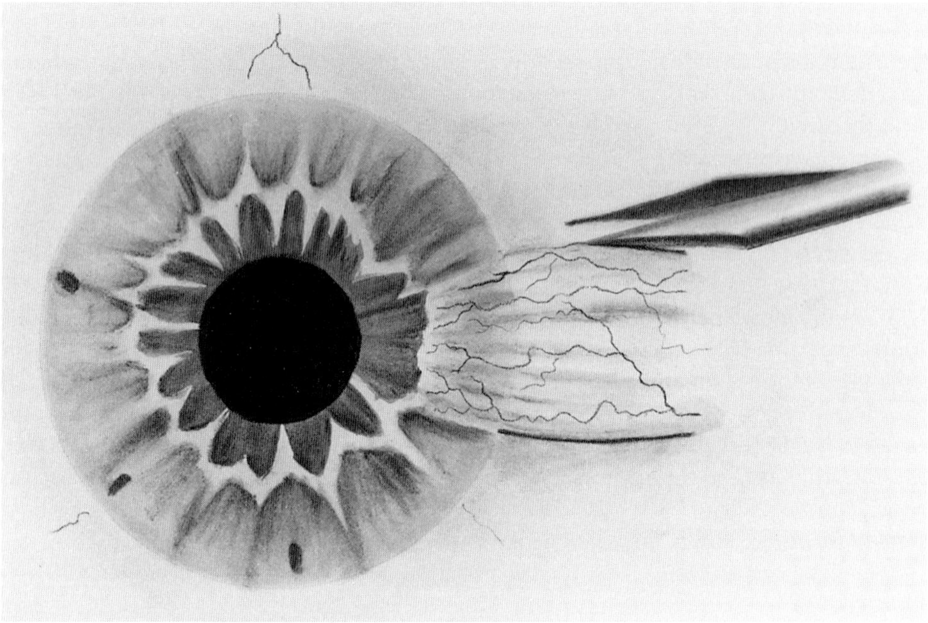

FIGURE 21-11 Excision of the pterygium body. Horizontal incisions are made at the superior and inferior extents of the body.

pterygia can be removed by virtually any technique, with little risk of recurrence. However, actively growing or fleshy pterygia are more likely to recur.

Preoperative Medications

No specific preoperative medications are necessary for the excision of a pterygium. If the pterygium is inflamed, a topical anti-inflammatory agent should be used preoperatively to reduce inflammation. Medications that decrease intraocular pressure should be avoided to facilitate dissection of the pterygium from the cornea or a lamellar keratectomy, if necessary.

Anesthesia

The type of anesthesia necessary for the excision of a pterygium depends on the size of the pterygium and the extent of the subconjunctival scar tissue, especially in cases of recurrent pterygia. For removal of a small primary pterygium, topical anesthetic such as 0.5 percent proparacaine is used. The topical anesthetic is supplemented with a subconjunctival injection of 2 percent lidocaine with epinephrine by means of a short 30-gauge needle. The lidocaine aids in anesthesia, the epinephrine provides hemostasis, and the body of the pterygium and surrounding conjunctiva are elevated by the injection.

Very fleshy or extensive pterygia may require retro- or peribulbar anesthesia combined with an eyelid block. These types of pterygia require more extensive dissection and subsequent reconstruction of the epibulbar surface and possibly the fornices. As with topical anesthesia, a subconjunctival injection of lidocaine with epinephrine is administered in addition to the retro- or peribulbar anesthesia, to provide hemostasis.

Excision of Primary Pterygia

An eyelid speculum that provides maximum exposure is placed in the fornices. Forced duction testing is performed to detect restriction of extraocular movement from the pterygium. Depending on the size of the pterygium and the extent of the anticipated dissection, sutures may be placed through partial-thickness cornea central to the limbus at the 12 o'clock and 6 o'clock positions to rotate the eye nasally or temporally to allow better surgical access to the pterygium. This is not necessary for small pterygia. Generally, ophthalmic surgeons prefer to perform surgery while sitting at the 12 o'clock position. However, some surgeons prefer to sit temporally when operating on pterygia.

Horizontal incisions superior and inferior to the body of the pterygium are made with sharp-tipped Westcott scissors (Figure 21-11). Blunt-tipped Westcott scissors are then placed through one of these incisions and are used to dissect the body of the pterygium from the sclera as the body is lifted with a large-toothed forceps (Figure 21-12). Depending on the size of the pterygium and the extent of scar tissue, the surgeon may elect to isolate and expose the horizontal rectus muscle with a muscle hook to avoid injuring it during the dissection. This is not necessary with small primary pterygia. A vertical incision is made at the peripheral extent of the pterygium, and the pterygium is reflected centrally (Figure 21-13). The underlying bed

FIGURE 21-12 Excision of the pterygium body. Dissection with Westcott scissors.

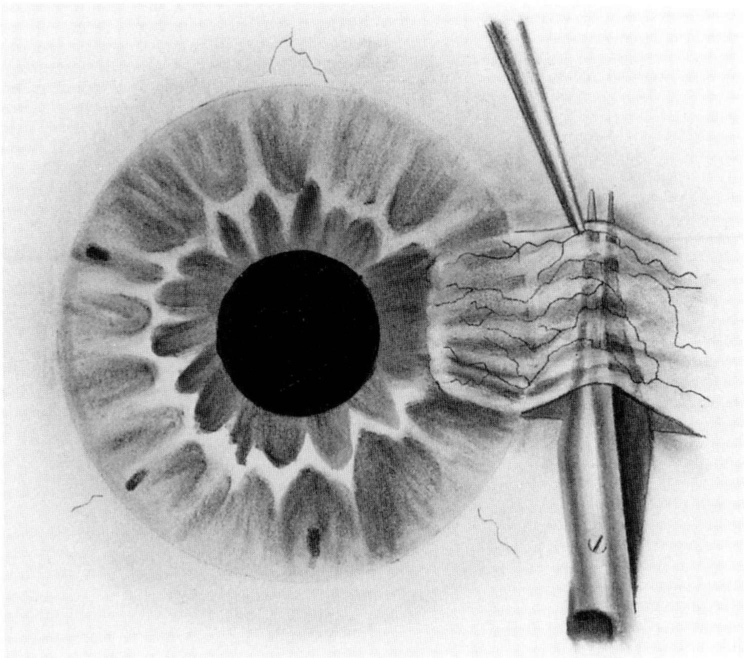

should reveal a clean episcleral surface, and the cut edges of conjunctiva and Tenon's capsule should be smooth, pale, and uninvolved. Any visible epibulbar scar tissue is dissected and excised. Light wetfield cautery is used to coagulate all bleeding vessels on the sclera.

As the body of the pterygium is pulled centrally, Westcott or Vannas scissors are used to dissect the pterygium from and sever its attachments to the limbus (Figure 21-14). The tips of the blades should be directed upward to avoid dissecting along a plane deeper than desired (i.e., into the cornea).

The body of the pterygium is grasped with a large-toothed forceps, and an attempt is made to avulse the head of the pterygium from the cornea by firmly pulling the pterygium centrally (Figure 21-15). Primary pterygia can usually be removed in this manner, which is the pre-

FIGURE 21-13 Excision of the pterygium body. Vertical incision at the peripheral extent of the body.

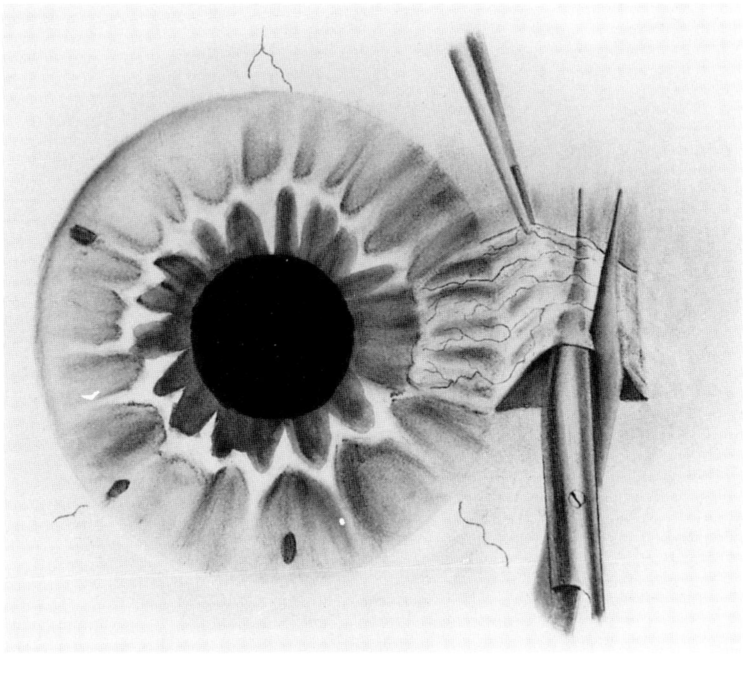

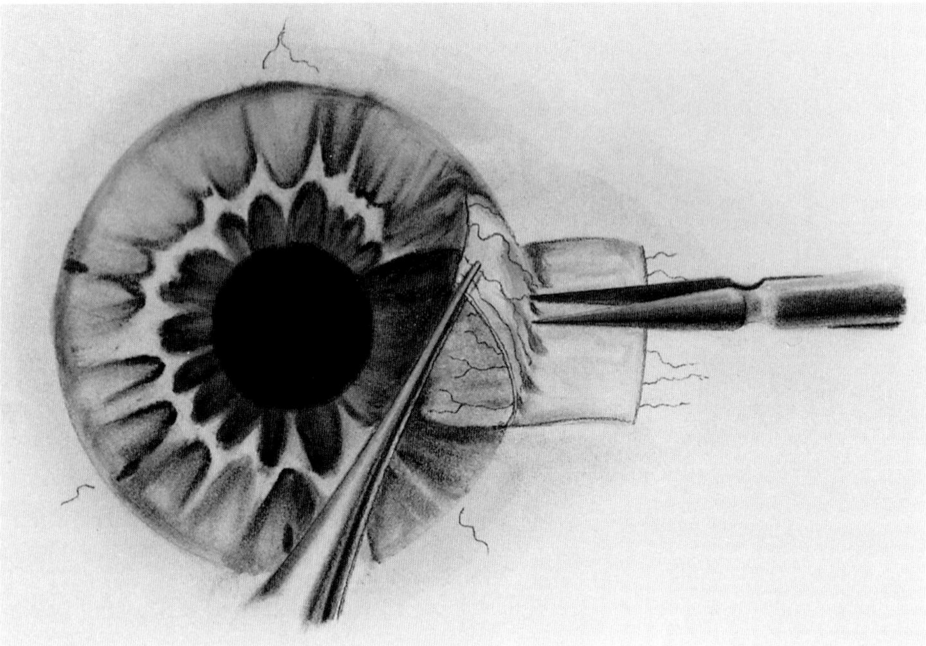

FIGURE 21-14 Excision of the pterygium body. Severing of limbal attachments.

ferred technique because it leaves a smoother corneal surface than that created by a lamellar keratectomy. If the head cannot be avulsed, it must be removed by lamellar keratectomy. As the body of the pterygium is grasped with a toothed forceps, a lamellar dissector is used to create a keratectomy beneath the head of the pterygium as smoothly and evenly as possible (Figure 21-16). The keratectomy usually extends to a depth just beneath Bowman's layer, although in some cases, a deeper keratectomy is necessary to remove the head.

The corneal epithelium at the central edge of the pterygium is scraped off with a blunt spatula or the flat surface of a blade to remove the gray zone, or cap. If the corneal bed is irregular, the flat surface of a blade can be used to scrape the bed. Alternatively, a diamond burr can be used to polish the corneal surface to a smooth config-

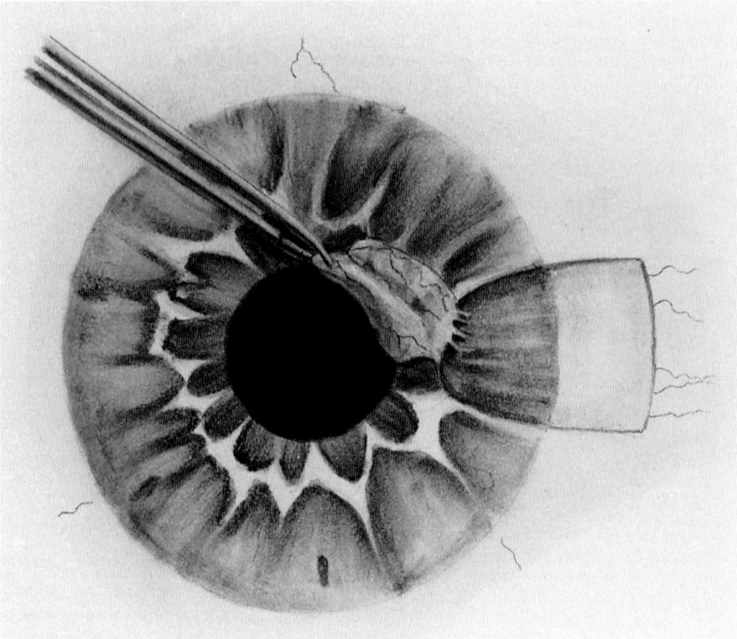

FIGURE 21-15 Avulsion of the pterygium head.

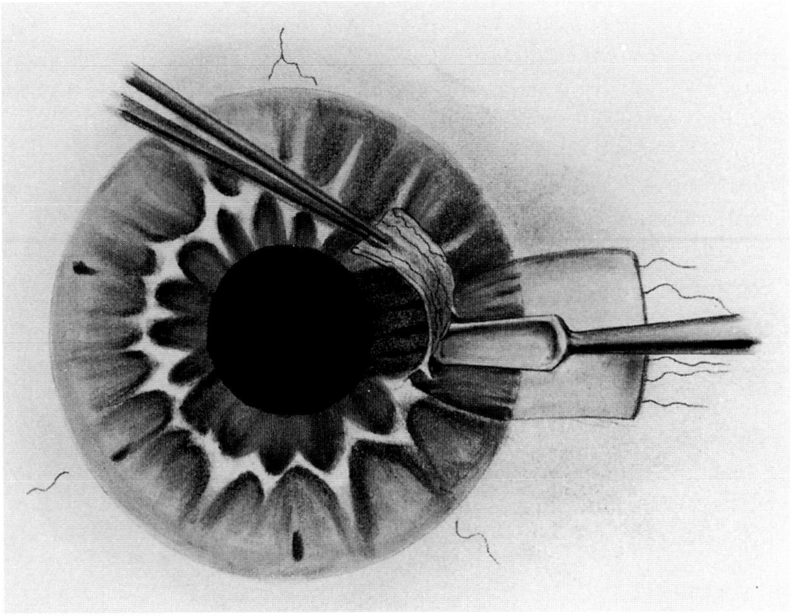

FIGURE 21-16 Lamellar keratectomy of the pterygium head.

uration[47] (Figure 21-17). A high-powered or battery-operated drill maneuvered in small circular motions is recommended. The least amount of tissue that creates a smooth surface should be removed. The surgeon should not hold the burr too long in one position, and should be careful not to remove more corneal tissue than is desired.

The scleral surface adjacent to the limbus is cleansed of tissue tags by scraping with the flat surface of a blade or a diamond burr. Light cautery is applied to close all vessels on the sclera adjacent to the limbus. Excessive cautery should be avoided because it predisposes the sclera to necrosis, especially if other adjunctive therapy, such as antimetabolites or β-radiation, is used.

To prepare a sliding conjunctival flap, the superior horizontal edge of the conjunctiva is lifted with a fine-toothed forceps and separated from the underlying Tenon's capsule with Westcott scissors. The conjunctiva is incised parallel to the limbus; the length of the incision is approximately

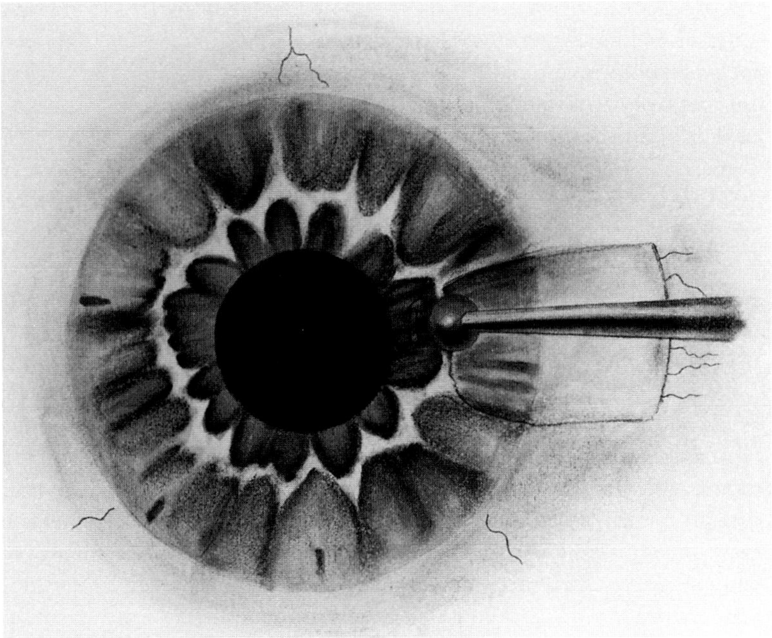

FIGURE 21-17 Polishing of the corneal surface with a diamond burr.

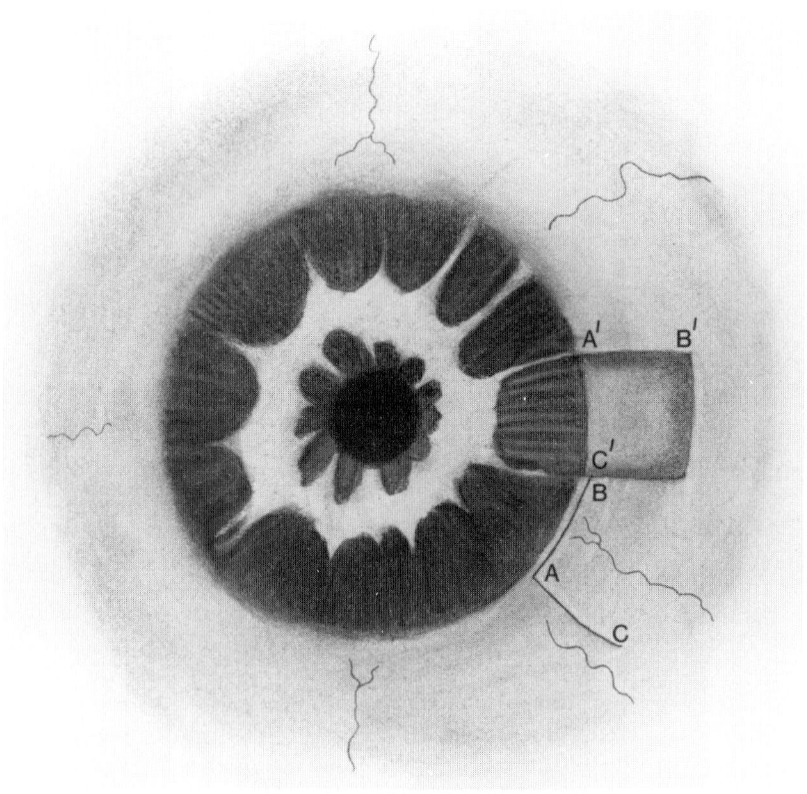

FIGURE 21-18 Incisions for a sliding conjunctival flap. *A* will be moved to *A′*, *B* to *B′*, and *C* to *C′*.

the length of the horizontal conjunctival defect (Figure 21-18). The incision is extended peripherally to the approximate length of the vertical conjunctival defect left by the pterygium excision. The flap is then brought inferiorly to cover the conjunctival defect. If the pterygium has a broad base and its excision leaves a large defect, the inferior conjunctiva can be dissected and mobilized in a similar manner to provide more conjunctiva to cover the defect. The conjunctival flap is sutured with interrupted 10-0 polyglactin sutures (Figure 21-19). The flap should cover the raw epibulbar surface, leaving approximately 1 mm of bare sclera adjacent to the limbus. Sutures can be placed at the central edge of the flap to secure it to the episclera and prevent its migration toward the cornea, if necessary.

Excision of Recurrent Pterygia

Most patients with stationary or atrophic pterygia do well with simple excision and sliding conjunctival flaps. However, if the same technique is used for an active or fleshy lesion, the pterygium usually recurs promptly. In a retrospective analysis, Hirst et al[48] found that the mean time to recurrence was 123 days after excision of a primary pterygium, 97 days after a second surgery, and 67 days after a third operation, regardless of the type of procedure.

In terms of surgical treatment, a recurrent pterygium is considerably different from a primary pterygium. In a recurrent pterygium, subconjunctival fibrous tissue is more abundant and is tightly bound to the underlying sclera. If the recurrent pterygium does not involve deep stroma, a superficial keratectomy can be performed, followed by polishing of the cornea with a diamond burr. If a deep lamellar keratectomy is required or the involved sector of cornea is thin from previous keratectomies, a peripheral inlay lamellar graft is indicated.[49–51]

Various adjunctive therapies may also be considered for a recurrent pterygium. One option is a conjunctival autograft. If the pterygium recurs a second time and requires surgery, a second conjunctival autograft may be performed. β-Radiation or antimetabolite therapy may also be considered. If a pterygium recurs after either β-radiation or antimetabolite therapy, additional β-radiation or antimetabolite therapy only increases the risk of scleral necrosis. Therefore, a conjunctival autograft is recommended for a recurrence after β-radiation or antimetabolite therapy.

Recurrent pterygia usually cannot be avulsed from the cornea and, therefore, must be dissected. It is best to first dissect the pterygium head from the cornea, because dissection of the pterygium body from the sclera causes

FIGURE 21-19 Sliding conjunctival flap sutured into place, leaving 1 mm of bare sclera adjacent to the limbus. *A* has been moved to *A′*, *B* to *B′*, and *C* to *C′*.

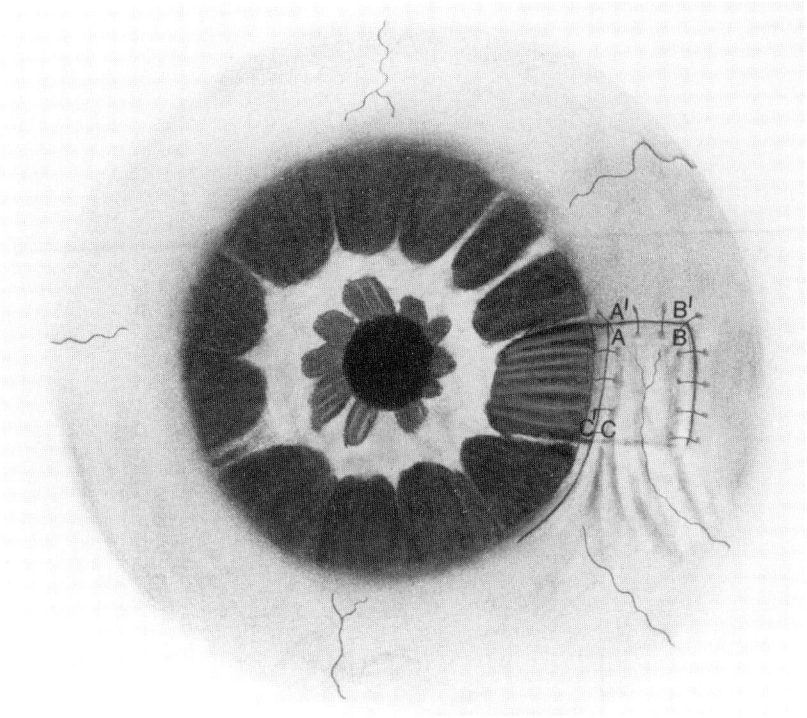

a moderate amount of bleeding, which can obscure the lamellar keratectomy. A sharp blade is used to make incisions into clear cornea approximately 0.75 mm in front of and parallel to the edges of the head of the pterygium (Figure 21-20). The depth of penetration is just beneath Bowman's layer. In some cases, deeper penetration is required before normal corneal tissue is reached. The head of the pterygium is grasped with a fine-toothed forceps, and a lamellar dissector is used to create a smooth and even keratectomy (Figure 21-21). The dissection should stop at the limbus and should not extend into the sclera. Vannas scissors are used to amputate the head of the

FIGURE 21-20 Incision of the cornea central to the pterygium head.

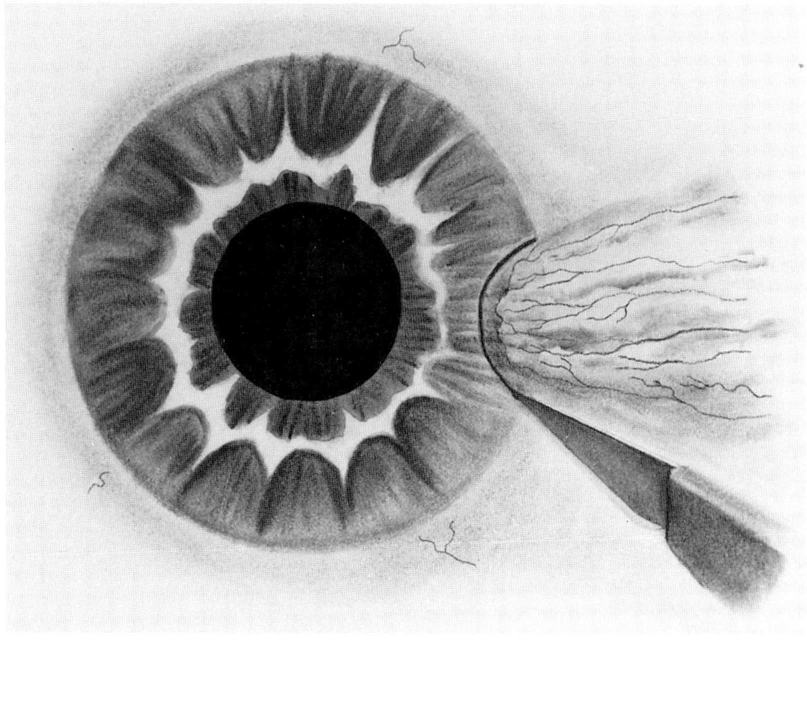

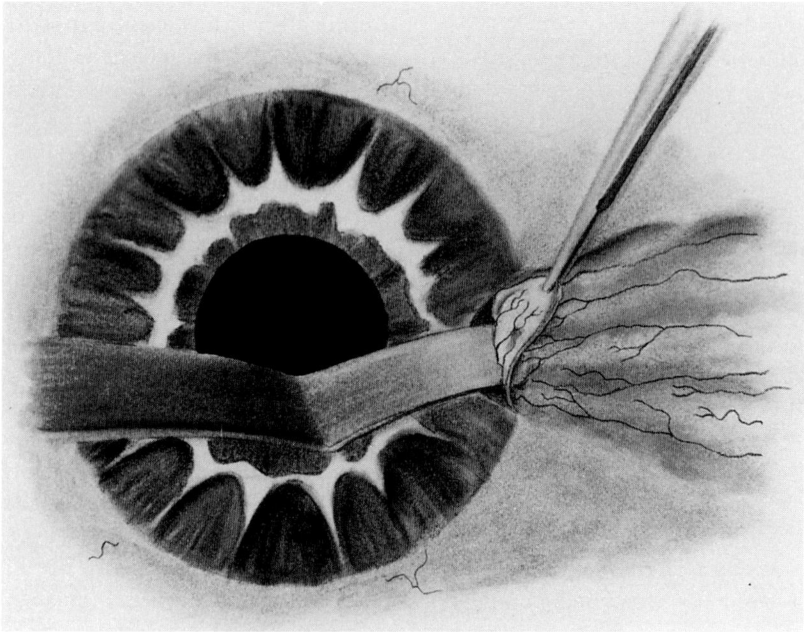

FIGURE 21-21 Lamellar keratectomy of the pterygium head.

pterygium and underlying lamellar tissue at a 45-degree angle to create a smooth transition between the keratectomy bed and the sclera (Figure 21-22).

If an inlay lamellar graft is anticipated, the lamellar keratectomy should have a regular shape. If the pterygium is small and not near the visual axis, a crescent-shaped keratectomy is performed (Figure 21-23). If the pterygium is large or near the visual axis, a trapezoid-shaped keratectomy is performed (Figure 21-24). The incisions of the keratectomy are deepened with a stainless steel blade and are made perpendicular to the corneal surface to create distinct edges to which the lamellar graft will be sutured (Figure 21-25). The head of the pterygium is then grasped with a fine-toothed forceps and a lamellar dissector is inserted into the depth of the central incision. The lamellar dissection is continued to the limbus and should not extend into the sclera. Vannas scissors are used to amputate the head of the pterygium and the underlying corneal

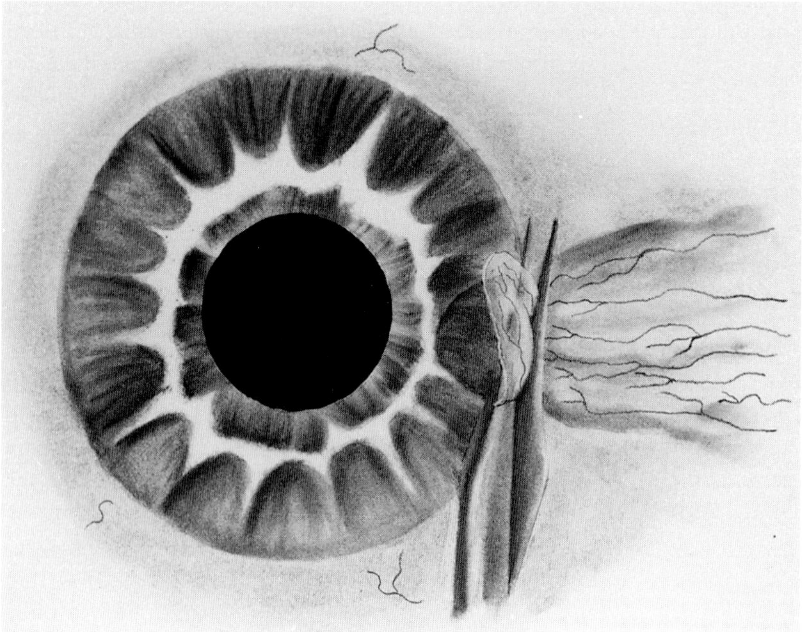

FIGURE 21-22 Excision of the pterygium head.

FIGURE 21-23 Crescent-shaped keratectomy (*A*) for a pterygium that has not invaded the cornea very far centrally. An inlay lamellar graft will be placed in the keratectomy bed, and conjunctiva will cover the episcleral defect (*C*), except for an area adjacent to the limbus (*B*).

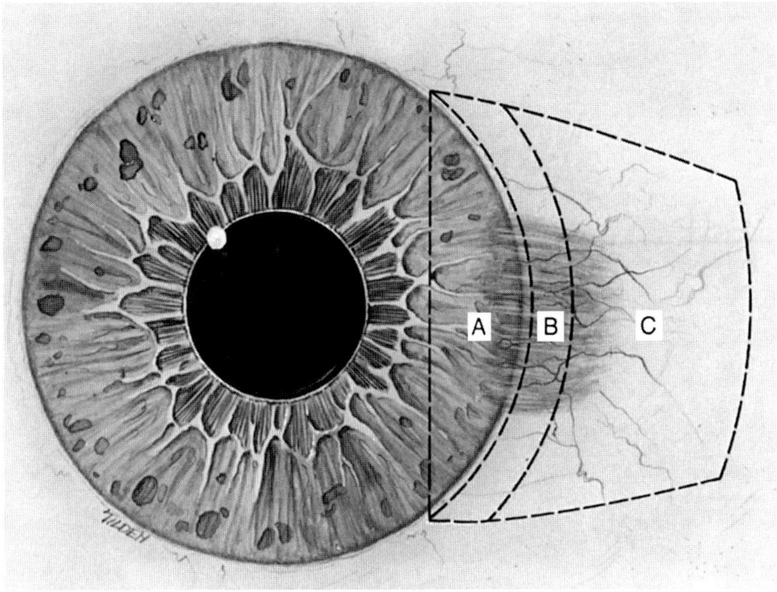

lamellar tissue perpendicular to the corneal surface to create a distinct edge to which the inlay lamellar graft is eventually sutured. The base of the keratectomy bed is inspected for any remnants of the pterygium which, if present, are removed by a deeper keratectomy.

The body of the pterygium is grasped with a large-toothed forceps and is dissected and excised from the sclera after the horizontal rectus muscle has been isolated (Figure 21-26). Dense fibrous scar tissue commonly forms under the body of a recurrent pterygium and attaches to the orbital rim. It is important to resect all of this tissue and any symblephara associated with it. After the dissection has been completed, bleeding vessels are lightly cauterized.

If a lamellar graft is required, donor lamellar tissue can be obtained as described in Chapter 31. The use of precarved donor lamellar tissue 9 to 12 mm in diameter and 0.3 mm in thickness has been described.[52] The graft is sutured to the limbal edge of the keratectomy bed with interrupted 10-0 nylon sutures and is then cut with straight scissors to match the shape of the keratectomy bed. Several more sutures are placed to secure the graft (Figures

FIGURE 21-24 Trapezoid-shaped keratectomy (*A*) for a pterygium that is near the visual axis. An inlay lamellar graft will be placed in the keratectomy bed, and conjunctiva will cover the episcleral defect (*C*), except for an area adjacent to the limbus (*B*).

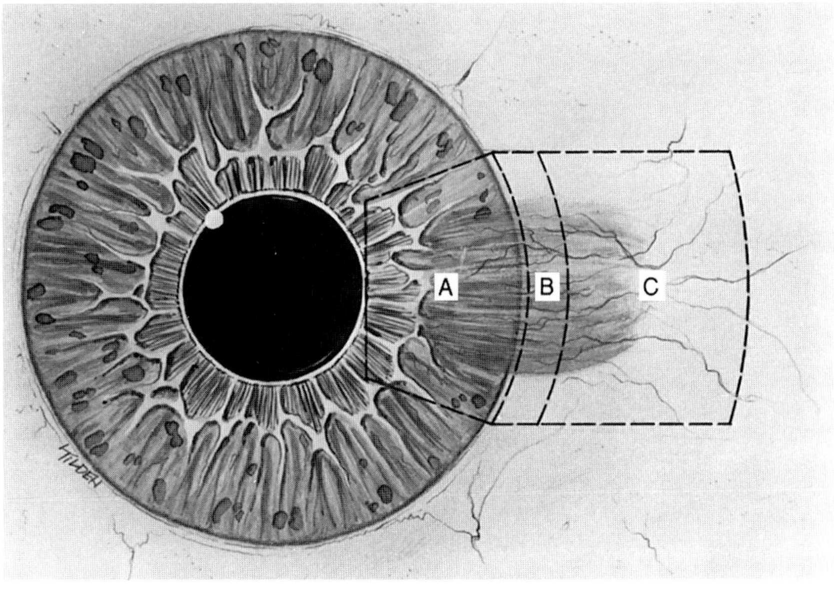

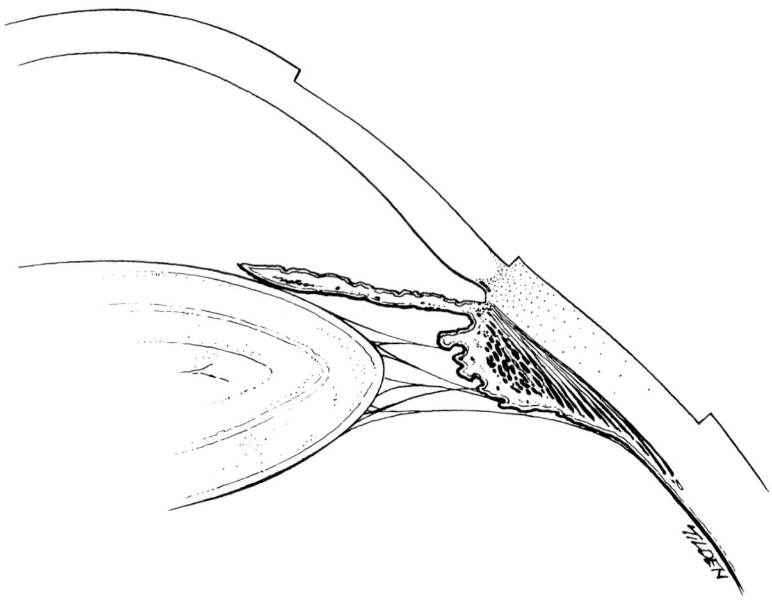

FIGURE 21-25 Dissection planes for removal of a recurrent pterygium for which an inlay lamellar graft is anticipated. The keratectomy bed should have well-defined edges to which the lamellar graft is sutured. The dissection plane is stepped up at the limbus so that the dissection does not extend into sclera.

21-27 and 21-28). If the central aspect of the keratectomy bed is close to the visual axis, a suture is placed parallel to the edge of the keratectomy to prevent possible decreased visual acuity or glare caused by a suture or the scar it induces in the visual axis.

A conjunctival autograft will cover exposed sclera and extraocular muscle, and will re-form any fornices that may have been obliterated by scar tissue. A conjunctival autograft is harvested by rotating the eye inferomedially to allow exposure of the superotemporal bulbar conjunctiva. Lidocaine with epinephrine may be injected subconjunctivally in the area where the graft is to be harvested to provide hemostasis and to hydraulically elevate the conjunctiva from Tenon's capsule. Calipers are used to measure the size of the required graft. The conjunctiva is dissected as thinly as possible, using sharp dissection with blunt-tipped Westcott scissors in a manner similar to that described in Chapter 29 for conjunctival flaps. This allows the donor site to heal rapidly without scarring or suturing. Autografts as large as 15 × 15 mm can be obtained easily. The surgeon may mark the epithelial surface of the conjunctival graft with gentian violet so that it can be

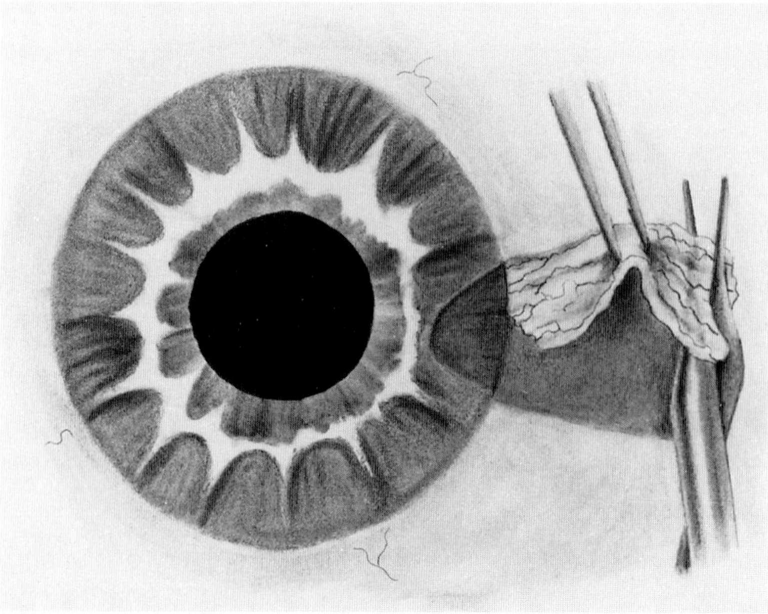

FIGURE 21-26 Dissection and excision of the pterygium body.

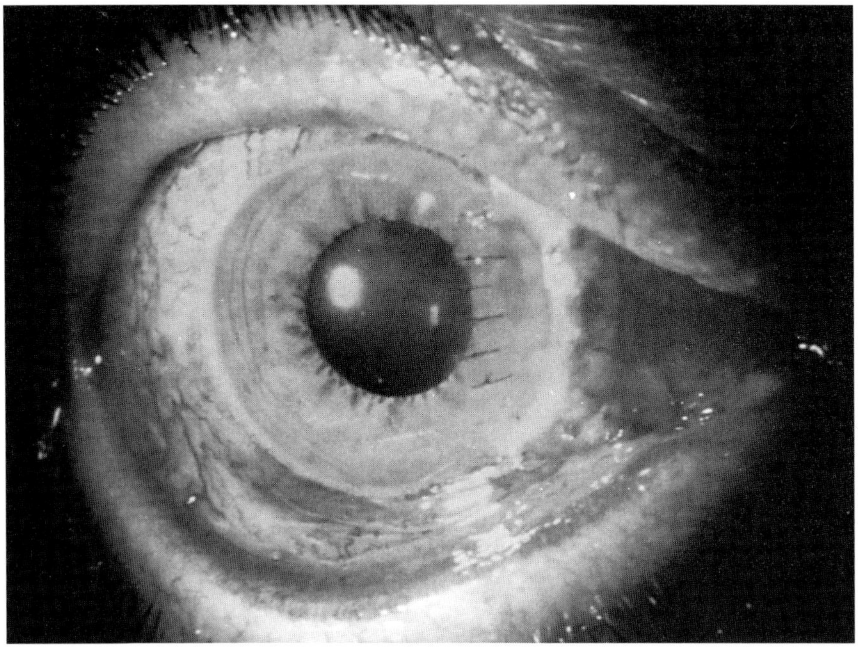

FIGURE 21-27 Crescent-shaped lamellar graft sutured in place.

readily identified to ensure that the graft is not inverted. Kenyon and co-workers[44] recommend marking the epithelial surface with cautery to outline the graft before excision, leaving the cautery marks within the graft to mark the epithelial surface. Shaw[53] recently described the use of a paper template to assist in the harvest of the graft. The template is custom cut to the shape and size of the conjunctival defect. The template is then placed over the area where the graft is to be harvested and the conjunctiva is outlined with cautery. As the conjunctiva is dissected, the template is slid under the conjunctiva. To maintain the proper orientation, the template holding the graft is transferred to the site of the pterygium excision. This ensures that the epithelial side is up and the graft is flat. The epithelium of the graft should have the same orientation as that of the host conjunctiva, with the limbal side corresponding to the position of the limbus in the host bed.[54] The graft is secured in place with interrupted 10-0

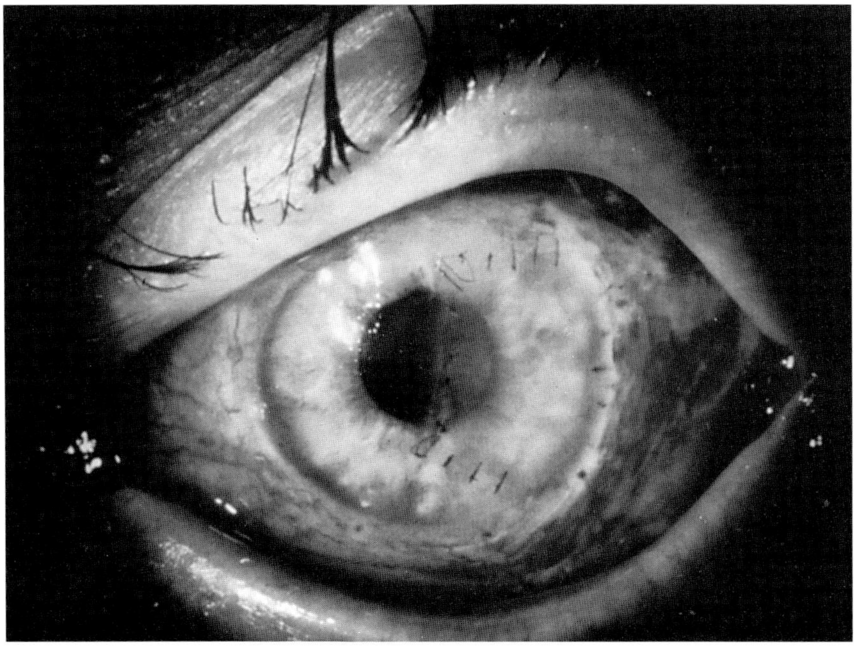

FIGURE 21-28 Trapezoid-shaped lamellar graft sutured in place. Note that the placement of the central sutures avoids the visual axis.

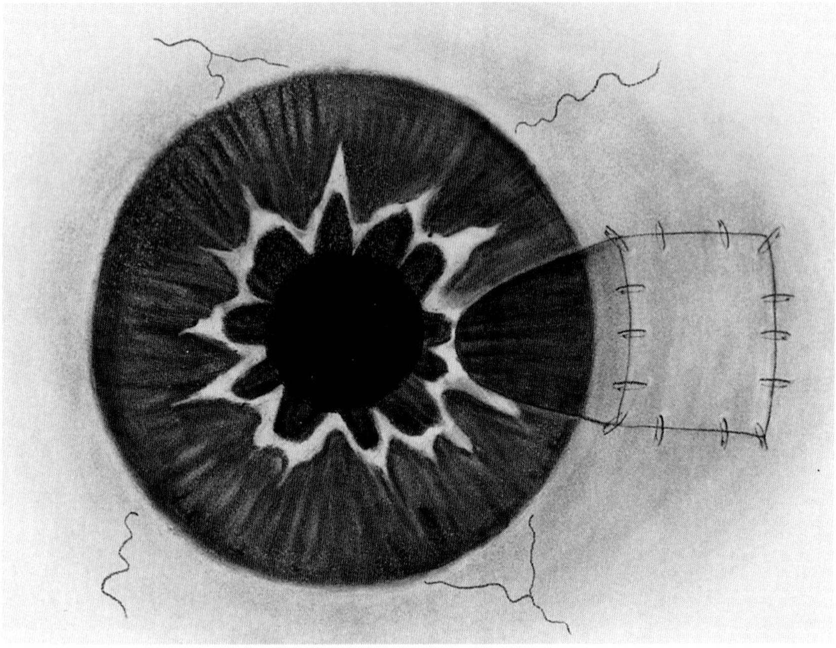

FIGURE 21-29 Conjunctival autograft sutured in place.

polyglactin sutures secured to the edges of the conjunctiva and the episclera (Figure 21-29). Free conjunctival autografts revascularize within 3 to 5 days.

Postoperative Care

At the conclusion of the procedure, 1 ml of methylprednisolone acetate (80 mg/ml) is injected into the inferior fornix beneath Tenon's capsule. A 12-hour collagen shield hydrated in 0.3 percent gentamicin or other topical antibiotic is placed over the cornea. Topical 5 percent homatropine is instilled, and a combination antibiotic and corticosteroid ointment is placed on the eye, which is then patched.

On the first postoperative day the patch is removed and the eye is examined for corneal re-epithelialization and inflammation. A topical combination corticosteroid and antibiotic ointment is instilled four times a day. A topical cycloplegic agent is instilled twice a day until the inflammation subsides. The ointment is continued for at least 1 week or until the corneal epithelium is completely healed, at which time a topical corticosteroid eye drop is started and tapered over several weeks until postoperative inflammation subsides.

Complications

Intraoperative complications are avoidable with proper care. Perforation of the cornea during the keratectomy is rare with microscopic visualization and maintenance of a superficial plane of dissection. If perforation does occur, the dissected tissue should be sutured when donor tissue is not available. When donor tissue is available, inlay lamellar keratoplasty should be performed. Perforation or dissection into the sclera can be avoided by taking care to observe the limbal junction and then shifting to a more superficial plane. Some degree of scarring is inevitable at the keratectomy site, but it is usually mild and does not interfere with vision unless the pupillary axis is involved. Minor amounts of astigmatism may occur with excision of lesions having considerable corneal involvement.

The area of bare sclera adjacent to the limbus where the pterygium was excised should be monitored for evidence of revascularization, which can be the first sign of pterygium recurrence. Two or three weeks after the removal of a pterygium, fine capillaries may be seen in some cases. These vessels appear to arise from the episcleral surface under the conjunctival flap. Many parallel vessels race forward toward the area of bare sclera in a brush-like fashion. If not treated, they often cross the bare area and extend into the cornea. In a matter of weeks, the vascularized region is covered by fibrous tissue similar in appearance to the original pterygium, so that the patient is left with a lesion as unsightly as the original one. Whether this lesion constitutes a true recurrence is academic. From the patient's point of view, the pterygium has grown back. Therefore, prompt action is required as soon as the brush-like vessels are detected. Various methods of adjunctive therapy may be applied at that time. The argon laser has been used successfully to treat these early recurring vessels without significant complications.[28]

Complications associated with conjunctival flaps or autografts are rarely encountered and tend to be minor.[54] Conjunctival graft edema generally occurs within the first 10 postoperative days, and is usually caused by excessive surgical manipulation, inadequate Tenon's capsule excision, or poor graft orientation. The edema generally resolves within 2 to 4 weeks. However, persistent graft edema may be reduced by pressure patching or, if severe, by puncturing the graft several times with a scalpel blade. Excessive graft edema can lead to delle formation. Conjunctival graft retraction can occur when the graft has excessive Tenon's capsule, is of inadequate size, or is of poor quality because of cicatricial processes, including trauma, prior surgery, infection, or inflammatory reaction. Necrosis of conjunctival autografts has been associated with avascular scleral beds resulting from β-radiation therapy or the use of mitomycin C.

Inadvertent inversion of the graft, such that the epithelium is apposed to the sclera, will cause the graft to fail. Epithelial cysts are another possible complication and are best treated with marsupialization. Hematomas are best prevented with the use of adequate but not excessive thermal cautery for hemostasis and pressure patching postoperatively. If the hematoma is large and beneath the graft, it can increase the tension on the sutures and cause wound dehiscence and possible displacement or loss of the graft. Small hematomas usually resolve within 3 weeks without treatment. Management of larger hematomas consists of drainage by puncturing the graft with a needle followed by a pressure patch in an attempt to prevent rebleeding.

Damage to the medial rectus muscle after pterygium excision has been reported.[55] Damage to the horizontal rectus muscle is prevented by careful dissection of the subconjunctival scar tissue and identification of the muscle prior to excision of scar tissue, especially in recurrent pterygia. Symptoms of injury to the horizontal rectus muscle include diplopia and restriction of ocular movement. Both of these symptoms can also occur with symblepharon formation. Symblepharon formation is prevented by covering the denuded areas completely with a conjunctival flap or autograft.

Adjunctive Therapy

Antimetabolites

Antimetabolites decrease the recurrence of pterygia by preventing the proliferation of abnormal tissue. Triethylene thiophosphoramide (thiotepa) and mitomycin C have been investigated for their ability to prevent pterygium recurrence.

Triethylene Thiophosphoramide (Thiotepa) Thiotepa is an alkylating, chemotherapeutic agent that has been used successfully in the prevention of pterygium recurrence.[56–59] It is a radiomimetic agent (mimicking ionizing radiation) related chemically and pharmacologically to the nitrogen mustards and inhibits capillary endothelial proliferation.[59]

Meacham[56] was the first to report the use of thiotepa in the prevention of pterygium recurrence in 1962. He transposed the head of the pterygium followed by topical application of a 1:2,000 dilution of thiotepa (15 mg thiotepa in 30 ml Ringer's solution) every 3 hours for 6 weeks. He reported no recurrences in 19 pterygia. Cassady[57] confirmed Meacham's findings, reporting only one recurrence (6 percent) in 17 cases of pterygia excised with the bare-sclera technique and treated with thiotepa for 6 to 8 weeks; the recurrence occurred in a patient who prematurely discontinued the thiotepa drops. Kleis and Pico[60] reported a recurrence rate of 8 percent with topical thiotepa compared with a rate of 31 percent in the control group. Other studies have reported recurrence rates from 0 to 16 percent with the use of various dosages of thiotepa.[61]

Although the results of early studies of topical thiotepa were promising, side effects from this medication began to be reported.[59,62–64] Initially, the side effects were neither serious nor irreversible. Joselson and Muller[62] reported that 39 of 46 eyes treated with thiotepa had extended postoperative hyperemia. In addition, one case had granuloma formation that required resection; three cases had severe conjunctival hypertrophy. Allergy to the drug also occurred. Reports of more serious side effects soon followed. Howitt and Karp[63] reported depigmentation of periorbital skin and eyelashes in a patient 1 year after excision of a pterygium followed by a 6-week course of topical thiotepa. A skin biopsy showed absence of melanin pigment. Asregadoo[58] also described depigmentation of eyelid skin and eyelashes in two patients treated with thiotepa, and black deposits in the fornix that caused irritation in one patient. Hornblass et al[64] described a patient who developed poliosis and periorbital skin depigmentation 6 years after using the drug. Avascularity of the conjunctiva and sclera have been reported as complications of thiotepa; a scleral hole, although possibly from cautery, has also been described.[58,65] Bacterial sclerokeratitis and endophthalmitis were reported 6 weeks postoperatively in a patient treated with topical thiotepa.[66] In view of the complications described with topical thiotepa and the lack of complications known to occur at that time (late 1970s) from β-radiation, it was recommended that thiotepa be used only in difficult recurrent pterygia after a trial of β-radiation therapy.[61]

Mitomycin C The treatment of pterygia with mitomycin C was introduced in Japan by Kunitomo and Mori[67] in 1963, but did not become popular in the Western world

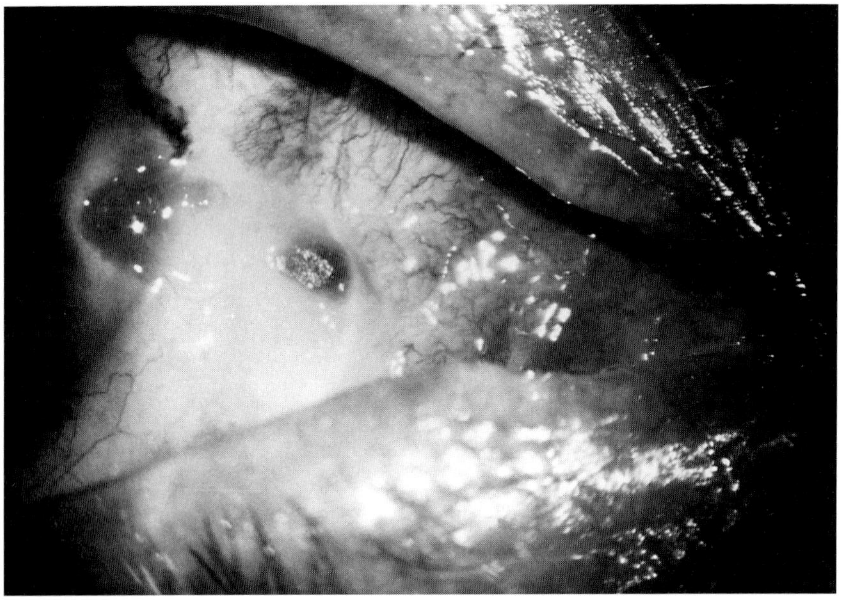

FIGURE 21-30 Corneal and scleral ulceration after pterygium excision with the bare-sclera technique and postoperative topical mitomycin C. The dark uvea is visible through the sclera.

until it was introduced in the Western literature by Singh et al[68] in 1988. Mitomycin C is produced by *Streptomyces caespitosus* and is a non-cell-cycle-specific alkylating agent that forms covalent bonds with guanine residues in DNA.[68,69] It inhibits the synthesis of DNA, RNA, and protein. Mitomycin C is extremely toxic and, like thiotepa, is radiomimetic.[70] Indeed, some of the complications seen with mitomycin C are also seen with β-radiation, including scleral ulceration.

After prior experience with the use of mitomycin C in the prevention of recurrent pterygia in India, Singh et al[68] performed controlled treatment trials in the United States. After the pterygium was excised with a bare-sclera technique, one drop of mitomycin C (either 0.1 percent or 0.04 percent) was applied topically every 6 hours for 2 weeks in addition to topical corticosteroids. The group that received the 0.1 percent concentration had a recurrence rate of 5 percent; the group that received the 0.04 percent concentration had no recurrences, giving an overall recurrence rate of 2.3 percent. Singh et al[71] continued to add patients to the study and later reported an even lower overall recurrence rate of 1.7 percent over a 7- to 21-month follow-up period.

At the same time, Hayasaka et al,[72] aware of the complications of topical 0.04 percent mitomycin C reported in the Japanese literature, compared a dose of 0.04 percent three times a day for 7 days with a dose of 0.02 percent twice a day for 5 days. Both dosages of mitomycin C were combined with a bare-sclera operative technique. They found a recurrence rate of 7 percent with the 0.02 percent concentration compared with 11 percent for the 0.04 percent concentration. Complications, however, were experienced more frequently with the higher (0.04 percent) concentration than with the lower (0.02 percent) concentration (26 percent vs. 3 percent). The complications consisted of mild discomfort, decreased vision, symblepharon formation, and scleral ulceration. Complications of the 0.02 percent concentration consisted of only mild discomfort. Hayasaka et al[73] later used the same low dose of mitomycin C (0.02 percent twice a day for 5 days) to treat patients with recurrent pterygia and found only a 5 to 9 percent recurrence rate over a 3- to 7-year follow-up period.

Frucht-Pery and Ilsar[74] compared even lower doses of mitomycin C combined with the bare-sclera technique. They reported a recurrence rate of 4 percent in patients receiving 0.02 percent mitomycin C twice daily for 5 days, and a recurrence rate of 8 percent in patients receiving 0.01 percent mitomycin C twice daily for 5 days. They subsequently combined a single intraoperative dose of 0.02 percent on a sponge applied for 5 minutes with the bare-sclera technique and found a recurrence rate of 5 percent, compared with 45 percent for the bare-sclera technique alone.[75]

Complications involving various dosages of topical mitomycin C combined with the bare-sclera technique include irritation, photophobia, delayed epithelial healing, avascularity of the sclera and cornea, scleral calcification, scleral ulceration, necrotizing scleritis, perforation, iridocyclitis, cataracts, punctal occlusion, infection, glaucoma, symblepharon formation, and loss of the eye[76–85] (Figure 21-30). There have been a few reports of complications even with low doses of mitomycin C combined with the bare-sclera technique. Yamanouchi et al[76] reported the development of scleromalacia in a patient treated with 0.04 percent topically once a day for 2 days. Rubinfeld et al[77] reported a patient who developed scleral melting after 0.02 percent was applied four times daily for 3 days. The apparent dose-dependent toxic nature of mitomycin C is consistent with its known pharmacologic properties.[69] As mitomycin C is considered a radiomimetic agent, it should be emphasized that long-term follow-up to monitor for complications is necessary.

In a review of several case reports involving mitomycin C combined with the bare-sclera technique, Rubinfeld[77,86] concluded that patients with conditions predisposed to ulceration or poor wound healing, such as Sjögren's syndrome, severe keratoconjunctivitis sicca, severe meibomian gland dysfunction, blepharitis, acne rosacea, atopic keratoconjunctivitis, neurotrophic keratitis, or herpes simplex viral keratitis, should not be considered for mitomycin C therapy.

Penna[89] noted that serious complications occurred with topical application of mitomycin C over several days in association with the bare-sclera operative technique. He suggested that the major cause of these complications is leaving the bare sclera vulnerable to the avascular effect of mitomycin C, leading to scleral or corneal necrosis and ulceration. Therefore, he recommended a single application of mitomycin C at the time of surgery, similar to the procedure used in filtering surgery, combined with closing the conjunctiva over the sclera after the pterygium has been excised. Subsequently, Cardillo et al[88] studied recurrence rates using various doses of topical mitomycin C applied intraoperatively or postoperatively combined with a sliding conjunctival flap. With intraoperative application for 3 minutes, recurrence rates were 7 percent using a 0.02 percent concentration and 4 percent using a 0.04 percent concentration. With topical application over several days after surgery, the recurrence rate was 4 percent with both the 0.02 percent concentration used three times a day for 7 days and the 0.04 percent concentration used three times a day for 14 days. Mean follow-up was 28 months. There were no complications.

Although a longer follow-up period is needed to monitor long-term complications, several recommendations can be derived from these findings. Given the complications associated with using mitomycin C in combination with the bare-sclera technique and the low recurrence rate and lack of complications associated with mitomycin C in combination with a sliding conjunctival flap, the bare-sclera technique should be avoided if the antimetabolite is to be used. If mitomycin C is combined with a conjunctival flap, a sliding flap rather than a free autograft is recommended; a sliding flap brings its own blood supply with it, whereas a free autograft requires 3 to 5 days to revascularize. In that mitomycin C can prevent revascularization, necrosis of the free graft may ensue. Also, because the difference in recurrence rates with 0.02 and 0.04 percent mitomycin C was not significant, the lower concentration should be used. Finally, because there was no significant difference between the recurrence rates for intraoperative versus postoperative application, intraoperative administration is preferred; this approach is more convenient for the patient and prevents complications resulting from improper use of the topical medication. Further studies are needed to identify the lowest dose and shortest period of intraoperative application that are effective and safe.

Patients receiving mitomycin C should be monitored closely for severe ischemia of the operative site, evidence of failure of epithelial healing, and ulceration. Damage to the sclera intraoperatively by excision of superficial scleral fibers or excessive cautery should be avoided in an attempt to prevent the scleral thinning associated with mitomycin C.[77,88,89] If areas of ischemia or ulceration develop, scleral patch grafts or lamellar or penetrating keratoplasty may be necessary. The use of topical corticosteroids and/or systemic agents, such as cyclophosphamide, should also be considered.[77] The avascular area should be covered by the transposition of a sliding conjunctival flap, rather than a free conjunctival autograft without an existing vascular supply. This may encourage revascularization and thereby arrest the ulcerative process.

β-Radiation

Like x-rays and γ-rays, β-radiation is an emission of high-speed electrons that induce ionizing radiation, which produces tissue damage. The penetration of β-radiation is limited, however. Only 10 percent of the surface dose penetrates a distance of 3 mm.[90] β-Radiation is highly selective in the type of tissue affected; collagen shows little change, while vascular walls and young, actively dividing vascular endothelial cells are very sensitive.[91] The purpose of β-radiation is to prevent the formation of new episcleral capillaries, which may act as a source of granulation tissue and recurrence.

Strontium 90 is the safest and most effective mode of applying β-radiation to the eye.[92,93] A federal license from the Nuclear Regulatory Commission (NRC) is required for a practitioner to apply strontium 90. However, in most institutions, a radiologist or a radiotherapist administers the radiation. The unit for strontium 90 is the roentgen equivalent physical, rep; 1 rep = 1.08 rad.

Controversy exists in the literature regarding the postoperative timing of the applications and the most effective dose of strontium 90. β-Radiation applied immediately after surgical excision of a pterygium inhibits early vascular budding and, thereby, controls vascular proliferation. The effect appears within hours and lasts for several weeks. In a prospective study, Aswad and Baum[94] found a 12.5 percent recurrence rate in patients who had immediate postoperative irradiation compared with a 33.3 percent recurrence rate in patients irradiated 4 days postoperatively. β-Radiation should be applied immediately postoperatively, before the patient leaves the operating room. This is also more convenient and economical for the patient.

There is considerable latitude in the literature concerning the dose of β-radiation. Although some authors have advocated 3,000 rep in divided doses of 1,000 rep per week, others have advocated single doses of 1,500 to 2,200 rep.[92,94,95] If β-radiation is used, we recommend 2,000 rep of strontium 90 applied immediately postoperatively.

The effectiveness of β-radiation becomes apparent when the results of series with and without irradiation are reviewed. Pico[21] observed a recurrence rate of 3 percent with and 8 percent without β-radiation. In Hilgers' series,[25] the recurrence rate was 8 percent with and 23 percent without β-radiation, whereas Cameron[2] cited higher rates: 16 percent with and more than 50 percent without. In a large study with a 10-year follow-up, Mackenzie et al[95] reported a recurrence rate of 12 percent with β-radiation. De Keizer et al[96] reported no recurrences with β-radiation for primary pterygia, and an 11 percent recurrence rate with β-radiation for recurrent pterygia, compared with a 67 percent recurrence rate after excision of primary pterygia with the bare-sclera technique.

β-Radiation has been combined with conjunctival flaps, conjunctival autografts, lamellar keratoplasty, and antimetabolites.[97,98] However, a combination of β-radiation and antimetabolites is not recommended because it may greatly increase the risk of serious complications, most notably scleral ulceration.

β-Radiation was used for decades to prevent the recurrence of pterygia before its complications were recognized.[97] Complications of postoperative irradiation following pterygium excision are known to occur as late as 3 to 20 years after treatment.[95,97] Complications associated with β-radiation include scleral ulceration, corneal ulceration, ptosis, symblepharon formation, iris atrophy, and cataract formation.[95,97] Scleral ulceration after β-radiation can lead to serious side effects, including infectious scleritis and endophthalmitis.[95,99,100] Infectious scleritis generally occurs 3 to 10 years after β-radiation, but has been reported as early as 2 weeks.[65] In a large study with at least 10 years of follow-up after doses of 1,800 to 2,200 rads of β-radiation in a single application, Mackenzie et al[95] reported a 13 percent incidence of some sign of scleral necrosis and a 4.5 percent incidence of severe scleral ulceration. These authors used applicators with a large surface area (6 mm by 11 to 12 mm rectangular or 10 to 16 mm diameter circular). Levine[101] proposed that reducing the surface area of the applicator might reduce the incidence of scleral necrosis and suggested using a kidney-shaped applicator measuring 3 mm by 8.5 mm at the limbus. Tarr and Constable[97] reported scleral ulceration in a patient treated with a single dose of 750 rads. They suggested that scleral necrosis is not a primary event but occurs secondary to scleral exposure either from leaving bare sclera at the time of pterygium excision or by conjunctival breakdown postoperatively. Based on this pathogenetic theory of scleral necrosis, if β-radiation is planned, the epibulbar defect created by pterygium excision should be covered with conjunctiva, except for a 3-mm area next to the limbus. The applicator should be applied only to this area of paralimbal bare sclera, without overlapping fields of exposure. From the observations of Mackenzie and others, it appears that scleral necrosis generally occurs as late as 3 to 10 years after irradiation.[95]

Although β-radiation can cause cataracts, they are rarely visually significant or progressive.[90,97,102] Ionizing radiation initially injures the equatorial epithelial cells of the lens, leading to typical peripheral sectorial opacities involving the posterior subcapsular region.[90,102] The most peripheral portion of the lens is approximately 3 mm from the limbal surface where the β-radiation is applied. At this depth, the dose is approximately 10 percent of the surface dose. The incidence of cataract formation and the extent of these changes appear to be dose dependent. The periphery is most vulnerable, with lens changes occurring with surface doses of 1,300 to 3,500 rep; the central area requires approximately 8,000 rep to show significant changes resulting in decreased visual acuity.[90] The onset of cataract formation generally ranges from 2 to 10 years after radiation.[90] Hilgers,[102] in a 5- to 7-year follow-up study, reported no lens opacities after fractionated doses of β-radiation totaling 1,000 to 3,000 rep, but 6 percent of eyes developed lens opacities after 3,000 to 5,000 rep. These opacities were localized and nonprogressive, and appeared clinically insignificant.

Lasers and Thermal Cautery

The theoretical use of the excimer laser as an adjunct to pterygium surgery is to polish the cornea after excision of the pterygium to create an ultrasmooth surface, which may re-epithelialize more quickly and uniformly and help to prevent recurrence of the pterygium. Krag and Ehlers[103] combined the bare-sclera technique with excimer laser ablation and found a high recurrence rate of 91 percent within the first year of follow-up. The high recurrence rate was attributed to the bare-sclera technique and not to any contributing factor of the excimer laser. Dausch et al[104] combined conventional surgical excision of a pterygium with a conjunctival autograft followed by excimer laser ablation of the cornea. They found a much lower recurrence rate of 12 percent during a 3-year follow-up period. However, these relatively good results do not indicate a reduction of pterygium recurrence rates compared with those obtained with conjunctival autografts alone. Removal of pterygia at or near the visual axis may result in decreased vision secondary to scarring or irregular astigmatism. After surgical removal of the pterygium, these patients may benefit from excimer laser phototherapeutic keratectomy for visual rehabilitation.

Caldwell[28] reported a high success rate in treating pterygia with the argon laser. He hypothesized that an angiogenic factor released by the cornea leads to neovascular tufts or membranes similar to those seen in the retina of diabetic patients. Early pterygia that have not encroached on the limbus or cornea (more correctly termed pingueculae), but are inflamed and elevated, can be treated effectively with the argon laser. Removal of the elevated mass with the laser re-establishes normal eyelid apposition to the cornea, thereby removing the proposed anoxic stimulus from the cornea. However, once there is elevation at the limbus or advancement onto the cornea, surgical excision of the pterygium is required. The excised pterygium bed is then observed for neovascular fronds weekly until the eye is white and uninflamed. Neovascular fronds are indicative of a possible recurrence; if they develop, they are treated extensively with the argon laser at an intensity high enough to close the vessels but not to burn the conjunctival epithelium. Damage to the epithelium would increase the stimulus for neovascularization. A 50-μm spot size with a 0.1 second exposure time at a power setting of 0.2 to 0.3 watts is recommended by Caldwell.[28]

The traditional use of thermal cautery alone to treat pterygia is controversial despite the fact that it was described as early as 1896 by Coe.[105] Ling[106] reported success with a technique involving hand-held thermal cautery applied extensively, without excision, to the noncorneal aspect of the pterygium. Cautery is currently generally applied after the pterygium is excised. Some authors augment their surgical technique with extensive cautery in the belief that blood vessels at the operative site induce recurrence. Others argue that aggressive cautery may induce exaggerated scar formation and stimulate recurrence. Because aggressive cautery can damage both the episclera and sclera, it should not be combined with adjunctive therapy that can also lead to scleral thinning, such as antimetabolites or β-radiation.[75]

REFERENCES

1. Rosenthal JW: Chronology of pterygium therapy. Am J Ophthalmol 36:1601, 1953
2. Cameron ME: Pterygium throughout the World. Charles C. Thomas, Springfield, IL, 1965
3. Hilgers JHC: Pterygium on the Island of Aruba. Klein Offset Drukkerij, Amsterdam, Poortpers NV, 1959
4. Dimitry TJ: Dust factor in production of pterygium. Am J Ophthalmol 20:40, 1937
5. Zehender W, cited by Parsons JHL: p. 106. In Pathology of the Eye. GP Putnam & Sons, London, 1904
6. Fuchs E: Über das Pterygium. Albrecht von Graefes Arch Ophthalmol 38:1, 1892
7. Stocker F: Eine pigmentierte Hornhautlinie beim Pterygium. Klin Monatsbl Augenheilkd 102:384, 1939
8. Hansen A, Norn M: Astigmatism and surface phenomena in pterygium. Acta Ophthalmol (Copenh) 58:174, 1980
9. Lin S, Reiter K, Dreher AW, et al: The effect of pterygia on contrast sensitivity and glare disability. Am J Ophthalmol 107:407, 1989
10. Holladay JT, Lewis JW, Allison ME, Ruiz RS: Pterygia as cause of post-cataract with-the-rule astigmatism. Am Intraocul Implant Soc J 11:176, 1985
11. Hochbaum DR, Moskowitz SE, Wirtschafter JD: A quantitative analysis of astigmatism induced by pterygium. J Biomech 10:735, 1977
12. Oldenburg JB, Garbus J, McDonnell JM, McDonnell PJ: Conjunctival pterygia: mechanism of corneal topographic changes. Cornea 9:200, 1990
13. Cogan DG, Kuwabara T, Howard J: The nonelastic nature of pingueculas. Arch Ophthalmol 61:388, 1959
14. Scarpa A, cited by Poncet F: Du pterygion. Arch Ophtalmol (Paris) 1:21, 1880–1881
15. Friede R: Die Pathogenese des echten Pterygiums. Acta Ophthalmol (Copenh) 27:507, 1949
16. Kamel S: The pterygium: its etiology and treatment. Am J Ophthalmol 38:682, 1954
17. Redslob E: Contribution a l'étude de la nature du pterygion. Ann Oculist 170:42, 1933
18. Austin P, Jakobiec FA, Iwamoto T: Elastodysplasia and elastodystrophy as the pathologic bases of ocular pterygia and pinguecula. Ophthalmology 90:96, 1983
19. Talbot G: Pterygium. Trans Ophthalmol Soc NZ 2:42, 1948
20. Blum HF: Carcinogenesis by Ultraviolet Light. Princeton University Press, Princeton, NJ, 1959
21. Pico G: Pterygium. Current concept of etiology and management. p. 280. In King JH, McTigue JW (eds): The Cornea. World Congress. Butterworths, Washington, 1965
22. Diponegoro RMA, Houwer AWM: A statistical contribution to the etiology of pterygium. Folia Ophthalmol Orient 2:195, 1936
23. Kerkenesov N: A pterygium survey of the far north coast of NSW. Trans Ophthalmol Soc Aust 16:110, 1956
24. Elliot R: The aetiology of pterygium. Trans Ophthalmol Soc NZ 13:22, 1961

25. Hilgers JHC: Pterygium. Am J Ophthalmol 50:635, 1960
26. Mackenzie FD, Hirst LW, Battistutta D, Green A: Risk analysis in the development of pterygia. Ophthalmology 99:1056, 1992
27. Barraquer JI: Etiologia y patogenia del pterigiom y de las excavaciones de la cornea de Fuchs. Arch Soc Am Oftalmol Optom 5:45, 1964
28. Caldwell DR, as quoted in Boyd BF: Highlights of Ophthalmology: Atlas and Textbook of Microsurgery and Laser Surgery, 30th Anniversary Edition. Vol. 1. Highlights of Ophthalmology. Panama City, Republic of Panama, 1985, p. 534
29. Stainer GA, Brightbill FS, Holm P, Lanx D: The development of pseudopterygia in hard contact lens wearers. Contact Lens 7:1, 1981
30. Honan PR: Complications associated with hard contact lenses. Ophthalmology 86:1102, 1979
31. Ehrlich D: The management of pterygium. Ophthalmic Surg 8:23, 1977
32. Rich AM, Keitzman B, Payne T, et al: A simplified way to remove pterygia. Ann Ophthalmol 6:739, 1974
33. Jaros PA, DeLuise VP: Pingueculae and pterygia. Surv Ophthalmol 33:41, 1988
34. Tower P: Corrugated silver wire for severing pterygium from the cornea. Am J Ophthalmol 33:1439, 1950
35. Gibson JBG: Brisbane survey of pterygium. Trans Ophthalmol Soc Aust 16:125, 1956
36. Desmarres LA: Traité Theorique et Practique des Maladies des Yeux. Vol. 2. G Baillière, Paris, 1855
37. Berens C, King JH: Atlas of Ophthalmic Surgery. JB Lippincott, Philadelphia, 1961
38. McReynolds JO: The nature and treatment of pterygia. JAMA 39:296, 1902
39. Wilson SE, Bourne WM: Conjunctival Z-plasty in the treatment of pterygium. Am J Ophthalmol 106:355, 1988
40. Stocker FW: Operation for removal of pterygium. Arch Ophthalmol 27:925, 1942
41. Alger LH: Etiology of pterygium recurrence. Am J Ophthalmol 57:450, 1964
42. Arruga H: Ocular Surgery. p. 323. McGraw-Hill, New York, 1962
43. Tomas T: Sliding flap of conjunctival limbus to prevent recurrence of pterygium. Refract Corneal Surg 8:394, 1992
44. Kenyon KR, Wagoner MD, Hettinger ME: Conjunctival autograft transplantation for advanced and recurrent pterygium. Ophthalmology 92:1461, 1985
45. Lewallen S: A randomized trial of conjunctival autografting for pterygium in the tropics. Ophthalmology 96:1612, 1989
46. Trivedi LK, Massey DB, Rohatgi R: Management of pterygium and its recurrence by grafting with mucous membrane from the mouth. Am J Ophthalmol 68:353, 1969
47. Small R: A technique for removal of pterygium. Ann Ophthalmol 9:349, 1977
48. Hirst LW, Sebban A, Chant D: Pterygium recurrence time. Ophthalmology 101:755, 1994
49. Pearlman G, Susal AL, Hushaw J, Bartlett RE: Recurrent pterygium and treatment with lamellar keratoplasty with presentation of a technique to limit recurrences. Ann Ophthalmol 2:763, 1970
50. Poirier RH, Fish JR: Lamellar keratoplasty for recurrent pterygium. Ophthalmic Surg 7:38, 1976
51. Laughrea PA, Arentsen JJ: Lamellar keratoplasty in the management of recurrent pterygium. Ophthalmic Surg 17:106, 1986
52. Busin M, Halliday BL, Arffa RC, et al: Precarved lyophilized tissue for lamellar keratoplasty in recurrent pterygium. Am J Ophthalmol 102:222, 1986
53. Shaw EL: A modified technique for conjunctival transplant. CLAO J 18:112, 1992
54. Starck T, Kenyon KR, Serrano F: Conjunctival autograft for primary and recurrent pterygia: surgical technique and problem management. Cornea 10:196, 1991
55. Raab EL, Metz HS, Ellis FD: Medial rectus injury after pterygium excision. Arch Ophthalmol 107:1428, 1989
56. Meacham C: Triethylene thiophosphoramide in the prevention of pterygium recurrence. Am J Ophthalmol 54:751, 1962
57. Cassady J: The inhibition of pterygium recurrence by thiotepa. Am J Ophthalmol 61:886, 1966
58. Asregadoo ER: Surgery, thiotepa, and corticosteroid in the treatment of pterygium. Am J Ophthalmol 74:960, 1972
59. Liddy B St. L, Morgan JF: Triethylene thiophosphoramide (thiotepa) and pterygium. Am J Ophthalmol 61:888, 1966
60. Kleis W, Pico G: Thio-tepa therapy to prevent postoperative pterygium occurrence and neovascularization. Am J Ophthalmol 74:371, 1973
61. Olander K, Haik KG, Haik GM: Management of pterygia: should thiotepa be used? Ann Ophthalmol 10:853, 1978
62. Joselson GA, Muller P: Incidence of pterygia recurrence in patients treated with thiotepa. Am J Ophthalmol 61:891, 1966
63. Howitt D, Karp E: Side effect of topical thiotepa. Am J Ophthalmol 68:473, 1969
64. Hornblass A, Adler R, Vukcevich W, Gombos GM: A delayed side effect of topical thiotepa. Ann Ophthalmol 6:1155, 1974
65. Harrison M, Kelly A, Ohlrich J: Pterygium: "thiotepa" versus beta radiation, a double blind trial. Trans Aust Coll Ophthalmol 1:64, 1969
66. Farrell PLR, Smith RE: Bacterial corneoscleritis complicating pterygium excision. Am J Ophthalmol 107:515, 1989
67. Kunitomo N, Mori S: Studies on the pterygium. Part 4. A treatment of the pterygium by mitomycin C instillation. Nippon Ganka Gakkai Zasshi 67:601, 1963
68. Singh G, Wilson MR, Foster CS: Mitomycin eye drops as treatment for pterygium. Ophthalmology 95:813, 1988
69. Gilman AG, Rall TW, Nies AS, Taylor P (eds): Goodman and Gilman's The Pharmacological Basis of Therapeutics. 8th Ed. Pergamon Press, New York, 1990, p. 1247
70. Bowman WC, Rand MJ (eds): Textbook of Pharmacology. 2nd Ed. Vol. 3. Blackwell, Oxford, 1980, p. 14

71. Singh G, Wilson MR, Foster CS: Long-term follow-up study of mitomycin eyedrops as adjunctive treatment for pterygia and its comparison with conjunctival autograft transplantation. Cornea 9:331, 1990
72. Hayasaka S, Noda S, Yamamoto Y, Setogawa T: Postoperative instillation of low-dose mitomycin C in the treatment of primary pterygium. Am J Ophthalmol 106:715, 1988
73. Hayasaka S, Noda S, Yamamoto Y, Setogawa T: Postoperative instillation of mitomycin C in the treatment of recurrent pterygium. Ophthalmic Surg 20:580, 1989
74. Frucht-Pery J, Ilsar M: The use of low-dose mitomycin C for prevention of recurrent pterygium. Ophthalmology 101:759, 1994
75. Frucht-Pery J, Islar M, Hemo I: Single dosage of mitomycin C for prevention of recurrent pterygium: preliminary report. Cornea 13:411, 1994
76. Yamanouchi U, Takaku I, Tsuda N, et al: Scleromalacia presumably due to mitomycin C instillation after pterygium excision. Jpn J Clin Ophthalmol 33:139, 1979
77. Rubinfeld RS, Pfister RR, Stein RM, et al: Serious complications of topical mitomycin C after pterygium surgery. Ophthalmology 99:1647, 1992
78. Dunn JP, Seamone CD, Ostler HB, et al: Development of scleral ulceration and calcification after pterygium excision and mitomycin therapy [letter]. Am J Ophthalmol 112:343, 1991
79. Ewing-Chow DA, Romanchuk KG, Gilmour GR, et al: Corneal melting after pterygium removal followed by topical mitomycin C therapy. Can J Ophthalmol 27:197, 1992
80. Singh G: Ocular toxicity of topical mitomycin as an adjunctive treatment for pterygium. Trans Pac Coast Otoophthalmol Soc Annu Meet 69:82, 1988
81. Fukamachi Y, Hikita N: Ocular complication following pterygium operation and instillation of mitomycin C. Nippon Ganka Kiyo 32:197, 1981
82. Yamanouchi U: A case of scleral calcification due to mitomycin C instillation after pterygium operation. Nippon Ganka Kiyo 29:1221, 1978
83. Yamanouchi U, Mishima K: Eye lesions due to mitomycin C instillation after pterygium operation. Nippon Ganka Kiyo 18:854, 1967
84. Gupta S, Basti S: Corneosclera, ciliary body, and vitreoretinal toxicity after excessive instillation of mitomycin-C [letter]. Am J Ophthalmol 114:503, 1992
85. Fujitani A, Hayasaka S, Shibuya Y, Noda S: Corneoscleral ulceration and corneal perforation after pterygium excision and topical mitomycin C therapy. Ophthalmologica 207:162, 1993
86. Rubinfeld RS: Mitomycin-C after pterygium surgery [reply]. Ophthalmology 100:977, 1993
87. Penna EP: Mitomycin-C after pterygium surgery [letter]. Ophthalmology 100:976, 1993
88. Cardillo JA, Alves MR, Ambrosio LE, et al: Single intraoperative application versus postoperative mitomycin C eye drops in pterygium surgery. Ophthalomolgy 102:1949, 1995
89. Singh G: Postoperative instillation of low-dose mitomycin C in the treatment of primary pterygium [letter]. Am J Ophthalmol 107:570, 1989
90. Thomas CI, Storaasli JP, Friedell HL: Lenticular changes associated with beta radiation of the eye and their significance. Radiology 79:588, 1962
91. Bloom W: Histopathology of Irradiation from External and Internal Sources. McGraw-Hill, New York, 1948
92. Cooper JS: Postoperative irradiation of pterygia: ten more years of experience. Ther Radiol 128:753, 1978
93. Griedell HL, Thomas CI, Krohmer JS: Beta-ray application to the eye. Am J Ophthalmol 33:525, 1950
94. Aswad MI, Baum J: Optimal time for postoperative irradiation of pterygia. Ophthalmology 94:1450, 1987
95. Mackenzie FD, Hirst LW, Kynaston B, Bain C: Recurrence rate and complications after beta irradiation for pterygia. Ophthalmology 98:1776, 1991
96. De Keizer RJW, Swart-Van den Berg M, Baartse WJ: Results of pterygia excision with Sr 90 irradiation, lamellar keratoplasty and conjunctival flaps. Doc Ophthalmol 67:33, 1987
97. Tarr KH, Constable IJ: Late complications of pterygium treatment. Br J Ophthalmol 64:496, 1980
98. Monselise M, Schwartz M, Politi F, Barishak YR: Pterygium and beta irradiation. Acta Ophthalmol (Copenh) 62:315, 1984
99. Tarr KH, Constable IJ: *Pseudomonas* endophthalmitis associated with scleral necrosis. Br J Ophthalmol 64:676, 1980
100. Moriarty AP, Crawford GJ, McAllister IL, Constable IJ: Severe corneoscleral infection. A complication of beta irradiation scleral necrosis following pterygium excision. Arch Ophthalmol 111:947, 1993
101. Levine DJ: Beta irradiation of pterygium [letter]. Ophthalmology 99:841, 1992
102. Hilgers JHC: Strontium 90 β-irradiation, cataractogenicity, and pterygium recurrence. Arch Ophthalmol 76:329, 1966
103. Krag S, Ehlers N: Excimer laser treatment of pterygium. Acta Ophthalmol (Copenh) 70:530, 1992
104. Dausch D, Klein RJ, Shröder E: Pterygium. p. 68. In Ophthalmic Excimer Laser Surgery. Europe Excimer Center, Strasbourg, 1991
105. Coe A: A new method of treating pterygium. Ann Ophthalmol 5:250, 1896
106. Ling RT: Treatment of pterygium using thermal cautery. Ophthalmic Surg 20:511, 1989

22

Ectatic Corneal Degenerations

LEO J. MAGUIRE

Keratoconus, pellucid marginal degeneration, and keratoglobus all exhibit corneal ectasia secondary to corneal stromal thinning and are unrelated to any obvious inflammatory process. Posterior keratoconus is a disorder of mesenchymal dysgenesis characterized by posterior corneal thinning without ectasia; it is included in this chapter primarily to distinguish it from keratoconus.

KERATOCONUS

Diagnosis and Natural History

Keratoconus is a noninflammatory corneal thinning disorder. In its most advanced stage, keratoconus is characterized by a localized conical protrusion of the cornea associated with an area of corneal stromal thinning. The stromal thinning is most apparent at the apex of the cone. The cone may be small or large, round or oval, and is located either near the visual axis or inferior to it[1,2] (Figures 22-1 and 22-2). Irregular astigmatism and high myopia caused by the steep conical protrusion often preclude adequate spectacle correction, forcing the patient to rely on contact lens correction or surgery to improve vision.

Other characteristics of keratoconus are apparent on slit lamp examination. A Fleischer ring is a corneal epithelial iron ring that partially or completely encircles the base of the cone. The color of the ring varies from yellow to brown, depending on the amount of ferritin deposited in the basal layer of the epithelium. The ring is best seen with cobalt blue illumination[3] (Figure 22-3). If the Fleischer ring is incomplete, the borders of the cone can be delineated by retroilluminating the cornea with a direct ophthalmoscope after the pupil has been dilated. The cone reflects the light internally, producing a dark area within the illuminated field (Figure 22-4).

Vogt's striae are fine vertical folds in the deep stroma and Descemet's membrane that parallel the steep axis of the cone[4,5] (Figure 22-5). Gentle digital pressure causes transient disappearance of the striae.[6]

Fine anterior stromal scars are common in keratoconus. These scars are caused by the repair of idiopathic breaks in Bowman's layer (Figure 22-6). Clinically less important findings include enlarged corneal nerves,[7] increased intensity of the corneal endothelial reflex, clear spaces in the anterior stroma,[8] and fine subepithelial fibrillary lines.[9] Patients may develop scarring at the apex of the cone when corrective contact lenses chronically abrade the corneal surface. Occasionally, a hyperplastic subepithelial layer (corneal nebula) develops as a reaction to contact lens wear. These opacities can cause severe glare as well as decreased vision. In some cases, a nebula can be removed surgically, avoiding the need for penetrating keratoplasty.[10]

Tears in Descemet's membrane cause acute stromal edema in the area of the cone (acute corneal hydrops)[11] (Figure 22-7). The edema usually resolves within 4 months but leaves a residual scar. The cone may flatten after the hydrops resolves, and visual acuity may improve if the scar is outside the visual axis.

Two external findings associated with advanced keratoconus are Munson's sign and Rizzuti's sign. Munson's sign is a V-shaped conformation of the lower eyelid produced by the ectatic cornea in downgaze (Figure 22-8). Rizzuti's sign is a sharply focused beam of light near the nasal limbus produced by lateral illumination of the cornea[12] (Figure 22-9). The beam is central to the limbus in moderate cases, and moves peripherally as the cone progresses.

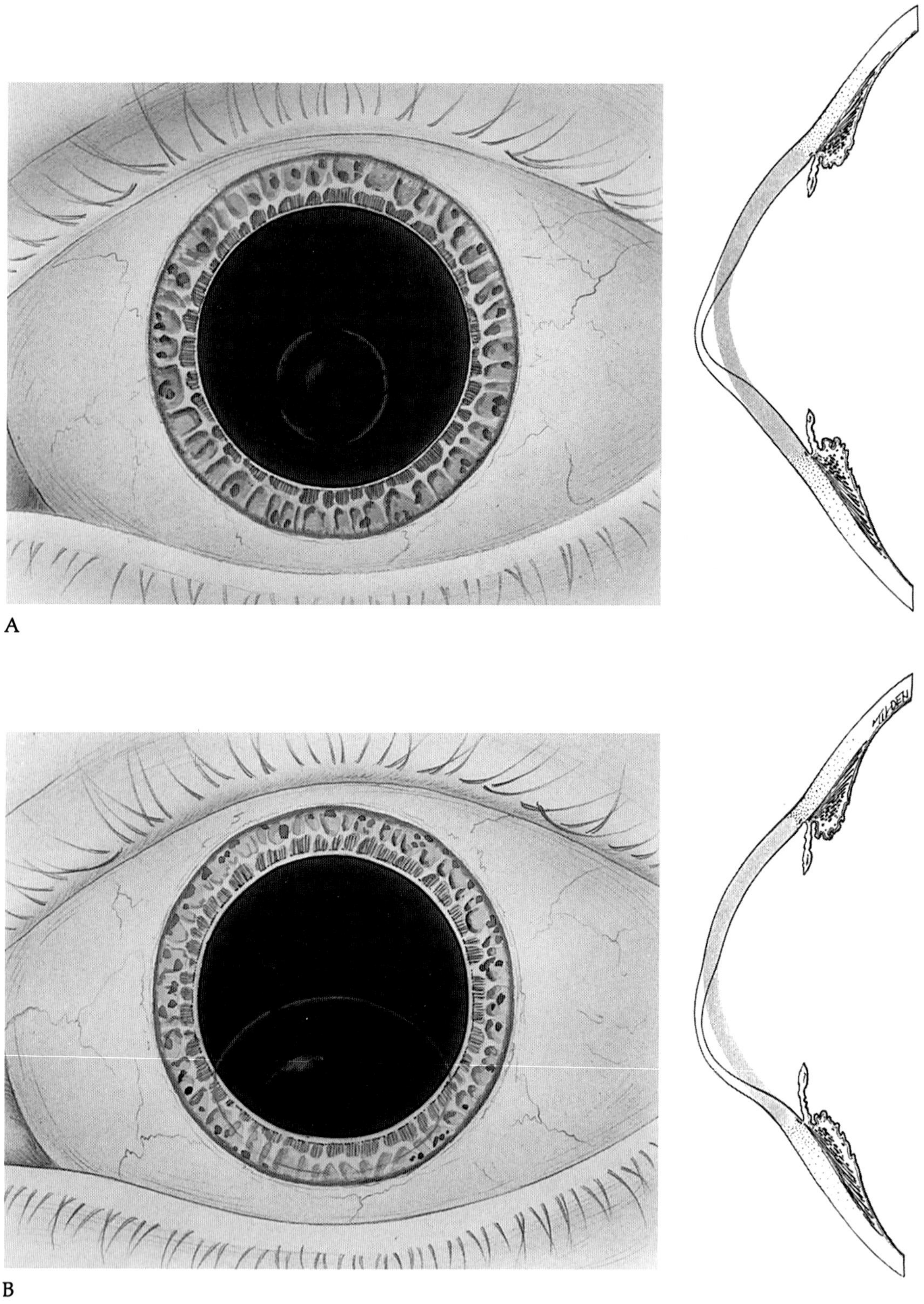

FIGURE 22-1 Advanced keratoconus is characterized by a localized conical protrusion of the cornea associated with an area of corneal stromal thinning most marked at the cone apex. The cone may be **(A)** round or **(B)** oval in shape. The Fleischer ring may partially or completely surround the cone.

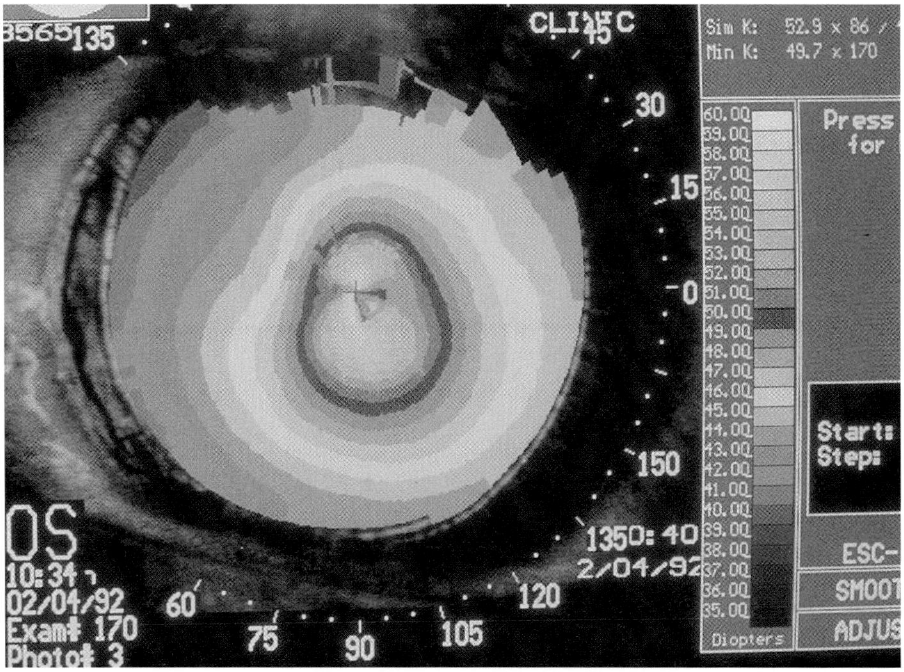

FIGURE 22-2 Videokeratograph of central keratoconus. The central cornea is markedly steep. Each color represents 1 diopter of power.

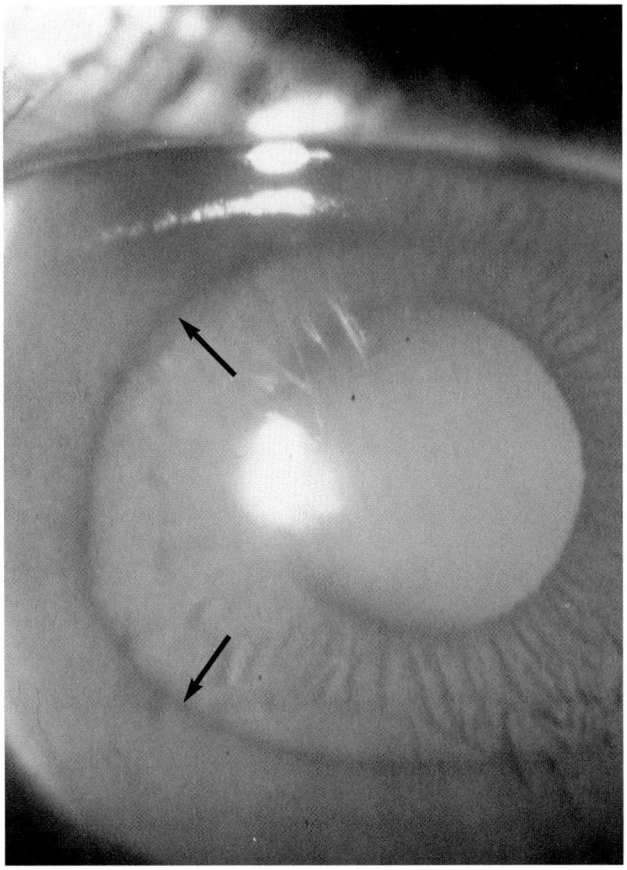

FIGURE 22-3 A large Fleischer ring (arrows) appears as a dark band with cobalt blue illumination.

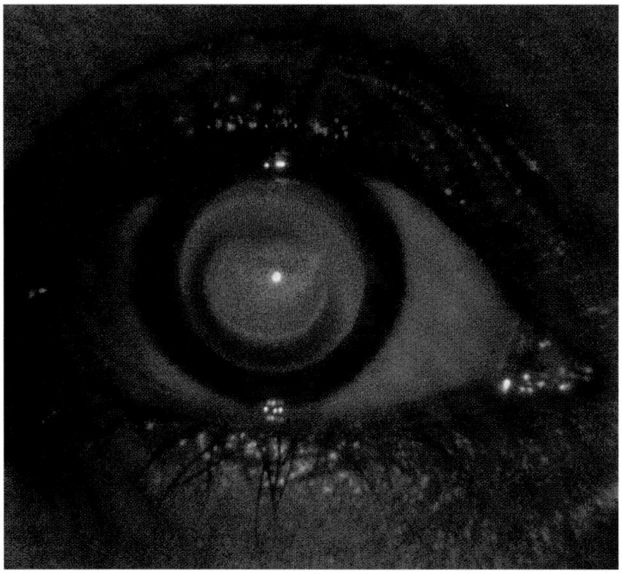

FIGURE 22-4 Corneal retroillumination is a useful technique to identify the extent of the cone. Retroillumination can often identify the presence of keratoconus before it is evident on slit lamp examination.

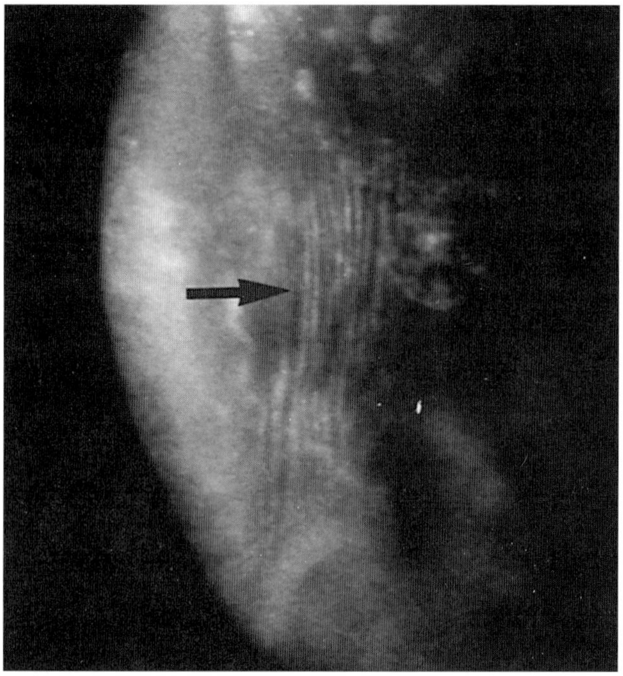

FIGURE 22-5 Vogt's striae (arrow) are found in the deep stroma and Descemet's membrane. They usually run parallel to the steep axis of the cone.

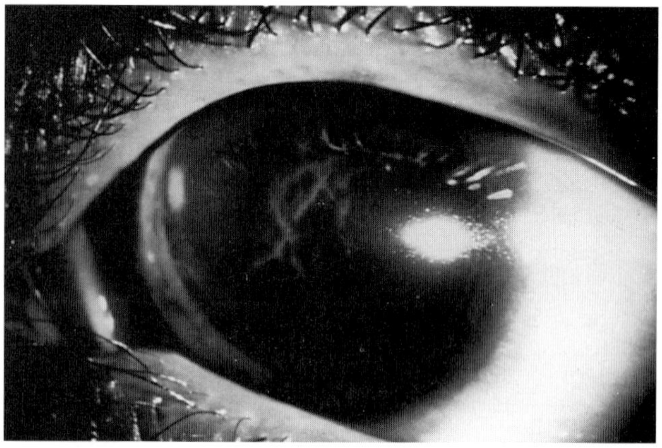

FIGURE 22-6 Anterior stromal scars caused by breaks in Bowman's layer.

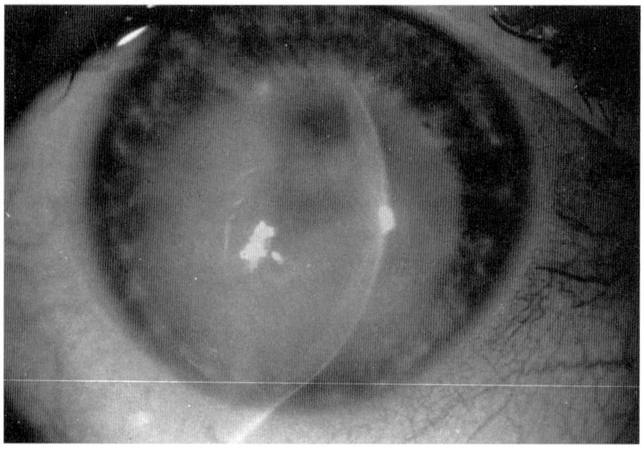

FIGURE 22-7 Corneal hydrops. Tears in Descemet's membrane cause focal corneal edema. Edema usually resolves in 4 months. Hydrops appears to occur more frequently in Down syndrome patients with keratoconus than in the rest of the keratoconus population.

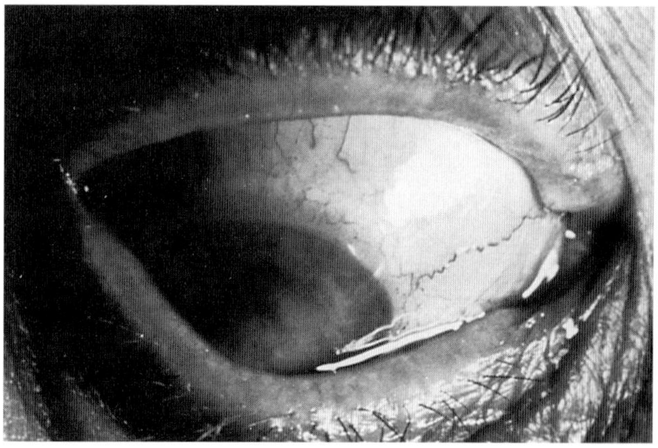

FIGURE 22-8 Munson's sign. The V-shaped conformation of the lower eyelid is produced by the ectatic cornea in downgaze.

When slit lamp examination and external findings of advanced keratoconus are present, diagnosis presents little difficulty. However, early diagnosis is not easy. Patients who develop keratoconus putatively begin life with a normal cornea, progress through an asymptomatic subclinical stage, and then, between puberty and 30 years of age, present with visual complaints or subtle signs consistent with the diagnosis. Keratoconus should be suspected in any adolescent or young adult with progressive myopic astigmatism. Thus far, the most effective way to identify early cases of keratoconus is with computer-based corneal topographic analysis[2,13,14] (Figure 22-10).

Amsler[15,16] documented the progression of keratoconus from minor distortions of the corneal surface to clinically recognizable cone formation. He divided keratoconus into the clinically recognizable stage and an earlier latent stage recognizable only by Placido disk examination of the corneal surface. At that time, diagnosing subclinical keratoconus was only of academic interest. However, in this age of keratorefractive surgery, it is essential to screen keratorefractive candidates for the condition to avoid potentially disastrous results.[15,17,18]

Often, keratoconus is subtle in at least one eye, and in most patients, involvement is asymmetrical. In Amsler's study[15] of 600 keratoconus patients, 22 percent had clinically recognizable keratoconus in both eyes, 26 percent had clinically recognizable keratoconus in one eye and latent keratoconus in the other eye, and 52 percent had latent keratoconus bilaterally.

Progression is highly variable and usually asymmetrical. The cone may remain stationary, progress rapidly over 3 to 5 years and arrest, or progress intermittently over an extended period of time. When Amsler reexamined 286 eyes 3 to 8 years after diagnosis, only 22 percent of the entire group, but 66 percent of the latent cases, had progressed.[16] Progression is most likely to occur between 10 and 20 years of age, slows between 20 and 30 years, and is less likely after 30 years (Figure 22-11). Many investigators believe progression is accelerated when patients vigorously rub their eyes.[19,20]

The need for penetrating keratoplasty to correct keratoconus was estimated at less than 20 percent over a 20-year period in the Mayo epidemiology study[21]; this percentage is probably lower now because contact lens fitting techniques have improved.[22,23]

Prevalence

The prevalence of keratoconus in the general population has been estimated to be between 4 and 600 per 100,000, but diagnostic criteria vary among studies.[21,24-29] The disorder occurs in all races. The female preponderance described in earlier studies is not a constant finding.[24,30-32]

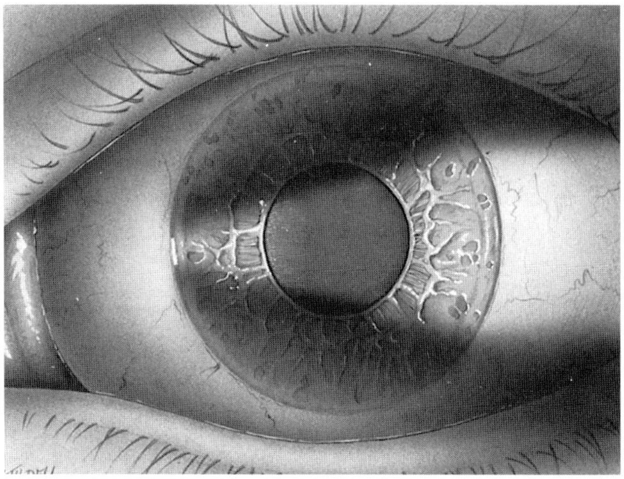

FIGURE 22-9 Rizutti's sign. Lateral illumination of the cornea produces a sharply focused beam of light near the nasal limbus in patients with advanced keratoconus.

Heredity

Heredity plays a significant role in at least a portion of keratoconus patients. Von Ammon first described the familial incidence of keratoconus in 1830; it has since been found that familial incidence varies from less than 5 percent to as high as 20 percent.[21,24,33-37]

Familial incidence may vary within a region.[24] Falls and Allen[33] reported a family with irregular dominant inheritance through two generations, reviewed 20 earlier cases in which dominant inheritance appeared likely, and reviewed reports of recessive transmission. A large epidemiologic study from Finland supports the idea of dominant inheritance in that region.[24] One case exists of a patient whose parents both had keratoconus. The patient developed severe keratoconus in early adolescence.[38]

Keratoconus has been reported in seven sets of monozygous twins. In five sets, both twins were affected.[39-42] In two sets, only one sibling was affected.[43,44] These cases illustrate how difficult the genetic study of keratoconus can be, because there are different degrees of penetrance, even in monozygous twins.

Topographic analysis of the corneal surface may help to explain the role of heredity in keratoconus. A pilot study that used such analysis to evaluate 28 family members of five patients with keratoconus found topographic abnormalities in 50 percent of the family members studied, which was significantly higher than in normal con-

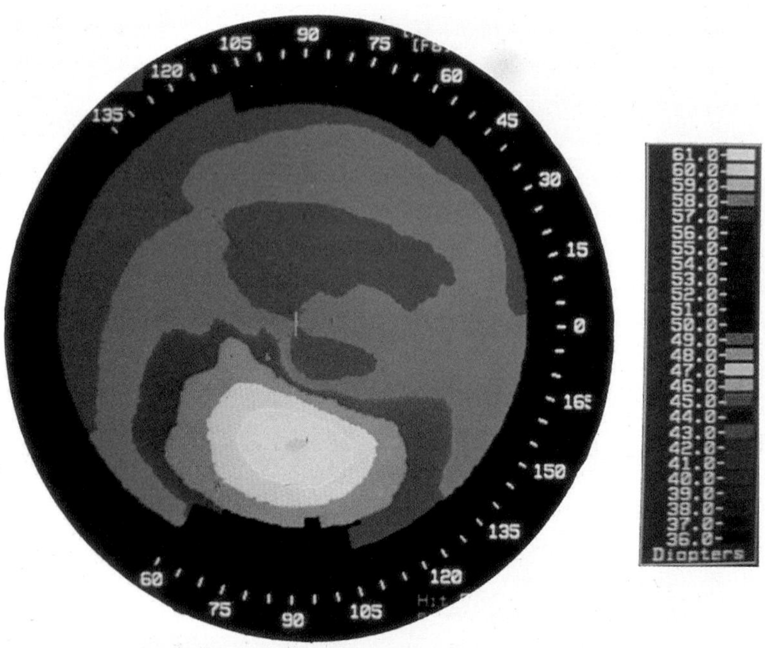

A

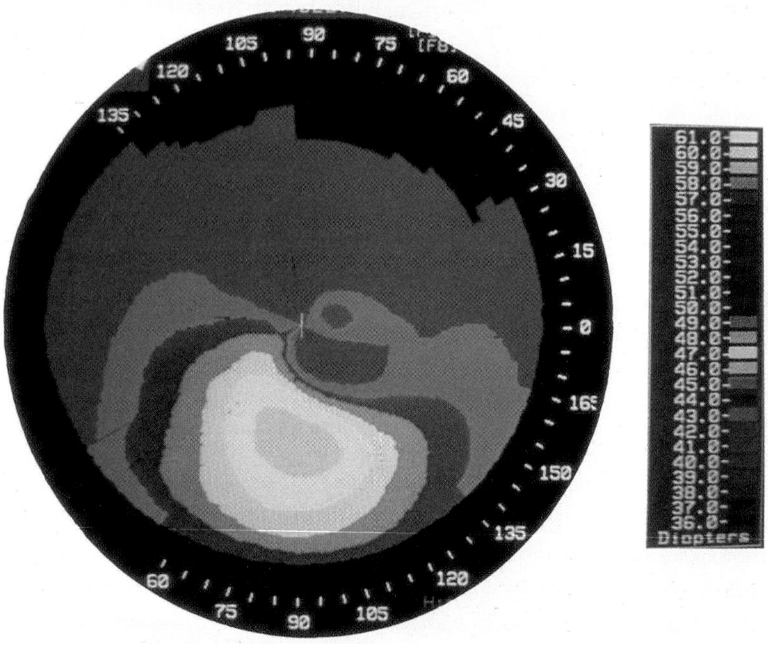

B

FIGURE 22-10 Videokeratographs illustrating progression of subclinical keratoconus. **(A)** At diagnosis, the patient showed no slit lamp evidence of keratoconus, and visual acuity was 20/20 with spectacle correction. Nevertheless, the color-coded map reveals the presence of the cone, which is displaced inferiorly, as is the case in approximately 75 percent of keratoconus patients. The power at the apex of the cone is less than 48 diopters. **(B)** Three months later, the patient was still symptom free, but the cone had progressed. *(continues)*

trols.[45] Another topographic study examined the parents of 12 patients with clinical disease; seven of the patients had at least one parent with evidence of subclinical keratoconus.[46] If larger studies confirm that family members of patients with clinically obvious keratoconus have a higher incidence of topographic abnormalities and that these abnormalities are consistent with keratoconus,[14] assumptions about the sporadic incidence of the disorder will have to be revised.

Histopathology

The earliest morphologic changes in keratoconus occur in the anterior portion of the cornea. Early cones exhibit

FIGURE 22-10 *(continued)* **(C)** Six months later (9 months after diagnosis), the patient began to notice spectacle blur as the cone continued to progress. **(D)** Two months later, the cone had progressed to the point where evidence of keratoconus was visible at the slit lamp. (Adapted with permission from LJ Maguire, J Lowry: Identifying progression of subclinical keratoconus by serial topography analysis. Am J Ophthalmol 112:41, 1991. Copyright by The Ophthalmic Publishing Company.)

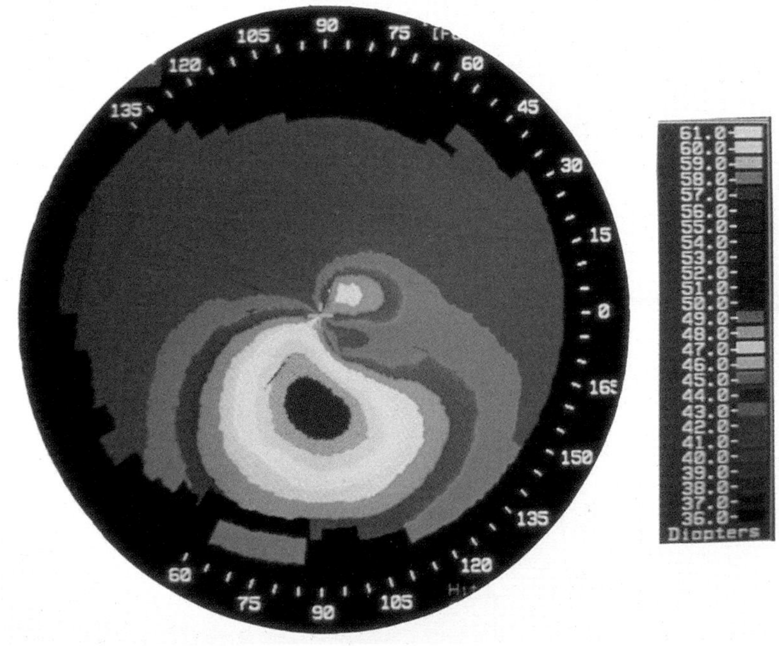

C

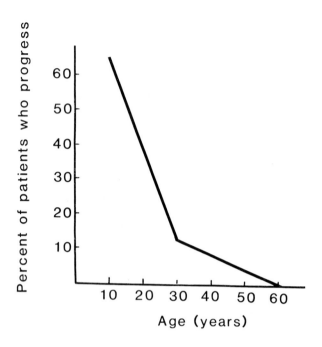

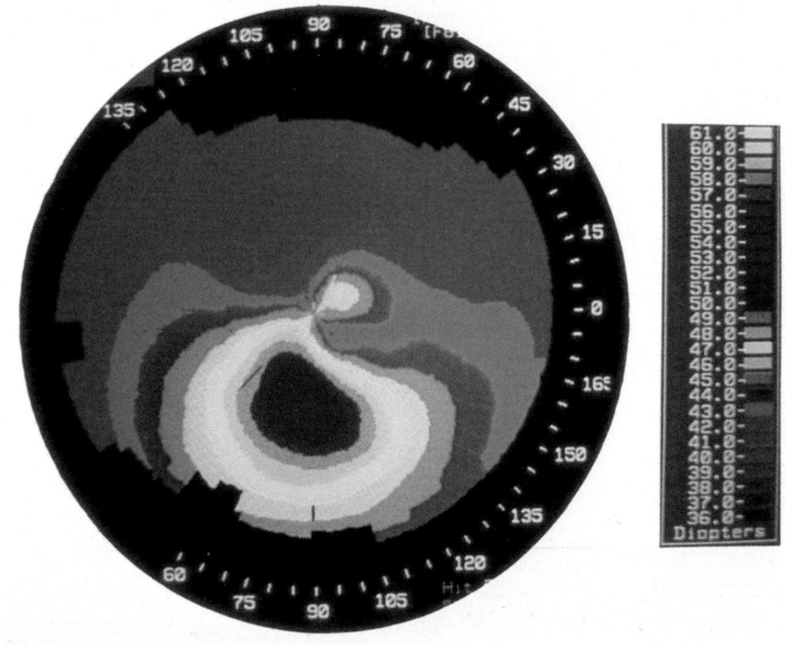

D

fibrillation and irregularity of Bowman's layer; interruptions of Bowman's layer are common[47–51] (Figure 22-12). The corneal scarring evident on slit lamp examination is caused by repair of these breaks with connective tissue formed by activated stromal keratocytes.[52] These keratocytes, as well as corneal epithelial cells, may project into the interruptions of Bowman's layer. The anterior stromal lamellae are thrown into characteristic Z-shaped folds in these areas.[53,54] These lamellae are surrounded by a periodic acid–Schiff positive granular substance[55] that appears to be produced by the keratocytes found in this area.[47,48,50,53,54,56–58] Stromal keratocytes in regions away from the cone are apparently normal.

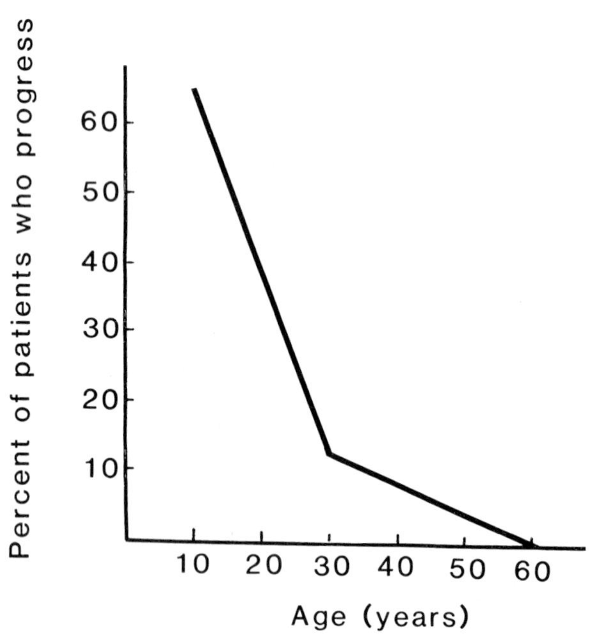

FIGURE 22-11 Chart from Amsler's long-term study of the relationship of age to the risk of keratoconus progression. (Adapted from M Amsler: Quelques donnees du probleme du keratocone. Bull Soc Belge Ophtalmol 129:331, 1961.)

The corneal epithelium tends to be thin and may exhibit loss of normal architecture in the area of the cone as the cone progresses. Specular microscopy may show enlarged, elongated, superficial epithelial cells.[59,60] Increased numbers of epithelial dark cells are seen with specular, light, and electron microscopy.[48,59,61] A Fleischer ring is produced by the collection of extracellular and intracellular ferritin in the epithelium at the periphery of the cone[51,59,62,63] (Figure 22-13).

The mechanism of stromal thinning is poorly understood. Contrary to previous beliefs,[50] the corneal lamellae are of normal thickness. Stromal thinning appears to be the result of a decrease in the number of lamellae in the area of the cone. Pouliquen et al[54] found an average of 140 lamellae within the central cone, 220 lamellae in the peripheral cone, and 340 lamellae in the unaffected stroma. No pathologic study has been able to demonstrate lysis of collagen fibrils. Based on work by Pataa et al[53] and Pouliquen et al,[54] Polack[64] suggested that alterations in stromal ground substance weaken interlamellar adhesions so that lamellae separate from one another, allowing focal stromal thinning without collagen lysis.

Descemet's membrane and the corneal endothelium are unaffected until the cone is well advanced. Endothelial cell density is usually normal, but a subpopulation of large, elongated cells, whose long axes are oriented toward the apex of the cone, may be seen.[65,66]

Histopathologic examination of acute corneal hydrops reveals severe stromal edema. Descemet's membrane separates from the posterior surface and retracts into scrolls, ledges, or ridges.[67] During the repair process, corneal endothelium extends over the anterior and posterior surfaces of the detached Descemet's membrane and denuded stroma; endothelial integrity is usually re-established 3 to 4 months after the acute event.[68] Rarely, hydrops may be followed by corneal perforation or pseudocyst formation.[69–72] Corneal perforation in keratoconus patients with no history of hydrops is rare.

Biochemical Studies

The literature on the biochemical basis of keratoconus is confusing and often contradictory.[73] Corneal stromal col-

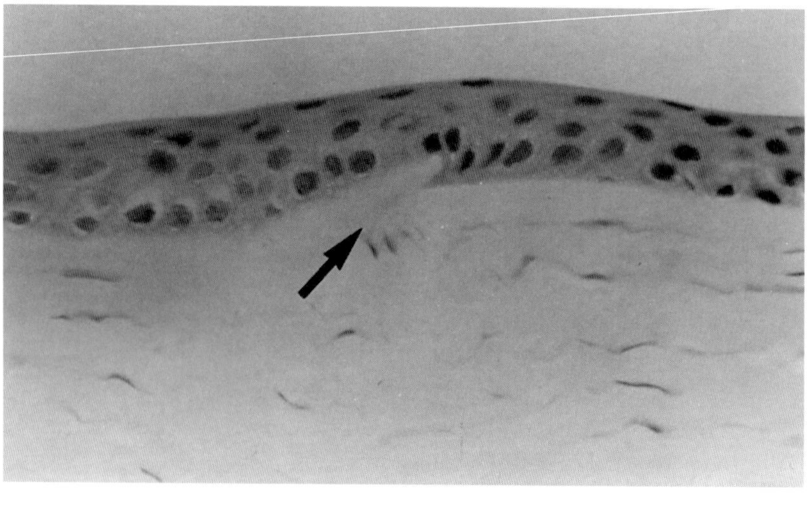

FIGURE 22-12 Corneal button from a patient with keratoconus demonstrating a break (arrow) in Bowman's layer (hematoxylin and eosin stain).

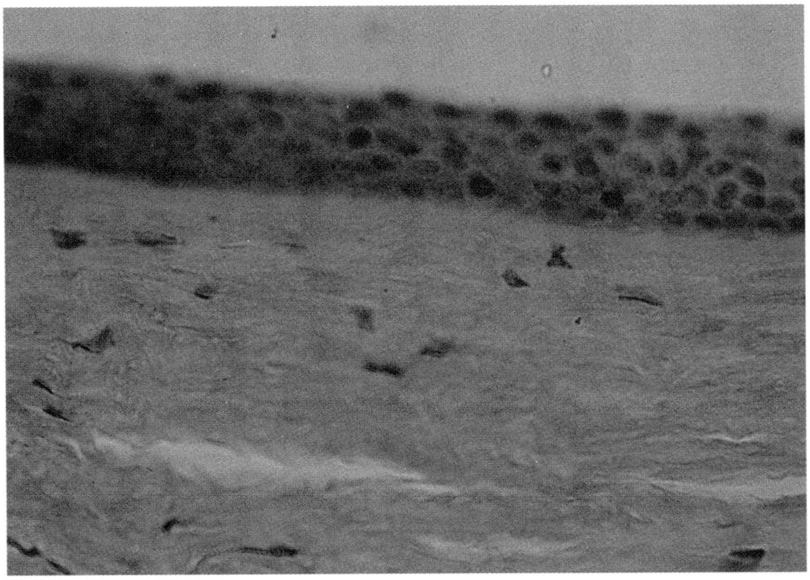

FIGURE 22-13 Light micrograph of a Fleischer ring demonstrating epithelial iron deposits with Prussian blue stain. (Courtesy of the Armed Forces Institute of Pathology Washington, DC, AFIP 10-79958.)

lagen cross-linking has been declared to be both normal[74–76] and reduced,[77] as have the rate and amount of collagen and glycosaminoglycan production.[55,78–85] Yue et al[86,87] presented evidence that earlier conflicting data on collagen synthesis may be the result of the heterogeneous nature of keratoconus. Tissue culture studies of corneal stromal keratocytes suggest that at least two biochemically distinct types of keratoconus exist. In one group, protein synthesis appears to be normal; in the second group, defects in RNA translation lead to reduced protein and collagen synthesis.[88] Abnormalities in corneal collagenase activity have also been suggested as a cause of corneal thinning.[74,89,90]

Degradation processes in keratoconus corneas may be abnormal. In one study, levels of α_1-proteinase inhibitors were 25 percent of normal in keratoconus epithelium and one-sixth of normal in stroma.[91] Lysosomal enzyme activity, important in tissue degradation processes, appears to be abnormal in keratoconus epithelium. Acid phosphatase, acid esterase, and acid lipase have been found in significantly higher amounts in the basal layer of keratoconus epithelium, compared with controls.[92]

Associated Conditions

Scleral Rigidity

Keratoconus may tend to develop in those patients who have low corneal tensile strength. Werb[93] observed the development of an intrascleral cyst caused by progressive dissection of the sclera in a patient with keratoconus and elevated intraocular pressure. Davies and Ruben[94] observed an anterior bowing of the lens-iris diaphragm in a number of keratoconus patients at the time of penetrating keratoplasty. Based on topographic studies, Edmund[95] concluded that tissue strength and ocular rigidity are significantly decreased in keratoconus patients. In one case, Hornblass and Sabates[96] questioned whether compression from an orbital and eyelid cavernous hemangioma contributed to the development of keratoconus. Several reports describing the development of keratoconus in hard contact lens wearers have questioned whether they had low scleral rigidity.[97–100]

Two in vivo studies of scleral rigidity that compared keratoconus patients with normal individuals found no statistically significant difference between the two groups.[101,102] However, two in vitro studies that compared axial tensile strength measurements of keratoconus corneas and normal corneas yielded contradictory results.[102,103] Poole[104] developed a mathematical model for evaluating the stress distribution within the cone. He found that as the apex of the cone is approached, corneal stress decreases significantly. This phenomenon explains the low incidence of corneal perforation in patients with keratoconus and no history of hydrops.

Corneal Warpage

Hard contact lens wear can lead to corneal warpage, that is, contact lens–induced distortions in corneal curvature, that can produce increased regular and irregular astigmatism and resultant spectacle blur[105–108] (see Ch. 27). Rowsey et al[109] proposed that warpage results from steepening of the inferior intermediate zone of the cornea caused by repeated trauma inflicted by the inferior edge of an improperly fitting contact lens. Topographic analysis in patients with warpage confirms this hypothesis and shows that the pattern of topographic abnormality in the area of trauma mimics that of keratoconus.[110] Unlike keratoconus, corneal warpage regresses over a period of months to a more normal topography once the patient discontinues contact lens wear. Furthermore, patients with corneal warpage do not develop corneal thinning or other biomicroscopic evidence of keratoconus.

However, some investigators believe that hard and even soft contact lens wear can cause keratoconus.[97–100,111–113] The most compelling evidence for this thesis was presented by Macsai and associates,[113] who compared 53 patients with a history of contact lens wear before the diagnosis of keratoconus with 146 keratoconus patients with no history of contact lens wear. They found that keratoconus associated with antecedent contact lens wear tended to be more central, have a later age of onset, and have lower keratometry readings than keratoconus in patients without a history of contact lens wear. Others suggest that these cases may represent patients who had subclinical central keratoconus at the time contact lens wear was begun and that diagnosis was delayed because central cones permit good spectacle-corrected vision longer than decentered cones.[14,45] Ironically, by the time keratoconus is diagnosed, contact lenses are usually necessary for good vision.

Atopy

Many investigators have studied the association of keratoconus with atopic disease,[24,40,114,115] and several studies that link keratoconus with atopic dermatitis, vernal conjunctivitis, asthma, and hay fever have been published.[26,116–129]

The incidence of keratoconus among patients with atopic dermatitis is relatively low. Brunsting et al[120] diagnosed keratoconus in only 6 of 1,158 patients with atopic dermatitis, and Roth and Kierland[121] reported 1 case in 492 patients. Spencer and Fisher[119] found only six patients with keratoconus and atopic dermatitis during a 3-year study. Copeman[26] found signs or past history of atopic eczema in 15 of 100 patients with keratoconus, and other forms of eczema in an additional 17 patients.

A number of scattered reports have described patients with vernal conjunctivitis and keratoconus[122,130]; Bietti and Ferraboschi[123] confirmed a statistically significant association between the two.

The incidence of asthma and hay fever in keratoconus patients is between 15 percent and 70 percent.[19,125–128] The incidence of atopy is higher in keratoconus patients than in normal controls.[114,129] In patients with keratoconus, particularly those with a history of atopy, IgE levels may be elevated.[131–133]

Down Syndrome

Down syndrome (trisomy 21) has been associated with a number of ocular abnormalities, including abnormal palpebral apertures, epicanthus, cataract, Brushfield spots, strabismus, nystagmus, and blepharoconjunctivitis. Although the incidence of keratoconus in patients with Down syndrome has been reported to be as low as zero,[134,135] most modern series report an incidence between 5 percent and 15 percent.[24,136–141] Studies comparing Down syndrome patients with other mentally retarded patients housed within the same institution reveal a marked difference in the incidence of keratoconus. Cullen and Butler[137] observed keratoconus in 8 of 43 Down syndrome patients, but in only 3 of 160 others; Walsh[140] found keratoconus in 7 of 91 Down syndrome patients, but in only 1 of 357 others. Patients with congenital rubella show a similar correlation between mental retardation and keratoconus, with a 4 percent incidence reported in one study.[142]

Corneal hydrops appears more commonly in Down syndrome patients with keratoconus than in the rest of the keratoconus population.[24,137,139,140] Walsh[140] examined seven patients and reported hydrops in at least one eye of four; in an examination of eight patients, Cullen[136] observed hydrops in at least one eye of five. Down syndrome patients have an increased risk of postoperative complications following penetrating keratoplasty because many rub their eyes excessively and cannot recognize and report early signs of rejection. These patients may have good results, however, if they can be induced to not rub their eyes and if their caregivers are observant.[143]

Retinal Disease

Keratoconus is associated with tapetoretinal degeneration,[144] especially Leber's congenital amaurosis, in which the incidence of keratoconus is between 30 percent and 50 percent in patients above the age of 15 years.[145–147] Keratoconus is less strongly associated with retinopathy of prematurity.[148,149]

Systemic Collagen Diseases

Given the natural history of keratoconus, it is possible that at least a subpopulation of keratoconus patients has systemic collagen disease. Studies differ on the association of keratoconus with mitral valve prolapse, with the largest studies finding no correlation.[114,150] False chordae tendineae of the left ventricle occur more frequently in patients with keratoconus than in controls.[151] Studies also differ on whether joint hypermobility is more common with keratoconus.[114,152] The possibility of an association between keratoconus and Marfan syndrome, osteogenesis imperfecta, and Ehlers-Danlos syndrome has been suggested. The association of keratoconus with Marfan syndrome is rare. Although scattered reports do exist,[153,154] two large series with a combined total of 302 patients with Marfan syndrome failed to identify one patient with keratoconus.[155,156] An association of Marfan syndrome with megalocornea was noted in both studies, however. The association of keratoconus with osteogenesis imperfecta appears even more tenuous, with only two cases reported in the modern literature.[157]

Ehlers-Danlos syndrome is a heterogeneous group of connective tissue diseases sharing the clinical features of tissue fragility, hyperextensible skin, hypermobility of joints, and a tendency to bleed easily. Seven clinical subtypes exist, differing mainly in the relative preponderance of the four clinical signs. Ehlers-Danlos syndrome type VI is characterized by ocular findings disproportionate to systemic findings. Spontaneous corneal and scleral perforations are common.[158,159] Some of these patients have a deficiency in lysyl hydroxylase, an enzyme important in the development of collagen cross-linkage.[160] Although none of the patients with known lysyl hydroxylase deficiency reported in the literature has developed keratoconus,[160,161] keratoconus, keratoglobus, microcornea, megalocornea, blue sclera, and retinal detachment have all been associated with the clinical syndrome.[157–159,162–169] Long-term administration of large doses of ascorbic acid may improve ocular and cutaneous integrity in this group.[170]

Management

Contact Lens Correction

When the keratoconus patient fails to obtain good visual acuity from spectacle correction, a contact lens is used to provide a regular refracting surface that masks the irregular astigmatism caused by the ectatic cornea. Contact lens fitting in keratoconus is, to a large extent, a matter of trial and error. The process can be frustrating and time consuming and requires patience and motivation on the part of both the patient and the ophthalmologist. The approach to contact lens fitting must be tailored to the individual patient, because fitting techniques vary, depending on the size, shape, location, and steepness of the cone. As a general rule, cones are increasingly difficult to fit as the ectasia increases. Round cones and cones located near the visual axis are less difficult to fit than oval cones and cones located closer to the limbus. General guidelines for fitting have been outlined by a number of authors.[171–176]

Belin's approach[176] is recommended for the practitioner with occasional experience with keratoconus. Four categories of lenses are used: (1) large-diameter rigid gas-permeable lenses, (2) aspheric lenses, (3) nipple cone lenses, and (4) Soper or McGuire lenses, which are designed specifically for keratoconus.

In the early to moderate stages of keratoconus, inferiorly displaced cones are associated with a much more uniform contour over the superior than the inferior corneal surface. Large-diameter rigid gas-permeable lenses can take advantage of this fact and provide a reasonable fit. A lens with a small optical zone and three peripheral posterior curves 0.50, 1.50, and 2.50 mm flatter than the central posterior curve can approximate a cone well, especially oval and globus cones. Belin recommends an initial trial fit with a lens with a central posterior curve equal to or 0.5 mm flatter than the flat keratometry reading. The ideal fluorescein pattern should show 2 to 5 mm of apical bearing and minimal inferior edge lift.

Posterior aspheric lenses allow a smooth transition in contour between the cornea and the central and peripheral portions of the lens. Such lenses are useful for moderate nipple cones and for inferiorly displaced cones when paracentral lens-corneal alignment with a spheric lens cannot be attained.

Spheric and aspheric lenses do not work well for nipple cones that have moderately severe to severe ectasia. Small- (8.0 to 8.5 mm) diameter nipple cone lenses with two peripheral curves are better suited for such cases. Keratometry readings underestimate the steepness of nipple cones. Topographic analysis can be used to help choose an initial base curve, or a base curve can be chosen that is 3 to 4 diopters steeper than keratometry readings. The fluorescein pattern can be evaluated to determine if a steeper or flatter lens is needed. Apical touch should be only 1 to 2 mm.

More ectatic cones require the bicurved Soper lens or the McGuire lens, with its steep central base curve and four graduated intermediate curves, to allow a better vault of the central ectasia.[176–178] Custom-fitted rigid gas-permeable scleral contact lenses may be another alternative for cases of severe ectasia.[179]

Surgical Treatment

Surgery for keratoconus is indicated when the patient is unable to obtain clear, comfortable vision without too much glare with contact lenses or if contact lenses cannot be comfortably worn most of the day.

Excision of Nebula As discussed previously, contact lenses may chronically rub the apex of a cone in highly ectatic cases and cause a subepithelial hyperplastic response called a *corneal nebula.* This tissue adheres loosely to the underlying stroma and can be removed surgically by scraping the surface with a #15 Bard-Parker blade, resulting in more comfortable lens wear and avoiding keratoplasty.[11] Although this procedure is worth considering, it is only occasionally successful.

Penetrating Keratoplasty Penetrating keratoplasty is the most commonly performed surgical procedure for the correction of keratoconus, and keratoconus continues to account for 8 to 34 percent of all penetrating keratoplasties performed throughout the world.[180-187] Over the past 30 years, most series with adequate postoperative follow-up report an incidence of graft clarity greater than 90 percent[34,181,188-205] (Table 22-1). Series with long-term follow-up suggest that graft survival remains above 90 percent even 4 to 5 years after surgery.[201,203] Postoperative best-corrected visual acuity is usually 20/40 or better in more than 80 percent of patients[181,189,192,193,195-198,202,203,206] (Table 22-2).

The incidence of graft rejection in keratoconus depends on the series and the criteria for rejection. Table 22-3 shows that graft reactions occur with considerable frequency (6 to 38 percent), but few grafts fail because of rejection (0 to 9.4 percent).[191-193,195-198,200-209]

The relationship between corneal graft rejection and the timing of penetrating keratoplasty in the second eye is unclear. Donshik et al[206] reported 27 percent graft rejection in 48 eyes undergoing bilateral penetrating keratoplasties performed 1 year apart, compared with 13 percent graft rejection in 76 patients undergoing unilateral keratoplasty. In nine of the bilateral cases, the second graft rejected first, and in four cases, the first graft rejected first. Three of the 13 patients ultimately had bilateral rejections. Ruedemann[34] reported rejection of the second graft in five of 15 patients who underwent bilateral penetrating keratoplasty. Other authors have noted no difference in the incidence of rejection between unilateral and bilateral grafts,[181,192,196,197,207,209-212] although most recommend separating bilateral surgeries by an interval of at least 1 year.

The assumption that keratoconus patients will have more postkeratoplasty astigmatism than other graft patients is not necessarily true[181,213,214]; however, astigmatism greater than 6.00 diopters occurs in 20 to 30 percent of patients.[192,196,197,200] Many theories have been proposed to explain this problem, including eccentric placement of the graft, failure to remove the peripheral portion of the cone during trephination, differences in graft/recipient bed diameters,[211] suturing techniques,[212] and distortion of the cornea by the central obturator of a corneal trephine.[215]

High myopia can be a problem after penetrating keratoplasty, and is caused in part by the tendency toward longer than normal axial lengths in keratoconus patients. Axial length measurements in these patients show a bimodal distribution, with a large peak with longer than normal lengths and a smaller peak with shorter than normal lengths.[216] This bimodal distribution may account for the wide variations in refractive error that occur after penetrating keratoplasty.[217] Theoretically, the incidence of postoperative myopia could be lowered by changing the relative diameters of the graft and recipient bed. Although some recommend a graft the same size or even 0.25 mm smaller than the recipient trephine cut,[216,218,219] such grafts can result postoperatively in a cornea with a bizarre tabletop shape that can be impossible to fit with a contact lens, if necessary. A better alternative is to thermally shrink the cone with cautery to create a cornea with a more normal shape before trephination. The techniques for penetrating keratoplasty for keratoconus are discussed in Chapter 34.

Urrets-Zavalia[220] described a curious complication of penetrating keratoplasty for keratoconus characterized by permanent mydriasis associated with iris atrophy and glaucoma. The finding has been confirmed by several reports,[94,200,221-224] with an incidence of zero[173,225,226] to 18 percent.[221] Mydriasis is usually noted within the first 48 hours after surgery. The pupil may be fixed and dilated, or sluggish and partially dilated. Paresis may be transient, but is usually permanent. Iris atrophy may be either focal or sectorial. Sectorial atrophy is common in permanently dilated pupils.[94] This complication has been attributed to the postoperative use of strong mydriatics and to ischemia of the iris sphincter muscle caused by pressure of the edge of the corneal wound on the iris as the lens-iris diaphragm bows anteriorly after the recipient cornea has been removed.[94] Shands and Lass[227] reported severe anterior segment inflammation lasting for up to a month in 2 of 80 grafts for keratoconus. These patients also had fixed pupils and iris atrophy. Patients were premedicated with indomethacin 50 mg twice a day before surgery in the second eye and had no complications.

Keratoconus can recur in grafts.[228-233] Most recurrent keratoconus is probably caused by incomplete excision of abnormal cornea, but in at least two cases,[228,229] keratoconus recurred in the graft many years after keratoplasty. Keratoconus in the donor corneal button and invasion of the graft by host keratocytes or epithelial cells have been suggested as possible explanations for this phenomenon.

Epikeratophakia (Onlay Lamellar Keratoplasty) In this technique, a plano lamellar graft lathed on a modified Barraquer cryolathe is sutured into a circular superficial keratectomy to flatten and reinforce thin corneal tissue in the area of the cone. Epikeratophakia is appropriate for those patients whose corneal scarring is sufficiently minimal to allow a preoperative visual acuity of 20/40 or better when a contact lens is worn for diagnostic purposes. Any scarring must be located far enough in the periphery so that it will not be displaced into the line of sight when the cone is compressed by the graft.

TABLE 22-1
Graft Clarity After Penetrating Keratoplasty for Keratoconus

Study	*No. of Eyes*	*Clear Grafts (%)*	*Follow-Up*
Robert, 1950[188]	20	85	>4 mo
Paton, 1954[189]	84	89	>2 mo
Hughes, 1960[190]	43	81	Average 21 mo
Anseth, 1967[192]	50	100	9 mo–8 yr
Buxton et al, 1969[191]	36	93	3–48 mo
Ruedemann, 1970[34]	48	81	NR
Keates and Falkenstein, 1972[193]	27	100	1–6 yr
Boruchoff et al, 1975[194]	48	93	7–42 mo
Moore and Aronson, 1978[195]	64	88	>1 yr
Richard et al, 1978[196]	50	98	>1 yr
Troutman and Gaster, 1980[197]	82	98	>6 mo
Paglen et al, 1982[198]	326	90	5–34 yr
Payne, 1982[181]	322	93	>6 mo
Bishop et al, 1986[199]	83	97	2 yr
Troutman and Lawless, 1987[200]	111	100	7 mo–3 yr
Epstein et al, 1987[201]	228	96	2 yr
	94	91	4 yr
Sharif and Casey, 1991[203]	100	93	4–16 yr (mean 6.1 yr)
Price et al, 1991[204]	124	100	1–84 mo (mean 22 mo)

Abbreviation: NR, not reported.

There are a number of advantages of epikeratophakia for the treatment of keratoconus[234–245] (see Ch. 32). The procedure is extraocular and there is no risk of endothelial graft rejection. Unlike inlay lamellar keratoplasty, epikeratophakia does not require extensive dissection of the host stroma, thereby minimizing the risk of inadvertent entry into the anterior chamber, as well as the potential for graft-host interface opacity. When the cone is close to the limbus, epikeratophakia may be used as a definitive surgical treatment or as a tectonic graft, followed by central penetrating keratoplasty as a secondary procedure.

Inlay Lamellar Keratoplasty Because inlay lamellar keratoplasty is technically difficult and offers less satisfactory visual results than penetrating keratoplasty, it is not often used to treat keratoconus[246–248] (see Ch. 31). Nevertheless, inlay lamellar keratoplasty is of value in some keratoconus patients, particularly those who are not candidates for penetrating keratoplasty because of anticipated postoperative self-inflicted trauma or poor compliance and who have too much central scarring for epikeratophakia.

Thermokeratoplasty In thermokeratoplasty, the cone is flattened by thermally shrinking the stromal collagen.[249–251] In an early study of 59 cases with postoperative follow-up of 2 to 24 months, most patients achieved visual acuities better than 20/30.[249] However, later studies reported inadequate visual improvement in the majority of cases and complications that included instability of the corneal curvature, persistent epithelial defects, corneal edema, and aseptic stromal necrosis.[252–255]

TABLE 22-2
Visual Acuity After Penetrating Keratoplasty for Keratoconus

Study	*No. of Eyes*	*Visual Acuity of 20/40 or Better (%)*
Paton, 1954[189]	84	41
Anseth, 1967[192]	50	100
Keates and Falkenstein, 1972[193]	27	84
Moore and Aronson, 1978[195]	62	88
Richard et al, 1978[196]	50	90
Donshik et al, 1979[206]	124	86
Troutman and Gaster, 1980[197]	82	92
Payne, 1982[181]	308	79
Paglen et al, 1982[198]	326	90
Kirkness et al, 1990[202]	198	91
Sharif and Casey, 1991[203]	100	81

Limited data exist on the results of penetrating keratoplasty following thermokeratoplasty, but Mandelberg et al[256] noted no statistical difference in the incidence of graft rejection between 17 keratoconus patients treated with thermokeratoplasty followed by penetrating keratoplasty and 44 controls treated with penetrating keratoplasty alone. Thermokeratoplasty is rarely used in the United States because the results are too variable.

TABLE 22-3
Graft Rejection After Penetrating Keratoplasty for Keratoconus

Study	No. of Eyes	Graft Reaction (%)	Graft Failure Secondary to Graft Rejection (%)
Anseth, 1967[192]	50	6	0
Buxton et al, 1969[191]	36	8.3	0
Keates and Falkenstein, 1972[193]	27	7.4	0
Chandler and Kaufman, 1974[207]	53	37.7	9.4
Moore and Aronson, 1978[195]	62	6.4	1.5
Richard et al, 1978[196]	50	10.0	0
Donshik et al, 1979[206]	124	18.5	3.2
Troutman and Gaster, 1980[197]	82	7.3	2.4
Alldredge and Krachmer, 1981[208]	29	18.0	NR
Paglen et al, 1982[198]	326	9.2	2.4
Malbran and Fernandez-Meijide, 1982[209]	105	15	0
Troutman and Lawless, 1987[200]	111	11.6	0
Epstein et al, 1987[201]	325	18.5	2.7
Sharif and Casey, 1991[203]	100	21	3
Price et al, 1991[204]	124	NR	0
Musch et al, 1991[205]	174	33	NR

Abbreviation: NR, not reported.

PELLUCID MARGINAL DEGENERATION

Pellucid marginal degeneration, a variant of keratoconus,[257-260] is an uncommon, but not rare, cause of corneal ectasia. It differs from keratoconus in that the corneal protrusion occurs inferiorly, above a narrow band of clear, nonvascularized, thinned corneal stroma that is concentric to the limbus. The band of thinning most commonly extends from the 4 o'clock to 8 o'clock positions, varies from 1 to 2 mm in width, and occurs 1 to 2 mm from the limbus. The corneal protrusion is steepest directly above the thinned area, giving a "beer belly" appearance when viewed in cross section (Figure 22-14) or seen in topographic studies[261] (Figure 22-15). The central cornea is of normal thickness. Vertical stress lines and hydrops may occur.[129] Rarely, the ectasia and thinning occur superiorly.[261] The area of stromal thinning is always epithelialized, clear, avascular, and without lipid deposition, thereby differentiating this condition from Mooren's ulcer and Terrien's marginal degeneration. Vascularization and scarring may occur in the thinned area after hydrops.[262] In patients in the western hemisphere, pellucid marginal degeneration has generally been reported to be an isolated clinical entity,[263] but 17 of 20 cases described in Japan occurred in conjunction with keratoconus in the same eye.[264]

Pellucid marginal degeneration most commonly presents between the ages of 20 and 40 years, and may progress slowly over a period of years. It occurs with equal frequencies in men and women. The disorder does not appear to be hereditary, although moderate to high astigmatism in family members of affected patients has been noted.[265,266]

The approach to therapy depends on the degree of corneal protrusion. Spectacle correction is almost always unsatisfactory because of large amounts of irregular corneal astigmatism. Contact lens correction may be attempted when corneal ectasia is mild. Barraquer[267] and Krachmer[262] recommend large, inferiorly decentered penetrating keratoplasty grafts for highly ectatic cases. However, penetrating keratoplasty for pellucid marginal degeneration is technically more difficult than penetrating keratoplasty for keratoconus, and has an increased risk of vascularization and corneal graft rejection because of the large size of the graft and its location near the limbus.[268]

Other surgical procedures have been advocated as alternatives to penetrating keratoplasty for cases of pellucid marginal degeneration with moderate degrees of corneal ectasia. Zucchini[257] reported improved vision in one eye with the use of diathermy. Hallermann[269] obtained good results with lamellar keratoplasty in five patients. Barraquer[267] obtained corneal flattening and slight astigmatic correction in six eyes by lamellar crescentic resection of the affected area and reapposition of normal-thickness cornea from each side of the resected area; Cameron[270] reported good results with this procedure in four of five eyes. Full-thickness crescentic resection was less effective.[267] Schanzlin et al[271] reported one case in which a lamellar crescentic resection of the involved thinned cornea was replaced by a freehand corneoscleral graft, resulting in a

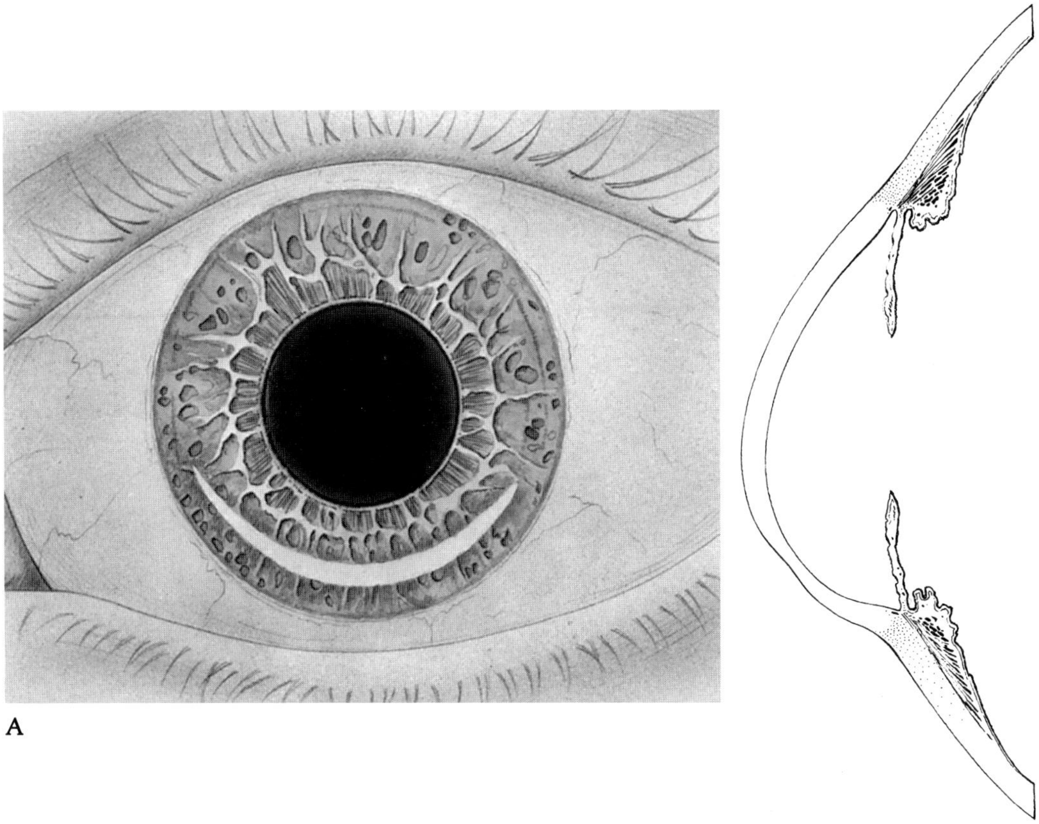

A

FIGURE 22-14 **(A)** In pellucid marginal degeneration, corneal ectasia occurs above a narrow band of clear, thin, nonvascularized cornea that parallels the inferior limbus. Corneal thickness is normal central and peripheral to the band of thinning. The cornea is steepest just above the area of thinning. **(B)** Pellucid marginal degeneration—slit lamp view. Note the area of corneal thinning (arrow).

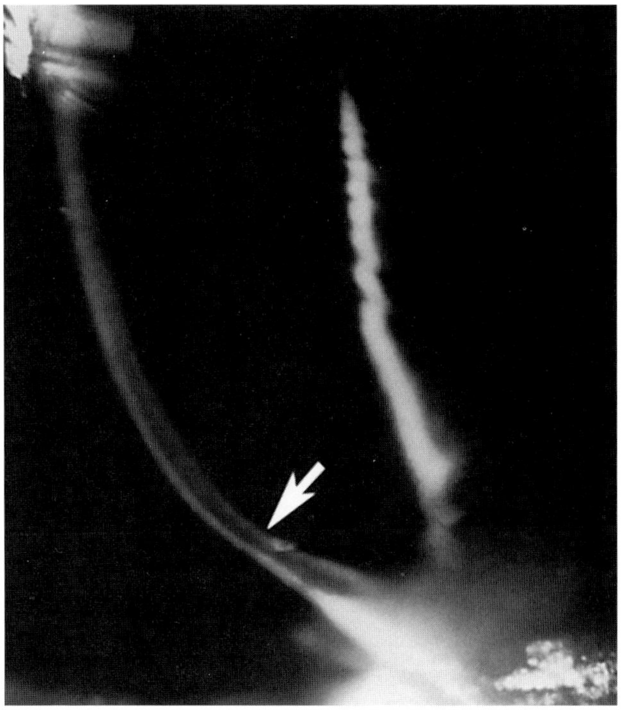

B

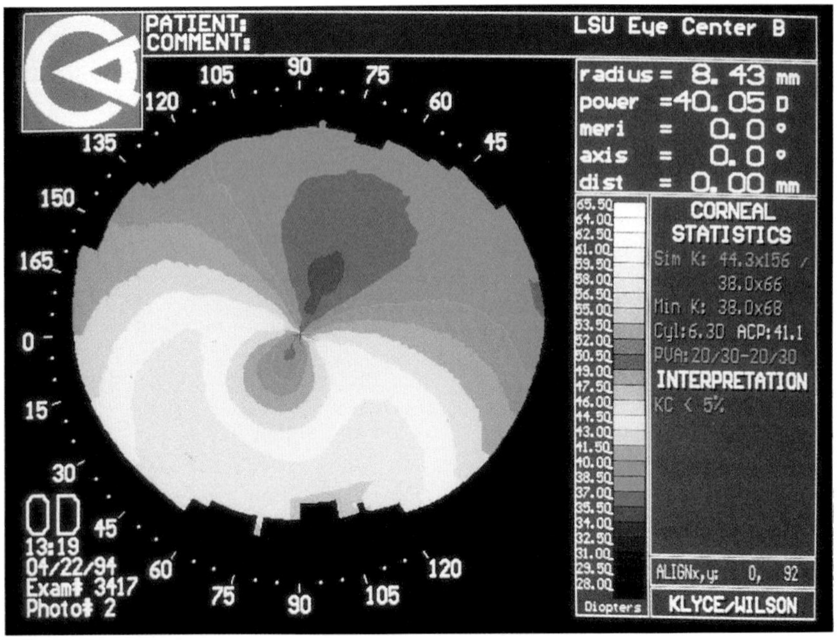

FIGURE 22-15 Videokeratograph of pellucid marginal degeneration, showing marked flattening of the central cornea along the 65-degree axis and marked steepening of the inferior cornea peripherally. Each color represents 1.5 diopters of power. (Courtesy of Stephen D. Klyce, Ph.D., and Naoyuki Maeda, M.D., New Orleans, LA.)

spectacle-corrected visual acuity of 20/25. A large epikeratophakia graft, extending to the limbus if necessary, has also been used for the surgical treatment of pellucid marginal degeneration.[272]

KERATOGLOBUS

Keratoglobus is an extremely rare, bilateral, corneal ectatic disorder characterized by a globoid protrusion of a clear, diffusely thin cornea of normal to moderately increased diameter. The corneal stroma is one-third to one-fifth normal thickness, and is most attenuated near the limbus (Figure 22-16). Although acquired keratoglobus has been described in a patient with Graves' ophthalmopathy,[273] the condition is almost always present at birth and tends to be nonprogressive. Acute hydrops may occur, and corneal perforation is frequent. Perforation occurred before the age of 20 years in seven eyes of five patients in one series[145] and eight eyes of five patients in two other reports.[274,275] Despite the frequent finding of high myopia, high astigmatism, and nystagmus, visual acuity may be as good as 20/60. The entity may appear as an isolated finding or may be associated with Leber's congenital amaurosis[145,274,276] or a syndrome of blue sclera, moderately extensible joints, and hearing and dental abnormalities clinically similar to Ehlers-Danlos syndrome type VI. Keratoglobus has no association with congenital glaucoma or megalocornea, two entities with which it may be confused.

Few pathologic studies of keratoglobus exist. Biglan and coworkers[163] examined two eyes with keratoglobus and blue sclera following corneal perforation. The first case demonstrated absence of Bowman's layer, stromal thinning to one-fifth normal thickness, normal-appearing stromal lamellae, and a thickened Descemet's membrane. The second case was similar to the first except for slight thickening of the corneal epithelium and generalized stromal fibrosis. Pathologic examination of the one reported case of acquired keratoglobus revealed corneal epithelium of variable thickness, with central thinning to a monolayer, a few focal breaks in Bowman's layer without the fibrillar changes associated with keratoconus, normal-appearing lamellae in a stroma one-third normal thickness, a few small breaks in Descemet's membrane, and normal endothelium.[273] The trabecular meshwork, optic nerve, and nerve fiber layer were normal in all three cases.

Keratoglobus and keratoconus may be genetically linked in some cases. Cavara[277] reported a father with keratoglobus and a son with keratoconus, and Greenfield et al[168] described a brother with keratoglobus and a sister with keratoconus. Both keratoglobus and keratoconus may be associated with Leber's congenital amaurosis or with the blue sclera syndrome, reviewed by Biglan et al.[163] Although some authors believe keratoglobus and keratoconus are variants of the same process, differences in age of onset, progression, slit lamp appearance, and risk of perforation warrant separate clinical classification.

Treatment of keratoglobus is difficult. Contact lenses are contraindicated because of the high risk of perfora-

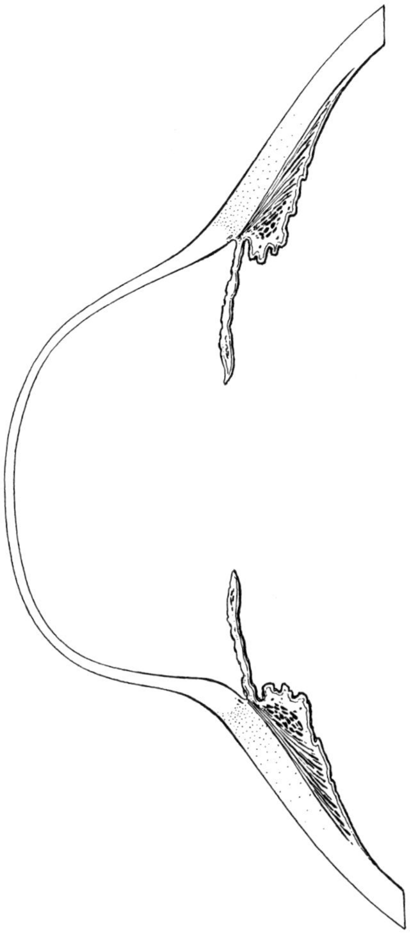

A

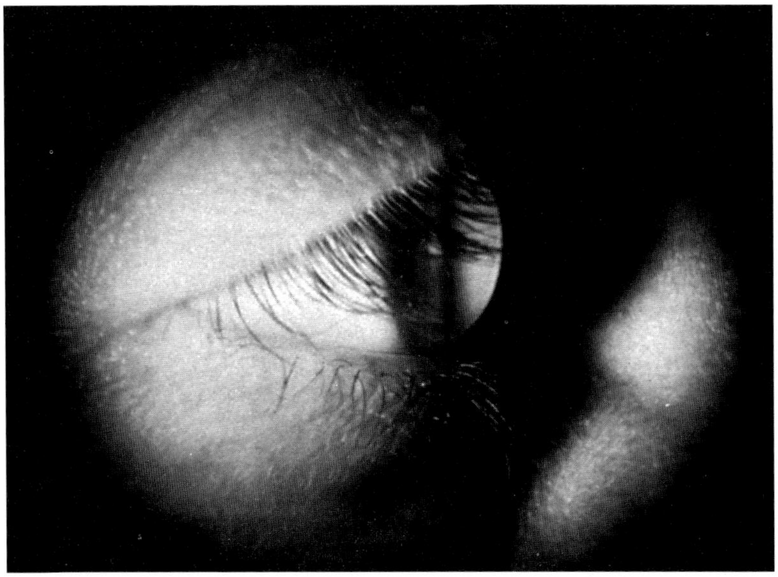

B

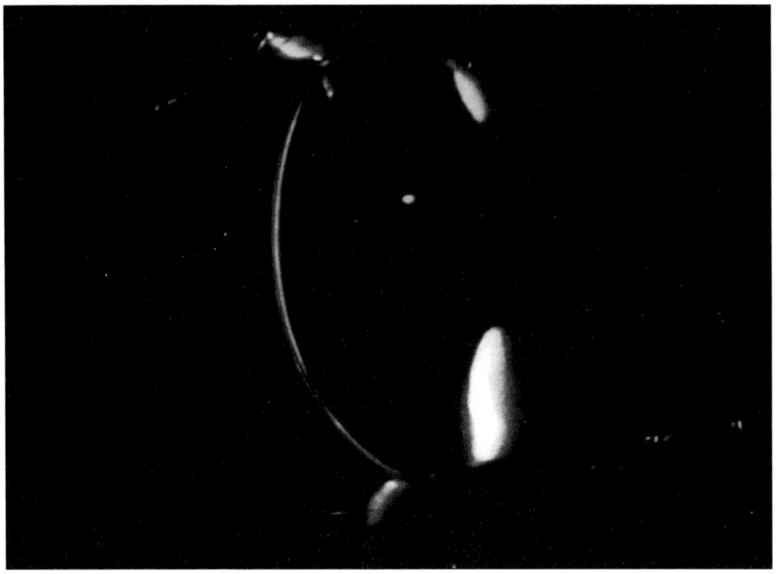

C

FIGURE 22-16 **(A)** Keratoglobus is characterized by the globoid protrusion of a clear, diffusely thin cornea. Corneal thickness is one-fifth to one-third normal. Corneal perforation is common after even minor trauma. **(B)** Keratoglobus—side view. **(C)** Keratoglobus—slit lamp view. Note the diffusely thin corneal stroma.

tion with even mild trauma. Penetrating keratoplasty is technically challenging and dangerous, given the diffuse thinness of the patient's cornea and sclera. Epikeratophakia with a graft that extends onto the sclera is probably the treatment of choice for these patients, either as a solitary procedure or in preparation for penetrating keratoplasty[278] (see Ch. 32).

POSTERIOR KERATOCONUS

Posterior keratoconus is a rare corneal abnormality characterized by a steep concavity of the posterior corneal surface in association with a normal anterior corneal curvature[279] (Figure 22-17). The posterior conical surface may be focal (keratoconus posticus circumscriptus)[275] or

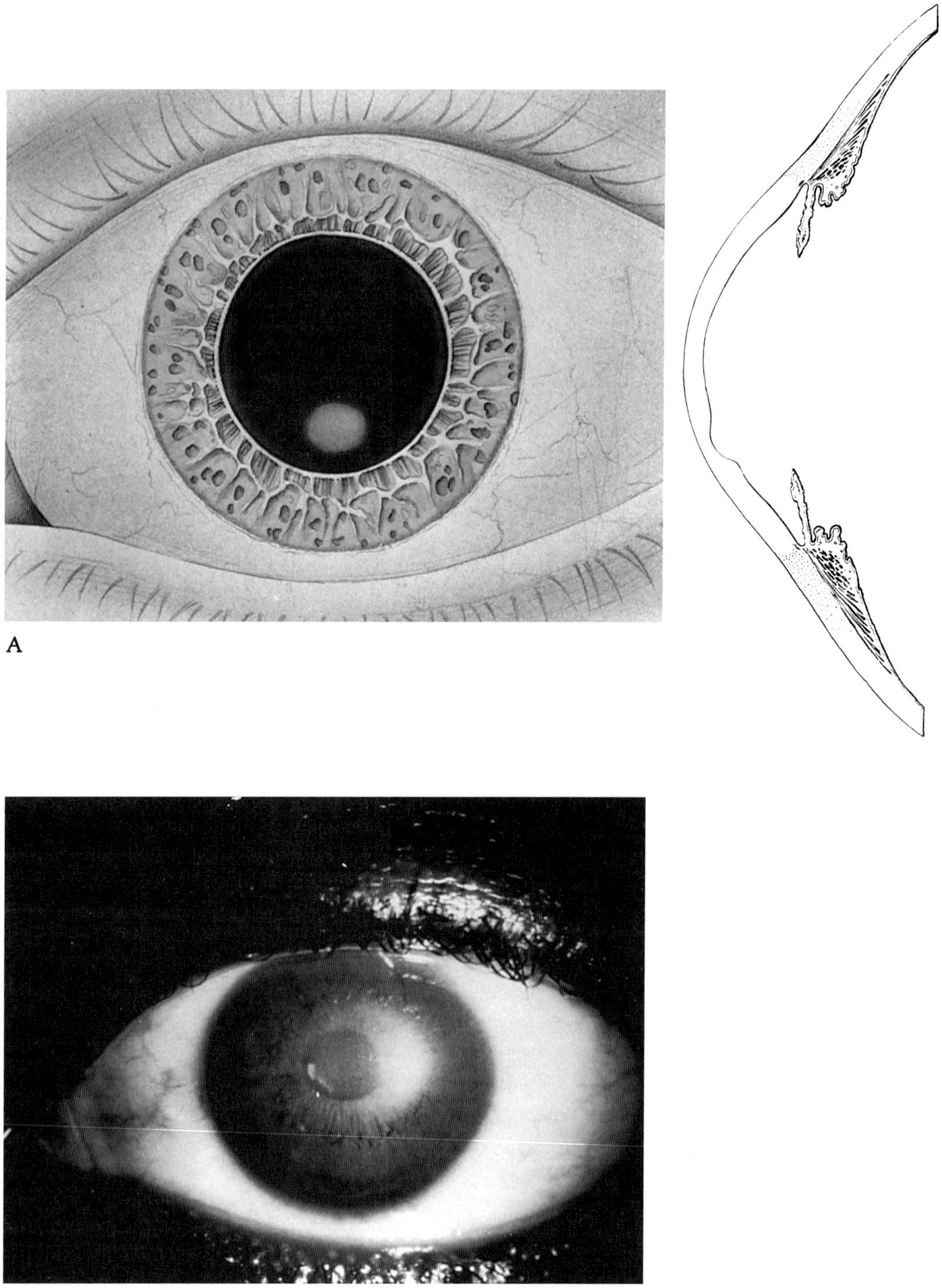

FIGURE 22-17 **(A)** Posterior keratoconus. The anterior corneal curvature is normal. The posterior corneal surface demonstrates a focal indentation. **(B)** Clinical photograph of posterior keratoconus. Mild stromal haze is visible in the affected area.

diffuse.[280,281] Unilateral cases are more common than bilateral cases.[282] Scarring is noted in the corneal stroma anterior to the area of posterior concavity. Bowman's layer is absent centrally. Descemet's membrane and corneal endothelium are always present, but are abnormal in the area of posterior concavity. Corneal guttae and larger Descemet's excrescences may be present within and just outside the perimeter of the affected area.[280,281–285] A thickened ring of Descemet's membrane occasionally surrounds the area.[282] Synechiae may occur between the iris and the affected area.[286] A number of patients observed soon after birth have demonstrated extremely close approximation of the lens to the affected posterior corneal surface, with spontaneous deepening of the anterior chamber within the first months of life.[287,288]

Ocular abnormalities most frequently associated with posterior keratoconus include choroidal and/or retinal sclerosis[281,283,289] and lens abnormalities.[283,287–290] Less frequently noted abnormalities are posterior polymorphous dystrophy,[286] retinal coloboma,[291] optic nerve hypoplasia,[284] ptosis,[291] and corneal epithelial iron rings surrounding the affected area.[284] Although posterior keratoconus is usually congenital, it has been reported following trauma.[292] The majority of cases are nonfamilial.[282,289,293,294] Posterior keratoconus associated with systemic abnormalities has been reported.[282,291,294] Systemic findings may include mental retardation, webbed neck, hypertelorism, superiorly displaced lateral canthi, short stature, and genitourinary abnormalities. There is little doubt that posterior keratoconus results from an abnormal development of the anterior chamber, and therefore, should be classified as a disorder of mesenchymal dysgenesis[295] (see Ch. 16).

REFERENCES

1. Perry HD, Buxton JN, Fine BS: Round and oval cones in keratoconus. Ophthalmology 87:905, 1980
2. Wilson SE, Lin DT, Klyce SD: Corneal topography of keratoconus. Cornea 10:2, 1991
3. Gass JD: The iron lines of the superficial cornea: Hudson-Stähle line, Stocker's line, and Fleischer's ring. Arch Ophthalmol 71:348, 1964
4. Vogt A: Reflexlinien durch Faltung spiegeln der Grenzflachen im Bereiche von Corneo, Linsenkapsel und Netzhaut. Albrecht von Graefes Arch Ophthalmol 99:296, 1919
5. Vogt A: Die Keratokonuslinien der Kegelspitze und ihre anatomische Grundlage. Klin Monatsbl Augenheilkd 98:577, 1937
6. Schmidt M: Die Natur und Entstehungsweise der Keratokonuslinien. Klin Monatsbl Augenheilkd 101:36, 1938
7. Kinoshita S, Tanaka F, Ohashi Y, et al: Incidence of prominent corneal nerves in multiple endocrine neoplasia. Am J Ophthalmol 111:307, 1991
8. Shapiro MB, Rodrigues MM, Mandel MR, Krachmer JH: Anterior clear spaces in keratoconus. Ophthalmology 93:1316, 1986
9. Bron AJ, Lobascher DJ, Dixon WS, et al: Fibrillary lines of the cornea. A clinical sign in keratoconus. Br J Ophthalmol 59:136, 1975
10. Moodaley L, Buckley RJ, Woodward EG: Surgery to improve contact lens wear in keratoconus. CLAO J 17:129, 1991
11. Terrien F: Ectasie transitoire au cours du keratocone. Arch Ophtalmol (Paris) 26:9, 1906
12. Rizzuti AB: Diagnostic illumination test for keratoconus. Am J Ophthalmol 70:141, 1970
13. Maguire LJ, Bourne WM: Corneal topography of early keratoconus. Am J Ophthalmol 108:107, 1989
14. Maguire LJ, Lowry J: Identifying progression of subclinical keratoconus by serial topography analysis. Am J Ophthalmol 112:41, 1991
15. Amsler M: Keratocone classique et keratocone fruste: arguments unitaires. Ophthalmologica 111:96, 1946
16. Amsler M: Quelques donnees du probleme du keratocone. Bull Soc Belge Ophtalmol 129:331, 1961
17. Mamalis N, Montgomery S, Anderson C, Miller C: Radial keratotomy in a patient with keratoconus. Refract Corneal Surg 7:374, 1991
18. Maguire LJ, Bourne WM: A multifocal lens effect as a complication of radial keratotomy. Refract Corneal Surg 5:394, 1989
19. Karseras AG, Ruben M: Aetiology of keratoconus. Br J Ophthalmol 60:522, 1976
20. Gritz DC, McDonnell PJ: Keratoconus and ocular massage. Am J Ophthalmol 106:757, 1988
21. Kennedy RH, Bourne WM, Dyer DA: A 48-year clinical and epidemiologic study of keratoconus. Am J Ophthalmol 101:267, 1986
22. Smiddy WE, Hamburg TR, Kracher GP, Stark WJ: Keratoconus. Contact lens or keratoplasty? Ophthalmology 95:487, 1988
23. Belin MW, Fowler WC, Chambers WA: Keratoconus. Evaluation of recent trends in the surgical and nonsurgical correction of keratoconus. Ophthalmology 95:335, 1988
24. Ihalainen A: Clinical and epidemiological features of keratoconus. Genetic and external factors in the pathogenesis of the disease. Acta Ophthalmol (Copenh) 178(suppl):1, 1986
25. Applebaum A: Keratoconus. Arch Ophthalmol 15:900, 1936
26. Copeman PW: Eczema and keratoconus. Br Med J 2:977, 1965
27. Duke-Elder S, Leigh AG: System of Ophthalmology. Diseases of the Outer Eye. Vol. 8, Part 2. Henry Kimpton, London, 1965
28. Franceschetti A: Keratoconus. In King JH, McTigue JW (eds): World Congress on the Cornea, 1st. Washington, DC. Butterworths, Washington, 1965

29. Hofstetter H: A keratoscopic survey of 13,395 eyes. Am J Optom Arch Am Acad Optom 36:3, 1959
30. Laqua H: Heriditare Erkrankungen beim Keratokonus. Klin Monatsbl Augenheilkd 159:609, 1971
31. Thomas CI: The Cornea. Charles C. Thomas, Springfield, IL, 1955
32. Palimeris G, Droutsas D, Chimonidou E, Moschos M: Some observations on the pathogenesis and management of keratoconus. p. 927. In Trevor-Roper P (ed): Sixth Congress of the European Society of Ophthalmology. Vol. 40. The Royal Society of Medicine and Academic Press, London, 1981
33. Falls HF, Allen AW: Dominantly inherited keratoconus. Report of a family. J Genet Hum 17:317, 1969
34. Ruedemann AD Jr: Clinical course of keratoconus. Trans Am Acad Ophthalmol Otolaryngol 74:384, 1970
35. Hammerstein W: Zur Genetik des Keratoconus. Albrecht von Graefes Arch Klin Exp Ophthalmol 190:293, 1974
36. Hallermann W, Wilson EJ: Genetische Betrachtungen uber den Keratokonus. Klin Monatsbl Augenheilkd 170:906, 1977
37. Redmond KB: The role of heredity in keratoconus. Trans Ophthalmol Soc NZ 27:52, 1968
38. Forstot SL, Goldstein JH, Damiano RE, Dukes DK: Familial keratoconus. Am J Ophthalmol 105:92, 1988
39. Etzine S: Conical cornea in identical twins. S Afr Med J 28:154, 1958
40. Franceschetti A, Lisch K, Klein D: Zwei eineiige Zwillingspaare mit konkordantem Keratokonus. Klin Monatsbl Augenheilkd 133:15, 1958
41. Woillez M, Razemon PH, Constantinides G: A propos d'un nouveau cas de keratocone ches des juneaux univitellins. Bull Soc Ophtalmol Fr 76:279, 1976
42. Hammerstein W: Konkordanter Keratoconus bei eineiigen Zwillingen. Ophthalmologica 165:449, 1972
43. Bourne WM, Michels VV: Keratoconus in one identical twin. Cornea 1:35, 1982
44. Harrison RJ, Klouda PT, Easty DL, et al: Association of keratoconus and atopy. Br J Ophthalmol 73:816, 1989
45. Rabinowitz YS, Garbus J, McDonnell PJ: Computer assisted corneal topography in family members of patients with keratoconus. Arch Ophthalmol 108:365, 1990
46. Gonzales V, McDonnell PJ: Computer-assisted topography in parents of patients with keratoconus. Arch Ophthalmol 110:1412, 1992
47. McTigue J: The human cornea. A light and electron microscopic study of the normal cornea and its alterations in various dystrophies. Trans Am Ophthalmol Soc 65:591, 1967
48. Teng C: Electron microscopic study of the pathology of keratoconus. Am J Ophthalmol 55:18, 1963
49. Caffi M: Histopathology of keratoconus. Ann Ottalmol Clin Ocul 92:429, 1966
50. Jakus M: Further observations on the fine structure of the cornea. Invest Ophthalmol 1:202, 1962
51. McPherson SD, Kiffney GT: Some histologic findings in keratoconus. Arch Ophthalmol 79:669, 1968
52. Pouliquen Y, Graf B, Hamada R, et al: Fibrocytes in keratoconus. Morphological appearance and change in the extracellular spaces. Optical and electron microscopic study. Arch Ophtalmol (Paris) 32:571, 1972
53. Pataa C, Joyon L, Roucher F: Ultra-structure du keratoconus. Arch Ophtalmol (Paris) 30:403, 1970
54. Pouliquen Y, Graf B, de Kozak Y, et al: Ètude morphologique et biochemique du keratocone. I. Ètude morphologique. Arch Ophtalmol (Paris) 30:498, 1970
55. Robert L, Schillinger G, Moczar M, et al: Ètude morphologique et biochimique du keratocone. II. Ètude biochimique. Arch Ophtalmol (Paris) 30:590, 1970
56. Pouliquen Y, Graf B, Frouin M, et al: Histological and ultrastructural interpretation of corneal lesions in keratoconus. Ber Zusammenkunft Dtsch Ophthalmol Ges 71:52, 1972
57. Gottinger W, Aubock L: Elektronenmikroskopische Befunde bei Keratokonus. Klin Monatsbl Augenheilkd 157:762, 1970
58. Pouliquen Y, Fauve J, Limon S, Bisson J: Les depots extracellulaires du stroma cornéen dans le keratocone. Ètude au microscope electronique. Arch Ophtalmol (Paris) 28:283, 1968
59. Lohman LE, Rao GN, Aquavella JV: In vivo microscopic observations of human corneal epithelial abnormalities. Am J Ophthalmol 93:210, 1982
60. Wong S, Rodrigues MM, Blackman HJ, et al: Color specular microscopy of disorders involving the corneal epithelium. Ophthalmology 91:1176, 1984
61. Pfister RR, Burstein NC: The normal and abnormal human corneal epithelial surface. A scanning microscopic study. Invest Ophthalmol Vis Sci 16:614, 1977
62. Iwamoto T, DeVoe AG: Electron microscopic study of the Fleischer ring. Arch Ophthalmol 94:1579, 1976
63. Barraquer-Somers E, Chan CC, Green WR: Corneal epithelial iron deposition. Ophthalmology 90:729, 1983
64. Polack FM: Contributions of electron microscopy to the study of corneal pathology. Surv Ophthalmol 20:375, 1976
65. Laing RA, Sandstrom MM, Berrospi AR, Leibowitz HM: The human corneal endothelium in keratoconus. A specular microscopic study. Arch Ophthalmol 97:1867, 1979
66. Matsuda M, Suda T, Manabe R: Quantitative analysis of endothelial mosaic patterns in anterior keratoconus. Am J Ophthalmol 98:43, 1984
67. Waring G, Laibson P, Rodrigues M: Clinical and pathologic alterations of Descemet's membrane with emphasis on endothelial metaplasia. Surv Ophthalmol 18:325, 1974
68. Stone DL, Kenyon KR, Stark WJ: Ultrastructure of keratoconus with healed hydrops. Am J Ophthalmol 82:450, 1976
69. Rubsamen PE, McLeish WM: Keratoconus with acute hydrops and perforation. Brief case report. Cornea 10:83, 1991
70. Lahoud S, Brownstein S, Laflamme MY, Poleski SA: Keratoconus with spontaneous perforation of the cornea. Can J Ophthalmol 22:230, 1987
71. Margo CE, Mosteller MW: Corneal pseudocyst following acute hydrops. Br J Ophthalmol 71:57, 1987
72. Musco PS, Aquavella JV: Cornea fistula. Ophthalmic Surg 18:574, 1987

73. Bron AJ: Keratoconus. Cornea 7:163, 1988
74. Kao WW, Vergnes JP, Ebert J, et al: Increased collagenase and gelatinase activities in keratoconus. Biochem Biophys Res Commun 107:929, 1982
75. Critchfield JW, Calandra AJ, Nesburn AB, Kenney MC: Keratoconus: I. Biochemical studies. Exp Eye Res 46:953, 1988
76. Zimmerman DR, Fischer RW, Winterhalter KH, et al: Comparative studies of collagens in normal and keratoconus corneas. Exp Eye Res 46:431, 1988
77. Cannon DT, Foster CS: Collagen cross-linking in keratoconus. Invest Ophthalmol Vis Sci 17:63, 1978
78. Buddecke E, Wollensak J: Saure Mucopolysaccharide und Glykoproteine der menschlichen Cornea in Abhangigkeit vom Lebensalter und bei Keratoconus. Albrecht von Graefes Arch Klin Exp Ophthalmol 171:105, 1966
79. Yue BY, Baum JL, Smith BD: Identification of collagens synthesized by cultures of normal human corneal and keratoconus stromal cells. Biochim Biophys Acta 755:318, 1983
80. Newsome DA, Foidart JM, Hassel JR, et al: Detection of specific collagen types in normal and keratoconus corneas. Invest Ophthalmol Vis Sci 20:738, 1981
81. Yue BY, Baum JL, Silbert JE: The synthesis of glycosaminoglycans by cultures of corneal stromal cells from patients with keratoconus. J Clin Invest 63:545, 1979
82. Bleckman H, Kresse H: Studies on the glycosaminoglycan metabolism of cultured fibroblasts from human keratoconus corneas. Exp Eye Res 30:215, 1980
83. Anseth A: Changes in the glycosaminoglycans in some human corneal disorders. Exp Eye Res 8:438, 1969
84. Praus P, Goldman GN: Glycosaminoglycans in human corneal buttons removed at keratoplasty. Ophthalmic Res 2:223, 1971
85. Funderburgh JL, Panjwani N, Conrad GW, Gaum J: Altered keratan sulfate epitopes in keratoconus. Invest Ophthalmol Vis Sci 30:2278, 1989
86. Yue BY, Sugar J, Benveniste K: Heterogenicity in keratoconus: possible biochemical basis. Proc Soc Exp Biol Med 175:336, 1984
87. Yue BY, Sugar J, Schrode K: Histochemical studies of keratoconus. Curr Eye Res 7:81, 1988
88. Yue BY, Sugar J, Benveniste K: RNA metabolism in cultures of corneal stromal cells from patients with keratoconus. Proc Soc Exp Biol Med 178:126, 1985
89. Rehany U, Lahau M, Shoshan S: Collagenolytic activity in keratoconus. Ann Ophthalmol 14:751, 1982
90. Rehany U, Shoshan S: In vitro incorporation of proline into keratoconic human corneas. Invest Ophthalmol Vis Sci 25:1254, 1984
91. Sawaguchi S, Twining SS, Yue BY, et al: Alpha-1 proteinase inhibitor levels in keratoconus. Exp Eye Res 50:549, 1990
92. Sawaguchi S, Yue BY, Sugar J, Gilboy JE: Lysosomal enzyme abnormalities in keratoconus. Arch Ophthalmol 107:1507, 1989
93. Werb A: Keratoconus. Br J Ophthalmol 56:565, 1972
94. Davies PD, Ruben M: The paretic pupil: its incidence and etiology after keratoplasty for keratoconus. Br J Ophthalmol 59:223, 1975
95. Edmund C: Corneal elasticity and ocular rigidity in normal and keratoconic eyes. Acta Ophthalmol (Copenh) 66:134, 1988
96. Hornblass A, Sabates WI: Eyelid and orbital cavernous hemangioma associated with keratoconus. Am J Ophthalmol 89:396, 1980
97. Hartstein J: Keratoconus that developed in patients wearing corneal contact lenses. Arch Ophthalmol 80:345, 1968
98. Brady HR: Keratoconus development in a contact lens wearer. Contact Lens Med Bull 5:23, 1972
99. Steahly LP: Keratoconus following contact lens wear. Ann Ophthalmol 10:1177, 1978
100. Hartstein J, Becker B: Research into the pathogenesis of keratoconus. A new syndrome: low ocular rigidity, contact lenses, and keratoconus. Arch Ophthalmol 84:728, 1970
101. Foster CS, Yamamoto GK: Ocular rigidity in keratoconus. Am J Ophthalmol 86:802, 1978
102. Andreassen TT, Simonsen AH, Oxlund H: Biomechanical properties of keratoconus and normal corneas. Exp Eye Res 31:435, 1980
103. Nash IS, Greene PR, Foster CS: Comparison of mechanical properties of keratoconus and normal corneas. Exp Eye Res 35:413, 1982
104. Poole TA: Calculations of stress distribution in keratoconus. N Y State J Med 73:1284, 1973
105. Hartstein J: Corneal warping. Am J Ophthalmol 60:1103, 1965
106. Levenson DS, Berry CV: Findings on follow-up of corneal warpage patients. CLAO J 9:126, 1983
107. Rubin ML: The tale of the warped cornea. A real-life melodrama. Arch Ophthalmol 77:711, 1967
108. Levenson DS: Changes in corneal curvature with long-term PMMA contact lens wear. CLAO J 9:121, 1983
109. Rowsey JJ, Reynolds AE, Brown R: Corneal topography. Corneascope. Arch Ophthalmol 99:1093, 1981
110. Wilson SE, Lin DTC, Klyce SD, et al: Topographic changes in contact lens-induced corneal warpage. Ophthalmology 97:734, 1990
111. Barry WE, Tredici TJ: Keratoconus in USAF personnel. Aerosp Med 43:1027, 1972
112. Nauheim JS, Perry AD: A clinicopathologic study of contact-lens related keratoconus. Am J Ophthalmol 100:543, 1985
113. Macsai MS, Varley GA, Krachmer JH: Development of keratoconus after contact lens wear. Patient characteristics. Arch Ophthalmol 108:534, 1990
114. Street DA, Vinokur ET, Waring GO, et al: Lack of association between keratoconus, mitral valve prolapse, and joint hypermobility. Ophthalmology 98:170, 1991
115. Tuft SJ, Kemeny DM, Dart JKG, Buckley RJ: Clinical features of atopic keratoconjunctivitis. Ophthalmology 98:150, 1991
116. François J: Dermatite atopique cataracte et keratocone. Ann Dermatol Syphiligr (Paris) 88:397, 1961
117. Longmore L: Atopic dermatitis, cataract, and keratoconus. Aust J Dermatol 11:139, 1970

118. Norins A, Field L: Atopic cataracts and keratoconus in one patient. Arch Dermatol 90:102, 1964
119. Spencer WH, Fisher TJ: The association of keratoconus with atopic dermatitis. Am J Ophthalmol 47:332, 1959
120. Brunsting L, Reed WR, Bair HL: Atopic eczema and keratoconus. Arch Dermatol 72:237, 1955
121. Roth JL, Kierland PR: The natural history of atopic dermatitis. Arch Dermatol 89:209, 1964
122. Tabbara K, Butrus S: Vernal conjunctivitis and keratoconus. Am J Ophthalmol 95:704, 1983
123. Bietti GB, Ferraboschi C: Sur l'association de keratocone avec le catarrhe printainer et sur son evidence statistique. Bull Mem Soc Fr Ophtalmol 71:185, 1958
124. Galin MR, Berger R: Atopy and keratoconus. Am J Ophthalmol 45:904, 1958
125. Gasset AR, Hison WA, Frias JL: Keratoconus and atopic diseases. Ann Ophthalmol 10:991, 1978
126. Sabiston DW: The association of keratoconus, dermatitis, and asthma. Trans Ophthalmol Soc NZ 18:66, 1966
127. Ridley F: Eye rubbing and contact lenses. Br J Ophthalmol 45:631, 1961
128. Ridley F: Contact lenses in the treatment of keratoconus. Br J Ophthalmol 40:295, 1956
129. Cameron JA, Al-Rajhi AA, Badr IA: Corneal ectasia in vernal keratoconjunctivitis. Ophthalmology 96:1615, 1989
130. Gonzales J de J: Keratoconus consecutive to vernal conjunctivitis. Am J Ophthalmol 3:127, 1920
131. Rahi A, Davies P, Ruben M, et al: Keratoconus and coexisting atopic disease. Br J Ophthalmol 61:761, 1977
132. Kemp EG, Lewis CJ: Immunoglobulin patterns in keratoconus with particular reference to total and specific IgE levels. Br J Ophthalmol 66:717, 1982
133. Easty D, Entwistle C, Fink A, Witcher J: Herpes simplex keratitis and keratoconus in the atopic patients. A clinical and immunological study. Trans Ophthalmol Soc UK 95:267, 1975
134. Eissler R, Longnecker LP: Common eye findings in mongolism. Am J Ophthalmol 54:398, 1962
135. Lowe RF: The eyes in mongolism. Br J Ophthalmol 33:131, 1949
136. Cullen TF: Blindness in mongolism (Down's syndrome) and keratoconus. Br J Ophthalmol 47:331, 1963
137. Cullen TF, Butler HG: Mongolism (Down's syndrome) and keratoconus. Br J Ophthalmol 47:321, 1963
138. Missiroli A, Vonni V: Sui segni oculari della syndrome di Down. Boll Ocul 49:123, 1970
139. Pierse D, Eustace P: Acute keratoconus in mongols. Br J Ophthalmol 55:50, 1971
140. Walsh SZ: Keratoconus and blindness in 469 institutionalized subjects with Down's syndrome and other causes of mental retardation. J Ment Defic Res 25:243, 1981
141. Shapiro MB, France T: The ocular features of Down's syndrome. Am J Ophthalmol 99:659, 1985
142. Boger WP, Peterson RA, Robb RM: Keratoconus and acute hydrops in mentally retarded patients with congenital rubella syndrome. Am J Ophthalmol 91:231, 1981
143. Frantz JM, Insler MS, Hagenah M, McDonald MB: Penetrating keratoplasty for keratoconus in Down's syndrome. Am J Ophthalmol 109:143, 1990
144. Bietti GB, Cambiaggi A, DelCastillo A: Sull analisi statistica dill associazione di malattie oculari. Boll Ocul 41:3, 1962
145. Alstrom CH, Olson O: Heredo-retinopathia congenitalis. Monohydribe recessiva autosomalis. Hereditas Genetiski Arkiv 43:1, 1957
146. Karel I: Keratoconus in congenital diffuse tapetoretinal degeneration. Ophthalmologica 155:8, 1968
147. Smith D, Oestreicher J, Musarella MA: Clinical spectrum of Leber's congenital amaurosis in the second to fourth decade of life. Ophthalmology 97:1156, 1990
148. Karel I: Akuti keratokonus jako komplikale retrolentarni fibroplasie. Cesk Oftalmol 25:347, 1969
149. Lorfel RS, Sugar HS: Keratoconus associated with retrolental fibroplasia. Ann Ophthalmol 8:449, 1976
150. Beardsley TL, Foulks GN: An association of keratoconus and mitral valve prolapse. Ophthalmology 89:35, 1982
151. Bermudez FJ, Ruiz C, Carreras B, Aneiros J: Association of keratoconus and false chordae tendineae in the left ventricle. Am J Ophthalmol 108:93, 1989
152. Robertson I: Keratoconus and the Ehlers-Danlos syndrome. A new aspect of keratoconus. Med J Aust 1:571, 1975
153. Austin MG, Schaefer RF: Marfan syndrome with unusual blood vessel manifestations; primary medionecrosis, dissection of the right inominate. Arch Pathol Lab Med 64:205, 1957
154. Storck H: Ein Fall von Arachnodaktylie (Dystrophia mesodermalis congenita), Typus Marfan. Dermatologica 104:322, 1952
155. Maumenee IH: The eye in the Marfan syndrome. Trans Am Ophthalmol Soc 79:684, 1981
156. Cross HE, Jensen AD: Ocular manifestations in the Marfan's syndrome and homocystinuria. Am J Ophthalmol 75:405, 1973
157. McKusick VA: Heritable Diseases of Connective Tissue. 4th Ed. CV Mosby, St. Louis, 1972
158. Blandau RJ: Morphogenesis and malformations of the skin. Birth Defects 17:155, 1981
159. Judisch F, Wariri M, Krachmer J: Ocular Ehlers-Danlos syndrome with normal lysyl hydrolase activity. Arch Ophthalmol 94:1489, 1976
160. Pinnell SR, Krane SM, Kensora J, Glimcher MJ: A heritable disorder of connective tissue hydroxylysine-deficient collagen disease. N Engl J Med 286:1013, 1972
161. Sussman M, Lichtenstein JR, Nigra TP, et al: Hydroxylysine-deficient skin collagen in a patient with a form of the Ehlers-Danlos syndrome. J Bone Joint Surg 56A:1228, 1974
162. Steinmann B, Gitzelmann R, Vogel A, et al: Ehlers-Danlos syndrome in two siblings with deficient lysylhydroxylase activity in cultured skin fibroblasts but only mild hydroxylysine deficiency in skin. Helv Paediatr Acta 30:255, 1975
163. Biglan AW, Brown SI, Johnson BC: Keratoglobus and blue sclera. Am J Ophthalmol 83:225, 1977

164. Babel J, Houber J: Keratocone et sclerotiques bleues dans une anomalie congenitale de tissu conjonctif. J Genet Hum 17:241, 1969
165. Gregoratos N, Bartoscocas C, Papas K: Blue sclera with keratoglobus and brittle cornea. Br J Ophthalmol 55:424, 1971
166. Hymas SW, Dar H, Newman E: Blue sclera keratoglobus. Br J Ophthalmol 53:53, 1969
167. Stein R, Lazar M, Adam A: Brittle cornea. A familial trait associated with blue sclera. Am J Ophthalmol 66:67, 1968
168. Greenfield G, Romano A, Stein R, et al: Blue sclera and keratoconus. Key features of a distinct heritable disorder of connective tissue. Clin Genet 4:8, 1973
169. May MA, Beauchamp GR: Collagen maturation defects in Ehlers-Danlos keratopathy. J Pediatr Ophthalmol Strabismus 24:78, 1987
170. Elas LJ, Miller RL, Pinnell SR: Inherited human collagen lysyl hydroxylase deficiency: ascorbic acid response. J Pediatr 92:378, 1978
171. Hartstein J: Basics of Contact Lenses. 3rd Ed. American Academy of Ophthalmology, San Francisco, 1979
172. Buxton JN: Contact lenses in keratoconus. Contact Intraocul Lens Med J 4:74, 1978
173. Krachmer JH, Feder R, Belin MW: Keratoconus and related noninflammatory corneal thinning disorders. Surv Ophthalmol 28:293, 1984
174. Buxton JN, Keates RH, Hoefle FB: The contact lens correction of keratoconus. In Dabezies OH (ed): Contact Lenses. The CLAO Guide to Basic Science and Clinical Practice. Grune & Stratton, Orlando, FL, 1984
175. Mannis MJ, Zadnik K: Contact lens fitting in keratoconus. CLAO J 15:282, 1989
176. Belin MW: Optical and surgical correction of keratoconus. Focal Points in Ophthalmology. American Academy of Ophthalmology, San Francisco, CA, 1988
177. Soper JW, Jarrett A: Results of a systemic approach to fitting keratoconus and corneal transplants. Contact Lens Med Bull 5:50, 1972
178. Caroline PJ, McGuire JR, Doughman DJ: Report on a new contact lens design for keratoconus. Contact Intraocul Lens Med J 4:69, 1978
179. Schein OD, Rosenthal P, Ducharme C: A gas permeable scleral contact lens for visual rehabilitation. Am J Ophthalmol 109:318, 1990
180. Arentsen JJ, Morgan B, Green WR: Changing indications for keratoplasty. Am J Ophthalmol 81:313, 1976
181. Payne JW: Primary penetrating keratoplasty for keratoconus: a long-term follow-up. Cornea 1:21, 1982
182. Smith RE, McDonald HR, Nesburn A, Minckler DS: Penetrating keratoplasty: changing indications, 1947–1978. Arch Ophthalmol 98:1226, 1980
183. Lindquist TD, McGlothan JS, Rotkis WM, Chandler JW: Indications for penetrating keratoplasty: 1980–1988. Cornea 10:210, 1991
184. Mamalis N, Craig MT, Coulter VL, et al: Penetrating keratoplasty 1981–1988: clinical indications and pathologic findings. J Cataract Refract Surg 17:163, 1991
185. Morris RJ, Bates AK: Changing indications for keratoplasty. Eye 3:455, 1989
186. Brady SE, Rapuano CJ, Arentsen JJ, et al: Clinical indications for and procedures associated with penetrating keratoplasty, 1983–1988. Am J Ophthalmol 108:118, 1989
187. Robin JB, Gindi JJ, Koh K, et al: An update of the indications for penetrating keratoplasty, 1979–1983. Arch Ophthalmol 104:87, 1986
188. Robert JE: Statistics on the results of keratoplasty. Am J Ophthalmol 33:21, 1950
189. Paton RT: Corneal transplantation: a review of 365 operations. Arch Ophthalmol 52:871, 1954
190. Hughes WF: The treatment of corneal dystrophies by keratoplasty. Am J Ophthalmol 50:1100, 1960
191. Buxton JN, Apisson JG, Hoefle FB: Corticosteroids in 100 keratoplasties. Am J Ophthalmol 67:46, 1969
192. Anseth A: Keratoplasty for keratoconus: a report of 50 operated eyes. Acta Ophthalmol (Copenh) 45:684, 1967
193. Keates RH, Falkenstein S: Keratoplasty in keratoconus. Am J Ophthalmol 74:442, 1972
194. Boruchoff SA, Jensen AD, Dohlman CH: Comparison of suturing techniques in keratoplasty for keratoconus. Ann Ophthalmol 7:433, 1975
195. Moore TE, Aronson SB: Results of penetrating keratoplasty in keratoconus. Adv Ophthalmol 37:106, 1978
196. Richard J, Paton D, Gasset A: A comparison of penetrating keratoplasty and lamellar keratoplasty in the surgical management of keratoconus. Am J Ophthalmol 86:807, 1978
197. Troutman RC, Gaster RN: Surgical advances and results of keratoconus. Am J Ophthalmol 90:131, 1980
198. Paglen PG, Fine M, Abbot RL, Webster RG: The prognosis for keratoplasty in keratoconus. Ophthalmology 89:651, 1982
199. Bishop VL, Robinson LP, Wechscer AW, Bierson FA: Corneal graft survival: a retrospective Australian study. Aust NZ J Ophthalmol 14:133, 1986
200. Troutman RC, Lawless MA: Penetrating keratoplasty for keratoconus. Cornea 6:298, 1987
201. Epstein RT, Seepor JA, Dreizen NG, et al: Penetrating keratoplasty for herpes simplex keratitis and keratoconus. Allograft rejection and survival. Ophthalmology 94:935, 1987
202. Kirkness CM, Ficker LA, Steble AD, Rice NS: The success of penetrating keratoplasty for keratoconus. Eye 4:673, 1990
203. Sharif KW, Casey TA: Penetrating keratoplasty for keratoconus: complications and long-term success. Br J Ophthalmol 75:142, 1991
204. Price FW Jr, Whitson WE, Mark RG: Graft survival in four common groups of patients undergoing penetrating keratoplasty. Ophthalmology 98:322, 1991
205. Musch DC, Schwartz AF, Fitzgerald-Shelton K, et al: The effect of allograft rejection after penetrating keratoplasty on central endothelial cell density. Am J Ophthalmol 111:739, 1991
206. Donshik PC, Cavanagh HD, Boruchoff SA, Dohlman CH: Effect of bilateral and unilateral grafts on the incidence of rejections in keratoconus. Am J Ophthalmol 87:823, 1979

207. Chandler JW, Kaufman HE: Graft reactions after keratoplasty for keratoconus. Am J Ophthalmol 77:543, 1974
208. Alldredge C, Krachmer JH: Clinical types of corneal transplant rejections. Arch Ophthalmol 99:599, 1981
209. Malbran ES, Fernandez-Meijide RE: Bilateral versus unilateral penetrating graft in keratoconus. Ophthalmology 89:38, 1982
210. Buxton J, Schuman M, Pecego J: Graft reactions after unilateral and bilateral keratoplasty for keratoconus. Ophthalmology 88:771, 1981
211. Perl T, Charlton KH, Binder PS: Disparate diameter grafting: astigmatism, intraocular pressure, and visual acuity. Ophthalmology 88:774, 1981
212. Troutman RC, Meltzer M: Astigmatism and myopia in keratoconus. Trans Am Ophthalmol Soc 70:265, 1972
213. Musch DC, Meyer RF, Sugar A: The effect of removing running sutures on astigmatism after penetrating keratoplasty. Arch Ophthalmol 106:488, 1988
214. Binder PS: The effect of suture removal on postkeratoplasty astigmatism. Am J Ophthalmol 105:637, 1988
215. Kaufman HE: Astigmatism after keratoplasty—possible cause and method of prevention. Am J Ophthalmol 94:556, 1982
216. Wilson SE, Bourne WM: Effect of recipient-donor trephine size disparity on refractive error in keratoconus. Ophthalmology 96:299, 1989
217. Meyer RF, Musch DC: Discussion of: effect of recipient-donor trephine size disparity on refractive error in keratoconus. Ophthalmology 96:304, 1989
218. Perry HD, Foulks GN: Oversize donor buttons in corneal transplantation surgery for keratoconus. Ophthalmic Surg 18:751, 1987
219. Girard LJ, Eguez I, Esnaola N, et al: Effect of penetrating keratoplasty using grafts of various sizes on keratoconic myopia and astigmatism. J Cataract Refract Surg 14:541, 1988
220. Urrets-Zavalia A: Fixed, dilated pupil, iris atrophy, and secondary glaucoma. A distinct clinical entity following penetrating keratoplasty in keratoconus. Am J Ophthalmol 56:257, 1963
221. Beretelson T, Seim V: Irreversible mydriasis following keratoplasty in keratoconus. Acta Ophthalmol (Copenh) 125(suppl):45, 1976
222. Gasset AR: Fixed dilated pupil following penetrating keratoplasty in keratoconus. Castroviejo syndrome. Ann Ophthalmol 9:623, 1977
223. Hammerstein W, Friedburg D: Ergebnisse der perforierenden Keratoplastik bei hereditaren Hornhauterkrankungen. Klin Monatsbl Augenheilkd 166:24, 1975
224. Pouliquen Y, Bellivet J, Lecoq PJ, Clay C: Keratoplastie transfixiante dans le traitement du keratocone. Arch Ophtalmol (Paris) 32:735, 1972
225. Buxton JN: Surgery in keratoconus, including thermokeratoplasty. In Symposium on Medical and Surgical Diseases of the Cornea, Transactions of the New Orleans Academy of Ophthalmology. CV Mosby, St. Louis, 1980
226. Pouliquen Y, Guimaraes R, Petroutsos G, Lacombe E: Is Urrets-Zavalia syndrome still a reality? J Fr Ophtalmol 6:325, 1983
227. Shands PR, Lass JH: Severe anterior segment inflammation following corneal surgery in keratoconus. Ophthalmic Surg 21:645, 1990
228. Nirankari VS, Karesh J, Bastion F, et al: Recurrence of keratoconus in donor cornea 22 years after successful keratoplasty. Br J Ophthalmol 67:32, 1983
229. Abelson MB, Collin HB, Gillette TE, Dohlman CH: Recurrent keratoconus after keratoplasty. Am J Ophthalmol 90:672, 1980
230. Jahne M: Keratokonusrezidiv nach Keratoplastik. Z Arztl Fortbild (Jena) 468:434, 1974
231. Fanta H: Akuter keratoconus. Ber Zusammenkunft Dtsch Ophthalmol Ges 71:46, 1972
232. Filderman IP: A suggested therapy for cases of keratoconus. J Am Optom Assoc 31:623, 1960
233. Matzen C: Das Endresultat von Keratoplastiken bei Keratokonus nach Langzeitbeobachtung. In Kruger KE, Tost M (eds): Augenheilkunde in Forchung and Praxis. Vol. 2. Martin Luther University, Halle-Wittenberg, 1972
234. Kaufman HE, Werblin TP: Epikeratophakia for the treatment of keratoconus. Am J Ophthalmol 93:342, 1982
235. Itoi M, Nakaji Y, Nakae T: Keratoconus: the Japanese experience. CLAO J 9:254, 1983
236. Fronterre A, Portesani GP: Epikeratoplasty for keratoconus. Report of 40 cases. Cornea 8:236, 1989
237. Dietze TR, Durrie DS: Indications and treatment of keratoconus using epikeratophakia. Ophthalmology 95:236, 1988
238. Steinert RF, Wagoner MD: Long-term comparison of epikeratoplasty and penetrating keratoplasty for keratoconus. Arch Ophthalmol 106:493, 1988
239. Lehtosalo J, Uusitalo RJ, Mianowizc J: Epikeratophakia for treatment of keratoconus. Acta Ophthalmol (Copenh) 182(suppl):74, 1987
240. Fronterre A, Portesani GP: Comparison of epikeratoplasty and penetrating keratoplasty for keratoconus. Refract Corneal Surg 7:167, 1991
241. Goosey JD, Prager TC, Goosey CB, et al: A comparison of penetrating keratoplasty to epikeratoplasty in the surgical management of keratoconus. Am J Ophthalmol 111:145, 1991
242. Lass JH, Lembach RG, Park SB, et al: Clinical management of keratoconus. A multicenter analysis. Ophthalmology 97:433, 1990
243. Carney LG, Lembach RG: Management of keratoconus: comparative visual assessments. CLAO J 17:52, 1991
244. McDonald MB, Koenig SB, Safir A, Kaufman HE: Onlay lamellar keratoplasty for the treatment of keratoconus. Br J Ophthalmol 67:615, 1983
245. McDonald MB, Kaufman HE, Durrie DS, et al: Epikeratophakia for keratoconus. The nationwide study. Arch Ophthalmol 104:1294, 1986
246. Malbran E: Lamellar keratoplasty in keratoconus. Int Ophthalmol Clin 6:99, 1966

23

Immunologic Disorders of the Cornea and Conjunctiva

JEFFREY B. ROBIN, RAJ DUGEL, AND STEVEN B. ROBIN

The ocular surface may be affected by a variety of disorders that result from normal or abnormal processes of the immune system, the basic components and mechanisms of which are described in Chapter 3. The unique location and structural components of the cornea and conjunctiva make these tissues susceptible to involvement in all types of immunologic reactions.[1] The conjunctiva and corneoscleral limbus are rich in blood vessels and lymphatics. Mucous-membrane-associated lymphoid tissue, which is important in antigen processing, appears to be present in the conjunctiva. Additionally, IgA, IgG, and IgM are present in high concentrations in the conjunctiva; IgG and IgA are also found in the cornea, although in lesser concentrations.[2] The presence of collagen and blood vessels in the sclera and limbus may predispose these tissues to involvement in systemic collagen-vascular diseases.

The exposure of the ocular surface to environmental antigens facilitates the production of type I, or immediate, hypersensitivity reactions. Clinically, these reactions appear to be the mechanism underlying allergic conjunctivitis; they are also partly responsible for vernal keratoconjunctivitis, giant papillary conjunctivitis, and atopic keratoconjunctivitis. Type II hypersensitivity reactions, characterized by the presence of tissue-fixed antibodies and complement, may be the underlying cause of cicatricial pemphigoid, pemphigus vulgaris, dermatitis herpetiformis, corneal immune rings, and Mooren's ulcer. Type III hypersensitivity reactions are characterized by the presence of circulating immune complexes and may be involved in the pathogenesis of bullous pemphigoid, Stevens-Johnson syndrome, Lyell's disease, Reiter syndrome, Mooren's ulcer, and the systemic vasculitides. Type IV hypersensitivity reactions involve cell-mediated immunity, and may be responsible to some degree for the pathogenesis of herpes simplex disciform keratitis, corneal graft rejection, phlyctenulosis, vernal keratoconjunctivitis, giant papillary conjunctivitis, and atopic keratoconjunctivitis.

This chapter describes the clinical manifestations of the many immunologic disorders that can involve the cornea and conjunctiva. It should be read in conjunction with Chapter 3.

ATOPIC DISORDERS OF THE OCULAR SURFACE

Exposure of the cornea and conjunctiva to the external environment enables environmental antigens to interact with these tissues. The ocular surface is especially well suited to react to antigenic stimuli. The presence of immunoglobulins in the conjunctiva (and to a lesser degree, in the cornea), as well as a wide range of leukocytes and macrophages, facilitates effector responses to antigenic stimuli. Antigens can be processed because of the presence of mucous-membrane-associated lymphoid tissue in the conjunctiva, as well as the extensive lymphatic channels that drain the conjunctiva and peripheral cornea.

The term *atopy* is used to describe type I hypersensitivity reactions induced by tissue-fixed IgE antibodies in response to environmental antigens. Approximately 15 percent of the general population demonstrates atopic phenomena.[1] The major atopic disorders are allergic rhinitis, bronchial asthma, and atopic dermatitides. Minor atopic diseases include food allergies, urticaria, and nonhereditary angioedema. Atopic phenomena are entirely or partially responsible for several disorders of the ocular surface. These include allergic conjunctivitis, vernal keratoconjunctivitis, giant papillary conjunctivitis, and atopic keratoconjunctivitis.

Allergic Conjunctivitis

Allergic conjunctivitis is one of the most common ocular immunologic disorders encountered in general ophthalmic practice. It results from a type I, immediate hypersensitivity reaction of the ocular surface to a variety of airborne antigens, including pollens, hay, grasses, and weeds. Symptoms of acute allergic conjunctivitis include rapid onset of ocular itching, redness, burning, and lacrimation. There is usually a concomitant allergic rhinitis or sinusitis. Commonly, there is a personal or family history of atopic phenomena, such as asthma, eczema, or seasonal rhinitis. Affected patients characteristically have marked injection of the conjunctival and episcleral vessels; they may also have mild accompanying chemosis and eyelid edema. The cornea is not involved in acute allergic conjunctivitis.

The pathogenesis of allergic conjunctivitis involves an immediate hypersensitivity reaction to an environmental antigen to which the patient has been previously exposed. The reaction is IgE-mediated and involves eosinophils and mast cells. The density of mast cells in the conjunctiva of allergic individuals is significantly greater than in normal individuals.[3] Mast cells degranulate and liberate many substances, including histamine[4] and tryptase. Histamine is responsible for many of the clinical symptoms and signs of allergic conjunctivitis.

In most cases, the diagnosis of allergic conjunctivitis may be made on the basis of a typical history and clinical signs. Additionally, conjunctival scrapings frequently demonstrate eosinophils, particularly in more severe cases.[5] However, in milder cases these scrapings are usually devoid of eosinophils.[4] These clinical findings correlate with the observations of Abelson et al[6] that eosinophils are frequently absent from conjunctival scrapings but are generally present in the deeper conjunctiva in rabbits with experimental allergic conjunctivitis. Thus, the presence of eosinophils in conjunctival scrapings may confirm the diagnosis of allergic conjunctivitis, but their absence does not exclude it. Tear tryptase levels may serve as an objective parameter of disease activity.[7]

Treatment of allergic conjunctivitis involves removal of the offending antigen, if known, from the patient's environment. If the antigenic agent is identified, recurrences may be avoided by desensitizing the patient. For acute relief, a variety of antihistamines and topical vasoconstricting agents may be used. Topical 0.05 percent levocabastine (Livostin), a potent histamine H_1-receptor antagonist, has shown promise in raising the threshold of early allergic response.[8] Combinations of antihistamines and topical vasoconstricting agents may be most efficacious.[9] Topical corticosteroids effectively inhibit the allergic response,[10] although the severity of symptoms rarely warrants their use. Topical nonsteroidal anti-inflammatory drugs such as 0.5 percent ketorolac (Acular), relieve the itching associated with allergic conjunctivitis. Topical cromolyn sodium (Crolom), an inhibitor of mast cell degranulation, is effective for the relief of symptoms and signs.[11] It has no effect, however, on the symptoms and signs caused by histamine that has already been released, and therefore, should be used prior to and during exposure to the offending antigen. Topical 0.1 percent lodoxamide (Alomide) is a second-generation mast cell stabilizing agent. Topical 0.1 percent olopatadine (Patanol) is both an inhibitor of histamine release and a relatively selective H_1-receptor antagonist recently approved for the treatment of allergic conjunctivitis.

Vernal Keratoconjunctivitis

Vernal keratoconjunctivitis (VKC) is a recurrent bilateral inflammation of the conjunctiva characterized by giant cobblestone papillae on the superior tarsal conjunctiva, a gelatinous hypertrophy of the limbal conjunctiva, and a typical epithelial keratopathy. Vernal keratoconjunctivitis is associated with prominent itching, photophobia, and a distinct ropy discharge that is rich in eosinophils. Although the distribution is worldwide, vernal keratoconjunctivitis occurs predominantly in the warm climates of the Middle East, the Mediterranean, and parts of South America.[12–14] In the northern hemisphere, as the name *vernal (spring)* implies, it is usually seasonal and tends to recur in the months of May and June. In tropical climates, vernal keratoconjunctivitis tends to be perennial.[1]

Vernal keratoconjunctivitis is a disease of youth; it rarely develops in patients before the age of 3 years or after the age of 25 years.[1,13–15] Its peak incidence occurs between the ages of 6 and 20 years. Before puberty, there is a 2:1 male preponderance, with equalization of this ratio thereafter.[12] Vernal keratoconjunctivitis is a chronic disease that typically lasts 4 to 10 years, although its duration may be as long as 24 years.[1,12,14,16,17] Two-thirds of patients with vernal keratoconjunctivitis have a family history of atopy (allergic rhinitis, bronchial asthma, eczema, and environmental allergies).[13,18] Ninety percent of patients with vernal keratoconjunctivitis have one or more of these atopic disorders.

Clinical Features

Itching is the predominant symptom of vernal keratoconjunctivitis. It may be intense, and frequently precedes

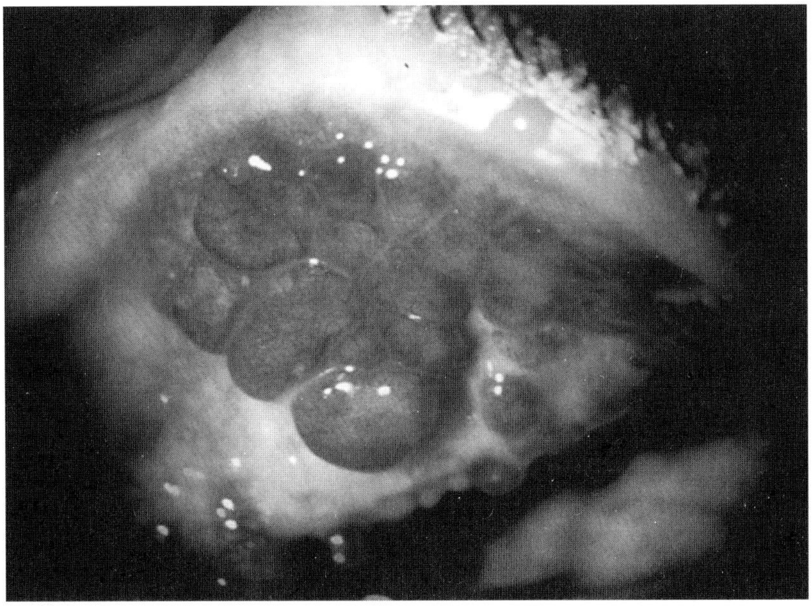

FIGURE 23-1 Giant cobblestone papillae of the superior tarsal conjunctiva in a patient with vernal keratoconjunctivitis.

any clinical manifestations of the disease. The absence of itching should make the diagnosis of vernal keratoconjunctivitis questionable. Additional symptoms may include eyelid heaviness, tearing, and photophobia.

Vernal keratoconjunctivitis is a bilateral disease and is divisible into two overlapping forms: palpebral and limbal. The palpebral form involves the superior tarsal conjunctiva with characteristic giant papillae. Although the inferior tarsal conjunctiva may show similar involvement, it is usually much less severely affected. In the early stages, the papillae may be small in size and number, and there is usually generalized conjunctival hyperemia. As the disease progresses, the papillae coalesce or enlarge into the characteristic giant papillae (Figure 23-1). They assume a flat top, which is presumably caused by pressure on the tarsal conjunctiva from the cornea, and are thus described as cobblestone papillae. These papillae initially involve the superior border of the tarsus but eventually progress to form a mosaic over the entire tarsal surface. In advanced cases, they can cause a mechanical ptosis (Figure 23-2). Although tarsal scarring is rare in patients with vernal keratoconjunctivitis, it can occasionally occur. The discharge of vernal keratoconjunctivitis is characteristic; it is yellow-white and has a ropy consistency (Figure 23-3). It covers the conjunctival surface and may be peeled off without inducing bleeding. The discharge consists of mucus, epithelial cells, neutrophils, and most notably, an abundance of eosinophils and free eosinophilic granules.[1,12,14]

The limbal form of vernal keratoconjunctivitis occurs more frequently in darker-skinned races,[1,19] and is characterized by elevated gelatinous excrescences along the limbus (Figure 23-4). These excrescences may be single or confluent; they usually occur at the superior limbus, although they may involve any quadrant. Discrete lumps that may be apparent within the gelatinous mass are essentially papillae; their color varies, depending on the amount of core vascularization. Additionally, whitish spots, known as Trantas dots, may be visible within the gelatinous mass. Trantas dots consist of degenerated eosinophils and epithelial cells. They may be present at any stage of the disease

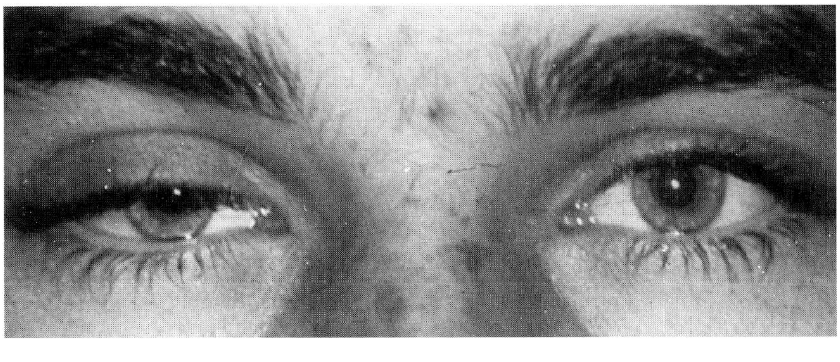

FIGURE 23-2 Ptosis of the right upper eyelid caused by giant papillae of the superior tarsal conjunctiva.

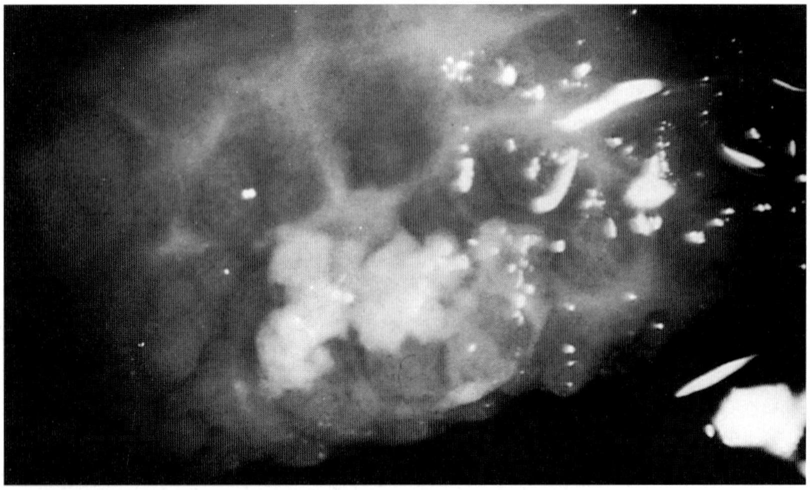

FIGURE 23-3 Thick discharge of vernal keratoconjunctivitis.

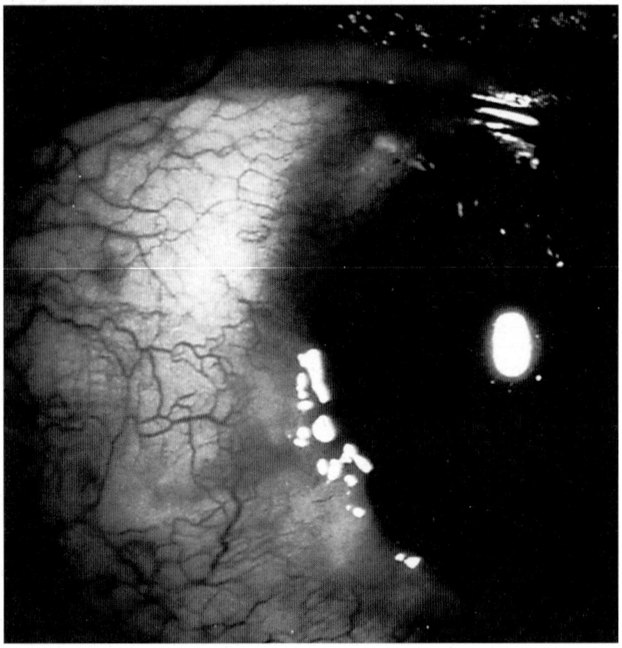

FIGURE 23-4 Limbal vernal keratoconjunctivitis.

and are evanescent, rarely lasting more than 1 week. Although they occur most commonly at the limbus, Trantas dots have been described in the palpebral and bulbar conjunctiva[1] (Figure 23-5). The appearance of tiny pits at the limbus and clear elevated cysts may follow the limbal form of vernal keratoconjunctivitis.[1] The pits represent areas of resolved limbal infiltrates and they appear as translucent spots in the normally opaque limbal conjunctiva. They are not true depressions and can thus be easily differentiated from Herbert's pits of trachoma. The limbal cysts that occur in vernal keratoconjunctivitis typically occur superiorly and contain clear colorless fluid.

In its mildest form, corneal involvement in vernal keratoconjunctivitis consists of prominent limbal vessels. In exceptionally severe cases, the limbal vessels may extend onto the cornea, resulting in a superficial fibrovascular pannus or destruction of Bowman's layer and scarring. Additionally, two types of vernal keratitis can occur.[20] First, a superficial keratitis, called *epithelial keratitis of Tobgy,*[21] manifests as a punctate, gray, flour-like dusting of the epithelium. The superior mid-peripheral cornea is predominantly involved; severe cases may affect the entire cornea.[20] These lesions stain with both fluorescein and rose bengal, and they represent areas of epithelial necrosis. Epithelial keratitis of Tobgy is generally associated with the palpebral form of vernal keratoconjunctivitis. These epithelial lesions tend to clear spontaneously within days to weeks.

The second type of corneal involvement in vernal keratoconjunctivitis is the vernal or shield ulcer, and is a relatively unusual complication of the disease. A shield ulcer has a characteristic appearance (Figure 23-6); it is transversely oval and is situated in the center of the superior third of the cornea. The lesion may rarely be found in the inferior cornea as well.[22] The ulcer is shallow and has white, shaggy epithelial edges. The underlying Bowman's layer may appear slightly opacified, and the superficial stroma shows variable cellular infiltration without vascularization. A shield ulcer is usually indolent and may persist for weeks or months without enlarging. It may result in corneal scarring, which most commonly appears as a gray, plaque-like opacity of Bowman's layer and superficial stroma. Shield ulcers tend to occur in very young patients and are usually present in the palpebral form of the disease, particularly when there are large cobblestone

FIGURE 23-5 Trantas dots in the bulbar conjunctiva.

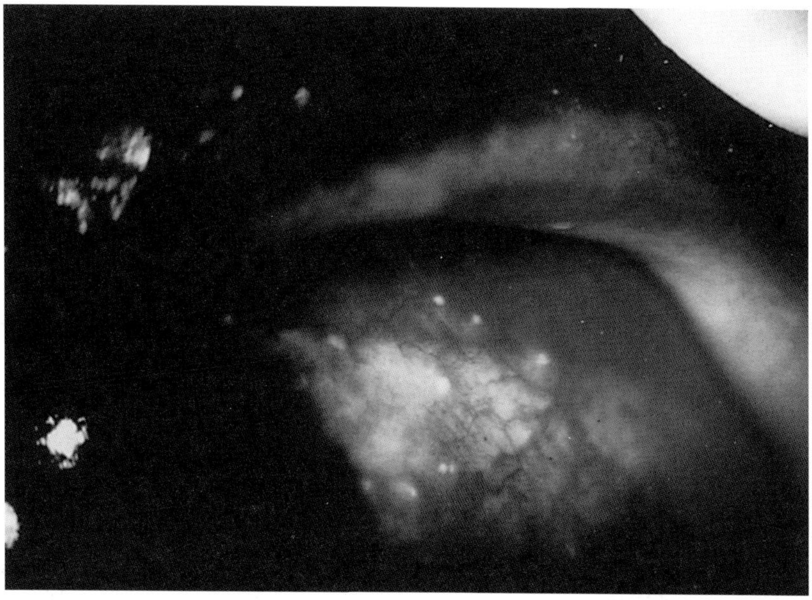

papillae. Although the cause of shield ulcers is unknown, their association with large papillae suggests a mechanical cause.

Degenerative corneal disorders occasionally occur in vernal keratoconjunctivitis. An arcus-like opacity parallel to and separated from the superior limbus may occur. This degenerative lesion is referred to as a vernal pseudogerontotoxon. It is peripherally located, grayish white, and resembles the involutional arcus of old age.[1] However, vernal pseudogerontotoxon tends to be irregular in width and is not as sharply delineated as arcus senilis. Myopic astigmatism and keratoconus have been noted to occur in long-standing cases of severe vernal keratoconjunctivitis. It is postulated that these disorders may result from chronic eye rubbing.[23,24]

Histopathology

Histopathologically, the early stages of vernal keratoconjunctivitis result in vascular engorgement and cellular infiltration of the conjunctival substantia propria. The cellular infiltration characteristically contains large numbers of eosinophils, as well as neutrophils, basophils, and mast cells.[1,12,25] Conjunctival scrapings of the superior tarsal conjunctiva characteristically show a large number of eosinophils. More than two eosinophils per high-power field is considered characteristic for vernal keratocon-

FIGURE 23-6 Characteristic shield ulcer in vernal keratoconjunctivitis.

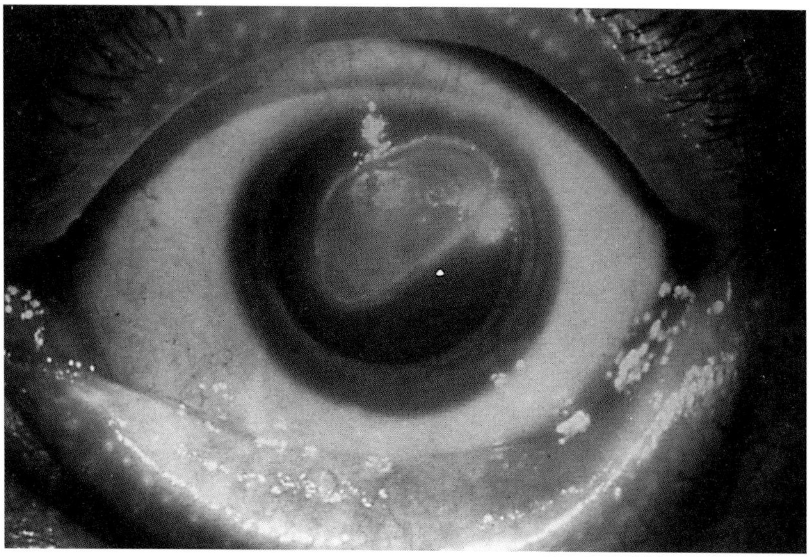

junctivitis.[5,9,19] Electron microscopy reveals a greater density of mast cells in the conjunctival epithelium and substantia propria than is evident on light microscopy.[26] Most of these mast cells are degranulated.[27,28] Lymphocytes and macrophages appear in the later stages.

In the palpebral form of vernal keratoconjunctivitis, hyperplasia of fibrous tissue in the substantia propria extends throughout the tarsal plate. This fibrous tissue hyperplasia is accompanied by new vessel formation, cellular infiltration, and formation of a subepithelial hyaline layer in the substantia propria,[12,14,29] and appears to form the fibrous cores of the cobblestone papillae. Following collagen proliferation in the substantia propria, the overlying conjunctival epithelium undergoes dramatic thickening, often becoming 10 cell layers thick. Characteristic epithelial infolding into the deeper conjunctival layers occurs. In the advanced stages of the disease, the papillae assume a circumvallate form and consist almost entirely of fibrous tissue. The overlying epithelium atrophies into only one cell layer and may become keratinized.

The limbal form of vernal keratoconjunctivitis shows essentially the same features as the palpebral form: cellular infiltration (most notably with eosinophils), fibrous tissue hyperplasia, hyaline degeneration, and epithelial proliferation. Fibrous tissue hyperplasia is less evident in the limbal form than in the palpebral form, where epithelial proliferation is more prominent. This accounts for the gelatinous character of the limbal lesions.

The vernal or shield ulcer consists of fibrin deposits adherent to Bowman's layer.[30]

Pathogenesis

Although the cause of vernal keratoconjunctivitis is unclear, evidence indicates that a type I hypersensitivity reaction plays a major role.[18,31,32] The cellular histopathology, however, suggests that other concurrent mechanisms may contribute. The atopic (IgE-mediated, type I reaction) nature of vernal keratoconjunctivitis is supported by the following:

1. Seasonal occurrence of the disease
2. Frequent personal and family history of atopy
3. Serum antibodies to environmental allergens in the majority of patients[14,15,32-34]
4. Positive skin tests to bacteria and fungi in 50 percent and 42 percent of patients, respectively[13]
5. Nearly universal local eosinophilia and frequent systemic eosinophilia[35]
6. Accumulations of conjunctival T cells showing helper functions for IgE synthesis[36]
7. Elevated serum levels of IgE and increased tear levels of IgE in some patients[16,33-38]
8. Elevated tear histamine levels[39-41] and elevated eosinophilic granule major basic protein in both tears[42] and conjunctival biopsy specimens[43] of acute cases
9. Conformance of animal models of vernal keratoconjunctivitis to a type I hypersensitivity reaction[44]
10. Alleviation of symptoms with topical agents that prevent mast cell degranulation[45-51]

Certain features of vernal keratoconjunctivitis, however, are not consistent with a type I reaction alone. Zavaro et al[16] found that 20 percent of patients with typical clinical findings had normal tear IgE levels and lacked any eosinophilic reaction. The preponderance of basophils and the reactive proliferation of fibroblasts and capillaries in the involved conjunctiva are suggestive of a type IV (cell-mediated) hypersensitivity reaction. Butrus et al[52] described three cases of vernal keratoconjunctivitis occurring in young patients with hyper-IgE syndrome (which is characterized by a severe deficiency of suppressor T cells and elevated levels of IgE). Such an association may indicate a T-cell–mediated immunologic mechanism (type IV, cell-mediated response) in the pathogenesis of this disorder.[19] Furthermore, subtype analysis of hyperplastic mast cell populations in the conjunctivas of patients with vernal conjunctivitis revealed an increased proportion of cells containing tryptase, but not chymase. These cells are thought to be T-cell dependent.[53] The possible relationship between suppressor T cells and serum IgE levels is discussed further in the section on atopic keratoconjunctivitis.

Diagnosis

Typical vernal keratoconjunctivitis (consisting of bilateral itching, giant papillae on the superior tarsal conjunctiva, and gelatinous hypertrophy of the limbal conjunctiva) is easy to diagnose. Laboratory tests are generally unnecessary, although tear tryptase levels may be used to monitor efficacy of therapy.[7] The difficulty arises in differentiating more subtle cases of this disorder from allergic conjunctivitis, atopic keratoconjunctivitis, trachoma, and giant papillary conjunctivitis (Table 23-1).

Similarly to vernal keratoconjunctivitis, allergic conjunctivitis may present with itching. Furthermore, the two disorders usually display a similar seasonal occurrence. However, the papillae in allergic conjunctivitis are much smaller, and chemosis is a prominent finding. The limbal and corneal changes that may be seen in vernal keratoconjunctivitis are not part of allergic conjunctivitis. Additionally, the concomitant nasal involvement in allergic conjunctivitis is not usually seen in vernal keratoconjunctivitis.

The salient differences between vernal keratoconjunctivitis and atopic keratoconjunctivitis are outlined by Smolin

TABLE 23-1
Features of Atopic Conjunctivitides

Disorder	*Superior Tarsus*	*Corneal Involvement*	*Other Features*	*Causes*
Vernal keratoconjunctivitis	Giant papillae	Limbal thickening, epithelial keratitis, fibrovascular pannus, Trantas dots, shield ulcer	Seasonal occurrence, other atopic diseases, children, young adults	Airborne antigens?
Allergic conjunctivitis	Papillae	None	Seasonal	Airborne antigens?
Atopic keratoconjunctivitis	Papillae, hyperemia, scarring	Epithelial keratitis, fibrovascular pannus, ulcerations	Dermatitis, cataract, hereditary, perennial (keratoconus)	Idiopathic
Giant papillary conjunctivitis	Giant papillae	None	Perennial	Foreign body

and O'Connor.[1] Vernal keratoconjunctivitis is a seasonal disorder, compared to atopic keratoconjunctivitis, which tends to be perennial. Vernal keratoconjunctivitis predominantly affects children and adolescents, whereas atopic keratoconjunctivitis affects adolescents and young adults. The conjunctival discharge in vernal keratoconjunctivitis is characteristically ropy and white, whereas in atopic keratoconjunctivitis it is usually watery and clear. Clinically, vernal keratoconjunctivitis exhibits giant papillae and involves primarily the superior tarsal conjunctiva; atopic keratoconjunctivitis is characterized by small papillae and affects predominantly the inferior forniceal and tarsal conjunctivas. Conjunctival scarring and contracture occur rarely in vernal keratoconjunctivitis, but are seen more frequently in severe cases of atopic keratoconjunctivitis.[54] The limbal gelatinous hypertrophy and cysts found in limbal vernal keratoconjunctivitis are not present in atopic keratoconjunctivitis. Trantas dots, which occur commonly in vernal keratoconjunctivitis, are rarely found in atopic keratoconjunctivitis. Vernal keratoconjunctivitis may have plaque-like (shield) superior corneal ulcers; this type of corneal ulceration is not a complication of atopic keratoconjunctivitis. The deep corneal neovascularization that occurs with severe atopic keratoconjunctivitis is rarely found in vernal keratoconjunctivitis. Conjunctival scrapings in vernal keratoconjunctivitis show an abundance of eosinophils and free eosinophilic granules. Both atopic keratoconjunctivitis and allergic conjunctivitis show fewer eosinophils and eosinophilic granules. Finally, atopic keratoconjunctivitis patients frequently have characteristic dermatologic changes that are not seen in vernal keratoconjunctivitis.

The early stages of trachoma (MacCallan classification, stage II) may be difficult to differentiate clinically from vernal keratoconjunctivitis, because both have a predilection for the superior tarsal conjunctiva and may manifest with a superior pannus and limbal pits. The presence of subconjunctival scarring, tarsal and limbal follicles, and the characteristic cellular morphology of conjunctival scrapings in trachoma help to differentiate this disease from vernal keratoconjunctivitis. Such scrapings may reveal neutrophils, lymphocytes, Leber's giant cells, and rarely, intracytoplasmic inclusion bodies in epithelial cells. Unlike in vernal keratoconjunctivitis, however, no eosinophils are found (see Ch. 14).

The differentiation between vernal keratoconjunctivitis and giant papillary conjunctivitis is usually evident from the history. Giant papillary conjunctivitis is associated with external ocular foreign bodies. Like vernal keratoconjunctivitis, it presents with itching, giant cobblestone papillae, and a ropy, white discharge. Unlike vernal keratoconjunctivitis, giant papillary conjunctivitis does not involve the cornea, although one case of limbal involvement has been reported.[55]

Treatment

In view of the tendency for vernal keratoconjunctivitis to be self-limited and to improve with a change in the season, treatment is directed toward reducing symptoms to tolerable levels rather than attempting to eradicate them altogether. Thus, patients should be instructed first to try general measures and then to use medications only if these measures are unsuccessful. Medications should be used in the smallest dosage and lowest frequency necessary to make symptoms bearable. Explanation of the risks and benefits of each drug, particularly topical corticosteroids, often results in improved patient cooperation with this therapeutic approach. Patients should also understand that treatment of vernal keratoconjunctivitis is palliative rather than curative.

Avoidance of known allergens and environmental irritants is the first measure in therapy. Permanent relocation to a cooler climate is the best, and sometimes the only effective therapy for vernal keratoconjunctivitis. If such a measure is not feasible, the patient's symptoms may be alleviated by maintaining a dust-free air-conditioned environment at home and at work. Patients should be instructed to minimize eye rubbing, as this may be associated with the development of keratoconus.

Desensitization appears to be of no significant clinical benefit. Cold compresses and periodic irrigation of the eyes with ice-cold saline or a weak alkaline solution, such as 8 percent monohydrated sodium carbonate, which tends to dissolve the ropy discharge, may provide temporary relief. When symptoms are secondary to corneal involvement, occlusive patching or a bandage soft contact lens may produce dramatic relief of symptoms and improvement of the keratitis.

Topical mucolytic agents such as acetylcysteine drops have been used to dissolve the discharge and thereby provide relief. The 10 percent solution is tolerated better than the 20 percent solution, although the drug itself may produce burning and stinging. Vasoconstrictors, such as naphazoline, reduce hyperemia and edema. They provide relief in mild cases of vernal keratoconjunctivitis but are ineffective in more severe cases. Topical antihistamines are of theoretical benefit in alleviating symptoms; however, their practical benefit is unproven and they may be irritating to the ocular surface. Oral antihistamines have no utility in the management of vernal keratoconjunctivitis.

Although its effects are variable, topical cromolyn sodium may alleviate symptoms and reduce the need for topical corticosteroids. Cromolyn sodium prevents the degranulation of mast cells by stabilizing the cell membranes.[45-51] Topical cromolyn sodium is most effective as a 4 percent solution, used four times daily.[49,51] Several weeks of uninterrupted use may be required before any beneficial effects are noted; therefore, the medication should be used continuously, even during periods of anticipated remission. Topical 0.1 percent lodoxamide, used four times daily, is a mast cell stabilizing agent approved for the treatment of vernal keratoconjunctivitis.

Topical corticosteroids provide the most effective and immediate relief of symptoms. Because of the side effects of chronic topical corticosteroid use and the young age of most patients with vernal keratoconjunctivitis, corticosteroids should be used in the lowest concentration and for the shortest period necessary. Pulse therapy, consisting of 1 percent prednisolone acetate or 0.1 percent dexamethasone sodium phosphate drops used every 2 hours for 1 week, followed by a rapid taper, usually alleviates symptoms sufficiently to permit control with nonsteroidal medications. Such pulse doses of topical corticosteroids may be required several times a year.

In severe cases of vernal keratoconjunctivitis, if topical corticosteroids prove inadequate or if the associated blepharospasm makes topical instillation impossible, a 2-week tapering course of oral corticosteroids may be helpful.[1] Other therapeutic agents reported to be effective in the treatment of vernal keratoconjunctivitis include aspirin[56] and topical cyclosporine.[57] In recalcitrant cases, cryosurgery of the affected palpebral conjunctiva may help ameliorate signs and symptoms.[58,59]

Shield ulcers are particularly difficult to treat. Sometimes vigorous scraping of the base of the ulcer combined with a bandage soft contact lens facilitates healing. It seems necessary both to rid Bowman's layer of the fibrin deposits and to lift the potentially abrasive tarsal conjunctival papillae off the ulcerated cornea as it heals. In particularly recalcitrant cases, a superficial keratectomy or excimer laser photoablation[60] may be necessary.

Giant Papillary Conjunctivitis

Giant papillary conjunctivitis (GPC) is an inflammatory reaction of the tarsal conjunctiva that has been associated with a variety of foreign bodies on the external ocular surface, including soft contact lenses,[61-63] hard contact lenses,[61,64,65] ocular prostheses,[66,67] extruded scleral buckles,[68] and exposed sutures after cataract extraction[69,70] or penetrating keratoplasty.[71] The condition was first noted by Spring[72] in 1974, and the complete syndrome was first described by Allansmith et al[61] in 1977.

Clinical Features

Patients with giant papillary conjunctivitis present with symptoms not unlike those of vernal keratoconjunctivitis: ocular itching and mucoid discharge. The degree of itching in giant papillary conjunctivitis is usually milder than that in vernal keratoconjunctivitis. Patients who wear contact lenses usually manifest some degree of lens intolerance, characterized by decreased wearing time and excessive lens movement.[61,72] In severe cases, patients may present with mechanical ptosis from the giant papillae.[64]

The clinical signs of giant papillary conjunctivitis are concentrated in the superior tarsal conjunctiva (Figure 23-7). By definition, the papillae are 1 mm or larger in diameter.[61] This results in a cobblestone appearance of the superior tarsal conjunctiva, much like that seen in the palpebral form of vernal keratoconjunctivitis. Visualization of the papillae can be enhanced by applying fluorescein to the tarsal surface and viewing it with the cobalt blue light of the slit lamp microscope. A ropy, whitish mucoid discharge is frequently found, usually concentrated in the inferior fornix and the nasal interpalpebral fissure.

Allansmith et al[61] outlined the progression of papillary changes in the superior tarsal conjunctiva of patients with

FIGURE 23-7 Giant papillary conjunctivitis caused by a soft contact lens.

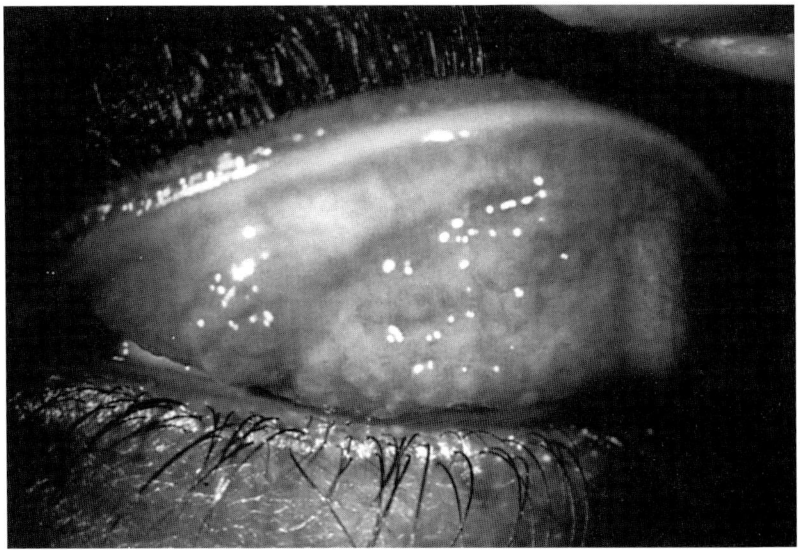

giant papillary conjunctivitis. In the earliest stages, small normal papillae become elevated and the conjunctiva thickens. As the disease progresses, the translucency of the conjunctiva is lost and the papillae become further elevated and enlarged. With further growth, the papillae eventually take on the classic flat top or cobblestone appearance. The spread of giant papillae, in most cases, appears to be from the superior tarsal border to the eyelid margin.[61,73] Of interest is the observation that the degree of symptoms varies among patients who have equivalent clinical signs.

Histopathology

The histopathologic findings of giant papillary conjunctivitis consist of a polymorphic infiltration in the affected conjunctiva.[61] Specifically, plasma cells, lymphocytes, mast cells, eosinophils, and basophils have been identified. The mast cells appear to be concentrated in the epithelium, whereas the eosinophils and basophils are found in both the epithelium and the substantia propria.[63] In specimens of tarsal conjunctiva from patients with either giant papillary conjunctivitis or vernal keratoconjunctivitis, the majority of mast cells are degranulated[27,28] and levels of eosinophil granule major basic protein are high.[43] Meisler et al[66] noted IgE-containing inflammatory cells in a biopsy specimen of tarsal conjunctiva from a patient with giant papillary conjunctivitis. These findings, as well as the observation that tear immunoglobulins (especially IgE) and tryptase are elevated in giant papillary conjunctivitis,[73] are consistent with the hypothesis that this disorder, like vernal keratoconjunctivitis, is a combination of an IgE-mediated, type I, immediate hypersensitivity reaction and a cell-mediated, type IV, delayed hypersensitivity reaction.

Pathogenesis

The stimuli for the giant papillary conjunctival reaction have been postulated as antigenic, secondary to proteins deposited on the foreign body. In a series of contact lens wearers,[61] lens deposits were noted in all of the patients who developed giant papillary conjunctivitis. However, the observation that not all patients with lens deposits develop this syndrome indicates that the individual response to these proteins is of primary importance. Mechanical trauma to conjunctival cells has been implicated as a likely stimulus for heightened neutrophil chemotactic activity, although specific chemotactic agents have yet to be identified.[75] Giant papillary conjunctivitis seems to be far more common with soft contact lens wear than with polymethyl methacrylate or rigid gas-permeable contact lens wear.

Diagnosis

Although giant papillary conjunctivitis presents a clinical picture similar to that of vernal keratoconjunctivitis, there are some important differences.[76] Patients with giant papillary conjunctivitis present with a milder degree of symptoms than do patients with vernal keratoconjunctivitis; furthermore, symptoms of giant papillary conjunctivitis usually respond rapidly to removal of the external ocular foreign body. Patients with giant papillary conjunctivitis do not have the atopic history commonly associated with vernal keratoconjunctivitis. Also, the seasonal nature of vernal keratoconjunctivitis is absent in giant papillary conjunctivitis. Finally, giant papillary conjunctivitis rarely involves the limbus[55] and does not show the corneal complications of vernal keratoconjunctivitis.

Treatment

The primary treatment for giant papillary conjunctivitis is removal of the foreign body. Symptoms may also be ameliorated by the use of topical cromolyn sodium.[77] In contact lens wearers, it is best to remove the lens, initiate topical treatment if symptoms persist, and begin again with a new lens once the symptoms have resolved. The morphologic appearance of the papillae may last for many months, even after symptoms have resolved. A trial of contact lens wear does not necessarily require that the papillae be gone. Proper lens hygiene is important in preventing protein buildup on the lens and exacerbation of giant papillary conjunctivitis. The recurrence rate may be less with disposable contact lenses, especially daily disposable contact lenses. Occasionally, the patient may have to switch to hard or rigid gas-permeable contact lenses.

Atopic Keratoconjunctivitis

Atopic dermatitis is a common, hereditary disorder that begins early in childhood and usually runs a chronic course.[78-80] In addition to characteristic skin changes, patients with atopic dermatitis may also have asthma, hay fever, urticaria, migraine headaches, and rhinitis. Additionally, atopic dermatitis is associated with a variety of ocular surface and lenticular abnormalities. Perhaps the common ectodermal origin of these ocular structures and the skin, as well as the close proximity between the ocular surface and the eyelid skin, explains this association.[81]

The association between atopic dermatitis and ocular surface disorders was first recognized by Hogan in 1953.[82] He described five similar cases of a distinct "keratoconjunctivitis" in male atopic dermatitis patients between the ages of 29 and 47 years. Ocular involvement in atopic dermatitis has an incidence of approximately 25 percent,[54,83] and usually develops many years after the onset of other atopic symptoms.[84] In most patients, the clinical signs of atopic keratoconjunctivitis improve with age and may even totally regress. Severe cases persist into later life.

Clinical Features

The symptoms of atopic keratoconjunctivitis are usually perennial, and may be worse in winter. Atopic keratoconjunctivitis is invariably bilateral. Affected patients note itching as the most prominent symptom. Other complaints include burning, tearing, and a clear or slightly mucoid discharge.

In atopic keratoconjunctivitis, the eyelid skin is scaly, indurated, excessively wrinkled, and inflamed; the process results in a leather-like appearance and consistency. Excessive tearing and rubbing may result in skin fissures at the lateral canthus, as well as excoriations of the eyelid skin. The eyelid margins are thickened and injected, with abundant crusting. Staphylococcal infections are frequent in patients with atopic dermatitis, and staphylococcal colonization of the eyelid margins is nearly universal.[85,86] Thus, atopic eyelid margin disease with superimposed bacterial infection may produce an ulcerative blepharitis.

Although hyperemia may be present, the conjunctiva in atopic keratoconjunctivitis is usually pale, with papillary hypertrophy of the superior and inferior tarsal regions.[1,54,85,86] Such papillary reactions may also involve the perilimbal conjunctiva and result in gelatinous limbal nodules. During acute exacerbations, the conjunctiva becomes hyperemic and chemotic, and has a distinctive, purplish-gray, smooth appearance. With severe and prolonged ocular surface involvement, contracture and scarring of the conjunctiva, especially in the inferior fornix, can occur. Symblephara can occur; one study noted this association in 27 percent of cases.[84]

The earliest corneal involvement in atopic keratoconjunctivitis is punctate epithelial keratitis confined in some cases to the inferior third of the cornea.[84,86] Chronic atopic keratoconjunctivitis may result in superficial and deep vascularization of the limbus and peripheral cornea, which is frequently accompanied by peripheral stromal scarring (Figure 23-8). In rare cases, the entire cornea may be involved by pannus formation and stromal vascularization.[82] Most of the corneal changes in atopic keratoconjunctivitis are secondary to keratinized eyelid margins. If the eyelid margins can be improved or kept off the cornea with a bandage soft contact lens in the early stages of the disease, the cornea will improve. Other reported corneal findings include intraepithelial microcysts, pseudogerontotoxon, Trantas limbal dots, indolent ovoid ulcers, marginal ulcers (infectious and sterile), and clear limbal epithelial inclusion cysts.[1,54,85,86] In addition, the cornea may be secondarily involved by entropion and trichiasis or by ocular surface infections. In one series, herpes simplex viral keratitis was found in 13 percent of patients with atopic keratoconjunctivitis.[84] There is an association between atopic dermatitis and keratoconus[84,87] (see Ch. 22). The keratoconus usually develops in young adulthood, after years of severe atopic disease. Intolerance of contact lenses because of the accompanying keratoconjunctivitis makes optical correction in these keratoconus patients particularly difficult.

Approximately 8 percent of all patients with atopic keratoconjunctivitis have characteristic lenticular changes.[84,88,89] The earliest opacities occur in the posterior subcapsular region and are polychromatic; later, anterior subcapsular opacities may occur. The latter are polygonal plaques, commonly referred to as shield cataracts. The lens opacities are usually bilateral, begin in adoles-

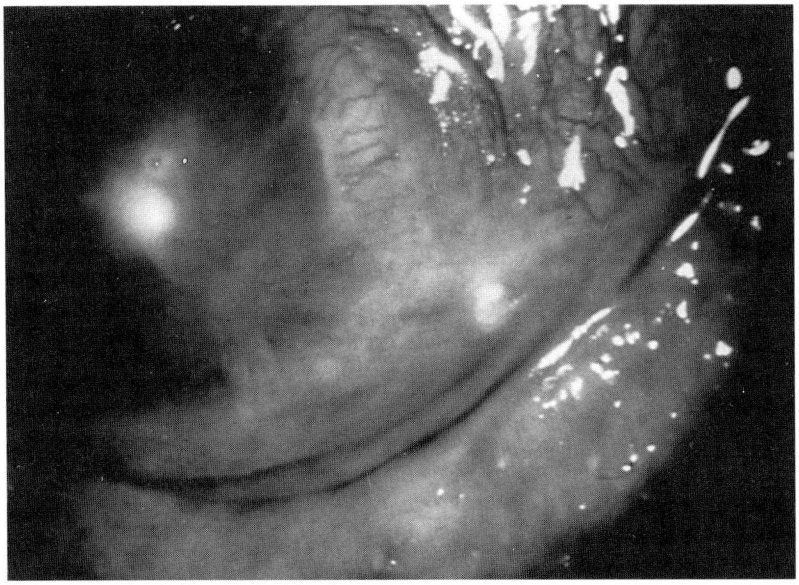

FIGURE 23-8 Corneal vascularization and scarring as a result of atopic keratoconjunctivitis.

cence, and tend to progress slowly. Chronic corticosteroid administration may accelerate cataract progression in these patients. An increased incidence of retinal detachment after cataract extraction in atopic dermatitis patients has been reported.[88,90] The cause of this phenomenon is not clear, but may be related to a mechanical origin, such as vigorous postoperative eye rubbing.

Laboratory Findings

Conjunctival scrapings in atopic keratoconjunctivitis demonstrate primarily eosinophils.[82] The number of eosinophils, however, is less than that seen in vernal keratoconjunctivitis. Furthermore, the free eosinophilic granules that are commonly found in vernal keratoconjunctivitis are not seen in atopic keratoconjunctivitis.[25] Mast cells are rarely noted in scrapings from patients with atopic keratoconjunctivitis. Elevated levels of serum and tear IgE,[91,92] as well as serum eosinophilia,[82] characteristically occur during exacerbations of atopic keratoconjunctivitis. During remissions, serum IgE levels usually decrease.[93]

Pathogenesis

The aforementioned findings (associated atopic disorders, local and systemic eosinophilia, and elevated tear and systemic IgE concentrations) provide evidence that atopic keratoconjunctivitis is caused, at least in part, by a type I hypersensitivity reaction. However, as in vernal keratoconjunctivitis, some of the immunologic findings implicate a cell-mediated, type IV hypersensitivity reaction.[94-100] In acute attacks of atopic keratoconjunctivitis, the level of B cells is elevated, while the level of T cells is depressed.[98] Additionally, atopic dermatitis patients manifest evidence of abnormal T-cell function,[97,99] which may account for their tendency to develop infections.[97] T cells, particularly suppressor T cells, regulate IgE production; the number of these circulating cells is inversely proportional to the serum IgE concentration. Gottlieb and Hanifin[98] suggest that in atopic dermatitis, the number of circulating suppressor T cells may be sufficiently decreased to allow interruption of the normal inhibitory controls on serum IgE production. This, in turn, may play a role in the development of atopy, since IgE regulates mast cell degranulation and histamine release. On the subcellular level, evidence suggests that atopic dermatitis may result from phosphodiesterase-mediated abnormalities in leukocytic cyclic AMP (cAMP).[100,101]

Treatment

The treatment of atopic keratoconjunctivitis, like that of vernal keratoconjunctivitis, is primarily symptomatic. Cold compresses and topical vasoconstrictors and antihistamines may help during acute exacerbations. Patients should be encouraged to avoid eyelid rubbing, which tends to perpetuate the itching cycle. Topical corticosteroids afford dramatic relief of symptoms; however, they must be used with caution because atopic keratoconjunctivitis patients tend to develop cataracts and are susceptible to ocular surface infections (particularly herpes simplex viral keratitis). Topical cromolyn sodium (4 percent) is beneficial in controlling severe symptoms.[54,102,103] As with vernal keratoconjunctivitis, patients with atopic keratoconjunctivitis can be treated chronically with cromolyn sodium; topical corticosteroids should be reserved for episodes of acute exacerbation.

Bandage soft contact lenses are useful in treating corneal changes caused by abnormal eyelid margins. Keratoepithelioplasty (transplantation of donor limbal epithelium) has not proven to be successful for those with serious superficial keratopathy.[104]

BULLOUS OCULOCUTANEOUS DISEASES

The ocular surface may be involved in a variety of immunologic disorders that produce bullous lesions of the skin and mucous membranes. That the ocular surface epithelial cells should be involved is not surprising, considering the immunochemical similarities between mucosal epithelium and cutaneous epidermis.[105] In particular, the epidermal antigens (pemphigus antigen, pemphigoid antigen, laminin, and type IV collagen) have all been demonstrated in squamous epithelial cells. The diseases that affect both skin and mucosal surfaces include cicatricial pemphigoid, bullous pemphigoid, dermatitis herpetiformis, pemphigus vulgaris, Stevens-Johnson syndrome, Lyell's disease, and Reiter syndrome.

Cicatricial Pemphigoid

Cicatricial pemphigoid (also referred to as benign mucous membrane pemphigoid, essential shrinkage of the conjunctiva, chronic cicatrizing conjunctivitis, or retracting conjunctivitis) is a presumed autoimmune disorder of unknown cause that affects a variety of mucosal surfaces and is believed to result from a type II hypersensitivity reaction.[106] Ocular involvement frequently results in severe surface changes that can cause significant visual impairment.

Cicatricial pemphigoid is chronic in nature and primarily affects patients over 60 years of age.[107–109] Women are affected twice as often as men. The basic lesions in cicatricial pemphigoid consist of subepithelial bullae without acantholysis; the bullae eventually are replaced by cicatrizing connective tissue, resulting in mucosal shrinkage. Ocular involvement occurs in the majority of patients with cicatricial pemphigoid. In a review of 65 such patients, 34 percent presented with ocular symptoms, whereas 88 percent had signs of cicatrizing conjunctival changes.[110] The oral mucosa is similarly involved in about 50 percent of patients.[109,111] Other less commonly affected sites include the nasal, esophageal, anal, and genital mucosae. Skin lesions are noted in fewer than 50 percent of all cicatricial pemphigoid patients; the head and neck are the most frequently involved cutaneous sites.

Clinical Features

Clinically, ocular cicatricial pemphigoid is characterized by a chronic progressive course.[112] At first, the disease may be unilateral; eventually, both eyes are affected, although the severity may remain markedly asymmetrical.

In the early stages, cicatricial pemphigoid presents as repeated episodes of mild to moderate conjunctival inflammation.[111–113] Conjunctival vascular injection, papillae formation, chemosis, and occasionally, ulcerations and vesicles are noted. Although bullae are frequently seen in the skin and mucous membrane areas, they are rarely apparent in the conjunctiva. In the earliest phases, shortening of the inferior fornix occurs. Concurrently, fine subepithelial scarring of the tarsal conjunctiva may be noted (Figure 23-9). Any elderly patient with a chronic, indolent conjunctivitis should be carefully examined for evidence of this early subepithelial scarring.

As the disease progresses, the chronic conjunctivitis continues and is unresponsive to topical lubricants, antibiotics, antivirals, and corticosteroids.[106–108,110–114] The fine subepithelial scar tissue enlarges, contracts, and leads to gradual shortening of the inferior fornix. The relentless scarring of the conjunctiva has its most untoward effects on the tear film. First, the bulbar conjunctiva is affected by a loss of goblet cells,[115,116] which results in a severe deficiency in the mucin layer of the tear film.[117] Later, the aqueous layer may be compromised by cicatrization of the lacrimal gland ducts.[107] The combined mucin and aqueous deficiencies result in xerosis and keratinization of the conjunctiva and frequently, the cornea. In addition, it has been suggested that lipid abnormalities in the tear film secondary to keratinization of the meibomian glands result in rapid break-up time and evaporation of the tear film.

The cornea is affected not only by the tear film abnormalities but also by the typical eyelid changes.[114] The progressive cicatrizing conjunctivitis characteristically leads to symblephara and entropion (Figure 23-10). The corneal epithelium may then be compromised by the resultant trichiasis and in severe cases, exposure keratopathy. The combination of an abnormal tear film, trichiasis, and exposure predisposes the cornea to keratinization, vascularization, chronic epithelial defects, sterile stromal melts, infectious ulcerations, and perforation (Figure 23-11).

Foster et al[113] catalogued the clinical courses of a large series of patients and subsequently described four clinical stages of ocular cicatricial pemphigoid. In stage 1, there is conjunctival inflammation, mucoid discharge, rose bengal staining of the conjunctiva, and subtle conjunctival subepithelial fibrosis. Stage 2 is marked by the onset of conjunctival shrinkage, most notably in the inferior fornix. Stage 3 consists of more advanced shrinkage, symblephara, keratopathy, corneal vascularization, trichiasis, and tear film abnormalities. Stage 4, marking end-stage disease, consists of severe keratoconjunctivitis sicca, keratinization, and ankyloblepharon.

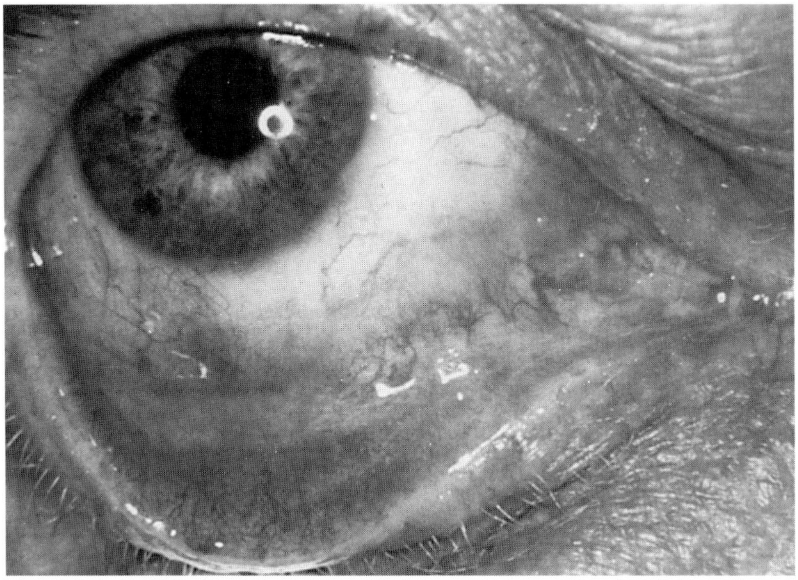

FIGURE 23-9 Early pemphigoid shows scarring of the conjunctiva.

Mondino[109] reported that the percentage of eyes that progress in disease severity increases with stages 2 and 3, relative to stage 1.

Histopathology

The histopathologic appearance of conjunctival biopsy specimens from patients with active cicatricial pemphigoid reveals a variety of changes. Subepithelial bullae are common in nonconjunctival areas.[108] The epithelium and substantia propria show a chronic inflammatory response, with lymphocytes and plasma cells predominating.[118] A decrease in the density of goblet cells is characteristic.[114,115] In more advanced cases, there is metaplasia of the conjunctival (and even corneal) epithelium to a parakeratinized or keratinized state.[119] Thoft et al[120] noted an increase in mitosis in the conjunctival epithelium. Subepithelial fibrosis leads clinically to conjunctival shrinkage. In tissue culture, conjunctival fibroblasts from patients with cicatricial pemphigoid are hyperproliferative, compared with normal controls.[121] Ultrastructural studies demonstrate a marked increase in desmosomes in the conjunctival epithelial cells, which is evidence for altered interepithelial adhesions.[122,123] Galbavy and Foster[124] noted a comparative decrease in these desmosomal changes in

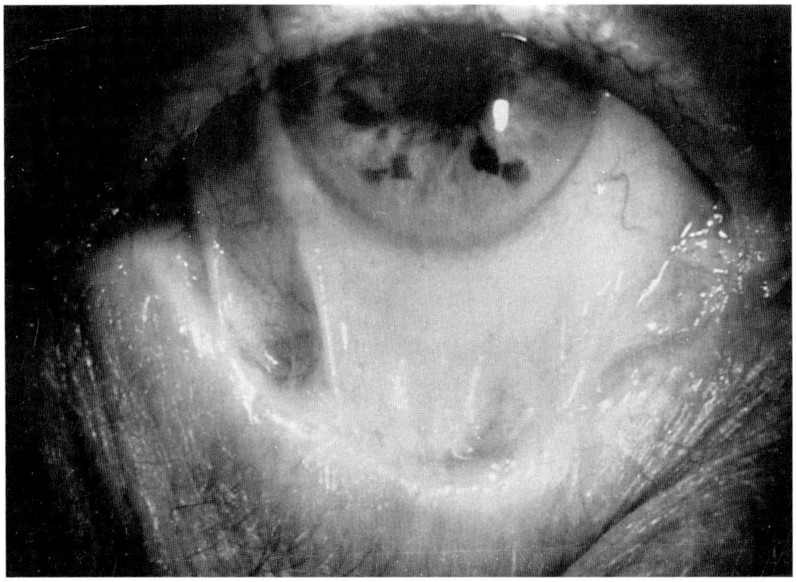

FIGURE 23-10 Advanced pemphigoid shows marked symblephara formation and shortening of the inferior fornix.

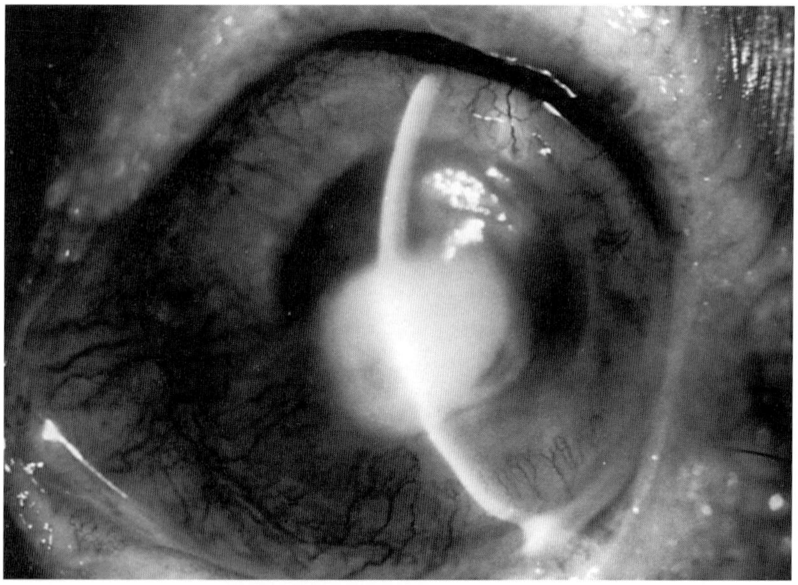

FIGURE 23-11 Corneal ulcer in a patient with pemphigoid. Note the peripheral corneal vascularization caused by dry eyes and trichiasis.

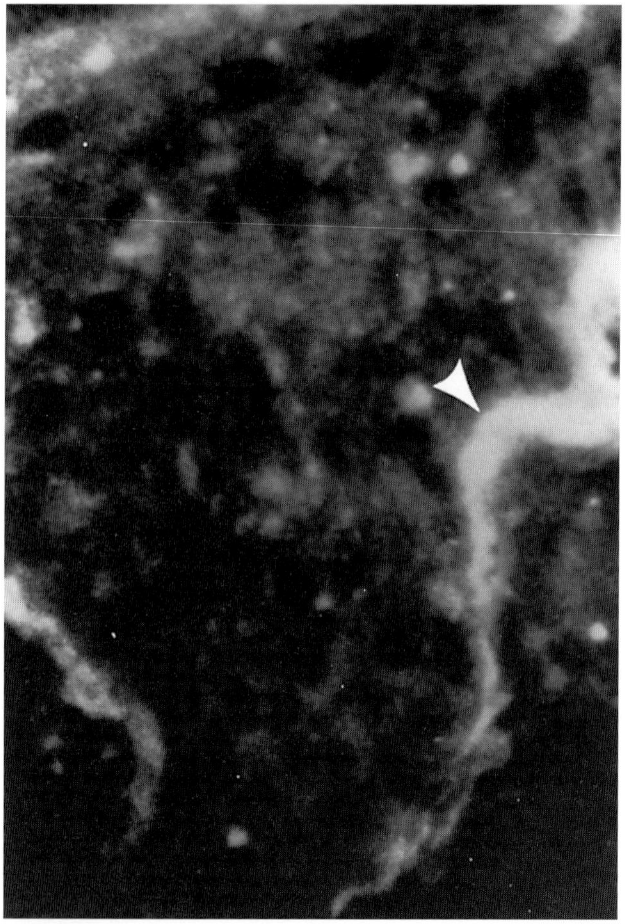

FIGURE 23-12 Direct immunofluorescence staining of a conjunctival biopsy specimen from a patient with pemphigoid demonstrating deposition of anti-basement-membrane zone antibodies and complement (arrowhead).

patients who had undergone successful immunosuppressive therapy. Additional changes observed in the conjunctival epithelium include duplication and thickening of the basal lamina, as well as thickening of the lamina propria and cellular infiltration. Scanning electron microscopic examination shows that ocular surface mucus is abnormally thickened in patients with active ocular cicatricial pemphigoid.[125]

Pathogenesis

Although the exact pathogenesis of cicatricial pemphigoid is unknown, all of the available evidence implicates some abnormality in the immunoregulatory system.[108,110–114,125–139] Although some of this evidence implicates cell-mediated mechanisms,[138,139] the classic immunopathologic finding in cicatricial pemphigoid is a deposition of immunoglobulins and/or complement components along the basement membrane zone of the affected mucosal epithelium[126–128,131,136,137] (Figure 23-12). Although IgG has been identified most frequently, IgA and IgM commonly occur.[108,127,136] The deposition of anti-basement-membrane zone antibodies and complement is usually linear and has been observed in 64 to 84 percent of biopsy specimens.[137] A case of granular deposition of IgA and complement has been reported.[136] This granular nature is more typical of immune complex (antigen-antibody-complement) deposition. One important observation is that circulating anti-basement-membrane zone antibodies are uncommon in cicatricial pemphigoid.[129,131,134] This is in contrast to bullous pemphigoid, which is a related blistering disorder that affects the skin more than the mucosal surfaces, and in which circulating anti-basement-membrane zone antibodies are the rule.[108] However, other circulating immunologic abnormalities can occur in cicatricial pemphigoid. In one series, anti-nuclear antibodies were noted in two-thirds of the patients.[129] Mondino et al[130] reported a decrease in both the percentage and absolute numbers of T and B cells in a large series of patients.

The immunologic abnormalities of cicatricial pemphigoid appear to be indicative of an autoimmune attack against the basal epithelial cells. Supporting this hypothesis is an animal model of cicatricial pemphigoid created by injecting the autoantibodies of bullous pemphigoid intrastromally in rabbit corneas.[135] However, there is not universal agreement on the sequence of immunologic events that causes cicatricial pemphigoid.

Diagnosis

The diagnosis of cicatricial pemphigoid is best made by observing the typical clinical findings of progressive conjunctival shrinkage. Serial photography of patients in primary gaze, upgaze, and downgaze is helpful for documenting progression. Mondino and Brown[133] described a grading system for conjunctival forniceal shrinkage: stage 0, no shrinkage; stage 1, shrinkage of 25 percent or less; stage 2, 25 to 50 percent shrinkage; stage 3, approximately 75 percent shrinkage; stage 4, total obliteration of the fornix. In advanced cases, the diagnosis is not difficult. However, in early cases, the clinical signs may be subtle. Any elderly patient with chronic conjunctivitis should be examined carefully for the early stages of subepithelial fibrosis; additionally, the skin and oral mucosa should be carefully examined. Cellulose acetate filter paper impression cytologic study of the conjunctival epithelium may help to confirm the diagnosis.[140] Immunopathologic examination of a conjunctival biopsy may demonstrate anti-basement-membrane zone antibodies and complement. However, a conjunctival biopsy (as well as other types of conjunctival surgery) may exacerbate disease activity, and is rarely indicated clinically. If a conjunctival biopsy is done, the risk of postoperative symblepharon formation may be minimized by taking a specimen of bulbar conjunctiva adjacent to the limbus instead of forniceal conjunctiva.[113] Alternatively, biopsy of any clinically uninvolved bulbar conjunctiva can be performed, with direct immunofluorescence staining of the specimen serving as a useful, but not absolute, diagnostic marker for the disease. Whether this technique also minimizes postoperative symblepharon formation is unclear.[141]

Cicatricial pemphigoid must be differentiated from a variety of disorders that can cause cicatrizing conjunctivitis. Bullous pemphigoid is a similar subepithelial cicatrizing disorder characterized by vesicular cutaneous lesions.[108] This disorder also primarily affects elderly patients; however, unlike cicatricial pemphigoid, there is no sex predilection. Additionally, mucosal involvement is uncommon and circulating anti-basement-membrane zone antibodies are usually found in bullous pemphigoid. A related vesicular disorder is dermatitis herpetiformis, which is characterized by a severe pruritic rash and infrequent mucosal involvement.

Other causes of cicatrizing conjunctivitis include chemical burns, radiation exposure, inflammatory bowel syndromes, adenovirus type 19 keratoconjunctivitis, β-hemolytic streptococcal conjunctivitis, and diphtherial conjunctivitis.[110,133] The cicatrization in these cases is generally nonprogressive, unlike that in cicatricial pemphigoid. Stevens-Johnson syndrome can also cause cicatrizing conjunctivitis; however, it is usually associated with an inciting agent, has associated typical skin lesions, and occurs in younger age groups. Additionally, several drugs produce pseudopemphigoid, a clinical picture identical to cicatricial pemphigoid.[110,142–155] These drugs include systemic practolol and topical epinephrine, echothiophate, pilocarpine, D-penicillamine, and idoxuridine. Pouliquen et al[147] demonstrated that the histopathologic and ultrastructural changes in cases of pseudopemphigoid were identical to those described in classic cicatricial pemphigoid. Kremer et al[156] observed intercellular immunoglobulin staining in the conjunctival epithelium in a patient with pseudopemphigoid.

Treatment

The treatment of cicatricial pemphigoid is difficult and frequently frustrating. These patients, in the early phases of their disease, are typically treated with a variety of topical agents (antibiotics, antivirals, and corticosteroids) for chronic conjunctivitis, all of which prove ineffective. Furthermore, topical corticosteroid treatment has been recognized as a risk factor in the development of microbial keratitis in these patients.[157] The primary goal of therapy is to inhibit the progression of conjunctival shrinkage. Other therapeutic goals include supplementation of the tear film, restoration of the normal eyelid-ocular surface anatomic relationship, and maintenance or re-establishment of a clear central cornea.

In 1971, Hardy et al[148] demonstrated that high-dose systemic corticosteroids effectively slow the rate of conjunctival cicatrization. The mucosal shrinkage, although slowed, does progress, however. In the mid-1970s, cyclophosphamide and azathioprine were first reported to be successful adjuncts to systemic corticosteroid therapy.[149–151] This initial experience was confirmed by Foster et al,[113] who noted cessation of inflammation and cicatrization in 14 of 15 patients treated with either cyclophosphamide or azathioprine in addition to prednisone. Mondino and Brown[133] evaluated immunosuppressive therapy in 57 patients. They noted that, although immunosuppression inhibited conjunctival shrinkage in the majority of patients, some cases eventually progressed despite therapy. They agreed that immunosuppressive agents were necessary therapeutic adjuncts; however, they recommended that because of the severity of potential side effects associated with these agents (alopecia, hemorrhagic cystitis, gastrointestinal distress, severe leukopenia, pulmonary fibrosis), immunosuppressive agents should be used only in patients with at least stage 2 cicatrization who have documented progression.

More recently, Tauber et al[158] reviewed the records of patients with ocular cicatricial pemphigoid treated with three different agents: diaminodiphenylsulfone (dapsone), cyclophosphamide, or azathioprine. They found that in patients with mild to moderate inflammation, dapsone had the lowest therapeutic failure rate, whereas in patients with intense inflammation, cyclophosphamide had the lowest therapeutic failure rate. Dapsone is relatively nontoxic, and seems safer than systemic corticosteroids or immunosuppressive agents; the main side effects are hemolysis and gastrointestinal complaints.[158–161] Dapsone should not be given to patients with glucose-6-phosphate dehydrogenase deficiency or a history of sulfa allergy. The mode of action of dapsone is unknown, but appears to be inhibition of migration of polymorphonuclear leukocytes.

There is a report documenting successful therapy of bullous pemphigoid and pemphigus vulgaris using cyclosporine[152]; however, its use in ocular cicatricial pemphigoid has been disappointing.[159]

Long-term follow-up of ocular cicatricial pemphigoid patients treated with various therapeutic agents has shown that approximately one-third of patients respond to therapy and remain free of inflammation (at least temporarily) after cessation of therapy, one-third remain free of inflammation as long as they continue to receive therapy, and one-third respond only partially to therapy.[159] A significantly higher rate of corneal infections has been reported in cicatricial pemphigoid patients whose disease has not been controlled with systemic immunosuppressive therapy.[157]

Patients with cicatricial pemphigoid should be aggressively treated with artificial tear preparations and lubricating ointments. Bandage soft contact lenses are an important management option in keratoconjunctivitis sicca, entropion, and trichiasis.[153] Because of the severe abnormalities of the tear film and ocular surface, patients are at high risk of corneal infections; the use of contact lenses increases this risk. The diagnosis and treatment of a potential infectious keratitis should, therefore, be pursued aggressively.

In general, eyelid or conjunctival surgery should not be performed unless absolutely necessary, because the trauma of surgery often seems to reactivate the disease, resulting in worse eyelid abnormalities and symblephara than were originally present. Therefore, eyelid or conjunctival abnormalities should not be treated surgically simply because they are there. If they result in incomplete eyelid closure or trichiasis, and are causing corneal disease that is threatening vision or the integrity of the globe, surgery is justified. Such surgery should be performed when the disease is relatively quiescent, if possible. Sometimes cicatricial pemphigoid is so asymmetrical that a tarsorrhaphy on the worse eye can relieve symptoms. The surgical correction of cicatricial eyelid abnormalities is discussed further in Chapter 6.

The treatment of end-stage corneal disease in patients with cicatricial pemphigoid is fraught with disaster. Because of ocular surface abnormalities, transplanted corneas fare no better than the patient's own cornea, making the prognosis for successful penetrating keratoplasty dismal.[162] Penetrating keratoplasty is useful only if the disease has become inactive, the eye is moist, and there are no eyelid abnormalities that will damage the corneal epithelium. Prosthokeratoplasty is the only hope for visual rehabilitation in many of these patients with end-stage disease (see Ch. 36).

Bullous Pemphigoid

Bullous pemphigoid is a blistering dermatosis that primarily affects the elderly and shows no sex predilection. Like cicatricial pemphigoid, the lesions in bullous pemphigoid consist of subepithelial bullae that eventually undergo replacement by scar tissue.[108] In contrast to cicatricial pemphigoid, as classically described, bullous pemphigoid nearly always affects the skin and rarely affects the mucous membranes.[154]

The characteristic immunopathologic abnormality of bullous pemphigoid consists of linear deposition of IgG and complement along the basement membrane zone of the epidermis or mucosal epithelium.[107,161] Additionally, the majority of patients demonstrate circulating anti-basement-membrane zone antibodies.[161,163,164] A subgroup of patients has been reported with a lower frequency of circulating antibodies and a higher incidence of mucosal involvement.[108] Furthermore, a British study[165] seeking to distinguish clinical bullous pemphigoid from cicatricial pemphigoid found mucous membrane involvement in 58 percent of patients with bullous pemphigoid, with fine conjunctival scarring sometimes present, and even frank symblephara in one patient. These findings emphasize the probability that bullous pemphigoid and cicatricial pemphigoid are parts of a spectrum of autoimmune subepithelial bullous diseases.

Treatment of bullous pemphigoid consists of oral corticosteroids,[166] immunosuppressive agents,[167,168] and sulfones.[169] Other effective approaches have been reported, including a combination of tetracycline and niacinamide,[155] plasmapheresis,[170] and cyclosporine.[151]

Dermatitis Herpetiformis

Dermatitis herpetiformis is another blistering dermatosis related to the pemphigoid disorders. Affected patients characteristically present with a pruritic erythematous or vesicular eruption distributed over the elbows, knees, and buttocks.[107] Patients frequently have an associated gluten enteropathy. Mucosal involvement in dermatitis herpetiformis, although uncommon, can produce an ophthalmic clinical picture similar to that of cicatricial pemphigoid.[110]

The characteristic immunopathologic finding in dermatitis herpetiformis is a granular deposition of anti-basement-membrane zone IgA. Treatment of dermatitis herpetiformis consists of oral sulfones.[110]

Pemphigus Vulgaris

Pemphigus vulgaris, or true pemphigus, is a chronic vesicular disease of the skin and mucous membranes. The primary lesions in pemphigus vulgaris are intraepithelial bullae that result from acantholysis of the epithelial cells.[166] Because of their intraepithelial location, these bullae are not replaced by fibrous tissue. Therefore, in pemphigus vulgaris the cutaneous and mucosal cicatrization characteristic of the pemphigoid disorders is not seen.

Pemphigus vulgaris is seen primarily in elderly men. The conjunctiva may be involved, along with the skin and other mucosal membranes. The resulting conjunctival bullae do not scar, and in contrast to pemphigoid, there are no long-term ocular surface complications.[171] The characteristic immunopathologic finding is circulating and fixed autoantibodies in the epithelial intercellular spaces.[111,171,172] Treatment of pemphigus vulgaris consists of oral corticosteroids or immunosuppressive agents. Cyclosporine has also been reported to be effective.[152]

Stevens-Johnson Syndrome

Stevens-Johnson syndrome, or erythema multiforme major, was first described in 1922.[173] It is an acute, potentially fatal, inflammatory vesiculobullous reaction of the skin and mucous membranes. Stevens-Johnson syndrome is commonly associated with an inciting drug or infectious agent, and most commonly occurs in children and young adults. Clinically, the hallmarks of the syndrome include fever, erythematous skin lesions, and inflammation of the mucous membranes, including the conjunctiva.

Clinical Features

In about one-half of the cases, Stevens-Johnson syndrome begins with a 1- to 14-day prodrome of fever, malaise, arthralgias, and symptoms of an upper respiratory infection.[174] Cutaneous and mucosal lesions then suddenly develop. Skin lesions consist of erythematous macules or papules, as well as vesicles; they usually develop symmetrically and diffusely, except on the scalp.[175-177] The trunk is usually spared, except in severe cases.[109] Hemorrhage into the vesicles produces the characteristic "iris" or "target" lesions.[178] Healing of the skin lesions occurs within days to weeks, and may result in scarring (Figure 23-13). Rarely, the skin of the eyelids may be involved. Other systemic complications include pneumonitis, septicemia, myocarditis, myositis, and glomerulonephritis.[108]

Mucosal involvement may include the conjunctiva, mouth, genitalia, and anus; the mouth is most commonly affected.[174,177] Characteristically, mucosal lesions are bullous and result in membrane or pseudomembrane formation with resultant cicatrization. The acute phase of Stevens-Johnson syndrome usually lasts from 2 to 6 weeks.[176,179] Unlike cicatricial pemphigoid, the disease is usually self-limited, but systemic manifestations occasionally can recur. A small set of Stevens-Johnson syndrome patients reported by Foster et al[180] displayed recurrent episodes of conjunctival inflammation unassociated with external aggravating factors or nonocular recurrent manifestations.

Acute ocular disease consists of a severe, bilateral, diffuse conjunctivitis that may be characterized as catarrhal, purulent, mucopurulent, hemorrhagic, membranous, pseudomembranous, or cicatrizing[175,176,181-184] (Figure 23-14). Ocular involvement occurs in 43 to 81 percent of patients, with 35 percent experiencing permanent visual sequelae.[175,183,185]

The chronic phases of Stevens-Johnson syndrome are the most difficult from the ophthalmic standpoint. The conjunctival inflammation frequently results in membranes, pseudomembranes, and cicatrization. There can be varying degrees of symblephara, entropion, trichiasis, tear film abnormalities, xerosis, keratinization, and corneal vascularization.[181,183] The resultant clinical picture can be similar to that of cicatricial pemphigoid, except that Stevens-Johnson syndrome usually does not actively progress after the acute phase. Tear film abnormalities may be of the aqueous or mucin varieties and result from cicatrization of the lacrimal ducts and destruction of the conjunctival goblet cells.[114,115,183]

The cornea can be affected by a combination of the tear film and eyelid abnormalities (Figure 23-15). The desiccation produced by the keratoconjunctivitis sicca commonly results in corneal pannus. Trichiasis may pro-

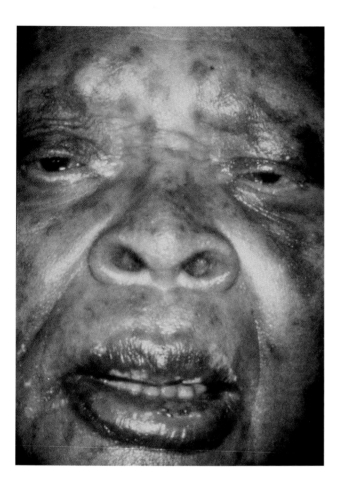

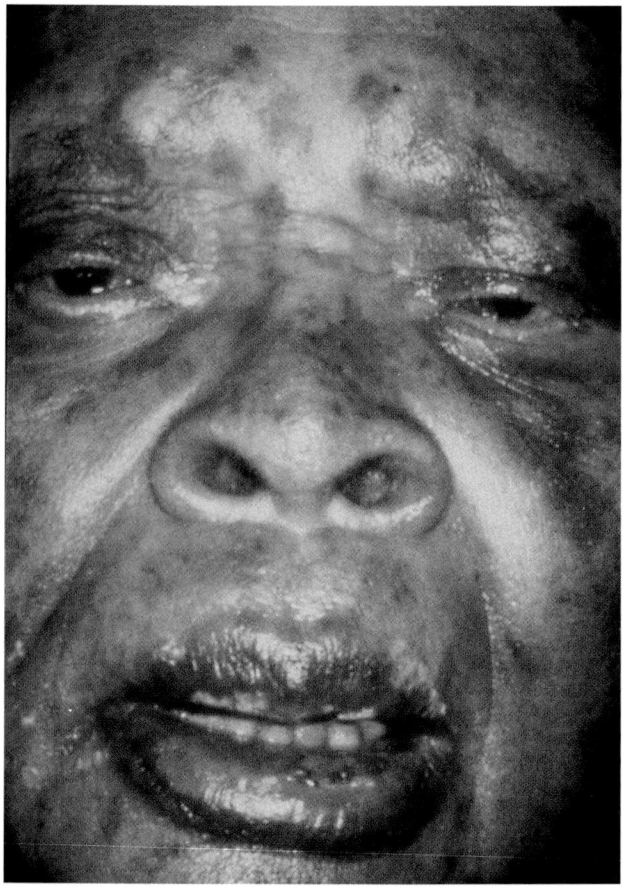

FIGURE 23-13 Scarring and depigmentation of the skin as a result of Stevens-Johnson syndrome.

duce corneal epithelial erosions and infections. The end result of these processes frequently involves varying degrees of corneal opacification, vascularization, keratinization, and thinning.

Histopathology

Histopathologically, the acute phase of Stevens-Johnson syndrome is characterized by nonspecific mononuclear cellular inflammation affecting the subepithelial layers of the skin and mucosa, including the conjunctiva.[186] An accompanying angiitis of the microvasculature in the affected areas is common. Conjunctival findings in the recurrent form include vasculitis, perivasculitis, immunoreactant deposition in vessel walls, vascular basement membrane anomalies, and a preponderance of helper T cells, macrophages, and Langerhans cells, none of which characterizes postacute Stevens-Johnson syndrome.[180] Cicatrization occurs in the affected mucosal tissues. In the conjunctiva, this subepithelial fibrosis may involve the lacrimal ducts. Additionally, the density of conjunctival goblet cells is decreased.[114]

Immunopathologic findings consist of the deposition of immune complexes in the microvasculature of the dermis and mucosal subepithelial tissues.[187] Additionally, circulating immune complexes have been found in several patients.[188-190]

Pathogenesis

Stevens-Johnson syndrome has been associated with a variety of potential causative factors.[185] Drugs[128] and infectious agents have been most commonly noted. Drugs associated with the syndrome include systemic or ophthalmic sulfonamides,[191-194] ampicillin,[195] isoniazid,[196] anticonvulsants,[197] salicylates,[198] penicillin,[199] and phenylbutazone.[200] Nevertheless, it is probably the patient's

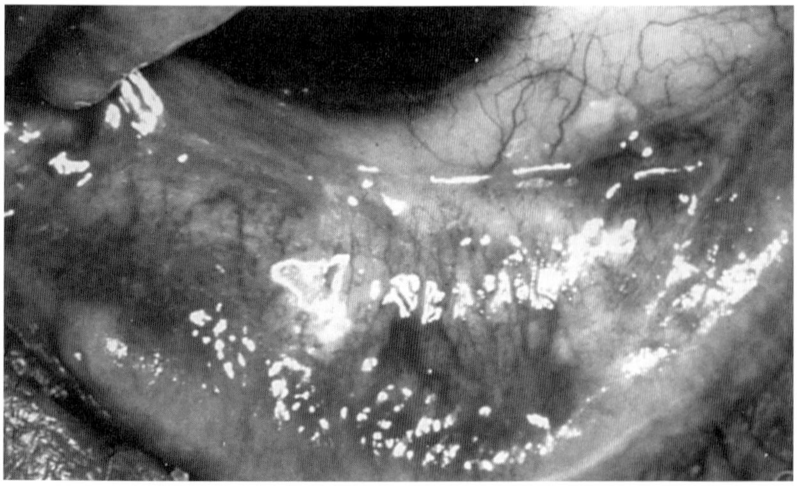

FIGURE 23-14 Acute conjunctivitis in Stevens-Johnson syndrome.

individual idiosyncratic reaction, and not the drug itself, that is primarily responsible. Infectious agents associated with the syndrome include streptococci, *Mycoplasma,* herpes simplex virus, and adenovirus.[184,201-203] In most cases, however, these agents appear to have been casually, and not causally, related to the development of the syndrome.

Studies of the genetic status of patients with Stevens-Johnson syndrome also indicate that certain individuals may be inclined to develop this disease in response to a variety of possible inciting agents. Mondino et al[204] demonstrated that these patients have a significantly increased incidence of HLA-B44 antigen compared with controls. This antigen also has an increased incidence among patients with cicatricial pemphigoid.[131] Perhaps certain patients, therefore, are genetically predisposed to cicatrizing mucous membrane disorders.

Treatment

Although corticosteroids were the first agents shown to be of some benefit in the treatment of Stevens-Johnson syndrome,[205-207] it soon became apparent that these drugs alone do not adequately control the disease in most cases.[208] Corticosteroids ameliorate somewhat the acute systemic manifestations of the disease. However, retrospective studies of patients with erythema multiforme suggest that patients treated with systemic corticosteroids had more complications and prolonged recovery times compared with those receiving only supportive care.[109] In the acute ophthalmic phase, topical corticosteroids may decrease inflammation. Nonetheless, symblephara usually form despite use of topical corticosteroids. During the acute phase of the disease, conjunctivitis produces raw conjunctival surfaces that tend to adhere to one another, and massive symblephara can form very quickly. Daily lysis of these symblephara is usually ineffective in preventing their recurrence. To prevent the raw bulbar and palpebral conjunctival surfaces from touching each other, ordinary household plastic wrap or a symblepharon ring with a bandage soft contact lens may be used. Plastic wrap is used to line the palpebral surface by placing one end in the fornix, and draping the sheet over the palpebral surface, eyelid margin, and skin. The protective film is anchored by mattress sutures that pass through the end that is in the fornix, the full thickness of the eyelid, and the end that is on the skin (Figure 23-16). The plastic wrap is left in place until the acute episode is over. In general, plastic wrap is better tolerated in children than a symblepharon ring and bandage soft contact lens.

Treatment of the chronic phase of Stevens-Johnson syndrome is similar to that of cicatricial pemphigoid. It is directed at supplementing the tear film and overcoming any corneal complications from trichiasis and entropion.

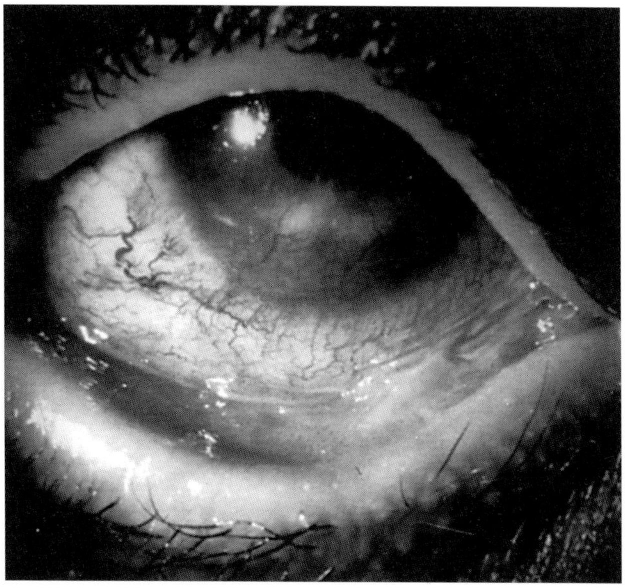

FIGURE 23-15 Inferior corneal vascularization and scarring caused by cicatricial changes from Stevens-Johnson syndrome.

Surgery to correct eyelid abnormalities can be undertaken without the risk of reactivation of the disease, unlike in cicatricial pemphigoid. Because of the compromised tear film and eyelid abnormalities, corneal infections should be suspected and treated aggressively. As with cicatricial pemphigoid, penetrating keratoplasty has a dismal prognosis. Prosthokeratoplasty may be successful in these severe cases. Successful keratoepithelioplasty for a persistent corneal epithelial defect has been reported in one patient.[104]

Lyell's Disease

Lyell's disease (toxic epidermal necrolysis, scalded skin syndrome) is a generalized necrosis of the skin that clinically resembles a severe thermal burn. It was first described by Lyell in 1956.[209] Epidermolysis is the hallmark lesion in Lyell's disease.[179] There is widespread necrosis of the epidermal cells with resultant loosening of the epidermis; large flaccid bullae result. These bullae differ in appearance from the tense bullae of Stevens-Johnson syndrome (which are produced by a subepidermal process). Commonly, the epidermis in Lyell's disease completely detaches in large areas, leaving a raw, denuded dermal surface. Patients can also experience severe fever and prostration. As in Stevens-Johnson syndrome, several pharmacologic and infectious agents have been associated causally with Lyell's disease.

Mucosal surfaces are involved in the majority of patients with Lyell's disease.[179,209-212] Conjunctival and oral mucous

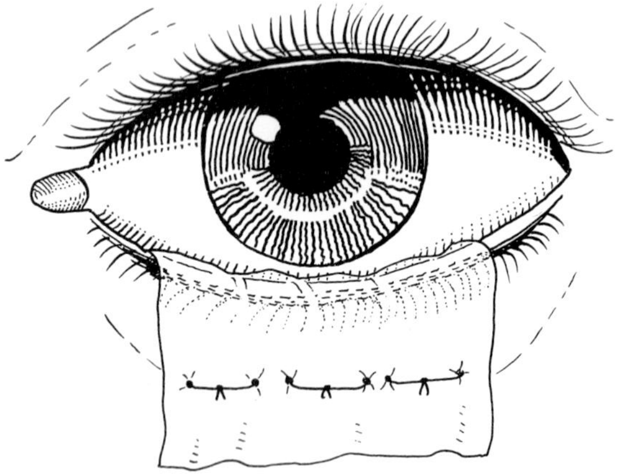

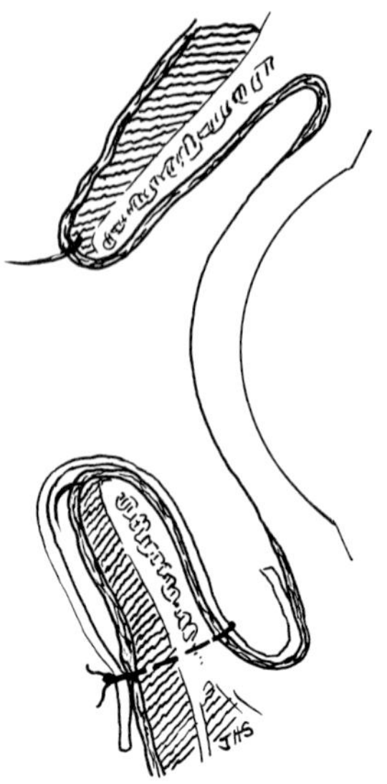

FIGURE 23-16 Placement of plastic wrap in the inferior fornix to prevent symblepharon formation.

membranes are most commonly affected. Conjunctival involvement in Lyell's disease is generally bilateral and occurs most commonly in those cases associated with staphylococcal infections.[213] The primary ocular lesion is a mucopurulent conjunctivitis. Pseudomembranous conjunctivitis, which is the hallmark of Stevens-Johnson syndrome, occurs less commonly in Lyell's disease. When it does occur, the resultant clinical picture may closely resemble that seen in end-stage cicatricial pemphigoid or Stevens-Johnson syndrome. Like Stevens-Johnson syndrome, Lyell's disease usually does not actively progress after the acute phase.

Treatment for Lyell's disease is similar to that for Stevens-Johnson syndrome. One important difference is that patients with associated staphylococcal infections should be treated aggressively with a penicillinase-resistant penicillin.[181]

Reiter Syndrome

Reiter syndrome is characterized by conjunctivitis, urethritis, arthritis, and mucocutaneous lesions.[214] It was first described by Brodie[215] in the 19th century and then later defined by Reiter[216] early in the 20th century. Demographically, the syndrome occurs worldwide and primarily affects young men. There is a correlation with previous exposure to venereal disease or dysentery.[217] Additionally, there is a high incidence of HLA-B27 genotype among patients with Reiter syndrome.

Joint involvement is the most common manifestation of Reiter syndrome; it occurs in more than 90 percent of patients, and accounts for the majority of associated morbidity.[218,219] Characteristically, the joints in the lower extremities are more frequently affected, but all articular and periarticular structures may be involved.

Other non-ophthalmic manifestations of Reiter syndrome include urethritis and mucocutaneous lesions. Mucocutaneous lesions occur in 30 to 100 percent of patients.[214,220–222] Most commonly, the genital and oral mucosae are affected. The most common genital lesion is balanitis. The oral lesions are usually red, painless macules that rarely ulcerate. The mucosal lesions are generally transient. The typical cutaneous lesion is keratoderma blenorrhagica.[214] Seborrheic or psoriatic dermatitis may also be seen.

Conjunctivitis is the second most common manifestation of Reiter syndrome, and the most common ophthalmic manifestation.[214,223–226] In a series from the Mayo Clinic,[214] 58 percent of Reiter syndrome patients had conjunctivitis. The conjunctivitis may be papillary or follicular, and an accompanying mucopurulent discharge is usually present. Rarely, cicatrization is noted.[214] Less common ophthalmic manifestations include iridocyclitis, which can be severe, episcleritis, scleritis, and keratitis. Keratitis generally manifests as subepithelial or anterior stromal opacities, frequently involving the peripheral cornea. The conjunctival and corneal changes in Reiter syndrome are generally self limited; occasionally, topical corticosteroids may be necessary for severe cases of keratitis.

The pathogenesis of Reiter syndrome is unknown. The characteristic multisystem involvement, as well as the association with certain infectious diseases and the HLA-B27 genotype, suggests that this disorder is the result of an unusual host response to an infectious agent or other unknown antigen.[214] It does not appear to be a direct infectious disorder; rather, it is the result of an immunologic response to the infecting organisms. One of the commonly associated organisms is *Chlamydia.* In those cases associated with chlamydial disease, systemic therapy with tetracycline or erythromycin is recommended.

SYSTEMIC VASCULITIDES

The ocular surface can be involved in many systemic vasculitides, which is not surprising considering the vascularity of the ocular surface and its high collagen content. Although the exact pathogeneses of these disorders are not known, it is generally agreed that aberrations in the host immunologic response play an important role. Ocular surface involvement is of great significance in systemic vasculitides, because in many of these disorders it may be the presenting manifestation.[227,228] Common ocular surface manifestations in systemic vasculitides include keratoconjunctivitis sicca, scleritis, episcleritis, and peripheral corneal disease (infiltrates, furrowing, ulcerations).

Rheumatoid Arthritis

Rheumatoid arthritis is the most common vasculitic disorder that involves the ocular surface. Classic rheumatoid arthritis is a multisystem disorder that affects 2.5 to 3 percent of adults.[229] Women are primarily affected, and the average age at onset is 35 to 40 years.

Clinical Features

The onset of rheumatoid arthritis is usually characterized by a period of nonspecific prodromal symptoms followed by mild joint pain. Some patients, however, have a fulminant initial course with a relatively sudden onset of severe joint pain accompanied by fever and chills. The peripheral joints, particularly the interphalangeal and metacarpophalangeal joints, are primarily involved.[230] Periarticular involvement, characterized by tenosynovitis, tendonitis, and muscular or bone atrophy, is also a prominent feature. Extra-articular findings are present in about 25 percent of patients; these include subcutaneous nodules, cardiac involvement, pulmonary disease, splenomegaly, and ocular disease.[229]

The characteristic ocular changes of rheumatoid arthritis include keratoconjunctivitis sicca, scleritis, episcleritis, and keratitis. Ocular involvement tends to occur in patients with more advanced disease, especially those with subcutaneous nodules, vasculitis, or cardiac involvement.[230,231] Keratoconjunctivitis sicca (secondary Sjögren's syndrome) is by far the most common ocular manifestation. Sialochemical analyses[232] and lacrimal gland biopsy specimens[233] have demonstrated changes consistent with Sjögren syndrome in 24 to 31 percent of patients with rheumatoid arthritis. Of these patients, 80 percent had clinical keratoconjunctivitis sicca.

Scleritis occurs in 0.67 to 6.3 percent of rheumatoid arthritis patients[234,235] (Figure 23-17). The development of scleritis is generally considered to be an ominous sign of systemic vasculitis; without aggressive treatment, most of these patients die within 5 years.[236,237] Episcleritis also commonly occurs in rheumatoid arthritis.[236,238] It can be nodular or diffuse, and generally does not carry the ominous implications that scleritis does.

Corneal involvement in rheumatoid arthritis is common and is most frequently the result of keratoconjunctivitis sicca. Corneal involvement can range from mild punctate epithelial keratitis to severe sterile or infectious stromal ulcerations (Figure 23-18). Corneal changes are also common in patients who have scleritis or episcleritis. The cornea is affected in 46 to 69 percent of rheumatoid arthritis patients with scleritis.[234,239,240] Most commonly, the cornea is involved by a direct extension of a paralimbal scleritic process. The patterns of corneal involvement in scleritis include sclerosing keratitis, acute stromal keratitis, furrowing, and keratolysis.[231,236,238,241]

Sclerosing keratitis is the most common of these patterns, and is characterized by thickening and opacification of the affected peripheral stroma.[234] The process generally extends centrally and is followed by superficial stromal vascularization. Acute stromal keratitis begins as superficial and midstromal peripheral infiltrates; usually, it develops in association with non-necrotizing scleritis. These infiltrates may coalesce; eventually the overlying epithelium may break down and the affected stroma may melt. Acute stromal keratitis generally resolves with treatment of the scleritis. Peripheral corneal furrowing usually begins in an area of sclerosing keratitis. It involves a well-circumscribed band of stromal thinning with intact overlying epithelium (Figure 23-19). The degree of thinning may be severe, but perforation is uncommon. Furrowing may occur even without an associated scleritis.[231,242,243] Keratolysis involves acute melting of clear corneal stroma. The process is usually fulminant, and severe thinning, with descemetocele formation or perforation, is the rule. Keratolysis usually occurs in patients with associated severe scleritis, either necrotizing or scleromalacia perforans.

Corneal involvement also occurs in approximately 15 percent of rheumatoid arthritis patients with episcleritis.[236,238] It most frequently manifests as peripheral stromal infiltration and edema in direct association with an area of paralimbal episcleritis. Additionally, if the paralimbal episcleritis is nodular and elevated, peripheral corneal dellen may result.

Pathogenesis

The exact pathogenesis of rheumatoid arthritis is unknown. It is thought that a combination of altered immunologic responses (to unknown antigens) and genetic susceptibil-

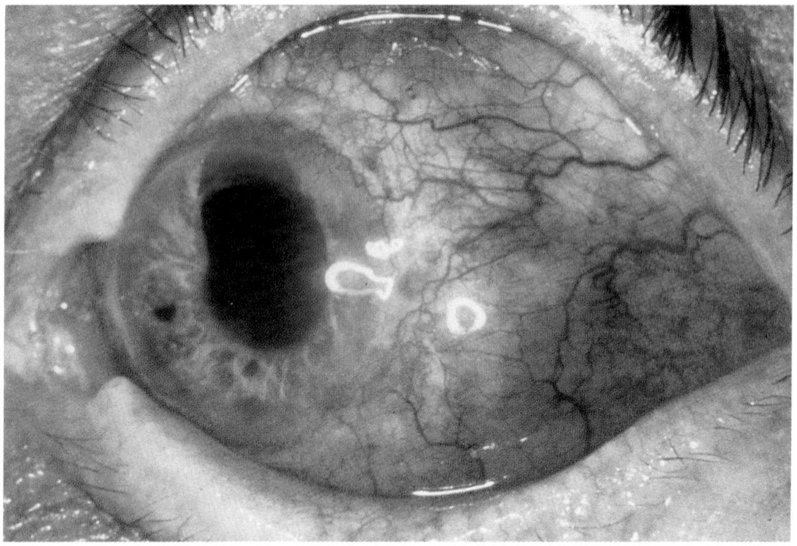

FIGURE 23-17 Scleromalacia associated with rheumatoid arthritis.

ity is involved. Immunologically, rheumatoid arthritis, like most of the systemic vasculitides, probably results from a type III (immune-complex-mediated) hypersensitivity reaction. As evidence, investigators have noted serum and synovial immune complexes, depressed levels of synovial fluid complement, serum autoantibodies, and serum cryoglobulins.[231]

Treatment

As with most of the systemic vasculitides, treatment of the ocular complications of rheumatoid arthritis is predicated on effective therapy of the systemic disease. In most cases, this involves the use of systemic corticosteroids and/or immunosuppressive agents to control ocular inflammation.[236,238,244–247] Topical corticosteroids are useful in controlling scleritis, episcleritis, sclerosing keratitis, and acute stromal keratitis; they should be avoided in cases of furrowing or keratolysis.[231,238,242,248] Other local measures include tear film replacement for keratoconjunctivitis sicca, bandage soft contact lenses for epithelial keratitis,[153] cyanoacrylate adhesive for severe stromal melting processes,[249] conjunctival resection for refractory cases of peripheral

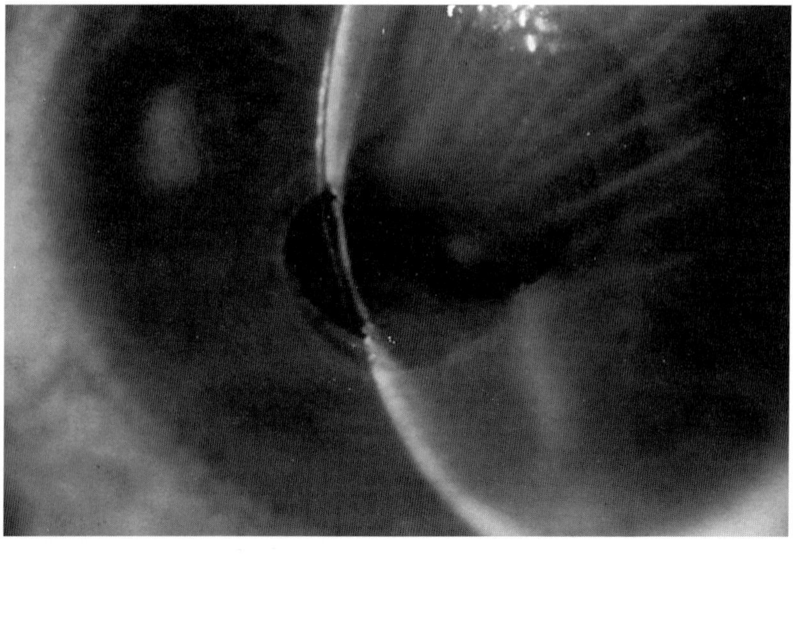

FIGURE 23-18 Marked corneal thinning in a patient with rheumatoid arthritis and dry eyes. The striae radiating from the area of thinning signify the severity of the thinning.

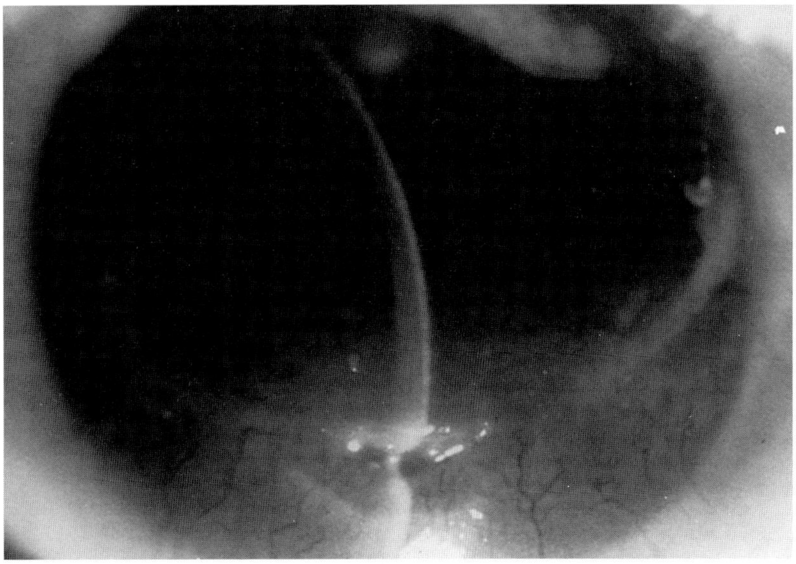

FIGURE 23-19 Peripheral corneal furrowing caused by rheumatoid arthritis.

corneal involvement,[243,250,251] and lamellar or penetrating keratoplasty to repair or prevent perforation or to restore a clear visual axis. Any surgical procedure should be deferred, if possible, until associated scleral inflammation is controlled. If the scleritis results in thinning of the sclera to the extent that it needs to be repaired, a patch graft of eye bank sclera may be used; however, the graft usually becomes involved by the disease process in much the same way as the patient's own sclera. An alternative is to use pretibial periosteum to reinforce both sclera and peripheral cornea, if necessary, because the periosteum does not melt (Figure 23-20). The technique for harvesting pretibial periosteum is described in Chapter 36.

Sjögren's Syndrome

Sjögren's syndrome is a multisystem disorder primarily seen in middle-aged women, although it has been recognized in men and women of all ages and even in children. It is characterized by keratoconjunctivitis sicca and xerostomia.[252] Two forms of the syndrome are recognized: keratoconjunctivitis sicca and xerostomia alone (primary) or in combination with a known vasculitic disease (secondary). The most common vasculitis associated with secondary Sjögren's syndrome is rheumatoid arthritis. However, several other systemic vasculitides and other autoimmune disorders can be associated with keratoconjunctivitis sicca.[253]

The primary ocular findings in Sjögren's syndrome are caused by the keratoconjunctivitis sicca (see Ch. 5). Additionally, patients may develop typical peripheral corneal changes, even in the primary form of the syndrome. Peripheral stromal infiltrates resembling those of staphylococcal marginal keratitis occur in approximately 10 percent of patients.[254] Peripheral corneal thinning and perforation can also occur; most of these cases involve secondary Sjögren's syndrome associated with rheumatoid arthritis.[255–259] Additionally, the use of topical corticosteroids appears to be associated with those cases that progress to perforation.

The pathogenesis of Sjögren's syndrome remains unknown, although it is probably related to an autoimmune or other immunologic aberration. In addition to its association with other known or suspected autoimmune disorders, a wide variety of immunologic abnormalities can be seen in Sjögren's syndrome, including hypergammaglobulinemia, Raynaud's phenomenon, impaired lymphocyte function, serum autoantibodies, and lymphoreticular neoplasms.[17,260] The keratoconjunctivitis sicca in Sjögren's syndrome results from an immunologic attack on the lacrimal gland. Histopathologically, plasma cells and lymphocytes are seen in the affected glands in acute exacerbations; following repeated attacks, the glandular tissue is replaced by fibrous tissue. Diagnosis of Sjögren's syndrome can be made by typical clinical findings and lacrimal or labial salivary gland biopsy.[261] In addition, impression cytology has been shown to be an effective diagnostic adjunct; squamous metaplasia of the temporal bulbar and inferior bulbar conjunctiva, extensive goblet cell loss of the temporal bulbar conjunctiva, mucous aggregates on the bulbar conjunctiva, and inflammatory cells intercalated with epithelial cells on the inferior tarsal conjunctiva all may occur in primary Sjögren's syndrome.[262]

Therapy for the ocular surface complications of Sjögren's syndrome is directed primarily at the keratoconjunctivitis sicca. It usually involves replenishment of the tear film with artificial tear preparations and lubricating ointments. Because patients are frequently unable to tolerate one or

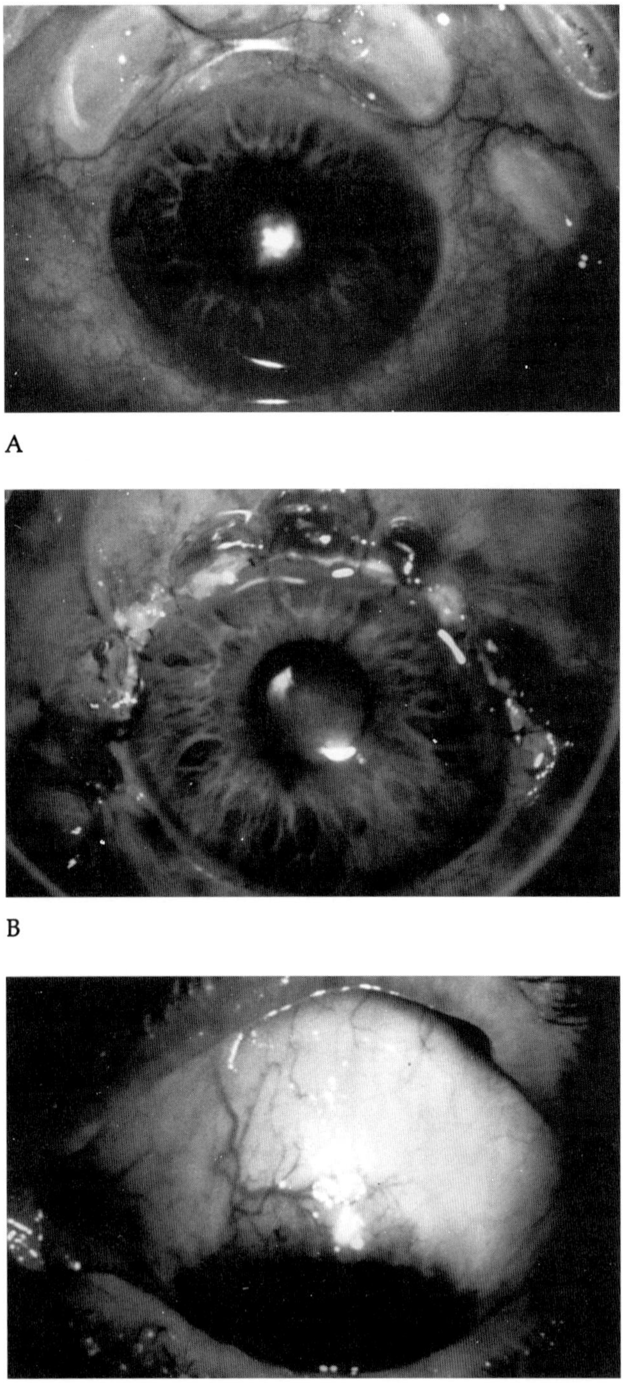

A

B

C

FIGURE 23-20 **(A)** Preoperative photograph of marked scleral necrosis in a patient with rheumatoid arthritis. **(B)** Intraoperative photograph of pretibial periosteum over the area of necrosis. **(C)** Postoperative photograph showing that the integrity of the eye has been maintained and there has been no necrosis of the periosteum.

more of the commercially available tear preparations, they should be encouraged to try different preparations, particularly those free of preservatives. Other measures for treatment include punctal occlusion, bandage soft contact lenses, and moist chambers (swim goggles). If there are peripheral corneal infiltrates, a short course of topical corticosteroids may help; corticosteroids should not be used in cases of peripheral corneal thinning. Severe corneal thinning or perforation may necessitate the use of cyanoacrylate adhesive or partial- or full-thickness keratoplasty.[259]

Systemic Lupus Erythematosus

Systemic lupus erythematosus (SLE) is a multisystem disorder that commonly affects the articular, mucosal, cutaneous, hematologic, pulmonary, renal, neurologic, and ocular systems. The skin is involved by an erythematous rash that can affect the face, neck, and extremities. Arthritis, polyarthralgias, pleuritis, pericarditis, lymphadenopathy, splenomegaly, and mucosal ulcerations may occur. Foster[263] has extensively reviewed the clinical, diagnostic, and differential diagnostic features of systemic lupus erythematosus. Burge et al[264] found linear deposition of an immunoreactant along the basement membrane zone in 42 percent of bulbar conjunctival biopsy specimens obtained from patients with systemic lupus erythematosus, a percentage similar to that seen in skin and lip mucosal biopsy specimens. The same study reported similar ocular findings in 50 percent of those with chronic cutaneous lupus erythematosus (CCLE), a much higher rate than was found at other CCLE biopsy sites.

Ocular complications include keratoconjunctivitis sicca, episcleritis, scleritis, epithelial keratitis, interstitial keratitis, peripheral corneal ulcerations, iridocyclitis, and retinal vasculitis. As with many of the systemic vasculitides, keratoconjunctivitis sicca is a common feature. Episcleritis and scleritis are not uncommon manifestations.[17,263] Burge et al[265] showed episcleritis to be present in 9 percent of patients with systemic lupus erythematosus, but not at all in those with chronic cutaneous lupus erythematosus. The presence of scleritis indicates underlying vasculitic activity. The cornea may be involved by a punctate epithelial keratitis that does not appear to be caused by tear film abnormalities. First reported by Gold et al[266] and later by Spaeth,[267] this punctate epithelial keratitis appears to be related to the severity of systemic lupus erythematosus activity. Band-shaped interstitial keratitis[268,269] and peripheral corneal ulcerations with vascularization and infiltration[17,238] have also been reported. Scleral, episcleral, and corneal inflammation respond well to topical corticosteroids.

Polyarteritis Nodosa

Polyarteritis nodosa is a chronic, idiopathic necrotizing vasculitis of medium and small arteries. First described in 1861,[270] it is seen most frequently in 20- to 40-year-old men.[263]

Clinical Features

The clinical manifestations of polyarteritis nodosa are diverse; they include fever, arthralgias, weight loss, malaise, glomerulonephritis, cutaneous nodules, peripheral neuropathy, cardiovascular disease, severe abdominal pain from mesenteric arteritis, hepatic infarction, and testicular pain. These various clinical findings are the result of diffuse vasculitis.

Ocular involvement occurs in approximately 20 percent of patients; the most common ocular findings include scleritis, choroidal vasculitis, retinal vasculitis, optic atrophy, exudative retinal detachment, papilledema, and keratitis.

Keratitis is bilateral and usually affects the peripheral cornea[271,272] (Figure 23-21). As with peripheral corneal involvement in many of the vasculitides, it begins with midstromal infiltrates. These infiltrates progress both circumferentially and centrally, and may eventually ulcerate. This progression is similar to that seen in Mooren's ulcer. In most cases, the peripheral keratitis is associated with an adjacent, highly destructive necrotizing scleritis.[273] Of importance is the observation that as in Wegener's granulomatosis, ocular involvement may be the presenting sign of the disease.

Histopathology and Pathogenesis

Histopathologic findings in the ocular lesions of polyarteritis nodosa are nonspecific. The ocular lesions appear to result from the deposition of immune complexes in the sclera and limbus, with subsequent complement activation and inflammatory cell migration.[263] The overall disease process appears to be the result of an immune-complex-mediated type III hypersensitivity reaction.

Treatment

Treatment of ocular involvement depends on adequate therapy of the systemic disease. The recommended therapeutic regimen is a combination of systemic corticosteroids and cyclophosphamide.[274] Local adjunctive measures include conjunctival resection, a bandage soft contact lens, cyanoacrylate adhesive, and partial- or full-thickness keratoplasty.

Wegener's Granulomatosis

Wegener's granulomatosis is one of the multisystem vasculitides categorized as a respiratory vasculitis. The classic clinicopathologic triad consists of (1) necrotizing granulomatous inflammation of the upper respiratory tract, (2) granulomatous inflammation of the lower respiratory tract, and (3) focal glomerulonephritis.[275,276] Additionally, most cases have an accompanying systemic vasculitis, particularly involving the smaller arteries and veins.

Clinical Features

There are two forms of Wegener's granulomatosis: the classic form and the limited form. The classic form affects males slightly more frequently than females. Although it can present at any age, the average age of onset is in the fourth or fifth decade. Patients usually present with symptoms referable to the upper respiratory tract.[275,277] Initial involvement may be subtle, with mild upper respiratory tract symptoms accompanied by night sweats or arthralgias. Occasionally, patients present with a fulminant onset, with rapidly progressive renal failure and respiratory insufficiency.

The respiratory mucosa is nearly always involved.[228,278] Characteristically, there is a diffuse, necrotizing granulomatous inflammation resulting in a shaggy, gray surface. The necrotic process eventually progresses to involve the nasal bone and cartilage, resulting in the typical saddlenose deformity and nasal-paranasal sinus fistulas. Extension of this necrotic inflammation can involve the orbits, buccal mucosa, and temporal fossa.

The lower respiratory mucosa is involved in more than 90 percent of cases. The characteristic findings are productive cough, hemoptysis, and transient pulmonary infiltrates and nodules on chest radiographs.

Glomerulonephritis generally occurs late in the course of the disease, and is frequently the terminal event. Clinically, azotemia and albuminuria are noted. Eventually, this process results in chronic renal failure.

In addition to the classic triad, a multisystem focal vasculitis is usually present. The most commonly involved organs are the spleen, heart, lungs, pancreas, and adrenal glands. Other clinical manifestations include arthralgias, hemorrhagic dermatitis, endocarditis, and polyneuritis.

Carrington and Liebow[279] described a series of patients with characteristic pulmonary involvement, but with only minimal disseminated disease. In particular, renal disease was notably absent. This limited form of Wegener's granulomatosis affects females more often than males, and has a milder course than does the classic form. The classic form of Wegener's granulomatosis generally progresses rapidly. When the condition is untreated, the 1-year mortality rate is 82 percent[280]; patients with the limited form have a greater life expectancy.

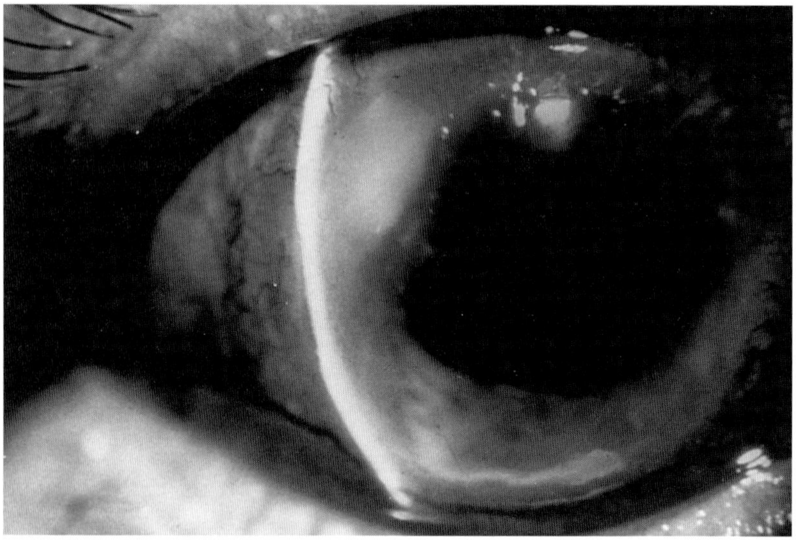

FIGURE 23-21 Peripheral keratitis in a patient with polyarteritis nodosa.

The incidence of ocular involvement in Wegener's granulomatosis is 28 to 45 percent,[277,280] and is the same in both the classic and limited forms of the disease.[281] Ocular manifestations include both secondary orbital involvement from contiguous sinus disease and primary focal disease. Of primary importance is the common observation that either contiguous or focal ocular involvement can be the presenting manifestation of Wegener's granulomatosis.[280]

Contiguous, or secondary, ocular disease presents as orbital inflammation and occurs in 18 to 22 percent of patients.[282] It accounts for nearly 50 percent of all the ocular involvement in Wegener's granulomatosis. Proptosis is the most common presenting sign; severe sinus involvement is invariably present. Severe cases may be accompanied by exposure keratopathy, restricted ocular motility, papilledema, and congested retinal vasculature. Orbital involvement is characteristically bilateral, thus differentiating it from the more common forms of orbital inflammation, such as pseudotumor.

Focal, or primary, ocular disease occurs independent of respiratory tract involvement, and may include the following: conjunctivitis, scleritis, episcleritis, keratitis, uveitis, retinal vasculitis, and retinal detachment.[277,280,283] Conjunctivitis and posterior segment involvement are uncommon.[284] Approximately 7 percent of patients with focal ocular disease have either infarctions of the retinal vasculature[271,282–288] or a retinal vasculitis.[280] Anterior segment changes are usually, but not always, bilateral. Corneal involvement begins as peripheral midstromal infiltrates (Figure 23-22). These may eventually ulcerate, as well as extend circumferentially or centrally.[285,286] Perforation of these ulcers has been noted.[287] The progression and appearance of these peripheral corneal lesions are similar to those of Mooren's ulcer. Scleritis is a common feature of focal ocular disease.[277,279,280,283] Scleral involvement typically occurs adjacent to an area of marginal keratitis.[271,287] It is usually nodular and necrotizing, similar to that seen in rheumatoid arthritis and other collagen vascular diseases.

Histopathology

The histopathology of peripheral corneal involvement in Wegener's granulomatosis consists of necrosis of the epithelium and superficial stroma, accompanied by formation of granulation tissue along the ulcer base. There is usually a mixed inflammatory cell infiltrate in the affected stroma; occasionally, epithelioid cells and giant cells are noted.[271,287,289,290] This necrotizing granulomatous inflammation may extend into the adjacent sclera and its underlying ciliary body. Discrete granulomas of the cornea are rare.

Pathogenesis

The cause of Wegener's granulomatosis is obscure. The primary respiratory tract involvement probably results from an aberrant immunologic response to an airborne antigen.[271,283,287,290,291] Systemic involvement may result from repeated antigenic exposure, leading to presentation of the antigen to the general circulation. Unlike in polyarteritis nodosa, there is little evidence linking Wegener's granulomatosis to humoral immune abnormalities, such as immune complexes or complement.[292] The laboratory findings are generally nonspecific; they include elevated erythrocyte sedimentation rate, hypergammaglobulinemia, positive rheumatoid factors, and

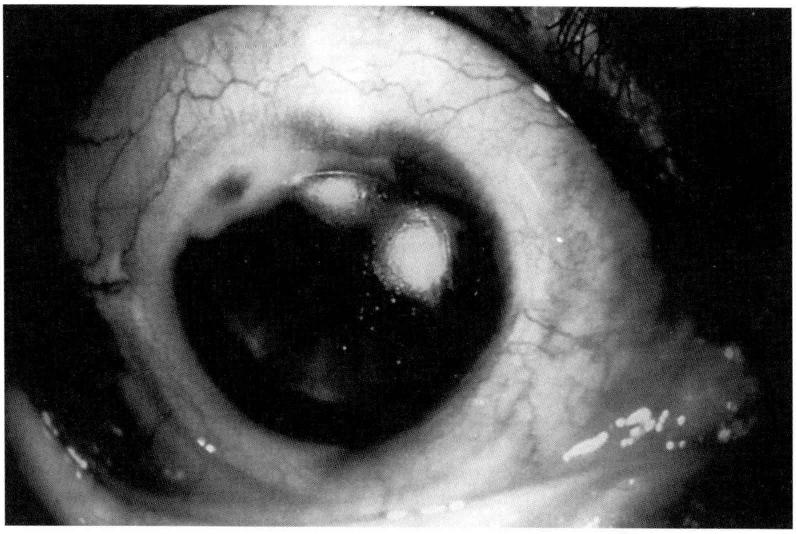

FIGURE 23-22 Peripheral keratitis in a patient with Wegener's granulomatosis.

occasionally, serum immune complexes.[293,294] However, given the similarities between Wegener's granulomatosis and known immune-complex–mediated disorders, such as polyarteritis nodosa, it is probable that circulating and/or tissue-fixed immune complexes play a prominent pathogenic role. There is also evidence that Wegener's granulomatosis may result, in part, from abnormalities in the cell-mediated immune system.[292,295] As with other vasculitides, the abnormal host immune response may be genetically mediated. Katz et al[296] noted a statistical correlation between the HLA-B8 genotype and Wegener's granulomatosis. The pathogenesis of peripheral corneal lesions appears to involve an occlusive vasculitis of the adjacent blood vessels.[287]

Diagnosis

The diagnosis of Wegener's granulomatosis is predicated on clinical suspicion. From the standpoint of ocular surface problems, the diagnosis of Wegener's granulomatosis should be considered in any patient with scleritis or peripheral corneal ulceration, either unilateral or bilateral. This is important, because the ocular manifestations may be the presenting signs of this potentially fatal disease. As mentioned above, there are few consistent serum abnormalities in Wegener's granulomatosis. Diagnostic assistance may be obtained from radiographic studies. In particular, sinus studies frequently are abnormal; mucosal thickening or obstruction is common. Chest radiographs may reveal nodular or cavitary pulmonary infiltrates. In suspected cases, diagnosis may be proven by biopsy of affected tissues.

All of the systemic vasculitides must be considered in the differential diagnosis of Wegener's granulomatosis. Final determination frequently rests on histopathologic examination, because Wegener's granulomatosis is one of the few vasculitides with a primarily granulomatous inflammatory response.[228] Allergic granulomatosis and hypersensitivity angiitis also are granulomatous vasculitides, but they are associated with a known history of exposure to foreign substances or atopy.

Treatment

Treatment of the ophthalmic manifestations of Wegener's granulomatosis depends on adequate therapy of the systemic disease; local treatment alone is generally unsuccessful. Corticosteroids, originally the mainstay of therapy, have been supplanted by immunosuppressive agents, particularly cyclophosphamide and azathioprine.[293] Cyclophosphamide used in combination with systemic corticosteroids produces remissions in more than 90 percent of patients.[297,298] Disease activity can be monitored by serial measurements of erythrocyte sedimentation rate. Local adjunctive measures include topical antibiotics, bandage soft contact lenses, conjunctival resection, cyanoacrylate adhesive or lamellar keratoplasty for impending or actual perforations, and penetrating keratoplasty for restoration of a clear visual axis.

Churg-Strauss Syndrome

Churg-Strauss syndrome, first described in 1951,[299] is characterized as one of the respiratory vasculitides. It is a multisystem syndrome characterized by fever, eosinophilia, and necrotizing vasculitis.[300] The cardinal systemic feature is asthma, which may precede the onset

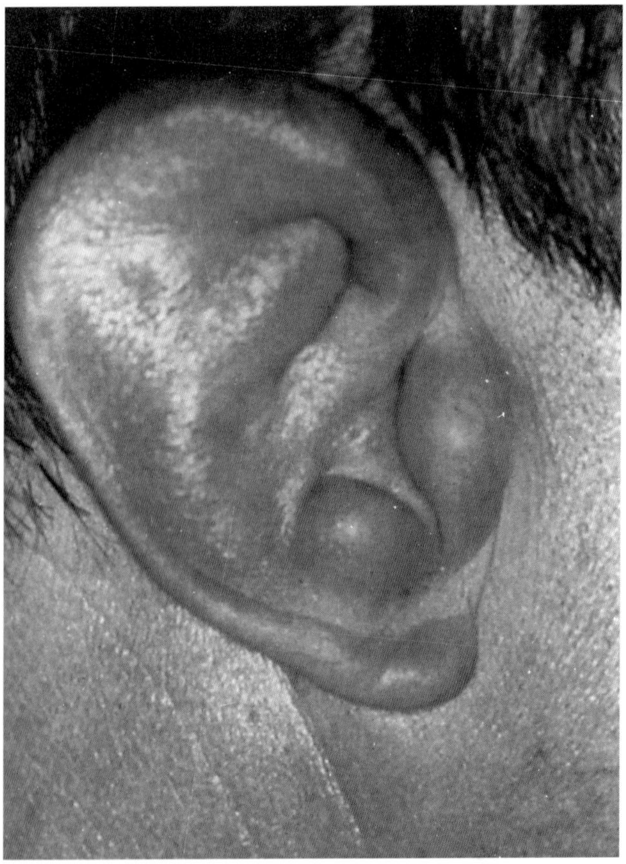

FIGURE 23-23 Inflammation of the ear cartilage caused by relapsing polychondritis.

of vasculitis by many years. Other allergic manifestations, particularly nasal polyps and allergic rhinitis, are also frequently noted. The manifestations of the active syndrome are variable. Involvement may include the gastrointestinal, prostatic, dermatologic, lymphatic, neurologic, articular, and pulmonary systems.

Laboratory findings include anemia, elevated erythrocyte sedimentation rate, eosinophilia, and hypergammaglobulinemia E.[301,302] Histopathologic findings are characterized by a necrotizing granulomatous vasculitis involving the small- and medium-size arteries.[299] The pathogenesis of the disease probably involves an immune-complex-mediated vasculitis that occurs in response to airborne antigens in susceptible patients.

Ocular involvement in Churg-Strauss syndrome is uncommon. Episcleritis,[303] marginal corneal ulceration,[301] and conjunctival granulomatous nodules[304-306] have been reported. Treatment involves high doses of systemic corticosteroids or, in rare cases, immunosuppressive agents.[301,307,308] When left untreated, Churg-Strauss syndrome is frequently fatal.

Relapsing Polychondritis

Relapsing polychondritis is an uncommon disorder that was first described in 1923.[309] It is characterized by recurrent inflammation of cartilaginous tissues. Nasal, auricular, costal, aortic, tracheal, and laryngeal cartilages are primarily affected; the auricular pinnae are the most commonly affected (Figure 23-23). Additionally, the joints can be affected. Other potential systemic features include myocardial disease, anemia, liver dysfunction, and airway obstruction.[310] Rare cases prove fatal as a result of respiratory obstruction or cardiac disease.

Ocular involvement occurs in approximately 60 percent of patients.[311] The episclera, sclera, cornea, conjunctiva, uveal tract, retina, and optic nerve may be involved. Episcleritis and/or scleritis (Figure 23-24) are the most common ocular manifestations, occurring in 30 to 60 percent of patients.[311-313] Corneal disease occurs in 11 percent of patients and primarily adjacent to areas of scleritis. Corneal changes include sclerosing keratitis, peripheral corneal edema, peripheral stromal infiltrates, and ulcerations[312-315] (Figure 23-25). Although marginal corneal involvement is generally associated with concomitant scleritis, cases have been reported in the absence of any scleral involvement.[316,317] Peripheral corneal thinning and ulceration may progress circumferentially to involve the entire periphery; perforation has been reported.[316,317] Anterior segment angiography has been performed in active relapsing polychondritis[310]; no evidence of ischemia or overt vasculitis was noted.

The pathogenesis of relapsing polychondritis is not known. The disease has been associated with other autoimmune disorders, such as Sjögren's syndrome. Evidence suggests that anticollagen antibodies may play an important role in the development of the clinical features of relapsing polychondritis.[318] The inciting factors for the development of these antibodies, however, remain unclear.

The treatment of relapsing polychondritis involves systemic corticosteroids, dapsone, azathioprine, and cyclophosphamide.[310,317,319-321] Ocular involvement may be ameliorated by the addition of topical corticosteroids.

Progressive Systemic Sclerosis (Scleroderma)

Progressive systemic sclerosis (PSS) is an idiopathic, multisystem disorder that primarily affects women.[322] The skin, esophagus, blood vessels, joints, kidneys, heart, and lungs are most commonly affected. Raynaud's phenomenon is a common presenting sign. Other clinical findings include

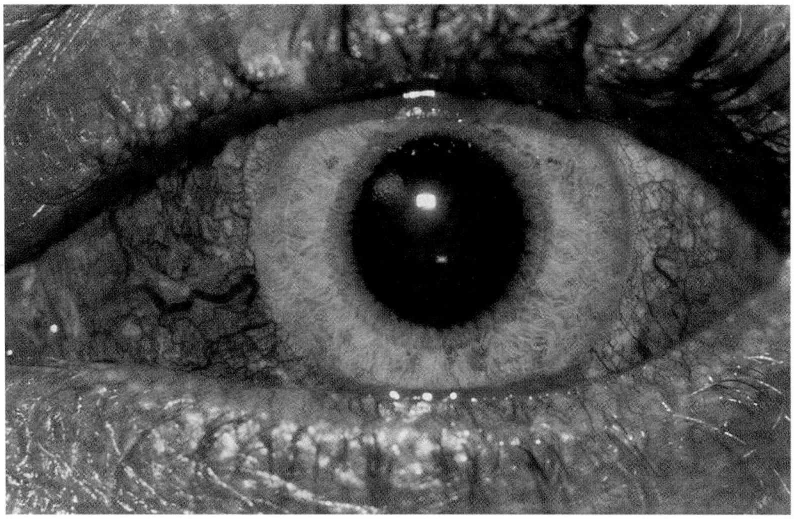

FIGURE 23-24 Diffuse scleritis in a patient with relapsing polychondritis. There is also an accompanying episcleritis.

digital edema, induration and contraction of the skin, esophageal dysfunction, polyarthralgia, calcinosis, pulmonary fibrosis, myocardial fibrosis, and renal failure.

Skin biopsy specimens from patients routinely show extensive T-cell infiltration and perivascular inflammation. Foster[263] believes that the pathogenesis of progressive systemic sclerosis involves sensitization to skin antigens and a subsequent proliferation of dermal fibroblasts, production of immature collagen, and vascular ingrowth. Additionally, vasculitis is a prominent finding in affected viscera. Patients frequently have circulating immune complexes and/or autoantibodies.

Ocular findings include keratitis, keratoconjunctivitis sicca, conjunctival shrinkage, choroidal vasculitis, and extraocular muscle myositis.[263,323,324] Secondary Sjögren's syndrome is particularly common, occurring in approximately 70 percent of patients.[325] Peripheral corneal furrows or ulcers not associated with keratoconjunctivitis sicca can occur.[326]

Miscellaneous Vasculitides

Some of the other vasculitides that may involve the ocular surface include cranial arteritis and Cogan syndrome. In cranial arteritis, marginal corneal ulcers and conjunctival ulcerations with scleromalacia have been reported.[327] These ocular surface lesions resolve with systemic corticosteroid therapy. Cogan syndrome is a vas-

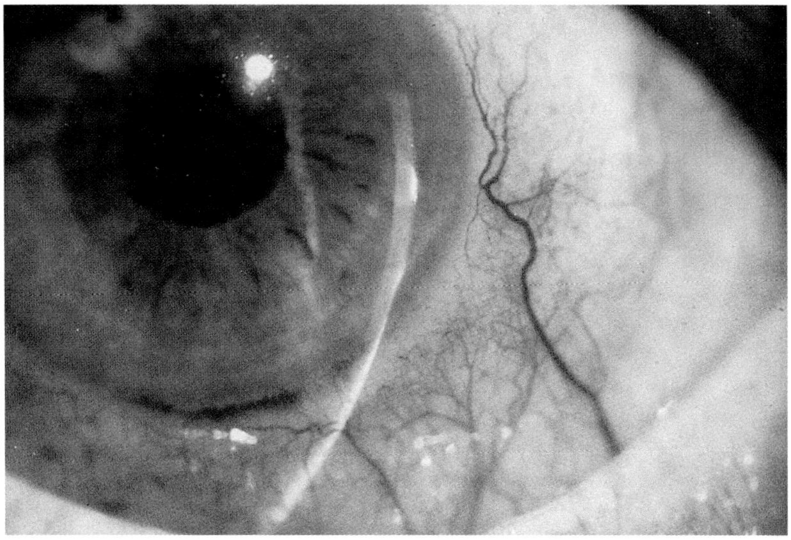

FIGURE 23-25 Peripheral corneal ulceration in a patient with relapsing polychondritis. Note the scleral thinning temporally.

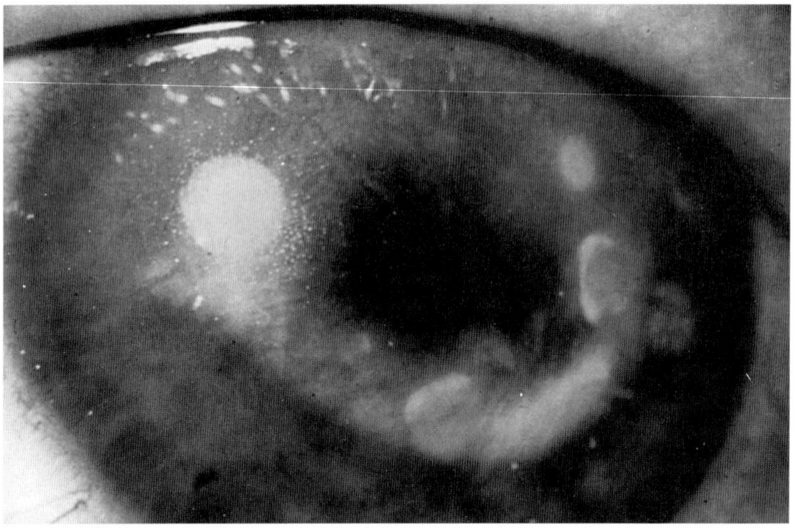

FIGURE 23-26 Interstitial keratitis in Cogan syndrome.

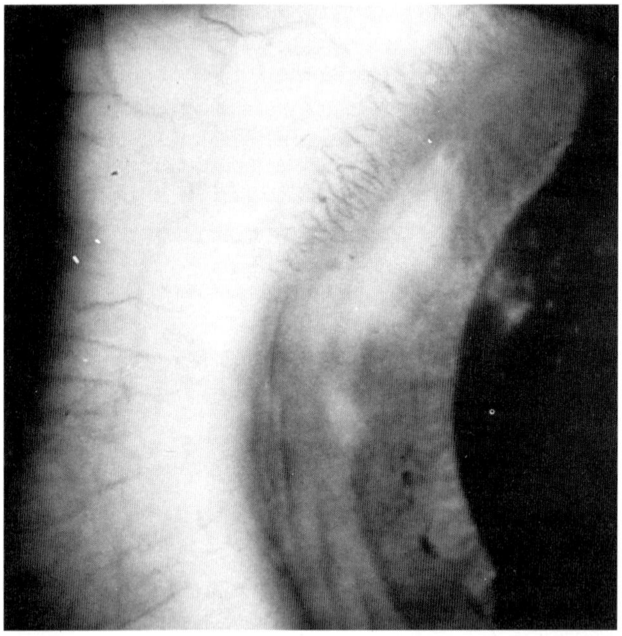

FIGURE 23-27 Marginal keratitis. There is a mild degree of vascularization.

culitis characterized by vertigo, deafness, and nonluetic interstitial keratitis[328] (Figure 23-26). Cobo and Haynes[329] reported that bilateral, peripheral, subepithelial nummular corneal opacities are the most common ocular findings in early Cogan syndrome. The treatment of corneal changes in this syndrome consists of topical corticosteroids, whereas the vertigo and deafness require use of systemic corticosteroids.

MISCELLANEOUS IMMUNOLOGIC DISORDERS

Marginal Keratitis

Marginal keratitis is a disorder of peripheral corneal infiltration and ulceration. It is commonly attributed to a local corneal hypersensitivity to toxins elaborated by bacteria colonizing the eyelid margins or conjunctiva. Although no epidemiologic statistics are available, the resulting catarrhal lesions probably represent the most common disorder of the peripheral cornea. Marginal keratitis usually occurs in middle-aged patients and is associated with a concomitant blepharoconjunctivitis. Unusually severe marginal keratitis can also be a feature in children with neutrophil dysfunction or Wiskott-Aldrich syndrome.[330,331]

Clinical Features

The lesions of marginal keratitis begin as one or more grayish, peripheral stromal infiltrates (Figure 23-27). Characteristically, these infiltrates are parallel to the limbus and are separated from it by a 1- to 2-mm area of uninvolved cornea (commonly referred to as the *clear zone*).[332,333] At this stage patients may complain of ocular redness, pain, foreign body sensation, and particularly, photophobia. These infiltrates, if untreated, may form marginal ulcerations by breakdown of the overlying epithelium. The natural course is generally benign, and the lesions eventually heal in 2 to 4 weeks with little, if any, vascularization. It is important to stress that the lesions of marginal keratitis are sterile. However, cultures of the eyelid margins and conjunctiva may reveal bacterial pathogens. Unless the associated blepharoconjunctivitis is controlled, the peripheral corneal lesions generally recur.

Pathogenesis

In 1946, Thygeson[332] first associated marginal keratitis with hypersensitivity reactions to chronic staphylococcal blepharitis or conjunctivitis. It was known by that time that staphylococci could adversely affect the ocular surface not only by direct infection but also by elaboration of toxins. In a series of patients with marginal keratitis, Chignell et al[333] were able to culture these bacteria from the eyelid margins of nearly 30 percent of patients (as opposed to 11 percent of unaffected controls). Other organisms that have been implicated in marginal keratitis include *Streptococcus pneumoniae, Haemophilus aegyptius, Bacillus* species, *Moraxella lacunata,* actinomycetes, *Neisseria gonorrhoeae, Escherichia coli,* and streptococci.[332,334]

The pathogenesis of marginal corneal infiltrates and ulcerations is thought to involve the deposition of antigen-antibody complexes in the peripheral corneal stroma.[335] The antigen is most likely an exotoxin elaborated by local bacteria. This was shown experimentally when Mondino et al[336,337] developed an animal model of catarrhal infiltrates by applying staphylococcal exotoxins onto the eyes of previously sensitized rabbits. They demonstrated that immune complexes were indeed deposited in the peripheral corneal stroma of these animals. It was their theory that immune complex deposition activates the classic complement pathway and leads to polymorphonuclear leukocyte infiltration with subsequent enzyme elaboration and ulceration.

Treatment

The treatment of marginal keratitis is twofold. First, because the lesions result from a local immunologic reaction, immune suppressants are effective. Topical corticosteroids, in low doses, are the agents of choice in the treatment of acute attacks. Long-term control, however, is based on reduction of the antigenic load by the use of topical antibiotics and eyelid hygiene. Similarly, oral tetracycline may help in cases associated with clinically evident meibomian gland disease.

A note of caution is necessary with regard to corticosteroid use. The peripheral corneal lesions of marginal keratitis can be confused with those of peripheral herpes simplex viral infections.[338] These herpetic lesions generally develop as ulcerations first, then progress to infiltrations; the typical dendritic appearance is not present in all cases. Therefore, if the history is in doubt, it is prudent to withhold corticosteroids until bacterial and viral culture results are obtained.

Phlyctenulosis

Phlyctenulosis is an inflammatory disorder involving the conjunctiva, limbus, and/or cornea. It is usually bilateral and primarily affects young children and young adults.

Clinical Features

Phlyctenules are pinkish white nodules that vary in size from pinpoint to several millimeters (Figure 23-28); they may be solitary or multiple. Generally, the limbus is affected first, although isolated involvement of the bulbar conjunctiva, tarsal conjunctiva, or even the cornea has been reported. The typical course of a phlyctenule is to become grayish, ulcerate, and heal completely within 10 to 15 days. Resolution of corneal lesions involves scarring and vascularization (Figure 23-29); conjunctival lesions do not scar. Phlyctenules involving the conjunctiva or limbus may migrate onto the cornea and spread centrally in a wandering fashion. These corneal migrations have a characteristic wedge-shaped leash of blood vessels from the most central extension back over the healed peripheral areas of previous involvement to the limbus. Stromal scarring is generally superficial, although deeper involvement may occur with staphylococcal phlyctenulosis. Corneal perforation rarely occurs in staphylococcal disease, but has been noted more commonly in tubercular disease[339] (Figure 23-30).

Patients with phlyctenulosis may have a wide range of symptoms. Isolated conjunctival lesions may cause only minimal ocular redness and foreign body sensation. Active corneal involvement, however, typically results in severe photophobia. Patients in areas of endemic tuberculosis should have a tuberculin skin test and, if necessary, a chest radiograph. In most areas of the United States, eyelid margin and conjunctival cultures are the only diagnostic tests required.

Pathogenesis

The pathogenesis of phlyctenulosis is believed to be similar to that of marginal keratitis, namely a local immunologic reaction of the ocular surface to bacteria-elaborated antigens. Immunologically, the pathogenesis of phlyctenulosis appears to be related to a cell-mediated type IV hypersensitivity reaction to these antigens. Prior exposure to these antigens is necessary for development of the cell-mediated response. Mondino et al,[336,337] in their animal model of marginal keratitis, were also able to create lesions similar to phlyctenules by applying staphylococcal exotoxin topically to previously sensitized rabbits. In the past, the presence of phlyctenules was closely linked to tuberculosis[334]; today, the most commonly associated microbial agent is *Staphylococcus aureus.*[336,337,340] Although other organisms have been implicated in the pathogenesis of phlyctenulosis (includ-

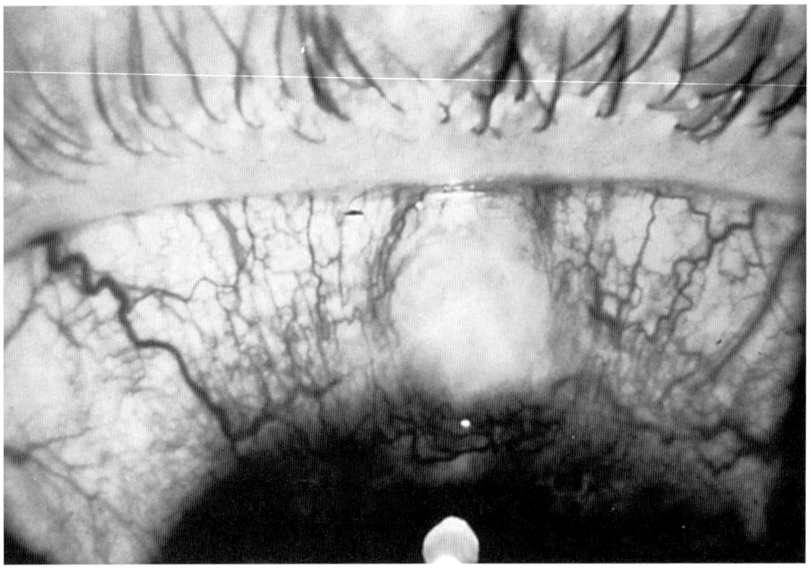

FIGURE 23-28 Limbal phlyctenule.

ing *Coccidioides imitis,* the lymphogranuloma venereum biovar of *Chlamydia trachomatis, Ascaris lumbricoides, Ancylostoma duodenale, Enterobius vermicularis, Entamoeba histolytica, Hymenolepis nana,* adenoviruses, and herpes simplex virus),[17,336,341] they are rarely associated with the disorder in the United States. In this country, phlyctenulosis is usually associated only with blepharitis.

Treatment

Treatment of phlyctenulosis should be directed at both the active disease and any predisposing condition. Any existing blepharoconjunctivitis should be aggressively treated with eyelid hygiene and topical antibiotics. Topical corticosteroids are the mainstay for treating the acute ocular lesions, particularly in tuberculosis-related disease.[340,342] Staphylococcal phlyctenulosis appears to be less responsive to these agents.[17] The efficacy of staphylococcal desensitization remains unproven. Phlyctenules may recur many times despite vigorous eyelid hygiene and treatment of previous phlyctenules with corticosteroids. Because of progressive corneal scarring, the prognosis for recurrent phlyctenulosis may be poor. In cases of central corneal involvement that has resulted in

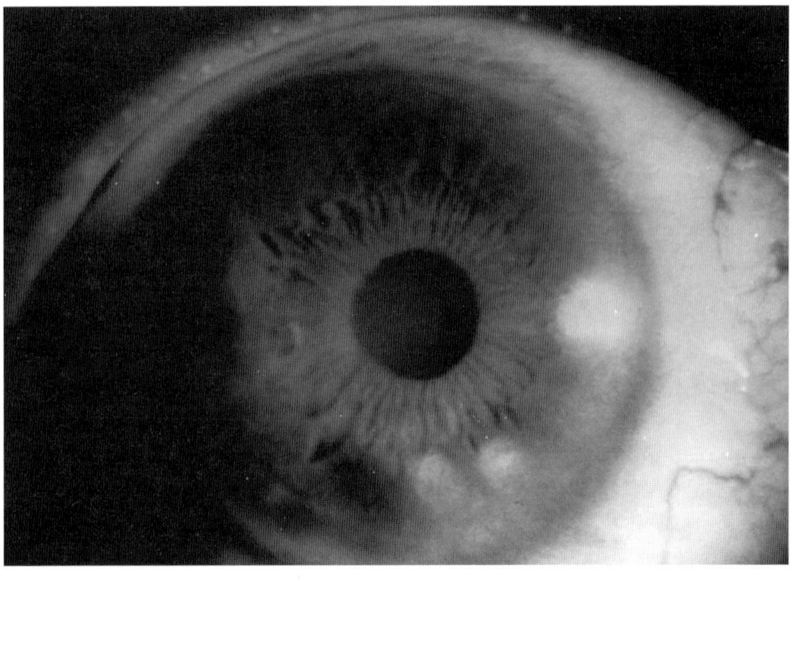

FIGURE 23-29 Three areas of corneal scarring caused by phlyctenulosis.

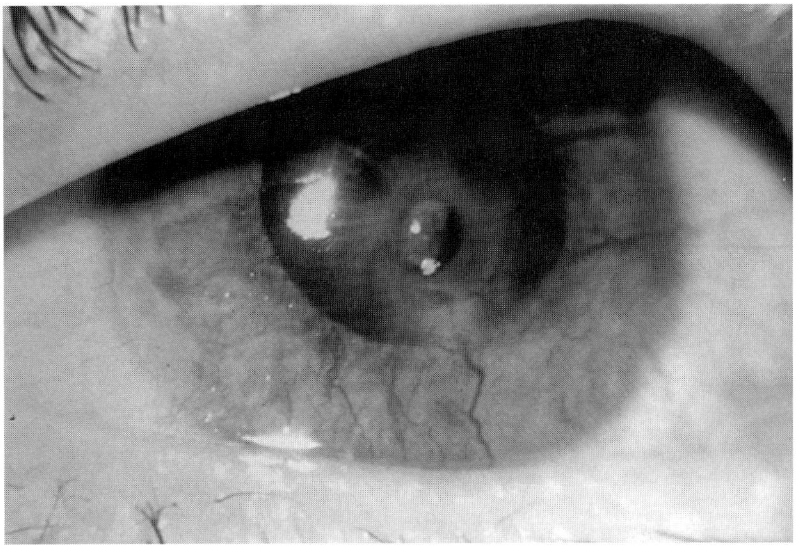

FIGURE 23-30 Corneal perforation from a phlyctenule. Note the leash of blood vessels inferiorly.

visually debilitating scarring, Smith et al[342] reported that penetrating keratoplasty can be effective.

Mooren's Ulcer

Mooren's ulcer is an idiopathic noninfectious ulceration of the peripheral cornea. In 1867, Mooren[343] described the disease in detail, thereby establishing it as a distinct clinical entity. Nettleship, in 1902, reviewed the cumulative literature on Mooren's ulcer, then totaling 78 cases.[344] Wood and Kaufman[345] categorized Mooren's ulcer into two clinical types. The first (or limited) type usually occurs in patients beyond their fourth decade of life, is usually unilateral, and responds well to medical therapy. The second (or "malignant") type occurs in younger patients (most frequently during the third decade of life), is usually bilateral, and is relentlessly progressive despite medical therapy. This latter type of ulcer was also described by Kietzman[346] in a series of 37 progressive cases of Mooren's ulcer in Nigerian men between the ages of 20 and 30 years. Subsequent reports[347,348] confirmed the frequency of the "malignant" form of Mooren's ulcer in young Nigerian males.

Clinical Features

Mooren's ulcer typically occurs in healthy men. Although it predominantly affects adults, one case has been reported in a 3-year-old child.[349] Patients complain of severe incapacitating pain, which occurs early in the course of the disease and is exacerbated by light. Visual acuity can become significantly diminished.

The clinical progression of Mooren's ulcer follows a typical course. It begins as an infiltrate in the peripheral anterior stroma, typically within the interpalpebral fissure. This is followed within weeks by loss of the overlying epithelium (Figure 23-31). Unlike staphylococcal marginal keratitis, there is no clear zone between the ulcer and the limbus. Some areas appear acutely inflamed, while other areas are in the progressive stages of healing. The central margin of the ulcer has a characteristic overhanging edge with intact overlying epithelium, a result of the central progression of the infiltrate occurring first in the deeper stroma, with the more anterior stroma and the epithelium following. The anterior one-half to one-third of the stroma is infiltrated and eventually melts, characteristically leaving a thinned residual stroma. Healing occurs with conjunctival vascularization over the residual peripheral stroma. The end result is a severely scarred cornea with resultant compromised visual acuity. Perforation is common in the "malignant" form of Mooren's ulcer, occurring in 36 percent of the cases in one series.[350]

In severe cases of Mooren's ulcer, the acute marginal inflammation may involve the entire cornea as well as the adjacent paralimbal tissue, with resultant scleritis, episcleritis, or conjunctival hyperemia. Although a mild anterior uveitis may be present, hypopyon in the absence of infection is rare. Cataract and secondary glaucoma are well-known complications of Mooren's ulcer.

Histopathology

The histopathology of Mooren's ulcer suggests an autoimmune process. The involved corneal stroma contains three distinct zones.[350] The superficial stroma is vascularized and infiltrated with neutrophils, plasma cells, and lymphocytes[350-352]; its collagen structure is disrupted. The

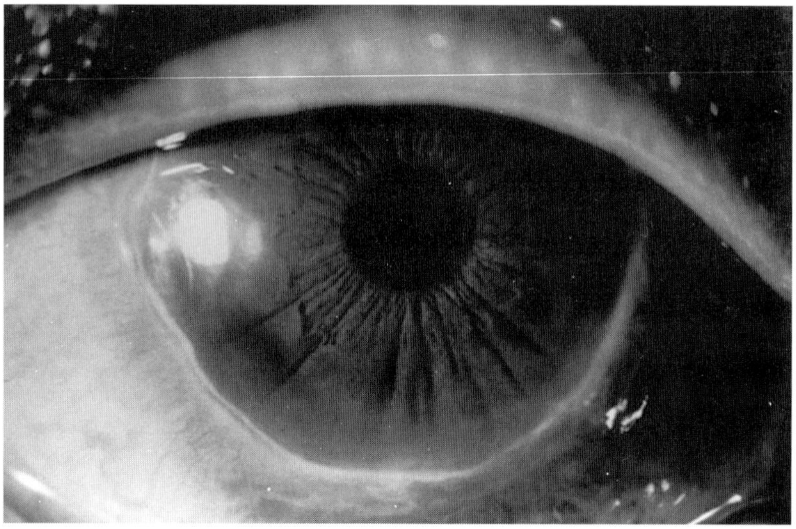

FIGURE 23-31 Mooren's ulcer.

midstroma shows collagen destruction, with fibroblastic hyperactivity. The deep stroma is characterized by macrophage infiltration. The leading edge of the ulcer shows disruption of the epithelial basement membrane and disorganization of the superficial stroma, together with heavy neutrophil infiltration. The adjacent conjunctiva is infiltrated with lymphocytes and plasma cells, as well as neutrophils, eosinophils, and mast cells.[352-354] Several investigators have described the presence of tissue-fixed autoantibodies and complement in the epithelial basement membrane and stroma of the involved cornea, as well as in the adjacent conjunctiva.[354-356]

Pathogenesis

The difference in clinical characteristics between the unilateral and bilateral types of Mooren's ulcer suggests a corresponding difference in their causes. The cause of unilateral Mooren's ulcer is unknown; affected patients have no associated systemic conditions. Several reports[347,348] of bilateral Mooren's ulcers occurring in Nigeria have implied an association with parasitic infection, especially systemic helminthiasis. Trojan[348] demonstrated the arrest of Mooren's ulcer in 14 Nigerian patients after treatment for systemic helminthiasis. Majekodunmi[347] demonstrated systemic helminth infections in four of his five Nigerian patients with Mooren's ulcer. However, the endemic prevalence of helminthiasis in these communities makes such implied causative associations conjectural. Although direct corneal infection by helminths has not been demonstrated, an immunologic mechanism has been hypothesized by which an antigen-antibody reaction may occur either to helminth toxins deposited on the cornea or to helminth-altered corneal antigens.[357]

Strong evidence suggests that Mooren's ulcer has an autoimmune cause. Because the disease is sometimes preceded by injury,[345,346] ocular surgery,[358-361] or infection,[347,348,362] Mooren's ulcer may represent an autoimmune response to altered corneal antigens. Serum antibodies against corneal and conjunctival tissue have been demonstrated by several investigators.[352,353,363-366] Elevated levels of circulating IgA[353,365] and immune complexes[363] have also been reported. Some investigators[351,365] have reported a possible role for cell-mediated autoimmunity in the pathogenesis of Mooren's ulcer.

Murray and Rahi[353] attributed the pathogenesis of Mooren's ulcer to a deficiency in circulating suppressor T cells. They suggested that the resultant imbalance in the helper/suppressor T-cell ratio may lead to antibody excess, chronic immune-complex–mediated inflammation, immune complex deposition in tissues, complement activation, neutrophil infiltration, and subsequent release of collagenolytic enzymes. Depressed suppressor T-cell function may also lead to production of autoantibodies, cytotoxic T cells, and lymphokine-producing T cells.

The pathogenesis of Mooren's-like marginal corneal ulceration following cataract extraction[358,360] is presumably related to surgical trauma.

Diagnosis

Mooren's ulcer is an idiopathic ocular condition, unassociated with any systemic disease. The presence of any circumferential marginal ulceration warrants the exclusion of associated systemic diseases, primarily the collagen vascular diseases and other vascular disorders. Ocular changes may be the first clinical presentation of these systemic disorders. Any case of noninfectious peripheral Mooren's-like ulceration should be evaluated with a thorough medical examination, as well as comprehensive laboratory investigations consisting of a complete blood count, measurement of erythrocyte sedimentation rate, antinuclear antibody and rheumatoid factor assays, liver function and chemistry panels, serology, chest radiography, and urinalysis, to exclude the possibility of an associated underlying vasculitic disease. Other systemic diseases that may uncommonly manifest with Mooren's-like ulceration include leukemia, gonorrhea, syphilis, and dysentery.

Mooren's ulcer can be distinguished easily from the primary (noninflammatory) peripheral corneal degenerations, primarily Terrien's marginal degeneration, pellucid marginal degeneration, and involutional marginal degeneration. The epithelium over these degenerative lesions usually remains intact, and pain is absent. Furthermore, these degenerations have a predilection for the vertical quadrants, in contradistinction to Mooren's ulcer, which usually begins in the horizontal interpalpebral fissure.

Staphylococcal marginal keratitis occasionally presents with peripheral corneal infiltration followed by epithelial breakdown. This entity can be differentiated from Mooren's ulcer by the presence of a lucent interval between the ulcer and the limbus, as well as the concurrent presence of blepharitis, the prompt response to topical corticosteroid therapy, the lack of progression over the follow-up period, and the lack of the severe debilitating pain that usually accompanies Mooren's ulcer.

Infectious peripheral corneal ulcers can be distinguished by a characteristic discharge, positive microbial culture results, and response to appropriate antibiotic therapy.

Treatment

Treatment of Mooren's ulcer is often unsatisfactory, especially in bilateral cases. The goal of therapy is to arrest the progression of the disease. Although initial management with topical cycloplegics and a bandage soft contact lens may alleviate the symptoms, the progression of the ulcer is usually unaffected. Topical corticosteroids are the next line of defense and their frequent use may arrest the progression of the unilateral limited or bilateral nonsimultaneous type of Mooren's ulcer[367–369]; however, these agents seldom affect the course of the bilateral, simultaneously active "malignant" type.

The role of systemic corticosteroids in the management of Mooren's ulcer has not been well outlined, although they are of theoretical value. Systemic immunosuppressive agents (such as azathioprine, methotrexate, and cyclophosphamide) have been tried when conventional medical management has failed to arrest the progression of these ulcers.[245,248,367,368] Although a therapeutic protocol has not yet been established, some reports of immunosuppressive therapy for Mooren's ulcer have been encouraging.[245,248] However, Brown and Mondino[368] have reported that nearly one-half of simultaneously bilateral cases are unresponsive to all medical therapy. The use of cyclosporine, although clinically unproven, is theoretically appealing because of its ability to increase the suppressor T-cell population.[353] A multitude of other therapies, including subconjunctival heparin, collagenase inhibitors,[370] and plasma exchange have been attempted, but none has been proven to be consistently effective in arresting the progression of the disease.

When maximal medical therapy fails, a resection of 4 mm of adjacent bulbar conjunctival tissue may halt the progression of the ulcer.[251,368,371–373] Brown[371] reported a 50 percent success rate with this procedure; however, its benefits are sometimes transient and the procedure may need to be repeated several times before the ulcer eventually heals. Furthermore, he noted that the lesion may recur at other sites in a majority of cases. Cryotherapy of the adjacent bulbar conjunctiva has been reported, but its clinical value is uncertain.[374] The therapeutic effects of such conjunctival destructive procedures may be accounted for by the elimination of inflammatory cells, immunoglobulins, complement, and collagenases from the limbal area; thus, the melting process may be interrupted long enough for the ulcer to become epithelialized. Following these conjunctival procedures, the eye should be fitted with a bandage soft contact lens for several weeks to promote epithelialization of the ulcer.

Other surgical procedures described for the acute phases of Mooren's ulcer are directed at arresting the melting process and maintaining the integrity of the eye. These include lamellar keratoplasty,[372,375–377] delimiting keratotomy,[378] cyanoacrylate application,[379–381] central lamellar keratectomy,[382] and conjunctival flaps.[383,384] In our experience, keratotomies, keratectomies, and conjunctival flaps are rarely beneficial. In cases of extreme peripheral thinning, a large tectonic onlay lamellar graft (epikeratophakia) is useful, and appears to be better than a large doughnut-shaped inlay lamellar graft.

Mooren's ulcer is one of the few conditions in which a lamellar patch graft may become involved by the disease process and melt (Figure 23-32). Other than intensive medical therapy and repeat lamellar grafts, there are no treatment options that are more satisfactory, although pretibial periosteum may be used to repair the thinned area if it does not involve the central cornea. Recurrence of thinning in Mooren's ulcer appears to be tissue specific, and the periosteum does not melt.

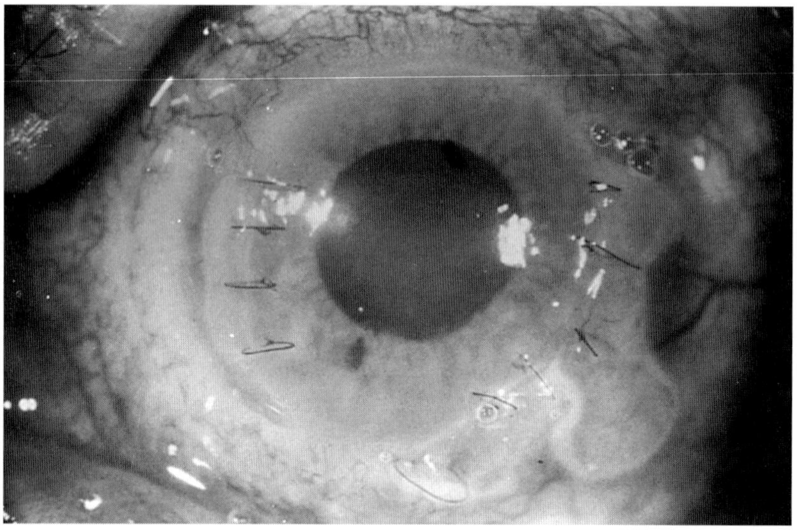

FIGURE 23-32 Melting of lamellar patch grafts in a patient with Mooren's ulcer.

When the inflammatory process has resolved, leaving behind a thinned scarred cornea, surgical restoration of the cornea and rehabilitation of visual acuity may be attempted. In cases of extreme corneal thinning, a large tectonic onlay lamellar graft (epikeratophakia) followed by a therapeutic small penetrating central graft may be necessary. This appears safer than a large tectonic penetrating graft because of the decreased likelihood of graft rejection and postoperative glaucoma.

REFERENCES

1. Smolin G, O'Connor GR: Ocular Immunology. Lea & Febiger, Philadelphia, 1981
2. Allansmith MR, McClellan BH: Immunoglobulins in the human cornea. Am J Ophthalmol 80:123, 1975
3. Morgan SJ, Williams JH, Walls AF, et al: Mast cell numbers and staining characteristics in the normal and allergic human conjunctiva. J Allergy Clin Immunol 87:111, 1991
4. Abelson MB, Madiwale N, Weston JH: Conjunctival eosinophils in allergic ocular disease. Arch Ophthalmol 101:631, 1983
5. Theodore FH: The significance of conjunctival eosinophilia in the diagnosis of allergic conjunctivitis. Ear Nose Throat J 30:653, 1951
6. Abelson MB, Udell IJ, Weston JH: Conjunctival eosinophils in compound 48/80 rabbit model. Arch Ophthalmol 101:631, 1983
7. Butrus SI, Ochsner KI, Abelson MB, Schwartz LB: The level of tryptase in human tears: an indicator of activation of conjunctival mast cells. Ophthalmology 97:1678, 1990
8. Azevedo M, Castel-Branco MG, Oliveira JF, et al: Double-blind comparison of levocabastine eye drops with sodium cromoglycate and placebo in the treatment of seasonal allergic conjunctivitis. Clin Exp Allergy 21:689, 1991
9. Abelson MB, Paradis A, George MA, et al: Effects of vasocon-A in the allergen challenge model of acute allergic conjunctivitis. Arch Ophthalmol 108:520, 1990
10. Calonge MC, Pastor JC, Herreras JM, González JL: Pharmacologic modulation of vascular permeability in ocular allergy in the rat. Invest Ophthalmol Vis Sci 31:176, 1990
11. Greenbaum J, Cockcroft D, Hargreave FE, et al: Sodium cromoglycate in ragweed-allergic conjunctivitis. J Allergy Clin Immunol 59:437, 1977
12. Beigelman MN: Vernal Conjunctivitis. University of Southern California Press, Los Angeles, 1950
13. Neumann E, Gutman MJ, Blumenkrantz N, Michaelson IC: A review of 400 cases of vernal conjunctivitis. Am J Ophthalmol 74:166, 1959
14. Allansmith MR: Vernal conjunctivitis. p. 1. In Duane TD (ed): Clinical Ophthalmology. Vol. 4. Harper & Row, Philadelphia, 1984
15. Allansmith M, Frick OL: Antibodies to grass in vernal conjunctivitis. J Allergy 34:535, 1963
16. Zavaro A, Baryishak YR, Samra Z, Sompolinsky D: Extrinsic and idiopathic vernal keratoconjunctivitis? Two cases with dissimilar immunopathology. Br J Ophthalmol 67:742, 1983
17. Grayson M: Diseases of the Cornea. 2nd Ed. CV Mosby, St. Louis, 1983
18. Frankland AW, Easty D: Vernal keratoconjunctivitis: an atopic disease. Trans Ophthalmol Soc UK 91:479, 1971
19. Beigelman MN: Dystrophy of the corneal epithelium in vernal catarrh. Am J Ophthalmol 15:95, 1932
20. Jones BR: Vernal keratitis. Trans Ophthalmol Soc UK 81:215, 1962

21. Tobgy AF: Keratitis epithelialis vernalis. Bull Ophthalmol Soc Egypt 28:104, 1935
22. Shuler JD, Levenson J, Mondino BJ: Inferior corneal ulcers associated with palpebral vernal conjunctivitis. Am J Ophthalmol 106:106, 1988
23. Tabbara KF, Butrus ST: Vernal keratoconjunctivitis and keratoconus. Am J Ophthalmol 95:704, 1983
24. Gormaz A, Eggers C: Vernal keratoconjunctivitis and keratoconus. Am J Ophthalmol 96:555, 1983
25. Allansmith MR, Abelson MB: Ocular allergies. p. 231. In Smolin G, Thoft RA (eds): The Cornea: Scientific Foundations and Clinical Practice. Little, Brown, Boston, 1983
26. Allansmith MR: The Eye and Immunology. CV Mosby, St. Louis, 1982
27. Allansmith MR, Baird RS: Percentage of degranulated mast cells in vernal conjunctivitis and giant papillary conjunctivitis associated with contact lens wear. Am J Ophthalmol 91:71, 1981
28. Henriquez AS, Kenyon KR, Allansmith MR: Mast cell ultrastructure: comparison in contact lens-associated giant papillary conjunctivitis and vernal conjunctivitis. Arch Ophthalmol 99:1266, 1981
29. Morgan G: The pathology of vernal conjunctivitis. Trans Ophthalmol Soc UK 91:467, 1971
30. Dherny P, Pouliquen Y, Foels MO, Salvoldelli M: The vernal plaque, a complication of so-called spring conjunctivitis. J Fr Ophtalmol 8:711, 1985
31. Jones BR: Allergic disease of the outer eye. Trans Ophthalmol Soc UK 9:441, 1971
32. Ballow M, Mendelson L: Specific immunoglobulin E antibodies in tear secretions of patients with vernal conjunctivitis. J Allergy Clin Immunol 66:112, 1980
33. Easty DL, Brickenshaw M, Merrett T, et al: Immunological investigations in vernal eye disease. Trans Ophthalmol Soc UK 100:98, 1980
34. Allansmith MR, Hahn GS, Simon MA: Tissue, tear, and serum IgE concentrations in vernal conjunctivitis. Am J Ophthalmol 81:506, 1976
35. Alimuddin M: Vernal conjunctivitis. Br J Ophthalmol 39:160, 1955
36. Maggi E, Biswas P, Del Prete G, et al: Accumulation of Th-2-like helper T cells in the conjunctiva of patients with vernal conjunctivitis. J Immunol 146:1169, 1991
37. Samra Z, Zavaro A, Baryishak Y, Sampolinsky D: Vernal keratoconjunctivitis: the significance of immunoglobulin E levels in tears and serum. Int Arch Allergy Appl Immunol 74:158, 1984
38. Brauninger GE, Centifanto YM: Immunoglobulin E in human tears. Am J Ophthalmol 72:558, 1971
39. Abelson MB, Soter NA, Simon MA, et al: Histamine in human tears. Am J Ophthalmol 83:417, 1977
40. Allansmith MR, Baird RS, Higginbotham EJ, Abelson MB: Technical aspects of histamine determination in human tears. Am J Ophthalmol 90:714, 1980
41. Abelson MB, Baird RS, Allansmith MR: Tear histamine levels in vernal conjunctivitis and other ocular inflammations. Ophthalmology 87:812, 1980
42. Udell IJ, Gleich GJ, Allansmith MR, et al: Eosinophil granule major basic protein and Carcot-Leyden crystal protein in human tears. Am J Ophthalmol 92:824, 1981
43. Trocme S, Kephart GM, Allansmith MR, et al: Conjunctival deposition of eosinophil granule major basic protein in vernal keratoconjunctivitis and contact lens-associated giant papillary conjunctivitis. Am J Ophthalmol 108:57, 1989
44. Khatami M, Donnelly JJ, John T, Rockey JH: Vernal conjunctivitis: model studies in guinea pigs immunized topically with fluoresceinyl ovalbumin. Arch Ophthalmol 102:1683, 1984
45. Easty DL, Rice NSE, Jones BR: Clinical trial of topical disodium cromoglycate in vernal keratoconjunctivitis. Clin Allergy 2:99, 1972
46. Tabbara KF, Arafat NT: Cromolyn effects on vernal keratoconjunctivitis in children. Arch Ophthalmol 95:2184, 1977
47. El Hennawi M: Clinical trial with 2% sodium cromoglycate (Opticrom) in vernal keratoconjunctivitis. Br J Ophthalmol 64:483, 1980
48. Baryishak YR, Zavaro A, Monselise M, et al: Veral keratoconjunctivitis in an Israeli group of patients and its treatment with sodium cromoglycate. Br J Ophthalmol 66:118, 1982
49. Vakil DV, Ayiomamitis A, Nizami RM: Treatment of seasonal conjunctivitis: comparison of 2% and 4% sodium cromoglycate ophthalmic solutions. Can J Ophthalmol 19:207, 1984
50. Hyams SW, Bialik M, Neumann E: Clinical trails of topical disodium cromoglycate in vernal keratoconjunctivitis. J Pediatr Ophthalmol 12:116, 1975
51. Foster CS, The Cromolyn Sodium Collaborative Study Group: Evaluation of topical cromolyn sodium in the treatment of vernal keratoconjunctivitis. Ophthalmology 95:194, 1988
52. Butrus SI, Leung DY, Gellis S, et al: Vernal conjunctivitis in the hyperimmunoglobulinemia E syndrome. Ophthalmology 91:1213, 1984
53. Irani AM, Butrus SI, Tabbara KF, Schwartz LB: Human conjunctival mast cells: distribution of MCT and MCTC in vernal conjunctivitis and giant papillary conjunctivitis. J Allergy Clin Immunol 86:34, 1990
54. Jay JL: Clinical features and diagnosis of adult atopic keratoconjunctivitis and the effect of treatment with sodium cromoglycate. Br J Ophthalmol 65:335, 1981
55. Meisler DM, Zaret CR, Stock EL: Trantas dots and limbal inflammation associated with soft contact lens wear. Am J Ophthalmol 89:66, 1980
56. Abelson MB, Butrus SI, Weston JH: Aspirin therapy in vernal keratoconjunctivitis. Am J Ophthalmol 95:502, 1983
57. BenEzra D, Pe'er J, Brodsky M, Cohen E: Cyclosporine eyedrops for the treatment of severe vernal keratoconjunctivitis. Am J Ophthalmol 101:278, 1986
58. Singh G: Cryosurgery in palpebral vernal catarrh. Ann Ophthalmol 14:252, 1982
59. Abiose A, Merz M: Cryosurgery in the management of vernal keratoconjunctivitis. Ann Ophthalmol 15:744, 1983

60. Cameron JA, Antonios SR, Badr IA: Excimer laser phototherapeutic keratectomy for shield ulcers and corneal plaques in vernal keratoconjunctivitis. J Refract Surg 11:31, 1995
61. Allansmith MR, Korb DR, Greiner JV, et al: Giant papillary conjunctivitis in contact lens wearers. Am J Ophthalmol 83:697, 1977
62. Fowler SA, Greiner JV, Allansmith MR: Soft contact lenses from patients with giant papillary conjunctivitis. Am J Ophthalmol 88:1056, 1979
63. Allansmith MR, Korb DR, Greiner JV: Giant papillary conjunctivitis induced by hard or soft contact lens wear: quantitative histology. Ophthalmology 85:766, 1979
64. Sheldon L, Biedner B, Geltman C, et al: Giant papillary conjunctivitis and ptosis in a contact lens wearer. J Pediatr Ophthalmol Strabismus 16:136, 1984
65. Korb DR, Allansmith MR, Greiner JV, et al: Prevalence of conjunctival changes in wearers of hard contact lenses. Am J Ophthalmol 90:336, 1980
66. Meisler DM, Krachmer JH, Goeken JA: An immunopathologic study of giant papillary conjunctivitis associated with an ocular prosthesis. Am J Ophthalmol 92:368, 1981
67. Srinivasan BD, Jakobiec FA, Iwamoto T, DeVoe AG: Giant papillary conjunctivitis with ocular prosthesis. Arch Ophthalmol 97:892, 1979
68. Robin JB, Regis-Pacheco LF, May WN, et al: Giant papillary conjunctivitis associated with an extruded scleral buckle [letter]. Arch Ophthalmol 105:619, 1987
69. Friedman T, Friedman Z, Neumann E: Giant papillary conjunctivitis. Ophthalmic Surg 15:139, 1984
70. Jolson AS, Jolson SC: Suture barb giant papillary conjunctivitis. Ophthalmic Surg 15:139, 1984
71. Sugar A, Meyer RF: Giant papillary conjunctivitis after keratoplasty. Am J Ophthalmol 91:239, 1981
72. Spring TF: Reaction to hydrophilic lenses. Med J Aust 1:499, 1974
73. Korb DR, Greiner JV, Finnermore VM, et al: Biomicroscopy of papillae associated with wearing of soft contact lenses. Br J Ophthalmol 67:733, 1983
74. Donshik PC, Ballow M: Tear immunoglobulins in giant papillary conjunctivitis induced by contact lenses. Am J Ophthalmol 96:460, 1983
75. Elgebaly SA, Donshik PC, Rahhal F, Williams W: Neutrophil chemotactic factors in the tears of giant papillary conjunctivitis patients. Invest Ophthalmol Vis Sci 32:208, 1991
76. Allansmith MR, Baird RS, Greiner JV: Vernal conjunctivitis and contact lens-associated giant papillary conjunctivitis compared and contrasted. Am J Ophthalmol 87:544, 1979
77. Meisler DM, Berzins UJ, Krachmer JH, Stock L: Cromolyn treatment of giant papillary conjunctivitis. Arch Ophthalmol 100:1608, 1982
78. Carr RD, Berke M, Becker SW: Incidence of atopy in the general population. Arch Dermatol 89:27, 1964
79. Roth H, Kierland R: The natural history of atopic dermatitis. Arch Dermatol 89:209, 1964
80. Hanifin JM, Lobitz WC: Newer concepts of atopic dermatitis. Arch Dermatol 113:663, 1977
81. Braude LS, Chandler JW: Atopic corneal disease. Int Ophthalmol Clin 24:145, 1984
82. Hogan MJ: Atopic keratoconjunctivitis. Am J Ophthalmol 36:937, 1953
83. Karel T, Myska F, Kvicalova E: Ophthalmological changes in atopic dermatitis. Acta Derm Venereol (Stockh) 45:381, 1985
84. Tuft SJ, Kemeny DM, Dart JKG, Buckley RJ: Clinical features of atopic keratoconjunctivitis. Ophthalmology 98:150, 1991
85. Rich LF, Hanifin JM: Ocular complications of atopic dermatitis and other eczemas. Int Ophthalmol Clin 25:61, 1985
86. Fridman SJ, Schroeter AL, Homburger HA: IgE antibodies to *Staphylococcus aureus*: prevalence in patients with atopic dermatitis. Arch Dermatol 121:869, 1985
87. Brunsting LA, Reed WB, Bair HL: Occurrence of cataracts and keratoconus with atopic dermatitis. Arch Dermatol 72:237, 1955
88. Hurlbut WB, Domonkos AN: Cataract and retinal detachment associated with atopic dermatitis. Arch Ophthalmol 52:852, 1954
89. Cowan A, Klaruder JV: Frequency of occurrence of cataracts in atopic dermatitis. Arch Ophthalmol 43:759, 1950
90. Coles RS, Laval J: Retinal detachments occurring in cataract associated with neurodermatitis. Arch Ophthalmol 48:30, 1952
91 Stone SP, Muller SA, Gleich GJ: IgE levels in atopic dermatitis. Arch Dermatol 108:806, 1973
92. Jansen CT, Haapalhi J, Hopsu-Havu VK: Immunoglobulin E in the human atopic skin. Arch Dermatol Forsch 246:299, 1973
93. Johansson SGO, Juhlin L: Immunoglobulin E in "healed" atopic dermatitis and after treatment with corticosteroids and azathioprine. Br J Ophthalmol 82:10, 1970
94. McGeady SJ, Buckley RH: Depression of cell-mediated immunity in atopic eczema. J Allergy Clin Immunol 56:39, 1975
95. Carapeto FJ, Winkelmann RK, Jordan RE: T and B lymphocytes in contact and atopic dermatitis. Arch Dermatol 112:1095, 1976
96. Rachelefsky GS, Opelz G, Mickey MR, et al: Defective T-cell function in atopic dermatitis. J Allergy Clin Immunol 57:50, 1976
97. Lobitz WC, Honeyman JF, Winkler NW: Suppressed cell-mediated immunity in two adults with atopic dermatitis. Br J Dermatol 86:317, 1972
98. Gottlieb BR, Hanifin JM: Circulating T-cell deficiency in atopic dermatitis. Clin Res 22:150, 1974
99. Hall TJ, Rycroft R, Brostoff J: Decreased natural killer cell activity in atopic eczema. Immunology 56:337, 1985
100. Parke CW, Kennedy S, Eisen AZ: Leukocyte and lymphocyte cyclic AMP responses in atopic eczema. J Invest Dermatol 65:302, 1976

101. Hanifin JM, Butler JM, Chan SC: Immunopharmacology of the atopic diseases. J Invest Dermatol 85(suppl):161, 1985
102. Ostler HB, Martin RG, Dawson DR: The use of sodium cromoglycate in the treatment of atopic ocular disease. p. 99. In Leopold IH, Burns RD (eds): Symposium on Ocular Therapy. John Wiley & Sons, New York, 1977
103. Allansmith MR, Ross RN: Ocular allergy and mast cell stabilizers. Surv Ophthalmol 30:229, 1986
104. Turgeon PW, Nauheim RC, Roat MI, et al: Indications for keratoepithelioplasty. Arch Ophthalmol 108:233, 1990
105. Cowen SJ, Anhalt GJ, Wicha MS, et al: Distribution of pemphigus and pemphigoid antigens, laminin, and type IV collagen in corneal epithelium. Invest Ophthalmol Vis Sci 21:879, 1981
106. Rook A, Wilkinson DS, Ebling FJG: Textbook of Dermatology. Vol. 2. Blackwell Scientific, Oxford, 1968
107. Leonard JN, Wright P, Haffenden GP, et al: Skin diseases and the dry eye. Trans Ophthalmol Soc UK 104:467, 1985
108. Person JR, Rogers RS: Bullous and cicatricial pemphigoid: clinical, histopathologic, and immunopathologic correlations. Mayo Clin Proc 52:54, 1977
109. Mondino BJ: Cicatricial pemphigoid and erythema multiforme. Ophthalmology 97:939, 1990
110. Wright P: Cicatrizing conjunctivitis. Trans Ophthalmol UK 105:1, 1986
111. Bean SF: Cicatricial pemphigoid. Int J Dermatol 14:23, 1975
112. Mondino BJ, Brown SI, Lempert S, et al: The acute manifestations of ocular cicatricial pemphigoid. Ophthalmology 86:543, 1979
113. Foster CS, Wilson LA, Ekins MB: Immunosuppressive therapy for progressive ocular cicatricial pemphigoid. Ophthalmology 88:340, 1982
114. Mondino BJ, Brown SI: Ocular cicatricial pemphigoid. Ophthalmology 88:95, 1981
115. Ralph RA: Conjunctival goblet cell density in normal subjects and in dry eye syndromes. Invest Ophthalmol 14:299, 1975
116. Nelson JD, Wright JC: Conjunctival goblet cell densities in ocular surface disease. Arch Ophthalmol 102:1049, 1984
117. Lemp MA, Dohlman CH, Kuwabara T, et al: Dry eye secondary to mucus deficiency. Trans Am Acad Ophthalmol Otolaryngol 75:1223, 1971
118. Norn MS, Kristensen EB: Benign mucous membrane pemphigoid II: cytology. Acta Ophthalmol (Copenh) 52:282, 1974
119. Anderson SR, Jensen OA, Kristensen EB, et al: Benign mucous membrane pemphigoid III: biopsy. Acta Ophthalmol (Copenh) 52:455, 1974
120. Thoft RA, Friend J, Kinoshita S, et al: Ocular cicatricial pemphigoid associated with hyperproliferation of the conjunctival epithelium. Am J Ophthalmol 98:37, 1984
121. Roat MI, Sossi G, Lo CY, Thoft RA: Hyperproliferation of conjunctival fibroblasts from patients with cicatricial pemphigoid. Arch Ophthalmol 107:1064, 1989
122. Carroll JM, Kuwabara T: Ocular pemphigus. Arch Ophthalmol 80:683, 1968
123. Brauner JG, Jimbow K: Benign mucous membrane pemphigoid: an unusual case with electronmicroscopic findings. Arch Dermatol 106:535, 1972
124. Galbavy EJ, Foster CS: Ultrastructural characteristics of conjunctiva in cicatricial pemphigoid. Cornea 4:127, 1986
125. Foster CS, Shaw CD, Wells PA: Scanning electron microscopy of conjunctival surfaces in patients with ocular cicatrical pemphigoid. Am J Ophthalmol 102:584, 1986
126. Furey N, West C, Andrews T, et al: Immunofluorescent studies of ocular cicatricial pemphigoid. Am J Ophthalmol 80:825, 1975
127. Rogers RSIII, Perry HO, Bean SF, et al: Immunopathology of cicatricial pemphigoid: studies of complement deposition. J Invest Dermatol 68:39, 1977
128. Mondino BJ, Ross AN, Rabin BS, Brown SI: Autoimmune phenomena in ocular cicatricial pemphigoid. Am J Ophthalmol 83:443, 1977
129. Waltman SR, Yarian D: Circulating autoantibodies in ocular pemphigoid. Am J Ophthalmol 77:891, 1974
130. Mondino BJ, Rao H, Brown SI: T and B lymphocytes in ocular cicatricial pemphigoid. Am J Ophthalmol 92:536, 1981
131. Griffith MR, Fukuyama K, Tuffanelli D, Silverman S Jr: Immunofluorescent studies in mucous membrane pemphigoid. Arch Dermatol 109:195, 1974
132. Mondino BJ, Brown SI, Rabin BS: HLA antigens in ocular cicatricial pemphigoid. Arch Ophthalmol 97:479, 1979
133. Mondino BJ, Brown SI: Immunosuppressive therapy in ocular cicatricial pemphigoid. Am J Ophthalmol 96:453, 1983
134. Dantzig PI: Circulating antibodies in cicatricial pemphigoid. Arch Dermatol 108:264, 1973
135. Anhalt GJ, Bahn CF, Labib RS, et al: Pathogenic effects of bullous pemphigoid autoantibodies on rabbit corneal epithelium. J Clin Invest 68:1097, 1981
136 Proia AD, Foulks GN, Sanfilippo FP: Ocular cicatricial pemphigoid with granular IgA and complement deposition. Arch Ophthalmol 103:1669, 1985
137. Harrist TJ, Mihm MC: Cutaneous immunopathology: the diagnostic use of direct and indirect immunofluorescence techniques in dermatologic disease. Hum Pathol 6:625, 1979
138. Rice BA, Foster CS: Immunopathology of cicatricial pemphigoid affecting the conjunctiva. Ophthalmology 97:1476, 1990
139. Sacks EH, Jakobiec FA, Wieczorek R, et al: Immunophenotypic analysis of the inflammatory infiltrate in ocular cicatricial pemphigoid: further evidence of a T-cell mediated disease. Ophthalmology 96:236, 1989
140. Nelson JD: Ocular surface impressions using cellulose acetate filter material: ocular pemphigoid. Surv Ophthalmol 27:76, 1982
141. Leonard JN, Hobday CM, Haffenden BR, et al: Immunofluorescent studies in ocular cicatricial pemphigoid. Br J Dermatol 118:209, 1988

142. Patten JT, Cavanagh HD, Allansmith MR: Induced ocular pseudopemphigoid. Am J Ophthalmol 83:443, 1977
143. Wright P: Skin reactions to practolol. Br Med J 2:560, 1974
144. Hirst LW, Werblin T, Novak M, et al: Drug-induced cicatrizing conjunctivitis simulating ocular pemphigoid. Cornea 1:121, 1982
145. Lass JH, Thoft RA, Dohlman CH: Idoxuridine-induced conjunctival cicatrization. Arch Ophthalmol 101:747, 1983
146. Norn MS: Pemphigoid related to epinephrine treatment. Am J Ophthalmol 83:138, 1977
147. Pouliquen Y, Patey A, Foster CS, et al: Drug-induced cicatricial pemphigoid affecting the conjunctiva: light and electron microscopic features. Ophthalmology 93:775, 1986
148. Hardy KM, Perry HO, Pingree GC, et al: Benign mucous membrane pemphigoid. Arch Dermatol 104:467, 1971
149. Dantzig PI: Immunosuppressive and cytoxic drugs in dermatology. Arch Dermatol 110:393, 1974
150. Dave VK, Vickers CFH: Azathioprene in the treatment of mucocutaneous pemphigoid. Br J Dermatol 90:183, 1974
151. Brody JH, Pirozzi DJ: Benign mucous membrane pemphigoid. Response to therapy with cyclophosphamide. Arch Dermatol 113:1598, 1977
152. Thivolet J, Barthelemey H, Rigot-Muller G, et al: Effects of cyclosporin on bullous pemphigoid and pemphigus. Lancet 1:334, 1985
153. Mackie IA: Contact lenses in dry eyes. Trans Ophthalmol Soc UK 104:477, 1985
154. Berk MA, Lorincz AL: The treatment of bullous pemphigoid with tetracycline and niacinamide. Arch Dermatol 122:670, 1986
155. Martí-Huguet T, Quintana M, Cabiró I: Cicatricial pemphigoid associated with D-penicillamine treatment [letter]. Arch Ophthalmol 107:1115, 1989
156. Kremer I, Rozenbaum D, Aviel E: Immunofluorescence findings in pseudopemphigoid induced by short-term idoxuridine administration [letter]. Am J Ophthalmol 111:375, 1991
157. Ormerod LD, Fong LP, Foster CS: Corneal infection in mucosal scarring disorders and Sjögren's syndrome. Am J Ophthalmol 105:512, 1988
158. Tauber J, de la Maza MS, Foster CS: Systemic chemotherapy for ocular cicatricial pemphigoid. Cornea 10:185, 1991
159. Neumann R, Tauger J, Foster CS: Remission and recurrence after withdrawal of therapy for ocular cicatricial pemphigoid. Ophthalmology 98:858, 1991
160. Fern AI, Jay JL, Young H, MacKie R: Dapsone therapy for the acute inflammatory phase of ocular pemphigoid. Br J Ophthalmol 76:332, 1992
161. Jordan RW, Trifthauser CT, Schroeter AL: Direct immunofluorescent studies of pemphigus and bullous pemphigoid. Arch Dermatol 103:486, 1971
162. Tugal-Tutkun I, Akova YA, Foster CS: Penetrating keratoplasty in cicatrizing conjunctival diseases. Ophthalmology 102:576, 1995
163. Tuffanelli CL: Cutaneous immunopathology: recent observations. J Invest Dermatol 65:143, 1975
164. Ahmed AR, Maize JC, Provost TT: Bullous pemphigoid: clinical and immunologic follow-up after successful therapy. Arch Dermatol 113:1043, 1977
165. Venning VA, Frith PA, Bron AJ, et al: Mucosal involvement in bullous and cicatricial pemphigoid: a clinical and immunopathologic study. Br J Dermatol 118:7, 1988
166. Lever WF: Pemphigus and pemphigoid: a review of the advances made since 1964. J Am Acad Dermatol 1:2, 1979
167. Greaves MW, Burton JL, Marks J, Dawber RP: Azathioprine in treatment of bullous pemphigoid. Br Med J 1:144, 1971
168. Krain LS, Landau JW, Newcomer VD: Cyclophosphamide in the treatment of pemphigus vulgaris and bullous pemphigoid. Arch Dermatol 106:657, 1972
169. Person JR, Rogers RS III: Bullous pemphigoid responding to sulfapyridine and the sulfones. Arch Dermatol 113:610, 1977
170. Goldberg NS, Robinson JK, Roenigk HH, et al: Plasmapheresis therapy for bullous pemphigoid [letter]. Arch Dermatol 121:1484, 1985
171. Bean SF, Holubar K, Gillett RB: Pemphigus involving the eyes. Arch Dermatol 111:1484, 1975
172. Herron BE: Immunologic aspects of cicatricial pemphigoid. Am J Ophthalmol 79:271, 1975
173. Stevens AM, Johnson FC: A new eruptive fever associated with stomatitis and ophthalmia. Am J Dis Child 24:526, 1922
174. Bianchine JR, Macarey PVJ, Lasagna L, et al: Drugs as etiologic factors in the Stevens-Johnson syndrome. Am J Med 44:390, 1968
175. Howard GM: The Stevens-Johnson syndrome. Ocular prognosis and treatment. Am J Ophthalmol 55:893, 1963
176. Patz A: Ocular involvement in erythema multiforme. Arch Ophthalmol 43:244, 1950
177. Ashby DW, Lazar T: Erythema multiforme exudativum major. Lancet 1:1091, 1951
178. Courson DB: Stevens-Johnson syndrome. Nonspecific parasensitivity reaction? JAMA 198:133, 1966
179. Ostler HB, Conant MA, Groundwater J: Lyell's disease, the Stevens-Johnson syndrome, and exfoliative dermatitis. Trans Am Acad Ophthalmol Otolaryngol 74:1254, 1970
180. Foster CS, Fong LP, Azar D, Kenyon KR: Episodic conjunctival inflammation after Stevens-Johnson syndrome. Ophthalmology 95:453, 1988
181. Dohlman CH, Doughman DJ: The Stevens-Johnson syndrome. Trans New Orleans Acad Ophthalmol 7:1254, 1970
182. Baum J: Clinical manifestations of dry eye states. Trans Ophthalmol Soc UK 104:415, 1985
183. Arstikaitis MJ: Ocular aftermath of Stevens-Johnson syndrome. Arch Ophthalmol 90:376, 1973
184. Kiernan JP, Schanzlin DJ, Leveille AS: Stevens-Johnson syndrome associated with adenovirus conjunctivitis. Am J Ophthalmol 92:543, 1981
185. Yetiv JZ, Bianchine JR, Owen JA: Etiologic factors of the Stevens-Johnson syndrome. South Med J 73:799, 1980
186. Bedi TR, Pincus H: Histopathological spectrum of erythema multiforme. Br J Dermatol 95:243, 1976

187. Kazmierowski JA, Wuepper KD: Erythema multiforme: immune complex vasculitis of the superficial cutaneous microvasculature. J Invest Dermatol 71:366, 1978
188. Swinehart JM, Weston WL, Huf JC, et al: Identification of circulating immune complexes in erythema multiforme. Clin Res 26:577A, 1978
189. Safai B, Good RA, Day NK: Erythema multiforme: report of two cases and speculation on immune mechanisms involved in the pathogenesis. Clin Immunol Immunopathol 7:379, 1977
190. Wuepper KD, Watson PA, Kazmierowski JA: Immune complexes in erythema multiforme and the Stevens-Johnson syndrome. J Invest Dermatol 74:368, 1980
191. Carroll OM, Bryan PA, Robinson RJ: Stevens-Johnson syndrome associated with long-acting sulfonamides. JAMA 195:179, 1981
192. Taylor GM: Stevens-Johnson syndrome following the use of an ultra-long-acting sulphonamide. S Afr Med J 42:501, 1968
193. Gottschalk HR, Stone OJ: Stevens-Johnson syndrome from ophthalmic sulfonamide. Arch Dermatol 112:513, 1976
194. Rubin Z: Ophthalmic sulfonamide-induced Stevens-Johnson syndrome [letter]. Arch Dermatol 113:235, 1977
195. McArthur JE, Dyment PG: Stevens-Johnson syndrome with hepatitis following therapy with ampicillin and cephalexin. N Z Med J 81:390, 1975
196. Bomb BS, Purohit SD, Bedi HK: Stevens-Johnson syndrome caused by isoniazid. Tubercle 57:229, 1976
197. Ritchie EB, Kolb W: Reaction to sodium diphenylhydantionate (Dilantin sodium): hemorrhagic erythema multiforme terminating fatally. Arch Dermatol Syphilol 46:856, 1942
198. Soll SN: Eruptive fever with involvement of the respiratory tract, conjunctivitis, stomatitis, and balanitis. Arch Intern Med 79:475, 1947
199. Scott TF: Hypersensitivity syndromes. Pediatr Clin North Am p. 771, August, 1956
200. Steel SJ, Moffat JL: Stevens-Johnson syndrome and granulocytopenia after phenylbutazone. Br Med J 1:795, 1954
201. Finland M, Jollife LS, Parker F Jr: Pneumonia and erythema multiforme exudativum. Am J Med 4:473, 1948
202. Fleming PC, Krieger E, Turner JAP, et al: Febrile mucocutaneous syndrome with respiratory involvement, associated with the isolation of *Mycoplasma pneumoniae.* Can Med Assoc J 97:1458, 1967
203. Foerster DW, Scott LV: Isolation of herpes simplex virus from a patient with erythema multiforme exudativum. N Engl J Med 259:473, 1958
204. Mondino BJ, Brown SI, Biglan AW: HLA antigens in Stevens-Johnson syndrome with ocular involvement. Arch Ophthalmol 100:1453, 1982
205. Bleier AH, Schwartz E: Cortisone in treating Stevens-Johnson syndrome. Am J Ophthalmol 34:618, 1951
206. Weeks VT, Lehman WX: Erythema multiforme exudativum treated with cortisone or ACTH. J Pediatr 44:508, 1954
207. Yaffess HS: Stevens-Johnson syndrome. US Armed Forces Med J 10:148, 1959
208. Claxton RC: A review of 31 cases of Stevens-Johnson syndrome. Med J Aust 50:963, 1963
209. Lyell A: Toxic epidermal necrolysis: an eruption resembling scalding of the skin. Br J Dermatol 68:355, 1956
210. Lyell A, Dick HM, Alexander JO: Outbreak of toxic epidermal necrolysis associated with staphylococci. Lancet 1:787, 1969
211. Björnberg A, Björnberg K, Gisslen H: Toxic epidermal necrolysis with ophthalmic complications. Acta Ophthalmol (Copenh) 42:1084, 1964
212. Abrahams I, McCarthy JT, Sanders SL: 101 cases of exfoliative dermatitis. Arch Dermatol 87:96, 1963
213. Lang R, Walker J: An unusual bullous eruption. S Afr Med J 30:97, 1956
214. Lee DA, Barker SM, Su WPD, et al: The clinical diagnosis of Reiter's syndrome: ophthalmic and nonophthalmic aspects. Ophthalmology 93:350, 1986
215. Brodie BC: Pathological and Surgical Observations of Diseases of the Joints. Longman, Hurst, Rees, Orme, and Brown, London, 1818
216. Reiter H: Über eine bisher unerkannte Spirochäteninfektion (Spirochaetosis arthritica). Dtsch Med Wochenschr 42:1535, 1916
217. Ford DK: Reiter's syndrome. Bull Rheum Dis 20:588, 1970
218. Popert AJ, Gill AJ, Laird SM: A prospective study of Reiter's syndrome; an interim report on the first 82 cases. Br J Vener Dis 43:280, 1967
219. Sharp JT: Reiter's syndrome: a review of clinical features and studies on etiology. Med Clin North Am 45:1325, 1961
220. Montgomery MM, Posker RN, Barton EM, et al: The mucocutaneous lesions of Reiter's syndrome. Ann Intern Med 51:99, 1959
221. Leirisalo M, Skylv G, Kousa M, et al: Followup study on patients with Reiter's disease and reactive arthritis, with special reference to HLA-B27. Arthritis Rheum 25:249, 1982
222. Hall WH, Finegold S: A study of 23 cases of Reiter's syndrome. Ann Intern Med 38:533, 1982
223. Ostler HB, Dawson CR, Schachter J, Engleman EP: Reiter's syndrome. Am J Ophthalmol 71:986, 1971
224. Mills RP, Kalina RE: Reiter's keratitis. Arch Ophthalmol 87:447, 1972
225. Dawson CR, Schachter J, Ostler HB, et al: Inclusion conjunctivitis and Reiter's syndrome in a married couple: *Chlamydia* infections in a series of both diseases. Arch Ophthalmol 83:300, 1970
226. Thygeson P: Historical review of oculogenital disease. Am J Ophthalmol 71:975, 1971
227. Robin JB, Schanzlin DJ, Verity SM, et al: Peripheral corneal disorders. Surv Ophthalmol 31:1, 1986
228. Robin JB, Schanzlin DJ, Meisler DM, et al: Ocular involvement in the respiratory vasculitides. Surv Ophthalmol 30:127, 1985
229. Koffler D: The immunology of rheumatoid diseases. Ciba Clin Symp 31:1, 1979
230. Fuerst DJ, Smith RE, Schanzlin DJ: Rheumatoid diseases. p. 364. In Smolin G, Thoft RA (eds): The Cornea: Scien-

tific Foundations and Clinical Practice. 3rd Ed. Little, Brown, Boston, 1994
231. Jayson MIV, Easty DL: Ulceration of the cornea in rheumatoid arthritis. Ann Rheum Dis 36:428, 1977
232. Ben-Aryheh H, Nahir M, Scharf Y, et al: Sialochemistry of patients with rheumatoid arthritis. Oral Surg 45:63, 1978
233. Erickson S, Sundmark E: Studies on the sicca syndrome in patients with rheumatoid arthritis. Acta Rheum Scand 16:60, 1970
234. McGavin DDM, Williamson J, Forrester JV, et al: Episcleritis and scleritis: a study of their clinical manifestations and association with rheumatoid arthritis. Br J Ophthalmol 60:192, 1976
235. Jayson MIV, Jones DED: Scleritis and rheumatoid arthritis. Ann Rheum Dis 30:343, 1971
236. Watson PG, Hayreh SS: Scleritis and episcleritis. Br J Ophthalmol 60:163, 1976
237. Foster CS, Forstot SL, Wilson LA: Mortality rate in rheumatoid arthritis patients developing necrotizing scleritis or peripheral ulcerative keratitis: effects of systemic immunosuppression. Ophthalmology 90:175, 1980
238. Watson PG, Hazelman B: The Sclera and Systemic Disorders. WB Saunders, Philadelphia, 1976
239. Lyne AJ: "Contact lens" cornea in rheumatoid arthritis. Br J Ophthalmol 54:410, 1970
240. Sevel D: Rheumatoid nodule of the sclera. Trans Ophthalmol Soc UK 85:357, 1965
241. Watson PG: Diseases of the episclera and sclera. Ch. 23, p. 1. In Duane TD (ed): Clinical Ophthalmology. Vol. 4. Harper & Row, Philadelphia, 1984
242. Brown SI, Grayson M: Marginal furrows: a characteristic corneal lesion of rheumatoid arthritis. Arch Ophthalmol 79:563, 1968
243. Scharf Y, Meyer E, Nahir M, Zonis S: Marginal mottling of cornea in rheumatoid arthritis. Ann Ophthalmol 16:924, 1984
244. Eiferman RA, Carothers DJ, Yankeelov JA: Peripheral rheumatoid ulceration and evidence for conjunctival collagenase production. Am J Ophthalmol 87:703, 1979
245. Foster CS: Immunosuppressive therapy for external ocular inflammatory disease. Ophthalmology 87:140, 1980
246. Jakobiec FA, Lefkowitch J, Knowles DM: B- and T-lymphocytes in ocular disease. Ophthalmology 87:140, 1980
247. Jampol LW, West C, Goldberg MF: Therapy of scleritis with cytotoxic agents. Am J Ophthalmol 86:266, 1978
248. Easty DL, Madden P, Hayson MIV, et al: Systemic immunosuppression in marginal keratolysis. Trans Ophthalmol Soc UK 98:410, 1978
249. Fogle JA, Kenyon KR, Foster CS: Tissue adhesive arrests stromal melting in the human cornea. Am J Ophthalmol 89:795, 1980
250. Feer RS, Krachmer JH: Conjunctival resection for the treatment of the rheumatoid corneal ulceration. Ophthalmology 91:111, 1984
251. Wilson FM II, Grayson M, Ellis FD: Treatment of peripheral corneal ulcers by limbal conjunctivectomy. Br J Ophthalmol 60:713, 1976
252. Sjögren H, Bloch KJ: Keratoconjunctivitis and the Sjögren's syndrome. Surv Ophthalmol 16:145, 1971
253. Moutsopoulos HM, Chuset TM, Mann DL, et al: Sjögren's syndrome (sicca syndrome): current issues. Ann Intern Med 92:212, 1980
254. Tabbara KF: Sjögren's syndrome. p. 477. In Smolin G, Thoft RA (eds): The Cornea: Scientific Foundations and Clinical Practice. Little, Brown, Boston, 1994
255. Chudwin DS, Daniels TE, Wara DW, et al: Spectrum of Sjögren's syndrome. Br J Ophthalmol 66:179, 1982
256. Cohen KL: Sterile corneal perforation after cataract surgery in Sjögren's syndrome. Br J Ophthalmol 66:179, 1982
257. Gudas PP, Altman B, Nicholson DH, Green WR: Corneal perforations in Sjögren's syndrome. Arch Ophthalmol 90:470, 1973
258. Krachmer JH, Laibson PR: Corneal thinning and perforation in Sjögren's syndrome. Am J Ophthalmol 78:917, 1974
259. Pfister RR, Murphy GE: Corneal ulceration and perforation associated with Sjögren's syndrome. Arch Ophthalmol 98:89, 1980
260. Anderson LG, Talal N: The spectrum of benign to malignant lymphoproliferation in Sjögren's syndrome. Clin Exp Immunol 10:199, 1972
261. Tabbara KF, Ostler HB, Daniels TE, et al: Sjögren's syndrome: a correlation between ocular findings and labial salivary gland histology. Trans Am Acad Ophthalmol Otolaryngol 78:467, 1974
262. Pflugfelder SC, Haung AJ, Feure W, et al: Conjunctival cytologic features of primary Sjögren's syndrome. Ophthalmology 97:985, 1990
263. Foster CS: Ocular manifestations of nonrheumatoid acquired vascular diseases. p. 385. In Smolin G, Thoft RA (eds): The Cornea: Scientific Foundations and Clinical Practice. Little, Brown, Boston, 1994
264. Burge SM, Frith PA, Millard PR, Wojnarowska F: The lupus band test in oral mucosa, conjunctiva and skin. Br J Dermatol 121:743, 1989
265. Burge SM, Frith PA, Juniper RP, Wojnarowska F: Mucosal involvement in systemic and chronic cutaneous lupus erythematosus. Br J Dermatol 121:727, 1989
266. Gold DH, Morris DA, Henkind P: Ocular findings in systemic lupus erythematosus. Br J Ophthalmol 56:800, 1972
267. Spaeth GK: Corneal staining in systemic lupus erythematosus. N Engl J Med 276:1168, 1967
268. Halmay O, Ludwig K: Bilateral band-shaped deep keratitis and iridocyclitis in systemic lupus erythematosus. Br J Ophthalmol 48:558, 1964
269. Reeves JA: Keratopathy associated with systemic lupus erythematosus. Arch Ophthalmol 74:159, 1965
270. Kussmaul A, Maier R: Huber eine bisher nicht beschriebene eigenthümiliche Artereinerkrankung (Periarteritis nodosa die mit Morbus Brightii und rapid fortschreitender allgeiner Muskellähung einhergeht). Dtsch Arch Klin Med 1:484, 1866
271. Cogan DG: Corneoscleral lesions in periarteritis nodosa and Wegener's granulomatosis. Trans Am Ophthalmol Soc 53:321, 1965

272. Moore JG, Sevel D: Corneoscleral ulceration in polyarteritis nodosa. Br J Ophthalmol 50:651, 1966
273. Harbert F, McPherson SD: Scleral necrosis in polyarteritis nodosa. Am J Ophthalamol 30:727, 1947
274. Fauci AS, Doppman JL, Wolff SM: Cyclophosphamide-induced remissions in advanced polyarteritis nodosa. Am J Med 64:890, 1978
275. Godman GC, Churg J: Wegener's granulomatosis. Pathology and review of the literature. Arch Pathol 58:533, 1954
276. Wegener F: Über generalisierte septische Gefasserkrankungen. Verh Dtsch Ges Pathol 29:202, 1936
277. Bullen CL, Liesegang TJ, McDonald TJ, DeRemee RA: Ocular complications of Wegener's granulomatosis. Ophthalmology 90:270, 1983
278. Wolff SM, Fauci AS, Horn RG, Dale DC: Wegener's granulomatosis. Ann Intern Med 81:513, 1974
279. Carrington CB, Liebow AA: Limited forms of angiitis and granulomatosis of Wegener's type. Am J Med 41:497, 1966
280. Straatsma BR: Ocular manifestations of Wegener's granulomatosis. Am J Ophthalmol 44:789, 1957
281. Coutu RE, Klein M, Lessell S, et al: Limited form of Wegener's granulomatosis. JAMA 246:2610, 1981
282. Haynes BF, Fishmann ML, Fauci AS, Wolff SM: The ocular manifestations of Wegener's granulomatosis: fifteen years experience and review of the literature. Am J Med 63:131, 1977
283. Spalton DJ, Graham EM, Page NGR, Sanders MD: Ocular changes in Wegener's granulomatosis. Br J Ophthalmol 65:553, 1981
284. Goder G, Dolter J: Wegenersche Granulomatose mit konjunktivalem Beginn. Ophthalmologica 162:321, 1971
285. Biglan AW, Brown SI, Cignetti FE, Linn JG: Corneal perforation in Wegener's granulomatosis treated with corneal transplantation. Case report. Ann Ophthalmol 9:799, 1979
286. Sevel D: Necrogranulomatous keratitis associated with Wegener's granulomatosis and rheumatoid arthritis. Am J Ophthalmol 63:250, 1967
287. Austin P, Green WR, Sallyer DC, et al: Peripheral corneal degeneration and occlusive vasculitis in Wegener's granulomatosis. Am J Ophthalmol 85:311, 1978
288. Greenberger MH: Central retinal artery closure in Wegener's granulomatosis. Am J Ophthalmol 63:515, 1967
289. Ferry AP, Leopold IH: Marginal (ring) corneal ulcer as presenting manifestation of Wegener's granulomatosis. Trans Am Acad Ophthalmol Otolaryngol 74:1276, 1970
290. Frayer WC: The histopathology of perilimbal ulceration in Wegener's granulomatosis. Arch Ophthalmol 64:58, 1960
291. Liebow AA: The J Burns Anderson Lecture—Pulmonary angiitis and granulomatosis. Am Rev Respir Dis 108:1, 1973
292. Shillitoe EJ, Lehner T, Lessof MJ, Harrison DFN: Immunological features of Wegener's granulomatosis. Lancet 1:282, 1974
293. Fauci AS, Wolff SM: Wegener's granulomatosis: studies in 18 patients and a review of the literature. Medicine 52:535, 1973
294. Howle SB, Epstein WV: Circulating immunoglobulin complexes in Wegener's granulomatosis. Am J Med 60:259, 1976
295. Niinaka T, Okochi T, Watanabe Y, et al: Lymphocyte functions in Wegener's granulomatosis. J Med 9:491, 1978
296. Katz P, Alling DW, Haynes BF, Fauci AS: Association of Wegener's granulomatosis with HLA-B8. Clin Immunol Immunopathol 14:268, 1979
297. Brubaker R, Font RL, Shepherd EM: Granulomatous sclerouveitis: regression of ocular lesions with cyclophosphamide and prednisone. Arch Ophthalmol 86:517, 1971
298. Fauci AS, Haynes BF, Katz P, Wolff SM: Wegener's granulomatosis: prospective and therapeutic experience with 85 patients for 21 years. Ann Intern Med 88:76, 1977
299. Churg J, Strauss L: Allergic granulomatosis, allergic angiitis and periarteritis nodosa. Am J Pathol 27:277, 1951
300. Rose GA, Spencer H: Polyarteritis nodosa. Q J Med 26:43, 1957
301. Chumbley LC, Harrison EG Jr, DeRemee RA: Allergic granulomatosis and angiitis (Churg-Strauss syndrome): report and analysis of 30 cases. Mayo Clin Proc 52:477, 1977
302. Crotty CP, DeRemee RA, Winkelmann RK: Cutaneous clinicopathologic correlation of allergic granulomatosis. J Am Acad Dermatol 5:571, 1981
303. Cury D, Breakey AS, Payne BF: Allergic granulomatous angiitis associated with uveoscleritis and papilledema. Arch Ophthalmol 55:261, 1956
304. Meisler DM, Stock EL, Wertz RD, et al: Conjunctival inflammation and amyloidosis in allergic granulomatosis and angiitis (Churg-Strauss syndrome). Am J Ophthalmol 91:216, 1981
305. Nissim F, Von der Valde J, Czernobilsky B: A limited form of Churg-Strauss syndrome: ocular and cutaneous manifestations. Arch Pathol Lab Med 106:305, 1982
306. Shields CL, Shields JA, Rozanski TI: Conjunctival involvement in Churg-Strauss syndrome. Am J Ophthalmol 102:601, 1986
307. Cooper BJ, Bacal E, Patterson R: Allergic angiitis and granulomatosis: prolonged remission induced by combined prednisone-azathioprine therapy. Arch Intern Med 138:367, 1978
308. Hoekstra JA, Fauci AS: The granulomatous vasculitides. Clin Rheum Dis 6:373, 1980
309. McKay DAR, Watson PG, Lyne AJ: Relapsing polychondritis and eye disease. Br J Ophthalmol 58:600, 1974
310. Zion VM, Brackup AH, Weingeist S: Relapsing polychondritis, erythema nodosum and sclerouveitis. Case report with anterior segment angiography. Surv Ophthalmol 19:107, 1974
311. Dolan DL, Lemmon GB, Teitelbaum SL: Relapsing polychondritis: analytical literature review and studies on pathogenesis. Am J Med 41:285, 1966
312. Anderson B: Ocular lesions in relapsing polychondritis and other rheumatoid syndromes. Am J Ophthalmol 64:35, 1967
313. Hughes RAC, Berry CL, Seifert M, Leesof MH: Relapsing polychondritis: three cases with a clinico-pathologic study and literature review. Q J Med 41:363, 1972

314. Harwood TR: Diffuse perichondritis, chondritis and iritis. Report of an autopsied case. Arch Pathol 65:81, 1958
315. Kaye RL, Sones DA: Relapsing polychondritis. Clinical and pathological features in fourteen cases. Ann Intern Med 60:653, 1964
316. Barth WF, Berson EL: Relapsing polychondritis, rheumatoid arthritis and blindness. Am J Ophthalmol 85:613, 1978
317. Matoba A, Plager S, Barber J, McCulley JP: Keratitis in relapsing polychondritis. Am J Ophthalmol 16:367, 1984
318. Meyer O, Cyna J, Dryll A, et al: Relapsing polychondritis—pathogenic role of anti-native collagen type II antibodies. J Rheumatol 8:820, 1981
319. Martin J, Roenigk HH, Lynch W, Tingwald FR: Relapsing polychondritis treated with dapsone. Arch Dermatol 112:1271, 1976
320. Bergaust B, Abrahamsen AM: Relapsing polychondritis: report of a case presenting multiple ocular complications. Acta Ophthalmol (Copenh) 47:174, 1969
321. Hoang-Xaun T, Foster CS, Rice BA: Scleritis in relapsing polychondritis. Response to therapy. Ophthalmology 97:892, 1990
322. Goetz RH: The pathology of progressive systemic sclerosis (generalized scleroderma with special reference to changes in viscera). Clin Proc (Cape Town) 4:337, 1945
323. Horan EC: Ophthalmic manifestations of progressive systemic sclerosis. Br J Ophthalmol 53:388, 1969
324. Manschot WA: Generalized scleroderma with ocular symptoms. Ophthalmologica 149:131, 1965
325. Kirkham TH: Scleroderma and Sjögren's syndrome. Br J Ophthalmol 53:131, 1969
326. Coyle EF: Scleroderma of the cornea. Br J Ophthalmol 40:239, 1956
327. Gerstle CC, Friedman AH: Marginal corneal ulceration (limbal guttering) as a presenting sign of temporal arteritis. Ophthalmology 87:1173, 1980
328. Cogan DG: Syndrome of nonsyphilitic interstitial keratitis and vestibuloauditory symptoms. Arch Ophthalmol 33:144, 1945
329. Cobo LM, Haynes BF: Early corneal findings in Cogan's syndrome. Ophthalmology 91:903, 1984
330. Palestine AG, Meyers SM, Fauci AS, Gallin JI: Ocular findings in patients with neutrophil dysfunction. Am J Ophthalmol 95:598, 1983
331. Guss RB, McCulley JP: Abnormal immune responses in the ocular presentation of Wiskott-Aldrich syndrome. Ann Ophthalmol 14:1058, 1982
332. Thygeson P: Marginal corneal infiltrates and ulcers. Trans Am Acad Ophthalmol Otolaryngol 51:198, 1946
333. Chignell AG, Easty DL, Chesterton JR, Thomsitt J: Marginal ulceration of the cornea. Br J Ophthalmol 54:433, 1970
334. Duke-Elder S: System of Ophthalmology. Vol. VII. Diseases of the Outer Eye. Part 2. Cornea and Sclera. CV Mosby, St. Louis, 1965
335. Friedlander MH: Ocular allergy and immunology. J Allergy Clin Immunol 63:51, 1979
336. Mondino BJ, Kowalski R, Ratajczak HV, et al: Rabbit model of phlyctenulosis and catarrhal infiltrates. Arch Ophthalmol 99:891, 1981
337. Mondino BJ, Kowalski RP: Phlyctenulae and catarrhal infiltrates. Occurrence in rabbits immunized with staphylococcal cell walls. Arch Ophthalmol 100:1968, 1982
338. Thygeson P: Marginal herpes simplex keratitis simulating catarrhal ulcer. Invest Ophthalmol 10:1006, 1971
339. Ostler HB: Corneal perforation in nontuberculous (staphylococcal) phlyctenular keratoconjunctivitis. Am J Ophthalmol 79:446, 1975
340. Thygeson PL: The etiology and treatment of phlyctenular keratoconjunctivitis. Am J Ophthalmol 9:446, 1975
341. Al-Houssaini MK, Khalifa R, Al-Ansary ATA, et al: Phlyctenular eye disease in association with *Hymenolepis nana* in Egypt. Br J Ophthalmol 63:627, 1979
342. Smith RE, Dippe DW, Miller SD: Phlyctenular keratoconjunctivitis. Results of penetrating keratoplasty in Alaska natives. Ophthalmic Surg 6:62, 1975
343. Mooren A: Ophthalmiatrische Beobachtungen. A Hirschwald, Berlin, 1867
344. Slansky HH, Dohlman CH: Collagenase and the cornea. Surv Ophthalmol 14:402, 1970
345. Wood TO, Kaufman HE: Mooren's ulcer. Am J Ophthalmol 71:417, 1971
346. Kietzman B: Mooren's ulcer in Nigeria. Am J Ophthalmol 65:679, 1968
347. Majekodunmi AA: Ecology of Mooren's ulcer in Nigeria. Doc Ophthalmol 49:211, 1980
348. Trojan HJ: Ulcus rodens (Mooren)—Aspekte der Atiologie, des Verlaufs und der Therapie. Klin Monatsbl Augenheilkd 174:166, 1972
349. Taylor SJ: Notes of a case of roden ulcer of the cornea in a child. Trans Ophthalmol Soc UK 22:98, 1902
350. Young RG, Watson PG: Light and electron microscopy of corneal melting syndrome (Mooren's ulcer). Br J Ophthalmol 66:341, 1982
351. Foster CS, Kenyon KR, Greineder J, et al: The immunopathology of Mooren's ulcer. Am J Ophthalmol 88:149, 1979
352. Brown SI: Mooren's ulcers. Histopathology and proteolytic enzymes of adjacent conjunctiva. Br J Ophthalmol 59:670, 1975
353. Murray PI, Rahi AHS: Pathogenesis of Mooren's ulcer: some new concepts. Br J Ophthalmol 68:182, 1984
354. Tabbara KF, Ostler HB: Mooren's ulcer. p. 269. In Trevor-Roper P (ed): Proceedings of the 6th Congress of European Ophthalmology, Royal Society of Medicine. Academic Press, London, 1980
355. Eiferman R, Hyndiuk R: IgE in limbal conjunctiva in Mooren's ulcer. Can J Ophthalmol 12:234, 1979
356. Eiferman R, Hyndiuk RA, Hensley GT: Limbal immunopathology of Mooren's ulcer. Ann Ophthalmol 10:1203, 1978
357. Ban der Gaag R, Abdillahi H, Stilma JS, Vetter JCM: Circulating antibodies against corneal epithelium and hookworm in patients with Mooren's ulcer from Sierra Leone. Br J Ophthalmol 67:623, 1983

358. Arentsen JJ, Christiansen JM, Maumenee AE: Marginal ulceration after intracapsular cataract extraction. Am J Ophthalmol 81:194, 1976
359. Salamon SM, Mondino BJ, Zaidman GW: Peripheral corneal ulcers, conjunctival ulcers, and scleritis after cataract surgery. Am J Ophthalmol 93:334, 1982
360. Joondeph HC, McCarthy WL, Rabb M, Constantaras A: Mooren's ulcer. Two cases occurring after cataract extraction and treated with hydrophilic lens. Ann Ophthalmol 8:187, 1976
361. Mondino BJ, Hofbauer JD, Foos RY: Mooren's ulcer after penetrating keratoplasty. Am J Ophthalmol 103:53, 1987
362. Mondino BJ, Brown SI, Mondzelewski JP: Peripheral corneal ulcers with herpes zoster ophthalmicus. Am J Ophthalmol 86:611, 1978
363. Berkowitz PT, Arentsen JJ, Felbeg NT, Laibson PR: Presence of circulating immune complexes in patients with peripheral corneal disease. Arch Ophthalmol 101:242, 1983
364. Brown SI, Mondino BJ, Rabin BS: Autoimmune phenomenon in Mooren's ulcer. Am J Ophthalmol 82:835, 1976
365. Mondino JB, Brown SI, Rabin BS: Cellular immunity in Mooren's ulcer. Am J Ophthalmol 85:788, 1978
366. Schaap OL, Feltkamp TEW, Breenbaart A: Circulating antibodies to corneal tissue in a patient suffering from Mooren's ulcer (ulcus rodens corneae). Clin Exp Immunol 5:365, 1969
367. Brown SI: What is Mooren's ulcer? Trans Ophthalmol Soc UK 98:390, 1978
368. Brown SI, Mondino BJ: Therapy of Mooren's ulcer. Am J Ophthalmol 98:1, 1984
369. Pandey R: Topical cortisone in the treatment of Mooren's ulcer. J All India Ophthalmol Soc 17:114, 1969
370. Brown SI: Collagenolytic enzymes in corneal pathology. Isr J Med Sci 8:1537, 1972
371. Brown SI: Mooren's ulcer: treatment by conjunctival excision. Br J Ophthalmol 59:675, 1975
372. Chihara E, Nishi R, Asayama K, Tsukahara I: Treatment of Mooren's ulcer by conjunctival excision. Ophthalmologica 179:258, 1979
373. Stilma JS: Conjunctival excision or lamellar scleral autograft in 38 Mooren's ulcers from Sierra Leone. Br J Ophthalmol 67:475, 1983
374. Aviel E: Combined cryoapplications and peritomy in Mooren's ulcer. Br J Ophthalmol 56:48, 1972
375. Grana PC: Therapeutic keratoplasty in Mooren's ulcer. Arch Ophthalmol 62:414, 1959
376. Rycroft BW, Tomantes GJ: Lamella corneal grafts—clinical reports on 62 cases. Br J Ophthalmol 36:337, 1952
377. Zu D: Mooren's ulcer treated by lamellar keratoplasty. Jpn J Ophthalmol 23:257, 1979
378. Ferguson CE, Carreno OB: Mooren's ulcer and delimiting keratotomy. South Med J 62:1170, 1969
379. Hirst LW, DeJuan E: Sodium hyaluronate and tissue adhesive in treating corneal perforations. Ophthalmology 89:1250, 1982
380. Hyndiuk RA, Hull DS, Kinkyoun JL: Free tissue patch and cyanoacrylate in corneal perforations. Ophthalmic Surg 5:50, 1974
381. Webster RG, Slansky HH, Refojo MF, et al: The use of adhesive for the closure of corneal perforations. Arch Ophthalmol 80:705, 1968
382. Brown SI, Mondino BJ: Penetrating keratoplasty in Mooren's ulcer. Am J Ophthalmol 89:255, 1980
383. Dean AC: Ulcus rodens of right eye treated by a conjunctival flap operation. Minn Med 13:44, 1930
384. Tyrrell F: Case of Mooren's ulcer treated with a conjunctival flap. Trans Ophthalmol Soc UK 37:235, 1917

24

Corneal Tumors

FREDERICK A. JAKOBIEC AND MACIE FINKELSTEIN

Tumors that affect the cornea are inseparable from those that affect the conjunctiva. The corneal epithelium is topographically continuous with the conjunctival epithelium. The former is composed of nonkeratinizing squamous cells with sparse antigen-processing Langerhans cells and dendritic melanocytes at the limbus,[1–3] whereas the latter has more nonsquamous cell types and a variably distributed density of mucin-producing goblet cells. The corneal epithelium sits on a nonvascularized collagenous layer called Bowman's layer, which is normally devoid of fibroblasts; the conjunctival epithelium sits on a delicate substantia propria, in which lymphocytes, blood vessels, lymphatic channels, and terminal nerve endings are dispersed. Consequently, the richer connective tissue base of the conjunctiva allows for a wider range of mesenchymal or connective tissue-related tumors than is encountered in the cornea.[4–6] When buccal mucous membrane grafts are placed next to the limbus, sebaceous glands (Fordyce nodules) may be transplanted that can create limbal masses not spontaneously produced by the autochthonous conjunctiva.[7]

The most common growth that encroaches on the cornea is a pterygium, an actinically induced modification of the substantia propria of the interpalpebral conjunctiva[8] in which fibroblasts grow into the peripheral cornea, destroying Bowman's layer and bringing in blood vessels (see Ch. 21). This condition is reactive rather than neoplastic, although occasionally the overlying epithelium associated with the fibrous growth may show evidence of actinic damage in the form of squamous dysplasia.[5,9] A congenital, isolated, temporal epibulbar lesion that appears to be a pterygium could be elastofibroma oculi with abundant mature elastic fibers intermixed with fibrous tissue.[10]

The most common true neoplasms of the cornea are those arising from disturbances of the squamous cells or from proliferations of the intraepithelial dendritic melanocytes. In this chapter, most of the emphasis is placed on these conditions; however, for completeness, congenital abnormalities, inflammatory and degenerative conditions that may simulate a neoplasm, and rare episcleral mesenchymal proliferations that overlap the limbus and thereby involve the cornea are also discussed.

CONGENITAL LESIONS

Congenital lesions usually affect the peripheral cornea but may encroach on the central cornea. Most congenital lesions are choristomas, which are tumor-like growths of elements not normally indigenous to the area in which they are found.

Dermoid and Dermolipoma

The prototypical choristoma is a dermoid or dermolipoma.[5] Dermoids usually involve the temporal epibulbar and limbal corneal areas (Figure 24-1). They are solid placoid tumors composed of thick dermis-like collagen, which may be embedded with sweat glands, hairs, sebaceous glands, and lobules of fat (Figure 24-2). If fine hairs project from the surface of the dermoid, the patient may experience a foreign body sensation. Occasionally, inherited bilateral ring dermoids can affect the entire corneal limbus.[11] In some rare variants, all of the corneal stroma is involved, leading to bilateral, congenital, white, corneal opacifications in which the stroma is disorganized and possesses adnexal glands.[12] A dermolipoma is a dermoid in which fat is prominent and cutaneous adnexal structures are usually absent. In Goldenhar syndrome, an epibulbar dermoid or dermolipoma coexists with vertebral body anomalies and a malformation of the pinna. Rarely, epibul-

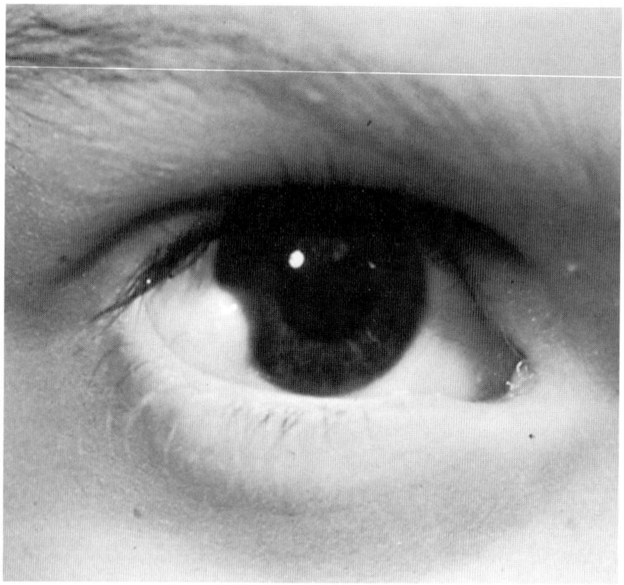

FIGURE 24-1 An epibulbar solid dermoid located characteristically in the inferotemporal quadrant with extension onto the peripheral cornea.

bar dermoids may also be associated with colobomas of the eyelids, abnormalities of closure of the fetal fissure, central nervous system disorders, and organoid cutaneous nevi.[5] Dermoids and dermolipomas grow with the patient and the eye but tend not to progress or undergo neoplastic degeneration. When the cornea is involved, a superficial lamellar keratectomy may be performed to remove the protruding mass and correct any associated astigmatism; however, the cornea underlying the lesion remains scarred. If the lesion extends toward the fornices or lateral canthus, the connective tissue may trail off into the orbital fat, with entanglements within extraocular muscles; excision of these lesions must be done cautiously so as not to damage the lacrimal gland or rectus muscles. The Proteus syndrome, a rare hamartomatous syndrome (the principal clinical findings of which include skeletal anomalies, gyriform hyperplasia of the hands and feet, subcutaneous tumors, epidermal nevi, and visceral abnormalities), is associated with epibulbar tumors. In one case, histology was reported as a fibrous hamartoma rather than a choristoma.[13,14]

Ectopic Lacrimal Gland

The second most common epibulbar choristoma[15] that may affect the cornea is ectopic lacrimal gland (Figure 24-3). If only lacrimal gland tissue is present, the lesion is called a *simple choristoma;* if there are other elements, such as cartilage, smooth muscle, sweat glands, hairs, or sebaceous glands, the lesion is called a *complex choristoma* (Figure 24-4). The frequent presence of smooth muscle bundles in these lesions suggests that they may be ectopias of the palpebral lobe of the lacrimal gland, which normally has a considerable amount of Müller's smooth muscle intermixed. In contrast to the porcelain white or yellowish appearance of dermoids and dermolipomas, ectopic lacrimal gland is fleshy and highly vascularized, with raised translucent nodules. The lesion may extend into the corneal stroma, and there may be associated superficial stromal scarring adjacent to the

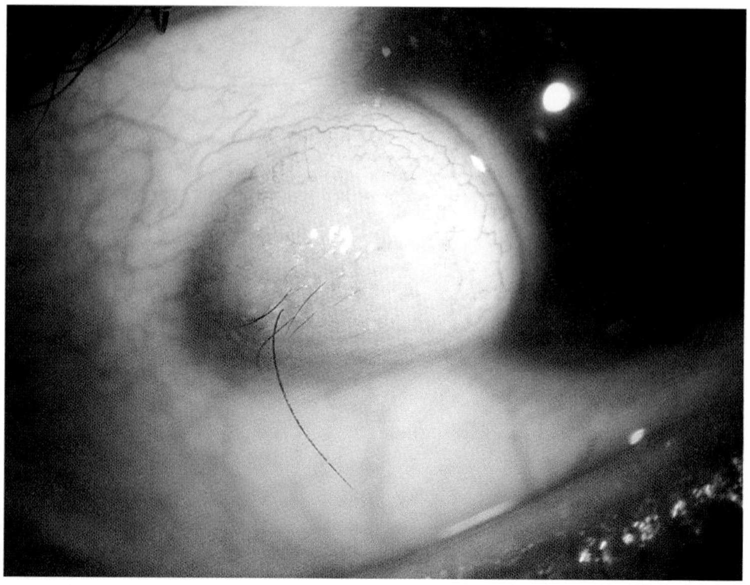

FIGURE 24-2 Limbal dermoid. A whitish yellow lesion with projecting hairs also has an associated nimbus of corneal sclerosis.

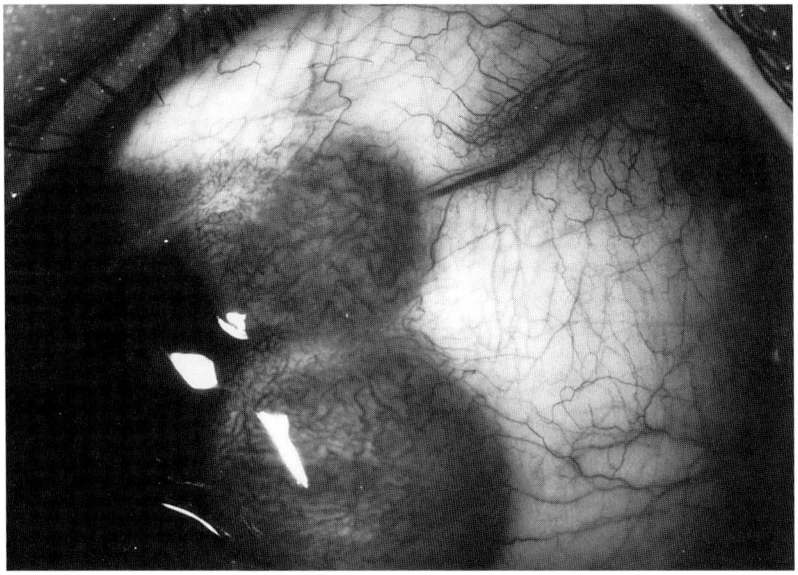

FIGURE 24-3 Two nodules of corneoscleral ectopic lacrimal gland tissue. Note the feeder vessel coming into the superior nodule from the lacrimal gland region.

lesion or at its leading margin (Figure 24-5). Lacrimal tissue itself may be found in the corneal stroma. The lesion can show mild growth, particularly during puberty, during which the parenchymal lacrimal elements may hypertrophy. The excision of the corneal component of the lesion may be more treacherous than the excision of solid dermoids, because the lacrimal tissue may extend deep into the corneal stroma. In these cases, judicious surgery should be aimed only at improving the cosmetic appearance rather than total removal. Although ectopic lacrimal gland of the orbit has been associated with tumors, such as vascular malformations, benign mixed tumors, and even rare adenocarcinomas, the potential for malignant degeneration of the epibulbar and corneal lesions is close to nil.

Osseous and Neuroglial Choristomas

Other epibulbar choristomas that contain elements in addition to those described above include osseous choristoma[16] and congenital epibulbar neuroglial choristoma.[17,18] Osseous choristoma tends to be a much more discrete lesion with sharper edges than those previously described; it usually spares the cornea. Epibulbar neuroglial choristomas probably represent ectopias of the anterior lip of the optic cup or vesicle. These are sta-

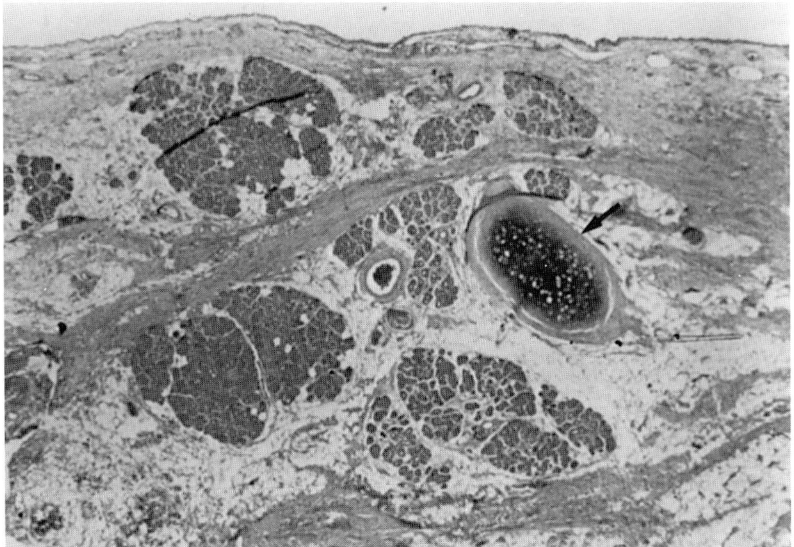

FIGURE 24-4 Histologic appearance of a lacrimal choristoma. Multiple lobules of lacrimal tissue are embedded in fibroadipose connective tissue. A focus of hyaline cartilage (arrow) is present. (Hematoxylin and eosin, × 40.)

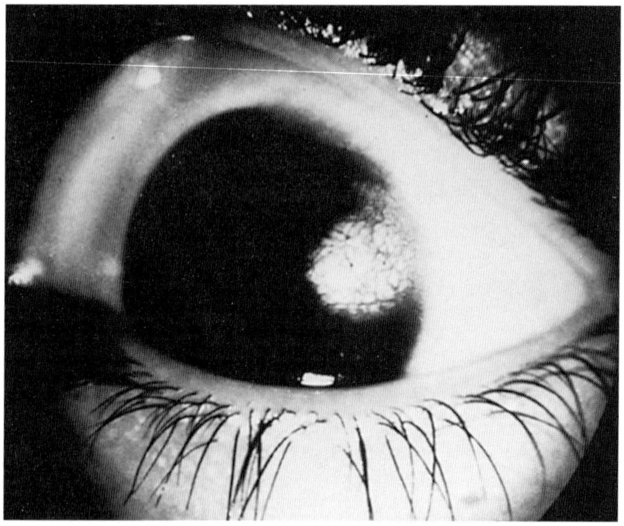

FIGURE 24-5 Typical superficial corneal sclerosis in a lacrimal choristoma.

tionary lesions that do not progress; surgery is indicated to rule out other lesions or for cosmetic improvement.

INFLAMMATORY TUMEFACTIONS AND MESENCHYMAL TUMORS

Pannus

The corneal epithelium normally sits on the acellular fibrous Bowman's layer with no interposed blood vessels or connective tissue. Blood vessels and associated fibroblasts may superficially grow into the cornea (pannus formation) from the limbal blood vessels as a result of inflammatory events (Figure 24-6). These events may be external to the eye, such as infections or irritations,[19] or internal to the eye, such as uveitis, phthisis bulbi, or glaucoma.[20] In infants, a pannus can become so exuberant as to simulate an epibulbar keloid or fibromatosis. This situation is most often encountered in buphthalmic glaucomatous eyes. Hyperplastic pannuses are not seen in adults, possibly because their fibroblasts are less reactive and proliferative than those of infants or children. Epicorneal deposition of amyloid plaques may create a clinical appearance similar to that of a hyperplastic pannus; however, it occurs later in life.[21,22] Some pannuses can bleed spontaneously and create the false impression of a melanoma or an expulsive hemorrhage.[20]

Pyogenic Granuloma

The presence of a fibrovascular pannus may be the basis for the development of a pyogenic granuloma[23-25] that involves the superficial aspect of the cornea (Figure 24-7). This rare corneal lesion is a reactive proliferation of "proud flesh" that is frequently the result of trauma or infection. Pyogenic granulomas usually occur over chalazia or on the conjunctival surface after strabismus surgery; they rarely occur spontaneously. There are only a few documented cases of pyogenic granulomas of the cornea. A corneal pyogenic granuloma can occur at the site of excision of a squamous dysplastic lesion and can be confused clinically with a recurrence of the dysplasia. The intense red appearance of a pyogenic granuloma and the rapidity with which it develops distinguish it from most true neoplasms, including amelanotic melanomas,

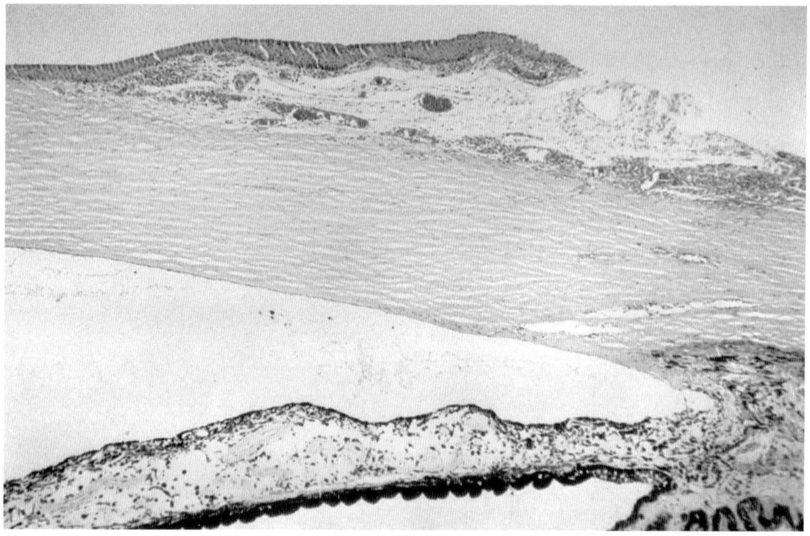

FIGURE 24-6 Pannus. Vascularized connective tissue is growing anterior to Bowman's layer, lifting up the corneal epithelium peripherally.

which grow more slowly and in which the vascular component is much less conspicuous.

Other circumstances conducive to pyogenic granuloma formation include extensive pannus resulting from earlier surgery, phthisis bulbi, and chemical burn. In these cases, the fibrovascular pannus overlying Bowman's layer (which may or may not be destroyed) provides the vascular supply for the exuberant proliferation of vascular endothelial cells and immature granulation tissue. Corneal pyogenic granulomas project as bulbous nodules through a collarette of surrounding epithelium that squeezes the base of the lesion, creating a pedunculated appearance. The term *pyogenic granuloma* is, strictly speaking, a misnomer, because granulomatous inflammation is not present. Rather, there are plump capillaries, among which are scattered lymphocytes, plasma cells, and occasionally, polymorphonuclear leukocytes, if the surface is eroded (Figure 24-8). Simple excision with cautery of the base of the lesion should be curative. With the increase in cases of acquired immunodeficiency syndrome (AIDS), Kaposi sarcoma should be included in the differential diagnosis of a corneal pyogenic granuloma.[26,27] There has been at least one unpublished case of Kaposi sarcoma involving the peripheral corneal stroma; however, Kaposi sarcoma more often involves the epibulbar, plical, or tarsal conjunctiva.

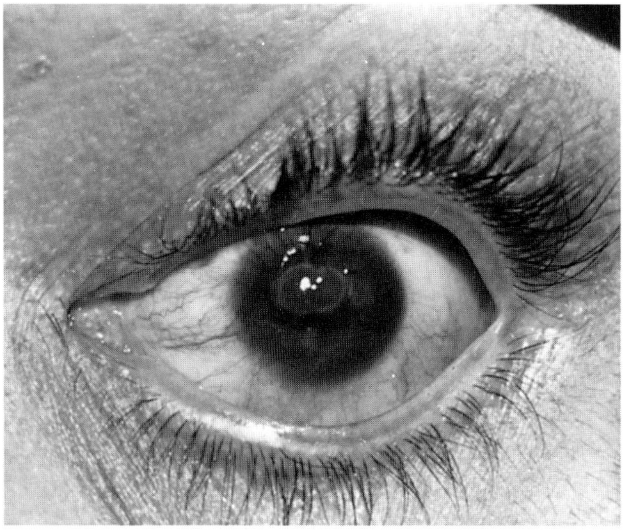

FIGURE 24-7 Epicorneal pyogenic granuloma in an eye that had prior trauma with subsequent pannus formation. (Reprinted with permission from JM Googe, G Mackman, MR Peterson, et al: Pyogenic granulomas of the cornea. Surv Ophthalmol 29:188, 1984.)

Fibrous Histiocytoma

Fibrous histiocytoma[28–32] may grow at the limbus and overlap the peripheral cornea (Figure 24-9); it has never been described centrally in the cornea without an episcleral or scleral origin. The lesion is cytologically bland but may extensively infiltrate the corneal stroma. Its color, which is yellowish to white, is the result of a mixture of fibroblasts and lipidized histiocytes (Figure 24-10). The biphasic cellular composition of spindled fibroblasts and rounded lipidized histiocytes is charac-

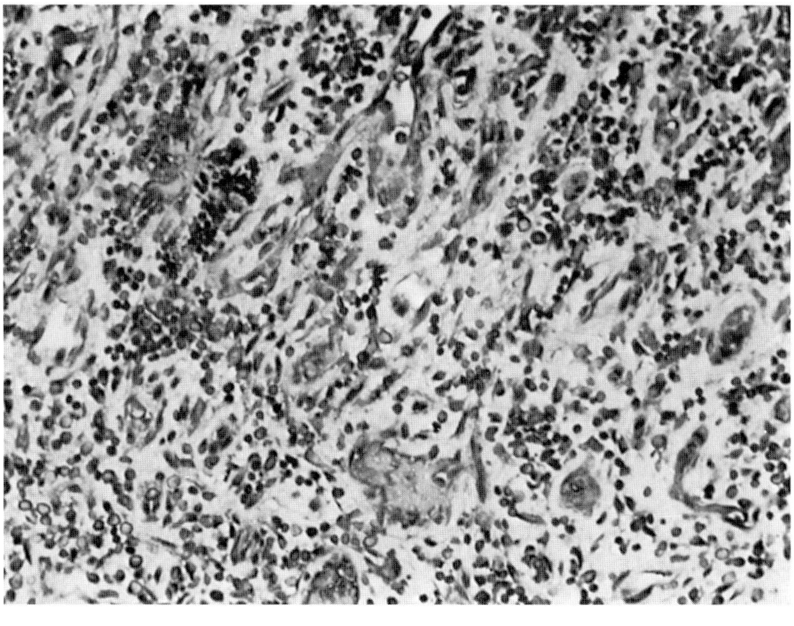

FIGURE 24-8 Histologic appearance of an epicorneal pyogenic granuloma. The lesion is composed of succulent capillaries and intermixed inflammatory cells, which are usually lymphocytes, plasma cells, and scattered polymorphonuclear leukocytes. (Hematoxylin and eosin, × 180.) (Courtesy of David J. Apple, M.D., Charleston, SC.)

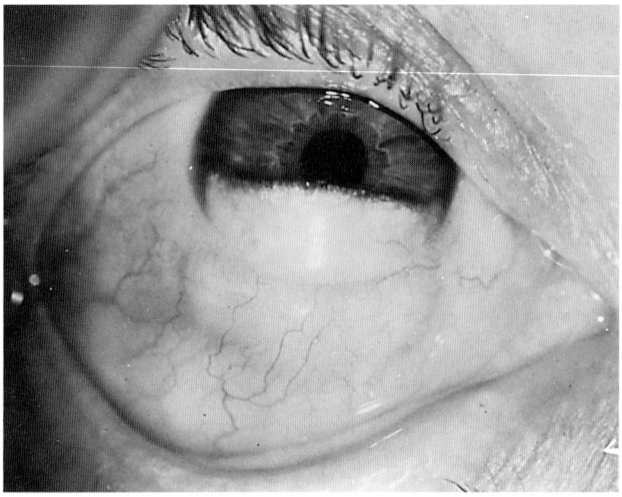

FIGURE 24-9 An infiltrative but cytologically benign corneoscleral fibrous histiocytoma that has extensively invaded the cornea. (Courtesy of Sigmund Schutz, M.D., New York, NY.)

teristic of the lesion, as is the storiform or cartwheel configuration of the bundles of cells. Electron microscopy (Figure 24-11) reveals the two populations of cells: fibroblasts with abundant rough endoplasmic reticulum, and histiocytic cells with smooth endoplasmic reticulum and lysozymes. The histiocytic cells may contain unusual curvilinear inclusions, which may be modifications of smooth endoplasmic reticulum. Both the fibroblasts and the histiocytic cells contain many lipid vacuoles.[31,32] Local excision is generally curative.

Corneal Myxoma

Corneal myxoma is an exceedingly rare primary corneal tumor. To date, there have been only three reported cases, two of which were associated with long-term corneal inflammation.[33] The third case involved a 44-year-old woman with a 5-year history of an avascular, grayish white corneal lesion. A subepithelial translucent mass measuring 8 mm by 4 mm, with ill-defined borders, was excised. Pathology revealed myxomatous tissue with a paucity of cells. Cellular components were fusiform, stellate, or spindle shaped. Special stains and electron microscopy confirmed the diagnosis of myxoma. This patient's tumor recurred 2 months after excision. Because this is the only reported case without antecedent corneal disease, the natural history of this lesion is unknown.

Nodular Fasciitis

Nodular fasciitis is a rapidly developing reactive proliferation of immature connective tissue[34] that often has a zonal architecture, with bundles of immature fibroblasts in some areas and pools of extracellular mucinous material in other areas. Lymphocytes, plasmacytes, and plump vascular endothelial cells are admixed. Most of these lesions can be managed by simple local excision, although they may rarely show locally aggressive growth with extension into the eye.

Granulomatous Lesions

Three lesions with granulomatous microscopic features may involve the corneal stroma: juvenile xanthogranu-

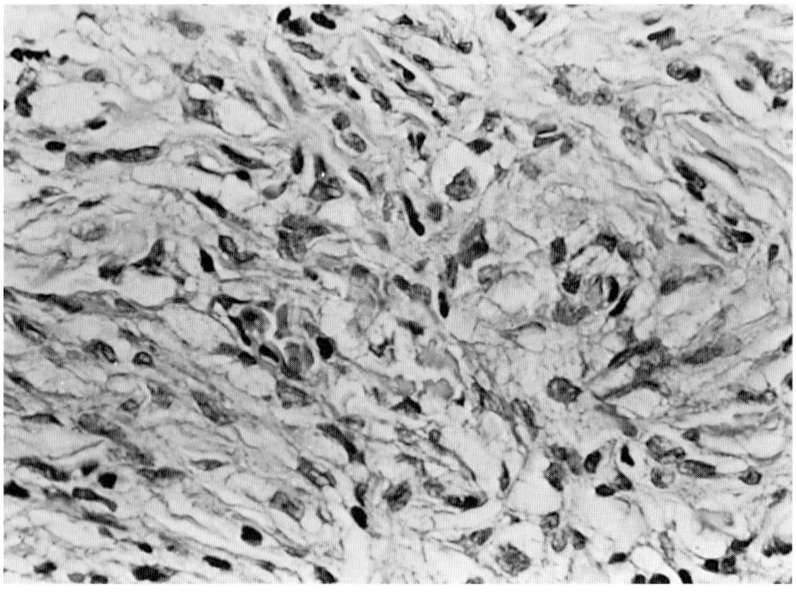

FIGURE 24-10 Characteristic pattern of a fibrous histiocytoma. Plump spindle cells and more ovoid lipidized histiocytes are featured. There is a vague storiform or cartwheel pattern to the lesion. The combination of spindled fibroblasts and rounded histiocytes accounts for the term *fibrous histiocytoma*. (Hematoxylin and eosin, × 280.)

FIGURE 24-11 Electron microscopic features of a benign corneoscleral fibrous histiocytoma. **(A)** A fibroblastic cell contains abundant rough endoplasmic reticulum (arrows), cytoplasmic filaments (*f*), dispersed lipid vacuoles (*li*), and elements of the Golgi apparatus (*g*). F_1 is the cell nucleus. Toward the bottom is a histiocytic cell with lysosomes (*ly*) and cytoplasmic filaments (*f*). (×11,000.) **(B)** A histiocyte with curvilinear membranous inclusions (arrows). The cytoplasm additionally contains lipid vacuoles (*li*) and dilated rough endoplasmic reticulum (*re*). Extracellular collagen fibers (*c*) are seen on the bottom right. (×18,000.)

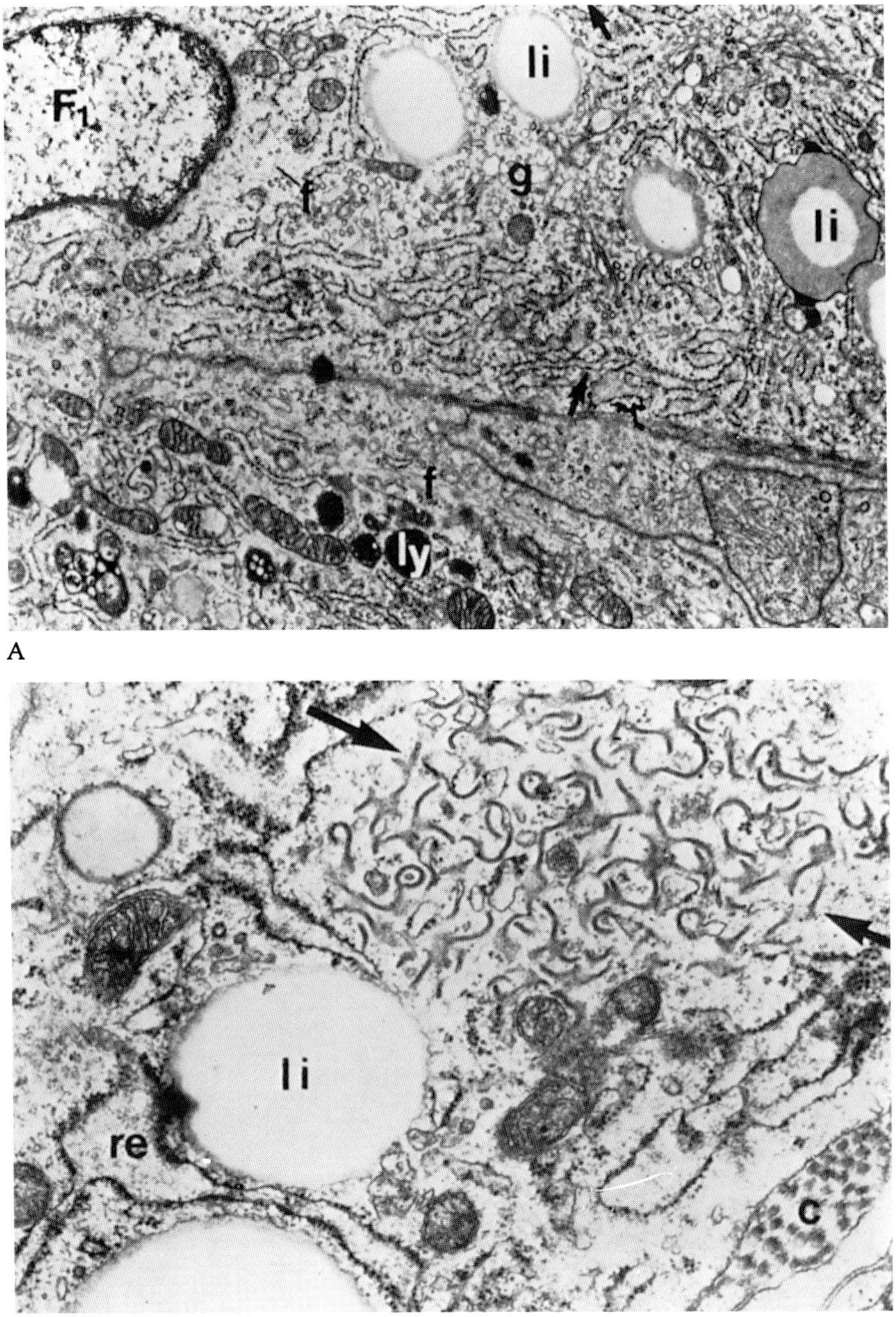

loma, sarcoidosis, and leprosy. Juvenile xanthogranuloma[35] typically affects the uveal tract but may affect the conjunctiva and the corneal stroma (Figure 24-12). Pathologically, the diagnostic feature is the presence of Touton giant cells, which exhibit a central annulus of nuclei enclosing an intensely eosinophilic cytoplasm, surrounded by peripheral vacuolated cytoplasm.

Sarcoid nodules normally involve the conjunctiva. If they involve the iris and a biopsy is performed through a corneal incision, the corneal stroma may be seeded with histiocytes that proliferate and produce intracorneal stromal nodules.

Leprosy is most likely to be confused with a fibrous histiocytoma, except that the abundant and highly vacuolated histiocytes in lepromatous lesions contain acid-fast bacilli.

Systemic vasculitis and bowel disease such as regional enteritis may produce episcleral nodules, corneal thin-

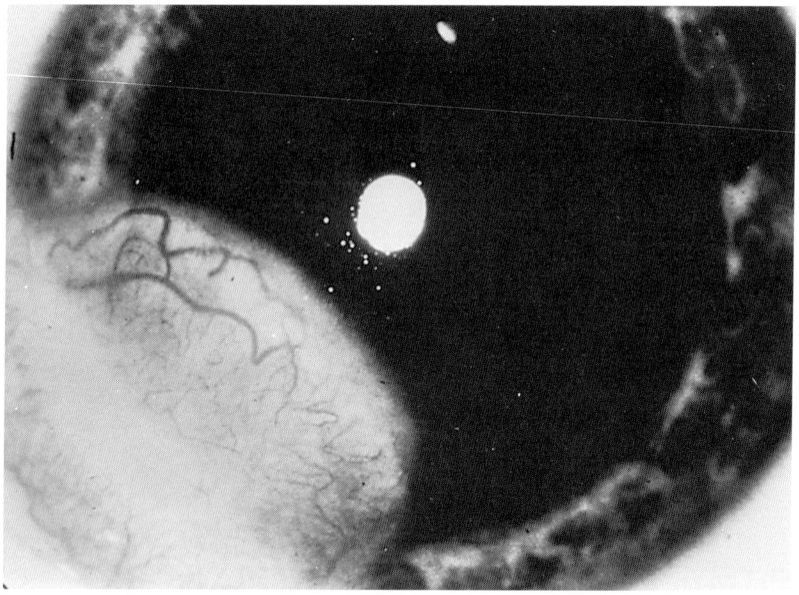

FIGURE 24-12 A peripheral corneal lesion in juvenile xanthogranuloma. The lesion has a vascularized and yellow appearance as a result of the presence of lipid.

ning, and occasionally, hyperplastic inflammatory masses or nodules.[36-40]

Intrastromal Cysts

Intrastromal corneal cysts (Figure 24-13) are unusual lesions.[41] They result from penetrating or perforating wounds to the cornea in which surface corneal epithelium is implanted in the midstroma and later proliferates between the collagenous lamellae to create an intrastromal cyst lined by desquamating corneal squamous epithelium (Figure 24-14). At some stage, there may be a fluid line as the desquamated material settles toward the inferior region of the cyst. When the cyst becomes completely filled, an evenly opalescent lesion is seen. These lesions tend to occur after corneal trauma in young individuals, in whom the epithelium appears to be more robust and capable of surviving and proliferating when implanted intrastromally.

Miscellaneous Conditions

Several other conditions affect the substantia propria of the conjunctiva, but because this layer is missing from the

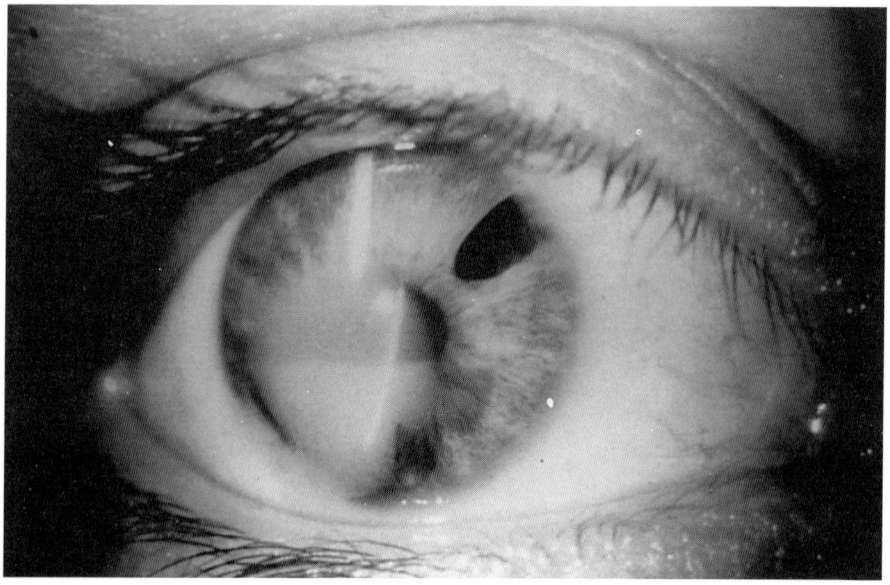

A

FIGURE 24-13 Post-traumatic intrastromal corneal cyst created by implantation of surface epithelium. **(A)** A fluid line can be discerned from the settling of cellular debris toward the inferior region of the cyst. *(continues)*

FIGURE 24-13 *(continued)*
(B) Several months later, the cyst has completely filled with desquamated debris so that the fluid line is no longer visible. (Reprinted with permission from SE Bloomfield, FA Jakobiec, T Iwamoto: Traumatic intrastromal corneal cyst. Ophthalmology 87:951, 1980. Courtesy of Ophthalmology.)

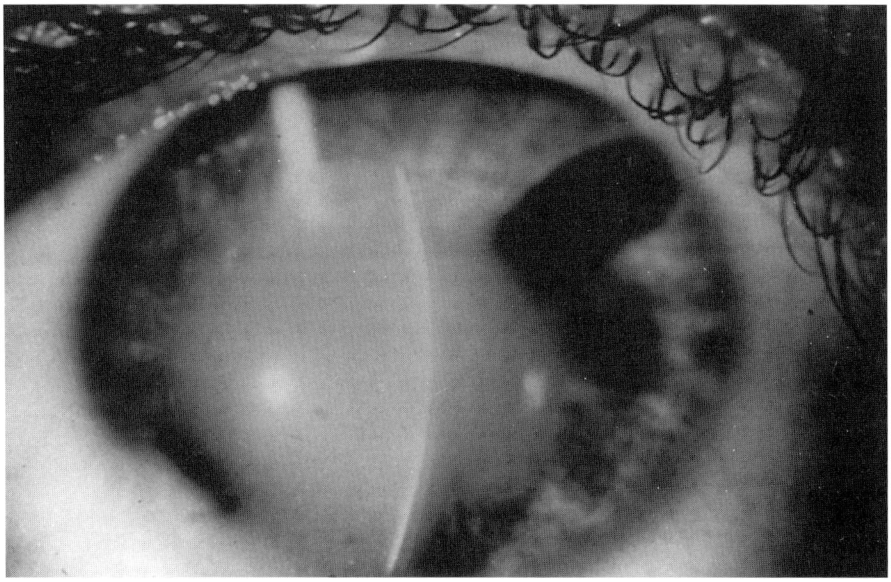

B

cornea, there tends to be no corneal involvement. Lymphoid hyperplasia is restricted to the substantia propria of the conjunctiva, with a propensity for involvement of the forniceal regions and sometimes extending onto the epibulbar surface. Extension into the cornea has not been reported. Peripheral nerve sheath tumors (neurofibromas and schwannomas)[42] may affect the substantia propria of the conjunctiva and can be located at the limbus but have not been reported centrally in the cornea. Non-neoplastic thickening of the corneal nerves may occur in the multiple endocrine neoplasia (MEN) syndrome, type IIb, which includes potentially fatal medullary carcinoma of the thyroid and pheochromocytoma.[43,44] Earlier reports of thickened corneal nerves in neurofibromatosis may not be accurate because of a failure to appreciate the distinct and separate nature of the multiple endocrine neoplasia syndrome. Thickened corneal nerves may also be seen in Refsum's disease. Because the normal cornea does not possess lymphatic channels or capillary channels lined with endothelium (although both of these may occur in inflamed or damaged corneas), primary vascular tumors have not been described in the corneal stroma. Hemangiopericytoma has been described in the conjunctiva,[45] but its analogue in the cornea has yet to be reported. In comparison

FIGURE 24-14 Histologic section through the cyst, which was located in the posterior third of the corneal stroma. Nonkeratinizing squamous epithelium without goblet cells lines the cyst. Descemet's membrane is present below. (Hematoxylin and eosin, × 240.) (Reprinted with permission from SE Bloomfield, FA Jakobiec, T Iwamoto: Traumatic intrastromal corneal cyst. Ophthalmology 87:951, 1980. Courtesy of Ophthalmology.)

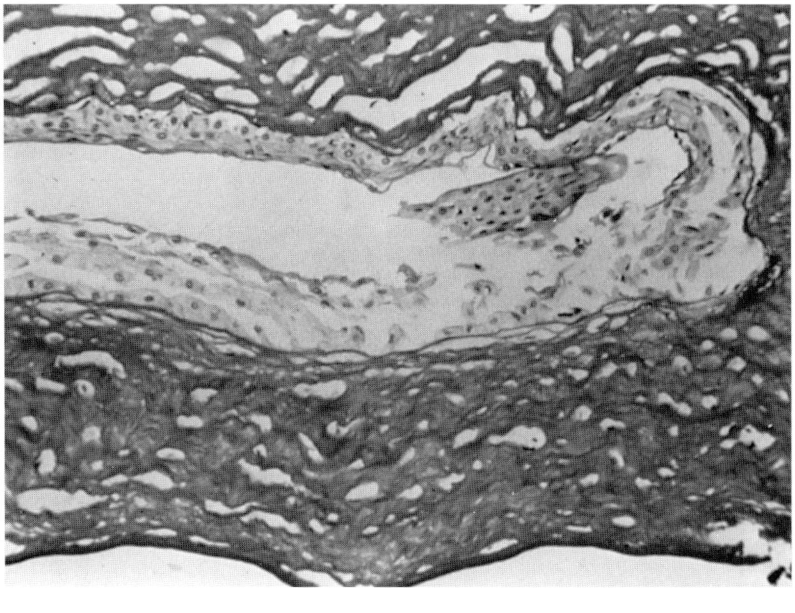

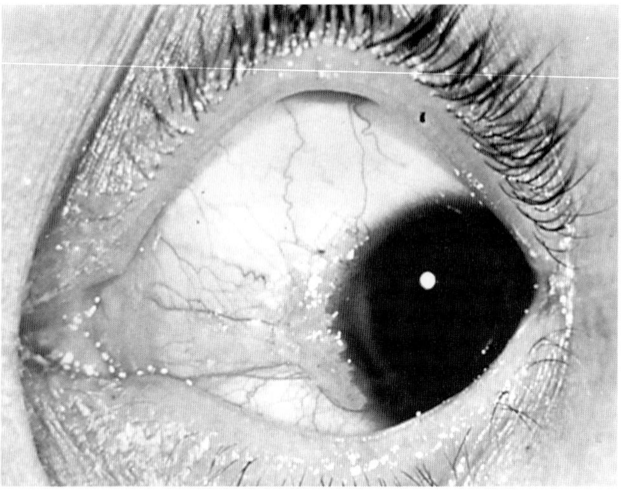

FIGURE 24-15 Juxtalimbal hyperplastic squamous lesion in benign hereditary dyskeratosis.

with the substantia propria, the corneal stroma is an extremely inert tissue, perhaps as a result of the widely spaced keratocytes that are normally in an indolent metabolic state. It is interesting to speculate whether the neural crest origin of the corneal fibroblasts or keratocytes[46,47] is related to the more lethargic reactive condition of these cells. Leukemia rarely affects the cornea, although ring ulcers may be seen in acute myelocytic leukemia.[48] There is one published case of a patient with known chronic lymphocytic leukemia who presented with subepithelial opacities in an eye with a previous penetrating keratoplasty.[49] On biopsy, using light and electron microscopy, the infiltrates were found to be sheets of lymphocytes.

SQUAMOUS EPITHELIAL TUMORS

Although the corneal epithelium is topographically continuous with the conjunctival epithelium, a major biologic transition zone occurs at the limbus. Here the substantia propria of the conjunctiva disappears, to become modified into Bowman's layer. Subtle electron microscopic differences exist between the conjunctival and corneal epithelia, although both are nonkeratinizing in type. Most important, the limbal region is a mitotically active zone. If the corneal epithelium is traumatically or surgically scraped off, the surrounding corneal epithelial cells slide to fill in the defect, but the replenishment of new corneal epithelial cells occurs in the mitotically active zone at the limbus. The location of this mitotic zone probably explains why most corneal epithelial proliferations and dysplasias begin at the limbus and spread either centrally onto the corneal surface or peripherally toward the conjunctival surface.

Benign Hereditary Dyskeratosis

Benign hereditary dyskeratosis is inherited as an autosomal dominant trait and appears within the first decade of life.[50,51] It is usually bilateral and affects a consanguineous kindred of individuals, all apparently descended from the Haliwa Indians in North Carolina, whose descendants now include triracial backgrounds. Some of the affected individuals have relocated, and the disease has subsequently appeared in other parts of the country.[52]

The lesions typically begin at the limbus or overlie the peripheral cornea and the contiguous conjunctiva in a V shape (Figure 24-15). They are hyperplastic and translucent, with foci of whiteness corresponding to keratinization of the surface. The lesions do not extend centrally toward the visual axis and do not threaten vision. The conjunctiva frequently has a vascularized and irritated appearance; a foreign body sensation may result from heaped up masses of abnormal epithelium. Associated lesions of the oropharynx and buccal mucosa may be observed. Even after complete local excision, the corneal lesions can recur because of an inherited genetic disorder of squamous cell maturation.

Histopathologically, the lesions are composed of acanthotic, or hyperplastic, epithelium (Figure 24-16) in which there is premature keratinization of individual cells (dyskeratosis) (Figure 24-17). There may be a mild degree of invasive acanthosis of the associated corneal pannus, but cytologic atypia apart from the dyskeratosis is not present. These lesions have no potential to evolve into true dysplasia or squamous cell carcinoma.

Squamous Papillomas

Squamous papillomas are so called because the surface squamous epithelium lies on connective tissue fronds, which are responsible for the papillary architecture.[5] If these connective tissue fronds emanate from a central stock, the lesion is referred to as pedunculated; if the connective tissue fronds are individually and broadly pulled up from the underlying connective tissue of the substantia propria or from a fibrovascular pannus of the cornea, the lesion is called sessile.

The major clinical clue that one is dealing with a squamous papilloma is the repeating fibrovascular cores, which appear as a geometrically arranged set of red dots throughout the lesion. As one looks at the lesion, the transparent surface squamous epithelium allows visualization of the underlying capillaries, which supply and nourish the

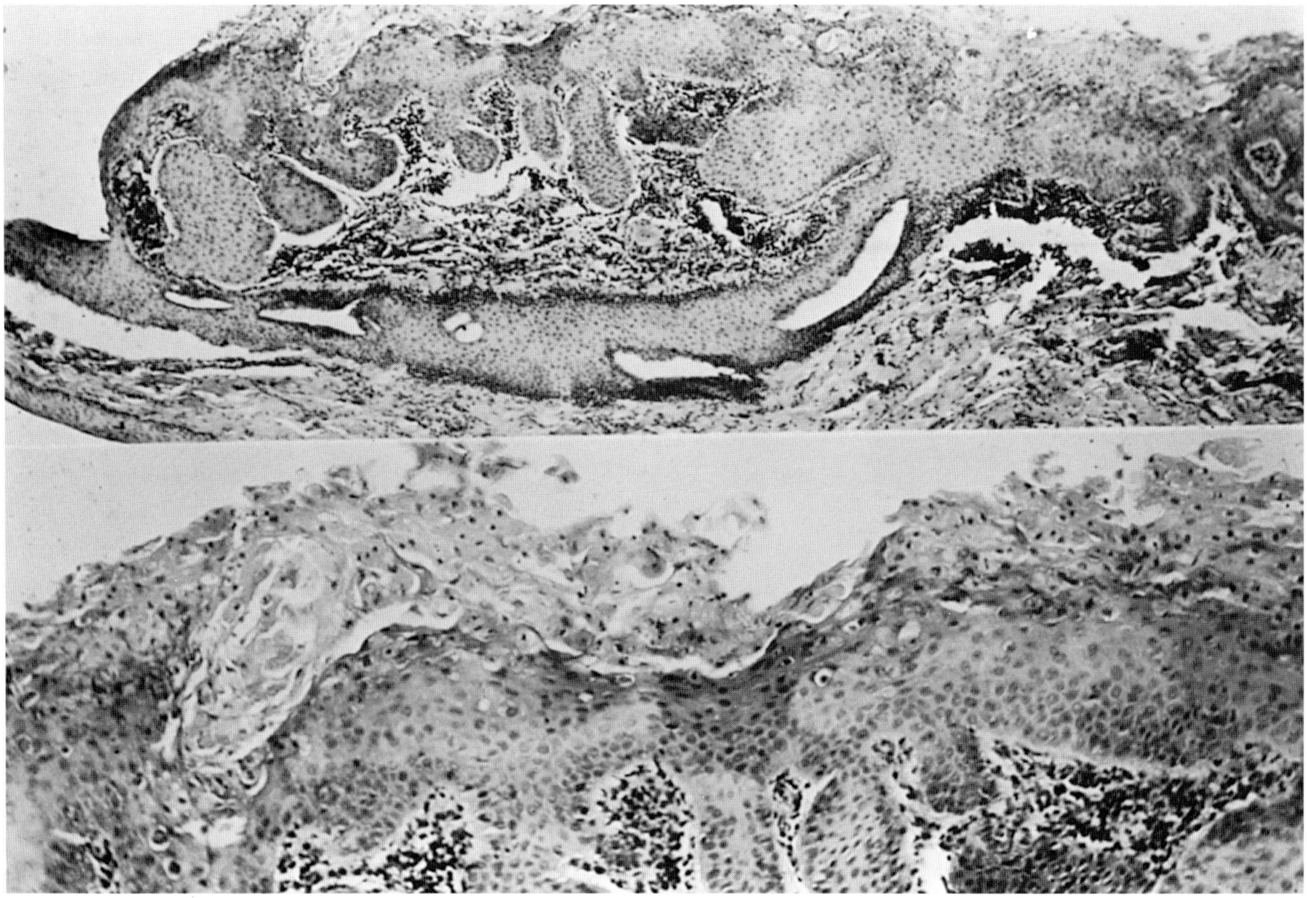

FIGURE 24-16 Benign invasive acanthosis is featured in hereditary dyskeratosis. With higher magnification in the bottom figure, a surface parakeratotic plaque can be seen. Parakeratosis represents the retention of nuclei in degenerating squamous cells. (Hematoxylin and eosin, top, × 40; bottom, × 220.)

FIGURE 24-17 Dyskeratosis is present in lesions of benign hereditary dyskeratosis. Note the mild mononuclear inflammation in the substantia propria beneath the acanthotic epithelium. Dyskeratotic cells stand out from their surrounding cells by virtue of a more eosinophilic cytoplasm and surrounding halo, due to inspissation of the cytoplasm from tonofilamentary conglutination. (Hematoxylin and eosin, × 260.)

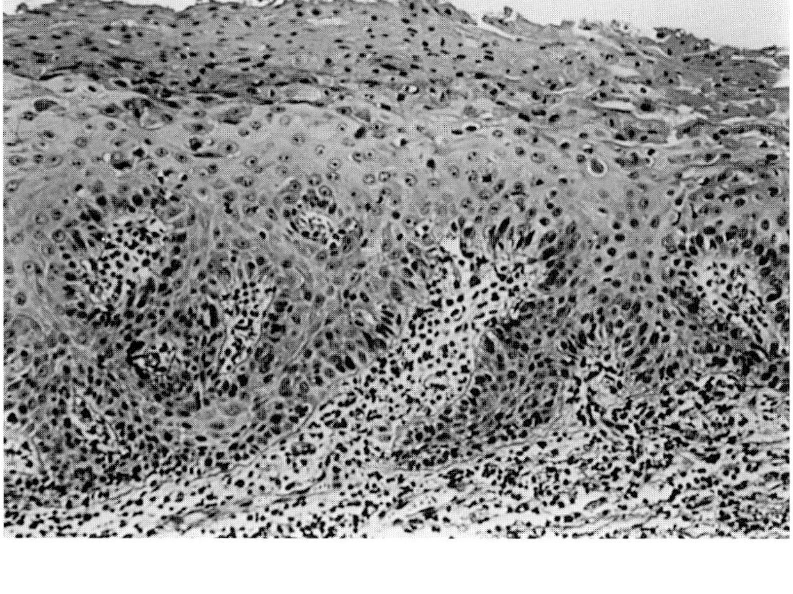

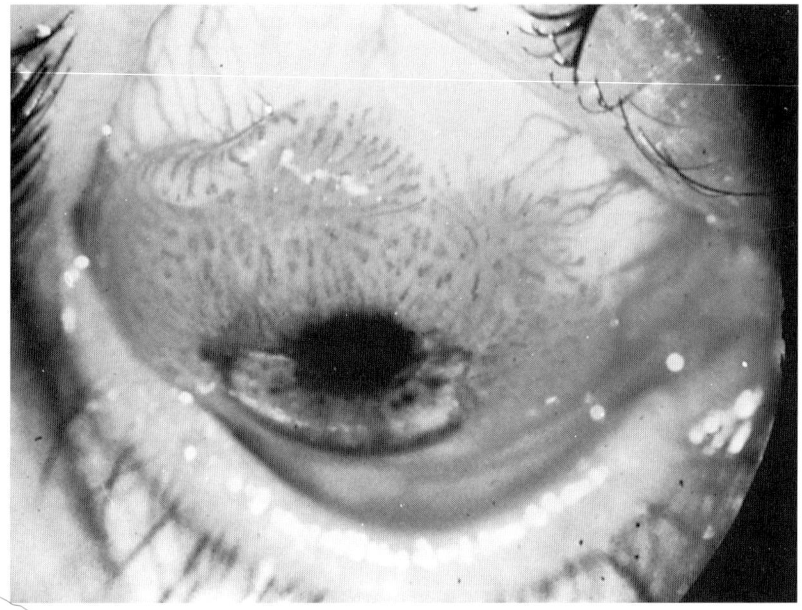

FIGURE 24-18 A papillary lesion with regularly distributed vascularity has significantly encroached on the cornea. This lesion was a papillary dysplasia rather than a benign squamous papilloma. The latter may drape on the cornea but does not infiltrate it or grow directly from the surface of the cornea.

connective tissue papillary cores. Consequently, the lesion has a red or frambesiform appearance, and the surface appears glistening and transparent except for possible focal areas of surface keratinization from irritation caused by rubbing of the eyelids. In black patients, the lesion may be partially pigmented because of benign melanocytes scattered throughout the lesion.[5]

Squamous papillomas may be found anywhere on the conjunctiva but sometimes develop at the limbus and may drape over the cornea. If the cornea is disproportionately involved, there is an obligatory underlying fibrovascular pannus, and squamous dysplasia should be suspected (Figure 24-18). Multiple benign lesions may be scattered throughout the conjunctiva; they have a particular propensity to develop in children, and papillomavirus has been incriminated as the causative agent[53] (see Ch. 13).

The surface covering of a papilloma is generally a nonkeratinizing squamous epithelium that is somewhat more thickened, or acanthotic, than that of the normal conjunctiva or cornea. There may be mucin-producing goblet cells scattered throughout the epithelium, as well as melanocytes if the lesion arises in a black individual. A squamous papilloma has virtually no potential for degeneration into a squamous cell carcinoma. There are papillary squamous dysplastic and carcinomatous lesions of the conjunctiva and cornea; in these instances, the surface epithelial cells microscopically display atypia and defects of polarity and maturation, as mentioned below.

Simple excision, with cryotherapy to the base of the excision and to the surrounding epithelium, can effect a cure. Recurrences are frequent, particularly in children, because there may be subclinically infected areas of the epithelium with the potential to spawn another papillary lesion. Additionally, excision of a viral papilloma may lead to seeding of the conjunctiva with virus, with recurrence of multiple lesions. Viral papillomas may regress spontaneously.

Pedunculated and sessile squamous papillomas grow in an exophytic fashion toward the outside, drawing up connective tissue fronds from the underlying substantia propria or fibrovascular tissue. An inverted or endophytic squamous papilloma is a rare variant of squamous papilloma that affects the conjunctiva. There is a report of three of these unusual lesions,[54] one of the tarsus and two of the caruncle. Two juxtalimbal lesions of the epibulbar surface have also been reported,[55] neither of which infiltrated the cornea. In these lesions, there are invasive lobules of benign-appearing squamous epithelium, with conspicuous cystic areas and intermixed mucin-producing goblet cells. These lesions appear to be indolent, and simple local excision is sufficient for cure. They are much less aggressive than inverted squamous papillomas arising in the lacrimal sac, the latter being similar to those of the nose and sinus mucosa, which can aggressively infiltrate underlying connective tissues and may even be associated with squamous cell carcinoma.

Pseudoepitheliomatous Hyperplasia

Pseudoepitheliomatous hyperplasia is a benign reactive proliferation of the epithelium of the conjunctiva and of the cornea if the limbus is involved.[5,56] The lesion typically develops rapidly over weeks to months and has a

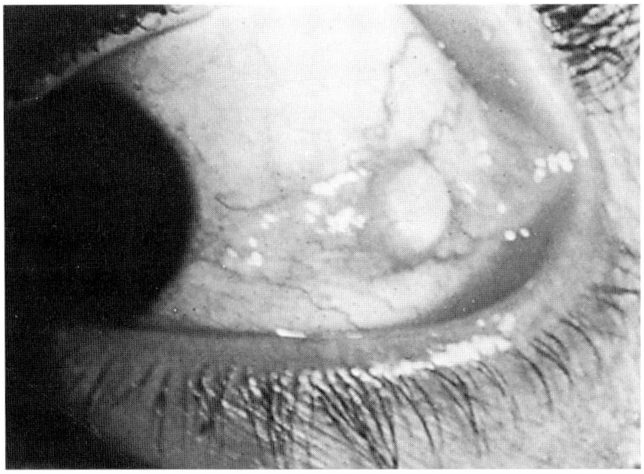

FIGURE 24-19 Epibulbar lesion of pseudoepitheliomatous hyperplasia. The lesion does not involve the limbus and, therefore, in all likelihood, is benign. The lesion develops rapidly over weeks to months, as opposed to the more insidious growth of a true dysplasia or neoplasm. The lesion is white because of the maturation present within it tending toward complete keratinization (leukoplakia).

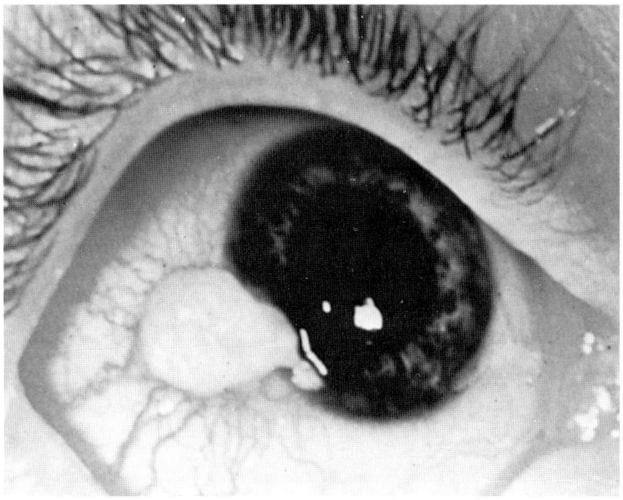

FIGURE 24-20 Lesion of pseudoepitheliomatous hyperplasia involving the limbus. If a history of rapid growth is not elicited from the patient, such a lesion with a limbal connection must be suspected of being squamous dysplasia. Most dysplastic lesions, however, are gelatinous rather than white, because they fail to exhibit much keratinization.

raised, whitened, hyperkeratotic surface. Some lesions may have incipient central umbilication or crater formation, similar to a keratoacanthoma. Pseudoepitheliomatous hyperplasia that develops away from the limbus (Figure 24-19) can generally be accurately diagnosed clinically, because most squamous dysplasias or carcinomas arise at the limbus. Pseudoepitheliomatous hyperplasia that develops at the limbus (Figure 24-20), however, cannot be distinguished clinically from squamous dysplasia, unless there is a history of rapid proliferation, particularly overlying a pinguecula or pterygium. Pseudoepitheliomatous hyperplasia lacks the regularly arranged red dots of capillaries seen in papillary cores of squamous papillomas or dysplasias.

Histopathologically, pseudoepitheliomatous hyperplasia is composed of piled up masses of squamous epithelium (Figure 24-21), which may be pushed down in an invasive acanthotic manner into the underlying tissue. Cytologic atypia is not marked, although there may be mitotic figures. A zone of lymphocytic infiltration is frequently found subjacent to the margins of the invading benign epithelium. There is no abrupt demarcation at the lateral edges of the lesion; rather, the lesion undergoes a transition into undisturbed surface epithelium, and the reactive cells have cytologic features similar to those of the uninvolved epithelium. This is in contrast to squamous dysplasia and carcinoma in situ, in which there is usually an abrupt demarcation between abnormal and normal epithelium. Keratoacanthoma is a more structured form of pseudoepitheliomatous hyperplasia, manifesting a cup-like growth pattern with a central collection of keratin and acanthotic lobules of epithelium (Figure 24-22).

Generally, simple excision is curative of all types of pseudoepitheliomatous hyperplasia, and even if these lesions recur, they are not formal precursors of precarcinomatous or carcinomatous conditions.

Squamous Dysplasia and Carcinoma In Situ

Neoplastic proliferations of the squamous epithelium have a predilection to arise at the limbus[57–59] because of the pronounced mitotic activity in this region. More than 95 percent of dysplastic lesions of the epibulbar surface have a portion of the lesion in contact with the limbus. Other dysplastic lesions may arise at the mucocutaneous junction of the eyelid margin or even medially in the caruncle area. Rare diffuse lesions are discovered so late in their course that a precise origin cannot be determined. Any proliferative squamous epithelial lesion attached to the limbus must be seriously considered as being dysplastic.

Because squamous dysplasia arises from a single cell that undergoes neoplastic transformation, it takes time for the proliferation to create a clinically detectable tumefaction; the lesion, therefore, evolves slowly. Patients may even be unaware of it at the time an ophthalmologist detects it. In this regard, squamous dysplasia differs

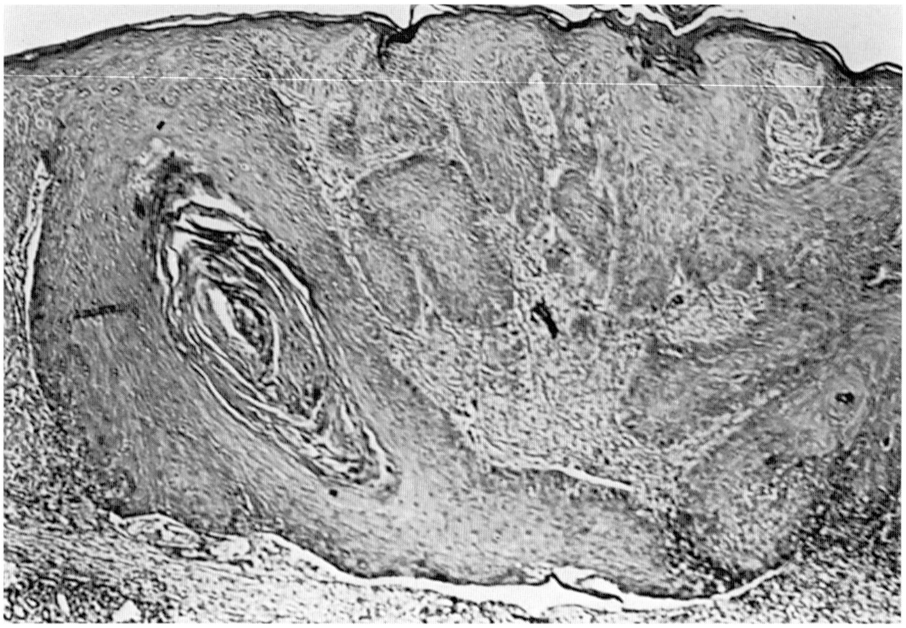

FIGURE 24-21 Microscopic appearance of invasive acanthosis in pseudoepitheliomatous hyperplasia. Note the keratin whorl in the lobule on the left. Keratinization accounts for the white appearance observed clinically. There is also mild mononuclear inflammation in the substantia propria. (Hematoxylin and eosin, × 90.)

from pseudoepitheliomatous hyperplasia in that the latter develops rapidly. Such rapid development may be caused by the simultaneous stimulation of a large number of cells in a focal area of epithelium, perhaps by inflammation, so that the clinical tumefaction forms more rapidly than it would if it were derived, as in the case of dysplasia, from a single cell.

Most dysplastic lesions are translucent or gelatinous; fewer than 10 percent are leukoplakic. Leukoplakia refers to the appearance of lesions that are white because of surface keratinization; however, this is not a pathologic diagnosis because pseudoepitheliomatous hyperplasia may also show surface keratinization. Some dysplastic lesions exhibit a distinct papillary character. Terms such as *Bowen's disease* and *dyskeratosis* used diagnostically should be abandoned; *squamous dysplasia* and *intraepithelial neoplasia* are much more inclusive and pathologically acceptable terms.

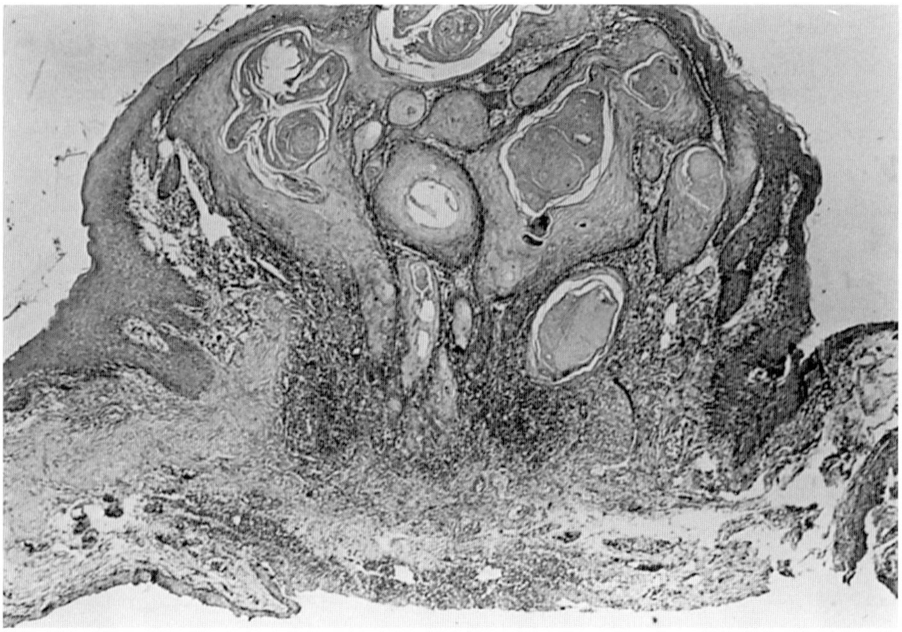

FIGURE 24-22 An epibulbar pseudoepitheliomatous hyperplasia with some of the features of a keratoacanthoma. In these more structured lesions, there is a cup-like growth pattern, with massive lobules of squamous acanthosis in the center along with keratin whorls. Note the mononuclear inflammation in the subjacent connective tissue. (Hematoxylin and eosin, × 60.)

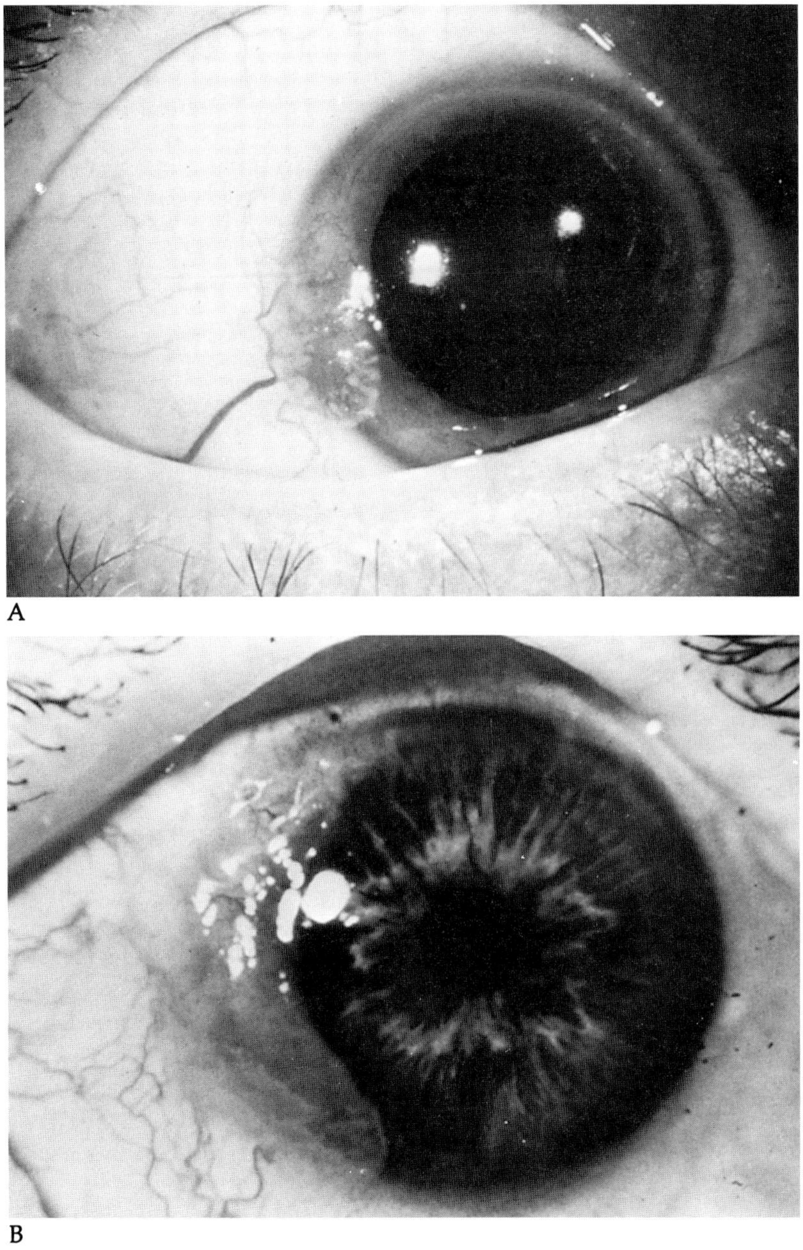

FIGURE 24-23 (A & B) Two typical lesions of squamous dysplasia involving the corneoscleral limbus. Most of these lesions are gelatinous because of the absence of significant keratinization.

Most dysplastic lesions arise in the interpalpebral zone at the limbus, either nasally or temporally, in older, fair-skinned individuals, more often in men (Figure 24-23). This phenomenon suggests that solar radiation and ultraviolet exposure may play a role in provoking the neoplastic transformation. Many lesions occur in association with either a pinguecula or a pterygium, which are also the result of stromal actinic damage and stimulation.[8] Several studies have shown an association between human papillomavirus type 16 and conjunctival squamous changes ranging from hypertrophic papillary change without dysplasia to invasive squamous cell carcinoma. One study used polymerase chain reaction and DNA hybridization techniques to demonstrate the presence of human papillomavirus type 16 in 75 percent of studied conjunctival squamous dysplasias and carcinomas.[60] Six control lesions (papillomas, pterygia) were negative. Interestingly, one patient with unilateral corneal dysplasia demonstrated the virus in cells swabbed from both corneas. There also have been several case reports of patients with bilateral squamous conjunctival tumors associated with human papillomavirus type 16.[61] One patient developed invasive

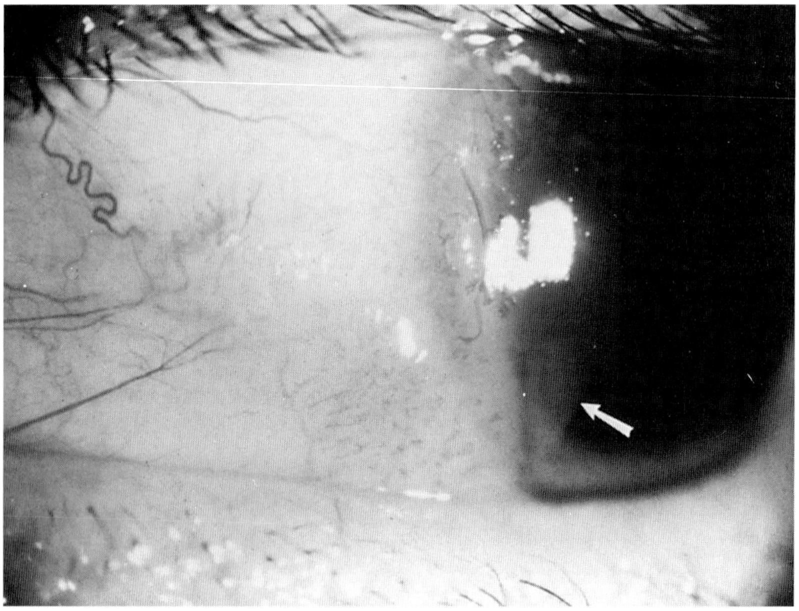

FIGURE 24-24 The temporal corneoscleral limbus and adjacent conjunctiva are involved by a thickened gelatinous and vascularized mass. Note that there is a frosting of nonvascularized dysplastic epithelium (arrow) extending away from the main mass toward the visual axis on the corneal surface.

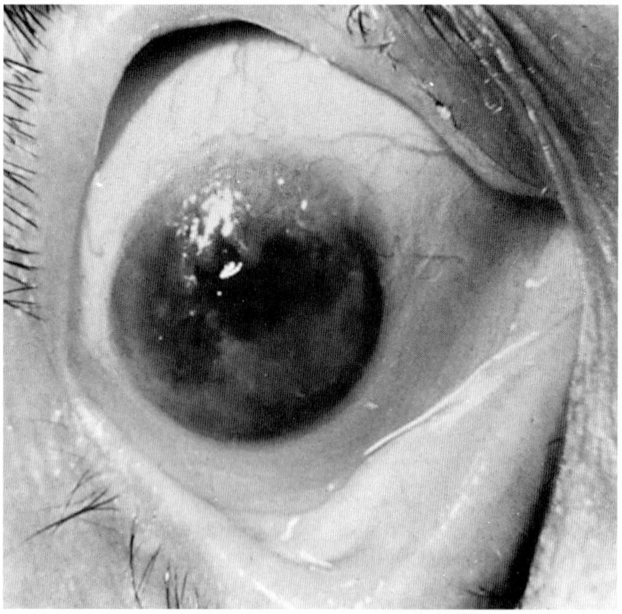

FIGURE 24-25 An advanced case of extensive squamous dysplasia of the corneal surface that has progressed to carcinoma in situ.

squamous cell carcinoma in one eye and orbit that required exenteration and areas of carcinoma in situ, dysplasia, and symblephara in the other eye. Multiple biopsy sites in both eyes were positive for human papillomavirus type 16, although one leukoplakic area in the exenterated eye was negative. A second patient presented with bilateral circumlimbal conjunctival changes. Multiple biopsies revealed severe dysplasia, carcinoma in situ, and invasive squamous cell carcinoma. One biopsy from each eye was tested and was positive for the virus. A third patient presented with bilateral superior tarsal papillary lesions. Biopsy revealed pseudoglandular invaginations of the surface epithelium and inflammatory cells without evidence of dysplasia. Again, both lesions were positive for the virus. These results raise interesting questions about the role of infectious agents in the etiology of conjunctival and corneal squamous pathology. The viral agent may act in concert with actinic exposure to promote disease, or it may be an independent factor. Studies to determine the incidence of human papillomavirus type 16 in normal conjunctiva, benign conjunctival lesions, and other dysplastic and malignant lesions are ongoing.

The corneal component of dysplastic lesions is often the result of a spreading of involved epithelium anterior to Bowman's layer beyond the main area of limbal thickening (Figure 24-24). This abnormal frosted epithelium is frequently not recognized by the examining clinician, and if it is not removed at the time of surgery, it can lead to a recurrence because it is composed of dysplastic cells. An important sign of squamous dysplasia is a fine underlying vascularity that has a hairpin configuration, although, rarely, it may be papillary as well. This hairpin vascularity can extend onto the cornea underlying the frosted epithelium; it is reflective of a neoplastic pannus that supports the metabolic needs of the neoplastic epithelium. With time, a large area of the corneal surface may become involved (Figure 24-25).

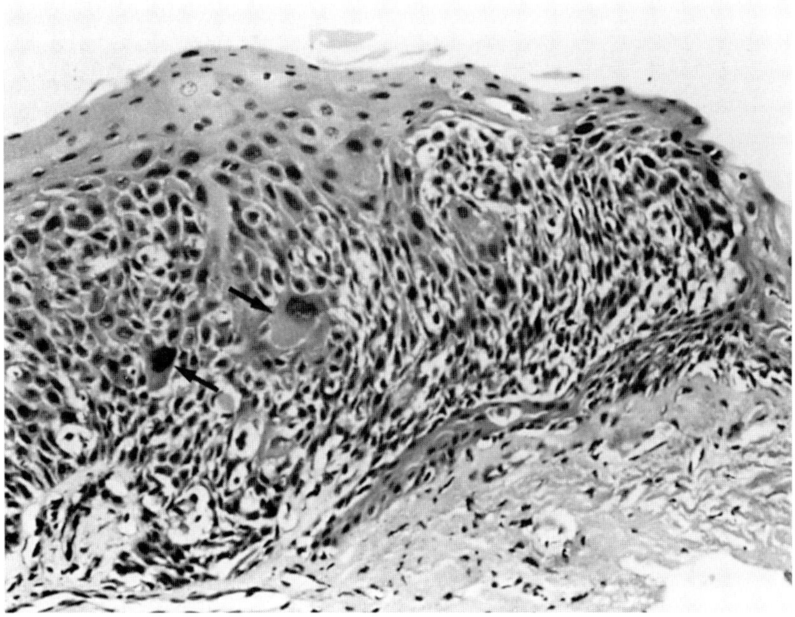

FIGURE 24-26 Histologic appearance of severe dysplasia involving approximately two-thirds of the thickness of the epithelium. There is a surface umbrella of more normal-appearing cells. Both small hyperchromatic and larger bizarre cells (arrows) are present within the lesion. (Hematoxylin and eosin, × 140.)

Unlike squamous papilloma and pseudoepitheliomatous hyperplasia, in which the epithelial constituents may be somewhat thickened and excessive but do not display neoplastic cytologic detail, squamous dysplasia and carcinoma in situ have anaplastic cells (Figures 24-26 and 24-27). The most important feature of an anaplastic cell is the high ratio of nuclear to cytoplasmic volume, which means that the nucleus occupies much more of the cell's volume than normal because of scanty cytoplasm or a large hyperchromatic nucleus. In contrast, squamous papilloma and pseudoepitheliomatous hyperplasia have a normal or low ratio of nuclear to cytoplasmic volume; the nuclei are widely separated by conspicuous amounts of eosinophilic cytoplasm. The cytologic atypia in dysplasia does not have to be bizarre; cells with a high ratio of nuclear to cytoplasmic volume in some dysplastic lesions are banal and monotonous in their appearance, but the nuclei are clearly more crowded than normal and are sharply delineated from the adjacent normal epithelium. In addition, there is a disturbance of polarity and maturation; the cells may be disorganized in their relationship and orientation to one another (dyspolarity), and toward the surface, there is frequently an absence of maturation. Isolated cells may be extremely bizarre, with large pleomorphic nuclei and multiple mitotic figures at all levels of the epithelium; sometimes, these cells have more conspicuous eosinophilic cytoplasm. If these cells show inspissation with retraction of the cell borders from surrounding squamous cells, they are referred to as neoplastic dyskeratotic cells; the nucleus is usually shriveled. These dyskeratotic cells may be seen at all levels of the epithelium; they are not seen when the cytoplasm is scant.

The distinction between squamous dysplasia and carcinoma in situ is merely one of degree: a partial-thickness replacement of the epithelium by atypical cells is called *dysplasia,* whereas a total replacement from the basement membrane to the outermost superficial cells is called *carcinoma in situ.* Both lesions, however, are restrained by an intact basement membrane and do not invade the underlying connective tissue. There is generally a sharp demarcation between the neoplastic cells and the benign epithelium at the lateral edges of the lesion where the cells abut uninvolved epithelium. This feature differs from that of squamous papilloma or pseudoepitheliomatous hyperplasia, wherein there is an imperceptible blending of the non-neoplastic, but hyperplastic, epithelium with the undisturbed adjacent epithelium. If the lesion has been caused by actinic damage, there may be evidence of elastotic degeneration of the underlying substantia propria. Suprabasilar clefting (acantholysis) of poorly adherent neoplastic epithelium may be seen in such actinically induced lesions. These are also the lesions most apt to have bizarre cells; they are frequently seen in corneal lesions associated with xeroderma pigmentosum.

Squamous dysplasia and carcinoma in situ represent a spectrum of slowly progressive lesions that need only be adequately excised locally. If there is no invasion of the underlying connective tissue, there is no potential for metastases, because metastases depend on either blood vessels or lymphatic channels, which are only present in the substantia propria of the conjunctiva. The management of these lesions depends on whether they are being encountered for the first time or represent recurrences of previously incompletely

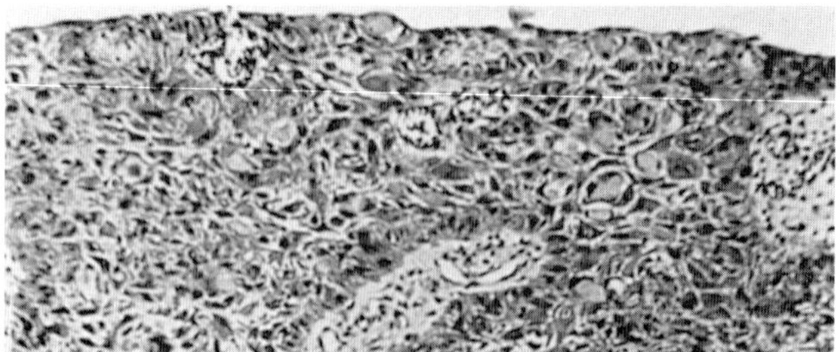

FIGURE 24-27 A carcinoma in situ has replaced the entire thickness of the corneal epithelium. Note the subjacent corneal stroma and Descemet's membrane at the bottom. Bowman's layer has been destroyed by the neoplastic pannus. (Hematoxylin and eosin, × 140.)

excised lesions. A lesion encountered for the first time should be widely locally excised down to the sclera; a surrounding area of apparently uninvolved conjunctiva should also be excised to secure adequate surgical margins. The application of either fluorescein or rose bengal stain assists in defining how widespread the disease is; dysplastic epithelium tends to stain diffusely, with fine stippling where the dysplastic cells are located, whereas normal corneal and conjunctival epithelium does not stain in this manner.

The thickened portion of the lesion at the limbus is generally excised first, followed by removal of the corneal epithelial component. Cocaine is placed on the corneal epithelium to soften it, and then a stainless steel blade (#64 Beaver blade) is used to scrape any frosted epithelium off Bowman's layer. Some normal epithelium in advance of where the frosted area ends is also scraped off. While scraping the frosted epithelium, one may encounter a fibrovascular pannus, which can also be dissected from Bowman's layer with a stainless steel blade. After corneal scraping, Bowman's layer may be scrubbed with absolute alcohol to devitalize fragments of cells that might have crumbled during scraping. Alternatively, the limbal area can be frozen with a retinal cryoprobe in a double or triple freeze-thaw technique.[62] A retinal cryoprobe allows control of the depth of the iceball to minimize damage to underlying tissues. The bed of the lesion should be frozen. Additionally, the cut conjunctival edges should be elevated with a subconjunctival injection of lidocaine and frozen.

Recurrent lesions are often more widespread and cause concern about the potential for conversion into invasive squamous cell carcinoma. Management involves the same surgical methods and maneuvers described above. Deep excision with lamellar keratoplasty may be necessary. Cryotherapy is applied more generously to the bed of excision as well as to the cut edges of conjunctiva. If there is any concern about invasion of the underlying connective tissues, a cutaneous cryogun, which has more energy, is used to ensure that the iceball goes through full-thickness sclera. Although there may be sectorial damage to the ciliary body, root of the iris, and trabecular meshwork, the eye can tolerate this. Postoperatively, the patient undergoes cycloplegia and is given 80 mg of oral prednisone each day. Cycloplegia is discontinued as soon as anterior segment inflammation has resolved. The oral prednisone dosage is tapered over 1 month.

For lesions that are extensive and diffuse at the time of discovery, the bulkiest portions of the lesion are removed by surgery, and the epithelium of the involved corneal areas is scraped off with a stainless steel blade; again, the proliferation is generally restrained by Bowman's layer. Thereafter, the conjunctiva is ballooned up with lidocaine, and double or triple freeze-thaw cryotherapy is applied to all involved conjunctival areas and to a generous surrounding area of apparently uninvolved epithelium. Eyes in which the lesion involves more than 50 percent of the limbus and cornea may have a poor visual prognosis after excision of the lesion and cryotherapy, secondary to surface abnormalities, corneal neovascularization, scarring, and inflammation. Some surgeons have obtained good visual results in these cases with limbal conjunctival autografting.[63]

Primary Corneal Epithelial Dysplasia and Epithelial Dysmaturation

There is an extremely unusual group of conditions that represent involvement of the corneal epithelium only, or a

FIGURE 24-28 Several large areas of nonvascularized, frosted, and dysplastic epithelium are present in the central cornea.

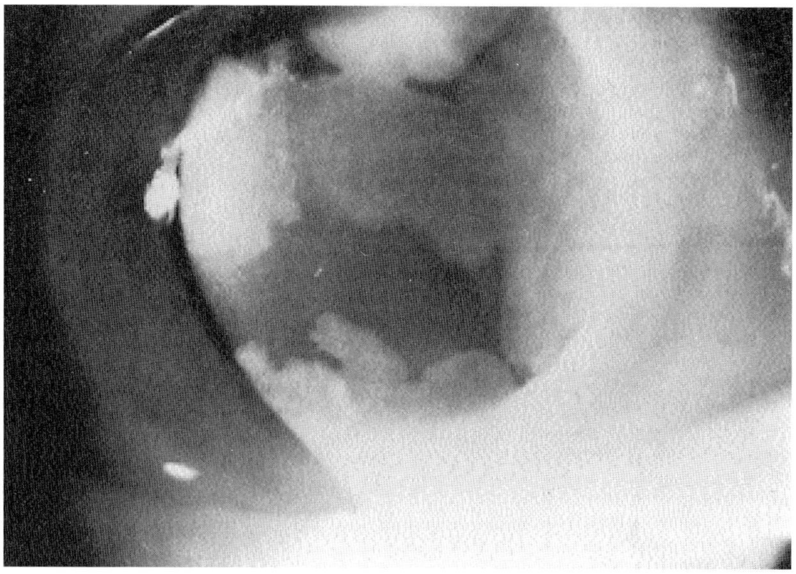

disproportionate involvement of the corneal epithelium from a small limbal lesion that has preferentially spread toward the cornea.[64] In such cases, there tends not to be a neoplastic fibrous pannus, but rather a wide field of frosted corneal epithelium (Figure 24-28) or individual islands of opalescent epithelium (Figure 24-29). In some of these lesions, cytologic features of unmistakable atypia are present. These lesions are called *primary corneal epithelial dysplasia*. In other lesions,[65] the nuclear/cytoplasmic volume ratio is either not grossly disturbed or is normal, there appears to be intact maturation, or there may be only slight differences from cell to cell in terms of the size of the nucleus (Figure 24-30). We prefer to term these lesions *corneal epithelial dysmaturation*. Both unilateral and bilateral, stationary and slowly progressive cases of epithelial dysmaturation have been noted (Figures 24-31 and 24-32), which distinguishes them from true, inexorably evolving dysplasia. All these cases, which one might conceive of as occupying a spectrum, are indolent and can be treated by scraping the corneal epithelium; any associated limbal tumefaction

FIGURE 24-29 Fimbriated and digitated extensions of dysplastic epithelium in the central cornea. (Reprinted with permission from GO Waring, AM Ross, MB Ekins: Clinical and pathologic description of 17 cases of corneal intraepithelial neoplasia. Am J Ophthalmol 97:547, 1984. Copyright by The Ophthalmic Publishing Company.)

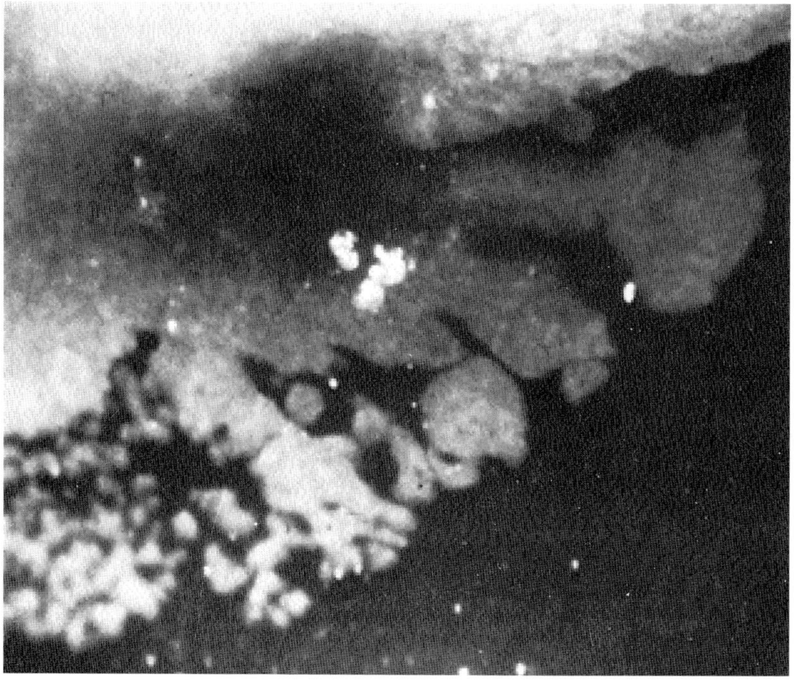

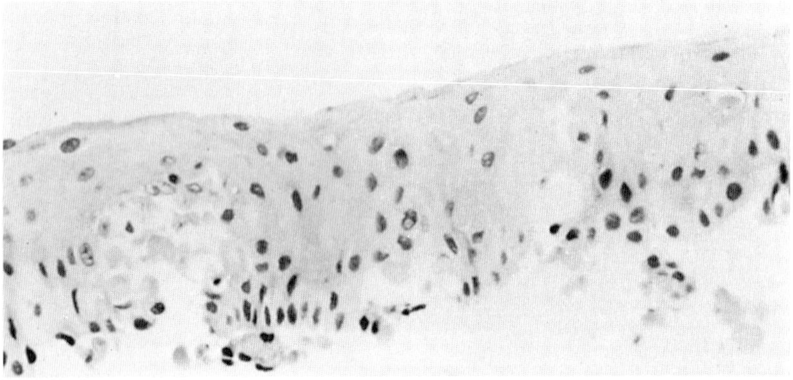

A

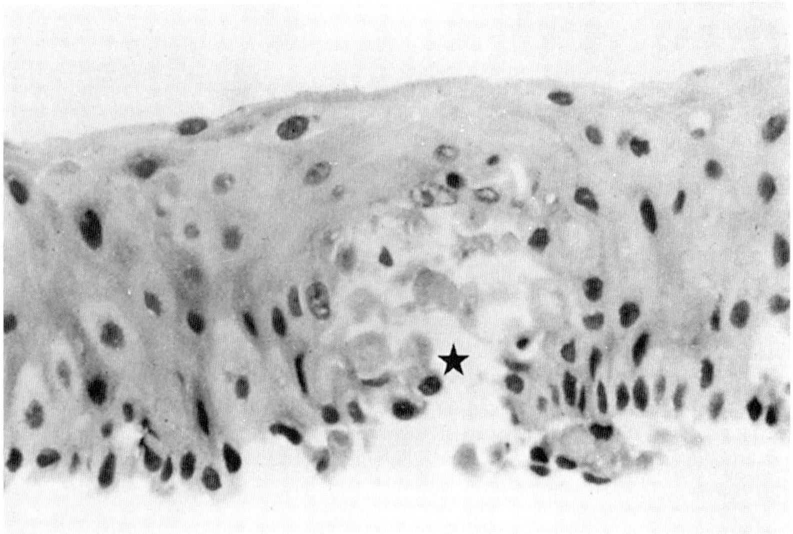

B

FIGURE 24-30 **(A)** A strip of corneal epithelium in a case of dysmaturation. Only subtle histologic features distinguish this condition from true dysplasia. Note the low nuclear/cytoplasmic ratio and the slight dyspolarity of cellular orientation and maturation. **(B)** A cavity lined by dyskeratotic or apoptotic cells (star). Note the bounteous cytoplasm widely separating the nuclei, which show only a mild degree of enlargement and irregularity. No mitotic figures are present. (Hematoxylin and eosin, A, × 110; B, × 190.) (Reprinted with permission from RJ Campbell, WM Bourne: Unilateral central corneal epithelial dysplasia. Ophthalmology 88:1231, 1981. Courtesy of Ophthalmology.)

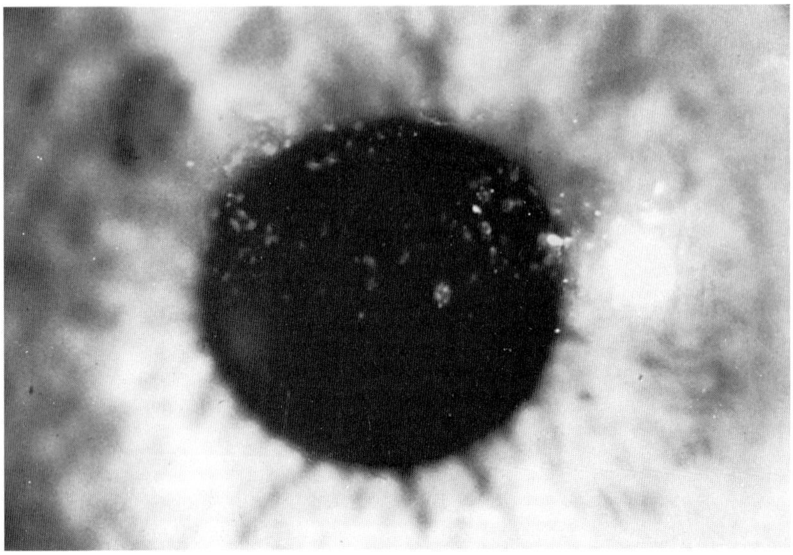

FIGURE 24-31 Multiple separate small areas of frosted epithelium in the visual axis. This lesion corresponds to the microscopic appearance shown in Figure 24-30. (Reprinted with permission from RJ Campbell, WM Bourne: Unilateral central corneal epithelial dysplasia. Ophthalmology 88:1231, 1981. Courtesy of Ophthalmology.)

should be widely excised, as mentioned above. Sometimes the opalescent islands and fingers spread over the corneal epithelium and can be mapped geographically over the course of months to years[64] (Figure 24-33). This feature is reminiscent of the waxing and waning spread of pigmentation seen in Reese's primary acquired melanosis.

Electron microscopy in cases of both primary corneal epithelial dysplasia (Figure 24-34) and epithelial dysmaturation (Figures 24-35 and 24-36) reveals a disorganization of the cytoplasmic tonofilaments, which are often clumped around the nucleus; large electron-dense granules that may be keratohyalin or tonofilamentary degeneration products; and disorganized desmosome formation.[64,65] The desmosomes can be found endocytosed into the cytoplasm of the tumor cells. Some of these features have been interpreted as representative of individual tumor cell death (apoptosis). Ultrastructural criteria appear not to be valid in making distinctions between the dysmaturational and the more dysplastic ends of the spectrum; such judgments are best made on the basis of clinical behavior, cellular atypia, and ratios of nuclear to cytoplasmic volume.

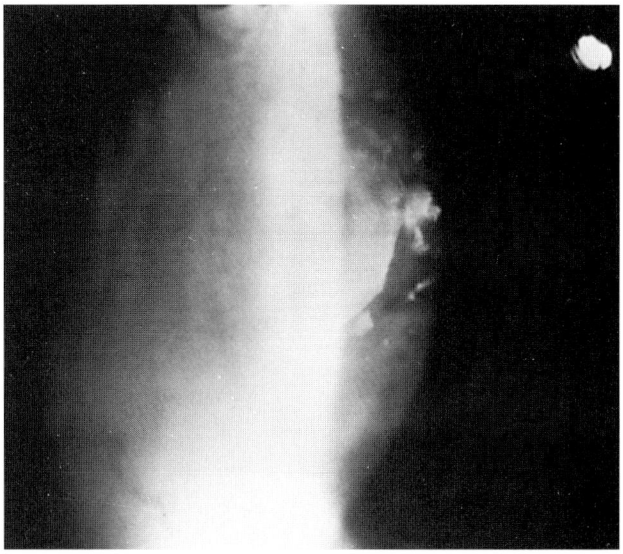

FIGURE 24-32 A patch of corneal epithelial frosting with an adjacent satellite lesion. In this case, there were symmetrically bilateral frosted areas in the nasal epithelium without any limbal thickening. The lesions remained stationary over several years. This is probably an example of epithelial dysmaturation.

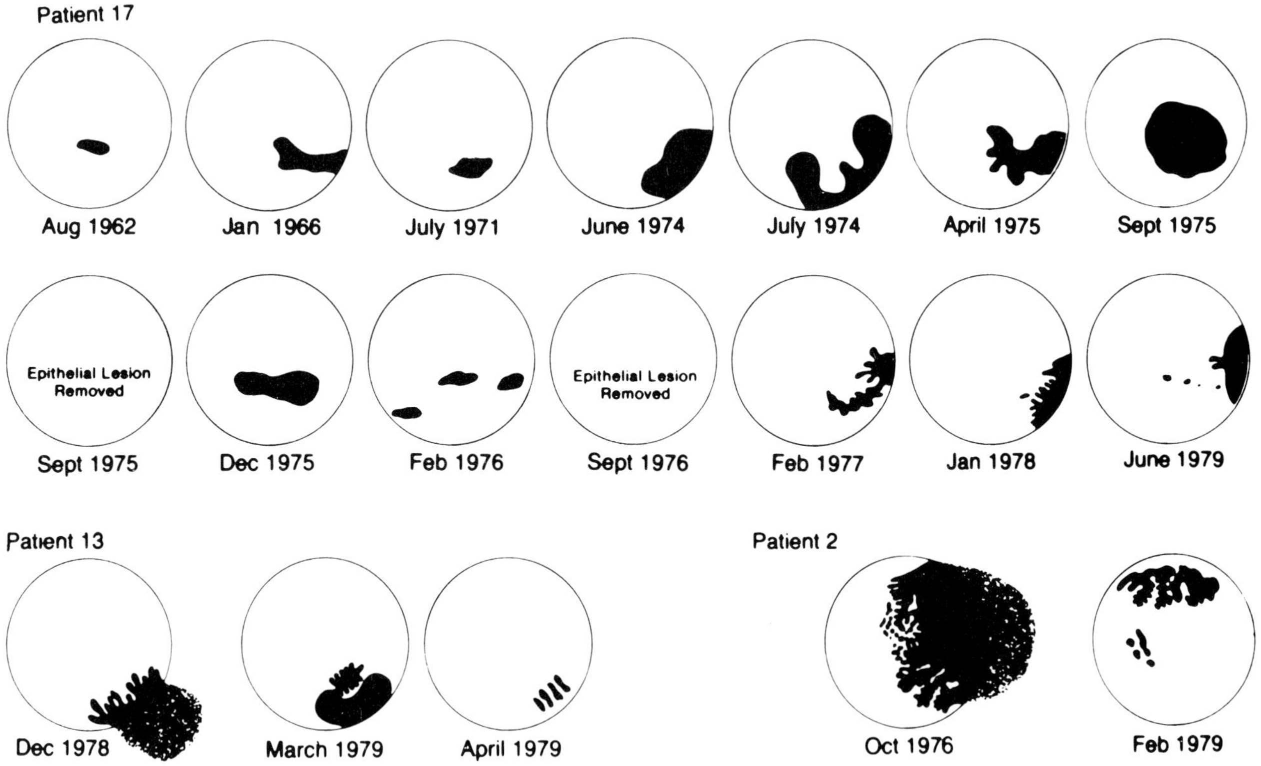

FIGURE 24-33 Corneal maps of several lesions of low-grade corneal epithelial dysplasia followed over time. There is a waxing and waning character to many of these lesions. These lesions can have an associated component of minimal limbal thickening. (Reprinted with permission from GO Waring, AM Ross, MB Ekins: Clinical and pathologic description of 17 cases of corneal intraepithelial neoplasia. Am J Ophthalmol 97:547, 1984. Copyright by The Ophthalmic Publishing Company.)

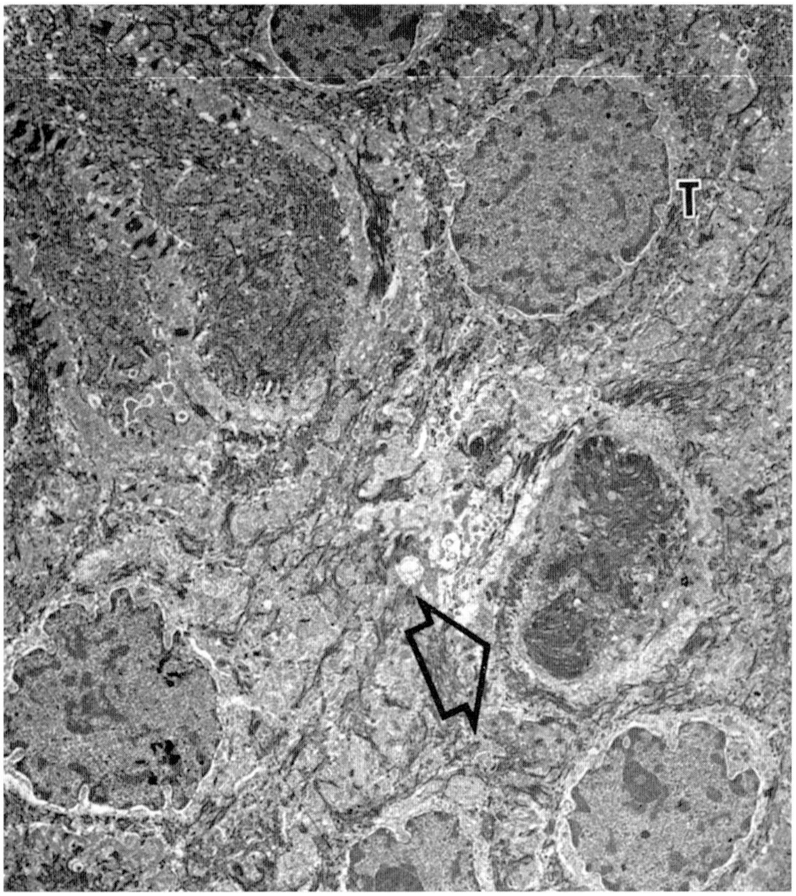

FIGURE 24-34 Electron micrograph of corneal intraepithelial dysplasia. Most of the tumor cells possess normal amounts of tonofilaments *(T)*. The large open arrowhead indicates a degenerating cell in which the tonofilaments are becoming conglutinated. (× 4,000.) (Reprinted with permission from GO Waring, AM Ross, MB Ekins: Clinical and pathologic description of 17 cases of corneal intraepithelial neoplasia. Am J Ophthalmol 97:547, 1984. Copyright by The Ophthalmic Publishing Company.)

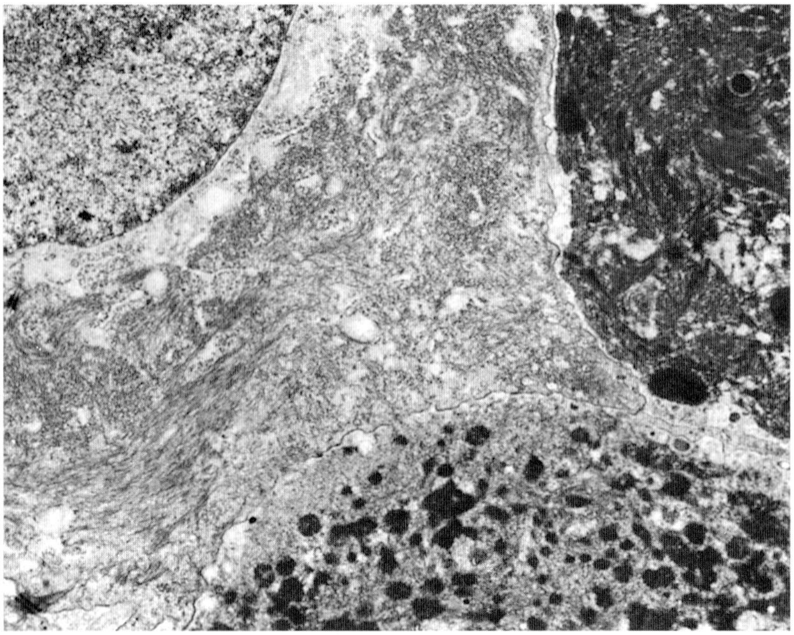

FIGURE 24-35 Electron micrograph of intraepithelial corneal dysmaturation. Two cells, shown toward the bottom right and the upper right, display tonofilamentary degeneration along with electron-dense granules, some of which may be keratohyalin and others that may be products of the degenerated tonofilaments. (× 15,000.) (Reprinted with permission from RJ Campbell, WM Bourne: Unilateral central corneal epithelial dysplasia. Ophthalmology 88:1231, 1981. Courtesy of Ophthalmology.)

FIGURE 24-36 **(A & B)** Corneal intraepithelial dysmaturation. Many intracytoplasmic desmosomes (arrow) are present, one of which is shown at higher magnification in Figure B, floating in a sea of tonofilaments. (A, × 22,000; B, × 75,000.) (Reprinted with permission from RJ Campbell, WM Bourne: Unilateral central corneal epithelial dysplasia. Ophthalmology 88:1231, 1981. Courtesy of Ophthalmology.)

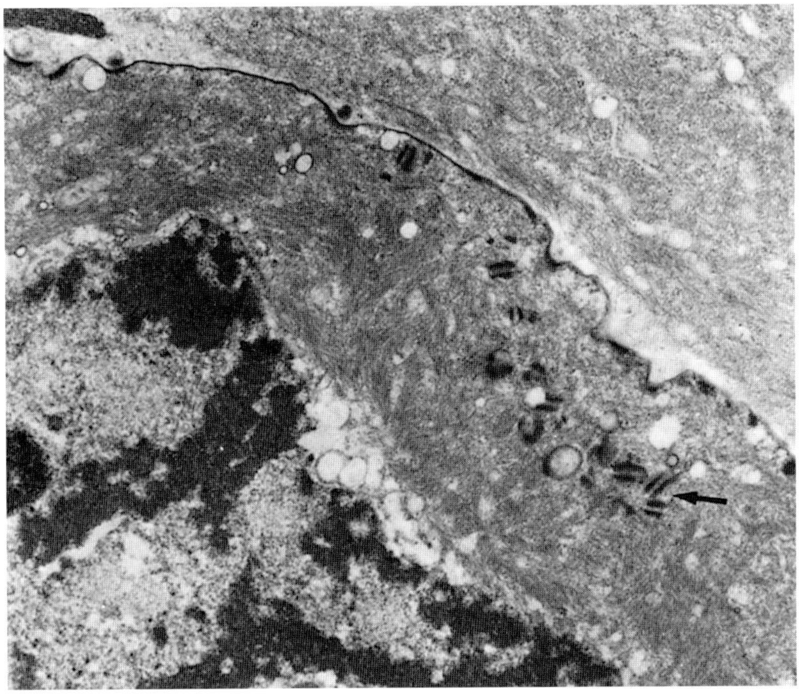

A

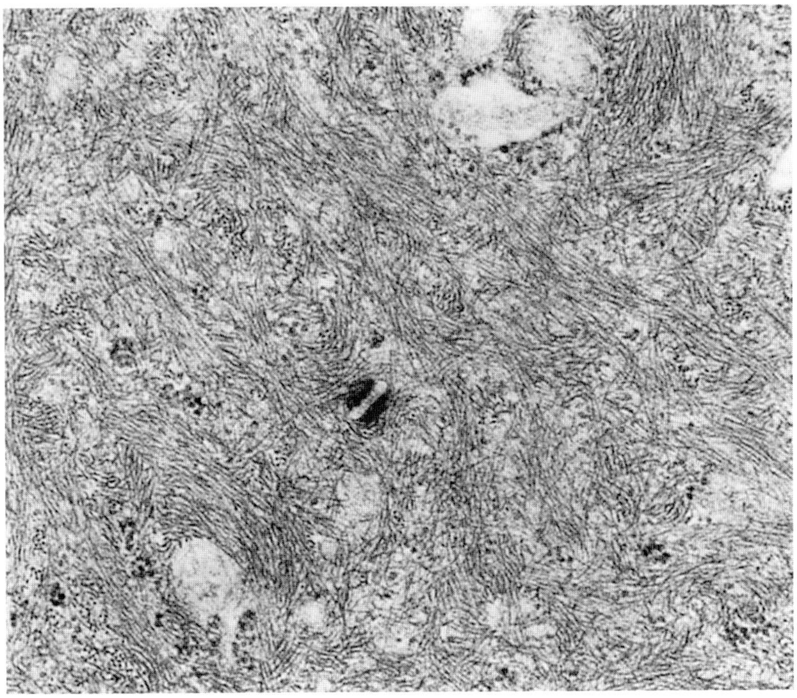

B

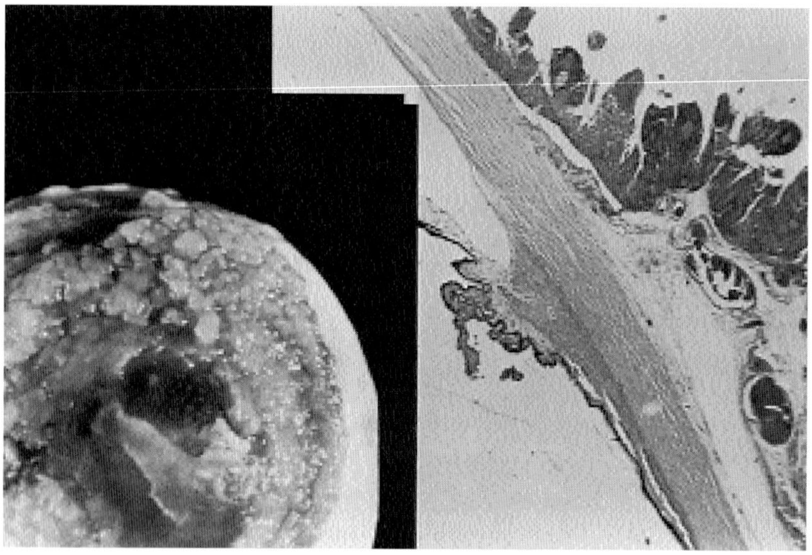

FIGURE 24-37 An extensive papillary squamous cell carcinoma in situ with focal microinvasion of the underlying connective tissue is shown in an enucleated globe on the left. The microscopic section on the right shows the papillary growth pattern extending onto the cornea toward the upper left. (Right, hematoxylin and eosin, × 60.) (Courtesy of the Armed Forces Institute of Pathology, Washington, DC.)

Invasive Squamous Cell Carcinoma

Either squamous dysplasia or carcinoma in situ over many years can breach the underlying basement membrane and invade the connective tissues (Figures 24-37 and 24-38). This event occurs more often on the conjunctival side than on the corneal side of the lesion, where Bowman's layer is reasonably resistant to such invasion. However, neoplastic cells can invade a softer neoplastic fibrous pannus underlying the corneal aspect of the lesion. These locally invasive lesions are still virtually incapable of regional or widespread metastases. In black patients, squamous cell carcinoma can be partially pigmented.[66] Wide local excision, coupled with either a superficial scleral lamellar excision or vigorous cryotherapy, should eradicate these lesions. Cryotherapy has reduced recurrence from 40 percent to less than 10 percent.[62] Only in very neglected cases is there likely to be deep corneal, intraocular, or rarely, even orbital invasion. Regional metastases with such advanced disease have been documented in only a few cases.[56] For lesions that invade the eye, enucleation is required; for lesions involving the orbit, exenteration is unavoidable. It is fortunate that these situations occur in fewer than 1 percent of cases.

Human immunodeficiency virus (HIV) infection has been reported in association with an aggressive conjunctival squamous cell carcinoma.[67] Atypical features in this case were the young age of the patient, rapid growth of the lesion, and marked pleomorphism, hyperchromasia, and mitotic activity on pathologic examination. In cases of atypical squamous cell carcinoma, immune suppression should be considered as a possible contributing factor.

Mucoepidermoid Carcinoma

In contrast to the desultory development of squamous dysplasia, carcinoma in situ, and eventual invasive squamous cell carcinoma, mucoepidermoid carcinoma is more aggressive from the outset.[68-70] This condition can occur anywhere in the conjunctiva and is not as severely restricted to the limbal zone as is typical squamous dysplasia or carcinoma in situ. The lesion is called *mucoepidermoid* because it consists of a mixture of squamous cells and mucin-producing goblet cells; the prominence of the mucin-producing goblet cells can confer a gelatinous appearance to the lesion. Mucoepidermoid carcinoma is more likely to invade the underlying connective tissues early, and intraocular invasion is also more likely to occur. Far more serious is the development of regional lymph node metastases, which characteristically are noted after recurrences. Epibulbar mucoepidermoid carcinoma is treated with wide local excision combined with cryotherapy.

Spindle Cell Carcinoma

Another highly malignant carcinoma of the epibulbar surface that may involve the limbus and the cornea is spindle cell carcinoma.[71,72] This tumor, which is capable of deep infiltration into the globe, is composed of elongated or fusiform cells that frequently do not obviously suggest an origin from the surface squamous epithelium. Instead, the appearance of a spindle cell melanoma, a fibrosarcoma, or even a leiomyosarcoma is suggested. Electron microscopy may identify cytoplasmic tonofilaments and desmosomes, and use of mon-

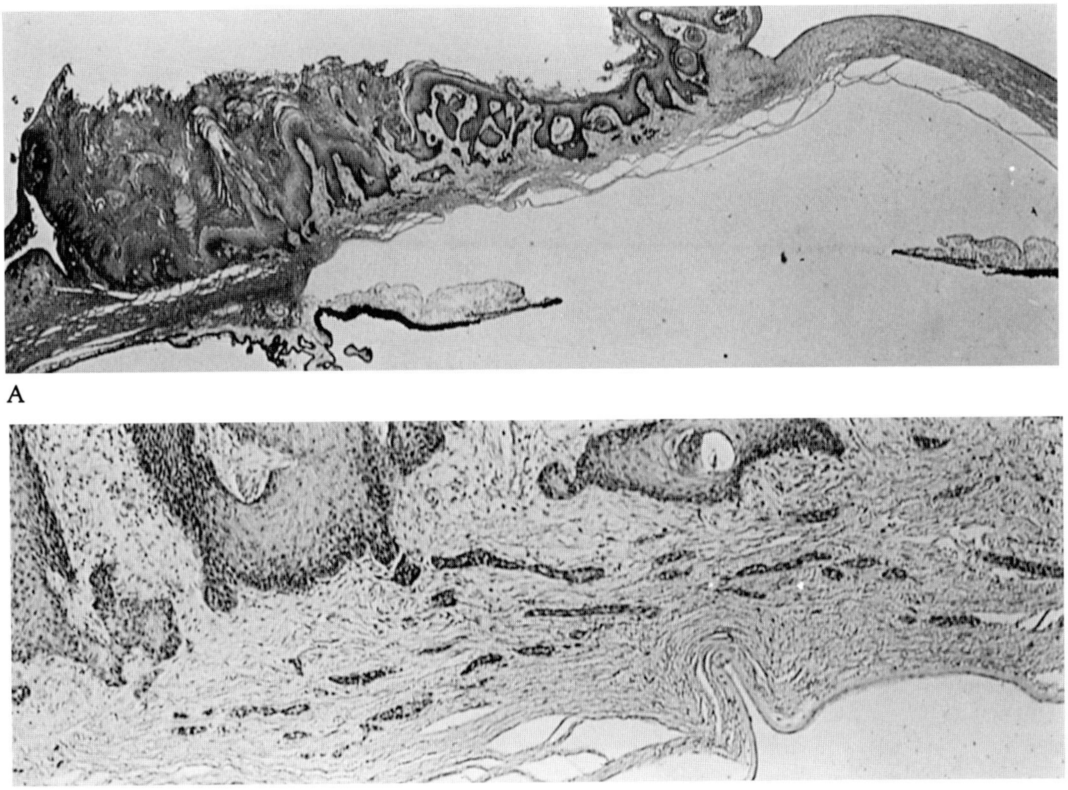

FIGURE 24-38 **(A)** Anterior segment of an enucleated eye with an infiltrating verrucous squamous cell carcinoma. **(B)** Small fingers of infiltrating malignant squamous cells extending into the deep corneal stroma toward Descemet's membrane. (Hematoxylin and eosin, A, × 60; B, × 200.) (Courtesy of the Armed Forces Institute of Pathology, Washington, DC.)

oclonal antibodies that identify cytokeratins can also be helpful.

MELANOCYTIC PROLIFERATIONS AND TUMORS

Melanocytes are scattered throughout all regions of the conjunctival epithelium in all races[1] but may be more numerous and are certainly more active in dark-skinned or black individuals. Intraepithelial melanocytes may extend into the limbal region of the corneal epithelium but are absent from the paracentral and central regions of the epithelium, unless there is a degenerative pannus, which tends to pull in conjunctival epithelium and associated melanocytes. Both a hemorrhagic pannus[20] and corneal deposits of epinephrine[73] can give the misleading clinical appearance of a pigmented melanocytic tumor of the cornea.

Benign Epithelial Melanosis

The most common condition of the intraepithelial conjunctival melanocyte is benign epithelial melanosis, which is most typically seen in black patients in the perilimbal and interpalpebral zone.[1,5] Streaks and whorls of pigment may extend into the peripheral corneal epithelium. The pigmentation fades toward the fornices, where there is lack of exposure and irritation from incident climatic factors or ultraviolet radiation. Benign epithelial melanosis, or racial melanosis, is a flat uninflamed condition that is virtually always bilateral and roughly symmetrical and has no potential for malignant degeneration. Rather than being a proliferative condition of intraepithelial melanocytes, it is a metabolic hyperactivity of the normally resident melanocytes, which manufacture more melanin granules than normal and inject them into the surrounding squamous epithelial cells.

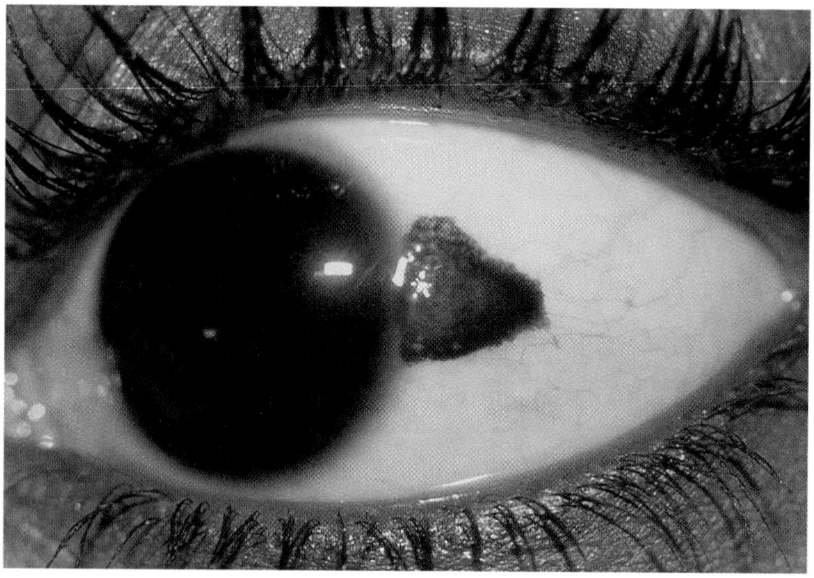

FIGURE 24-39 Juxtacorneal pigmented conjunctival nevus. Such lesions are freely movable upon the sclera, except where they are hinged at the limbus.

Benign Melanocytic Nevi

The most common proliferative condition of the conjunctival melanocyte is a nevus.[1,5] Conjunctival nevi are located on the surface of the globe, plica, caruncle, or eyelid margin (Figure 24-39). They rarely occur on the tarsal conjunctiva or in the fornix. Pigmented lesions of the tarsal or forniceal conjunctiva, therefore, should be excised as suspected malignant melanomas until proved otherwise. Conjunctival nevi are freely movable over the surface of the globe because the cells of the subepithelial component do not descend deeper than the substantia propria. Twenty to 30 percent of nevi may be nonpigmented (Figure 24-40).

Conjunctival nevi generally appear within the first two decades of life and represent proliferations of abnormal but nonmalignant melanocytes that have retracted their dendritic processes and rounded up. These modified melanocytes create small clusters of cells on the undersurface of the epithelium that are separated from the substantia propria by the epithelial basement membrane. The clusters formed by these rounded melanocytes are referred to as *junctional nests* or *thèques* (Figure 24-41). Junctional nests are observed in the earlier stages of the lesion, within the first two decades of life (junctional nevi); thereafter, the cells drop down into the underlying connective tissue to form nests in the substantia propria

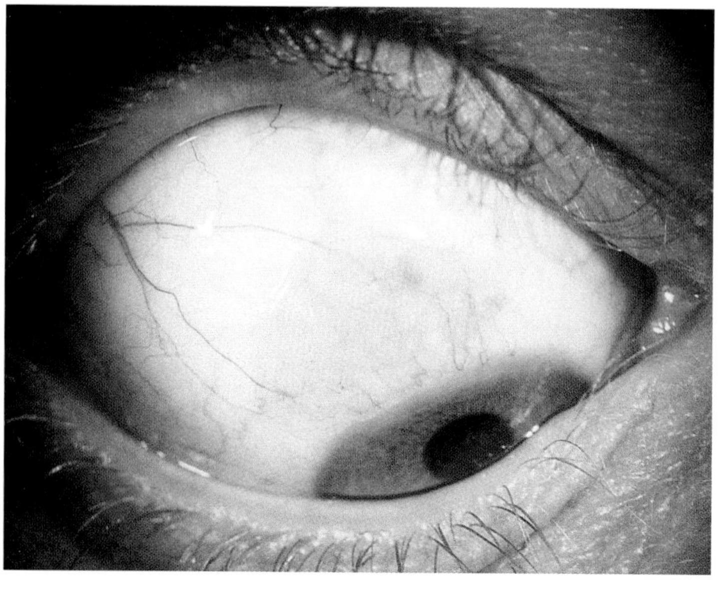

FIGURE 24-40 Amelanotic conjunctival nevus.

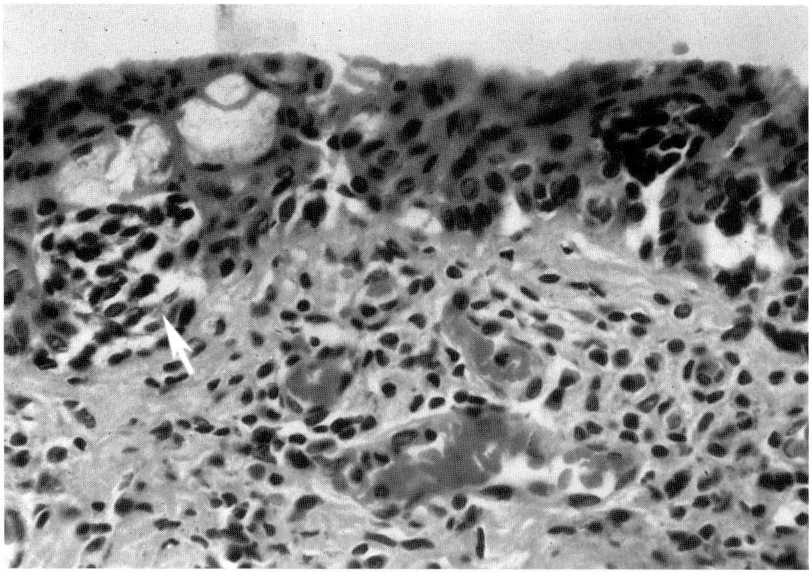

FIGURE 24-41 Nests of small melanocytes are scattered throughout the epithelium in a junctional nevus, which normally occurs in the first decade of life. A cluster of nevus cells (arrow) is called a *thèque*.

of the conjunctiva (compound nevi) (Figure 24-42). Finally, in the second, third, and fourth decades of life, the junctional cellular component disappears, and most of the lesion is located in the subepithelial substantia propria (subepithelial nevi). Conjunctival nevi frequently contain diagnostic epithelial inclusion cysts (Figure 24-43). Any lesion in an adult that is completely composed of junctional nests should be considered to be primary acquired melanosis.

Conjunctival nevi have a predilection for the limbus and, therefore, may overlap the peripheral cornea. However, because there is no substantia propria in the cornea, strictly corneal nevi are unknown, although deep scleral or corneal melanocytes can be seen in congenital melanosis oculi. Because nevi progressively thicken with time, there may be a disturbance of the precorneal tear film, leading to peripheral corneal lipid deposition.

Approximately 20 percent of conjunctival melanomas arise from pre-existing nevi or in association with them. In children and adolescents, the histologic features of conjunctival nevi may be alarming, with atypia and significant junctional activity. There is a report of an 11-year-old patient who presented with a changing congenital conjunctival nevus. Biopsy showed junctional activity with intraepithelial nests, and spindle and epithelioid cells with pleomorphic nuclei. After excision, the patient presented with multifocal conjunctival melanoma and later developed metastatic disease. Although such cases are rare, it is important to consider malignancy in a changing conjunctival lesion in a child.[74]

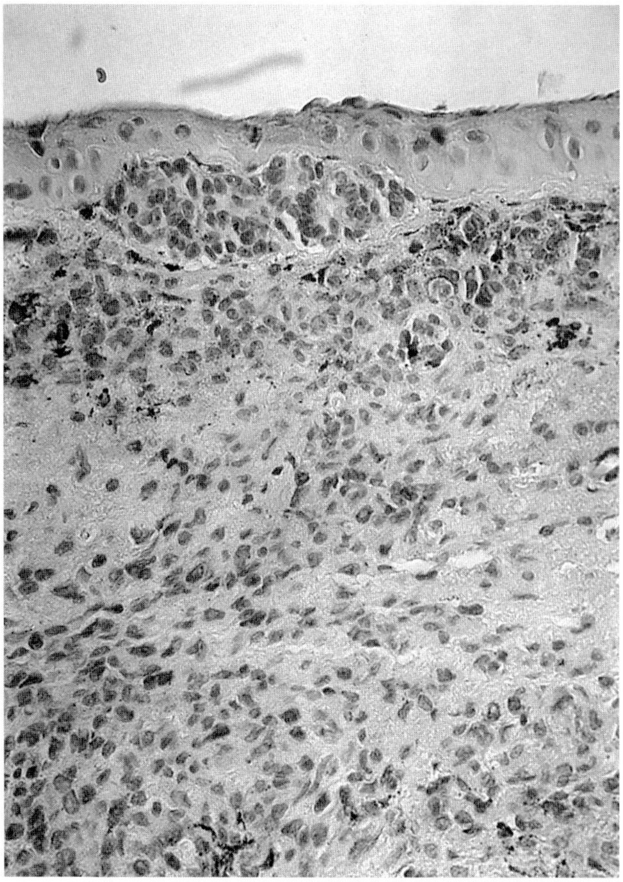

FIGURE 24-42 In a compound nevus, there are nests of nevus cells within the epithelium as well as in the underlying substantia propria.

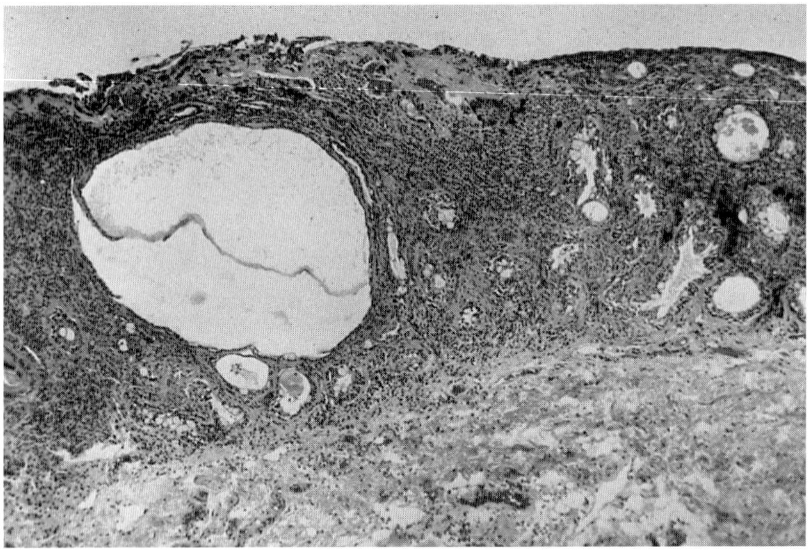

FIGURE 24-43 Conjunctival nevus with numerous intralesional cysts composed of conjunctival epithelium, a characteristic that is distinctive to conjunctival nevi and is not present in dermal nevi.

Primary Acquired Melanosis

Adults, but usually not children, may be affected by primary acquired melanosis, which is a proliferative lesion of the intraepithelial conjunctival melanocytes.[1,5,75–77] This condition is always unilateral and begins as flat golden brown areas of conjunctival pigmentation that may wax and wane and spread in various directions on the conjunctival surface over many years and even decades (Figure 24-44). If the condition extends toward the limbus, corneal involvement with epithelial pigmentation may be observed.

Primary acquired melanosis must be distinguished from the nonproliferative benign epithelial melanosis that is seen predominantly in dark-skinned or black individuals and, as mentioned above, is the result of increased production of melanin granules. In primary acquired melanosis, there is a proliferation of intraepithelial melanocytes. In contrast to the situation in squamous dysplasia, when primary acquired melanosis extends onto the corneal epithelium, there is not apt to be any subjacent fibrovascular pannus.

The risk with primary acquired melanosis is that in some cases, nodules of invasive malignant melanoma may develop (Figures 24-45 and 24-46). Sixty to 70 percent of conjunctival melanomas arise from primary acquired melanosis. These nodules may be seen anywhere within the area of flat conjunctival pigmentation and may also arise at the lim-

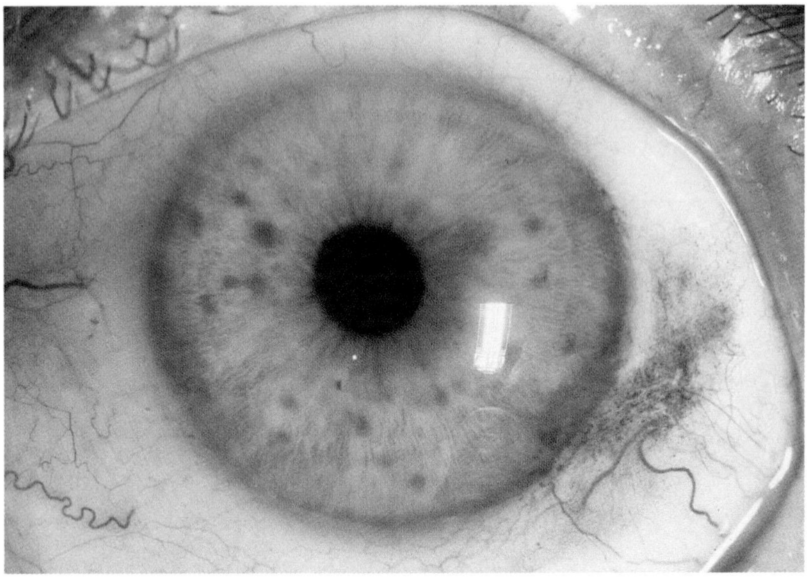

FIGURE 24-44 Small focus of primary acquired melanosis of the conjunctiva and peripheral cornea.

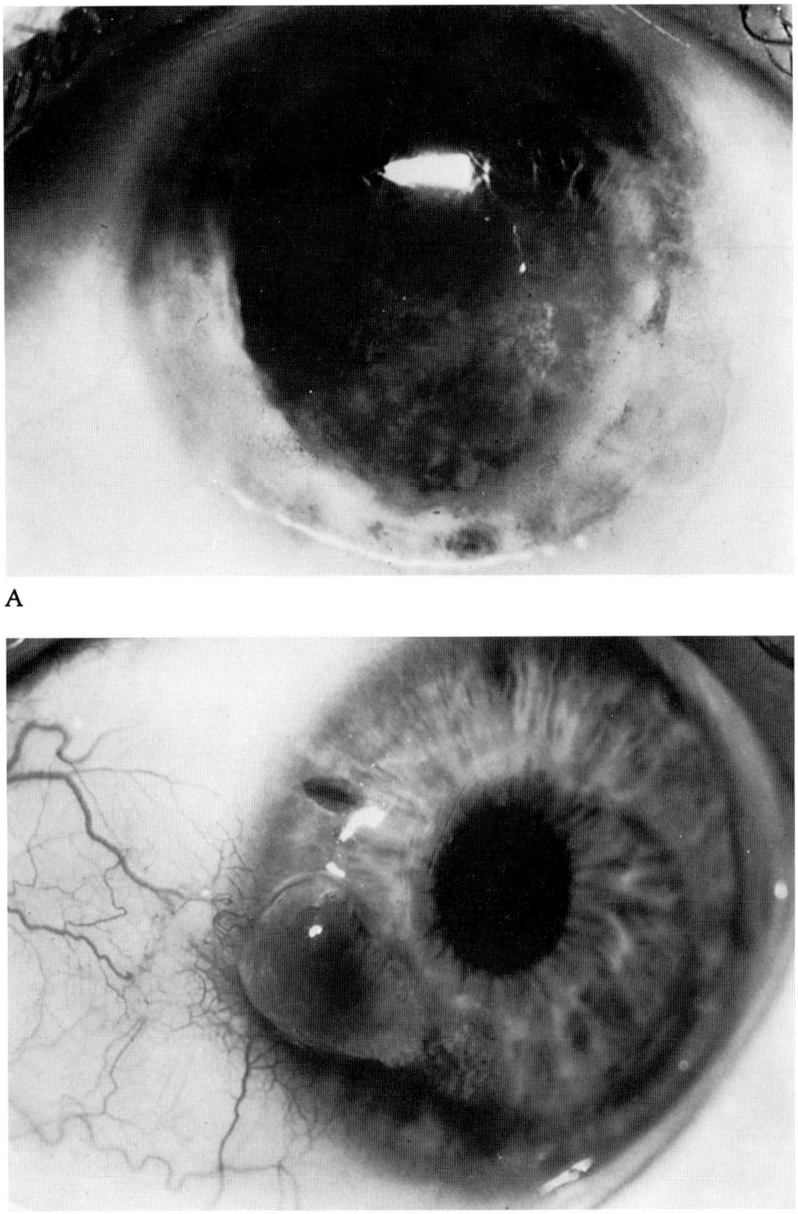

FIGURE 24-45 **(A)** Appearance of a post-herpetic cornea that also had a golden brown pigmentation to the corneal epithelium. **(B)** Nodular malignant melanoma arising in the corneal wound after penetrating keratoplasty. Intraepithelial dysplastic melanocytes had been displaced into the wound during surgery and spawned a nodular melanoma several years later.

bus. A strictly corneal nodule is extremely rare. To define the likelihood of the progression of primary acquired melanosis toward nodules of malignant melanoma, multiple biopsies of the different areas of pigmentation are taken. Both light and electron microscopy can be used to evaluate the severity of the intraepithelial melanocytic proliferation and the extent of individual cell atypia.[1,76] Primary acquired melanosis is divided into those cases that do not show cytologic atypia and have a low likelihood of subsequent nodule formation and those that exhibit atypia and have a high likelihood of invasive nodule formation. If the melanocytes are restricted to the basement membrane region of the epithelium, retain their dendritic shape, and contribute their pigment to the surrounding basilar and suprabasilar squamous epithelial cells, there is little likelihood of subsequent invasion. However, if epithelioid cells are conspicuous and if there is evidence of spread of individual cells to higher levels of the epithelium (pagetoid or buckshot appearance), the chance of invasive malignant melanoma eventually developing approaches 90 percent.

For lesions of primary acquired melanosis that show atypia, either wide local excision of small areas or cryother-

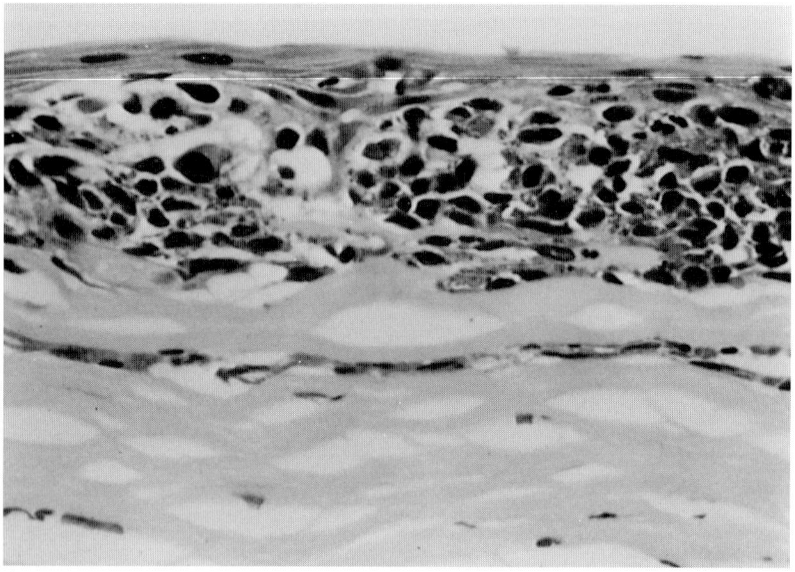

A

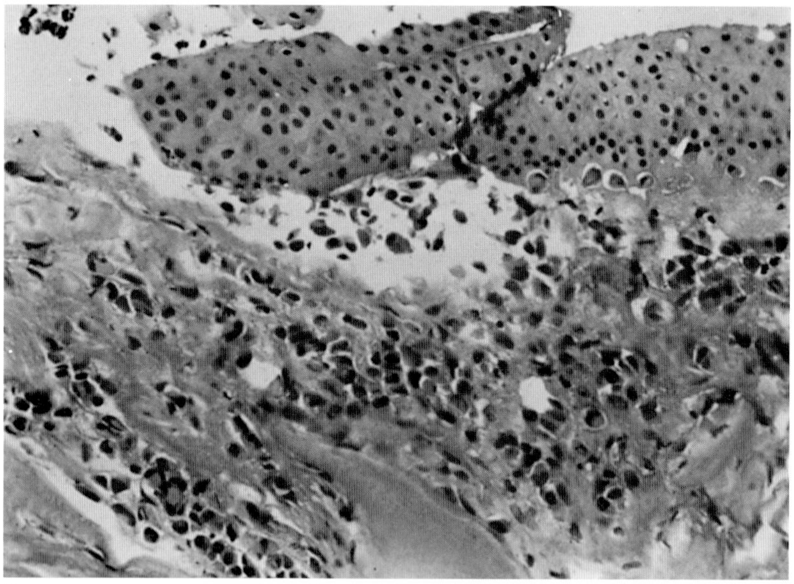

B

FIGURE 24-46 (A) Microscopic appearance of the corneal button obtained by keratoplasty on the cornea shown in Figure 24-45A. Note the confluent nests of atypical epithelioid intraepithelial melanocytes, separated from the stroma below by an intact Bowman's layer. (B) Infiltrating malignant melanoma cells can be seen in the superficial corneal stroma, adjacent to the nodular lesion shown in Figure 24-45B. (Hematoxylin and eosin, A, × 280; B, × 200.)

apy of large areas of pigmentation can be performed.[78-80] With respect to cryotherapy, one waits for the biopsy sites to heal and then injects lidocaine into the substantia propria to balloon up the conjunctiva. Two or three freeze-thaw applications are administered to the pigmented and surrounding nonpigmented areas to provide a zone of safety; the ballooned-up conjunctiva prevents the iceball from damaging underlying intraocular structures. Involved corneal epithelium, if present, is scraped off Bowman's layer, and alcohol or cryotherapy is applied to the region as previously described.

Invasive Malignant Melanoma

Malignant melanoma of the conjunctiva and cornea is a raised, pigmented, or nonpigmented lesion that appears in adult life[1,5,75,77] (Figure 24-47). We have never seen a melanoma of the conjunctiva develop in the first two decades of life, although we have seen histopathologic material on two such cases. Neither of these cases involved the cornea. Conjunctival melanomas can arise in previously unblemished and unpigmented regions (about 10 percent of cases), from a pre-existing nevus (about 20 percent of cases), or

FIGURE 24-47 **(A)** Malignant melanoma of the limbal conjunctiva with extension onto the peripheral cornea. **(B)** The microscopic appearance shows large epithelioid cells with increased nuclear/cytoplasmic volume ratio and prominent nucleoli.

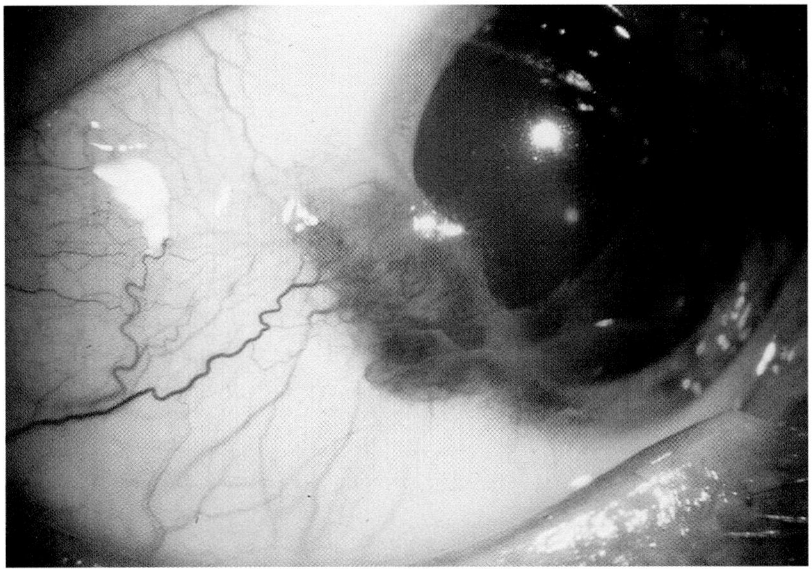

A

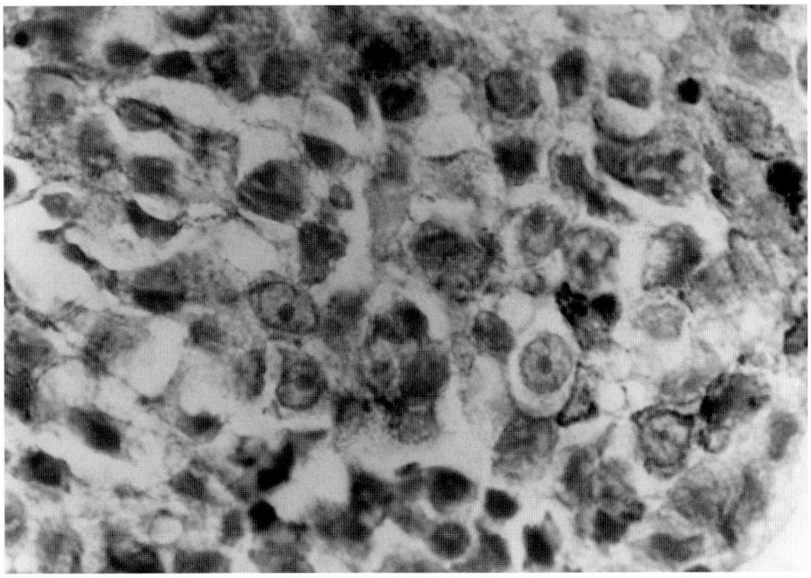

B

from the flat spreading pigmentation of primary acquired melanosis with atypia (60 to 70 percent of cases).

Conjunctival melanomas may extend onto the peripheral limbus. Most melanomatous nodules at the limbus affect the peripheral cornea; some grow circumferentially around the limbus. Rarely, a melanomatous nodule may be located more centrally in the cornea (Figure 24-48). At least one case of a paracentral corneal melanoma nodule occurred in a healed penetrating keratoplasty scar in a herpetic cornea that had concurrently been involved with extensive primary acquired melanosis with atypia[80] (see Figures 24-45 and 24-46). There has been one reported case of a "black cornea" in a 39-year-old white woman with a 9-year history of recurrent conjunctival melanoma arising from primary acquired melanosis.[81] The patient had contiguous extension of her melanoma involving the anterior two-thirds of the corneal stroma. It is possible for iris melanomas to become so bulky as to involve the cornea by direct extension. In one instance, a patient presented with a 10-year history of presumed iris melanoma that had perforated the cornea and protruded through the eyelid margins. Fifteen months after enucleation, this patient developed metastatic disease.[82]

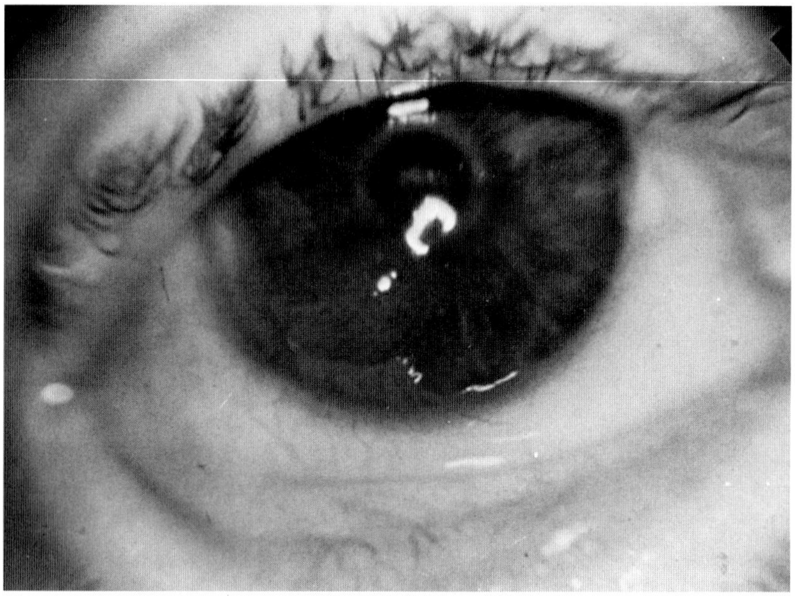

FIGURE 24-48 An extraordinary case of an epicorneal pigmented and vascularized nodule of malignant melanoma. (Courtesy of Frederick T. Fraunfelder, M.D., Portland, OR.)

The overall prognosis for conjunctival melanomas seems to be better than that for cutaneous melanomas, with a 70 to 80 percent survival rate at 10 years. The prognosis for conjunctival malignant melanoma has to do in part with location; lesions of the limbus and epibulbar surface have a better prognosis than those of the caruncle, fornices, or palpebral conjunctiva. The thickness of the invasive nodules is also of prognostic importance; lesions measuring 1.5 mm or less in total thickness tend to do well and usually do not metastasize, whereas those measuring progressively over 2 mm in thickness have an increasing likelihood of regional or distant metastases.[75,76] Before metastasizing to the lungs or distant sites, most conjunctival melanomas metastasize to the regional lymph nodes—either to the preauricular, the submandibular, or the cervical chains. Few ophthalmic surgeons recommend radical surgery in the form of a parotidectomy or cervical lymph node dissection unless there is clinically obvious evidence of concurrent disease in these sites at the time of initial ocular presentation, which is rare.

In an adult, all raised or enlarged pigmented lesions with a history of change should be excised as suspected malignant melanoma. Any nevus that has increased in vascularity, size, or solidity or that has become fixed to the underlying sclera (nevi are always freely movable over the sclera except at the fixation point at the limbus) should be suspected of being a malignant melanoma. The treatment of conjunctival or corneal melanomatous nodules is by wide local excision, including the performance of a superficial lamellar keratectomy or superficial sclerectomy if there is a fixation to the deeper tissues. The bed of excision, as well as the surrounding conjunctiva or cornea away from the nodule, is treated with cryotherapy. If there are widespread flat areas of primary acquired melanosis, these should be treated as described in the section on squamous dysplasia.[78-80]

PAGETOID SEBACEOUS CELL CARCINOMA

It may seem strange to discuss sebaceous cell carcinoma of the eyelids in a chapter devoted to corneal tumors, but the ability of sebaceous carcinoma cells to spread in a pagetoid fashion enables them to reach the corneal epithelium.[83] Corneal epithelial involvement can be an important part of the initial presentation of advanced sebaceous cell carcinoma of the eyelid.

Sebaceous cell carcinoma normally begins in the meibomian glands, the glands of Zeis, or the sebaceous glands associated with the small hairs in the caruncle. These carcinoma cells may erupt into the contiguous connective tissue, where they form nodules, but they may also creep along epithelial surfaces, which is referred to as the intraepithelial pagetoid pattern. The tumor cells may spread along the eyelid margin, along the tarsus, through the forniceal epithelium, and finally onto the epibulbar and corneal surfaces (Figure 24-49). Corneal epithelial involvement leads to irregular staining of the corneal surface and sometimes to neoplastic pannus formation. When extensive pagetoid disease develops, there is a unilateral red eye appearance. Any patient who presents with a chronic unilateral red eye with or without eyelid thickening and with or without eyelash loss should be considered to have a sebaceous cell carcinoma.

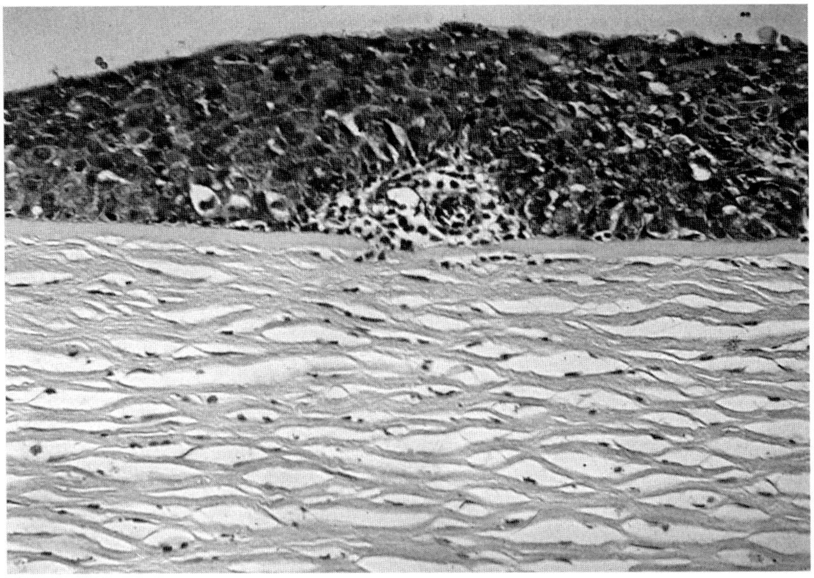

FIGURE 24-49 Sebaceous cell carcinoma of the corneal epithelium. Sebaceous carcinoma cells are replacing the corneal epithelium. Note that the cells continue to respect the underlying Bowman's layer. Many of the sebaceous carcinoma cells show vacuolated cytoplasm. (Courtesy of the Armed Forces Institute of Pathology, Washington, DC.)

There are rare cases of strictly pagetoid conjunctival sebaceous cell carcinoma without eyelid involvement. These cases probably represent a malignant sebaceous metaplasia of the conjunctival epithelium. The pathogenesis of this metaplasia is more understandable if one realizes that sebaceous cell carcinoma may arise primarily in the lacrimal gland, which embryologically is an outpouching of the conjunctiva, and if one also realizes that the adnexal structures of the caruncle, including the sebaceous glands embedded therein, are also embryologically derived from surface epithelium of the conjunctiva.[7]

Whenever there is suspicion of extensive pagetoid spread throughout the conjunctiva and corneal epithelium, multiple biopsies must be performed. These should be done to map the full extent of the pagetoid extension. Corneal scrapings may also identify intraepithelial pagetoid cells of sebaceous cell carcinoma. In contrast to squamous dysplasia, which may spread diffusely throughout the conjunctival and corneal epithelia and replace the basal cell region upward, sebaceous carcinoma cells may allow normal epithelium to survive in the basal region, with the atypical cells occurring at higher levels of the epithelium. When this pattern is seen and the cells have highly anaplastic and large nuclei, sebaceous cell carcinoma should be suspected. The cells should be studied for vacuolated frothy cytoplasm. Sebaceous carcinoma cells are very easily rubbed off the conjunctival substantia propria. Consequently, when a biopsy shows extensive denudation of the epithelium with only a few adherent cells, the possibility of sebaceous cell carcinoma should be considered, because squamous dysplastic cells are generally firmly adherent to the underlying substantia propria.

The management of sebaceous cell carcinoma with extensive pagetoid disease of the conjunctiva and cornea is generally exenteration, although cryotherapy may be applied to the areas of extensive pagetoid disease if only one-half of the conjunctiva is involved. In such cases, the nodular, invasive, sebaceous cell carcinoma of the involved portion of the eyelid is also widely excised.

CYTOLOGIC AND BIOPSY TECHNIQUES

Cytologic techniques have become popular in the diagnosis of inflammatory and neoplastic conditions of the conjunctiva and cornea.[5,84–86] It is easy to use a stainless steel blade after topical instillation of anesthetic drops to obtain scrapings of the corneal or conjunctival epithelium. The material obtained from these scrapings is spread immediately on a cytologic slide with the scalpel blade or a platinum spatula. An assistant should immediately spray the cytologic smear on the slide without allowing it to air dry. Spray fixatives or alcohol dips are excellent for preserving the cells. If air drying is allowed to occur before a spray fixative is used, shrinkage and artifacts will be introduced, making cytologic interpretation more difficult, if not impossible.

Because the information from a conjunctival biopsy is more reproducible and rewarding than that from cytologic scrapings and because the conjunctiva is so accessible to small surgical biopsies, biopsies are recommended when possible. Small snips of conjunctiva can be taken under topical or local anesthesia without the need for suture placement. For example, in widespread areas of primary acquired melanosis, up to 10 small biopsies can be done without placing a single suture. Each biopsy specimen is put into a separate bottle accompanied by a map, so that the pathologist can report accurately which areas are involved and which are not. Similar methods pertain to extensive diffuse squamous cell dysplasia or carcinoma in situ, as well as to extensive areas of pagetoid extension of sebaceous cell carcinoma. In performing such biopsies, one should not pick up and drop the tissue multiple times with a toothed forceps, which can squeeze the tissue and result in a valueless specimen due to crush artifact. It is preferable to grasp one edge of the specimen, tent it up, and then use Westcott scissors to make one graceful snip. Although one end of the specimen may be somewhat crushed by having been grasped with the forceps, the remainder of the specimen will not be crushed and will allow an accurate pathologic interpretation.

A corneal biopsy of stromal lesions can be performed with a topical anesthetic such as 0.5 percent proparacaine, 0.5 percent tetracaine, or 4 percent lidocaine solution that contains no preservatives. A circular sponge saturated with the anesthetic may be placed around the limbus to provide additional anesthesia so the eye can be fixated with a forceps in this area if necessary. The biopsy site is outlined with either a stainless steel blade or a trephine to include the area of pathology and a partial-thickness incision made to a depth that includes the lesion. Fixation of the tissue to be excised with a forceps should be avoided, if possible, because the forceps can crush the tissue and make the biopsy specimen difficult to interpret. Instead, one edge of the incision is retracted with a cellulose sponge. A lamellar keratectomy is performed with a stainless steel blade. When the keratectomy is almost complete, the specimen is grasped gently with a forceps, the keratectomy is completed, and the specimen is placed in fixative. The forceps with the specimen should be swished in the fixative until the specimen floats off. Placement of the specimen on a cellulose sponge and immersing the sponge in the fixative makes the specimen difficult to find. Donor tissue does not need to be placed in the biopsy site unless the excision is deep enough to affect the integrity of the cornea. Postoperatively, the patient is treated with a topical antibiotic and a cycloplegic agent until the epithelium has covered the biopsy site.

REFERENCES

1. Jakobiec FA: The ultrastructure of conjunctival melanocytic tumors. Trans Am Ophthalmol Soc 82:599, 1984
2. Sacks E, Rutgers J, Jakobiec FA, et al: A comparison of conjunctival and extra-ocular dendritic cells utilizing new monoclonal antibodies. Ophthalmology 93:1089, 1986
3. Sacks E, Wieczorek R, Jakobiec FA, Knowles DM II: Lymphocyte subpopulations in the normal conjunctiva. Ophthalmology 93:1276, 1986
4. Elsas FJ, Green WR: Epibulbar tumors in childhood. Am J Ophthalmol 79:1001, 1975
5. Spencer WH, Zimmerman LE: Conjunctiva. p. 109. In Spencer WH (ed): Ophthalmic Pathology: An Atlas and Textbook. Vol. I. WB Saunders, Philadelphia, 1985
6. Grossniklaus HE, Green WR, Luckenbach M, Chan CC: Conjunctival lesions in adults: a clinical and histopathologic review. Cornea 6:78, 1987
7. Levinson AW, Jakobiec FA, Reifler DM, Hornblass A: Ectopic epibulbar Fordyce nodules in a buccal mucous membrane graft. Am J Ophthalmol 100:724, 1985
8. Austin P, Jakobiec FA, Iwamoto T: Elastodysplasia and elastodystrophy as the pathologic bases of ocular pterygia and pinguecula. Ophthalmology 90:96, 1983
9. Clear AS, Chirambo MC, Hutt MSR: Solar keratosis, pterygium, and squamous cell carcinoma of the conjunctiva in Malawi. Br J Ophthalmol 63:102, 1979
10. Austin P, Jakobiec FA, Iwamoto T, Hornblass A: Elastofibroma oculi. Arch Ophthalmol 101:1575, 1983
11. Mattos J, Contreras F, O'Donnell FE: Ring dermoid syndrome: a new syndrome of autosomal dominantly inherited, bilateral, annular limbal dermoids with corneal and conjunctival extension. Arch Ophthalmol 98:1059, 1980
12. Henkind P, Marinoff G, Manas A, et al: Bilateral corneal dermoids. Am J Ophthalmol 76:972, 1973
13. Burke JP, Bowell R, O'Doherty N: Proteus syndrome: ocular complications. J Pediatr Ophthalmol Strabismus 25:99, 1988
14. Bouzas EA, Krasnewich D, Koutroumanidis M, et al: Ophthalmologic examination in the diagnosis of Proteus syndrome. Ophthalmology 100:334, 1993
15. Pokorny KS, Hyman BM, Jakobiec FA, et al: Epibulbar choristomas containing lacrimal tissue: clinical distinction from dermoids and histologic evidence of an origin from the palpebral lobe. Ophthalmology 94:1249, 1987
16. Dreizen NG, Schachat AP, Shields JA, Augsburger JJ: Epibulbar osseous choristoma. J Pediatr Ophthalmol Strabismus 20:247, 1983
17. Hutchinson DS, Green WR, Iliff CE: Ectopic brain tissue in a limbal dermoid associated with a scleral staphyloma. Am J Ophthalmol 76:984, 1973
18. Emamy J, Ahmadian H: Limbal dermoid with ectopic brain tissue. Arch Ophthalmol 95:2201, 1977
19. Bloomfield SE, Jakobiec FA, Theodore FH: Contact-lens induced keratopathy: a severe complication extending the spectrum of keratoconjunctivitis in contact lens wearers. Ophthalmology 91:290, 1984
20. Crowell D, Jakobiec FA: Hemorrhagic corneal pannus simulating a spontaneous expulsive hemorrhage. Ophthalmology 88:693, 1981

21. Knowles D, Jakobiec FA, Rosen M, Howard G: Amyloidosis of the orbit and adnexae. Surv Ophthalmol 19:367, 1975
22. Spencer WH: Ophthalmic Pathology: An Atlas and Textbook. 3rd Ed. Vol. I. WB Saunders, Philadelphia, 1985
23. Ferry AP, Zimmerman LE: Granuloma pyogenicum of limbus: simulating recurrent squamous cell carcinoma. Arch Ophthalmol 74:229, 1965
24. Boockvar W, Wessely Z, Ballen P: Recurrent granuloma pyogenicum of limbus. Arch Ophthalmol 91:42, 1974
25. Googe JM, Mackman G, Peterson MR, et al: Pyogenic granulomas of the cornea. Surv Ophthalmol 29:188, 1984
26. Howard G, Jakobiec FA, DeVoe AG: Kaposi's sarcoma of the conjunctiva. Am J Ophthalmol 79:420, 1975
27. Weiter J, Jakobiec FA, Iwamoto T: Kaposi sarcoma of the conjunctiva: clinical, pathologic, and ultrastructural features. Am J Ophthalmol 89:546, 1979
28. Albert DM, Smith RS: Fibrous xanthomas of the conjunctiva. Arch Ophthalmol 80:474, 1968
29. Grayson M, Pieroni D: Solitary xanthoma of the limbus. Br J Ophthalmol 54:562, 1970
30. Jakobiec FA: Fibrous histiocytoma of the corneoscleral limbus. Am J Ophthalmol 78:700, 1974
31. Faludi JE, Kenyon KR, Green WR: Fibrous histiocytoma of the corneoscleral limbus. Am J Ophthalmol 80:619, 1975
32. Iwamoto T, Jakobiec FA, Darrell RW: Fibrous histiocytoma of the corneoscleral limbus: the ultrastructure of a distinctive inclusion. Ophthalmology 88:1260, 1981
33. Lo GG, Biswas J, Rao NA, Font RL: Corneal myxoma: case report and review of the literature. Cornea 9:174, 1990
34. Font RL, Zimmerman LE: Nodular fasciitis of the eye and adnexa: a report of 10 cases. Arch Ophthalmol 75:475, 1966
35. Cogan DG, Kuwabara T, Parke D: Epibulbar nevo-xantho-endothelioma. Arch Ophthalmol 59:717, 1958
36. Austin P, Green WR, Sallyer DC, et al: Peripheral corneal degeneration and occlusive vasculitis in Wegener's granulomatosis. Am J Ophthalmol 85:311, 1978
37. Ashton N, Cook C: Allergic granulomatous nodules of the eyelid and conjunctiva. Am J Ophthalmol 87:1, 1979
38. Cameron ME, Greer H: Allergic conjunctival granulomas. Br J Ophthalmol 64:494, 1980
39. Purcell JJ, Birkenkamp R, Tsai CC: Conjunctival lesions in periarteritis nodosa: a clinical and immunopathologic study. Arch Ophthalmol 102:736, 1984
40. Blase WP, Knox DL, Green WR: Granulomatous conjunctivitis in a patient with Crohn's disease. Br J Ophthalmol 68:901, 1984
41. Bloomfield SE, Jakobiec FA, Iwamoto T: Traumatic intrastromal corneal cyst. Ophthalmology 87:951, 1980
42. Perry HD: Isolated episcleral neurofibroma. Ophthalmology 89:1095, 1982
43. Robertson DM, Sizemore GW, Gordon H: Thickened corneal nerves as a manifestation of multiple endocrine neoplasia. Trans Am Acad Ophthalmol Otolaryngol 79:772, 1975
44. Spector B, Klintworth GK, Wells SA: Histologic study of the ocular lesions in multiple endocrine neoplasia syndrome type IIb. Am J Ophthalmol 91:204, 1981
45. Grossniklaus HE, Green WR, Wolfe SM, Iliff NT: Hemangiopericytoma of the conjunctiva: two cases. Ophthalmology 93:265, 1986
46. Ozanics V, Jakobiec FA: Prenatal development of the eye and its adnexa. p. 11. In Jakobiec FA (ed): Ocular Anatomy, Embryology, and Teratology. Harper & Row, Philadelphia, 1982
47. Nodon DM: Periocular mesenchyme: neural crest and mesodermal interactions. p. 97. In Jakobiec FA (ed): Ocular Anatomy, Embryology, and Teratology. Harper & Row, Philadelphia, 1982
48. Kincaid M, Green W: Ocular and orbital involvement in leukemia. Surv Ophthalmol 27:211, 1983
49. Eiferman R, Levartovsky S, Schulz J: Leukemic corneal infiltrates. Am J Ophthalmol 105:319, 1988
50. Yanoff M: Hereditary benign intraepithelial dyskeratosis. Arch Ophthalmol 79:291, 1968
51. Reed JW, Cashwell LF, Klintworth GK: Corneal manifestations of hereditary benign intraepithelial dyskeratosis. Arch Ophthalmol 97:297, 1979
52. McLean IW, Riddle PJ, Scruggs JH, Jones DB: Hereditary benign intraepithelial dyskeratosis: a report of two cases from Texas. Ophthalmology 88:164, 1981
53. Lass JH, Grove AS, Papale JJ, et al: Detection of human papillomavirus DNA sequences in conjunctival papilloma. Am J Ophthalmol 96:670, 1983
54. Streeten BW, Carrillo R, Jamison R, et al: Inverted papilloma of the conjunctiva. Am J Ophthalmol 88:1062, 1979
55. Jakobiec FA, Harrison W, Aronian D: Inverted mucoepidermoid papillomas of the epibulbar conjunctiva. Ophthalmology 94:283, 1987
56. Zimmerman LE: The cancerous, precancerous, and pseudocancerous lesions of the cornea and conjunctiva. Corneoplastic surgery. p. 547. Proc 2nd Ann Intl Corneoplastic Conference. Pergamon Press, London, 1969
57. Ash JE, Wilder HC: Epithelial tumors of the limbus. Am J Ophthalmol 25:926, 1942
58. Pizzarello L, Jakobiec FA: Bowen's disease of the conjunctiva: a misnomer. p. 553. In Jakobiec FA (ed): Ocular and Adnexal Tumors. Aesculapius, Birmingham, AL, 1978
59. Erie JC, Campbell RJ, Liesegang TJ: Conjunctival and corneal intraepithelial and invasive neoplasia. Ophthalmology 93:176, 1986
60. McDonnell J, Mayr A, Martin WJ: DNA of human papillomavirus type 16 in dysplastic and malignant lesions of the conjunctiva and cornea. N Engl J Med 320:1442, 1989
61. Odrich MG, Jakobiec FA, Lancaster WD, et al: A spectrum of bilateral squamous conjunctival tumors associated with human papillomavirus type 16. Ophthalmology 98:628, 1991
62. Fraunfelder FT, Wingfield D: Management of intraepithelial conjunctival tumors and squamous cell carcinomas. Am J Ophthalmol 95:359, 1983

63. Copeland R, Char D: Limbal autograft reconstruction after conjunctival squamous cell carcinoma. Am J Ophthalmol 110:412, 1990
64. Waring GO, Ross AM, Ekins MB: Clinical and pathologic description of 17 cases of corneal intraepithelial neoplasia. Am J Ophthalmol 97:547, 1984
65. Campbell RJ, Bourne WM: Unilateral central corneal epithelial dysplasia. Ophthalmology 88:1231, 1981
66. Jauregvi HO, Klintworth GR: Pigmented squamous cell carcinoma of the cornea and conjunctiva: a light microscopic, histochemical and ultrastructural study. Cancer 38:778, 1976
67. Winward K, Curtin V: Conjunctival squamous cell carcinoma in a patient with human immunodeficiency virus infection. Am J Ophthalmol 107:554, 1989
68. Rao NA, Font RL: Mucoepidermoid carcinoma of the conjunctiva: a clinicopathologic study of five cases. Cancer 38:1699, 1976
69. Brownstein S: Mucoepidermoid carcinoma of the conjunctiva with intraocular invasion. Ophthalmology 88:1226, 1981
70. Herschorn BJ, Jakobiec FA, Hornblass A, et al: Mucoepidermoid carcinoma of the palpebral mucocutaneous junction: a clinical, light microscopic, and electron microscopic study of an unusual tubular variant. Ophthalmology 90:1437, 1983
71. Wise AC: A limbal spindle-cell carcinoma. Surv Ophthalmol 12:244, 1967
72. Cohen BH, Green WR, Iliff NT, et al: Spindle cell carcinoma of the conjunctiva. Arch Ophthalmol 98:1809, 1980
73. Ferry AP, Zimmerman LE: Black cornea: a complication of topical use of epinephrine. Am J Ophthalmol 58:205, 1964
74. Croxatto J, Guillermo I, Ugrin C, et al: Malignant melanoma of the conjunctiva: report of a case. Ophthalmology 94:1281, 1987
75. Folberg R, McLean IW, Zimmerman LE: Conjunctival melanosis and melanoma. Ophthalmology 91:673, 1984
76. Folberg R, McLean IW, Zimmerman LE: Primary acquired melanosis of the conjunctiva. Hum Pathol 16:129, 1985
77. Silvers DN, Jakobiec FA, Freeman TR, et al: Melanoma of the conjunctiva: a clinicopathologic study. p. 583. In Jakobiec FA (ed): Ocular and Adnexal Tumors. Aesculapius, Birmingham, AL, 1978
78. Jakobiec FA, Brownstein S, Wilkinson RD, et al: Combined surgery and cryotherapy for diffuse malignant melanoma of the conjunctiva. Arch Ophthalmol 98:1390, 1980
79. Brownstein S, Jakobiec FA, Wilkinson RD, et al: Cryotherapy for precancerous melanosis (atypical melanocytic hyperplasia) of the conjunctiva. Arch Ophthalmol 99:1224, 1981
80. Jakobiec FA, Brownstein S, Albert W, et al: The role of cryotherapy in the management of conjunctival melanoma. Ophthalmology 89:502, 1982
81. Paridaens A, Kirkness C, Garner A, Hungerford J: Recurrent malignant melanoma of the corneal stroma: a case of "black cornea." Br J Ophthalmol 76:444, 1992
82. Margo C, Groden L: Iris melanoma with extensive corneal invasion and metastases. Am J Ophthalmol 104:543, 1987
83. Rao NA, McLean IW, Zimmerman LE: Sebaceous carcinoma of eyelids and caruncle. Correlation of clinicopathologic features with prognosis. p. 461. In Jakobiec FA (ed): Ocular and Adnexal Tumors. Aesculapius, Birmingham, AL, 1978
84. Jakobiec FA, Chattock A: The role of cytology and needle biopsies in the diagnosis of ophthalmic tumors and simulating conditions. p. 341. In Jakobiec FA (ed): Ocular and Adnexal Tumors. Aesculapius, Birmingham, AL, 1978
85. Jakobiec FA, Chattock A: Aspiration cytodiagnosis of lid tumors. Arch Ophthalmol 97:1907, 1979
86. Stenson S: Cytologic diagnosis. The anterior segment cytopathology. p. 90. In Karcioglu ZA (ed): Laboratory Diagnosis in Ophthalmology. Macmillan, New York, 1987

25

Corneal Trauma

CAROLYN M. PARRISH AND JOHN W. CHANDLER

The cornea is continually exposed to minor trauma from chemicals and particles in the atmosphere. Occasionally, significant trauma occurs. The specialized optical functions and anatomic structures of the cornea mandate that all corneal trauma be managed promptly and correctly. The anatomy, biochemistry, physiology, microbiology, and immunology of the cornea, as well as the clinical aspects of corneal trauma, must be understood if wound healing and visual rehabilitation following corneal trauma are to be optimized.

This chapter discusses the various causes of corneal trauma, including radiant, chemical, and mechanical trauma. The pathogenesis, clinical course, and management of the various types of trauma are described. Corneal trauma resulting from ocular surgery is discussed in Chapter 26. Management of the types of infectious keratitis that may occur in conjunction with trauma is discussed in Chapters 8, 9, and 15.

CORNEAL WOUND HEALING AFTER TRAUMA

Corneal anatomy and physiology are discussed in detail in Chapter 1. Trauma damages various corneal structures. Four basic lesions are commonly encountered in corneal trauma: epithelial defects, epithelial and superficial stromal defects, deep stromal defects, and full-thickness defects. Each lesion involves specialized wound healing events.

Epithelial Defects

Corneal abrasions result from the removal of some or all of the layers of the epithelium, leaving Bowman's layer intact. Epithelial defects heal by the sliding and proliferation of adjacent epithelial cells. The process begins with the flattening and sliding of wing layer cells adjacent to the defect, which leads to covering of the abraded area with a thin layer of epithelial cells in 24 to 96 hours. The epithelial cells surrounding the abrasion begin to replicate within 24 hours after trauma and eventually restore the epithelial layer to its normal thickness. Large defects may require conjunctival epithelium for repair. Whereas corneal epithelium may cover an abrasion in 1 to 4 days, conjunctival epithelium may require 1 to 2 weeks or more.

Although corneal epithelial cells can divide, there is good evidence in animals and some evidence in man that the limbal cells are the stem cells that divide to restore wounded corneal epithelium.[1-4] Without an intact corneal limbus, corneal epithelial healing may be impaired and recurrent or persistent epithelial defects may develop. When the limbal cells are absent, cells that are normally present in conjunctiva, but not in cornea, migrate over the cornea and only very slowly differentiate into corneal epithelium. Conjunctivalization can lead to superficial stromal vascularization.[5,6] In patients with 360-degree limbal damage, as occurs in some chemical burns, Stevens-Johnson syndrome, and, rarely, long-term contact lens wear, among other conditions, corneal epithelial healing is deficient and recurrent corneal ulcers are common. A variety of techniques have been developed for the transplantation of limbal epithelial cells (see Ch. 28).[7] When the cells are transplanted from the normal fellow eye, the surgical procedure is relatively simple and straightforward, and a number of surgical techniques have proven satisfactory. The value of limbal transplantation from unrelated donors is less clear, however. Most reports are subjective, single case reports, and most of the transplants have required a variety of immunosuppressive regimens to prevent rejection of the donor graft.[8]

The healing of an epithelial abrasion requires a number of specialized and coordinated biological interactions. The basement membrane of normal corneal epithelium anchors the basal cells to the underlying stroma. The basal cells of normal corneal epithelium have hemidesmosomes that are essential for firm attachment to the stroma (see Ch. 1). Hemidesmosomes are usually lacking in areas of recurrent epithelial erosions.[9]

At the level of the basement membrane, three other components can be identified.[10] Bullous pemphigoid antigen is a 220,000 dalton glycoprotein that can be demonstrated by electron microscopy in the lamina lucida, just beneath the basal cell plasma membrane. Laminin is another noncollagenous glycoprotein that appears to be located in the lamina lucida. Beneath the lamina lucida is an electron-dense layer, the lamina densa, which is closest to the corneal stroma and is composed of type IV collagen. When the epithelium is abraded gently, it separates between the bullous pemphigoid antigen and laminin. This reaction suggests that this zone of the basement membrane is the weakest and is the area most likely to give way under stress.

Before any abrasion is covered with epithelium, it is coated with another glycoprotein, fibronectin. Fibronectin is present in serum and is produced by a variety of cells, including liver cells, vascular endothelium, several types of epithelium, macrophages, and fibroblasts. The fibronectin present acutely in corneal abrasions is probably from serum. The in situ production of fibronectin begins 2 to 4 days after trauma, by which time most epithelial defects are covered with epithelial cells. It is thought that fibronectin forms a matrix that provides a platform for the migration (sliding) of epithelial cells adjacent to the abrasion.[11,12]

Sliding epithelial cells undergo intracellular reorganization that probably allows them to move over the fibronectin-coated surface. In normal corneal epithelium, intracytoplasmic actin filaments are most dense just beneath the microplicae of the superficial corneal epithelial cells. After a corneal abrasion, actin filaments are present in the leading edges of sliding epithelial cells.[13] It appears that the actin filaments track across the fibronectin matrix to cover the epithelial defect. The deposition of fibronectin on the defect and the reorganization of actin filaments within the epithelial cells are key elements in the healing of abrasions. Following this process, new bullous pemphigoid antigen and laminin are produced.[10]

Keratocytes in the stroma become metabolically active in the region of a corneal epithelial abrasion.[14] What the stromal keratocytes contribute to successful epithelial wound healing is uncertain, however.

Thus, the healing of a simple corneal epithelial abrasion involves a number of complex active processes, any disturbance of which may lead to incomplete wound healing. Infection or drugs can destroy fibronectin or prevent its production, interfere with the function of actin filaments, or inhibit epithelial cell mitosis. For example, epithelial wound healing is inhibited by medications containing benzalkonium chloride.[15] It is important to realize that virtually all eye drops can be toxic to the epithelium. Aminoglycosides, such as gentamicin and tobramycin, are very toxic to the epithelium, but other antibiotics and corticosteroid preparations are also toxic and should be given as seldom as possible if epithelial healing is critical.

Epithelial and Superficial Stromal Defects

A combined epithelial and superficial stromal defect leads to the loss of Bowman's layer, and possibly the loss of anterior stroma. The process of epithelial wound healing is the same as for an epithelial abrasion. However, the underlying stroma is usually rough and is not an ideal structural platform for epithelial wound healing. Bowman's layer and normal stroma are not regenerated. They may be replaced by collagenous scar tissue or the defect may be filled in by thickened epithelium that forms a facet.

Deep Stromal Defects

Deep stromal defects are repaired in a similar fashion, except that the deposition of collagenous scar tissue is a component of the wound healing process. Although it usually takes many weeks for a corneal stromal wound to heal completely, changes in the adjacent viable stromal keratocytes, including changes in shape, hypertrophy, and the development of many large nucleoli, begin to take place almost immediately.[16,17] The changes within the stroma during scar formation are complex. Normal corneal stroma is composed of type I collagen, whereas corneal scars contain large quantities of type III collagen.[18] The relative concentrations of various glycosaminoglycans in the stroma surrounding the collagen fibrils change during the formation of scars.[19] Again, other concurrent conditions, as well as drug therapies, may alter the rate of formation or the structural composition of the scar. For example, failure of corneal epithelium to cover a wound[20] or immediate application of topical corticosteroids[21] delays the initiation of stromal wound healing.

Full-Thickness Defects

The repair of trauma affecting all layers of the cornea involves wound healing mechanisms similar to those already described. When the posterior cornea is lacerated, Descemet's membrane tends to scroll, and the cut ends roll anteriorly toward the stroma. Yanoff and Fine[22] described six phases of wound healing after a perforating injury to the cornea.

The phase immediately after the injury shows anterior and posterior wound gape caused by retraction of collagen in these areas. Fibrinogen in the aqueous humor cleaves to fibrin on contact with the cut portions of the stroma and forms a fibrin plug. Stromal edema begins.

A leukocytic phase begins approximately 30 minutes after the injury. Polymorphonuclear leukocytes migrate into the damaged area via the tears, aqueous humor, and limbal blood vessels. These cells are mildly phagocytic and release a variety of enzymes. Approximately 12 to 24 hours after the injury, mononuclear cells accumulate at the limbus and may migrate to the wound, especially if the wound is near the limbus. Mononuclear cells migrate very slowly through the stroma. Their function is speculative, but they may participate in phagocytosis.

Epithelial wound healing begins approximately 1 hour after injury and involves sliding and proliferation as described above. Early and accurate wound reapproximation aids epithelial wound healing. Epithelium migrates more rapidly over sloping or gradually inclined defects than it does over steps or sharp discontinuities. If there is an anterior wound gape, the epithelium usually fills in the area until stromal healing fills the defect with scar tissue and the epithelium retracts. Early epithelial wound healing is an important step in stromal wound healing. The clinician must be attentive to the promotion of early epithelial wound healing in the proper management of perforating injuries of the cornea. If the wound is left open or is filled with intraocular structures, such as iris, lens remnants, or vitreous, the possibility of epithelial ingrowth and the ultimate destruction of the eye is enhanced.[23]

The fibroblastic phase of wound healing begins approximately 12 hours after injury and is related to the onset of successful epithelial wound healing. The stromal keratocytes adjacent to the corneal laceration are activated and become similar to fibroblasts. They produce typical scar glycosaminoglycans and type III collagen. If the laceration is near the limbus, monocytes may undergo metaplastic changes and participate in the fibroblastic phase.

The corneal endothelial phase of wound healing begins at 24 hours and involves sliding of endothelial cells. Over several weeks, the endothelial cells that cover the area of injury secrete a new Descemet's membrane.

The late phase of wound healing begins 1 week after injury. The cellularity of the wound decreases. The collagen fibrils that were originally secreted in haphazard directions become oriented more like normal type I corneal collagen. The scar contracts, especially if good wound apposition was achieved immediately after the injury.

MODULATORS OF WOUND HEALING

Trauma to the cornea sets in motion a molecular response at the nuclear level.[24,25] Sequences of gene expression control and direct the response of the cells of the individual layers of the cornea. Exogenous modifiers secreted after wounding, such as growth factors in the tears, come into direct contact with corneal cells.[26,27] Changes in the composition and amounts of extracellular matrix proteins that are found shortly after wounding may be important to provide a suitable lattice or substrate for the migration and restoration of the corneal epithelium and also modulate the response of the stromal keratocytes.[28,29] The observation that components of the extracellular matrix, such as fibronectin and tenascin, are found in the cornea after re-epithelialization is complete suggests an ongoing role after the initial healing processes. Conversely, some molecules found in the cornea after wounding, such as the matrix metalloproteinases, may be the cause of delayed re-epithelialization and eventual corneal melting.[30]

Wounding of the cornea is followed by epithelial reorganization and transformation of the cells to a motile form. These events occur during the early phase of the response to wounding, called the *latent phase*, in which there is no cellular activity other than reorganization of the epithelium into a leading edge in preparation for cellular migration.[31] These early events are important, as they stimulate the production of new genetic information that may in turn be used to regulate genes that encode structural proteins, enzymes, and growth factors, as well as growth factor receptors, all of which can greatly modify the eventual outcome of the response to injury.

The effects of growth factors on corneal cells have been studied extensively in vivo and in vitro; nevertheless, clear evidence of therapeutic efficacy in humans is lacking.[32–36] Epithelial and endothelial cells respond to a variety of growth factors, including epidermal growth factor (EGF) and basic fibroblast growth factor (FGF-2). Platelet-derived growth factor (PDGF) and epidermal growth factor have been suggested to promote endothelial cell wound closure in organ-cultured human corneas and wounded feline corneas in vivo.[37,38]

Keratocytes have the primary role in stromal healing after trauma or surgical wounds. Cell signaling molecules modulate the biosynthetic response of the fibroblastic keratocytes, which in turn affects the mechanical resistance and optical quality of the cornea; the activity of these cells can lead to appropriate healing, inadequate healing (as in wound dehiscence), or even scar formation (as may be seen after excimer laser ablation of the cornea). Fibronectin, a product of the fibroblasts, is a component of the migratory substrate of epithelial cells and is essential for proper reepithelialization. Platelet-derived growth factor-beta (PDGF-β) may enhance gene expression for the production of fibronectin by fibroblasts. Laminin and type IV collagen are components of the epithelial basement membrane. Growth factors, such as transforming growth factor β-1, may modulate the association of integrin subunits and specific interactions of fibroblasts with type I collagen, as well as with type IV collagen and laminin. At the same time, inflammatory mediators produced in response to corneal wounding may stimulate the production of metalloproteinases, which can degrade these basement membrane components and lead to failure of epithelialization.[30,39] Other studies have shown that platelet-derived growth factor and fibroblast growth factor (but not epidermal growth factor) induce the expression of intermediate filaments, such as vinculin, in fibroblasts. In addition to having a direct effect on the structure of keratocytes, growth factors may also modulate the regulatory effect of the extracellular matrix on these cells, thereby modifying the corneal response to the wound and affecting the outcome of the recovery process.

FACTORS INVOLVED IN CORNEAL WOUND HEALING

A number of factors can enhance, prevent, retard, or complicate corneal wound healing. The clinician must consider these factors and their interplay with wound healing mechanisms in the management of corneal trauma.

Age

In general, young people heal rapidly and may have completely healed wounds in several days to a few weeks. In contrast, elderly people may take longer to heal an identical wound. Reduced tear flow, more common in the elderly, may contribute to the reduction in healing rate.

Nutrition

Malnutrition greatly retards wound healing. Nutrition that provides protein, ascorbic acid, and vitamin A appears essential for wound healing. In severe vitamin A deficiency, corneal ulceration is common.

Cause of the Trauma

The exact nature of the trauma obviously influences wound healing. These influences are discussed in the sections on specific causes of corneal trauma.

Wound Apposition

Excellent and prompt realignment of the corneal layers, along with avoidance of distortion or malapposition by sutures, enhances normal wound healing. Poor apposition results in gaping of the anterior and/or posterior aspects of the wound, and makes the normal progression of wound healing unlikely. Poor wound apposition also increases the possibility of infection and incarceration or adhesion of tissues to the wound.

Infection

Microorganisms interfere with the healing of corneal wounds. They may enhance the inflammatory response, which may, in turn, retard wound healing or cause further collagen degradation and corneal cell death. Microorganisms may also produce enzymes that degrade glycosaminoglycans and/or collagen (see Chs. 8 and 9).

Inflammation

Various types of trauma elicit different inflammatory responses that may alter wound healing. For instance, an inflammatory response to retained foreign material may induce giant cells and other cells that produce an exuberant scar. In contrast, total suppression of the early inflammatory response with topical corticosteroids may significantly retard corneal wound healing.[21] Thus, control of the inflammatory response must be carefully monitored.

Vascularization

There appear to be multiple mechanisms leading to corneal vascularization. The presence of an inhibitor to vascularization in normal cornea has been postulated but never proved.[40] Acute inflammation with polymorphonuclear leukocytes is capable of causing experimental corneal vascularization,[41] as is prostaglandin E_1.[42] However, other models have been developed in which acute inflammation is avoided, and vascularization still develops.[43] Trauma near or involving the limbus is frequently associated with vascularization. Corneal necrosis, poor wound apposition, and iris adhesion to the wound also predispose to vascularization. It is clear that the presence of necrotic corneal tissue incites neovascularization and the removal of necrotic tissue decreases the response. Proliferating vascular endothelium is an in situ source of fibronectin[44] and may assist in epithelial wound healing when other sources do not provide sufficient fibronectin.

Keratitis Sicca and Exposure

Keratitis sicca retards corneal healing. It is a primary and frequent cause of epithelial ulcers and exposure keratitis (especially when accompanied by lagophthalmos) and is often difficult to treat. Unpreserved artificial tears and ointments are useful and punctal occlusion and tarsorrhaphy may be necessary, especially in patients with ocular burns or conjunctival cicatrization (see Ch. 5).

Sensory Innervation

The mechanisms by which intact corneal sensory nerves assist in corneal wound healing have not been elucidated. However, experimental sensory denervation[45] and clinical experience document that sensory innervation plays an important role. Without sensory innervation, cellular migration and adhesion are greatly impaired. Sensory innervation also affects tear production; dry eye is common in denervated corneas and also slows the re-innervation process.

Intraocular Pressure and Corneal Edema

Increased intraocular pressure may prevent scar shrinkage during the healing of stromal wounds. In traumatized or scarred corneas, it is often difficult to obtain accurate measurements of intraocular pressure by Goldmann applanation tonometry; better results are achieved with electronic applanation tonometry (Tono-Pen). Corneal edema also causes bullae, which may rupture and impede epithelial migration.

INJURIES CAUSED BY RADIANT ENERGY

Radiant energy is emitted in a spectrum ranging from very long wavelengths, as in sound waves, to very short wavelengths, as in gamma rays and cosmic rays (Figure 25-1). The biological effects caused by particular forms of radiant energy, including varying degrees of damage, are governed by the characteristics of both the energy form and the target tissue. Several types of radiant energy may cause damage to the cornea, including microwaves, infrared radiation, lasers, ultraviolet light, and x-rays. The nature of these injuries and their treatment are described below.[46,47]

Short Wave Diathermy

Short wave diathermy may cause tissue damage or death by sufficiently raising tissue temperature to cause coagulation of proteins and other intracellular damage. Short wave diathermy is not often used about the face or eyes, and when it is, the temperature is rarely permitted to exceed a level that damages tissue. Experimentally, corneal epithelial edema and opacification and, with extremely high temperatures, stromal opacification and necrosis, have been produced. A diathermy burn can be diagnosed on the basis of a careful history and observation of burns on the surrounding skin. Management may range from treatment of an abrasion to that of corneal melting; however, clinical cases will likely require no more than topical antibiotics, cycloplegia, and occlusive patching to heal the corneal epithelium.

Microwaves

Microwave radiant energy causes thermal damage similar to that caused by short wave diathermy. In some tissues, especially the lens, repeated exposure causes cumulative damage. Exposure to the eyes may lead to skin burns, conjunctival hyperemia, and loss of corneal epithelium, as well as stromal edema, opacification, and possibly necrosis with melting.

Infrared Radiation

Pathologic thermal effects are common sequelae of the exposure of ocular tissues to infrared radiant energy, especially wavelengths of 900 to 1,000 nm. Thermal damage from infrared radiation can be caused by a short-duration, high-energy flash burn or a longer, lower energy exposure, such as a solar burn. High-energy burns tend to damage the skin and cornea, whereas low-energy burns tend to damage the retina and/or lens and spare the skin and cornea.

Infrared flash burns are caused by the flashback of large artillery and by the flash of a nuclear bomb. These types of injuries also include ultraviolet exposure. The burns are identical to those caused by other types of thermal exposure. The skin of the face and eyelids becomes erythematous and may proceed through the stages of a severe sunburn, with blistering, peeling, and eventual resolution. In severe flash burns, full-thickness burns occur and lead to severe scarring. In most flash burns, the blink reflex protects the eyes from damage. However, when the cornea is involved, the intense heat destroys the epithelium and coagulates the intra- and extracellular proteins of the stroma and endothelium. Corneal necrosis leads to sloughing, thinning, scarring, and vascularization. Most severe

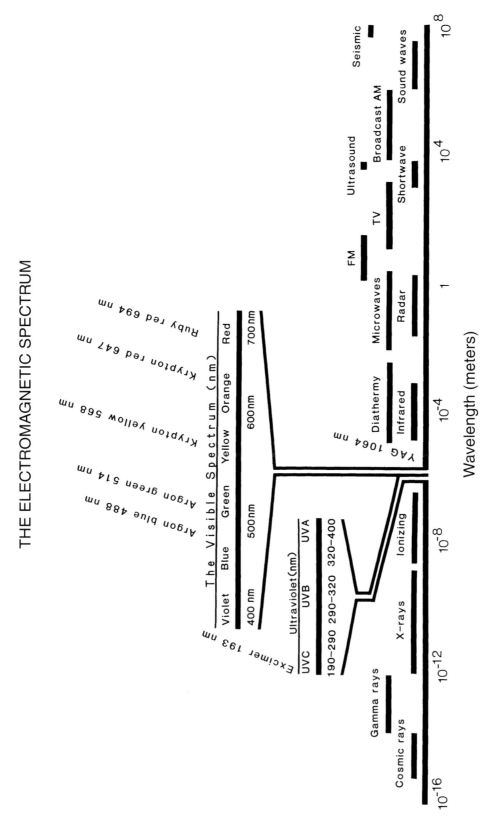

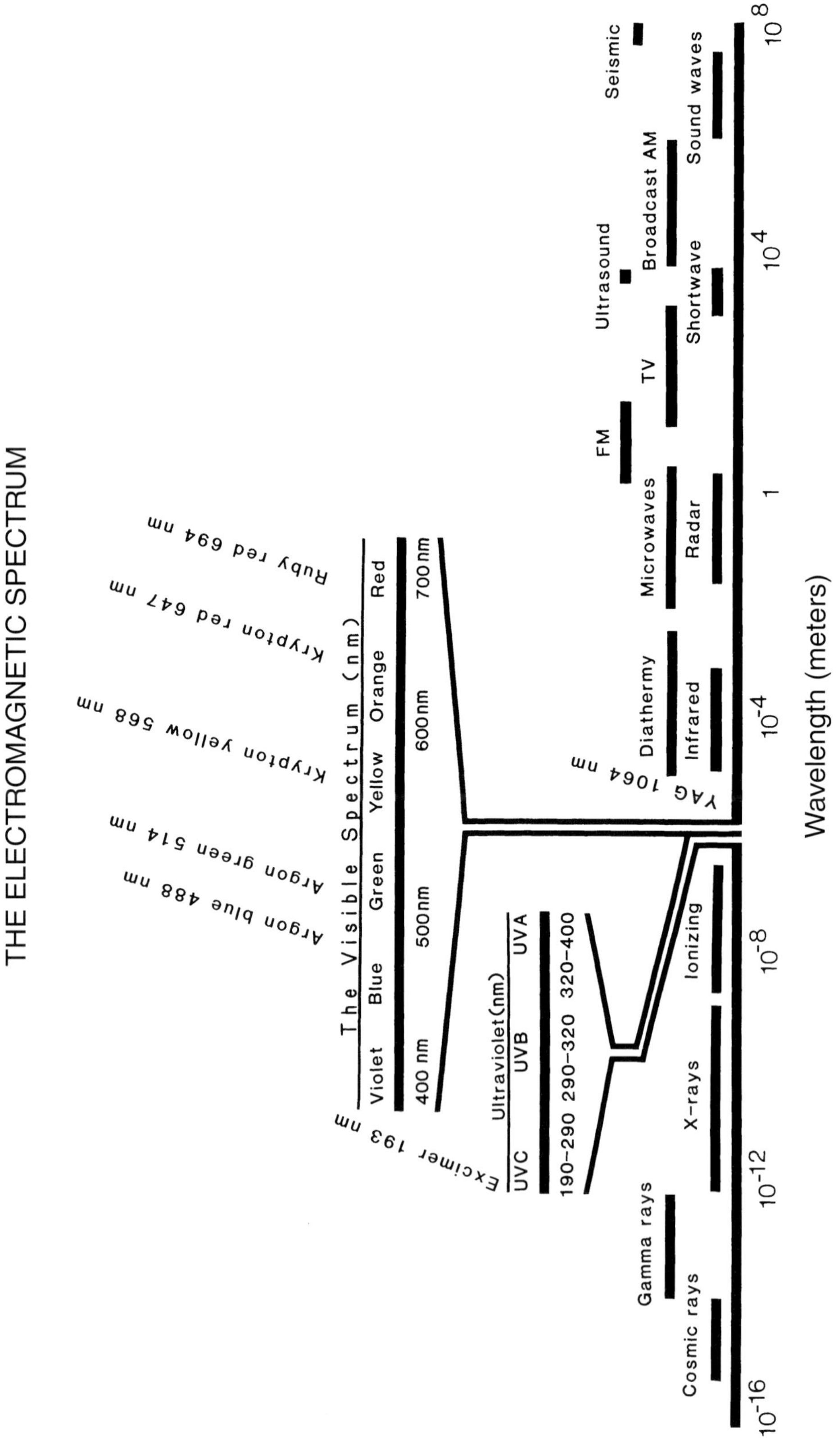

FIGURE 25-1 Radiant energy chart.

flash burns are the result of proximity to a nuclear explosion. Management may be complicated in such situations by other extensive bodily injuries. The corneal problems may require a conjunctival flap and/or penetrating keratoplasty to restore viable tissue to the anterior segment.

In lower intensity, longer, or repeated infrared exposures, chronic blepharitis with degenerative and hyperemic changes of the eyelid margins is common. Occasionally, corneal stromal opacities are noted, especially in association with cataracts, for example, in glassblowers. Infrared energy may also account, at least in part, for retinal solar burns. Corneal damage is not usually seen in these types of solar infrared exposures. Corneal edema can result from endothelial damage caused by infrared absorption and heating of the tissue during xenon arc photocoagulation.[48] Contact lenses impede the dissipation of heat in the cornea; saline irrigation promotes heat loss.[49] Thus, photocoagulation treatment through contact lenses should be accompanied by frequent irrigations of the ocular surface with saline or balanced salt solution.

Lasers

Lasers for industrial and biomedical uses can cause corneal trauma as well as severe retinal burns. Most of the reported laser-related corneal injuries have occurred during photocoagulation therapy for retinal vascular diseases, but such damage is uncommon.[48] Argon laser treatment can cause incidental epithelial erosions, corneal edema that may progress to bullous keratopathy, and corneal neovascularization.[50,51] Even when there are no obvious corneal complications, argon laser panretinal photocoagulation may cause a small decrease in endothelial cell density.[52] This decrease is probably the result of a significant elevation of corneal temperature. Argon laser iridotomy and trabeculoplasty do not cause corneal damage unless the cornea, especially the endothelium, is hit directly.[53–55] If the cornea is damaged by the argon laser, management is directed toward the corneal problem. There are no unique modalities of treatment for argon laser damage.

The neodymium:yttrium-aluminum-garnet (Nd:YAG) laser is used primarily in the treatment of opacifications in the ocular media, especially the posterior lens capsule after phacoemulsification or extracapsular cataract extraction. If the laser beam is focused on the corneal endothelium, the endothelial cells and Descemet's membrane sustain significant damage. Focus of the beam from 0.9 mm to as much as 3.5 mm away from the endothelium causes localized damage to the endothelium but not to Descemet's membrane. Some studies suggest that Q-switched lasers have a more restricted range of damage from the plane of focus than do mode-locked lasers.

Carbon dioxide lasers are becoming increasingly popular for cosmetic skin resurfacing. Protection of the patient's globe with a metal shield is essential to prevent corneal damage directly from the laser beam or indirectly from reflected laser energy. Operating room personnel should also wear glasses to protect their eyes.[56–58]

Interactions of the excimer laser with corneal tissue are discussed in Chapter 40.

Ultraviolet Radiation

Just beyond the blue-violet end of the visible spectrum is the ultraviolet (UV) radiant spectrum of 190 to 400 nm. Different portions of the ultraviolet spectrum are UVA (320 to 400 nm), UVB (290 to 320 nm), and UVC (190 to 290 nm). The absorption of ultraviolet radiation by the cornea is nearly 100 percent for wavelengths less than 290 nm (UVC). In contrast, the corneal absorption of wavelengths greater than 320 nm and less than 1,300 nm is 10 to 20 percent.[59] In other words, the cornea transmits 80 to 90 percent of visible light (Figure 25-2). Exposure to ultraviolet radiation results in characteristic changes in cells as a result of changes in proteins. Clinical and pathologic changes are evident 6 to 8 hours after exposure. At the tissue and cellular level, several changes are noted, including inhibition of mitosis, fragmentation of nuclei, eosinophilic staining resulting from changes in protein, and loss of cellular adhesion.

The clinical findings associated with ultraviolet photokeratitis are the result of excessive exposure to radiation with a wavelength of approximately 290 nm, except in cases of exposure to artificial ultraviolet sources. Snowblindness and welder's arc burns are well known. Other exposure sources are sunlamps, malfunctioning mercury vapor lamps, accidental replacement of UVA (black light) lamps with UVB lamps, and UVC (germicidal) lamps. In all cases, the onset of symptoms is 8 to 24 hours after exposure and is characterized by pain, foreign body sensation, and photophobia. The findings on examination are skin erythema, tearing, conjunctival hyperemia, corneal epithelial irregularities, edema, and punctate epithelial erosions. The signs and symptoms resolve during a period of 24 to 48 hours.

The findings on histologic examination of the corneal epithelium include loss of cell layers as a result of excessive desquamation and intracellular edema.[60] In some experimental studies, changes in stromal hydration[61] and endothelial morphology[62] have also been noted. Two clinical studies[63,64] using specular microscopy also suggested that ultraviolet exposure can damage the corneal endothelium. Although corneal studies have not been performed, the possibility exists that concurrent treatment with pho-

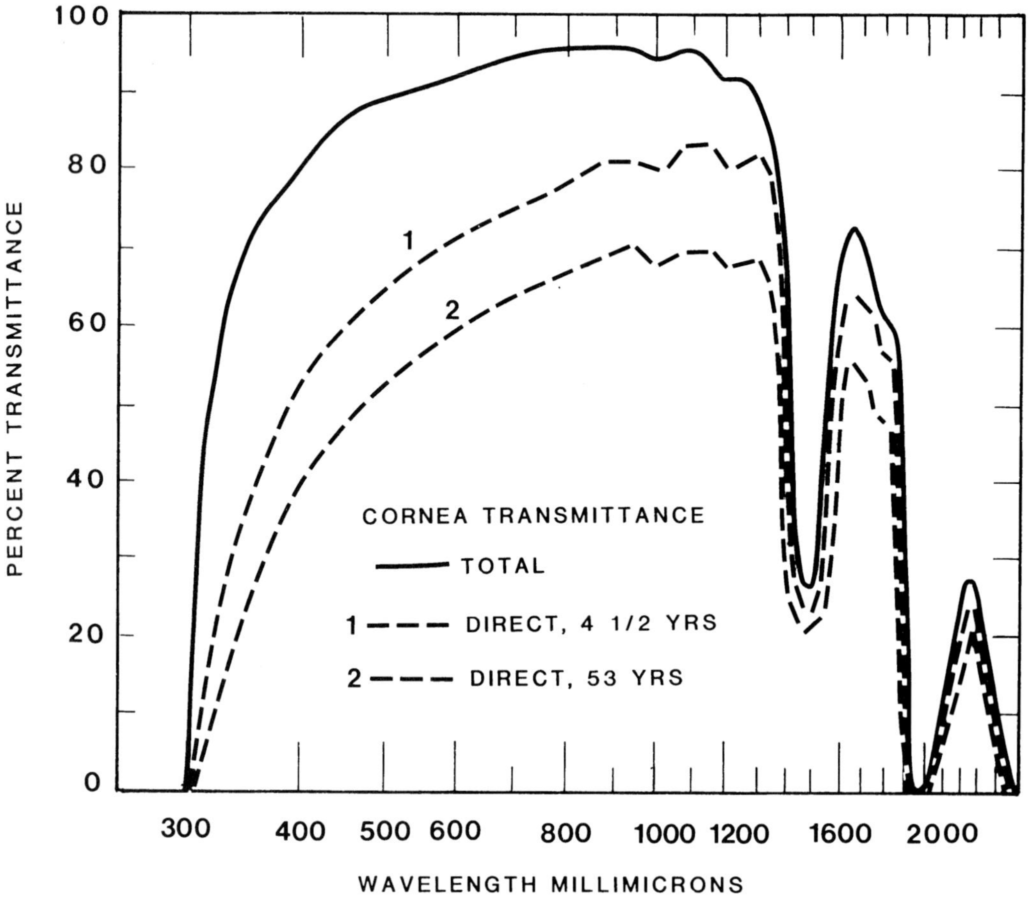

FIGURE 25-2 Transmittance of the cornea. (Redrawn from EA Boettner, JR Wolter: Transmission of the ocular media. Invest Ophthalmol 1:776, 1962.)

tosensitizing drugs increases the risk of ultraviolet-induced corneal damage.

Ultraviolet photokeratitis is a preventable condition. Public awareness and proper use of ultraviolet absorbing glasses, goggles, and occluders are needed. In patients with ultraviolet keratitis, treatment is aimed at promoting comfort until the symptoms subside. Oral analgesics, occlusive eye patches, and short-acting cycloplegics are useful. As an alternative to patching, a darkened room and cool compresses are palliative. The patients should be told what to expect in terms of the duration of symptoms and reassured that the prognosis for visual recovery is excellent.

Ionizing Radiation

Accidental exposure to ionizing radiation may be associated with nuclear explosions, x-rays, and radioisotopes. The amount of exposure is related to the amount of energy, the type of rays being emitted, and the proximity to the ionizing source. Exposure to ionizing radiation affects multiple tissues and organs. In general, the shorter the wavelength, the higher the quantum of energy that affects the exposed tissue. Longer wavelengths penetrate less, and, thus, cause a more intense reaction in superficial layers. In contrast, shorter wavelengths penetrate to deeper tissues and may not cause extensive damage to superficial tissues. The tissue destruction produced by ionizing radiation may be the result of direct killing of cells, cellular DNA changes that produce lethal or other abnormal mutations, or radiation damage to blood vessels, with secondary ischemic necrosis. Because description of malignant transformation resulting from accidental exposure to ionizing radiation is outside the scope of this chapter, only the effects of ionizing radiation on the cornea and the management of acute and semi-acute exposure are discussed here.

In most cases of ocular exposure to ionizing radiation, both the conjunctiva and cornea are involved. Acute changes in the conjunctiva include edema and chemosis

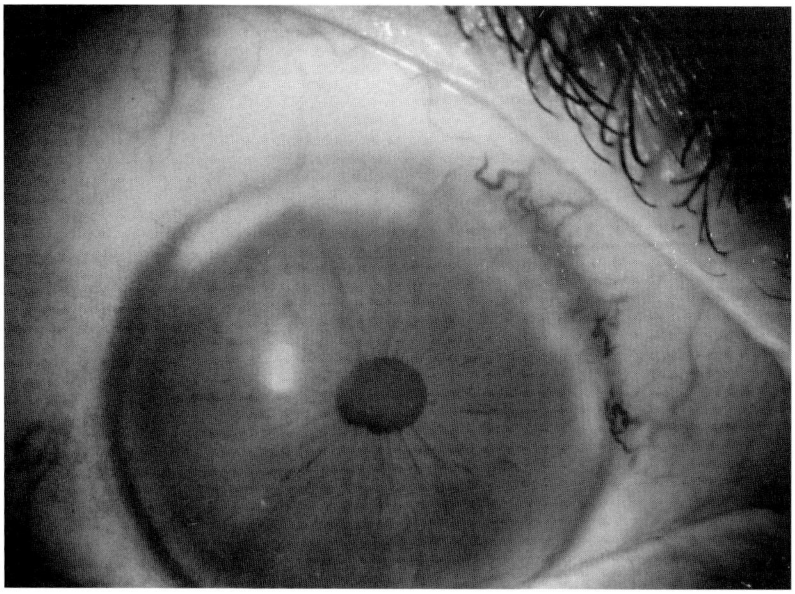

FIGURE 25-3 Radiation keratitis in a patient who received radiation therapy for acne. Note the superior telangiectatic vessels and corneal scarring.

with tearing. Later, there may be scarring, shrinkage, loss of tear production, and alterations in blood vessels, with large telangiectatic changes. If radioactive material is embedded in the conjunctiva, necrosis of this tissue and the underlying sclera occurs. Acute changes in the cornea after exogenous exposure to ionizing radiation are typified by punctate epithelial erosions. If the exposure is related to an explosion involving ionizing radiation, there may be a perforation associated with immediate radiation necrosis.

Management of the acute problems includes removal of foreign bodies, especially those that are radioactive. A bandage soft contact lens, tissue adhesive, or penetrating keratoplasty may be required. Poor wound healing is a hallmark of ionizing radiation injuries. The late changes in the conjunctiva preclude its use for a flap. If the opposite eye has not been injured, it is reasonable to use a contralateral autologous conjunctival flap.

The later complications of ionizing radiation injuries are related to lack of tears, loss of corneal sensation, loss of corneal epithelium and its failure to heal, secondary microbial keratitis, vascularization, and keratitis (Figure 25-3). Chronic radiation keratitis and iritis are rare but devastating. Management includes artificial tears, tarsorrhaphy, contralateral autologous conjunctival flap, and other appropriate supportive measures. The prognosis for penetrating keratoplasty in these situations is poor.

CHEMICAL INJURIES

Chemical burns of the cornea constitute true emergencies in the sense that the immediate management, if appropriate, may be the single most important factor in determining the outcome. The rapid dilution of the corrosive chemical by any benign, well-tolerated liquid, such as water, is the key to successful treatment. Therefore, the general public must be educated about the necessity of rapid irrigation in the management of chemical injuries.

Chemical injuries occur in home, industrial, leisure, war, and agricultural settings. Occasionally, they occur in a medical setting, for instance, in the treatment of a conjunctival papilloma with silver nitrate applicator sticks. The chemical may be a solid, liquid, or gas. The circumstances surrounding the injury, for example, exposure to pressurized liquid ammonia or a flake of sodium hydroxide, may play a key role in the outcome. Additionally, the chemical and physical properties of the substance determine the nature of the biological insult to a tissue. Rapid identification of the chemical and knowledge of the pathogenesis of the chemical injury help the physician to anticipate problems and complications. Toxicology books, ocular toxicology and pharmacology texts, poison control centers, package labels and inserts, and the product information divisions of manufacturers are all useful sources of information about the chemical. The person accompanying a chemical burn patient should be told to bring the container that identifies the chemical, especially when it is an uncommon agent.

In general, chemicals can be characterized as acidic or alkaline, and organic or inorganic. Various types of chemicals interact with cellular and extracellular components in specific ways. For example, alkali injuries raise the concentration of hydroxyl ions, which causes several changes, including saponification of fatty acids, loss of glycosaminoglycans in the stroma, and swelling of collagen fibrils. Other chemical groups bind to proteins, inactivate enzymes, tie up or destroy sulfhydryl groups, or interact with other normal components of tissues in a detrimental fashion. While knowledge of the chemical identity of an agent may help to understand the pathogenesis of an injury and allow the formulation of appropriate treatment and accurate prognosis, the clinical findings in injuries caused by different kinds of chemical agents are often indistinguishable.

An important parameter for the management of chemical burns is the establishment of a classification of severity. Several classifications have been proposed[65–68]; however, these classifications are, at best, generalizations, as each chemical burn is unique. The classification by Roper-Hall[68] appears to be the most useful because it is semiquantitative, and the clinical course and prognosis correlate well with the assigned severity (Table 25-1; Figure 25-4). This classification was developed for evaluating alkali burns, but it is also useful for classifying other chemical burns. Additionally, damage to other structures, such as the eyelids and/or accessory lacrimal glands or ducts, can alter the prognosis from good to poor.

Alkali Burns

Alkaline chemicals are the cause of many severe ocular injuries. The initial workup and subsequent management require complete evaluation of the involved structures and a thorough understanding of the pathogenesis of these injuries.

Alkaline Chemicals

The most caustic alkaline chemicals are ammonium hydroxide, sodium hydroxide, potassium hydroxide, calcium hydroxide, and magnesium hydroxide. Ammonium hydroxide is formed by the interaction of ammonia and water. Ammonia is extremely hydrophilic, and exposure to ammonia gas can burn parts of the body that are covered with water, such as mucous membranes or a wet extremity, while dry parts of the body may escape serious injury. Ammonia gas can be liquefied under high pressure. Chemical and fertilizer plants use this technique to make anhydrous ammonia, which is then used for other chemical processes. If tanks or lines containing anhydrous ammonia rupture, anyone in the path of the spray is exposed to a forceful stream of extremely hydrophilic ammonia. Even relatively small amounts can combine with tears and cause devastating ocular injuries. More commonly, people suffer chemical injuries with solutions containing 5 to 29 percent ammonia. These solutions can also produce significant injuries because ammonia is lipophilic as well as hydrophilic, and it penetrates into and through the epithelial cells and underlying tissue. In the cornea, this leads to rapid penetration into the anterior chamber, with exposure of the corneal endothelium, trabecular meshwork, iris, lens, and ciliary body.

Sodium hydroxide crystals or solutions also rapidly penetrate tissues and cause severe injuries. This chemical is commonly referred to as *lye* or *caustic soda* and is used in industry to clean vats, tanks, pipes, and other utensils; in the home to open clogged plumbing; and in manufacturing and processing in chemical and research industries. Potassium hydroxide (caustic potash) is used for similar purposes and has similar chemical properties.

Calcium hydroxide is a commonly encountered chemical that is present in lime, plaster, cement, and whitewash. Injury with this chemical is common and is likely to involve dispersion of particles on the conjunctiva and cornea. Calcium hydroxide does not penetrate through epithelial surfaces as readily as the other hydroxides because it combines with cell membranes to form precipitated soaps. This phenomenon causes corneal opacification, which may improve with time.

Magnesium hydroxide is a component of some fireworks, such as sparklers, as well as road flares. This substance enhances the damage caused by thermal burns when it comes in contact with the skin or eyes.

There are a number of other hydroxide-containing substances that cause ocular chemical burns. Grant and Shuman's *Toxicology of the Eye*[69] is an excellent source of further information on this subject.

Pathogenesis

The pathophysiologic basis for tissue damage caused by alkali burns is the result of the interaction of hydroxyl ions and chemical structures in tissues. In high concen-

TABLE 25-1
Classification of Chemical Burns

Grade	*Prognosis*	*Clinical Findings*
I	Good	Corneal epithelial damage; no ischemia
II	Good	Cornea hazy; iris details visible; ischemia less than one-third at limbus
III	Guarded	Total loss of corneal epithelium; stromal haze obscures iris details; ischemia of one-third to one-half at limbus
IV	Poor	Cornea opaque; iris and pupil obscured; ischemia affects more than one-half at limbus

Source: Adapted from MJ Roper-Hall: Thermal and chemical burns. Trans Ophthalmol Soc UK 85:631, 1965.

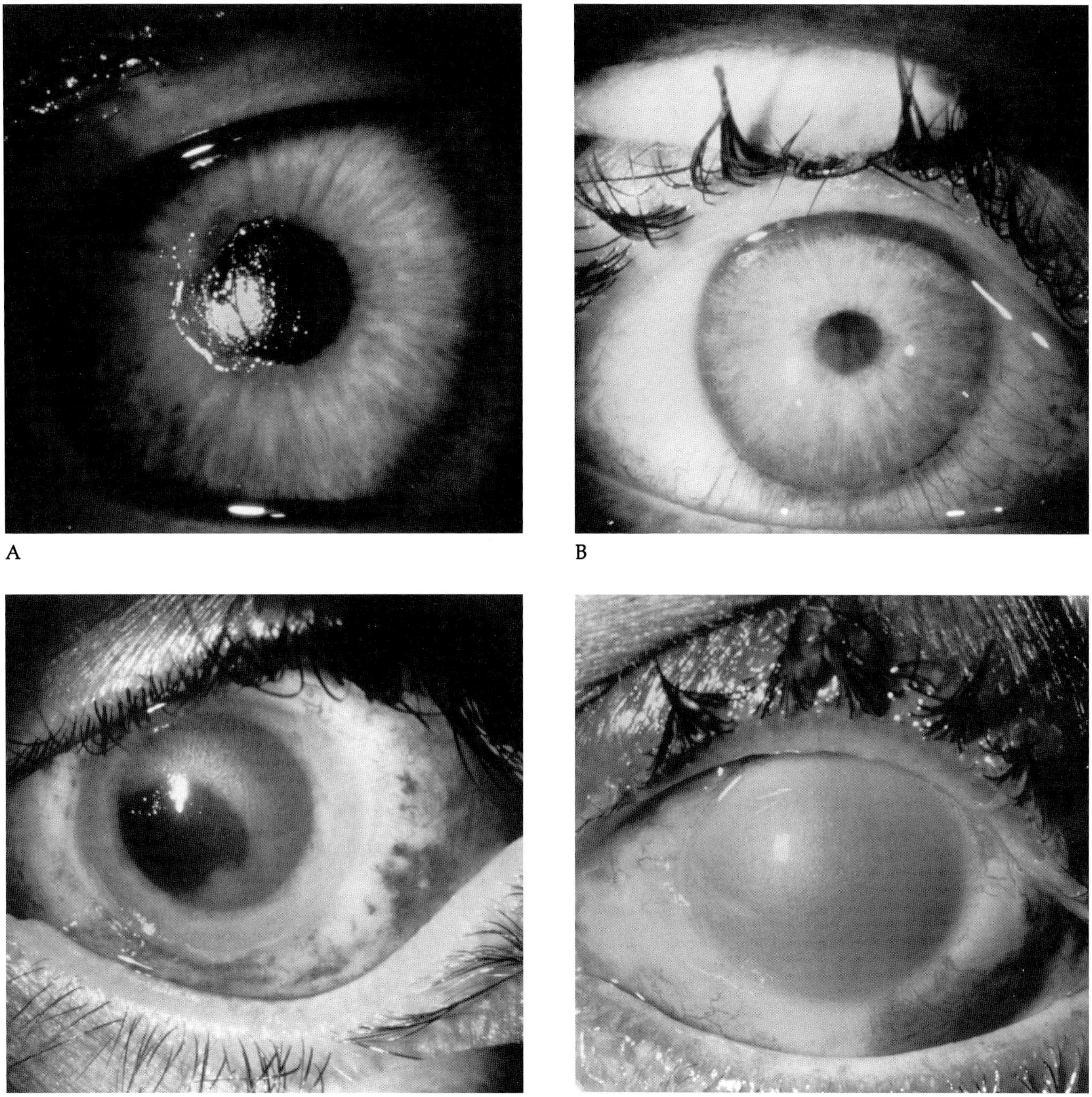

FIGURE 25-4 Chemical burns. (A) Grade I burn. Only the corneal epithelium is damaged. (B) Grade II burn. There is slight corneal haze, but iris details are clear. The limbus is partially ischemic. (C) Grade III burn. The stromal haze is obscuring some details. The interpalpebral limbus is ischemic. (D) Grade IV burn. The cornea is totally opaque. The limbus is markedly ischemic.

trations, alkaline compounds cause saponification of fatty acids in cell membranes, which leads to cell death by disrupting the structural integrity of the cell. This mechanism destroys epithelium and deeper cellular structures. However, an alkaline solution can penetrate a cell layer without disrupting it by virtue of its lipophilic characteristics. Alkali also causes significant alterations of the extracellular matrix. Hydroxyl ions bind to glycosaminoglycans and cause them to disappear.[70] Additionally, hydroxyl ions modify collagen. Individual fibrils

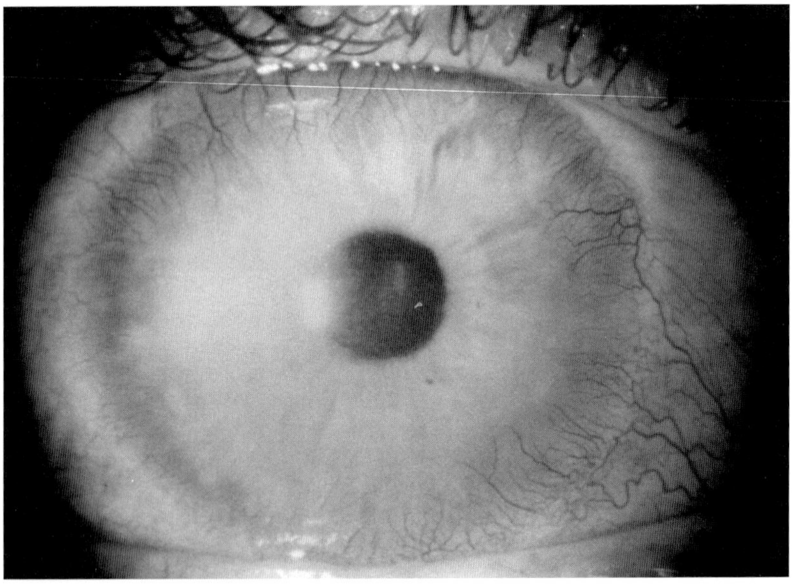

FIGURE 25-5 Corneal neovascularization and slight stromal scarring in an eye burned with anhydrous ammonia.

swell, either because of the direct action of the chemical or after the loss of glycosaminoglycans. The altered collagen is thought to be more susceptible to degradative enzymes. These chemical reactions appear to occur in all cells and tissues, and seem to be responsible for damage to conjunctiva, cornea, trabecular meshwork, iris, ciliary body, and lens, as well as coagulation of blood vessels.

Clinical Findings

The clinical course after a corneal alkali burn can be divided into three distinct stages that are characterized by tissue changes and responses. The acute stage lasts for 1 week after injury. Most of the damage results from the rapid saponification of fatty acids in cell membranes. Cells and structures of the corneal and conjunctival epithelium, goblet cells, stromal keratocytes, corneal extracellular matrix, trabecular meshwork and vascular endothelium, and ciliary body and lens epithelium may be killed or severely damaged. Depending on the severity of the burn, some or all of these structures may be involved. In mild burns, the corneal and conjunctival epithelium may have defects, and the blood vessels may be spared. In severe burns, the epithelium is destroyed, and there is immediate ischemia as a result of damage to blood vessels. In cases with visible damage to limbal vessels and limbal avascularity, there is probably also ciliary body necrosis, which may indicate a poor prognosis for the eye. The cornea is edematous and hazy, the anterior chamber is filled with fibrin, and the lens becomes cataractous. The pH of the aqueous humor increases within minutes and may remain elevated for a few hours. This increase in pH is accompanied by a decrease in glucose and ascorbate levels. Thus, there is early cell death, ischemia, and alterations of nutrients. As a result of these factors and other changes, such as changes in prostaglandin levels, the intraocular pressure may rise shortly after the injury. Over the next few days, the intraocular pressure should be measured frequently, because it can vary from hypotony to marked elevation. Within the first 2 days, the damaged tissues become infiltrated with polymorphonuclear leukocytes and monocytes. By the end of the acute stage, fibroblasts begin to enter the damaged tissue.

The early reparative stage (1 to 3 weeks after injury) is characterized by replacement of destroyed cells and extracellular matrix. In grade I or II chemical burns, regeneration of conjunctival and corneal epithelium is completed. At the same time, neovascularization of the cornea may begin (Figure 25-5). The corneal stroma may become clear in association with the invasion of fibroblasts, as well as bursts of collagen and glycosaminoglycan synthesis. Iritis may result from direct iris necrosis, but if a hypopyon develops, ciliary body necrosis may be present. The iritis begins to clear after 2 to 3 weeks, and iris and ciliary body vessels may recanalize. In severe burns (grades III and IV), the regeneration of epithelium may not progress, the stroma may remain hazy, inflammatory cells may persist, and dead corneal endothelium may be replaced with a fibrous retrocorneal membrane. Friable granulation tissue and early fibrosis occur in the severely damaged iris and ciliary body. In this early reparative stage, severely burned corneas develop the first major complication: failure of re-epithelialization and stromal ulceration (Figure 25-6). Lack of epithelial healing may occur even when most of the limbal tissue remains intact to provide a source of cells for epithelial healing. This healing problem may represent alter-

FIGURE 25-6 Severe peripheral neovascularization and central stromal ulceration in an alkali-burned eye.

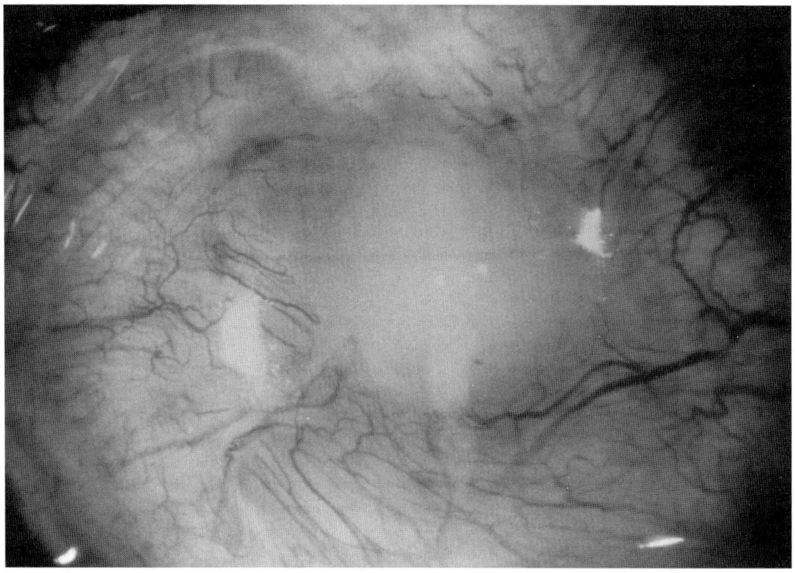

ation of the surface over which the epithelium must migrate. Stromal ulceration has been attributed to the action of digestive enzymes such as collagenases, metalloproteinases, and other proteases released from regenerating corneal epithelium and polymorphonuclear leukocytes. There is evidence that the plasminogen activator-plasmin system is operative.[71-74] Plasminogen is present in the cornea, as is latent intracellular plasminogen activator. Alkali burns cause release of active plasminogen activator, which converts plasminogen to plasmin. Plasmin, in turn, activates latent collagenase. The active form of plasminogen activator also degrades fibrin, fibronectin, and laminin. Aprotinin is an inhibitor of this system but its therapeutic value is unclear. Similarly, metalloproteinase inhibitors have been tested, but their clinical value is uncertain. In general, the major effort should be directed toward healing the epithelium, because once the epithelium heals, stromal ulceration stops.

The late reparative stage (3 weeks after injury and later) is characterized by completion of healing in burns with a good prognosis (grades I and II) and complications in those with a guarded or poor prognosis (grades III and IV). In alkali burns with a good prognosis, the epithelium remains intact and no stromal ulceration occurs. However, neovascularization of the stroma is likely. The range of other adverse changes in the eye is great and may include tear film abnormalities, secondary glaucoma, synechia formation, iris atrophy, and secondary cataract. Burns with a guarded or poor prognosis cause more severe changes that may threaten the salvation of the injured eye. In these eyes, epithelial defects persist, and in the second or third week, stromal ulceration begins. The ulceration usually occurs in areas where there is no stromal neovascularization. It is hypothesized that antiproteases in blood prevent stromal ulceration in areas that have become vascularized.[66] The corneal and conjunctival surfaces are often covered with thick fibrovascular tissue. In areas of ulceration, collagen is degraded faster than it is synthesized. Collagen degradation is most likely the result of the activity of multiple proteolytic enzymes released by dead cells, actively replicating cells, and white blood cells that have invaded the injured tissues. Progressive ulceration with descemetocele formation or perforation is catastrophic. Additionally, the death of corneal nerves creates the potential for neurotrophic keratitis.

Other adverse extraocular problems also become manifest. Eyelid scarring with lagophthalmos, ectropion or entropion, and exposure keratitis complicate the epithelial resurfacing problems. Burned areas on the eyelid margins may become keratinized. Symblepharon formation may begin where two surfaces devoid of epithelium touch (Figure 25-7). As the fibrovascular tissue begins to contract, the mobility of the globe is reduced (Figure 25-8). Finally, the components of the tear film are abnormal or absent. Loss of goblet cells results in absence of the mucin layer. Occlusion of meibomian gland orifices in the eyelids results in an abnormal or absent lipid component. The obliteration of the accessory lacrimal glands depletes the normal basal secretion of the aqueous component. Depending on the amount of damage to the lacrimal gland ducts, there may be a total absence or a vast excess of reflex tearing.

Treatment

The treatment of alkali burns is based on prevention, early intervention, and management of the sequelae. Ammo-

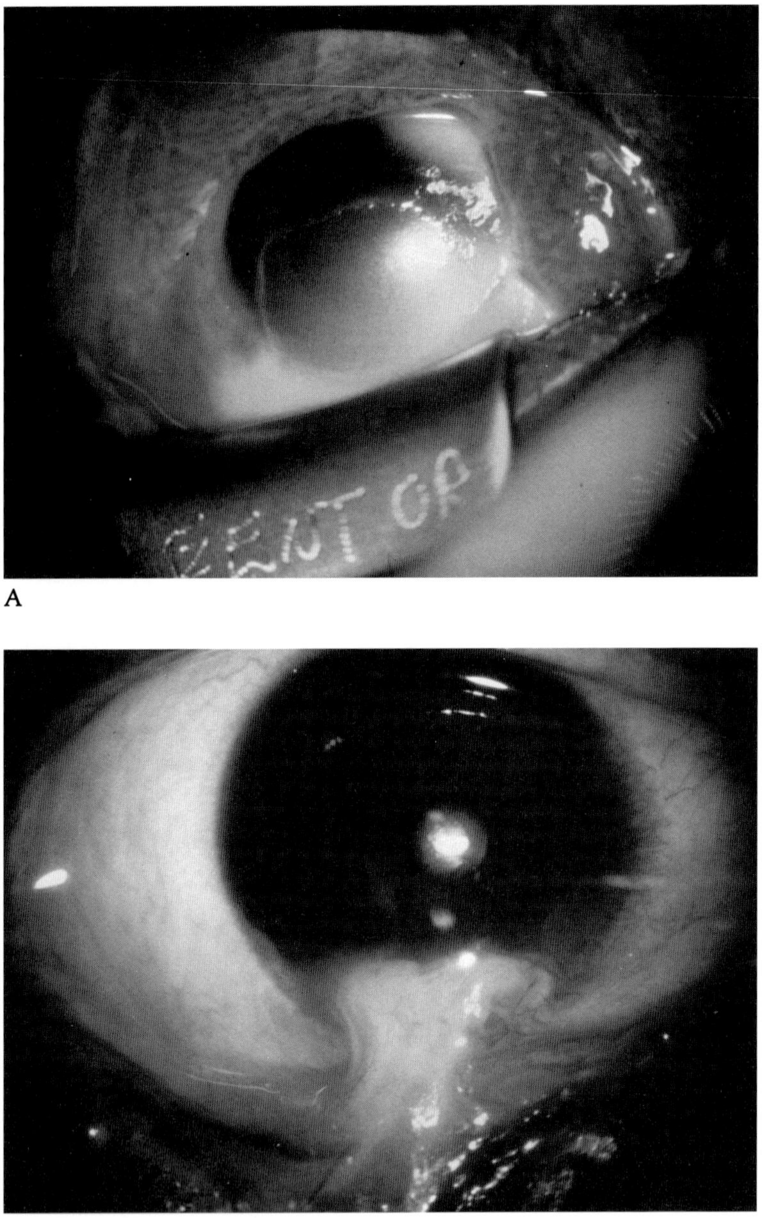

A

B

FIGURE 25-7 **(A)** Corneal and conjunctival epithelial surface defects immediately after an alkali burn. **(B)** The apposition of the two raw surfaces led to the formation of a symblepharon.

nia, and to a lesser extent sodium hydroxide and potassium hydroxide, penetrate tissues so rapidly that there is no opportunity to prevent sequelae to the extent possible with other types of chemical burns. Public education has been an important factor in the prevention and early management of alkali burns. Similarly, industrial safety precautions, including eye protection and equipment for immediate ocular irrigation, have improved the final outcome in many chemical burn accidents.

The treatment of ocular alkali burns within the first 2 to 3 minutes after the injury is most important. The immediate initiation of ocular surface irrigation with any nontoxic liquid is essential. Dilution of the chemical is the key factor. Therefore, it is mandatory that the eyelids be opened wide and the cornea and all of the conjunctival surface be bathed in large volumes of fluid. This treatment should be done at the site of the injury, and only then should the patient be rapidly transported to a medical facility, where irrigation should immediately be resumed with saline. Intravenous tubing is easily available, and can be used safely to irrigate the ocular surface. The pH of the conjunctival cul-de-sacs should be monitored and the irrigation continued until the pH is neutral, or for a minimum of 30 min-

FIGURE 25-8 **(A)** A nasal symblepharon developed after a calcium hydroxide burn despite the use of a bandage soft contact lens. **(B)** There is marked restriction of lateral gaze.

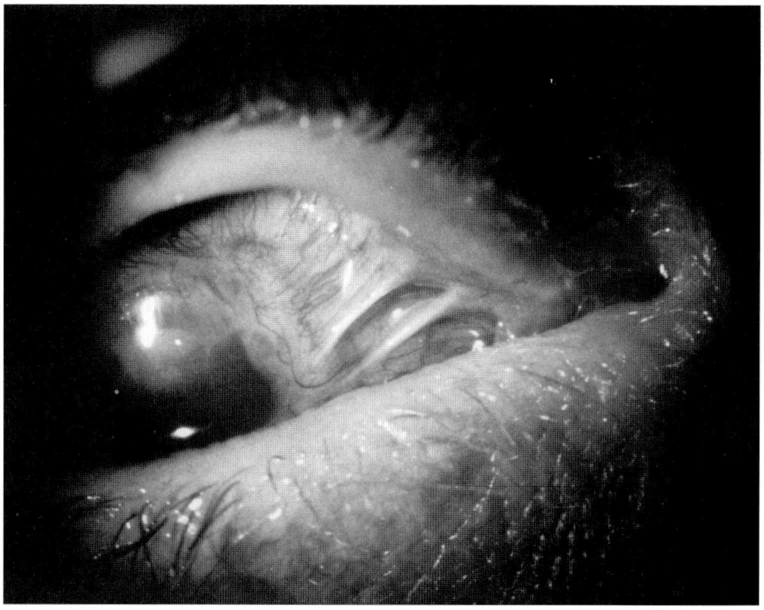

A

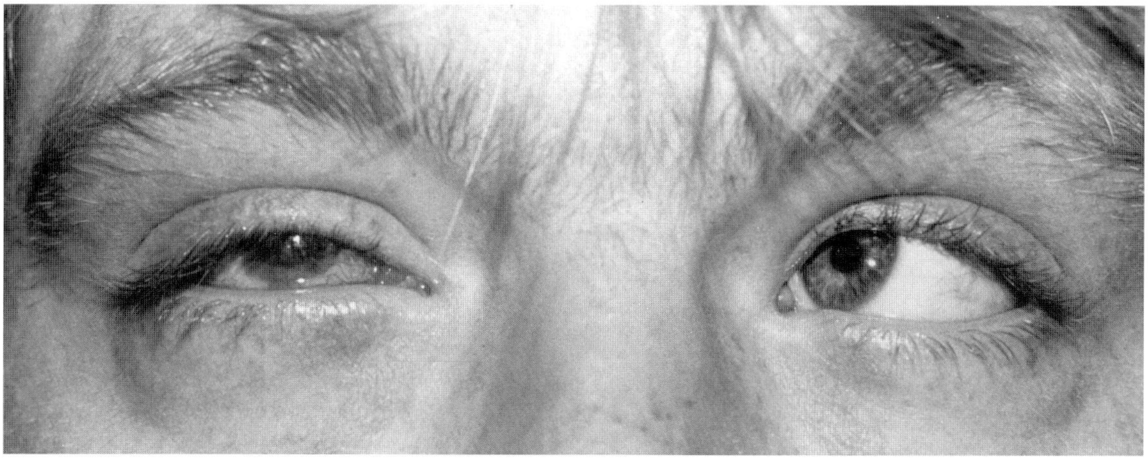

B

utes. Topical anesthesia and separation of the eyelids with retractors assist in effective irrigation. Any visible particulate matter must be removed with irrigation, a cotton-tipped applicator, or forceps. In addition, the eyelids should be everted and examined for particulate matter and the fornices should be swabbed with a moist cotton-tipped applicator. Materials containing calcium hydroxide can be especially difficult to remove mechanically. Irrigation with 0.01 to 0.05 M ethylenediaminetetraacetic acid (EDTA) can be used to chelate calcium hydroxide.[75] Once irrigation has been discontinued, the pH should be monitored every 10 to 15 minutes for another 60 minutes to ensure that residual material does not turn the pH basic again.

Various types of specialized equipment have been described for the irrigation of chemical burns, but none has been shown to be superior to the methods just described. Anterior chamber paracentesis, as well as anterior chamber irrigation, has also been suggested. However, the risks attendant on such procedures are not definitely outweighed by the benefits.

Therapy for the acute stage (immediate to 1 week) begins as soon as the emergency measures are completed. A thorough examination of the injured eye is mandatory for grad-

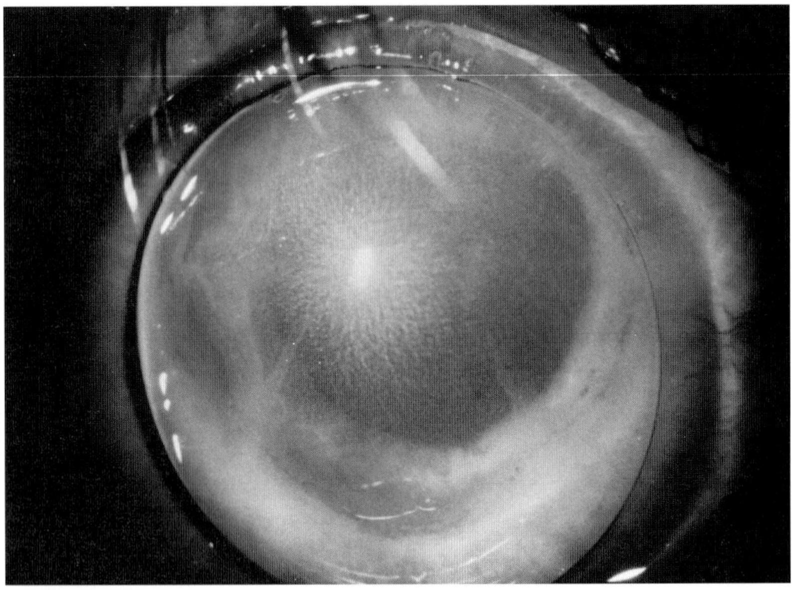

FIGURE 25-9 A bandage soft contact lens and symblepharon ring may prevent symblepharon formation caused by the apposition of two de-epithelialized surfaces. However, they do not prevent the formation and contraction of subepithelial scar tissue.

ing severity and planning therapy. The key goals of therapy during this stage are promotion of epithelial healing, avoidance of stromal ulceration, and early treatment of potential complicating problems. A topical antibiotic should be used two to four times daily as prophylaxis against infection. In the absence of infection, potent antibiotics, such as aminoglycosides and chloramphenicol, should be avoided, as they may inhibit epithelial healing. A fluoroquinolone antibiotic twice a day is usually sufficient. A cycloplegic agent, such as 1 percent atropine, should be started to help reduce the pain associated with ciliary spasm and prevent the formation of synechiae. Intraocular pressure may increase significantly and should be monitored carefully. Timolol, latanoprost, and/or carbonic anhydrase inhibitors may be used.

The degree of severity and the presence or absence of other damage dictate what additional measures should be instituted. In grade I or II injuries, the only other measure may be application of a pressure patch or bandage soft contact lens. Occasionally, these injuries also require artificial tears. Daily examinations to monitor epithelial healing and the clearing of the conjunctival ischemia and/or stromal haze will determine if further treatment is needed. In more severe or complicated injuries (grades III and IV), damage to the eyelid margins or exposure keratitis may require the use of lubricating ointments in association with patching or a contact lens. Marked anterior segment inflammation is an indication for potent topical corticosteroids (e.g., prednisolone acetate or dexamethasone sodium phosphate) for the first week after injury, even in cases in which the epithelium is not intact.[76] The anti-inflammatory activity of corticosteroids may assist corneal epithelial wound healing because the epithelial cells adhere poorly to an inflamed stroma. Some recommend that topical corticosteroids be discontinued 7 to 10 days after the injury. Several reports have claimed that corticosteroids either inhibit or potentiate tissue collagenase activity.[72,76–78]

Sodium citrate, plasminogen inhibitors, collagenase inhibitors, and metalloproteinase inhibitors are being tested for the prevention of stromal ulceration, but none has been clearly shown to be useful.

Significant alkali burns cause decreased ascorbate levels in the aqueous humor, and many of the changes in the cornea resemble those seen in scurvy.[79] In experimental alkali burns, the incidence of ulceration and perforation can be reduced by the topical and/or parenteral administration of ascorbate. A 10 percent solution of ascorbate can be made up in artificial tears and applied topically on an hourly basis 12 to 14 times a day. The therapy must be instituted before ulceration begins.[80] The human systemic dosage is unknown but is probably 1 to 2 g per day.

The prevention of symblephara is critical. Even when damage to the globe cannot be prevented, if the eyelids are normal, symblephara do not form, and, if the tear film is adequate, penetrating keratoplasty may have a reasonable chance of success, whereas dry eyes and symblepharon formation with trichiasis usually prevent successful penetrating keratoplasty and restoration of vision.

Daily lysis of adhesions between the palpebral and bulbar conjunctiva with an ointment-coated glass rod to prevent symblephara is usually unsuccessful. In mild burns, especially in adults, a scleral lens or symblepharon ring combined with a bandage soft contact lens (Figure 25-9) can minimize the chance of raw conjunctival surfaces sticking together and reduce symblepharon formation, and should be left in place for 2 weeks. In more extensive burns or in children, lining the inner eyelids and fornices with a thin flexible plastic, such as plastic food wrap, which can be sutured in place and left for 2 weeks, is very effective but must be used early if it is to be successful in preventing symblepharon formation (see Ch. 23).[81]

Treatment of an alkali burn during the early reparative stage is largely a continuation of the acute stage management. Most of the effort is directed toward healing the corneal epithelium and preventing ulceration. Adequate treatment of tear film abnormalities (qualitative and quantitative) with artificial tears is important. Bandage soft contact lenses protect the corneal epithelium from abnormal eyelids and help manage exposure keratitis. The early reparative stage is the stage during which some advocate that topical corticosteroids should be avoided.

If ulceration occurs or a perforation is impending, a thin conjunctival flap, conjunctival transplant from the contralateral eye, or mucous membrane graft is indicated. The choice of a specific procedure depends on the concomitant findings. A conjunctival flap should not be performed if the conjunctival epithelium is necrotic. If only one eye is involved and the ipsilateral conjunctiva is abnormal, a conjunctival transplant can be performed using autologous tissue from the contralateral eye.[82] If both eyes are involved and no source of normal autologous conjunctiva is available, mucous membrane grafts are indicated.[83]

If a perforation occurs as a result of stromal ulceration, the possible contribution of microbial keratitis must be considered. Smears and cultures are mandatory. Intensive topical antibiotics should be used before surgical treatment. For small perforations, tissue adhesive may be used.[84] With larger perforations, a lamellar or full-thickness patch graft is indicated (see Chs. 31 and 32).[85] The graft may be covered by conjunctiva for protection. The success rates of these procedures are low. In the postoperative period, careful examination and management of all the attendant complications of alkali burns must be continued.

Therapy during the late reparative stage and beyond is similar to previous management. If deficiencies in the aqueous and/or mucin layers of the tear film persist, long-term therapy with artificial tears is required. When the epithelium is healed or a conjunctival flap is in place, use of topically applied corticosteroids may be reinstituted.

Acid Burns

Acid burns of the eye can be as catastrophic as alkali burns and demand the same comprehensive care.

Acidic Chemicals

Sulfuric acid is probably the major cause of significant ocular acid burns. It is the acid found in automotive batteries and is also widely used in industry. Exposure of the ocular surface to concentrated sulfuric acid is especially devastating because this form of the acid is extremely hydrophilic. The reaction between concentrated sulfuric acid and water in the cornea is exothermic, and thermal and chemical damage occur as well. Lesser concentrations of sulfuric acid cause mild to moderate chemical burns of the eye.

Sulfurous acid burns occur when sulfur dioxide gas (used as a refrigerant, bleach, or preservative for fruits and vegetables) comes in contact with water, as in the tear film and the corneal stroma. Sulfurous acid denatures protein and inactivates intracellular enzymes. It also causes damage to nerves, which results in anesthesia. Thus, ocular injuries with this chemical may not look or feel bad initially but worsen with time.

Hydrochloric acid is usually used in concentrations of 32 to 38 percent. It is also used in swimming pools as muriatic acid in weaker concentrations. Vapors from the acid are irritating and cause profuse reflex tearing. If the acid comes in contact with the eye, severe ocular damage occurs. Nitric acid burns are similar, except that corneal epithelial opacities are yellowish rather than white.

Hydrofluoric acid has unique properties that can cause severe chemical burns. Although it is a weak acid, it is a strong solvent. As an acid, it is used in concentrations varying from 0.5 to 70 percent. In other solutions, it is mixed with chemicals such as acetic acid or nitric acid. Hydrofluoric acid is especially efficient in dissolving cell membranes. This characteristic, plus its small molecular size, aids in its deep penetration into ocular tissues.

Chromic acid is used as a cleaning agent, for example, in washing laboratory glassware and in the chrome plating industry. Exposure to small amounts of chromic acid causes chronic conjunctival injection and brownish discoloration, whereas more extensive exposure causes severe ocular damage. Acetic acid (vinegar, glacial acetic acid) is a common, relatively weak inorganic acid, high concentrations (80 to 90 percent) of which can cause severe ocular damage.

Pathogenesis

The pathogenesis of acid burns is related to the coagulation and precipitation of proteins. The degree of damage to protein depends on the affinity between the protein and the anion of a particular acid and on the pH change caused by the hydrogen ions.[86] Because most proteins in tissues, including the cornea, are capable of binding an acid and buffering its effect, most acid burns remain localized.[87]

Coagulated corneal epithelial cells may also serve as a barrier to prevent deeper penetration of acids.

In the corneal stroma, acids cause shortening of collagen fibrils and precipitation of glycosaminoglycans. The changes in the glycosaminoglycans probably cause loss of stromal clarity. An acute increase in intraocular pressure occurs after acid burns and is presumably the result of collagen shrinkage. The pH of the aqueous humor decreases and the protein and prostaglandin levels increase.[88] Stromal ulceration is not common after acid burns, and the level of damage to cellular enzyme systems caused by acids is probably less than that caused by alkali. Acids do not appear to cause a predictable defect in collagen synthesis. However, severe acid burns involving the ciliary body lead to decreased corneal and aqueous humor ascorbate levels and a localized scorbutic state similar to that seen in severe alkali burns.[89]

Clinical Findings

The damage after an acid burn should be thoroughly evaluated and classified according to the Roper-Hall[68] scheme. The same prognostic predictions as for an alkali burn are valid. The degree of ocular damage depends on the type, concentration, and quantity of acid, its pH, and the duration of exposure. Other features of a particular acid, such as its hydrophilic or lipophilic nature and its affinity for a particular protein, also play roles in the severity of ocular damage.

Treatment

The treatment of acid burns is similar to that of alkali burns.

NONPERFORATING MECHANICAL INJURIES

Abrasion of the Corneal Epithelium

Abrasion of the corneal epithelium is a common ocular injury in which epithelial cells are lost but Bowman's layer remains intact. If Bowman's layer is not disrupted, no corneal scarring will result. Abrasions are often caused by foreign bodies; glancing blows by twigs, fingers, or other objects; contusive force; and ill-fitting or overworn contact lenses. Symptoms include sudden onset of foreign body sensation, lacrimation, and photophobia. Blepharospasm and pain are often intense and can be aggravated by blinking and movement of the eye. Depending on the location of the abrasion, visual acuity may be normal or decreased.

Examination is facilitated by instillation of a topical anesthetic. Slit lamp examination should be performed to observe for fluorescein staining of epithelial defects and to rule out the presence of foreign bodies in the conjunctiva, including the fornices, or the cornea. If there is a sharp edge to the epithelial defect, re-epithelialization is typically prompt. In contrast, the presence of loose epithelium with edema and a grayish appearance often signifies a defect that will heal slowly.

Objectives of therapy are pain relief, prevention of secondary infection, and promotion of corneal re-epithelialization. Treatment usually includes instillation of a short-acting cycloplegic agent and a topical antibiotic ointment four times a day. A collagen shield soaked in an antibiotic solution may be placed if microbial contamination is likely. Nonsteroidal anti-inflammatory drops, such as 0.5 percent ketorolac four times a day, significantly relieve pain, and bandage soft contact lenses may provide additional relief if bacterial contamination has been ruled out.[90] Patching sometimes relieves discomfort but it is not necessary, especially for small abrasions. The eye should be re-examined in 24 to 36 hours to detect potential complications, such as secondary infection. Treatment should be continued until the epithelium has healed. The rapid regenerative capacity of the corneal epithelium allows most small abrasions to heal without sequelae in 24 to 48 hours. Larger epithelial defects may require a longer period for complete re-epithelialization.[91–94] Some plants, such as *Dieffenbachia*, contain toxins that can cause a focal keratitis that responds to topical corticosteroids. Fungal keratitis must be excluded before the initiation of topical corticosteroids in any patient who has sustained a corneal abrasion from vegetable matter.

Post-Traumatic Recurrent Corneal Erosion

Most corneal epithelial defects heal rapidly with few complications. One exception is recurrent corneal erosion syndrome (Figure 25-10). This clinical entity is characterized by recurrent attacks of pain, photophobia, and lacrimation, especially during sleep or in the morning on waking.

Erosive attacks may occur after trauma, as discussed here, spontaneously, or in certain inherited corneal dystrophies, such as map-dot-fingerprint, Reis-Bücklers', or lattice dystrophies[95,96] (see Ch. 18). Abrasions with paper, fingernails, or plants are likely to cause recurrent erosions. When precipitated by injury, the disorder is usually unilateral, and the recurrences appear in the same corneal area as the trauma. The inherited forms tend to be bilateral and symmetrical, and develop in multiple corneal locations. Lagophthalmos causes epithelial damage due to exposure that is easily confused with a recurrent erosion and must be ruled out in all cases.

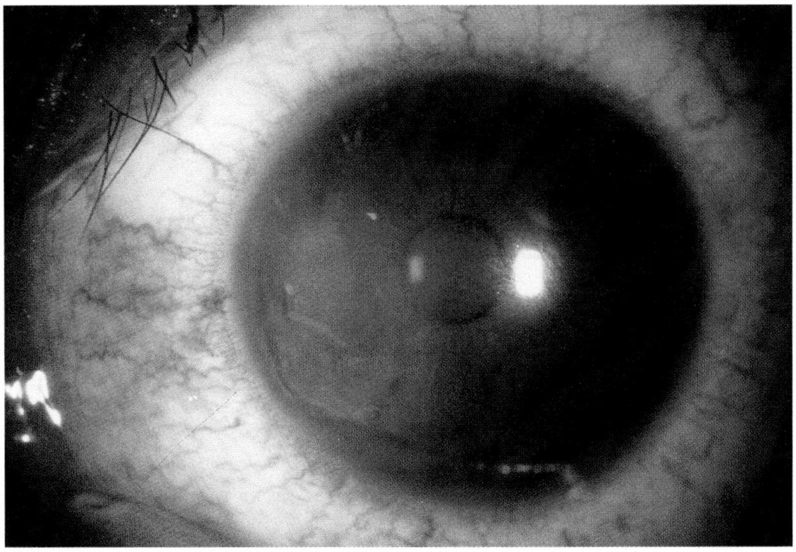

A

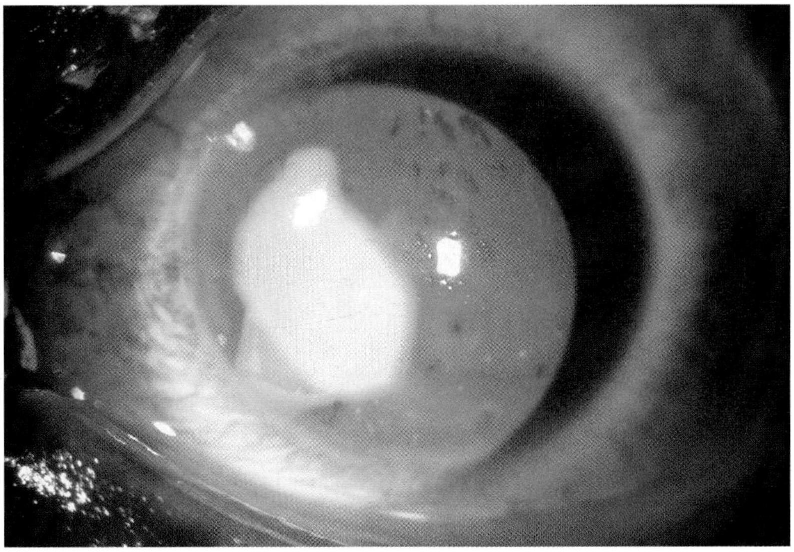

B

FIGURE 25-10 **(A)** Recurrent epithelial erosion after a traumatic abrasion. Note the hazy appearance of the surrounding epithelium. **(B)** Fluorescein staining outlines the area of erosion.

The cause of recurrent erosions is poor adhesion between the epithelium and Bowman's layer. Abnormalities of the basement membrane, with absence of the hemidesmosomes that normally anchor the basal epithelial cells to the basement membrane, have been found in traumatic and spontaneous cases.[9,97] In one study of post-traumatic recurrent corneal erosions, the stroma was also affected; numerous leukocytes and relatively few keratocytes were seen by light and electron microscopy.[98]

Various treatment regimens are available for recurrent erosions. Conventional therapy includes pressure patching, bandage soft contact lens wear, ointments instilled at bedtime, artificial tears as required, mild corticosteroids (e.g., fluorometholone), and occasionally debridement of loose epithelium. In these patients, previously asymptomatic blepharitis, dry eyes, or both constitute major impediments to successful healing of recurrent erosions and must be managed aggressively. Occasionally, erosions recur. When the treatment modalities described above fail, a technique of microcautery of the superficial portion of Bowman's layer in the area of a traumatic recurrent erosion[99] or a method of anterior stromal punctures

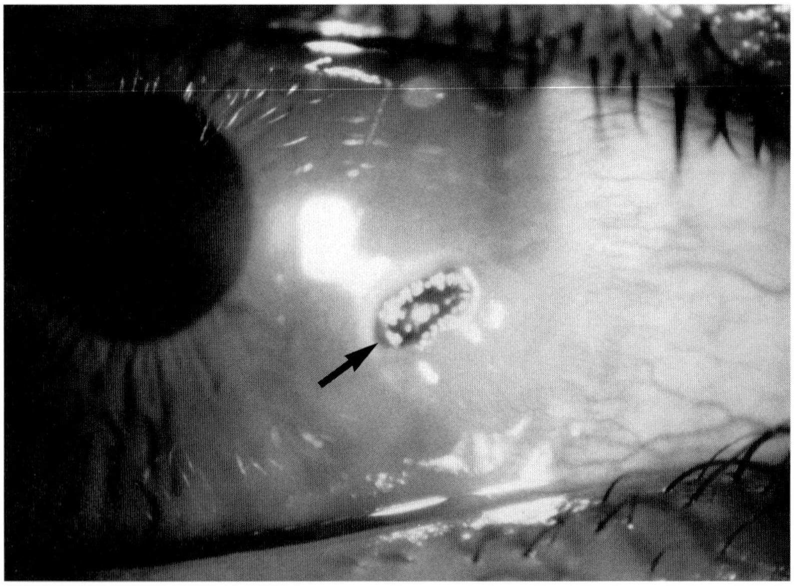

FIGURE 25-11 Retained superficial metallic foreign body (arrow) caused edema, inflammation, and vascularization of the adjacent cornea.

with a 20-gauge needle[100] may be tried. The reported success of these approaches makes them attractive options in the treatment of recalcitrant recurrent erosions. These procedures should not be used on the central cornea, however, because they may leave scars that cause glare. Minimal phototherapeutic keratectomy with the excimer laser is an excellent way to treat medically resistant erosions (see Ch. 30).

Corneal Foreign Bodies

A variety of substances can lodge on or within the cornea, including windblown grit, fragments of insects, fragments of glass, thorns, and metallic filings. The composition of the foreign material determines whether the object remains inert or causes a local inflammatory response.

In general, substances such as glass, sand, and certain minerals are well tolerated and may remain within the stroma for long periods. Other materials, including many metals, vegetable matter, and insect parts, are poorly tolerated and can lead to focal edema, inflammatory reaction, vascularization, and necrosis[91,94] (Figure 25-11). There are exceptions to this generalization, however, including reports of a nonedematous keratopathy associated with microscopic intracorneal glass fragments,[101] and a bee stinger that remained inert.[102]

The goals of treatment are to remove the foreign body, relieve discomfort, avoid secondary infection, and minimize corneal scarring. Most corneal foreign bodies involving the epithelium and superficial stroma are easily removed at the slit lamp microscope after instillation of a topical anesthetic. A moist, cotton-tipped applicator or fine-gauge needle may be used. Care is taken to avoid disrupting deeper layers of the cornea, which can lead to unnecessary scarring. Deep corneal foreign bodies that have penetrated the anterior chamber or whose removal may lead to perforation are managed as intraocular foreign bodies. Their removal requires microsurgical procedures with local or general anesthesia as indicated. Rigid materials with a direct entry path may be grasped through the route of penetration. Softer foreign bodies or those with tangential routes may be more readily removed via a direct stab wound. Special care should be taken to prevent converting a corneal foreign body into an intraocular foreign body.

Deeply embedded foreign bodies are treated as indicated based on the ophthalmologist's knowledge of the nature of the foreign body and observation of its behavior and the reaction of the cornea. An embedded foreign body is removed unless removal presents a greater threat to the health of the eye than allowing it to remain. Deep corneal foreign bodies that require microsurgical removal are cultured at the time of surgery. An antibiotic-soaked collagen shield or subconjunctival injection of antibiotics is used at the completion of surgery.

Metallic foreign bodies often leave rust rings that are more easily removed 72 to 96 hours after initial removal of the foreign body (Figure 25-12). Fine needles, spuds, and dental burs have been used for this purpose. Following instillation of a topical anesthetic, rust rings are easily lifted off with a 25-gauge needle. Rust rings may retard healing or cause irritation. However, aggressive removal may cause additional scarring, and most residual rust rings will eventually be absorbed. Galin and his col-

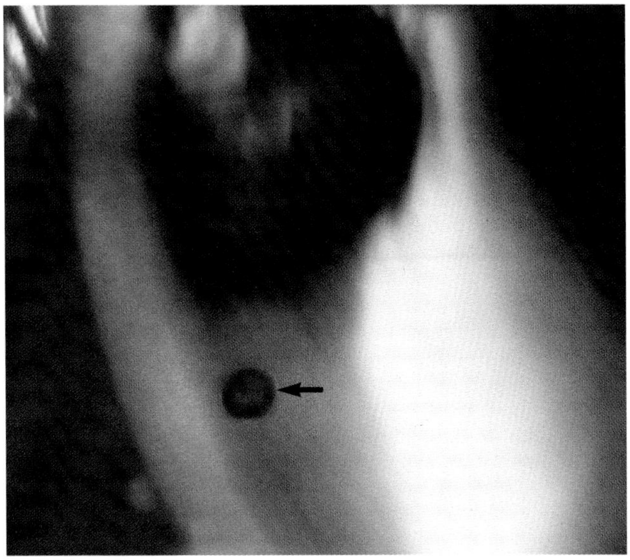

FIGURE 25-12 Dense rust ring (arrow) from a metallic foreign body.

leagues[103,104] reported chemical removal of rust rings with a chelating agent, deferoxamine mesylate. This therapy, which has not gained widespread acceptance, is effective only as long as re-epithelialization has not occurred.

Treatment after corneal foreign body removal is similar to that described for a corneal abrasion. Patients should be re-examined in 24 to 36 hours and subsequently until the cornea is completely re-epithelialized.[91-94] Special attention must be paid to detect early signs of microbial keratitis or endophthalmitis.

Occasionally, patients present with corneal necrosis surrounding foreign bodies that have been in place for prolonged periods. Some may even have descemetoceles or perforations. These foreign bodies are easily lifted off of the cornea. Small defects that are not infected can be closed with tissue adhesive and a bandage soft contact lens. Large defects may require lamellar or penetrating keratoplasty. Topical cycloplegics and antibiotics and frequent re-examinations are required.

Blunt Trauma

Injuries to the globe and its surrounding tissues occur frequently and are commonly produced by trauma with a blunt object. A contusive injury results from a direct blow to the eye that usually does not lacerate the tissue surface. A variety of blunt objects may cause a contusive injury. A concussive injury is caused by a violent jar or shake, rather than by an object directly striking the eye. A blow to the head can cause a concussive injury to the eye by tissue conduction of the waves of force. Similar ocular injuries may occur during an explosion, through conduction of airwaves.[93,94] The results of contusive and concussive injuries are variable. Although sometimes only the cornea is involved in an ocular contusion, damage to both anterior and posterior segment structures can also occur, as shown in Table 25-2. The extent of such injuries is often not obvious on initial examination. Careful follow-up is necessary in most cases to evaluate the total damage. The ophthalmologist should be aware that an injury by a blunt instrument or BB pellet severe enough to rupture the globe is likely to result in retinal damage incompatible with good vision. Injuries from automobile air bags also produce blunt trauma and have become more frequent.[105-111]

One particular entity associated with blunt trauma is traumatic posterior annular keratopathy, or traumatic

TABLE 25-2
Ocular Effects of Blunt Trauma

Eye Part	*Effect of Trauma*
Eyelids/conjunctiva	Ecchymosis
	Subconjunctival hemorrhage
	Laceration
Cornea	Abrasions
	Edema
	Tears in Descemet's membrane
	Traumatic corneal endothelial rings
Iris/ciliary body	Traumatic iritis/uveitis
	Traumatic mydriasis/miosis
	Iris sphincter tears
	Iridodialysis
	Hyphema
	Cyclodialysis
	Glaucoma (acute, late)
	Angle recession
Lens	Vossius ring
	Phakodonesis
	Subluxation
	Luxation
	Contusion cataract
Vitreous	Hemorrhage
Choroid	Rupture/tear
	Hemorrhage
	Detachment
Retina	Edema
	Hemorrhage
	Detachment
	Tear
Optic nerve	Atrophy
	Avulsion
Sclera	Rupture
Orbit	Fractures
	Hemorrhage

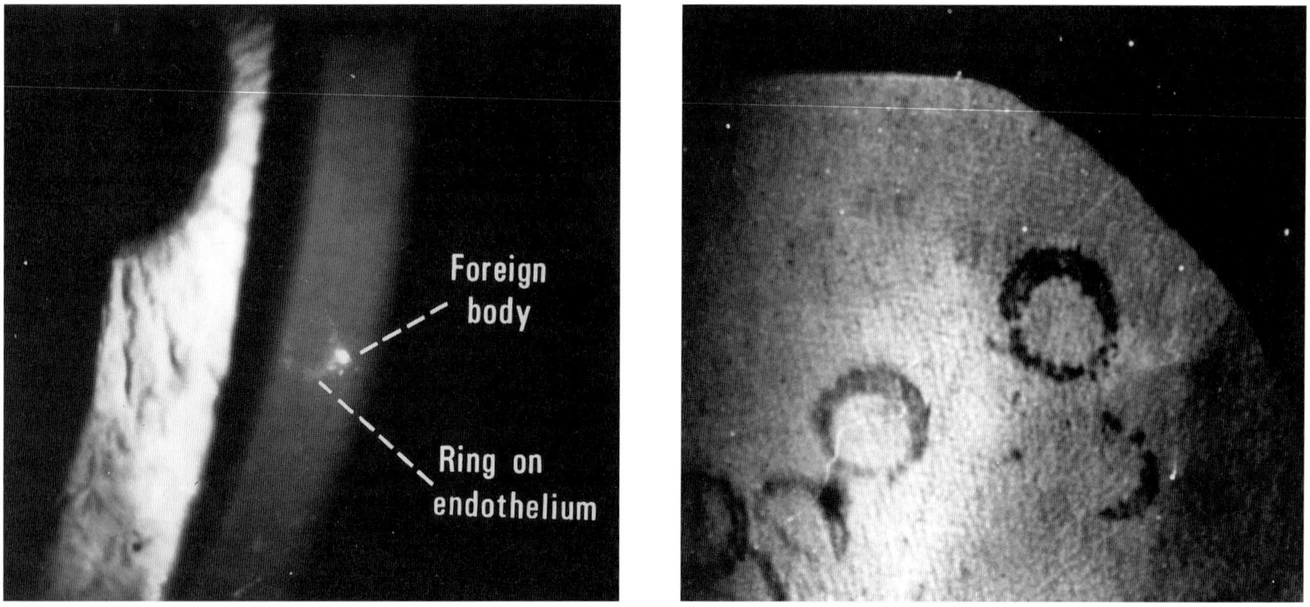

FIGURE 25-13 **(A)** Traumatic corneal endothelial ring. (Reprinted with permission from WF Maloney, M Colvard, WM Bourne, R Gardon: Specular microscopy of traumatic posterior annular keratopathy. Arch Ophthalmol 97:1647, 1979. Copyright 1979, American Medical Association.) **(B)** Specular photomicrograph of traumatic endothelial rings. (Reprinted with permission from GW Cibis, TA Weingeist, JH Krachmer: Traumatic corneal endothelial rings. Arch Ophthalmol 96:485, 1978. Copyright 1978, American Medical Association.)

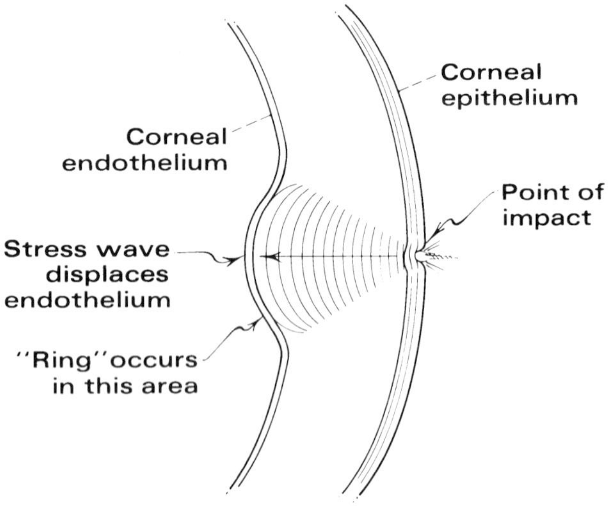

FIGURE 25-14 Pathogenesis of a traumatic corneal endothelial ring. (Reprinted with permission from WF Maloney, M Colvard, WM Bourne, R Gardon: Specular microscopy of traumatic posterior annular keratopathy. Arch Ophthalmol 97:1647, 1979. Copyright, 1979, American Medical Association.)

corneal endothelial rings.[112-115] These rings are whitish-gray and occur directly posterior to the impact of a foreign body (Figure 25-13). The intervening stroma is normal. The rings appear within several hours of a contusive injury and disappear within a few days. Specular microscopy has shown the rings to be composed of disrupted and swollen endothelial cells.[115] Experiments in animal models have also shown that the rings consist of disrupted and swollen endothelial cells to which fibrin and leukocytes adhere.[114] The pathogenesis of the rings is thought to be a concussive injury caused by the transfer of force from the impact site to the endothelium (Figure 25-14).

Tears in Descemet's membrane with central corneal hydrops are not uncommon with blunt trauma[116] (Figure 25-15). Sometimes the tear is visible through the edematous cornea. The condition is not helped by corticosteroids and frequently resolves in 6 weeks. If it has not resolved by 3 months, penetrating keratoplasty will probably be required.

Traumatic Hyphema

Although a hyphema is not a corneal injury, it frequently accompanies a corneal injury and deserves special attention during management of corneal trauma.

Pathogenesis

Blunt trauma causes an indentation of the anterior surface of the eye, as well as a sudden increase in intraocular pressure, stretching of limbal tissues, posterior and peripheral movement of aqueous humor, and retrodisplacement of the iris and lens. These mechanical deformations can tear the iris and/or ciliary body, usually in the anterior chamber angle.[117] The most common source of bleeding, reported in 71 to 94 percent of cases,[118,119] is a tear in the anterior face of the ciliary body, with resultant angle recession. The circular and oblique ciliary muscle fibers are torn from the longitudinal (meridional) fibers, which remain attached to the scleral spur.[22] Such an injury may disrupt the major arterial circle of the iris and arterial branches to the ciliary body. Postcontusion angle deformity is often noted when healing is completed. These residual changes are characterized by deepening of the anterior chamber locally, with posterior retraction of the angle recess, iris root, anterior ciliary processes, and circular and oblique ciliary muscle fibers.[120]

In traumatic cyclodialysis, the longitudinal ciliary muscle fibers are completely separated from the scleral spur, producing a cleft in the supraciliary space. Occasionally, a hyphema results. In contrast, iridodialyses (disinsertions of the iris root) and tears of the iris stroma or iris sphincter generally cause little or no bleeding, and are uncommon causes of hyphema.[22]

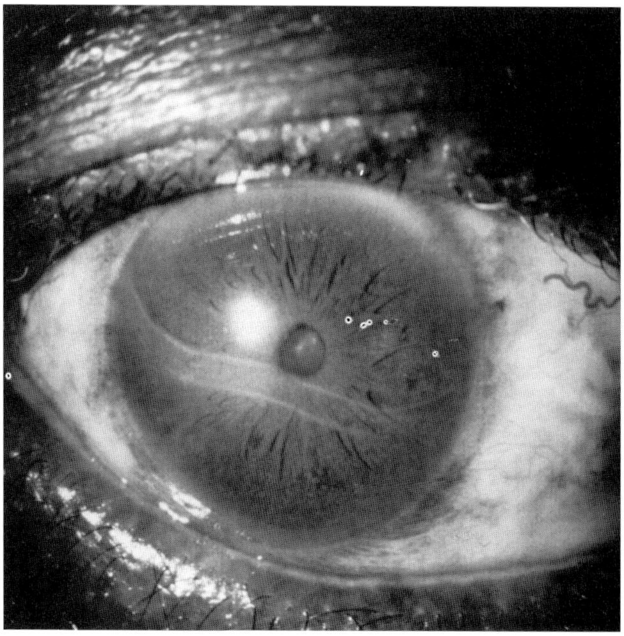

FIGURE 25-15 Rupture of Descemet's membrane. Note the parallel and continuous edges of the rupture.

Clinical Findings

The amount of blood present in the anterior chamber may vary from free-floating erythrocytes in the aqueous humor to large amounts that settle to the dependent portion of the anterior chamber, forming a layered hyphema (Figure 25-16). Total hyphemas that fill the anterior chamber and clot are often dark brown, black, or purple, and are referred to as *eight-ball* or *black-ball hyphemas.*

Classification of hyphemas can be useful in the clinical assessment of the severity of injury and its prognosis. Classification is also a useful guideline for management. It can be based on several variables, the most important of which appears to be the size of the initial hyphema. Edwards and Layden[121] used this variable as follows:

FIGURE 25-16 Traumatic hyphema.

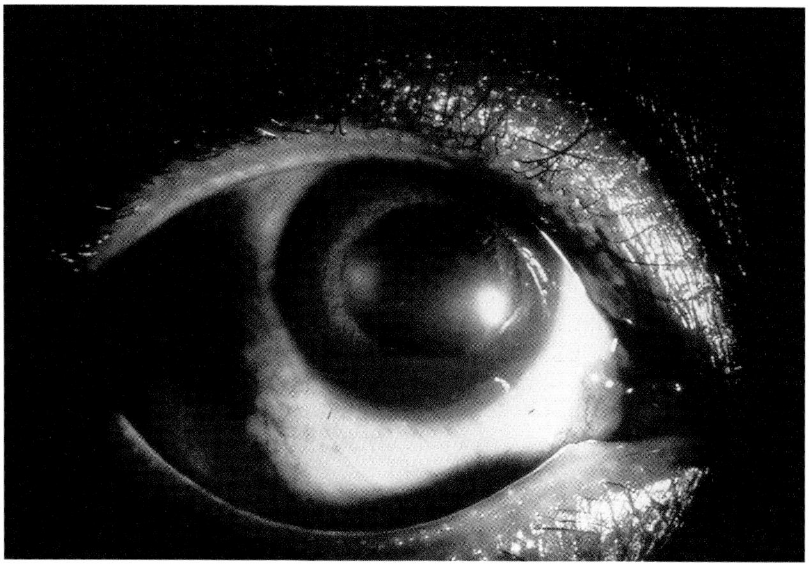

Grade I: hyphema that occupies less than one-third of the anterior chamber
Grade II: hyphema that occupies one-third to one-half of the anterior chamber
Grade III: hyphema that occupies one-half or more of the anterior chamber

Increased severity, poor prognosis, and complications are associated with larger hyphemas. Small hyphemas usually resolve in 4 to 5 days.[122] Grade II or III hyphemas are more frequently associated with rebleeding, glaucoma, corneal blood staining, delayed clearing of the blood, and poor visual results.[118,123] The chance of recovering visual acuity of 20/50 or better is 75 to 90 percent with grade I hyphemas, 65 to 70 percent with grade II hyphemas, and 25 to 50 percent with grade III hyphemas.[121,122] Thus, more aggressive therapy is required for grade II and grade III hyphemas.

Significant complications of hyphemas include secondary hemorrhage, glaucoma (acute or late), and corneal blood staining. The overall incidence of rebleeding after traumatic hyphemas is 20 to 25 percent.[91,122] However, the incidence ranges from 0 to 54 percent, depending on the severity of the initial hemorrhage, the treatment, and the series of patients reported.[121,122,124–127] Twenty-five percent of patients with a grade I hyphema have a secondary hemorrhage, compared with 65 percent of patients with a grade III hyphema. The majority of rebleeds occur 2 to 5 days after initial trauma, and nearly all occur before day 7.[119,122,124–127] Rebleeding worsens the prognosis because secondary hyphemas are usually larger than primary ones.[121,122,128,129] Approximately one-third of rebleeds are of grade III severity. The incidence of glaucoma with rebleeds is approximately 50 percent. The pathogenesis of rebleeding is unknown. Theories include bleeding of fragile new capillaries, or a possible relationship to fibrinolysis and retraction of clots and protein aggregates that had initially occluded the traumatized vessels.[125,126]

Three studies have indicated a markedly higher rate of secondary hemorrhage in black patients compared with that in white patients.[130–132] Other studies have failed to demonstrate a notable difference in hemorrhage rates between whites and blacks. Traumatic hyphema studies performed in areas with predominately white populations (e.g., Great Britain, Canada, Northern Europe, Minnesota, Australia) have all demonstrated secondary hemorrhage rates of less than 10 percent.[133–138]

Increased intraocular pressure may develop acutely after traumatic hyphema as a result of pupillary block by clotted blood and/or the tamponade effect of the red blood cells on the outflow pathway. Blood in the anterior chamber exits through the trabecular meshwork.[129,139,140] Although the iris is a source of fibrinolysin,[141] which frees erythrocytes from fibrin clots and allows them to escape via the trabecular meshwork, it is insignificant in absorbing blood. Approximately 6 to 10 percent of patients with traumatic hyphemas develop late glaucoma in association with postcontusion deformity of the angle.[22,91] The glaucoma may appear many years after the initial injury and is usually associated with recession of at least one-half of the angle.

Damage may occur in an otherwise healthy optic nerve if the intraocular pressure remains above 50 mmHg for more than 5 days, above 45 mmHg for more than 1 week, or above 35 mmHg for more than 2 weeks.[142] The risks increase for elderly patients and those with vascular disease.

Even small hyphemas in patients with sickle cell hemoglobinopathies can cause marked intraocular pressure elevations[143] because of the difficulty the elongated, rigid sickled erythrocytes have in traversing the corneoscleral meshwork, juxtacanalicular connective tissue, and inner wall of Schlemm's canal[144] (Figure 25-17). These patients are particularly susceptible to complications of high pressures because of sickling in vessels of the optic nerve and retina.[145–148] Sickle cell hyphemas, therefore, must be monitored closely and treated aggressively.

Corneal blood staining results from impregnation of the corneal stroma with hemoglobin and small amounts of hemosiderin (Figure 25-18). Predisposing factors include prolonged duration of a hyphema,[149] a large amount of blood in the anterior chamber, increased intraocular pressure, and dysfunction of the corneal endothelium.[91] Damage to Descemet's membrane and the endothelium may hasten the development of blood staining and may allow it to occur with normal intraocular pressure.[119,149,150] Corneal edema in the presence of a hyphema signifies that blood staining is imminent. Blood staining is likely to develop in any eye with a grade III hyphema when the intraocular pressure stays above 25 to 30 mmHg for more than 6 days.[91,122] Initially, the deep stroma shows a tan or rust color that is visible only on slit lamp microscopy. Later, the blood staining can affect the full thickness of the stroma and cause substantial loss of vision, the extent of which depends on both the location and intensity of the staining. In most cases, the blood staining clears eventually, beginning in the periphery and progressing centrally. The phagocytic process is slow and may take months to several years. Sometimes, if staining is severe or if the clot organizes to a retrocorneal fibrotic mass, penetrating keratoplasty is preferable to inaction. This is especially true for children, in whom loss of binocularity and amblyopia are risks.

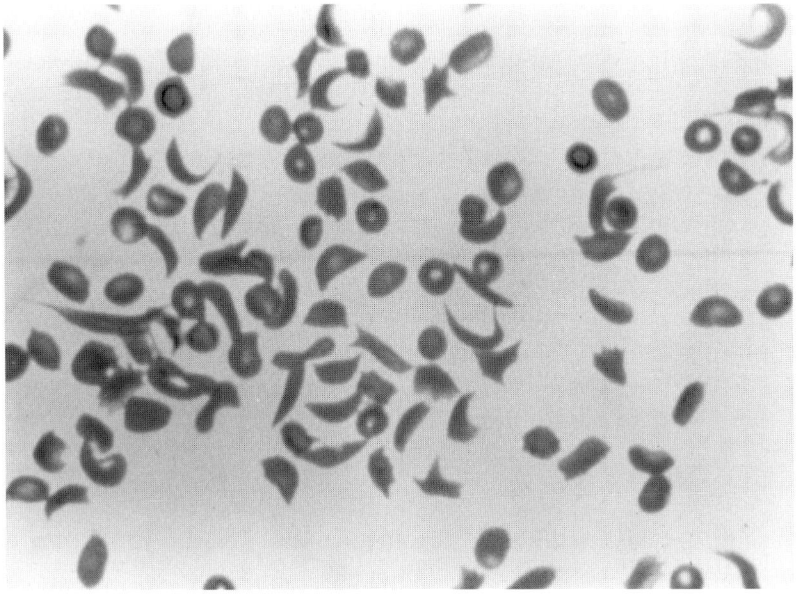

FIGURE 25-17 Elongated and rigid sickled red blood cells recovered from the anterior chamber of a patient with sickle cell hemoglobinopathy and traumatic hyphema.

Treatment

Although there is disagreement regarding treatment of hyphemas, goals include prevention of secondary hemorrhage, control of intraocular pressure, and prevention of corneal blood staining. Diseases or drugs (e.g., aspirin, anticoagulants) that contribute to abnormal bleeding or clotting should be identified during the initial history and physical examination. Aspirin ingestion at the time of injury is associated with increased incidence of rebleeding.[127,151,152] A screening test for sickle hemoglobin or a hemoglobin electrophoresis should be performed in all black patients. Gonioscopy should be avoided until the danger of rebleeding has passed.

Although some patients are hospitalized, especially those who are uncooperative or who have rebleeds or glaucoma, most small hyphemas are treated with relative inactivity or bed rest at home.

Medical Treatment A variety of drugs have been used in the treatment of traumatic hyphemas, including cycloplegics, miotics, sympathomimetics, corticosteroids, vitamins, calcium, rutin, estrogens, antifibrinolytic agents, carbonic anhydrase inhibitors, and osmotics. Havener[142] reviewed the subject in detail and concluded that "the spontaneous course of hyphema is totally unchanged by any form of medical management." For almost every study claiming to show benefits derived from a specific agent,

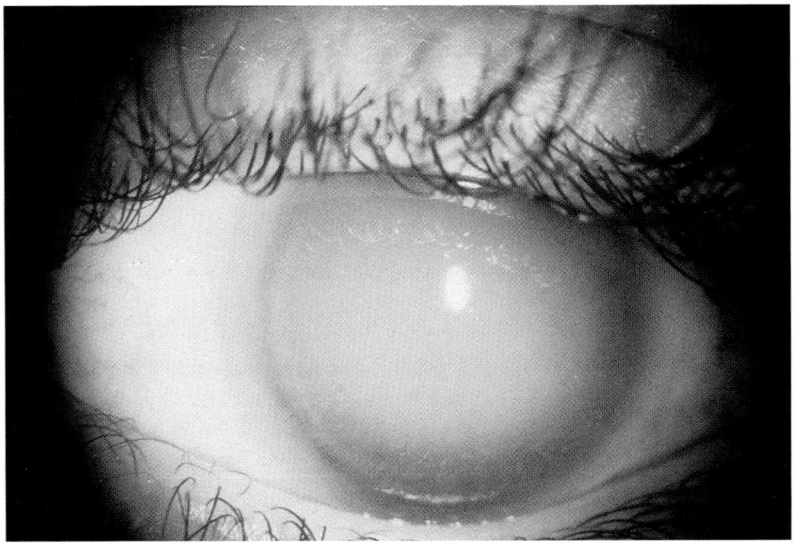

FIGURE 25-18 Corneal blood staining after a traumatic hyphema.

there is at least one contradictory study that shows a deleterious or no effect. Most authors agree that the final outcome depends more on the nature and severity of the injury than on any medical treatment prescribed by the physician. However, appropriate medications are indicated to treat complications.

There has been considerable controversy about the use of cycloplegics and miotics, and neither is of established value for routine use.

One controversy in the medical management of traumatic hyphemas is the use of aminocaproic acid (Amicar) to prevent secondary hemorrhage. Aminocaproic acid, an antifibrinolytic agent, competitively inhibits activation of profibrinolysin (plasminogen) to fibrinolysin (plasmin). This action prevents or delays clot dissolution and presumably allows more time for the traumatized vessels to regain their integrity without the occurrence of secondary hemorrhage, but the clinical value is uncertain.

In three randomized, double-masked studies, treatment with aminocaproic acid markedly decreased the risk of secondary hemorrhage in patients with traumatic hyphema.[125,153,154] Comparable findings were obtained in European studies,[155,156] in which different antifibrinolytic agents, such as tranexamic acid, were evaluated in human clinical trials. However, other studies did not show that treatment with aminocaproic acid is beneficial.[133,157] The rate of secondary hemorrhage (and therefore the risk to each patient) is so variable that confusion exists about the necessity of treatment.

Common side effects of aminocaproic acid are nausea and vomiting. Palmer et al[132] compared two dose regimens of aminocaproic acid for the treatment of traumatic hyphemas. They found that 50 mg/kg four times a day for 5 days (one-half the dose used by McGetrick et al[153]) had no adverse effect on the reduced rate of recurrent hemorrhage, was more cost-effective, and substantially reduced the more serious side effects of dizziness, hypotension, and syncope. The incidence of nausea and vomiting was approximately the same with both dose regimens. Aminocaproic acid is contraindicated if there is evidence of an active intravascular clotting process and in pregnancy. Based on animal studies, it should be used cautiously in patients with cardiac, hepatic, or renal disease.

A potent topical corticosteroid (e.g., prednisolone acetate or dexamethasone sodium phosphate) may be given four times a day to control inflammation. Latanoprost is used once a day, or timolol is used twice a day if the intraocular pressure is elevated. If marked elevations of intraocular pressure are present, topical or systemic carbonic anhydrase inhibitors may also be given. If necessary, osmotic agents may be used to treat intraocular pressure elevations that are unresponsive to timolol, latanoprost, and carbonic anhydrase inhibitors. Carbonic anhydrase inhibitors should be used with caution in patients with sickling hemoglobinopathies because they can cause hemoconcentration, systemic acidosis, and elevated levels of ascorbic acid, all of which can increase sickling. Osmotic agents should also be used with caution if at all in such patients because of their tendency to cause intracellular dehydration and exacerbate intravascular sickling.

Surgical Treatment As with medical therapy, there is no general agreement regarding the indications or optimal time for surgical intervention in the treatment of a hyphema. Surgery for a hyphema is not an innocuous procedure. Some studies[123,126,158] suggest that surgical intervention may actually worsen the prognosis. Surgical risks include damage to the cornea, iris, or lens; inadvertent extraction of the iris; rebleeding; prolapse of intraocular contents; increased inflammation and synechia formation; and postoperative glaucoma.[159]

Various criteria have been proposed as indications for surgery. Medically uncontrolled, elevated intraocular pressure that has reached a dangerous level is an obvious and undisputed indication for surgery. Goldberg[160] noted that in patients with sickle cell hemoglobinopathy, even moderate elevations of intraocular pressure produced rapid deterioration of the visual field. Therefore, surgical intervention is indicated earlier in this group.

In 1970, Sears[161] recommended waiting 4 days before removal of a total or black-ball hyphema. By this time, the clot is retracted and encapsulated by fibrin and has fewer connections to surrounding tissue, which allows easier removal. Subsequent pathologic evidence[162] supports this view. Read,[158] in 1975, recommended surgery under three conditions: when corneal blood staining is present; when a total hyphema is not more than 50 percent resolved at 6 days and the intraocular pressure is 25 mmHg or more; or when a hyphema remains unresolved for 9 days. Anterior synechiae are likely to develop after this time.[119] In 1983, Weiss et al[163] recommended that cases of total hyphema undergo prompt surgery unless the intraocular pressure is well controlled medically and there is evidence that spontaneous resolution of the hyphema is underway. In that most of their cases of total hyphema (73 percent in the reported series) eventually underwent surgery, they suggested that early surgery might reduce the incidence of optic nerve damage and corneal blood staining.

There is no single, universally accepted procedure for the surgical management of a hyphema. The simplest procedure is paracentesis[164] or release of blood through a small limbal incision. If these approaches are unsuccessful, an attempt may be made to irrigate blood from the anterior chamber, which usually requires enlarging the incision. An irrigating/aspirating instrument may be used through a single limbal incision. Vitrectors should be avoided unless there is good visualization. Fibrinolytic agents, such as tissue plasminogen activator (tPA), urokinase,[126] or fibrinolysin, have been used for irrigation, with varying degrees of success in cases where the blood is partially clotted. Thrombin may be injected intracamerally if rebleeding is apparent.

A large limbal incision is preferred by many[91,159] when dealing with a black-ball hyphema. If the clot does not prolapse spontaneously, it may be manually expressed with gentle pressure over the inferior limbus or gently rolled from the eye with a cellulose sponge or lens loop. A cryoprobe has been used to extract the clot,[161] but care must be taken to avoid incorporating the iris. Parrish and Bernardino[164] had good success performing a simple iridectomy, which was associated with complete absorption of the blood and relief of the associated glaucoma. They postulated that an iridectomy relieves the pupillary and/or angle block caused by the clot, thus re-establishing the aqueous humor circulation necessary for absorption of blood from the anterior chamber.

Should active bleeding occur during surgical manipulation, attempts are made to identify and cauterize the source. Most often, bleeding is from the ciliary body and cannot be directly reached. If thrombin does not stop the bleeding, diathermy can be applied to the overlying sclera.[91,165] A large air bubble placed in the anterior chamber can also be used to tamponade the bleeding.

PERFORATING INJURIES

Although perforating injuries vary considerably in type and severity, they carry a high risk of significant and permanent visual morbidity. Perforating injuries are a leading cause of unilateral vision loss in young adults.[166] A penetrating injury is one in which a tissue or structure is partially torn or cut. It has an entrance wound but no exit wound. In contrast, a perforating injury results in a tissue or structure that is torn or cut through completely, and has both an entrance and an exit wound. Therefore, a perforating injury of the cornea is a penetrating injury of the globe.

Perforating injuries of the cornea account for one-half to two-thirds of all penetrating injuries of the globe. Recovery from such injuries depends on three factors: degree of initial damage from both direct trauma and retinal contusion, efficacy of early treatment, and satisfactory management of complications.[167] Immediate complications after a perforating injury include iris prolapse, hemorrhage, cataract formation, various degrees of lens disruption, vitreous loss, and combinations of these.[168] Infections also pose a threat in the early period after injury.

Pathophysiology

Perforating injuries, including rupture of the globe by blunt trauma, cause varying amounts of initial damage. This damage may be so severe that the eye cannot be salvaged. Secondary complications may also lead to loss of the eye.

Faulty wound healing, which is a major cause of secondary complications, is frequently associated with loss of ocular structures, poor apposition of wound edges, and/or incarceration of intraocular tissues in the wound. Faulty wound healing, often accompanied by tissue or vitreous incarceration in the wound, may result in a dense, vascularized corneal scar, chronic wound leak, epithelial ingrowth, peripheral anterior synechiae, and intraocular fibrous tissue proliferation involving anterior segment structures. If tissue is left incarcerated in the wound, there is chronic edema of the scar, which thickens over time and vascularizes, often converting a non–visually disabling scar into a blinding one. Involvement of the vitreous may lead to its contraction and organization, producing transvitreal membranes and intravitreal fibrous proliferation. Complicated retinal detachments or cyclitic membrane formation may follow, resulting in ciliary body detachment, hypotony, and phthisis bulbi.

Microbial endophthalmitis can occur after any perforating injury, including those associated with metallic intraocular foreign bodies. The addition of specific antimicrobial agents to the physician's armamentarium has greatly decreased the incidence of postinjury infections and has improved the prognosis for useful vision.

Chronic intraocular inflammation is common in eyes after perforating injuries. A disrupted lens capsule is often associated with intraocular inflammation. Complicated wound healing in injuries with uveal or vitreous incarceration may cause traction on the iris or ciliary body and lead to chronic inflammation, as does intraocular hemorrhage. Chronic inflammation contributes to the development of secondary complications, including pupillary membranes, peripheral anterior synechiae, intraocular fibrosis, and vitreous organization. In rare instances, sympathetic ophthalmia may occur.

Other complications that may result in loss of the eye include glaucoma caused by mechanical damage to the anterior chamber angle structures or obstruction of the angle by inflammatory debris and/or erythrocytes. Large amounts of intravitreal blood may cause ocular

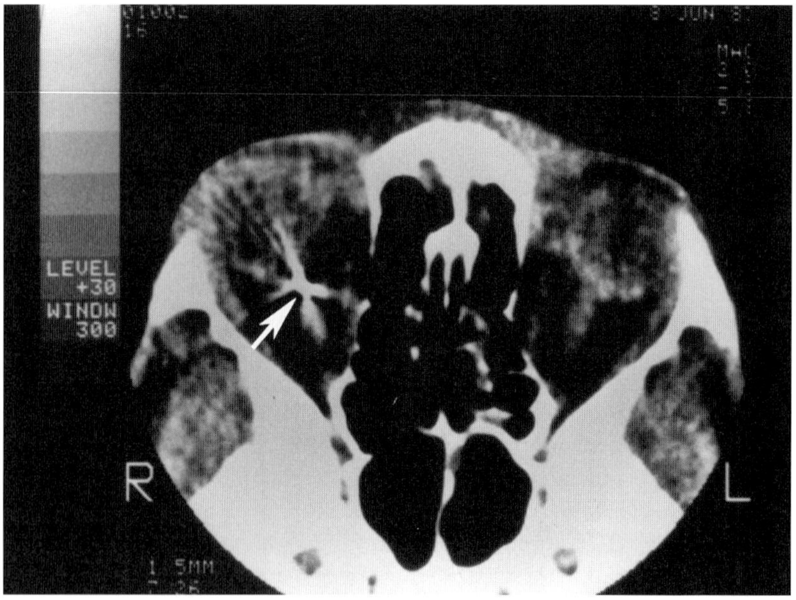

FIGURE 25-19 Axial computed tomography demonstrating a foreign body in the right optic nerve (arrow).

hemosiderosis, with cataract formation and retinal damage. Intraocular foreign bodies may result in toxic damage to ocular tissues or mechanical damage from contraction of the vitreous.

Preoperative Management

Examination and Assessment

Intraocular damage after a corneal laceration often cannot be adequately assessed during the initial examination because the patient is uncooperative or details are obscured by edema, chemosis, hemorrhage, and media opacities. Blunt trauma serious enough to cause even a small rupture carries a guarded prognosis.

During the preoperative examination, pressure on the globe must be meticulously avoided. Pressure exerted while opening the eyelids must be applied to the brow, not the globe itself, to avoid extrusion of the intraocular contents. Further damage can be avoided during the preoperative period by relieving blepharospasm with analgesics or a facial nerve block and by taping a protective shield over the eye. The shield should rest on the bony orbit and not on the eyelids. A minimal eye examination should include visual acuity, estimation of intraocular pressure, examination of the anterior segment, and an attempt to examine the posterior segment. If the examination is painful or might endanger the integrity of the globe, the entire evaluation of the extent of injury is completed after the patient is under general anesthesia. Measurement of visual acuity must always be performed, however, especially for medicolegal reasons.

In any perforating injury, it is important to determine the presence or absence of an intraocular foreign body. If the media are clear, the simplest and most reliable way to detect a foreign body, or lack thereof, is by direct and indirect ophthalmoscopy. Computerized axial tomography is superior to a simple radiograph in that it detects foreign bodies with greater sensitivity and provides better tissue localization (Figure 25-19).

Tetanus Prophylaxis

After perforating injuries, tetanus immunization in the form of intramuscular tetanus toxin is recommended. The American College of Surgeons' Committee on Trauma recommends an initial immunizing dose or a booster for previous immunization unless the patient has completed the initial immunizing series within the last 5 years.

Prophylactic Antibiotics

There is no unanimity regarding the administration of prophylactic antibiotics. Paton and Goldberg[91] recommended that broad-spectrum parenteral antibiotics be started promptly and continued for at least 3 days after surgery, in addition to subconjunctival antibiotics injected at the completion of surgery. If prophylactic antibiotics are given, both gram-positive and gram-negative organisms should be covered. For example, intravenous administration of an aminoglycoside, such as gentamicin, 3 mg/kg/day in three divided doses, and a cephalosporin, such as cephalothin, 1.5 g every 6 hours, provides such coverage. If prophylactic antibiotics are used, a culture should be obtained first. Dosages of antibiotics need to be modified for children and patients with impaired renal function. Other types of infection should be considered; for instance, wood or plant foreign bodies are most likely to be contaminated with fungus.

Surgical Management

Surgical repair should be performed as soon as the condition of the patient and operating room facilities are optimal. With delay, corneal wounds become increasingly edematous, making suturing more difficult. Lens damage and tissue prolapse often result in a fibrinous reaction, and the risk of intraocular hemorrhage increases. Although surgery should not be deferred any longer than necessary, repair should not be attempted without the assistance of personnel trained in the use of ocular microsurgical instruments and techniques.

General anesthesia is preferred to avoid the increased orbital pressure that may occur with retrobulbar anesthesia. The anesthesiologist should be aware of the status of the open eye to avoid inducing squeezing, coughing, or other manipulations that may result in loss of intraocular contents. The use of succinylcholine should be avoided, because it causes an initial co-contraction of the extraocular muscles and may potentiate the loss of intraocular contents. If general anesthesia is contraindicated because of the patient's general health, injection of 0.5 to 1 ml of anesthetic over each rectus muscle combined with a Nadbath nerve block can be used. Injection of anesthetic for a Van Lint block commonly causes the patient to squeeze the eyelids and should be avoided.

Perforating injuries of the cornea and sclera vary both in the mechanism of injury and in the extent of resulting tissue damage. Thus, as in other forms of trauma surgery, there can be no standard technique of repair. It is, therefore, important to stress the principles of reconstruction rather than the details.

The primary repair should be the definitive reconstruction as far as possible. The same techniques of repair are applicable to corneal, scleral, and combined corneoscleral injuries. The basic objectives are adequate wound closure; removal of all abnormal tissue and foreign material from within the wound; reformation of the anterior chamber; and thorough exploration of the eye to rule out posterior rupture, intraocular foreign body, and retinal detachment. Excised tissue is difficult to identify at the time of surgery and should be submitted for pathologic examination. If all excised tissue is not necessary for pathologic study, it should be cultured. The importance of removing all material from the wound, especially lens capsule and vitreous, cannot be overemphasized and the surgeon should not hesitate to make limbal incisions and use a viscoelastic substance to make certain the wound is free of incarcerated tissue. Incarcerated tissue makes a corneal scar dense and wide and often leads to an avoidable visual handicap.

Primary enucleation of a traumatized eye is reserved for the most severe derangement of the globe (e.g., direct bullet injury or explosion). Salvaging the globe and obtaining useful vision have been reported after severe ocular injuries. If there is no chance for useful vision after surgery, enucleation can be performed later. Enucleation within 2 weeks is believed to prevent sympathetic ophthalmia. Even an unsuccessful attempt to repair the eye provides psychological benefits to the patient, who has the added time to adjust to the severity of the injury and the reassurance that every effort was made to save the eye.

The preferred suture for corneal wounds is 10-0 nylon. The depth of the sutures should be as close to Descemet's membrane as possible without perforation. Sutures placed too shallowly cause posterior gaping, which results in a scar that may become edematous and increase in thickness and density with time. It also leaves an irregular posterior surface to which iris can adhere during healing, forming anterior synechiae, and leads to flattening of the corneal curvature.

Corneal wounds without tissue edema can generally be repaired with interrupted sutures, with tissue bites 1 to 2 mm from each wound edge. Marked edema requires larger bites, up to 2.5 mm on each side. The suture loosens postoperatively unless it extends beyond the area of edema on each side of the wound and is tied tightly. When larger tissue bites are needed, a needle with a larger radius of curvature is advantageous. With such a needle, the wound can be closed by completing the arc of the needle's curvature, rather than by dragging the needle through the tissues in an attempt to make a wider bite than the arc of the needle allows. The knots are buried by rotating them into the stroma to minimize discomfort and vascularization.

Puncture Wounds

Puncture wounds (less than 2.0 mm) that perforate the cornea usually heal without being sutured. These injuries can sometimes be managed with a bandage soft contact lens, patching, and/or tissue adhesive as discussed below.

Corneal Lacerations

Penetrating corneal lacerations usually do not need suturing unless there is anterior gaping of the wound. Perforating lacerations require suturing unless they are self sealing. Shelved lacerations are more likely to be self sealing than lacerations with vertical edges.

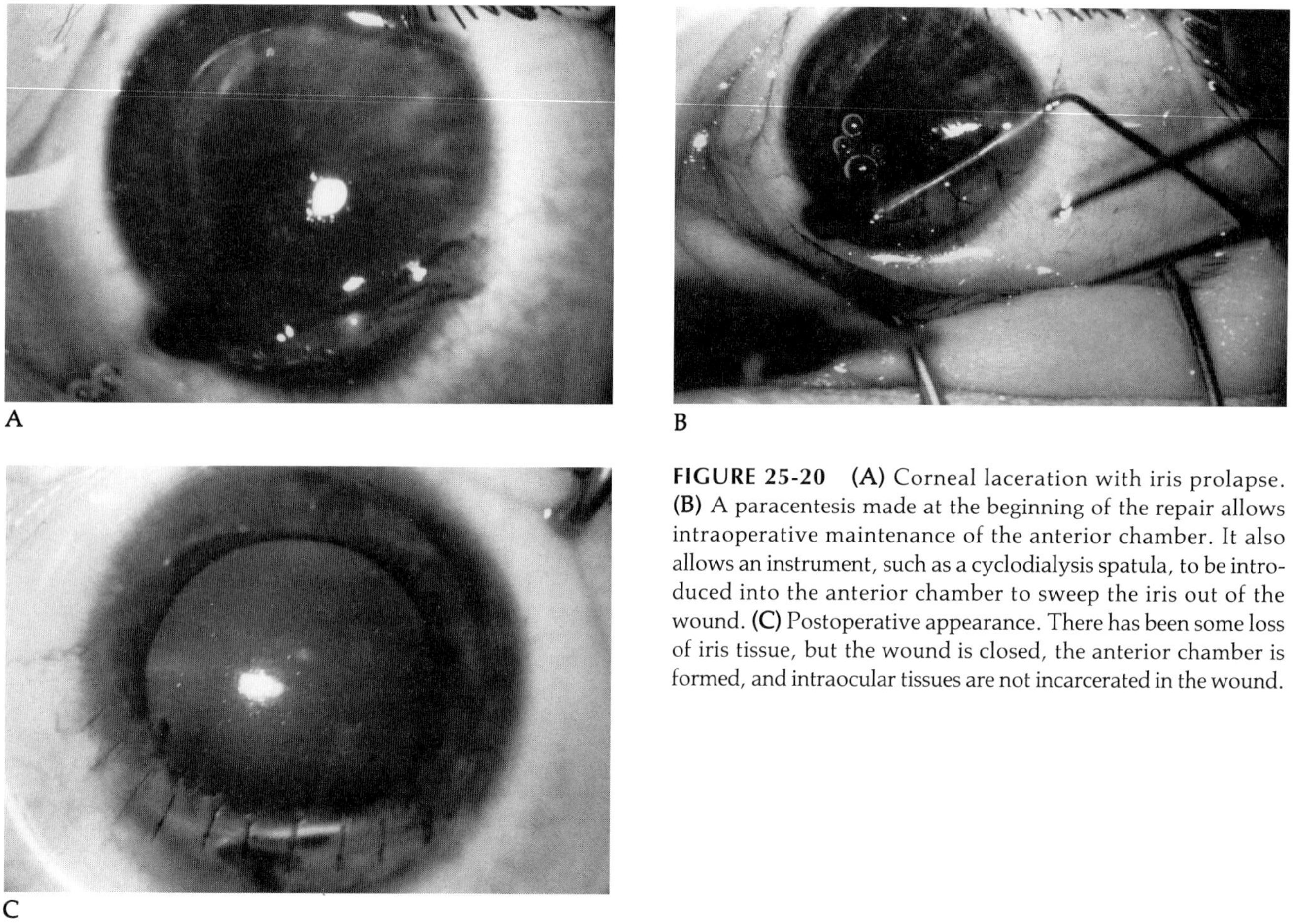

FIGURE 25-20 (A) Corneal laceration with iris prolapse. (B) A paracentesis made at the beginning of the repair allows intraoperative maintenance of the anterior chamber. It also allows an instrument, such as a cyclodialysis spatula, to be introduced into the anterior chamber to sweep the iris out of the wound. (C) Postoperative appearance. There has been some loss of iris tissue, but the wound is closed, the anterior chamber is formed, and intraocular tissues are not incarcerated in the wound.

Adequate corneal exposure is obtained with a speculum or eyelid sutures, and the globe is immobilized with fixation sutures or a Flieringa ring. Distortion of the globe must be avoided to ensure accurate wound apposition. Careful inspection is performed to confirm the type and extent of injury. Painstaking assessment of the structural damage sustained by the injured globe is an essential first stage in primary reconstruction. Care is taken not to cause additional insult to the tissues. Corneal lacerations may be classified as linear, stellate, or avulsing.

Linear Lacerations Linear lacerations are closed with interrupted sutures. Opposing wound edges are matched carefully. Linear displacement of the wound edge during suturing is undesirable and may create postoperative astigmatism.

When the laceration is limited to the cornea, the anterior chamber is formed at the beginning of the operation. It is helpful to perform a paracentesis with a knife through the peripheral cornea before repairing the wound. This procedure creates a useful opening through which balanced salt solution, air, or a viscoelastic substance can be injected to maintain or reform the anterior chamber while corneal sutures are placed (Figure 25-20). It also allows introduction of instruments to free incarcerated tissue. This technique enables repair of the laceration with reconstruction of the normal corneal contour and provides a method of freeing adherent iris from the posterior aspects of the wound. Air helps delineate the presence and location of vitreous in the anterior chamber. Before completion of the surgical repair, air or the viscoelastic substance should be removed and replaced with balanced salt solution. This eliminates the risks of air-block glaucoma and anterior synechiae that can occur with air posterior to the iris and lessens the likelihood of marked elevations of intraocular pressure caused by large amounts of intracameral viscoelastic substance. It also permits more accurate assessment of the wound closure for leaks.

Stellate Lacerations When a laceration is irregular or stellate, more complex suture patterns provide better apposition of the corneal fragments. Matching of irregular wound edges is best accomplished by visually aligning the irregular portions first and placing deep interrupted sutures to firmly fix the matched areas. The remainder of the wound is then closed with a purse string suture or a horizontal mattress suture, both of which are useful in irregular wounds. A single purse string suture may be the only closure necessary for a complex stellate laceration. A running suture can virtually never be used in such cases, because the ideal reapproximation of tissue is more difficult.

Avulsing Lacerations Debridement of the wound is inadvisable in an avulsing injury, because small, attached, or even free pieces of lacerated cornea can be used as autografts to seal the wound. If watertight suturing cannot be achieved, cyanoacrylate adhesive with a contact lens or donor cornea or sclera may be used to ensure adequate wound closure. It is advisable for all ophthalmologists to have immediate access to frozen sclera, whole eyes, or precarved lyophilized tissue for such emergencies. These tissues can be used as patch grafts to obtain wound integrity until a subsequent penetrating keratoplasty is performed if necessary.

Adjunctive Techniques for Wound Closure

Bandage Soft Contact Lens Soft contact lenses may be used as a primary treatment modality for small corneal lacerations (less than 3 mm). According to Leibowitz,[169] the indications for the use of a bandage soft contact lens to treat corneal lacerations include small wounds with well-approximated edges and no incarcerated uveal tissue or extruded lens material. In his series of cases selected on the basis of these criteria, wound healing progressed uneventfully, with excellent visual results. It is recommended that patients undergoing this mode of therapy be hospitalized to allow aggressive use of antibiotics and close observation.

Adhesives Since the 1970s, the use of tissue adhesive (cyanoacrylate) has become an important closure technique in corneal disease.[92,170] Because of the effectiveness of appositional suturing, the use of tissue adhesive in large lacerations is limited. For a stellate laceration, a purse string suture will usually close the wound, but adhesive applied over the sutures may occasionally be necessary.[93]

The main use of tissue adhesive in trauma is as the primary bonding agent to seal small corneal perforations[170] (Figure 25-21). Because of the potential toxicity of the material, it should not be used in cases in which it can enter the anterior chamber. The wound should be of limited size, with good apposition of the wound edges and no tissue incarceration. Before placement of the tissue adhesive, the site of the perforation must be meticulously dried with a cellulose sponge. If there is marked egress of aqueous humor, air or a viscoelastic substance can be injected into the anterior chamber through a separate limbal puncture. The smallest amount of tissue adhesive that seals the perforation is applied. A bandage soft contact lens is placed, which protects the adhesive from the blinking action of the eyelids and lessens the foreign body sensation. The adhesive usually sloughs spontaneously in several weeks to months, by which time fibroblastic scar tissue has generally sealed the perforation.

Another use of tissue adhesive is the temporary sealing of traumatized tissues during lamellar or penetrating keratoplasty. This maneuver makes the globe firm enough that a trephine incision can be made or a superficial keratectomy performed. In a situation in which the anterior segment is collapsed, the volume can be replaced temporarily with air or a viscoelastic substance, and the hole sealed with tissue adhesive. The initial steps of lamellar or penetrating keratoplasty can then be more easily accomplished. Alternatively, a suction trephine, such as the Barron radial vacuum trephine, can be used in cases of penetrating keratoplasty for corneal perforation.

Keratoplasty For corneal perforations that cannot be closed with sutures and are too large to be sealed with tissue adhesive, a lamellar patch graft is indicated if the perforation is in the corneal periphery and does not involve the visual axis. Donor cornea (fresh or from a frozen whole globe stored at −70°C) or sclera (fresh or frozen) can be used for the patch (Figure 25-22). The techniques of inlay and onlay lamellar keratoplasty are discussed in Chapters 31 and 32. Penetrating keratoplasty may be necessary if there has been extensive tissue loss (see Ch. 34).

Corneoscleral Lacerations

If a corneal laceration approaches the limbus, a conjunctival peritomy and exploration are necessary to ensure that the laceration has not extended into the sclera. Lacerations are often much larger than anticipated. Every corneal laceration approaching the limbus should be presumed to extend into the sclera until proved otherwise.

The principles of scleral repair are similar to those described for corneal lacerations. The first suture should realign the limbus. The limbus is usually a readily identifiable landmark, and its closure helps to ensure proper wound alignment. For limbal and corneal sutures, 9-0 or 10-0 nylon is used. For sclera, 9-0 nylon sutures are used. Scleral sutures should not be full thickness, because such sutures can incarcerate the uvea. Interrupted sutures are the most suitable for closure of a scleral laceration. The scleral wound edges must be matched carefully. Incarceration of uveal tissue in the wound is undesirable and should be avoided. Surface diathermy or cryotherapy may be applied around the area of injury after the laceration has been sutured.

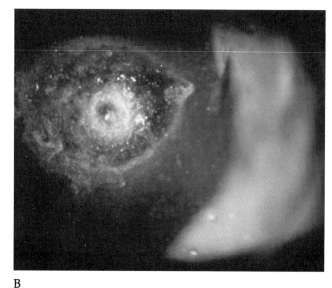

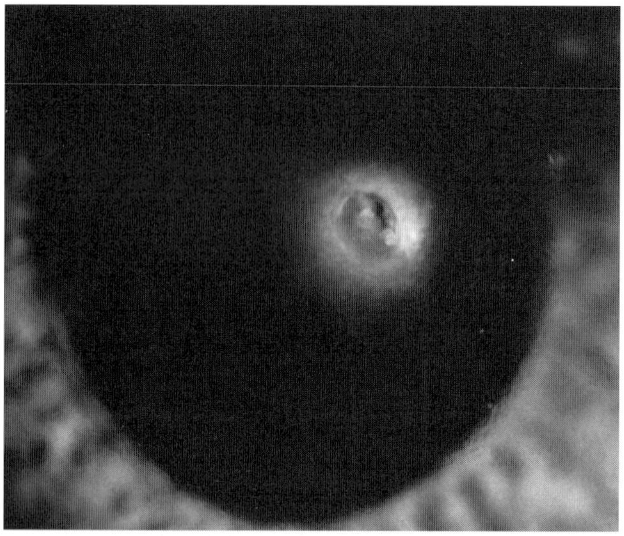
A

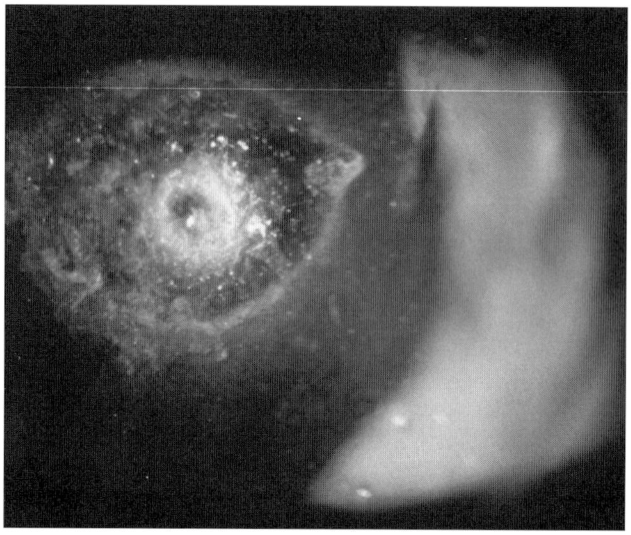
B

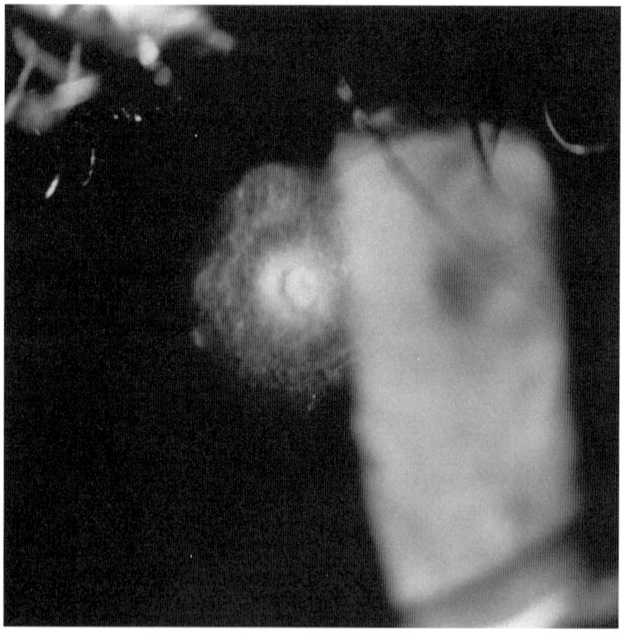
C

FIGURE 25-21 **(A)** Small paracentral traumatic corneal perforation. **(B)** Because of the proximity to the visual axis, tissue adhesive was applied to seal the perforation. A lamellar patch graft would have distorted the cornea in the visual axis, and penetrating keratoplasty would have carried more risks. **(C)** The adhesive spontaneously sloughed in 4 months, leaving the perforation sealed but surrounded by an area of stromal haze. Visual acuity was 20/40. Visual acuity eventually improved to 20/25.

If a scleral laceration results in loss of tissue or sufficient damage to the wound edges such that proper wound closure with sutures is not possible, a hinged scleral flap or scleral patch graft from eye bank sclera may be used. The donor sclera may be cut with a trephine or by a freehand technique to the required size and shape. The lacerated tissues are approximated as closely and accurately as possible and sutured with nylon suture. The split- or full-thickness scleral patch graft is then sutured over the damaged area.

In injuries involving perforation of the globe, the anterior entrance site should be repaired on the basis of the surgical principles just described. Small posterior exit wounds are usually self sealing, but larger wounds generally require repair. Management of iris, ciliary body, lens, and vitreous prolapse is discussed below.

Management of Associated Structural Damage

Corneal trauma is frequently accompanied by anterior and posterior segment injuries such as iris prolapse or laceration, lens disruption, and vitreous incarceration. There is sufficient evidence that repair of associated anterior segment abnormalities at the time of primary corneal repair offers many advantages. Intraocular inflammation is reduced, synechiae and secondary membranes are less readily formed, and the incidence of glaucoma is reduced. The endothelium is protected from contact with various intraocular structures, and visualization of the posterior segment is made possible. The need for further surgery may be obviated. Advances in mechanical microsurgical instrumentation have made intraocular repair possible, and the corneal surgeon should not hesitate to undertake simultaneous anterior segment repair.

Iris When iris tissue is incarcerated in a corneal wound, the pupil assumes a characteristic pear-shaped appearance, with peaking toward the wound. If the iris remains deep within the wound without reaching the surface of the globe, it should be reposited rather than excised. A variety of techniques can be used to reposit the iris.

Irrigation of the wound with acetylcholine hydrochloride or carbachol can be useful in releasing the iris. Injection of air or a viscoelastic substance through a limbal incision 90 degrees from the wound and the use of an iris repositor are also helpful. If the iris can easily be reposited by freeing it from the sphincter toward the periphery, the small risk of iridodialysis can be avoided; however, inserting a cyclodialysis spatula under the cornea near the iris root around the length of the adhesion, pushing down on the spatula, and moving it centrally is often most effective. Reformation of a round pupil indicates that no adhesions remain.

If the injury extends to the limbus, a small peripheral iridectomy may be performed at the lateral extent to prevent formation of anterior synechiae. A peripheral iridectomy is recommended when there is peripheral incarceration of the iris. The iridectomy may be made within or peripheral to the incarcerated portion of iris. If a large amount of fibrin or inflammatory debris is present, a peripheral iridectomy helps prevent late reincarceration and synechia formation.

In corneal lacerations with iris prolapse, the iris may be safely reposited if it appears clean and viable. Any epithelium that has grown over the iris must be removed before repositing the iris. Iris that is frankly necrotic or contaminated with foreign material should be excised to reduce the possibility of contaminating the anterior chamber with pathogenic organisms. The designation of a specific time after which iris should not be reposited, such as 12, 24, or 36 hours after injury, is inappropriate. The decision should be based on the surgeon's judgment as to the general appearance of the eye and the ease with which the iris can be reposited.

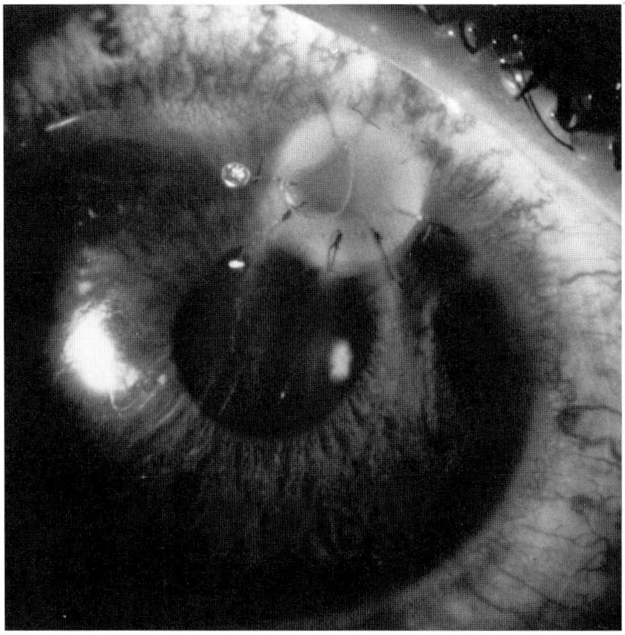

FIGURE 25-22 Patch graft for a peripheral corneal perforation. A small air bubble can be seen trapped under the bandage soft contact lens.

If the wound is clean and the iris can be reposited with minimal trauma, it is advisable to do so. Repositing the iris becomes particularly important if the prolapse occurs in the inferior quadrants, where an iridectomy would likely result in a photophobic, uncomfortable eye. It is less significant in a superior quadrant prolapse, in which the eyelid provides adequate coverage of an iridectomy.

No attempt should be made to reposit iris or other uveal tissue at any time after injury in an inflamed eye that has foreign material in the anterior chamber. Similarly, if the prolapsed iris is difficult to reposit after repeated manipulation, excision is indicated. Sometimes it may be difficult to differentiate iris from ciliary body. Therefore, excision should be limited to prolapsed uveal tissue that is definitely iris; the remainder should be reposited.

When the iris is severely lacerated or when an extensive iridectomy is necessary to remove necrotic tissue, surgical repair of the iris defect should be considered at the time of primary repair if sufficient iris tissue remains. If the primary laceration does not provide adequate exposure for iris repair, the laceration may be extended, or preferably, the corneal laceration closed and a separate limbal incision made. One or two interrupted 10-0 polypropylene sutures can be used to re-establish the pupil. Sutures should be placed near the midportion of the iris. Sutures at the iris sphincter should be avoided, because a small, nondilating pupil results.

Ciliary Body Prolapsed ciliary body should be reposited, with rare exception. Excision may be necessary if the ciliary body is severely traumatized, necrotic, or markedly contaminated. Cyclectomy may also be required to control bleeding that persists from a lacerated ciliary body. Transscleral diathermy should encircle any portion of ciliary body to be excised to minimize the complications of hemorrhage and ciliary body detachment.[171]

Trauma to uveal tissue, especially the ciliary body, is thought to predispose to sympathetic ophthalmia. Involvement of the ciliary body in a combined corneoscleral laceration decreases the prognosis for salvage of the globe and visual recovery. Painstaking repair and anterior segment reconstruction are necessary to prevent fibrous ingrowth. The eye should be evaluated within 8 to 10 days postoperatively to determine whether the globe is salvageable or should be enucleated to minimize the chance of sympathetic ophthalmia.[91]

Lens Small lacerations of the lens that may be self sealing (e.g., lacerations less than 2 mm) or simple opacities of the lens are not indications for immediate lensectomy. It is possible that the subsequent cataract may be minimal and localized and cause no vision loss. Small metallic foreign bodies have remained lodged in the lens for many years without subsequent cataract formation.

If definite lens rupture occurs, resulting in an opaque lens and flocculent lens fibers, the lens material should be removed during primary repair of the laceration. Several methods may be used for lens removal. If the laceration is large, the lens material may be aspirated directly through the corneal wound. If exposure is inadequate, the corneal laceration should be repaired first and the lens extracted with an irrigation/aspiration cannula or a phacoemulsification instrument through a separate limbal incision. A pars plana lensectomy and vitrectomy constitute an alternative approach for removal of lens fragments and vitreous. No matter which technique is used, the posterior aspect of the cornea should be free of all adherent material.

A critical problem in lens removal may be poor visualization of anterior chamber anatomy due to fibrin, lens material, and/or hemorrhage. The possibility exists that anterior or posterior segment structures could be incorporated into the lens fragments that are to be aspirated. Therefore, great caution is necessary when performing such procedures during the primary surgical repair.

Complete visual rehabilitation should be considered at the time of the initial repair. Depending on the degree of disruption of the anterior segment, an intraocular lens may be implanted at the time of cataract extraction.

Vitreous Prolapsed vitreous should be meticulously cleaned from a corneoscleral or scleral laceration. A partial vitrectomy may be necessary, especially when vitreous is mixed with ruptured lens material. Depending on associated injuries, an anterior segment or pars plana approach may be more appropriate. When a laceration extends posterior to the ora serrata, cryotherapy or diathermy may be used to help prevent retinal detachment, and vitrectomy may be necessary.

The role of damaged vitreous in the proliferation of intraocular fibrous tissue and secondary vitreoretinal complications is well documented.[172–174] Condensed vitreous that often forms along the path of a penetrating injury provides a scaffold for fibrous proliferation.[175] Vitrectomy performed soon after injury prevents intravitreal fibrous proliferation except on the retinal surface in the immediate vicinity of the scleral wound.[176]

It is generally recommended that vitrectomy for severe posterior segment damage be performed between 4 and 10 days after primary repair. This timing is thought to be optimal to avoid the hazards of immediate intervention (i.e., uncontrolled hemorrhage) while removing damaged tissue before serious sequelae occur.[177] This also permits spontaneous separation of the posterior vitreous face from the retina, facilitating removal of the posterior vitreous.

Prognosis

Although prognosis for penetrating injuries involving the anterior segment has improved over the past few decades,[178–181] injuries with contusions and those involving the posterior segment continue to have a poor prognosis when managed by current methods.

REFERENCES

1. Huang AJW, Tseng SCG, Kenyon KR: Morphogenesis of rat conjunctival goblet cells. Invest Ophthalmol Vis Sci 29:969, 1988
2. Tseng SCG: Concept and application of limbal stem cells. Eye 3:141, 1989
3. Chen JJY, Tseng SCG: Corneal epithelial wound healing in partial limbal deficiency. Invest Ophthalmol Vis Sci 31:1301, 1990
4. Huang AJW, Tseng SCG: Corneal epithelial wound healing in the absence of limbal epithelium. Invest Ophthalmol Vis Sci 32:96, 1991
5. Kruse FE, Chen JJY, Tsai RJF, Tseng SCG: Conjunctival transdifferentiation is due to the incomplete removal of limbal basal epithelium. Invest Ophthalmol Vis Sci 31:1903, 1990
6. Tseng SCG, Li D-Q: Comparison of protein kinase C subtype expression between normal and aniridic human ocular surfaces: implications for limbal stem cell dysfunction in aniridia. Cornea 15:168, 1996

7. Tsai RJ-F, Tseng SCG: Human allograft limbal transplantation for corneal surface reconstruction. Cornea 13:389, 1994
8. Tseng SCG, Zhang S-H: Limbal epithelium is more resistant to 5-fluorouracil toxicity than corneal epithelium. Cornea 14:394, 1995
9. Goldman JM, Dohlman CH, Kravitt BA: The basement membrane of the human cornea in recurrent epithelial erosion syndrome. Trans Am Acad Ophthalmol Otolaryngol 73:471, 1969
10. Fujikawa LS, Foster CS, Gipson IK, Colvin RB: Basement membrane components in healing rabbit corneal epithelial wounds: immunofluorescence and ultrastructural studies. J Cell Biol 98:128, 1984
11. Clark RAF, Winn HJ, Dvorak HF, Colvin RB: Fibronectin beneath re-epithelializing epidermis in vivo: sources and significance. J Invest Dermatol 80(suppl):26s, 1983
12. Nishida T, Nakagawa S, Awata T, et al: Fibronectin promotes epithelial migration of cultured rabbit cornea in situ. J Cell Biol 97:1683, 1983
13. Gipson IK, Keezer L: Effects of cytochalasins and colchicine on the ultrastructure of migrating corneal epithelium. Invest Ophthalmol Vis Sci 22:643, 1982
14. Weimar V: Activation of the corneal stromal cells to take up the vital dye neutral red. Exp Cell Res 18:1, 1959
15. O'Brien WJ, DeCarlo JD, Stern M, Hyndiuk RA: Effects of Timoptic on corneal re-epithelialization. Arch Ophthalmol 100:1331, 1982
16. Weimer VL: The transformation of corneal stromal cells to fibroblasts in corneal wound healing. Am J Ophthalmol 44(Part II):173, 1957
17. Weimar V, Haraguchi K: The development of enzyme activities in corneal connective tissue cells during the lag phase of wound repair: 1.5 nucleotidase and succinic dehydrogenase. Invest Ophthalmol 4:853, 1965
18. Newsome DA, Foidart J-M, Hassal JR, et al: Detection of specific collagen types in normal and keratoconus corneas. Invest Ophthalmol Vis Sci 20:738, 1981
19. Funderburgh JL, Stenzel-Johnson PR, Chandler JW: Corneal glycosaminoglycan synthesis in long-term organ culture. Invest Ophthalmol Vis Sci 24:208, 1983
20. Gassett AR, Dohlman CH: The tensile strength of corneal wounds. Arch Ophthalmol 79:592, 1968
21. Sugar J, Chandler JW: Experimental corneal wound strength: effect of topically applied corticosteroids. Arch Ophthalmol 92:248, 1974
22. Yanoff M, Fine BS: Ocular Pathology: A Text and Atlas. Harper & Row, Philadelphia, 1982
23. Jensen P, Minckler DS, Chandler JW: Epithelial ingrowth. Arch Ophthalmol 95:837, 1977
24. Beuerman RW, Thompson HW: Molecular and cellular responses of the corneal epithelium to wound healing. Acta Ophthalmol (Copenh) 70:7, 1992
25. Thompson H, Thompson J, Lockyer J, Beuerman RW: Protooncogene expression during corneal wound healing. p. 59. In Beuerman RW, Crossen CE, Kaufman HE (eds): Healing Processes in the Cornea. Portfolio Publications Co., The Woodlands, TX, 1989
26. van Setten G-B: Epidermal growth factor in human tear fluid: increased release but decreased concentrations during reflex tearing. Curr Eye Res 9:79, 1990
27. Li Q, Weng J, Mohan RR, et al: Hepatocyte growth factor and hepatocyte growth factor receptor in the lacrimal gland, tears, and cornea. Invest Ophthalmol Vis Sci 37:727, 1996
28. Tervo K, van Setten G-B, Beuerman RW, et al: Expression of tenascin and cellular fibronectin in the rabbit cornea after anterior keratectomy. Invest Ophthalmol Vis Sci 32:2912, 1991
29. Vaheri A, Salonen E-M, Vartio T: Fibronectin in formation and degradation of the pericellular matrix. p. 111. In Evered D, Whelan J (eds): Fibrosis. Ciba Foundation Symposium. Pitman, London, 1985
30. Fini ME, Parks WC, Rinehart WB, et al: Role of matrix metalloproteinases in failure to re-epithelialize after corneal injury. Am J Pathol 149:1287, 1996
31. Crosson CE, Klyce S, Beuerman RW: Epithelial wound closure in the rabbit cornea. Invest Ophthalmol Vis Sci 27:464, 1986
32. Assouline M, Chew SJ, Thompson HW, Beuerman R: Effect of growth factors on collagen lattice contraction by human keratocytes. Invest Ophthalmol Vis Sci 33:1742, 1992
33. Brazzell RK, Stern ME, Aquavella JV, et al: Human recombinant epidermal growth factor in experimental corneal wound healing. Invest Ophthalmol Vis Sci 32:336, 1991
34. Kandarakis AS, Page C, Kaufman HE: The effect of epidermal growth factor on epithelial healing after penetrating keratoplasty in human eyes. Am J Ophthalmol 98:411, 1984
35. Stern ME, Waltz KM, Beuerman RW, et al: Effect of platelet-derived growth factor on rabbit corneal wound healing. Wound Rep Reg 3:59, 1995
36. Kopecky EA, Rootman DS: Antimetabolite interactions with epidermal growth factor. Curr Eye Res 15:247, 1996
37. Hoppenreijs VP, Pels E, Vrensen GF, Treffers WF: Effects of platelet-derived growth factor on endothelial wound healing of human corneas. Invest Ophthalmol Vis Sci 35:150, 1994
38. Raphael B, Kerr NC, Shimizu RW, et al: Enhanced healing of cat corneal endothelial wounds by epidermal growth factor. Invest Ophthalmol Vis Sci 34:2305, 1993
39. Tao Y, Bazan HE, Bazan NG: Platelet-activating factor induces the expression of metalloproteinases-1 and -9, but not -2 or -3, in the corneal epithelium. Invest Ophthalmol Vis Sci 36:345, 1995
40. Campbell FW, Michaelson IC: Blood vessel formation in the cornea. Br J Ophthalmol 33:248, 1949
41. McCracken JS, Burger PC, Klintworth GK: Morphologic observations on experimental corneal vascularization in the rat. Lab Invest 41:519, 1979
42. Ben Ezra D: Neovasculogenic ability of prostaglandins, growth factors, and synthetic chemoattractants. Am J Ophthalmol 86:455, 1978

43. Sholley MM, Gimbrone MA, Cotran RS: The effects of leukocyte depletion on corneal neovascularization. Lab Invest 38:32, 1978
44. Ruoslahti E, Engvall E, Hayman EG: Fibronectin: current concepts of its structure and function. Coll Relat Res 1:95, 1981
45. Beuerman RW, Schimmelpfennig B: Sensory denervation of the rabbit cornea affects epithelial properties. Exp Neurol 69:196, 1980
46. Geeraets WJ, Williams RC, Chen C, et al: The loss of light energy in retina and choroid. Arch Ophthalmol 64:606, 1960
47. Kutscher CF: Ocular effects of radiant energy. Trans Am Acad Ophthalmol Otolaryngol 50:230, 1946
48. Pfister RR, Schepens CL, Lemp MA, Webster RG: Photocoagulation keratopathy. Arch Ophthalmol 86:94, 1971
49. deGuillebon H, Pfister R, Govignon J, et al: Corneal temperature measurements during retinal photocoagulation. Arch Ophthalmol 85:712, 1971
50. Sweng HC, Little HL, Hammond AH: Complications of argon laser photocoagulation. Trans Am Acad Ophthalmol Otolaryngol 78:195, 1974
51. Kanski JJ: Anterior segment complications of retinal photocoagulation. Am J Ophthalmol 79:424, 1975
52. Pardos GJ, Krachmer JH: Photocoagulation: its effect on the corneal endothelial density of diabetics. Arch Ophthalmol 99:84, 1981
53. Smith J, Whitted P: Corneal endothelial changes after argon laser iridotomy. Am J Ophthalmol 98:153, 1984
54. Traverso C, Cohen EJ, Groden LR, et al: Central corneal endothelial cell density after argon laser trabeculoplasty. Arch Ophthalmol 102:1322, 1984
55. Hirst LW, Robin AL, Sherman S: Corneal endothelial changes after argon-laser iridotomy and panretinal photocoagulation. Am J Ophthalmol 93:473, 1982
56. Baker SS, Muenzler WS, Small RG, Leonard JE: Carbon dioxide laser blepharoplasty. Ophthalmology 91:238, 1984
57. Friedman NR, Saleeby ER, Rubin MG, et al: Safety parameters for avoiding acute ocular damage from the reflected CO_2 (10.6 mm) laser beam. J Am Acad Dermatol 17:815, 1987
58. Goldberg RA: The carbon dioxide laser in ocular plastic surgery and sliced bread. Arch Ophthalmol 114:1131, 1996
59. Lerman S: Radiant Energy and the Eye. Macmillan, New York, 1980
60. Zuclich JA: Ultraviolet induced damage in the primate cornea and retina. Curr Eye Res 3:27, 1984
61. Foulks GN, Friend J, Thoft RA: Effects of ultraviolet radiation on corneal epithelial metabolism. Invest Ophthalmol Vis Sci 17:694, 1978
62. Ringvold A, Davanger M, Olsen EG: Changes of the corneal epithelium after ultraviolet radiation. Acta Ophthalmol (Copenh) 60:41, 1982
63. Olsen EG, Ringvold A: Human cornea endothelium and ultraviolet radiation. Acta Ophthalmol (Copenh) 60:54, 1982
64. Karai I, Matsumura S, Takise S, et al: Morphological change in the corneal endothelium due to ultraviolet radiation in welders. Br J Ophthalmol 68:544, 1984
65. Hughes FW Jr: Alkali burns of the eye. I. Review of the literature and summary of present knowledge. Arch Ophthalmol 35:423, 1946
66. Hughes FW Jr: Alkali burns of the eye. II. Clinical and pathologic course. Arch Ophthalmol 36:189, 1946
67. Ballen PH: Treatment of chemical burns of the eye. Eye Ear Nose Throat Mon 43:57, 1964
68. Roper-Hall MJ: Thermal and chemical burns. Trans Ophthalmol Soc UK 85:631, 1965
69. Grant WM, Schuman JS: Toxicology of the Eye. 4th Ed. Charles C. Thomas, Springfield, IL, 1993
70. Cejkova J, Lojda Z, Obenberger J, Havrankova E: Alkali burns of the rabbit cornea. II. A histochemical study of glycosaminoglycans. Histochemistry 45:71, 1975
71. Berman M, Leary R, Gage J: Evidence for a role of the plasminogen activator-plasmin system in corneal ulceration. Invest Ophthalmol Vis Sci 19:1204, 1980
72. Berman M, Winthrop S, Ausprunk D, et al: Plasminogen activator (urokinase) causes vascularization of the cornea. Invest Ophthalmol Vis Sci 22:191, 1982
73. Berman M, Manseau E, Law M, Aiken D: Ulceration is correlated with degradation of fibrin and fibronectin at the corneal surface. Invest Ophthalmol Vis Sci 24:1358, 1983
74. Wang H-M, Berman M, Law M: Latent and active plasminogen activator in corneal ulceration. Invest Ophthalmol Vis Sci 26:511, 1985
75. Grant WM, Kern HL: Action of alkalies on the corneal stroma. Arch Ophthalmol 54:931, 1955
76. Donshik PC, Berman MB, Dohlman CH: Effect of topical corticosteroids on ulceration in alkali-burned corneas. Arch Ophthalmol 96:2117, 1978
77. Brown SI, Weller CA, Vidrich AM: Effects of corticosteroids on corneal collagenase of rabbits. Am J Ophthalmol 70:744, 1970
78. Koob TJ, Jeffrey JJ, Eisen AZ: Regulation of human skin collagenase activity by hydrocortisone and dexamethasone in organ culture. Biochem Biophys Res Commun 61:1083, 1974
79. Pfister RR, Paterson CA: Ascorbic acid in the treatment of alkali burns of the eye. Ophthalmology 87:1050, 1980
80. Pfister RR, Paterson CA, Hayes SA: Effect of topical 10% ascorbate solution on established corneal ulcers after severe alkali burns. Invest Ophthalmol Vis Sci 22:382, 1982
81. Kaufman HE, Thomas EL: Prevention and treatment of symblepharon. Am J Ophthalmol 88:419, 1979
82. Thoft RA: Indications for conjunctival transplantation. Ophthalmology 89:335, 1982
83. Ballen PH: Mucous membrane grafts in chemical (lye) burns. Am J Ophthalmol 55:302, 1963
84. Webster RG Jr, Slansky HH, Refojo MF: The use of adhesives for the closure of perforations: a report of two cases. Arch Ophthalmol 80:705, 1968
85. Dohlman CH, Boruchoff SA, Sullivan GH: A technique for the repair of perforated corneal ulcers. Arch Ophthalmol 77:519, 1967
86. Friedenwald JS, Hughes WF Jr, Herrmann H: Acid burns of the eye. Arch Ophthalmol 35:98, 1946

87. Friedenwald JS, Hughes WF Jr, Herrmann H: Acid-base tolerance of the cornea. Arch Ophthalmol 31:279, 1944
88. Paterson CA, Eakins KE, Paterson E, et al: The ocular hypertensive response following experimental acid burns in the rabbit eye. Invest Ophthalmol Vis Sci 18:67, 1979
89. Pfister RR, Paterson CA: Additional clinical and morphological observations on the favorable effect of ascorbate in experimental ocular alkali burns. Invest Ophthalmol Vis Sci 16:478, 1977
90. Donnenfeld ED, Selkin BA, Perry HD, et al: Controlled evaluation of a bandage contact lens and a topical nonsteroidal antiinflammatory drug in treating traumatic corneal abrasions. Ophthalmology 102:979, 1995
91. Paton D, Goldberg MF: Management of Ocular Injuries. WB Saunders, Philadelphia, 1976
92. Runyon TE: Concussive and Penetrating Injuries of the Globe and Optic Nerve. CV Mosby, St. Louis, 1975
93. Gombos GM: Trauma—Part I. Nonpenetrating and nonperforating injuries of the eyeball. p. 92. In Gombos GM (ed): Handbook of Ophthalmologic Emergencies (A Guide for Emergencies in Ophthalmology). Medical Examination Publishing Company, Flushing, NY, 1974
94. Webster RG: Corneal injuries. p. 413. In Smolin G, Thoft RA (eds): The Cornea: Scientific Foundations and Clinical Practice. Little, Brown, Boston, 1983
95. Bron AJ, Tripathi RC: Corneal disorders. p. 281. In Goldberg MF: Genetic and Metabolic Eye Diseases. Little, Brown, Boston, 1983
96. Rice NSC, Ashton N, Jay B, Blach RK: Reis-Bücklers' dystrophy: a clinico-pathological study. Br J Ophthalmol 52:577, 1968
97. Tripathi RC, Bron AJ: Ultrastructural study of nontraumatic corneal erosion. Br J Ophthalmol 56:73, 1972
98. Isakow I, Romem M, Dabush S, et al: Post traumatic recurrent corneal erosion. I. Clinical and histological studies. Metab Pediatr Syst Ophthalmol 6:349, 1982
99. Wood TO: Recurrent erosions. Trans Am Ophthalmol Soc 82:851, 1984
100. McLean EN, MacRae SM, Rich LF: Recurrent erosion. Treatment by anterior stromal puncture. Ophthalmology 93:784, 1986
101. Mannis MJ, Fiori CE, Krachmer JH, et al: Keratopathy associated with intracorneal glass. Arch Ophthalmol 99:850, 1981
102. Smolin G, Wong I: Bee sting of the cornea: case reports. Ann Ophthalmol 14:342, 1982
103. Galin MA, Harris LS, Papariello GJ: Nonsurgical removal of corneal rust stains. Arch Ophthalmol 74:674, 1965
104. Harris LS, Galin MA, Mittag TW: Nonsurgical removal of corneal rust stains. Part II. Clinical trials. Am J Ophthalmol 71:854, 1971
105. Kuhn F, Morris R, Witherspoon CD, et al: Air bag: friend or foe? Arch Ophthalmol 111:1333, 1993
106. Rosenblatt MA, Freilich B, Kirsch D: Air bag–associated ocular injury. Arch Ophthalmol 111:1318, 1993
107. Fukagawa K, Tsubota K, Kimura C, et al: Corneal endothelial cell loss induced by air bags. Ophthalmology 100:1819, 1993
108. Driver PJ, Cashwell LF, Yeatts RP: Airbag-associated bilateral hyphemas and angle recession [letter]. Am J Ophthalmol 118:250, 1994
109. Gault JA, Vichnin MC, Jaeger EA, Jeffers JB: Ocular injuries associated with eyeglass wear and airbag inflation. J Trauma 38:494, 1995
110. Geggel HS, Griggs PB, Freeman MI: Irreversible bullous keratopathy after air bag trauma. CLAO J 22:148, 1996
111. Baker RS, Flowers CW Jr, Smith A, Casey R: Corneoscleral laceration caused by air-bag trauma. Am J Ophthalmol 121:709, 1996
112. Payrau P, Raynaud G: Lesions of the cornea by blast: microscopic penetrating foreign bodies: posterior velvety rings. Ann Oculist 198:1054, 1965
113. Forstot SL, Gasset AR: Transient traumatic posterior annular keratopathy of Payrau. Arch Ophthalmol 92:527, 1974
114. Cibis GW, Weingeist TA, Krachmer JH: Traumatic corneal endothelial rings. Arch Ophthalmol 96:485, 1978
115. Maloney WF, Colvard M, Bourne WM, Gardon R: Specular microscopy of traumatic posterior annular keratopathy. Arch Ophthalmol 97:1647, 1979
116. Lesher MP, Durrie DS, Stiles MC: Corneal edema, hyphema, and angle recession after air bag inflation. Arch Ophthalmol 111:1320, 1993
117. Hoskins RD: Secondary glaucoma. p. 376. In Heilmann K, Richardson KT (eds): Glaucoma. Conceptions of a Disease. Pathogenesis, Diagnosis, Therapy. WB Saunders, Philadelphia, 1978
118. Blanton FM: Anterior chamber angle recession and secondary glaucoma: a study of the after-effects of traumatic hyphema. Arch Ophthalmol 72:39, 1964
119. Read J, Goldberg MJ: Comparison of medical treatment for traumatic hyphema. Trans Am Acad Ophthalmol Otolaryngol 78:799, 1974
120. Wolff SM, Zimmerman LE: Chronic secondary glaucoma associated with retrodisplacement of iris root and deepening of the anterior chamber angle secondary to contusion. Am J Ophthalmol 54:547, 1962
121. Edwards WC, Layden WE: Traumatic hyphema. A report of 184 consecutive cases. Am J Ophthalmol 75:110, 1973
122. Shammas HF, Matta CS: Outcome of traumatic hyphema. Ann Ophthalmol 7:701, 1975
123. Edwards WC, Layden WE: Monocular versus binocular patching in traumatic hyphema. Am J Ophthalmol 76:359, 1973
124. Gilbert HD, Jensen AD: Atropine in the treatment of traumatic hyphema. Ann Ophthalmol 5:1297, 1973
125. Crouch ER Jr, Frenkel M: Aminocaproic acid in the treatment of traumatic hyphema. Am J Ophthalmol 81:355, 1976
126. Rakusin W: Traumatic hyphema. Am J Ophthalmol 74:284, 1972
127. Crawford JS, Lewandowski RL, Chan W: The effect of aspirin on rebleeding in traumatic hyphema. Am J Ophthalmol 80:543, 1975
128. Thygeson P, Beard C: Observations on traumatic hyphema. Am J Ophthalmol 35:977, 1952

129. Cahn PH, Havener WH: Factors of importance in traumatic hyphema, with particular reference to and study of routes of absorption. Am J Ophthalmol 55:591, 1963
130. Spoor TC, Kwitko GM, O'Grady JM, et al: Traumatic hyphema in an urban population. Am J Ophthalmol 109:23, 1990
131. Skalka HW: Recurrent hemorrhage in traumatic hyphema. Ann Ophthalmol 10:1153, 1978
132. Palmer DJ, Goldberg MF, Frenkel M, et al: A comparison of two dose regimens of epsilon aminocaproic acid in the prevention and management of secondary traumatic hyphemas. Ophthalmology 93:102, 1986
133. Kraft SP, Christianson MD, Crawford JS, et al: Traumatic hyphema in children. Ophthalmology 94:1232, 1987
134. Kearns P: Traumatic hyphaema: a retrospective study of 314 cases. Br J Ophthalmol 75:137, 1991
135. Bengtsson E, Ehinger B: Treatment of traumatic hyphema. Acta Ophthalmol (Copenh) 53:914, 1975
136. Agapitos PJ, Noel LP, Clarke WN: Traumatic hyphema in children. Ophthalmology 94:1238, 1987
137. Varnek L, Daisgaard C, Hansen A, Klie F: The effect of tranexamic acid on secondary hemorrhage after traumatic hyphema. Acta Ophthalmol (Copenh) 58:787, 1980
138. Sjolie AK, Mortensen KK: Traumatic hyphema treated ambulatory and without antifibrinolytic drugs. Acta Ophthalmol (Copenh) 58:125, 1980
139. Shabo Al, Maxwell DS: Observations on the fate of blood in the anterior chamber: a light and electron microscopic study of the monkey trabecular meshwork. Am J Ophthalmol 73:25, 1972
140. Horven I: Erythrocyte passage into Schlemm's canal. Am J Ophthalmol 74:168, 1974
141. Dandolfi M, Kwaan HC: Fibrinolysis in the anterior segment of the eye. Arch Ophthalmol 77:99, 1967
142. Havener WH: Ocular Pharmacology. 4th Ed. CV Mosby, St. Louis, 1978
143. Goldberg MF: Sickled erythrocytes, hyphema, and secondary glaucoma: I. The diagnosis and treatment of sickled erythrocytes in human hyphemas. Ophthalmic Surg 10:17, 1979
144. Goldberg MF, Tso MOM: Sickled erythrocytes, hyphema and secondary glaucoma: VIII. The passage of sickled erythrocytes out of the anterior chamber of the human and monkey eye. Light and electron microscopic studies. Ophthalmic Surg 10:89, 1979
145. Michelson PE, Pfaffenbach D: Retinal arterial occlusion following ocular trauma in youths with sickle-trait hemoglobinopathy. Am J Ophthalmol 74:494, 1972
146. Sorr EM, Goldberg RE: Traumatic central retinal artery occlusion with sickle cell trait. Am J Ophthalmol 80:648, 1975
147. Radius RL, Finkelstein O: Central retinal artery occlusion (reversible) in sickle trait with glaucoma. Br J Ophthalmol 60:428, 1976
148. Wax MB, Ridley ME, Magargal LE: Reversal of retinal and optic disc ischemia in a patient with sickle cell trait and glaucoma secondary to traumatic hyphema. Ophthalmology 89:845, 1982
149. Broderick JD: Corneal blood staining after hyphema. Br J Ophthalmol 56:589, 1972
150. Beyer TL, Hirst LW: Corneal blood staining at low pressures. Arch Ophthalmol 103:654, 1985
151. Ganley JP, Greiger JM, Clement JR, et al: Aspirin and recurrent hyphema after blunt ocular trauma. Am J Ophthalmol 96:797, 1983
152. Gorn RA: The detrimental effect of aspirin on hyphema rebleed. Ann Ophthalmol 11:351, 1979
153. McGetrick JJ, Jampol LM, Goldberg MF, et al: Aminocaproic acid decreases secondary hemorrhage after traumatic hyphema. Arch Ophthalmol 101:1031, 1983
154. Kutner B, Fourman S, Brein K, et al: Aminocaproic acid reduces the risk of secondary hemorrhage in patients with traumatic hyphema. Arch Ophthalmol 105:206, 1987
155. Uusitalo RJ, Saari MS, Aine E, et al: Tranexamic acid in the prevention of secondary hemorrhage after traumatic hyphema. Acta Ophthalmol (Copenh) 59:539, 1981
156. Bramsen T: Fibrinolysin and traumatic hyphema. Acta Ophthalmol (Copenh) 57:447, 1979
157. Kennedy RH, Brubaker RF: Traumatic hyphema in a defined population. Am J Ophthalmol 102:123, 1988
158. Read J: Traumatic hyphema: surgical versus medical management. Ann Ophthalmol 7:659, 1975
159. Wilson FM: Traumatic hyphema: pathogenesis and management. Ophthalmology 87:910, 1980
160. Goldberg MF: The diagnosis and treatment of secondary glaucoma in sickle cell patients. Am J Ophthalmol 87:43, 1979
161. Sears ML: Surgical management of black ball hyphema. Trans Am Acad Ophthalmol Otolaryngol 74:820, 1970
162. Wolter JR, Henderson JW, Talley TW: Histopathology of a black ball blood clot removed four days after total traumatic hyphema. J Pediatr Ophthalmol 8:15, 1971
163. Weiss JS, Parrish RK, Anderson DR: Surgical therapy of traumatic hyphema. Ophthalmic Surg 14:343, 1983
164. Parrish R, Bernardino V Jr: Iridectomy in the surgical management of eight-ball hyphema. Arch Ophthalmol 100:435, 1982
165. Gilbert HD, Smith RE: Traumatic hyphema: treatment of secondary hemorrhage with cyclodiathermy. Ophthalmic Surg 7:31, 1976
166. Barr CC: Prognostic factors in corneoscleral lacerations. Arch Ophthalmol 101:919, 1983
167. Roper-Hall MJ: Perforating ocular injuries: prognosis. Proc R Soc Med 60:597, 1967
168. Faulborn J, Atkinson A, Olivier D: Primary vitrectomy as a preventive surgical procedure in the treatment of severely injured eyes. Br J Ophthalmol 61:202, 1977
169. Leibowitz HM: Hydrophilic contact lenses in corneal disease. IV. Penetrating corneal wounds. Arch Ophthalmol 88:602, 1972
170. Boruchoff SA, Refojo MF, Slansky HH, et al: Clinical applications of adhesives in corneal surgery. Trans Am Acad Ophthalmol Otolaryngol 74:499, 1969

171. Paton D, Craig J: Management of iridodialysis. Ophthalmic Surg 4:38, 1973
172. Cleary PE, Ryan SJ: Method of production and natural history of experimental posterior penetrating eye injury in the rhesus monkey. Am J Ophthalmol 88:212, 1979
173. Cleary PE, Ryan SJ: Histology of wound, vitreous, and retina in experimental posterior penetrating eye injury in the rhesus monkey. Am J Ophthalmol 88:221, 1979
174. Cox MS, Freeman HM: Retinal detachment due to ocular penetration. I. Clinical characteristics and surgical results. Arch Ophthalmol 96:1354, 1978
175. Topping TM, Abrams GW, Machemer R: Experimental double-perforating injury of the posterior segment in rabbit eyes. The natural history of intraocular proliferation. Arch Ophthalmol 97:735, 1979
176. Abrams GW, Topping TM, Machemer R: Vitrectomy for injury. The effect on intraocular proliferation following perforation of the posterior segment of the rabbit eye. Arch Ophthalmol 97:743, 1979
177. Ryan SJ, Allen AW: Pars plana vitrectomy in ocular trauma. Am J Ophthalmol 88:483, 1979
178. Snell AC Jr: Perforating ocular injuries. Am J Ophthalmol 28:263, 1945
179. Moncrief WF, Scheribel KJ: Penetrating injuries of the eye: a statistical survey. Am J Ophthalmol 28:1212, 1945
180. Edmund J: The prognosis of perforating eye injuries. Acta Ophthalmol (Copenh) 46:1165, 1968
181. Eagling EM: Perforating injuries of the eye. Br J Ophthalmol 60:732, 1976

26

Corneal Changes from Ocular Surgery

ELISABETH J. COHEN AND CHRISTOPHER J. RAPUANO

The cornea is at risk for a variety of complications during and after ocular surgery. This chapter reviews these complications and describes the adverse responses of the conjunctiva and the corneal epithelium, stroma, Descemet's membrane, and endothelium to various surgical procedures.

EPITHELIAL CHANGES

Intraoperative Epithelial Defects

Epithelial defects can develop during or after any ocular surgery. Drops used to prepare the eye for surgery, including topical antibiotics, cycloplegic or dilating agents, anesthetics, and disinfectants such as povidone iodine, are usually well tolerated in the small amounts commonly used. Care must be taken not to inadvertently instill agents meant for skin disinfection into the eye. Chlorhexidine gluconate (Hibiclens) is not used as a skin disinfectant near the eye because it can cause a severe chemical burn and corneal edema if it comes into contact with the conjunctiva or cornea[1,2] (Figure 26-1).

It is important to ensure that the eyelids are closed during ocular massage. In patients undergoing general anesthesia for ocular surgery, lubricating or antibiotic ointment is placed on the fellow eye and the eyelids are taped closed to protect the epithelium.

The epithelium of the operated eye tends to become dry during surgery because of exposure and should be moistened with physiologic saline during the course of the procedure. Direct trauma can also damage the epithelium. Care is taken to avoid unnecessarily touching the epithelium with surgical instruments. Moistening the cornea facilitates picking up sutures to be tied without damaging the epithelium.

If the epithelium sloughs or becomes hazy to the point of preventing visualization of the anterior or posterior segment, the affected portion can be gently removed with a cellulose sponge or blunt spatula. Only as much epithelium as is necessary to permit adequate visualization is removed. Diabetic patients undergoing pars plana vitrectomy are at particular risk of developing epithelial problems that can lead to persistent postoperative epithelial defects.[3,4] Diabetic patients can also develop recurrent epithelial erosions after a contact lens is used for laser photocoagulation of the retina (Figure 26-2).

At the conclusion of surgery, instillation of an antibiotic ointment and application of an eye patch are routine, unless topical anesthesia has been used, in which case the eye can be left unpatched and the patient instructed to blink frequently until corneal sensation returns. Collagen shields have been advocated at the end of surgery.[5] When rehydrated in an antibiotic solution, collagen shields provide a depot of antibiotic during the early postoperative period, but they have not been shown to protect the epithelium more effectively than a standard patch. If a viscoelastic substance is used, it may be helpful to place the remainder on the surface of the eye at the end of the case.

Postoperative Epithelial Defects

Pre-existing ocular disorders, the surgery itself, and postoperative events can contribute to the development of postoperative epithelial defects. Improper patching that permits the eyelids to open under the patch can cause severe surface damage and is a special risk in children. Patients with pre-existing ocular surface disorders, including dry eyes, exposure, decreased corneal sensation, and ocular pemphigoid, are prone to the development of persistent epithelial defects. Early recognition of these risk factors is

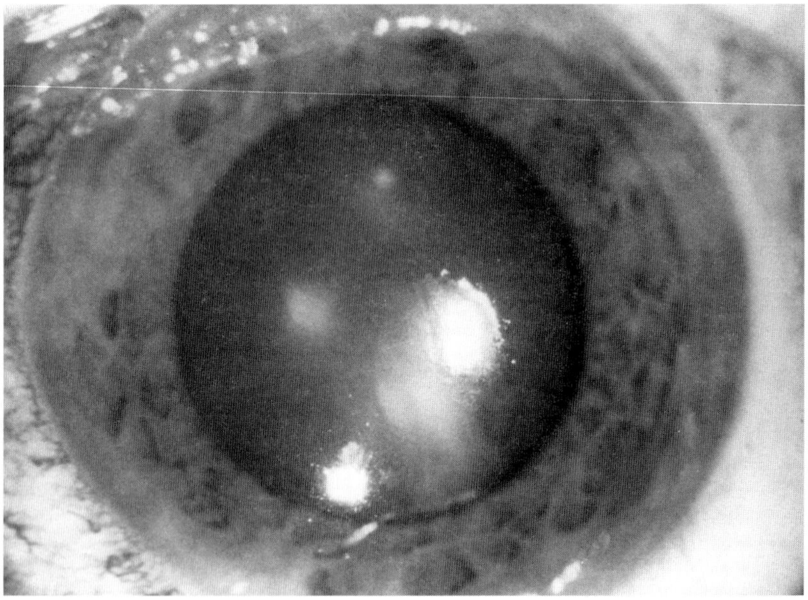

FIGURE 26-1 Chlorhexidine gluconate (Hibiclens) injury resulting in a chemical burn with corneal scarring.

important in preventing and treating these defects. Frequent ocular lubrication with preservative-free artificial tears during the day and a lubricating and/or bland antibiotic ointment at bedtime is used from the outset in patients with underlying ocular surface disorders. The status of the epithelium is considered in the selection of postoperative antibiotics. If the epithelium appears compromised or the patient is at increased risk for epithelial problems because of a pre-existing ocular surface disorder, a relatively bland antibiotic ointment, such as erythromycin, is preferred to relatively toxic aminoglycoside eye drops. Treatment with subconjunctival 5-fluorouracil after glaucoma filtering procedures can cause persistent epithelial defects.[6]

Any epithelial defect present at the end of surgery must be treated aggressively. Patients with epithelial defects have increased corneal edema because the barrier function of the epithelium is gone. Chronic defects, especially those that persist for 3 weeks or more, can be complicated by stromal melting and, rarely, perforation. If there is any stromal involvement, healing will result in corneal

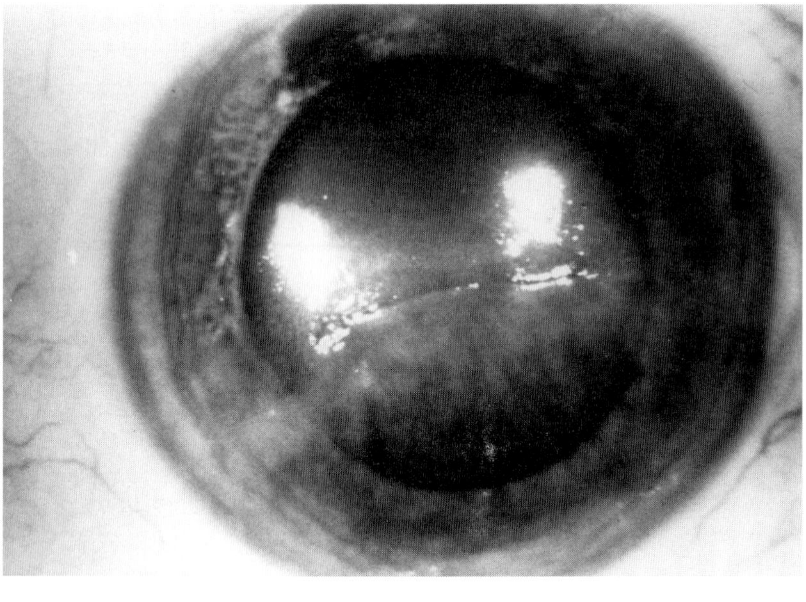

FIGURE 26-2 Persistent corneal epithelial defect in a diabetic patient after multiple laser retinal photocoagulation procedures.

FIGURE 26-3 Fluorescein staining of a cornea with superficial punctate keratopathy caused by toxicity from topical medications. The keratopathy is more prominent inferiorly.

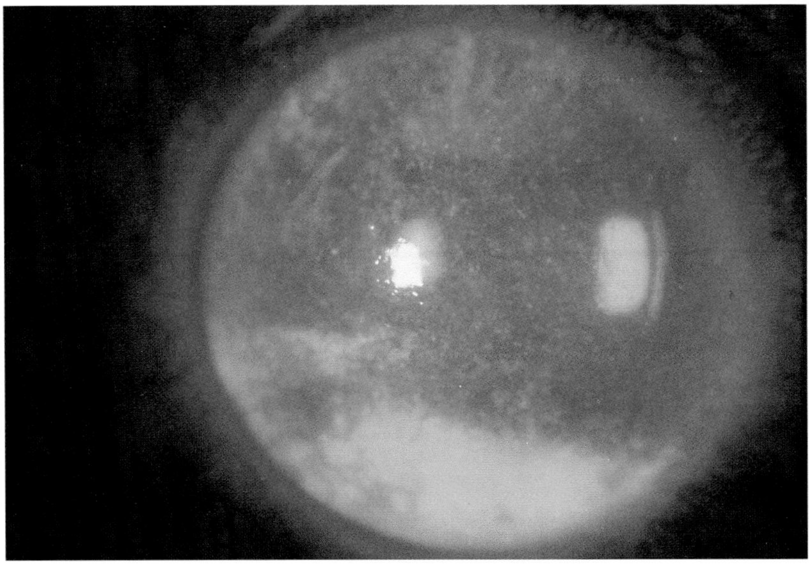

scarring, which may cause decreased visual acuity. Patients with dry eyes are especially susceptible to the development of sterile corneal ulcers.[7,8] Compared with fresh defects, defects that are 3 or more weeks old seem to heal much more slowly and are more resistant to therapy, so early vigorous treatment is important.

Corneas with persistent epithelial defects are at risk of becoming infected. Therefore, if there is any stromal infiltrate beneath the defect, corneal scrapings for smears and cultures should be obtained.

Treatment of postoperative epithelial defects includes frequent use of a bland antibiotic ointment, pressure patching, or application of a bandage soft contact lens. Bandage lenses are more effective than collagen shields in healing persistent epithelial defects after penetrating keratoplasty.[9] Any topical medications that can be reduced should be reduced because of possible toxic effects. If healing does not occur within 1 to 2 weeks, consideration is given to performing a temporary tarsorrhaphy as described in Chapter 6. Patients with corneal exposure, especially if combined with decreased corneal sensation, are not good candidates for a bandage soft contact lens and are more apt to require a tarsorrhaphy. In refractory cases, a conjunctival flap may be necessary (see Ch. 29).

Superficial Punctate Keratopathy

Superficial punctate keratopathy, or *SPK*, is relatively common after ocular surgery. A frequent cause is toxicity from topical medications, in which case the keratopathy and conjunctival hyperemia are more prominent inferiorly, where the medication is instilled, than superiorly (Figure 26-3). Toxic keratitis is often associated with a pseudodendritiform pattern of superficial punctate keratopathy. This condition must be differentiated from herpes simplex keratitis because treatment with topical antiviral medications aggravates the condition. Elimination of toxic medications and the use of preservative-free artificial tears are usually sufficient treatment. If not properly treated, superficial punctate keratopathy can evolve into a corneal erosion.[10]

Superficial punctate keratopathy is common after penetrating keratoplasty because the donor corneal epithelium is fragile. Also, closure of the keratoplasty wound with tight sutures can create a large tissue roll that results in an uneven or disrupted tear film. Relatively loose closure of the wound may prevent this problem but risks creating a wound that leaks.

Filamentary Keratitis

Filamentary keratitis may occur after ocular surgery.[11] The filaments—strands of epithelial cells and mucus—tend to occur superiorly near a cataract wound or near a penetrating keratoplasty wound and can cause a painful foreign body sensation. Patching may contribute to the development of filaments. Initial treatment consists of discontinuing patching and frequent lubrication with preservative-free artificial tears, ointment, or both. Filaments can be removed easily with forceps, but they quickly reform. A bandage soft contact lens can be effective treatment in refractory cases but must be worn for several months to prevent filament recurrence. Topical acetylcysteine can be used in stubborn cases.

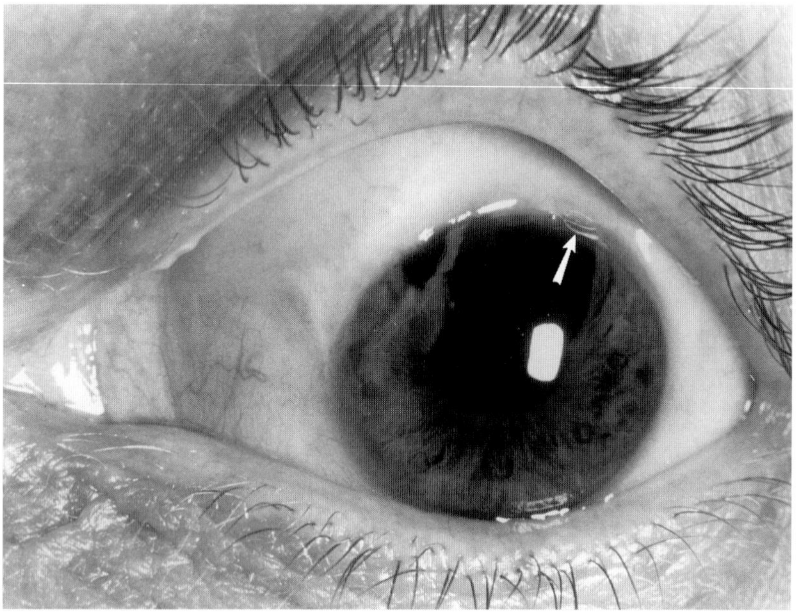

FIGURE 26-4 Postoperative delle (arrow) caused by elevation of the adjacent conjunctiva and a break in the tear film. (Courtesy of Stephen R. Waltman, M.D., Belleville, IL.)

Epithelial Edema

Epithelial edema may be caused by endothelial dysfunction or by increased intraocular pressure. In the former case, it is associated with stromal edema; in the latter case, the stroma is typically compact. Dystrophic basement membrane changes can develop in areas where there is, or has been, epithelial edema. If the edema is marked, bullae can form and rupture.

STROMAL CHANGES

Stromal changes from ocular surgery are less common than epithelial or endothelial changes, and most develop postoperatively. Stromal edema caused by endothelial dysfunction is discussed in the section on endothelial changes.

Dellen

Dellen are thin areas of the cornea caused by stromal dehydration. The overlying epithelium is intact, which distinguishes dellen from ulcers and stromal necrosis. Dellen develop adjacent to areas of limbal or conjunctival elevation where there is poor wetting of the cornea by the tear film (Figure 26-4). Dellen can occur after any type of ocular surgery, including cataract, glaucoma, and strabismus procedures. As long as the epithelium remains intact, dellen are not associated with the risk of corneal perforation. However, if the epithelium breaks down, dellen can progress to stromal necrosis or become infected. Dellen resolve rapidly with lubrication and patching. Lubricating ointment at bedtime is helpful to prevent recurrence while the paralimbal elevation persists.

Microbial Keratitis

Microbial keratitis can occur after any ocular surgery and is usually caused by problems with epithelial healing or by problems with sutures (Figure 26-5). Infections can develop around loose or broken sutures and after suture removal. As with any case of suspected microbial keratitis, multiple scrapings of the affected area are taken for smears and cultures. Sutures removed from the infected area are cultured because they contain material from deep within the cornea. Suture abscesses are usually caused by staphylococcal or streptococcal organisms, but they can be caused by a wide variety of organisms, especially in patients who have undergone penetrating keratoplasty. Suture abscesses can progress to endophthalmitis. Microbial keratitis is treated with intensive broad-spectrum topical antibiotics, as described in Chapter 8.

Patients who use extended-wear soft contact lenses to correct aphakia after cataract extraction are at increased risk for microbial keratitis, as are any patients who use extended-wear lenses.[12] When such patients present with corneal edema, epithelial defects, ocular inflammation, or a hypopyon years after cataract

FIGURE 26-5 Suture abscess caused by *Streptococcus pneumoniae* after cataract extraction through a clear corneal incision. A hypopyon is present inferiorly.

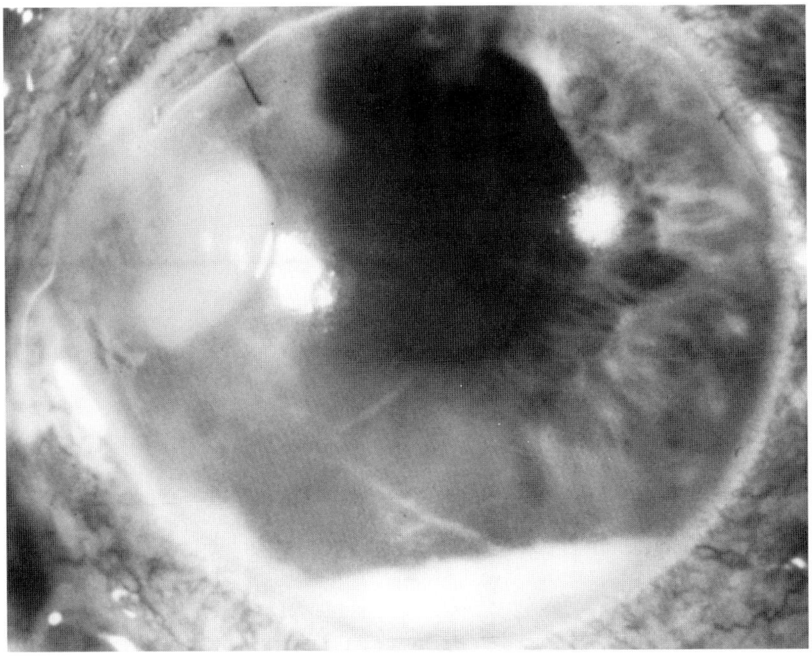

removal, one should suspect that the problem is contact lens related and look carefully for a corneal infiltrate (Figure 26-6). If the cataract wound is intact, endophthalmitis is unlikely.

Band Keratopathy

The introduction of new agents for use during surgery can be accompanied by unexpected complications. Intracameral viscoelastic substances with an elevated phosphate concentration, for example, an early formulation of sodium hyaluronate and chondroitin sulfate (Viscoat) that is no longer used, caused acute band keratopathy[13,14]; changes in the constituents eliminated the problem. Superficial stromal calcification and endothelial damage can occur after the use of intraocular silicone oil in vitrectomy procedures for retinal detachment repair.[15,16] Anterior stromal calcification may develop rarely in association with persistent epithelial defects after penetrating keratoplasty (Figure 26-7).

FIGURE 26-6 Several small corneal ulcers in a patient who wore an extended-wear contact lens for the correction of aphakia.

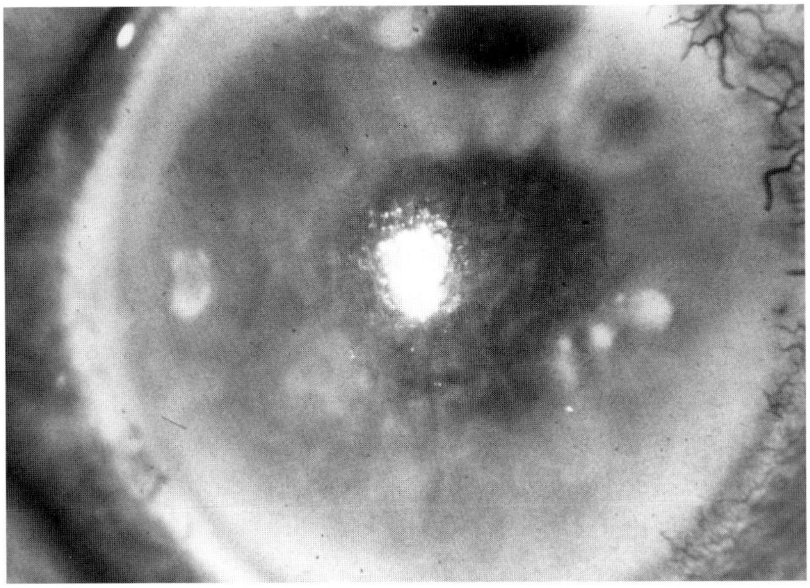

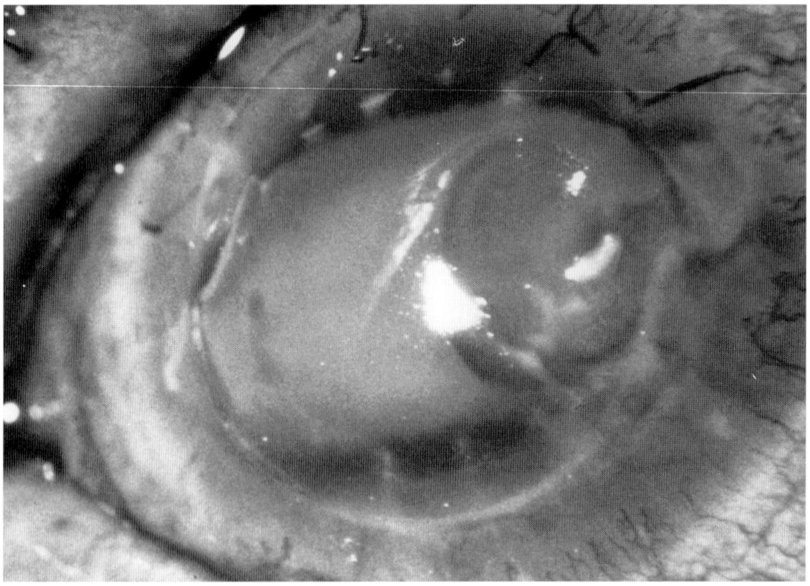

FIGURE 26-7 Marked stromal calcification in a corneal graft.

CHANGES IN DESCEMET'S MEMBRANE

Descemet's Membrane Detachment

A Descemet's membrane detachment appears as a sharply demarcated area of corneal edema. The detached membrane resembles a scroll protruding into the anterior chamber, although it is not usually visible because of the edema. Detachments can occur at the time of entry into the anterior chamber and may be enlarged when scissors are used to extend the wound, when instruments are introduced into the eye for phacoemulsification or irrigation and aspiration, or when an intraocular lens is implanted (Figure 26-8). Inadvertent injection of viscoelastic substances anterior to Descemet's membrane has been reported to cause disciform detachments of Descemet's membrane.[17,18] During removal of the recipient cornea in penetrating keratoplasty for bullous keratopathy, Descemet's membrane can separate completely from the stroma and be left behind in the eye. If the problem is unrecognized and the membrane is not removed, the donor corneal endothelium will be apposed to the membrane and the graft will likely fail (Figure 26-9).

Management of Descemet's membrane detachments depends on the cause and extent of the detachment. Small,

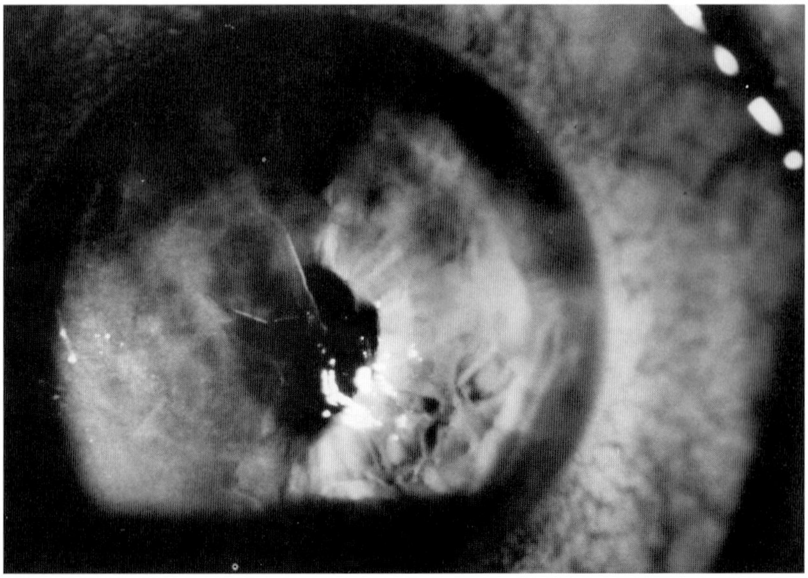

FIGURE 26-8 Descemet's membrane detachment and edema following phacoemulsification. Corneal edema is present temporally. The scroll of detached Descemet's membrane is seen centrally.

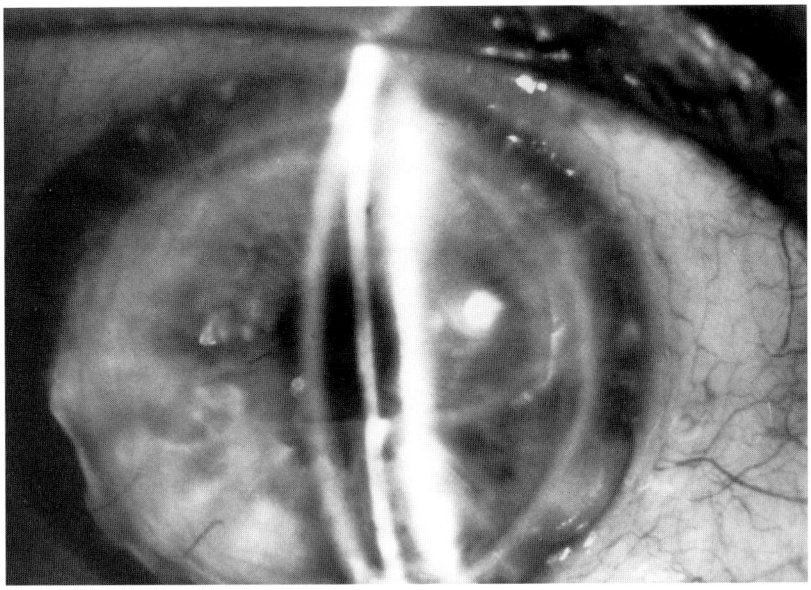

FIGURE 26-9 Retained Descemet's membrane after penetrating keratoplasty.

peripheral detachments are not clinically significant and can be watched for potential enlargement. Detachments caused by viscoelastic substances may gradually resolve.[18] When large detachments with scrolled flaps occur, surgical repair is recommended, although the situation is not urgent because the corneal endothelial cells remain viable on the detached membrane. Mechanical damage to Descemet's membrane and the endothelial cells must be avoided during repair. To flatten the detached membrane, air is injected into the anterior chamber in an area where the flap is hinged so that the scrolled membrane is pushed to unroll and reapproximate the surface of the posterior stroma (Figure 26-10). Viscoelastic substances should not be used for this purpose because they can get between the flap and the stroma and cause further detachment. A spatula may be used to gently help unroll the flap, if necessary. The air bubble is left in the anterior chamber to act as a tamponade. If detachment recurs within a few days (after the air bubble has dissipated), the process is repeated and full-thickness 10-0 nylon sutures are placed to hold the membrane in position.[19]

ENDOTHELIAL CHANGES

Endothelial Cell Loss

Endothelial cell loss is the most important corneal change that occurs during and after ocular surgery. Corneal edema caused by endothelial cell loss after cataract extraction and intraocular lens implantation is one of the most common indications for penetrating keratoplasty[20–22] (see Ch. 34).

In humans, corneal endothelial cells are essentially amitotic after birth, and there is a gradual decrease in endothelial cell density with age.[23,24] Operative trauma, postoperative inflammation, and endothelial dystrophy contribute to

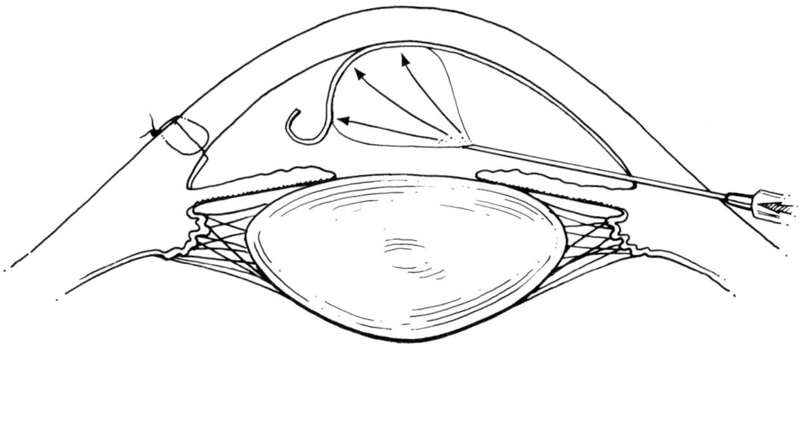

FIGURE 26-10 Injection of air intracamerally through a needle inserted at the limbus to reapproximate a detached Descemet's membrane to the posterior stromal surface.

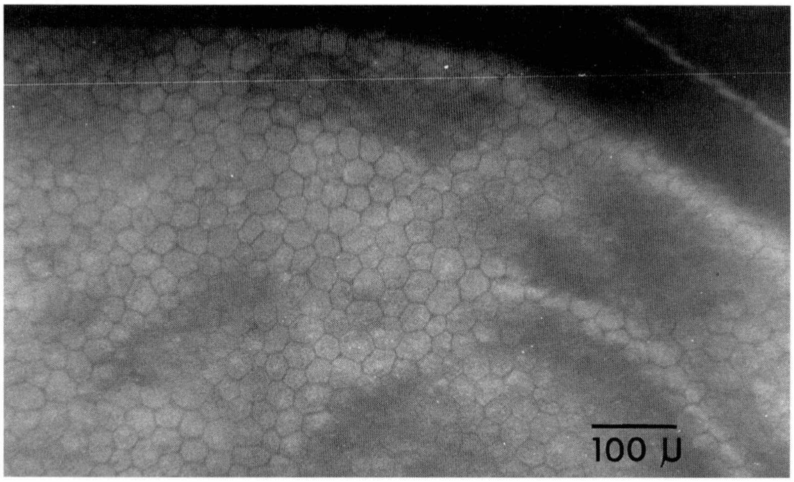

FIGURE 26-11 Endothelial specular photomicrograph. The endothelial cell density is approximately 1,200 cells/mm^2.

endothelial cell loss. Healing of the corneal endothelium involves cell enlargement and migration. Therefore, endothelial trauma reduces endothelial cell density and compromises the barrier and pump functions of the endothelial cells.

Endothelial cell density does not necessarily correlate with endothelial cell function. Morphometric analysis of endothelial cells to determine variability of cell size (polymegethism) and shape (pleomorphism) appears to be a more sensitive indicator of endothelial functional reserve than is endothelial cell density.[25-27] Corneal thickness, as measured by optical or ultrasonic pachymetry, is also a better indicator of endothelial cell function than is endothelial cell density. The normal central corneal thickness in humans is approximately 500 μm. Stromal edema becomes clinically apparent when the thickness increases to 600 μm. Epithelial edema, with marked reduction in visual acuity, occurs when the thickness approaches 700 μm. Although the cell density at which corneal decompensation occurs may vary from patient to patient, it is believed that below approximately 500 cells/mm^2, corneal edema is inevitable.

The corneal endothelium can usually be seen using the slit lamp microscope with specular reflection and a magnification of 16× to 40×.[28] A grid can be inserted into one of the oculars to estimate endothelial cell density. However, the specular microscope is the standard instrument used to view the corneal endothelium. This microscope was developed by Maurice[29] for in vitro research studies and was adapted by Bourne et al[30] and Laing et al[31] for clinical use. Currently, contact and noncontact specular microscopes with wide-field viewing capability are available. Specular photomicroscopy is an important clinical research tool and provides information that can be helpful in decision making regarding patient care (Figure 26-11). For example, if the endothelial cell density is low (less than 1,000 cells/mm^2), the patient is not a good candidate for elective surgical intervention, such as secondary intraocular lens implantation, because of the risk of decreasing the density further and causing postoperative corneal decompensation. The confocal microscope may also provide qualitative and quantitative information about the endothelial cell layer, and can be used to view the endothelium in edematous corneas, for which the specular microscope cannot be used[32] (Figure 26-12).

There are many causes of intraoperative endothelial cell loss. Direct contact between surgical instruments or an intraocular lens and the endothelium may destroy endothelial cells, as discussed below. The introduction of viscoelastic substances, beginning with Healon in 1980, has facilitated maintenance of the anterior chamber during surgery and avoidance of direct mechanical trauma to the endothelium.[33,34] Bending of the cornea also contributes to endothelial cell loss. Corneal bending is less with extracapsular cataract extraction or phacoemulsification than with intracapsular cataract extraction.

Residual detergent present on phacoemulsification tips and reusable cannulas is toxic to the endothelium and can cause postoperative corneal edema.[35] Irrigating solutions used in the anterior chamber are an important potential cause of endothelial cell loss. Even preservative-free pharmacologic agents can contain potentially harmful buffers, as observed in the case of epinephrine.[36] Balanced salt solution (BSS) has an ionic composition, osmolarity, and pH similar to those of aqueous humor and contains a citrate-acetate buffer. BSS Plus is composed of Ringer's solution with a bicarbonate buffer (identical to the buffer in aqueous humor), glutathione (a reducing agent that may protect endothelial cells from the damaging effects of oxidants and free radicals), and dextrose (an energy source). In animal studies, BSS Plus caused minimal

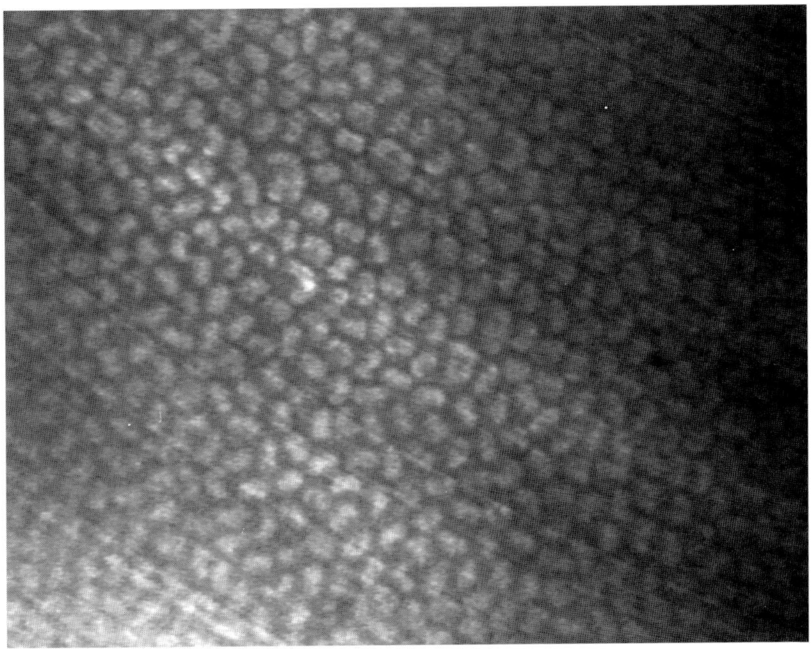

FIGURE 26-12 Confocal image of the human corneal endothelium. The endothelial cells are bright polygonal objects with dark borders where the lateral margins of the cells overlap. The overall appearance is very similar to that of a specular microscopic view; however, with the confocal microscope, the image can be taken from various planes across the endothelium. (Original magnification × 250). (Courtesy of Roger W. Beuerman, Ph.D., New Orleans, LA.)

changes in endothelial morphology regardless of the irrigation time, whereas BSS caused a significant increase in polymegethism and pleomorphism, especially after prolonged irrigation.[37] In other experimental studies, BSS Plus was shown to be less harmful to the barrier function of the endothelium than a citrate-acetate-buffered solution.[38] There is debate, however, as to the clinical significance of these findings and whether the possible advantages of BSS Plus justify the additional expense. BSS Plus is recommended for patients with endothelial dystrophy or corneal grafts who are undergoing intraocular surgery. It is also recommended for procedures in which the irrigation time is anticipated to be longer than 30 minutes.[39]

Surgical technique can contribute to intraoperative endothelial damage. When complications arise in the course of cataract surgery, increased endothelial cell loss is likely to occur. In the absence of a known history of intraoperative complications, suggestive signs include a distorted pupil, broken posterior capsule, vitreous in the anterior chamber, and the presence of an intraocular lens most likely used as a backup, such as an anterior chamber intraocular lens.

Intraoperative endothelial damage is usually not apparent during surgery but manifests beginning on the first postoperative day. Patients with preoperative endothelial cell dysfunction are more likely to develop postoperative corneal edema from intraoperative damage than are patients with a normal endothelium. In patients with corneal edema immediately after surgery, topical corticosteroids should be used to reduce any postoperative inflammation that might contribute to further endothelial damage. Frequently, the edema will resolve over several weeks, but if it has not cleared within 2 to 3 months, it is likely to be irreversible.

Endothelial Cell Loss after Cataract Surgery

The normal endothelial cell density in patients undergoing cataract surgery is approximately 2,000 to 2,500 cells/mm^2.[40] Endothelial cell loss following various techniques of cataract extraction has been studied intensively. The greatest endothelial cell loss occurs near the cataract wound,[41] and approximately 3 months are required for endothelial cell density to stabilize after cataract surgery.[41,42] In the 1970s, when intracapsular cataract extraction was the standard procedure, endothelial cell loss was 5 to 15 percent in uncomplicated cases.[43,44] Endothelial cell loss superiorly near the wound is greater after intracapsular cataract surgery than it is after extracapsular cataract extraction with or without posterior chamber intraocular lens implantation.[41]

Planned extracapsular cataract extraction became popular in the late 1970s and early 1980s. The development of highly successful posterior chamber intraocular lenses that required the presence of the posterior capsule for insertion paralleled the shift from intracapsular to extracapsular cataract extraction as the standard technique. Planned extracapsular cataract extraction was associated with an endothelial cell loss of approximately 12 percent.[45] Since 1980, the use of viscoelastic substances has reduced cell loss to less than 10 percent.

Interest in phacoemulsification began in the mid-1970s. The smaller wound required for phacoemulsification com-

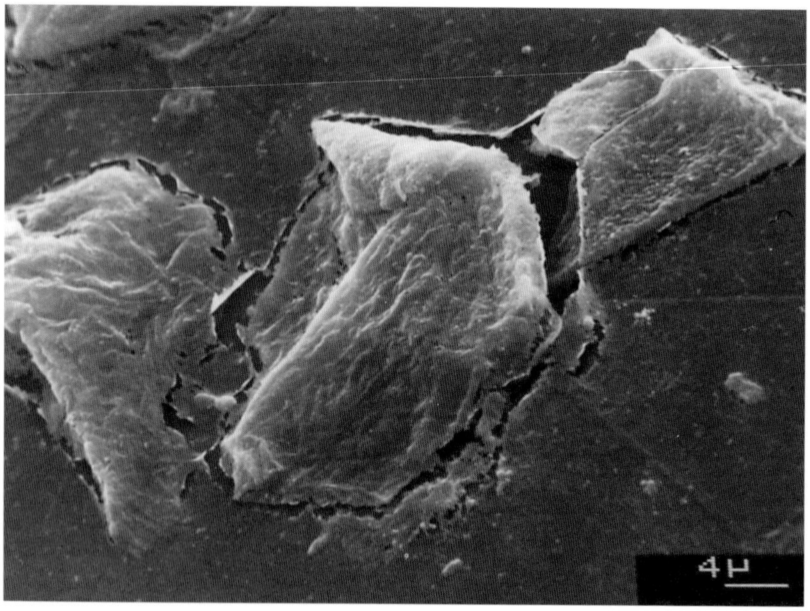

FIGURE 26-13 Scanning electron micrograph of an intraocular lens that has touched the corneal endothelium. Endothelial cells are adherent to the lens surface. (Reproduced with permission of the Authors and Editors of Transactions of the Ophthalmological Society of the United Kingdom. HE Kaufman, JI Katz: Effect of intraocular lenses on the corneal endothelium. Trans Ophthalmol Soc UK 97:265, 1977.)

pared with that needed for intracapsular cataract extraction was thought to facilitate more rapid postoperative rehabilitation. Early cases, however, with phacoemulsification performed in the anterior chamber, were complicated by more postoperative corneal edema than occurred after intracapsular cataract extraction. Even experienced surgeons reported an endothelial cell loss of more than 30 percent after phacoemulsification,[46] and older patients had more cell loss than younger patients, presumably because older patients had harder nuclei, requiring longer emulsification times.[47,48] Later, the procedure was modified so that phacoemulsification was performed in the posterior chamber, which was associated with much less endothelial cell loss.[49] In the 1990s, the procedure was modified further to incorporate smaller incisions, smaller openings in the anterior capsule by capsulorrhexis, and endocapsular phacoemulsification, which resulted in even less endothelial cell loss.[50,51]

Endothelial Cell Loss after Intraocular Lens Implantation

In the 1970s, when intraocular lenses came into common use, it was quickly recognized that endothelial cell loss was greater after cataract extraction and intraocular lens implantation than after cataract extraction alone.[52,53] The initial studies were performed on iris-supported lenses implanted at the time of intracapsular cataract extraction. Results were variable, but most series reported a cell loss of approximately 40 percent after apparently uncomplicated procedures.[43]

Damage caused by direct contact between the intraocular lens and the endothelium was significant. In the late 1970s, Kaufman et al[54] provided experimental scanning electron microscopic data demonstrating that endothelial cells adhered to polymethyl methacrylate intraocular lenses on contact (Figure 26-13) and that endothelial cells were damaged and killed when they touched an intraocular lens (Figure 26-14). In clinical studies, a direct relationship was shown between the amount of intraoperative contact between the intraocular lens and the endothelial cells and the severity of endothelial cell loss.[55,56] In looking back on the early experience with intraocular lenses, it is important to remember that viscoelastic substances were not available in the 1970s, and it was difficult for the surgeon to maintain the anterior chamber with an air bubble and prevent contact between the intraocular lens and the endothelium while implanting an iris-supported lens.

Both immediate and progressive endothelial cell loss were documented following implantation of iris-supported intraocular lenses[57] (Figure 26-15). Iris-supported lenses were associated with increased long-term cell loss after both intracapsular and extracapsular cataract extraction, compared with losses after intracapsular cataract extraction without intraocular lens implantation.[58] Factors contributing to ongoing endothelial cell loss included the movement of the intraocular lens-iris diaphragm, with intermittent touch between the intraocular lens and the endothelium, and low-grade inflammation. Many patients with iris-supported lenses have impressive amounts of iridodonesis that can be appreciated on slit lamp microscopy when the eye moves.

The amount of ongoing damage to the endothelium varied with the type of iris-supported lens. Lenses with metal (platinum) loops were associated with more endothelial cell loss than other lenses. Years later, when patients with iris-supported intraocular lenses developed pseudophakic bullous keratopathy and underwent penetrating keratoplasty, it was shown that corneal grafts were more likely to fail when a Copeland Maltese cross-style lens was left in place than when iris-clip lenses were left in place.[59] This suggests that ongoing endothelial cell loss was greater with the rigid Copeland lens than with iris-clip lenses.

In the late 1970s and early 1980s, rigid and closed-loop anterior chamber intraocular lenses increased in popularity relative to iris-supported lenses.[60] Initially these lenses were thought to represent an advance in intraocular lens design; however, in terms of long-term endothelial cell loss, this proved not to be the case. In the "epidemic" of pseudophakic bullous keratopathy,[61] anterior chamber intraocular lenses in general and closed-loop anterior chamber lenses in particular accounted for most of the cases[62] (Figure 26-16). These lenses can cause uveitis-glaucoma-hyphema, or *UGH,* syndrome, which necessitates their removal. Chronic low-grade inflammation caused by closed-loop lenses contributes not only to progressive endothelial cell loss and eventually corneal decompensation but also to chronic cystoid macular edema. Patients considering penetrating keratoplasty and removal of a closed-loop lens should be aware that postoperative visual acuity may be limited by this complication.

Some broadening of the indications for intraocular lens implantation probably resulted in implantation of anterior chamber lenses in patients younger than those who had received iris-supported lenses, thus providing more time for long-term endothelial cell loss to result in corneal

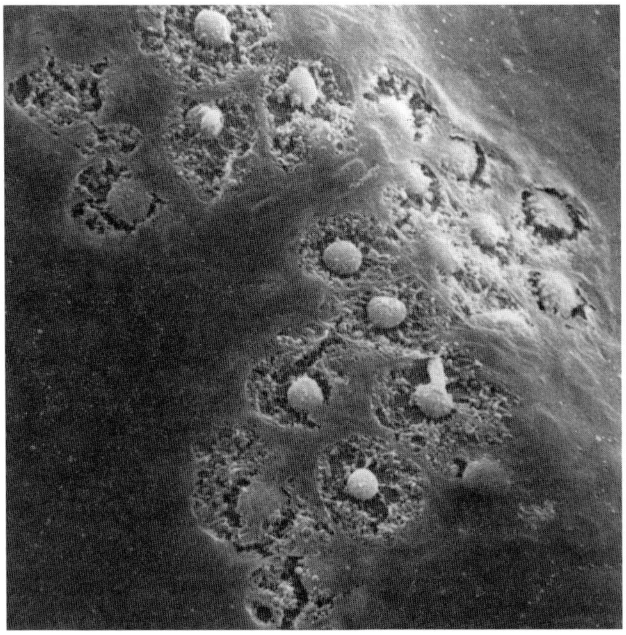

FIGURE 26-14 Scanning electron micrograph of human corneal endothelium after contact with an intraocular lens. Stripping of endothelial cell membranes has exposed the nuclei of several cells. Normal endothelial cells are seen on the lower right. (Reprinted with permission from J Katz, HE Kaufman, EP Goldberg, JW Sheets: Prevention of endothelial damage from intraocular lens insertion. Trans Am Acad Ophthalmol Otolaryngol 83:OP204, 1977. Courtesy of Ophthalmology.)

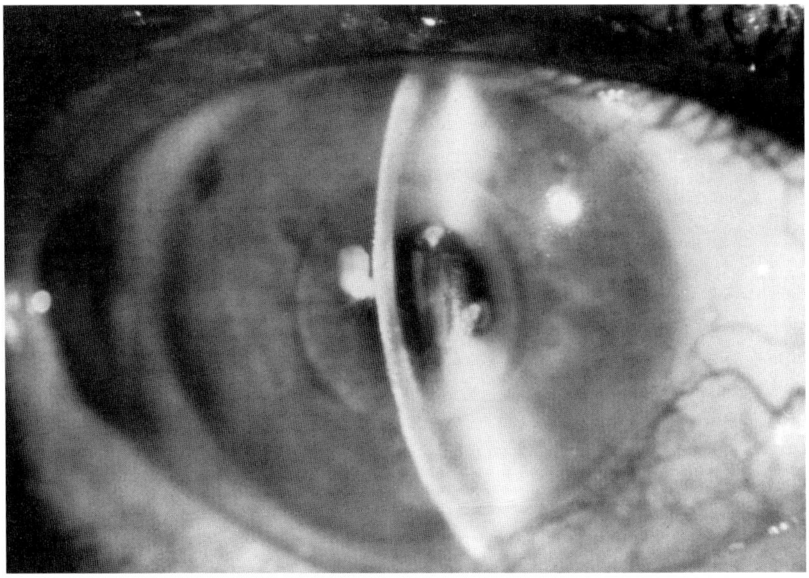

FIGURE 26-15 Pseudophakic bullous keratopathy associated with an iris-supported Medallion lens.

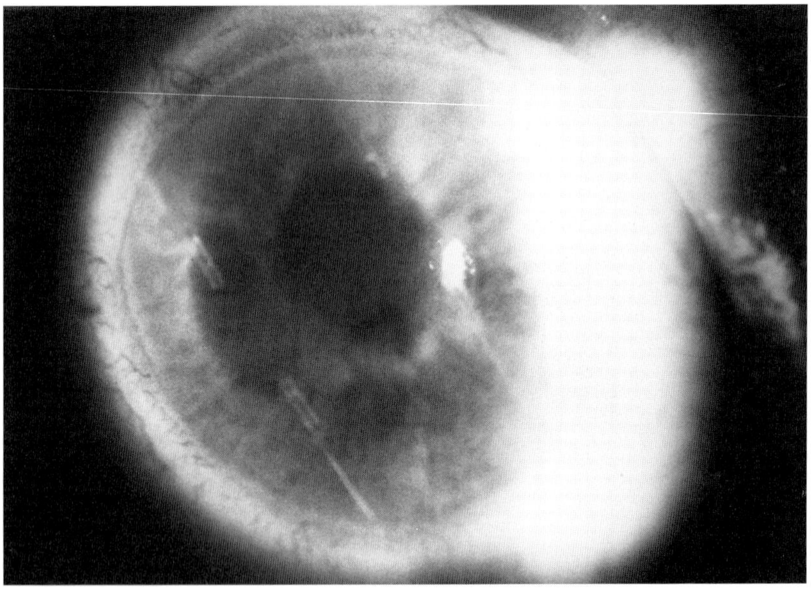

FIGURE 26-16 Pseudophakic bullous keratopathy associated with a closed-loop Leiske anterior chamber intraocular lens.

decompensation. However, corneal decompensation occurred even sooner after implantation of closed-loop anterior chamber lenses than after implantation of iris-supported lenses.[62] In addition, corneal graft failure occurred more rapidly when closed-loop anterior chamber lenses were left in place than when iris-supported lenses were left in place.[59] This suggests that closed-loop anterior chamber lenses cause greater ongoing endothelial cell loss than do iris-supported lenses. Rigid anterior chamber lenses were associated with a lower rate of graft failure than closed-loop anterior chamber lenses after penetrating keratoplasty.[59] The exchange of iris-supported lenses for Stableflex anterior chamber lenses before problems with closed-loop anterior chamber lenses were recognized led to progressive endothelial cell loss and increased rates of graft failure.[63,64]

It is important not to lump all anterior chamber lenses together with regard to their effect on the endothelium. Even within one type of lens, manufacturing techniques can affect lens safety.

Open-loop anterior chamber lenses should be considered separately from closed-loop anterior chamber lenses. Evidence is accumulating that one-piece open-loop anterior chamber lenses are well tolerated and safe for primary implantation at the time of cataract surgery when there is insufficient capsular support for a posterior chamber lens, for secondary implantation after cataract surgery, and for intraocular lens exchange at the time of penetrating keratoplasty.[64-66] The Kelman Multiflex-style anterior chamber lens with four-point fixation seems to be especially well tolerated.

Posterior chamber intraocular lens implantation after extracapsular cataract extraction or phacoemulsification is well tolerated by the corneal endothelium.[67] Corneal decompensation, when it occurs, usually happens soon after surgery because of surgical trauma, pre-existing endothelial dystrophy, or both.[68,69] Progressive endothelial cell loss and delayed corneal decompensation are not significant problems with posterior chamber lenses in the absence of pre-existing endothelial cell dysfunction or surgical complications.

Endothelial cell loss after secondary intraocular lens implantation depends on the type of lens implanted and whether there are surgical complications. Preoperative evaluation of endothelial cell density is indicated because these eyes already have reduced endothelial cell reserve compared with unoperated eyes. There is no absolute cell density below which surgery is contraindicated, but the risk of corneal decompensation increases with cell densities below 1,000 to 1,200 cells/mm^2.

Prevention of Endothelial Cell Loss

Meticulous uncomplicated surgery is the best way to minimize endothelial cell loss. Physiologic irrigating solutions are used routinely, and the debate regarding BSS versus BSS Plus is discussed above. The use of viscoelastic substances has been a major advance in reducing surgical trauma. Healon was the first viscoelastic substance shown to reduce endothelial cell loss in patients undergoing implantation of iris-supported lenses.[70] Sodium hyaluronate (AMO Vitrax Solution, AmVisc, AmVisc Plus, Healon, Healon GV, ProVisc), sodium hyaluronate

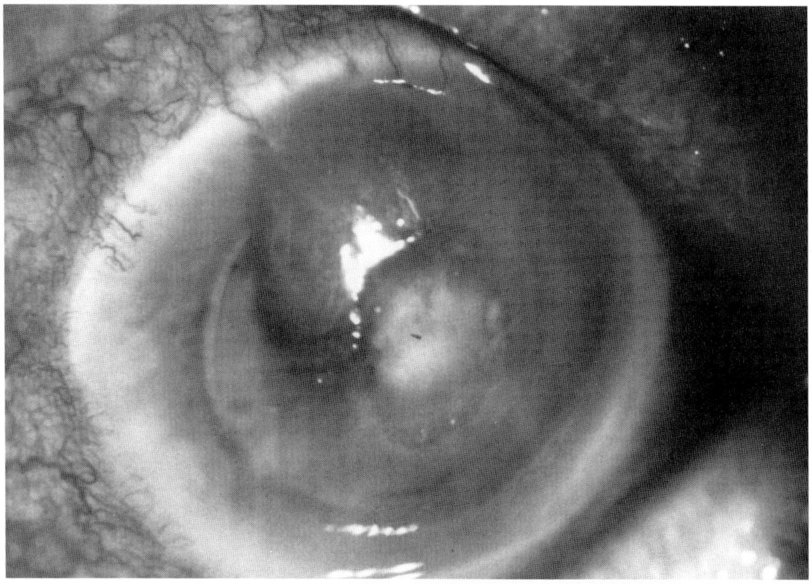

FIGURE 26-17 *Candida* corneal ulcer in a patient treated with a bandage soft contact lens for pain caused by pseudophakic bullous keratopathy, which occurred after secondary implantation of a closed-loop anterior chamber intraocular lens.

and chondroitin sulfate (Viscoat, DuoVisc), and hydroxypropyl methylcellulose (Ocucoat) are currently available viscoelastic agents that protect the endothelium comparably. Their use is associated with transient elevation of intraocular pressure several hours postoperatively, which may require medical treatment.[71-73] This problem is reduced, but not eliminated, by aspirating the viscoelastic substance at the end of surgery.

Treatment of Corneal Edema from Endothelial Cell Loss

Treatment of corneal edema caused by endothelial dystrophies is discussed in Chapter 19. Aspects that are helpful in the treatment of postoperative corneal edema from endothelial cell loss are reviewed here. Although 5 percent sodium chloride has some value in the treatment of early epithelial edema in Fuchs' dystrophy, it has limited value in the treatment of postoperative corneal decompensation. In acute postoperative corneal decompensation, inflammation is usually present, and a regimen of intensive topical corticosteroids should be tried. Low-grade inflammation may also be present in delayed corneal decompensation and should be treated similarly. If there is no response to topical corticosteroids, they should be tapered rapidly. Patients with advanced bullous keratopathy may have pain from the bullae, which may be reduced by the use of a bland antibiotic or lubricating ointment. Bandage soft contact lens wear can reduce pain on a temporary basis but should not be used long term because the lenses require regular care and periodic replacement, and their use can be complicated by microbial keratitis[74] (Figure 26-17). In patients with good visual potential, penetrating keratoplasty can be performed, with clear grafts obtained in more than 75 percent of cases.[59,62,64,75,76] The techniques for penetrating keratoplasty are described in Chapter 34. In patients with poor visual potential from a posterior segment abnormality, a total conjunctival flap is indicated (see Ch. 29).

Vitreous Touch to the Corneal Endothelium

Vitreous touch to the corneal endothelium is not an indication for vitrectomy. Many patients with vitreous touch do not develop corneal decompensation whether or not the vitreous face is intact. If there is localized, peripheral corneal edema in the area of vitreous touch, a vitrectomy may be indicated, but additional surgery carries the risk of further endothelial damage. If visually significant corneal edema is present, penetrating keratoplasty and vitrectomy are necessary for visual rehabilitation.

Brown-McLean Syndrome

Brown-McLean syndrome usually occurs after intracapsular cataract extraction, and consists of peripheral corneal edema associated with orange punctate pigmentation of the endothelial surface underlying the areas of edema[77,78] (Figure 26-18). The edema typically spares the superior and central cornea, and usually does not progress.[79] Brown-McLean syndrome has also been reported after extracapsular cataract extraction, phacoemulsification,

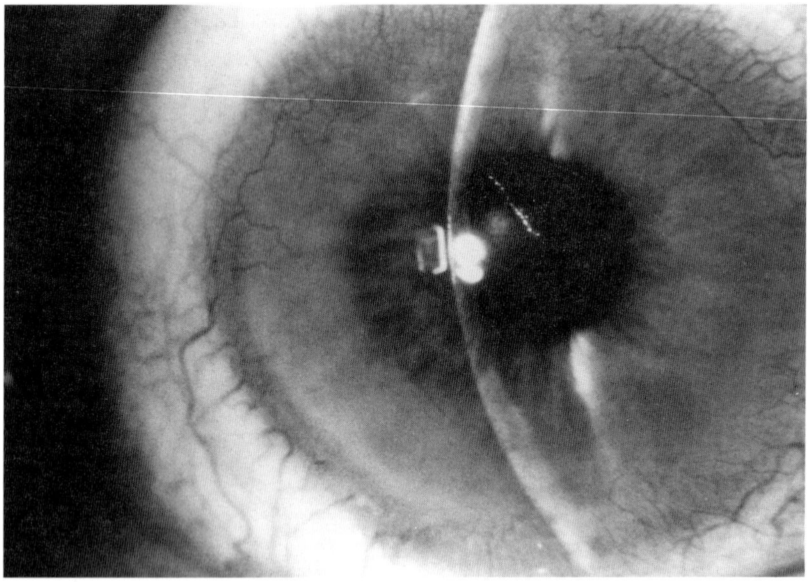

FIGURE 26-18 Peripheral corneal edema in Brown-McLean syndrome. The central cornea is thin and clear.

and pars plana lensectomy and vitrectomy, and in patients who have had no previous ocular surgery but have a subluxated lens or a lens that has spontaneously resorbed.[80]

Despite the presence of peripheral corneal decompensation, the central endothelial cell density has been reported to be as high as 2,150 cells/mm^2.[80] Light and electron microscopic studies have shown the central cornea to be relatively normal. In the periphery, disintegrated endothelial cells with an abnormal posterior collagenous layer of Descemet's membrane have been reported.[81]

Treatment consists of a trial of topical corticosteroids. In patients who do not respond and in whom peripheral cornea edema causes discomfort, a peripheral annular inlay conjunctival flap may be placed. Penetrating keratoplasty is indicated in the occasional patient in whom the central cornea becomes edematous.

CORNEAL WOUND PROBLEMS

In normal healing of a cataract wound, endothelial cell migration and laying down of new Descemet's membrane precedes stromal healing. If this series of events is disrupted, epithelial or fibrous ingrowth may occur or filtering blebs may develop.

Epithelial Ingrowth

Epithelial ingrowth is a rare, but disastrous, complication of intraocular surgery. Surface epithelium is thought to grow into the eye through a poorly healed wound or by way of full-thickness suture tracts. It occurs most often after cataract surgery or penetrating keratoplasty.[82,83] Epithelial ingrowth can also complicate removal of iris inclusion cysts.[84] The incidence of epithelial ingrowth has decreased in recent years, most likely because of advancements in microsurgical techniques and improved wound closure.

Patients with epithelial ingrowth present with tearing, photophobia, pain, and decreased visual acuity, usually within 1 year of surgery. Epithelium may be seen as an undulating line on the posterior surface of the cornea (Figure 26-19). Corneal thickness is normal unless there are other causes of edema, such as elevated intraocular pressure. Epithelial ingrowth invariably progresses, which can be documented by measuring the distance between the line and the limbus on successive visits over several weeks. The epithelium can also grow posteriorly over the anterior chamber angle, anterior and posterior iris surfaces, and ciliary body. The extent of iris involvement can be determined by applying argon laser photocoagulation burns to the surface of the iris; areas of epithelium turn white.[85] It is important to examine the wound carefully for Seidel-positive fistulas. The intraocular pressure may be low if a fistula is present and high if the fistula has sealed over and the anterior chamber angle is involved. Fistulas can leak intermittently, causing the intraocular pressure to fluctuate.

Treatment of epithelial ingrowth is difficult and the prognosis is poor. The goal is to destroy or remove all areas of epithelial proliferation as soon as the diagnosis is made and to prevent recurrences thereafter. If a fistula is present, it

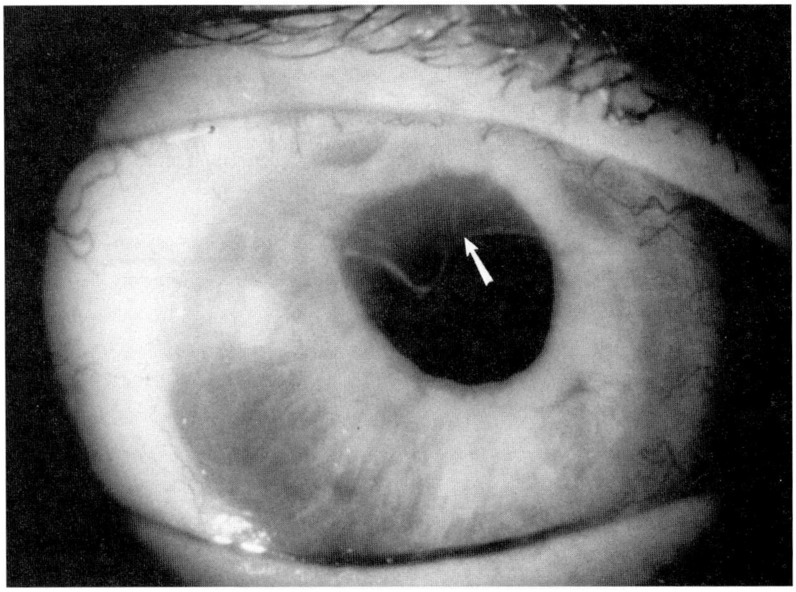

FIGURE 26-19 Epithelial ingrowth (arrow) advancing from a cataract incision toward the central cornea.

is excised and closed, usually with a scleral flap or graft.[86] The epithelium on the posterior surface of the cornea can be peeled off or destroyed by transcorneal cryotherapy after an air bubble is injected into the anterior chamber; both may be necessary. The currently preferred surgical technique for removal of involved areas of iris and ciliary body is by a pars plana vitrectomy approach followed by injection of intraocular air and transcorneal and transscleral cryotherapy of the involved cornea, anterior chamber angle, and ciliary body.[87] This procedure causes corneal decompensation in the area of cryotherapy, but penetrating keratoplasty can be performed later if eradication of the epithelial ingrowth has been successful. Setons have been used to control refractory glaucoma in patients with inoperable epithelial ingrowth[88] and in patients who have had extensive ingrowth eradication surgery. Because the degradation of vision in eyes with epithelial ingrowth is usually slow and the chance of obtaining functional reading vision is poor if the ingrowth is extensive, the surgeon must seriously consider whether the cost and discomfort of surgery, coupled with the chance of vision worsened by the surgery, make palliative therapy a better option.

Filtering Blebs

Occasionally, filtering blebs occur spontaneously after cataract surgery and usually heal without treatment in 6 to 12 months.[89] In most cases, repair is unnecessary. Patients with these blebs may have low intraocular pressure and are at risk for bleb infections. They are likely to have astigmatism, with the flat axis in the same meridian as the bleb. The application of trichloroacetic acid or cryotherapy to the bleb can cause inflammation and promote scarring.[89] One can also open the bleb and resuture the wound. A scleral flap may be used to seal the wound, if necessary.

Hyphema

Hyphemas can occur immediately or months after cataract surgery. It is important to distinguish microhyphemas from uveitis, because the causes, treatments, and significance differ. Use of the red-free (green) light on the slit lamp microscope is helpful in distinguishing red blood cells from white blood cells; red blood cells tend to disappear from view, whereas white cells remain visible.

Bleeding from the wound may be complicated by a transient elevation in intraocular pressure, but is usually self limited and without sequelae. Posterior scleral incisions are associated with hyphemas more frequently than are anterior incisions. Recurrent hyphemas may be caused by vascularization of the wound[90] and can be diagnosed by gonioscopy or fluorescein angiography. Vessels in the wound can be treated by transscleral cryotherapy or diathermy, or argon or neodymium:yttrium-aluminum-garnet (Nd:YAG) laser photocoagulation to control recurrent bleeding.[91]

Hyphemas caused by irritation from an intraocular lens may require removal of the lens. This problem occurred more often with closed-loop anterior chamber lenses as part of the uveitis-glaucoma-hyphema (UGH) syndrome than with other types of lenses.

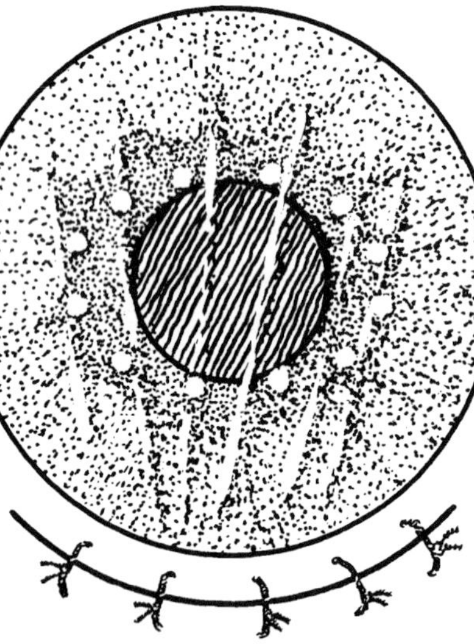

FIGURE 26-20 Wound compression from tight sutures causing peripheral corneal flattening and central corneal steepening. Reflection from a keratoscope shows an oval, with the shorter diameter in the steep meridian. (Courtesy of Stephen R. Waltman, M.D., Belleville, IL.)

Postoperative Astigmatism

Astigmatism occurs when light rays are not refracted by the eye equally in all meridians. The distortion originates primarily from the cornea, although the lens may contribute. Regular astigmatism occurs when the steep and flat meridians are 90 degrees apart, and can usually be corrected with cylindrical lenses. Irregular astigmatism occurs when the principal meridians are not 90 degrees apart or when the corneal distortion is such that the mires are so irregular that exact corneal curvature measurements cannot be determined by keratometry. Irregular astigmatism can often be corrected with a hard contact lens but not with spectacles. Surgically induced astigmatism is the difference between preoperative and postoperative astigmatism and is generally caused by corneal deformation.[92]

Astigmatism is classically measured by refraction or keratometry. Refraction measures the astigmatism of the whole eye; keratometry measures only corneal astigmatism. Keratometry measures the radius of curvature of the principal meridians of the central 3 mm of the cornea and converts these measurements to diopters of refractive power. The difference in power between the two meridians is the amount of astigmatism. Refractive astigmatism and corneal astigmatism, as measured by keratometry, correlate well after cataract extraction and intraocular lens implantation.[92]

Keratoscopy, in which multiple concentric rings of light are projected on the cornea, is also used to evaluate astigmatism. In photokeratoscopy, the reflection of these rings is recorded on film. Videokeratography, which involves computerized quantification and manipulation of photokeratoscopic data, provides a variety of information on corneal shape in a clinically useful format (see Ch. 46).

Any ocular surgery can potentially affect corneal astigmatism. Retinal detachment surgery increases refractive astigmatism by 2 diopters or more in almost one-third of patients.[93] Strabismus surgery can also induce astigmatism; more astigmatism is induced when nonadjacent rectus muscles are operated on.[94] The two most common procedures associated with postoperative astigmatism in adults, however, are cataract surgery and penetrating keratoplasty.

Astigmatism after Cataract Surgery

Postoperative astigmatism has always been a potential complication of cataract surgery. Until recently, however, it was not considered an important problem. In the past, visual rehabilitation after cataract surgery was with aphakic spectacles, which could correct significant amounts of postoperative astigmatism. With the advent of microsurgical techniques, aphakic soft contact lenses, intraocular lenses, and small incision cataract surgery, prevention of postoperative astigmatism has become more important. Today the goal of cataract surgery is to obtain good visual acuity without optical aids.[95]

Numerous studies have detailed the natural and modified course of astigmatism after cataract surgery.[96–104] With a superior extracapsular cataract incision, the vertical meridian is steep early in the postoperative course. Over weeks to years, the vertical meridian gradually flattens.

The pathophysiologic mechanisms of postoperative cataract astigmatism have been described by Jaffe and Clayman[105] and corroborated by others.[106,107] The two most important factors are wound compression and wound gape. Wound compression is caused by tight sutures and early postoperative wound edema. The peripheral cornea is flattened and the central cornea is steepened in the meridian of the wound, resulting in with-the-rule astigmatism (Figure 26-20). Wound gape is caused by loosely tied sutures, early degradation of sutures, or early suture removal. The peripheral cornea is steepened and the central cornea is flattened in the meridian of the wound, resulting in against-the-rule astigmatism (Figure 26-21). Typically, the meridian 90 degrees away from the wound undergoes an equal but opposite change that keeps the spherical equivalent roughly the same.[107] Wound misalignment or a decentered or tilted intraocular lens can cause significant postoperative astigmatism, but these complications are uncommon. Preoperative corneal astigmatism is another factor that affects postoperative corneal astigmatism; the two are often correlated.[99]

Many aspects of cataract surgery have been shown to have an effect on postoperative astigmatism, including the location, size, and shape of the incision; suture material and technique; use of cautery; and intraocular pressure at the time of suturing. Anterior cataract incisions induce more astigmatism early in the postoperative course and also change the axis of astigmatism significantly more than posterior incisions.[108,109] Thrasher and Boerner[108] found minimal induced astigmatism in both a 6.5-mm incision phacoemulsification group and a 9.5-mm incision extracapsular cataract extraction group when a posterior incision was used. Other studies have shown less induced astigmatism with 3.0- to 6.5-mm incisions than with 10.0- to 11.0-mm incisions.[110–112] One study compared (1) phacoemulsification with implantation of a foldable silicone intraocular lens through a 4.0-mm incision, (2) phacoemulsification with implantation of a polymethyl methacrylate intraocular lens through a 6.0-mm incision, and (3) extracapsular cataract extraction with implantation of a polymethyl methacrylate intraocular lens through a 10.0-mm incision.[111] At 3 and 6 months postoperatively, significantly less surgically induced astigmatism was found in the two groups with small incisions than in the group with the larger incision. Steinert et al[113] compared surgically induced astigmatism after phacoemulsification with implantation of a foldable silicone intraocular lens through a 4-mm posterior incision and phacoemulsification with implantation of a polymethyl methacrylate intraocular lens through a 6.0- to 6.5-mm posterior incision. They found significantly less surgically induced astigmatism in the smaller incision group at 1 day, 1 week, and 2 weeks, but not at 3 months postoperatively.

Along with smaller and more posterior incisions, scleral tunnels or scleral pocket incisions are being used in cataract surgery in an attempt to reduce postoperative astigmatism and achieve rapid wound stabilization.[104,114] Masket[115] demonstrated that deep suturing of superior scleral pocket incisions resulted in less surgically induced early with-the-rule astigmatism and less late against-the-rule slippage when compared with appositional suturing of the incisions. Small incisions can also be closed with horizontal mattress sutures, which also produce less surgically induced astigmatism and less late wound slippage than closure with radial sutures.[112,116] Some surgeons are performing cataract surgery through unsutured scleral or clear corneal tunnel incisions. These incisions are constructed such that they are sealed by the intraocular pressure and not by sutures. Sutureless incisions cause peripheral corneal flattening in the area of the incision.[117]

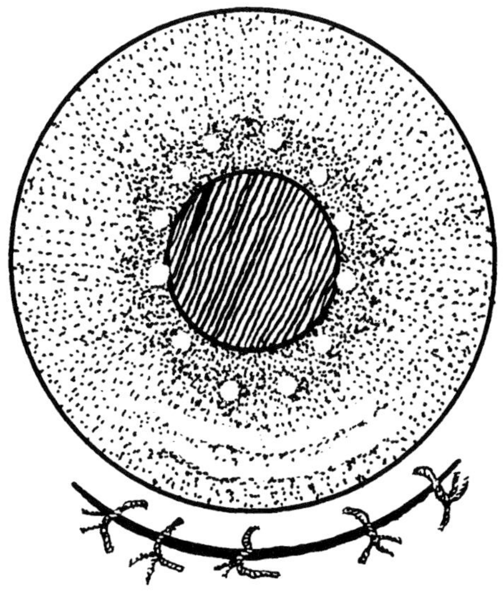

FIGURE 26-21 Wound gape causing peripheral corneal steepening and central corneal flattening. Reflection from a keratoscope shows an oval, with the longer diameter in the flat meridian. (Courtesy of Stephen R. Waltman, M.D., Belleville, IL.)

Clinically, the surgically induced astigmatism is minimal, especially if the incision is small.[118] Occasionally, however, wound slippage may occur and result in an unacceptable amount of astigmatism. Some studies[119] have found less postoperative astigmatism with scleral incisions, whereas others[120] have found less with clear corneal incisions.

Many different suture materials have been used in cataract surgery. Absorbable sutures, such as polyglactin, tend to degrade early in the postoperative course, causing wound gape and against-the-rule astigmatism in some patients. Silk sutures often spontaneously loosen and cause against-the-rule astigmatism. Nylon, which is frequently used to close cataract incisions, is considered a nonabsorbable suture and does not degrade early; however, it loses its tensile strength slowly over months to years.[95] Typically, by the time the nylon biodegrades, the wound is stable, but not always. Polypropylene and polyester degrade very slowly, if at all. Cravy[103] showed more against-the-rule slippage with nylon than with polyester over a 2-year period and postulated that biodegradation of the nylon was the cause. Masket[121] found no significant difference in surgically induced astigmatism with 10-0 nylon or 10-0 polyester 4 months postoperatively.

Astigmatism after Penetrating Keratoplasty

Technical advances and improvements in eye banking and corneal preservation have improved the long-term

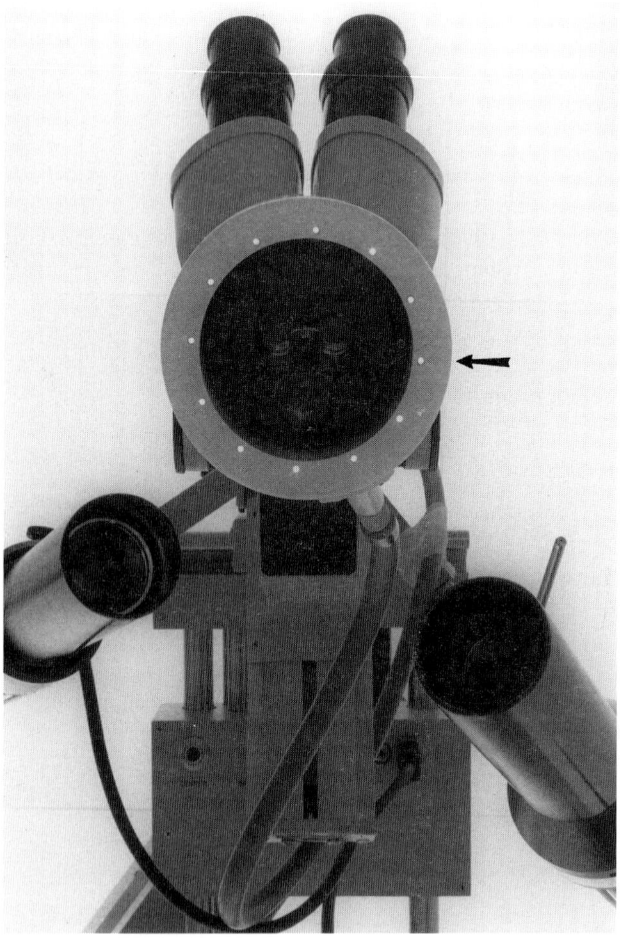

FIGURE 26-22 Troutman keratometer (arrow) attached to an operating microscope as seen by the patient. The surgeon can estimate the degree of astigmatism by observing the shape made by the reflection of the 12 lights from the anterior corneal surface.

success of penetrating keratoplasty, and postoperative astigmatism is now an important factor affecting visual acuity in these patients. Numerous factors affect corneal curvature after penetrating keratoplasty, including size and shape of the recipient opening and donor corneal button, suture type and pattern, and wound healing.

Of these factors, the suture pattern is perhaps the most controversial. The patterns include all interrupted sutures, a combination of interrupted and running sutures, and single or double running sutures. A single running suture technique with early postoperative suture adjustment has been shown to reduce early postoperative astigmatism.[122] However, no one suture pattern has been shown to consistently produce significantly less final astigmatism than any other.[123,124]

Prevention of Postoperative Astigmatism

An evaluation of corneal curvature intraoperatively is often advocated as a way to prevent postoperative astigmatism caused by cataract surgery or penetrating keratoplasty. These measurements are typically performed either quantitatively, as with a Terry keratometer, or qualitatively, as with an intraoperative keratoscope consisting of a circle of lights (Figure 26-22). An intraoperative videokeratoscope, such as the PAR system, can also be used. Lindstrom and Destro[110] found a significant decrease in postoperative astigmatism at 6 to 8 weeks in both small incision and routine extracapsular cataract surgery cases in which the Terry keratometer was used. They also demonstrated that fewer sutures needed to be cut postoperatively to reduce astigmatism in cases performed with the Terry keratometer than needed to be cut in cases performed without this device. Others have found only a small beneficial effect of the use of the Terry keratometer on the final postoperative astigmatism.[125,126]

Treatment of Postoperative Astigmatism

In the early postoperative period, suture removal and suture adjustment have been the primary modalities for reducing astigmatism. Early on, sutures perform a critical role in holding the wound together, but if they are tight, they may cause wound compression and astigmatism. Wound healing and stability are multifactorial processes, depending on such factors as size of the wound and number of sutures in place, distance of the wound from the limbus, amount of inflammation and vascularization, host healing response, and amount and duration of postoperative corticosteroid use. The more poorly the wound is healed, for example, from intensive and prolonged corticosteroid use, the greater the effect of suture removal. In fact, wound slippage that causes flattening of the cornea in the meridian in which the wound is located may be promoted by extended corticosteroid use.[96]

A tight suture causes corneal flattening in the area of the suture and steepening centrally in the meridian of the suture. Wound gape causes the reverse. When postoperative astigmatism is encountered, it is important to determine whether it is the result of wound compression or wound gape. If a tight suture is present in an area of wound compression, then cutting that suture can decrease astigmatism centrally.[92,96,127] Cataract sutures, which are often cut and left in place, should be cut away from the knot just where the suture enters the cornea so the suture end retracts into the cornea. Penetrating keratoplasty sutures, which are often removed, should be cut and pulled so the knot does not traverse the keratoplasty wound.

Ideally, suture removal should be performed when healing is sufficiently advanced so that the absence of the suture does not result in dehiscence of the wound, but not so late that the removal of the suture has no effect on astigmatism. For a typical cataract wound in a patient taking minimal to no corticosteroids, the best time for suture removal appears to be between 4 and 8 weeks postoperatively.[92,99,125] For penetrating keratoplasty wounds, single running sutures can be adjusted as early as the first postoperative week. Depending on the number of sutures, individual interrupted sutures can usually be removed after a few months if a running suture is in place.[128] If visual acuity is good, running sutures are generally left in place unless they become vascularized or loosen. Removal of a running suture can be complicated by large changes in astigmatism and wound slippage or dehiscence, and should be delayed until at least 12 to 18 months after surgery, especially if there are no other sutures in place.[129] Sutures should not be adjusted or removed to reduce astigmatism before it is possible to obtain a reasonably accurate evaluation of the corneal curvature by photokeratoscopy or videokeratography.

After the early postoperative period, typically 4 to 12 weeks for cataract surgery and 3 to 12 months for penetrating keratoplasty, optical correction is attempted. Spectacle correction is usually successful if the astigmatism is not marked and anisometropia is not significant. Small amounts of myopia and astigmatism after cataract surgery have been shown to yield good uncorrected distance and near visual acuities.[130,131] A hard contact lens can be used to correct anisometropia and moderate amounts of astigmatism. With smaller and smaller incisions being used for cataract surgery, surgically induced astigmatism is becoming less prevalent, and some surgeons are attempting to correct preoperative astigmatism at the time of cataract surgery.[132–135]

When postoperative astigmatism is not adequately corrected by suture manipulation or removal, spectacles, or contact lenses, surgical correction may be necessary to improve vision.[136] If wound gape is causing flattening in that meridian, reopening and resuturing the wound may be the best way to correct astigmatism.[137] Corneal wedge resections can also be used to correct central flattening in that meridian.[138] Corneal relaxing incisions, with or without compression sutures, can be used to flatten a steep meridian.[139–141] If astigmatism is present, especially in an ametropic patient, photoastigmatic refractive keratectomy with the excimer laser may be the best method of correction for binocular vision. Astigmatic keratotomy for postoperative astigmatism is discussed in Chapter 38 and photoastigmatic refractive keratectomy is discussed in Chapter 42.

CORNEAL CHANGES FROM LASER SURGERY

Laser treatments to the eye can be complicated by damage to the cornea. Any time a goniolens is used to perform a laser treatment there is potential for an epithelial abrasion. A bandage soft contact lens placed between the cornea and the goniolens can be used to prevent epithelial breakdown, especially in predisposed patients, such as those with diabetes mellitus or recurrent erosions.[142] The epithelium can also be damaged by a direct laser burn, especially if the eye moves or the laser beam is not correctly focused. Epithelial damage from a laser is treated in the same manner as a corneal abrasion and typically heals without scarring.

Laser treatment can also cause endothelial damage. Reversible and irreversible corneal decompensation, presumably caused by endothelial damage, has been reported after xenon arc retinal photocoagulation[143–145]; it was suggested that heat from the burn site was the culprit.[143,144] The focus of the laser beam for retinal photocoagulation is far from the cornea, however. Two studies showed minimal endothelial damage after retinal photocoagulation with the argon laser.[146,147] Because the wavelength of argon laser light is absorbed less by the cornea than that of xenon arc light, less direct damage is likely.

The argon laser is also used to perform trabeculoplasty and peripheral iridotomy. Although damage does not always occur, the potential for endothelial damage during these procedures is not difficult to imagine, because the laser energy is focused close to the cornea.[148,149] Endothelial damage has been demonstrated 6 months after argon laser trabeculoplasty.[150] Among the possible causes are a direct laser burn to the peripheral endothelium; heat generated by laser shots to the anterior chamber angle; aqueous, air bubbles, or cellular debris propelled against the endothelium by the laser shot; and increased intraocular pressure. Similar mechanisms could be responsible for endothelial damage from argon laser peripheral iridotomy; such damage has been shown in human eyes 3 months after the laser procedure.[150] Corneal decompensation was described in 11 eyes of 9 patients between 3 months and 6 years after argon laser peripheral iridotomy.[151,152]

The Nd:YAG laser is also used commonly for peripheral iridotomy and posterior capsulotomy and less commonly for lysis of vitreous strands or membranes and cyclophotocoagulation. Mild endothelial damage has been demonstrated after Nd:YAG iridotomy and capsulotomy,[153–155] but one study found no decrease in central endothelial cell density 1 week after the capsulotomy procedure.[156] In another study, however, a small (2.3

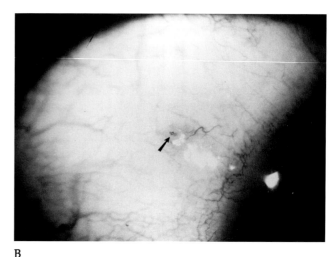

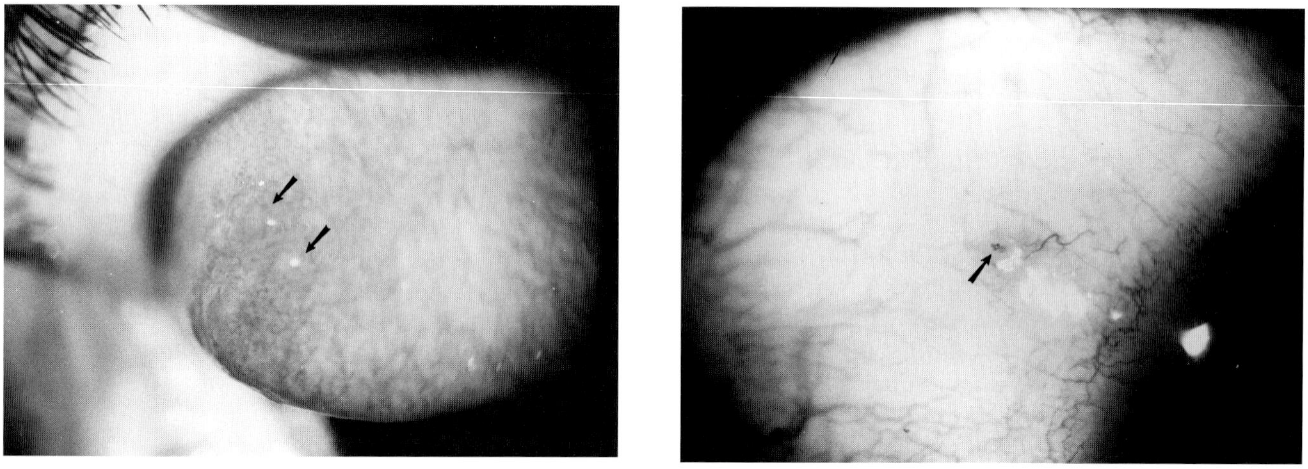

A B

FIGURE 26-23 **(A)** Giant papillae (arrows) on the superior tarsal conjunctiva postoperatively. **(B)** Examination of the bulbar conjunctiva reveals the inciting agent: an exposed suture (arrow). (Courtesy of Stephen R. Waltman, M.D., Belleville, IL.)

percent) but statistically significant decrease was noted after an average of 38 days. Endothelial damage has been observed after Nd:YAG lysis of vitreous strands.[157] Hypotony and focal scleral thinning have been reported after Nd:YAG cyclophotocoagulation.[158-160]

The corneal response to the excimer laser is described in Chapter 40. Potential complications include persistent or recurrent epithelial defects, corneal haze and scarring, and significant refractive changes.[161] Minimal or no endothelial cell damage has been demonstrated after 193-nm excimer laser ablation.[162,163]

CONJUNCTIVAL CHANGES

Giant Papillary Conjunctivitis

Giant papillary conjunctivitis, or *GPC*, should be considered in any patient who develops postoperative conjunctivitis accompanied by itching and a mucoid discharge. The disorder is thought to be caused by an allergic reaction to the protein coating on foreign bodies in the eye, including contact lenses, ocular prostheses, and exposed sutures.[164,165] It is diagnosed by everting the upper eyelid and looking for giant papillae on the tarsal conjunctiva (Figure 26-23). Suture-related giant papillary conjunctivitis is prevented by burying or covering the suture knots with conjunctiva. Treatment consists of burying the suture knots, if possible, or removing the exposed sutures if wound healing permits. Giant papillary conjunctivitis is refractory to treatment if the cause is not recognized.

Allergic or Toxic Conjunctivitis

Allergic or toxic reactions to topical medications can cause postoperative conjunctivitis. In contact hypersensitivity reactions, a lichenified rash develops on the eyelids. In other drug reactions, a follicular response of the inferior palpebral conjunctiva is characteristic. Aminoglycosides are particularly toxic when used on a chronic basis. Treatment involves discontinuing the offending medication.

REFERENCES

1. MacRae SM, Brown B, Edelhauser HF: The corneal toxicity of presurgical skin antiseptics. Am J Ophthalmol 97:221, 1984
2. Phinney RB, Mondino BJ, Hofbauer JD, et al: Corneal edema related to accidental Hibiclens exposure. Am J Ophthalmol 106:210, 1988
3. Schultz RD, Van Horn DL, Peters MA, et al: Diabetic keratopathy. Trans Am Ophthalmol Soc 79:180, 1981
4. Hatchell DL, Pederson HF, Faculjak ML: Susceptibility of the corneal epithelial basement membrane to injury in diabetic rabbits. Cornea 1:227, 1982
5. Poland DE, Kaufman HE: Clinical uses of collagen shields. J Cataract Refract Surg 14:489, 1988
6. Knapp A, Heuer DK, Stern GA, et al: Serious corneal complications of glaucoma filtering surgery with postoperative 5-fluorouracil. Am J Ophthalmol 103:183, 1987
7. Radtke N, Meyers S, Kaufman HE: Sterile corneal ulcers after cataract surgery in keratoconjunctivitis sicca. Arch Ophthalmol 96:51, 1978

8. Maffett MJ, Johns KJ, Parrish CM, et al: Sterile corneal ulceration after cataract extraction in patients with collagen vascular disease. Cornea 4:279, 1990
9. Groden LR, White W: Porcine collagen corneal shield treatment of persistent epithelial defects following penetrating keratoplasty. CLAO J 16:95, 1990
10. Zabel RW, Mintsioulis G, MacDonald IM: Corneal toxic changes after cataract extraction. Can J Ophthalmol 24:311, 1989
11. Dodds HT, Laibson PR: Filamentary keratitis following cataract extraction. Arch Ophthalmol 88:609, 1972
12. Glynn S, Schein OD, Seddon JM: The incidence of ulcerated keratitis among aphakic contact lens wearers in New England. Arch Ophthalmol 109:104, 1991
13. Nevyas AS, Raber IM, Eagle RC, et al: Acute band keratopathy following intracameral Viscoat. Arch Ophthalmol 105:958, 1987
14. Binder PS, Deg JK, Kohl S: Calcific band keratopathy after intraocular chondroitin sulfate. Arch Ophthalmol 105:1243, 1987
15. Sternberg P, Hatchell DL, Foulks GN, et al: The effect of silicone oil on the cornea. Arch Ophthalmol 103:90, 1985
16. Beekhius WH, Van Rij G, Zivojnovic R: Silicone oil keratopathy: indications for keratoplasty. Br J Ophthalmol 69:247, 1985
17. Graether JM: Detachments of Descemet's membrane by the injection of sodium hyaluronate. J Ocul Ther Surg 3:178, 1981
18. Hoover DL, Giangiacomo J, Benson RL: Descemet's membrane detachment by sodium hyaluronate. Arch Ophthalmol 103:805, 1985
19. Vastine DW, Weinberg RS, Sugar J, et al: Stripping of Descemet's membrane associated with intraocular lens implantation. Arch Ophthalmol 101:1042, 1983
20. Robin JB, Gindi JJ, Koh K, et al: An update of the indications for penetrating keratoplasty: 1979 through 1983. Arch Ophthalmol 104:87, 1986
21. Brady SE, Rapuano CJ, Arentsen JJ, et al: Clinical indications for and procedures associated with penetrating keratoplasty: 1983–1988. Am J Ophthalmol 108:118, 1989
22. Lindquist TD, McGlothan JS, Rotkis WM, et al: Indications for penetrating keratoplasty: 1980–1988. Cornea 10:210, 1991
23. Waring GO 3rd, Bourne WM, Edelhauser HF, Kenyon KR: The corneal endothelium: normal and pathologic structure and function. Ophthalmology 89:531, 1982
24. Yee RW, Matsuda M, Schultz RD, et al: Changes in the normal corneal endothelial cellular pattern as a function of age. Curr Eye Res 4:671, 1985
25. Rao GN, Aquavella JV, Goldberg SH, Berk SL: Pseudophakic bullous keratopathy: relationship to preoperative corneal endothelial status. Ophthalmology 91:1135, 1984
26. Matsuda M, Suda T, Manabe R: Serial alterations in endothelial cell shape and pattern after intraocular surgery. Am J Ophthalmol 98:313, 1984
27. Matsuda M, Miyake K, Inaba M: Long-term corneal endothelial changes after intraocular lens implantation. Am J Ophthalmol 105:248, 1988
28. Holladay JT, Bishop JE, Prager TC: Quantitative endothelial biomicroscopy. Ophthalmic Surg 14:33, 1983
29. Maurice DM: Cellular membrane activities in the corneal endothelium of the intact eye. Experientia 24:1094, 1968
30. Bourne WM, McCarey BE, Kaufman HE: Clinical specular microscopy. Trans Am Acad Ophthalmol Otolaryngol 81:743, 1976
31. Laing RA, Sandstrom MM, Leibowitz HM: In vivo photomicrography of the corneal endothelium. Arch Ophthalmol 93:143, 1975
32. Laird JA, Beuerman RW, Kaufman SC: Quantification of confocal images of human corneal endothelium. Proceedings. SPIE, San Jose, CA, January, 1996. Ophthalmic Technologies VI 2673:224, 1996
33. Pape LG, Balazs EA: The use of sodium hyaluronate (Healon) in human anterior segment surgery. Ophthalmology 87:699, 1980
34. Miller D, Stegman R: The use of Healon in intraocular lens implantation. Int Ophthalmol Clin 22:177, 1982
35. Breebart AC, Nuyts RMMA, Pels E, et al: Toxic endothelial cell destruction of the cornea after routine extracapsular cataract surgery. Arch Ophthalmol 108:1121, 1990
36. Edelhauser HF, Hyndiuk RA, Zeeb A, et al: Corneal edema and the intraocular use of epinephrine. Am J Ophthalmol 93:327, 1982
37. Glasser DB, Matsuda M, Ellis JG, et al: Effects of intraocular irrigating solutions on the corneal endothelium after in vivo anterior chamber irrigation. Am J Ophthalmol 99:321, 1985
38. Araie M: Barrier function of corneal endothelium and the intraocular irrigating solutions. Arch Ophthalmol 104:435, 1986
39. MacRae S: Intraocular drugs used in cataract surgery and their effect on the corneal endothelium. Refract Corneal Surg 7:249, 1991
40. Hoffer KJ, Kraff MC: Normal endothelial cell count range. Ophthalmology 87:861, 1980
41. Schultz RO, Glasser DB, Matsuda M, et al: Response of the corneal endothelium to cataract surgery. Arch Ophthalmol 104:1164, 1986
42. Galin MA, Lin LL, Fetherolf E, et al: Time analysis of corneal endothelial cell density after cataract extraction. Am J Ophthalmol 88:93, 1979
43. Bourne WM, Kaufman HE: Cataract extraction and the corneal endothelium. Am J Ophthalmol 82:44, 1976
44. Drews RC, Waltman SR: Endothelial cell loss in intraocular lens placement. J Am Intraocul Implant Soc 4:14, 1978
45. Kraff MC, Sanders DR, Lieberman HL: Specular microscopy in cataract and intraocular lens patients: a report of 564 cases. Arch Ophthalmol 98:1782, 1980
46. Sugar J, Mitchelson J, Kraff M: The effect of phacoemulsification on corneal endothelial cell density. Arch Ophthalmol 96:446, 1978

47. Waltman SR, Cozean CH Jr: The effect of phacoemulsification on the corneal endothelium. Ophthalmic Surg 10:31, 1979
48. Graether JM, Davison JA, Harris GW, et al: A comparison of the effects of phacoemulsification and nucleus expression on endothelial cell density. J Am Intraocul Implant Soc 9:420, 1983
49. Cozean CH Jr, Waltman SR: The effects of posterior chamber phacoemulsification and secondary Kelman anterior chamber lens implantation on the corneal endothelium. J Am Intraocul Implant Soc 7:237, 1981
50. Hayashi K, Nakao F, Hayashi F: Corneal endothelial cell loss after phacoemulsification using nuclear cracking procedures. J Cataract Refract Surg 20:44, 1994
51. Dick HB, Kohnen T, Jacobi FK, Jacobi KW: Long-term endothelial cell loss following phacoemulsification through a temporal clear corneal incision. J Cataract Refract Surg 22:63, 1996
52. Bourne WM, Kaufman HE: Endothelial damage associated with intraocular lenses. Am J Ophthalmol 81:482, 1976
53. Forstot SL, Blackwell WL, Jaffe NS, et al: The effect of intraocular lens implantation on the corneal endothelium. Trans Am Acad Ophthalmol Otolaryngol 83:195, 1977
54. Kaufman HE, Katz J, Valenti J, et al: Endothelial damage with intraocular lenses: contact adhesions between surgical materials and tissue. Science 198:525, 1977
55. Kaufman HE, Katz JI: Endothelial damage from intraocular lens insertion. Invest Ophthalmol 15:996, 1976
56. Sugar J, Mitchelson J, Kraff M: Endothelial trauma and cell loss from intraocular lens insertion. Arch Ophthalmol 96:449, 1978
57. Kraff MC, Sanders DR, Lieberman HL: Monitoring for continuing endothelial cell loss with cataract extraction and intraocular lens implantation. Ophthalmology 89:30, 1982
58. Cheng H, McPherson K, Bron AJ (Oxford Cataract Treatment and Evaluation Team): Long-term corneal endothelial cell loss after cataract surgery. Arch Ophthalmol 104:1170, 1986
59. Speaker MG, Lugo M, Laibson PR, et al: Penetrating keratoplasty for pseudophakic bullous keratopathy. Ophthalmology 95:1260, 1988
60. Stark WJ, Whitney CE, Chandler JW, et al: Trends in intraocular lens implantation in the United States. Arch Ophthalmol 104:1769, 1986
61. Waring GO 3rd: The 50-year epidemic of pseudophakic corneal edema. Arch Ophthalmol 107:657, 1989
62. Cohen EJ, Brady SE, Leavitt K, et al: Pseudophakic bullous keratopathy. Am J Ophthalmol 106:264, 1988
63. Sugar A, Meyer RF, Heidemann D: Specular microscopic follow-up of corneal grafts for pseudophakic bullous keratopathy. Ophthalmology 92:325, 1985
64. Sugar A: An analysis of corneal endothelial and graft survival in pseudophakic bullous keratopathy. Trans Am Ophthalmol Soc 87:762, 1989
65. Lim ES, Apple DJ, Tsai JC, et al: An analysis of flexible anterior chamber lenses with special reference to the normalized rate of lens explantation. Ophthalmology 98:243, 1991
66. Lass JH, DeSantis DM, Reinhart WJ, et al: Clinical and morphometric results of penetrating keratoplasty with one piece anterior chamber or suture-fixated posterior chamber lenses in the absence of lens capsule. Arch Ophthalmol 108:1427, 1990
67. Hayashi K, Hayashi H, Nakao F, Hayashi F: Corneal endothelial cell loss in phacoemulsification surgery with silicone intraocular lens implantation. J Cataract Refract Surg 22:743, 1996
68. Arentsen JJ, Donoso R, Laibson PR: Penetrating keratoplasty for the treatment of pseudophakic corneal edema associated with posterior chamber lens implantation. Ophthalmic Surg 18:514, 1987
69. Lugo M, Cohen EJ, Eagle RC: The incidence of preoperative endothelial dystrophy in pseudophakic bullous keratopathy. Ophthalmic Surg 19:16, 1988
70. Miller DM, Stegmann R: Use of sodium hyaluronate in human IOL implantation. Ann Ophthalmol 13:811, 1980
71. Barron BA, Busin M, Page C, et al: Comparison of the effects of Viscoat and Healon on postoperative intraocular pressure. Am J Ophthalmol 100:377, 1985
72. Glasser DB, Edelhauser HF: Toxicity of surgical solutions. Int Ophthalmol Clin 29:179, 1989
73. Liesegang TJ: Viscoelastic substances in ophthalmology. Surv Ophthalmol 34:268, 1990
74. Kent HD, Cohen EJ, Laibson PR, et al: Microbial keratitis and corneal ulceration associated with therapeutic soft contact lenses. CLAO J 16:49, 1990
75. Waring GO 3rd, Stulting RD, Street D: Penetrating keratoplasty for pseudophakic corneal edema with exchange of intraocular lenses. Arch Ophthalmol 105:58, 1987
76. Busin M, Arffa RC, McDonald MB, et al: Intraocular lens removal during penetrating keratoplasty for pseudophakic bullous keratopathy. Ophthalmology 94:505, 1987
77. Brown SI, McLean JM: Peripheral corneal edema after cataract extraction: a new clinical entity. Trans Am Acad Ophthalmol Otolaryngol 73:465, 1969
78. Brown SI: Peripheral corneal edema after cataract extraction. Am J Ophthalmol 70:326, 1970
79. Tuft SJ, Kerr Muir M, Sherrard ES, Buckley RJ: Peripheral corneal edema following cataract extraction (Brown-McLean syndrome). Eye 6:502, 1992
80. Gothard TW, Hardten DR, Lane SS, et al: Clinical findings in Brown-McLean syndrome. Am J Ophthalmol 115:729, 1993
81. Reed JW, Cain LR, Weaver RG, Oberfeld SM: Clinical and pathologic findings of aphakic peripheral corneal edema: Brown-McLean syndrome. Cornea 11:577, 1992
82. Weiner MJ, Trentacost J, Pon DM, et al: Epithelial downgrowth. A clinicopathological review. Br J Ophthalmol 73:6, 1989
83. Feder RS, Krachmer JH: The diagnosis of epithelial downgrowth after keratoplasty. Br J Ophthalmol 99:697, 1985
84. Orlin SE, Raber IM, Laibson PR, et al: Epithelial downgrowth following the removal of iris inclusion cysts. Ophthalmic Surg 22:330, 1991

85. Maumenee AE: Treatment of epithelial downgrowth and intraocular fistula following cataract extraction. Trans Am Ophthalmol Soc 62:153, 1964
86. Anseth A, Dohlman CH, Albert DM: Epithelial downgrowth fistula repair and keratoplasty. Refract Corneal Surg 7:23, 1991
87. Stark WJ, Michels RG, Maumenee AE, Cupples H: Surgical management of epithelial ingrowth. Am J Ophthalmol 85:772, 1978
88. Fish A, Heuer DK, Baerveldt G, et al: Molteno implantation for secondary glaucomas associated with advanced epithelial ingrowth. Ophthalmology 97:557, 1990
89. Yannuzzi LA, Theodore FH: Cryotherapy of post cataract blebs. Am J Ophthalmol 76:217, 1973
90. Swan KC: Hyphema due to wound vascularization after cataract extraction. Arch Ophthalmol 89:87, 1973
91. Kramer TR, Reay HB, Lynch MG, et al: Transscleral Nd:YAG photocoagulation for cataract incision vascularization associated with recurrent hyphema. Am J Ophthalmol 107:681, 1989
92. Kronish JW, Forster RK: Control of corneal astigmatism following cataract extraction by selective suture cutting. Arch Ophthalmol 105:1650, 1987
93. Goel R, Crewdson J, Chignell AH: Astigmatism following retinal detachment surgery. Br J Ophthalmol 67:327, 1983
94. Thompson WE, Reinecke RD: The changes in refractive status following routine strabismus surgery. J Pediatr Ophthalmol 17:372, 1980
95. Swinger CA: Postoperative astigmatism. Surv Ophthalmol 31:219, 1987
96. Stainer GA, Binder PS, Porker WT, et al: The natural and modified course of post-cataract astigmatism. Ophthalmic Surg 13:822, 1982
97. Gorn RA: Surgically induced corneal astigmatism and its spontaneous regression. Ophthalmic Surg 16:162, 1985
98. Wishart MS, Wishart PK, Gregor ZJ: Corneal astigmatism following cataract extraction. Br J Ophthalmol 70:825 1986
99. Axt JC: Longitudinal study of postoperative astigmatism. J Cataract Refract Surg 13:381, 1987
100. Richards SC, Brodstein RS, Richards WL, et al: Long-term course of surgically induced astigmatism. J Cataract Refract Surg 14:270, 1988
101. Parker WT, Clorfeine GS: Long-term evolution of astigmatism following planned extracapsular cataract extraction. Arch Ophthalmol 107:353, 1989
102. Cory CC: Prevention and treatment of post implantation astigmatism. J Cataract Refract Surg 15:58, 1989
103. Cravy TV: Long-term corneal astigmatism related to selected elastic, monofilament, nonabsorbable sutures. J Cataract Refract Surg 15:61, 1989
104. Masket S: Keratorefractive aspects of the scleral pocket incision and closure method for cataract surgery. J Cataract Refract Surg 15:70, 1989
105. Jaffe NS, Clayman HM: The pathophysiology of corneal astigmatism after cataract extraction. Trans Am Acad Ophthalmol Otolaryngol 79:615, 1975
106. Van Rij G, Waring GO: Changes in corneal curvature induced by sutures and incisions. Am J Ophthalmol 98:773, 1984
107. Bartholomew RS: Post-cataract astigmatism: its control and correction. Aust N Z J Ophthalmol 16:215, 1988
108. Thrasher BH, Boerner CF: Control of astigmatism by wound placement. Am Intraocul Implant Soc J 10:176, 1984
109. Jaffe NS, Jaffe MS, Jaffe GF: Cataract Surgery and its Complications. CV Mosby, St. Louis, 1990
110. Lindstrom RL, Destro MA: Effect of incision size and Terry keratometer usage on postoperative astigmatism. Am Intraocul Implant Soc J 11:469, 1985
111. Neumann AC, McCarty GR, Sanders DR, et al: Small incisions to control astigmatism during cataract surgery. J Cataract Refract Surg 15:78, 1989
112. Shepard JR: Induced astigmatism in small incision cataract surgery. J Cataract Refract Surg 15:85, 1989
113. Steinert RF, Brint SF, White SM, et al: Astigmatism after small incision cataract surgery. Ophthalmology 98:417, 1991
114. Kansas PG: Modified pocket incision: a simplified technique for astigmatism control and wound closure. J Cataract Refract Surg 15:93, 1989
115. Masket S: Deep versus appositional suturing of the scleral pocket incision for astigmatic control in cataract surgery. J Cataract Refract Surg 13:131, 1987
116. Werblin TP: Refractive stability after cataract extraction using a 6.5-millimeter scleral pocket incision with horizontal or radial sutures. J Refract Corneal Surg 10:339, 1994
117. Hayashi K, Hayashi H, Nakao F, Hayashi F: The correlation between incision size and corneal shape changes in sutureless cataract surgery. Ophthalmology 102:550, 1995
118. Kohnen T, Dick B, Jacobi KW: Comparison of the induced astigmatism after temporal clear corneal tunnel incisions of different sizes. J Cataract Refract Surg 21:417, 1995
119. Nielsen PJ: Prospective evaluation of surgically induced astigmatism and astigmatic keratotomy effects of various self-sealing small incisions. J Cataract Refract Surg 21:43, 1995
120. Gross RH, Miller KM: Corneal astigmatism after phacoemulsification and lens implantation through unsutured scleral and corneal tunnel incisions. Am J Ophthalmol 121:57, 1996
121. Masket S: Comparison of suture materials for closure of the scleral pocket incision. J Cataract Refract Surg 14:548, 1988
122. Van Meter WS, Gassier JR, Solomon KD, et al: Post keratoplasty astigmatism control: single continuous suture adjustment versus selective interrupted suture removal. Ophthalmology 98:177, 1991
123. Musch DC, Meyer RF, Sugar A, et al: Corneal astigmatism after penetrating keratoplasty: the role of suture technique. Ophthalmology 96:698, 1989
124. Stainer GA, Binder PS: Controlled reduction of post keratoplasty astigmatism. Ophthalmology 89:668, 1982
125. Perl T, Binder PS, Earl K: Post-cataract astigmatism with and without the use of the Terry keratometer. Ophthalmology 91:489, 1984
126. Jacobi KW, Strobel J: Control of post operative astigmatism. Trans Ophthalmol Soc UK 104:715, 1985

127. Roper-Hall MJ: Control of astigmatism after surgery and trauma. Br J Ophthalmol 66:556, 1982
128. Binder PS: The effect of suture removal on post keratoplasty astigmatism. Am J Ophthalmol 105:637, 1988
129. Musch DC, Meyer RF, Sugar AI: The effect of removing running sutures on astigmatism after penetrating keratoplasty. Arch Ophthalmol 106:488, 1988
130. Datiles MB, Gancayco T: Low myopia with low astigmatic correction gives cataract surgery patients good depth of focus. Ophthalmology 97:922, 1990
131. Sawusch MR, Guyton DL: Optimal astigmatism to enhance depth of focus after cataract surgery. Ophthalmology 98:1025, 1991
132. Osher RH: Paired transverse relaxing keratotomy: a combined technique for reducing astigmatism. J Cataract Refract Surg 15:32, 1989
133. Davison JA: Transverse astigmatic keratotomy combined with phacoemulsification and intraocular lens implantation. J Cataract Refract Surg 15:38, 1989
134. Maloney WF, Grindle L, Sanders D, et al: Astigmatism control for the cataract surgeon: a comprehensive review of surgically tailored astigmatism reduction. J Cataract Refract Surg 15:45, 1989
135. Shepherd JR: Correction of pre-existing astigmatism at the time of small incision cataract surgery. J Cataract Refract Surg 15:55, 1989
136. Gelendev H: Management of corneal astigmatism after cataract surgery. Refract Corneal Surg 7:99, 1991
137. Cravy TV: Modification of post cataract astigmatism by wound revision. Int Ophthalmol Clin 23:111, 1983
138. Lugo M, Donnenfeld ED, Arentsen JJ: Corneal wedge resection for high astigmatism following penetrating keratoplasty. Ophthalmic Surg 18:650, 1987
139. Mandel MR, Shapiro MB, Krachmer JH: Relaxing incisions with augmentation sutures for the correction of post-keratoplasty astigmatism. Am J Ophthalmol 103:441, 1987
140. Thornton SP: Astigmatic keratotomy: a review of basic concepts with case reports. J Cataract Refract Surg 16:430, 1990
141. Buzard KA: Paired relaxing incisions for the control of astigmatism. Cornea 10:38, 1991
142. Arentsen JJ, Tasman W: Using a bandage contact lens to prevent recurrent corneal erosion during photocoagulation in patients with diabetes. Am J Ophthalmol 92:714, 1981
143. Pfister RR, Schepens CL, Lemp MA, Webster RG: Photocoagulation keratopathy. Arch Ophthalmol 86:94, 1971
144. Kanski JJ: Anterior segment complications of retinal photocoagulation. Am J Ophthalmol 79:424, 1975
145. MacKay CJ, Koester CJ, Campbell CJ: The corneal endothelium following photocoagulation: induced decompensation. Ann Ophthalmol 15:346, 1983
146. Pardos GJ, Krachmer JH: Photocoagulation: its effect on the corneal endothelial cell density of diabetics. Arch Ophthalmol 99:84, 1981
147. Hirst LW, Robin AL, Sherman S, et al: Corneal endothelial changes after argon-laser iridotomy and panretinal photocoagulation. Am J Ophthalmol 93:473, 1982
148. Traverso C, Cohen EJ, Groden LR, et al: Central corneal endothelial cell density after argon laser trabeculoplasty. Arch Ophthalmol 102:1322, 1984
149. Thoming C, Van Buskirk EM, Samples JR: The corneal endothelium after laser therapy for glaucoma. Am J Ophthalmol 103:518, 1987
150. Hong C, Kitazawa Y, Tanishima T: Influence of argon laser treatment of glaucoma on corneal endothelium. Jpn J Ophthalmol 27:567, 1983
151. Jeng S, Lee JS, Huang SC: Corneal decompensation after argon laser iridectomy—a delayed complication. Ophthalmic Surg 22:565, 1991
152. Schwartz AL, Martin NF, Weber PA: Corneal decompensation after argon laser iridectomy. Arch Ophthalmol 106:1572, 1988
153. Sherrard ES, Kerr Muir MG: Damage to the corneal endothelium by Q-switched Nd:YAG laser posterior capsulotomy. Trans Ophthalmol Soc UK 104:524, 1985
154. Wishart PK, Sherrard ES, Nagasubramanian S, et al: Corneal endothelial changes following short pulsed laser iridotomy and surgical iridectomy. Trans Ophthalmol Soc U K 105:541, 1986
155. Canning CR, Capon MRC, Sherrard ES, et al: Neodymium:YAG laser iridotomies—short-term comparison with capsulotomies and long-term followup. Graefes Arch Clin Exp Ophthalmol 226:49, 1988
156. Kraff MC, Sanders DR, Lieberman HL: Intraocular pressure and the corneal endothelium after neodymium:YAG laser posterior capsulotomy. Arch Ophthalmol 103:511, 1985
157. Nirankari VS, Richards RD: Complications associated with the use of the neodymium:YAG laser. Ophthalmology 92:1371, 1985
158. Levy NS, Bonney RC: Transscleral YAG cyclocoagulation of the ciliary body for persistently high intraocular pressure following penetrating keratoplasty. Cornea 8:178, 1989
159. Maus M, Katz LJ: Choroidal detachment, flat anterior chamber, and hypotony as complications of neodymium:YAG laser cyclophotocoagulation. Ophthalmology 97:69, 1990
160. Fiore PM, Melamed S, Krug JH: Focal scleral thinning after transscleral Nd:YAG cyclophotocoagulation. Ophthalmic Surg 20:215, 1989
161. Sher NA, Bowers RA, Zabel RW, et al: Clinical use of the 193-nm excimer laser in the treatment of corneal scars. Arch Ophthalmol 109:491, 1991
162. Amano S, Shimizu K: Corneal endothelial changes after excimer laser photorefractive keratectomy. Am J Ophthalmol 116:692, 1993
163. Carones F, Brancato R, Venturi E, Morico A: The corneal endothelium after myopic excimer laser photorefractive keratectomy. Arch Ophthalmol 112:920, 1994
164. Sugar A, Meyer RF: Giant papillary conjunctivitis after keratoplasty. Am J Ophthalmol 91:239, 1981
165. Nirankari VS, Karesh JW, Richards RD: Complications of exposed monofilament sutures. Am J Ophthalmol 95:515, 1983

27

Corneal Changes from Contact Lenses

OLIVER H. DABEZIES, JR., STEPHEN D. KLYCE, JOHN F. MORGAN, JACK HARTSTEIN, PETER C. DONSHIK, GUY J. BOSWALL, WILLIAM H. EHLERS, RAYMOND M. STEIN, AND DONALD J. DOUGHMAN

After the introduction of polymethyl methacrylate contact lenses in 1948,[1] contact lenses became a practical modality for the correction of refractive errors. By the early 1960s, more than a half million people were wearing hard contact lenses. With the introduction of daily-wear soft lenses in the late 1960s and extended-wear soft lenses in the 1980s, the number of people wearing contact lenses increased dramatically. It is estimated that there are now 25 million contact lens wearers in the United States alone.[2]

As might be anticipated, a growing incidence of complications has accompanied the increased use of contact lenses. This chapter discusses these complications, which include corneal warpage, hypersensitivity and toxicity reactions to preservatives in contact lens care products, corneal neovascularization, changes in the corneal epithelium and anterior stroma, microbial keratitis, and changes in the posterior stroma and endothelium. Giant papillary conjunctivitis is discussed in Chapter 23.

CORNEAL WARPAGE

Astigmatic changes are fairly common in contact lens wearers. One study reported astigmatic changes in 70 percent of contact lenses wearers[3]; in addition to regular astigmatism, some patients also developed irregular astigmatism. Contact lens wear can induce corneal warpage, which is a distortion of the cornea resulting in irregular astigmatism.[4]

Many contact lens wearers are not aware that they have corneal warpage because they are asymptomatic as long as they wear their lenses. However, when they replace their lenses with eyeglasses, they notice a decrease in vision, referred to as *spectacle blur.*

The clinical signs of corneal warpage include a change in refraction, a change in keratometry readings, and a decrease in spectacle-corrected visual acuity. Videokeratography illustrates pronounced irregular astigmatism and abnormal corneal power distribution. Patients with corneal warpage can obtain normal (20/20) vision only by wearing hard or rigid gas-permeable contact lenses, which provide an optically smooth surface.

Contact lens-induced corneal warpage is either deliberate or inadvertent. Deliberate warpage occurs with orthokeratology and other corneal molding techniques; inadvertent warpage occurs with the cosmetic wear of contact lenses, especially hard lenses.

Deliberate Warpage

At one time, patients with myopia were fitted with hard contact lenses that were flatter than the cornea in an attempt to permanently flatten the cornea and thereby decrease the myopia. This technique, called *orthokeratology,* is of little practical use in the treatment of myopia. Although one study documented that contact lenses can flatten the cornea and decrease myopia,[5] the change was not permanent and continued contact lens wear was necessary to maintain the effect.

The use of contact lenses to flatten the cornea has also been advocated in the management of keratoconus. Some maintain that better vision can be obtained when the lens is fitted slightly flatter than the cone so that it lightly touches the apex of the cone. Such a fit can flatten the cone to some extent; however, central anterior stromal scarring may be induced.

Contact lenses may help mold the corneas of patients who have undergone penetrating keratoplasty. Astigmatism is common after penetrating keratoplasty; the

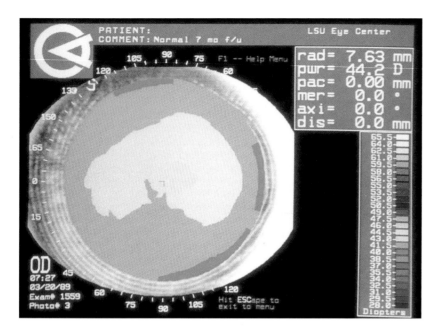

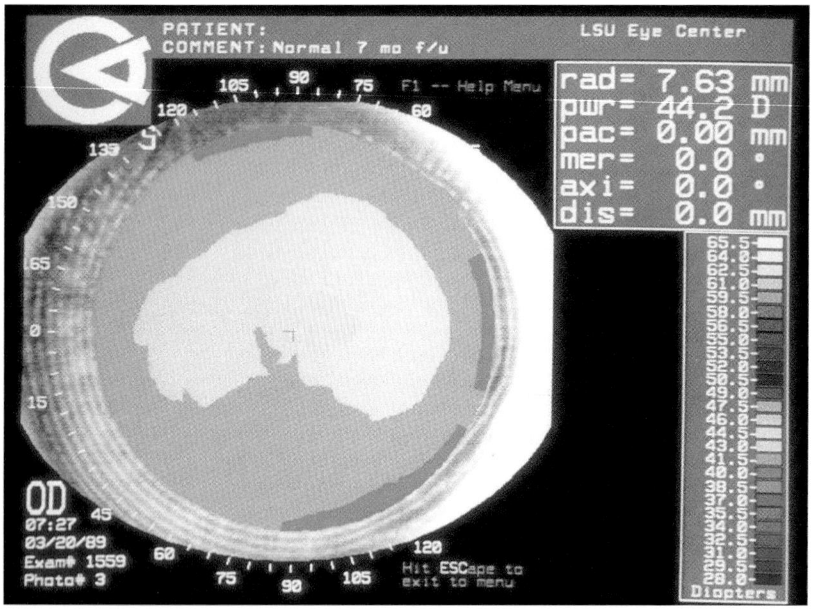

FIGURE 27-1 Videokeratograph of a normal cornea that is radially asymmetrical. Note that the central area of the cornea is light green (steeper) superiorly and dark green (flatter) inferiorly.

average amount is 4 diopters, but many patients have more. Irregular astigmatism is also common. Contact lens wear in the early postoperative period may decrease astigmatism and improve the regularity and optical qualities of the graft. The hypothesis is that the contact lens, by providing a splint (or mold), forces the cornea into a more spherical shape as the wound heals. Support for this hypothesis has been shown retrospectively in a series of keratoconus graft patients[6] and in a more general series,[7] although a conclusive demonstration awaits a larger clinical trial.

Inadvertent Warpage

Contact lens wear for cosmetic purposes can cause inadvertent corneal warpage because pressure is exerted by the contact lens (which has a spherical posterior surface) on the cornea (which does not have a spherical anterior surface).

It was once thought that the cornea was radially symmetrical. However, videokeratography has shown that normal corneas are radially asymmetrical, aspherical, and distinctive from individual to individual[8] (Figure 27-1). Because most contact lenses are radially symmetrical, a parallel fitting relationship between the contact lens and the cornea is not always possible. This disparity between the shape of the contact lens and the contour of the cornea is probably the main cause of inadvertent corneal warpage. The consequences of inadvertent corneal warpage have been studied with videokeratography[9,10] (Figure 27-2).

Various authors[11–15] have expressed concern that contact lenses can induce or promote keratoconus. In all likelihood, these were cases in which decentered contact lenses caused corneal warpage. Because this condition can mimic keratoconus, it is called *pseudokeratoconus.* Pseudokeratoconus is especially likely to occur with a superior-riding hard contact lens on a cornea with pre-existing with-the-rule astigmatism. In this case, the contact lens can flatten the superior cornea and steepen the inferior cornea (Figure 27-3).

Although corneal warpage can mimic keratoconus, early keratoconus is sometimes actually present. The two conditions can be differentiated only by discontinuing contact lens wear and performing follow-up examinations with videokeratography until the corneal topography stabilizes. If the irregular astigmatism persists or becomes more prominent, keratoconus is present. However, if the irregular astigmatism improves, then pseudokeratoconus is the correct diagnosis. Videokeratography can detect early keratoconus well before any other clinical symptoms or signs occur (see Ch. 22).

If inadvertent corneal warpage occurs, contact lens wear should be discontinued. The average time for corneal stabilization is 5 weeks for soft lenses, 10 weeks for rigid gas-permeable lenses, and 15 weeks for polymethyl methacrylate lenses.[10] If a patient chooses to continue contact lens wear in the presence of corneal warpage, the refraction and keratometry readings should not be used for keratorefractive surgery. Not permitting the corneal power to stabilize can add an element of unpredictability of 1 to 2 diopters to a refractive surgical result.

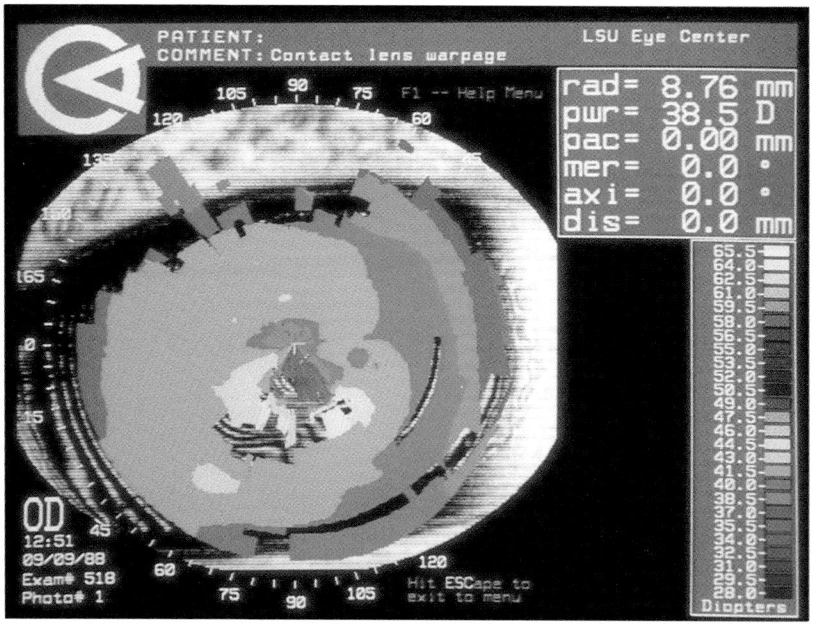

FIGURE 27-2 Videokeratograph of irregular corneal warpage caused by contact lens wear. Note that the two halves of the blue "bowtie" are skewed in relation to each other. This patient wore a flat-fitting contact lens.

HYPERSENSITIVITY AND TOXICITY REACTIONS

Chemical preservatives in contact lens care products can cause hypersensitivity and/or toxicity reactions[16–25] (Table 27-1). A hypersensitivity reaction (cell-mediated delayed hypersensitivity) occurs when an antigen is reintroduced and causes sensitized T cells to produce a variety of effects, including direct cytotoxicity against cells bearing the offending antigen and elaboration of lymphokines, which then have various secondary effects. A hypersensitivity reaction is not dose related. It may develop to any of the preservatives used in contact lens care products, particularly mercurials such as thimerosal (Figure 27-4). Thimerosal is found in 15 percent of ophthalmic drug solutions, 21 percent of polymethyl methacrylate contact lens care products, 44 percent of rigid gas-permeable contact lens care products, and 24 percent of soft contact lens care products.

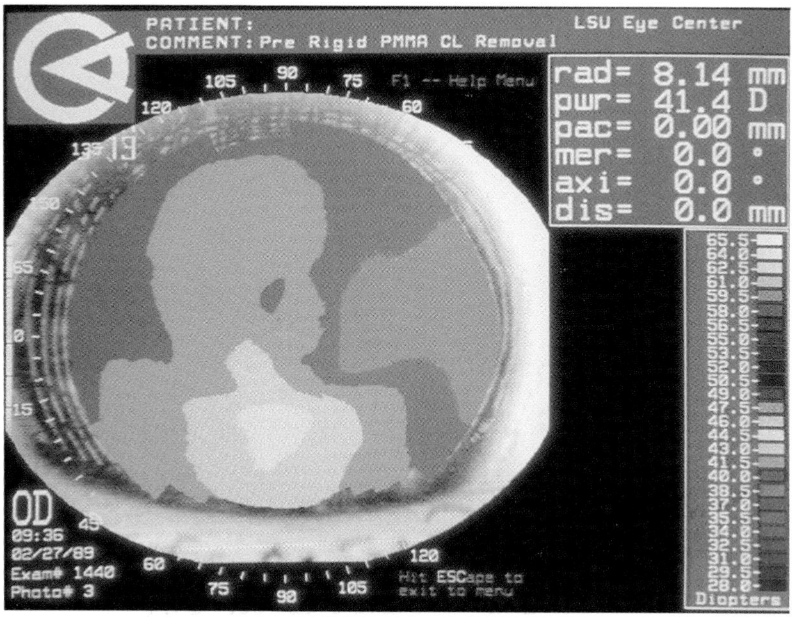

FIGURE 27-3 Videokeratograph of pseudokeratoconus caused by contact lens-induced warpage. Note the relative flattening (blue, dark green) superiorly and the relative steepening (light green, yellow) inferiorly. This patient wore a superior-riding hard contact lens.

TABLE 27-1
Hypersensitivity and Toxicity Reactions to Preservatives in Contact Lens Care Products

Preservative	*Hypersensitivity Reaction*	*Toxicity Reaction*	*Lens Care Product Containing Preservative*
Alkyl triethanol ammonium chloride	–	+	Soft contact lens soaking solutions
Benzalkonium chloride	–	++	PMMA contact lens care products; RGP contact lens care products
Chlorbutanol	–	+	Hard contact lens care products
Chlorhexidine	–	++	RGP contact lens soaking solutions
Hydrogen peroxide	–	++	Soft contact lens disinfectants
Polyaminopropyl biguanide	–	–	RGP contact lens soaking solutions; preserved saline and soaking solutions for soft contact lenses
Polyquaternium 1	–	–	Saline solution; contact lens surfactant cleaner
Sodium dichloroisocyanate	–	–	
Sorbate	+	–	
Thimerosal	++++	–	PMMA, RGP, and soft contact lens care products

Abbreviations: PMMA, polymethyl methacrylate; RGP, rigid gas-permeable.

Unlike a hypersensitivity reaction, a toxicity reaction is dose related. Preservatives kill microorganisms by disrupting the integrity of their enzyme systems or cell walls or their ability to replicate. Preservatives sometimes damage corneal cells, particularly the metabolically active epithelial cells, and produce a toxicity reaction. Toxicity reactions occur most frequently with benzalkonium chloride and chlorhexidine, especially when contact lens solutions that contain such preservatives are used by soft contact lens wearers (Figure 27-5).

CORNEAL NEOVASCULARIZATION

Although contact lens wear normally causes dilation and slight radial extension of the limbal blood vessels into the cornea, these vessels do not have the branching pattern of proliferating new blood vessels; this phenomenon is not considered to be a form of corneal neovascularization. (Figure 27-6). In one study,[26] the average radial extension of vessels into the cornea in soft contact lens wearers was 1.02 mm (±0.47 mm) superiorly and 0.39 mm (±0.25 mm) inferiorly.

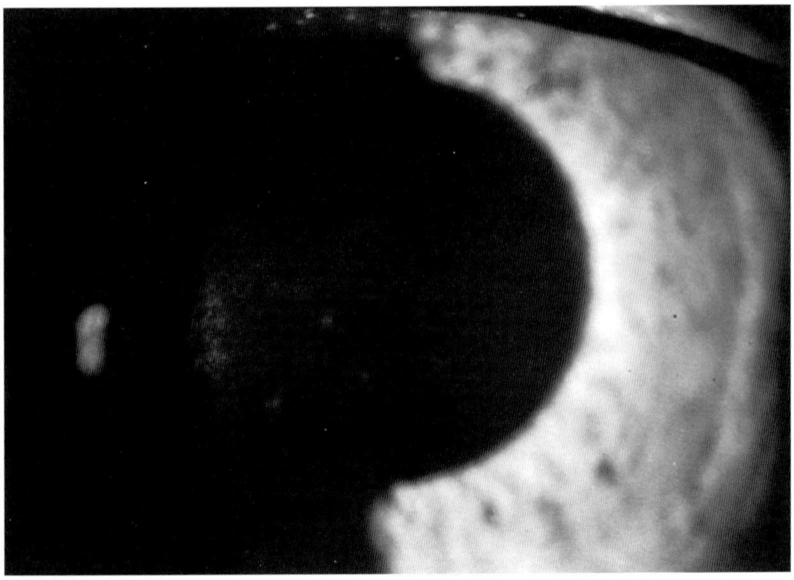

FIGURE 27-4 Keratopathy caused by hypersensitivity reaction to thimerosal. Note the punctate subepithelial opacities.

True corneal neovascularization is the formation of new blood vessels that extend in a branching pattern into the cornea (Figure 27-7). It occurs in 7 to 8 percent of patients who wear extended-wear soft lenses[27] and in 1 to 2 percent of patients who wear daily-wear hard lenses.[28] Corneal neovascularization can be divided into two grades.[29] Grade 1 is vessel encroachment on the cornea that does not exceed 0.4 mm with daily-wear hard lenses, 0.6 mm with daily-wear soft lenses, or 1.4 mm with extended-wear soft lenses. Grade 2 is vessel encroachment that exceeds grade 1 and extends up to but does not enter the entrance pupil.

The cause of neovascularization in contact lens wearers is not known, but a variety of metabolic factors may be involved. Contact lenses can cause hypoxia, which may result in the accumulation of lactic acid and, subsequently, stimulation of neovascularization. Substances that could inactivate normally present angiogenic suppression factors may play a role, such as the corneal factor that restrains division and migration of cells of the pericorneal vascular plexus.[30]

The risks of corneal neovascularization may be minimized by fitting a lens that provides minimal interference with corneal physiology (i.e., a lens with high oxygen permeability) or fitting a lens that has good movement to avoid limbal compression.

If corneal neovascularization has already begun, the patient should (1) change to a lens care system that either does not contain preservatives or has preservatives that do not cause hypersensitivity or toxicity reactions; (2) change from extended-wear lenses to daily-wear lenses; (3) reduce lens wearing time; or (4) change from

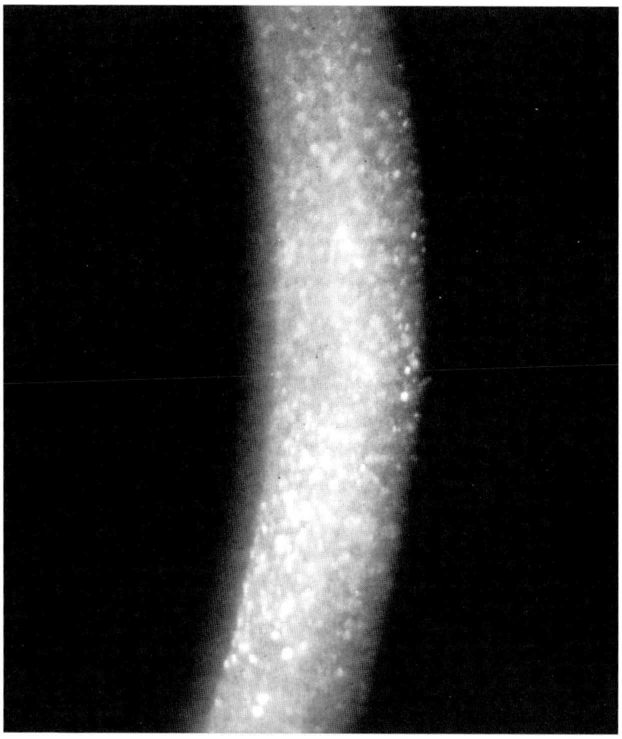

FIGURE 27-5 Superficial punctate keratitis in a contact lens wearer who had a toxicity reaction to a lens care solution.

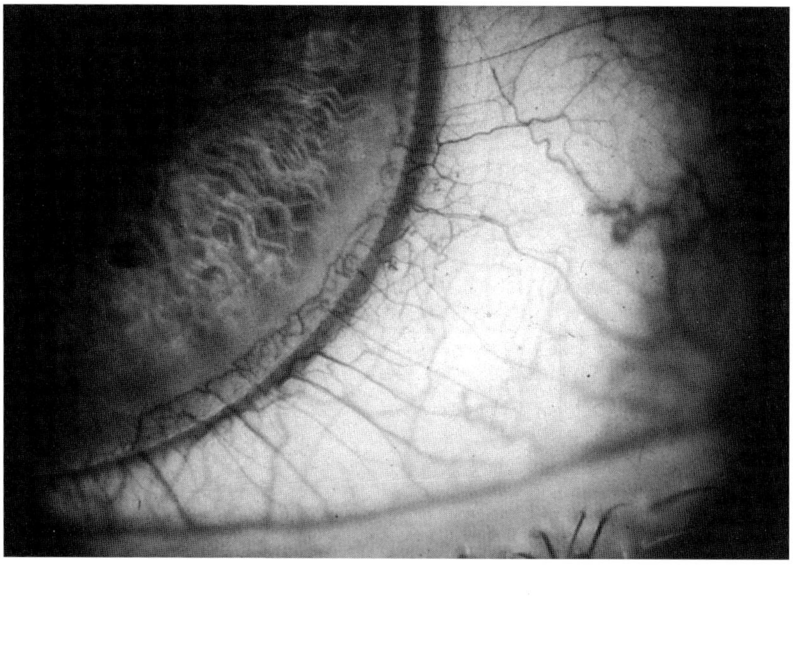

FIGURE 27-6 Normal vascular response to contact lens wear. There is dilation of normal limbal blood vessels with slight radial extension into the cornea.

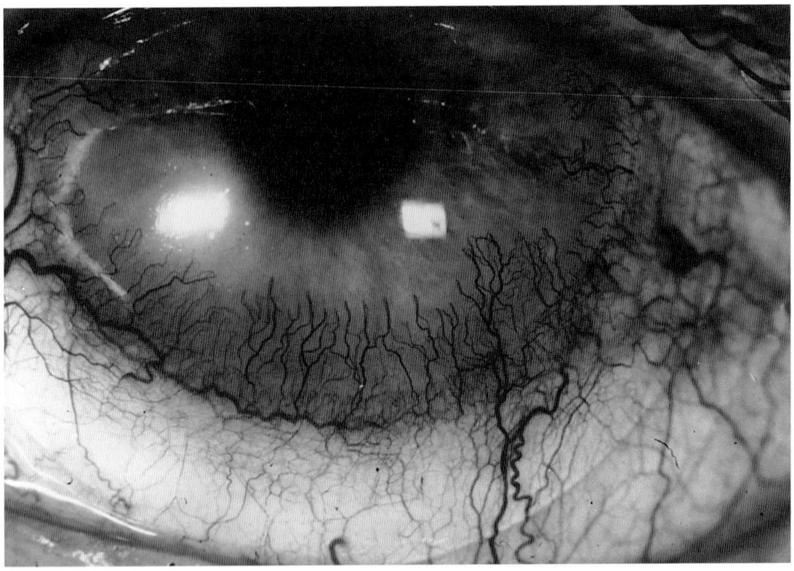

FIGURE 27-7 Abnormal vascular response (neovascularization) to contact lens wear. New blood vessels extend into the cornea in a branching pattern.

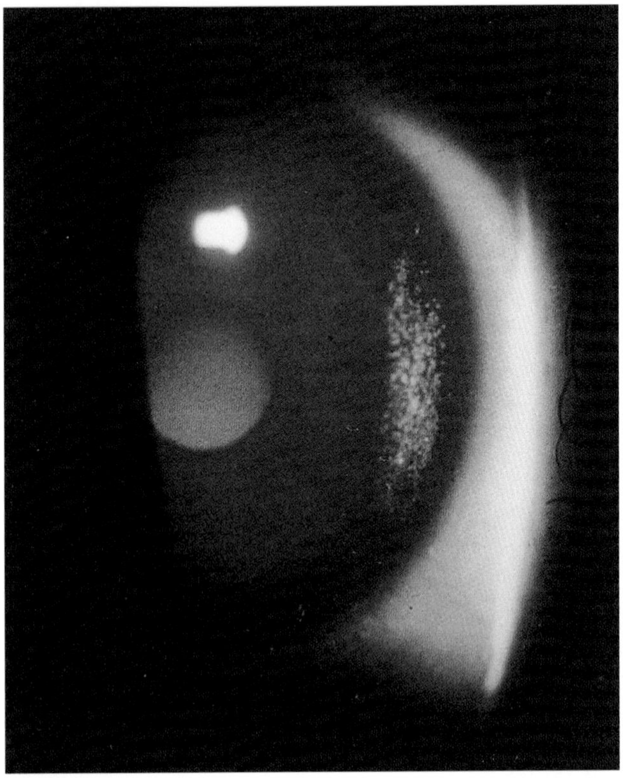

FIGURE 27-8 Corneal staining at the 3-o'clock position in a contact lens wearer.

soft to hard lenses. If these measures fail to control the neovascularization, the patient should discontinue contact lens wear.

CHANGES IN THE CORNEAL EPITHELIUM AND ANTERIOR STROMA

Mechanical Damage

Contact lens wear often causes mechanical damage to the corneal epithelium. The pattern of damage is different for soft and hard lenses.

With soft lenses, arcuate epithelial staining is often seen. This staining typically occurs nasally, where surface microabrasions produce fine fluorescein uptake at the site of the arc of contact between the edge of the contact lens and the cornea. Occasionally, there is delle formation because of poor focal wetting in this area.

With hard contact lenses, staining at the 3- and 9-o'clock positions often develops at the points of contact between the contact lens and the cornea (Figure 27-8). It may be caused by lens edge-ocular surface friction, poorly finished or blended lens edges, or poor wetting at the slope created by the angle between the peripheral lens and the corneal surface.

Superficial Punctate Keratitis

The most common pattern of epithelial keratitis seen in contact lens wearers is a fine, diffuse, superficial punctate keratitis (SPK). The epithelial lesions may or may not stain with fluorescein. The keratitis can be attributed to

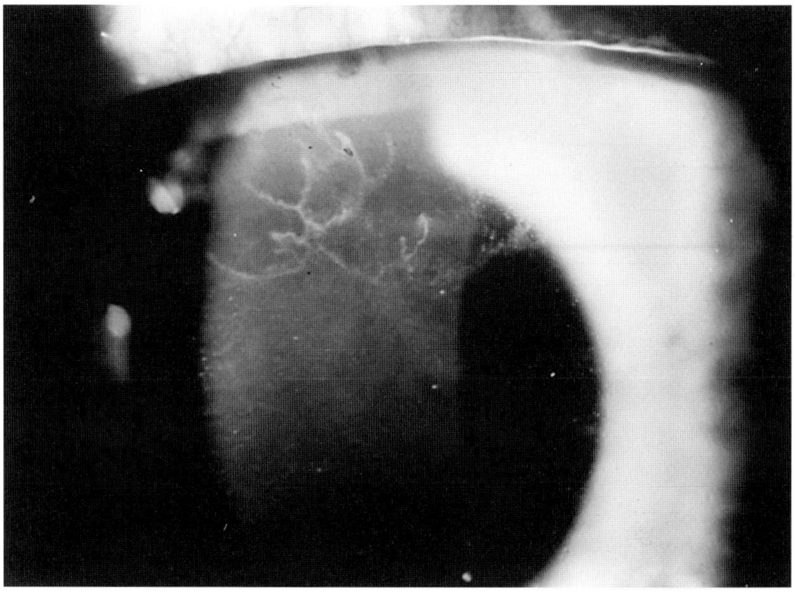

FIGURE 27-9 Contact lens–related pseudodendrite caused by thimerosal. Note the branching epithelial lesion.

several mechanisms, including improper lens fit, which produces ocular surface damage, and hypersensitivity or toxicity reactions to lens care products.

Epithelial Hyperplasia

Prolonged contact lens wear can cause hyperplasia of the epithelium and basement membrane, which can mimic carcinoma in situ. These changes usually regress with discontinuation of contact lens wear.

Pseudodendrites

Dendrite-like epithelial lesions have been associated with contact lens wear[31] (Figure 27-9) and may involve one or both eyes. The lesions may be single or multiple and are most commonly seen at the periphery of the cornea. They usually do not have the terminal bulbs and prominent arborizations of dendrites caused by herpes simplex virus. Corneal sensation may be diminished, but this is more likely the normal adaptive hypesthesia present in many contact lens wearers. Often, there is associated conjunctival hyperemia, but a follicular reaction is not typical.

Contact lens-related pseudodendrites are usually attributed to a hypersensitivity reaction to preservatives in lens care products, particularly thimerosal. Viral cultures are negative, and the lesions do not respond to topical antiviral agents. It is important to differentiate a pseudodendrite from a true dendrite caused by herpes simplex virus, because antiviral medications are not only ineffective in nonherpetic processes, they are also toxic to the epithelium.

Pseudodendrites generally improve when contact lens wear is discontinued. Topical corticosteroids may hasten resolution. Once the pseudodendrite has resolved, most patients can resume successful contact lens wear, provided that the lens care regimen is modified to eliminate the offending agents.

Superior Limbic Keratoconjunctivitis

Superior limbic keratoconjunctivitis (SLK) can be seen in contact lens wearers[32–34] and is similar to the idiopathic disorder described by Theodore.[35,36] One or both eyes may be involved.

Symptoms include a gradual decrease in contact lens tolerance with a persistent foreign body sensation under the upper eyelid. On slit lamp examination, there is a fine, diffuse, papillary pattern on the superior tarsal conjunctiva with intense fluorescein uptake (Figure 27-10). The superior bulbar conjunctiva also stains intensely with fluorescein, and there is prominent hyperemia in this area, with engorgement of the vertical blood vessels (Figure 27-11). The superior limbal conjunctiva may thicken, and there may be a coarse epithelial keratitis involving the superior third of the cornea. Filaments are occasionally seen. With long-standing disease, the epithelial keratitis can progress centrally, with accompanying superficial neovascularization and corneal scarring.

In contradistinction to idiopathic superior limbic keratoconjunctivitis, there is no recognized association between contact lens-related superior limbic keratoconjunctivitis and thyroid dysfunction. Contact lens–related

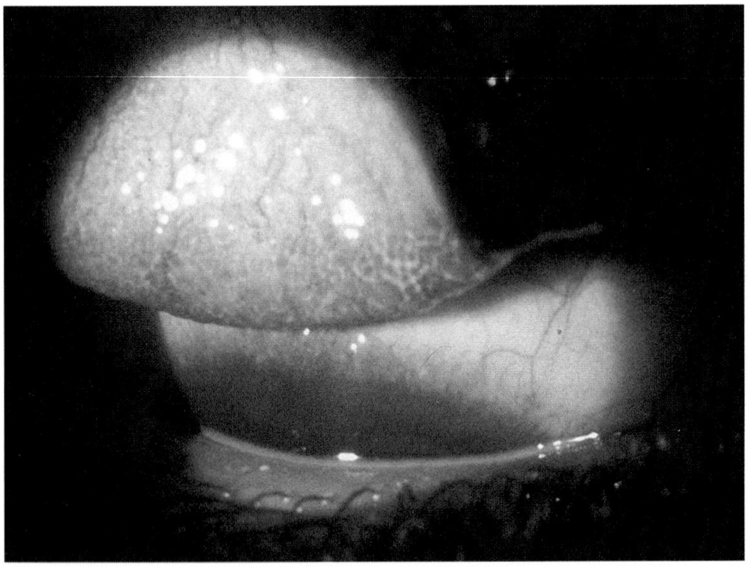

FIGURE 27-10 Contact lens–related superior limbic keratoconjunctivitis. Note the fine, diffuse, papillary pattern on the superior tarsal conjunctiva and the intense fluorescein uptake.

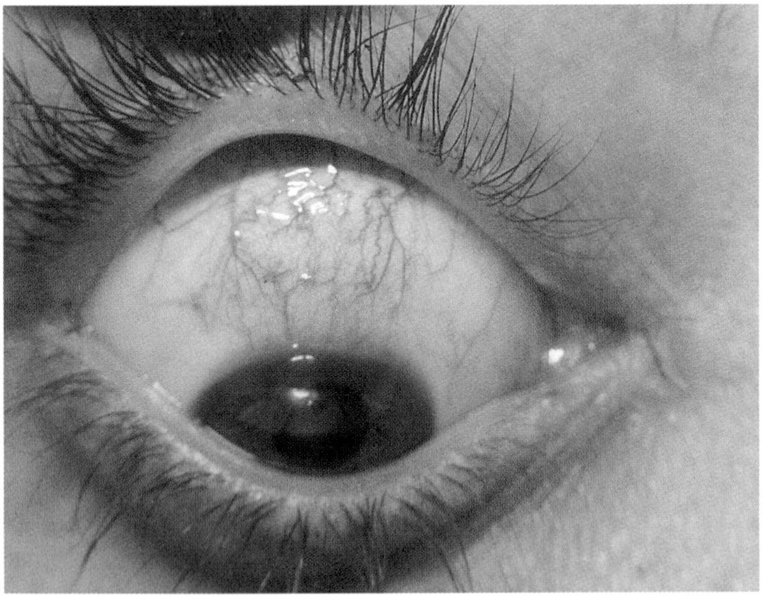

FIGURE 27-11 Contact lens–related superior limbic keratoconjunctivitis. Note the intense local hyperemia of the superior bulbar conjunctiva.

superior limbic keratoconjunctivitis is generally milder than the idiopathic form.

Among the causative factors implicated in contact lens-related superior limbic keratoconjunctivitis are hypersensitivity reactions to preservatives in lens care products, particularly thimerosal, and improper lens fit (large-diameter lenses with eccentric fit and excessive movement).

Mild cases typically respond to discontinuation of contact lens wear. Topical corticosteroids may hasten the resolution of the keratitis. If the keratitis has spread centrally, there may be marked decrease in vision, incapacitating pain, and photophobia.[37] In these cases, improvement is slow, regardless of treatment. In some cases, surgery may be required. Among the surgical procedures recommended for both contact lens-related and idiopathic superior limbic keratoconjunctivitis are silver nitrate cautery of the involved tarsal conjunctiva, diathermy, and conjunctival resection. Paradoxically, one of the treatments for idiopathic superior limbic keratoconjunctivitis is the use of a bandage soft contact lens. In

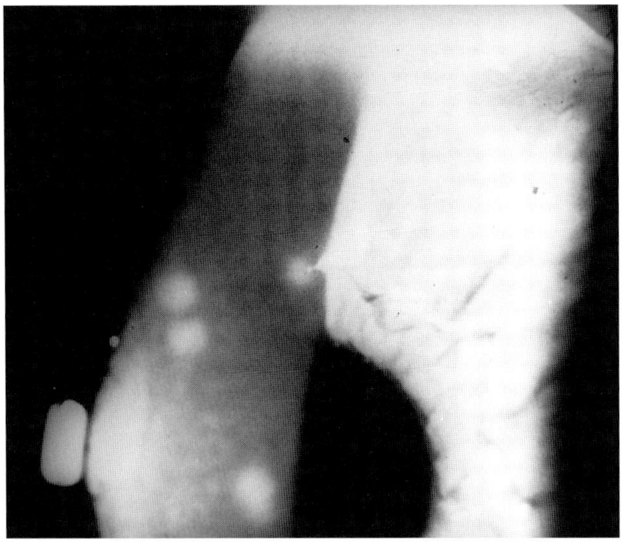

FIGURE 27-12 Contact lens-induced nummular keratitis. Note the multiple coin-shaped corneal epithelial lesions. The patient was a soft contact lens wearer who used a lens care solution containing thimerosal.

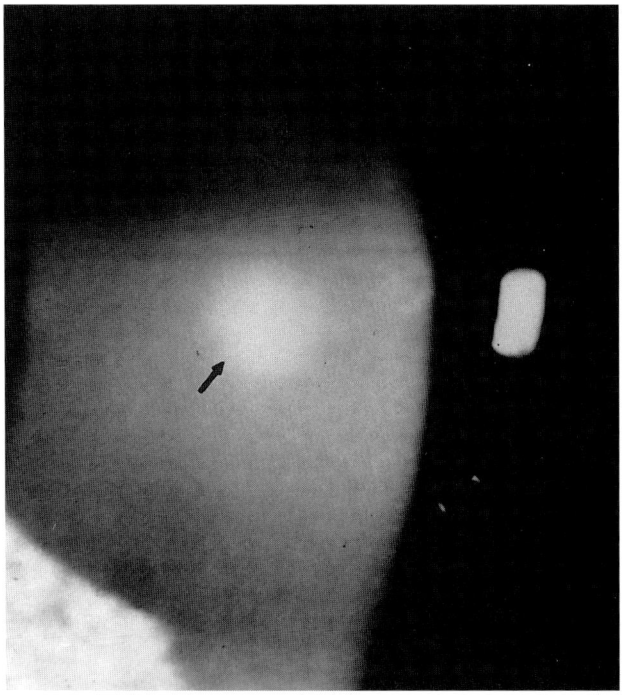

FIGURE 27-13 White spot. Note the round infiltrate in the superficial cornea (arrow).

the most severe cases, in which the epithelial keratitis is advanced and vision is compromised, penetrating keratoplasty may be required.

In patients with mild to moderate contact lens-related superior limbic keratoconjunctivitis, successful return to contact lens wear is often possible with the appropriate modifications in the contact lens fit and care regimen.

Nummular Keratitis

A nummular, or coin-shaped, keratitis has been described as a complication of soft contact lens wear[38] (Figure 27-12). It has been attributed to a hypersensitivity reaction to preservatives in lens care products, particularly thimerosal. The pattern of the keratitis is reminiscent of that seen in epidemic keratoconjunctivitis (EKC).[39]

The most common complaint with nummular keratitis is blurred vision, which is often aggravated by glare. Foreign body sensation and photophobia may also be reported.

The infiltrates of nummular keratitis develop in the deep epithelial and subepithelial layers of the cornea; they are generally located more peripherally than the lesions of epidemic keratoconjunctivitis, which tend to develop centrally. Nummular infiltrates usually do not stain with fluorescein, although there may be overlying fluorescein stippling from focal wetting abnormalities. The nummular lesions are multiple and may coalesce, causing a marked decrease in vision. A moderately severe conjunctivitis usually accompanies nummular keratitis. Follicles are not typical, and there is no associated preauricular lymphadenopathy, unlike in epidemic keratoconjunctivitis.

With discontinuation of contact lens wear, nummular keratitis tends to resolve spontaneously, although topical corticosteroids may hasten the resolution. A short course of corticosteroids is usually adequate; corticosteroid dependence, which is typical in the treatment of epidemic keratoconjunctivitis, does not develop.

Most patients can successfully resume contact lens wear after the keratitis resolves, with appropriate modification of the lens care regimen.

White Spots

Although microbial keratitis is the most serious corneal complication of contact lens wear, white spots are more common.[40] White spots represent single or multiple round infiltrates in the superficial cornea, with surrounding edema and inflammation (Figure 27-13). The epithelial surface may or may not be intact. There is

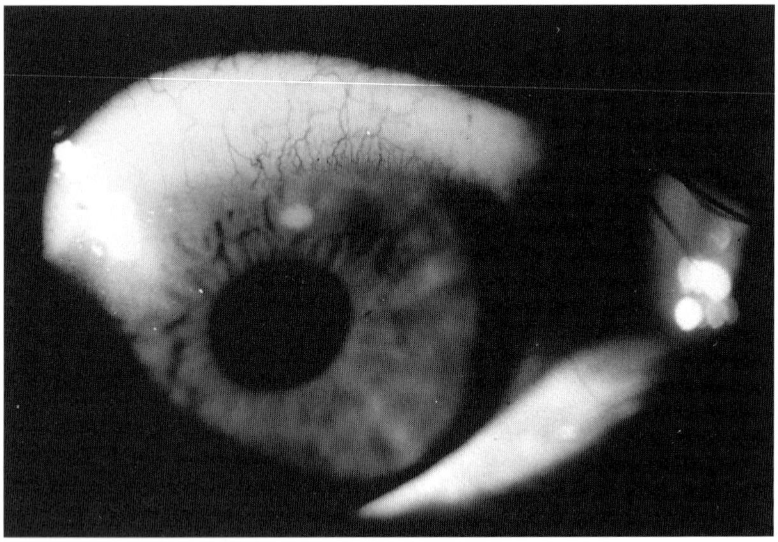

FIGURE 27-14 Peripheral corneal infiltrate in the superior cornea. There is an area of clear cornea between the infiltrate and the limbus.

usually some degree of conjunctival hyperemia, and mild iritis may occur.

Patients typically complain of irritation and a foreign body sensation, which is aggravated by eye or eyelid movement. Photophobia is also common.

White spots are generally attributed to a hypoxic or hypersensitivity reaction. However, similar changes may be seen in the early stages of microbial keratitis, particularly if there is disruption of the corneal epithelium.

White spots can be difficult to manage. In the early stages, it may not be possible clinically to distinguish between infectious and noninfectious causes. Cultures of the cornea should be taken if the epithelium is disrupted. If the epithelium is intact, however, it is usually preferable to avoid disturbing it.

Noninfectious white spots typically respond well to a topical antibiotic/corticosteroid preparation and temporary discontinuation of contact lens wear. If there is any suspicion of infection, corneal scrapings should be obtained for culture, and treatment for microbial keratitis should be initiated. Generally, corticosteroids should be withheld until the infection is eradicated.

Once the keratitis has resolved, contact lens wear can be resumed. There is usually some residual scarring at the sites of the infiltrates. White spots have a tendency to recur in many patients.

Peripheral Corneal Infiltrates

Peripheral corneal infiltrates are a fairly common finding in contact lens wearers, especially those who wear extended-wear lenses, and account for 12.5 percent of all contact lens-related problems.[41,42]

The most common presenting symptoms are ocular discomfort, foreign body sensation, tearing, photophobia, and conjunctival hyperemia.

Characteristically, peripheral corneal infiltrates are small (1 to 2 mm), grayish white lesions located in the epithelium and anterior stroma (Figure 27-14). There is minimal disruption of the overlying epithelium. Epithelial edema or superficial punctate keratitis is found in half of the cases. There is usually an area of clear cornea between the infiltrate and the limbus. Although any area of the cornea can be involved, there is a predilection for the superior cornea. Most patients have a single infiltrate, but multiple infiltrates are not uncommon. Anterior chamber inflammation is absent or minimal. Although the infiltrates are often considered to be sterile,[43] cultures are positive in a significant number of patients.

The pathophysiology of peripheral corneal infiltrates is not well understood. Hypersensitivity and toxicity reactions to preservatives in contact lens care products have been postulated as possible causes.[38] However, in one series,[44] most patients were not using a chemical disinfecting system.

Suchecki et al[44] noted that these infiltrates are similar to the peripheral infiltrates associated with staphylococcal blepharitis. However, an earlier study by this same group[45] found no correlation between contact lens-associated infiltrates and the presence of blepharitis. Also, staphylococcal infection was not common in those patients who had positive cultures.

The contact lenses of most patients who have peripheral corneal infiltrates are coated with protein deposits.[44] It is postulated that these deposits elicit an antigen-antibody reaction. The immune complexes then penetrate the cornea, resulting in a stromal infiltrate. In addition, bacteria might also be responsible for the development of this reaction by causing either a hypersensitivity[46] or toxicity[47] reaction.

The findings that these infiltrates are associated more often with extended-wear lenses than daily-wear lenses and are more common with soft lenses than hard lenses suggest that hypoxia may be an aggravating factor.

In addition, it has been postulated that leukocytes in the tear film, which appear as a result of diapedesis through conjunctival vessels secondary to physical irritation or possibly an immune response, can be trapped beneath the contact lens, where they may cause damage to epithelial cells, epithelial ulcers, and anterior stromal infiltrates.[48,49] It has also been shown that both injury to the conjunctival epithelial cells by contact lenses and protein deposits on the lenses can cause the release of neutrophilic chemotactic factor, which can attract cells such as polymorphonuclear leukocytes, mast cells, eosinophils, and basophils.[50]

If the infiltrate is smaller than 1 mm and the overlying epithelium is intact, anterior chamber inflammation is absent, and there is no significant ocular pain, it is not necessary to scrape the infiltrate for stains and cultures. Contact lens wear should be discontinued, and the patient should be treated with topical antibiotics for 1 to 3 days. If the infiltrate does not resolve, topical corticosteroids can be added for an additional week. In most cases, the infiltrate regresses slowly but often leaves a faint subepithelial scar.

If the infiltrate is larger than 1 mm and there is an epithelial defect, anterior chamber inflammation, or pain, microbial keratitis must be considered, and appropriate scrapings should be obtained for stains and cultures. The patient should be started on fortified antibiotic eye drops until culture results are available. If the cultures indicate the absence of a significant pathogen, topical corticosteroids can be instituted.

After the resolution of peripheral infiltrates, the patient may be refitted with contact lenses, preferably either daily-wear soft or rigid gas-permeable contact lenses unless there are strong mitigating circumstances for the continuation of extended-wear lenses. If the patient had previously been wearing daily-wear soft lenses, then use of a frequent-replacement disposable contact lens system should be considered.

MICROBIAL KERATITIS

Microbial keratitis is the most serious complication of contact lens wear. Such infections may occur with soft or hard lenses but are more frequent with soft lenses, especially extended-wear soft lenses. Large-scale studies indicate that the relative risk of microbial keratitis is 10 to 15 times greater with extended-wear lenses than with daily-wear soft lenses,[51–54] and the risks with daily-wear and extended-wear disposable lenses are similarly high.[55,56] Despite appropriate management, corneal scarring and decreased vision may occur.

A variety of factors increase the risk of microbial keratitis in contact lens wearers, including (1) microbial contamination of the lens, lens care products, or case; (2) lack of hand washing before lens manipulation; (3) lens overwear; (4) swimming while wearing contact lenses; and (5) external ocular diseases, such as dry eyes or blepharitis.

Although any organism can cause microbial keratitis in a contact lens wearer, *Pseudomonas aeruginosa* and *Acanthamoeba* are two organisms particularly associated with contact lens wear for cosmetic purposes. *Serratia marcescens* is a pathogen found almost exclusively in contact lens wearers and virtually never infects the cornea in the absence of a contact lens. A description of *Pseudomonas* and *Acanthamoeba* keratitis as they relate to contact lens wear is given below. Diagnostic studies and treatment are discussed in Chapters 8 and 15.

Pseudomonas aeruginosa

Pseudomonas aeruginosa is the most common organism encountered in contact lens-related microbial keratitis. The organism is ubiquitous and can proliferate on contact lenses without a breach in lens care or hygiene. Although lens contamination from poor lens care is the major causative factor, a traumatic epithelial defect, lens deposits, and prolonged wear are important predisposing factors. Corneal trauma may occur during lens insertion or removal or as a result of hypoxia, toxicity reactions to preservatives in lens care products, lens deposits, or entrapment of debris between the contact lens and the cornea.

Soft lenses, especially extended-wear lenses, have been associated with a greater frequency of *Pseudomonas* keratitis. The polymer matrix of these lenses is apparently suited to the adherence of *Pseudomonas*. Lens deposits, which increase with time, enhance the adherence of organisms. Infection is more common with mucin-coated lenses than with noncoated lenses.[57]

Pseudomonas keratitis should be suspected in any contact lens patient with the acute onset of severe pain, regardless of the size of the infiltrate. Clinical findings may include an ulcer covered by thick, adherent mucopurulent discharge, a wide area of surrounding stromal edema, a ring infiltrate surrounding the ulcer (Wessely ring), and in advanced cases, a hypopyon (Figure 27-15). Although these features may be seen in *Pseudomonas* infections, they are not pathognomonic and can also be seen in other bacterial ulcers. *Pseudomonas* keratitis is discussed further in Chapter 8.

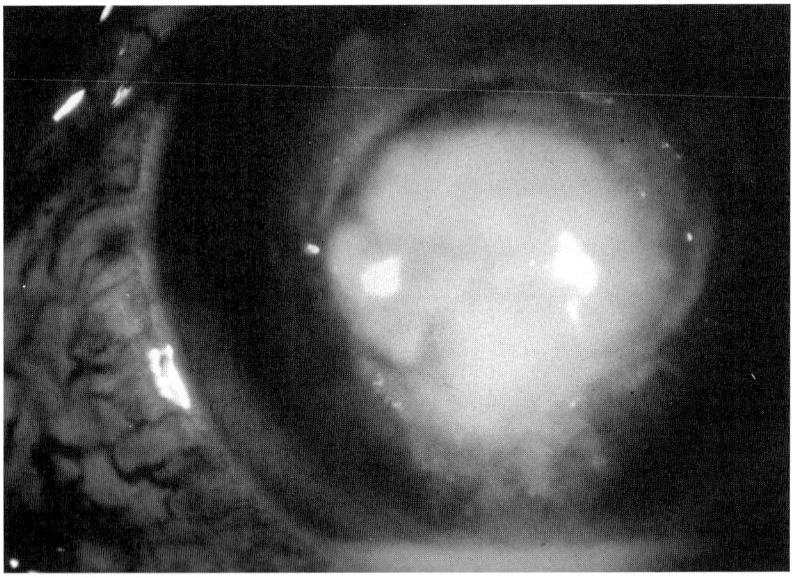

FIGURE 27-15 *Pseudomonas* corneal ulcer in association with contact lens wear. Note the corneal ulcer covered with mucopurulent discharge and the surrounding stromal edema, ring infiltrate, and hypopyon.

Acanthamoeba

Acanthamoeba is an uncommon but increasingly prevalent infection[58,59] with the potential to cause severe ocular damage. The organism has been identified in saliva, soil, and almost all types of water, including distilled water used in the preparation of homemade saline.

The risk factors for *Acanthamoeba* keratitis include (1) use of homemade saline made from distilled water and salt tablets; (2) swimming with contact lenses; (3) ocular exposure to hot tub or tap water; and (4) chemical, rather than thermal, disinfection of contact lenses.

The clinician must be aware of the early clinical symptoms and signs so a diagnosis can be made early in the disease course and treatment initiated. Delayed diagnosis or improper treatment may result in severe scarring, corneal perforation, and loss of the eye.[59]

Early clinical signs of *Acanthamoeba* keratitis include severe pain out of proportion to the clinical findings, irregularity of the epithelium, and patchy stromal infiltrates.

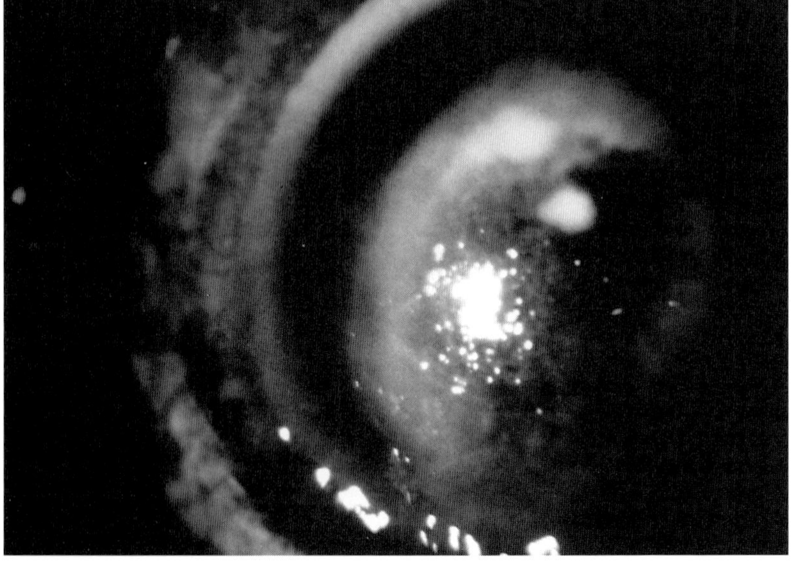

FIGURE 27-16 *Acanthamoeba* corneal ulcer in association with contact lens wear. Note the stromal ring infiltrate.

Late clinical signs (Figure 27-16) include a stromal ring infiltrate, infiltrates along corneal nerves (radial keratoneuritis), elevated nonbranching corneal epithelial lines, and absence of neovascularization. *Acanthamoeba* keratitis is discussed further in Chapter 15.

CHANGES IN THE POSTERIOR STROMA

Corneal metabolism is dependent on oxygen, the major source of which is atmospheric oxygen. Contact lenses, particularly polymethyl methacrylate lenses, are a significant physical barrier to corneal oxygenation.[60] As a result of hypoxia, edema occurs in the posterior stroma and causes striae, folds in the posterior stroma and Descemet's membrane, endothelial buckling, and sometimes, loss of stromal transparency.

Striae

Contact lens-induced striae appear as fine, wispy, white, vertical lines in the posterior stroma[61,62] (Figure 27-17). The striae are reversible. However, they recur each time a lens that causes sufficient hypoxia is worn, usually appearing 4 to 6 hours after lens wear is begun and disappearing 1 to 2 hours after lens wear is discontinued.[63] Normally, the collagen fibrils are loosely arranged in the posterior stroma. When there is corneal edema, the fibrils are compressed so they reflect, rather than transmit, light.[64] Striae are best seen by direct or indirect focal illumination.

Studies[42,64-67] have documented that striae occur in soft contact lens wearers when there is a 6 to 8 percent increase in corneal thickness. In one study,[66] striae also occurred in 10 percent of polymethyl methacrylate lens wearers when the increase in corneal thickness was 6.4 percent and in 2 percent of rigid gas-permeable lens wearers when the increase in corneal thickness was 4.5 percent.

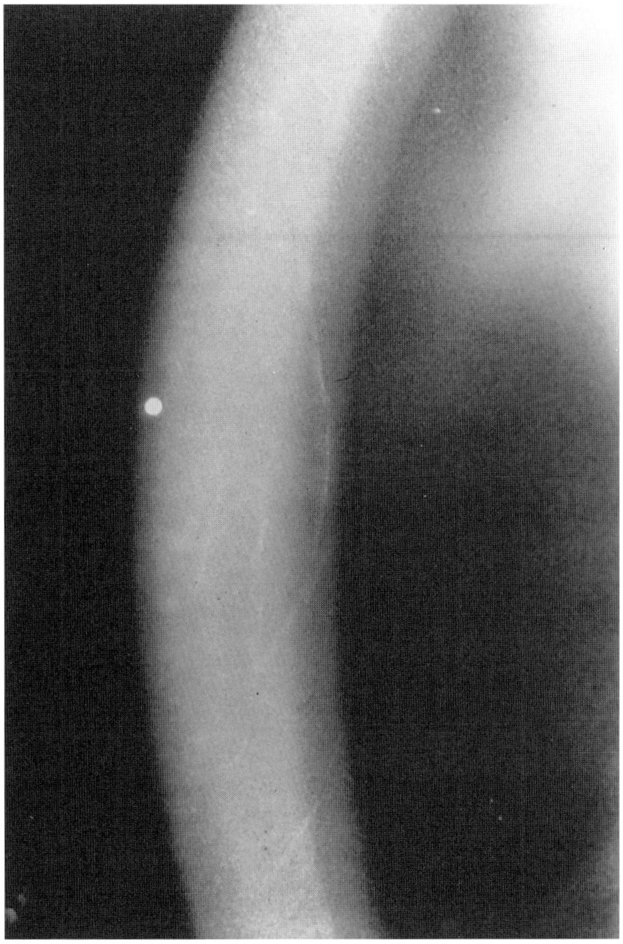

FIGURE 27-17 Vertical corneal striae in a soft contact lens wearer. Note the white vertically oriented lines in the posterior stroma. (Courtesy of Steve Zantos, Ph.D., Bausch and Lomb, Rochester, NY.)

Folds in the Posterior Stroma and Descemet's Membrane

Folds are dark, deep-appearing, criss-cross lines in the posterior stroma and Descemet's membrane[68] (Figure 27-18). They are a manifestation of progressive corneal edema and occur when there is an 8 to 10 percent increase in corneal thickness.[69]

Endothelial Buckling

Endothelial buckling manifests as dark, deep-appearing grooves visible in the endothelial mosaic (Figure 27-19). They represent a physical buckling of the posterior stroma, Descemet's membrane, and endothelium[42] and are best seen by specular reflection. Buckling occurs when there is a 10 to 15 percent increase in corneal thickness.[42,69]

Loss of Stromal Transparency

Loss of stromal transparency gives a hazy, milky appearance to the cornea (Figure 27-20) that partially obscures the fine iris details. The haziness is attributed to separation of the collagen fibrils, which disrupts the regular optical geometry of the stromal lamellae. Loss of stromal transparency is best observed with sclerotic scatter and occurs when there is a 20 to 25 percent increase in corneal thickness.[69]

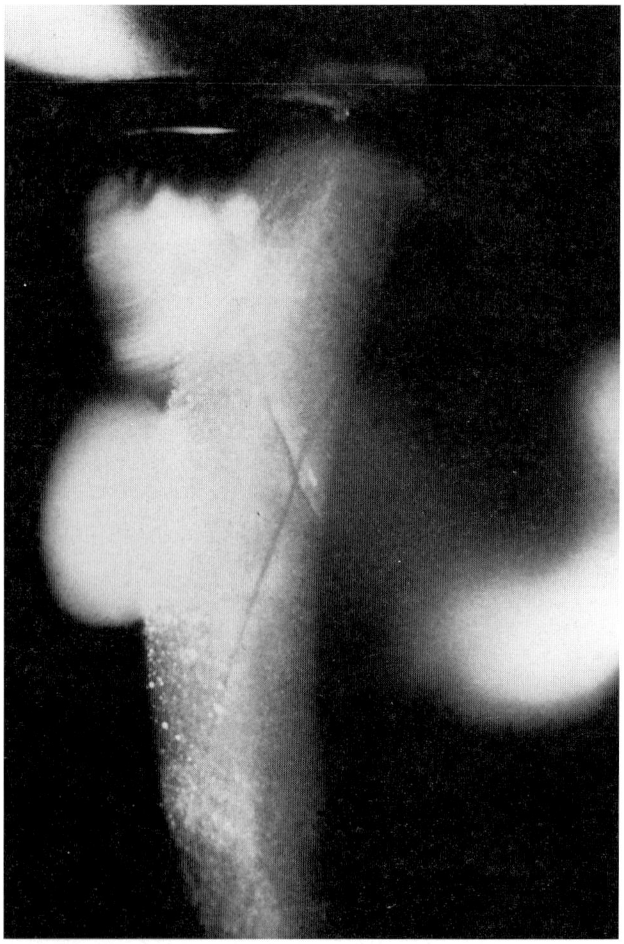

FIGURE 27-18 Folds in the posterior stroma and Descemet's membrane. Note the dark criss-crossing lines at the level of the posterior stroma and Descemet's membrane. (Courtesy of Steve Zantos, Ph.D., Bausch and Lomb, Rochester, NY.)

CHANGES IN THE ENDOTHELIUM

Endothelial Blebs

The development of the specular microscope in the 1970s allowed clinicians to observe the corneal endothelium of contact lens wearers. With this instrument, Zantos and Holden[68] noted that endothelial blebs developed immediately after insertion of soft contact lenses in unadapted (beginning) contact lens wearers. Endothelial blebs appear as black, nonreflecting, blister-like eruptions that bulge posteriorly (Figure 27-21). With the slit lamp microscope, they are best seen using high magnification and specular reflection. Although blebs were first reported with extended-wear soft lenses, they have now been reported with all types of lenses except silicone lenses.[68,70–72]

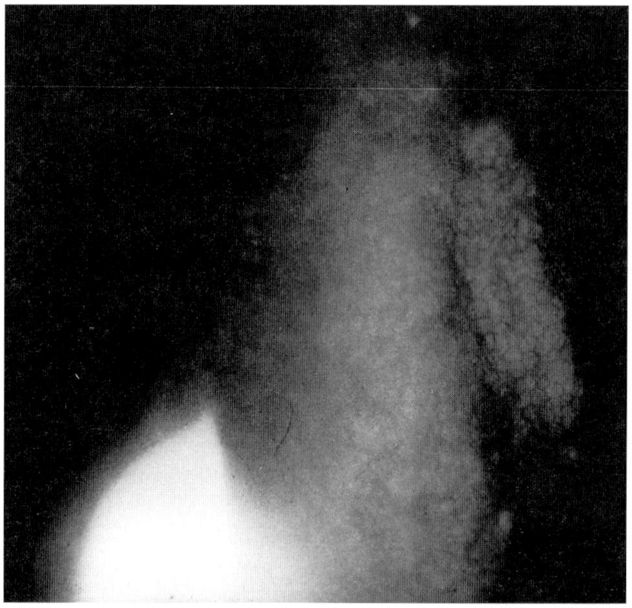

FIGURE 27-19 Endothelial buckling. Dark deep-appearing grooves are visible in the endothelial mosaic.

Endothelial blebs begin to develop within minutes after a contact lens is inserted. They are transient, however, and disappear after 30 to 60 minutes of lens wear. An adaptation to the bleb response can occur. In one study,[73] the authors evaluated the endothelial bleb response in unadapted extended-wear soft lens wearers over 7 days. Each day, the response on awakening peaked at 30 seconds and then decreased to a baseline level. After 4 to 5 days, the bleb response on awakening was barely perceptible. Thus, continued wear caused the endothelium to lose its ability to respond.

Histologic examination of the human corneal endothelium indicates that blebs represent changes in the contour of the posterior endothelial cell membranes associated with swelling of the cells.[74] The cause of bleb formation is not known. It is postulated that the initial corneal hypoxia results in an accumulation of carbon dioxide in the stroma, causing a pH shift toward acidity. The pH shift also spreads to the endothelium, and it is this shift in pH that causes bleb formation.[75]

Endothelial Polymegethism

Variation in endothelial cell size is referred to as *polymegethism* (Figure 27-22). Although contact lens-induced polymegethism was first reported with daily-wear polymethyl methacrylate lenses,[76,77] it was later noted to occur also with soft lenses.[78] Subsequently, it was observed that polymegethism is greater with extended-wear soft lenses than daily-wear soft lenses. Hirst et al[79] studied long-term hard contact lens wearers and found that the longer patients had worn lenses, the greater the amount of polymegethism. Hypoxia was thought to be the probable cause of polymegethism. Indirect evidence for this hypothesis was the observation of polymegethism in a young patient with unilateral ptosis who had never worn a contact lens.[80] Cessation of contact lens wear does not reverse contact lens-induced polymegethism.[81-83]

Dutt et al[84] studied 11 extended-wear soft contact lens wearers with an average of 4 years of wear. Using fluorophotometry and quantitative specular microscopy, they found a significant increase in corneal endothelial permeability as well as increased corneal thickness, suggesting decreased endothelial cell function. These data showed that there may be functional as well as morphologic defects in the corneal endothelium of long-term extended-wear patients.

Polymegethism begins to develop about the same time that the endothelium loses its ability to show the bleb response. It has been hypothesized that initial hypoxia causes the bleb response and that longer-lasting hypoxia causes structural changes in the endothelium.[81]

Because of these findings, contact lens materials were developed with oxygen permeabilities higher than those of polymethyl methacrylate or hydrogel materials. Silicone and fluorocarbon polymers led to the development of rigid gas-permeable contact lenses with high oxygen permeabilities.[85] One study showed no evidence of progression of polymegethism or pleomorphism after 7 to 24 months of rigid gas-permeable contact lens wear.[86]

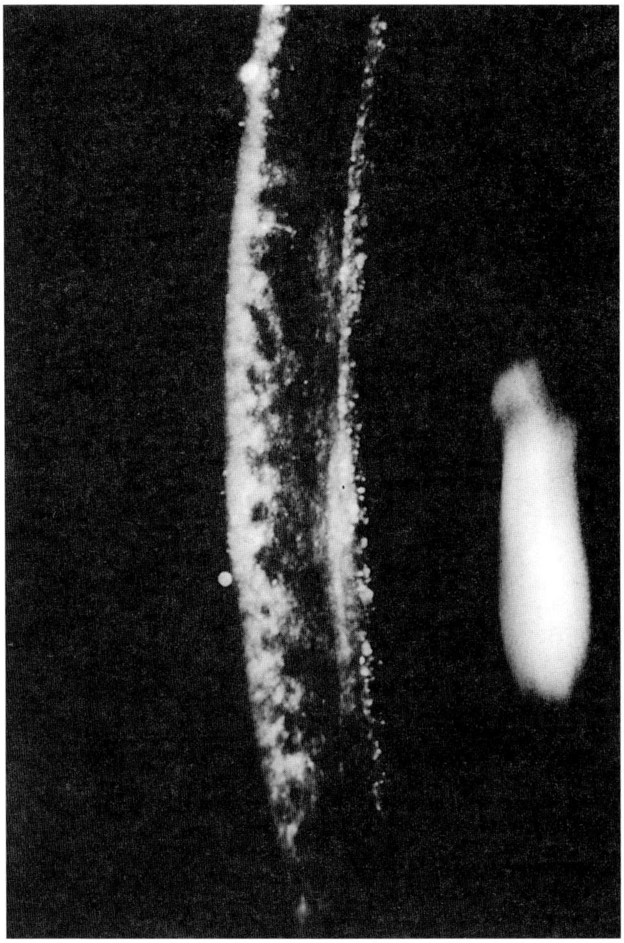

FIGURE 27-20 Loss of stromal transparency. Note the hazy, milky appearance of the cornea.

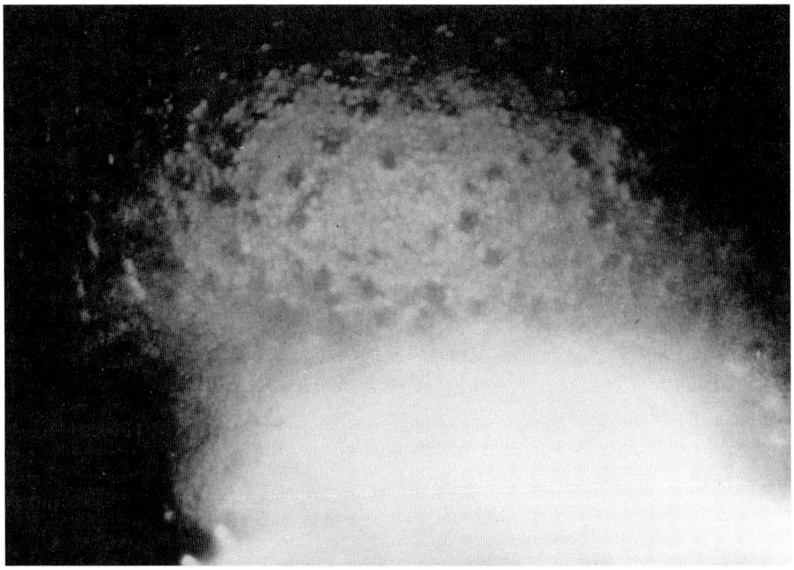

FIGURE 27-21 Endothelial blebs. Note the black blister-like eruptions that bulge toward the anterior chamber.

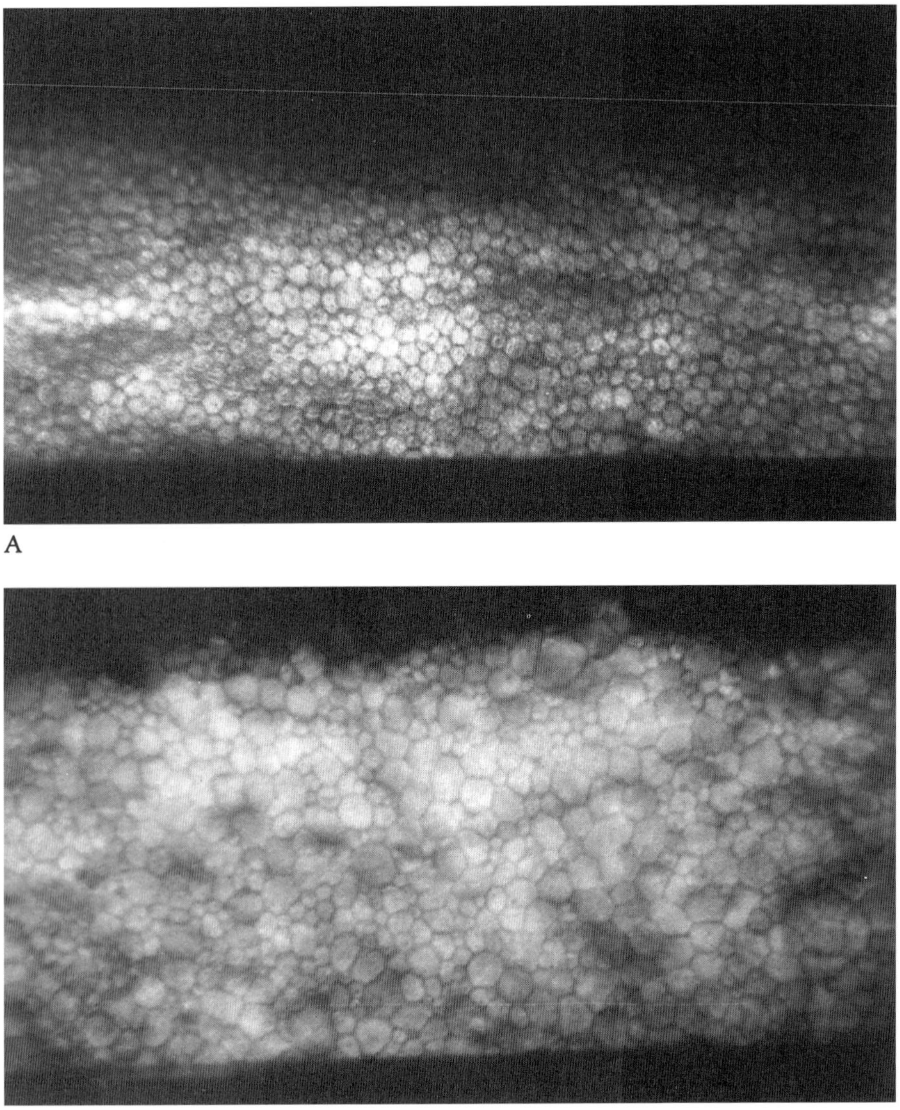

A

B

FIGURE 27-22 **(A)** Specular photomicrograph of the endothelium of a normal patient. Note the uniform endothelial cell size. (Courtesy of Scott MacRae, M.D., Portland, OR.) **(B)** Specular photomicrograph of the endothelium of a long-term contact lens wearer. Note the variation in endothelial cell size. (Courtesy of Scott MacRae, M.D., Portland, OR.)

It is not known whether contact lens-induced changes in corneal endothelial morphology can lead to eventual corneal decompensation. However, it is only prudent to assume that endothelial failure may occur with time unless the situation is reversed. Therefore, the use of contact lenses with high oxygen permeability, worn as daily wear, with good movement and frequent replacement, should be encouraged to minimize these effects.[81]

REFERENCES

1. Nugent MW: The corneal lens—a new type of plastic lens. A preliminary report. Ann West Med Surg 2:241, 1948
2. Barr JT: Contact lenses and vision: the annual report. Contact Lens Spectrum 12(1):21, 1997
3. Miller D: Contact lens-induced corneal curvature and thickness changes. Arch Ophthalmol 80:430, 1968
4. Hartstein J: Corneal warping due to wearing of corneal contact lenses. A report of 12 cases. Am J Ophthalmol 60:1103, 1965
5. Polse KA, Brand RJ, Vastine DW, Schwalbe JS: Corneal change accompanying orthokeratology. Plastic or elastic? Results of a randomized controlled clinical trial. Arch Ophthalmol 101:1873, 1983
6. Woodward EG, Moodaley LC, Lyons C, et al: Post keratoplasty dimensional and refractive change in contact lens and spectacle corrected cases. Eye 4:689, 1990
7. Wilson SE, Friedman RS, Klyce SD: Contact lens manipulation of corneal topography after penetrating keratoplasty: a preliminary study. CLAO J 18:177, 1992
8. Dingeldein SA, Klyce SD: The topography of normal corneas. Arch Ophthalmol 107:512, 1989

9. Wilson SE, Lin DTC, Klyce SD, et al: Topographic changes in contact lens-induced corneal warpage. Ophthalmology 97:734, 1990
10. Wilson SE, Lin DTC, Klyce SD, et al: Rigid contact lens decentration—a risk factor for corneal warpage. CLAO J 16:177, 1990
11. Hartstein J: Keratoconus that developed in patients wearing corneal contact lenses. Report of four cases. Arch Ophthalmol 80:345, 1968
12. Hartstein J, Becker B: Research into the pathogenesis of keratoconus. A new syndrome: low ocular rigidity, contact lenses, and keratoconus. Arch Ophthalmol 84:728, 1970
13. Gasset AR, Houde WL, Garcia-Bengochea M: Hard contact lens wear as an environmental risk in keratoconus. Am J Ophthalmol 85:339, 1978
14. Nauheim JS, Perry HD: A clinicopathologic study of contact-lens-related keratoconus. Am J Ophthalmol 100:543, 1985
15. Macsai MS, Varley GA, Krachmer JH: Development of keratoconus after contact lens wear. Patient characteristics. Arch Ophthalmol 108:534, 1990
16. Browne RK, Anderson AN, Charvez BW, Azzarello RJ: Ophthalmic response to chlorhexidine digluconate in rabbits. Toxicol Appl Pharmacol 32:621, 1975
17. Burstein NL: Preservative cytotoxic threshold for benzalkonium chloride and chlorhexidine digluconate in cat and rabbit corneas. Invest Ophthalmol Vis Sci 19:308, 1980
18. Foulkes DM: Some toxicological observations on chlorhexidine. J Peridont Res 12(suppl):55, 1973
19. Josephson JE, Caffery B: Sorbic acid revisited. J Am Optom Assoc 57:188, 1986
20. Morgan JF: Complications associated with contact lens solutions. Ophthalmology 86:1107, 1979
21. Morgan JF: Opti-Soft for the care of soft contact lenses: a triphasic, one year evaluation. CLAO J 13:268, 1987
22. Morgan JF, Perry DL, Stein JM, Randeri KJ: The margin of safety of Polyquarternium-1 preserved lens care solutions: a phase 1 clinical study. CLAO J 14:76, 1988
23. Shaw EL: Allergies induced by contact lens solutions. Contact Intraocul Lens Med J 6:273, 1980
24. Stern ME, Edelhauser HF, Krebs SJ, et al: A comparison of corneal and endothelial toxicity of common preservatives. ARVO abstract. Invest Ophthalmol Vis Sci 156(suppl):32, 1983
25. Wilson LA, McNatt J, Reitschel RL: Delayed hypersensitivity to thimerosal in soft contact lens wearers. Ophthalmology 88:804, 1981
26. Stark WJ, Martin NF: Extended-wear contact lenses for myopic correction. Arch Ophthalmol 99:1963, 1981
27. Dohlman CH, Boruchoff A, Mobilia EF: Complications in use of soft contact lenses in corneal disease. Arch Ophthalmol 90:367, 1973
28. Dixon JM: Corneal vascularization due to corneal contact lenses: the clinical picture. Trans Am Ophthalmol Soc 65:393, 1967
29. Ephron N, Carney LF: Models of extended performance for the static, dynamic, and closed-lid wear hydrogel contact lenses. Aust J Optom 64:223, 1981
30. Maurice DM, Zauberman H, Michaelson IC: The stimulus to neovascularization in the cornea. Exp Eye Res 5:168, 1966
31. Margulies LJ, Mannis MJ: Dendritic corneal lesions associated with soft contact lens wear. Arch Ophthalmol 101:1551, 1983
32. Stenson S: Superior limbic keratoconjunctivitis associated with soft contact lens wear. Arch Ophthalmol 101:402, 1983
33. Sendele DD, Kenyon KR, Mobilia EF: Superior limbic keratoconjunctivitis in contact lens wearers. Ophthalmology 90:616, 1983
34. Miller RA, Brightbill FS, Slama S: Superior limbic keratoconjunctivitis in soft contact lens wearers. Cornea 1:293, 1982
35. Theodore FH: Superior limbic keratoconjunctivitis. Eye Ear Nose Throat Mon 42:25, 1963
36. Theodore FH, Ferry AP: Superior limbic keratoconjunctivitis. Clinical and pathological correlations. Arch Ophthalmol 84:481, 1970
37. Bloomfield SE, Jakobiec FA, Theodore FH: Contact lens induced keratopathy: a severe complication extending the spectrum of keratoconjunctivitis in contact lens wearers. Ophthalmology 91:290, 1984
38. Mondino BJ, Groden LR: Conjunctival hyperemia and corneal infiltrates with chemically disinfected soft contact lenses. Arch Ophthalmol 98:1767, 1980
39. Binder PS, Rasmussen DM, Gordon M: Keratoconjunctivitis and soft contact lens solutions. Arch Ophthalmol 99:87, 1981
40. Stenson SM (ed): Contact Lenses: A Guide to Selection, Fitting, and Management of Complications. Appleton & Lange, E. Norwalk, CT, 1987
41. Ruben M: Acute eye disease secondary to contact-lens wear. Report of a census. Lancet 1:138, 1976
42. Zantos SG, Holden BA: Ocular changes associated with continuous wear of contact lenses. Aust J Optom 61:418, 1978
43. Stein RM, Clinch TE, Cohen EJ, et al: Infected vs sterile corneal infiltrates in contact lens wearers. Am J Ophthalmol 105:632, 1988
44. Suchecki JK, Ehlers WH, Donshik PC: Peripheral corneal infiltrates associated with contact lens wear. CLAO J 22:41, 1996
45. Boswall GJ, Ehlers WH, Luistro A, et al: A comparison of conventional and disposable extended wear contact lenses. CLAO J 19:158, 1993
46. Friedlaender MH: Ocular allergy and immunology. J Allergy Clin Immunol 63:51, 1979
47. Thygeson P: Marginal corneal infiltrates and ulcers. Trans Am Acad Ophthalmol Otolaryngol 51:198, 1946
48. Josephson JE, Caffery BE: Proposed hypothesis for corneal infiltrates, microabrasions, and red eye associated with extended wear [letter]. Optom Vis Sci 66:192, 1989

49. Elegbaly SA, Gillies C, Farouhar F, et al: An in vitro model of leukocyte mediated injury to the corneal epithelium. Curr Eye Res 4:31, 1985
50. Ehlers WH, Fishman JB, Donshik PC, et al: Neutrophil chemotactic factors derived from conjunctival epithelial cells: preliminary biochemical characterization. CLAO J 17:65, 1991
51. Bates AK, Morris RJ, Stapleton F, et al: 'Sterile' corneal infiltrates in contact lens wearers. Eye 3:803, 1989
52. Poggio EC, Abelson M: Complications and symptoms in disposable extended wear lenses compared with conventional soft daily wear and soft extended wear lenses. CLAO J 19:31, 1993
53. Schein OD, Glynn RJ, Poggio EC, et al: The relative risk of ulcerative keratitis among users of daily-wear and extended-wear soft contact lenses. A case-control study. N Engl J Med 321:773, 1989
54. MacRae S, Herman C, Stulting RD, et al: Corneal ulcer and adverse reaction rates in premarket contact lens studies. Am J Ophthalmol 111:457, 1991
55. Buehler PO, Schein OD, Stamler JF, et al: The increased risk of ulcerative keratitis among disposable soft contact lens users. Arch Ophthalmol 110:1555, 1992
56. Matthews TD, Frazer DG, Minassian DC, et al: Risks of keratitis and patterns of use with disposable contact lenses. Arch Ophthalmol 110:1559, 1992
57. Stern GA: *Pseudomonas* keratitis and contact lens wear: the lens/eye is at fault. Cornea 9(suppl):S36, 1990
58. Stehr-Green JK, Bailey TM, Visvesvara GS: The epidemiology of *Acanthamoeba* keratitis in the United States. Am J Ophthalmol 107:331, 1989
59. Moore MB: *Acanthamoeba* keratitis [editorial]. Arch Ophthalmol 106:1181, 1988
60. Feldman GL: Physiologic aspects of contact lens wear. p. 18. In Girard LS, Soper JW, Sampson WG (eds): Corneal Contact Lenses. CV Mosby, St. Louis, 1970
61. Sarver MD: Striate corneal lines among patients wearing hydrophilic contact lenses. Am J Optom 48:762, 1971
62. Polse KA, Sarver MD, Harris MG: Corneal edema and vertical striae accompanying the wearing of hydrogel lenses. Am J Optom 52:185, 1975
63. Polse KA, Mandell RB: Etiology of corneal striae accompanying hydrogel lens wear. Invest Ophthalmol 15:553, 1976
64. Kame RT: Clinical management of hydrogel induced edema. Am J Optom Physiol Optics 53:468, 1976
65. Mandell RB: Corneal edema from hard and hydrogel lenses. Contacto 20:8, 1976
66. Kamiya C: Study of vertical striae and horizontal striae in contact lens wearers. Contacto 24:9, 1986
67. La Hood D, Grant T: Striae and folds as indicators of corneal edema. Optom Vis Sci 67(suppl):196, 1990
68. Zantos SG, Holden BA: Transient endothelial changes soon after wearing soft contact lenses. Am J Optom Physiol Opt 54:856, 1978
69. Effron N: Clinical management of corneal edema. Contact Lens Spectrum 1:13, 1986
70. Barr JT, Schoessler JP: Corneal endothelial response to rigid contact lenses. Am J Optom Physiol Opt 57:267, 1980
71. Antti V, Jukka M, Jukka S, et al: Contact lens induced transient changes in corneal endothelium. Acta Ophthalmol (Copenh) 59:552, 1981
72. Schoessler JP, Woloschak MJ, Mauger TF: Transient endothelial changes produced by hydrophilic contact lenses. Am J Optom Physiol Opt 59:764, 1982
73. Williams L, Holden BA: The bleb response of the endothelium decreases with extended wear contact lenses. Clin Exp Optom 69:90, 1986
74. Antti V, Holden BA, Jukka M: The ultrastructure of contact lens induced changes. Acta Ophthalmol (Copenh) 62:320, 1984
75. Holden BA, Williams L, Zantos SG: The etiology of transient endothelial changes in the human cornea. Invest Ophthalmol Vis Sci 26:1354, 1985
76. Schoessler JP, Woloschak MJ: Corneal endothelium in veteran PMMA contact lens wearers. Int Contact Lens Clin 8:19, 1981
77. Caldwell DR, Kastl PR, Dabezies OH, et al: The effects of long-term hard lens wear on corneal endothelium. Contact Intraocul Lens Med J 8:87, 1982
78. Schoessler JP: Corneal endothelial polymegethism associated with extended wear. Int Contact Lens Clin 10:148, 1983
79. Hirst LW, Auer C, Cohn J, et al: Specular microscopy of hard contact lens wearers. Ophthalmology 91:1147, 1984
80. Schoessler JP, Orsborn GN: A theory of corneal endothelial polymegethism and aging. Curr Eye Res 6:301, 1987
81. Holden BA, Sweeney DF, Vannas A, et al: Contact lens induced endothelial polymegathism. ARVO abstract. Invest Ophthalmol Vis Sci 26(suppl):275, 1985
82. MacRae SM, Matsuda M, Shellans S, Rich LF: The effects of hard and soft contact lenses on the corneal endothelium. Am J Ophthalmol 102:50, 1986
83. Sibug ME, Datiles MB III, Kashima K, et al: Specular microscopy studies on the corneal endothelium after cessation of contact lens wear. Cornea 10:395, 1991
84. Dutt RM, Stocker EG, Wolff CH, et al: A morphologic and fluorophotometric analysis of the corneal endothelium in long-term extended wear soft contact lens wearers. CLAO J 15:121, 1989
85. Keates RH, Ihlenfeld JV, Isaacson WB: An introduction to fluoropolymer contact lenses: a new class of materials. CLAO J 10:332, 1984
86. Nieuwendaal CP, Kok JH, De Moor EA, et al: Corneal endothelial cell morphology under permanent wear of rigid contact lenses. Int Ophthalmol 15:313, 1991

28

Surgical Procedures to Restore the Corneal Epithelium

DOUGLAS J. COSTER

Ocular surface disorders are common and pose a serious threat to vision. The pattern and severity of pathologic changes that occur on the external eye in these disorders are variable; however, there are common pathways by which these disorders progress to threaten vision (Figure 28-1). Clinically, there may be a deficiency in the tear film, conjunctival inflammation with subsequent loss of normal cellular maturation that results in dysplasia and metaplasia of the conjunctival epithelium, and submucosal fibrosis of the conjunctiva that results in symblepharon formation and entropion. The cornea may also be affected, manifesting as epithelial metaplasia and inability of the epithelium to replenish itself, resulting in relapsing or indolent ulceration. In severe cases, there may be vascularization and scarring of the cornea. In some cases, the pathology is confined largely to the cornea; in others, all elements of the ocular surface are affected (Figure 28-2). When the cornea is involved, either in isolation or as part of a more widespread process, vision is invariably affected.

Aside from treatment of tear film abnormalities and suppression of inflammation with topical corticosteroids and systemic immunosuppressive agents, there is no effective medical treatment for many of the disorders of the ocular surface, with the possible exception of retinoic acid for epithelial metaplasia with keratinization.[1,2] In recent years, various surgical procedures have been developed to treat disorders of the ocular surface. These procedures are based on an increasing understanding of the growth and differentiation of the corneal epithelium.

THE LIMBUS AND REPLENISHMENT OF THE CORNEAL EPITHELIUM

The role of the limbus in repair of the corneal epithelium has been recognized for many years,[3] and the concept that there is a population of cells at the limbus responsible for corneal epithelial replenishment was proposed in 1971.[4] Subsequently, more formal proposals for the role of limbal epithelial stem cells have been offered and attempts to specifically characterize these cells have been made.[5–9]

All tissues with the ability to replenish themselves rely on stem cells to accomplish this task. Hemopoietic stem cells are the most accessible, the most studied, and consequently the best understood. Limbal epithelial stem cells have proved more difficult to isolate and are best understood by extrapolation from what is known about other stem cells and the basal epithelial cells of the limbus.

All stem cells share some traits. They represent a small subpopulation of cells, usually 0.5 to 10 percent of the total cell population.[10,11] A stem cell is defined in terms of its high capacity for self-renewal that persists throughout life.[12] Other shared characteristics include a high proliferation potential, a long cell cycle time, and the capacity to divide asymmetrically. Asymmetrical division means that one of the daughter cells remains a stem cell while the other daughter cell becomes slightly more differentiated. The latter cell is called a *transient amplifying cell* and has limited proliferative potential. It is the first generation on the path to terminal differentiation.[7]

There are some important questions about stem cells that remain unanswered, such as what induces them to divide and what causes the daughter cell that continues to be a stem cell to remain in immediate proximity to the place where division took place. Schofield[13] proposed that stem cells exist in a microniche that promotes their maintenance in an undifferentiated state. After cell division, only one of the progeny can reenter the niche, while the other enters an environment that encourages cell division and differentiation.

It has been suggested that the palisades of Vogt represent an epithelial stem cell niche at the limbus.[14,15] These

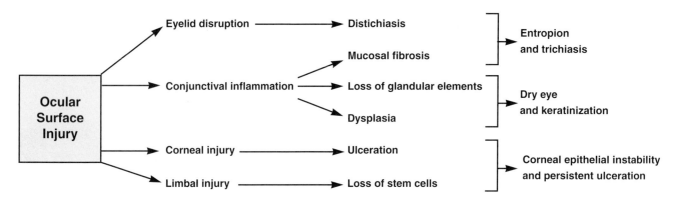

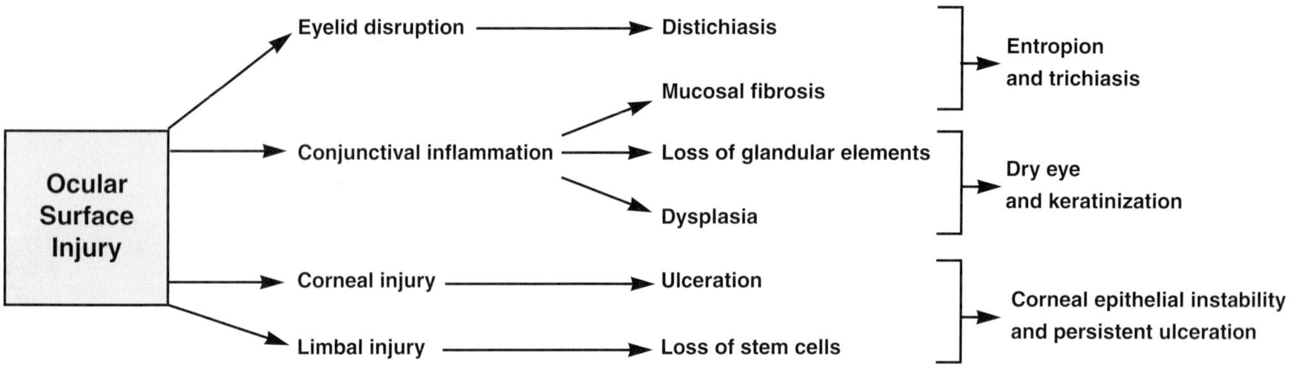

FIGURE 28-1 Patterns of ocular surface disease. Mechanisms generating corneal disease are emphasized.

palisades are a series of radially orientated fibrovascular ridges that are most obvious along the superior and inferior limbus. Between the palisades are areas of thickened epithelium. The palisades contain specialized blood vessels. Goldberg and Bron[16] suggested that the thick layer of interpalisadal epithelium may serve as a repository of cells ready to migrate onto the cornea to replace diseased or destroyed corneal epithelial cells and that the palisadal vessels nourish these cells.

Efforts to positively identify epithelial stem cells at the limbus have not yielded convincing results, and the evidence for the presence of these cells is largely circumstantial.[17] The failure of some cells to express keratin markers, which can be demonstrated in more differentiated cells, is the strongest evidence.[7] Limbal basal epithelial cells retain tritiated thymidine for long periods, suggesting a long cell cycle time,[6] and they proliferate faster in culture than do central corneal epithelial cells.[8,18,19] Furthermore, ablation of the limbus by surgery or other methods results in abnormal epithelialization of the cornea with impaired reparative capacity,[20,21] which can be overcome by transplantation of the limbus.[22] Finally, the healing of a central corneal epithelial defect involves increased cell division in the basal epithelial cells of the limbus.[8,9] As circumstantial as the evidence is, there is an increasing acceptance of the concept of the limbal epithelial stem cell, which has been important as a basis for the evolution of limbal transplantation procedures for the correction of corneal epithelial abnormalities.

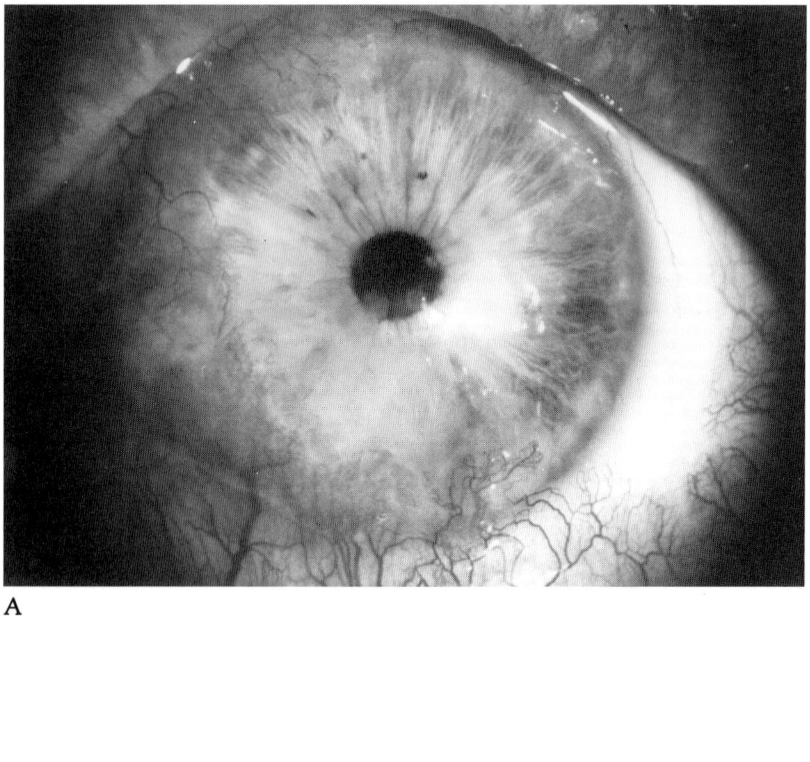

A

FIGURE 28-2 **(A)** Limbal epithelial failure after repeated resection of limbal carcinoma. *(continues)*

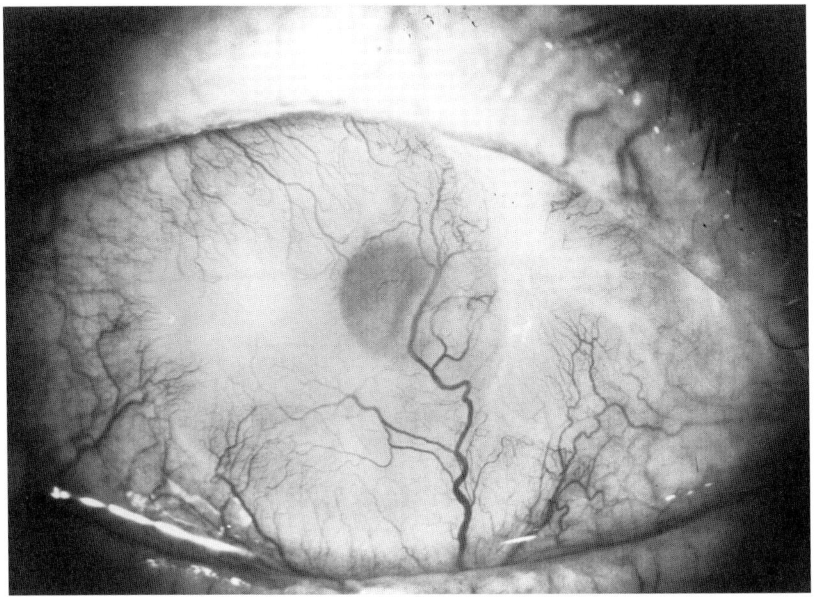
B

FIGURE 28-2 *(continued)* (B) Stevens-Johnson syndrome with corneal involvement.

CLINICAL MANIFESTATIONS OF LIMBAL FAILURE

The cornea may be affected as part of an extensive process involving the external eye, or it may be affected in relative isolation with minimal changes in other components of the external eye. When the cornea is affected in relative isolation, many of the changes can be attributed to limbal epithelial stem cell deficiency. The effects of this deficiency on the cornea are perhaps best illustrated in patients who have had extensive resections of limbal neoplasms and adjunctive cryotherapy of the limbus. The central cornea usually shows changes that range from mild to severe. In some patients, the changes are so extreme that the integrity of the globe is threatened.

In the mildest form, there is an observable change in the limbal architecture, with loss of the palisades of Vogt. In more severe cases, the central corneal epithelium is abnormal, which manifests clinically as superficial staining with rose bengal or fluorescein. Beyond this, patients develop superficial vascularization of the cornea. At this level of pathology, epithelial defects, either transient or indolent, may occur. With such severe epithelial disease, stromal inflammation and subsequent scarring are common. Focal inflammation in the stroma underlying an epithelial defect may proceed to necrosis and perforation, which is the most severe complication of ocular surface disease.

Apart from acquired deficiencies of limbal epithelial stem cells resulting from the surgical treatment of tumors, contact lens wear, or mucosal inflammatory disorders such as Stevens-Johnson syndrome and ocular pemphigoid, there are other corneal disorders that may be caused by abnormalities in limbal stem cells. The keratopathy associated with aniridia has many of the features described above, with instability of the corneal epithelium, superficial corneal vascularization, and corneal scarring. It is likely that the primary defect in the related conditions of epithelial dysplasia, carcinoma in situ, and invasive squamous cell carcinoma are at the level of the limbal epithelial stem cell. Another hypothesis, originally proposed in the first paper to allude to the importance of basal epithelial cells at the limbus,[4] is that pterygium occurs because a focal loss of stem cells encourages conjunctivalization of the cornea.

INDICATIONS

The surgical treatment of ocular surface disorders is most applicable to patients with a predominantly corneal element to their disease. Surgery to replace or replenish the corneal epithelium may be indicated in two situations: (1) when the corneal epithelium is unstable, resulting in a poor refracting surface or recurrent or indolent ulceration; or (2) when penetrating keratoplasty is required, but the condition of the corneal epithelium and limbus is such that postoperative re-epithelialization of the graft is likely to be a problem (e.g., in a graft for a chemical burn).

Patients who are likely to benefit from corneal epithelial replacement are those who have changes predominantly or exclusively in the cornea and limbus. When there is extensive disease of the external eye with severe tear

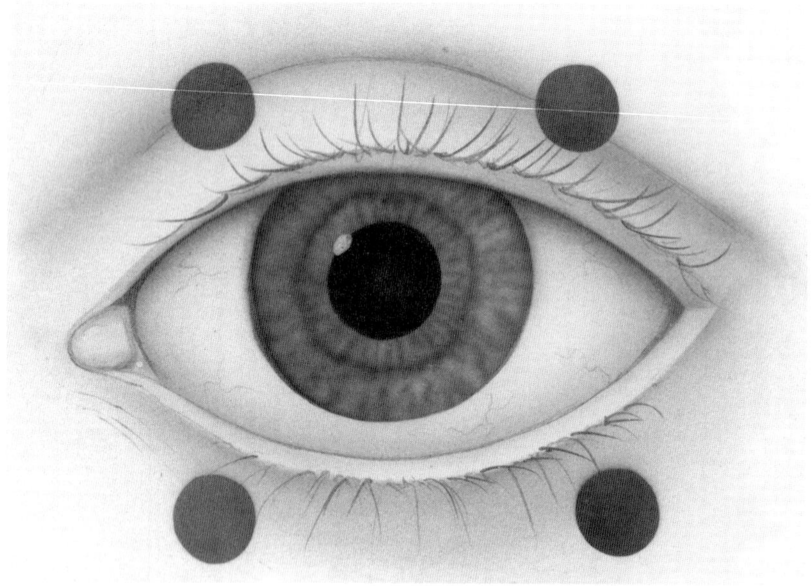

A

FIGURE 28-3 Conjunctival autografting as described by Thoft. **(A)** Donor eye. Four grafts 5 mm in diameter (gray circles) are taken from the bulbar conjunctiva of the uninvolved fellow eye. The sites are located beneath the upper and lower eyelids. *(continues)*

film deficiency, eyelid disease, and conjunctival metaplasia with keratinization, corneal epithelial replacement procedures are less likely to be successful.

PREOPERATIVE EVALUATION

Patients who are to undergo corneal epithelium replacement need to be evaluated for a suitable donor site. Whenever possible, the contralateral eye should be used. This necessitates careful examination of the proposed donor site to ensure that there are no subtle signs of limbal or corneal disease. If there are, the functional reserve capacity of the epithelial replacement system may be impaired, jeopardizing not only the grafted eye but also the donor eye. Often there is no satisfactory donor site in the contralateral eye. Ocular surface disease is commonly bilateral, and those with bilateral disease are usually the most incapacitated and in greatest need of surgery. For these patients, an allograft is required.

SURGICAL PROCEDURES

A number of surgical procedures have been proposed for patients who need replacement of the corneal epithelium.

Conjunctival Autografts

The use of conjunctival grafts to treat abnormalities of the corneal epithelium began with Thoft in 1977.[23] He described a series of cases in which small pieces of bulbar conjunctiva were taken from one eye and grafted onto the peripheral cornea of the fellow eye, which had abnormal corneal epithelium as a result of ocular surface disease (Figure 28-3). This procedure was predicated on the basis of conjunctival transdifferentiation, which postulates that conjunctival epithelium can transform into corneal epithelium under appropriate conditions. A stable ocular surface was obtained in 19 of the 22 cases reported.[23,24] Despite these excellent results, considerable doubt remains as to whether conjunctival epithelium can acquire the characteristics of corneal epithelium, and whether it is possible that the epithelium on the cornea after surgery in these cases actually came from limbal stem cells that were retained at the limbus of the grafted eye and became functional again.

Limbal Autografts

As an understanding of the role of the limbus in epithelial replacement grew, limbal transplantation became a preferred procedure for restoring the corneal epithelium. In 1989, Kenyon and Tseng[22] described transplantation of the peripheral cornea, limbus, and conjunctiva from a normal eye to treat limbal deficiency in the fellow eye of patients with unilateral ocular surface disease (Figure 28-4). A stable corneal surface was achieved in 20 of 21 cases, with no complications in the donor eye.

The major limitation of limbal autografting is that it is applicable only in patients with unilateral disease because there must be a normal contralateral eye to serve as a

FIGURE 28-3 *(continued)* **(B)** Recipient eye. A 360-degree peritomy is made 5 mm posterior to the limbus, and conjunctiva and Tenon's capsule are excised from the peritomy to the limbus. Superficial vascularized scar tissue is removed from the cornea. Each graft is anchored to the limbus with interrupted 10-0 nylon sutures. A purse string 10-0 nylon suture placed through the apices of the grafts pulls the grafts into direct contact with the cornea. (Adapted from RA Thoft: Conjunctival transplantation. Arch Ophthalmol 95:1425, 1977.)

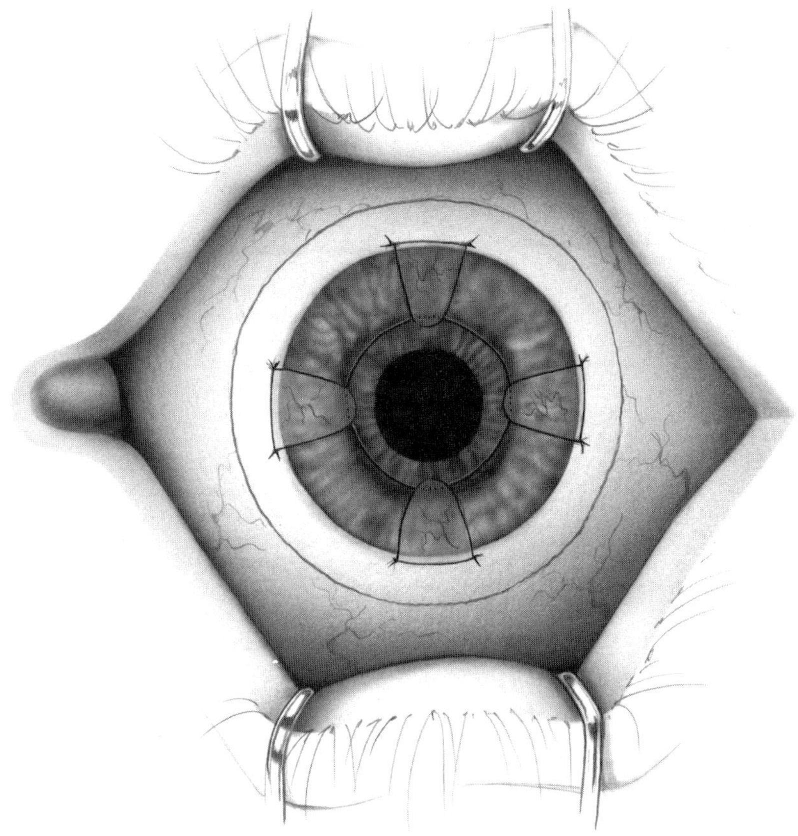

B

donor site. Disorders affecting the ocular surface tend to be bilateral, and the neediest cases are those with poor vision from bilateral disease. For these patients, allografts rather than autografts are required.

Epithelial Allografts

The first epithelial allografts were reported by Thoft in 1984.[25] He described a procedure he termed *keratoepithelioplasty,* in which lenticles of peripheral cornea were taken from deceased donors and sewn into the peripheral corneas of recipients with ocular surface disorders (Figure 28-5). Of the 11 patients followed, seven achieved a stable epithelium. Although Thoft intended to graft corneal epithelium without involving the limbus, it is likely that the grafts included some limbal elements.

Turgeon et al[26] described a procedure similar to keratoepithelioplasty but involving intentional transplantation of limbal tissue. The results of this procedure were similar to those of keratoepithelioplasty. A further modification of keratoepithelioplasty reported by Tsai and Tseng[27] in 1994 consisted of taking superficial peripheral cornea, limbus, and conjunctiva from a cadaveric whole globe and grafting them into the recipient eye. They termed this procedure *allograft limbal transplantation.* Oral and topical cyclosporine were used in all cases. The procedure was considered successful in five of the six patients reported. This and similar techniques have been widely used in recent years.

Two other techniques have evolved as part of these surgical developments: the combination of limbal grafts with penetrating keratoplasty for patients with severely affected corneas, and the use of allogeneic grafts from living related donors. Penetrating keratoplasty is notoriously unsuccessful when the recipient ocular surface is significantly abnormal. Pfister,[28] Tsubota et al,[29] and Coster et al[30] have reported the transplantation of limbus and central cornea in such patients (Figure 28-6). They reported successes in groups of patients for whom long-term improvement would be unlikely with penetrating keratoplasty alone. The transplantation of conjunctiva and limbus from living related donors has also been used in patients with limbal failure.[31,32] The results reported are remarkably good, although the follow-up is short.

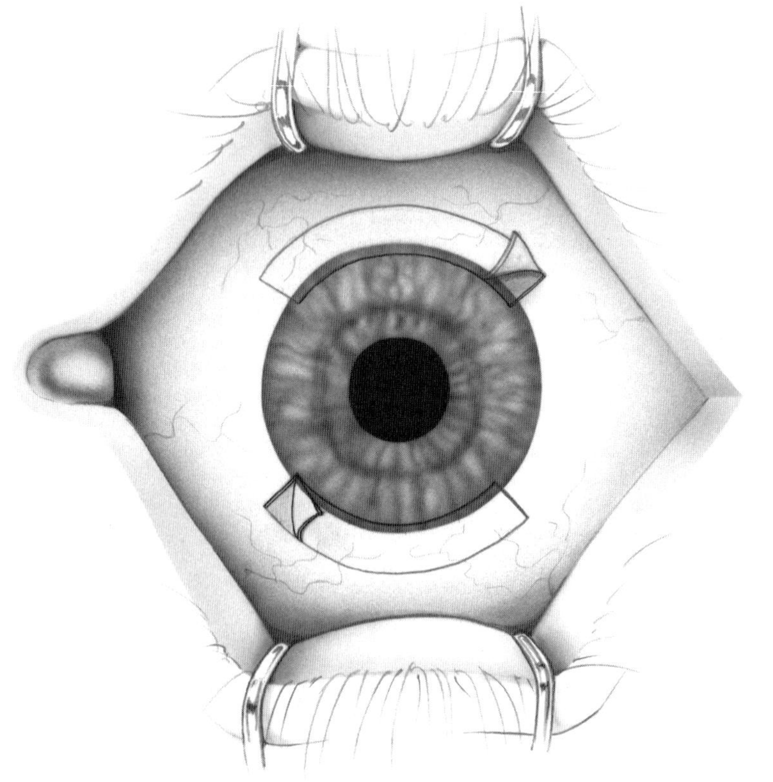

A

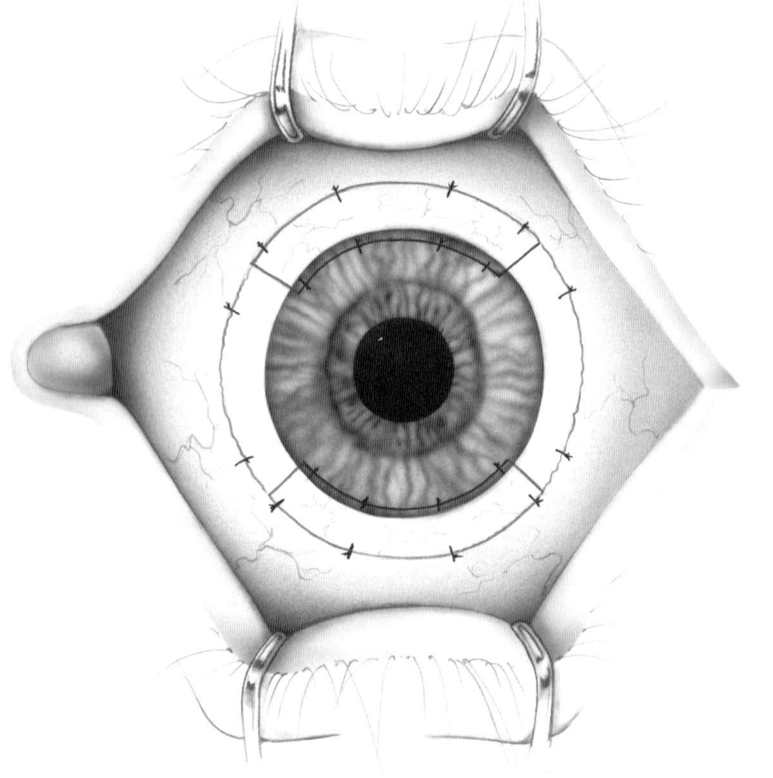

B

FIGURE 28-4 Limbal autografting as described by Kenyon and Tseng. **(A)** Donor eye. Two 4-clock-hour sectorial grafts of limbal tissue are taken from the uninvolved fellow eye. Each graft extends 0.5 mm into clear cornea centrally and 2 mm into bulbar conjunctiva peripherally. **(B)** Recipient eye. Superficial vascularized scar tissue is removed from the cornea. A 360-degree peritomy is made 2 mm posterior to the limbus, and conjunctiva and Tenon's capsule are excised from the peritomy to the limbus. The margins of the recipient conjunctiva are secured with four interrupted 8-0 polyglactin sutures. Each graft is secured with 10-0 nylon sutures at the corneal margin and 8-0 polyglactin sutures at the conjunctival margin. (Adapted from KR Kenyon, SC Tseng: Limbal autograft transplantation for ocular surface disorders. Ophthalmology 96:709, 1989.)

FIGURE 28-5 Keratoepithelioplasty as described by Thoft. **(A)** Donor eye. Four 4 × 6–mm lenticles consisting of epithelium and superficial stroma are carved from the corneal surface. **(B)** Recipient eye. A 360-degree peritomy is made 5 mm posterior to the limbus, and conjunctiva and Tenon's capsule are excised from the peritomy to the limbus. Superficial vascularized scar tissue is removed from the cornea. The lenticles are placed around the limbus and secured with interrupted 10-0 nylon sutures. (Adapted from RA Thoft: Keratoepithelioplasty. Am J Ophthalmol 97:1, 1984.)

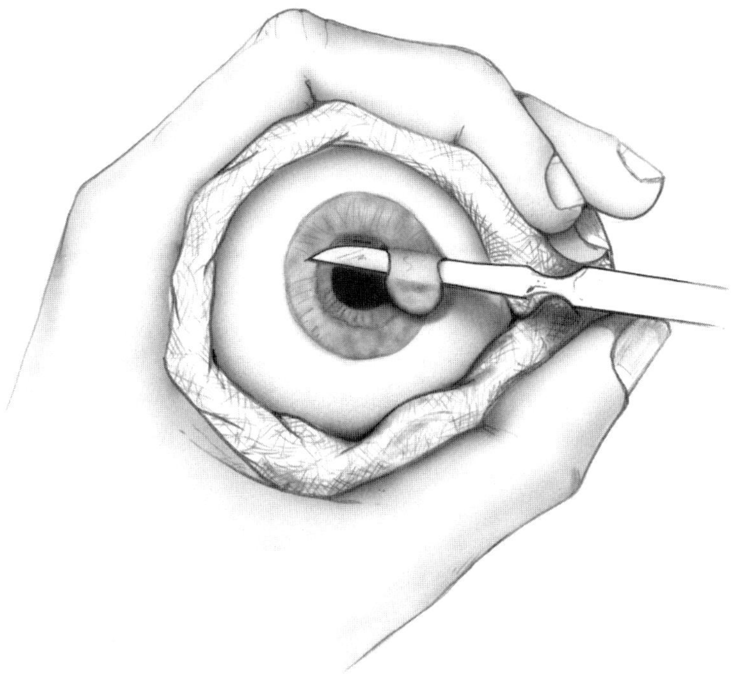

A

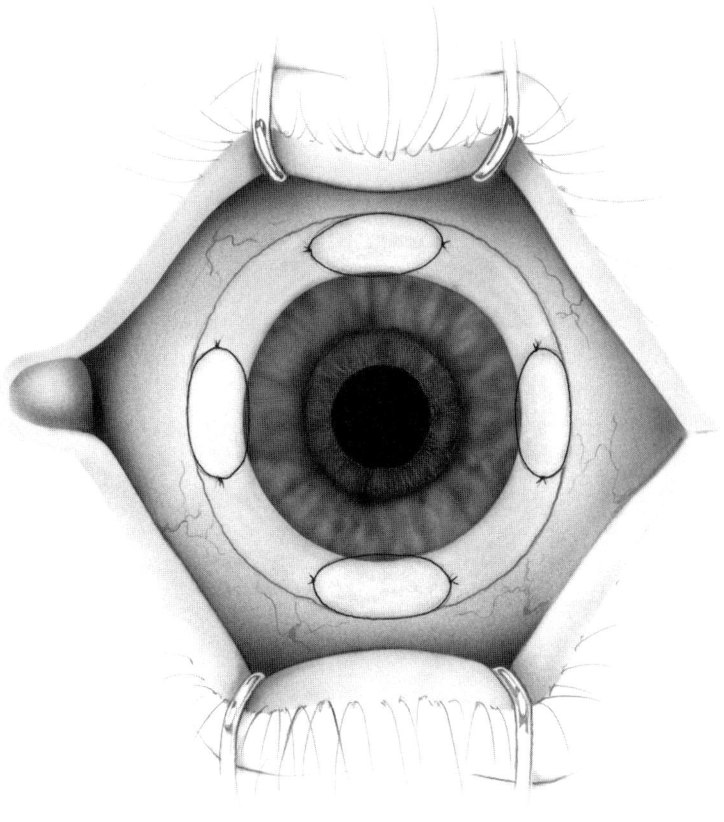

B

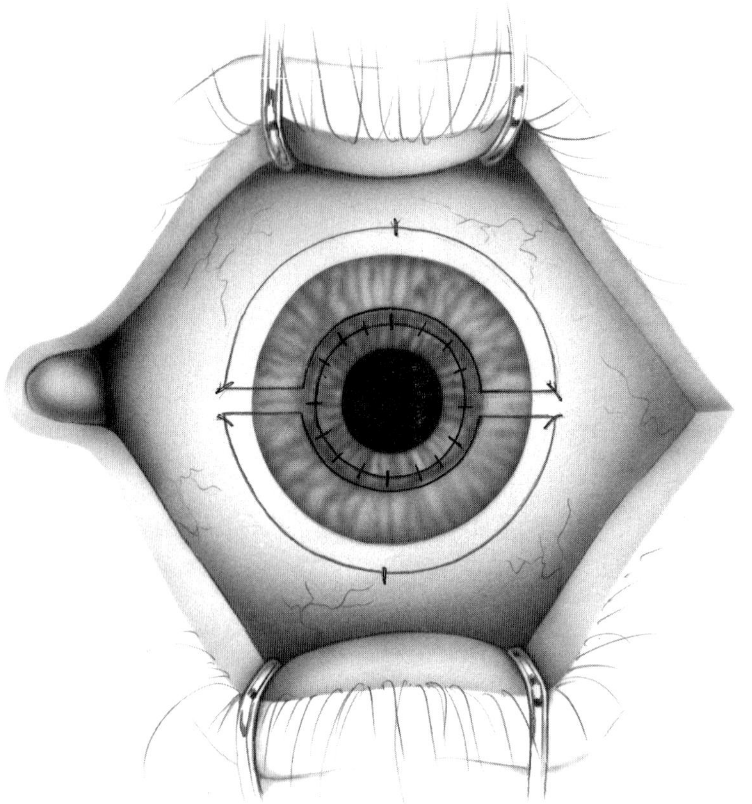

FIGURE 28-6 Combined penetrating keratoplasty and limbal allografting as described by Tsubota et al. Vascularized limbal scar tissue is excised to expose bare limbus. Penetrating keratoplasty is performed in the usual manner. The donor rim is cut in half, and a lamellar dissection of the cornea and sclera is performed to create two grafts consisting of Bowman's layer, a small amount of corneal stroma, and corneal and limbal epithelium. The grafts are secured at the limbus with interrupted 10-0 nylon sutures. (Adapted from K Tsubota, I Toda, H Saito, et al. Reconstruction of the corneal epithelium by limbal allograft transplantation for severe ocular surface disorders. Ophthalmology 102:1486, 1995.)

SURGICAL TECHNIQUE FOR LIMBAL TRANSPLANTATION

Because surgical procedures to replace the corneal epithelium are new and evolving, it is unwise to be emphatic about the optimal technique. Although some surgeons have had excellent results with conjunctival transplantation, a general preference for limbal transplantation has emerged. Most surgeons now prefer to use limbal and conjunctival tissue rather than conjunctival or corneal tissue alone. This reflects a widespread belief in the notion of limbal epithelial stem cells and the need to transfer this population of cells in the graft. Another reason for including the limbus is related to surgical technique. By excising superficial peripheral cornea, it is possible to accurately inlay the graft bearing the limbal epithelium flush with the surface of the recipient. At the same time, a frill of 2 to 3 mm of conjunctiva can be sutured to the recipient conjunctiva so that a smooth ocular surface is achieved over which the eyelids can move without discomfort or disruption of the graft.

When possible, limbal autografts are used, but if there is a problem in obtaining sufficient limbus from the contralateral eye, allografting is necessary. It is generally agreed that no more than 180 degrees of limbus can be taken from the contralateral donor without creating limbal deficiency and epithelial abnormalities on the donor cornea. This limits the extent of limbus grafted in these cases to two 90-degree sectors, which are usually sewn into the superior and inferior limbus. Allografting is not limited in this way, and a 360-degree or doughnut-shaped graft can be used. The principles of surgery are the same whether an autograft or allograft is used.

Most limbal grafts can be performed with local anesthesia. For some patients, however, the resection and repair may be complicated to the extent that the surgery may last 2 hours or more. For these patients, general anesthesia may be advisable.

A limbal peritomy is made, and abnormal corneal epithelium and fibrous tissue are removed. The abnormal tissue can usually be peeled off the stroma, leaving a smooth stromal surface. Occasionally, the abnormal tissue is scarred to the underlying stroma—especially if there has been previous corneal surgery—and must be dissected off. It is important to remove any islands of abnormal epithelium to facilitate re-epithelialization from the donor.

A peripheral keratectomy is performed to create a bed into which the graft is placed. The cornea is marked with a 9-mm trephine and is incised to quarter depth with a

FIGURE 28-7 Limbal transplantation as described by Kruse. **(A)** After removal of superficial vascularized corneal scar tissue, an incision is made in the peripheral cornea to approximately 25 percent depth, and a lamellar dissection is performed peripherally to 1 mm beyond the limbus. An identical graft is cut from the donor eye. *(continues)*

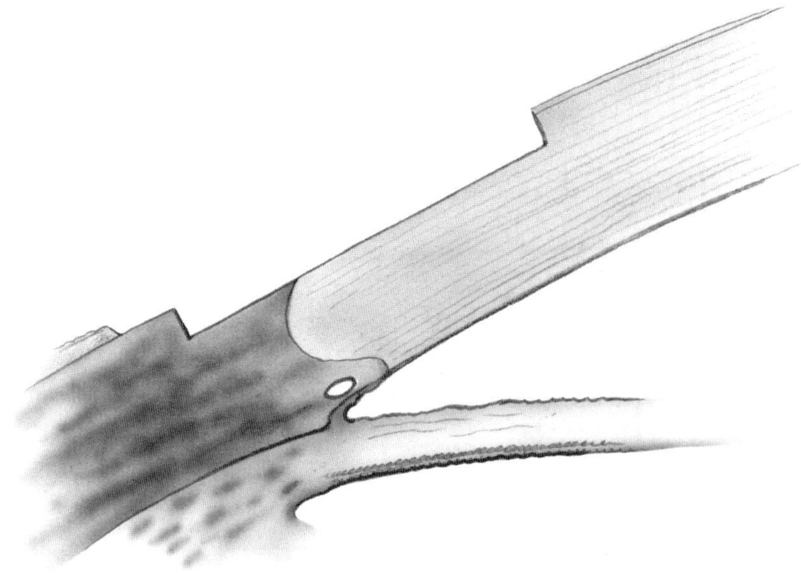

A

diamond knife. For an allograft, the incision is circumferential; for an autograft, two 90-degree incisions are made. A superficial lamellar keratectomy is done from the edge of the incision peripherally to 1 mm beyond the limbus[33] (Figure 28-7).

An allograft is prepared from a whole eye, with the goal of excising a graft that matches the bed prepared in the recipient eye. It is usually necessary to make the eye bank aware of the specific requirements for the donor eye. In general terms, these requirements are the same as those for penetrating keratoplasty; however, the donor eye should be enucleated in a manner to preserve as much conjunctiva as possible and should be stored in a moist chamber at 4°C for no more than 24 hours. Because excision of the graft from the donor eye can be difficult, two donor eyes should be available.

The donor eye is wrapped in gauze and held by an assistant. Careful excision of the donor graft is achieved using a technique similar to that described above for the recipient bed. The assistant can help in this procedure by maintaining pressure on the globe, which makes the keratectomy easier to perform, and by rotating the donor eye so that its position is optimal for the surgeon. Any excess conjunctiva or Tenon's capsule is excised before the graft is cut free from the rest of the eye.

Once the graft is obtained, it is transferred to the recipient eye. The graft is positioned in the keratectomy bed to optimize the fit, ensuring that any variations in the thickness of the graft and the depth of the keratectomy bed are matched as well as possible and that the surface of the graft is level with the surface of the recipient cornea.

The corneal edge of the graft is sutured with interrupted 10-0 nylon sutures, usually four in each quadrant, and the knots are buried. The scleral edge of the graft is then sutured with eight 10-0 nylon sutures. Finally, the conjunctiva of the graft is sutured to the edge of the recipient conjunctiva with eight 8-0 polyglactin sutures after any excess conjunctiva has been trimmed from the graft.

A similar procedure is used for autografts. The graft is harvested from the normal contralateral eye in two 90-degree sectors and is sutured into identical defects prepared in the recipient cornea.

POSTOPERATIVE CARE

Topical antibiotics are used for 7 days. Stromal inflammation impairs epithelial replacement.[34] Therefore, it is important to suppress local inflammation by ensuring that the graft is well positioned on the ocular surface and that the suture knots are buried. Topical corticosteroids, such as 0.5 percent prednisolone phosphate eye drops, are used to suppress inflammation in the early postoperative period and for long-term immunosuppression in patients with allografts. Sutures are removed at 3 to 6 months, or earlier if they loosen, protrude, or attract mucus.

Allograft rejection is common in animal models and in patients not receiving immunosuppression.[35] For this reason, systemic immunosuppression is recommended in patients with allografts. How much is required and for how long remain to be determined. Current practice in many places is to treat with both topical medication (cortico-

FIGURE 28-7 *(continued)* **(B & C)** The graft is inlaid into the corneoscleral bed. The corneal and scleral margins are secured with interrupted 10-0 nylon sutures. The conjunctival margin of the graft is apposed to the conjunctival margin of the recipient with interrupted 8-0 polyglactin sutures. (Adapted from FE Kruse: Stem cells and corneal epithelial regeneration. Eye 8:170, 1994.)

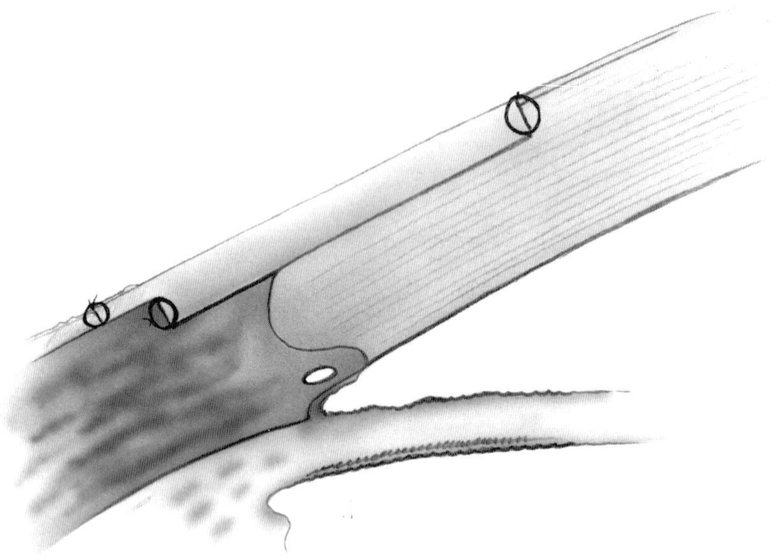

B

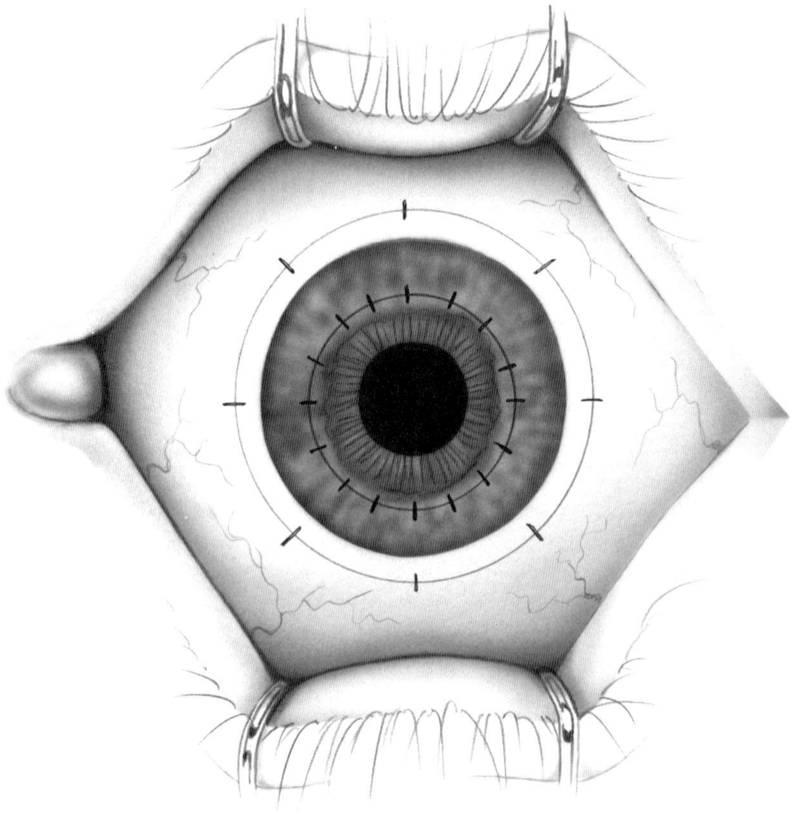

C

steroids) and systemic medication.[27,30] In our center, we use triple systemic therapy with prednisolone, cyclosporine, and azathioprine. The prednisolone is continued for 3 weeks; the cyclosporine and azathioprine are continued for 1 year unless intolerable side effects develop, in which case they are discontinued sooner. All patients receiving systemic immunosuppression develop some side effects, but these are usually mild. However, there is the potential for life-threatening complications. Patients must be carefully assessed to ensure that they do not have co-morbidities that put them at additional risk. Chronic infections, neoplasms, hypertension, and renal disease are examples of conditions that can complicate immunosuppression.

COMPLICATIONS

Postoperative complications of limbal transplantation are usually not serious because the procedure is extraocular.

Failure of Engraftment

The most disappointing complication of limbal transplantation is failure of engraftment. This may occur because the graft is not viable at the time of surgery or cannot be sustained for one reason or another in its new environment, or because of allograft rejection. Failed engraftment results in the reappearance of the clinical manifestations of the disorder for which the graft was placed, but these are usually no worse than they were before surgery.

Surprisingly, clinical success can be maintained long term despite the absence of donor cells in the central cornea or over the limbal graft.[36] This result is difficult to explain other than by assuming that either long-term immunosuppression improves the function of the recipient limbal epithelium, or that the surgery altered the microenvironment of the limbus, encouraging more normal growth and differentiation of the recipient limbal epithelial cells.[37]

Allograft Rejection

Allograft rejection is to be expected, although the pattern of clinical expression is somewhat unusual. Histologically, conjunctiva resembles skin, but the patterns of allograft rejection are different in the two tissues. Allogeneic skin grafts reject with ischemic necrosis. Rejection of an allogeneic limbal graft is more subtle.

Normally, anastomosis of the microvasculature of the limbal graft to the underlying and surrounding tissues occurs within a few days of grafting, and flow in the conjunctival vessels is observed after 3 or 4 days. In the case of rejection, however, the vessels soon become engorged, with stagnation of flow and swelling of the tissue. This phase is temporary, lasting 4 to 5 days, after which vascular flow is resumed. There is no obvious tissue necrosis. This pattern of rejection is observed in patients and in animal models. In the experimental situation, the frequency and severity of rejection episodes are reduced by the application of topical corticosteroids.[35]

The occurrence of allograft rejection raises a number of questions. Presumably the viability of the cells within the allograft is affected by the rejection, but the impact this has on engraftment is unknown. An issue that arises as a consequence of this is the role of immunosuppression, which has not been resolved. A wide range of approaches to immunosuppression have been employed in patients with limbal allografts, ranging from the use of topical corticosteroids to systemic immunosuppression with corticosteroids, cyclosporine, and azathioprine. Although long-term success has been observed in patients who use nothing other than topical corticosteroids, there is an increasing tendency for surgeons to prescribe systemic immunosuppression. How much immunosuppression is required and for how long are not known.

Complications in the Donor

Postoperative epithelial abnormalities on the donor cornea have been reported in patients with contact lens–associated epitheliopathy.[38] This suggests that dysfunction of limbal epithelial stem cells may be subclinical and that harvesting a limbal graft from such an eye can jeopardize the corneal epithelial integrity of the donor eye.

RESULTS

There is no doubt that the surgical procedures described above to restore the corneal epithelium can produce improvements for patients who would be otherwise untreatable. Whether the success is sustained over years rather than months is not yet apparent. At least one group has reported a deterioration in outcome in patients with ocular surface disease when they were assessed again at 2 years, after achieving excellent results at 6 months. As yet, these results have not been published. The need for long-term evaluation is perhaps not surprising in view of the lengthy persistence of donor epithelium after penetrating keratoplasty.

Despite the promise of various procedures advocated for corneal epithelial replacement, a number of important issues demand clarification. The literature pertaining to the biology of the limbus and the corneal epithelium is limited, and so, too, are the clinical reports of the various procedures advocated. What is reported raises many questions, and there is an urgent need for more formal clinical studies. Many of the issues important for contemporary clinical practice can only be surmised because of a lack of coherent clinical data.

REFERENCES

1. Tseng SCG, Maumenee AE, Stark WJ, et al: Topical retinoid treatment for various dry-eye disorders. Ophthalmology 92:717, 1985
2. Tseng SCG: Topical retinoid treatment for dry eye disorders. Trans Ophthalmol Soc UK 104:489, 1985
3. Mann I: A study of epithelial regeneration in the living eye. Br J Ophthalmol 28:26, 1944
4. Davanger M, Evensen A: Role of the pericorneal papillary structure in renewal of corneal epithelium. Nature 229:560, 1971
5. Tseng SCG: Concept and application of limbal stem cells. Eye 3:141, 1989
6. Cotsarelis G, Cheng S-Z, Dong G, et al: Existence of slow-cycling limbal epithelial basal cells that can be preferentially stimulated to proliferate: implications on epithelial stem cells. Cell 57:201, 1989
7. Schermer A, Galvin S, Sun T-T: Differentiation-related expression of a major 64K corneal keratin in vivo and in culture suggests limbal location of corneal epithelial stem cells. J Cell Biol 103:49, 1986
8. Ebato B, Friend J, Thoft RA: Comparison of central and peripheral human corneal epithelium in tissue culture. Invest Ophthalmol Vis Sci 28:1450, 1987
9. Zieske JD, Bukusoglu G, Yankauckas MA: Characterization of a potential marker of corneal epithelial stem cells. Invest Ophthalmol Vis Sci 33:143, 1992
10. Potten CS, Morris RJ: Epithelial stem cells in vivo. J Cell Sci 10(suppl):45, 1988
11. Gordon JI, Schmidt GH, Roth KA: Studies of intestinal stem cells using normal, chimeric, and transgenic mice. FASEB J 6:3039, 1991
12. Hall PA, Watt FM: Stem cells: the generation and maintenance of cellular diversity. Development 106:619, 1989
13. Schofield R: The stem cell system. Biomed Pharmacother 37:375, 1983
14. Gipson IK: The epithelial basement membrane zone of the limbus. Eye 3:132, 1989
15. Townsend WM: The limbal palisades of Vogt. Trans Am Ophthalmol Soc 86:721, 1991
16. Goldberg MF, Bron AJ: Limbal palisades of Vogt. Trans Am Ophthalmol Soc 80:155, 1982
17. Zieske JD: Perpetuation of stem cells in the eye. Eye 8:163, 1994
18. Ebato B, Friend J, Thoft RA: Comparison of limbal and peripheral human corneal epithelium in tissue culture. Invest Ophthalmol Vis Sci 29:1533, 1988
19. Lindberg K, Brown ME, Chaves HV, et al: In vitro propagation of human ocular surface epithelial cells for transplantation. Invest Ophthalmol Vis Sci 34:2672, 1993
20. Chen JJY, Tseng SCG: Abnormal corneal epithelial wound healing in partial-thickness removal of limbal epithelium. Invest Ophthalmol Vis Sci 32:2219, 1991
21. Huang AJW, Tseng SCG: Corneal epithelial wound healing in the absence of limbal epithelium. Invest Ophthalmol Vis Sci 32:96, 1991
22. Kenyon KR, Tseng SC: Limbal autograft transplantation for ocular surface disorders. Ophthalmology 96:709, 1989
23. Thoft RA: Conjunctival transplantation. Arch Ophthalmol 95:1425, 1977
24. Thoft RA: Indications for conjunctival transplantation. Ophthalmology 89:335, 1982
25. Thoft RA: Keratoepithelioplasty. Am J Ophthalmol 97:1, 1984
26. Turgeon PW, Nauheim RD, Roat MI, et al: Indications for keratoepithelioplasty. Arch Ophthalmol 108:233, 1990
27. Tsai RJF, Tseng SCG: Human allograft limbal transplantation for corneal surface reconstruction. Cornea 13:389, 1994
28. Pfister RR: Corneal stem cell disease; concepts, categorization, and treatment by auto- and homotransplantation of limbal stem cells. CLAO J 20:64, 1994
29. Tsubota K, Toda I, Saito H, et al. Reconstruction of the corneal epithelium by limbal allograft transplantation for severe ocular surface disorders. Ophthalmology 102:1486, 1995
30. Coster DJ, Aggarwal RK, Williams KA: Surgical management of ocular surface disorders using conjunctival and stem cell allografts. Br J Ophthalmol 79:977, 1995
31. Kwitko S, Marinho D, Barcaro S, et al. Allograft conjunctival transplantation for bilateral ocular surface disorders. Ophthalmology 102:1020, 1995
32. Kenyon KR, Rapoza PA: Limbal allograft transplantation for ocular surface disorders. AAO abstract. Ophthalmology 102(suppl):101, 1995
33. Kruse FE: Stem cells and corneal epithelial regeneration. Eye 8:170, 1994
34. Tsai RFJ, Tseng SCG: Effect of stromal inflammation on the outcome of limbal transplantation for corneal surface reconstruction. Cornea 14:439, 1995
35. Swift GJ, Aggarwal RK, Davis GJ, et al: Survival of rabbit limbal stem cell allografts. Transplantation 62:568, 1996
36. Williams KA, Brereton HM, Aggarwal R, et al: Use of DNA polymorphisms and the polymerase chain reaction to examine the survival of a human limbal stem cell allograft. Am J Ophthalmol 120:342, 1995
37. Coster DJ: Doyne Lecture. Influences on the development of corneal transplantation. Eye 8(Pt 1):1, 1994
38. Jenkins C, Tuft S, Liu C, et al. Limbal transplantation in the management of chronic contact-lens–associated epitheliopathy. Eye 7:629, 1993

29

Conjunctival Flaps

BRADLEY P. GARDNER

Conjunctival flaps were introduced as early as 1877 to treat corneal injuries and disease.[1] The surgical technique at that time involved dissecting both conjunctiva and Tenon's capsule and securing them on the cornea with interrupted sutures. Such thick flaps were only temporarily beneficial because the sutures cheesewired through the flap, and the flap retracted off the cornea. In 1954, Haik[2] introduced an incisionless flap, which was created by suturing together folds of conjunctiva from the superior and inferior fornices to cover the cornea. This technique was also plagued by retraction of the flap as the sutures cut through the tissue.

In 1958, Gundersen[3] introduced the thin conjunctival flap. His technique involved dissecting conjunctiva from Tenon's capsule, which decreased the likelihood of retraction of the flap. Although modifications of Gundersen's technique have subsequently been described, he is credited with developing the basic procedure, which is still referred to as the *Gundersen flap*.[4]

There are two types of conjunctival flaps: total (Gundersen) and partial (Figures 29-1 and 29-2).

INDICATIONS

The indications for conjunctival flaps have diminished over the years because more effective ways to treat disorders of the ocular surface have been developed.[5,6] Advances in antimicrobial agents, ocular lubricants, bandage soft contact lenses, tissue adhesives, and conjunctival, corneal, and oculoplastic surgical techniques have reduced the need for conjunctival flaps. However, these therapies are not effective in every case, and in certain situations, such as poor patient compliance, they are not practical. Thus, conjunctival flaps continue to be indicated.

Restoration of Ocular Surface Integrity

Nonhealing sterile corneal ulcers unresponsive to medical therapy are the most common indication for conjunctival flaps.[7,8] Such ulcers are caused by a variety of disorders, including dry eyes, exposure keratopathy, neurotrophic keratitis, corneal anesthesia, sterilized infectious keratitis, chemical burns, and other forms of trauma. Under adverse conditions, the vascularity of the conjunctival flap enhances the potential for survival of the ocular surface.

Penetrating keratoplasty has replaced the conjunctival flap as the treatment of choice for bullous keratopathy.[9] However, in an eye with a posterior segment abnormality that limits visual potential, a conjunctival flap is more convenient, more comfortable, and safer than prolonged treatment with hyperosmotic agents or a bandage soft contact lens.

A conjunctival flap should not be used to control pain in a blind eye unless the pain is caused by a disorder of the corneal surface. For example, pain from bullous keratopathy can be relieved with a conjunctival flap, but pain associated with end-stage glaucoma may not be relieved with a conjunctival flap and is best treated by other methods.

A conjunctival flap may be considered in the treatment of certain cases of fulminant corneal graft rejection unresponsive to medical therapy.[7] If the patient is relatively asymptomatic and the eye is not inflamed, a conjunctival flap is not indicated. However, if the eye is inflamed and painful, a conjunctival flap can provide symptomatic relief and help quiet the eye in preparation for future penetrating keratoplasty.

Marginal corneal thinning secondary to Mooren's ulcer or a systemic collagen-vascular disease is better managed

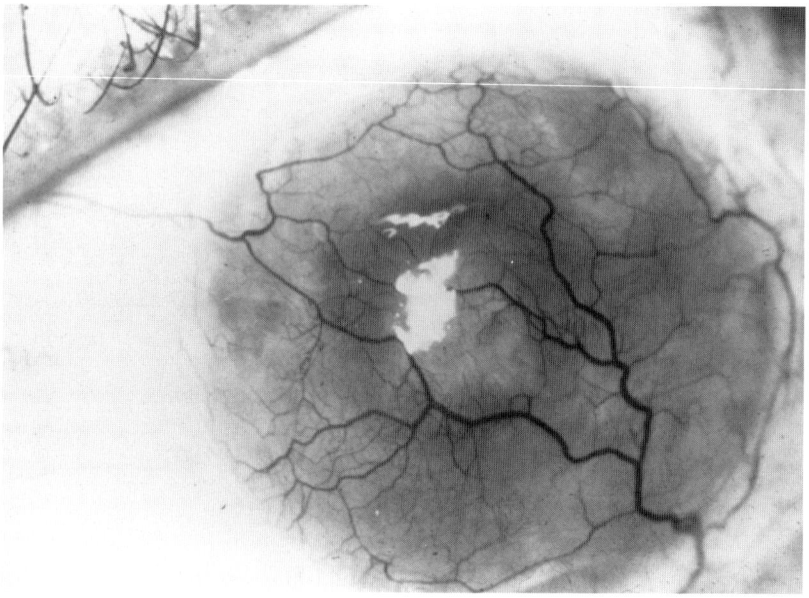

FIGURE 29-1 Total conjunctival flap. The flap is thin, which allows visualization of anterior chamber structures.

with conjunctival recession or resection accompanied by systemic immunosuppressive therapy than with a conjunctival flap. Paton and Milauskas[4] reported a 100 percent failure rate of conjunctival flaps used for the treatment of Mooren's ulcer.

A conjunctival flap should not be considered the sole treatment for impending or actual corneal perforation.[10-12] A flap may impede leakage of aqueous humor and help to reform the anterior chamber; however, it does not seal the perforation but rather forms a filtering bleb. Saini et al[13] reported long-term uncomplicated healing of corneal perforations in only 30 percent of eyes treated with conjunctival flaps compared with 92 percent of eyes treated with tissue adhesive or penetrating or lamellar keratoplasty. However, where penetrating or lamellar keratoplasty is not feasible or donor tissue and other resources are not available, a conjunctival flap can help to maintain the integrity of the eye and prevent infection.

Corneal ulceration caused by exposure or dry eyes can lead to perforation. A lamellar or full-thickness patch graft used to seal the perforation will have the same fate as the original cornea unless the graft is protected by a conjunctival flap (Figure 29-3). Similarly,

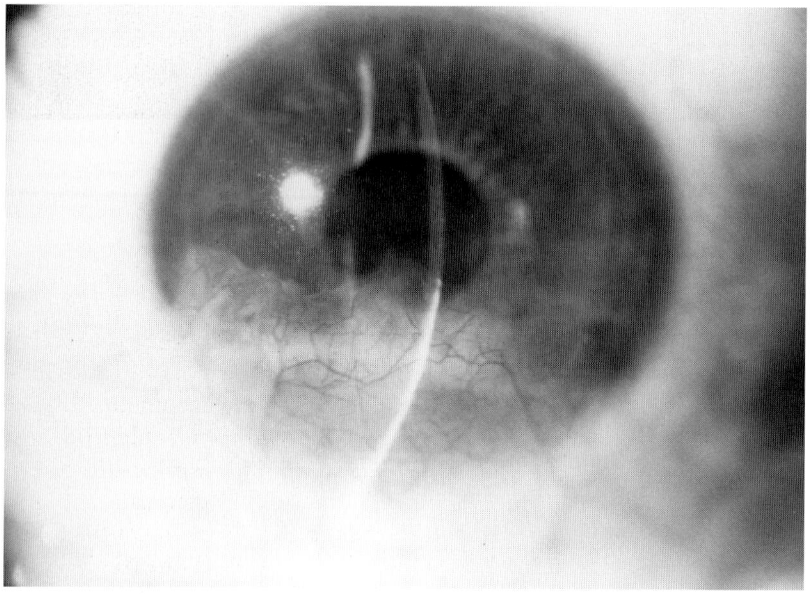

FIGURE 29-2 Partial conjunctival flap. Such a flap is used for localized lesions. A partial flap permits better visual acuity than does a total flap.

FIGURE 29-3 (A) Corneal perforation caused by dry eyes. (B) A lamellar patch graft was placed and covered with a partial conjunctival flap to protect the graft and prevent reperforation.

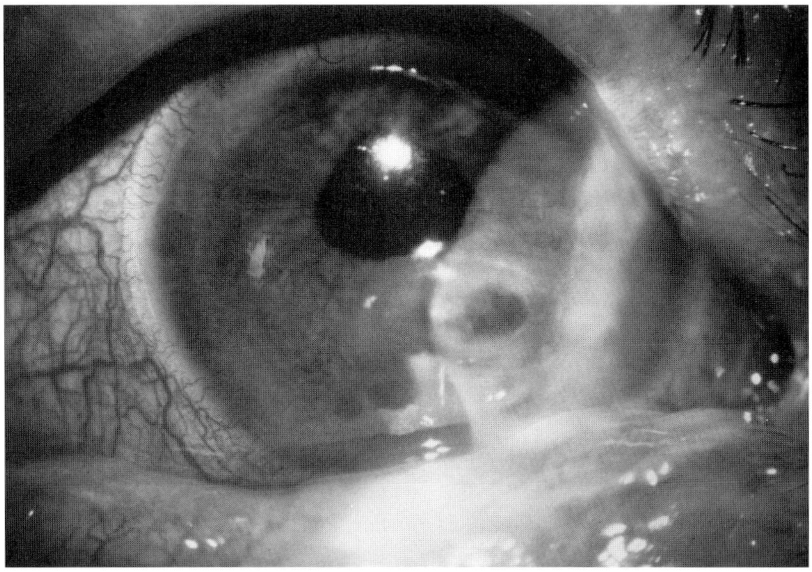

A

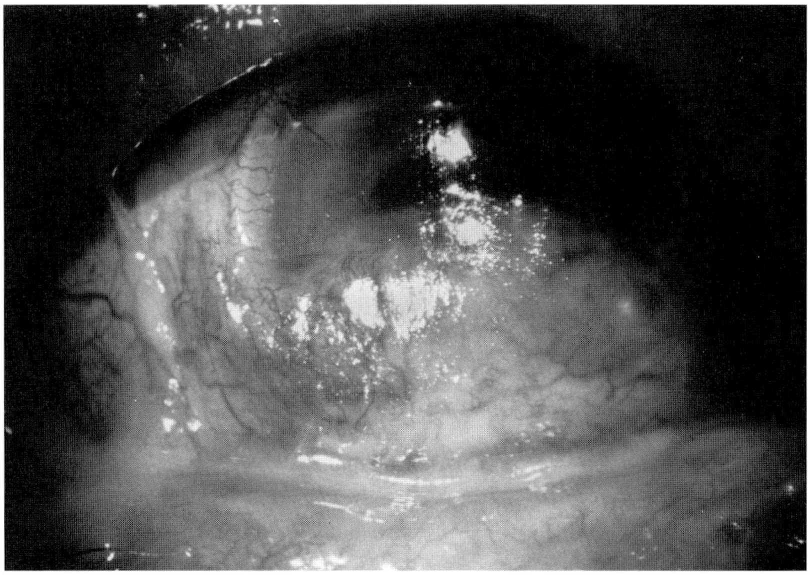

B

a lamellar patch graft used to treat an impending or actual perforation from active herpes simplex viral keratitis is more likely to be successful when covered by a conjunctival flap.

A conjunctival flap may be placed to prepare the ocular surface for a cosmetic scleral shell in a disfigured blind or phthisical eye. Such a shell can erode the corneal epithelium. The epithelium of the conjunctiva is less subject to erosion than that of the cornea, and a conjunctival flap creates a surface more tolerant of the shell.

The use of conjunctival flaps in pterygium surgery is described in Chapter 21.

Resistant Microbial Infections

Corneal ulcers caused by various microbial organisms that are resistant to medical therapy may be treated with a conjunctival flap. Although the corneal stroma contains elements of the humoral immune system (immunoglobulins), it lacks elements of the cell-mediated immune system (T cells).[14] A conjunctival flap provides blood vessels and lymphatic channels that increase exposure of the invading organisms to immunologic defenses.

Successful treatment of medically resistant bacterial keratitis with conjunctival flaps has been reported[15]; how-

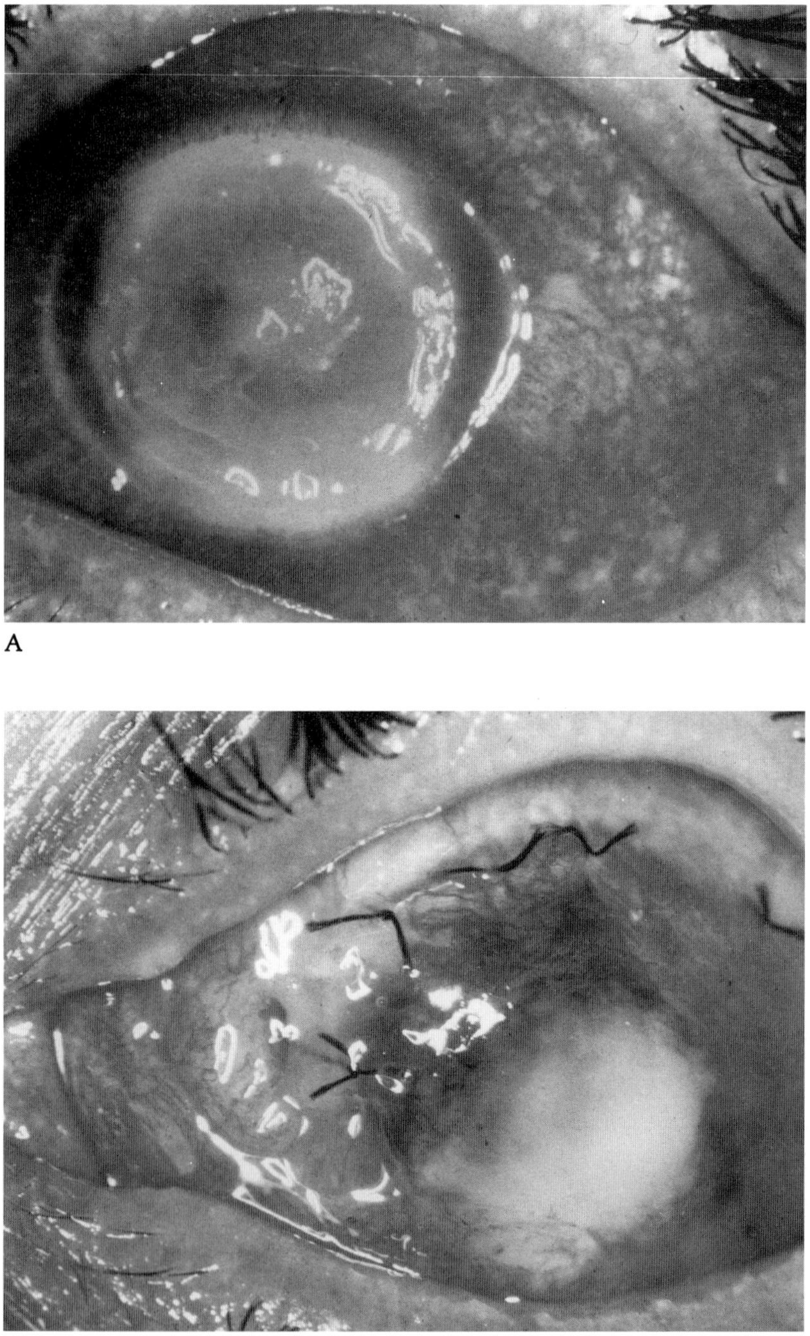

A

B

FIGURE 29-4 **(A)** Severe necrosis of the corneal stroma. **(B)** Treatment with a conjunctival flap without removal of the necrotic corneal tissue led to necrosis of the flap. (Courtesy of William M. Townsend, M.D., San Juan, PR.)

ever, bacterial keratitis is generally not treated with a conjunctival flap unless the infected area has first been sterilized with antibiotics and is free of necrotic corneal tissue. In general, a flap that is placed on necrotic tissue will not survive because the flap becomes avascular at the site of the necrosis. A hole then forms and consumes the flap (Figure 29-4). Therefore, any visible necrotic tissue should be removed before the flap is placed.

Advances in antifungal agents have made medical therapy the treatment of choice for most cases of fungal keratitis. However, the frequent use of topical, subconjunctival, and/or systemic antifungal agents for several weeks is generally necessary. Some patients cannot or will not comply with such an intensive treatment regimen. Even in patients who can comply, a lamellar keratectomy combined with a conjunctival flap is often an excellent

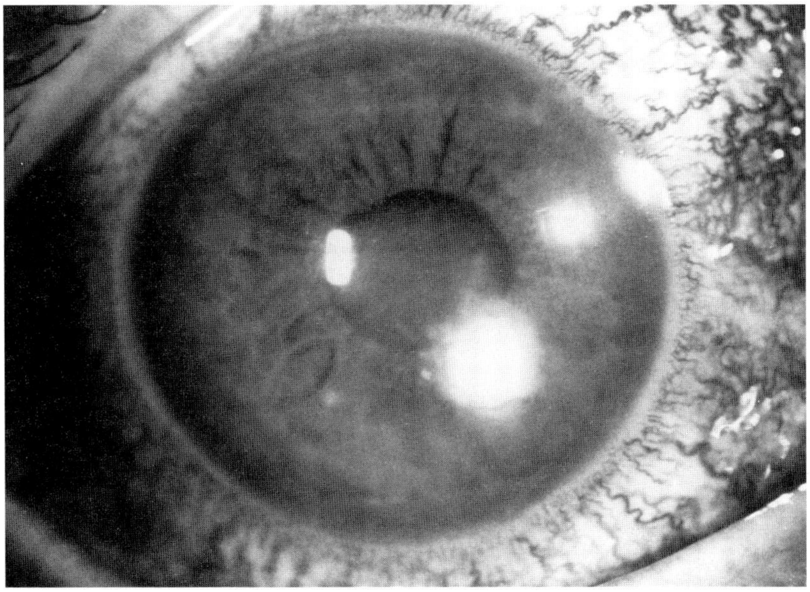

A

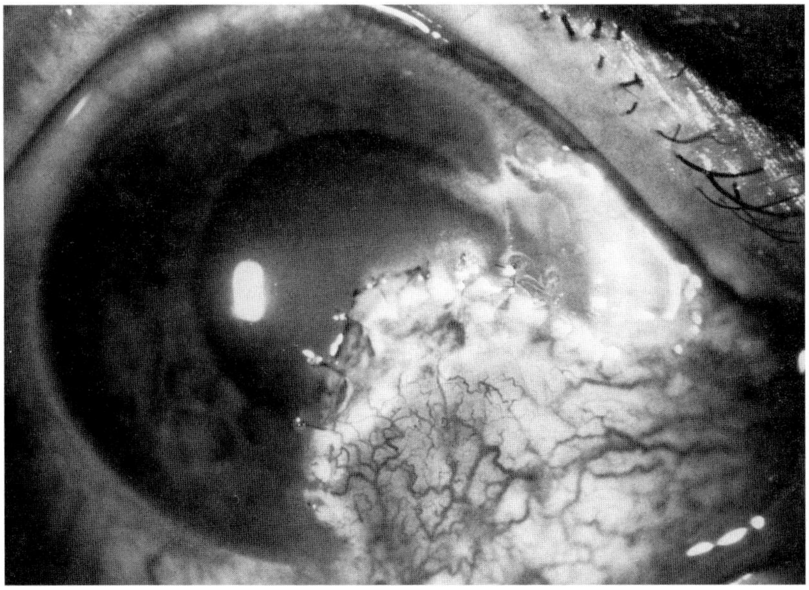

B

FIGURE 29-5 **(A)** Fungal keratitis caused by *Curvularia*. **(B)** The infection was resistant to treatment with antifungal agents. A lamellar keratectomy was performed followed by placement of a partial conjunctival flap, which controlled the infection. Visual acuity after the flap healed was 20/30 -2.

alternative to medical therapy, especially if the infection is peripheral.

There is usually time for a trial of medical therapy early in the course of fungal keratitis, but lack of response or progression of the keratitis is an indication for surgical intervention. If the infection is peripheral, a lamellar keratectomy is performed to remove all necrotic material, and a partial conjunctival flap is placed in the keratectomy bed (Figure 29-5).[16] If the infection is central, penetrating keratoplasty is indicated. If the infection is more extensive and involves both the central and peripheral cornea, a lamellar keratectomy and total conjunctival flap are performed (Figure 29-6), followed by penetrating keratoplasty after the infection and inflammation have resolved.

Herpes zoster and herpes simplex viral keratitis can cause recurrent and long-standing corneal inflammation, persistent nonhealing epithelial defects, and stromal ulceration. Medical therapy consisting of antivirals,

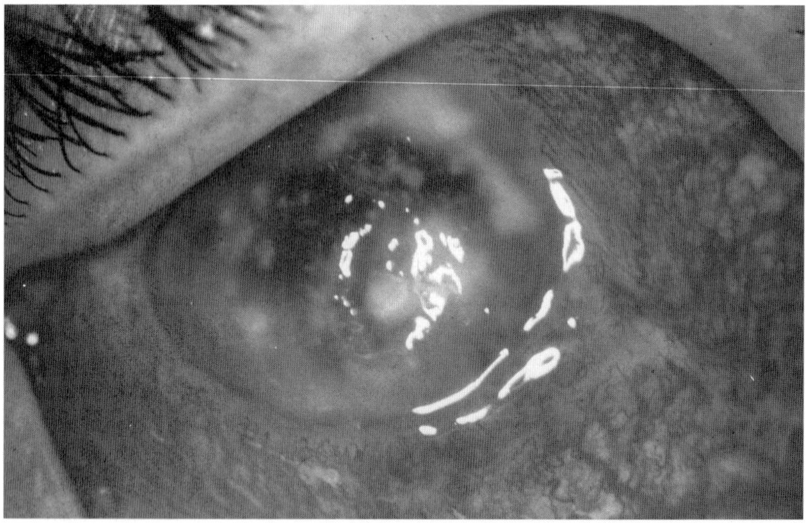

A

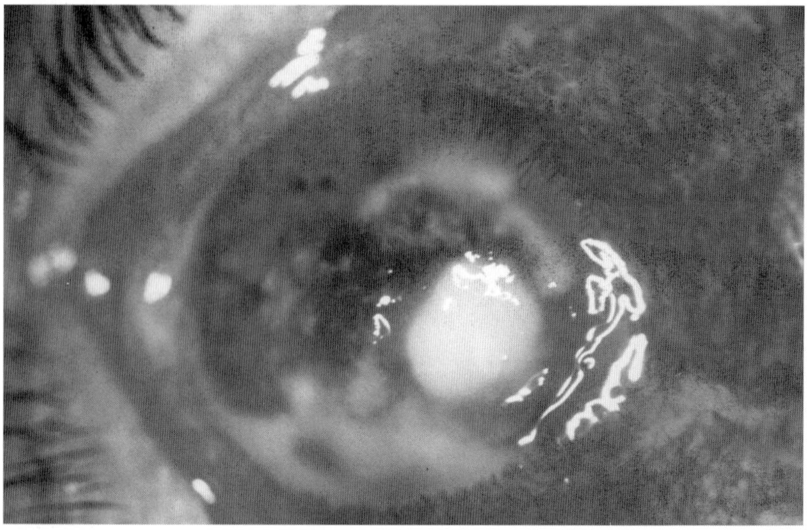

B

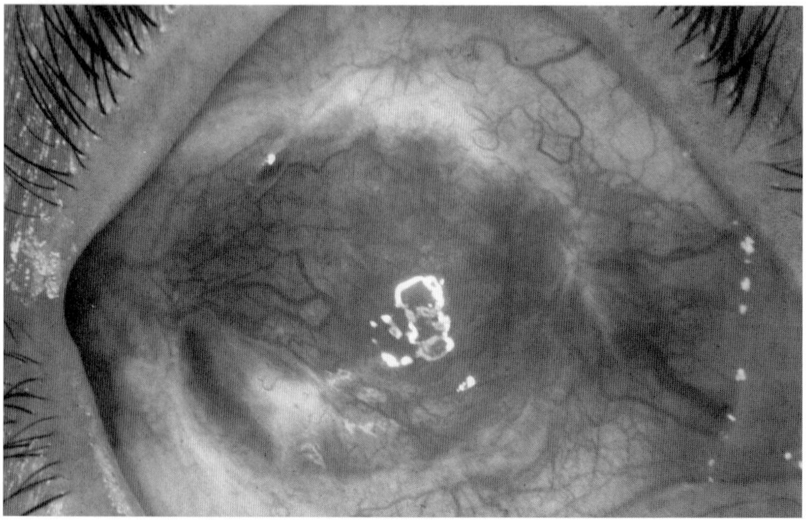

C

FIGURE 29-6 **(A)** Fungal keratitis. Note the severity of involvement, with deep stromal infiltrates. **(B)** Three weeks later, a stromal abscess can be seen despite treatment with topical amphotericin B. **(C)** Six months after a conjunctival flap was placed, the eye is quiet and free of infection. (Courtesy of William M. Townsend, M.D., San Juan, PR.)

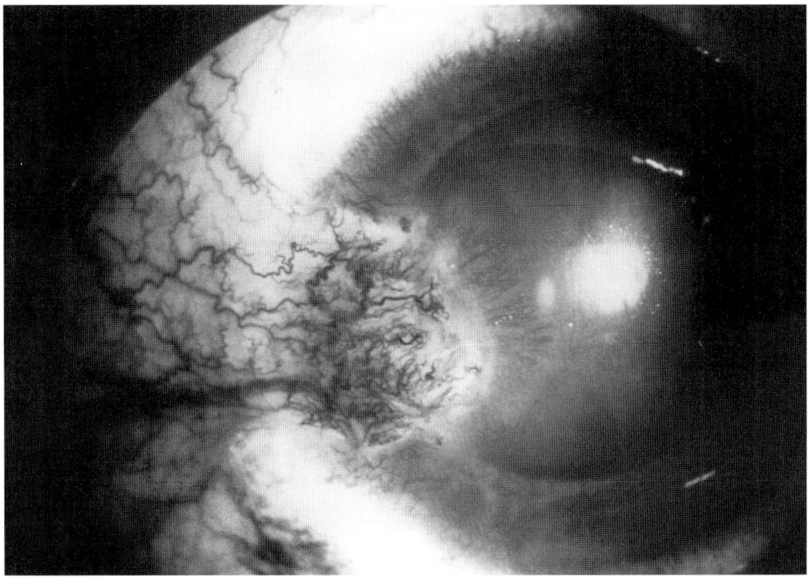

FIGURE 29-7 Partial conjunctival flap for herpes simplex ulcerative keratitis resistant to medical therapy.

corticosteroids, ocular lubricants, and bandage soft contact lenses is effective in most patients. Prolonged morbidity is common, however, especially if the eye is dry and desensitized. Frequent instillation of topical medications and multiple office visits often become more burdensome to the patient than the keratitis itself.[17] A conjunctival flap may help a patient whose life is dominated by the keratitis become more comfortable without the need for constant medical attention. A lamellar keratectomy to remove necrotic cornea followed by a conjunctival flap can relieve inflammation, pain, and other symptoms in as little as 1 week (Figure 29-7). The flap shortens the recovery time, and penetrating keratoplasty can be postponed until the disease is inactive. The results of penetrating keratoplasty in eyes with active herpetic infection are poor. Polack and Kaufman[18] reported clear grafts for at least 1 year in only 45 percent of eyes with active herpetic keratitis compared with 100 percent in eyes with inactive disease.

It is possible, but rare, for inflammation to recur after placement of a conjunctival flap for herpetic keratitis.[19] Brown et al[17] described two patients with herpes zoster keratitis and seven patients with herpes simplex keratitis treated with conjunctival flaps; the keratitis did not recur during follow-up of 1 to 6 years. In another study by Paton and Milauskas,[4] conjunctival flaps were performed in 36 eyes for chronic herpetic stromal keratitis; persistent inflammation and erosion of the flap occurred in only four eyes.

Conjunctival flaps are ineffective in the treatment of *Acanthamoeba* keratitis.[20]

PREOPERATIVE EVALUATION AND MEDICATIONS

Preoperatively, the conjunctiva intended for a flap should be examined and its mobility determined. This is accomplished by applying a topical anesthetic and attempting to move the conjunctiva with a cotton-tipped applicator. Conjunctiva attached to the globe by scar tissue is difficult to mobilize without creating buttonholes. Failure to detect conjunctival scarring preoperatively increases the risk of intraoperative complications and makes the procedure difficult, if not impossible, to perform. Preparations to obtain cultures and pathology specimens, if needed, should be made before surgery.

No specific preoperative medications are required for a conjunctival flap unless the flap is performed for infectious keratitis, in which case antimicrobial agents are given. A firm eye is preferable for surgery, especially if a lamellar keratectomy is to be performed. Medications that lower the intraocular pressure should not be given, and external pressure on the eye should be avoided.

ANESTHESIA

Conjunctival flaps can be performed with retrobulbar or peribulbar anesthesia, supplemented with a subconjunctival injection of anesthetic if necessary. It can be difficult to obtain adequate local anesthesia in inflamed eyes. In these patients, periocular injections are usually more effective than a retrobulbar injection; however, general

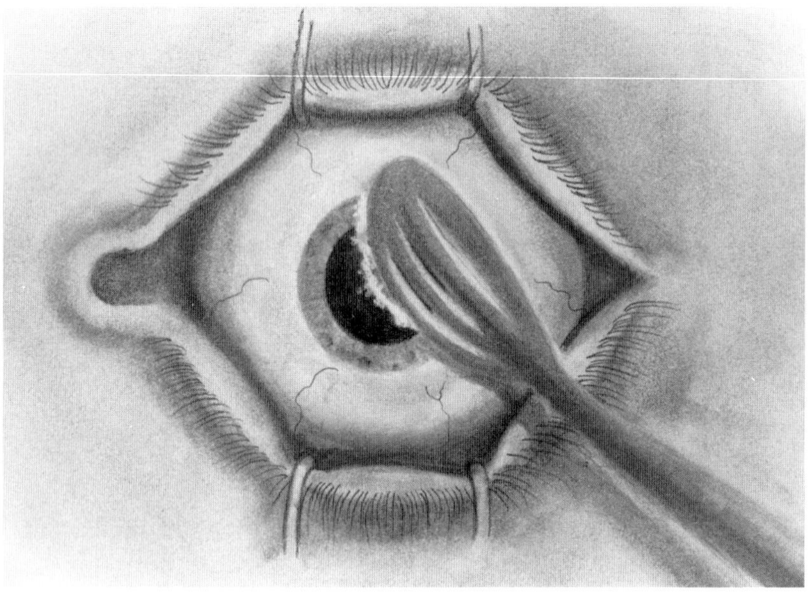

FIGURE 29-8 Removal of the corneal epithelium with a Paton spatula.

anesthesia may have to be used. General anesthesia is preferred in children and uncooperative adults.

SURGICAL TECHNIQUES

Although the indications and surgical techniques for total and partial conjunctival flaps differ, there are common surgical principles shared by both.[21] First, the flap should consist of conjunctiva only, and should be thin enough so that the cornea beneath the flap is visible. If Tenon's capsule is included in the flap, the flap will be thick and cosmetically unacceptable, and will have a greater chance of retracting off the cornea. Second, there should be no tension on the flap because tension can cause the flap to retract or tear. Relaxing incisions should be placed in the conjunctiva surrounding the flap to relieve tension, even if the incisions appear to compromise the vascular supply of the flap. Third, there should be no buttonholes in the flap. Fourth, the flap should cover the entire area of corneal abnormality. Finally, necrotic corneal tissue in the area to be covered by the flap must be completely removed by lamellar keratectomy; failure to do so will result in consumption of the flap by the necrotic process.

Total Conjunctival Flap (Gundersen Flap)

The most commonly used total conjunctival flap is the thin flap described by Gundersen[3] or a modification thereof.[4] A total conjunctival flap is indicated when the abnormality involves a large area of the corneal surface.

The corneal epithelium is removed, because retained epithelium can proliferate beneath the flap, form epithelial inclusion cysts, and separate the flap from the cornea. The epithelium may be removed mechanically with a blunt spatula (Paton spatula) (Figure 29-8), a surgical blade (#15 Bard-Parker or #64 Beaver blade), or a dry cellulose sponge. A cellulose sponge saturated with absolute alcohol or 4 percent cocaine without preservatives may be rubbed on the epithelium to loosen it so it can be removed more easily (Figure 29-9). Care is taken to prevent the alcohol or cocaine from flowing onto and destroying the conjunctival epithelium. The corneal epithelium should be removed from the ocular surface as soon as it is loosened to prevent it from later becoming trapped beneath the flap.

If the flap is to be temporary, Bowman's layer is left undisturbed. If the flap is to be permanent, Bowman's layer may be scarified with a blade to increase adherence of the flap to the cornea (Figure 29-10). All necrotic corneal tissue should be removed by lamellar keratectomy to prevent necrosis of the flap. Lamellar keratectomy also aids in adherence of the flap to the cornea.

Superior conjunctiva is usually used for a total conjunctival flap; however, inferior or temporal conjunctiva can be used, if necessary. There is usually not enough nasal conjunctiva for a total flap. The superior conjunctiva is best exposed by rotating the eye inferiorly with a traction suture placed through partial-thickness cornea at the superior limbus or by placing a suture through the superior rectus muscle. If a superior rectus muscle suture is used, it should be high enough in the fornix to avoid damaging conjunctiva intended for the flap. The amount

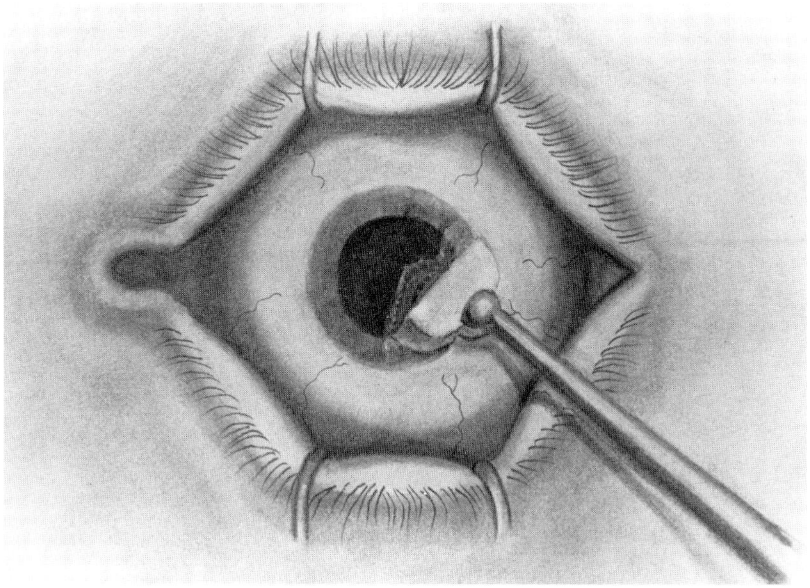

FIGURE 29-9 Loosening of the corneal epithelium with a cellulose sponge saturated with absolute alcohol. The tip of the sponge has been cut off to make the sponge stiffer.

of conjunctiva needed for the flap is determined by measuring the vertical diameter of the cornea and adding a few millimeters. Generally, 15 mm is sufficient to cover the entire cornea. The superior extent of the flap should not involve palpebral conjunctiva; otherwise, a symblepharon will form between the palpebral and bulbar surfaces that are devoid of epithelium.

Conjunctiva may be hydraulically separated from Tenon's capsule with a subconjunctival injection of lidocaine and epinephrine. In addition to facilitating the surgical dissection, the lidocaine aids anesthesia and the epinephrine aids hemostasis. The needle should be inserted bevel-up in an area of conjunctiva not intended for the flap; otherwise a buttonhole will form in the flap. The injection is directed toward the conjunctiva intended for the flap (Figure 29-11). The needle may be safely advanced once the conjunctiva has been separated from the underlying tissues. A moist cotton-tipped applicator may be gently rolled across the conjunctiva to help disperse the fluid.

A conjunctival incision is made with sharp-tipped Westcott scissors at the superior extent of the flap, and is extended temporally and nasally parallel to the superior limbus (Figure 29-12). Serrated nontoothed forceps (Bonaccolto forceps) grasp the conjunctiva well without creat-

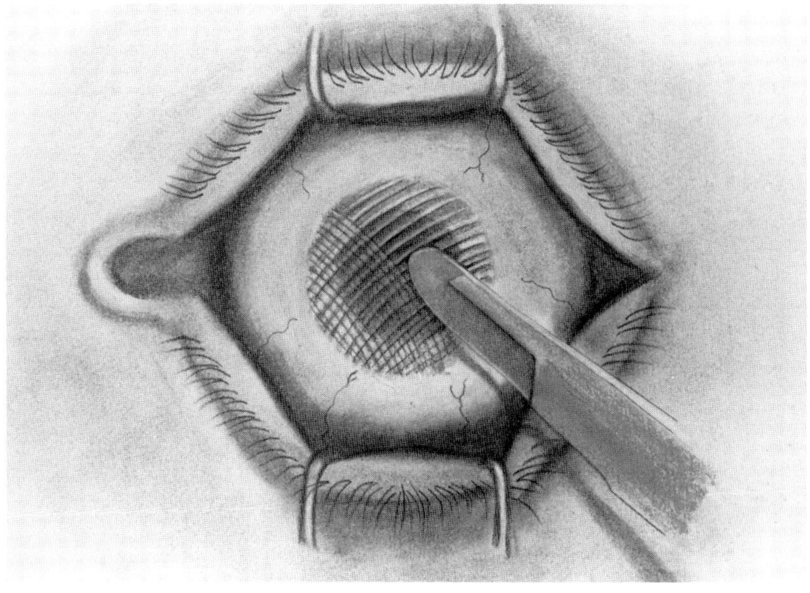

FIGURE 29-10 Scarification of Bowman's layer with a #64 Beaver blade.

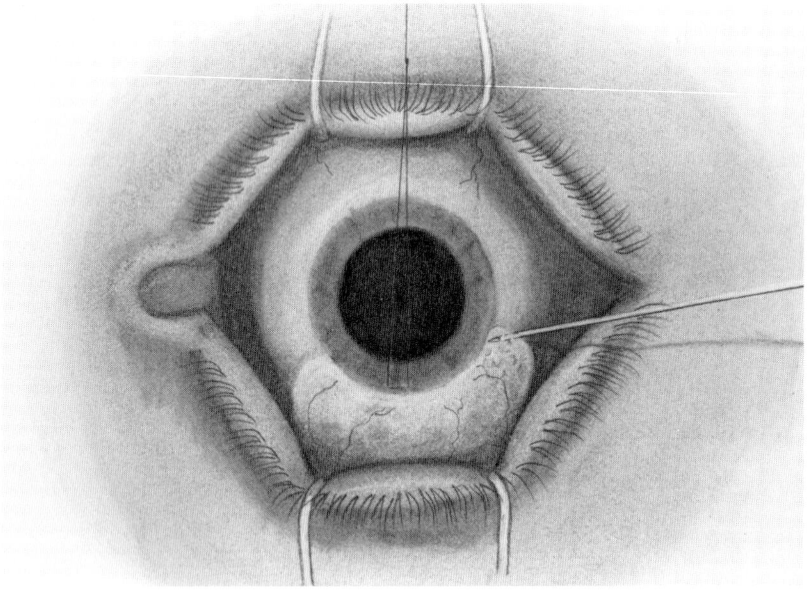

FIGURE 29-11 Hydraulic separation of conjunctiva from Tenon's capsule by injection of lidocaine with epinephrine. The needle is inserted bevel-up in an area of conjunctiva not intended for the flap.

ing holes. Toothed forceps tear the conjunctiva, and smooth forceps do not grasp well.

The conjunctiva is sharply dissected from Tenon's capsule. Blunt dissection is not recommended because this method easily tears the conjunctiva. Opened, blunt-tipped Westcott scissors are placed against the undersurface of the conjunctiva, the conjunctiva is draped over the scissors, and the scissors are lifted against the conjunctiva and closed, with care taken not to let conjunctiva fall between the blades of the scissors (Figure 29-13). This procedure is preferable to lifting the conjunctiva and severing attachments to Tenon's capsule under direct visualization because it is safer, with less chance of buttonhole formation, and it is easier to obtain a thin flap. The dissection is continued to the limbus, and then temporally and nasally.

Sharp-tipped Westcott scissors are inserted under the flap and a hole is made through the superior limbal conjunctiva (Figure 29-14). The scissors are then withdrawn, one blade is placed through the hole, and a 360-degree limbal conjunctival peritomy is performed (Figure 29-15). This frees the superior limbal conjunctiva so it can be pulled over the cornea to the inferior limbus, and provides an inferior edge of conjunctiva to which the flap can be sutured. It is important to separate the inferior con-

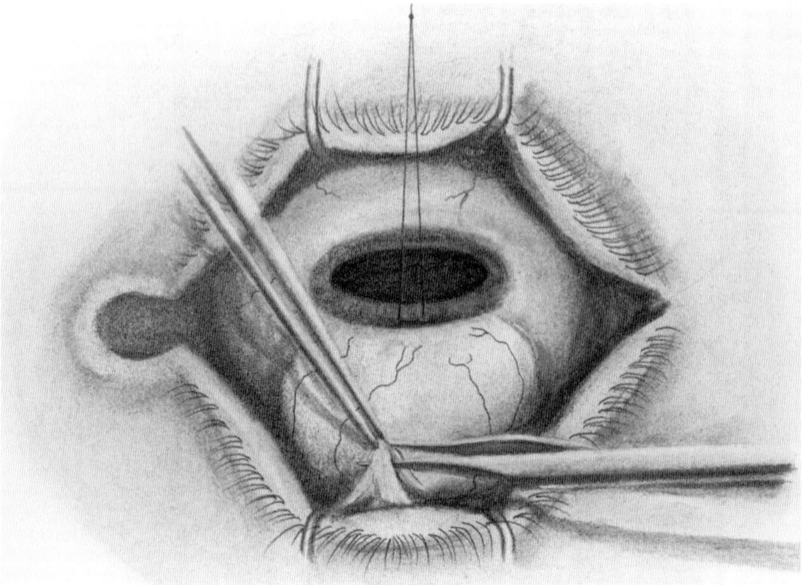

FIGURE 29-12 Incision of the conjunctiva at the superior extent of the intended flap.

FIGURE 29-13 Conjunctival dissection. **(A)** Opened, blunt-tipped Westcott scissors are placed against the undersurface of the conjunctiva. **(B)** The conjunctiva is draped over the scissors. *(continues)*

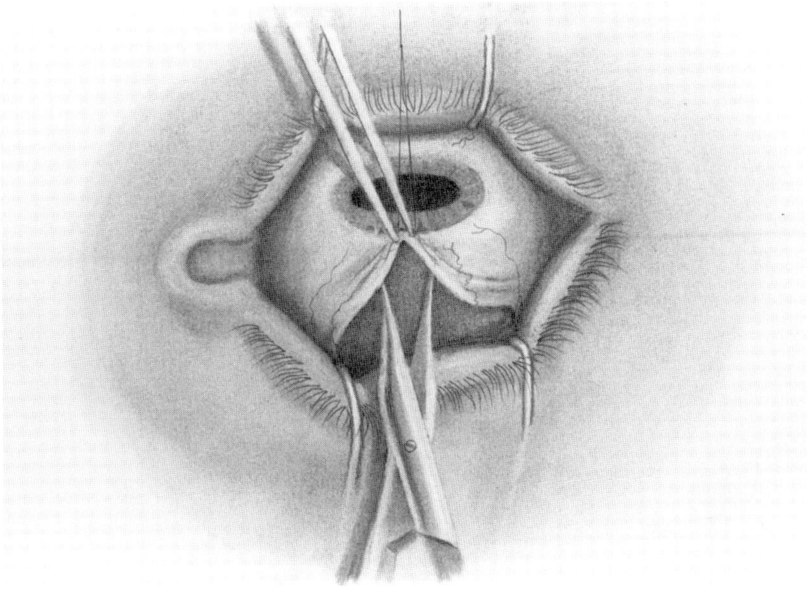

A

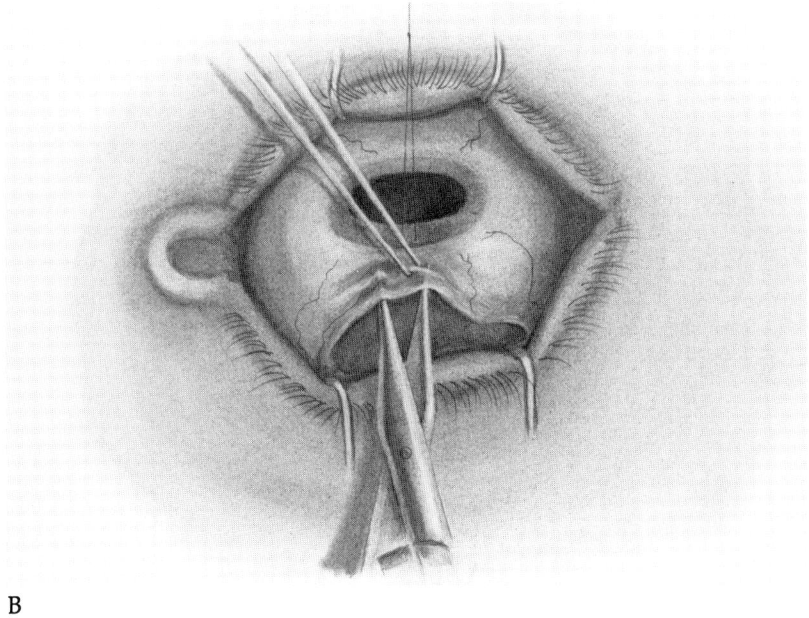

B

junctiva from the limbus to prevent the incursion of limbal epithelial cells beneath the flap.

Any conjunctiva remaining at the limbus is excised with Vannas scissors. The corneal surface and limbus are scrubbed with a cellulose sponge saturated with absolute alcohol to destroy any viable epithelial cells, while care is taken to avoid damaging the epithelium of the flap with the alcohol. Finally, the ocular surface is copiously irrigated with balanced salt solution to remove the alcohol. Hemostasis is obtained with wet-field cautery.

The superior traction suture is removed. The superior limbal conjunctiva is moved to the inferior limbus, and the superior forniceal conjunctiva is moved to the superior limbus (Figure 29-16). The superior epibulbar surface is left bare of conjunctiva, but will re-epithelialize.

The flap should be inspected for inversion, size, tension, buttonholes, and thickness. The flap should not be inverted or twisted on its pedicles and should lie flat on the cornea. Initially, the flap may appear to be too small because the edges have rolled underneath; once the edges are unrolled,

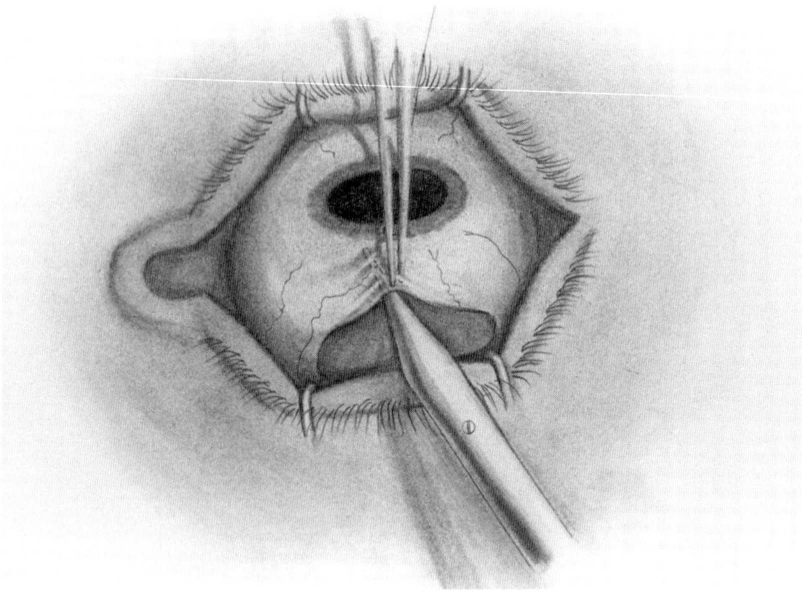

C

FIGURE 29-13 *(continued)* (C) The scissors are closed, severing the connections between the conjunctiva and Tenon's capsule.

however, there is usually adequate conjunctiva to cover the cornea. If not, the existing flap may be converted to a partial flap, if appropriate, or another larger flap may be created from the inferior or temporal conjunctiva. If there is tension on the flap, additional dissection is performed temporally and nasally until the tension is released. Relaxing incisions may be necessary for this purpose. If the relaxing incisions are ineffective, one of the two vascular pedicles of the flap may have to be severed. Severance of a pedicle does not adversely affect the survival of the flap; a flap with a small vascular pedicle or even a flap with no vascular pedicle generally survives.

Any buttonhole in the flap should be moved off the cornea, if possible, because it will enlarge and destroy the flap. Care is taken not to enlarge a buttonhole by manipulating the conjunctiva. If a buttonhole cannot be moved off the cornea and is small, it is closed with interrupted 10-0 nylon sutures that pass through the edges of the hole and underlying partial-thickness cornea (Figure 29-17). This maneuver anchors the conjunctiva surrounding the hole to the cornea. If the hole is large, a new flap may have to be dissected from the inferior or temporal conjunctiva.

After the flap is inspected, it is anchored to the epibulbar surface with interrupted sutures. Polyglactin or

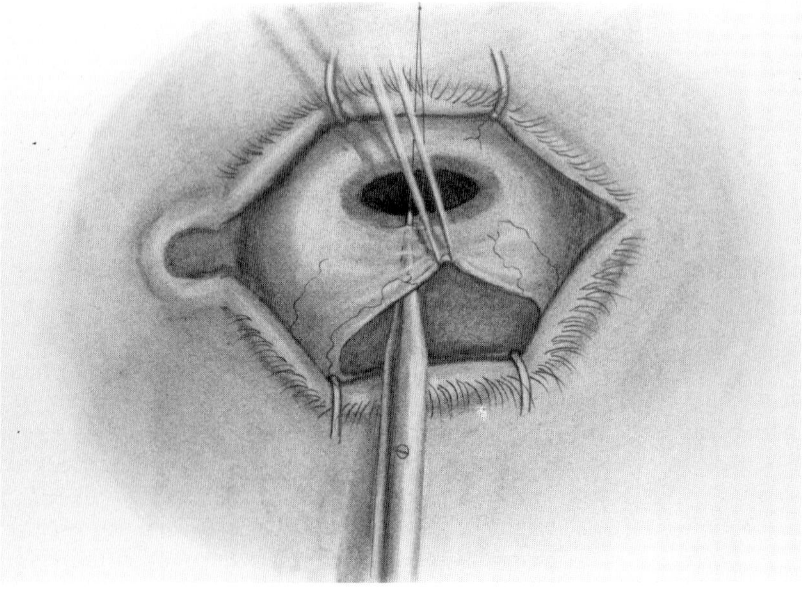

FIGURE 29-14 Creation of a hole in the limbal conjunctiva with sharp-tipped Westcott scissors.

FIGURE 29-15 Limbal peritomy.

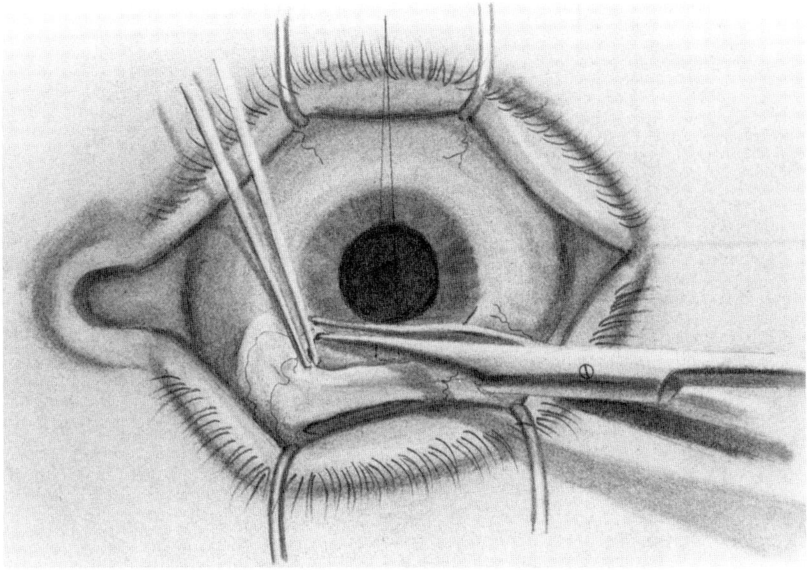

chromic sutures (8-0) are usually preferred because they dissolve and do not need to be removed. In addition, they produce a mild localized inflammatory reaction that aids in adhesion of the flap to the epibulbar surface. In an inflamed eye, however, absorbable sutures may dissolve too quickly, allowing the flap to retract off the cornea. In this situation, nylon sutures or a combination of nylon and either polyglactin or chromic sutures is preferred.

The sutures are placed through the edges of the flap. It is important to be certain that the edges are completely unrolled and lying flat to prevent epithelial cell proliferation under the flap. The inferior limbal sutures are placed first and pass through the edge of the flap, superficial limbal tissue, and the edge of the inferior limbal conjunctiva. The superior edge of the flap is then sutured to superficial epibulbar tissue such that the flap is snug but not tightly stretched over the cornea (Figure 29-18).

Partial Conjunctival Flaps

A partial conjunctival flap is indicated when the corneal lesion does not involve the entire cornea. A focal central or peripheral lesion is amenable to treatment with a partial flap. An obvious advantage of a partial flap is that,

FIGURE 29-16 (A) Translocation of the superior conjunctiva over the cornea. *(continues)*

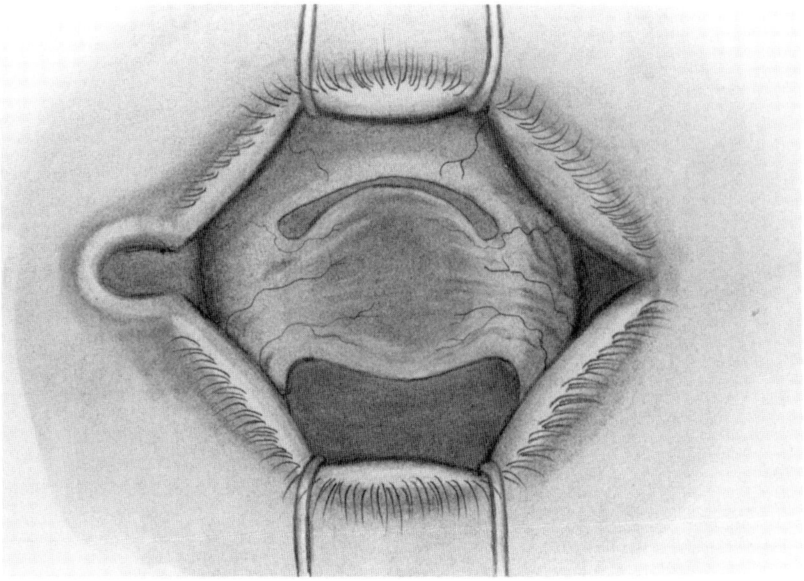

A

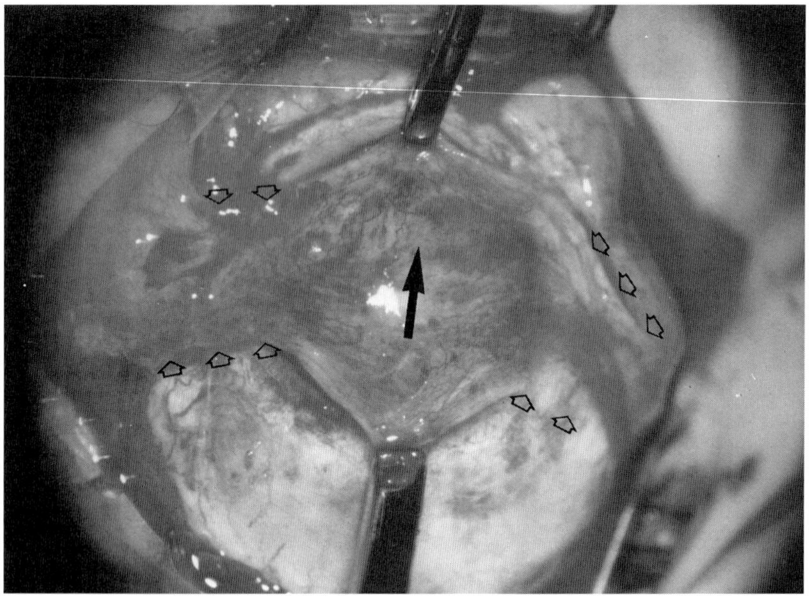

B

FIGURE 29-16 *(continued)* **(B)** The conjunctival flap is slid inferiorly (arrow) such that the superior limbal conjunctiva is at the inferior limbus and the superior forniceal conjunctiva is at the superior limbus. The "bridge" of the flap is indicated by open arrows.

depending on the location of the lesion, the visual axis may remain clear, allowing the patient better vision than would be achieved with a total flap. A partial flap also permits better visualization of the anterior chamber and monitoring of anterior chamber inflammation and depth than does a total flap.

There are three types of partial conjunctival flaps: hood or advancement flap, bipedicle or bucket-handle flap, and single pedicle or racquet flap.[5,8,22] A hood flap is indicated for a peripheral corneal lesion that does not involve the visual axis, for example, a sterile ulcer caused by exposure or a herpetic or fungal ulcer. A bipedicle flap is used to cover a focal central or paracentral lesion. A single pedicle flap is useful for a small limbal lesion or a small paracentral lesion close to, but not involving, the visual axis.

Most partial conjunctival flaps are inlay flaps, whereas total conjunctival flaps are onlay flaps. Partial flaps sutured to a cornea that has been merely debrided of epithelium have a high risk of retraction. Lamellar keratectomy not only removes necrotic corneal tissue, but increases adhesion of the flap to the cornea and prevents retraction of the flap.

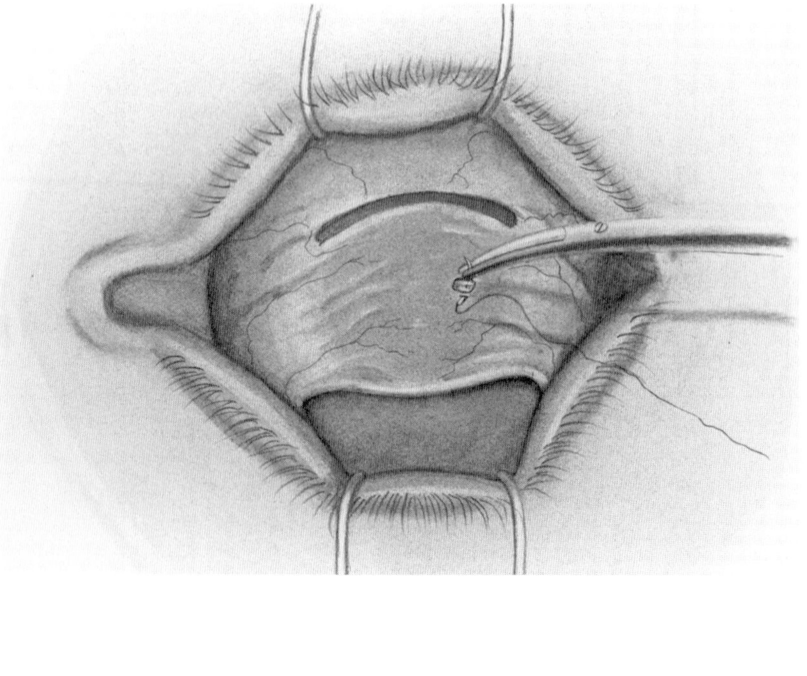

FIGURE 29-17 Closure and anchorage of a buttonhole to the underlying cornea.

FIGURE 29-18 (A) Total conjunctival flap sutured in place. (B) The inferior edge of the flap (white arrowhead) is sutured to the superficial epibulbar tissue and to the edge of the inferior conjunctiva. The superior edge of the flap (black arrowhead) is sutured only to superficial epibulbar tissue. The area superiorly from which the flap was obtained is left bare of conjunctiva (asterisks).

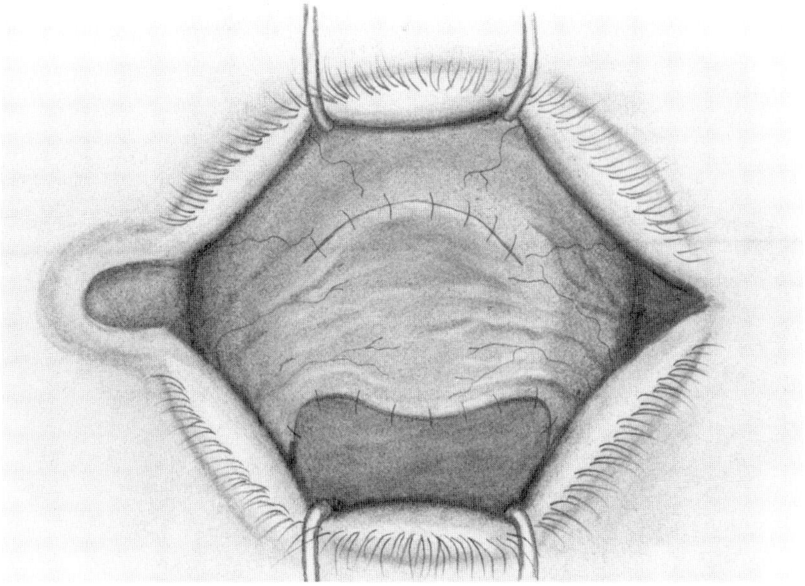

A

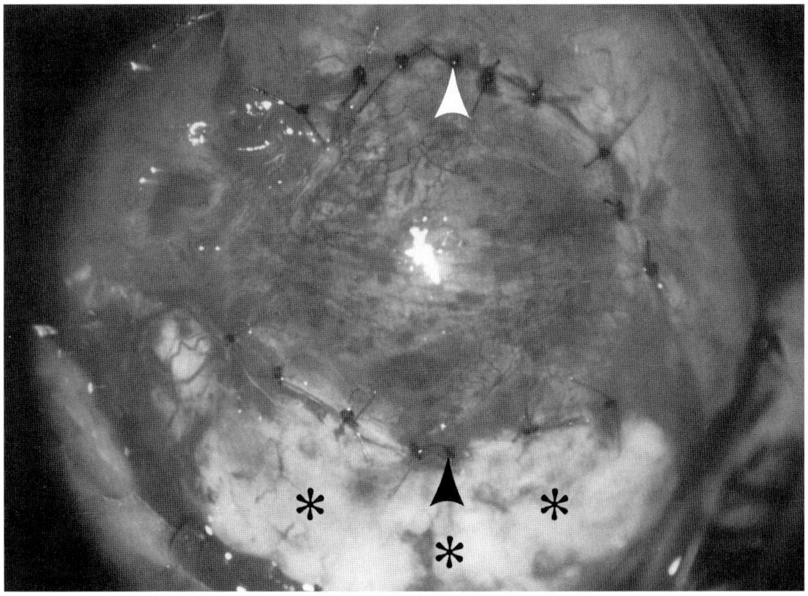

B

Hood Flap

A hood flap is constructed from conjunctiva adjacent to the area of a peripheral corneal lesion (Figure 29-19). For example, a flap for a sterile inferior corneal ulcer from lagophthalmos is fashioned from the inferior conjunctiva. The area of cornea to be covered by the flap is first debrided of epithelium, as described above, and is then outlined centrally with a stainless steel or diamond blade held perpendicular to the corneal surface, and the cornea is incised to a depth that includes all necrotic tissue. This incision provides an edge to which the flap will be sutured. A lamellar keratectomy is performed with a crescent blade to remove necrotic cornea and may extend to 90 percent of the corneal thickness, if necessary. As the lamellar keratectomy approaches the limbus, it should taper anteriorly to provide a gradual transition zone from the keratectomy bed to the sclera (Figure 29-20).

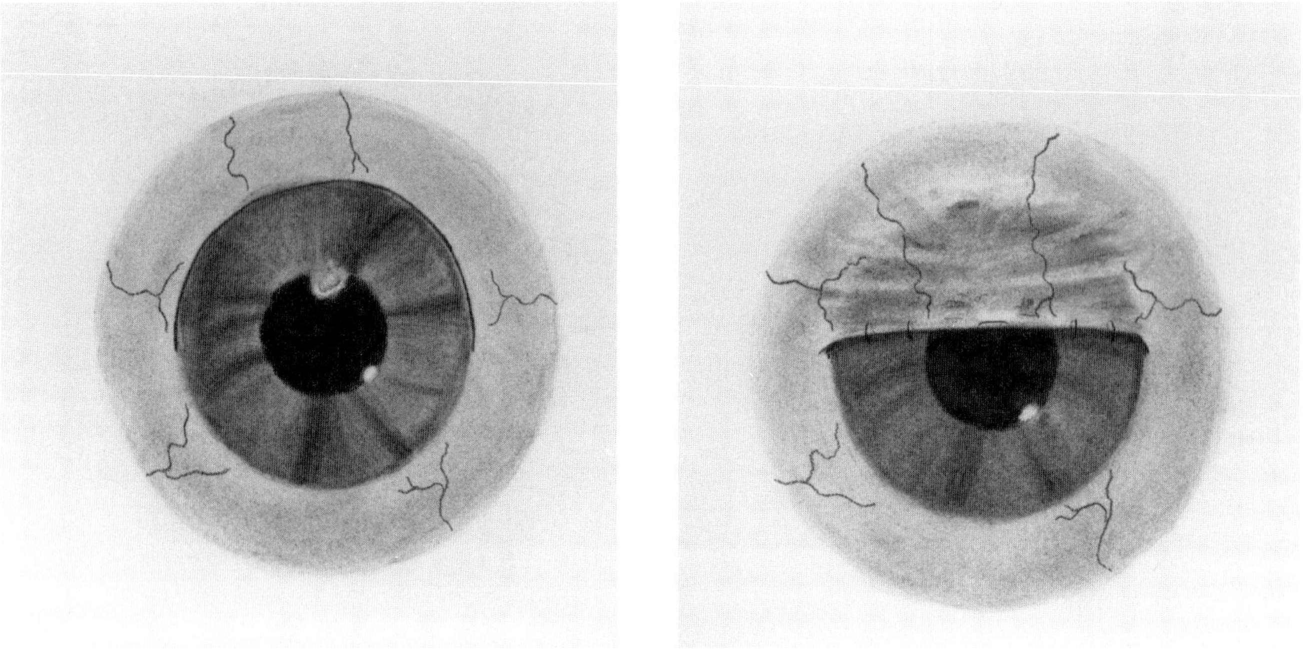

A B

FIGURE 29-19 Hood flap. (A) A lamellar keratectomy is performed, and the conjunctiva adjacent to the lesion is incised and dissected from Tenon's capsule. (B) The flap is pulled over the lesion and sutured in place. Note the horizontal placement of the central suture such that it avoids the visual axis.

Conjunctiva adjacent to the keratectomy bed is usually used to create the flap. However, if the conjunctiva in that area is inadequate or scarred, conjunctiva from a different area may be used. The conjunctiva is hydraulically separated from Tenon's capsule. The conjunctiva is grasped with a Bonaccolto forceps, and sharp-tipped Westcott scissors are used to perform a limbal peritomy, extending a few millimeters on either side of the keratectomy bed. Any remnants of epithelium or conjunctiva attached to the limbus are excised. The conjunctiva is sharply dissected from Tenon's capsule with blunt-tipped Westcott scissors, as described above, from the limbus toward the periphery.

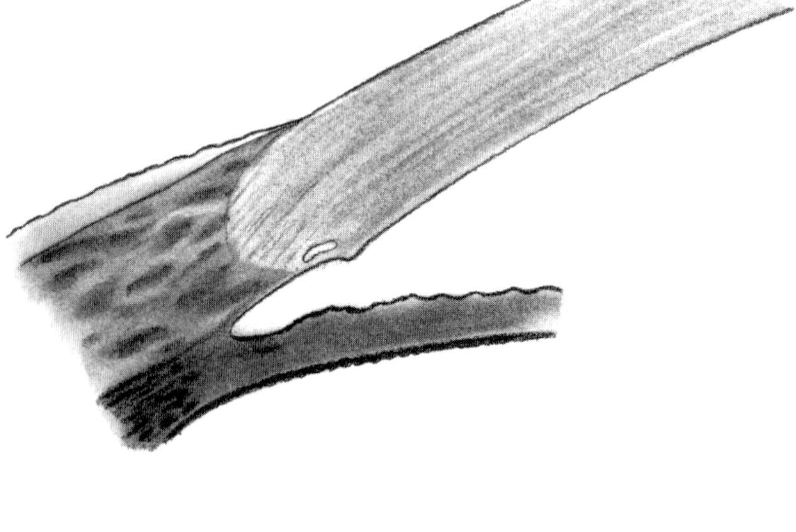

FIGURE 29-20 Side view of the keratectomy bed prepared for a partial inlay conjunctival flap. A lamellar keratectomy has been performed, creating a sharp central edge and a tapered peripheral edge.

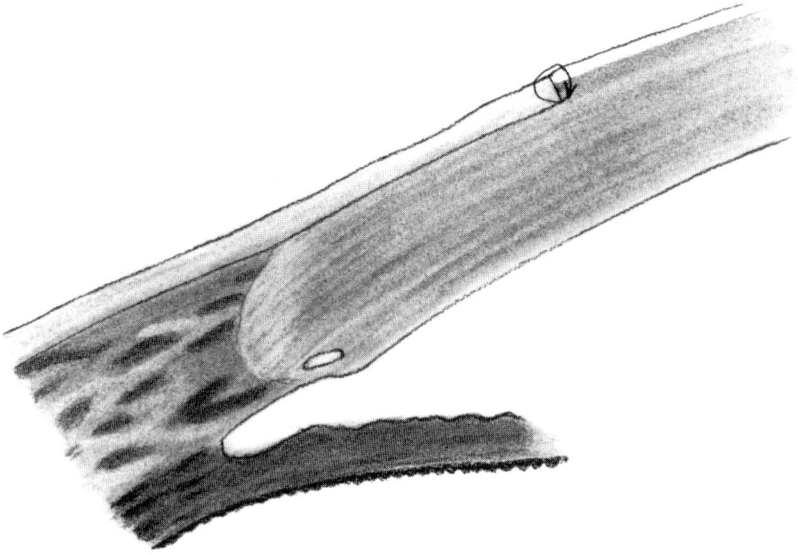

FIGURE 29-21 Partial flap sutured in place in the keratectomy bed.

The flap is placed in the keratectomy bed and sutured to the edges of the bed with interrupted 10-0 nylon sutures (Figure 29-21). The sutures are placed first through the flap and then through the base of the keratectomy bed to exit the corneal surface approximately 1 mm from the edge of the bed. The sutures should be close to each other to prevent retraction of the flap. If the flap comes close to the visual axis, the central suture may be placed through the conjunctiva, through the cornea at the base of the keratectomy bed parallel to the edge of the bed, and then back through the conjunctiva (see Figure 29-19). This avoids placement of a suture through the visual axis. However, if the cornea at the base of the keratectomy bed is thin, placement of such a suture risks corneal perforation.

Because partial flaps have a greater tendency to retract than do total flaps, it is important to inspect the flap for tension and to release any tension by making a relaxing incision in the peripheral conjunctiva. This converts the flap from a hood flap to a bipedicle, or bridge, flap (Figure 29-22).

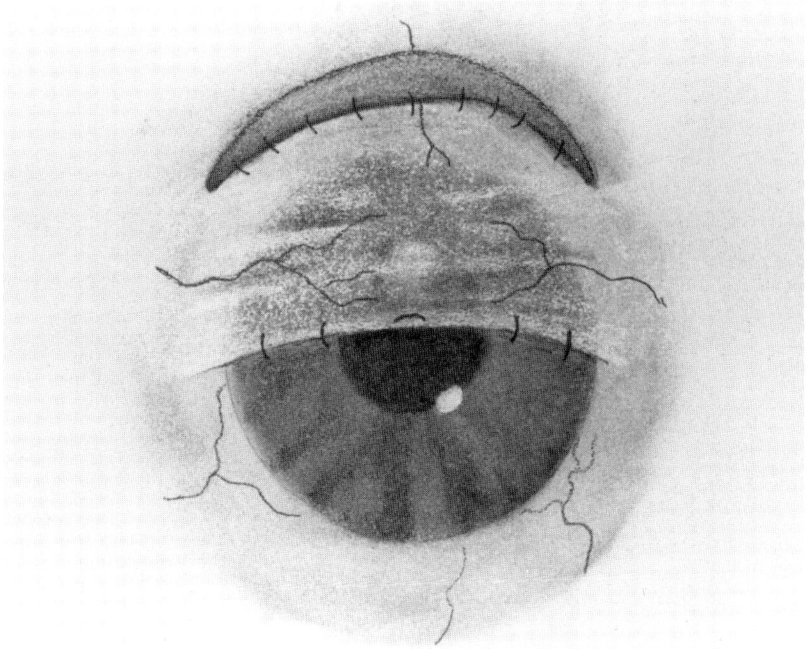

FIGURE 29-22 Inferior bipedicle flap. An incision has been made in the inferior conjunctiva to release tension, and the inferior edge of the flap has been sutured to adjacent epibulbar tissue.

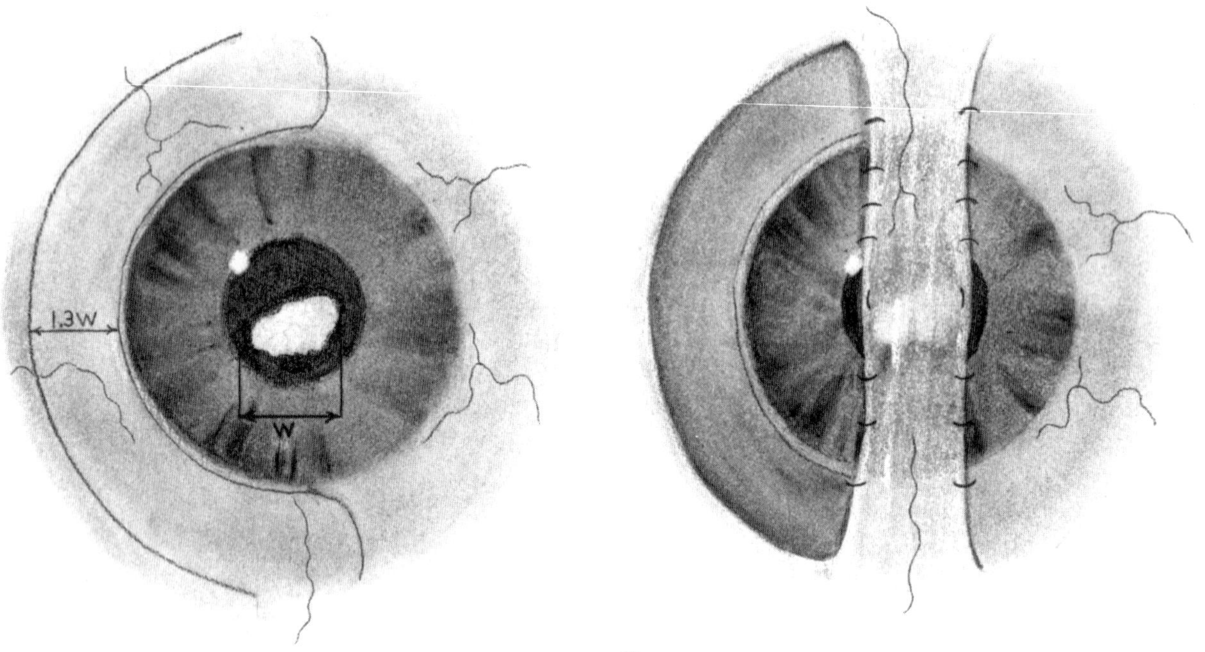

FIGURE 29-23 Vertical bipedicle flap. **(A)** The width of conjunctiva for the flap should be approximately 1.3 times the width (*W*) of the lesion. **(B)** The temporal conjunctiva has been dissected, translocated, and sutured in place.

Bipedicle Flap

The surgical technique for a bipedicle flap is similar to that for a total conjunctival flap. In effect, a total conjunctival flap is usually a bipedicle flap. The primary difference is that a partial bipedicle flap is just large enough to cover the corneal lesion. The corneal epithelium is debrided and a lamellar keratectomy is performed in the area of the cornea to be covered by the flap, as described in the previous section. The lesion is measured, and 20 to 30 percent is added. This measurement is used to mark the temporal conjunctiva intended for the flap. The temporal conjunctiva is used to create a vertical flap so that the blinking action of the eyelids does not mechanically dislodge the flap. A vertical incision is made at the temporal extent of the flap, and the conjunctiva is dissected and mobilized as described above in the section on total conjunctival flaps. The flap is placed in the keratectomy bed, inspected, and secured with interrupted 10-0 nylon sutures (Figure 29-23).

Single Pedicle Flap

A single pedicle flap is constructed from conjunctiva adjacent to the corneal lesion.[22] The corneal epithelium is debrided and a lamellar keratectomy is performed as described above in the section on hood flaps. The area to be covered by the flap is measured, and 20 to 30 percent is added. The area of conjunctiva to be mobilized is marked with a surgical marking pen or cautery. The conjunctiva is hydraulically separated and sharply dissected from Tenon's capsule. The flap is placed in the keratectomy bed and sutured with interrupted 10-0 nylon sutures (Figure 29-24).

POSTOPERATIVE MEDICATIONS AND CARE

Immediately postoperatively, one drop of 1 percent atropine and an antibiotic ointment are applied topically, and the eye is patched. The patch is removed 24 hours later and a topical antibiotic eye drop or ointment is used until the sutures dissolve or are removed. In the case of herpetic or fungal keratitis, the lamellar keratectomy and conjunctival flap are usually sufficient treatment, and neither antiviral nor antifungal medications, which may irritate the flap, are generally necessary postoperatively.

Inflammation is almost always a concomitant of an indication for a conjunctival flap, but the signs may not be visible by slit lamp examination once the flap is in place.

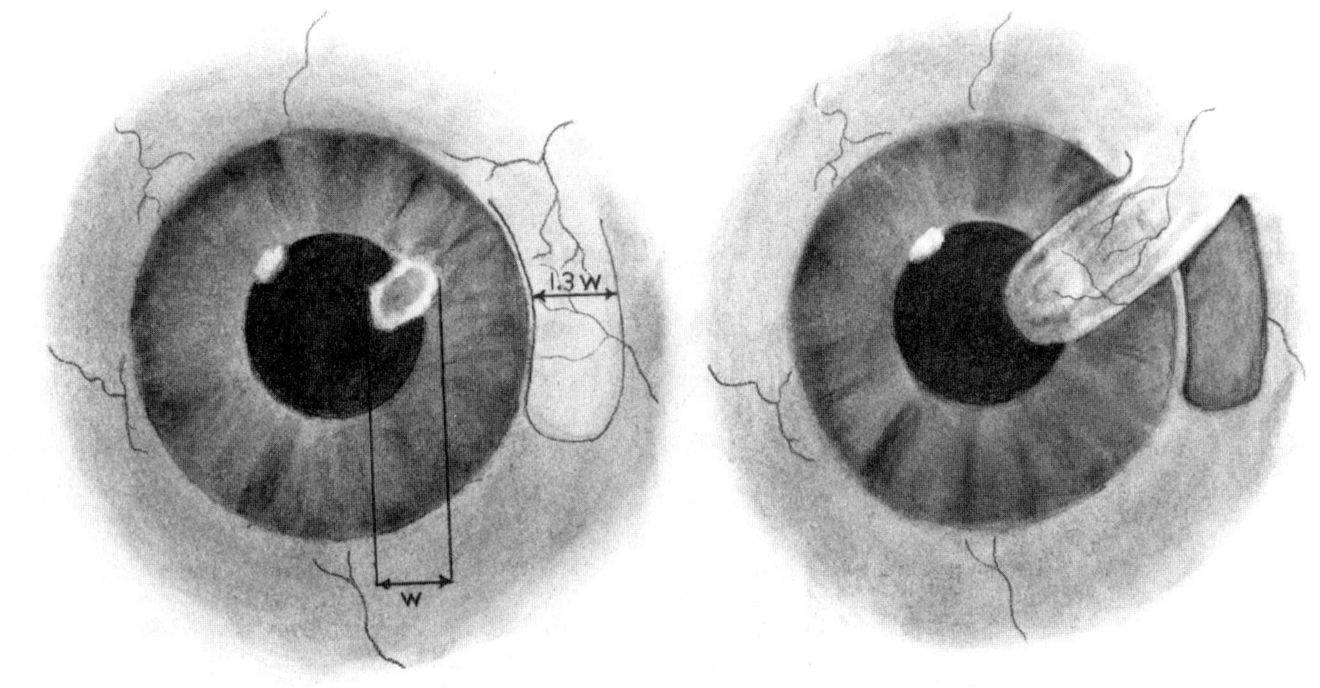

A B

FIGURE 29-24 Single pedicle flap. **(A)** The width of conjunctiva for the flap should be approximately 1.3 times the width (*W*) of the lesion. **(B)** The conjunctiva adjacent to the lesion has been dissected, translocated, and sutured in place.

A strong topical cycloplegic agent, such as 1 percent atropine, is continued for several weeks postoperatively and is then tapered, depending on the patient's symptoms. Some patients may require atropine indefinitely. Although rarely needed, topical corticosteroids and, in more severe cases, systemic corticosteroids may be used to control inflammation if the conjunctival flap was performed for a noninfectious disorder.

Intraocular pressure may be difficult to measure in an eye with a conjunctival flap. The Tono-Pen may allow accurate measurement of intraocular pressure in such an eye, especially if the flap is partial. Medications may be required to control intraocular pressure postoperatively. A conjunctival flap is not as permeable as the cornea and constitutes more of a barrier to topical medications, possibly decreasing their efficacy. Therefore, a systemic carbonic anhydrase inhibitor may be required to treat elevated intraocular pressure.

COMPLICATIONS

Although the construction of conjunctival flaps is relatively straightforward, it can be fraught with intraoperative and postoperative complications. Most complications can be avoided by careful preoperative examination of the conjunctiva intended for the flap, and most important, by meticulous attention to surgical detail. However, even the most experienced surgeon can encounter complications.

If the indication for a conjunctival flap is unresponsive ulcerative keratitis, a lamellar keratectomy must be performed to remove all necrotic tissue. Necrosis of the flap resulting from an inadequate keratectomy and/or perforation resulting from persistent inflammation will require surgical repair with resection of all necrotic tissue, formation of a new flap, and, in the case of perforation, a lamellar or full-thickness patch graft.

Tension on the flap may cause the flap to retract and cheesewire through the sutures. If retraction is noticed postoperatively, it may be possible to undermine the flap, release the tension, and suture the flap back into place. The earlier this problem is detected postoperatively, the easier it is to correct.

Overlooked buttonholes in the flap will enlarge and destroy the flap (Figure 29-25). If a hole is noticed postoperatively, it should be repaired by undermining the edges of the hole, removing any epithelium that has grown onto the cornea through the hole, and suturing the edges

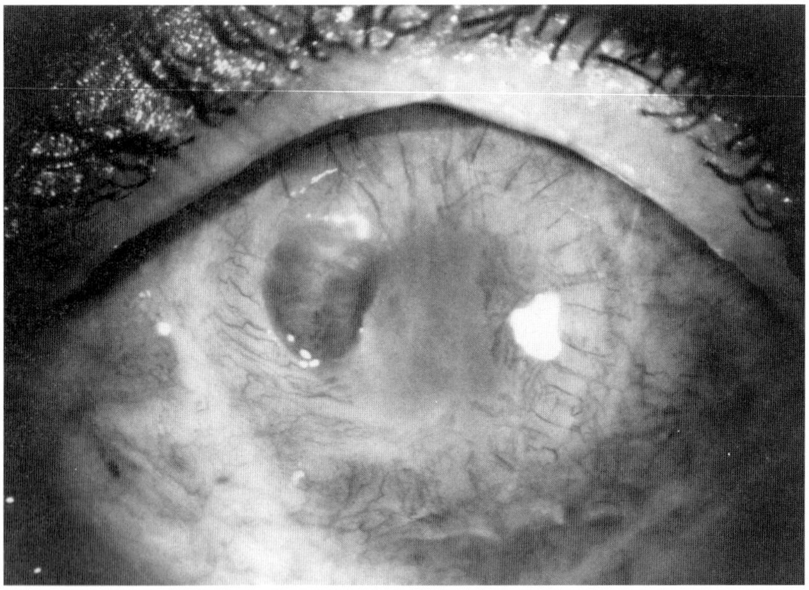

FIGURE 29-25 Large hole in a total conjunctival flap.

of the hole to each other and to the underlying cornea as described in the section on surgical techniques. The smaller the hole is at the time of discovery, the easier it is to repair. Large holes usually require construction of a new flap.

Retained epithelium under a conjunctival flap can proliferate and separate the flap from the cornea or form epithelial cysts (Figure 29-26). Epithelial cysts may regress spontaneously or may become large enough to require excision via marsupialization.

An inflamed eye requiring a conjunctival flap is at increased risk of a subconjunctival hemorrhage. This is usually controlled intraoperatively by a subconjunctival injection of lidocaine with epinephrine and by wet-field cautery. Hemorrhages occurring postoperatively under the flap generally resolve and do not need to be evacuated. A pressure dressing placed on the eye at the end of the procedure helps prevent postoperative hemorrhage.

Ptosis after a total conjunctival flap may be transient from ocular discomfort in the early postoperative period or may be permanent. Eyelid surgery may occasionally be necessary to correct the problem.

Symblepharon formation is rare following a conjunctival flap procedure. However, if the surgeon is aggressive in obtaining a large flap and removes palpebral

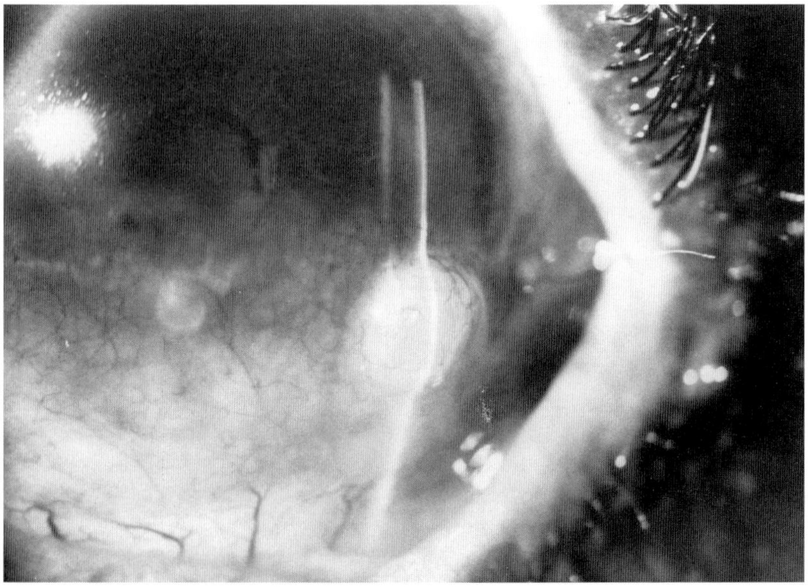

FIGURE 29-26 Epithelial inclusion cysts in a partial conjunctival flap.

FIGURE 29-27 Total conjunctival flap on the right cornea. **(A)** On close inspection, the blood vessels of the flap appear prominent. **(B)** From a distance, the blood vessels are not as noticeable, and the flap is cosmetically acceptable.

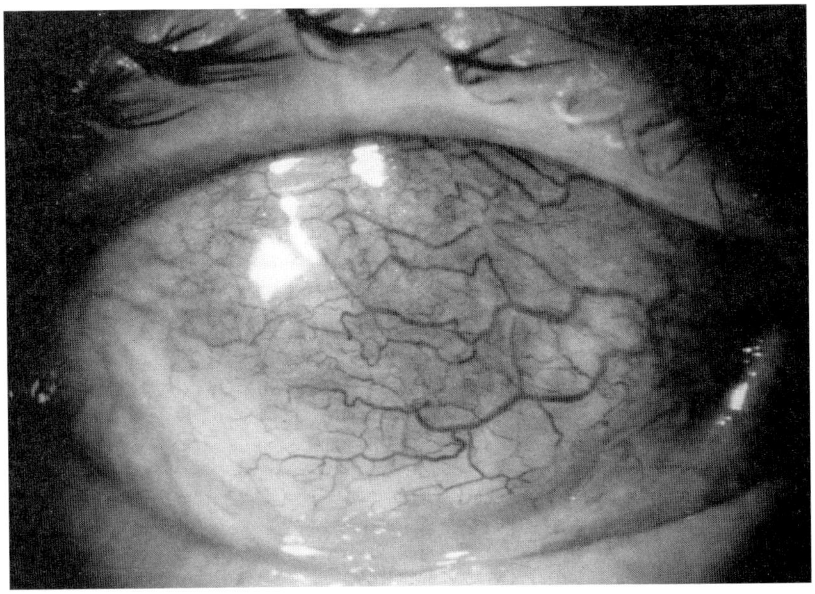

A

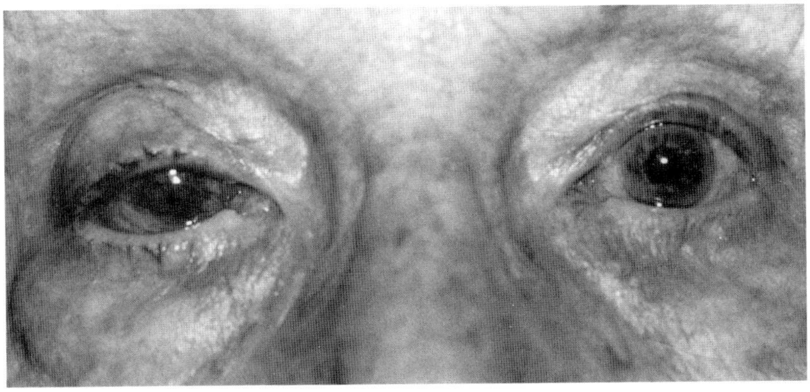

B

conjunctiva in addition to the adjacent bulbar conjunctiva, the two nonepithelialized surfaces left apposed to one another can form adhesions. To prevent this complication, palpebral conjunctiva should not be used. A symblepharon can be corrected surgically if necessary.

The most obvious disadvantage of a conjunctival flap is poor transparency, especially in the first few weeks postoperatively. This problem makes it difficult to monitor corneal or anterior chamber inflammation. Although conjunctival flaps alone are contraindicated for actual or impending perforations, progression of the underlying disease can result in a corneal perforation, which may not be detectable through the flap and which can cause scarring of the anterior chamber angle and severe glaucoma. Partial flaps should be used when possible because they allow better visualization of the anterior chamber than do total flaps.

A total conjunctival flap generally impairs vision, although visual acuity as good as 20/100 has been reported. In most patients in whom a conjunctival flap is indicated, vision is usually not the primary concern. If the lesion does not encroach on the visual axis, a partial flap should be used when possible so as not to obstruct the visual axis. Partial flaps not involving the visual axis may be left in place indefinitely and may not require future surgical procedures for visual rehabilitation, unlike total conjunctival flaps.

Cosmetically, the eye never looks entirely normal with a conjunctival flap. However, after a thin conjunctival flap is healed, it is usually noticeable only on close inspection, and most patients who are prepared preoperatively will accept the result (Figure 29-27). If the patient is unhappy, a cosmetic contact lens can create a more normal appearance.

Mobilization of the conjunctiva leads to scar formation in the area where the surgery was performed, which may complicate or decrease the chance for success of subsequent procedures such as glaucoma filtration surgery.

If a conjunctival flap is left in place for a long period of time, vascularization or opacification of the underlying cornea may occur. Although the conjunctival flap is easily removed, corneal vascularization may increase the risk of failure of a subsequent corneal graft. However, penetrating keratoplasty in an eye that has had a conjunctival flap is usually successful (depending on the indication for the flap), but should not be done until the eye is quiet and the flap has been in place for at least 6 months. Removal of the flap and penetrating keratoplasty can be performed in a single procedure (see Ch. 34).

REFERENCES

1. Schöler: Jahresberichte uber die Wirksamkeit der Augen-Klinik, in den Jahren 1874-1880, H. Peters, Berlin, 1875-1881
2. Haik GM: A fornix conjunctival flap as a substitute for the dissected conjunctival flap: a clinical and experimental study. Trans Am Ophthalmol Soc 52:497, 1954
3. Gundersen T: Conjunctival flaps in the treatment of corneal disease with reference to a new technique of application. Arch Ophthalmol 60:880, 1958
4. Paton D, Milauskas AT: Indications, surgical technique, and results of thin conjunctival flaps on the cornea. Int Ophthalmol Clin 10:329, 1970
5. Reinhart WJ: Conjunctival flap surgery. p. 63. In Bruner WE, Stark WJ, Maumenee AE (eds): Manual of Corneal Surgery. Churchill Livingstone, New York, 1987
6. Donzis PB, Mondino BJ: Management of noninfectious corneal ulcers. Surv Ophthalmol 32:94, 1987
7. Insler MS, Pechous B: Conjunctival flaps revisited. Ophthalmic Surg 6:455, 1987
8. Mannis MJ: Conjunctival flaps. Int Ophthalmol Clin 28:165, 1988
9. Gundersen T: Surgical treatment of bullous keratopathy. Arch Ophthalmol 64:260, 1960
10. Arentsen J, Laibson PR, Cohen EJ: Management of corneal descemetoceles and perforations. Ophthalmic Surg 16:29, 1985
11. Lin DTC, Webster RG, Abbot RL: Repair of corneal lacerations and perforations. Int Ophthalmol Clin 28:63, 1988
12. Portnoy SL, Insler MS, Kaufman HE: Surgical management of corneal ulceration and perforation. Surv Ophthalmol 34:47, 1989
13. Saini JS, Sharma A, Grewal SP: Chronic corneal perforations. Ophthalmic Surg 23:399, 1992
14. Williams DM, Weiner MH, Drutz DJ: Immunologic studies of disseminated infection with *Aspergillus fumigatus* in the nude mouse. J Infect Dis 143:726, 1981
15. Baxton JN, Fox ML: Conjunctival flaps in the treatment of refractory *Pseudomonas* corneal abscess. Ann Ophthalmol 18:315, 1986
16. Sanitato JJ, Kelley CG, Kaufman HE: Surgical management of peripheral fungal keratitis (keratomycosis). Arch Ophthalmol 102:1506, 1984
17. Brown DD, McCulley JP, Bowman RW, Halstead MA: The use of conjunctival flaps in the treatment of herpes keratouveitis. Cornea 11:44, 1992
18. Polack FM, Kaufman HE: Penetrating keratoplasty in herpetic keratitis. Am J Ophthalmol 73:908, 1972
19. Lesher MP, Lohman LE, Yeakly W, Lass J: Recurrence of herpetic stromal keratitis after a conjunctival flap surgical procedure. Am J Ophthalmol 114:231, 1992
20. Auran JD, Starr MB, Jakobiec FA: *Acanthamoeba* keratitis: a review of the literature. Cornea 6:2, 1987
21. Kaufman HE, McDonald MB, Barron BA, Wilson SE: Conjunctival flaps. p. 197. In Wright KW, Ryan SJ Jr (eds): Color Atlas of Ophthalmic Surgery. Corneal and Refractive Surgery. JB Lippincott, Philadelphia, 1992
22. Cies WA, Odeh-Nasrala N: The racquet conjunctival flap. Ophthalmic Surg 7:31, 1976

30

Phototherapeutic Keratectomy

EDWARD W. TRUDO, WALTER J. STARK, AND DIMITRI T. AZAR

Trokel and colleagues introduced excimer laser surgery of the cornea in 1983.[1] They showed that the 193-nm wavelength emission of the argon-fluoride excimer laser ablated corneal tissue of bovine eyes with microscopic precision. The use of the excimer laser in human patients was first reported 5 years later.[2] In contrast to excision of tissue with a stainless steel or diamond blade, photoablation removes corneal tissue with minimal alteration of the adjacent collagen lamellae.[3-5]

Removal of diseased corneal tissue with the excimer laser is termed *phototherapeutic keratectomy* or *PTK* (Figure 30-1). This procedure has the potential to improve visual function by reducing or eliminating corneal opacities and smoothing the anterior corneal surface. Increased corneal clarity and decreased surface irregularity contribute to improved visual acuity. Patients may also benefit from delaying or eliminating the need for penetrating or lamellar keratoplasty.

INDICATIONS

The most rewarding results of phototherapeutic keratectomy are obtained when the diseased tissue is located in the anterior one-fifth of the cornea. However, patients with disease and scars extending deeper into the cornea may also benefit from phototherapeutic keratectomy because removal of the entire opacity is often not necessary to achieve visual improvement. The treatment plan requires that the corneal tissue remaining after phototherapeutic keratectomy have a thickness of at least 250 μm. Some of the disorders treated with phototherapeutic keratectomy are listed in Table 30-1. Phototherapeutic keratectomy is successful in the primary treatment of granular, lattice, and Reis-Bücklers' dystrophies (Figures 30-2 and 30-3), and in the treatment of their recurrence in penetrating keratoplasty grafts. It is also effective in removing superficial surgical and nonsurgical scars but is less beneficial for deeper opacifications. Phototherapeutic keratectomy has also been used to treat epithelial dystrophies and recurrent epithelial erosions, and to smooth an irregular corneal surface after pterygium removal or chelation of band keratopathy with ethylenediaminetetraacetic acid (EDTA). Its use in keratoconus is limited to the removal of superficial scars because of corneal thinning in keratoconus.

Phototherapeutic keratectomy is not indicated in cases of recently active herpes simplex keratitis because the 193-nm beam may reactivate latent virus.[6,7] Treatment of active microbial keratitis is not recommended because of the failure to eradicate all viable organisms.[8-10] Other relative contraindications include significant blepharitis, severe dry eyes, lagophthalmos, and systemic immunosuppression, all of which may impair corneal healing and increase the likelihood of postoperative infection. Phototherapeutic keratectomy is also not routinely recommended for patients with uncontrolled uveitis or corneal neovascularization, or for pregnant women.

The indications and treatment goals are patient specific. The surgeon must document and discuss with the patient whether the goal is to improve visual acuity, decrease symptoms, or improve contact lens fitting. A clear understanding of the intended goal is important so that patient expectations will be realistic and achievable.

PREOPERATIVE EVALUATION

All patients require a thorough preoperative history and ophthalmologic examination. The history includes assess-

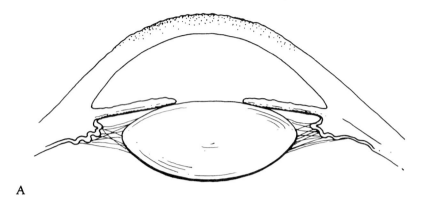

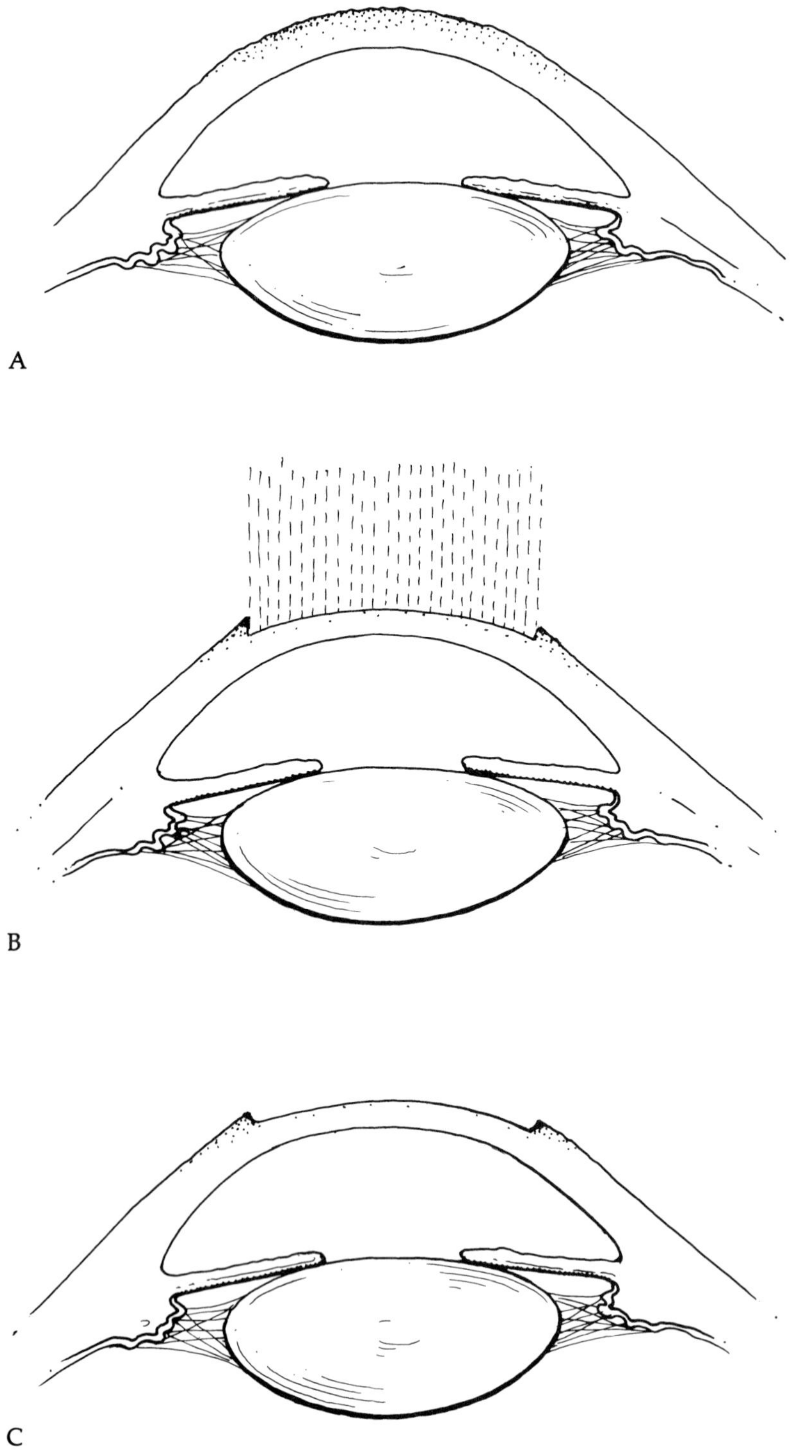

FIGURE 30-1 Phototherapeutic keratectomy. **(A)** Cornea with surface irregularity and opacities in the anterior stroma. **(B)** Excimer laser photoablation of the anterior corneal layers. **(C)** Most of the central opacities have been removed, and the anterior corneal surface is more regular.

ment for diabetes, collagen-vascular disease, ocular hypertension or glaucoma, herpetic eye disease, seasonal allergy, antihistamine use, and the use of medications that affect the cornea (e.g., amiodarone or sumatriptan).

The examination includes measurement of uncorrected and best spectacle-corrected visual acuities. Best-corrected visual acuity is measured by placing a hard contact lens on the cornea, which masks irregular astigmatism, and performing an overrefraction. If the contact lens provides adequate visual improvement, irregular astigmatism and not corneal opacification per se is responsible for the decreased vision. Such patients are offered

TABLE 30-1
Disorders Treated with Phototherapeutic Keratectomy

Postinfectious scars
Post-traumatic scars
Irregular corneal surface after pterygium removal
Shield ulcer from vernal keratoconjunctivitis
Corneal dystrophies
Epithelial and basement membrane dystrophies
Recurrent epithelial erosion
Meesmann's dystrophy
Reis-Bücklers' dystrophy
Stromal dystrophies
Granular dystrophy
Lattice dystrophy
Avellino dystrophy
Schnyder's dystrophy
Corneal degenerations
Band keratopathy
Salzmann's nodular degeneration
Amyloidosis
Keratoconus (superficial scarring)

a trial of contact lens wear as an alternative to phototherapeutic keratectomy. The ocular adnexa is inspected for evidence of rosacea, lagophthalmos, and incomplete blink. Evaluation for blepharitis, tear film insufficiency, and meibomian gland disease is important, because any ocular surface disorder can lead to delayed re-epithelialization and subsequent corneal haze or infection postoperatively. Ocular surface disorders and exposure keratopathy must be corrected before phototherapeutic keratectomy is performed.

The conjunctiva is evaluated for subepithelial fibrosis and chronic or allergic conjunctivitis. Each layer of the cornea is examined, with particular attention to the contour of the epithelial surface and the presence of any epithelial facets. In addition to noticing any obvious scars or dystrophies, the surgeon inspects the stroma for subtle ghost vessels or herpetic stromal scarring. Inspection of Descemet's membrane and the endothelium is essential because significant endothelial disease leads to poor epithelial healing after phototherapeutic keratectomy. The diameter of the pupil is measured under both light and dim conditions. Because corticosteroids are often prescribed after surgery, baseline intraocular pressure and lens opacities are recorded. A dilated funduscopic examination is important to exclude retinal disorders contributing to decreased vision.

Further testing includes keratometry, videokeratography, and pachymetry. Optical pachymetry, as described by Stark et al,[11] is invaluable for measuring scar or disease depth. Topical fluorescein and/or rose bengal staining, Schirmer tear testing, and estimation of visual potential with a laser interferometer or potential acuity meter are performed as indicated.

At the preoperative visit, patients are instructed to not wear makeup, mascara, eyeliner, perfume, or cologne on the day of surgery, because these substances can interfere with the operation and effectiveness of the laser. A prescription for a mild sedative to be taken approximately 30 minutes preoperatively is provided as needed. Sedation should be such that the patient is relaxed but still able to maintain fixation during the procedure.

SURGICAL TECHNIQUES

On the day of treatment, the surgeon ensures that the laser is calibrated by the method recommended by the manufacturer and that all required instruments are available. After receiving a topical anesthetic, the patient is prepped and draped; the procedure is performed under sterile conditions.

The corneal epithelium is removed by laser ablation or by mechanical scraping with a blade or spatula, depending on the smoothness of the epithelial surface. Epithelium fills in microscopic valleys of any mildly irregular underlying tissue and provides an excellent smoothing surface. Therefore, unless the epithelium is very irregular, it is left in place and transepithelial ablation is performed. If the surface under the epithelium is irregular, a masking agent, such as methylcellulose, can be used to fill in the valleys, effectively shielding these areas from ablation. Laser ablation then removes the elevated areas (Figure 30-4). The treatment bed does not have to be made absolutely smooth because residual subtle irregularities will be filled in by epithelium postoperatively, producing a relatively smooth anterior surface.

The surgeon programs the excimer laser for an ablation depth that will remove the majority of the anterior stromal opacities. Talamo et al[12] suggested treatment strategies based on the lesion elevation and distribution (Figure 30-5). Minimization of corneal stromal exposure to air during treatment is important, because prolonged exposure leads to stromal dehydration and may increase the tissue ablation rate. It is also important not to ablate too deeply, as this will create considerable flattening of the central cornea and induce a hyperopic shift.[5,13]

The treatment of central elevated nodules is particularly challenging. Azar et al[14] reported a technique in which the epithelium overlying the nodule, as well as a small amount of epithelium surrounding the peak, is scraped away. This results in an annular furrow around the elevated lesion. The

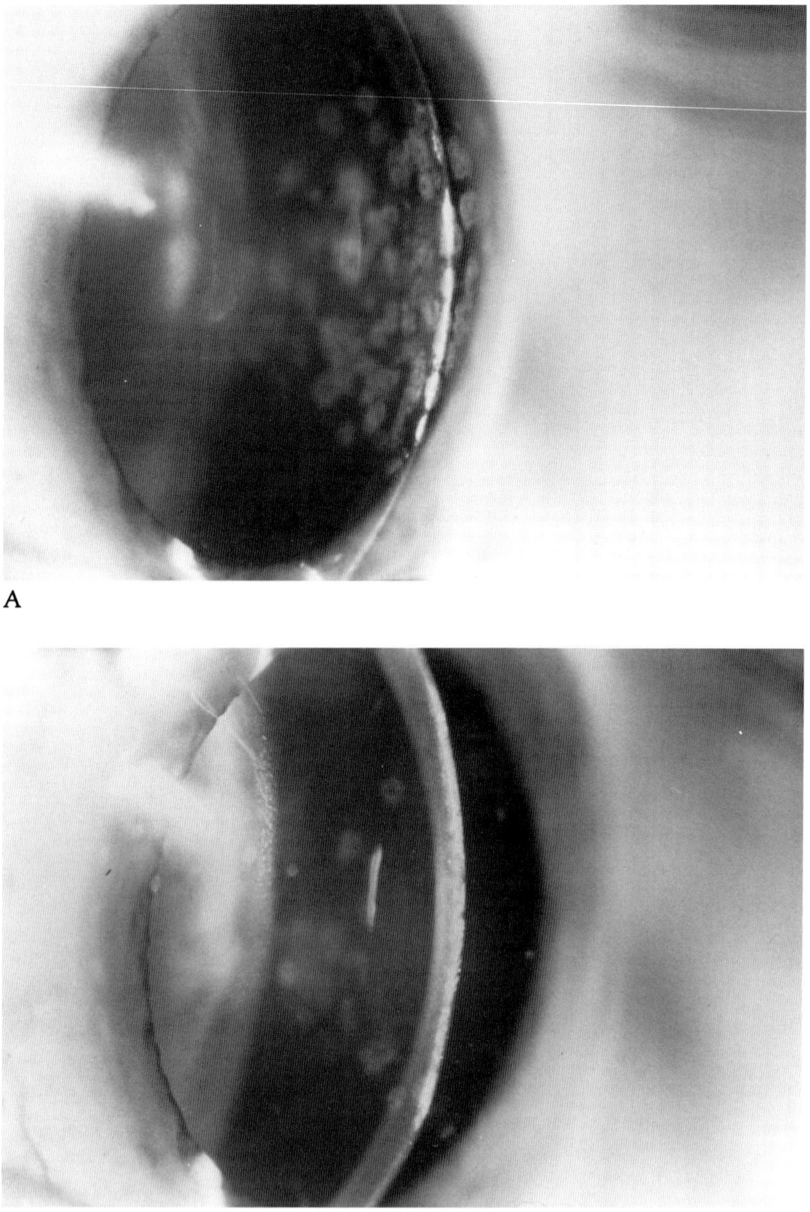

A

B

FIGURE 30-2 **(A)** Clinical photograph of granular dystrophy before phototherapeutic keratectomy. Best-corrected visual acuity was 20/50. **(B)** Postoperative appearance. The patient attained a best-corrected visual acuity of 20/25 at 12 months after phototherapeutic keratectomy and 20/20 at 60 months.

furrow is then filled with masking fluid to allow laser debulking of the opacity or nodule. Before complete excision of the opacity, a 6-mm diameter ablation is performed by a transepithelial technique. This procedure allows leveling of the residual lesion using masking agents.

The initial therapy of recurrent corneal erosions consists of patching, hypertonic drops and ointment, and bandage soft contact lenses. Surgical treatment can be performed in an office setting by epithelial debridement or anterior stromal puncture. Phototherapeutic keratectomy adds another option to the treatment regimen. Laser treatment is limited to approximately 5 μm of Bowman's layer. Minimal refractive change usually occurs under these circumstances.

POSTOPERATIVE CARE

One major goal during the early postoperative period is rapid re-epithelialization of the cornea. Early protocols specified the instillation of a topical cycloplegic agent, an

FIGURE 30-3 **(A)** Clinical photograph of Reis-Bücklers' dystrophy before phototherapeutic keratectomy. Best-corrected visual acuity was 20/70. **(B)** Postoperative appearance. Best-corrected visual acuity was 20/25.

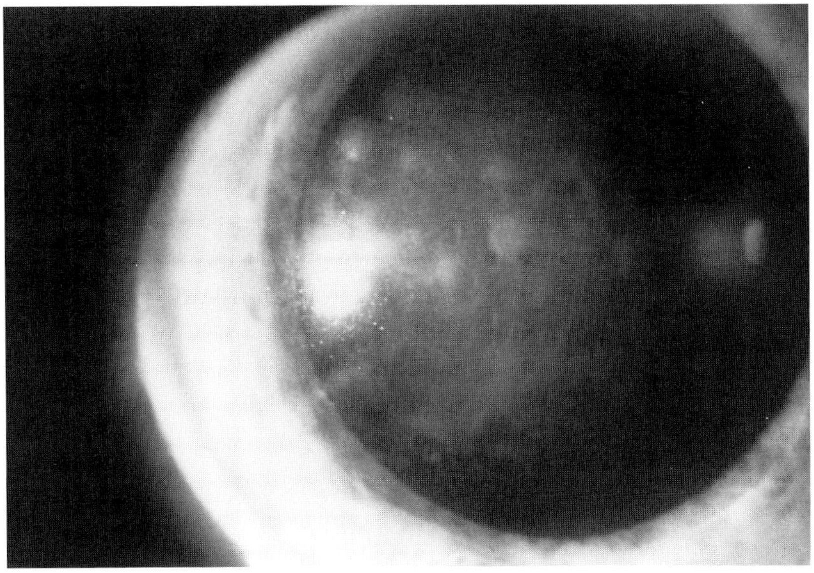

A

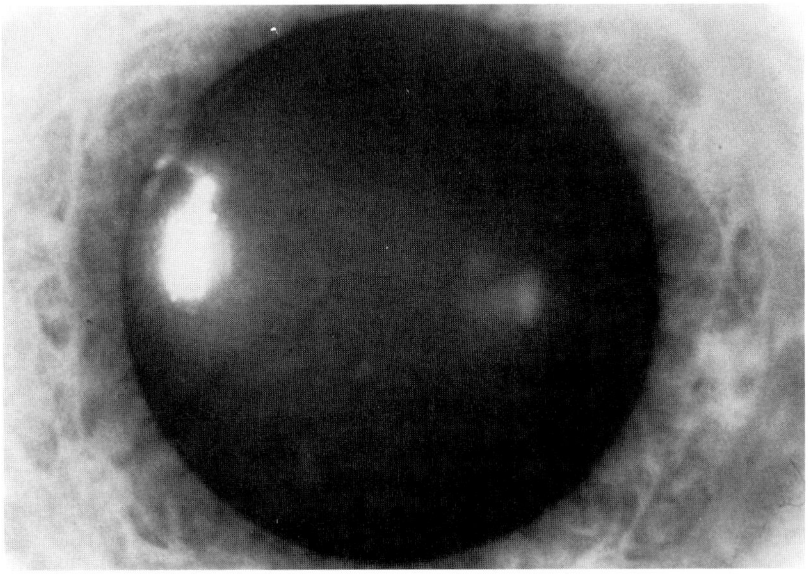

B

antibiotic eye drop, and a combination antibiotic-corticosteroid ointment at the end of the procedure, followed by patching the eyelids closed. An alternative approach, first described for the treatment of corneal abrasions, is the use of a bandage soft contact lens.[15] The lens is placed on the eye at the end of the procedure, and a topical antibiotic eye drop is used four times a day until re-epithelialization occurs. The contact lens remains in place until the epithelial defect is healed.

The second major goal is reduction of pain. For this purpose, patients are given a prescription for an oral analgesic, such as acetaminophen with codeine, to be used as needed. Also, a topical nonsteroidal anti-inflammatory drug may be used four times a day for the first few days. Although nonsteroidal anti-inflammatory drugs decrease pain, there have been reports of noninfectious infiltrates in excimer laser keratectomy patients treated for more than 24 hours with these drugs.[16]

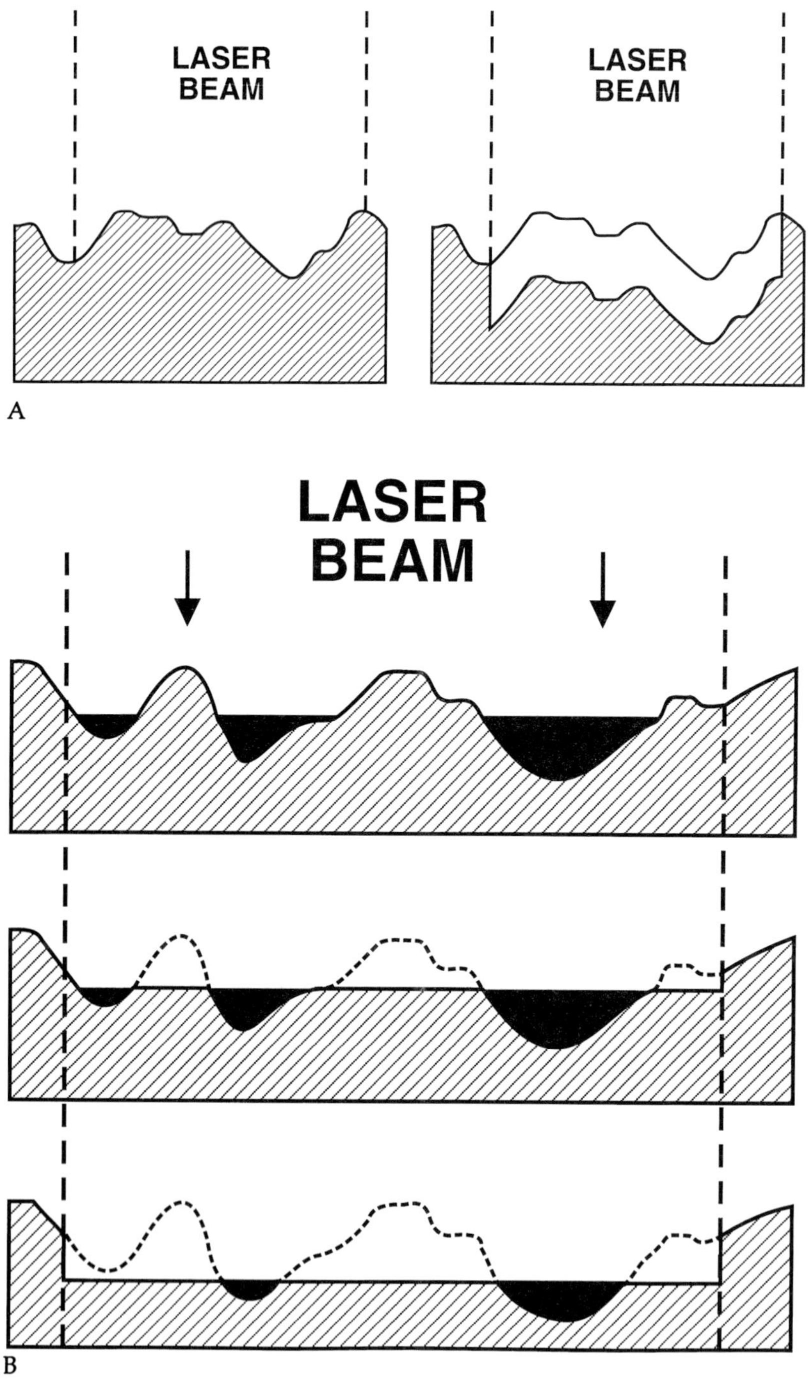

FIGURE 30-4 **(A)** Excimer laser keratectomy removes a precise amount of corneal tissue. Any irregular surface is reproduced at a deeper level in the corneal stroma. **(B)** A surface modulator (masking agent) shields the stromal valleys, allowing selective photoablation of the exposed tissue peaks. This results in a much smoother stromal surface after ablation.

Postoperative examinations are performed on the first postoperative day and then every few days to assess the patient's level of comfort, measure visual acuity and intraocular pressure, and evaluate the status of the epithelial defect and any evidence of infiltrates, corneal haze, or stromal edema. Once the epithelial defect has healed, the patient uses a mild topical corticosteroid, such as 0.1 percent fluorometholone eye drops, four times a day, tapered over 1 to 6 months. Intraocular pressure is monitored for evidence of corticosteroid-associated elevation. In patients with elevated intraocular pressure, corticosteroids may be discontinued and topical glaucoma medications given. Preservative-free artificial tears are an important adjunct for both patient comfort and epithelial healing. Follow-up

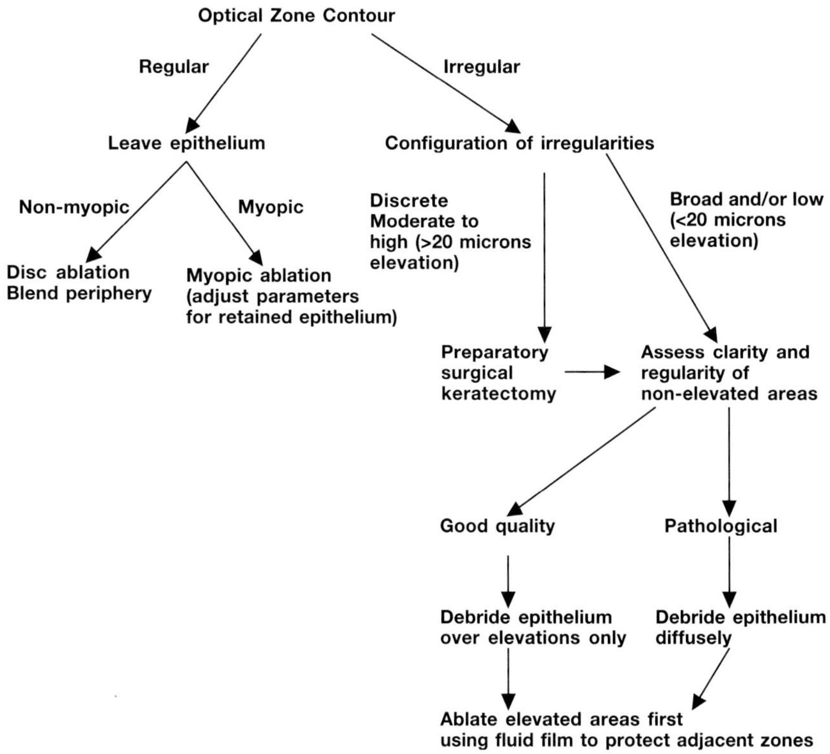

FIGURE 30-5 Treatment strategies for phototherapeutic keratectomy of superficial scars and irregularities. (Reprinted with permission from JH Talamo, RF Steinert, CA Puliafito: Clinical strategies for excimer laser therapeutic keratectomy. Refract Corneal Surg 8:319, 1992.)

examinations are routinely scheduled for 1 month, 3 months, 6 months, 1 year, and 2 years after surgery.

COMPLICATIONS

Complications after phototherapeutic keratectomy are infrequent. Table 30-2 lists complications reported in five major series.[5,13,17–19]

Delayed Re-Epithelialization

Re-epithelialization of the cornea occurs in most patients within the first week after phototherapeutic keratectomy. Sher et al[13] reported delayed epithelial healing in one of 33 patients; this patient eventually required a tarsorrhaphy and penetrating keratoplasty. Corneal healing was delayed more than 2 weeks in two of 27 phototherapeutic keratectomy–treated patients in the study by Stark et al[5]; one patient with Salzmann's nodular degeneration healed within 3 weeks, and one patient with a history of excessive alcohol intake healed in 4 weeks. Delayed epithelial healing of more than 7 days occurred in nine of 48 patients in the study by Zuckerman et al,[19] and delayed healing of 1 month or longer occurred in 3 percent of patients in the study by Maloney et al.[17] Delayed re-epithelialization often occurs in patients with diabetes, poor diet, or excessive alcohol intake. An inadequate or unstable tear film and chronic blepharitis are the most common local disorders associated with delayed epithelial healing.

A persistent epithelial defect places the patient at risk for increased stromal haze and corneal infection. Treatment includes eyelid hygiene, preservative-free artificial tears, punctal occlusion, and a bandage soft contact lens. In recalcitrant cases, a temporary tarsorrhaphy may be necessary.

Corneal Infiltrates

Postoperative corneal infiltrates often pose a diagnostic challenge and may have several causes. Bacterial keratitis, although uncommon, can have devastating effects on postoperative vision. Fulton et al[20] reported a bacterial ulcer 3 days after phototherapeutic keratectomy in a patient who was not treated prophylactically with antibiotics after surgery. Scrapings from a cornea with a suspected infection should be cultured, and the eye should be treated aggressively with appropriate antibiotics. The preoperative detection and treatment of blepharitis, the use of sterile technique, and the enhancement of corneal re-epithelialization decrease the risk of infection.

Another cause of corneal infiltrates in the postoperative period is reactivation of herpes simplex keratitis.[6,7,17–19,21] It has been recommended that patients with a history of herpes simplex keratitis be disease free for 1

TABLE 30-2
Complications after Phototherapeutic Keratectomy

Study	Number of Eyes	Complications	
		Number (%)	Diagnosis
Sher et al, 1991[13]	33	1 (3.0)	Delayed re-epithelialization (period undefined)
Stark et al, 1992[5]	27	2 (7.4)	Delayed re-epithelialization greater than 2 weeks
		2 (7.4)	Increased intraocular pressure
Maloney et al, 1996[17]	232	—[a] (3)	Delayed re-epithelialization of 1 month or more
		1 (0.5)	Bacterial keratitis
		3 (1.3)	Herpes simplex keratitis recurrence
		1 (0.5)	Iritis
		2 (0.9)	Graft rejection
Starr et al, 1996[18]	45	3 (6.6)	Increased intraocular pressure
		3 (6.6)	Herpes simplex keratitis recurrence
Zuckerman et al, 1996[19]	48	9 (19)	Delayed re-epithelialization of greater than 7 days
		2 (4.4)	Herpes simplex keratitis recurrence
		1 (2)	Episcleritis
		1 (2)	Angle closure after cycloplegia

[a] Percentage only given.

year before phototherapeutic keratectomy. Patients with a history of herpetic eye disease are treated prophylactically with preoperative and postoperative oral acyclovir or valacyclovir, along with a topical antiviral agent, such as trifluridine. Herpetic keratitis occurring after phototherapeutic keratectomy is treated as it would be in any patient who has herpetic keratitis.

Finally, noninfectious infiltrates are seen after phototherapeutic keratectomy in patients treated with a bandage soft contact lens and a topical nonsteroidal anti-inflammatory drug. These infiltrates usually resolve when the nonsteroidal anti-inflammatory drug is stopped and topical corticosteroids are begun, after an infectious cause has been excluded.

Stromal Haze

Stromal haze is common after most excimer laser procedures. It usually increases for the first few months after surgery, then diminishes by the sixth postoperative month. Activated keratocytes and new collagen deposition have been implicated in stromal haze formation during this period; the keratocytes may remain active for up to 18 months. If haze worsens, topical corticosteroids are increased and the cornea is closely observed.

Corneal Graft Rejection

Graft rejection has been reported in patients who have undergone phototherapeutic keratectomy after penetrating keratoplasty.[20,22,23] It is important to recognize diagnostic differences between the corneal edema, inflammation, and stromal haze expected after phototherapeutic keratectomy and the early signs of graft rejection. Prompt treatment of a rejection episode is mandatory.

Hyperopia

In contrast to photorefractive keratectomy, phototherapeutic keratectomy is designed to create a plano ablation. However, it appears that, in fact, hyperopia is probably the most frequent side effect of this procedure, and is now considered to be both expected and predictable. Significant amounts of induced hyperopia were observed in many of the early phototherapeutic keratectomy studies.[5,13,24] Gartry et al[25] suggested three reasons for this hyperopic shift: (1) greater disease density in the peripheral cornea, as in band keratopathy, results in corneal ablation that is deeper centrally than peripherally; (2) removal of the central portions of the corneal lamellae leads to centrifugal contracture and central corneal flattening; and (3) centrifugal spray of debris and ablation debris creates a shield that blocks the peripheral beam. Alternatively, increased obliquity of the incident laser beam falling on the peripheral cornea may result in less peripheral ablation.[26] Corneal wound healing with early epithelial hyperplasia at the treatment zone border and late new collagen deposition may also be factors in induced hyperopia.[14,27,28]

Surface modulating agents and alterations in photoablation techniques have been shown to reduce the hyperopic shift. Because the amount of hyperopic shift correlates directly with the ablation depth, surface modulating agents reduce the shift by allowing removal of elevated diseased tissue while minimizing ablation of the surrounding stroma. Stark et al[5] described a technique in which, after the initial plano treatment is completed, the eye is moved in a circular fashion such that a 2-mm diameter laser beam is delivered along the edge of the treatment zone, resulting in a peripheral taper with an ablation depth of approximately 20 μm. The initial results of this modified taper method showed a significant reduction in induced hyperopia. Sher et al[13] described two different methods that reduce the hyperopic effect. In the smoothing technique, the surgeon moves the eye in a circular fashion under a beam of varying aperture size. In the combined ablation technique, a second hyperopic ablation is performed to the peripheral portion of the central cornea after the phototherapeutic ablation has been completed.

RESULTS

In a review of the results of phototherapeutic studies published between 1991 and 1995 (Table 30-3), Azar et al[14] found that the best outcomes occurred with anterior corneal dystrophies and Salzmann's nodular degeneration, whereas less satisfactory and more variable outcomes were seen for treatment of herpetic keratitis and postinfectious scars.[5,13,24,29-37] In the early studies,[5,13,24] at least 50 percent of treated patients experienced improved visual acuity and avoided more invasive surgery (Table 30-4). Stark et al[5] showed visual acuity improvement in 78 percent of eyes with either spectacle or contact lens correction. Sher et al[13] reported an increase in best spectacle-corrected visual acuity in 48 percent of eyes treated by phototherapeutic keratectomy and Campos et al[24] showed visual acuity improvement in half of the treatment group in their 1993 study. More recent studies showed gains in 45 to 72 percent of patients.[17-19,29] Maloney et al[17] reported the findings of a prospective multicenter trial of phototherapeutic keratectomy in which 45 percent of 232 eyes with at least 12 months of follow-up had improved best spectacle-corrected visual acuity. These authors reported that the treatment was most effective in eyes with hereditary corneal dystrophies, Salzmann's nodular degeneration, and corneal scars, and least effective in eyes with calcific band keratopathy.

In these studies, fewer than 20 percent of patients experienced decreased best-corrected visual acuity after phototherapeutic keratectomy. Rapuano and Laibson[29]

TABLE 30-3
Efficacy of Phototherapeutic Keratectomy in the Treatment of Various Corneal Disorders

Corneal Disorder	*Percent Success*	*References*
Reis-Bücklers' dystrophy	100	5, 13, 29, 31–37
Lattice dystrophy	90–100	5, 24, 35, 37
Granular dystrophy	66–100	5, 24, 29, 31, 35, 37
Salzmann's nodular degeneration	60–100	5, 13, 29, 31, 32
Post-traumatic scar	50–66	13, 24, 30
Herpetic keratitis	25–80	13, 30
Postinfectious scar	33–100	13, 24, 35

Source: Data from DT Azar, S Jain, WJ Stark: Phototherapeutic keratectomy. p. 501. In Azar DT (ed): Refractive Surgery. Appleton & Lange, Stamford, CT, 1996.

TABLE 30-4
Best-Corrected Visual Acuity after Phototherapeutic Keratectomy

		Effect on Best-Corrected Visual Acuity[a]		
Study	*Number of Eyes*	*Increased (%)*	*Unchanged (%)*	*Decreased (%)*
Sher et al, 1991[13]	33	48	36	15
Stark et al, 1992[5]	27	78	15	7
Campos et al, 1993[24]	18	50	33	17
Rapuano and Laibson, 1994[29]	20	45	50	5
Maloney et al, 1996[17]	232	45	46	9
Starr et al, 1996[18]	45	71	14	15
Zuckerman et al, 1996[19]	48	72	13	15

[a] Best-corrected visual acuity is with spectacles for Sher et al,[13] Campos et al,[24] Maloney et al,[17] Starr et al,[18] and Zuckerman et al,[19] and with spectacles or contact lenses for Stark et al[5] and Rapuano and Laibson.[29]

reported only one of 20 treated eyes (5 percent) with decreased vision after phototherapeutic keratectomy. Sher et al,[13] Starr et al,[18] and Zuckerman et al[19] each reported a decrease in best-corrected visual acuity in 15 percent of eyes, and Campos et al[24] reported a decrease in 17 percent of eyes. The percentage of patients whose vision remained unchanged after excimer treatment varied from 13 percent to 50 percent in these studies.[5,13,17–19,24,29]

The future of phototherapeutic keratectomy holds promise for an improved understanding of postexcimer healing in the human cornea, the etiology and modulation of induced hyperopia, and the development of diverse treatment techniques to maximally benefit specific disease entities. In the interim, phototherapeutic keratectomy remains a safe and effective surgical procedure with the option of retreatment and no serious adverse effects on the outcome of future lamellar or penetrating keratoplasty, if such surgery becomes necessary.

REFERENCES

1. Trokel SL, Srinivasan R, Braren B: Excimer laser surgery of the cornea. Am J Ophthalmol 96:710, 1983
2. L'Esperance FA, Taylor DM, Del Pedro RA, et al: Human excimer laser corneal surgery: preliminary report. Trans Am Ophthalmol Soc 86:208, 1988
3. Marshall J, Trokel S, Rothery S, et al: A comparative study of corneal incisions induced by diamond and steel knives and two ultraviolet radiations from an excimer laser. Br J Ophthalmol 70:482, 1986
4. Wu WC, Stark WJ, Green WR: Corneal wound healing after 193-nm excimer laser keratectomy. Arch Ophthalmol 109:1426, 1991
5. Stark WJ, Chamon W, Kamp MT, et al: Clinical follow-up of 193-nm ArF excimer laser photokeratectomy. Ophthalmology 99:805, 1992
6. Pepose JS, Laycock KA, Miller JK, et al: Reactivation of latent herpes simplex by excimer laser photokeratectomy. Am J Ophthalmol 114:45, 1992
7. Vrabec MP, Anderson JA, Rock ME, et al: Electron microscopic findings in a cornea with recurrence of herpes simplex keratitis after excimer laser phototherapeutic keratectomy. CLAO J 20:41, 1994
8. Gottsch JD, Gilbert ML, Goodman DF, et al: Excimer laser ablative treatments of microbial keratitis. Ophthalmology 98:146, 1991
9. Keates RH, Drago PC, Rothchild EJ: Effect of excimer laser on microbiological organisms. Ophthalmic Surg 19:715, 1988
10. Eiferman RA, Forgey DR, Cook YD: Excimer laser ablation of infectious crystalline keratopathy. Arch Ophthalmol 110:18, 1992
11. Stark WJ, Gilbert ML, Gottsch JD, Munnerlyn C: Optical pachometry in the measurement of anterior corneal disease: an evaluative tool for phototherapeutic keratectomy. Arch Ophthalmol 108:12, 1990
12. Talamo JH, Steinert RF, Puliafito CA: Clinical strategies for excimer laser therapeutic keratectomy. Refract Corneal Surg 8:319, 1992
13. Sher NA, Bowers RA, Zabel RW, et al: Clinical use of the 193-nm excimer laser in the treatment of corneal scars. Arch Ophthalmol 109:491, 1991
14. Azar DT, Jain S, Stark WJ: Phototherapeutic keratectomy. p. 501. In Azar DT (ed): Refractive Surgery. Appleton & Lange, Stamford, CT, 1996
15. Donnenfeld ED, Selkin BA, Perry HD, et al: Controlled evaluation of a bandage contact lens and a topical nonsteroidal anti-inflammatory drug in treating traumatic corneal abrasions. Ophthalmology 102:979, 1995
16. Sher NA, Krueger RR, Teal P, et al: Role of corticosteroids and nonsteroidal anti-inflammatory drugs in the etiology of stromal infiltrates after excimer photorefractive keratectomy. J Refract Corneal Surg 10:587, 1994
17. Maloney RK, Thompson V, Ghiselli G, et al: A prospective multicenter trial of excimer laser phototherapeutic keratectomy for corneal vision loss. Am J Ophthalmol 122:149, 1996
18. Starr M, Donnenfeld E, Newton M, et al: Excimer laser phototherapeutic keratectomy. Cornea 15:557, 1996
19. Zuckerman SJ, Aquavella JV, Park SB: Analysis of the efficacy and safety of excimer laser phototherapeutic keratectomy in the treatment of corneal disease. Cornea 15:9, 1996
20. Fulton JC, Cohen EJ, Rapuano CJ: Bacterial ulcer 3 days after excimer laser phototherapeutic keratectomy. Arch Ophthalmol 114:626, 1996
21. Fagerholm P, Ohman L, Orndahl M: Phototherapeutic keratectomy in herpes simplex keratitis. Acta Ophthalmol (Copenh) 72:457, 1994
22. Hersh PS, Jordan AJ, Mayers M: Corneal graft rejection episode after excimer laser phototherapeutic keratectomy. Arch Ophthalmol 11:735, 1993
23. Epstein RJ, Robin JB: Corneal graft rejection episode after excimer laser phototherapeutic keratectomy [letter]. Arch Ophthalmol 112:157, 1994
24. Campos M, Nielsen S, Szerenyi K, et al: Clinical follow-up of phototherapeutic keratectomy for treatment of corneal opacities. Am J Ophthalmol 115:433, 1993
25. Gartry D, Kerr-Muir M, Marshall J: Excimer laser treatment of corneal surface pathology: a laboratory and clinical study. Br J Ophthalmol 75:258, 1991
26. Goodman GL, Trokel SL, Stark WJ, et al: Corneal healing following laser refractive keratectomy. Arch Ophthalmol 107:1799, 1989
27. Azar DT, Spurr-Michaud SJ, Tisdale AS, et al: Reassembly of the corneal epithelial adhesion structures following human epikeratoplasty. Arch Ophthalmol 109:1279, 1991
28. Chamon W, Azar DT, Stark WJ, et al: Phototherapeutic keratectomy. Ophthalmol Clin North Am 6:399, 1993
29. Rapuano CJ, Laibson PR: Excimer laser phototherapeutic keratectomy for anterior corneal pathology. CLAO J 20:253, 1994

30. Fagerholm P, Fitzsimmons TD, Örndahl M, et al: Phototherapeutic keratectomy: long-term results in 166 eyes. Refract Corneal Surg 9(suppl):S76, 1993
31. Rapuano CJ, Laibson PR: Excimer laser phototherapeutic keratectomy. CLAO J 19:235, 1993
32. Hersh PS, Spinak A, Garrana R, Mayers M: Phototherapeutic keratectomy: strategies and results in 12 eyes. Refract Corneal Surg 9(suppl):S90, 1993
33. Rogers C, Cohen P, Lawless M: Phototherapeutic keratectomy for Reis-Bücklers' corneal dystrophy. Aust N Z J Ophthalmol 21:247, 1993
34. Lawless MA, Cohen PR, Rogers CM: Retreatment of undercorrected photorefractive keratectomy for myopia. J Refract Corneal Surg 10(suppl):S174, 1994
35. Hahn TW, Sah WJ, Kim JH: Phototherapeutic keratectomy in nine eyes with superficial corneal diseases. Refract Corneal Surg 9(suppl):S115, 1993
36. McDonnell PJ, Seiler T: Phototherapeutic keratectomy with excimer laser for Reis-Bücklers' corneal dystrophy. Refract Corneal Surg 8(suppl):306, 1992
37. Orndahl M, Fagerholm P, Fitzsimmons T, Tengroth B. Treatment of corneal dystrophies with excimer laser. Acta Ophthalmol (Copenh) 72:235, 1994

31

Inlay Lamellar Keratoplasty

WARREN HAMILTON AND THOMAS O. WOOD

In the early 1980s, the term *inlay lamellar keratoplasty* would have been redundant because all lamellar keratoplasties were inlay lamellar keratoplasties. With the development of epikeratophakia, the term *onlay lamellar keratoplasty* was introduced to differentiate this procedure from inlay lamellar keratoplasty. In inlay lamellar keratoplasty, a portion of the anterior stromal lamellae of the patient's cornea is removed (lamellar keratectomy) and replaced with partial-thickness donor cornea (lamellar graft) consisting of stroma, Bowman's layer, and, in some cases, epithelium. In onlay lamellar keratoplasty, a partial-thickness donor cornea is placed on a de-epithelialized cornea in which a small peripheral keratectomy and/or peripheral lamellar dissection has been done. Onlay lamellar keratoplasty is described in Chapter 32. Inlay lamellar keratoplasty is described in this chapter and in Chapter 21 for the treatment of pterygia.

The goal in inlay lamellar keratoplasty is to replace abnormal corneal tissue or to add corneal tissue to strengthen the cornea. Inlay lamellar keratoplasty has been used for the treatment of corneal perforations, corneal thinning disorders, pterygia, and any corneal disorder that involves only the anterior layers of the cornea. In the past, inlay lamellar keratoplasty was more successful than penetrating keratoplasty for the treatment of anterior corneal abnormalities because the surgical techniques for ensuring proper wound closure in penetrating keratoplasty were inchoate, and the importance of healthy donor corneal endothelium was not recognized. Unlike penetrating keratoplasty, lamellar keratoplasty (both inlay and onlay) does not require living corneal tissue.

The disadvantages of inlay lamellar keratoplasty include reduced visual acuity as a result of interface irregularities caused by uneven lamellar dissection of the recipient cornea and, in some cases, the donor tissue, and/or opacities in the donor-recipient interface. Visual acuities after inlay lamellar keratoplasty can range from 20/20 to 20/60; most are about 20/30. When inlay lamellar keratoplasty is performed infrequently, it is technically more difficult than penetrating keratoplasty.[1,2]

INDICATIONS

The high success rate of penetrating keratoplasty in recent years and the introduction of excimer laser phototherapeutic keratectomy have resulted in fewer indications for inlay lamellar keratoplasty. In general, inlay lamellar keratoplasty is used to add substance to a thinned or perforated cornea, as occurs in peripheral degeneration, stromal necrosis, a descemetocele, or after pterygium removal, and, rarely, to treat selected cases of keratoconus. It is also used to treat anterior stromal scars and irregularities of the anterior corneal surface; however, excimer laser phototherapeutic keratectomy has become the preferred treatment for most of these cases (see Ch. 30).

Inlay lamellar keratoplasty can be used tectonically in corneal thinning disorders to restore corneal thickness and maintain the integrity of the globe. In cases of perforation, descemetocele, or peripheral degeneration, an inlay lamellar patch graft can be fashioned to conform to the stromal defect to reinforce the thinned area (Figure 31-1).

In the case of a descemetocele caused by an infection, inlay lamellar keratoplasty should be performed only after the infection is under control[3–6]; otherwise, the infection will consume the graft. A superficial keratectomy is usually required to remove a recurrent pterygium, and an inlay lamellar graft may be required to replace the excised cornea if the keratectomy is deep,[7–9] as described in Chapter 21 (Figure 31-2). Postpterygium surgical scars and lim-

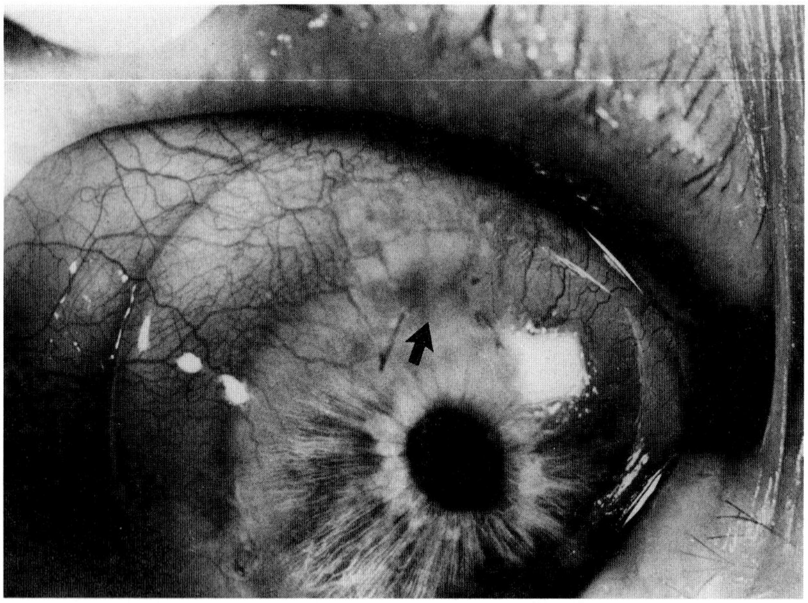

FIGURE 31-1 Perforated peripheral ulcer associated with rheumatoid arthritis was treated with a lamellar patch graft (arrow) and bandage soft contact lens.

bal abnormalities, such as dermoids and tumors, can also be excised and the corneal defect repaired with an inlay lamellar graft. It should be remembered that most dermoids extend deep into the cornea and sclera and should be approached with caution.

Scars or deposits of abnormal material in the anterior corneal stroma can usually be removed by excimer laser phototherapeutic keratectomy. However, if the keratectomy leaves an irregular corneal surface, or if a manual keratectomy is required and the underlying cornea is thin, inlay lamellar keratoplasty is indicated.

The calcium deposition in band keratopathy can usually be removed by chelation with ethylenediaminetetraacetic acid (EDTA)[10] or by a manual superficial keratectomy.[11] Phototherapeutic keratectomy with the excimer laser also effectively removes band keratopathy. An inlay lamellar graft can be placed if the corneal surface is irregular. Salzmann's nodular degeneration has been treated with inlay lamellar keratoplasty, but a manual superficial keratectomy of the large nodules may be sufficient. Combined superficial keratectomy and excimer laser phototherapeutic keratectomy are performed by

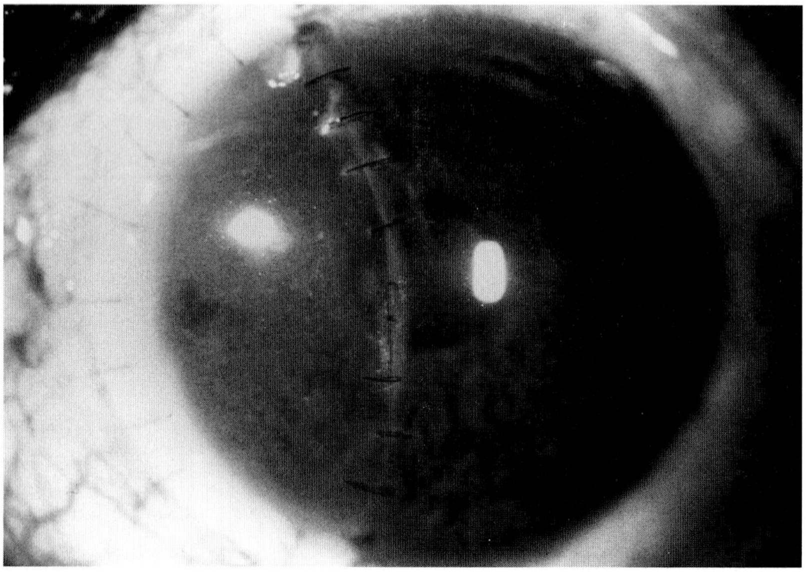

FIGURE 31-2 Large inlay lamellar graft for treatment of a recurrent pterygium. The central suture has been placed in a manner such that it does not encroach on the center of the pupil.

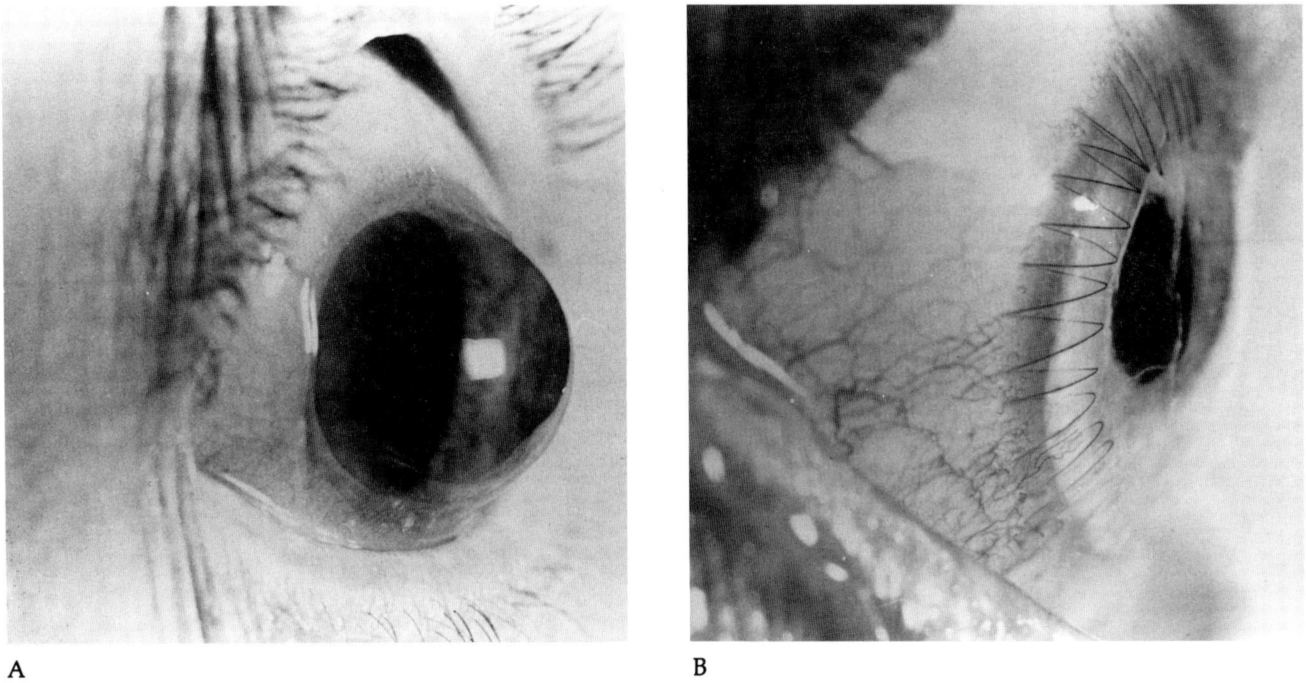

FIGURE 31-3 **(A)** Large cone with extreme peripheral thinning. **(B)** Postoperative inlay lamellar keratoplasty. Note the flattening effect of the graft. The vertical epithelial line represents epithelial rejection, which does not affect graft clarity.

some surgeons to treat this disorder. Severe Reis-Bücklers' dystrophy usually responds to dissection of the fibrous membrane from the surface of the cornea[12] or to excimer laser phototherapeutic keratectomy. Inlay lamellar keratoplasty has also been used to treat other corneal dystrophies that involve predominately the anterior stroma; however, excimer laser phototherapeutic keratectomy is increasingly being used for these disorders as well.

The treatment of keratoconus in most patients consists initially of spectacles and later of contact lenses. Surgery is indicated when contact lenses no longer are tolerated or do not provide acceptable vision.[1,13] Surgical treatment includes penetrating keratoplasty (see Ch. 34), onlay lamellar keratoplasty (see Ch. 32), or inlay lamellar keratoplasty.[14] Penetrating keratoplasty is the most common surgical procedure used to treat keratoconus and gives excellent visual results.[2,15] Onlay lamellar keratoplasty (epikeratophakia) can be used in patients who can no longer wear contact lenses and who have no corneal scarring within 1 mm of the visual axis, or to add corneal substance in anticipation of penetrating keratoplasty.[16,17]

Although inlay lamellar keratoplasty is rarely indicated for the treatment of keratoconus today, historically the procedure had some advantages over penetrating keratoplasty. Lamellar keratoplasty does not perforate the cornea and, therefore, has fewer intraocular complications. A lamellar graft can flatten the entire cone, even if the cone extends to the limbus (Figure 31-3). Criteria for the selection of donor tissue for lamellar keratoplasty are less rigid than those for penetrating keratoplasty because the viability of the graft does not depend on the presence of donor corneal endothelial cells. The incidence of graft rejection is lower with lamellar keratoplasty compared to penetrating keratoplasty, because endothelial rejection does not occur.[1,2,13,18–21] In cases of stromal or epithelial rejection, the recipient cornea clears because the corneal endothelial cells of the recipient are not affected by the rejection episode.

In 1979, Vancea and Schwartzenberg[19] cited inlay lamellar keratoplasty as the preferred treatment for keratoconus. Richard et al[1] and Gasset[18] advocated choosing between inlay lamellar keratoplasty and penetrating keratoplasty on the basis of the clinical situation. Wood[2] suggested reserving inlay lamellar keratoplasty for large eccentric cones and for patients who are poor candidates for penetrating keratoplasty. With improvements in microsurgical techniques, penetrating keratoplasty has become safer and more successful in most patients. Since the introduction of onlay lamellar keratoplasty, inlay lamellar keratoplasty in keratoconus is reserved for eyes with deep central scarring in patients who are not good candidates for penetrating keratoplasty.

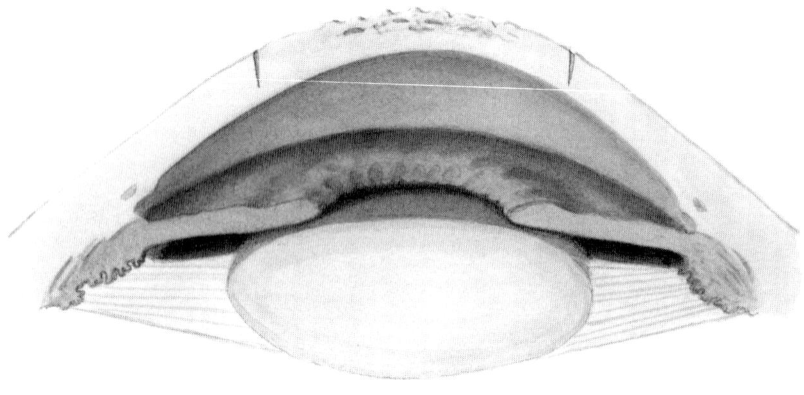

FIGURE 31-4 A partial thickness trephine cut is made to delineate the cornea to be excised.

SURGICAL TECHNIQUES

The sizes of the keratectomy bed and donor graft vary with the disorder requiring surgery. In disorders that cause opacification or irregularities of the central cornea, the keratectomy bed is usually 7.0 to 8.0 mm in diameter (Figure 31-4). In keratoconus, the bed should extend at least 0.5 mm beyond the edge of the cone; occasionally a 9- to 10-mm bed is required.[2] In an eye with necrotic stroma or a perforation, the diameter of the trephine should be large enough to encompass all of the necrotic stroma and cut into healthy cornea (Figure 31-5).

The trephine is centered on the area of abnormality, and the cut is made to a depth of 0.2 to 0.3 mm, depending on the condition of the cornea. In trephining the recipient cornea in keratoconus, it is important that the obturator of the trephine be retracted into the shaft of the trephine. This prevents flattening the apex of the cone and altering the shape of the recipient bed. Alternatively, a trephine without an obturator, such as the Barron radial vacuum trephine may be used. In eyes that are extremely soft, a shallow trephine mark can be made initially and deepened with a stainless steel blade. If a large keratectomy bed is required, the Barron radial vacuum trephine may be used. In the case of a noncircular keratectomy, the area of the keratectomy is outlined with a diamond blade or stainless steel blade, with care taken to make the incisions perpendicular to the corneal

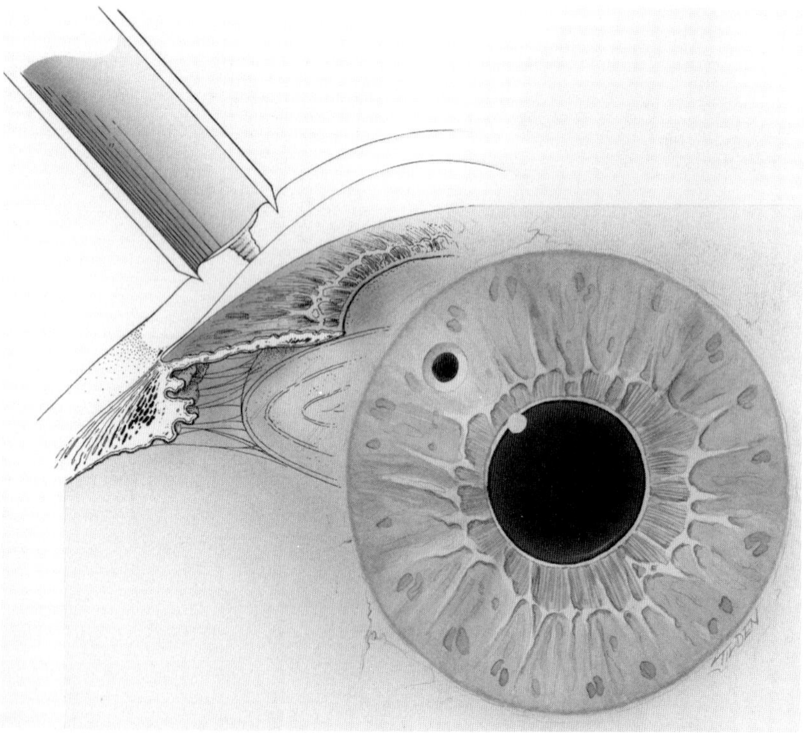

FIGURE 31-5 Trephination of the recipient cornea around the site of a necrotic corneal perforation.

surface to provide a distinct edge to which the graft can be sutured.

Lamellar keratectomy can be performed either by peeling off the diseased portion of the cornea[18,20,22] or by dissecting it with an instrument.[2,19,23–26] In both techniques, the area to be excised is cut with a trephine or blade as described above. In the peeling technique, a spatula or knife is used to dissect 2 to 3 mm horizontally into the desired plane (Figure 31-6). The lamellar flap is then grasped with two forceps and slowly but steadily pulled from the periphery toward the center, until the entire flap has been removed.[18,20,22] The cornea should be kept dry during the lamellar dissection; otherwise, fluid is absorbed by the stroma, which distorts the tissue and makes it difficult to maintain the dissection in the appropriate plane. The excised lamellar flap is left in place while the donor tissue is prepared.

There are several methods of performing the lamellar dissection with an instrument. The initial cut is made as above. The lamellar dissection is then performed using Castroviejo scissors, a cyclodialysis spatula, a surgical knife, or a stainless steel blade[19,24,25] (Figure 31-7). Another method of instrument dissection involves an automated blade (microkeratome).[24]

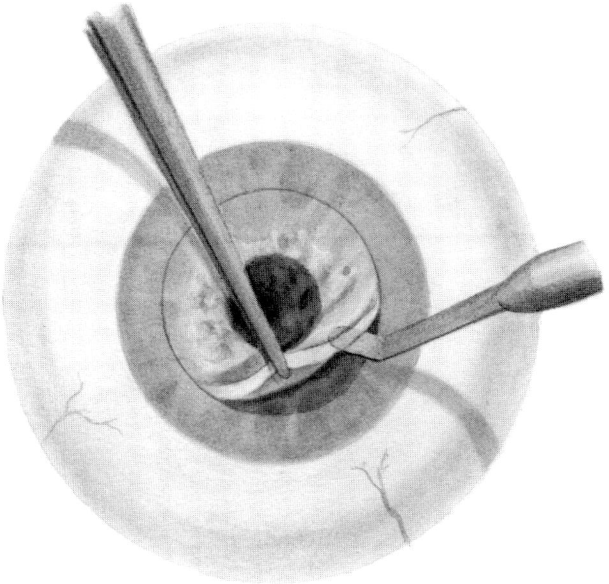

FIGURE 31-6 Peeling technique. After instrument dissection of the peripheral lamellar bed, as shown here, the lamellar flap is grasped with forceps and slowly peeled from the eye.

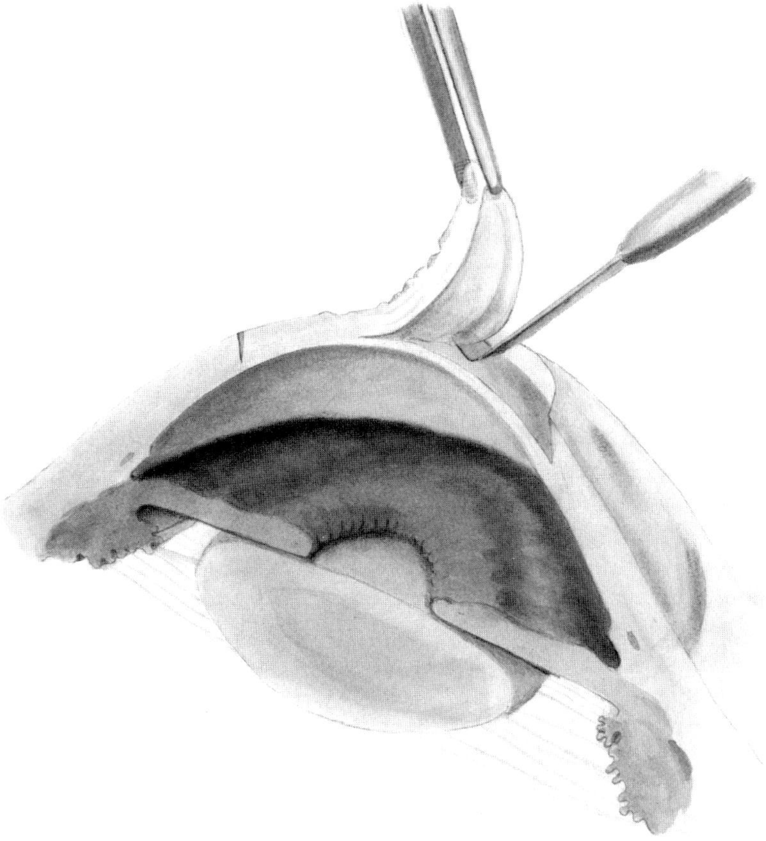

FIGURE 31-7 Instrument dissection of the entire lamellar bed.

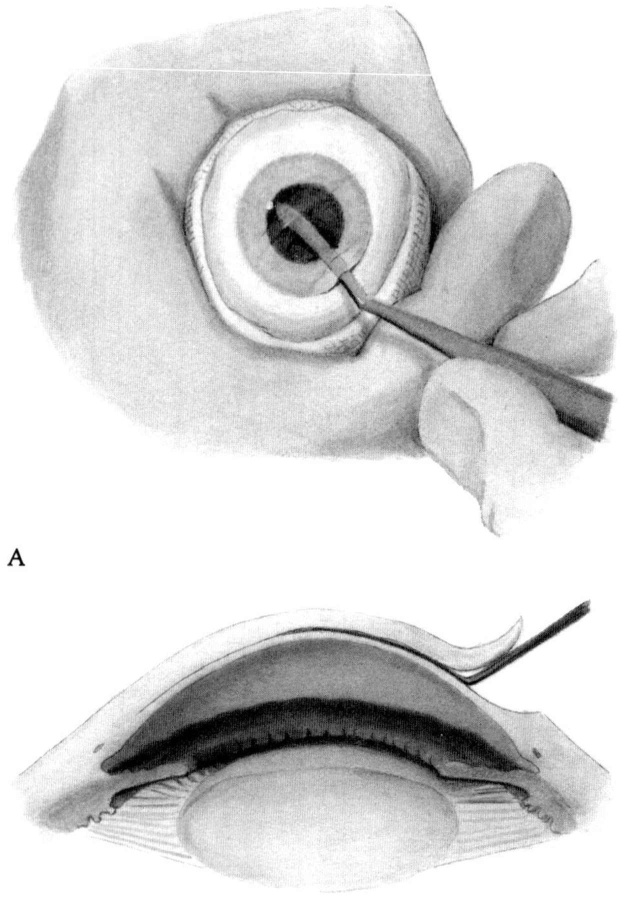

A

B

FIGURE 31-8 Lamellar dissection of the donor graft. (A) Top view. (B) Cross-sectional view. The whole globe is wrapped in gauze and held in the hand. A cyclodialysis spatula is used to perform the lamellar dissection.

Donor lamellar tissue can be prepared from a whole eye, donor corneal tissue, or precarved lyophilized tissue. It is easier to dissect a lamellar graft from a whole eye than from a donor cornea. A whole eye can be stored at -70°C, thawed, and used in an emergency or when living donor tissue is not available. To obtain the graft, a small cut is made at the limbus with a stainless steel blade. When the desired depth is reached, a cyclodialysis spatula is used to perform a lamellar dissection of the entire donor cornea (Figure 31-8). The proper size trephine is then used to cut the lamellar graft from the donor eye (Figure 31-9).

If donor tissue is available only in the form of a cornea with a few millimeters of attached sclera, as for penetrating keratoplasty, the graft is punched from the endothelial surface with a trephine, and the endothelium, Descemet's membrane, and part of the posterior stroma (how much depends on the desired thickness of the graft) are dissected away from the donor cornea, leaving the remainder as the lamellar graft.[18] Descemet's membrane should not be left on a lamellar graft because it inhibits healing of the graft to the recipient cornea. Except in keratoconus, the donor graft should be cut slightly larger than the keratectomy bed to facilitate apposition of the edge of the graft to the edge of the keratectomy bed without compression of the underlying cornea and shallowing of the anterior chamber. Because the objective in keratoconus is to flatten the cornea, the donor graft for this disorder should have the same diameter as the recipient keratectomy bed.

The donor lamellar graft is placed in the keratectomy bed and secured with interrupted or running 10-0 nylon sutures (Figures 31-10 and 31-11). In keratoconus, removal of aqueous humor is occasionally necessary to obtain adequate wound closure.

If a noncircular graft is required, it must be fashioned freehand to fit the keratectomy bed. This is best done by cutting one side of the graft and suturing this side to an edge of the keratectomy bed. Another side of the graft is then cut and this side is sutured into place. The sequence of cutting and suturing is repeated until the graft has been tailored to fit the keratectomy bed.

At the end of the procedure, a topical antibiotic ointment is applied, and an eye pad and shield are placed.

POSTOPERATIVE CARE

The eye pad and shield are removed 24 hours postoperatively, and the eye is examined for re-epithelialization, inflammation, and intraocular pressure elevation. Re-epithelialization of the graft is encouraged with patching, a bandage soft contact lens, or a temporary tarsorrhaphy,

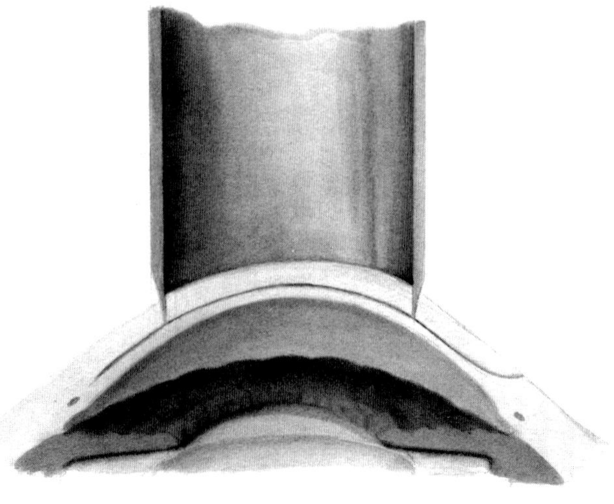

FIGURE 31-9 Trephination of the donor lamellar graft.

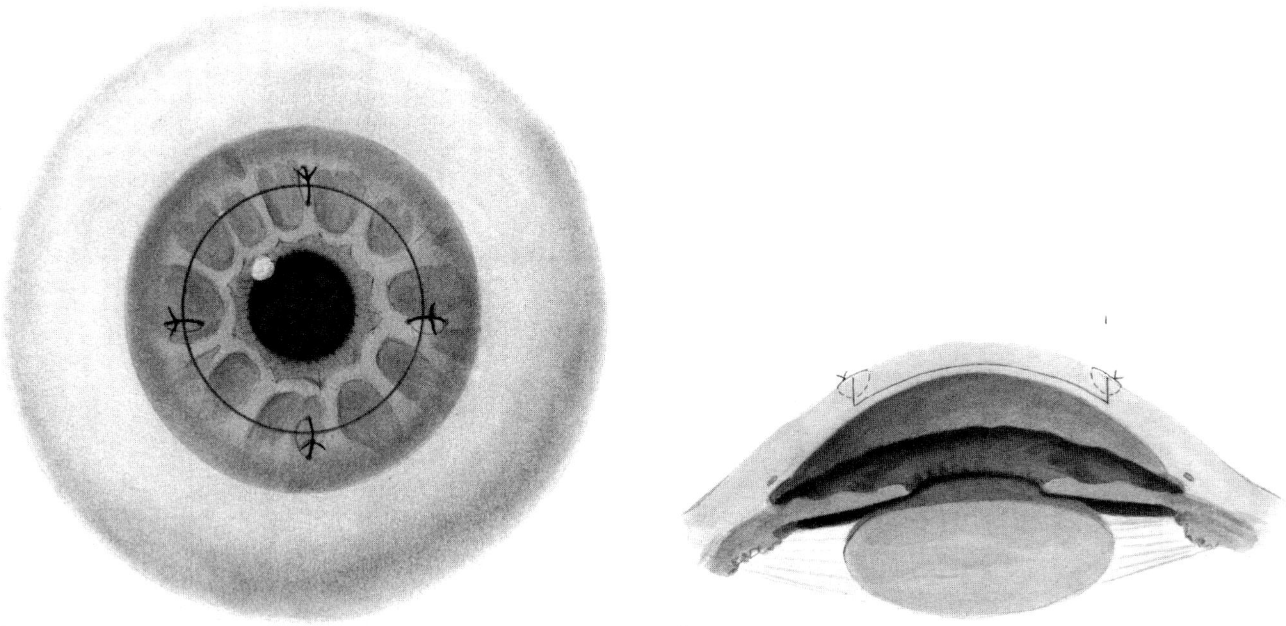

A

B

FIGURE 31-10 **(A)** Top and **(B)** cross-sectional views of suturing the lamellar graft with interrupted sutures. Only the cardinal sutures are shown here. A total of 12 or 16 sutures are usually required to secure a graft of this size.

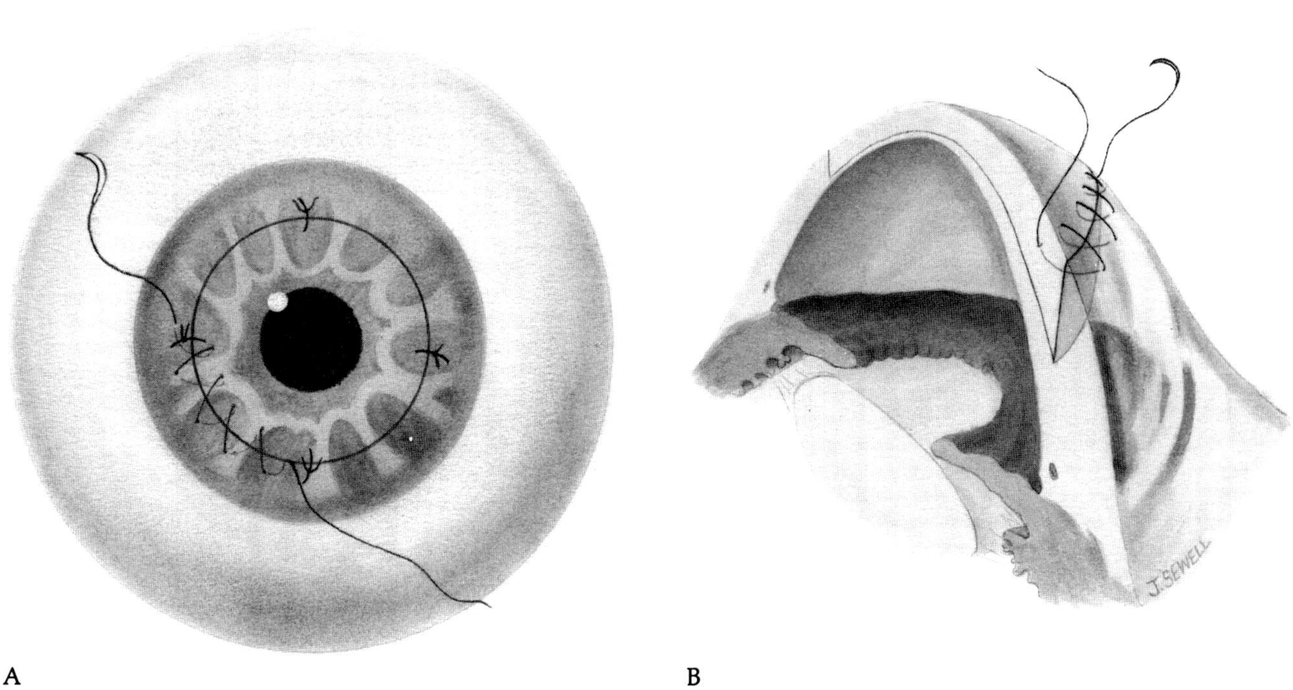

A

B

FIGURE 31-11 **(A)** Top and **(B)** cross-sectional views of suturing the lamellar graft with a running suture.

if necessary. A topical antibiotic eye drop or ointment is used four times a day for 1 week or until the epithelium has healed. Topical corticosteroid eye drops may be used four times a day for several weeks, if needed, to treat inflammation, or in an attempt to decrease scarring of the interface. Sutures are removed as soon as they loosen or become vascularized.

COMPLICATIONS

Corneal perforation is the most important intraoperative complication of inlay lamellar keratoplasty. It usually can be prevented by careful lamellar dissection of the recipient cornea with a blunt instrument. If perforation occurs, however, the procedure usually can be completed using careful sharp dissection of the remaining portion of the bed. The donor lamellar graft should be secured such that the interface between the recipient cornea and lamellar graft is tight. Otherwise, aqueous humor may percolate through the perforation and accumulate in the interface.

Uneven dissection can result in a rough keratectomy bed or posterior graft surface, creating a structurally and optically poor donor-recipient interface.

Incorporation of foreign particles into the keratectomy bed is a common problem. Care must be taken to keep glove powder, cellulose sponge material, lint, and epithelial cells from the interface. The graft can be anchored with three or four sutures, followed by irrigation of the interface with several milliliters of filtered balanced salt solution and removal of any debris with suction.

Imperfect coaptation of the edges of the lamellar graft and recipient cornea can result in astigmatism and epithelialization of the interface.[18,20,24-26]

REFERENCES

1. Richard JM, Paton D, Gasset AR: A comparison of penetrating and lamellar keratoplasty in the surgical management of keratoconus. Am J Ophthalmol 86:807, 1978
2. Wood TO: Lamellar transplants in keratoconus. Am J Ophthalmol 83:543, 1977
3. Van Loenen Martinet AHJ: Twenty therapeutic lamellar corneal grafts for herpes simplex. Trans Ophthalmol Soc UK 92:859, 1972
4. Laibson PR: Surgical approaches to the treatment of active keratitis. Int Ophthalmol Clin 13:65, 1973
5. Moretti JF: *Pseudomonas* corneal ulcer treated by full-thickness graft in a lamellar bed. Ann Ophthalmol 13:233, 1981
6. Morrison JC, Swan KC: Full-thickness lamellar keratoplasty. Ophthalmology 89:715, 1982
7. Reeh MJ: Corneoscleral lamellar transplant for recurrent pterygium. Arch Ophthalmol 86:296, 1971
8. Charieux J: Atypical lamellar grafts. Trans Ophthalmol Soc UK 92:3, 1972
9. Laughera PA, Arentsen JJ: Lamellar keratoplasty in the management of recurrent pterygium. Ophthalmic Surg 17:106, 1986
10. Breinin EM, DeVoe AG: Chelation of calcium with EDTA in band keratopathy and corneal calcium affectations. Arch Ophthalmol 52:846, 1954
11. Wood TO, Walker GG: Treatment of band keratopathy. Am J Ophthalmol 80:553, 1975
12. Wood TO, Fleming JC, Dotson RS, Cotton MS: Treatment of Reis-Bücklers' corneal dystrophy by removal of subepithelial fibrous tissue. Am J Ophthalmol 85:360, 1978
13. Soliman MM, Ayoub M: Lamellar keratoplasty in keratoconus. Bull Ophthalmol Soc Egypt 68:95, 1975
14. Benson WH, Goosey CB, Prager TC, Goosey JD: Visual improvement as a function of time after lamellar keratoplasty for keratoconus. Am J Ophthalmol 116:207, 1993
15. Wood TO, Tuberville AW: Phakic keratoplasty: results in keratoconus. p. 200. In Brightbill FS (ed): Corneal Surgery: Theory, Technique, and Tissue. CV Mosby, St. Louis, 1986
16. Kaufman HE, Werblin TP: Epikeratophakia for the treatment of keratoconus. Am J Ophthalmol 93:342, 1982
17. McDonald MB, Kaufman HE, Durrie DS, et al: Epikeratophakia for keratoconus. The nationwide study. Arch Ophthalmol 104:1294, 1986
18. Gasset AR: Lamellar keratoplasty in the treatment of keratoconus: conectomy. Ophthalmic Surg 10(2):26, 1979
19. Vancea PP, Schwartzenberg T: Lamellar keratoplasty in keratoconus. Albrecht von Graefes Arch Klin Exp Ophthalmol 212:55, 1979
20. Malbran E, Stefani C: Lamellar keratoplasty in corneal ectasias. Indications, surgical technique, results and complications. Ophthalmologica 164:50, 1972
21. Malbran E, Stefani C: Lamellar keratoplasty in corneal ectasias. Refractive results. Ophthalmologica 164:59, 1972
22. Polack FM: Lamellar keratoplasty. Arch Ophthalmol 86:293, 1971
23. Fine M: Techniques of keratoplasty. Int Ophthalmol Clin 10:289, 1970
24. Barraquer JI: Lamellar keratoplasty (special techniques). Ann Ophthalmol 4:437, 1972
25. Anwar M: Dissection technique in lamellar keratoplasty. Br J Ophthalmol 56:711, 1972
26. Smirmaul H, Casey TA: A clear view trephine and lamellar dissector for corneal grafting. Am J Ophthalmol 90:92, 1980

32

Onlay Lamellar Keratoplasty

MARGUERITE B. McDONALD

Two types of lamellar keratoplasty are used in the treatment of various pathologic corneal conditions: (1) inlay lamellar keratoplasty, which restores integrity to the globe in selected cases of perforation or replaces corneal tissue that has been lost or resected; and (2) onlay lamellar keratoplasty, which reinforces thin, ectatic corneas in patients with keratoconus, keratoglobus, or pellucid marginal degeneration (Figure 32-1). The uses of inlay lamellar grafts are described in Chapters 21 and 31. This chapter is confined to a discussion of the uses of onlay lamellar grafts originally developed by Kaufman and Werblin.[1] For a complete overview of the ectatic disorders that can be treated with onlay lamellar grafts, see Chapter 22.

The advantages of onlay lamellar keratoplasty over penetrating keratoplasty, for patients who are candidates for the procedure, are (1) onlay lamellar keratoplasty is an extracellular procedure and, as such, avoids serious, vision-threatening complications or permanent vision loss that can be associated with any intraocular procedure (e.g., penetrating keratoplasty); (2) an onlay lamellar graft is removable, which permits penetrating keratoplasty to be performed later if the onlay lamellar graft is not successful; and (3) the risk of rejection with an onlay lamellar graft is nil.[2,3] The advantages of onlay lamellar keratoplasty over inlay lamellar keratoplasty are (1) the preparation of the recipient bed is technically easier and less time-consuming, (2) the risk of corneal perforation is virtually nonexistent, and (3) the procedure is reversible. This chapter describes patient selection, surgical techniques, results, and complications of onlay lamellar keratoplasty for keratoconus, keratoglobus, and pellucid marginal degeneration.

KERATOCONUS

Indications

The primary indication for onlay lamellar keratoplasty for keratoconus is moderately advanced keratoconus in a patient who is intolerant to contact lens wear and who has no central corneal scarring within 1 mm of the visual axis. Candidates for this procedure should be able to demonstrate a best-corrected visual acuity of 20/40 or better with a hard contact lens placed on the eye for diagnostic purposes.

Because keratoconus is a disorder most often seen in relatively young and active patients, even moderate progression of the disorder can produce visually crippling disability. These patients cannot function if they are unable to wear their hard contact lenses for most of their waking hours; they lose the ability to read, work, drive, and carry out their daily activities. Therefore, patients with moderately advanced keratoconus who cannot wear contact lenses for enough hours of the day to satisfy their living requirements are candidates for onlay lamellar keratoplasty.

Because an onlay lamellar graft does not replace diseased tissue, the underlying cornea must be free of scarring in the central optical zone. Existing scars must be at least 1 mm from the visual axis because the flattening and folding of the ectatic cornea by the onlay graft may push paracentral scars into the optical zone, resulting in poor vision.

The best contact-lens–corrected visual acuity is measured without a pinhole, to prevent misleading results based on an artificial situation. A pinhole greatly reduces glare from paracentral scars. If, for example, a patient sees 20/400 with spectacles, 20/60 with a hard contact lens and over-refraction, and 20/30 with a pinhole, the patient is not a

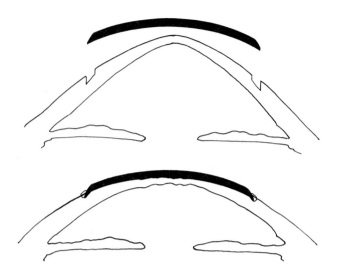

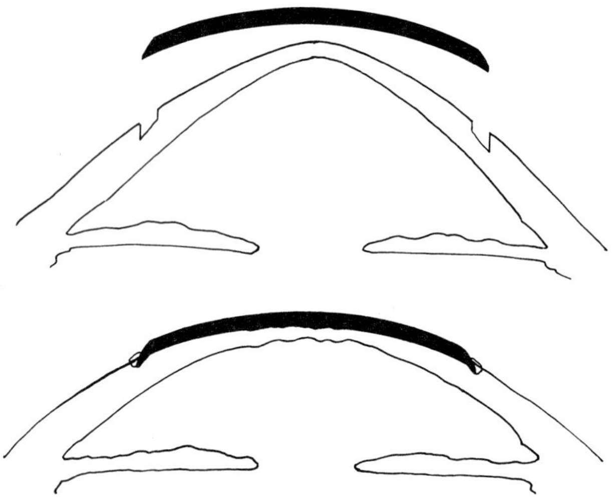

FIGURE 32-1 Onlay lamellar keratoplasty for ectatic corneal disorders is performed by suturing lamellar tissue into a peripheral keratectomy. This results in flattening and reinforcement of the ectatic cornea.

candidate for onlay lamellar keratoplasty, because the best possible postoperative visual acuity will be no better than the contact-lens-corrected visual acuity (i.e., 20/60).

Other potential candidates for onlay lamellar keratoplasty are keratoconus patients who have had penetrating keratoplasty in one eye, followed by repeated episodes of graft rejection requiring large amounts of corticosteroids over long periods of time. Some studies have shown that patients with keratoconus who have recurrent graft rejection episodes and/or repeat penetrating keratoplasty for a failed graft caused by graft rejection in one eye may have the same problems with penetrating keratoplasty in the other eye.[4] Topical corticosteroids often produce glaucoma and secondary cataract; their use may be avoided with onlay lamellar keratoplasty rather than penetrating keratoplasty. Additionally, patients whose lifestyle takes them far from medical care may be better off with a lamellar graft that carries no risk of endothelial rejection.

Patients with Down syndrome, who demonstrate an increased incidence of keratoconus, are also candidates for onlay lamellar keratoplasty.[5] This extraocular procedure may be preferred in such patients, who may cooperate poorly with postoperative care and who may be insufficiently articulate to make known the appearance of early symptoms of graft rejection. Self-inflicted or accidental damage to a lamellar graft is less serious and less vision threatening than similar injury to a penetrating graft. Early intervention with a lamellar graft may be preferable to multiple painful episodes of contact lens abrasions and/or hydrops leading to scarring, such that the only surgical alternative is penetrating keratoplasty. Less long-term postoperative care is required with a lamellar graft, which is preferable for an institutionalized patient.

Preoperative Evaluation

Before surgery, a complete ophthalmic examination is performed, including keratometry measurements, videokeratography, and refraction with a hard contact lens without a pinhole. All scars are noted and their distance from the visual axis is measured.

If there is a question as to the distance of a paracentral scar from the visual axis, the patient can be taken to minor surgery and asked to fixate on the filament of the operating microscope. The surgeon marks the visual axis (using the system most appropriate to the type of operating microscope) by making a small mark on the epithelium with a surgical marking pen. Using the reticle of a slit lamp microscope, the distance from the proximal end of the scar to the visual axis is then measured.

Occasionally, the tip of the cone is so irregular that the patient finds it difficult to fixate exactly on the filament of the microscope. In this case, the patient will make rapid fixation movements in a searching pattern, which means that the light rays are so diffracted by the cone that the patient does not know where to look. One possibly helpful maneuver is to place a plano soft contact lens on the cone, which may reduce the diffraction of light and enable the patient to fixate. The surgeon can then measure the distance of the scar from the visual axis with calipers. If there is any doubt about the proximity of a corneal scar to the visual axis, however, onlay lamellar keratoplasty should not be attempted and penetrating keratoplasty is recommended.

Tissue

Although some institutions are equipped to make onlay lamellar tissue, commercial tissue can be ordered from Cryo-Optics. The tissue is shipped in a vial containing a corneal preservation medium (Optisol). The lamellar tissue for the average keratoconus patient should have a diameter of 10 mm, a central thickness of 0.3 mm, and a 0.25-mm wide circumferential wing that tapers to 0.13 mm in thickness at the peripheral edge. The tissue has no optical power; in the optical zone, Bowman's layer and the posterior stromal surface are parallel. Tissue can be ordered in diameters up to 12 mm, but a 10-mm diameter is usually sufficient to prevent the development of permanent recipient folds over the visual axis, and a 10-mm graft in a 9-mm bed produces a marked reduction in myopia. Some investigators have cut an appropriate correction into the lamellar tissue by excimer laser photoablation and then attached the tissue to the recipient cornea with no attempt to flatten the cone.

Surgical Techniques

The patient is given local or general anesthesia; the choice depends on patient and physician preferences, as well as the general health of the patient. The eye is prepped and draped, and the eyelids are separated with a speculum. I prefer Jaffe specula. Silk (4-0) bridle sutures are placed through the superior and inferior rectus muscles, and the ends of the sutures are clamped to the drape with hemostats. The two rectus muscle sutures are used to stabilize the eye and to position it in later stages of the procedure.

The central corneal epithelium is removed with a Paton spatula. A cuff of epithelium 0.5 mm wide is left at the limbus to aid re-epithelialization of the graft surface after surgery. The surgical field is irrigated with balanced salt solution that is dispensed from a 20-ml syringe with a 20-μm Millipore filter and cannula. Aspiration is accomplished using an infant feeding tube attached to suction. Irrigation and aspiration are performed frequently during the removal of the epithelium to remove debris.

For a procedure involving a 10.0-mm graft (currently the most common size that I use), a 9.0-mm Barron radial vacuum trephine is used to cut the patient's cornea. This trephine is described and illustrated in Chapter 34. Before the trephine is used, the blade is observed under the operating microscope and positioned evenly with the inner wall of the vacuum chamber. The blade is then retracted three quarter-turns from this position so that it will not interfere with the establishment of suction. The trephine is placed on the eye such that the cone is enveloped within the blade. Perforation may occur if there is keratoconic tissue beneath the blade of the trephine. It is, therefore, important to ensure that the entire cone is surrounded by the blade. The cross hairs of the trephine may be cut and removed if they come into contact with the apex of the cone. After the trephine has been positioned, the plunger of the 5-ml syringe attached to the trephine is pushed in all the way, and the trephine is pressed gently on the cornea. The plunger is released abruptly to establish suction. The plunger usually stops at the 4.0-ml mark on the syringe if suction has been obtained. The trephine is gently supported by the struts at the top of the trephine with no upward or downward pressure applied. The plastic spokes on top of the blade assembly are slowly rotated clockwise five quarter-turns: three quarter-turns to reach the corneal surface, and two quarter-turns to make the cut. It is important not to confuse quarter-turns with full-turns, as this may result in a cut that is too deep, or even in corneal perforation.

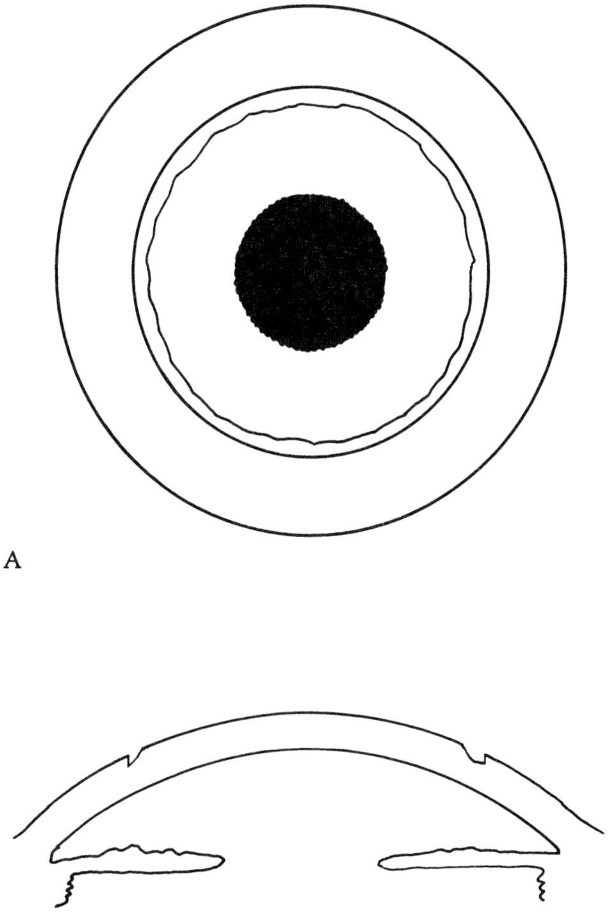

A

B

FIGURE 32-2 An annular keratectomy is performed by grasping the central edge of the trephine cut and excising an annular, wedge-shaped rim of tissue 0.5 mm wide using Vannas scissors held at a 45-degree angle. **(A)** Top view. **(B)** Cross-sectional view.

The plunger of the syringe attached to the trephine is pushed in all the way, which releases suction, the trephine is removed from the cornea, and the cut is inspected. The cut should be approximately 0.15 mm deep and should completely surround but not invade the cone. Even if the cut is somewhat decentered (i.e., closer to the limbus on one side than the other), there is no problem as long as the cone has been completely encircled. The 16 radial impressions made by the trephine peripheral to the cut are marked with a methylene blue or gentian violet surgical marking pen. These marks are used as a guide for suture placement.

The central edge of the trephine cut is grasped with a 0.12-mm forceps, and a circumferential 0.5-mm wide wedge of tissue is resected with curved Vannas scissors held at a 45-degree angle (Figure 32-2). This results in an annular

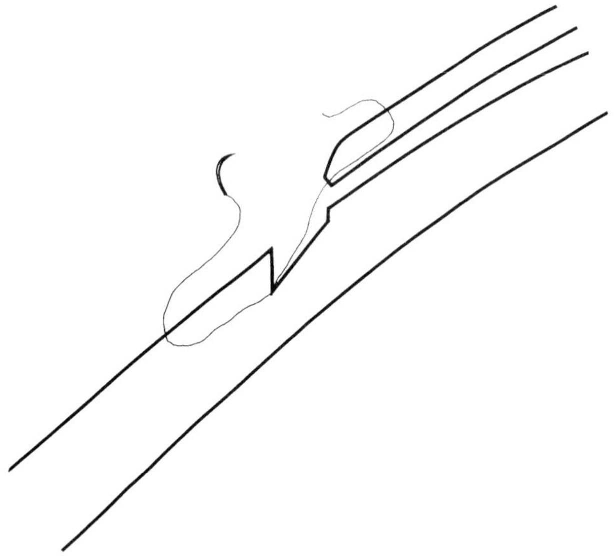

FIGURE 32-3 Sutures enter the lamellar tissue 0.75 mm central to the peripheral edge, exit near the bottom of the wing, enter the cornea at the depth of the annular keratectomy, and exit the cornea 1 mm peripheral to the keratectomy.

keratectomy 0.5 mm wide, with the deepest part of the keratectomy on the peripheral edge nearest the limbus.

The field is irrigated and aspirated again for debris. The lamellar tissue is grasped with a Polack forceps, which is a double-toothed forceps that is ideal for transferring the tissue across the surgical field because it provides a secure hold on the tissue. Under high magnification, the tissue is inspected for debris. The stromal surface is rinsed with a gentle stream from the irrigating syringe; visible debris can be dislodged by gently stroking the surface of the tissue with the blunt cannula of the syringe if necessary. The infant feeding tube is held by the assistant at the opposite edge of the tissue to aspirate the irrigation fluid and accompanying debris. This procedure is repeated for the Bowman's layer side of the tissue, for the surface of the recipient bed, and once more for the stromal side of the tissue.

The tissue is attached to the recipient cornea with 16 interrupted 10-0 nylon sutures. For the first suture, the lamellar tissue is grasped firmly with a Polack forceps and the needle is passed between the two prongs of the forceps, 0.75 mm central to the edge of the tissue. Once the tissue is engaged with the point of the needle, the needle is turned 90 degrees so that it traverses the stroma of the wing, splitting the wing and emerging as close to the posterior surface as possible (Figure 32-3). The peripheral aspect of the keratectomy is grasped with a 0.12-mm forceps at the superior radial mark, and the needle is passed into the base of the keratectomy and peripherally for a distance of 1 mm, then turned to emerge from the surface of the recipient cornea. This tucks the edge of the graft into the annular keratectomy. The suture is tied with a triple throw followed by two single throws, with as much tension as can be generated without breaking the suture.

The superior suture is placed first, followed by the inferior suture, and then the nasal and temporal sutures. Care is taken to distribute the tissue evenly as these sutures are placed. Immediately before the triple throw is cinched, on every second suture, the assistant presses firmly on the anterior surface of the tissue with a Paton spatula to flatten the cone so that the surgeon can tie the suture with maximal tension, ensuring that the edge of the graft is apposed to the peripheral edge of the keratectomy (Figure 32-4). During suturing, the intermittent compression on the center of the cornea flushes aqueous humor out through the trabecular meshwork, and the eye is softened, which allows the cone to flatten and the sutures to be tightly tied. These brief periods (5 to 10 seconds) of compression present no danger of compromising the vascular circulation to the optic nerve and retina. There is usually no difficulty in apposing the edge of the lamellar tissue to the peripheral edge of the keratectomy.

The next four sutures are placed equidistant between the first four sutures. Eight additional sutures are then placed equidistant between the first eight sutures. Sixteen sutures are usually sufficient to secure the graft. The wing of the graft should not protrude above the edge of the keratectomy at any point. If the edge of the graft appears to be protruding in any areas, additional sutures are placed in these areas. Protrusion of the wing leads to a flattening in that meridian and increases postoperative astigmatism. Properly performed, this suturing technique flattens the cone, reducing myopia and regular astigmatism.

The sutures are rotated to bury the knots in the recipient cornea. The knots are passed into the graft and into the recipient cornea or through the recipient cornea only with a small reverse direction tug given to the sutures, so that the knots lie just beneath the corneal surface and the ends of the sutures stream behind, forming small arrows pointing toward the surface. In this position, the knots are not irritating to the patient and will not pass through the surgical wound or the graft at the time of suture removal, thereby avoiding a possible iatrogenic dehiscence of the wound. Because of the tension on the sutures, at least half of them may break at the time of rotation; these are replaced until they can be rotated successfully.

By the end of the procedure, multiple wrinkles and folds are visible in the recipient cornea under the graft; these

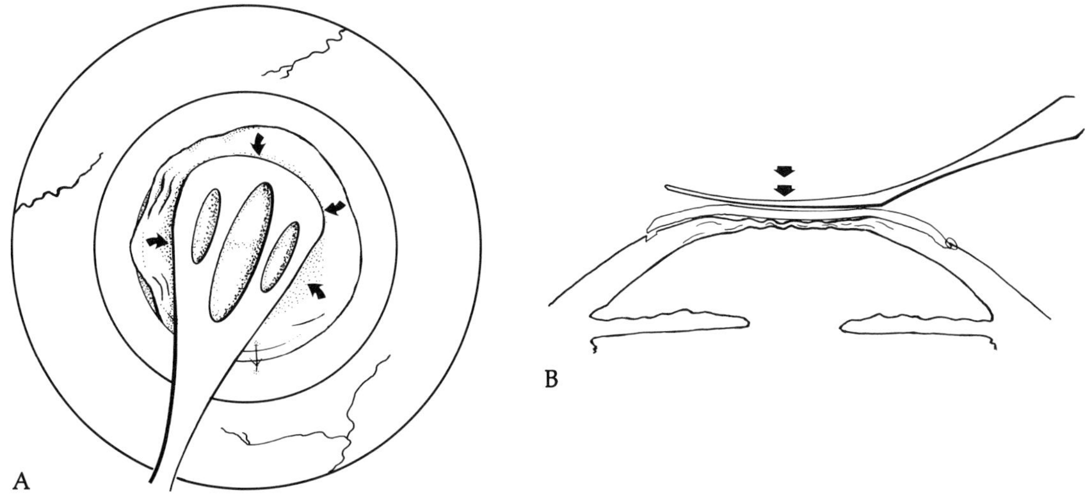

FIGURE 32-4 A Paton spatula is used to flatten the ectatic corneal tissue as the lamellar tissue is sutured into place. **(A)** Top view. **(B)** Cross-sectional view.

are the result of the compression and flattening of the cone and usually disappear within 6 weeks after surgery.

Methylprednisolone acetate (80 mg) is injected sub-Tenon's, and topical ciprofloxacin and 1 percent cyclopentolate eye drops are instilled. Long-acting cycloplegic agents are not used in patients with keratoconus because of reports of permanent pupillary dilation. The rectus muscle sutures and eyelid speculum are removed, a bandage soft contact lens is placed on the graft, the eyelids are closed, and an eye pad and a metal or plastic eye shield are applied.

For patients who cannot return for frequent follow-up visits, a temporary tarsorrhaphy can be placed at the end of the procedure, instead of a bandage soft contact lens, to aid in re-epithelialization.

Postoperative Care

The morning after surgery, the eye is examined for the presence of epithelium, and topical ciprofloxacin and 1 percent cyclopentolate are begun and continued twice a day. For patients who tolerate the bandage lens, this examination is repeated every 48 hours until the surface of the graft is completely covered with epithelium. Patients for whom the bandage lens is uncomfortable can have the lens removed and a pressure patch applied. In this case, the eye should be examined every 24 hours. When the epithelium is intact, the bandage lens or patch is removed, and the topical medications are discontinued. A bland antibiotic ointment, such as erythromycin, or a lubricating ointment without preservatives is applied four times a day and tapered over the course of 1 month.

Patients who have had a tarsorrhaphy need only be examined on the first day after surgery to be certain that the eyelids are tightly closed and again at 3 weeks after surgery to take down the tarsorrhaphy.

Topical corticosteroids are not used unless an intense allergic reaction to the sutures develops (sterile abscesses and neovascularization appearing within the first postoperative week around the sutures, with severe iritis) or if moderate or severe anterior chamber inflammation is seen. If needed, 0.1 percent dexamethasone sodium phosphate is applied topically four times a day for 1 week, and tapered thereafter.

The sutures are removed 3 months after surgery. Loose or neovascularized sutures are removed before that time, as necessary. Often the edge of the graft that is closest to the limbus heals first, and the sutures in that quadrant become neovascularized or loose, sometimes as early as 3 weeks after surgery in a young patient. Removal of sutures in one quadrant creates the appearance of an astigmatic graft, but this condition usually resolves when the remainder of the sutures are removed. Young patients, particularly those younger than 18 years of age, heal much more rapidly and may need to have all of the sutures removed by 4 weeks after surgery.

When any sutures are removed, the eye is usually patched for 24 to 48 hours to permit any epithelial defects to heal. If the sutures to be removed are loose and can be cut and removed without creating more than a pinpoint epithelial defect, patching can be avoided. In this case, erythromycin ointment is applied four times a day and tapered over the following 2 to 3 days.

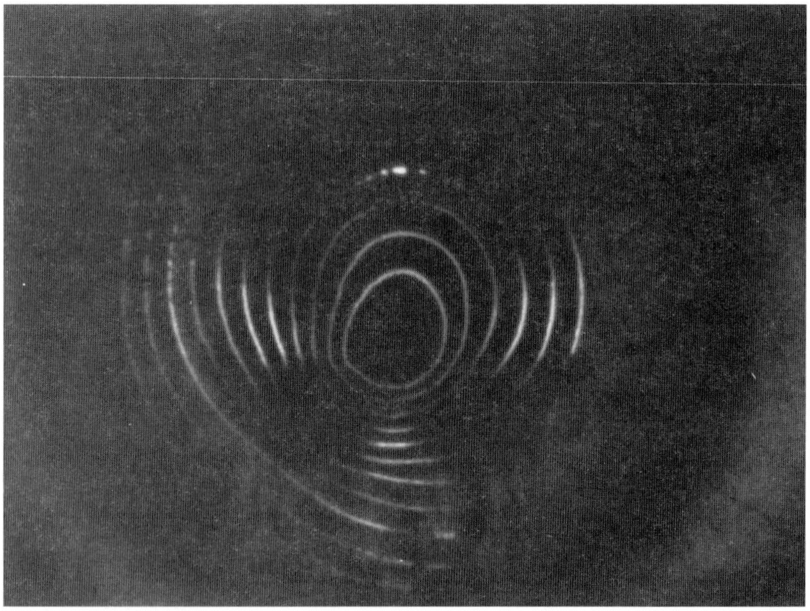
A

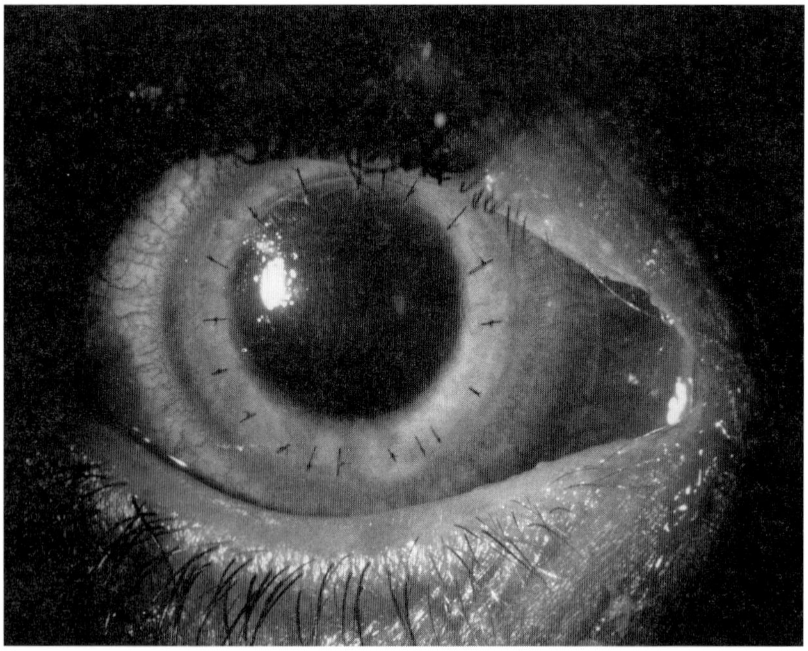
B

FIGURE 32-5 Onlay lamellar keratoplasty for keratoconus. **(A)** Preoperative photokeratograph shows severe irregular astigmatism. Keratometry readings were 49.25 by 64.50 diopters at 128 degrees. Best-corrected visual acuity was 20/80 with spectacles and 20/30 with a hard contact lens. **(B)** Onlay lamellar keratoplasty 1 day after surgery. *(continues)*

One month after the last suture has been removed (usually 4 months after surgery), the patient is fitted with a contact lens or spectacles. Most patients can wear a hard or rigid gas-permeable contact lens comfortably. Some choose spectacle correction, and some prefer soft contact lenses, but most have enough residual astigmatism to require a hard or rigid gas-permeable lens for optimal correction (Figure 32-5).

Results

In the first published results of the nationwide study of onlay lamellar keratoplasty for keratoconus,[3] the mean flattening by keratometry was 9 diopters, and the mean decrease in myopia, in terms of spherical equivalent, was 5 diopters. As a result, virtually all 82 patients with more than 30 days of follow-up demonstrated improved uncor-

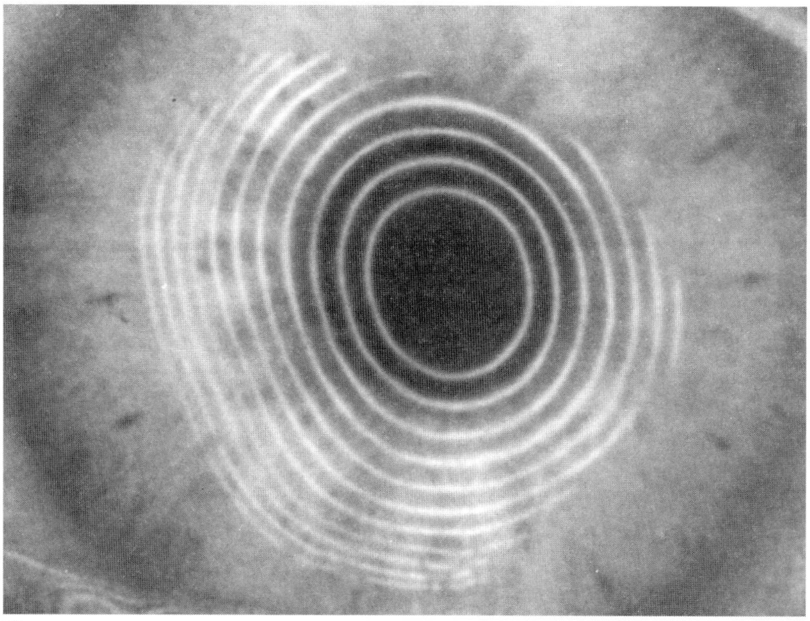

C

FIGURE 32-5 *(continued)* **(C)** Postoperative photokeratograph taken 3 months after surgery with some sutures still in place shows marked improvement of the irregular astigmatism. The central mires are regular, and there is residual against-the-rule astigmatism. Visual acuity was 20/40 with spectacles. One year after surgery, keratometry readings were 40.00 by 41.00 diopters at 90 degrees. Best-corrected visual acuity was 20/30 -1 with spectacles and 20/25 -1 with a hard contact lens.

rected visual acuity, some by as much as three or four Snellen lines. Most patients returned to within one line of their preoperative best-corrected visual acuity, 78 percent achieved 20/40 or better best-corrected visual acuity, and 10 percent required no postoperative overrefraction at all. In another study involving six eyes,[6] average corneal flattening was 6 diopters postoperatively; five of the six eyes demonstrated 20/40 or better spectacle-corrected visual acuity and three of the six eyes had 20/20 contact-lens–corrected visual acuity. Dietze and Durrie[7] reported their results in 19 patients. The mean decrease in myopia was 4.64 diopters. One year after surgery, all patients had a best-corrected visual acuity of 20/40 or better.

Three studies comparing onlay lamellar keratoplasty with penetrating keratoplasty for keratoconus with 1 to 6 years of follow-up[8–10] reported that the percentages of patients with 20/40 or better best-corrected visual acuity were similar, but in general, there were fewer patients with 20/20 visual acuity in the epikeratophakia groups, possibly as a result of decreases in contrast sensitivity.[9] A 1992 report described results in 16 keratoconus patients who received fresh, free-hand dissected lamellar tissue.[11] With 1 to nearly 4 years of follow-up, 14 (87.5 percent) had corrected visual acuities of 20/40 or better. A retrospective study of 10 consecutive patients with 5 years of follow-up showed long-term stability of best-corrected visual acuity, refractive astigmatism, and keratometric astigmatism; mean spectacle acuity was 20/30, but no patients had achieved best-corrected visual acuity of 20/20 at the end of the follow-up period.[12]

Complications

The medical complications of onlay lamellar keratoplasty are essentially the same as those of epikeratophakia for aphakia or myopia (see Ch. 39): failure to re-epithelialize the graft surface and chronic epithelial defects.[13]

Occasionally, fine blood vessels that reach the sutures before removal will recanalize and fill with blood, or new vessels will appear. This is usually the result of a poorly fitted contact lens, generally a lens that is too tight. A loose lens tends to slide off the visual axis or pop out of the eye, whereas a tight lens causes neovascularization and complaints of soreness, redness, and blurred vision. A tight lens should be discontinued immediately; a new lens can be fitted when the eye is quiet and the refraction has remained stable for two visits at least 1 week apart.

Optical complications include poor visual acuity and scarring in the graft. Poor visual acuity may be the result of poor patient selection, such as a case in which a paracentral scar in the patient's cornea is moved into the visual axis as the cone is compressed by the graft. Rarely, poor vision is due to a graft that has residual processing damage causing central haze, or a central subepithelial scar caused by delayed re-epithelialization. Correction of astigmatism after onlay lamellar keratoplasty for keratoconus by means of radial keratotomy[14] or relaxing incisions has been reported.[15]

In the nationwide study,[3] 11 of 177 grafts were removed. Three patients had repeat onlay lamellar keratoplasty, five (including one who had repeat onlay lamellar keratoplasty) underwent penetrating keratoplasty, and four had no further surgery.

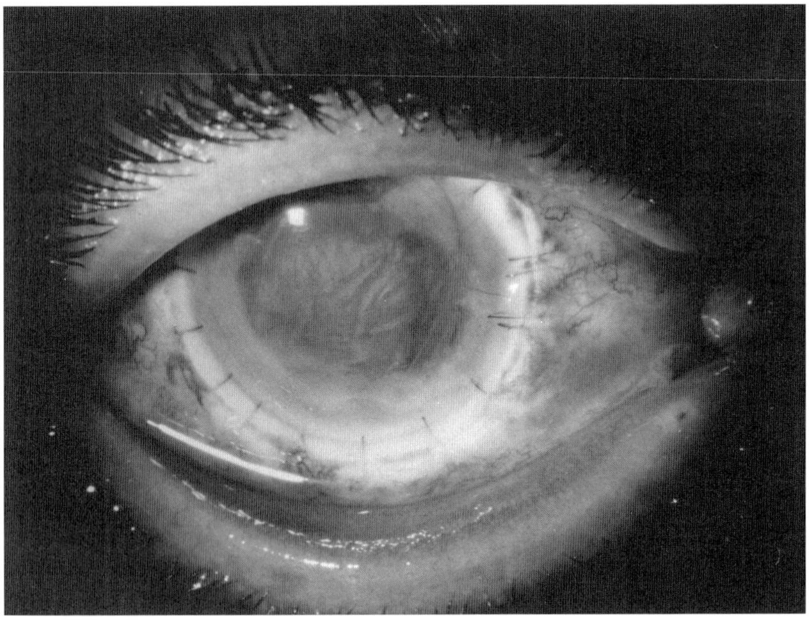

FIGURE 32-6 Onlay lamellar keratoplasty for keratoglobus. The 12-mm plano graft was sutured near the limbus. Note the numerous striae in the underlying cornea. A reefing suture is visible nasally.

In most patients, if penetrating keratoplasty becomes necessary, the onlay graft is removed before corneal transplantation is performed. Occasionally, if the underlying cornea is very thin, penetrating keratoplasty is performed through both the onlay graft and the underlying cornea, with the onlay graft providing tectonic support.

The results of subsequent penetrating keratoplasty are not compromised by prior onlay lamellar keratoplasty in patients with keratoconus. Successful penetrating keratoplasty has been reported in two patients who had onlay lamellar grafts, one[16] after a 3-year interval of deteriorating visual acuity and progressive contact lens intolerance and the other[17] after a 6-year interval and the development of progressive myopia. In a study at the Louisiana State University Eye Center,[18] 7 (8 percent) of 86 patients who underwent onlay lamellar keratoplasty for keratoconus subsequently had penetrating keratoplasty. Follow-up evaluation revealed that all patients achieved clear grafts and 20/40 or better best-corrected visual acuity.

KERATOGLOBUS

Patients with keratoglobus may have a corneal thickness of less than 0.1 mm and are poor candidates for penetrating keratoplasty. Often, such patients are left with no therapeutic option other than lamellar keratoplasty when contact lens wear becomes impossible. Onlay lamellar keratoplasty may be performed as part of a one- or two-step procedure (onlay lamellar keratoplasty alone or onlay lamellar keratoplasty followed by penetrating keratoplasty). In some patients, it may be feasible to flatten and reinforce the bulging cornea with a large onlay lamellar graft, much like the keratoconus procedure (Figure 32-6). If there is no central scarring, or if the scars can be manipulated out of the visual axis, the onlay graft may be all that is needed. If, however, there is severe central scarring, which is common in these eyes, the onlay graft is allowed to heal into place, and penetrating keratoplasty is performed 6 months later. The additional thickness of the large onlay graft provides more substantial tissue to which the smaller penetrating graft can be sutured.

Indications

Patients with keratoglobus usually have extremely thin, extremely steep corneas, with no areas of normal cornea. The central and peripheral corneal thicknesses are virtually the same. Scarring may be central, midperipheral, and/or peripheral, and is generally severe. Patients with keratoglobus who cannot be fitted with contact lenses, whose scarring precludes good vision, and who are not eligible for penetrating keratoplasty are candidates for onlay lamellar keratoplasty.

The preoperative examination for these patients is the same as for keratoconus patients, as described in the section above on preoperative evaluation, except that there is no visual acuity requirement because these patients have no alternative. However, careful counseling regarding the potential limits of visual rehabilitation should be undertaken to dispel unrealistic expectations on the part of the patient.

Surgical Techniques

The surgical procedure is similar to that for keratoconus, with a few exceptions. Extra care is taken during the removal of the epithelium because it is relatively easy to perforate the thin cornea. If a two-step procedure is planned, a blade can be used to scarify the surface of the recipient cornea very carefully after the epithelium has been removed. This scarification will help the onlay graft to adhere to the cornea, which will facilitate later penetrating keratoplasty. Ordinarily, for keratoconus patients, the onlay tissue heals to the cornea only in the area of the peripheral keratectomy; this leaves the central cornea clear and preserves the reversibility of the procedure, permitting the onlay tissue to be removed if necessary with no residual damage to the central cornea. In cases in which penetrating keratoplasty is to be performed after onlay lamellar keratoplasty, the scarification is of no visual consequence. If there is some doubt as to whether penetrating keratoplasty will be needed, only the midperiphery should be scarified, leaving the visual axis free; in the event that penetrating keratoplasty is not needed, vision will not be impaired by central scarification.

For this procedure, a lamellar graft 12 mm or 13 mm in diameter is placed in an 11-mm or 12-mm recipient bed, respectively. Although precut lamellar tissue is desirable, a full-thickness corneal donor graft can be used after the endothelium and Descemet's membrane are scraped off with a stainless steel blade (#15 Bard-Parker blade). The edge of the graft can be thinned so it is not elevated above the level of the recipient cornea after it is sutured in place.

A circular impression is made on the eye with the trephine just inside the limbus. Using this impression as a guide, the surgeon scratches down with a stainless steel blade (#64 or #75 Beaver blade) to a depth of 0.1 mm for 360 degrees. The central edge of the cut is grasped with a toothed forceps, and a wedge-shaped section of tissue 0.5 mm wide is resected around the cut with Vannas scissors. The keratectomy should be shallow centrally and 0.1 mm deep peripherally.

After the annular keratectomy is completed, but before the graft is sutured into place, an additional maneuver may be used to compress the ectatic cornea. Because the graft flattens the cornea to a great extent, it may throw the cornea into random folds that are too large to redistribute themselves after surgery, as occurs in keratoconus patients. Therefore, reefing sutures are used to pull the excess corneal tissue into folds in the periphery, resulting in a flattened and smooth central cornea (Figure 32-7).

In this procedure, four double-armed 10-0 nylon sutures, one in each quadrant, are used. The needle at each end of the suture is passed in a radial and nonpenetrating fash-

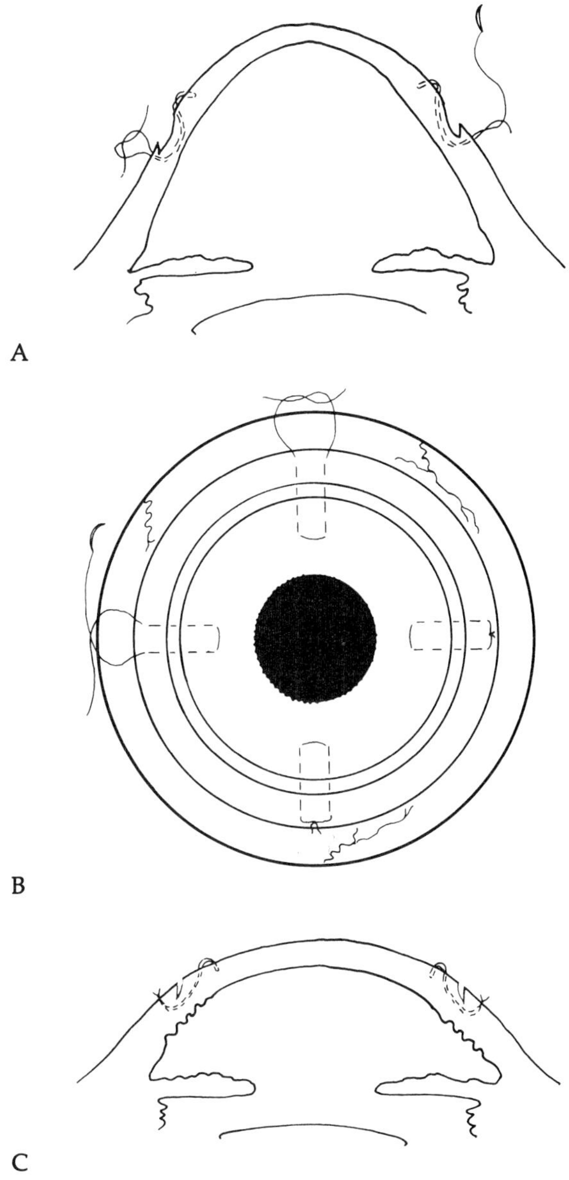

FIGURE 32-7 Reefing sutures. Mattress sutures are placed in the midperipheral cornea and tightened to throw the peripheral cornea into folds. The sutures are called reefing sutures because the peripheral cornea is bunched together, much like a reefed sail. Four sutures can be used to flatten and smooth the central cornea. Two sutures placed 90 degrees apart can be used to move a central scar away from the visual axis. **(A)** Reefing sutures are placed approximately 1 mm central to the keratectomy, with the two arms of the suture approximately 1 mm apart. They exit peripheral to the keratectomy. **(B)** Top view of four reefing sutures placed at 90 degree intervals. **(C)** Tightening the reefing sutures creates folds in the periphery and flattens the cornea. The onlay graft is placed on top of the smooth cornea and sutured into the peripheral keratectomy.

ion through the corneal stroma and pushed down below the depth of the keratectomy to emerge in the sclera just peripheral to the keratectomy. These sutures are tied tightly after a paracentesis is performed near the limbus to reduce the intraocular pressure, permitting the cornea to be flattened. The ends of the reefing sutures are left long so that these sutures can be removed 3 weeks after surgery.

After the reefing sutures are tied, the lamellar tissue is sutured in place. Twenty to 24 sutures are usually required because of the larger diameter of the graft compared with the graft used for keratoconus; 9-0 nylon may provide stronger force, but the suture knots are more difficult to bury compared with 10-0 nylon sutures. The knots are buried with the head of the knot just under the surface of the sclera so that they can be removed without disturbing the wound.

Postoperative medications are the same as for keratoconus patients, except that glaucoma medications are given at the end of the surgery. One drop of timolol is applied to the eye at the end of the case, and 500 mg of acetazolamide is given intravenously if there are no contraindications. Another 500-mg dose is given that evening and the next morning. The change in the architecture of the anterior chamber angle caused by suturing the graft over the trabecular meshwork and the shallowing of the anterior chamber tend to precipitate a sudden rise in intraocular pressure, especially if the graft is not at least 1 mm larger in diameter than the recipient bed. The intraocular pressure may be 50 mmHg or higher the morning after surgery. Occasionally, oral glycerin and intravenous mannitol, as well as topical glaucoma medications and oral acetazolamide are required for 24 to 72 hours after surgery. When the eye re-equilibrates with the shallower anterior chamber, intraocular pressure returns to normal.

Because limbal sutures must be removed sooner than corneal sutures, the first few sutures in keratoglobus patients are often removed within 7 to 10 days after surgery. The indications for suture removal are the same as in keratoconus: neovascularization approaching the surgical wound and loosening of the sutures. Nearly all of the sutures are removed by 2 months, especially in young patients; in teenagers, all sutures may be removed by 1 month after surgery. If sutures are not loose or causing vascularization, they are left in place for 3 months.

If best-corrected visual acuity is 20/40 or better 1 month after the sutures are removed, penetrating keratoplasty may not be needed. Often, best-corrected visual acuity is between 20/40 and 20/60 because there was scarring in the cornea that is now located in the visual axis. In such a case, the surgeon and the patient can decide, on the basis of the patient's needs and expectations, whether to proceed with penetrating keratoplasty.

Penetrating keratoplasty is performed no sooner than 6 months after onlay lamellar keratoplasty. The only major differences between penetrating keratoplasty after onlay lamellar keratoplasty and a primary penetrating keratoplasty for keratoconus are in the trephination and the suturing. Care is taken during trephination not to make two surgical wounds that overlap but do not coincide. The use of the Barron radial vacuum trephine and proceeding slowly are recommended to avoid this problem. Also, every other interrupted suture is passed beneath the recipient cornea (through-and-through sutures) and the alternating sutures are passed at the pre-Descemet's level in the recipient cornea. The deep sutures prevent the bottom layer of the onlay lamellar graft-cornea "sandwich"(i.e., the patient's cornea) from hanging down into the anterior chamber.

Whether keratoglobus patients have the one-step or the two-step procedure, they are generally able to be fitted with contact lenses postoperatively. Because keratoglobus combined with corneal surgery inevitably produces at least a moderate amount of regular and irregular astigmatism, vision is usually better with a hard or rigid gas-permeable contact lens.

Successful bilateral onlay lamellar keratoplasty for keratoglobus in a patient with severe diurnal variation in visual acuity has been described.[19] In another study,[20] five of six cases of onlay lamellar keratoplasty for keratoglobus associated with blue sclera were successful in providing tectonic support. Failure of re-epithelialization required removal of the graft in one eye. The three patients who were old enough for visual assessment showed improvement in best-corrected visual acuity. Reported complications of onlay lamellar keratoplasty for keratoglobus include peripheral interface opacities with no visual consequences[20] and massive epithelial cysts requiring replacement of the graft.[21]

PELLUCID MARGINAL DEGENERATION

Pellucid marginal degeneration can be treated with onlay lamellar keratoplasty (Figure 32-8). I consider pellucid marginal degeneration to be a type of keratoconus involving a massively decentered, inferior, "low-hanging" cone. The technique is the same as described for keratoconus, except that the inferior part of the graft is actually sutured into the sclera at the area of the limbus. The sutures near the limbus are removed early (1 to 2 months after surgery), as in keratoglobus patients. The postoperative course is similar to that of keratoconus patients. After surgery, these patients are able to resume daily contact lens wear for visual correction.[22]

FIGURE 32-8 Onlay lamellar keratoplasty for pellucid marginal degeneration. **(A)** Preoperative photokeratograph shows marked flattening in the vertical meridian centrally and marked steepening in the vertical meridian peripherally in the area of corneal thinning. The keratometry readings were 28.62 by 51.62 diopters at 170 degrees. (Reprinted with permission from LJ Maguire, SD Klyce, MB McDonald, HE Kaufman: Corneal topography of pellucid marginal degeneration. Ophthalmology 94:519, 1987. Courtesy of Ophthalmology.) **(B)** Postoperative clinical appearance shows that the onlay graft has been decentered inferiorly to support the inferior ectatic corneal tissue. Because the graft is closer to the limbus inferiorly, the inferior sutures have been removed first. *(continues)*

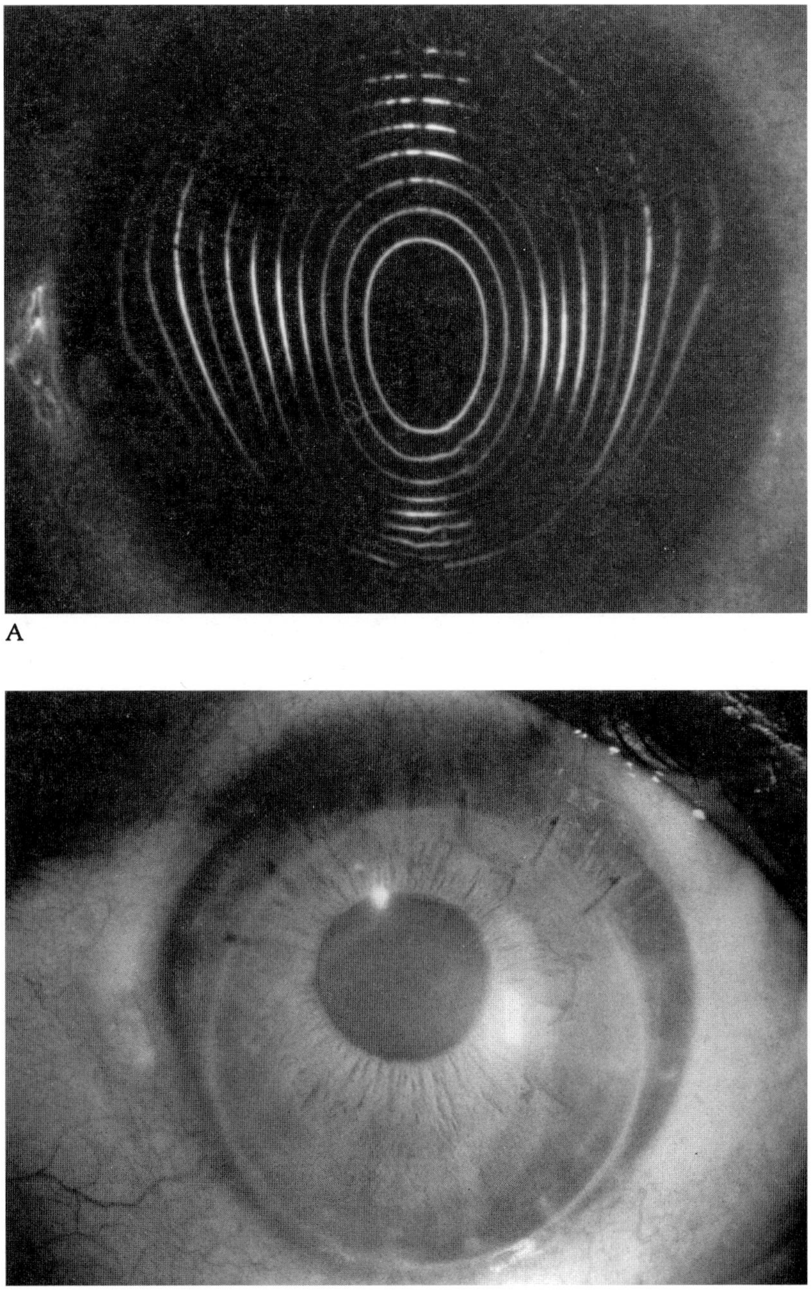

A

B

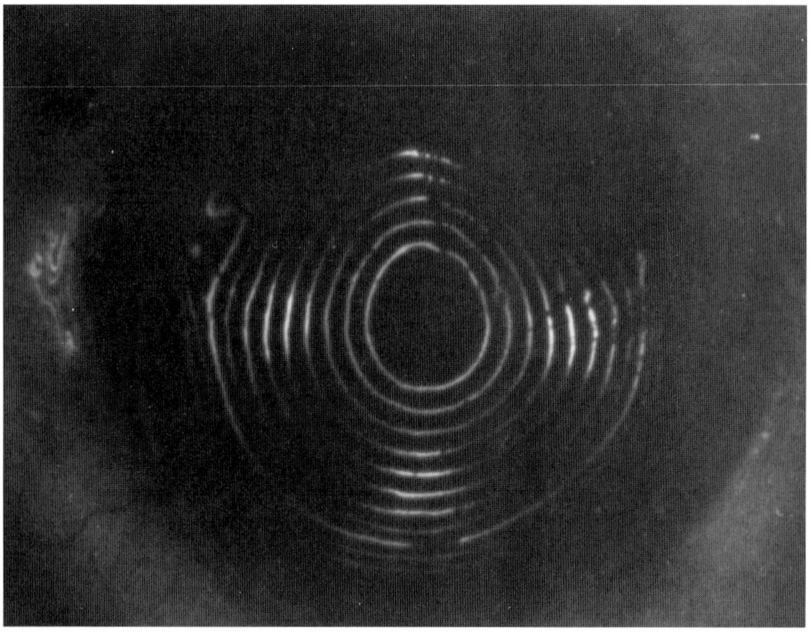

C

FIGURE 32-8 *(continued)* **(C)** Postoperative photokeratograph shows marked improvement of the astigmatism. There is still a slight amount of central flattening in the vertical meridian, and moderate irregular astigmatism is present. The keratometry readings were 43.75 by 48.00 diopters at 10 degrees. The patient was able to resume contact lens wear with a visual acuity of 20/25.

REFERENCES

1. Kaufman HE, Werblin TP: Epikeratophakia for the treatment of keratoconus. Am J Ophthalmol 93:342, 1982
2. McDonald MB, Koenig SB, Safir A, Kaufman HE: Onlay lamellar keratoplasty for the treatment of keratoconus. Br J Ophthalmol 67:615, 1983
3. McDonald MB, Kaufman HE, Durrie DS, et al: Epikeratophakia for keratoconus: the nationwide study. Arch Ophthalmol 104:1294, 1986
4. Donshik PC, Cavanagh HD, Boruchoff SA, Dohlman CH: Effect of bilateral and unilateral grafts on the incidence of rejections in keratoconus. Am J Ophthalmol 87:823, 1979
5. Høvding G, Haugen OH, Bertelsen T: Epikeratophakia for keratoconus in mentally retarded patients: the use of fresh, free-hand made lamellar grafts. Acta Ophthalmol (Copenh) 70:730, 1992
6. Lass JH, Stocker EG, Fritz ME, Collie DM: Epikeratoplasty: the surgical correction of aphakia, myopia, and keratoconus. Ophthalmology 94:912, 1987
7. Dietze TR, Durrie DS: Indications and treatment of keratoconus using epikeratophakia. Ophthalmology 95:236, 1988
8. Steinert RF, Wagoner MD: Long-term comparison of epikeratoplasty and penetrating keratoplasty for keratoconus. Arch Ophthalmol 106:493, 1988
9. Fronterre A, Portesani GP: Comparison of epikeratoplasty and penetrating keratoplasty for keratoconus. Refract Corneal Surg 7:167, 1991
10. Goosey JD, Prager TC, Goosey CB, et al: A comparison of penetrating keratoplasty to epikeratoplasty in the surgical management of keratoconus. Am J Ophthalmol 111:145, 1991
11. Høvding G, Bertelsen T: Epikeratophakia for keratoconus: long-term results using fresh, free-hand made lamellar grafts. Acta Ophthalmol (Copenh) 70:461, 1992
12. Waller SG, Steinert RF, Wagoner MD: Long-term results of epikeratoplasty for keratoconus. Cornea 14:84, 1995
13. Frangieh GT, Kenyon KR, Wagoner MD, et al: Epithelial abnormalities and sterile ulceration of epikeratoplasty grafts. Ophthalmology 95:213, 1988
14. Casebeer JC, Shapiro DR: Radial keratotomy in intact epikeratoplasty graft. Refract Corneal Surg 9:133, 1993
15. Fronterre A, Portesani GP: Relaxing incisions with compression sutures to reduce astigmatism after epikeratoplasty. Refract Corneal Surg 6:413, 1990
16. Goodman GL, Peiffer RL, Werblin TP: Failed epikeratoplasty for keratoconus. Cornea 5:29, 1986
17. Jaeger MJ, Berson P, Kaufman HE, Green WR: Epikeratoplasty for keratoconus. A clinicopathologic case report. Cornea 6:131, 1987
18. Frantz JM, Limberg MB, Kaufman HE, McDonald MB: Penetrating keratoplasty after epikeratophakia for keratoconus. Arch Ophthalmol 106:1224, 1988
19. Maguen E, Nesburn AB: Bilateral epikeratoplasty for variable diurnal vision and keratoglobus. J Refract Surg 3:12, 1987
20. Cameron JA, Cotter JB, Risco JM, Alvarez H: Epikeratoplasty for keratoglobus associated with blue sclera. Ophthalmology 98:446, 1991
21. al-Rajhi AA, al-Kharashi SA: Epithelial inclusion cysts following epikeratoplasty. J Refract Surg 12:516, 1996
22. Fronterre A, Portesani GP: Epikeratoplasty for pellucid marginal degeneration. Cornea 10:450, 1991

33

Corneal Preservation for Penetrating Keratoplasty

STEVEN E. WILSON AND WILLIAM M. BOURNE

Advances in corneal preservation have been paralleled by improvements in graft survival and increases in the number of penetrating keratoplasties. Further advances that extend the time corneal tissue can be preserved, augment the viability of preserved tissue, and improve tissue selection guidelines are needed to meet the increasing demand for donor corneas. This chapter provides information about the history of eye banking and corneal preservation, criteria for donor cornea selection, techniques for the assessment of endothelial cell viability, and methods of corneal preservation.

HISTORY OF EYE BANKING AND CORNEAL PRESERVATION

The first successful penetrating keratoplasty in a human was reported by Zirm in 1906.[1] The donor tissue came from the eye of an 11-year-old boy who had a perforating scleral injury that spared the cornea but required enucleation. The recipient had bilateral corneal opacification from a lye burn. Two grafts were obtained from the donor cornea, and the recipient underwent bilateral penetrating keratoplasty. Remarkably, one of the grafts remained clear for several years.

In the 1930s, the first corneal transplants from cadaver eyes were reported by Filatov[2] of Russia. He obtained whole eyes within a few hours of the donor's death, rinsed them in brilliant green solution, and stored at them at 4°C in glass jars for up to 56 hours before surgery. This procedure was the first known attempt at storage of donor corneal tissue, and Filatov is considered to be the father of modern eye banking. The first eye bank in the United States, the Eye-Bank for Sight Restoration, was founded in New York City in 1944 by ophthalmologist R. Townley Paton.

Subsequent methods developed to preserve donor corneas included drying,[3] formalin fixation,[4] freezing,[5] freeze-drying,[6,7] and liquid paraffin storage.[8] None of these approaches provided adequate preservation, however, and transplants performed with corneas preserved using these methods often ended in failure.

Stocker[9] was the first to recognize the importance of the corneal endothelium in the regulation of corneal hydration. This crucial observation, reported in the early 1950s, led to the emphasis on the maintenance of endothelial cell viability that has dominated research on corneal preservation to the present day.

In the same general time period, cryopreservation was under investigation as a means of achieving long-term preservation. Eastcott et al[10] were the first to report successful transplantation of cryopreserved corneas in humans. They pretreated the cornea in glycerol and then froze it in a mixture of alcohol and carbon dioxide. Nearly a decade later, Smith et al[11] introduced the use of dimethyl sulfoxide (DMSO) as a cryoprotectant for cultured rabbit corneal endothelium. Shortly thereafter, Mueller et al[12–14] successfully transplanted full-thickness animal and human corneas that had been preserved by injection of a solution containing dimethyl sulfoxide into the anterior chambers of whole eyes, then freezing the eyes in a solution containing glycerol.

A cryopreservation method developed by Capella et al[15] involved passing an extirpated cornea with a rim of sclera through a series of solutions with increasing concentrations of dimethyl sulfoxide followed by freezing and storage for up to 1 year. Thawing required a carefully monitored warming period. This method was technically demanding and resulted in less than optimal endothelial cell preservation. It was used successfully by a number of eye banks for several years, but the care required and the possibility of error resulted in this procedure being largely supplanted by simpler techniques (i.e., short- and intermediate-term preservation in corneal storage media).

The modern era of corneal storage began in early 1974 with the development of McCarey-Kaufman (M-K) medium.[16] This preservation solution consists of tissue culture medium, dextran, buffer, and antibiotics. Corneas can be stored successfully in this medium for up to 4 days at refrigerator temperatures (4°C). A modification of M-K medium is still used by eye banks throughout the world because of its simplicity and low cost.

A few years later, an organ-culture method for long-term preservation of corneas at 34 to 37°C was introduced by a group at the University of Minnesota, including Doughman, Lindstrom, and others.[17-21] The culture medium, which was composed of Eagle's minimum essential medium, calf serum, antibiotics, antifungal agents, and later chondroitin sulfate, allowed corneal preservation for more than 30 days.[18-22] The procedure is technically complex, however, which has precluded widespread use.

Based on studies in Japan in the 1960s suggesting the value of chondroitin sulfate in preservation media,[23-26] Kaufman et al[27] introduced K-Sol for storage of corneas at 4°C for up to 2 weeks.[27,28] K-Sol contained 2.5 percent chondroitin sulfate in tissue culture medium, with gentamicin and *N*-2-hydroxyethylpiperazine-*N'*-2-ethanesulfonic acid (HEPES) buffer. Although this medium is no longer available, most of the storage media in use in the United States today, including Dexsol and Optisol, are descendants of this formulation.

CRITERIA FOR DONOR CORNEA SELECTION

In the United States, eye banks commonly participate as the service agency in the procurement and distribution of corneal tissue. The Eye Bank Association of America (EBAA) promulgates medical standards designed to ensure that the recipient receives donor tissue of the highest quality and that the donor is free of diseases that could be transmitted to the recipient. This document, which is reviewed annually and approved by the Eye Banking Committee of the American Academy of Ophthalmology, is available from the Eye Bank Association of America, Washington, DC. The Eye Bank criteria for corneal donation are provided in Table 33-1, and some are discussed in the sections that follow.

A new problem that will become increasingly important is the screening of donor corneas that have had refractive surgery. Corneas that have had radial keratotomy can be easily detected by slit lamp microscopy and should be excluded. Corneas that have had photorefractive keratectomy or laser-assisted in situ keratomileusis, however, are frequently undetectable unless corneal curvature is measured with a portable keratometer. Although these corneas, including the corneal endothelium, are healthy, their use for transplantation can result in high hyperopia in the recipient. The 1996 Eye Bank Association of American medical standards document has added these forms of surgery as contraindications for use of donor tissue for penetrating keratoplasty.

Age Criteria

Upper Age Limit

Several studies have reported decreases in corneal endothelial cell density,[29-32] variations in endothelial cell size (polymegethism)[29,30,32] and shape (pleomorphism),[29,32,33] and alterations of endothelial cell function[30] with age. A number of clinical studies of penetrating keratoplasty, however, have detected no correlation between donor age and graft clarity[34-39] or donor age and endothelial cell loss over time after surgery.[38,39] A statistically significant positive correlation between donor age and endothelial cell layer fragility, as measured by intraoperative endothelial cell loss, has been reported,[29] and a retrospective case-control study of causes of primary graft failure found an increased risk with tissue from donors 70 years of age or older.[40]

Faced with these inconclusive findings, the Eye Bank Association of America has left the upper limit of donor age to the discretion of the medical directors of individual eye banks. Most medical directors have established an upper age limit of between 60 and 75 years for corneal donors. This criterion is arbitrary, however, and the argument can be made that endothelial cell density and morphology are the critical factors, regardless of the age of the donor. However, we prefer that the age of the donor not be significantly older than the age of the recipient, especially if the recipient is a child.

Lower Age Limit

Prenatal and infant corneas are steep; the average curvature at 40 weeks gestation is approximately 50 diopters.[41] Several studies have noted high myopia postoperatively when infant donor corneas are used.[42-44] Although some recommend the use of infant donor corneas in recipients in whom corneal steepening is desired to correct a refractive error, such as aphakia, we do not recommend this.

TABLE 33-1
Eye Bank Association of America Medical Standards for Donor Corneas

Donor Age

Since no definite relationship has been established between the quality of donor tissue and age, the upper and lower age limits are left to the discretion of the medical director.

Interval between Death, Enucleation, Excision and Preservation

Acceptable time intervals from death, enucleation or excision to preservation may vary according to the circumstances of death and interim means of storage of the body. It is generally recommended that corneal preservation occur as soon as possible after death.

Contraindications for Tissue for Penetrating Keratoplasty

Tissue from donors with the following are potentially health threatening for the recipient(s) or pose a risk to the success of the surgery and shall not be offered for surgical purposes:

1. Death of unknown cause
2. Death with neurologic disease of unestablished diagnosis
3. Creutzfeldt-Jakob disease
4. Subacute sclerosing panencephalitis
5. Progressive multifocal leukoencephalopathy
6. Congenital rubella
7. Reyes syndrome
8. Active viral encephalitis or encephalitis of unknown origin or progressive encephalopathy
9. Active septicemia (bacteremia, fungemia, viremia)
10. Active bacterial or fungal endocarditis
11. Active viral hepatitis
12. Rabies
13. Intrinsic eye disease
    a. Retinoblastoma
    b. Malignant tumors of the anterior ocular segment or known adenocarcinoma in the eye of primary or metastatic origin
    c. Active ocular or intraocular inflammation: conjunctivitis, scleritis, iritis, uveitis, vitreitis, choroiditis, retinitis
    d. Congenital or acquired disorders of the eye that would preclude a successful outcome for the intended use, e.g., keratoconus, keratoglobus, or a central donor corneal scar for an intended penetrating keratoplasty
    e. Pterygia or other superficial disorders of the conjunctiva or corneal surface involving the central optical area of the corneal button
14. Prior intraocular or anterior segment surgery
    a. Refractive corneal procedures, e.g., radial keratotomy, lamellar inserts
    b. Laser photoablation surgery
    c. Corneas from patients with anterior segment surgery (e.g., cataract, intraocular lens, glaucoma filtration surgery) may be used if screened by specular microscopy and meet the Eye Bank's endothelial standards
    d. Laser surgical procedures such as argon laser trabeculoplasty, retinal and panretinal photocoagulation do not necessarily preclude use for penetrating keratoplasty but should be cleared by the medical director
15. Leukemias
16. Active disseminated lymphomas
17. Hepatitis B surface antigen positive donors
18. Recipients of human pituitary-derived growth hormone (pit-hGH) during the years from 1963-1985
19. HTLV-I or HTLV-II infection
20. Hepatitis C seropositive donors
21. HIV seropositive donors
22. HIV or high risk for HIV: Persons meeting any of the following criteria should be excluded from donation: Behavioral/History Exclusionary Criteria (May, 1994 CDC Guidelines)
    a. Men who have had sex with another man in the preceding 5 years
    b. Persons who report nonmedical intravenous, intramuscular, or subcutaneous injection of drugs in the preceding 5 years
    c. Persons with hemophilia or related clotting disorders who have received human-derived clotting factor concentrates
    d. Men and women who have engaged in sex for money or drugs in the preceding 5 years
    e. Persons who have had sex in the preceding 12 months with any person described in items a–d above or with a person known or suspected to have HIV infection
    f. Persons who have been exposed in the preceding 12 months to known or suspected HIV-infected blood through percutaneous inoculation or through contact with an open wound, non-intact skin, or mucous membrane
    g. Inmates of correction systems (This exclusion is to address issues such as difficulties with informed consent and increased prevalence of HIV in this population.)

TABLE 33-1 *(continued)*

Specific Exclusionary Criteria for Pediatric Donors:

h. Children meeting any of the exclusionary criteria listed above for adults should not be accepted as donors
i. Children born to mothers with HIV infection or mothers who meet the behavioral or laboratory exclusionary criteria for adult donors (regardless of their HIV status) should not be accepted as donors unless HIV infection can definitely be excluded in the child as follows: Children more than 18 months of age who are born to mothers with or at risk for HIV infection, who have not been breast fed within the last 12 months, and whose HIV antibody tests, physical examination, and review of medical records do not indicate evidence of HIV infection can be accepted as donors
j. Children 18 months of age or younger who are born to mothers with or at risk for HIV infection or children of mothers with or at risk of HIV infection who have been breast fed within the last 12 months should not be accepted as donors regardless of their HIV test results

Laboratory and Other Medical Exclusionary Criteria

k. Persons who cannot be tested for HIV infection because of refusal, inadequate blood samples (e.g., hemodilution that could result in false-negative tests), or any other reasons
l. Persons with a repeatedly reactive screening assay for HIV-1 or HIV-2 antibody regardless of the results of supplemental assays
m. Persons whose history, physical examination, medical records, or autopsy reports reveal other evidence of HIV infection or high-risk behavior, such as a diagnosis of AIDS, unexplained weight loss, night sweats, blue or purple spots on the skin or mucous membranes typical of Kaposi's sarcoma, unexplained lymphadenopathy lasting more than 1 month, unexplained temperature higher than 100.5°F (38.6°C) for more than 10 days, unexplained persistent diarrhea, male-to-male sexual contact, sexually transmitted diseases, or needle tracks or other signs of parenteral drug abuse.

Abbreviations: CDC, Centers for Disease Control and Prevention; HIV, human immunodeficiency virus; HTLV, human T-cell leukemia virus.
Source: Information from Medical Advisory Board: Eye Bank Association of America Medical Standards, October 1996. Eye Bank Association of America, Washington, DC.

Better methods to correct aphakia exist, such as secondary intraocular lens implantation, and the postoperative topography of eyes that have had transplantation of infant corneas is unnatural, with a steeper than normal central curvature and a flatter than normal peripheral curvature. These eyes are often impossible to fit with a contact lens, if necessary, and binocular vision may not be possible unless the clear graft is replaced with a cornea of more normal curvature. In addition, corneas from young donors are flexible and have a tendency to fold over on themselves, which results in damage to the donor endothelium. For these reasons, we suggest that tissue from donors less than 3 years of age be used only in emergencies. The Eye Bank Association of America makes no recommendation on lower age limit for corneal donor tissue.

Medical Criteria

Detailed information about the transmission of diseases from the donor to the recipient by corneal transplantation has been published.[45–50] This chapter, therefore, provides only a summary of the current understanding of the risks of disease transmission.

Transmission of Bacteria and Fungi

Bacterial and fungal endophthalmitis are infrequent but serious complications of penetrating keratoplasty. Although studies correlating infection in the donor with infection in the recipient are few, there are enough data to confirm a definite risk. In a retrospective evaluation of 1,876 penetrating keratoplasties performed at a single institution,[51] three of four cases that developed bacterial endophthalmitis grew the same organism from the donor corneoscleral rim as from the aqueous humor and vitreous of the recipient. A more recent report involving 1,010 penetrating keratoplasties found three cases of bacterial endophthalmitis, all caused by streptococci, and one case of *Candida albicans* endophthalmitis. In all cases except one case of streptococcal endophthalmitis, the same organism was cultured from the donor rim.[52] Another report described the development of *C. albicans* in two patients who received corneas from the same donor.[53] Also, a number of cases of bacterial and fungal endophthalmitis after penetrating keratoplasty with corneas from septic donors have been published.[54–58] These reports support the recommendation by the Eye Bank Association of America for exclusion of tissue from donors with bacterial or fungal sepsis.

Despite the inclusion of antibiotics in all currently available preservation media, cases of endophthalmitis continue to be reported. In the majority of cases, infection is attributable to organisms resistant to gentamicin; *Streptococcus viridans* is the most commonly reported pathogen.[59] In the study mentioned above involving 1,010 penetrating keratoplasties,[52] 14 percent of the donor rim cultures were positive for organisms; a large percentage of the gram-positive bacteria were resistant to gentamicin.

An investigation of supplementation of corneal storage medium with 1 of 11 different antibiotics showed that streptomycin was the most effective against gentamicin-resistant strains of various gram-positive bacteria, although efficacy was much reduced at 4°C.[60] However, it should be noted that, in general, the antibiotics in corneal preservation solutions have little effect during storage at 4°C but are soaked up by the tissue and released after transplantation, achieving the bactericidal effect in the eye.[61,62] A formulation of Optisol containing streptomycin in addition to gentamicin, called *Optisol GS*, became commercially available in 1992. The efficacy and safety of vancomycin in preservation media has been investigated,[63–65] but to date this antibiotic has not been included in a commercially available preservation medium because of its short (less than 2 years) shelf life.

Amphotericin[66] has been considered as an antifungal supplement, but toxicity proved to be an insurmountable problem.

Transmission of Viruses

The two most prevalent viral infections that preclude corneal tissue donation are hepatitis and human immunodeficiency virus (HIV), the causative agent of acquired immunodeficiency syndrome (AIDS). The possibility of transmission of hepatitis B virus from an infected donor to the recipient by corneal transplantation was suggested by a study in which hepatitis B surface antigen was detected in washings of ocular tissue from corneal donors who had hepatitis B surface antigen present in the serum.[67] In addition, a 1986 memorandum from the Eye Bank Association of America described a case of possible transmission of hepatitis B virus from an infected donor to a recipient by corneal transplantation. For these reasons, the Eye Bank Association of America requires that a Food and Drug Administration (FDA)–approved screening test be negative for hepatitis B surface antigen before tissue is released for use.

Hepatitis C virus (formerly one of the non A–non B viruses) is transmitted by routes similar to those of hepatitis B virus. Although there have been no reported cases of the transmission of this virus by corneal transplantation, the Eye Bank Association of America requires that all potential donors have a negative screening or confirmatory test for hepatitis C virus.

There have been no reported cases of HIV transmission by corneal transplantation; however, the virus has been identified in tears,[68] conjunctival epithelium,[69] and corneal tissue[70] of patients with AIDS. In the latter report, HIV was isolated from both corneas of an AIDS patient that had been preserved in M-K medium for 4 days. There is also a report of corneal transplantation inadvertently performed with tissue from two HIV-infected donors.[71] Neither donor had developed AIDS by the time of death. Three recipients of the corneas from these donors had no detectable HIV antibodies for up to 5 years after corneal transplantation. The fourth recipient refused HIV testing but showed no clinical signs of HIV disease. However, two recipients of kidneys from these donors developed acute HIV infection 2 to 4 weeks after transplantation and had seroconversion of HIV antibodies 50 to 56 days after transplantation. Another case of an HIV-seronegative donor with no known risk factors for HIV infection had a similar outcome; recipients of solid organs and fresh frozen bone seroconverted, whereas the two recipients of the corneas and all tested recipients of lyophilized tissue remained HIV-negative.[72] The authors of one of the articles[71] pointed out that HIV could possibly be transmitted by corneal tissue from a donor with a more advanced stage of AIDS in that HIV is neurotropic and the cornea has a rich nerve supply.

The United States Public Health Service has recommended that all potential organ donors be tested for HIV antibodies in the blood or serum.[73] Pepose et al[74] reported 94 to 97 percent sensitivity and 99 percent specificity for antibody detection in cadavers with autopsy-proven AIDS by three commercially available enzyme-linked immunosorbent assay (ELISA) kits, and 97.1 percent sensitivity for the Western blot method. Positive tests were obtained from AIDS patients even when the blood sample was drawn up to 35 hours after death. The Eye Bank Association of America specifies that all potential corneal donors have a negative screening test for HIV-1 and HIV-2 antibodies before the cornea is released for transplantation.

Because HIV antibodies are not detected by ELISA in 3 to 6 percent of cadavers with autopsy-proven AIDS[74] and because of the months- to years-long incubation period after infection with HIV during which HIV antibodies are often undetectable, persons at high risk for HIV infection are excluded from corneal donation by the Eye Bank Association of America. High risk groups include homosexual and bisexual men, intravenous drug abusers, hemophiliacs, heterosexual partners of persons with AIDS or at risk for AIDS, prostitutes and their sexual partners, and inmates of correctional institutions.[75–79]

Rabies and Creutzfeldt-Jakob disease have been transmitted from donor to recipient by corneal transplantation.[80] Both of these viruses are neurotropic and are presumably transmitted via corneal nerves. Transmission of these diseases by corneal transplantation has led the Eye Bank Association of America to exclude all potential donors with neurologic diseases of unknown etiology, as well as donors who received human pituitary-derived growth hormone between 1963 and 1985, which may have been contaminated with the Creutzfeldt-Jakob disease virus.

Although persons with known human T-cell leukemia virus type 1 (HTLV-1) or type 2 (HTLV-2) infection are excluded as cornea donors, serologic testing for these viruses is not required.

Transmission of Malignancies

There is one documented case of transmission of retinoblastoma from donor to recipient by corneal transplantation.[81] Patients with retinoblastoma commonly have malignant cells in the anterior chamber and some of these cells may adhere to the donor corneal endothelium.[82] Therefore, the Eye Bank Association of America specifies that corneas from eyes with retinoblastoma should not be used for transplantation.

Corneas from eyes enucleated for choroidal melanoma are frequently used for transplantation; there have been no reported cases of transmission of melanoma by corneal transplantation and a retrospective study comparing outcomes with tissue from eyes with primary choroidal melanoma and normal eyes showed no evidence of tumor transmission.[83] There have been no reported cases of transmission of systemic malignancies by corneal transplantation[84]; therefore donors with systemic malignancies need not be excluded, even if there is metastatic disease. It is, however, our practice to use these corneas only if the melanoma or metastatic disease does not involve the ciliary body or more anterior structures of the eye.

Death-to-Enucleation Time Criteria

With the decomposition of uveal and other ocular tissues postmortem, it is likely that the aqueous humor provides an increasingly toxic environment for corneal endothelial cells because of changes in pH, release of lysosomal enzymes, and changes in electrolyte and oxygen concentrations. A study of changes in the composition of aqueous humor of rabbit eyes after death showed a 30 percent decrease in glucose concentration after 4 hours at 3°C, complete absence of glucose after 2 hours at 37°C, and a marked increase in potassium concentration after 4 hours at either 3°C or 37°C.[85] Lactic acid levels increased quickly at either temperature, but the change was greater at 37°C. It is unknown at what point these changes have an adverse effect on the viability of endothelial cells.

A clinical study of 240 consecutive transplants detected no difference in graft clarity when donor eyes were enucleated less than 4 hours, 5 to 10 hours, or more than 10 hours postmortem.[34] Graft clarity, however, is a relatively insensitive indicator of endothelial cell preservation. Other studies have monitored more sensitive indicators of endothelial cell viability, such as temperature reversal[86–88] and nitroblue tetrazolium staining,[89] and reported conflicting results relative to the time from death to enucleation.

With no definitive data relating the length of time the donor eye can remain in the cadaver without significant damage to the corneal endothelium, the Eye Bank Association of America leaves this decision to the discretion of the eye bank medical directors. We recommend that the donor eye be enucleated within 6 hours of death.

TECHNIQUES FOR ASSESSING ENDOTHELIAL CELL VIABILITY

Most techniques developed to evaluate the efficacy of various methods of corneal preservation are purported to monitor, directly or indirectly, endothelial cell viability in terms of changes in cell morphology or certain metabolic processes. However, some of these changes may be reversible, and normal morphology or metabolism may be observed in the presence of other irreversible damage to the cells. Several of the commonly used techniques for monitoring endothelial cell viability are described in the sections that follow. A more detailed description has been published elsewhere.[47]

Staining Techniques

One of the more popular techniques is cellular staining that differentiates viable from nonviable endothelial cells. The most commonly used stains are trypan blue, alizarin red, and nitroblue tetrazolium.

Trypan blue staining of endothelial cells was first described by Stocker et al.[90] In this simple and inexpensive technique, trypan blue is applied to the corneal endothelium for a few minutes and rinsed off. The stain is excluded from cells with intact plasma membranes but penetrates cells with damaged plasma membranes and stains the nuclei (Figure 33-1). The percentage of nonviable cells is then determined by counting the stained cells under light microscopic observation. Trypan blue staining may be combined with alizarin red staining.[91] Alizarin red stains intercellular spaces, which makes the endothelial cells easier to visualize and count. The major drawbacks to trypan blue staining are that cells that take up the stain are damaged but not necessarily dead, and severely damaged nuclei may not stain.

Nitroblue tetrazolium stain is reduced by corneal endothelial cell enzymes (including dehydrogenases and diaphorases) in the presence of the appropriate substrate, resulting in precipitation of a dark blue complex (diformazan) that can be identified by light microscopy.

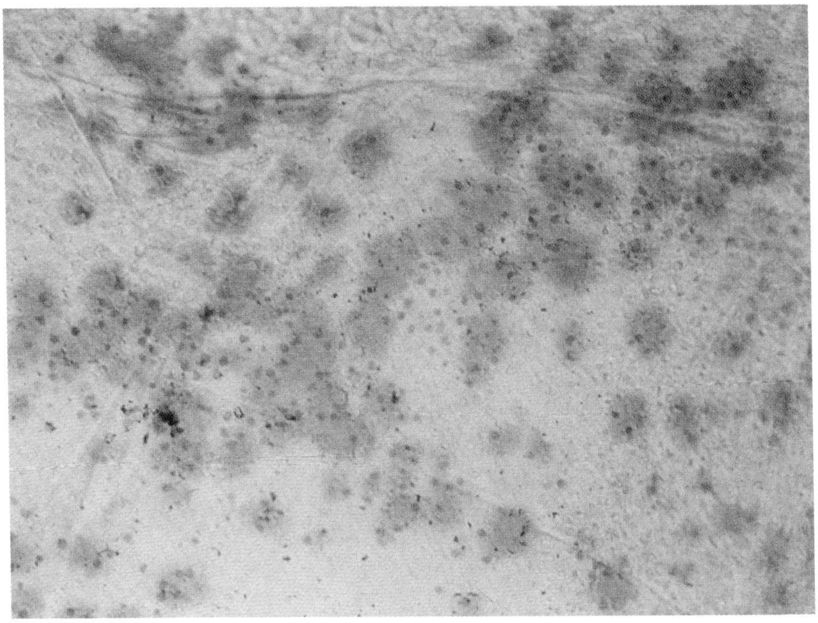

FIGURE 33-1 Trypan blue staining shows several areas of cell damage. The dye stains the nuclei of damaged endothelial cells. Viable endothelial cells do not stain. (Courtesy of Emily D. Varnell, New Orleans, LA.)

Cytoplasmic (α-glycerophosphate dehydrogenase), intramitochondrial (succinate dehydrogenase), and cytoplasmic and intramitochondrial (malate dehydrogenase) enzymes can participate in this reaction.[92] Like trypan blue staining, nitroblue tetrazolium staining is used as an exclusion assay, in which nonviable cells are stained.[93–95] Capella et al[15] reported that the results obtained with nitroblue tetrazolium staining did not parallel the results obtained in transplantation studies, however. They modified the procedure by adding a rapid freeze-thaw treatment that disrupted the plasma membranes of all the cells before staining[96] on the theory that, after thawing, cells that were normal before freezing would still contain enzymes and be stained, whereas cells that were damaged and had lost their intracellular contents before freezing would have no enzymes and would remain unstained. Other investigators have suggested that cells with severe changes in intracellular morphology incompatible with viability could retain enzymes at the time of freezing to give a false-positive staining result.[7,97]

The literature describing the use of nitroblue tetrazolium is confusing.[98] Some consider staining indicative of cell damage; others consider staining indicative of cell viability. Neither completely intact nor severely damaged cells stain, but for different reasons. With intact cells, nitroblue tetrazolium cannot reach the enzymes; in severely damaged cells, the enzymes have been lost. Damage sufficient to render the membranes permeable to nitroblue tetrazolium, but without much loss of enzymes will produce staining and the assay is then similar to an exclusion assay. Gross increases in permeability, however, prevent staining owing to loss of the enzymes.

Acridine orange is a fluorescent dye that penetrates viable cells, intercalates with double-stranded DNA, and fluoresces green when viewed with a fluorescence microscope (Figure 33-2). It was first used to stain viable corneal endothelial cells by Smith et al.[11] Another fluorescent dye, ethidium bromide,[99] penetrates only nonviable cells, intercalates into DNA, and fluoresces red (Figure 33-3). The combination of acridine orange and ethidium bromide allows for differential staining of viable and nonviable cells. As with other staining techniques, however, plasma membrane damage compatible with viability may allow entry of ethidium bromide and the marking of living cells as nonviable, and viable cells stained with acridine orange may have damage to an unmonitored system that results in eventual cell death.

Temperature Reversal

Davson[100] and Harris and Nordquist[101] first described the temperature reversal phenomenon as a corneal thinning response that occurs when the cornea is rewarmed after cooling and is related to resumption of the active pumping function of the corneal endothelium.[102] Specular microscopic methods for accurately monitoring the thickness of the cornea were developed by Hoefle[103] and Dikstein and Maurice.[104]

Temperature reversal testing has been used extensively to monitor endothelial cell viability during corneal

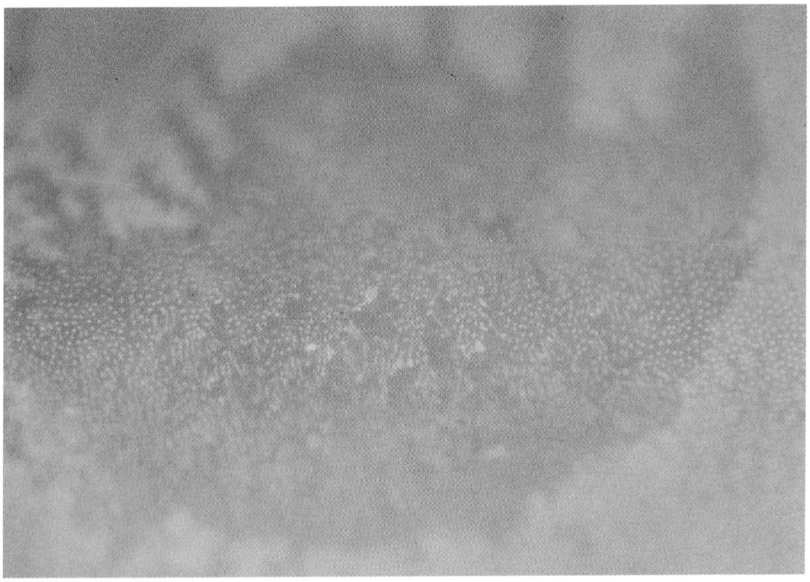

FIGURE 33-2 Acridine orange stains viable cells in the periphery but not dead cells in the center.

preservation because it monitors a function of the corneal endothelium that is a primary determinant of corneal graft survival.[105] One technical difficulty is the frequent presence of folds in Descemet's membrane in postmortem corneas that can hamper the accurate measurement of corneal thickness.[106,107] Also, discrepancies have been noted between temperature reversal testing and clinical results. In one study, corneas stored in M-K medium for 3 to 6 days failed temperature reversal testing although they could be used successfully for penetrating keratoplasty.[108] It is likely that osmotically active molecules, such as dextran in M-K medium and chondroitin sulfate in Optisol, which are able to pass into the corneal stroma, alter the regulation of corneal hydration and interfere with the mechanism of temperature reversal testing.[109,110]

Transmission Electron Microscopy

Transmission electron microscopy can be used to monitor the effect of corneal preservation on the subcellular morphology of corneal endothelial cells, including mitochondrial swelling, changes in the morphology of the endoplasmic reticulum, intracellular vacuolization, damage to the nuclear and plasma membranes, alterations in the character of the nucleoplasm and chromatin,

FIGURE 33-3 Ethidium bromide stains nonviable cells in the center but not viable cells in the periphery.

enlargement of the intercellular spaces, and disruption of the adhesions between endothelial cells and Descemet's membrane.[111-113] The primary limitations of this technique are the expense, confusion of artifacts with actual changes, and the small number of cells that are analyzed.

Alterations, such as complete cellular disorganization, mitochondrial disruption, and complete karyolysis, are indicators of cell death. It is frequently difficult to determine whether other changes noted by transmission electron microscopy would be irreversible and lead to cell death after corneal transplantation. For example, freeze-thaw changes, such as condensed mitochondria with enlarged cristae, swollen endoplasmic reticulum, and broken outer nuclear membranes, are reversible if the tissue is incubated in Kinsey medium before fixation for electron microscopy.[113,114]

Specular Microscopy

Specular microscopy in conjunction with morphometric analysis is most commonly used to monitor the efficacy of corneal preservation. Endothelial cell density, variations in cell size (polymegethism), variations in cell shape (pleomorphism), and the number of sides per cell can be determined in enucleated eyes[115] or in isolated corneas.[116] Donor corneal endothelium can be evaluated before transplantation to identify corneas with abnormal cell densities or cell structures.[105,115,117] An advantage is that specular microscopic evaluation can be performed in vitro before transplantation and in vivo at appropriate intervals after transplantation.

The major limitation of this method is technical difficulty. Relatively expensive instruments and a well-trained technician are needed. Optimally, a minimum of 50 cells are digitized for each examination to determine the cell density and morphologic parameters.[29] Interpretation of data is difficult unless there is an appropriate study design. Damage that occurs from surgical trauma at the donor-recipient junction results in a significant decrease in central endothelial cell density because of migration of cells from the center to the periphery, even in the absence of cell losses caused by corneal preservation.[29,38] This factor varies with the surgeon and the surgical technique. It is, therefore, imperative that studies be performed with prospective concurrent controls and that different surgeons in multicenter trials perform similar proportions of cases in experimental and control groups.

It is assumed that the best method of preservation produces the least central endothelial cell loss. We believe cell losses caused by corneal preservation should be assessed as soon as the graft is clear enough to allow reliable specular microscopy.[118,119] In the early postoperative period, central endothelial cell densities are less affected by redistribution of the cells toward the donor-recipient junction to repair surgical trauma and are more likely to reflect changes from preservation alone. We recommend 2 months after surgery as the appropriate time to perform specular microscopy for this purpose. With the ability to observe deeper corneal layers through edematous tissue, confocal microscopy may, in the future, be useful for monitoring endothelial cell density and morphology.

Clinical Results

Although clinical success is the ultimate goal of research on corneal preservation, it is a relatively insensitive measurement of the efficacy of a method of preservation in maintaining endothelial cell viability. Many studies have included clear grafts with endothelial cell densities as low as 300 to 500 cells/mm^2.[39,120-122] Transplanted corneas with endothelial cell densities this low are likely to fail with longer follow-up, however, because of further cell losses that occur with age[29-32]; insults, such as graft rejection, trauma, or glaucoma[105]; and normal attrition.[105] Therefore, the goal of corneal preservation should be to provide the largest number of viable endothelial cells in a clear graft.

METHODS OF CORNEAL PRESERVATION

The goal of research on corneal preservation is to develop a simple preservation medium that can indefinitely maintain viability of 100 percent of the corneal epithelium, keratocytes, and endothelium, and prevent microbial contamination. Although methods of corneal preservation have improved considerably since the 1960s, none has achieved this goal. In the following sections, the advantages and limitations of the primary methods of corneal preservation are discussed. Table 33-2 provides the compositions of some of the preservation media that have been developed for clinical use.

Moist Chamber Storage

Moist chamber storage, which was the primary method of corneal storage until the mid-1970s, continues to be used in many parts of the world. Antibiotic solutions are applied to the eye at the time of enucleation and the whole eye is stored at 4°C in a sealed chamber that contains a small amount of saline to moisten the air that surrounds the tissue (Figure 33-4). Although this is the simplest method for storing corneas, it is limited by a relatively short preservation time. It is generally accepted that the

TABLE 33-2
Constituents of Corneal Preservation Solutions

	M-K Medium	*Minnesota System Organ Culture Medium*	*K-Sol*	*CSM*	*Dexsol*	*Optisol and Optisol GS*
Base medium	TC-199	MEM (Eagle's)	TC-199	MEM	MEM	MEM, TC-199
Buffer system	Bicarbonate, HEPES	HEPES	HEPES	HEPES	Bicarbonate, HEPES	Bicarbonate, HEPES
Chondroitin sulfate	—	1.35%	2.50%	1.35%	1.35%	2.50%
Dextran	5% dextran 40	—	—	—	1% dextran 40	1% dextran 40
Antibiotic	Gentamicin	Gentamicin	Gentamicin	Gentamicin	Gentamicin	Gentamicin (Optisol GS: gentamicin and streptomycin)
Other components	—	10% defined fetal bovine serum, Earle's salts without L-glutamine, L-glutamine, nonessential amino acids, 2-mercaptoethanol (antioxidant)	—	Mercaptoethanol, nonessential amino acids	Sodium pyruvate, nonessential amino acids[a], additional antioxidants[a]	Sodium pyruvate, nonessential amino acids,[a] additional antioxidants,[a] ATP precursors, ascorbic acid, vitamin B_{12}

Abbreviations: TC-199, tissue culture medium 199; MEM, minimum essential medium; HEPES, *N*-2-hydroxyethylpiperazine-*N*′-2-ethanesulfonic acid.
[a] Exact components proprietary.

maximum storage time should not exceed 48 hours, because the endothelium of the cornea remains in contact with aqueous humor that is contaminated by increasing amounts of autolytic products from the uvea and other ocular tissues, which are likely to be toxic.[85,123] This time limitation has become a significant issue with the requirement for screening of donor tissue for HIV, hepatitis B virus, and hepatitis C virus.

The 48-hour limit for storage in a moist chamber has been supported by studies performed in rabbits[95] and humans.[112,124] In rabbit eyes, nitroblue tetrazolium staining showed a 25 to 30 percent decrease in viable corneal endothelial cells after 48 hours of moist chamber storage.[95] In human eyes stored in moist chambers, irreversible changes in endothelial cell morphology were demonstrated by transmission electron microscopy as early as 24 hours after enucleation,[112] and a loss of 44 percent of endothelial cell viability was shown by various staining techniques after 2 days of storage.[124] Moist chamber storage is dangerous if there is any likelihood that the cornea will become warmer than 4°C during transit, because no nutrients are available and the endothelium will die.

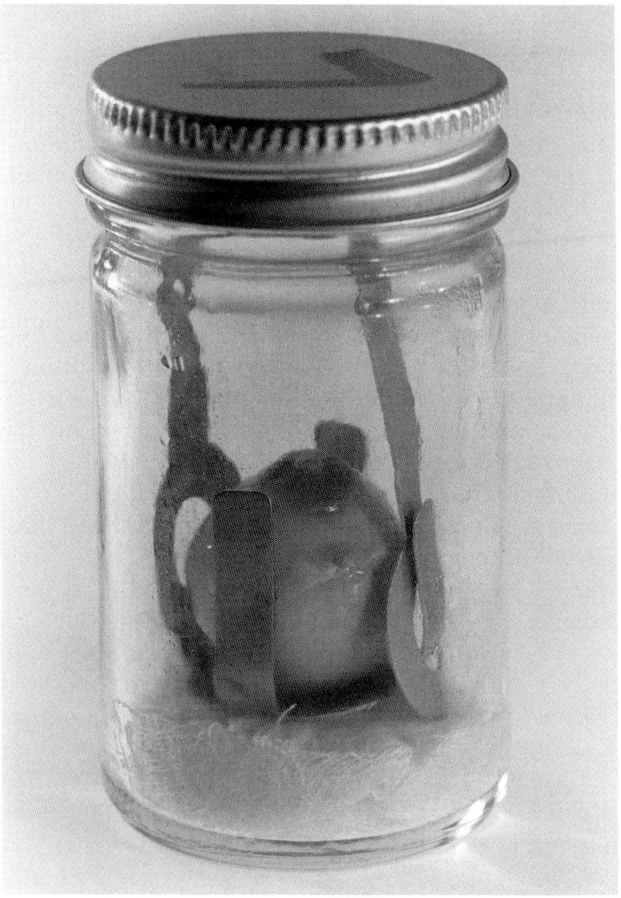

FIGURE 33-4 Eye in moist chamber. The saturated gauze in the bottom of the jar provides a moist environment. The eye is positioned so that nothing is touching the cornea.

Cryopreservation

Cryopreservation has been under development for the past 40 years as a method to provide indefinite preservation of corneal tissue. Thus far, these developments have not resulted in a method that is technically simple and effective in maintaining endothelial cell viability. Research continues, however, because of the potential advantages of cryopreservation, including unlimited storage time and elimination of the time-dependent endothelial cell deterioration and loss of stromal proteoglycans that occur during storage at 4°C or 34°C.[125]

Cryopreservation methods that have been used clinically have, with minor variations, been similar to those reported by Capella et al[15,96] and O'Neill et al.[94] In the method described by Capella et al,[15] the cornea must be preserved within 8 hours of death and soon after enucleation.[113] Dimethyl sulfoxide levels are increased in a series of steps to a final concentration of 7.5 percent. The tissue is then frozen to -80°C and stored at -196°C. Other critical factors include different freezing rates during different phases of the process and a rapid thawing technique that is used to prepare the cornea for transplantation. The thawing of cryopreserved corneas must be carefully controlled because agents such as dimethyl sulfoxide can be toxic if the temperature rises above 37°C.

Cryopreservation damages the corneal endothelium, which limits its efficacy. Loss of endothelial cell viability has been attributed to increasing solute concentrations in the liquid phase during freezing, the formation of ice crystals, and changes in pH and osmolality.[94,126-128] Glycerol, polyvinyl pyrrolidone, and dimethyl sulfoxide have been evaluated as cryoprotectants,[129] but only dimethyl sulfoxide has been used clinically with any frequency.

Changes in endothelial subcellular morphology caused by cryopreservation have been demonstrated by transmission electron microscopy.[111,113,130-132] Some of these changes are thought to be reversible.[113,114,132] In vitro studies have suggested that there is breakdown of the endothelial barrier function after cryopreservation,[133,134] and clinical studies have reported that, on average, cryopreserved corneas require a longer period to clear following transplantation compared with moist chamber- or M-K-preserved corneas.[135]

Specular microscopic studies of cryopreserved corneas have reported mean endothelial cell densities of 817, 1,028, and 678 cells/mm^2 at 1 year, 7 to 9 years, and 15 years after transplantation, respectively.[122,136,137] Mean endothelial cell loss of 55 percent was reported in cryopreserved grafts after 1 year, in comparison with losses of 21 to 22 percent in M-K medium-stored corneas and 40 to 44 percent in corneas transplanted fresh from donor eyes with malignant choroidal melanoma.[135] Clinical success rates for cryopreserved and moist chamber-preserved corneas were not different in many reported studies.[138]

Under appropriate conditions, solidification without crystallization can occur during cooling. This process is called *vitrification.*[139,140] Vitrification requires high concentrations of cryoprotectants but has the theoretical advantage of allowing the preservation of tissue to occur at very low temperatures without intracellular or extracellular ice formation, which is the major source of endothelial cell damage. Glycerol,[141] 1,2-propanediol,[142] and 2,3-butanediol[143] were examined as potential cryoprotectants for corneal vitrification, but the results showed that effective concentrations of single cryoprotectants would be toxic to the endothelium. Combinations of cryoprotectants or their addition at lower temperatures, at which they are less toxic,[144] may be useful, but preliminary studies of vitrification as a method of corneal preservation have reported less than optimal results.[141–143]

McCarey-Kaufman (M-K) Medium

The first medium introduced for corneal preservation was M-K medium.[16] M-K medium was designed for short-term preservation of corneas at 4°C for a maximum of 4 days. The original formulation included tissue culture medium 199 (TC-199), 5 percent dextran, bicarbonate buffer, and gentamicin. The current formulation contains 0.025 M HEPES buffer instead of the bicarbonate buffer and phenol red as a pH indicator.[145] This latter formulation is available commercially.

The superiority of M-K medium to moist chamber storage, particularly after 48 hours, was demonstrated with trypan blue staining,[123,146,147] electron microscopy,[123,146] and specular microscopy.[148] Endothelial cell viability diminishes in corneas stored in M-K medium after 4 to 5 days.[123,146,147,149,150] Movement of dextran from M-K medium into the stroma[151,152] appears to temporarily alter the normal leak-pump relationship of the endothelium that is responsible for maintaining corneal hydration, which has likely played a role in the disparate results that have been reported in temperature reversal testing.[108,152,153] Experimentally, dextran is taken up from the medium by corneal endothelial cells, keratocytes, and epithelial cells[154] but is apparently eluted over a relatively short period of time when the cornea is placed in a series of Kreb's Ringer bicarbonate solutions without dextran.[155]

Clinical studies have reported good success rates with corneas stored in M-K medium.[36,146,153,156–158] One study found no difference in clinical results between tissue stored in a moist chamber for 24 hours and tissue stored in M-K medium for a mean of 48 hours.[159] In a study of 198 eyes receiving donor tissue stored in M-K medium for an average of 46 hours, mean endothelial cell loss 2 months after corneal transplantation was 20 percent.[29] Some studies described good clinical results with tissue stored in M-K medium for as long as 5 to 7 days,[36,153] although it is generally accepted that storage time in M-K medium should not exceed 4 days. One study reported that optimal results are obtained with storage times of less than 2 days,[160] but such a short storage time is not always compatible with the requirement for donor serology testing for HIV and hepatitis viruses. Primary graft failure rates between 0 percent and 4.3 percent were reported in three large studies of corneal preservation with M-K medium.[29,36,161] These rates are similar to those for other methods of preservation.

Organ Culture

The organ culture method for long-term corneal preservation was introduced by Doughman and colleagues in 1976,[17,18] and variations have been described by other investigators in the United States and Europe.[162–167] In the original Doughman technique, the cornea was placed in a 20-ml Petri dish that contained organ culture medium, and the medium was changed three times a week, which increased the risk of microbial contamination. Eventually, a closed system was introduced so that changes in the medium were not required.[22] The latter method is similar to one developed by Sperling in Denmark.[162] The system eventually adopted by Doughman and Lindstrom included organ culture medium with chondroitin sulfate, and is called the *Minnesota system.*[22,168,169]

The formulation of the Minnesota system organ preservation medium is provided in Table 33-2. The medium includes 10 percent decomplemented fetal bovine serum and 1.35 percent chondroitin sulfate (molecular weight 50,000). Initially, the globe is decontaminated in 1.0 percent povidone-iodine for 3 minutes, rinsed for 1 minute in normal saline, and flushed with saline. A limbal swab is taken for culture. The cornea is excised and placed with the epithelial surface down in 15 ml of the medium. The tissue is maintained in the Petri dish for 2 to 3 days at 34°C in 5 percent CO_2 in a water-jacketed incubator with one or two changes of the medium. A spinal needle bent into the shape of a hook is passed through the scleral rim and the cornea is suspended in 130 ml of organ culture medium in a sterile sealed bottle and maintained at 34°C. Seven days after organ culture, 10 ml of the medium are withdrawn from the bottle and cultured for bacteria and fungi. If no growth is detected in any of the microbiologic cultures after 10 days and the medium in the closed bottle containing the cornea is clear, the system is considered sterile and the cornea is available for transplantation. Corneas stored in this manner can be stored for up to 35 days.

Transmission electron microscopy demonstrated that epithelial and endothelial cellular morphology are well maintained during organ culture for periods of 35 days or longer.[18,19,20,165,170,171] A specular microscopic study showed a dramatic difference in mean central endothelial cell losses (7.9 percent vs. 28.7 percent) 2 months after transplantation with donors that had been stored in organ culture medium either containing or lacking chondroitin sulfate, respectively.[169] No statistically significant difference in mean central endothelial cell loss was noted between corneas stored for a mean of 21 days in organ culture medium containing 1.35 percent chondroitin sulfate at 34°C (9 percent) and those stored a mean of 39 hours in M-K medium at 4°C (7 percent).[168]

Early studies reported significant problems with persistent epithelial defects in corneas stored in organ culture medium. Epithelial preservation reportedly improved with the addition of chondroitin sulfate[19] and coating of the graft with sodium hyaluronate before transplantation.[169] Primary graft failure rates of 0 percent,[18,22] 2 percent,[164] and 3 percent[29] have been reported for organ culture methods of preservation.

The advantage of organ culture is the long storage time at higher temperature, which allows detection and possibly elimination of infectious agents and time for other types of manipulations, such as addition of growth factors or other molecular biological agents, to enhance the density and survival of the endothelial cells. The disadvantages are the technical complexity and equipment required, which have limited the use of the procedure, particularly since intermediate-term preservation solutions, which provide similar advantages, have become available.

Media Containing Chondroitin Sulfate

K-Sol

The first commercially available chondroitin sulfate–containing corneal preservation medium was K-Sol, which was developed by Kaufman and coworkers for storage of corneas at 4°C for up to 2 weeks.[27,28] The original formulation contained TC-199, 0.025 M HEPES buffer, and 2.5 to 10 percent chondroitin sulfate (see Table 33-2) with no fetal calf serum. A concentration of 2.5 percent chondroitin sulfate was found to be superior to a concentration of 2.0 percent chondroitin sulfate in maintaining rabbit endothelium in corneas preserved at 4°C for 12 days.[172] Gel exclusion chromatography was used to remove polymers of chondroitin sulfate that had a molecular mass of less than 10,000 daltons. These smaller polymers were found to penetrate more readily into the corneal stroma, increasing osmotic pressure and causing excessive corneal swelling.

A number of studies of the in vitro and in vivo efficacy of K-Sol corneal storage were published. Two studies found little or no difference in endothelial survival in corneas stored for 1 to 2 weeks in K-Sol compared with corneas stored for 2 to 3 days in M-K medium.[173,174] In another study in dogs and humans, less disruption of endothelial cells was detected by scanning electron microscopy in corneas stored in chondroitin sulfate–containing medium for 14 days at 4°C (3 percent) than was detected in paired corneas stored in M-K medium for the same time (45 percent).[175] Farge et al[176] reported mean in vitro endothelial cell losses of 5.8 percent after 1 week and 7.4 percent after 13 days of storage in K-Sol.

Clinical studies also reported good endothelial preservation with K-Sol. Kaufman et al[27] showed that storage in K-Sol for up to 2 weeks provided preservation similar to that obtained with storage in M-K medium for 2 to 3 days. Another study described an endothelial cell loss of 6 percent 2 months after transplantation in 37 corneas stored in K-Sol at 4°C for 1 to 13 days (mean 6.8 days).[160] In that study, endothelial cell loss after storage in M-K medium for 1 to 81 hours (mean 39 hours) was also 6 percent. In both the K-Sol and M-K groups, there was a significant positive correlation between the length of preservation and endothelial cell loss 2 months after corneal transplantation, but only corneas stored for more than 10 days in K-Sol or more than 2 days in M-K medium were found to have cell losses greater than 30 percent. Primary graft failure was noted in two corneas stored in K-Sol for 6 and 8 days and in one cornea stored in M-K medium for 85 hours.

Keates and Rabin[177] reported no difference in clinical success with corneas transferred to K-Sol for 6 to 144 hours after initial storage in M-K medium for 7 to 84 hours or corneas stored in K-Sol alone. There was also no difference between the two groups in terms of endothelial cell loss. This study suggests that transfer from M-K medium to a chondroitin sulfate–containing medium does not adversely affect the tissue. Care should be taken, however, in applying these data to other chondroitin sulfate–containing media because unforeseen interactions could occur between the components of different formulations. Therefore, methods for transfer between different media should be individually investigated before being adopted for general use by eye banks.

K-Sol is no longer available commercially. Contamination of the medium with *Propionibacterium acnes* was detected in cultures of five corneoscleral rims in 1988.[178] The contamination was subsequently shown to have occurred during manufacture. K-Sol was withdrawn from the market at that time and has not been reintroduced.

Chondroitin Sulfate Corneal Storage Medium

The formulation of chondroitin sulfate corneal storage medium (CSM) (see Table 33-2) was originally developed to provide optimal intermediate-term preservation at 4°C and long-term preservation at 34°C. Several studies of CSM preservation have been reported.[179–182] Specular microscopy showed that mean endothelial cell loss in grafts stored in CSM at 4°C for 1 to 7 days was 10.2 percent, 12.8 percent, and 17.9 percent at 3, 6, and 12 months after corneal transplantation, respectively.[179] Endothelial cell viability determined with trypan blue and alizarin red staining was similar for tissue stored in CSM or K-Sol for 7 to 10 days. Corneas stored in K-Sol for 14 to 22 days had progressively more endothelial cell damage compared with corneas stored in CSM for the same period of time.[179] No significant difference in endothelial cell density or coefficient of variation of cell size was found 3, 6, or 12 months after transplantation in paired corneas stored for 8 to 97 hours in K-Sol or CSM[180]; there was a trend toward a greater decrease in mean endothelial cell density in the K-Sol group (27 percent) compared with the CSM group (17 percent) at 12 months, but the difference was not statistically significant.

Another study reported no difference in mean endothelial cell loss 4 months after corneal transplantation between corneas stored in CSM and those stored in CSM containing 1 percent dextran.[181] The addition of dextran to CSM resulted in a significant decrease in corneal thickness at the time of surgery. By 1 week after corneal transplantation, there was no difference in mean corneal thickness between the corneas stored in medium with or without dextran, however. Another study found no difference in the maintenance of endothelial morphology monitored by scanning electron microscopy between corneas stored in CSM or K-Sol at 4°C for 14 days.[182] CSM is no longer available from a commercial supplier.

Optisol and Dexsol

Optisol and Dexsol both contain chondroitin sulfate and 1 percent dextran (see Table 33-2). Differences include the base media and a higher concentration of chondroitin sulfate in Optisol (2.5 percent) than in Dexsol (1.35 percent). Optisol also contains other components, such as ascorbic acid, vitamin B_{12}, and adenosine triphosphate (ATP) precursors, that are not present in Dexsol. Optisol GS, first marketed in 1992, is identical to Optisol except that it contains streptomycin as well as gentamicin.

Based at least in part on reports that human endothelial cells can undergo mitosis under appropriate conditions, including the presence of various growth factors,[183–186] a formulation of Dexsol containing insulin (10 μg/ml) and human epidermal growth factor (10 ng/ml), called *Procell,* was evaluated in a multi-center clinical trial in comparison with the original formulation of Dexsol.[187,188] The results showed no significant differences in graft clarity, complication rate, endothelial cell loss, or other endothelial morphometric parameters. This formulation was marketed for a short time but is no longer commercially available.

Preliminary reports suggested that Optisol is superior to M-K medium, K-Sol, and CSM.[189,190] In vitro and open label clinical studies showed that Optisol preserved corneal endothelial cells for up to 2 weeks at 4°C.[191] A subsequent masked clinical study comparing paired corneas stored in Optisol or Dexsol for 20 to 134 hours found all grafts clear and no significant difference in postoperative clinical or endothelial morphometric parameters after 1 year.[192] Dexsol, Optisol, and Optisol GS are currently commercially available in the United States.

PROCURING DONOR CORNEAS

As a first step to optimal corneal preservation, it is important that proper techniques be used in procuring and processing corneal tissue. The donor cornea is obtained either by enucleation of the eye or by removal of the cornea with a rim of sclera in situ.

Enucleation

Sterile technique is used throughout the enucleation procedure. The eyelids are washed with soap, and the fornices are flushed with saline and antibiotics. The face is draped in a sterile fashion and an eyelid speculum is inserted. A conjunctival peritomy is made at the limbus, and adhesions between the sclera and Tenon's capsule are lysed by blunt dissection with scissors in all four quadrants of the orbit. The extraocular muscles are isolated with a muscle hook and excised from the globe at their insertions. The eye is lifted anteriorly and the optic nerve is cut with curved enucleation scissors. The enucleated eye is placed in a sterile moist chamber and flooded with or immersed in antimicrobial solution.[193]

Removing the Cornea

The majority of eye banks in the United States use a short-term or intermediate-term preservation medium, which

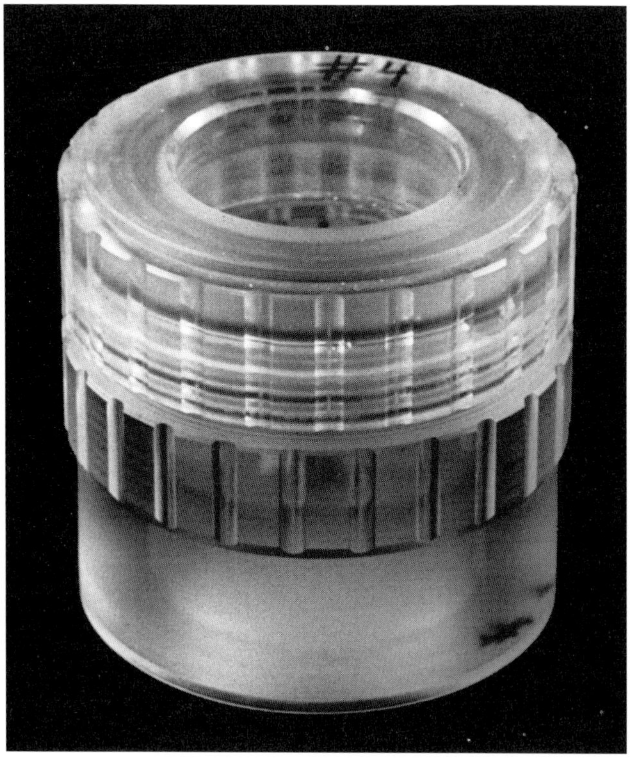

FIGURE 33-5 Modern corneal storage vial.

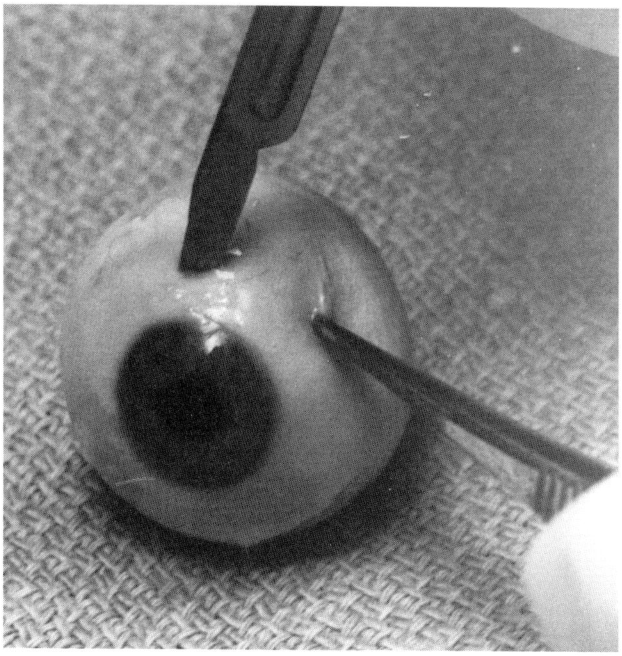

FIGURE 33-6 Removal of cornea. The sclera is incised with a blade 3 mm posterior to the limbus.

requires that the cornea with a rim of sclera be removed from the enucleated eye (Figure 33-5). Some eye banks remove only the cornea with a rim of sclera from the donor, and leave the remainder of the eye in situ.

A blade is used to make a full thickness incision in the sclera 3 mm posterior to the limbus (Figure 33-6). The incision is extended for 360 degrees with scissors; the inner blade of the scissors is placed in the supraciliary space so that only the sclera is cut (Figure 33-7). The scleral edge is lifted with forceps and separated from its attachment to the iris and choroid at the scleral spur (Figure 33-8). Thus, the anterior chamber is opened for the first time and the cornea and scleral rim are removed from the eye simultaneously. The cornea should not be bent or folded during this procedure to avoid traumatic damage to the endothelial cells. The cornea and scleral rim are then placed in preservation medium.

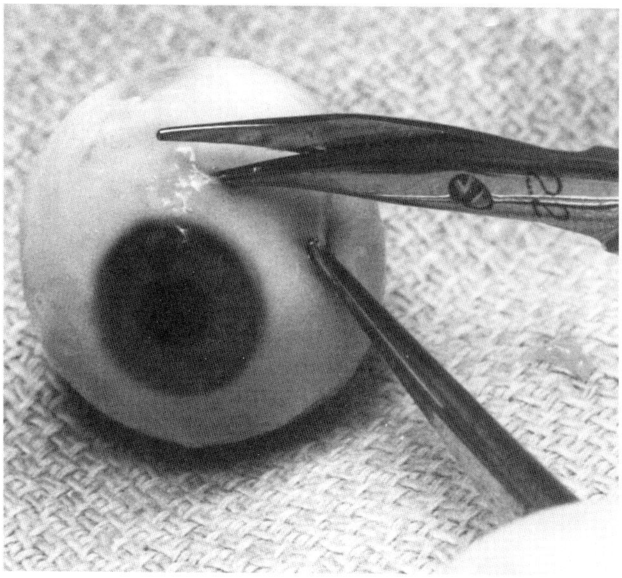

FIGURE 33-7 Removal of cornea. The sclera is cut with scissors for 360 degrees with the inner blade in the supraciliary space so that the underlying choroid is not cut.

EXAMINING THE DONOR CORNEA

Slit Lamp Examination

Enucleated eyes should be examined with a slit lamp microscope (Figure 33-9) to identify corneal abnormalities, such

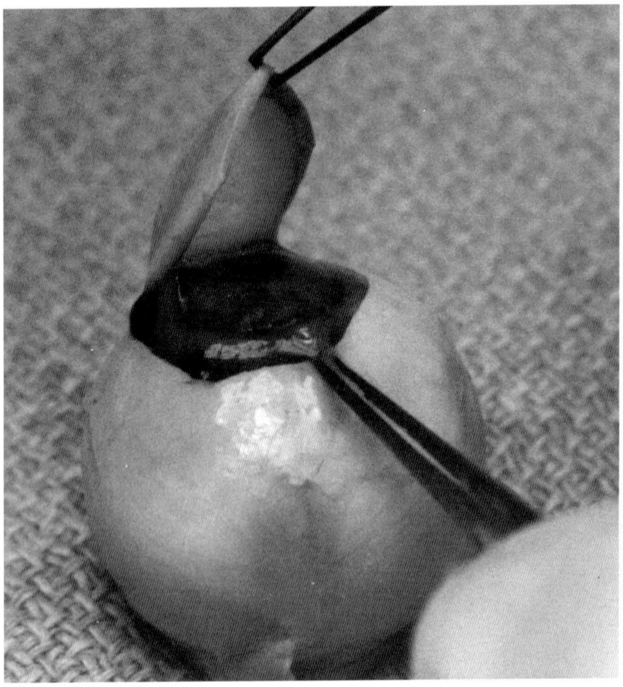

FIGURE 33-8 Removal of cornea. The cornea with its rim of sclera is removed from the eye by lifting the scleral edge with forceps and separating it from its attachment to the iris at the scleral spur.

as stromal opacities or infiltrates, vascularization, keratic precipitates, corneal guttae, or dot-like opacities indicative of nonviable endothelial cells,[194] that would make the cornea unsuitable for transplantation. Isolated corneas can be examined in their storage containers with a slit lamp microscope[195] (Figure 33-10).

Specular Microscopy

Endothelial cells on the donor cornea should be examined by specular microscopy. With intact donor eyes, the endothelium must be viewed through the corneal epithelium and stroma[23,106,107,117,194,196]; the view is often compromised by the postmortem epithelial and stromal edema. Confocal microscopy has the potential to solve this problem but has not yet achieved widespread use. If the donor cornea is removed and stored in preservation medium, the endothelial cells can be viewed directly from the posterior surface[116,197] (Figure 33-11). A video camera attached to the specular microscope permits immediate cell measurements from the image on the video monitor.

Specular microscopy of donor corneal endothelium can identify abnormalities that may be missed by slit lamp examination, such as early corneal guttae, pleomorphism, or polymegethism. Pseudoguttae can usually be distinguished from true guttae by warming the tissue to room temperature in the preservation medium for approximately 1 hour. Pseudoguttae caused by endothelial cell edema that develops at 4°C will usually resolve, while true guttae will remain.

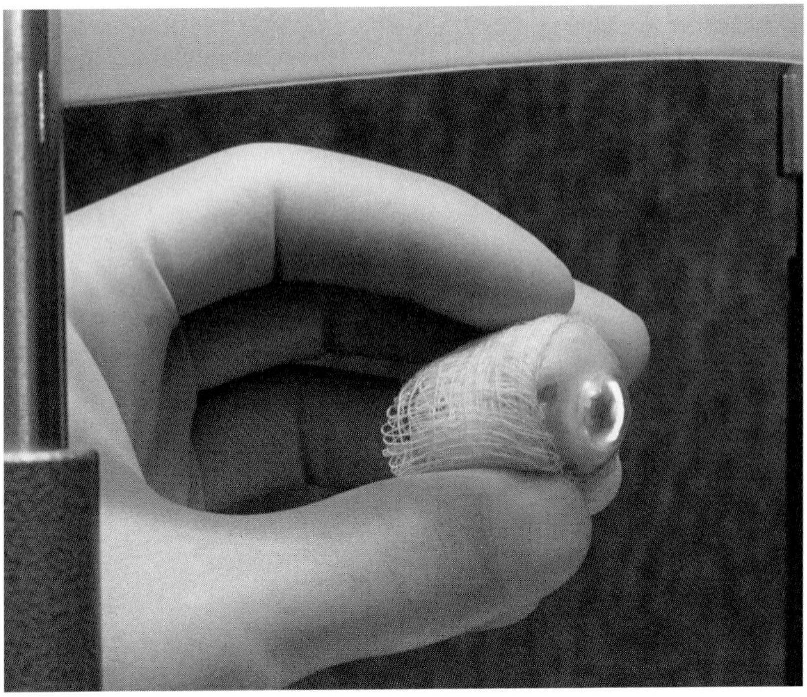

FIGURE 33-9 Examination of an enucleated eye with a slit lamp microscope. Sterility is maintained by the examiner wearing a sterile glove. The eye is easier to hold if a sterile piece of gauze is wrapped around the posterior segment.

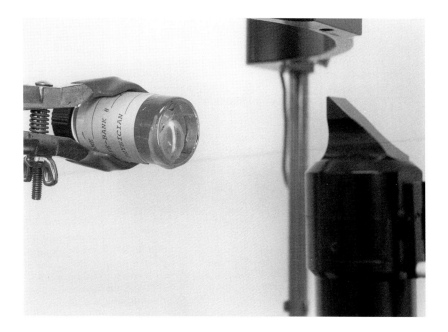

FIGURE 33-10 Examination of an isolated cornea with a slit lamp microscope. The cornea can be tipped on end and examined as shown here, or a mirror system can be used.

FUTURE DEVELOPMENTS

Many authors have reported attempts to transplant corneal endothelial cells that have been grown in tissue culture,[198–204] but results have been variable. There has been one report of transplantation of a donor button that was augmented with cultured human corneal endothelial cells into a human.[203] In that report, the donor cornea was transplanted 13 days after seeding; the paired nonseeded cornea was used as a control. Corneal endothelial cell densities determined at the time of transplantation by staining of the donor rims with alizarin red revealed counts of 3,068 cells/mm^2 in the enhanced cornea and 2,124 cells/mm^2 in the control cornea. Two months after transplantation, the central endothelial cell density in the eye that received the enhanced cornea was 2,800 cells/mm^2. Long-term results in these eyes were not reported in the literature. Further investigation will be needed to deter-

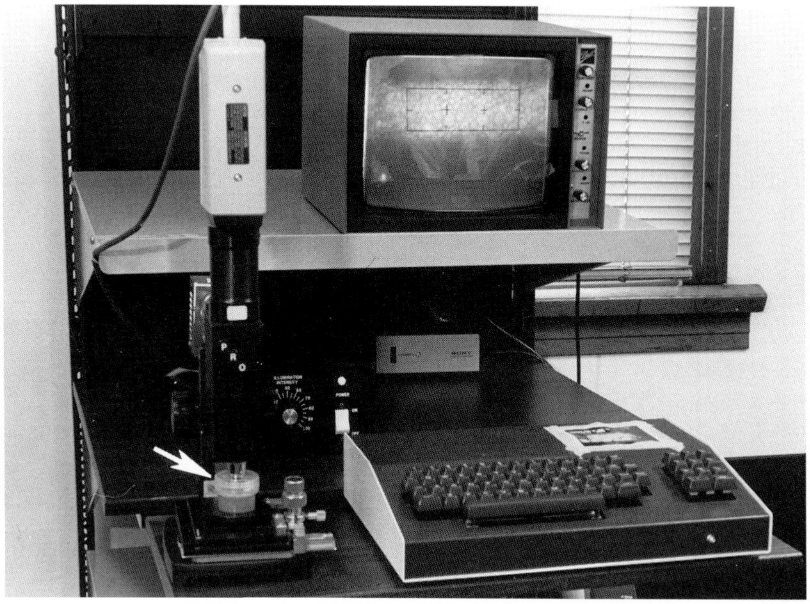

A

FIGURE 33-11 **(A)** Examination of the endothelium by specular microscopy. The cornea is in the container at the lower left (arrow), and the endothelial cells are displayed on the video monitor. *(continues)*

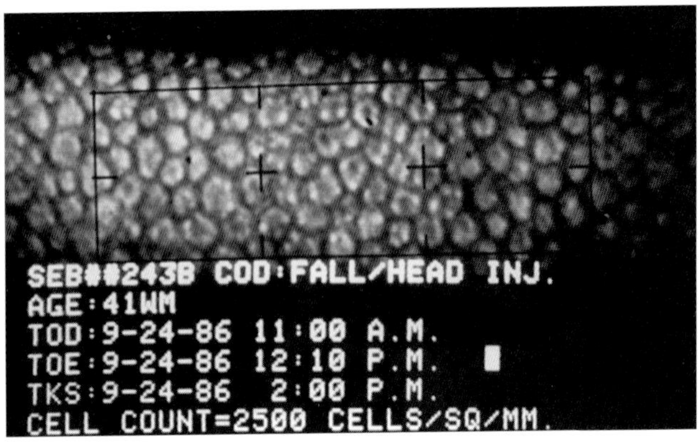

B

FIGURE 33-11 *(continued)* **(B)** A Polaroid picture can be taken of the video monitor for permanent documentation of the density and morphology of the donor endothelial cells. Other information about the donor can also be recorded.

mine if this approach to increasing the availability and quality of corneal tissue for transplantation is feasible.

Human corneal endothelial cells have been shown to produce messenger ribonucleic acids (mRNAs) and proteins, such as epidermal growth factor, basic fibroblast growth factor (FGFb), transforming growth factor beta (TGF-β), hepatocyte growth factor (HGF), keratinocyte growth factor (KGF), and interleukin-1 alpha (IL-1α), in tissue culture.[205-207] Bovine corneal endothelial cells have been shown to produce basic fibroblast growth factor mRNAs and protein.[208,209] Further work is needed to determine whether these putatively endogenous growth factors have an effect on human endothelial cell proliferation, and to evaluate whether exogenous growth factors can be used to modulate human endothelial cell metabolism, proliferation, and/or viability.[210] Eventually, it may be possible to use this knowledge to more directly and precisely stimulate the mitosis of corneal endothelial cells.

Another promising area of research with potential clinical applications is genetic engineering of endothelial cells. It is possible to trigger and modulate proliferation of corneal endothelial cells in culture by engineering them to express oncogenes.[211,212] These cells are unlikely to have clinical use in corneal endothelial transplantation because of uncertainties about the safety of the oncogenes. However, because the oncogenes work by altering the functions of endogenous proteins that are associated with the cell cycle, it should be possible to manipulate endothelial cell proliferation in culture, and possibly in vivo, by introducing carefully controlled regulatory elements. Indeed, the cornea may well be the ideal organ for genetic engineering because of its accessibility and the availability of noninvasive techniques to monitor endothelial morphology and function.

REFERENCES

1. Zirm E: Eine erfolgreiche totale Keratoplastik. Albrecht von Graefes Arch Ophthalmol 64:580, 1906
2. Filatov VP: Transplantation of the cornea. Arch Ophthalmol 13:321, 1935
3. Filatov VP, Bajenova MA: Culture of dried corneal tissue. Arch Ophtal and Rev Gin Ophtal 1:385, 1937
4. Oeutman AF: Formalinized cornea and keratoplasty in rabbits' eyes. Ophthalmologica 99:418, 1940
5. Smelser GK, Ozanics V: Effect of quick freezing of very low temperatures of donor tissue in corneal transplants. Proc Soc Exp Biol Med 62:274, 1946
6. Katzin HM: Preservation of corneal tissue by freezing and dehydration. Am J Ophthalmol 30:1128, 1947
7. Leopold IH, Adler FH: Use of frozen dried corneas as transplant material. Arch Ophthalmol 37:268, 1947
8. Bürki E: Ueber ein neues Verfahren zur Konserviering von Hornhautgewebe. Ophthalmologica 114:288, 1947
9. Stocker FW: The endothelium of the cornea and its clinical implications. Trans Am Ophthalmol Soc 51:669, 1953
10. Eastcott HHG, Gross AG, Leigh AG, North DP: Preservation of corneal grafts by freezing. Lancet 1:237, 1954
11. Smith AU, Ashwood-Smith MJ, Young MR: Some in vitro studies on rabbit corneal tissue. Exp Eye Res 2:71, 1962
12. Mueller FO: Techniques for full-thickness keratoplasty in rabbits using fresh and frozen corneal tissue. Br J Ophthalmol 48:377, 1964
13. Mueller FO, Casey TA, Trevor-Roper PD: Use of deep-frozen human cornea in full-thickness grafts. Br Med J 2:473, 1964
14. Mueller FO, Smith AU: Some experiments on grafting frozen corneal tissue in rabbits. Exp Eye Res 2:237, 1963
15. Capella JA, Kaufman HE, Robbins JE: Preservation of viable corneal tissue. Arch Ophthalmol 74:669, 1965
16. McCarey BE, Kaufman HE: Improved corneal storage. Invest Ophthalmol Vis Sci 13:165, 1974
17. Doughman DJ, Harris JE, Schmitt MK: Penetrating keratoplasty using 37°C organ cultured cornea. Trans Am Acad Ophthalmol Otolaryngol 81:778, 1976
18. Doughman DJ: Prolonged donor cornea preservation in organ culture: long-term clinical evaluation. Trans Am Ophthalmol Soc 78:567, 1980
19. Doughman DJ, Van Horn D, Harris JE, et al: The ultrastructure of the human organ-cultured cornea. Arch Ophthalmol 92:516, 1974
20. Lindstrom RL, Doughman DJ, Van Horn DL, et al: A metabolic and electron microscopic study of human organ-cultured cornea. Am J Ophthalmol 82:72, 1976
21. Summerlin MT, Miller GE, Harris JE, Good RA: The organ-cultured cornea. An in vitro study. Invest Ophthalmol 12:176, 1973

22. Lindstrom RL, Doughman DJ, Skelnik DL, Mindrup EA: Minnesota system corneal preservation. Br J Ophthalmol 70:47, 1986
23. Kuwahara Y, Sakanoue M, Hayashi M, et al: Studies on the long-term preservation of the cornea for penetrating keratoplasty. Nippon Ganka Gakkai Zasshi 69:1751, 1965
24. Mizukawa T, Manabe R: Recent advances in keratoplasty with special reference to the advantages of liquid preservation. Nippon Ganka Kiyo 19:1310, 1968
25. Mizukawa T, Mimura Y, Morisue T: Corneal transplantation. J Jpn Med Assoc 58:957, 1967
26. Nakano T: Studies on the viability of the cornea stored for penetrating keratoplasty under various experimental conditions: Report III. Oxygen consumption of rabbit corneas stored in newly devised preservation medium containing various macromolecular colloids. Nippon Ganka Gakkai Zasshi 70:662, 1966
27. Kaufman HE, Varnell ED, Kaufman S: Chondroitin sulfate in a new cornea preservation medium. Am J Ophthalmol 98:112, 1984
28. Kaufman HE, Varnell ED, Kaufman S, et al: K-Sol corneal preservation. Am J Ophthalmol 100:299, 1985
29. Bourne WM: Morphologic and functional evaluation of the endothelium of transplanted human corneas. Trans Am Ophthalmol Soc 81:403, 1983
30. Carlson KH, Bourne WM, Brubaker RF: Variations in human endothelial cell morphology and permeability to fluorescein with age. Exp Eye Res 47:27, 1988
31. Rao GN, Shaw EL, Arthur EJ, Aquavella JV: Endothelial cell morphology and corneal deturgescence. Ann Ophthalmol 11:885, 1979
32. Yee RW, Matsuda M, Schultz RO, Edelhauser HF: Changes in the normal corneal endothelial pattern as a function of age. Curr Eye Res 4:671, 1985
33. Rao GN, Aquavella JV, Goldberg SH, Berk SL: Pseudophakic bullous keratopathy. Relationship to preoperative corneal endothelial status. Ophthalmology 91:1135, 1984
34. Abbott RL, Forster RK: Determinants of graft clarity in penetrating keratoplasty. Arch Ophthalmol 97:1071, 1979
35. Forster RK, Fine M: Relation of donor age to success in penetrating keratoplasty. Arch Ophthalmol 85:42, 1971
36. Harbour RC, Stern GA: Variables in McCarey-Kaufman corneal storage. Ophthalmology 90:136, 1983
37. Jenkins MS, Lempert SL, Brown SI: Significance of donor age in penetrating keratoplasty. Ann Ophthalmol 11:974, 1979
38. Culbertson WM, Abbott RL, Forster RK: Endothelial cell loss in penetrating keratoplasty. Ophthalmology 89:600, 1982
39. Linn JG Jr, Stuart JC, Warnicki JW, et al: Endothelial morphology in long-term keratoconus corneal transplants. Ophthalmology 88:761, 1981
40. Wilhelmus KR, Stulting RD, Sugar J, Khan MM: Primary graft failure: a national reporting system. Medical Advisory Board of the Eye Bank Association of America. Arch Ophthalmol 113:1497, 1995
41. Donzis PB, Insler MS, Gordon RA: Corneal curvatures in premature infants. Am J Ophthalmol 99:213, 1985
42. Koenig S, Graul E, Kaufman HE: Ocular refraction after penetrating keratoplasty with infant donor corneas. Am J Ophthalmol 94:534, 1982
43. Wood TO, Nissenkorn L: Infant donor corneas for penetrating keratoplasty. Ophthalmic Surg 12:500, 1981
44. Pfister RR, Breaud S: Aphakic refractive penetrating keratoplasty using newborn donor corneas. Ophthalmology 90:1207, 1983
45. Gandhi SS, Lamberts DW, Perry HD: Donor to host transmission of disease via corneal transplantation. Surv Ophthalmol 25:306, 1981
46. Payne JW: Donor selection. p. 6. In Brightbill FS (ed): Corneal Surgery: Theory, Technique, and Tissue. CV Mosby, St. Louis, 1986
47. Wilson SE, Bourne WM: Corneal preservation. Surv Ophthalmol 33:237, 1989
48. O'Day DM: Diseases potentially transmitted through corneal transplantation. Ophthalmology 96:1133, 1989
49. O'Day DM: Donor tissue. p. 549. In Brightbill FS (ed): Corneal Surgery: Theory, Technique, and Tissue. 2nd ed. Mosby–Year Book, St. Louis, 1993
50. Koenig SB: Donor age. p. 555. In Brightbill FS (ed): Corneal Surgery: Theory, Technique, and Tissue. 2nd ed. Mosby–Year Book, St. Louis, 1993
51. Leveille AS, McMullan FD, Cavanagh HD: Endophthalmitis following penetrating keratoplasty. Ophthalmology 90:38, 1983
52. Kloess PM, Stulting RD, Waring GO III, Wilson SA: Bacterial and fungal endophthalmitis after penetrating keratoplasty. Am J Ophthalmol 115:548, 1993
53. Insler MS, Urso LF: *Candida albicans* endophthalmitis after penetrating keratoplasty. Am J Ophthalmol 104:57, 1987
54. Beyt BW Jr, Waltman SR: Cryptococcal endophthalmitis after corneal transplantation. N Engl J Med 298:825, 1978
55. Khodadoust AA, Franklin RM: Transfer of bacterial infection by donor cornea in penetrating keratoplasty. Am J Ophthalmol 87:130, 1979
56. Larsen PA, Lindstrom RL, Doughman DJ: *Torulopsis glabrata* endophthalmitis after keratoplasty with an organ cultured cornea. Arch Ophthalmol 96:1019, 1978
57. Le Francois M, Baum JL: *Flavobacterium* endophthalmitis following keratoplasty. Use of a tissue culture medium-stored cornea. Arch Ophthalmol 94:1907, 1976
58. Shaw EL, Aquavella JV: Pneumococcal endophthalmitis following grafting of corneal tissue from a (cadaver) kidney donor. Ann Ophthalmol 9:435, 1977
59. Baer JB, Nirankari VS, Glaros DS. Streptococcal endophthalmitis from contaminated donor corneas after keratoplasty. Arch Ophthalmol 106:517, 1988
60. Hwang DG, Nakamura T, Trousdale MD, Smith TM: Combination antibiotic supplementation of corneal storage medium. Am J Ophthalmol 115:299, 1993
61. Barza M, Baum JL, Kane A: Comparing radioactive and trephine-disk bioassays of dicloxacillin and gentamicin in ocular tissues in vitro. Am J Ophthalmol 83:530, 1977

62. Yau CW, Busin M, Kaufman HE: Ocular concentrations of gentamicin after penetrating keratoplasty. Am J Ophthalmol 101:44, 1981
63. Hwang DG, Nakamura T, Smith TM, Trousdale MD: Improved antibiotic supplementation of Dexsol corneal storage medium. ARVO abstract. Invest Ophthalmol Vis Sci 31(suppl):267, 1990
64. Steinemann TL, Kaufman HE, Beuerman RW, et al: Vancomycin-enriched corneal storage medium. Am J Ophthalmol 113:555, 1993
65. Lindquist TD, Roth BP, Fritsche TR: Stability and activity of vancomycin in corneal storage medium. Cornea 12:222, 1993
66. Unterman SR, Parelman JJ, Padumane KR, et al: Endothelial toxicity of amphotericin B in K-Sol. Presented at the 28th Annual Scientific Session of the Eye Bank Association of America, New Orleans, LA, 1989
67. Raber IM, Friedman HM: Hepatitis B surface antigen in corneal donors. Am J Ophthalmol 104:255, 1987
68. Fujikawa LS, Palestine AG, Nussenblatt RB, et al: Isolation of human T lymphotropic virus type III from the tears of a patient with the acquired immunodeficiency syndrome. Lancet 2:529, 1985
69. Fujikawa LS, Salahuddin SZ, Ablashi D, et al: Human T-cell leukemia/lymphotropic virus type III in the conjunctival epithelium of a patient with AIDS. Am J Ophthalmol 100:507, 1985
70. Salahuddin SZ, Palestine AG, Heck E, et al: Isolation of the human T-cell leukemia/lymphotropic virus type III from the cornea. Am J Ophthalmol 101:149, 1986
71. Schwarz A, Hoffmann F, L'age-Stehr J, et al: Human immunodeficiency virus transmission by organ donation. Transplantation 44:21, 1987
72. Simonds RJ, Holmberg SD, Hurwitz RL, et al: Transmission of human immunodeficiency virus type 1 from a seronegative organ and tissue donor. N Engl J Med 326:726, 1992
73. Centers for Disease Control: Testing donors of organs, tissues, and semen for antibody to human T-lymphotropic virus type III/lymphadenopathy-associated virus. MMWR 34:294, 1985
74. Pepose JS, Pardo F, Kessler JA, et al: Screening cornea donors for antibodies against human immunodeficiency virus. Ophthalmology 94:95, 1987
75. Centers for Disease Control: Recommendations for preventing transmission of infection with human T-lymphotropic syndrome in the United States. MMWR 34:681, 1985
76. Feorino PM, Jaffe HW, Palmer E, et al: Transfusion-associated acquired immunodeficiency syndrome. Evidence for persistent infection in blood donors. N Engl J Med 312:1293, 1985
77. L'age-Stehr J, Scharz A, Offermann G, et al: HTLV-III infection in kidney transplant recipients. Lancet 2:1361, 1985
78. Peterman TA, Jaffe HW, Feorino PM, et al: Transfusion-associated acquired immunodeficiency syndrome in the United States. JAMA 254:2913, 1985
79. Schuman JS, Orellana J, Friedman AH, Teich SA: Acquired immunodeficiency syndrome (AIDS). Surv Ophthalmol 31:384, 1987
80. Duffy P, Wolf J, Collins G, et al: Possible person-to-person transmission of Creutzfeldt-Jakob disease. N Engl J Med 290:692, 1974
81. Mata B: The uses of cornea from gliomatous eyes in corneal transplantation. Nippon Ganka Gakkai Zasshi 43:1963, 1939
82. Haik BG, Dunleavy SA, Cooke C, et al: Retinoblastoma with anterior chamber extension. Ophthalmology 94:367, 1987
83. Harrison DA, Hodge DO, Bourne WM: Outcome of corneal grafting with donor tissue from eyes with primary choroidal melanomas: a retrospective cohort comparison. Arch Ophthalmol 113:753, 1995
84. Wagoner MD, Dohlman CH, Albert DM, et al: Corneal donor material selection. Ophthalmology 88:139, 1981
85. Bito LZ, Salvador EV: Intraocular fluid dynamics. II. Post mortem changes in solute concentrations. Exp Eye Res 10:273, 1970
86. McKinnon JR, Walters GD: Cadaver storage time. An important factor in donor cornea survival. Arch Ophthalmol 94:217, 1976
87. Breslin CW, Ng W: The endothelial function of donor corneas. Effects of delayed enucleation and refrigeration. Invest Ophthalmol 15:732, 1976
88. Schimmelpfennig BH: Evaluation of endothelial viability in human donor corneas. Arch Ophthalmol 100:472, 1982
89. Casey TA, Gibbs D: Complications in corneal grafting. Trans Ophthalmol Soc UK 92:517, 1972
90. Stocker FW, King EH, Lucas DO, Georgiade N: A comparison of two different staining methods for evaluating corneal endothelial viability. Arch Ophthalmol 76:883, 1966
91. Taylor MJ, Hunt CJ: Dual staining of corneal endothelium with trypan blue and alizarin red S: importance of pH for the dye-lake reaction. Br J Ophthalmol 65:815, 1981
92. Baum JL: A histochemical study of corneal respiratory enzymes. Arch Ophthalmol 70:59, 1963
93. Mueller FO: Experiments on canine corneal donor material stored in liquid nitrogen. Br J Ophthalmol 52:649, 1968
94. O'Neill P, Mueller FO, Trevor-Roper PD: On the preservation of corneae at –196°C for full-thickness homografts in man and dog. Br J Ophthalmol 51:13, 1967
95. Pena-Carrillo J, Polack FM: Histochemical changes in the endothelium of corneas stored in moist chambers. Arch Ophthalmol 72:811, 1964
96. Robbins JE, Capella JA, Kaufman HE: A study of endothelium in keratoplasty and corneal preservation. Arch Ophthalmol 73:242, 1965
97. Kuming BS: The assessment of endothelial viability. South Afr Med J 43:1083, 1969
98. Pegg DE: Viability assays for preserved cells, tissues, and organs. Cryobiology 26:212, 1989
99. Kolb MJ, Bourne WM: Supravital fluorescent staining of the corneal endothelium with acridine orange and ethidium bromide. Curr Eye Res 5:485, 1986

100. Davson H: The hydration of the cornea. Biochem J 59:24, 1955
101. Harris JE, Nordquist LT: The hydration of the cornea. I. The transport of water from the cornea. Am J Ophthalmol 40:100, 1955
102. Mishima S, Kudo T: In vitro incubation of rabbit cornea. Invest Ophthalmol 6:329, 1967
103. Hoefle FB: Human corneal donor material. In-vitro studies. Arch Ophthalmol 82:361, 1969
104. Dikstein S, Maurice DM: The metabolic basis to the fluid pump in the cornea. J Physiol 221:29, 1972
105. Wilson SE, Kaufman HE: Graft failure after penetrating keratoplasty. Surv Ophthalmol 34:325, 1990
106. McCarey BE, McNeill JL: Specular microscopic evaluation of donor corneal endothelium. Ann Ophthalmol 9:1279, 1977
107. Sherrard ES: An application of the temperature reversal effect: a possible method to evaluate donor cornea for penetrating keratoplasty. Exp Eye Res 15:667, 1973
108. McCarey BE: In vitro specular microscope perfusion of M-K- and moist-chamber-stored human corneas. Invest Ophthalmol Vis Sci 16:743, 1977
109. Breslin CW, Kaufman HE, Centifanto YM: Dextran flux in M-K medium-stored human corneas. Invest Ophthalmol Vis Sci 16:752, 1977
110. Hull DS, Green K, Bowman K: Dextran uptake into, and loss from, corneas stored in intermediate-term preservative. Invest Ophthalmol 15:663, 1976
111. Fong LP, Hunt CJ, Taylor MJ, Pegg DE: Cryopreservation of rabbit corneas: assessment by microscopy and transplantation. Br J Ophthalmol 70:751, 1986
112. Schaeffer EM: Ultrastructural changes in moist chamber corneas. Invest Ophthalmol 2:272, 1963
113. Schultz RO: Laboratory evaluation of cryopreserved corneal tissue. Trans Am Ophthalmol Soc 69:563, 1971
114. Van Horn DL, Edelhauser HF: Reversibility of ultrastructural freeze-thaw induced injury. Arch Ophthalmol 87:422, 1972
115. Hoefle FB, Maurice DM, Sibley RC: Human corneal donor material. Arch Ophthalmol 84:741, 1970
116. Bourne WM: Examination and photography of donor corneal endothelium. Arch Ophthalmol 94:1799, 1976
117. Bigar F, Schimmelpfennig B, Gieseler R: Routine evaluation of endothelium in human donor corneas. Albrecht von Graefes Arch Klin Exp Ophthalmol 200:195, 1976
118. Schwartz AE, Bourne WM: Endothelial cell loss after keratoplasty. p. 300. In Brightbill FS (ed): Corneal Surgery: Theory, Technique, and Tissue. 2nd ed. Mosby–Year Book, St. Louis, 1993
119. Bourne WM: The endothelial cell assay method for the evaluation of corneal preservation. p. 111. In Cavanagh HD (ed): The Cornea: Transactions of the World Congress III. Raven Press, New York, 1988
120. Andersen J, Ehlers N: Corneal transplantation using long-term cultured donor material. Acta Ophthalmol (Copenh) 64:93, 1986
121. Bourne WM, Kaufman HE: The endothelium of clear corneal transplants. Arch Ophthalmol 94:1730, 1976
122. Neubauer L, Smith RS, Leibowitz HM, Laing RA: Endothelial findings in cryopreserved corneal transplants. Ann Ophthalmol 16:980, 1984
123. Friedland BR, Forster RK: Comparison of corneal storage in McCarey-Kaufman medium, moist chamber, or standard eye-bank conditions. Invest Ophthalmol 15:143, 1976
124. Means TL, Geroski DH, Hadley A, et al: Viability of human corneal endothelium following Optisol-GS storage. Arch Ophthalmol 113:805, 1995
125. Bourne WM: Corneal preservation: past, present, and future. Refract Corneal Surg 7:60, 1991
126. Farrant J: Mechanism of cell damage during freezing and thawing and its prevention. Nature 205:1284, 1965
127. Mazur P: Freezing of living cells: Mechanisms and implications. Am J Physiol 247:C125, 1984
128. Rowe AW: Biochemical aspects of cryoprotective agents in freezing and thawing. Cryobiology 3:12, 1966
129. Meryman HT: Cryoprotective agents. Cryobiology 8:173, 1971
130. McCarey BE, Edelhauser HF, Van Horn DL: The effect of cryoprotection and cryodamage on corneal rehydration and endothelial structure. Cryobiology 10:298, 1973
131. Taillebourg O, Payrau P, Pouliquen Y, Faure JP: Corneal cryopreservation. Ophthalmic Res 5:342, 1973
132. Van Horn DL, Schultz RO, Edelhauser HF: Corneal cryopreservation. Alterations in endothelial intercellular spaces. Am J Ophthalmol 68:454, 1969
133. Madden PW, Easty DL: Assessment and interpretation of corneal endothelial cell morphology and function following cryopreservation. Br J Ophthalmol 66:136, 1982
134. Taylor MJ, Hunt CJ, Sherrard ES: Assessment of corneal endothelial integrity by specular microscopy after cryopreservation. p. 437. In The Cornea in Health and Disease, Proceedings of the 6th Congress of the European Society of Ophthalmology, Royal Society of Medicine International Congress and Symposium Series no. 40. Academic Press and RSM, London, 1981
135. Ruusuvaara P: The fate of preserved and transplanted human corneal endothelium. Acta Ophthalmol (Copenh) 58:440, 1980
136. Ehlers N, Sperling S, Olsen T: Post-operative thickness and endothelial cell density in cultivated, cryopreserved human corneal grafts. Acta Ophthalmol (Copenh) 60:935, 1982
137. Schultz RO, Matsuda M, Yee RW, et al: Long-term survival of cryopreserved corneal endothelium. Ophthalmology 92:1663, 1985
138. Bourne WM: Corneal cryopreservation. p. 46. In Blodi FC (ed): Current Concepts in Ophthalmology. CV Mosby, St. Louis, 1974
139. Fahy GM: Vitrification: a new approach to organ transplantation. Prog Clin Biol Res 224:305, 1986
140. Fahy GM, Levy DI, Ali SE: Some emerging principles underlying the physical properties, biological actions, and utility of vitrification solutions. Cryobiology 24:196, 1987
141. Brunette I, Nelson LR, Bourne WM: Tolerance of human corneal endothelium to glycerol. Cryobiology 26:513, 1989

142. Rich SJ, Armitage WJ: Propane-1,2-diol as a potential component of a vitrification solution for corneas. Cryobiology 27:42, 1990
143. Bourne WM, Nelson LR: Two systems for testing corneal endothelial tolerance to cryoprotectants. ARVO abstract. Invest Ophthalmol Vis Sci 32(suppl):1062, 1991
144. Armitage WJ, Moss SJ, Easty DL: Effects of osmotic stress on rabbit corneal endothelium. Cryobiology 25:425, 1988
145. Waltman SR, Palmberg PF: Human penetrating keratoplasty using modified M-K medium. Ophthalmic Surg 9:48, 1978
146. Aquavella JV, Van Horn DL, Haggerty CJ: Corneal preservation using M-K medium. Am J Ophthalmol 80:791, 1975
147. Van Horn DL, Schultz RO, DeBruin J: Endothelial survival in corneal tissue stored in M-K medium. Am J Ophthalmol 80:642, 1975
148. Neubauer L, Laing RA, Leibowitz HM: Specular microscopic appearance of damaged and dead endothelial cells in corneas following short-term storage. Arch Ophthalmol 102:439, 1984
149. Holtmann HW, Stein HJ, Dardenne MU: Experiments on corneal preservation (short-time storage). Ophthalmic Res 8:124, 1976
150. Nayak SK, Binder PS: The growth of endothelium from human corneal rims in tissue culture. Invest Ophthalmol Vis Sci 25:1213, 1984
151. Bigar F, McCarey BE, Kaufman HE: Improved corneal storage: penetrating keratoplasties in rabbits. Exp Eye Res 20:219, 1975
152. Breslin CW, Sherrard ES, Marshall J, Rice NSC: Evaluation of McCarey-Kaufman technique of corneal storage. Arch Ophthalmol 94:1545, 1976
153. Bigar F, Kaufman HE, McCarey BE, Binder PS: Improved corneal storage for penetrating keratoplasties in man. Am J Ophthalmol 79:115, 1975
154. Van der Want JJL, Pels E, Schuchard Y, et al: Electron microscopy of cultured human corneas: osmotic hydration and the use of a dextran fraction (Dextran T5000) in organ culture. Arch Ophthalmol 101:1920, 1983
155. Graham CR, Gottsch JD, Chacko VP, Stark WJ: Dextran efflux from McCarey-Kaufman-stored corneas as measured by nuclear magnetic resonance. Cornea 8:98, 1989
156. McCarey BE, Meyer RF, Kaufman HE: Improved corneal storage for penetrating keratoplasties in humans. Ann Ophthalmol 8:1488, 1976
157. Polack FM: Penetrating keratoplasty using MK stored corneas and Na hyaluronate (Healon). Trans Am Ophthalmol Soc 80:248, 1982
158. Stark WJ, Maumenee AE, Kenyon KR: Intermediate-term storage for penetrating keratoplasty. Am J Ophthalmol 79:795, 1975
159. Stainer GA, Brightbill FS, Calkins B: A comparison of corneal storage in moist chamber and McCarey-Kaufman medium in human keratoplasty. Ophthalmology 88:46, 1981
160. Bourne WM: Endothelial cell survival on transplanted human corneas preserved at 4°C in 2.5% chondroitin sulfate for one to 13 days. Am J Ophthalmol 102:382, 1986
161. Mascarella K, Cavanagh HD: Penetrating keratoplasty using McCarey-Kaufman preserved corneal tissue. South Med J 72:1268, 1979.
162. Sperling S: Human corneal endothelium in organ culture. The influence of temperature and medium of incubation. Acta Ophthalmol (Copenh) 57:269, 1979
163. Easty DL, Carter CA, Lewkowicz-Moss SJ: Corneal cell culture and organ culture. Trans Ophthalmol Soc UK 105:385, 1986
164. Keates RH: Organ culture corneal preservation. A preliminary report. Dev Ophthalmol 11:44, 1985
165. Pels E, Schuchard Y: Organ culture and endothelial evaluation as a preservation method for human corneas. p. 93. In Brightbill FS (ed): Corneal Surgery: Theory, Technique, and Tissue. CV Mosby, St. Louis, 1986
166. Völker-Dieben HJ, D'Amaro J, Kok-van Alphen CC, Pels E: Survival of organ-cultured donor corneas. p. 632. In Brightbill FS (ed): Corneal Surgery: Theory, Technique, and Tissue. 2nd ed. Mosby–Year Book, St. Louis, 1993
167. Pels L, Schuchard Y: Organ culture in the Netherlands. p. 622. In Brightbill FS (ed): Corneal Surgery: Theory, Technique, and Tissue. 2nd ed. Mosby–Year Book, St. Louis, 1993
168. Bourne WM, Lindstrom RL, Doughman DJ: Endothelial cell survival on transplanted human corneas preserved by organ culture with 1.35% chondroitin sulfate. Am J Ophthalmol 100:789, 1985
169. Doughman DJ, Lindstrom RL, Skelnick DL, et al: Long-term organ culture for corneal storage: Minnesota system. p. 614. In Brightbill FS (ed): Corneal Surgery: Theory, Technique, and Tissue. 2nd ed. Mosby–Year Book, St. Louis, 1993
170. Doughman DJ, Van Horn D, Harris JE, et al: Endothelium of the human organ cultured cornea: an electron microscopic study. Trans Am Ophthalmol Soc 71:304, 1973
171. Van Horn DL, Doughman DJ, Harris JE, et al: Ultrastructure of human organ cultured cornea: II. Stroma and epithelium. Arch Ophthalmol 93:275, 1975
172. Yau C, Kaufman HE: A medium-term corneal preserving medium (K-Sol). Arch Ophthalmol 104:598, 1986
173. Busin M, Yau C, Avni I, Kaufman H: Comparison of K-Sol and M-K medium for cornea storage: results of penetrating keratoplasty in rabbits. Br J Ophthalmol 70:860, 1986
174. Stein RM, Bourne WM, Campbell RJ: Chondroitin sulfate for corneal preservation at 4°C. Arch Ophthalmol 104:1358, 1986
175. Stein RM, Laibson PR: Comparison of chondroitin sulfate to McCarey-Kaufman medium for corneal storage. Am J Ophthalmol 104:490, 1987
176. Farge EJ, Fort RA, Wilhelmus KR, et al: Morphologic changes of K-Sol preserved human corneas. Cornea 8:159, 1990
177. Keates RH, Rabin B: Extending corneal storage with 2.5% chondroitin sulfate (K-Sol). Ophthalmic Surg 19:817, 1988
178. Sieck EA, Enzenauer RW, Cornell M, Butler C: Contamination of K-Sol corneal storage medium with *Propionibacterium acnes*. Arch Ophthalmol 107:1023, 1989
179. Lindstrom RL, Skelnik DL, Mindrup EA, et al: Corneal preservation at 4°C with chondroitin sulfate containing

medium. ARVO abstract. Invest Ophthalmol Vis Sci 28(suppl):167, 1987
180. Lass JH, Reinhart WJ, Bruner WE, et al: Comparison of corneal storage in K-Sol and chondroitin sulfate corneal storage medium in human corneal transplantation. Ophthalmology 96:688, 1989
181. Lass JH, Reinhart WJ, Skelnik DL, et al: An in vitro and clinical comparison of corneal storage with chondroitin sulfate corneal storage medium with and without dextran. Ophthalmology 97:96, 1990
182. Saggau DD, Bourne WM: A comparison of two preservation media (CSM and K-Sol) by scanning electron microscopy of preserved endothelium. Arch Ophthalmol 107:429, 1989
183. Laing RA, Neubauer L, Oak SS, et al: Evidence for mitosis in the adult corneal endothelium. Ophthalmology 91:1129, 1984
184. Squires EL, Weimer VL: Stimulation of repair of human corneal endothelium in organ culture by mesodermal growth factor. Arch Ophthalmol 98:1462, 1980
185. Cipolla L, Whitehouse A, Eiferman R, Schultz G: Stimulation of human corneal endothelial cell mitosis in vitro by human cord serum. ARVO abstract. Invest Ophthalmol Vis Sci 26(suppl):52, 1985
186. Couch JM, Cullen P, Casey TA, Fabre JW: Mitotic activity of corneal endothelial cells in organ culture with recombinant human epidermal growth factor. Ophthalmology 94:1, 1987
187. Lindstrom RL: Advances in corneal preservation. Trans Am Ophthalmol Soc 88:555, 1990
188. Lass JH, Musch DC, Gordon JF, Laing RA: Epidermal growth factor and insulin use in corneal preservation: results of a multi-center trial. The Corneal Preservation Study Group. Ophthalmology 101:352, 1994
189. Laing RA, Hirokawa K, Yang ZR, Oak SS: Maintenance of corneal endothelium in storage media. ARVO abstract. Invest Ophthalmol Vis Sci 31(suppl):268, 1990
190. Farge EJ, Fort RA, Brown ES, et al: Experimental evaluation of new preservation media. ARVO abstract. Invest Ophthalmol Vis Sci 31(suppl):475, 1990
191. Lindstrom RL, Kaufman HE, Skelnik DL, et al: Optisol corneal storage medium. Am J Ophthalmol 114:345, 1992
192. Lass JH, Bourne WM, Sugar A, et al: A randomized, prospective, double-masked clinical trial of Optisol vs Dexsol corneal storage media. Arch Ophthalmol 110:1401, 1992
193. Binder PS, Stainer G, Peri T: Eye banking 1981–1982—recommended guidelines. J Ocular Ther Surg 2:125, 1983
194. Brown RM, Trevor-Roper PD: A clinical method for assessment of endothelial viability in donor corneae. Br J Ophthalmol 52:882, 1968
195. Cowden JW: Slit-lamp attachment for examination of donor corneas in McCarey-Kaufman medium. Arch Ophthalmol 97:953, 1979
196. Abbott RL, Forster RK: Clinical specular microscopy and intraocular surgery. Arch Ophthalmol 97:1476, 1979
197. McCarey BE: Noncontact specular microscopy. Ophthalmology 86:1848, 1979
198. Jumblatt MM, Maurice DM, McCulley JP: Transplantation of tissue-cultured corneal endothelium. Invest Ophthalmol Vis Sci 17:1135, 1978
199. Maurice DM, McCulley JP, Perlman MP: Donor endothelium from tissue culture. ARVO abstract. Invest Ophthalmol Vis Sci 16(suppl):102, 1977
200. Gospodarowicz D, Greenburg G, Alvarado J: Transplantation of cultured bovine corneal endothelial cells to rabbit cornea: clinical implications for human studies. Proc Natl Acad Sci USA 76:464, 1979
201. Gospodarowicz D, Greenburg G, Alvarado J: Transplantation of cultured bovine corneal endothelial cells to species with nonregenerative endothelium. Arch Ophthalmol 97:2163, 1979
202. Bahn CF, MacCallum DK, Lillie JH, et al: Complications associated with bovine corneal endothelial cell-lined homografts in the cat. Invest Ophthalmol Vis Sci 22:73, 1982
203. Skelnick DL, Lindstrom RL, Mindrup EA: Endothelium. Cell growth in organ culture. p. 620. In Brightbill FS (ed): Corneal Surgery: Theory, Technique, and Tissue. CV Mosby, St. Louis, 1986
204. Insler MS, Lopez JG: Heterologous transplantation versus enhancement of human corneal endothelium. Cornea 10:136, 1991
205. Wilson SE, Lloyd SA: Growth factor and growth factor receptor mRNA production by cultured human corneal endothelial cells. ARVO abstract. Invest Ophthalmol Vis Sci 32(suppl):953, 1991
206. Wilson SE, Shultz GS, Chegini N, et al: Epidermal growth factor, transforming growth factor alpha, transforming growth factor beta, acidic fibroblast growth factor, basic growth factor, and interleukin-1 proteins in the cornea. Exp Eye Res 59:63, 1994
207. Wilson SE, Walker JW, Chwang EL, He YG: Hepatocyte growth factor, keratinocyte growth factor, their receptors, fibroblast growth factor receptor-2, and the cells of the cornea. Invest Ophthalmol Vis Sci 34:2544, 1993
208. Schweigerer L, Ferrara N, Haaparanta T, et al: Basic fibroblast growth factor: Expression in cultured cells derived from corneal endothelium and lens epithelium. Exp Eye Res 46:71, 1988
209. Sato Y, Murphy PR, Sato R, Friesen HG: Fibroblast growth factor release by bovine endothelial cells and human astrocytoma cells in culture is density dependent. Mol Endocrinol 3:144, 1986.
210. Sabatier P, Rieck P, Daumer ML, et al: Effects of human recombinant basic fibroblast growth factor on endothelial wound healing in organ culture of human corneas. J Fr Ophtalmol 19:200, 1996
211. Wilson SE, Lloyd SA, He YG, McCash CS: Extended life of human corneal endothelial cells transfected with the SV40 large T antigen. Invest Ophthalmol Vis Sci 34:2112, 1993
212. Wilson SE, Weng J, Blair S, et al: Expression of E6/E7 or SV40 large T antigen-coding oncogenes in human corneal endothelial cells indicates regulated high-proliferative capacity. Invest Ophthalmol Vis Sci 36:32, 1995

34

Penetrating Keratoplasty

Bruce A. Barron

The cornea is the most commonly transplanted solid tissue[1,2] (Table 34-1); more than 34,000 penetrating keratoplasties are performed each year in the United States. Penetrating keratoplasty is also one of the most successful transplant procedures. Although the relative "immunologic privilege" of the cornea accounts for much of the high success rate, advances in corneal preservation, surgical techniques, and pre- and postoperative care are significant factors.

The term *penetrating keratoplasty* is actually a misnomer for a procedure that replaces full-thickness cornea. Although the term *perforating keratoplasty* is more accurate and is used by some to refer to the procedure, it has not become common parlance.

HISTORY

The first report of successful penetrating keratoplasty in a human was almost 100 years ago, when Eduard Konrad Zirm performed bilateral penetrating keratoplasties in Alois Glogar, a patient who sustained alkali burns while cleaning his chicken coop with lime.[3] Since then, a better understanding of corneal anatomy and physiology (especially with regard to the importance of the corneal endothelium); the elucidation of the principles of immunology; advances in corneal preservation; the introduction of microsurgical methodology, technology, and instrumentation; and the development of anti-inflammatory and immunosuppressive agents and antibiotics have resulted in an overall success rate greater than 90 percent.[4] Some of the milestones in the development of penetrating keratoplasty are listed in Table 34-2.[5-9]

INDICATIONS AND PATIENT SELECTION

Penetrating keratoplasty is indicated in four basic conditions: (1) loss of corneal integrity, (2) opacification of the deep layers of the central cornea resulting in decreased visual acuity, (3) abnormal curvature of the anterior corneal surface that cannot be corrected with optical aids, and/or (4) central infectious keratitis that is unresponsive to medical therapy and is extending toward the periphery. These conditions are common final pathways to surgery for many of the corneal disorders for which penetrating keratoplasty is performed.

Table 34-3 lists the indications for penetrating keratoplasty from various reports published over the past 5 years.[1,4,10-15] The most common indication varies from report to report, depending on the time period studied, the method by which the data were collected (e.g., retrospective clinical or histopathologic review of consecutive cases, information from registries, or responses to surveys), the locale from which the data were obtained, and the patient population base and the surgeons' practice patterns. Among the eight reports included in Table 34-3, five listed pseudophakic bullous keratopathy as the most common indication (23 to 39 percent),[1,4,10,14,15] two listed keratoconus (24 to 31 percent),[11,12] and one listed corneal graft failure (41 percent).[13] Several of the reports noted changes in the frequencies of indications over time. Of the 27,017 cases of penetrating keratoplasty with recipient diagnoses reported to the Eye Bank Association of America in 1996, pseudophakic bullous keratopathy was the most common indication for the procedure (24.9 percent), followed by corneal endothelial dystrophies (14.0 percent) and corneal ectasias such as keratoconus (12.2 percent).[1]

TABLE 34-1
Numbers of Transplants in the United States in 1996

Tissue	*Number of Transplants*[a]
Cornea	34,668
Kidney	10,799
Liver	3,715
Heart	2,140
Pancreas	918
Heart-lung	38

[a] In this table, simultaneous kidney-pancreas transplants are counted twice, both in kidney transplants and in pancreas transplants. Double kidney, double lung, and heart-lung transplants are counted as one transplant. All other multi-organ transplants are included in the total for each individual organ transplanted.
Source: Data from Eye Bank Association of America: 1996 Eye Banking Statistical Report. Eye Bank Association of America, Washington, DC, 1996; and United Network for Organ Sharing: 1996 Annual Report. United Network for Organ Sharing, Richmond, VA, 1996.

The major goals of penetrating keratoplasty are to improve visual acuity, maintain the integrity of the eye, and/or decrease pain. In some patients, procedures other than penetrating keratoplasty may be more appropriate to achieve these goals, such as excimer laser phototherapeutic keratectomy, photorefractive keratectomy, or photoastigmatic refractive keratectomy; inlay or onlay lamellar keratoplasty; partial or total conjunctival flaps; or prosthokeratoplasty. The circumstances for which these procedures might be preferable to penetrating keratoplasty are outlined in the chapters in which each of these procedures is discussed.

Patient compliance is important in any ophthalmic procedure; it is essential in penetrating keratoplasty. Postoperative follow-up is more involved for this procedure than for most intraocular surgical procedures. Penetrating keratoplasty is contraindicated when it is thought that the patient or, in the case of an infant or child, the parents are likely to be noncompliant with instructions for postoperative care and follow-up. In these cases, a perfect surgical result can become a worse problem than the disorder for which penetrating keratoplasty was performed.

PREOPERATIVE EVALUATION

One of the most important objectives of the preoperative evaluation is to identify any underlying disorders responsible for the corneal abnormality for which penetrating keratoplasty is indicated. If these disorders are not identified and treated aggressively, the graft will succumb to the same fate as the original cornea.

A complete history is taken in an attempt to identify systemic diseases, such as collagen-vascular diseases, that can cause corneal abnormalities. A comprehensive ophthalmologic examination is performed, with an emphasis on the external eye. The position and function of the eyelids are evaluated. Entropion, ectropion, lagophthalmos, or trichiasis are treated before or in concert with penetrating keratoplasty, as described in Chapter 6. Tear function is assessed and any abnormalities are treated as described in Chapter 5. The palpebral and tarsal conjunctiva are examined to look for scarring and cicatricial changes.

Slit lamp microscopy of the cornea is performed to assess clarity and integrity. The extent of the disease process in the cornea is measured, and the location and size of the graft are planned. Central and peripheral corneal thicknesses are measured by optical or ultrasonic pachymetry. The recipient cornea adjacent to the anticipated site of trephination must be thick enough to support sutures and sustain wound closure.

Many corneal disorders for which penetrating keratoplasty is indicated are associated with other anterior segment abnormalities, such as peripheral anterior synechiae, a distorted and/or displaced pupil, and glaucoma. Preoperative glaucoma and peripheral anterior synechiae are associated with an increased risk of graft failure.[16] In an eye with an irregular cornea, intraocular pressure must be measured with an electronic applanation tonometer such as the Tono-Pen; the Goldmann applanation tonometer cannot be used because the mires are too irregular. If the cornea is sufficiently clear, visual fields may be measured with a Goldmann or automated perimeter; otherwise, the fields can be crudely assessed with a hand-held light as the test object. Coexistent corneal disease and glaucoma may be managed either by drainage surgery and subsequent penetrating keratoplasty, or by combined drainage surgery and penetrating keratoplasty. Kirkness et al[17] reported that achieving and maintaining a clear graft and normal intraocular pressure was more likely with combined surgery than with separate surgeries (50 percent vs. 27 percent at 5 years).

Slit lamp microscopy of the lens is performed after dilation of the pupil to look for opacities. Coexistent corneal diseases and cataracts are common. An early cataract will progress after penetrating keratoplasty, and the likelihood of cataract formation subsequent to penetrating keratoplasty increases greatly after age 50 years, regardless of the indication for penetrating keratoplasty.[18] Therefore, a cataract, even an early one, in a patient older than 50 years of age should be removed at the time of penetrating keratoplasty. Usually, cataract extraction cannot be performed before penetrating keratoplasty because visualization through the cornea is poor, and cataract extraction after penetrating keratoplasty, when visual-

TABLE 34-2
Highlights in the Development of Penetrating Keratoplasty

Date	*Individual*	*Country*	*Contribution*
130–200	Galen	Greece	Advocated superficial keratectomy
1789	G.P. deQuengsy	France	Suggested replacing an opaque cornea with a thin glass disk set in a silver ring
1796	E. Darwin	England	Suggested cutting out a portion of an opaque cornea to allow healing with the formation of a "transparent scar"
1813	K. Himly	Germany	Suggested replacing an opaque cornea in one animal with a clear cornea from another animal
1824	F. Reisinger	Germany	Suggested replacing an opaque human cornea with a clear animal cornea; suggested the term *keratoplasty*
1837	S.L.L. Bigger	Ireland	Successfully performed penetrating allograft in animals
1844	R.S. Kissam	United States	Reported unsuccessful penetrating keratoplasty from a pig to a human
1846	W. Morton	United States	Introduced ether anesthesia
1884	C. Koller	Austria	Introduced cocaine as a topical anesthetic for ocular surgery
1867	J. Lister	England	Introduced principles of antiseptic surgery
1870s–1880s	A. von Hippel	Germany	Advocated lamellar keratoplasty; reported first successful transplantation of a portion of corneal tissue in a human (a full-thickness rabbit cornea into a lamellar bed of a human); invented the circular trephine
1872	H. Power	England	Advocated penetrating keratoplasty; suggested use of allogeneic donor tissue because of requirement to match the donor and recipient corneal thicknesses
1906	E.K. Zirm	Czechoslovakia	Reported first successful penetrating keratoplasty in a human
1910s–1930s	A. Elschnig	Czechoslovakia	Performed 180 corneal transplants, with 22 percent showing improvement in visual acuity; defined indications, techniques, and complications of penetrating keratoplasty
1910s–1950s	V. Filatov	Russia	Performed systematic study of penetrating keratoplasty; devised numerous instruments and surgical innovations; suggested using cadaver corneas as donor tissue
1930s–1950s	R. Castroviejo	United States	Devised numerous instruments and surgical techniques, including the square-graft technique
1944	R.T. Paton	United States	Founded the first eye bank in the United States
1968	D. Maurice	United States	Developed the specular microscope
1974	B. McCarey H. Kaufman	United States	Developed corneal storage medium

Source: Data from DM Albert: Corneal surgery. In DM Albert, DD Edwards (eds): The History of Ophthalmology. Blackwell Science, Cambridge, 1996; MJ Mannis, JH Krachmer: Keratoplasty: a historical perspective. Surv Ophthalmol 25:333, 1981; L Forstot, HE Kaufman: Corneal transplantation. Annu Rev Med 28:21, 1977; S Duke-Elder, AG Leigh: Diseases of the outer eye. p. 648. In S Duke-Elder (ed): System of Ophthalmology. Vol. III, Part 2. CV Mosby, St. Louis, 1965; and AJ Altman, DM Albert, GA Fournier: Cocaine's use in ophthalmology: our 100-year heritage. Surv Ophthalmol 29:300, 1985.

ization is good, may damage the graft. Pineros et al[19] found no statistically significant difference in outcome and refractive status after either triple procedures (penetrating keratoplasty, extracapsular cataract extraction, and posterior chamber intraocular lens implantation) or nonsimultaneous procedures (penetrating keratoplasty followed by extracapsular cataract extraction and posterior chamber intraocular lens implantation) in patients with Fuchs' endothelial dystrophy and visually significant cataracts. Performing a cataract extraction and penetrating keratoplasty at two separate times subjects the patient to two operations, increases costs, and delays visual rehabilitation. Therefore, the procedures should be performed simultaneously.

Intraocular lens power is calculated preoperatively using one of several formulas.[20] Preoperative keratometry measurements from a diseased cornea are less precise than those from a normal cornea and may not correlate with postoperative keratometry measurements from the graft. An average keratometry measurement (44 diopters), preoperative keratometry measurements from the diseased or fellow cornea, or an average of postoperative keratometry measurements from other patients who have undergone penetrating keratoplasty for similar diagnoses

TABLE 34-3
Indications for Penetrating Keratoplasty

	Hyman et al, 1992[10]	*Mamalis et al, 1992*[11]	*Price et al, 1993*[4]	*The Australian Corneal Graft Registry, 1993*[12]	*Sharif et al, 1993*[13]	*Haamann et al, 1994*[14]	*Flowers et al, 1995*[15]	*Eye Bank Association of America, 1996*[1]
Time period	1985–1988	1981–1990	1982–1990	1985–1991	1971–1990	1984–1993	1989–1993	1996
Location	Maryland	Utah	Indiana	Australia	England	Denmark	California	United States
Number of transplants	3,941	999	1,819	3,460	3,555	180	1,104	27,017
Indications (%)								
Pseudophakic bullous keratopathy	22.8	23.0	38.6	17	2	28.3	24.8	24.9
Aphakic bullous keratopathy	9.6	5.6	11.9	5	5.9	10.0	6.4	5.3
Keratoconus and other ectasias	12.9	24.2	10.0	31	16.8	6.7	7.1	12.2
Graft failure	16.9	13.1	6.6	14	40.8	11.1	21.3	10.5
Related to rejection	—	—	—	—	12.9	—	—	4.1
Unrelated to rejection	—	—	—	—	27.9	—	—	6.4
Corneal dystrophies								
Endothelial	13.0	5.8	19.5	5	3.9	13.9	4.8	14.0
Other	2.0	2.4	0.8	2	5.3	3.9	2.2	3.2
Corneal degenerations	3.1	—	—	1.5	0.4	—	0.1	4.0
Keratitis	12.6	3.0	4.0	5.6	16.7	13.9	2.9	6.2
Microbial	—	—	—	—	—	—	—	0.9
Viral	2.9	3.0	1.2	—	11.7	—	2.3	1.5
Syphilitic	—	—	2.8	—	5	—	0.6	0.4
Noninfectious	9.7	—	—	—	—	—	—	3.4
Trauma								
Mechanical	1.1	0.8	—	—	2.9	4.4	2.4	1.9
Chemical	0.6	1.3	—	—	1.2	1.1	1.0	0.3
Congenital abnormalities	0.8	0.5	—	<1	—	—	2.8	0.8
Other	4.3[a]	19.8[b]	8.6[c]	19.0[d]	0.1[e]	6.7[f]	22.9[g]	16.7
Unknown	0.2	0.4	—	1	2.9	—	1.4	—

[a] Includes ulcerative conditions (2.4%), previous pseudophakic bullous keratopathy (1.2%), and other (0.7%).
[b] Includes scarring (8.2%), ulcerative conditions (5.7%), chronic keratitis (3.1%), and other (2.8%).
[c] Includes scarring (6.4%), active ulcerative conditions or perforations (0.7%), and other (1.5%).
[d] Includes scarring and opacification (11%), unspecified bullous keratopathy (3%), ulcerative conditions (3%), astigmatism (<1%), and other (2%).
[e] Infection.
[f] Includes scarring (2.8%), ulcerative conditions (1.7%), and other (2.2%).
[g] Includes scarring (11.1%), ulcerative conditions (5.8%), chronic keratitis (1.0%), silicone oil keratopathy (0.6%), trachoma (0.2%), and other (4.2%).

may be used in the formula to calculate the power of the intraocular lens. The myopia induced by an oversized graft (see below) must be taken into account when calculating the power.

As discussed above, pseudophakic bullous keratopathy is one of the most common indications for penetrating keratoplasty. Preoperatively, the type of intraocular lens already in place is determined and a decision is made regarding its removal. The surgical report from the operation in which the intraocular lens was implanted is helpful. Some patients carry a card describing the type and power of intraocular lens implanted. An attempt is made to visualize the position of the haptics of anterior chamber intraocular lenses by gonioscopy, although corneal opacification may make this examination difficult.

Corneal opacification also makes it difficult to visualize the retina. B-scan ultrasonography is indicated if the retina cannot be seen. Various devices have been developed to assess visual potential in eyes with opaque media, such as the laser interferometer and Potential Acuity Meter, or PAM. However, sometimes the media are too opaque for their use and sometimes the predicted visual acuity is falsely high or low. Color perception indicates the presence of some cone function and can be tested by asking the patient to identify the colors of bottle caps held over the tip of a penlight.

PREOPERATIVE MEDICATIONS

Preoperative medications for penetrating keratoplasty are similar to those for any intraocular procedure and are divided into four groups: mydriatic and miotic agents, osmotic agents, corticosteroids, and antimicrobial agents.

Topical mydriatic agents, such as 0.5 percent tropicamide, 2.5 percent phenylephrine, and 1 percent cyclopentolate, are used when cataract extraction or posterior chamber intraocular lens implantation, repositioning, or removal is anticipated. A topical miotic agent, such as 2 or 4 percent pilocarpine, is used when protection of the lens, posterior capsule, vitreous face, or posterior chamber intraocular lens by the iris is desired. It is also used when an anterior chamber intraocular lens is to be implanted, repositioned, or removed, and a vitrectomy is not anticipated.

Posterior pressure is undesirable in penetrating keratoplasty, as in most intraocular procedures, because it can cause the iris, lens, and vitreous to move anteriorly. This risk may be reduced by lowering the pressure in the eye and orbit preoperatively by administration of a systemic osmotic agent, application of external pressure, and proper positioning of the patient. If there are no contraindications, a 20 percent solution of mannitol (20 g/100 ml) is given intravenously over the hour preceding surgery at a dosage of 1 to 2 g/kg, to a maximum of 100 grams. Mannitol is contraindicated in patients with limited cardiac reserve and should be avoided in elderly patients because it can cause excessive shrinkage of the brain and rupture of fragile subdural veins. The diuretic effect of mannitol can be disruptive. If the eye is intact, external pressure is applied to the eye manually or with a Honan intraocular pressure reducer for at least 10 minutes. This procedure is performed before the administration of general anesthesia or after the injection of peribulbar or retrobulbar anesthetics. Positioning of the patient in the reverse Trendelenburg position—that is, with the head above the feet—lowers intraocular and orbital pressures by decreasing venous pressure. These preoperative maneuvers are helpful but not always successful in decreasing posterior pressure. Most posterior pressure is caused by scleral collapse and can be prevented by suturing a scleral support ring onto the sclera, as described below. Hyperventilation helps decrease posterior pressure by producing hypocapnia. This effect occurs when the end-tidal CO_2 is approximately 25 mmHg, which is most easily achieved in patients under general anesthesia.

Preoperative systemic corticosteroids, such as prednisone at a dosage of 1 mg/kg, may be considered in patients who are at high risk for corneal graft rejection or who have active or inactive keratitis or uveitis that could flare postoperatively. Patients at high risk for corneal graft rejection include those who have had a previously rejected graft and those with stromal vascularization.[21] Inflammation at the time of penetrating keratoplasty is associated with graft failure,[22,23] and patients with active inflammation should not undergo elective penetrating keratoplasty until the inflammation is controlled. In patients with active bacterial, fungal, or viral keratitis requiring penetrating keratoplasty, systemic corticosteroids are started preoperatively to control inflammation. Systemic corticosteroids are also started preoperatively in patients with luetic interstitial keratitis or herpes simplex keratitis, even if the disease is quiescent. Systemic corticosteroids are fraught with side effects, and patients taking them must be closely monitored. These side effects occur more frequently with high doses and long-term administration (1 to 2 months or longer).

I do not routinely give preoperative antibiotics unless the cornea is infected, in which case appropriate antibacterial, antifungal, antiparasitic, and/or antiviral agents are given. Penetrating keratoplasty should be postponed, if possible, until the infection is under control. A corneal perforation from an infected ulcer is generally treated with antibiotics for 24 hours before penetrating keratoplasty is performed. In patients with a history of herpes simplex

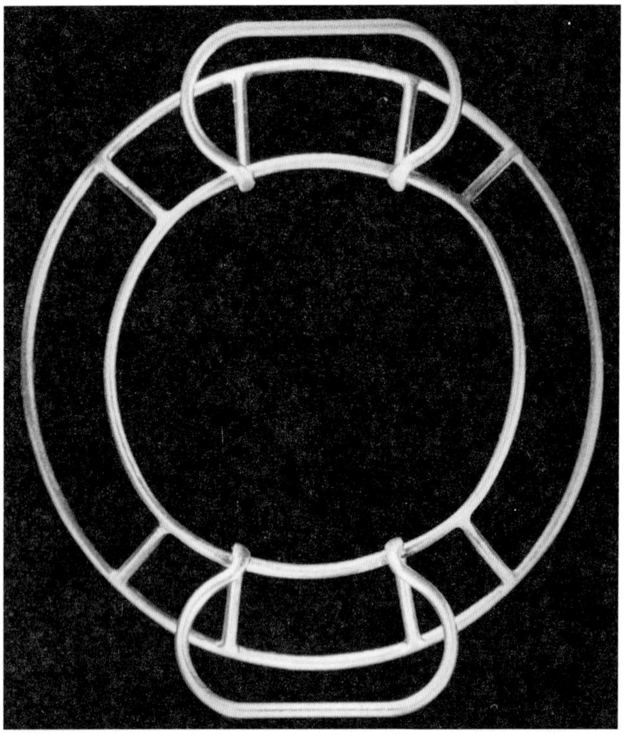

FIGURE 34-1 McNeill-Goldman scleral and blepharostat ring.

keratitis, long-term prophylactic oral acyclovir has been reported to decrease the recurrence of herpetic keratitis and reduce corneal graft failure.[24-26] Oral acyclovir (400 mg 5 times a day) or valacyclovir (500 mg 3 times a day) may be started a few days preoperatively in these patients.

ANESTHESIA

Penetrating keratoplasty can be performed with local or general anesthesia, depending on the patient's age and ability to cooperate, and the condition of the eye. Local anesthesia is obtained with an eyelid block and a peribulbar or retrobulbar injection of a mixture of 5 ml of 2 percent lidocaine without epinephrine, 5 ml of 0.5 or 0.75 percent bupivacaine, and 1 ml (150 USP units) of hyaluronidase (Wydase), as in any intraocular procedure. General anesthesia is indicated in infants, children, and uncooperative adults. General anesthesia is also indicated when the eye is inflamed because local anesthesia is difficult to obtain, and when the cornea is perforated because pressure on the eye from a peribulbar or retrobulbar injection is undesirable. In the latter case, an injection of anesthetic over each rectus muscle can safely be given if general anesthesia is contraindicated.

SURGICAL TECHNIQUES

Supporting the Sclera

The most common cause of posterior pressure and anterior displacement of the iris, lens, and vitreous after the recipient cornea has been removed is scleral collapse. Scleral collapse is more common in infants and young patients, myopic patients, and patients with keratoconus, and can create so much posterior pressure that the lens and vitreous may extrude from the eye. Scleral collapse also occurs in patients who are aphakic, especially if a vitrectomy has been performed. In these patients, the problem is not so much posterior pressure as collapse of the recipient corneal rim, which makes suturing the donor cornea difficult. It is prudent to support the sclera in all patients because once the sclera starts to collapse, it is difficult to reverse the process without extrusion of the intraocular contents.

A variety of scleral support rings have been developed to prevent scleral collapse. The two most commonly used are the McNeill-Goldman scleral and blepharostat ring and the Flieringa ring. The McNeill-Goldman scleral and blepharostat ring consists of two metal rings connected by four struts; two blepharostats are attached to the anterior ring (Figure 34-1).[27] It is available in two sizes: an adult size (with an anterior ring diameter of 17 mm and a posterior ring diameter of 24 mm) and a pediatric size (with an anterior ring diameter of 14 mm and a posterior ring diameter of 23 mm). The Flieringa ring is a simple metal ring that is available in several diameters. The size and placement of any scleral support ring must be such that the ring does not interfere with concomitant surgical procedures, such as transscleral fixation of an intraocular lens.

The McNeill-Goldman scleral and blepharostat ring is placed on the eye so that the anterior ring is against the bulbar conjunctiva, the posterior ring is in the fornices, and the blepharostats are anterior to the eyelids. Insertion of the ring is aided by a muscle hook. After insertion, the positions of the anterior and posterior rings are examined. If the anterior ring rests against the eye, the ring is sutured in place as described below. If the anterior ring has to be pushed posteriorly to touch the bulbar conjunctiva and causes the posterior ring to indent the eye (Figure 34-2), the McNeill-Goldman scleral and blepharostat ring is removed and an alternative method for separating the eyelids and supporting the sclera is used, such as an eyelid speculum and a Flieringa ring.

If the McNeill-Goldman scleral and blepharostat ring fits, the anterior ring is centered on the cornea and sutured to the sclera with interrupted 5-0 dacron sutures on a steeply curved spatula side-cutting needle, such as the D1 needle. Four sutures placed in the oblique quadrants are usually sufficient to support the sclera. Proper placement of the sutures is important because improperly placed sutures can distort the cornea and lead to postoperative astigmatism.[28] The sutures should be short, radially oriented, and placed directly beneath the anterior ring. The eye is fixated by grasping the conjunctiva and episclera next to a strut with a 0.3-mm forceps. The needle is passed through conjunctiva, episclera, and superficial sclera beneath the ring from the periphery toward the center (Figure 34-3A). Because the sclera is usually not directly visualized, the needle must be passed by feel, which is accomplished by holding the tip of the needle perpendicular to the sclera, engaging the sclera, turning the needle parallel to the scleral surface, and following the curve of the needle until it exits the sclera. After the needle has been passed, it is reloaded in the needle holder such that the hub can be looped beneath the anterior ring on the other side of the strut (Figure 34-3B). The suture is then tied with a double-throw and two single-throws (Figure 34-3C). Wrapping the suture around the strut stabilizes the eye and keeps the suture from sliding around the ring. The second suture is placed in a similar manner 180 degrees from the first suture. The third and fourth sutures are placed 90 degrees from the first two sutures (Figure 34-3D). It is necessary to wrap only one suture, usually the first one, around a strut. Occasionally, a subconjunctival hemorrhage may occur while suturing the ring to the eye. Most are self limited, but some may enlarge, creating a paralimbal mass and exerting pressure on the globe. The hematoma can be drained by incising the conjunctiva with scissors. The conjunctival incision does not need to be closed with sutures.

If the McNeill-Goldman blepharostat and scleral ring does not fit, it is removed, an eyelid speculum is placed, and a Flieringa ring is sutured to the eye in a manner similar to that described above (Figure 34-4). Once again, improperly placed sutures can distort the cornea, which may become apparent only after the recipient corneal button has been excised (Figure 34-5). An eyelid speculum is chosen that does not compress the globe (which can increase intraocular pressure) or distort the cornea (which can result in increased postoperative astigmatism).[29] It is possible to induce up to 6 diopters of astigmatism by compression of the eye with a speculum.[30] Bridle sutures of 4-0 silk may be passed through the superior and inferior rectus muscles to stabilize the eye.

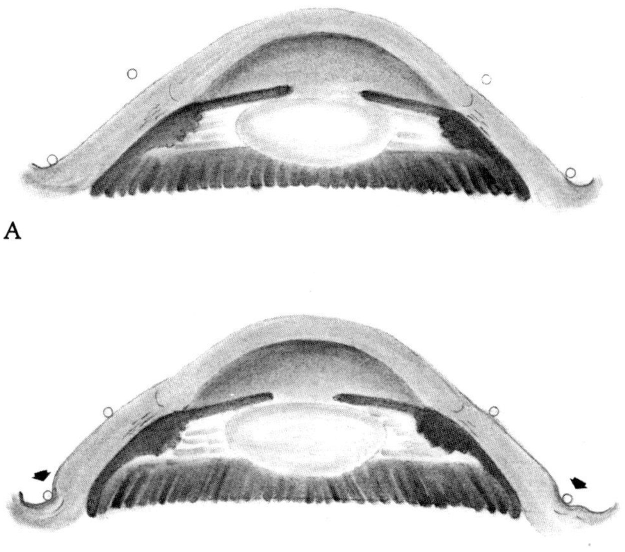

A

B

FIGURE 34-2 Schematic cross-sectional view of the McNeill-Goldman scleral and blepharostat ring. **(A)** The anterior ring is away from the globe. **(B)** The anterior ring has been pushed posteriorly to touch the globe, but the posterior ring is indenting the eye (arrowheads).

Centering the Graft

The location and size of a corneal graft depend, to some extent, on the corneal disorder for which penetrating keratoplasty is indicated. Although refractive surgical procedures, such as excimer laser photorefractive keratectomy, are centered on the center of the entrance pupil,[31] penetrating keratoplasty is centered on the geometric center of the cornea. A decentered graft has a higher risk of rejection, can cause more postoperative astigmatism,[32] and can damage a portion of the anterior chamber angle and trigger the formation of peripheral anterior synechiae. A decentered graft is indicated in certain situations, however. In a cornea with a peripheral perforation from a large infectious ulcer, a decentered graft that encompasses the perforation and area of ulceration but clears the pupil is preferred to a graft that encompasses the same area but, to be centered, is larger. If a previous decentered graft has failed, the previous keratoplasty wound is ignored and the second graft is centered on the geometric center of the cornea.

The geometric center of the cornea can be located by measuring the horizontal and vertical diameters of the cornea with calipers, halving each measurement, and finding the point at which the line bisecting the horizontal diameter intersects the line bisecting the vertical diameter. However, a careful visual estimation of the geometric center is usually sufficiently accurate. If the cornea is

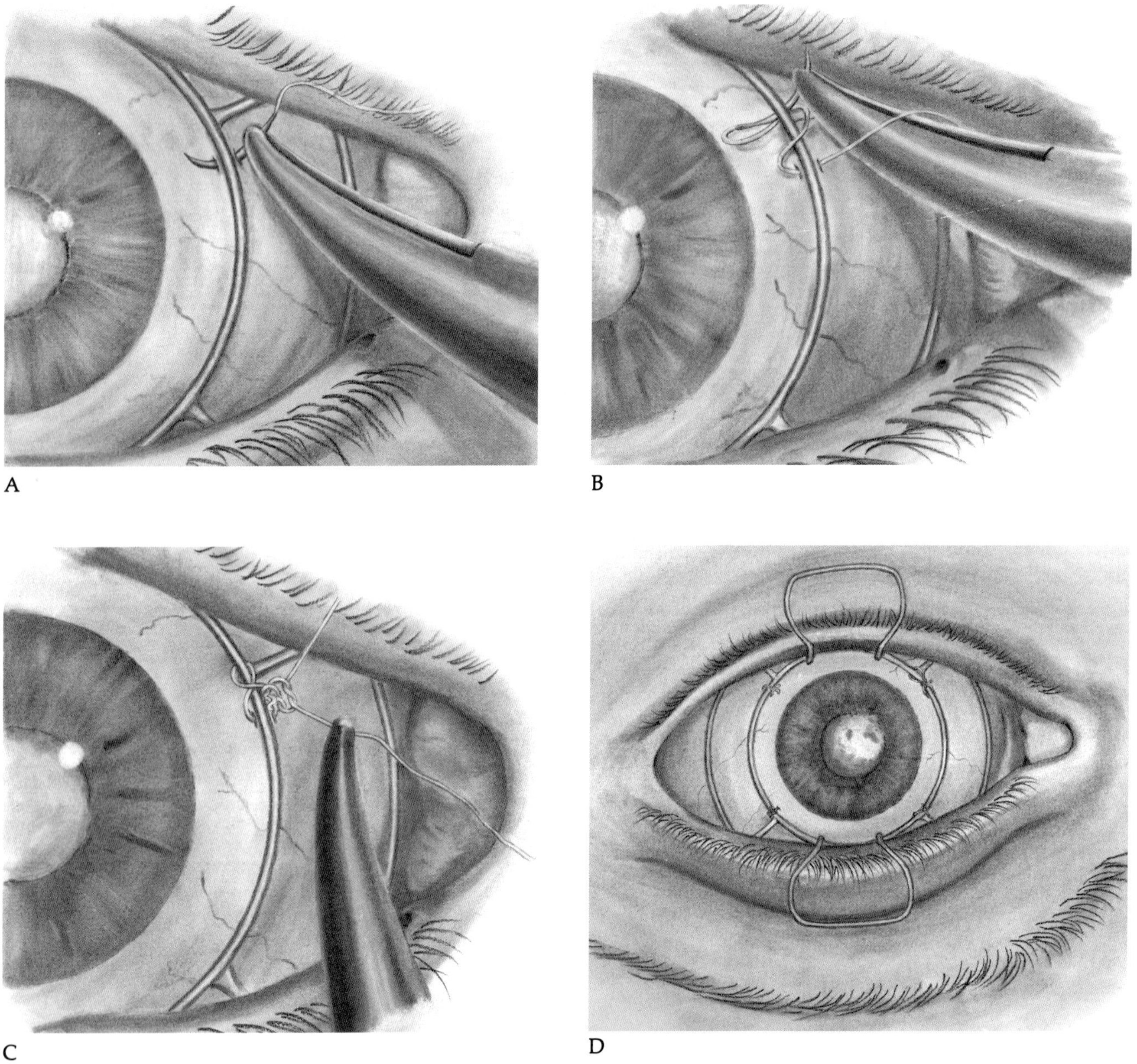

FIGURE 34-3 Suturing of the McNeill-Goldman scleral and blepharostat ring. **(A)** The suture bite is short, radially oriented, and placed directly beneath the anterior ring. **(B & C)** The suture is passed beneath the ring on the other side of the strut and tied with a double-throw and two single-throws. **(D)** Four sutures are usually sufficient to support the sclera.

scarred and the limbus cannot be identified, the eye can be transilluminated or the insertions of the rectus muscles can be located and the limbus identified by the spiral of Tillaux. A centration mark is made on the anterior corneal surface with a surgical marking pen containing gentian violet (Figure 34-6).

Trephining the Recipient Cornea

The area of recipient cornea to be excised depends on the corneal disorder for which penetrating keratoplasty is indicated. This area is measured intraoperatively with calipers to determine the diameter of trephine needed to

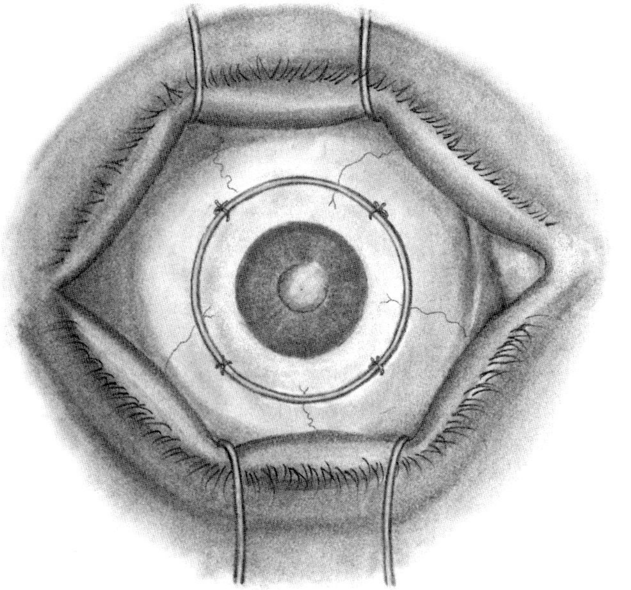

FIGURE 34-4 Flieringa ring sutured in place.

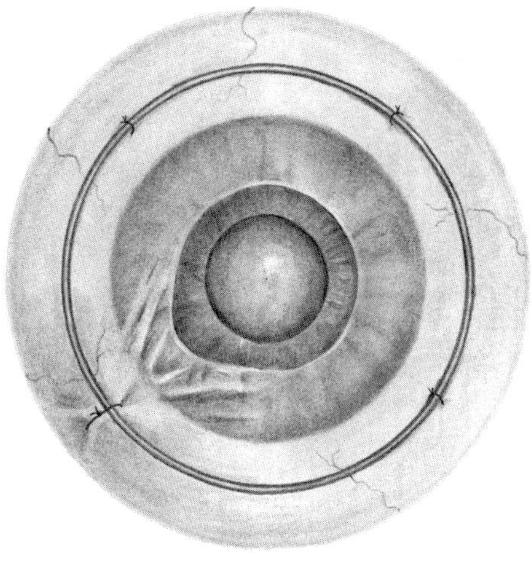

FIGURE 34-5 Distortion of the recipient corneal opening caused by a long and tight scleral support suture.

cut the recipient cornea. In general, the larger the diameter of the cut (and hence, the larger the graft), the greater the incidence of graft failure from rejection. Price et al[16] found that as the difference between the horizontal corneal diameter of the recipient and the trephination size decreased and approached 2.8 mm, the graft failure rate from rejection significantly increased. The smaller the diameter of the cut, the greater the amount of astigmatism reflected in the central cornea from irregularities of the keratoplasty wound. The most common diameters of trephines used to cut the recipient cornea are 7.0 to 8.0 mm. A larger trephine is used to excise necrotic cornea in certain cases, such as infectious keratitis; a smaller trephine is used in pediatric cases.

Some surgeons use a large trephine in cases of keratoconus to excise a larger amount of the cone. I prefer to apply cautery to the apex of the cone to shrink the collagen tissue until the cornea assumes a more normal shape before trephination. This pulls thin abnormal tissue into the center where it can be excised with the trephine. It also creates a more normal recipient bed, which decreases the likelihood of postoperative myopia and astigmatism, and the potential for creating a cornea with a tabletop topography (flat centrally and steep peripherally) that can be difficult to fit with a contact lens. The cone is shrunk by lightly touching the cornea with a hand-held disposable cautery, starting in the center and spiraling toward the periphery, always staying within the area to be excised with the trephine (Figure 34-7).

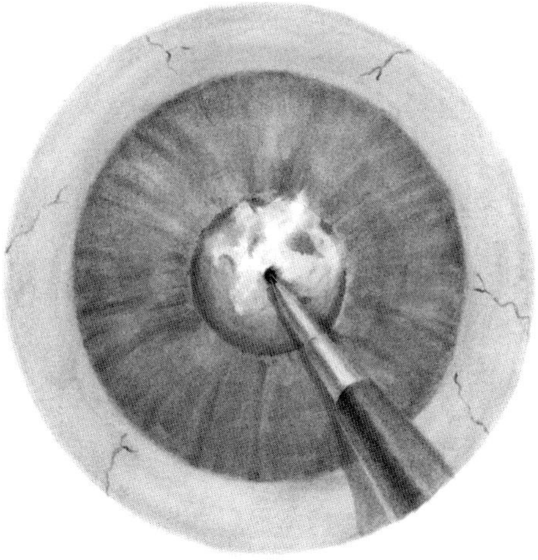

FIGURE 34-6 Marking the geometric center of the cornea.

If the cornea is vascularized, any superficial vessels may be scraped off peripherally and cauterized at the limbus to decrease bleeding during trephination and to keep vessels away from the graft. Cautery should not be applied to the cornea itself to close vessels because it can damage

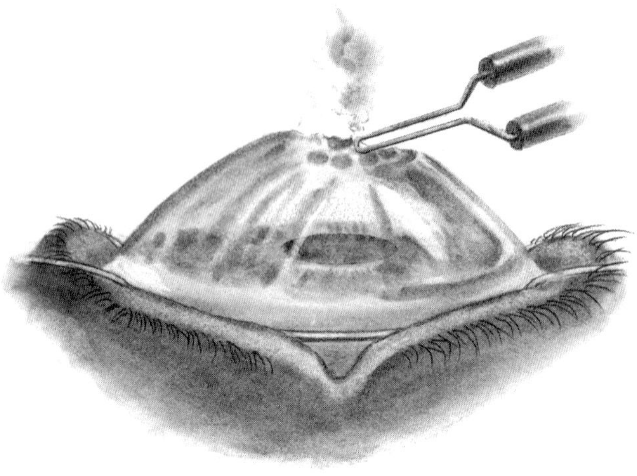

FIGURE 34-7 Cauterization of a cone.

tissue and cause problems with wound healing. If the cornea has previously had a total conjunctival flap, the peripheral portion of the flap that will not be excised with the trephine is peeled off the cornea, if possible. Usually a flap is most easily mobilized 2 mm central to the limbus, but if dissection is difficult, the flap is ignored and trephination is performed through it.

A variety of trephines have been developed in an attempt to create a perfect cut in the recipient cornea. The "standard" trephine is a circular stainless steel blade that can be used alone or placed on a handle (Figure 34-8). If the blade is used alone, it is positioned on the cornea by aligning the center of the blade, which must be approximated because there are no cross hairs, with the centration mark on the cornea and checking the amount of cornea surrounding the blade. The blade is held as perpendicular to the corneal surface as possible and is rotated between the thumb and forefinger. A better cut results if the trephine is held with the hand above the trephine rather than lateral to the trephine.

The blade may be placed on a hollow handle, in which case it is used as described above, or on a handle with an internal obturator (Figure 34-9). The obturator limits the depth of the cut, but necessitates positioning the blade solely by checking the amount of cornea surrounding the blade. The obturator can distort the cornea and cause an irregular, noncircular cut if it comes into contact with the corneal apex before the blade touches the cornea, a situation that occurs most commonly in keratoconus (Figure 34-10).[33]

Because proper tissue distribution is important in preventing postoperative astigmatism, an 8- or 16-spoke radial marker inked with gentian violet may be used to mark the recipient cornea for suture placement. This can be done before the trephine is placed on the eye or after a partial thickness cut has been made.

The Barron radial vacuum trephine, which fixates the cornea by suction during trephination, has become popular in the United States and is the trephine I use. This trephine consists of a body and a blade assembly (Figures 34-11 and 34-12). The body contains two plastic struts for holding and stabilizing the trephine, and a circular vacuum chamber with 16 radial spokes that mark the recipient cornea for suture placement. The inner wall of the vacuum chamber is recessed slightly relative to the outer wall to account for the anterior corneal curvature. The vacuum chamber is connected by a silicone tube to a 5-ml syringe with a spring-loaded plunger. The blade assembly contains a blade, cross hairs for centering the trephine, and four plastic spokes for turning the blade. The inner wall of the body and the outer wall of the blade assembly are threaded so they fit together in a nut-and-bolt fashion. The blade is lowered or raised by turning the spokes clockwise or counterclockwise, respectively. For each spoke (90 degrees) turned, the blade is lowered or raised approximately 0.06 mm. The Barron radial vacuum

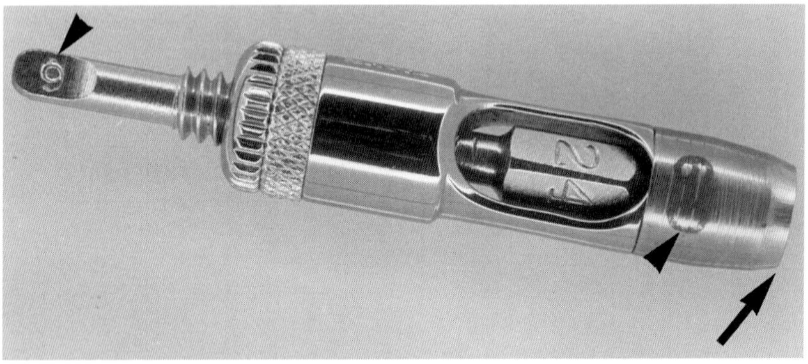

A

FIGURE 34-8 **(A)** Castroviejo trephine consisting of a circular blade (arrow) on a handle. The number (diameter) on the blade should correspond to the number at the end of the handle (arrowheads). The internal obturator can be set a given distance from the edge of the blade by turning the screw on the handle. When the donor corneal tissue is punched by hand, the obturator is fully retracted to prevent it from touching the endothelium. *(continues)*

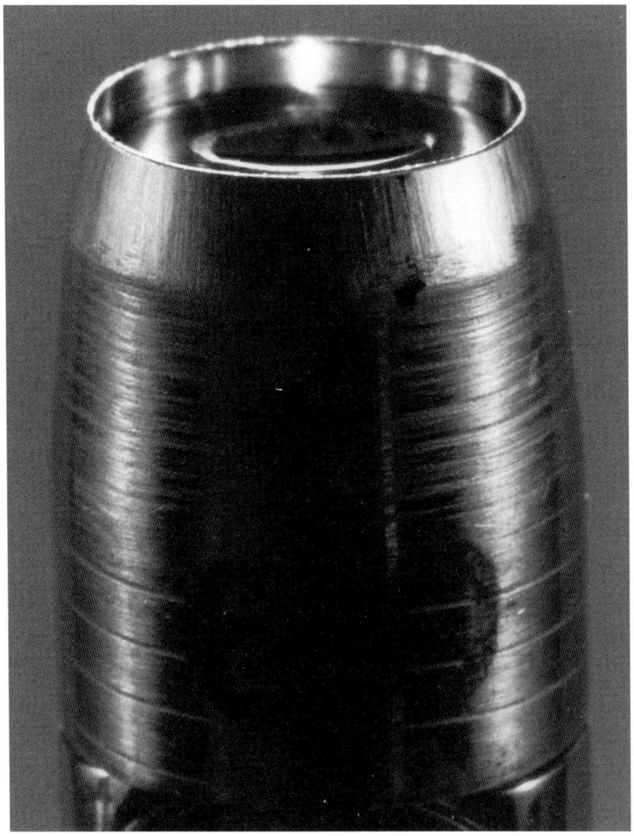

B

FIGURE 34-8 *(continued)* **(B)** Close examination of the tip of the trephine reveals the blade and internal obturator.

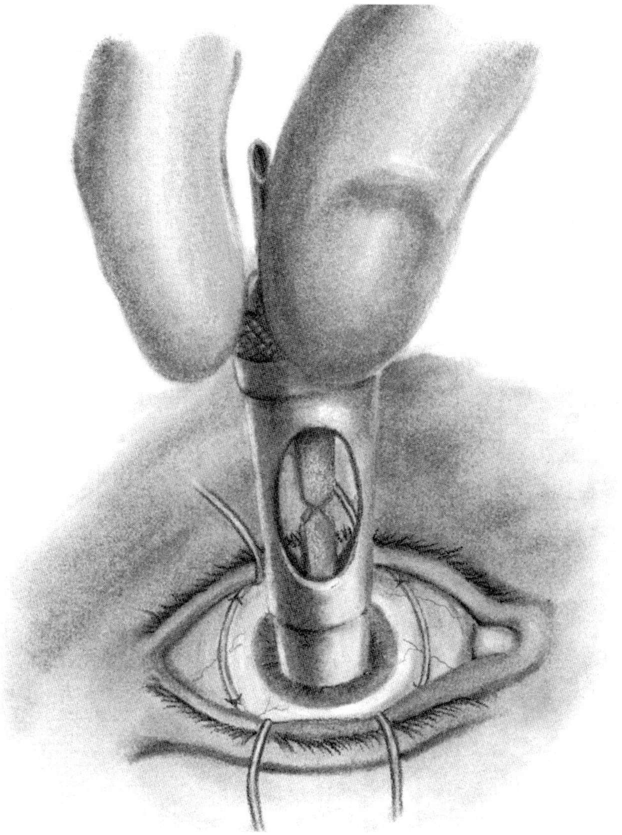

FIGURE 34-9 Trephination of the cornea with the Castroviejo trephine.

trephine is available in diameters of 6.0 to 9.0 mm, in 0.5-mm increments, as well as a diameter of 7.75 mm.

Before placement on the cornea, the trephine is examined under the microscope and the edge of the blade is aligned with the inner wall of the vacuum chamber (Figure 34-13A). This position is called the *zero position*. The blade is then retracted approximately 0.18 mm by turning the spokes 270 degrees (three spokes), which prevents the blade from hitting the cornea and interfering with suction as the trephine is placed on the eye (Figure 34-13B).

The plunger of the syringe is pushed in all the way, the cross hairs of the trephine are aligned with the centration mark on the cornea, the trephine is pressed evenly on the corneal surface, and the plunger is released abruptly (Figure 34-14). If suction has been obtained, the plunger stops at about the 4-ml mark on the syringe. If the plunger rebounds all the way out, suction has not been obtained and the above process is repeated. Failure to obtain suction can be caused by uneven pressure on the trephine, slow release of the plunger, or an irregular corneal surface. Irregularities of the corneal surface can be reduced

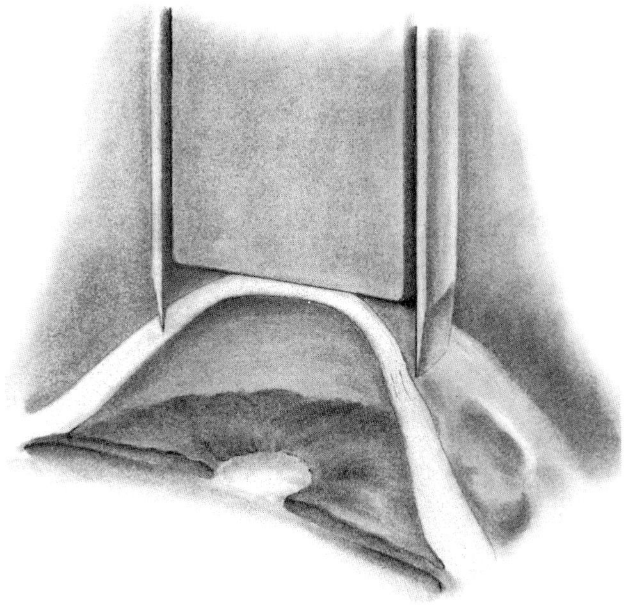

FIGURE 34-10 Corneal distortion caused by premature contact of the internal obturator with the central cornea.

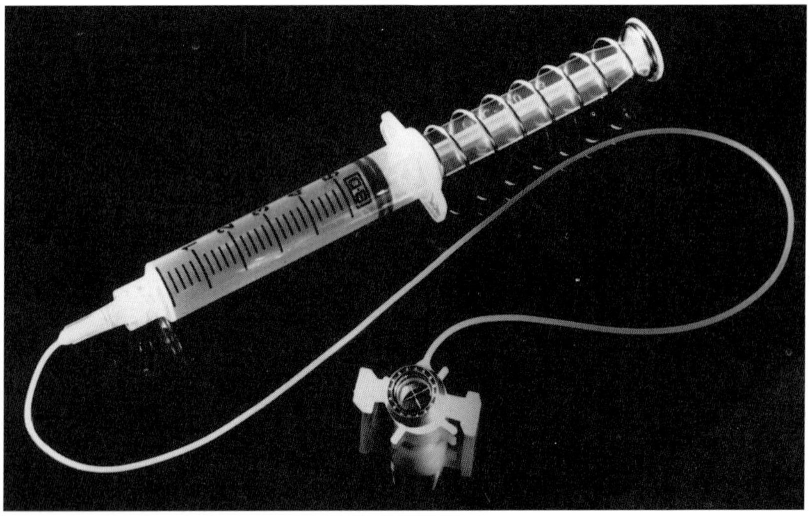

FIGURE 34-11 Barron radial vacuum trephine.

by moistening the surface with balanced salt solution, coating the surface with a viscoelastic substance, or removing bullous epithelium or scar tissue.

After suction has been obtained, the position of the trephine on the cornea is assessed by confirming that the cross hairs and centration mark are aligned and by checking the amount of cornea surrounding the outer wall of the vacuum chamber. If the eye must be moved during this assessment, the scleral support ring or the conjunctiva is grasped with a forceps; the trephine should not be grasped because it can become dislodged. If the position

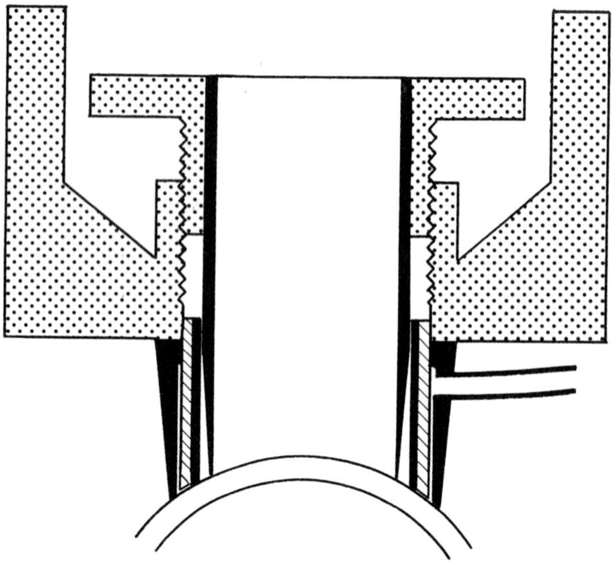

FIGURE 34-12 Schematic cross-sectional view of the Barron radial vacuum trephine.

of the trephine is not satisfactory, the plunger is pushed in to break the suction, the trephine is removed and repositioned, and the plunger is released.

The trephine is stabilized by gently holding the struts, and the cornea is cut by turning the spokes clockwise (Figure 34-15). Care is taken to avoid squeezing the struts, which can cause binding of the blade assembly, and to avoid lifting, pressing, or torquing the trephine, which can cause the blade to cut unevenly. The suction orients the trephine perpendicular to the cornea. As the blade is lowered, the trephine is steadied but its angle to the cornea should not be forcibly changed. The initial 270-degree (three-spoke) turn lowers the blade to the zero position. Because of the anterior corneal curvature, the cornea is cut slightly when the blade is lowered to this position. The number of spokes to turn further depends on the desired depth of cut and the corneal thickness: fewer for a shallow cut or a thin cornea and more for a deep cut or a thick cornea. It is recommended that the cornea be cut as close to Descemet's membrane as possible, without entering the anterior chamber. The barrel of the trephine should be watched as the blade is lowered because if the anterior chamber is inadvertently entered, aqueous humor will appear in the barrel. If this occurs, the plunger of the syringe is pushed in all the way, which releases suction, and the trephine is removed from the eye. Once the anterior chamber has been entered, further cutting with any type of trephine risks damaging the iris and lens.

After the cut has been made, the trephine is removed from the eye by pushing the plunger of the syringe in all the way, which releases the suction. The anterior surface of the cornea is dried to reveal the 16 radial impressions made by the trephine, and each impression is marked with a surgical marking pen containing gentian violet (Fig-

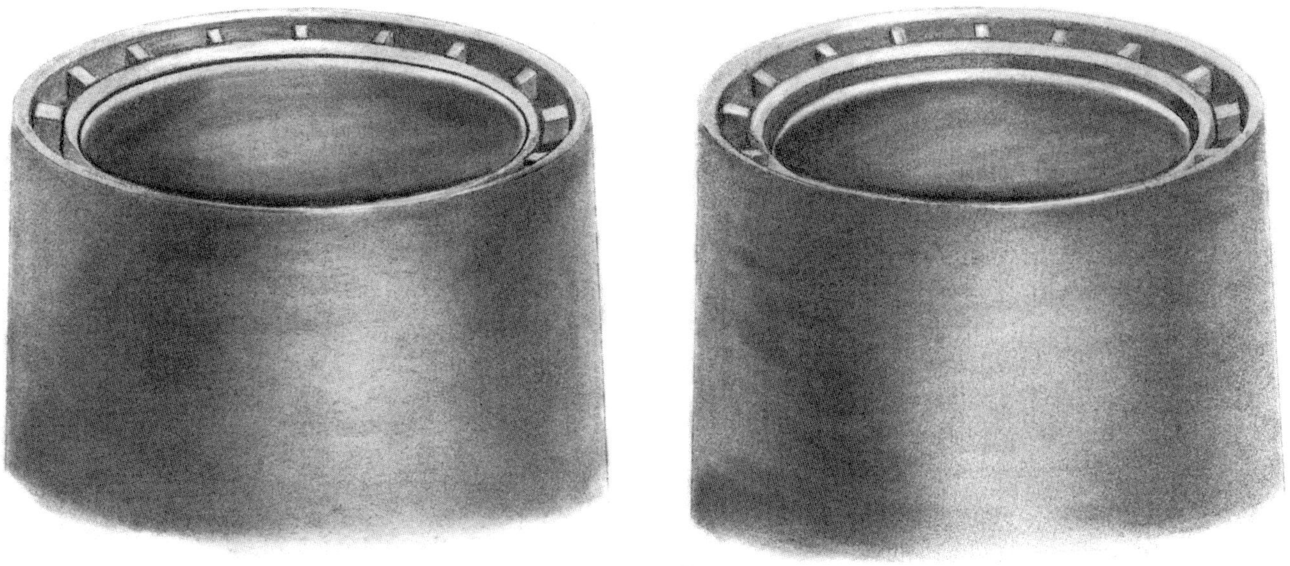

A B

FIGURE 34-13 **(A)** Alignment of the blade of the Barron radial vacuum trephine with the inner wall of the vacuum chamber. **(B)** Retraction of the blade three quarter-turns.

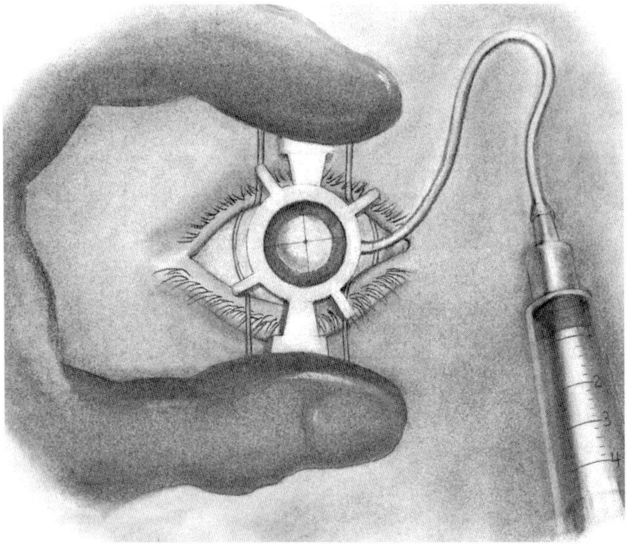

FIGURE 34-14 Placement of the Barron radial vacuum trephine on the cornea. The cross hairs are aligned with the centration mark.

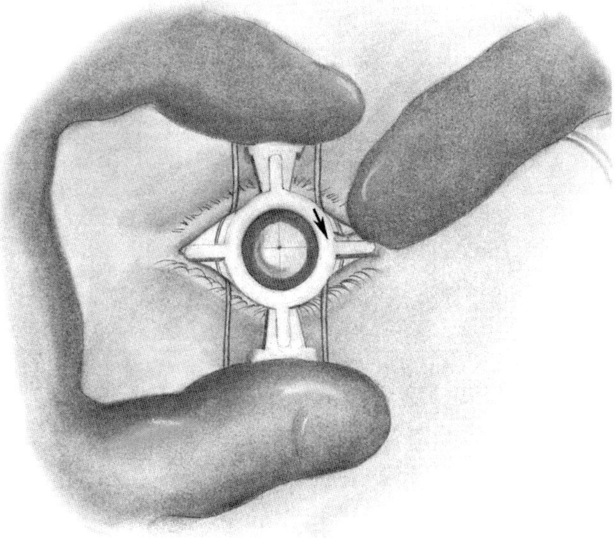

FIGURE 34-15 Trephination of the cornea with the Barron radial vacuum trephine. The blade is lowered by turning the spokes clockwise.

ures 34-16 and 34-17). Each impression starts 0.2 mm from the edge of the cut and is 0.5 mm in length.

The Barron radial vacuum trephine is particularly useful in perforated corneas. Ng et al[34] reported that in corneas with large perforations, suction trephines are easier to use, result in less anterior chamber collapse, cause less corneal distortion, and create a sharper, deeper, and more perpendicular incision than free blades. If the perforation is small, viscoelastic substance may be injected through the perforation to deepen the anterior chamber and protect the iris and lens, but if the perforation is large, the viscoelastic substance will escape and no benefit will be

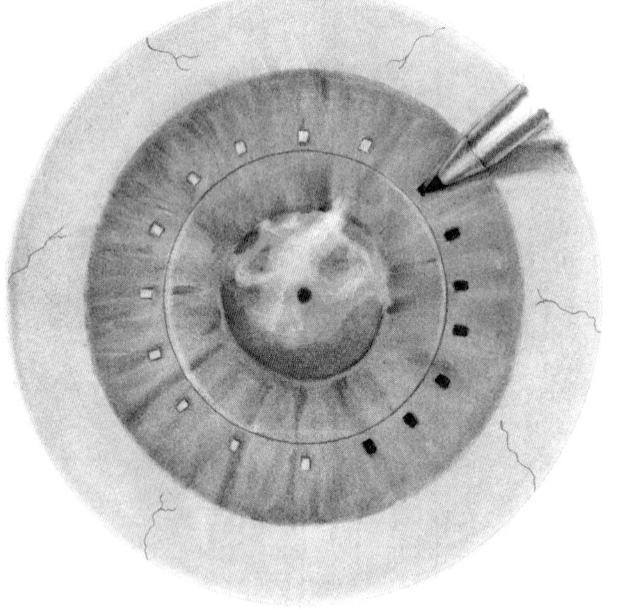

FIGURE 34-16 Marking of the radial impressions made by the Barron radial vacuum trephine for even suture placement.

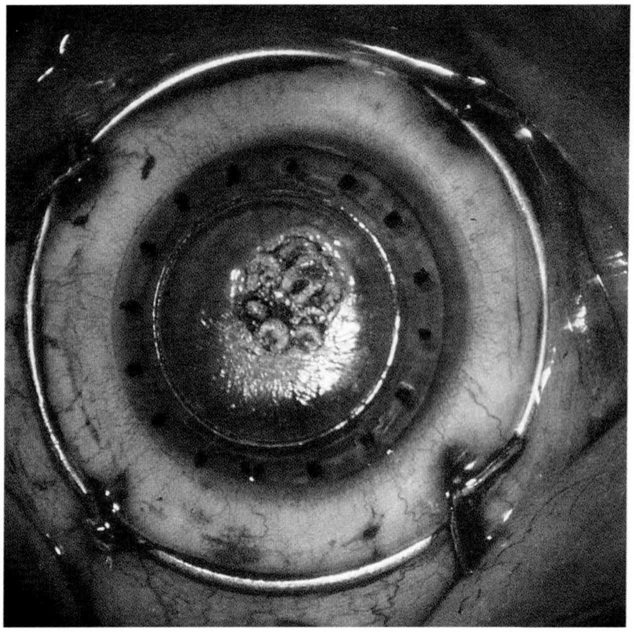

FIGURE 34-17 Recipient cornea marked with the Barron radial vacuum trephine. The cone has been cauterized.

obtained. Care is taken to avoid applying undue external pressure on the eye with the trephine and to be certain to cut only partial thickness. The iris and lens are frequently in contact with the posterior corneal surface in these cases and will be damaged if the cut is full thickness.

Cutting the Donor Cornea

It is recommended that the donor cornea be cut after the recipient cornea has been trephined but before the anterior chamber is entered. This allows the surgeon to assess the location and size of the trephine cut and the integrity of the surrounding corneal tissue before committing to a specifically sized graft. In cases of corneal necrosis, it is not uncommon to select a trephine with a diameter that appears sufficiently large to excise the area of necrotic tissue, only to discover after trephination that portions of the cornea peripheral to the trephine cut are too necrotic to support sutures. If the donor cornea has been cut, the surgeon is usually forced to accept the trephine cut, although a larger-diameter cut may have been more appropriate. Some argue that cutting the donor cornea before trephining the recipient cornea lessens the risk of extrusion of the intraocular contents because it decreases the time the eye is open. Full-thickness trephination is not necessary to assess corneal integrity, however. Partial-thickness trephination allows the eye to remain closed while the surgeon grasps the peripheral edge of the trephine cut with a forceps, assesses the integrity of the surrounding corneal tissue, and enlarges the trephine cut, if necessary, before cutting the donor cornea.

Guidelines for the selection and preservation of donor corneal tissue are discussed in Chapter 33. Some surgeons advocate the use of the patient's own cornea as the donor cornea (autograft) in select cases to eliminate the risk of graft rejection.[35] Autokeratoplasty is sometimes performed when one eye is blind but has a normal cornea and the other eye requires a corneal transplant. Because autokeratoplasty is somewhat difficult to perform without damaging endothelial cells, and because the prognosis of allografts is usually so good, autografts are usually reserved for cases in which the eye requiring penetrating keratoplasty has had multiple graft failures from graft rejection.

A rotating autograft is sometimes performed when a small scar impinges on the center of the cornea but the rest of the cornea is normal. The scar can be rotated out of the way by making a large eccentric trephine cut and rotating the corneal button such that the scar is moved to a more peripheral location (Figure 34-18). The optical results are generally better with standard penetrating keratoplasty with an allograft, but a rotating autograft may be used for high-risk cases.

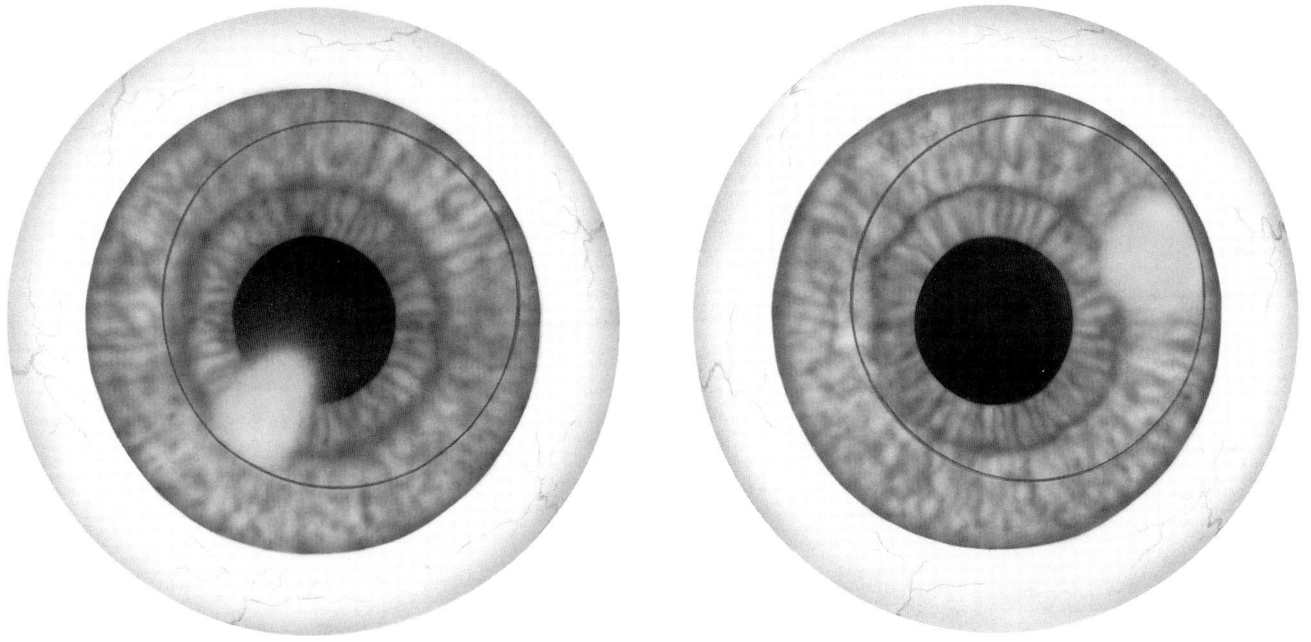
A B

FIGURE 34-18 Rotating autokeratoplasty. **(A)** Eccentric trephination of a paracentral corneal opacity. **(B)** Rotation of the graft such that the opacity is moved peripherally.

Some surgeons recommend the use of infant corneas in patients in whom postoperative corneal steepening is desired to correct a hypermetropic refractive error such as aphakia.[36] There are better methods to correct aphakia, however, such as secondary intraocular lens implantation, and the postoperative topography of such a cornea is bizarre, with a central curvature that is markedly steeper than normal and a peripheral curvature that is relatively flat. These corneas are often impossible to fit with a contact lens.

Most donor corneal tissue in the United States is preserved in a corneal preservation medium, such as Optisol, in the form of the cornea with a few millimeters of attached sclera. Although artificial anterior chambers have been devised that allow the donor cornea to be cut from the epithelial surface, most surgeons cut the donor cornea from the endothelial surface with a circular stainless steel blade.

The diameter of the blade depends on the diameter of the trephine used to cut the recipient cornea and the status of the lens and anterior chamber angle. If the diameter of the trephine is larger than 9 mm or smaller than 7 mm, a blade 1 mm larger in diameter is recommended. If the trephine diameter is between 7 mm and 9 mm and the eye is aphakic, a blade 0.5 mm larger is recommended; if the eye is phakic or pseudophakic, a blade 0.25 mm larger is recommended. If the donor corneal button is too large, however, postoperative corneal steepening occurs, which induces myopia. With a recipient bed of 7.5 mm, a 0.5-mm oversized graft induces about 4 diopters of myopia; with an 8-mm recipient bed, a 0.5-mm oversized graft induces about 2.5 diopters of myopia. With a 7.5-mm bed, a 0.25-mm oversized graft does not usually induce any refractive error. Some surgeons recommend a same-sized graft[37,38] or a 0.25-mm undersized graft[39] in patients with keratoconus. A graft the same size as or smaller than the recipient opening decreases myopia but can result in a flat cornea that usually cannot be fit with a contact lens. When the donor cornea is sutured to the recipient cornea, some of the tissue is incorporated into a tissue roll, and if the donor cornea is too small, the anterior chamber may shallow and the intraocular pressure may increase, especially in an aphakic eye or an eye with a shallow anterior chamber preoperatively.[40-43]

A variety of cutting blocks and trephines have been developed for cutting the donor cornea from the posterior surface. The cutting blocks are made of Teflon, nylon, or paraffin, and have a concave depression, or well, in which the donor cornea is placed with the epithelial surface down and centered. The diameters and radii of curvature of these wells vary.

The "standard" trephine for cutting the donor cornea consists of a circular stainless steel blade on a handle (Fig-

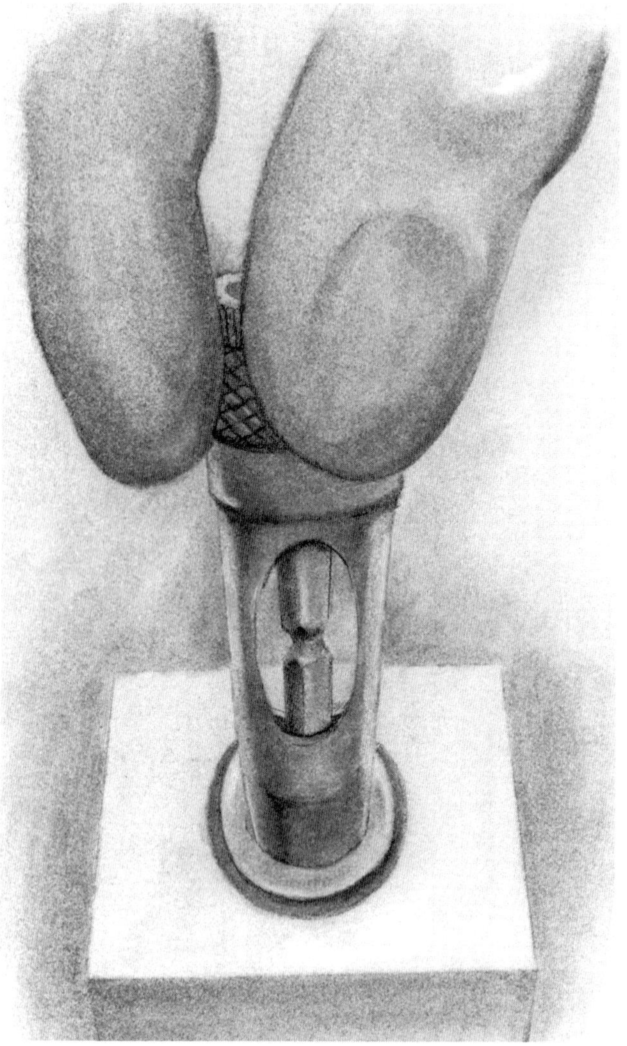

FIGURE 34-19 Punching of the donor cornea with the Castroviejo trephine. With this technique, it is difficult to ensure that the trephine is perpendicular to and centered on the cutting block and to prevent the donor cornea from sliding as it is being cut.

ure 34-19). It is important that the blade is secured properly on the handle, and that the obturator, if present, is fully retracted to prevent contact with the endothelium. Cutting the donor cornea by rotating the blade causes more endothelial damage than punching the cornea by pressing on the blade. If the blade is not held perpendicular to or centered on the cutting block, or if the donor cornea slips in the well as it is being cut, the tissue may be cut obliquely, resulting in an irregular or oval button that has a beveled or ragged edge. These irregularities can distort the wound and cause postoperative astigmatism.

As the trephine is lifted from the well, the corneoscleral rim usually remains on the blade and the corneal button remains in the well. If the corneal button remains in the barrel of the blade, the blade is removed from the handle and balanced salt solution, corneal preservation medium, or a viscoelastic substance is gently squirted into the barrel to dislodge the button so that it falls into the well or an edge becomes dislodged that can be grasped with a forceps. A metal cover is placed over the cutting block to prevent evaporation of the preservation medium and desiccation of the tissue and contamination with foreign material from the air.

One device available for punching the donor cornea is the Barron vacuum donor cornea punch, which not only cleanly cuts the cornea but also marks the cornea for suture placement (Figure 34-20). This punch consists of a nylon cutting block, seating ring, and blade. The cutting block has four holes into which steel guideposts of the blade fit to ensure that the blade is perpendicular. The well of the cutting block has a diameter of 19 mm and a radius of curvature of 25.4 mm, except for the central 11 mm, which has a radius of curvature of 10 mm. The well has a central positioning hole, as well as four additional holes and a circular trough 12 mm in diameter that are connected by a silicone tube to a 5-ml syringe with a spring-loaded plunger. The syringe creates suction that holds the cornea in place as it is cut and ensures that the corneal button remains in the well, and not in the blade, after the cut has been made. When inked with gentian violet, the four holes in the well mark the cornea for accurate placement of the cardinal sutures. The Barron vacuum donor cornea punch is available in diameters of 6.0 mm, 6.5 to 9.0 mm in 0.25-mm increments, and 9.5 mm.

To use the punch, the tip of a surgical marking pen is placed into each of the four holes in the well of the cutting block and the pen is twisted until the sides of each hole are evenly coated with gentian violet. The plunger of the syringe is pushed in all the way and held. The donor cornea is placed in the well and centered. The guideposts of the seating ring are inserted into the holes in each corner of the cutting block and the seating ring is pressed down gently. The plunger of the syringe is released abruptly. The seating ring is removed, and the guide posts of the blade are inserted into the holes in each corner of the cutting block. The thumb is placed directly over the blade, and the blade is pressed down firmly and then lifted and removed. The scleral rim of the donor cornea is grasped and removed from the well, which releases suction and leaves the marked corneal button in the well (Figure 34-21). To prevent the corneal button from sliding, which can smudge the marks, the cutting block is not moved until it is time for the button to be sutured in place.

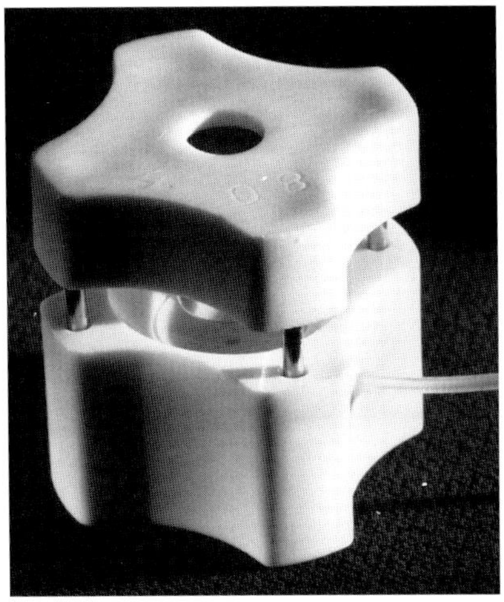

FIGURE 34-20 Barron vacuum donor cornea punch.

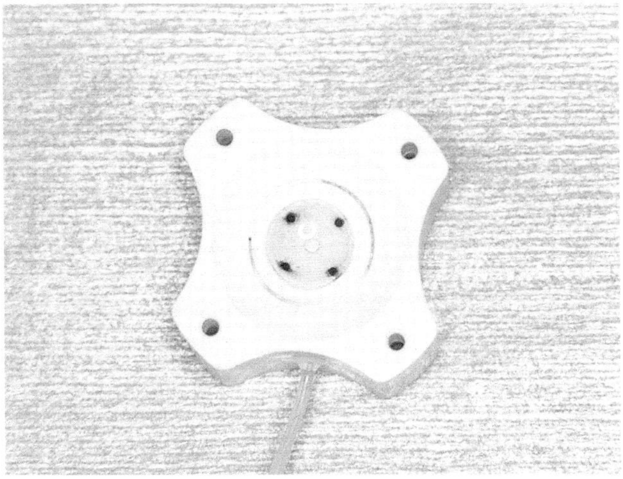

FIGURE 34-21 Donor corneal button marked with the Barron vacuum donor cornea punch.

Removing the Recipient Cornea

The anterior chamber is entered by grasping the central edge of the trephine cut with a 0.12-mm forceps, inserting a stainless steel blade perpendicularly bevel-up through the cut into the anterior chamber and making a full-thickness incision along the trephine cut as the blade is lifted and withdrawn from the eye (Figure 34-22). The incision should be large enough to allow insertion of corneal scissors into the anterior chamber. The most convenient location at which to enter the anterior chamber is the 9 o'clock position for right-handed surgeons and the 3 o'clock position for left-handed surgeons. Egress of aqueous humor ensures that a full-thickness incision has been made. If aqueous humor is not seen, it is possible that Descemet's membrane has detached from the posterior stroma. Such a detachment occurs most commonly in patients with bullous keratopathy. If the detachment is not recognized, Descemet's membrane can be stripped entirely from the corneal button, inadvertently left in the eye, and cause the graft to fail.[44]

A viscoelastic substance may be injected through the incision to deepen the anterior chamber and protect the iris and lens as the incision is completed with corneal scissors. Corneal scissors are curved to the right or to the left; the posterior blade is longer than the anterior blade, and the tips are blunt to protect the iris and lens.

There is some debate regarding the ideal shape of the recipient corneal opening. Some surgeons think the walls of the opening should be beveled, with the posterior opening smaller than the anterior opening, so that a ledge is created on which the donor cornea can rest, much like the top of a jack-o'-lantern. Other surgeons, myself included, think the walls of the opening should be perpendicular. This is accomplished by inserting the posterior blade of the scissors at an angle through the incision into the anterior chamber, hugging the posterior corneal surface centrally, and rotating the scissors so they are perpendicular to the cornea (Figure 34-23). The cornea is cut full thickness along the trephine cut by closing the scissors as upward pressure is applied, which prevents the scissors from plunging posteriorly and damaging the iris and lens. This maneuver is

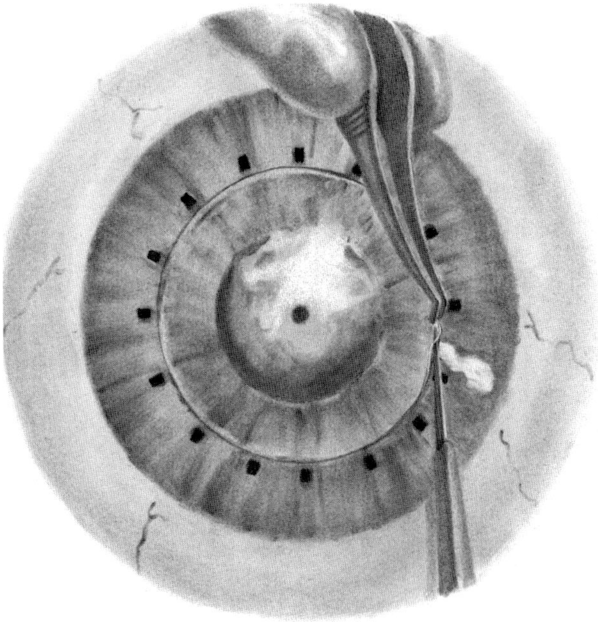

FIGURE 34-22 Entry into the anterior chamber with a stainless steel blade. Egress of aqueous humor must be seen to ensure that the cut is full thickness.

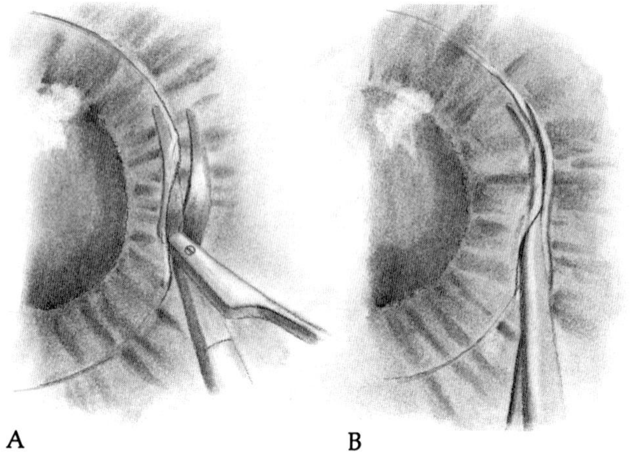

FIGURE 34-23 Excision of the recipient cornea. (A) Opened corneal scissors are inserted at an angle into the anterior chamber to avoid traumatizing the iris. (B) The scissors are rotated so that they are perpendicular to the cornea, lifted slightly, and closed.

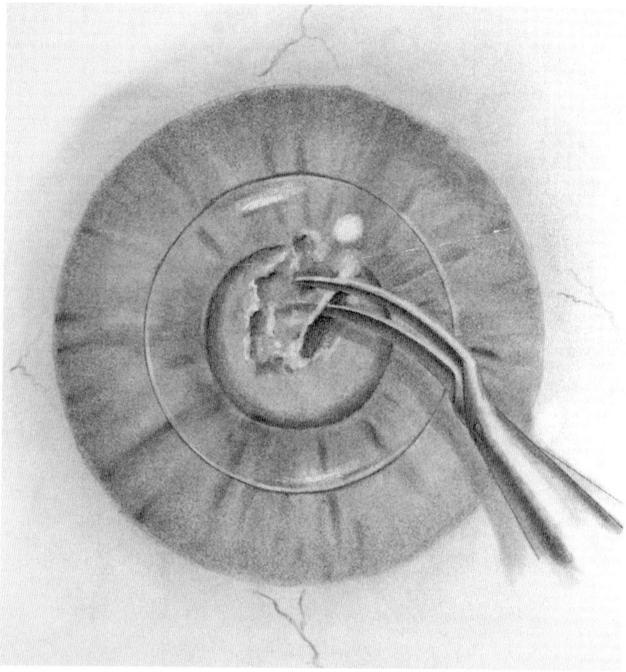

FIGURE 34-24 Excision of a perforated cornea. Scissors are inserted into the anterior chamber through the perforation and a full-thickness cut is made toward the trephine cut.

repeated until the inferior half of the cornea is cut; the superior half is cut in a similar fashion with scissors curved in the opposite direction. The scissors are withdrawn from the anterior chamber each time they are closed and are reinserted as described above. Stabilization of the cornea with a forceps may not be necessary during the early stage of cutting; however, after half of the cornea has been cut, the cornea must be stabilized with a forceps. Before the corneal button is removed, any iris or vitreous attachments to the posterior corneal surface are severed with scissors. After the corneal button has been removed, it is placed epithelial surface down on a wet instrument wipe and kept moist until the donor cornea is in place. It should not be removed from the sterile field in case a disaster befalls the donor cornea and it is needed to close the eye.

In a perforated cornea, the anterior chamber is frequently shallow, and entering the anterior chamber through the trephine cut with a stainless steel blade risks damaging the iris and lens. In these cases, a viscoelastic substance is injected through the perforation into the anterior chamber, and the cornea is cut by inserting the posterior blade of corneal scissors through the perforation, hugging the posterior corneal surface, and cutting radially toward the trephine cut, like the spoke of a wheel (Figure 34-24). The cornea is then cut along the trephine cut as described above.

The opening in the recipient cornea is examined to ensure that the edges are perpendicular. Tags of corneal tissue can cause postoperative astigmatism and should be removed by grasping the tag with a 0.12-mm forceps, pulling it centrally, and excising it with Vannas scissors (Figure 34-25). It is important to hold the scissors perpendicular to the cornea and, because the tips of these scissors are sharp, to avoid nicking the iris and lens.

Concomitant Intraocular Procedures

Cataract Extraction

Although some surgeons advocate closed-system phacoemulsification for cataract extraction combined with penetrating keratoplasty,[45] my preferred method is open-sky extracapsular cataract extraction through the recipient corneal opening, unless there is an indication for intracapsular cataract extraction, such as subluxation of the lens. It is critically important that all precautions to decrease posterior pressure be taken in cases in which cataract extraction is planned.

An anterior capsulotomy can be created by making multiple punctures in the anterior capsule with a stainless steel blade or needle, grasping the anterior capsule with a forceps, and removing it from the eye (Figure 34-26). Alternatively, the capsule may be cut with Vannas scissors, or a capsulorrhexis may be created with a bent 25-gauge needle or a capsulorrhexis forceps. As with any capsulorrhexis for extracapsular cataract extraction, relaxing incisions

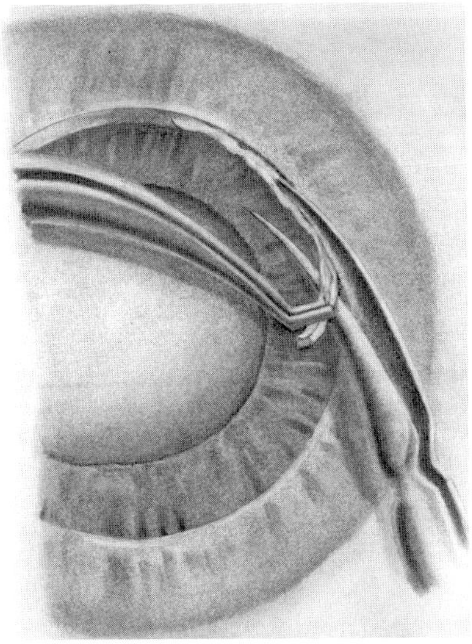

FIGURE 34-25 Excision of tags of corneal tissue with Vannas scissors.

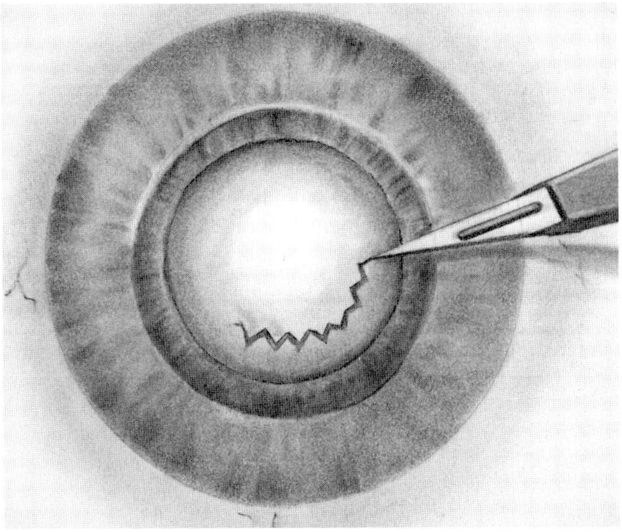

FIGURE 34-26 Anterior capsulotomy.

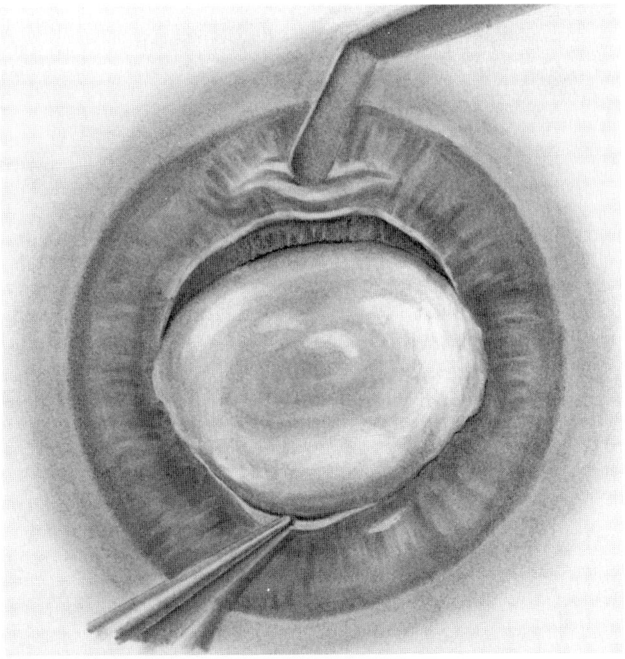

FIGURE 34-27 Expression of the nucleus.

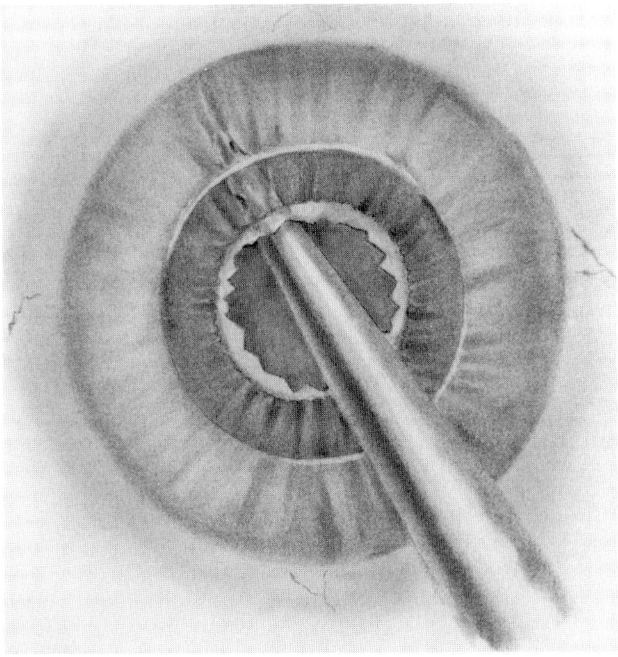

FIGURE 34-28 Aspiration of cortex.

must be made in the anterior capsule to prevent rupture of the capsule during expression of the lens nucleus.

The lens nucleus is expressed by grasping the superior edge of the recipient corneal opening with a 0.12-mm forceps and pressing posteriorly. Pressure is applied at the inferior limbus with the thin end of a Paton spatula or lens loop. This causes the inferior pole of the nucleus to move anteriorly. The spatula is then placed behind the nucleus, and the nucleus is tumbled out of the eye (Figure 34-27).

The lens cortex is removed with an automated or manual irrigating/aspirating instrument (Figure 34-28). The technique for removing cortex through a penetrating keratoplasty opening differs from that for removing it through a cataract incision in two ways. First, the irrigating/aspi-

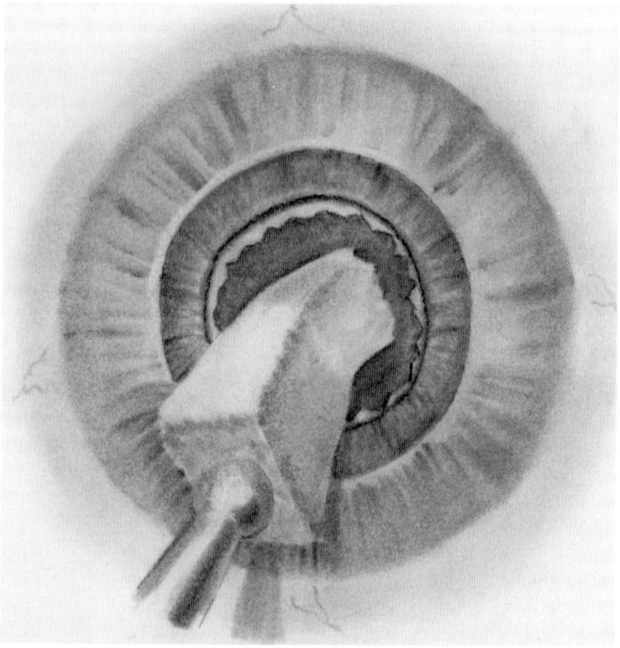

FIGURE 34-29 Polishing of the posterior capsule with a wet cellulose sponge.

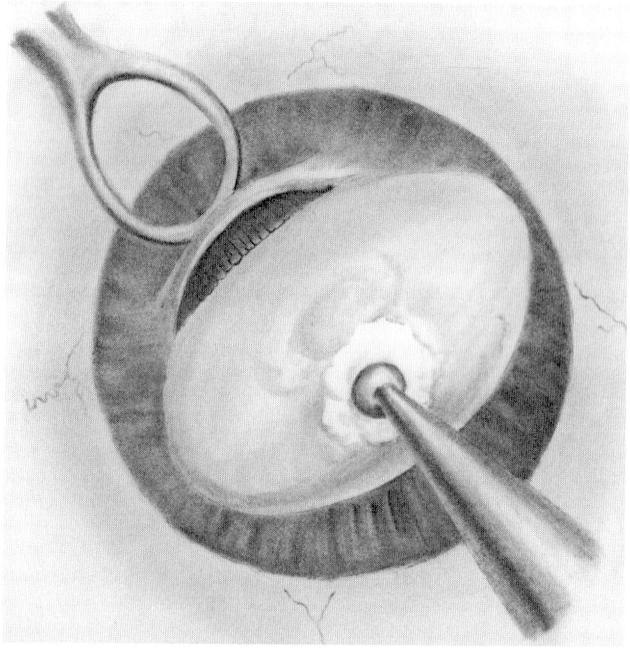

FIGURE 34-30 Intracapsular cataract extraction with a cryoprobe.

rating instrument must be gently pressed posteriorly when it is behind the iris to create an exit path for the irrigating solution. Otherwise, irrigating solution can accumulate behind the iris and push the peripheral posterior lens capsule posteriorly and the central posterior lens capsule anteriorly. Second, the irrigating/aspirating instrument is used as a forceps to remove cortex. That is, once cortex has been engaged in the aspirating port, it is removed from the eye by removing the instrument and wiping away the cortex with the thumb and forefinger; the cortex need not be completely aspirated through the port. It is faster to remove cortex in this manner than to wait for it to be completely aspirated. After the cortex has been removed, the posterior capsule is inspected and can be polished by gently wiping it with a wet cellulose sponge (Figure 34-29).

If an intracapsular cataract extraction is indicated, the anterior capsule is dried with a cellulose sponge, a cryoprobe is applied and frozen to the anterior capsule, and the lens is removed by gently pulling anteriorly with the cryoprobe and pushing posteriorly with a lens loop at the limbus (Figure 34-30).

Intraocular Lens Removal

As discussed in the section on indications and patient selection, pseudophakic bullous keratopathy is one of the most common indications for penetrating keratoplasty.[1,4,10,14,15] In a given region, the type of intraocular lens most commonly seen in association with pseudophakic bullous keratopathy depends not only on the problems of lens design in general but also on local practice patterns (i.e., the types of lenses that are implanted most often by surgeons in that area). The types of intraocular lenses associated with pseudophakic bullous keratopathy reported in recent publications are listed in Table 34-4[10,11,13–15,46–48] and include anterior chamber lenses in 31 to 75 percent of cases, iris-supported lenses in 2 to 62 percent of cases, and posterior chamber lenses in 7 to 26 percent of cases in various studies.

In pseudophakic bullous keratopathy, the decision must be made whether to remove the intraocular lens and, if so, whether to replace it with another lens at the time of penetrating keratoplasty. If bullous keratopathy is caused solely by surgical trauma during implantation of an intraocular lens, the lens may be left in place; if it is caused by the intraocular lens itself, the lens should be removed. In general, all rigid anterior chamber intraocular lenses (such as the Choyce lens), all closed-loop anterior chamber intraocular lenses (such as the Azar 91Z, Leiske, Hessburg, and Stableflex lenses), all iris-supported intraocular lenses, and any intraocular lens associated with the uveitis-glaucoma-hyphema, or UGH, syndrome are removed unless the removal would unduly traumatize the eye, in which

TABLE 34-4
Types of Intraocular Lenses Associated with Pseudophakic Bullous Keratopathy

	Hyman et al, 1992[10]	*Mamalis et al, 1992*[11]	*Chu et al, 1992*[46]	*Sharif et al, 1993*[13]	*Haamann et al, 1994*[14]	*Agrawal et al, 1994*[47]	*Flowers et al, 1995*[15]	*Kwartz et al, 1995*[48]
Time period	1985–1988	1981–1990	NR	1971–1990	1984–1993	1987–1993	1989–1993	1980–1992
Location	Maryland	Utah	Texas	England	Denmark	India	California	England
Type of intraocular lens (% of pseudophakic bullous keratopathy cases)								
Anterior chamber	56	51.3	69	75.0	66.7	32.1	67.9	31
Iris-supported	10.7	25.7	23	13.9	7.8	41.9[a]	2.2	62
Posterior chamber	20.9	19.6	8	11.1	25.5	21.0	25.2	7
Unknown	12.2	3.5					4.7	

Abbreviation: NR, not reported.
[a] Iris claw lens.

case the intraocular lens is left in place. In most cases, the lens is replaced with a posterior chamber intraocular lens (supported by the posterior capsule, if possible, or fixated in the iridociliary sulcus with transscleral sutures or to the iris with iris sutures) or a modern anterior chamber intraocular lens, such as a Kelman Multiflex–style lens.

Most intraocular lenses can be removed safely through the penetrating keratoplasty opening. It is important to remember that many lenses associated with pseudophakic bullous keratopathy were implanted in eyes with vitreous loss, and vitreous can be adherent to the lens. When the lens is removed, the surgeon must have scissors in hand and be ready to cut adherent vitreous to prevent traction on the vitreous and retina. It is also important to remember that iris can be adherent to these lenses.

Anterior Chamber Intraocular Lens Removal Although solid anterior chamber intraocular lenses, such as the Choyce lens, are rigid and larger than the penetrating keratoplasty opening, they can usually be removed through the opening if the opening is distorted into an oval. One end of the lens is grasped with a forceps and lifted through the opening (Figure 34-31). As this end is lifted, the other end is observed to ensure that it does not press posteriorly into the iris and ciliary body. If the lens cannot be removed through the opening without excessive pressure, a separate incision is made at the limbus in the area of one of the footplates, and the lens is removed through this incision.

Closed-loop anterior chamber intraocular lenses are more difficult to remove because of the anterior synechiae and fibrous tissue that usually cocoon the haptics in the anterior chamber angle.[49] Attempts to remove the lens by tugging on it may tear the iris or ciliary body, resulting in marked bleeding, iridodialysis, cyclodialysis, or avulsion of uveal tissue. Dissection of the fibrous tissue is difficult and bloody, and can damage the iris and ciliary body. The best way to free the haptics is to cut both sides of each haptic with scissors and slide the haptics through the fibrotic tunnels (Figure 34-32). Although the haptics usually deform and slide through the tissue easily, it is best to cut one side of each haptic close to the optic so it is easy to see and manipulate and the other side close to the anterior chamber angle. The long end of each haptic is then grasped with a forceps and gently rotated so that the short end passes through the tunnel of tissue. The shape of the haptics should be followed as the haptics are removed to minimize trauma. If the haptic cannot be safely removed, it is cut as short as possible and left in the angle.[49]

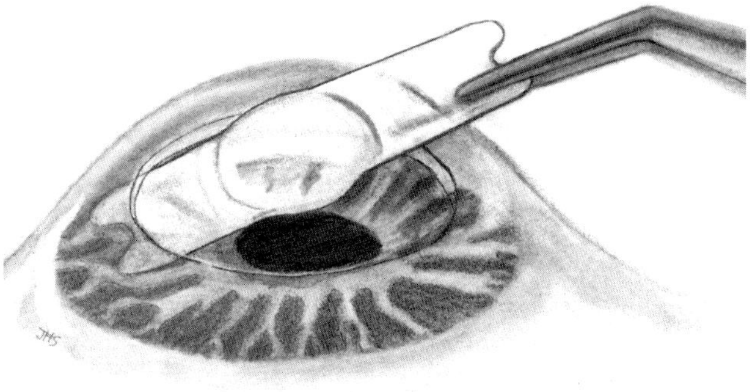

FIGURE 34-31 Removal of a Choyce anterior chamber intraocular lens through the penetrating keratoplasty opening.

The most difficult anterior chamber intraocular lens to remove is the Stableflex lens, which has four closed haptics, all of which can be anchored in the angle by synechiae.[49] Each haptic must be cut and rotated through the synechiae (Figure 34-33). The Hessburg lens is also difficult to remove because of the acute angle of curvature of the haptics.

Some anterior chamber intraocular lenses, such as the Kelman Omnifit lens, have a positioning hole in the haptic that can become encapsulated in uveal tissue. Care is

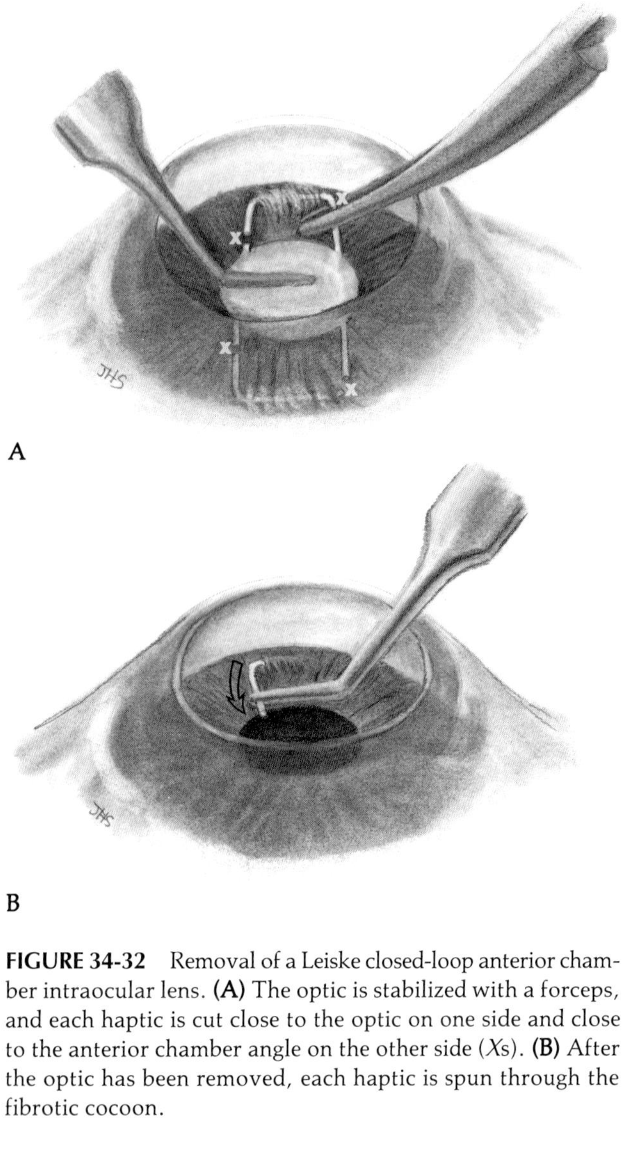

A

B

FIGURE 34-32 Removal of a Leiske closed-loop anterior chamber intraocular lens. **(A)** The optic is stabilized with a forceps, and each haptic is cut close to the optic on one side and close to the anterior chamber angle on the other side (*X*s). **(B)** After the optic has been removed, each haptic is spun through the fibrotic cocoon.

taken in removing these lenses because if the encapsulating tissue is pulled out with the loop, extensive tissue damage, bleeding, and a severe iridodialysis may occur.[49]

Iris-Supported Intraocular Lens Removal A variety of iris-supported intraocular lenses that were implanted before the introduction of modern anterior and posterior chamber intraocular lenses can cause bullous keratopathy and should be removed through the penetrating keratoplasty opening. Although iris-supported intraocular lenses tend to be easier to remove than some of the anterior chamber intraocular lenses because they are not fibrosed in the anterior chamber angle, they can be adherent to iris and vitreous and must be dissected free.

Posterior Chamber Intraocular Lens Removal In general, a modern posterior chamber intraocular lens that

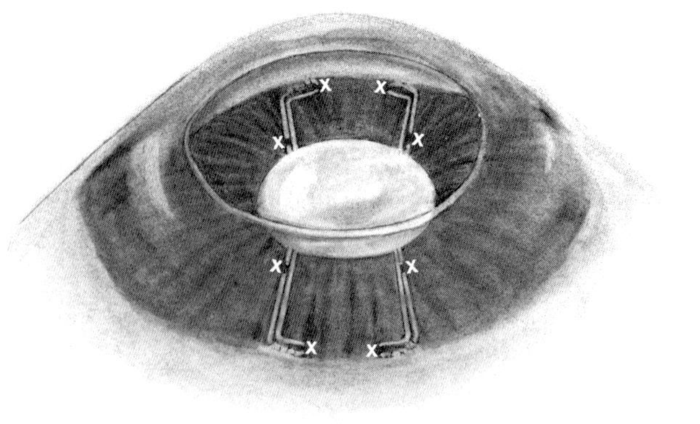

FIGURE 34-33 Removal of a Stableflex closed-loop anterior chamber intraocular lens. The haptics are cut at the *X*s, the optic is removed, and each haptic is spun through the synechiae.

does not appear to be causing problems is left in place. If removal is indicated, an intraocular lens hook is placed posterior to the lens and the lens is gently rotated to free the haptics from the capsular bag and/or iridociliary sulcus. If the lens rotates easily, it is lifted anteriorly with the hook and spun out of the eye through the penetrating keratoplasty opening. If the lens does not rotate, the haptics are cut peripherally, the optic removed, and the ends of the haptics left in place.[49] Difficulty in rotating the lens is caused by encapsulation of the haptics in fibrous tissue. Retained haptics do not appear to have as much of a detrimental effect on the eye as their traumatic removal, which can cause massive bleeding, damage to the ciliary body, vitreous loss, and retinal detachment. It is important to learn as much as possible about the design of the lens preoperatively; some lenses have notches or positioning holes in one or both haptics, which makes their removal more difficult.

Intraocular Lens Implantation

Some surgeons recommend the use of an infant cornea to create a steep graft and treat aphakia.[36] However, as discussed above, aphakia is best corrected with an intraocular lens if there are no contraindications. Some argue that because a contact lens is frequently required postoperatively to correct astigmatism in an eye with a corneal graft, the contact lens can also correct the aphakia. Although this may have been true in the past, when instruments, techniques, and intraocular lenses were less refined, it is not as often the case today. The understanding, prevention, and correction of postkeratoplasty astigmatism are advancing, and whereas a contact lens may be necessary in some patients for good visual acuity even after intraocular lens implantation, many patients have satisfactory visual acuity without a contact lens. It is often not possible to know before surgery if a contact lens will be necessary postoperatively. Even in patients who may require a contact lens, attempts should be made intraoperatively to provide the best postoperative uncorrected visual acuity possible. As much as is feasible should be done to correct any refractive error, including aphakia, at the time of penetrating keratoplasty.

Any of the modern posterior chamber intraocular lenses can be implanted in an eye with an intact posterior capsule. Implantation of a posterior chamber intraocular lens through a penetrating keratoplasty opening is similar to implantation through a cataract incision (Figure 34-34). The haptics are placed in the capsular bag, if possible. If the intraocular lens is implanted at the time of cataract extraction, a small amount of viscoelastic substance is injected to separate the anterior and posterior capsules. Care is taken not to inject too much of the substance because it can accumulate behind the iris and push the peripheral posterior capsule posteriorly and the central posterior capsule anteriorly. If the intraocular lens is implanted secondarily, the capsular bag is usually fibrosed, and attempts to open it risk breaking the capsule and losing vitreous. In the latter case, the haptics are placed in the iridociliary sulcus. The optic is grasped with a smooth forceps and the inferior haptic placed in the capsular bag or iridociliary sulcus. The superior haptic is then grasped at the tip, positioned, and released. The superior iris can be retracted with a Graether collar button to increase visualization, if necessary. A posterior chamber intraocular lens can be implanted in the iridociliary sulcus in an eye with a ruptured posterior capsule if the rupture is central, an anterior vitrectomy has been performed through the rupture, and the peripheral capsular rim is intact.

In the absence of capsular support, an anterior chamber intraocular lens may be implanted or a posterior chamber intraocular lens may be sutured to the peripheral iris or in the iridociliary sulcus, depending on the presence of anterior segment abnormalities.[48,50–62] In a retrospective review of these three techniques, Davis et al[50] found no significant difference in postoperative visual acuity, central corneal thickness, and intraocular pressure with single-piece four-point fixation anterior chamber lenses, iris-sutured posterior chamber lenses, or transsclerally sutured posterior chamber lenses. In a prospective, randomized study of 176 consecutive patients with pseudophakic bullous keratopathy, Schein et al[56] reported a greater risk of adverse outcomes (i.e., increased intraocular pressure, cystoid macular edema, dislocation of the intraocular lens, or graft failure) with transscleral fixation than with iris fixation of a posterior chamber intraocular lens. The risk of adverse outcomes with a Kelman Multiflex–style anterior chamber intraocular lens was intermediate and was not distinguishable statistically from the risks of either transscleral fixation or iris fixation of a posterior chamber intraocular lens. In a retrospective study of 122 eyes that underwent secondary intraocular lens implantation without capsular support at the time of penetrating keratoplasty, Brunette et al[59] reported a trend toward a better outcome with posterior chamber intraocular lenses than with anterior chamber intraocular lenses. It should be noted, however, that only 3.3 percent of the secondary anterior chamber intraocular lenses implanted in this study were Kelman Multiflex–style lenses. A recent review of the literature showed equivalent long-term results with penetrating keratoplasty and intraocular lens exchange using the Kelman Multiflex–style anterior chamber intraocular lens or a sutured posterior chamber intraocular lens.[58] Unless there is a contraindication, implantation of a Kelman Multiflex–style anterior chamber intraocular lens is recommended because suture fixation of a posterior chamber intraocular lens is technically so much more difficult to perform and takes so much longer than implantation of an anterior chamber intraocular lens.

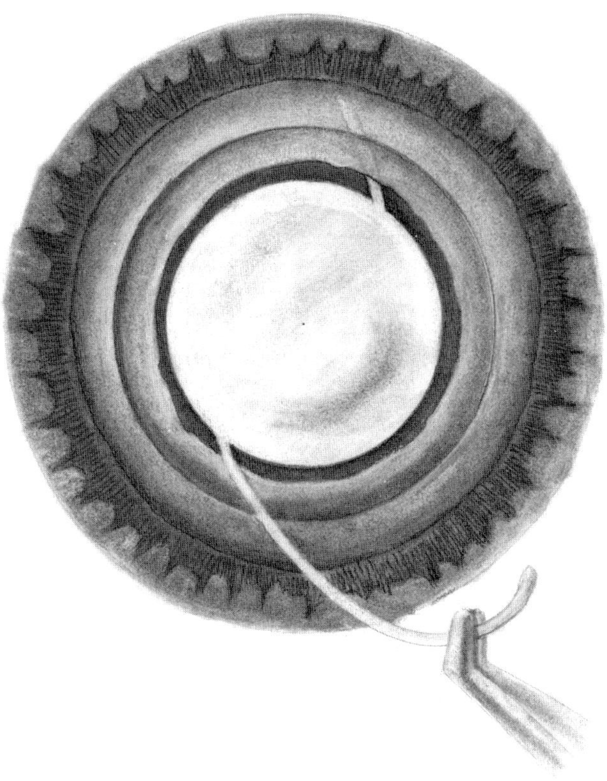

FIGURE 34-34 Implantation of a posterior chamber intraocular lens.

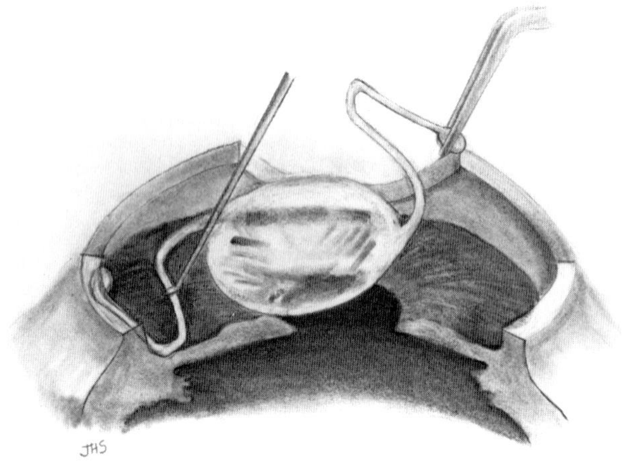

FIGURE 34-35 Implantation of a Kelman Multiflex–style anterior chamber intraocular lens. The inferior haptic is stabilized as the superior haptic is inserted.

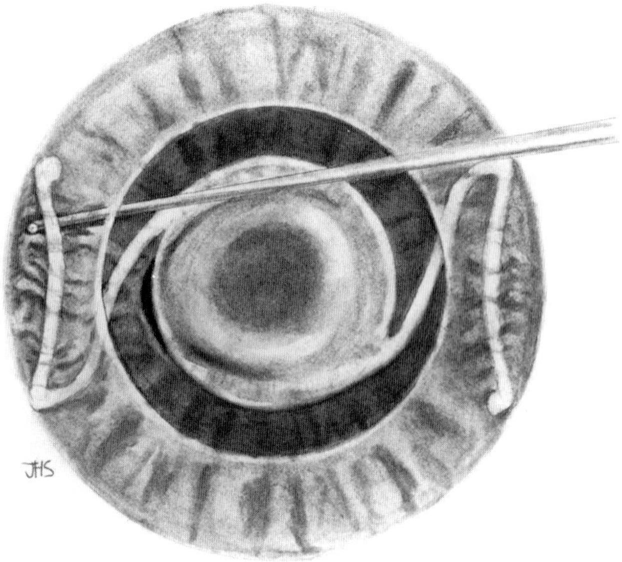

FIGURE 34-36 Release of iris entrapped by an anterior chamber intraocular lens haptic.

A Kelman Multiflex–style anterior chamber intraocular lens is the preferred lens for implantation in the anterior chamber. After a vitrectomy has been performed, a miotic agent, such as acetylcholine chloride, is instilled into the anterior chamber if the pupil is dilated. The optic of the intraocular lens is grasped with a smooth forceps and the inferior haptic is placed through the penetrating keratoplasty opening and slid down the peripheral cornea into the inferior angle. The superior haptic is then grasped, placed through the penetrating keratoplasty opening, and positioned in the superior angle. Care is taken not to transfer pressure to the inferior haptic as the superior haptic is placed, which could result in entrapment of the inferior iris and/or damage to the inferior iris root. Stabilization of the inferior haptic as the superior haptic is placed prevents pressure from being transferred to the inferior haptic and traumatizing the inferior angle (Figure 34-35).

A conscious effort is made to place the haptics in the anterior chamber angle without trapping iris between the haptics and the angle. If it becomes apparent by pupillary distortion that the peripheral iris is caught between the haptic and the anterior chamber angle, an intraocular lens hook is placed beneath the haptic and the haptic is compressed and lifted anteriorly, which releases the iris (Figure 34-36). The haptic is then placed back into the angle and released. Alternatively, an iris sweep can be placed between the haptic and iris, and the incarcerated iris freed by gently pushing it posteriorly.

If implantation of an intraocular lens is desirable and there is a contraindication to an anterior chamber intraocular lens, such as glaucoma, a posterior chamber intraocular lens can be sutured to the peripheral iris or in the iridociliary sulcus. As stated above, Schein et al[56] reported better results with iris fixation than with transscleral fixation.

A single-piece polymethyl methacrylate posterior chamber intraocular lens with two or four positioning holes in the optic is preferred to suture to the iris. After a vitrectomy has been performed, a double-armed 10-0 polypropylene suture on a blood vessel (BV) needle is passed through the positioning hole(s) and then through the midperipheral iris in a mattress fashion. Another suture is placed through the other positioning hole(s) and iris in a similar manner. The lens is placed posterior to the iris, with an attempt to position the haptics in the iridociliary sulcus. Upward tension is applied to the suture ends, and the sutures are tied and trimmed (Figure 34-37).

A single-piece polymethyl methacrylate posterior chamber intraocular lens with an eyelet in each haptic is the preferred lens to suture in the iridociliary sulcus. So that the knots of the sutures are covered at the end of the case, two conjunctival peritomies are made at the beginning of the case in the area where the sutures will exit the eye, usually at the 6 and 12 o'clock positions. The 3 o'clock and 9 o'clock positions should be avoided because the long posterior ciliary arteries and nerves are located in these regions. To provide additional coverage of the knots, two partial-thickness scleral flaps measuring 2 to 3 mm × 2 to 3 mm may be created. Some surgeons do not use scleral flaps, preferring instead to rotate the suture knots into the sclera. It is important that the sutures be covered because erosion through the conjunctiva can cause irritation and create a pathway for bacteria to enter the eye.

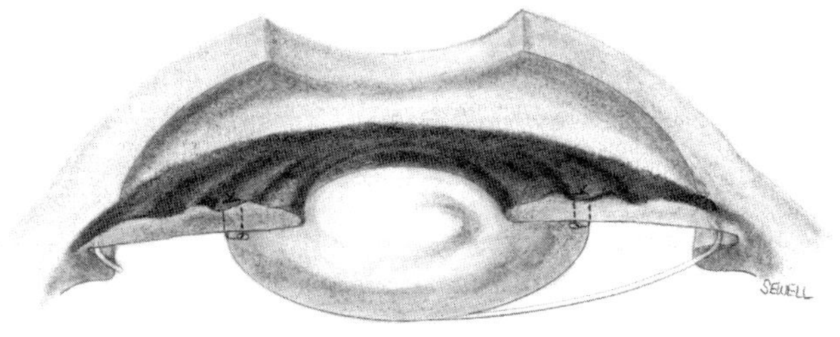

FIGURE 34-37 Posterior chamber intraocular lens sutured to the iris.

After a vitrectomy has been performed, a double-armed 9-0 or 10-0 polypropylene suture on spatula side-cutting needles or long curved needles (Ethicon CIF-6) is passed through the eyelet of the haptic. Each needle is then inserted through the penetrating keratoplasty opening, posterior to the iris, and out through the sclera approximately 1 mm posterior to the limbus. The needles should exit the sclera approximately 2 mm from each other. This procedure is repeated for the other haptic (Figure 34-38A). The optic of the intraocular lens is grasped with a forceps and each haptic is positioned in the iridociliary sulcus as the sutures are drawn taut. The sutures are then tied with a triple-throw, followed by two or three single-throws (Figure 34-38B). The positions of the optic and haptics are examined. The iris can be retracted, if necessary, to better visualize the position of the haptics. If the optic is decentered or tilted, one or both sutures may have to be replaced. When the intraocular lens is in good position, the suture knots are rotated into the sclera or the scleral flaps are brought over the knots and secured with two interrupted 10-0 nylon sutures. The conjunctiva is secured to the limbus with absorbable sutures.

After any intraocular lens is implanted, a viscoelastic substance is placed on the anterior surface of the lens to maintain the anterior chamber and protect the donor corneal endothelium should the cornea come into contact with the lens. A complication of viscoelastic substances is postoperative elevation of intraocular pressure, which can be lessened, but not eliminated, by removal of the substance at the end of the case. Removal is usually less complete than in routine cataract extraction because the configuration of a penetrating keratoplasty wound does not allow atraumatic insertion of an irrigating/aspirating instrument. Most of the viscoelastic substance can be removed by inserting a small cannula on a syringe filled with balanced salt solution through the keratoplasty wound into the anterior chamber, aspirating the substance, removing the cannula from the eye, squirting the substance out of the cannula, reinserting the cannula into the eye, deepening the anterior chamber with balanced salt

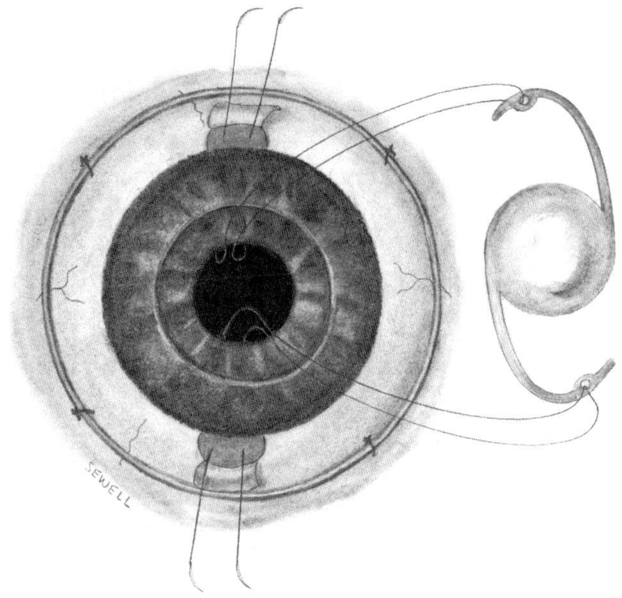

A

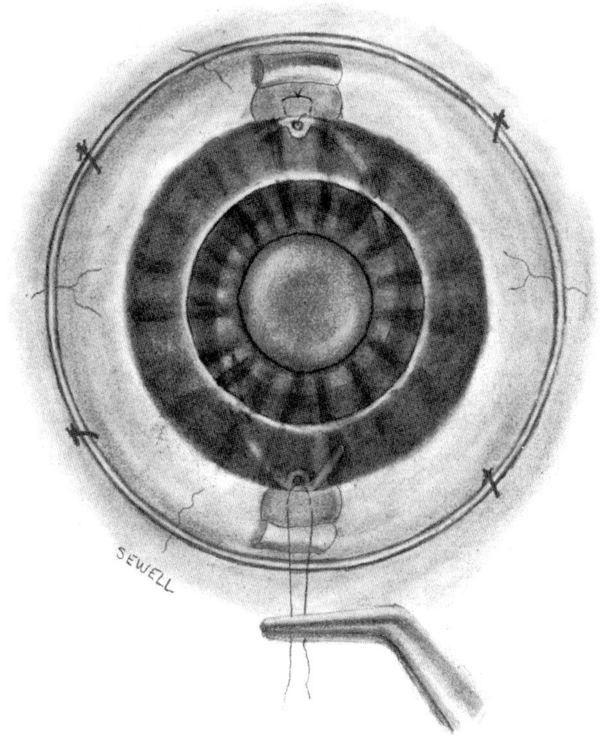

B

FIGURE 34-38 Transscleral fixation of a posterior chamber intraocular lens. **(A)** The sutures have been placed through the eyelets of the intraocular lens, and the needles have been passed through the pupil, posterior to the iris, and out through the sclera 1 mm posterior to the limbus. **(B)** The haptics are placed in the iridociliary sulcus as the sutures are drawn taut and tied.

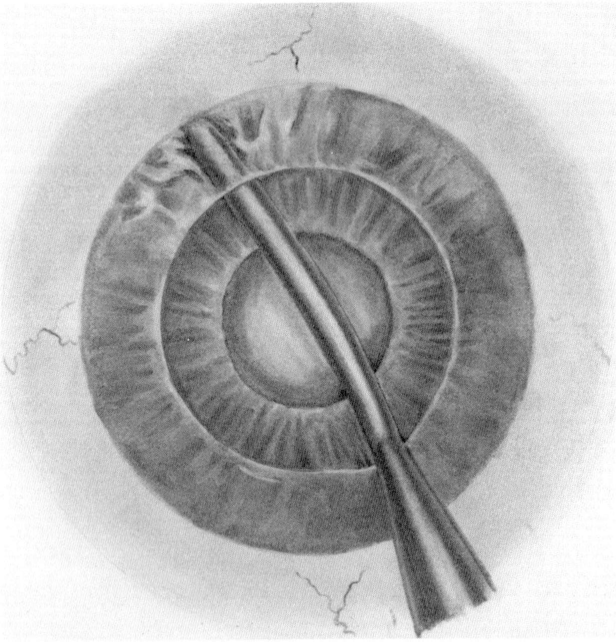

FIGURE 34-39 Blunt dissection of peripheral anterior synechiae with an iris spatula.

solution, and aspirating more substance. This process is repeated several times to remove as much viscoelastic substance as possible, taking care not to collapse the anterior chamber or damage the endothelium of the graft. Invariably, a small amount of viscoelastic substance remains in the eye at the end of the case, and pressure lowering medications must be administered intraoperatively and postoperatively until the substance has left the eye.

Vitrectomy

Many eyes undergoing penetrating keratoplasty have had vitreous loss and an inadequate vitrectomy. If a corneal graft is to survive, a vigorous core vitrectomy must be done. This procedure can be performed through the penetrating keratoplasty opening in an open-sky technique.

Any vitrector may be used. The tip of the vitrector is inserted through the penetrating keratoplasty opening and pupil into the midvitreous cavity, and the vitreous is cut and aspirated until there is no evidence of any vitreous strands in the anterior chamber. Enough of a vitrectomy is done so that if a posterior vitreous detachment occurs postoperatively, vitreous will not prolapse anteriorly and come into contact with the endothelium of the graft. Repeated vitrectomy after filling the eye with balanced salt solution permits removal of vitreous that can float anteriorly. Vitreocorneal touch is a not uncommon cause of late graft failure and is frequently misdiagnosed as a graft rejection. After the vitrectomy, a cellulose sponge is inserted into the anterior chamber angle and on the iris surface to check for vitreous strands, which are cut with Vannas scissors. If vitreous remains on the iris surface, it can pull the iris toward the cornea and cause the formation of broad anterior synechiae postoperatively.

The above technique is not recommended if a deep vitrectomy is indicated because, although the anterior sclera is supported by the scleral support ring, the posterior sclera can collapse and push the choroid and retina anteriorly. In these cases, a temporary keratoprosthesis is placed and a closed-system vitrectomy is done through the pars plana, as described in Chapter 36.

Iridoplasty

Many corneal disorders for which penetrating keratoplasty is indicated are associated with iris abnormalities, such as peripheral anterior synechiae and pupillary distortion. An attempt should be made to correct these abnormalities at the time of penetrating keratoplasty to maximize graft survival, decrease the incidence of glaucoma, obtain an optimal optical pathway, and provide a cosmetically acceptable pupil. Because the keratoplasty wound is often irregular and astigmatic, a small central pupil permits optics superior to those obtained with a large pupil, which allows light passing through the wound to reach the retina.

Peripheral anterior synechiae should be dissected from the cornea. They obliterate the anterior chamber angle, which increases the risk of glaucoma. They can also distort the pupil. If left alone, synechiae can progress circumferentially and zip the anterior chamber angle closed. They can also adhere to the graft, which increases the risk of graft rejection.

A viscoelastic substance may be used to hydraulically dissect the synechiae from the cornea. This procedure is frequently unsuccessful, however, and an attempt can be made to bluntly dissect the synechiae by pushing the iris adjacent to the synechiae posteriorly with an iris spatula or opened Castroviejo scissors (Figure 34-39). If there is a space between the synechiae and iris root, a cyclodialysis spatula can be inserted into the space and swept centrally toward the pupil. The spatula usually tears off the synechiae; rarely, however, the synechiae adhere to the cornea and the iris root tears from its insertion, creating an iridodialysis. One can usually tell when the synechiae are too firmly attached to be broken and can abandon the maneuver before creating an iridodialysis. If the synechiae cannot be broken by blunt dissection, they are sharply dissected from the cornea with scissors (Figure 34-40).

Synechiae may be associated with a fibrovascular membrane on the iris, which should be peeled off with a smooth forceps. Fibrous tissue on the iris seems to give it a "memory," and synechiae frequently reform postoperatively if the anterior chamber is not deep or the iris diaphragm is not taut. A viscoelastic substance may be left in the anterior chamber angle at the end of the case to separate the iris from the cornea during the early postoperative period. Although this is a temporary maneuver that can cause transient elevation of intraocular pressure, it is helpful in inflamed eyes because it keeps the iris away from the cornea as the inflammation is brought under control. An important consideration for preventing the reformation of synechiae is to create a taut iris diaphragm as described below.

A distorted pupil may be caused by or contribute to the formation of anterior synechiae, and should be repaired at the time of penetrating keratoplasty. Restoration of a taut iris diaphragm that will remain away from the cornea is as important as creation of a pupil of normal size and shape. Either 10-0 nylon or 10-0 polypropylene can be used to suture the iris. Nylon is easier to work with and does not appear to biodegrade inside the eye as it does outside the eye, unless it is chafed by an intraocular lens. Both kinds of sutures are available on a round, tapered BV needle, which tears the iris less than a spatula side-cutting needle. The suture is placed by grasping one edge of iris with a smooth forceps, passing the needle through full-thickness iris, releasing the iris and grasping the needle with the forceps, releasing the needle from the needle holder, and pulling the needle out of the eye. The other edge of the iris is sutured in a similar manner. This technique causes less tension on and tearing of the iris than if the needle is passed through both edges of the iris without being regrasped. The surgeon must never let go of the needle while it is inside the eye because it can fall posteriorly. The suture is tied with a double-throw followed by two single-throws, and the ends are cut on the knot with Vannas scissors. A stainless steel blade is not used for this purpose because too much countertraction is necessary, which may tear the suture out of the iris. As many sutures as are needed are placed in various locations in the iris to restore the pupil and iris diaphragm to as normal a condition possible.

Although sector iridectomies were common in the past when the preferred method for cataract extraction was by an intracapsular technique, they are rarely indicated today. A sector iridectomy is closed by placing interrupted sutures in the midperipheral iris. The peripheral iris is left open to function as a peripheral iridectomy (Figure 34-41).

If the pupil is updrawn, the inferior sphincter is cut with scissors, and the superior opening is closed with interrupted sutures (Figure 34-42). If the pupil is extremely updrawn, a hole may be made in the iris centrally and the updrawn pupil left undisturbed to function as a peripheral iridectomy.

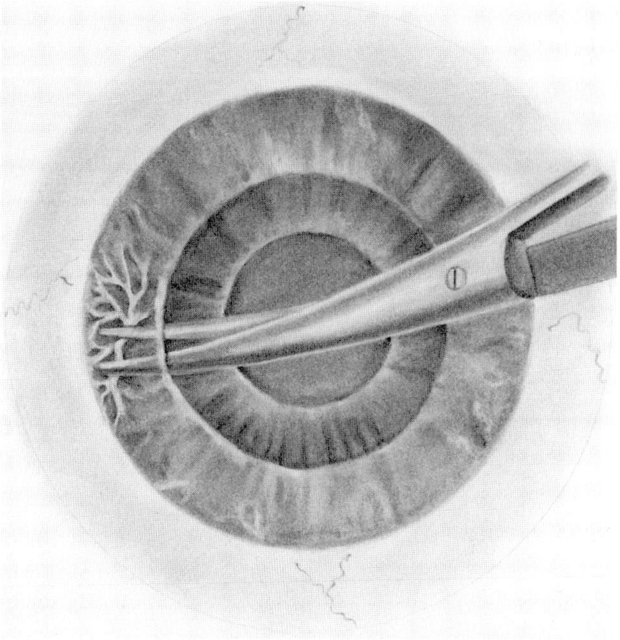

FIGURE 34-40 Sharp dissection of peripheral anterior synechiae with scissors.

A peripheral iridectomy is usually not routinely performed unless there is pupillary block, a narrow anterior chamber angle, a ruptured posterior capsule, inflammation, or peripheral anterior synechiae that cannot be dissected from the cornea. In the latter case, an iridectomy is performed on either side of the synechiae in an attempt to prevent the synechiae from progressing circumferentially. If a peripheral iridectomy is indicated, a forceps is placed through the penetrating keratoplasty opening, and peripheral iris is grasped, brought anteriorly (taking care not to create an iridodialysis), and cut with scissors (Figure 34-43). To ensure that the iridectomy is full-thickness, the excised iris is examined for pigment epithelium by rubbing it between the thumb and forefinger and looking for pigment. In an aphakic or pseudophakic eye, a peripheral iridotomy rather than a peripheral iridectomy may be created by inserting Vannas scissors near the anterior chamber angle and cutting a hole in the peripheral iris.

An iridodialysis is repaired by first making a conjunctival peritomy in the area of the dialysis. A double-armed 10-0 polypropylene suture on spatula side-cutting needles is used in a mattress fashion to approximate the iris to the iris root (Figure 34-44). The needles are passed through peripheral iris and full-thickness sclera, and the suture is tied externally with a triple-throw followed by two single-throws. The conjunctiva is then brought over the knot and

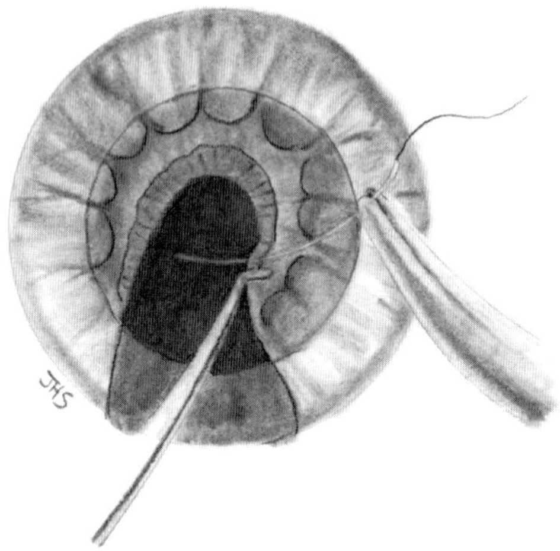

A

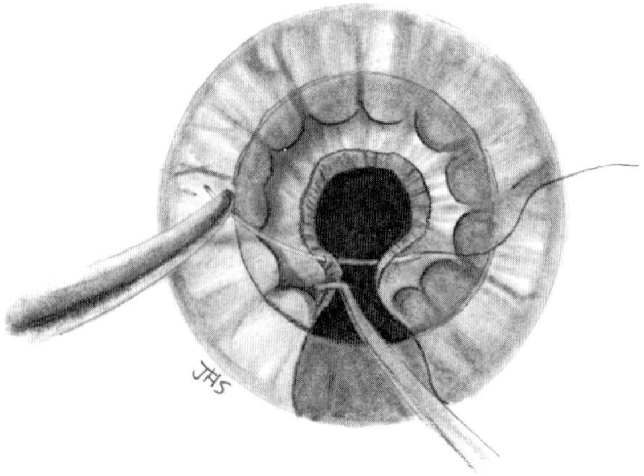

B

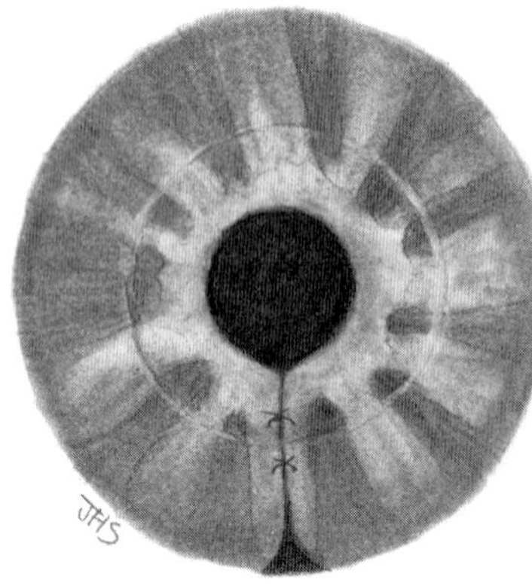

C

FIGURE 34-41 Closure of a sector iridectomy. **(A & B)** The iris on each side of the iridectomy is grasped, and a suture on a BV needle is placed. **(C)** Additional sutures are placed to close the iridectomy centrally. The peripheral portion is left open to function as a peripheral iridectomy.

anchored to the limbus with absorbable sutures. The knot can be buried under a scleral flap in a manner similar to that used for suturing a posterior chamber intraocular lens in the iridociliary sulcus, but this is usually not necessary.

Suturing the Donor Cornea

The donor cornea is brought into the field of the microscope in the well of the cutting block. A Paton spatula, which has slits that allow drainage of excess preservation medium (Figure 34-45), is placed under the donor corneal button, and the button is scooped out of the well and brought to the inferior limbus.

The edge of the button is placed on the inferior limbus and the spatula is rotated quickly to stand the button on end (Figure 34-46). It is important to rotate the spatula quickly so the button does not slide off, and to rest the button on the limbus. The Paton spatula is slid down the button so that it, too, rests on the limbus. The spatula is then rotated slightly further so the anterior layers of the button can be grasped with a forceps. Some surgeons flip the button completely over into the recipient corneal opening. However, the button can sink into the opening, and if the eye has little iris, is aphakic, and has had a vitrectomy, the button can even sink into the vitreous cavity. With the button standing on end, the anterior corneal layers are grasped with a Polack double corneal forceps, which has two tips and provides greater stability than a forceps with only one tip (Figure 34-47). If the button has been marked, as with the Barron vacuum donor cornea punch, it is grasped at one of the marks. Inversion of the corneal button has been reported,[63] but the epithelial and endothelial surfaces are easily identified by the orientation of the button in the well, the curvature of the button, and the marks on the epithelial surface.

After the button has been grasped, it is laid flat in the plane of the cornea and brought to the superior edge of the recipient corneal opening. The Paton spatula is exchanged for a needle holder, and the button is sutured to the recipient cornea with 10-0 nylon suture on a spatula side-cutting needle, such as the Ethicon TG160-6 or CS-160-6 needle. The needle is passed between the two tips of the Polack forceps, entering the button anteriorly through the central edge of one of the marks made by the Barron vacuum donor cornea punch (which is 0.85 mm from the edge of the button), and exiting just anterior to Descemet's membrane (Figure 34-48). If a Polack forceps is not available and the button is grasped with a 0.12-mm forceps, the needle must be placed immediately beneath the forceps teeth or the button will twirl. Twirling can also occur if the button is not grasped firmly. If this happens, an assistant can stabilize the button by grasp-

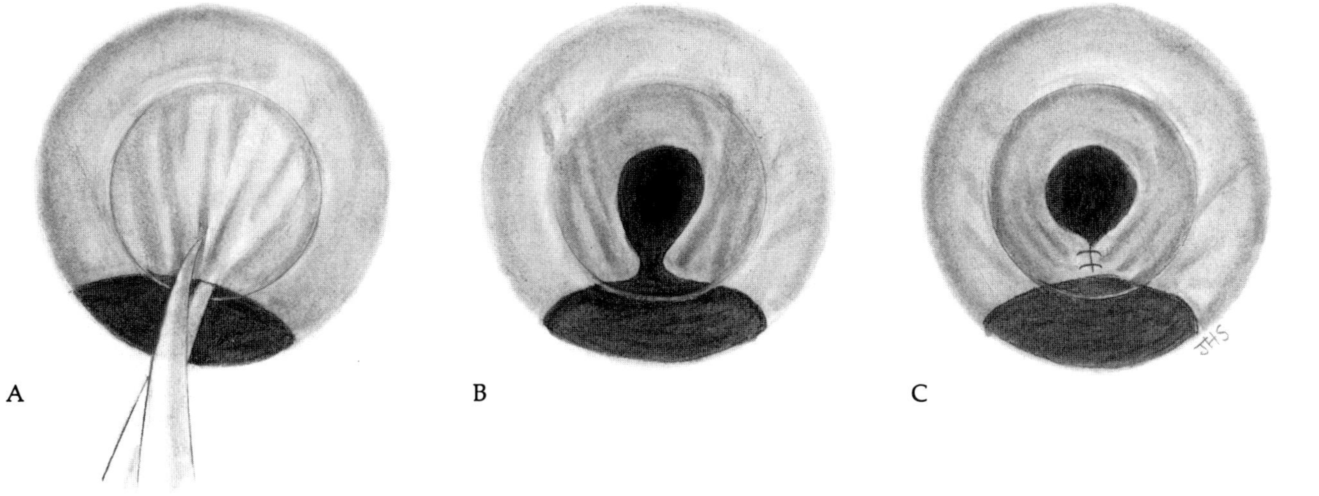

FIGURE 34-42 Pupilloplasty of an updrawn pupil. **(A & B)** Scissors are inserted through the pupil and used to cut the iris. **(C)** Sutures are placed to create a central pupil. The original pupil functions as a peripheral iridectomy.

ing the anterior layers of the inferior edge with a forceps. After the needle has been passed through the button, the button is released from the Polack forceps, which are exchanged for a 0.12-mm forceps. The edge of the recipient corneal opening is then grasped with these forceps, and the needle is passed through the recipient cornea at one of the radial marks made by the Barron radial vacuum trephine, entering just anterior to Descemet's membrane and exiting 1 mm from the edge. In cases in which the recipient corneal rim is too thin to support sutures, the needle is passed peripherally until normal tissue is reached, even if it has to be passed into sclera. The suture is tied with a triple-throw, followed by two single-throws.

The second suture is the most important suture in penetrating keratoplasty because it establishes distribution of the tissue. If improperly placed, this suture can cause severe postoperative astigmatism. Marks on the donor corneal button and recipient corneal rim eliminate the guesswork in placing this suture (Figure 34-49). The edge of the button is grasped with a 0.12-mm forceps at the inferior mark, and the needle is passed through the button as described above. The edge of the recipient corneal opening is then grasped at

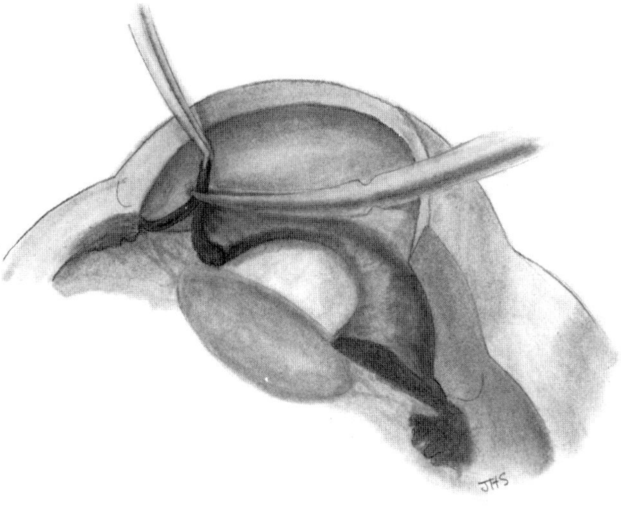

FIGURE 34-43 Peripheral iridectomy.

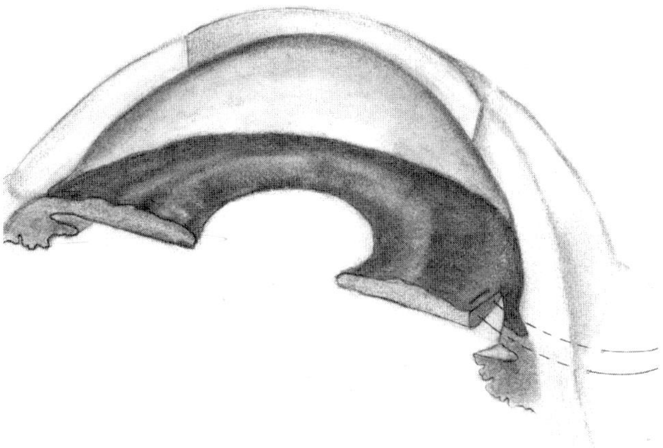

FIGURE 34-44 Repair of an iridodialysis.

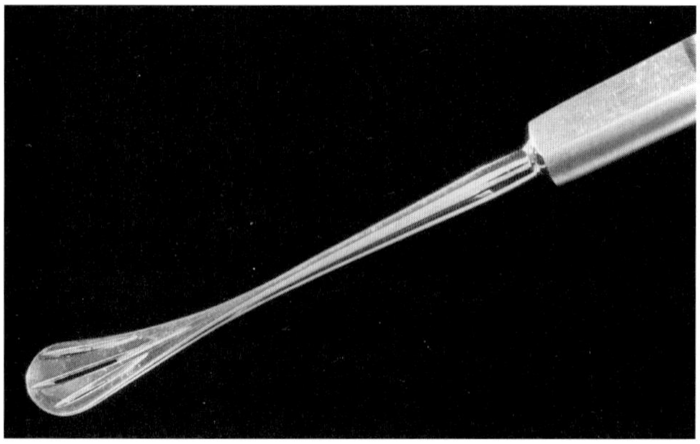

FIGURE 34-45 Paton spatula.

the radial mark 180 degrees from the first suture, and the needle is passed through the recipient cornea as described above. The third and fourth sutures are placed through the marks 90 degrees from the first two sutures. Collectively, the first four sutures are known as *cardinal sutures.*

After this point, the type and number of sutures to place and the pattern of their placement are the subject of considerable debate and vary with the corneal disorder for which penetrating keratoplasty is performed, patient considerations such as age and the amount of stress to which the graft will be subjected postoperatively, and surgeon preferences. Nylon and polyester sutures are most commonly used. Nylon is easy to work with but hydrolyzes over time and can spontaneously break, which may result in an increase in postoperative astigmatism.[64] Polyester (Mersilene) is strong and does not hydrolyze, which is advantageous in cases in which it is desirable to leave sutures in place, such as patients with low postoperative astigmatism.[65,66] However, polyester is difficult to work with; is inelastic, which can make postoperative suture manipulation difficult; and can cause tissue-related complications, such as cheesewiring through tissue and marked scarring along the loops of the sutures.[67,68] Polypropylene does not hydrolyze but is too elastic.

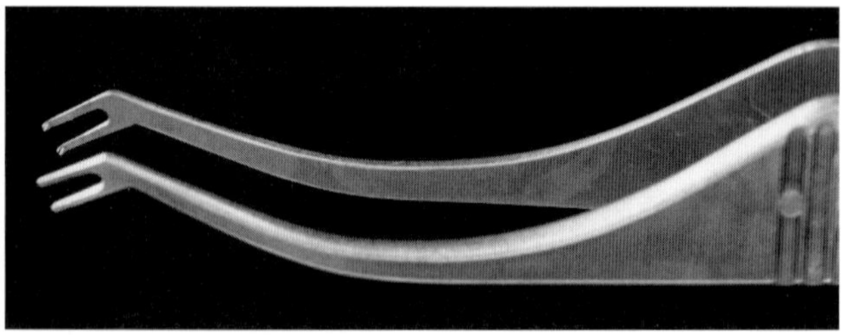

FIGURE 34-47 Polack forceps.

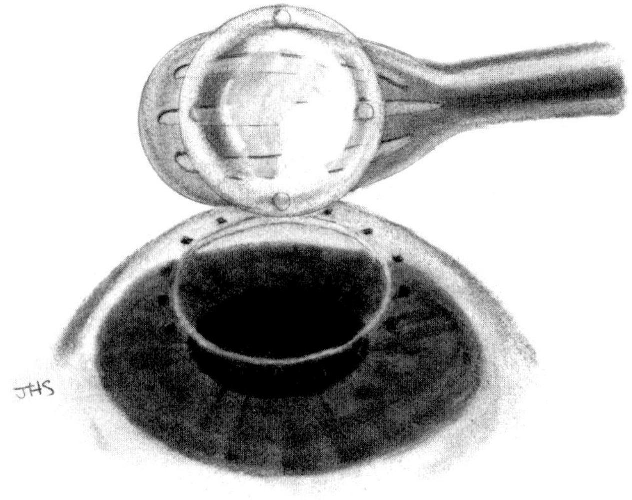

FIGURE 34-46 Positioning of the donor corneal button so that it can be grasped with a forceps.

Interrupted sutures, a single running suture, a combination of interrupted sutures and a single running suture, or double running sutures may be used (Figure 34-50). There are certain situations in which interrupted sutures are indicated, as discussed below. Otherwise, any suture pattern may be used. No one pattern has proved superior to the others, although a great deal has been written about

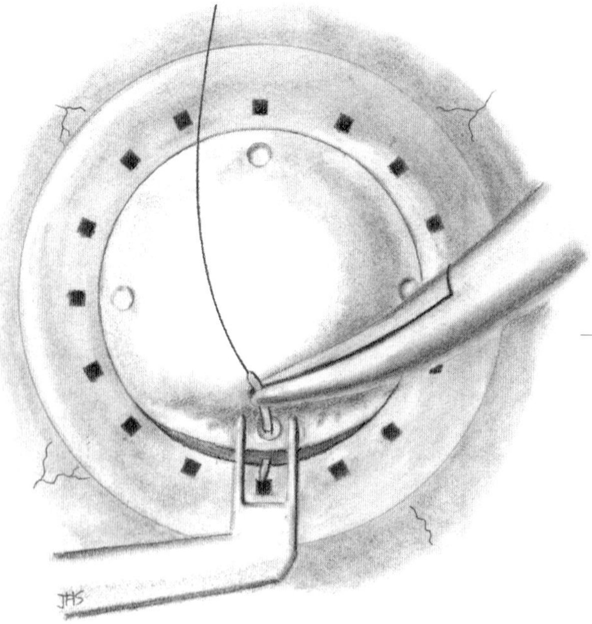

FIGURE 34-48 Placement of the first cardinal suture.

the subject, particularly with regard to the amount of postoperative astigmatism associated with the different patterns.[69-80] One must be discriminating in reading this literature, because many of the reported studies are retrospective, nonrandomized, and/or uncontrolled.

In a prospective randomized study, Filatov et al[74] compared a 24-bite single running 10-0 nylon suture followed by postoperative suture adjustment with a combination of eight interrupted 10-0 nylon sutures and a 16-bite running 10-0 nylon suture followed by selective postoperative removal of interrupted sutures. At approximately 9 months postoperatively, patients with the single running suture had less astigmatism than patients with combined interrupted and running sutures (2.7 diopters vs. 3.9 diopters). However, long-term (approximately 4 years) follow-up showed no significant difference in astigmatism regardless of suture technique or whether the sutures remained in place or were removed.[79]

Interrupted sutures are recommended in infants and children and in corneas that are vascularized or of uneven thickness. Infant corneas are thin and elastic, which makes wound closure difficult. Vascularized corneas have different rates of wound healing in different areas, especially if the vessels are unevenly distributed. This problem necessitates removal of some sutures before others, which can be done only if interrupted sutures are used; a running suture is contraindicated because it cannot be partially removed safely

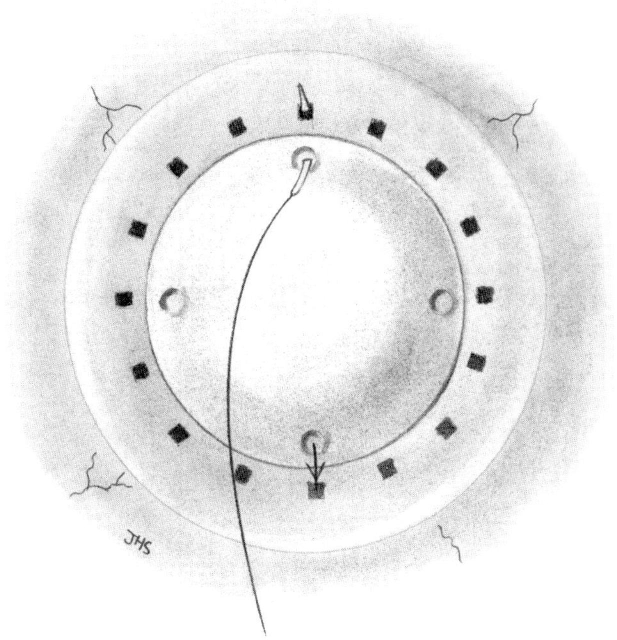

FIGURE 34-49 Placement of the second cardinal suture. Marks on the donor and recipient corneas ensure even tissue distribution.

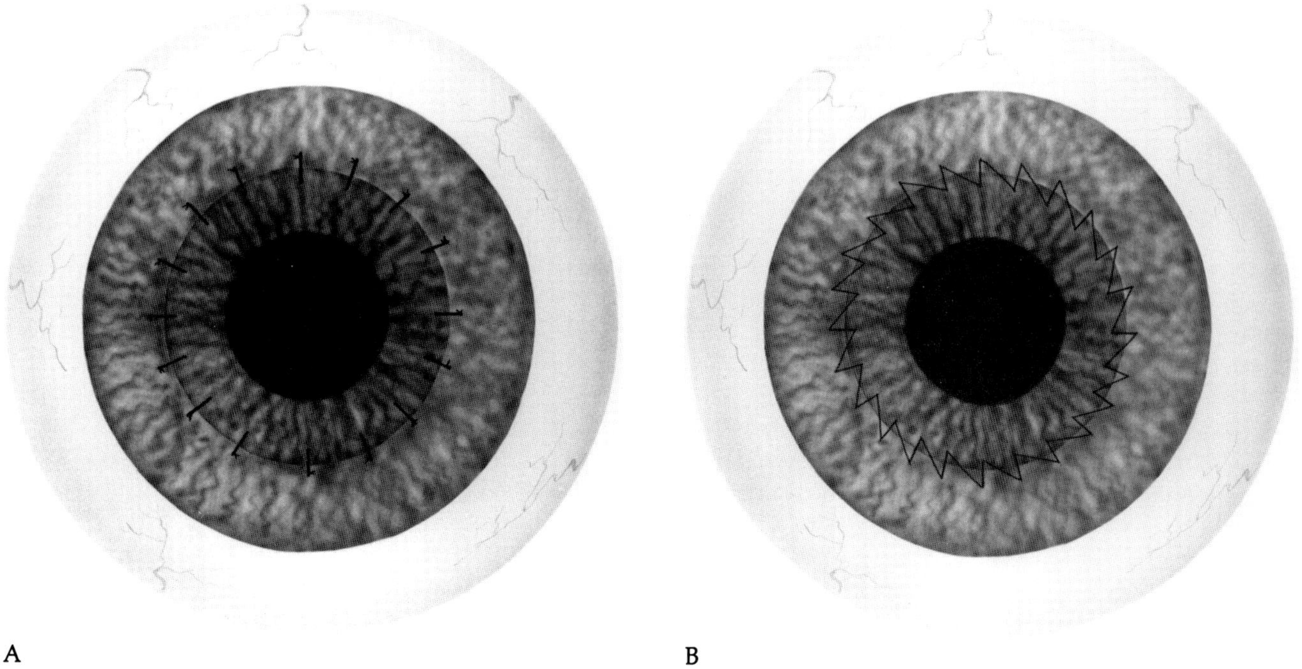

A B

FIGURE 34-50 Suture patterns. **(A)** Interrupted sutures. **(B)** Single running suture. *(continues)*

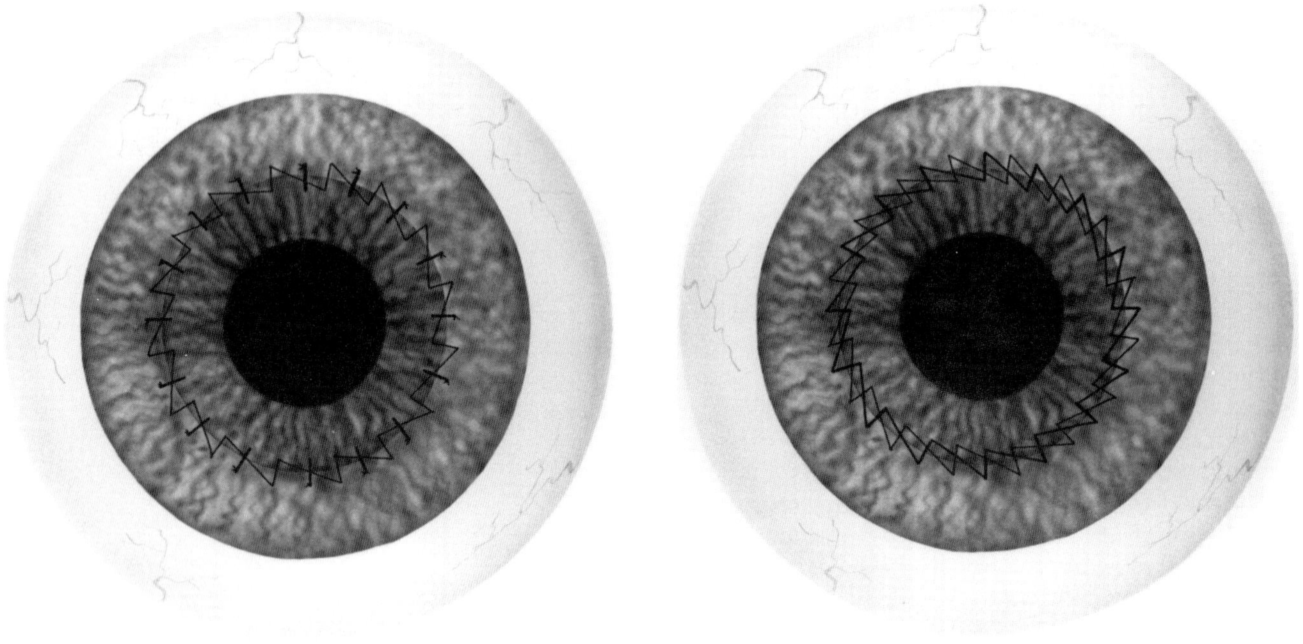

C D

FIGURE 34-50 *(continued)* **(C)** Combined interrupted and single running sutures. **(D)** Double running sutures.

if one area of the wound develops early vascularization. A similar situation occurs in corneas of uneven thickness; if a running suture is used and loosens or pulls through the tissue, the entire wound is in jeopardy. Interrupted sutures are also indicated in corneas in which the integrity of the wound should not depend on one knot, such as in eyes undergoing concomitant posterior segment surgery after the graft has been sutured in place, or in eyes that may be subjected to postoperative trauma, as could occur in uncooperative patients. A stronger suture, such as 9-0 nylon, may also be used in these eyes.

Interrupted sutures are placed in a manner similar to that used for the cardinal sutures. The needle of the 10-0 nylon suture enters the donor cornea approximately 1 mm from the edge, exits just anterior to Descemet's membrane, enters the recipient cornea just anterior to Descemet's membrane, and exits approximately 1 mm from the edge of the recipient corneal opening. If the recipient cornea is thin, the needle should exit at a point where the tissue is thick enough to support the suture, even if it is at the limbus or beyond. Otherwise, the suture will tear through the tissue. Although some surgeons place full-thickness sutures, these sutures cause more endothelial trauma than partial-thickness sutures, and aqueous humor may leak through the suture tracts postoperatively. In thin recipient corneas, full-thickness sutures frequently tear through the recipient cornea and leave large holes that leak and are difficult to close. If interrupted sutures alone are used, a total of 16 are usually placed, with the second four sutures equidistant between the first four (cardinal) sutures and the second eight sutures equidistant between the first eight sutures. More sutures may be required for larger grafts or in cases in which the recipient cornea is thin. If interrupted sutures are combined with a running suture, a total of 8, 12, or 16 are usually placed.

The ends of the sutures are trimmed, if necessary, by grasping the ends with a tying forceps and pulling them across a stainless steel blade. The sutures are then grasped with the forceps and rotated until the knots are buried just beneath the epithelium of the recipient cornea. Burying the knots results in less postoperative irritation than leaving them exposed, decreases the stimulus for suture-induced superficial corneal neovascularization, and allows intraoperative assessment of the stability of the knots; if the knots can be buried without unraveling, they are unlikely to unravel thereafter. Some surgeons routinely bury the knots in the donor cornea. This technique is not recommended because when the sutures are removed postoperatively, the knots either pass through the keratoplasty wound or the donor cornea, which can create traction on the graft and result in dehiscence of the wound. However, if the recipient cornea is thin and attempts to bury the knots cause tearing of the tissue and the creation of full-thickness holes, the knots should be buried in the donor cornea. Such tears may be closed with an 11-0 nylon suture placed perpendicular to the original suture or by replacing the suture with one that has a longer bite in the recipient cornea that extends beyond the tear. If the tears cannot be closed with sutures, cyanoacrylate glue can be applied, followed by placement of a bandage soft contact lens.

In a combined interrupted and running suture technique, an 11-0 nylon or polyester suture is placed by grasping the recipient cornea and passing the needle into the wound and through the recipient cornea. Sixteen equally spaced radial bites of 1-mm donor cornea and 1-mm recipient cornea are taken around the circumference of the graft. Placement of the running suture is more quickly performed if care is taken after each bite to grasp the needle such that the suture does not lock and the needle is positioned properly in the needle holder for the next bite as it is pulled out of the recipient cornea. On the last bite, the needle is passed through the donor cornea only and out of the wound in the area where the suture was started. If a single running suture technique is used, a 10-0 nylon suture is placed after the cardinal sutures are in position, and 24 bites are taken instead of 16. If a double running suture technique is used, an 11-0 nylon or polyester suture is placed between each bite of a 16-bite 10-0 nylon suture as described above.

Some disadvantages of running sutures are that suboptimal bites cannot be replaced and if the needle becomes dull, placement of the remaining bites is difficult. If a running suture breaks, it can be spliced to another suture by passing the needle of the new suture through the donor and recipient corneas, pulling the suture through until the end is visible, and tying it to the end of the previous suture with a triple-throw followed by two single-throws. Passing the new suture through the cornea before tying it to the previous suture stabilizes the suture. The ends are cut close to the knot with Vannas scissors, and the knot is buried in the wound. It is important to bury the knot at this time to ensure that it is stable and can be buried without unraveling.

A running suture is tightened by grasping the suture between each bite with a smooth forceps with round edges, such as the Harms-Tubingen tying forceps, and pulling the suture taut. It is important that the forceps be held parallel to the suture to minimize the risk of breaking the suture. If the suture has been spliced, it is tightened in each direction from the knot so the knot stays buried. If a single or double running suture technique is used, the cardinal sutures are removed before the suture is tightened. A running 10-0 suture should be tight enough so there is no slack and the wound is watertight but not so tight that it creates a large tissue roll. A running 11-0 suture should be tightened just enough to remove slack but not distort the wound. This second suture is not meant to provide wound closure but to stabilize the wound after the 10-0 suture has been

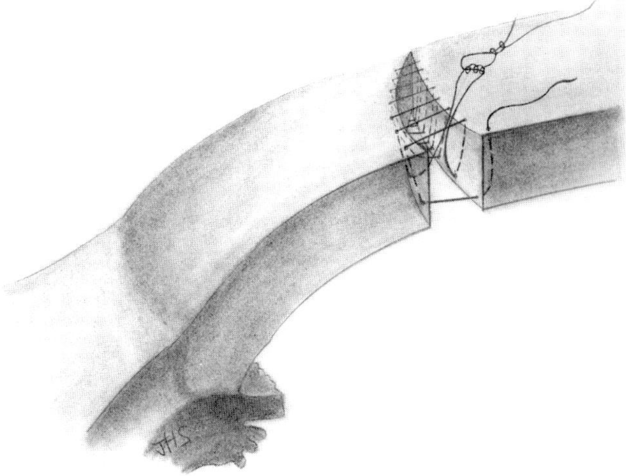

FIGURE 34-51 Tying of the running suture. The knot is buried in the wound.

removed postoperatively. A running suture is tied with a triple-throw followed by two single-throws, and the ends are cut with Vannas scissors. The knot is automatically buried in the wound because of the technique of starting and finishing the suture in the wound (Figure 34-51). It may be desirable to test the wound for leaks, as described below, after the triple-throw has been placed but before the suture is tied, so that if the wound is not watertight the suture can be retightened.

After the sutures have been placed, the wound is checked to be sure it is watertight, which is done by drying the surface of the wound with a cellulose sponge, pressing at the limbus, and observing the wound for leakage of aqueous humor. Topical fluorescein (Seidel's test) aids in this evaluation. It is important to recognize that intracameral viscoelastic substance can temporarily plug a leak so that the leak is not recognized until after surgery, when the viscoelastic substance has left the eye.

Leaks in the wound are repaired with sutures. If interrupted sutures have been used, additional interrupted sutures are placed at the site of the leak. If a running suture has been used, placement of interrupted sutures at the site of the leak may lead to the postoperative complication of leaks in other areas of the wound. The leak indicates that the running suture is too loose; placement of interrupted sutures at the site of the leak will close the leak, but slack in the running suture often works its way to another area postoperatively, causing that area to leak. Wound leaks caused by a loose running suture can be repaired in one of four ways. First, if the suture has not been tied, it can be retightened. Second, the suture can be retightened and any slack anchored to the limbus with a 10-0 nylon reefing suture. This type of repair is suboptimal and is not recommended unless there are conditions that prohibit keeping the patient under anesthesia any longer. Third, interrupted sutures can be placed around the entire wound. Fourth, the running suture can be intentionally broken at the knot and unraveled from the wound on both sides until the ends are long enough to splice and tie to another suture. The spliced suture is then placed in a running fashion and tied to the original suture after the suture has been tightened. In my opinion, there is no place for the use of tissue adhesives in the repair of wound leaks unless the leaks cannot be repaired with sutures.

Running sutures may be adjusted intraoperatively in an attempt to decrease astigmatism. In a prospective randomized clinical trial comparing astigmatism after penetrating keratoplasty with and without intraoperative suture adjustment, Serdarevic et al[78] reported less postoperative astigmatism with intraoperative suture adjustment. Before suture adjustment, the scleral support ring is removed and the eyelid speculum is lifted so it is not pressing on the eye. The cornea is moistened with balanced salt solution and the anterior corneal surface is examined with a keratoscope. The epithelial surface of the graft must be regular enough to obtain a reflection of suitable quality to assess the topography of the graft. If the reflection is circular, the surface is spherical. If the reflection is oval, the surface is astigmatic; the shortest diameter of the oval is in the steep meridian, and the longest is in the flat meridian. The suture is grasped in the flat meridian with a smooth forceps with round edges, such as the Harms-Tubingen tying forceps, and tightened in both directions so that the tension is redistributed and the suture is loosened in the previously steep meridian (Figure 34-52). It is important that the forceps be held parallel to the suture to minimize the risk of breaking the suture. The anterior corneal surface is re-examined with the keratoscope, and the suture is readjusted if necessary until the reflection is circular.

POSTOPERATIVE CARE

Antimicrobials

An antibiotic-soaked collagen shield is placed on the cornea at the end of the case, which both protects the corneal epithelium and provides antibiotic coverage during the early postoperative period. Topical antibiotic drops, such as ciprofloxacin or ofloxacin, are used four times a day for 1 week postoperatively or until the epithelium is healed. As an alternative, erythromycin ointment may be used. Prolonged use of topical aminoglycoside drops can be toxic to the epithelium and should be avoided.

If penetrating keratoplasty is performed for uncontrolled infectious keratitis, antimicrobials are used for longer periods of time postoperatively. In bacterial keratitis, broad spectrum topical antibiotics, such as a fluoroquinolone (ciprofloxacin or ofloxacin) and/or fortified tobramycin (14 mg/ml) and cefazolin (50 mg/ml), or an antibiotic based on culture and sensitivity results, if available, are used. The frequency depends on the activity of the keratitis, and varies from every 30 minutes to four times a day. These drops are generally tapered over a 2- to 3-week period postoperatively. Systemic antibiotics, initially intravenously and then orally, are recommended as well, especially in cases of corneal perforation. In filamentous fungal keratitis, topical natamycin and oral fluconazole are used postoperatively for several weeks. Although fungal elements are frequently found in the anterior chamber and are not totally removed from the recipient cornea at the time of penetrating keratoplasty, most of these eyes do well and endophthalmitis almost never occurs. In *Acanthamoeba* keratitis, topical polyhexamethylene biguanide, propamidine isethionate, and neomycin are used as frequently as every hour and are tapered over several months. In herpes simplex keratitis, even in quiescent eyes, topical trifluridine drops are used with a frequency equal to that of topical corticosteroid application and are tapered on a drop-per-drop basis with the corticosteroids. Postoperative prophylactic topical antiviral therapy decreases the rates of recurrent herpetic keratitis and allograft rejection.[81] It also appears that postoperative prophylactic oral acyclovir therapy decreases the rates of recurrent herpetic keratitis and graft failure.[24–26] Oral acyclovir (400 mg five times a day) or valacyclovir (500 mg three times a day) may be started 1 to 2 days before surgery, continued for 1 to 3 weeks, and then decreased to a maintenance dose (400 mg twice a day for acyclovir or 500 mg twice a day for valacyclovir) for several months.

Corticosteroids

At the end of the case, 0.5 to 1 ml of methylprednisolone acetate (80 mg/ml) is injected subconjunctivally in the inferior fornix. The injection should be far enough away from the interpalpebral conjunctiva so it is not cosmetically visible. Subconjunctival corticosteroids are not given in eyes with fungal or herpes simplex keratitis, or in eyes known to develop elevated intraocular pressure in response to corticosteroids. Topical corticosteroid drops, such as 1 percent prednisolone acetate or 0.1 percent dexamethasone sodium phosphate, are used four to six times a day and tapered over several months unless

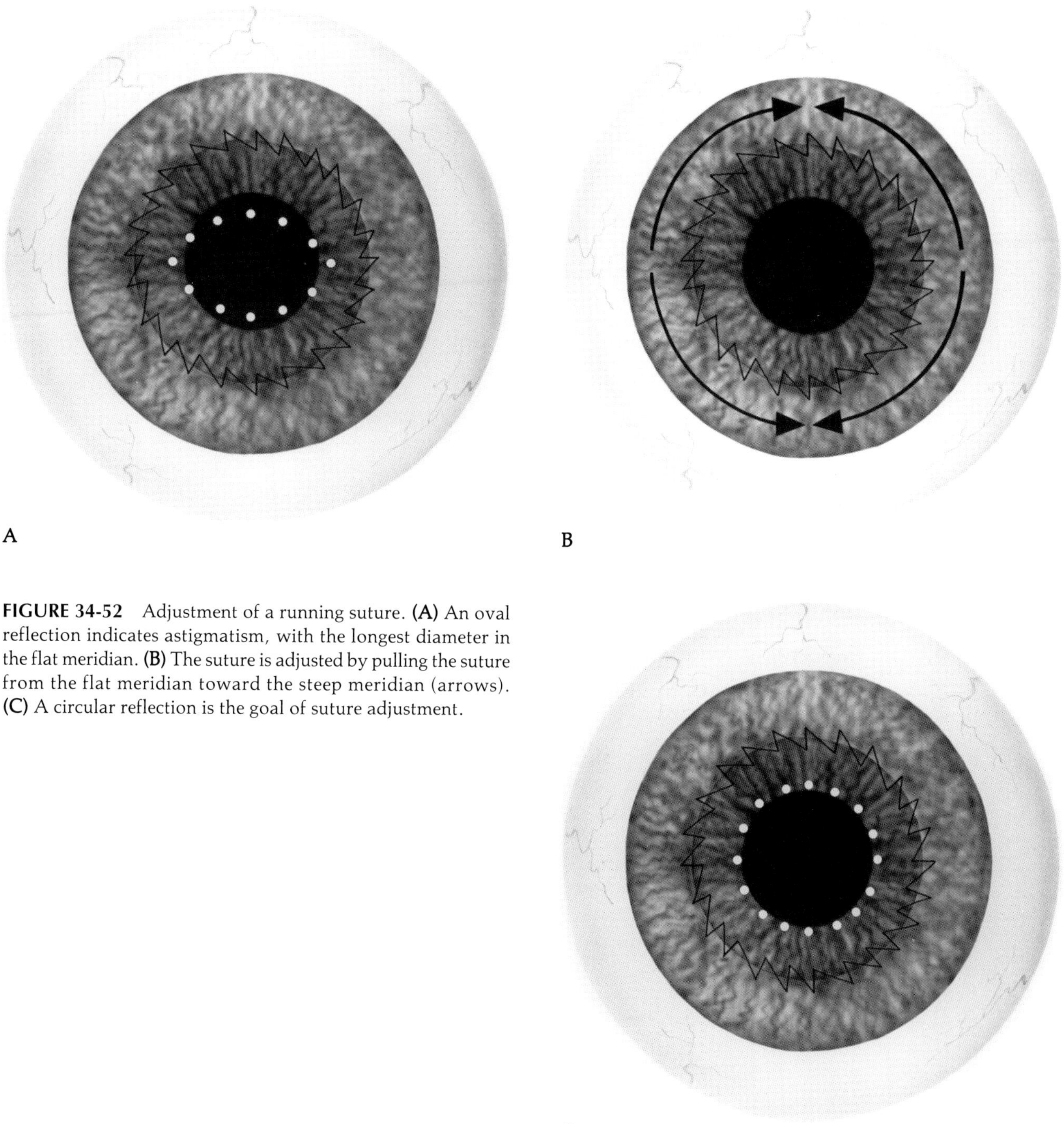

A

B

C

FIGURE 34-52 Adjustment of a running suture. (A) An oval reflection indicates astigmatism, with the longest diameter in the flat meridian. (B) The suture is adjusted by pulling the suture from the flat meridian toward the steep meridian (arrows). (C) A circular reflection is the goal of suture adjustment.

the patient is at high risk for graft rejection, in which case they are used more frequently for a longer period of time. If the patient develops increased inflammation in the anterior chamber, keratic precipitates on the graft, or increased corneal thickness, the dosage of topical corticosteroids is increased. Topical corticosteroids are tapered more rapidly in phakic eyes than in aphakic or pseudophakic eyes because of the risk of cataract formation. In aphakic or pseudophakic eyes, topical corticosteroids are continued once a day indefinitely if there are no contraindications, especially if the graft is at high risk for rejection.

Systemic corticosteroids are prescribed if the patient is at high risk for graft rejection or there is marked inflammation and there are no contraindications. Prednisone at a dosage of 1 mg/kg/day is started 1 to 2 days before surgery and tapered over 2 to 3 weeks.

Mydriatic and Cycloplegic Agents

Mydriatic agents are used to prevent the formation of posterior synechiae; cycloplegic agents are used to relax the ciliary body and decrease postoperative discomfort. Whether to dilate or constrict the pupil depends on the disorder for which penetrating keratoplasty is performed, the phakic status of the eye, and the amount of intraocular inflammation. Strong agents, such as atropine, should be avoided in patients with keratoconus because of reports of permanent pupillary dilation following their use (Urrets-Zavalia syndrome).[82] Wide dilation of the pupil in an eye with a posterior chamber intraocular lens increases the risk of formation of synechiae to the posterior capsule and capture of the edge of the lens by the iris. Wide dilation in an eye with a large graft can cause the iris to crowd the anterior chamber angle and adhere to the posterior edge of the wound. Constriction of the pupil is often done after implantation of an anterior chamber intraocular lens.

Glaucoma Medications

Intraocular pressure should be measured at each postoperative examination in all postkeratoplasty patients. Measurement of intraocular pressure usually must be done with an electronic applanation tonometer, such as the Tono-Pen, because the irregular surface of the graft precludes Goldmann applanation tonometry, and Schiøtz tonometry is unreliable. In a study involving penetrating keratoplasty in cadaver eyes, Menage et al[83] found a minified Goldmann applanation tonometer more accurate than the Tono-Pen in measuring intraocular pressure. Geyer et al[84] reported that the Tono-Pen tends to overestimate the actual intraocular pressure in an unpredictable manner, especially when the intraocular pressure is less than 9 mmHg.

In a prospective study of 155 consecutive patients undergoing penetrating keratoplasty, Chien et al[85] reported intraocular pressure elevation (30 mmHg or higher) in the immediate postoperative period in 18 patients (12 percent). There was an increased risk of pressure elevation in patients with a history of glaucoma, in patients who had a vitrectomy at the time of penetrating keratoplasty, and in patients who underwent penetrating keratoplasty combined with extracapsular cataract extraction and intraocular lens implantation. Sekhar et al[86] found preexisting glaucoma, regrafting, aphakia, and pseudophakia to be significant risk factors for the development of glaucoma following penetrating keratoplasty. Kirkness and Ficker[87] found that the risk of postkeratoplasty glaucoma varied with the indication for which penetrating keratoplasty was performed. Keratoconus and the stromal dystrophies (granular, macular, and lattice) were associated with the lowest risk and the anterior chamber cleavage syndromes with the highest risk. Combined cataract or lens implant surgery was also found to be a risk factor, with anterior vitrectomy, anterior segment reconstruction, and anterior chamber intraocular lens removal representing a greater risk than extracapsular cataract extraction and posterior chamber intraocular lens implantation.

High intraocular pressure after penetrating keratoplasty does not cause epithelial edema in the early postoperative period. On the contrary, the graft tends to be thinner and clearer than normal. The elevated pressure appears to press fluid out of the graft.

In patients at increased risk for developing elevated intraocular pressure, intravenous acetazolamide (500 mg) and topical timolol drops are given at the end of the case if there are no contraindications. Postoperatively, various glaucoma medications are used as necessary to control the intraocular pressure.

Protecting the Epithelium

An epithelial defect after penetrating keratoplasty must be recognized promptly and treated aggressively if the graft is to survive. In one study of factors associated with epithelial defects after penetrating keratoplasty, only a diagnosis of diabetes in the donor and a long death-to-enucleation time were associated with an increased risk of epithelial defects.[88] In another study, the only factor that had a statistically significant association with the degree of postoperative epithelial defect was the time interval from corneal preservation to surgery.[89] In this study, the mean preservation time was 78 hours in patients with no postoperative epithelial defect, 109 hours in patients with a partial epithelial defect, and 137 hours in patients with a total epithelial defect. It is important to realize that graft failure in patients with chemical burns, pemphigoid, Stevens-Johnson syndrome, or severe dry eyes is usually caused by abnormalities of the ocular surface. In these patients, only donor corneal tissue with healthy epithelium should be used for penetrating keratoplasty.

Intraoperative protection of the epithelium includes keeping the cornea moist with balanced salt solution, covering the anterior surface with a viscoelastic substance, and avoiding contact between the surgical instruments and the epithelium. In patients with severe dry eyes, the puncta of the upper and lower eyelids may be closed with a hand-held cautery at the time of penetrating keratoplasty if they have not been closed previously.

It takes several months for the epithelium of the graft to appear morphologically normal.[90] During this time, the epithelium should be protected with an artificial tear preparation. Drops and ointments that contain no preservatives are preferred because preservatives can be toxic to the epithelium. The chronic use of aminoglycoside eye drops should be avoided. Topical nonsteroidal anti-inflammatory drugs are also toxic to the corneal epithelium after penetrating keratoplasty.[91]

In patients at risk for epithelial healing problems, it is important to treat any epithelial defect, no matter how small, as an emergency. A defect occurring in the early postoperative period will usually heal fairly promptly with patching or a bandage soft contact lens. If the defect persists for more than 1 week, it becomes subacute and heals more slowly and with more difficulty. A defect that persists for more than 2 weeks is a serious problem; if the defect persists for more than 3 weeks, there is a risk of stromal melting. For late or persistent defects, a temporary tarsorrhaphy with a suture tied in a bow knot is performed as described in Chapter 6. It is not clear why a tarsorrhaphy works better than a bandage lens in some patients, but it does. The eye is examined weekly by untying the bow knot and opening the eyelids. If the epithelium has not healed completely, the suture is retied. The tarsorrhaphy is left in place as long as re-epithelialization is progressing. An epithelial defect associated with a large tissue roll that disrupts the tear film may be resistant to the above methods of treatment. If combined interrupted and running sutures are used, the interrupted sutures adjacent to the area of the defect may be removed in an attempt to reduce the tissue roll and produce a more even tear film distribution.

Adjusting and Removing Sutures

If a running suture is placed with the intent to adjust it in the early postoperative period, topographic analysis of the cornea is done within 1 week to 1 month of surgery, and the steep and flat meridians are identified. With the patient positioned at the slit lamp microscope, the cornea is anesthetized with topical 0.5 percent proparacaine. The suture is grasped with a Tennant tying forceps at the flat meridian and tightened in both directions so it is redistributed and loosened at the previously steep meridian, as illustrated by Figure 34-52. The platforms of the tying forceps are held parallel to the suture to prevent breaking the suture. Topographic analysis is repeated and the suture is readjusted if necessary.

About the only steadfast rule for removing sutures after penetrating keratoplasty is to remove any suture that is broken, loose, or associated with blood vessels crossing the keratoplasty wound. Sutures may be removed as soon as the wound is healed, but they are frequently left in place beyond this point to control astigmatism. However, there are risks that the sutures can loosen, break, or attract vessels, which can precipitate an infection or graft rejection. The healing status of the wound is not always clear from its clinical appearance. Healing depends on the age and health of the patient and the condition of the eye. Sutures are removed as early as 2 weeks in infants but may be left in place for 1 year or longer in the elderly. Although no set times for safe suture removal apply to every patient, general guidelines are given below for adults.

If an interrupted suture technique is used, the sutures are generally selectively removed 6 months to 1 year after surgery. If a combined interrupted and running suture technique is used, the interrupted sutures are selectively removed in the steep meridian starting at 3 months postoperatively. The running suture is left in place indefinitely or removed at 1 year, depending on the refractive status of the eye and whether the suture is attracting vessels; if the running suture appears to be causing astigmatism, it is removed. If a single running suture technique is used, the suture is adjusted and left in place indefinitely or removed at 1 year. If a double running suture technique is used, the 10-0 nylon suture is removed at 3 months postoperatively and the 11-0 suture is left in place indefinitely or removed at 1 year. It should be emphasized that these suggestions are merely guidelines. There is a growing tendency among surgeons to leave sutures in place indefinitely if an acceptable refractive outcome is achieved and the sutures are not causing any problems, because corneal astigmatism can change unpredictably and by large amounts when sutures are removed even years after penetrating keratoplasty.[92]

Sutures can be removed with topical anesthesia. Interrupted sutures are removed by cutting each suture in the middle with a stainless steel blade, grasping the peripheral end with a jeweler's forceps, and yanking the suture peripherally through the recipient cornea. A quick pull is more effective and less traumatic than a slow one. If the suture cannot be removed through the recipient cornea, an attempt can be made to remove it through the donor cornea, but this risks elevating the edge of the graft if the keratoplasty wound is not healed. Sometimes the suture ends break and the suture must be left buried in the cornea.

If interrupted sutures are combined with a running suture, the interrupted sutures can be removed selectively postoperatively in an attempt to decrease astigmatism, with the running suture left to stabilize the wound. Care is taken not to cut the running suture; the blade is held

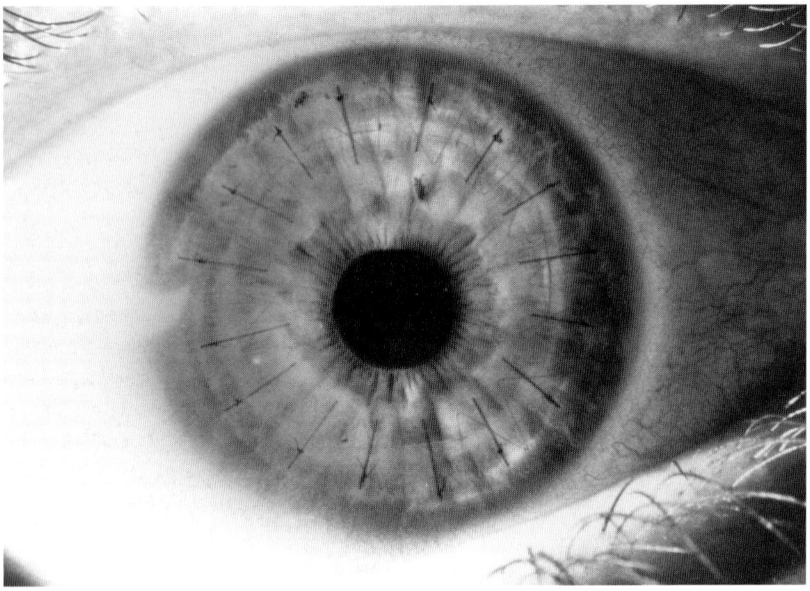

A

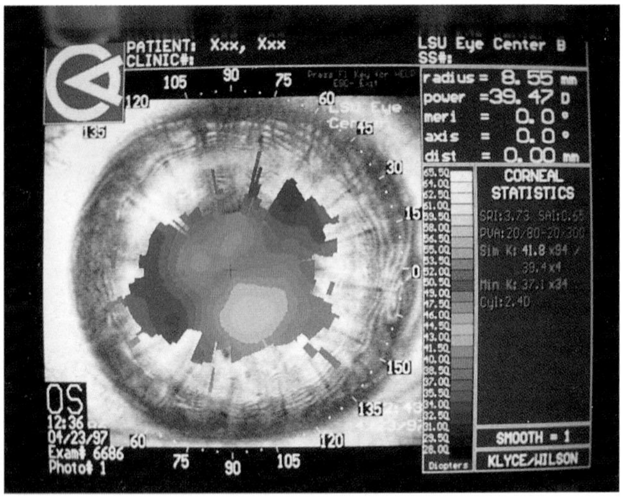

B

FIGURE 34-53 **(A)** Clear corneal graft in a patient with recurrent herpes simplex keratitis that resulted in a descemetocele. A combined interrupted 10-0 nylon and running 11-0 nylon suture technique was used. Visual acuity without correction was 20/40. With a refraction of $-0.75 + 1.75 \times 110$, visual acuity was 20/25. **(B)** Videokeratograph of the cornea demonstrates 2.4 diopters of asymmetrical astigmatism.

parallel to the anterior loop of the adjacent running suture, and the interrupted suture is cut in a direction such that if the eye moves or the blade slips, the running suture will not be cut.

A running suture is removed by cutting every other loop with a stainless steel blade, grasping each piece between the cuts with a jeweler's forceps, and pulling the pieces out of the cornea.

It is not uncommon to create small epithelial defects while removing sutures. A topical antibiotic is given four times a day for several days in an attempt to prevent infection. In addition, topical corticosteroids are increased for a week or two in an attempt to stave off a graft rejection.

RESULTS

The goal of penetrating keratoplasty is to obtain a clear graft through which the patient can see well (Figure 34-53). In the past, penetrating keratoplasty was considered successful if the graft survived and remained clear; any other accomplishments were considered as lagniappe. Today, in the era of refractive surgery, a clear graft in an eye that is emmetropic postoperatively defines the ultimate goal of penetrating keratoplasty. This is not to say that a clear graft is easily obtainable in all patients; that goal is still a challenge in patients with chemical burns, pemphigoid, Stevens-Johnson syndrome, or severe dry eyes.

Graft failure is usually classified as primary or secondary. Primary graft failure occurs when dysfunction of the donor corneal endothelium leads to persistent corneal edema after penetrating keratoplasty. Causes are related to the status of the donor cornea and include pre-existing abnormalities; damage during retrieval, processing, and storage; and surgical trauma. The incidence of primary graft failure is thought to be approximately 1 percent, although incidences of 0 to 10 percent have been reported.[93] In a retrospective case-control study, Wilhelmus et al[93] found no clearly defined donor tissue or eye bank procedural factor that accounted for most cases of primary graft failure, although advanced donor age and prolonged corneal preservation may increase the risk.

Secondary graft failure is defined as failure occurring 2 weeks or more after penetrating keratoplasty in a graft that was initially clear. Secondary graft failure occurs in less than 10 percent of all cases of penetrating keratoplasty.[4] Price et al[4] found endothelial decompensation as a result of immunologic graft rejection the most common cause of secondary graft failure (27 percent), but ocular surface disorders caused nearly as many failures (25 percent). Graft failures from ocular surface disorders tended to occur earlier than those from endothelial decompensation. Secondary graft failure is associated with patient-related factors such as history of previous graft failure; immunologic graft rejection; deep stromal vascularization; ocular surface disorders; coexistent ocular diseases, such as glaucoma; and concomitant intraocular procedures.[4,16,22,94] The disorder for which penetrating keratoplasty is performed is of prognostic value, mainly because of the concomitant patient-related risk factors described above. Grafts for keratoconus, stromal dystrophies, and central Fuchs' dystrophy have the best prognosis; those for chemical burns, pemphigoid, Stevens-Johnson syndrome, and severe dry eyes have the worst prognosis.[4,22,95–97]

The complications of penetrating keratoplasty, including immunologic graft rejection, are discussed in Chapter 35.

REFERENCES

1. Eye Bank Association of America: 1996 Eye Banking Statistical Report. Eye Bank Association of America, Washington, DC, 1996
2. United Network for Organ Sharing: 1996 Annual Report. United Network for Organ Sharing, Richmond, VA, 1996
3. Zirm E: Eine erfolgreiche totale Keratoplastik. Archiv für Ophthalmol 64:580, 1906
4. Price FW Jr, Whitson WE, Collins KS, Marks RG: Five-year corneal graft survival. A large, single-center patient cohort. Arch Ophthalmol 111:799, 1993
5. Albert DM: Corneal surgery. p. 225. In Albert DM, Edwards DD (eds): The History of Ophthalmology. Blackwell Science, Cambridge, 1996
6. Mannis MJ, Krachmer JH: Keratoplasty: a historical perspective. Surv Ophthalmol 25:333, 1981
7. Forstot L, Kaufman HE: Corneal transplantation. Annu Rev Med 28:21, 1977
8. Duke-Elder S, Leigh AG: Diseases of the outer eye. p. 648. In Duke-Elder S (ed): System of Ophthalmology. Vol. III, Part 2. CV Mosby, St. Louis, 1965
9. Altman AJ, Albert DM, Fournier GA: Cocaine's use in ophthalmology: our 100-year heritage. Surv Ophthalmol 29:300, 1985
10. Hyman L, Wittpenn J, Yang C: Indications and techniques of penetrating keratoplasties, 1985-1988. Cornea 11:573, 1992
11. Mamalis N, Anderson CW, Kreisler KR, et al: Changing trends in the indications for penetrating keratoplasty. Arch Ophthalmol 110:1409, 1992
12. The Australian Corneal Graft Registry: 1990 to 1992 report. Aust N Z J Ophthalmol 21(2 suppl):1, 1993
13. Sharif KW, Casey TA: Changing indications for penetrating keratoplasty, 1971–1990. Eye 7:485, 1993
14. Haamann P, Jensen OM, Schmidt P: Changing indications for penetrating keratoplasty. Acta Ophthalmol (Copenh) 72:443, 1994
15. Flowers CW, Chanq KY, McLeod SD, et al: Changing indications for penetrating keratoplasty, 1989–1993. Cornea 14:583, 1995
16. Price FW Jr, Whitson WE, Johns S, Gonzales JS: Risk factors for corneal graft failure. J Refract Surg 12:134, 1996
17. Kirkness CM, Steele AD, Ficker LA, Rice NS: Coexistent corneal disease and glaucoma managed by either drainage surgery and subsequent keratoplasty or combined drainage surgery and penetrating keratoplasty. Br J Ophthalmol 76:146, 1992
18. Martin TP, Reed JW, Legault C, et al: Cataract formation and cataract extraction after penetrating keratoplasty. Ophthalmology 101:113, 1994
19. Pineros OE, Cohen EJ, Rapuano CJ, Laibson PR: Triple vs nonsimultaneous procedures in Fuchs' dystrophy and cataract. Arch Ophthalmol 114:525, 1996
20. Flowers CW, McLeod SD, McDonnell PJ, et al: Evaluation of intraocular lens power calculation formulas in the triple procedure. J Cataract Refract Surg 22:116, 1996
21. Hill JC: The relative importance of risk factors used to define high-risk keratoplasty. Ger J Ophthalmol 5:36, 1996
22. Williams KA, Roder D, Esterman A, et al: Factors predictive of corneal graft survival. Report from the Australian Corneal Graft Registry. Ophthalmology 99:403, 1992
23. Killingsworth DW, Stern GA, Driebe WT, et al: Results of therapeutic penetrating keratoplasty. Ophthalmology 100:534, 1993
24. Barney NP, Foster CS: A prospective randomized trial of oral acyclovir after penetrating keratoplasty for herpes simplex keratitis. Cornea 13:232, 1994
25. van Rooij J, Rijneveld WJ, Remeijer LJ, Beekhuis WH: A retrospective study on the effectiveness of oral acyclovir to prevent herpes simplex recurrence in corneal grafts. Eur J Ophthalmol 5:214, 1995
26. Simon AL, Pavan-Langston D: Long-term oral acyclovir therapy. Effect on recurrent infectious herpes simplex keratitis in patients with and without grafts. Ophthalmology 103:1399, 1996
27. McNeill JI, Goldman KN, Kaufman HE: Combined scleral ring and blepharostat. Am J Ophthalmol 83:592, 1977
28. Olson RJ: The effect of scleral fixation ring placement and trephine tilting on keratoplasty wound size and donor shape. Ophthalmic Surg 12:23, 1981.
29. Sugiura T, Inamochi K, Soya K, Miyata K: Corneal distortion induced by speculum: studies with computer-assisted corneal topography. Nippon Ganka Gakkai Zasshi 100:520, 1996
30. Olson RJ: Corneal transplantation techniques. p. 743. In Kaufman HE, Barron BA, McDonald MB, Waltman SR (eds): The Cornea. Churchill Livingstone, New York, 1988

31. Uozato H, Guyton DL: Centering corneal surgical procedures. Am J Ophthalmol 103:264, 1987
32. van Rij G, Cornell M, Waring GO, et al: Postoperative astigmatism after central vs eccentric penetrating keratoplasties. Am J Ophthalmol 99:317, 1985
33. Kaufman HE: Astigmatism after keratoplasty—possible cause and method of prevention. Am J Ophthalmol 94:556, 1982
34. Ng JD, Nekola M, Parmley VC, et al: Comparison of three corneal trephines for use in therapeutic penetrating keratoplasties for large corneal perforations. Ophthalmic Surg 26:209, 1995
35. Price FW Jr, Hanna SI: Bilateral penetrating autokeratoplasty. J Refract Surg 11:494, 1995
36. Chen JQ: Refractive evaluation of donor corneas from the newborn in aphakic penetrating keratoplasty. Chung Hua Yen Ko Tsa Chih 29:224, 1993
37. Goble RR, Hardman Lea SJ, Falcon MG: The use of the same size host and donor trephine in penetrating keratoplasty for keratoconus. Eye 8:311, 1994
38. Spadea L, Bianco G, Mastrofini MC, Balestrazzi E: Penetrating keratoplasty with donor and recipient corneas of the same diameter. Ophthalmic Surg Lasers 27:425, 1996
39. Girard LJ, Esnaola N, Rao R, et al: Use of grafts smaller than the opening for keratoconic myopia and astigmatism. J Cataract Refract Surg 18:380, 1992
40. Olson RJ, Kaufman HE: A mathematical description of causative factors and prevention of elevated intraocular pressure after keratoplasty. Invest Ophthalmol Vis Sci 16:1085, 1977
41. Zimmerman T, Krupin T, Grodzki W: Size of donor corneal button and outflow facility in aphakic eyes. Ann Ophthalmol 11:809, 1979
42. Zimmerman T, Olson RJ, Waltman SR, et al: Transplant size and elevated intraocular pressure postkeratoplasty. Arch Ophthalmol 96:2231, 1978
43. Bourne W, Davison J, O'Fallon W: The effects of oversize donor buttons on postoperative intraocular pressure and corneal curvature in aphakic penetrating keratoplasty. Ophthalmology 89:242, 1982
44. Brown SI, Dohlman CH, Boruchoff SA: Dislocation of Descemet's membrane during keratoplasty. Am J Ophthalmol 60:43, 1965
45. Malbran ES, Malbran E, Buonsanti J, Adrogue E: Closed-system phacoemulsification and posterior chamber implant combined with penetrating keratoplasty. Ophthalmic Surg 24:403, 1993
46. Chu MW, Font RL, Koch DD: Visual results and complications following posterior iris-fixated posterior chamber lenses at penetrating keratoplasty. Ophthalmic Surg 23:608, 1992
47. Agrawal V, Vagh MM, Sangwan V, Rao GN: Penetrating keratoplasty for pseudophakic bullous keratopathy. Indian J Ophthalmol 42:75, 1994
48. Kwartz J, Leatherbarrow B, Dyer P, et al: Penetrating keratoplasty for pseudophakic corneal oedema. Br J Ophthalmol 79:435, 1995
49. Apple DJ, Kincaid MC, Mamalis N, Olson RJ: Intraocular Lenses: Evolution, Designs, Complications, and Pathology. Williams & Wilkins, Baltimore, 1989
50. Davis RM, Best D, Gilbert GE: Comparison of intraocular lens fixation techniques performed during penetrating keratoplasty. Am J Ophthalmol 111:743, 1991
51. Hill JC: Transsclerally-fixated posterior chamber intraocular implants without capsular support in penetrating keratoplasty. Ophthalmic Surg 23:320, 1992
52. Heidemann DG, Dunn SP: Transsclerally sutured intraocular lenses in penetrating keratoplasty. Am J Ophthalmol 113:619, 1992
53. Holland EJ, Daya SM, Evangelista A, et al: Penetrating keratoplasty and transscleral fixation of posterior chamber lens. Am J Ophthalmol 114:182, 1992
54. Althaus C, Sundmacher R: Transscleral suture fixation of posterior chamber intraocular lenses through the ciliary sulcus: endoscopic comparison of different suture techniques. Ger J Ophthalmol 1:117, 1992
55. Hardten DR, Holland EJ, Doughman DJ, et al: Clinical and anatomical study of the effect of transscleral fixation of posterior chamber lenses on early postkeratoplasty astigmatism. Cornea 12:282, 1993
56. Schein OD, Kenyon KR, Steinert RF, et al: A randomized trial of intraocular lens fixation techniques with penetrating keratoplasty. Ophthalmology 100:1437, 1993
57. Rijneveld WJ, Beekhuis WH, Hassman EF, et al: Iris claw lens: anterior and posterior iris surface fixation in the absence of capsular support during penetrating keratoplasty. J Refract Corneal Surg 10:14, 1994
58. Koenig SB, Apple DJ, Hyndiuk RA: Penetrating keratoplasty and intraocular lens exchange: open-loop anterior chamber lenses versus sutured posterior chamber lenses. Cornea 13:418, 1994
59. Brunette I, Stulting RD, Rinne JR, et al: Penetrating keratoplasty with anterior or posterior chamber intraocular lens implantation. Arch Ophthalmol 112:1311, 1994
60. Price FW Jr, Wellemeyer M: Transscleral fixation of posterior chamber intraocular lenses. J Cataract Refract Surg 21:567, 1995
61. Kandarakis AS, Doulas KG, Amariotakis AG: Penetrating keratoplasty and transsclerally suture-fixated intraocular lenses. J Refract Surg 12(suppl):S304, 1996
62. Bellucci R, Pucci V, Morselli S, Bonomi L: Secondary implantation of angle-supported anterior chamber and scleral-fixated posterior chamber intraocular lenses. J Cataract Refract Surg 22:247, 1996
63. Ohlrich S, Hirst LW, Harrison M, et al: Inadvertent corneal button inversion during penetrating keratoplasty. Cornea 11:586, 1992
64. Frueh BE, Feldman ST, Feldman RM, et al: Running nylon suture dissolution after penetrating keratoplasty. Am J Ophthalmol 113:406, 1992
65. Frueh BE, Brown SI, Feldman ST: 11-0 Mersilene as running suture for penetrating keratoplasty. Am J Ophthalmol 114:675, 1992
66. Ramselaar JA, Beekhuis WH, Rijneveld WJ, et al: Mersi-

lene (polyester), a new suture for penetrating keratoplasty. Doc Ophthalmol 82:89, 1992
67. Frucht-Pery J: Mersilene sutures for corneal surgery. Ophthalmic Surg 26:117, 1995
68. Bertram BA, Drews-Botsch C, Gemmill M, et al: Complications of Mersilene sutures in penetrating keratoplasty. Refract Corneal Surg 8:296, 1992
69. McNeill JI, Kaufman HE: A double running suture technique for keratoplasty: earlier visual rehabilitation. Ophthalmic Surg 8:58, 1977
70. McNeill JI, Wessels IF: Adjustment of single continuous suture to control astigmatism after penetrating keratoplasty. Refract Corneal Surg 5:216, 1989
71. Lin DTC, Wilson SE, Reidy JJ: An adjustable single running suture technique to reduce postkeratoplasty astigmatism. A preliminary report. Ophthalmology 97:934, 1990
72. Assil KK, Zarnegar SR, Schanzlin DJ: Visual outcome after penetrating keratoplasty with double continuous or combined interrupted and continuous suture wound closure. Am J Ophthalmol 114:63, 1992
73. Hope-Ross MW, McDonnell PJ, Corridan PG, et al: The management of post-keratoplasty astigmatism by postoperative adjustment of a single continuous suture. Eye 7:625, 1993
74. Filatov V, Steinert RF, Talamo JH: Postkeratoplasty astigmatism with single running suture or interrupted sutures. Am J Ophthalmol 115:715, 1993
75. Clinch TE, Thompson HW, Gardner BP, et al: An adjustable double running suture technique for keratoplasty. Am J Ophthalmol 116:201, 1993
76. Murta JN, Amaro L, Tavares C, Mira JB: Astigmatism after penetrating keratoplasty. Role of the suture technique. Doc Ophthalmol 87:331, 1994
77. Høvding G: Suture adjustment in penetrating keratoplasty. Acta Ophthalmol (Copenh) 72:246, 1994
78. Serdarevic ON, Renard GJ, Pouliquen Y: Randomized clinical trial comparing astigmatism and visual rehabilitation after penetrating keratoplasty with and without intraoperative suture adjustment. Ophthalmology 101:990, 1994
79. Filatov V, Alexandrakis G, Talamo JH, Steinert RF: Comparison of suture-in and suture-out postkeratoplasty astigmatism with single running suture or combined running and interrupted sutures. Am J Ophthalmol 122:696, 1996
80. Chell PB, Hope-Ross MW, Shah P, McDonnell PJ: Long-term follow-up of a single continuous adjustable suture in penetrating keratoplasty. Eye 10:133, 1996
81. Moyes AL, Sugar A, Musch DC, Barnes RD: Antiviral therapy after penetrating keratoplasty for herpes simplex keratitis. Arch Ophthalmol 112:601, 1994
82. Urrets-Zavalia A: Fixed, dilated pupil, iris atrophy, and secondary glaucoma. A distinct clinical entity following penetrating keratoplasty in keratoconus. Am J Ophthalmol 56:257, 1963
83. Menage MJ, Kaufman PL, Croft MA, Landay SP: Intraocular pressure measurement after penetrating keratoplasty: minified Goldmann applanation tonometer, pneumatonometer, and Tono-Pen versus manometry. Br J Ophthalmol 78:671, 1994
84. Geyer O, Mayron Y, Loewenstein A, et al: Tono-Pen tonometry in normal and in post-keratoplasty eyes. Br J Ophthalmol 76:538, 1992
85. Chien AM, Schmidt CM, Cohen EJ, et al: Glaucoma in the immediate postoperative period after penetrating keratoplasty. Am J Ophthalmol 115:711, 1993
86. Sekhar GC, Vyas P, Nagarajan R, et al: Post-penetrating keratoplasty glaucoma. Indian J Ophthalmol 41:181, 1993
87. Kirkness CM, Ficker LA: Risk factors for the development of postkeratoplasty glaucoma. Cornea 11:427, 1992
88. Chou L, Cohen EJ, Laibson PR, Rapuano CJ: Factors associated with epithelial defects after penetrating keratoplasty. Ophthalmic Surg 25:700, 1994
89. Kim T, Palay DA, Lynn M: Donor factors associated with epithelial defects after penetrating keratoplasty. Cornea 15:451, 1996
90. Tsubota K, Mashima Y, Murata H, et al: Corneal epithelium following penetrating keratoplasty. Br J Ophthalmol 79:257, 1995
91. Shimazaki J, Saito H, Yang HY, et al: Persistent epithelial defect following penetrating keratoplasty: an adverse effect of diclofenac eyedrops. Cornea 14:623, 1995
92. Mader TH, Yuan R, Lynn MJ, et al: Changes in keratometric astigmatism after suture removal more than one year after penetrating keratoplasty. Ophthalmology 100:119, 1993
93. Wilhelmus KR, Stulting RD, Sugar J, et al: Primary corneal graft failure. A national reporting system. Medical Advisory Board of the Eye Bank Association of America. Arch Ophthalmol 113:1497, 1995
94. Bradley BA, Vail A, Gore SM, et al: Penetrating keratoplasty in the United Kingdom: an interim analysis of the corneal transplant follow-up study. Clin Transpl p. 293, 1993
95. Pineros O, Cohen EJ, Rapuano CJ, Laibson PR: Long-term results after penetrating keratoplasty for Fuchs' endothelial dystrophy. Arch Ophthalmol 114:15, 1996
96. Tugal-Tutkun I, Akova YA, Foster CS: Penetrating keratoplasty in cicatrizing conjunctival diseases. Ophthalmology 102:576, 1995
97. Buxton JN, Buxton DF, Westphalen JA: Penetrating keratoplasty. Indications and contraindications. In Brightbill FS (ed): Corneal Surgery: Theory, Technique, and Tissue. 2nd ed. CV Mosby, St. Louis, 1993

35

Complications of Penetrating Keratoplasty

MICHAEL J. HODKIN

Despite significant advances in corneal preservation, surgical techniques, and postoperative care, a myriad of potential complications threatens the success of penetrating keratoplasty. These complications may occur intraoperatively, within several weeks postoperatively, or months to years later. As important as mastering the techniques for performing penetrating keratoplasty is the ability to recognize and treat these complications.

INTRAOPERATIVE COMPLICATIONS

Suprachoroidal Hemorrhage

Suprachoroidal hemorrhage, the rupture of a choroidal blood vessel with uncontrolled bleeding into the suprachoroidal space, is one of the most dreaded complications of penetrating keratoplasty. The result may be expulsion of the intraocular contents through the recipient corneal opening (Figure 35-1). Although this complication is rare, the incidence in penetrating keratoplasty is higher than for other intraocular procedures and may be as high as 1 percent.[1,2]

The mechanism of suprachoroidal hemorrhage during penetrating keratoplasty is unknown but may be related to sudden and prolonged decompression of the globe, resulting in an increased transmural pressure gradient in the affected choroidal blood vessel or traction on the vitreous or on fragile blood vessels. Risk factors include glaucoma, previous ocular surgery, trauma, inflammation, hypertension, tachycardia, high myopia, and intraoperative Valsalva maneuver. Elevated episcleral venous pressure created by the retrobulbar injection of an excessive amount of anesthetic may also increase the risk.[1] Price et al[2] found a higher incidence of suprachoroidal hemorrhage in eyes with anterior chamber intraocular lenses.

The initial signs of a suprachoroidal hemorrhage include increased posterior pressure, bulging of vitreous anteriorly, and/or direct observation of a developing choroidal detachment. Emergent treatment is occlusion of the recipient corneal opening, with a finger if necessary, to seal the eye and provide a tamponade. A temporary keratoprosthesis can also be used to plug the opening but is usually not available quickly enough to be of any use. One or more stab incisions (sclerotomies) are made into the suprachoroidal space with a stainless steel blade to drain the hemorrhage. The incisions should be T-shaped for adequate drainage because linear incisions are likely to self-seal if not held open. The donor corneal button is sutured in place as rapidly as possible with a strong suture such as 8-0 nylon. A suprachoroidal hemorrhage does not necessarily doom the eye if it is recognized promptly and treated appropriately.[2] The visual prognosis is relatively good if the hemorrhage is limited and the retina does not detach.[3] The prognosis is poor if the hemorrhage is extensive and there is a retinal detachment.

Preventive measures include lowering intraocular pressure preoperatively with a hyperosmotic agent and external massage, controlling blood pressure and heart rate, preventing a Valsalva maneuver (including bucking under general anesthesia), and keeping the patient's head elevated above the level of the chest.[1,4]

EARLY POSTOPERATIVE COMPLICATIONS

Epithelial Defect

The barrier function of an intact corneal epithelium is critical to the survival of a corneal graft.[5] Epithelial growth merits careful monitoring, because persistent epithelial defects can lead to infectious ulceration, stromal melting,

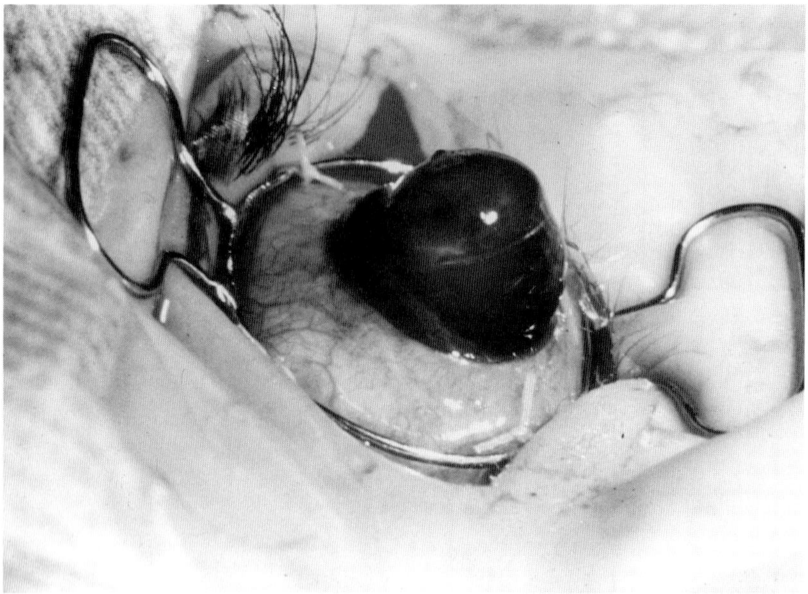

FIGURE 35-1 Extrusion of the lens and vitreous through a penetrating keratoplasty opening.

perforation, and graft failure[6] (Figure 35-2). The time to complete epithelialization of a corneal graft is usually 4 to 6 days[7] but may be as long as 12 days.[8]

Preoperatively, it is important to ensure that the eyelids adequately cover and protect the cornea. Significant entropion, ectropion, lagophthalmos, or other eyelid dysfunction that causes corneal exposure should be corrected before penetrating keratoplasty. A marginally dry eye may be improved by thermal punctal occlusion, which may be performed at the time of penetrating keratoplasty.

Intraoperatively, donor corneal epithelial loss can be prevented by keeping the cornea moist with balanced salt solution; excessive irrigation should be avoided, however. A viscoelastic substance may be placed on the graft to provide a barrier to desiccation and trauma.

Some surgeons routinely remove the donor corneal epithelium in an attempt to decrease the rate of graft rejection. Removal of this antigenic cell layer may be effective in decreasing the rate of epithelial rejection; however, it may create the problem of a persistent epithelial defect in an otherwise uncomplicated case. Although recipient lim-

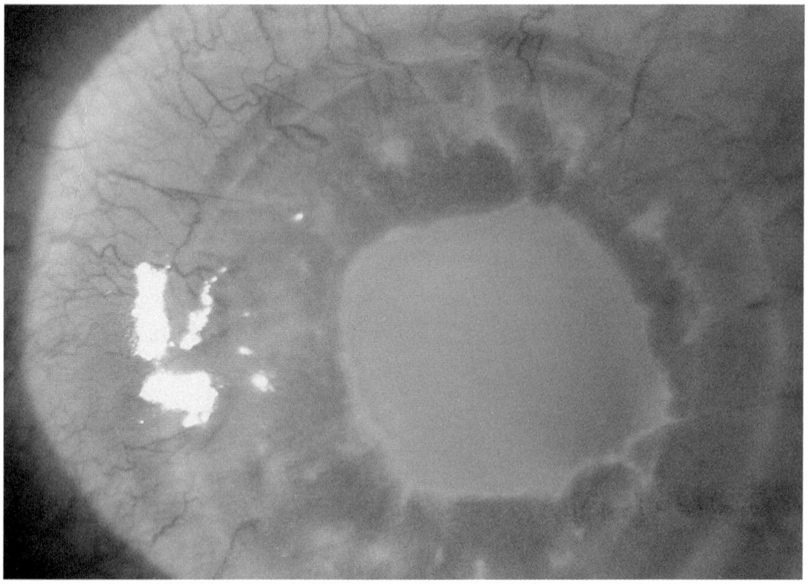

FIGURE 35-2 Persistent epithelial defect after penetrating keratoplasty caused by dry eyes.

bal epithelium eventually divides and migrates to replace donor corneal epithelium, a graft that is lacking most or all of the epithelium may have delayed epithelialization postoperatively.[8] This is especially true in eyes with compromised healing ability, as occurs with ocular pemphigoid, Stevens-Johnson syndrome, chemical or radiation burns, dry eyes, rosacea keratitis, and even chronic blepharitis. Because the likelihood of donor corneal epithelial loss increases with storage time, it is critical to use fresh donor tissue in these high risk cases.[9] In these cases, a bandage soft contact lens may be placed at the end of surgery to help protect the epithelium. Some surgeons advocate performing a temporary tarsorrhaphy at the end of surgery in such cases.

Dellen can cause postoperative epithelial and stromal ulceration. They develop as a result of localized dry spots from uneven tear wetting caused by a nearby anatomic irregularity. A large tissue roll from tight sutures or an ectatic wound from misalignment of the donor and recipient corneas or from dehiscence of the wound following premature suture removal is usually the cause. If lubrication with a bland ointment and placement of a bandage soft contact lens fail to promote healing, surgical correction to smooth the irregularity is indicated.

Reactivated latent herpes simplex virus, even in a patient with no prior history of herpetic eye disease, can cause a chronic epithelial defect after penetrating keratoplasty.[10,11] Because of false-negatives, multiple cultures may be necessary to confirm the diagnosis.[12]

An antibiotic-soaked collagen shield may be placed on the cornea at the end of surgery, followed by an eye patch and shield.[13,14] Although somewhat counterintuitive, it has been shown in a prospective study that patching beyond the usual 24-hour postoperative period does not shorten epithelial healing time.[15] After removal of the eye patch, topical antibiotics are started as prophylaxis against infection. Erythromycin ointment is probably the antibiotic least toxic to growing epithelium and is, therefore, a good choice. Most topical medications, especially trifluridine, aminoglycosides, and nonsteroidal anti-inflammatory drugs, impede epithelial healing to some degree. Therefore, the benefit of a topical medicine should be weighed against its possible adverse effect on epithelial healing. Patients with dry eyes or other ocular surface disorders are most susceptible to poor healing. Systemic medications should be substituted in these cases, if possible.

If epithelialization is not complete by 1 week postoperatively, a bandage soft contact lens is placed. The lens presumably promotes healing by protecting the migrating epithelial cells from mechanical abrasion by the eyelids. Because of the reported increased risk of infectious keratitis from prolonged bandage soft contact lens wear,[16] concurrent topical antibiotic coverage is recommended. Frequent application of unpreserved artificial tears or punctal occlusion should also be considered if there is any evidence of tear deficiency. If by the second postoperative week healing is still not complete, a temporary tarsorrhaphy is performed as described in Chapter 6.[17] The tarsorrhaphy is opened and the graft is examined weekly until epithelial healing is complete. Other potential therapies, such as topical application of epidermal growth factor[7,18] or fibronectin,[19] have not been shown to be effective. Keratoepithelioplasty[20] may be useful in unilateral ocular surface disorders, such as burns, in which an autograft can be obtained from the uninvolved fellow eye. The procedure is less useful in bilateral ocular surface disorders because of the requirement for an allograft, which is at risk for rejection (see Ch. 28).

Infection

Keratitis

Although the majority of graft infections occur 6 months or more after penetrating keratoplasty, some may occur much sooner. The usual signs include a corneal infiltrate with an overlying epithelial defect in an inflamed eye. A reactive hypopyon may also be present. The routine methods for diagnosis and treatment should be followed as described in the chapters on infectious keratitis and in the section below on late and recurrent graft infections.

Endophthalmitis

Endophthalmitis is rare after penetrating keratoplasty, with a reported incidence of 0.10 to 0.70 percent.[21] A nationwide survey of 40,351 Medicare beneficiaries admitted to United States hospitals for penetrating keratoplasty between 1984 and 1987 showed a 0.77 percent rehospitalization rate for endophthalmitis within 6 months of surgery, which was five times higher than the rate after cataract surgery.[22] Penetrating keratoplasty with concomitant anterior vitrectomy increased the risk to 1.03 percent. Risk factors for endophthalmitis include aphakia, which facilitates the spread of organisms into the vitreous cavity,[23,24] as well as previous inflammation, surgery, or corticosteroid use.[23]

A recent review noted that at least 59 cases of endophthalmitis immediately after penetrating keratoplasty have been reported in the literature.[21] Of these, 44 were caused by bacteria, 12 were caused by fungi, and 3 were of undetermined cause. Of 46 donor rim cultures performed in these cases, 33 of 34 positive cultures isolated an organism of the same genus and species as the organism that caused the endophthalmitis. Of 15 reported sensitivities, 13 indicated resistance of the organism to gentamicin,

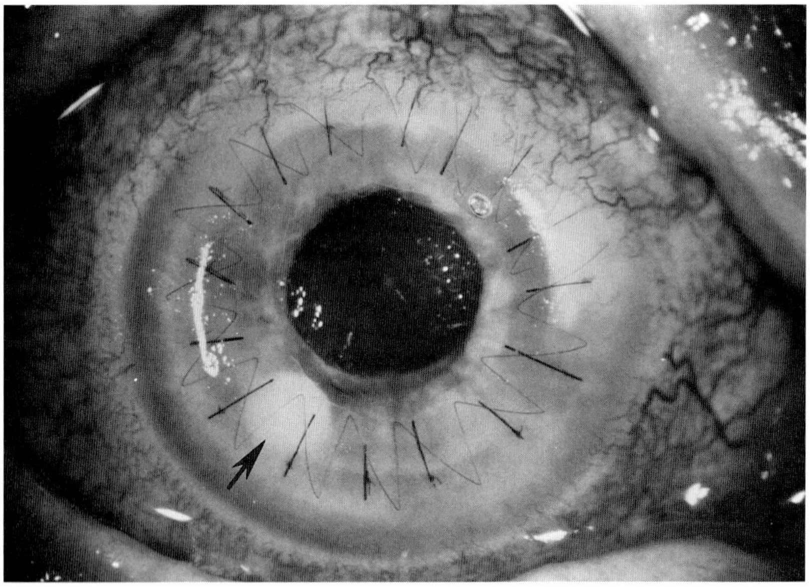

FIGURE 35-3 Intracameral *Candida* abscess after penetrating keratoplasty for herpes zoster keratitis. Cultures of the donor corneal rim grew *Candida*.

which had been present in the corneal storage medium. Resistant organisms included mostly streptococcal and staphylococcal species; however, resistant *Klebsiella pneumoniae, Pseudomonas aeruginosa, Enterococcus faecalis,* and *Flavobacterium meningosepticum* were also isolated. The most commonly reported fungal organisms were *Candida albicans* and *Torulopsis glabrata,* but cases of *Aspergillus flavus, Cryptococcus neoformans,* and *Cephalosporium* were noted as well (Figure 35-3).

To help prevent bacterial infections caused by organisms resistant to gentamicin, the addition of antibiotics with a spectrum of activity broader than that of gentamicin, such as vancomycin[25,26] or streptomycin,[27] to corneal storage media has been advocated; a formulation of Optisol containing both gentamicin and streptomycin (Optisol GS) has been available commercially since 1992 (see Ch. 33). The prophylactic effect of antibiotics in corneal storage media may result in part from their leaching out of the corneal stroma into the anterior chamber for several hours after penetrating keratoplasty.[25] In addition, because antibiotics kill bacteria most effectively during their growth phase at room temperature, removal of the donor tissue from the refrigerator at least 1 hour before surgery is advised.[21,22,28] Some recommend culturing all donor rims to identify patients at risk for developing endophthalmitis[21]; however, the cost-effectiveness of this practice is questionable because rates of positive donor rim cultures are much higher (12 to 39 percent) than the incidence of endophthalmitis (1 percent or less).[29]

Aside from contaminated donor tissue, other possible sources of infectious organisms are the eyelids and conjunctiva. The instillation of topical 5 percent povidone-iodine solution into the cul-de-sac preoperatively may reduce the incidence of endophthalmitis caused by external ocular flora.[30]

The classic symptoms of endophthalmitis, such as pain, decreased visual acuity, chemosis, and hyperemia, may be camouflaged by the background postoperative inflammation.[23] It is therefore critical to examine patients within 1 day of surgery and again within 1 week to assess for more objective signs, such as a graft infiltrate, hypopyon, or vitreous clouding. If endophthalmitis is suspected, the usual diagnostic and therapeutic measures are performed, including immediate tap of the anterior chamber and vitreous cavity and intravitreal injection of antibiotics. Referral to a retinal specialist for a vitrectomy may be indicated.

Wound Leak

An anterior chamber that is deep at the conclusion of penetrating keratoplasty but is shallow or flat on the first postoperative day usually signifies a wound leak. A shallow anterior chamber can also be caused by leaking suture tracts from full-thickness sutures or by cheesewiring of sutures through thin or necrotic tissue. A flat anterior chamber is particularly alarming because contact between the endothelium of the graft and the iris, natural lens, intraocular lens, or vitreous results in endothelial cell damage. The intraocular pressure is usually low, but may be normal or even high. Testing of the wound with topical fluorescein (Seidel's test) usually reveals the site of the leak. This test may be negative, however, if iris is incarcerated in the wound at the site of the leak and acts as a plug or if the anterior chamber is so shallow that there is little aqueous humor left to exit through the leak.

The most likely cause of a wound leak is a broken, loose, or misplaced suture. Occasionally, a suture knot may unravel, which is more common when the suture is not squarely tied, the ends of the suture are trimmed too close to the knot, or the knot is not buried in the cornea. A loose suture may result in a wound that leaks only when the intraocular pressure increases, such as during a Valsalva maneuver. Loose sutures tend to collect mucus and other tear film debris, which is a helpful identifying sign during examination.

A wound leak brisk enough to cause a flat anterior chamber requires immediate resuturing of the wound. Other therapies, such as application of a bandage soft contact lens, may be tried initially in cases in which the leak is slow and the anterior chamber is formed. These therapies are rarely effective, however, and require frequent follow-up that is usually more bothersome for the patient than resuturing of the wound.

Resuturing of a penetrating keratoplasty wound can be done under topical anesthesia. The patient is more comfortable if the eye is not fixated with a forceps. The manner in which the wound is resutured depends on the pattern of sutures used at the time of penetrating keratoplasty. If interrupted sutures were used, additional interrupted sutures are placed in the area of the leak. If a running suture was used, the tension in the suture may be redistributed by tightening the suture in the area of the leak and loosening the suture in other areas. If this maneuver does not close the leak, or closes the leak but creates a leak in another area, the suture may be broken at the knot and unraveled from the wound on both sides until the ends are long enough to splice and tie to another suture. The spliced suture is placed in a running fashion and tied to the original suture after the entire suture has been tightened. Alternatively, interrupted sutures may be placed around the entire circumference of the wound. If interrupted sutures are placed only in the area of the leak, the running suture can loosen in another area and cause a leak there.

Leaks caused by full-thickness sutures usually close spontaneously within the first postoperative week. Leaks caused by cheesewiring of sutures through thin or necrotic tissue are difficult to repair with additional sutures. In these cases, tissue adhesive may be used to seal the leaks, followed by application of a bandage soft contact lens.

Iris Incarceration

Iris incarceration in a penetrating keratoplasty wound is secondary to either a wound leak or a misplaced suture. Incarcerated iris should be freed because it can serve as a focus for chronic inflammation, graft rejection, or closure of the anterior chamber angle.[31,32] If the incarceration is minimal and is associated with a wound leak, sealing of the leak may be curative. Miotic or mydriatic agents rarely free incarcerated iris. Argon laser iridoplasty can be performed in an attempt to release the iris without having to enter the eye. If these measures fail, a viscoelastic substance is injected into the anterior chamber and the iris is swept out of the wound with an iris or cyclodialysis spatula introduced through another area of the wound or through a separate limbal incision. It is often easiest to insert the spatula between the iris root and the incarceration and gently press posteriorly and sweep centrally. The risk of causing an iridodialysis is small. The viscoelastic substance is useful in keeping the iris away from the wound after it has been reposited, but can caused elevated intraocular pressure. If the iris cannot be swept out of the wound, it may have been impaled by the suture in that area, in which case the suture must be removed and replaced. Prolapsed iris can usually be reposited after any epithelium that has grown over the surface is removed. Rarely, necrotic iris may have to be excised, but if possible, a round pupil should be maintained.

Hyphema

Hyphemas seen on the first postoperative day are not uncommon in patients in whom the recipient cornea is heavily vascularized and in patients in whom there has been significant intraoperative manipulation of the iris, such as lysis of peripheral anterior synechiae, iridoplasty, or removal of a closed-loop anterior chamber intraocular lens.

Therapy involves treating any associated intraocular pressure elevation with glaucoma medications and suppressing intraocular inflammation with topical corticosteroids. Corticosteroids also help prevent the formation of synechiae between the iris and the cornea at the site of the organizing clot. If the hyphema is small, resorption usually occurs without surgical intervention. If the hyphema is large, especially if it fills the entire anterior chamber, lavage may be necessary if no improvement occurs within several days. Rarely, it may be necessary to evacuate an organized clot by opening the penetrating keratoplasty wound. The use of thrombolytic agents, such as urokinase, streptokinase, or tissue plasminogen activator (tPA), to dissolve blood clots or antifibrinolytic agents, such as aminocaproic acid, to prevent rebleeds has not been adequately studied in penetrating keratoplasty. However, tissue plasminogen activator appears safe and effective for the treatment of severe fibrinous inflammation in the anterior chamber.[33,34]

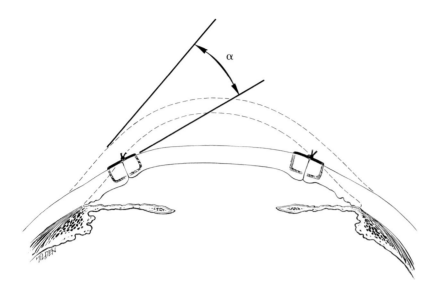

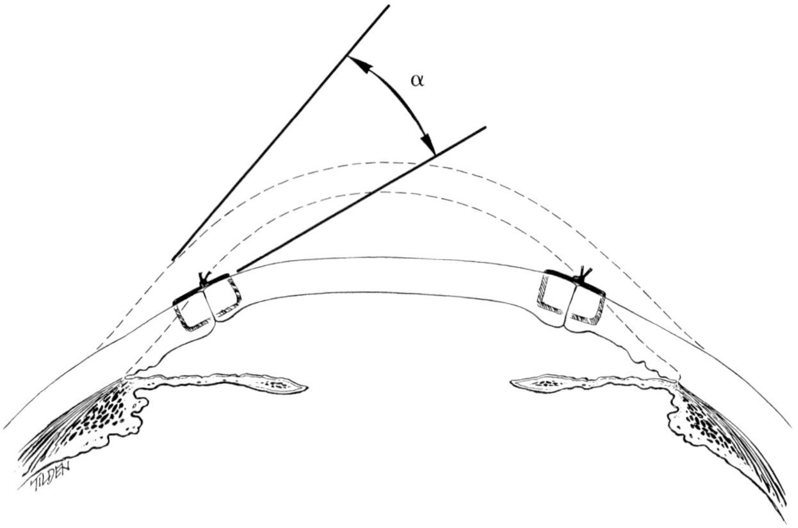

FIGURE 35-4 Crowding of the anterior chamber angle can occur if the sutures are tight or if the same size trephine is used to cut the recipient cornea and donor cornea.

High Intraocular Pressure

Measurement of the intraocular pressure in an eye with a corneal graft is discussed in Chapter 34. An abnormally thin graft on the first postoperative day is often a sign of increased intraocular pressure; the pressure essentially squeezes fluid out of the graft stroma and the lack of epithelial tight junctions prevents epithelial edema in newly healed epithelium.[35] Conversely, an abnormally edematous graft may be a sign of decreased intraocular pressure. Aphakic patients and those with a history of glaucoma are particularly at risk for early postoperative intraocular pressure elevation.[36]

Several surgical factors can contribute to elevated intraocular pressure. Residual viscoelastic substance in the anterior chamber is one of the most common causes of postoperative intraocular pressure elevation.[37] One study showed that both Healon and Viscoat caused intraocular pressure elevation after penetrating keratoplasty; the intraocular pressure peaked later and the elevation was sustained longer in the Healon group than in the Viscoat group.[38] By 72 hours postoperatively, however, mean intraocular pressure in both groups was less than preoperative values. Irrigation and aspiration of the viscoelastic substance at the end of surgery removes most of the substance and helps to some extent to prevent postoperative intraocular pressure elevation. Too vigorous an irrigation and aspiration should be avoided, however, because it can damage the endothelium of the graft.

Crowding of the anterior chamber angle is another cause of increased intraocular pressure, and can occur if the diameter of the donor corneal button is small in relation to the diameter of the recipient corneal opening, or if the graft is sutured too tightly (Figure 35-4). Anterior chamber angle crowding is especially significant in aphakic eyes, in which the propensity for immediate and long-term glaucoma after penetrating keratoplasty may be related to trabecular meshwork collapse from loss of lenticular support.[39] Cutting the donor corneal button with a trephine 0.5 mm larger in diameter than that used to cut the recipient cornea helps maintain an open angle and is recommended in aphakic eyes.[36,40] This much oversizing is not recommended in phakic or pseudophakic eyes, however, because the resultant corneal steepening induces myopia[41,42]; in these eyes, the donor corneal button should be cut with a trephine no more than 0.25 mm larger in diameter than that used to cut the recipient cornea. Inadvertent overtightening of the sutures can be avoided by maintaining a consistently deep anterior chamber during suture placement.

Therapeutic measures for reduction of postoperative intraocular pressure elevation include topical glaucoma medications, such as β-adrenergic antagonists (e.g., timolol), adrenergic agonists (e.g., epinephrine), an α_2-adrenergic agonist (apraclonidine), a carbonic anhydrase inhibitor (dorzolamide), and a prostaglandin analog (latanoprost). Topical parasympathomimetic agents should probably be avoided because they cause breakdown of the blood-aqueous barrier.[43] Oral or intravenous carbonic anhydrase inhibitors are usually effective and well tolerated. Some surgeons advocate routine administration of an oral carbonic anhydrase inhibitor on the first postoperative night and again on awakening the next morning when a viscoelastic substance has been used intraoperatively. Hyperosmotic agents, such as mannitol, glycerin, and isosorbide, are reserved for intraocular pressure elevations unresponsive to other agents.

High intraocular pressure in association with a shallow anterior chamber suggests the possibility of pupillary block. Pupillary block can occur as a result of the formation of posterior synechiae between the iris and the natural lens or an intraocular lens. In an aphakic eye, formation of posterior synechiae between the iris and vitreous face or entrapment of an air bubble posterior to the pupil may be the cause. Treatment includes the administration of glaucoma medications, vigorous pharmacologic dilation of the pupil and, if an air bubble is the culprit, positioning of the patient such that the bubble moves away from the pupil. A peripheral iridotomy may be created by a laser if the view permits; otherwise, a surgical iridectomy may be necessary. As in cataract surgery, an iridectomy is not routinely made during penetrating keratoplasty except in aphakic eyes, eyes with an anterior chamber intraocular lens, and eyes with severe inflammation.

Far more common than pupillary block, however, is a situation in which there is a diffuse wound leak and the iris moves anteriorly, which both plugs the leak and closes the anterior chamber angle. The wound is Seidel-negative and the intraocular pressure is high. Treatment consists of repairing the wound and repositing the iris.

Low Intraocular Pressure

In my experience, low intraocular pressure (less than 10 mmHg) is more common than high intraocular pressure in the early postoperative period after penetrating keratoplasty. In most cases, the low intraocular pressure probably occurs as a result of postoperative iridocyclitis and the accompanying decrease in aqueous humor production by the ciliary body. Hyposecretion of aqueous humor may be diagnosed by observing intense fluorescence in the anterior chamber 24 hours after the instillation of topical fluorescein drops. As the inflammation decreases with time (1 to 2 weeks) and topical corticosteroid treatment, normal aqueous humor production resumes and the intraocular pressure returns to normal.[44]

Apart from a wound leak (discussed above), other causes of postoperative hypotony include choroidal detachment, cyclodialysis cleft, scleral perforation, and retinal detachment. A choroidal detachment is usually associated with iridocyclitis and hypotony; which is cause and which is effect, however, remains unclear. Most choroidal detachments resolve spontaneously without sequelae. Commonly used treatment regimens include topical and systemic corticosteroids, as well as topical cycloplegic agents. If the anterior chamber remains flat or peripheral anterior synechiae begin to form, drainage of suprachoroidal fluid with reconstitution of the anterior chamber is indicated.

A cyclodialysis cleft is a separation of the ciliary body from the scleral spur, which effectively creates a drainage path between the anterior chamber and the supraciliary space. Apparently, even a tiny cleft is enough to channel all of the aqueous humor into the supraciliary space. It is difficult to identify the cleft with gonioscopy because graft edema associated with the hypotony prevents adequate visualization. If the cause of hypotony is determined to be a cleft and if resolution does not occur spontaneously, various surgical methods for closure may be considered.[45]

Scleral perforation may occur during retrobulbar anesthesia or during suturing of the scleral support ring. Several series describing scleral perforations caused by peribulbar or retrobulbar injections during cataract surgery have been published.[46,47] If perforation of the sclera occurs during suturing of the scleral support ring, as evidenced by pigmented uveal tissue, cryotherapy is usually all that is required if the perforation is less than 5 mm posterior to the limbus; a more posterior perforation may require a local buckling procedure.

Because the view of the retina is often obscured by the poor optics of a new corneal graft, low intraocular pressure may be the only sign of a retinal detachment.[48] Ultrasonography is indicated in such cases. It is important to realize that repair of the retinal detachment does not lead to immediate resolution of the hypotony.[49] Retinal detachment after penetrating keratoplasty is discussed further in the section below on late postoperative complications.

Primary Graft Failure

Primary graft failure occurs when dysfunction of the donor corneal endothelium leads to persistent corneal edema after penetrating keratoplasty. Because an intact endothelial pump is critical for corneal deturgescence, graft thickness is a sensitive index of endothelial function and can be measured by optical or ultrasonic pachymetry and followed over successive examinations. To make the diagnosis of primary graft failure, other causes of corneal edema must be excluded, such as hypotony, a large epithelial defect, and severe inflammation. Primary graft failure is uncommon, with a reported incidence of less than 5 percent.[40,50] Hyposecretion of aqueous humor by the ciliary body with accompanying hypotony and corneal edema that simulates primary graft failure is more common, especially in previously traumatized eyes.

Most cases of primary graft failure can be attributed to poor donor tissue, inadequate preservation, or surgical trauma. In selecting donor tissue, most eye banks follow the criteria established by the Eye Bank Association of America[51] (see Table 33-1 in Ch. 33). However, two criteria are left to the discretion of the medical directors of local eye banks because absolute guidelines are not given: an upper time interval from death to enucleation and an upper age limit for donors. For the death-to-enucleation time interval, the medical standards of the Eye Bank Association of America offer a general recommendation that corneal preservation occur as soon as possible after death. Less specific is the recommendation concerning the upper age limit for corneal donors. Although an inverse correlation between age and endothelial cell density is well documented,[52] it appears that the important factors are the endothelial cell density and morphology of the individual donor tissue, regardless of age. Nonetheless, many eye banks have arbitrarily established an upper age limit of between 60 and 75 years for corneal donors.

The corneal preservation medium used by most eye banks (Optisol) can generally preserve the endothelium for at least 10 days and the epithelium for at least 5 days. However, endothelial cell loss may occur inadvertently during some eye banking and tissue preservation procedures. Donor tissue may be damaged during procurement by excessive distortion of the cornea or by accidental endothelial contact with other surfaces. If such damage is localized, it could escape detection by specular microscopy because only a few areas of the endothelium are sampled on each cornea.

Contact between surgical instruments or other surfaces and the endothelial surface of the graft during penetrating keratoplasty results in endothelial cell damage and loss. A viscoelastic substance applied around the recipient corneal opening and injected into the anterior chamber provides protection against endothelial cell contact during transfer of the donor corneal button and subsequent suturing. Endothelial cell damage may occur from excessive irrigation of the anterior chamber with balanced salt solution. Finally, tainted irrigation fluids, viscoelastic substances, or intraocular medications may be responsible for primary graft failure, especially if a clustering of cases occurs.[40]

Once a diagnosis of primary graft failure has been made, the graft should be exchanged for another graft as soon as possible to permit rapid visual rehabilitation. Because primary graft failure is a relatively uncommon event, it should be investigated; the donor button should be submitted for pathologic evaluation and the eye bank that provided the tissue notified.

LATE POSTOPERATIVE COMPLICATIONS

Infection

Microbial Keratitis

The probability of developing an infection in any tissue is a balance between the virulence of the organism and the susceptibility of the host. Increased susceptibility of a corneal graft to infection commonly results from breaches in the epithelial barrier, possibly in conjunction with increased bacterial colonization of the ocular surface. Risk factors include persistent epithelial defects, loose, broken, or manipulated sutures, contact lens wear, and chronic use of topical corticosteroids and antibiotics. Corticosteroids impair host defense mechanisms and healing, promote microbial superinfection, and suppress inflammation. The chronic use of topical antibiotics alters the normal ocular flora and promotes infection by resistant organisms.[53] Contamination of ocular medication bottles, especially with *Serratia marcescens*, may provide a source of organisms for ocular infections.[54] Other deleterious factors in penetrating keratoplasty patients include diminished corneal sensation and poor visual acuity, which can contribute to delayed diagnosis and treatment of microbial keratitis.[55]

The incidence of microbial keratitis after penetrating keratoplasty is approximately 5 percent or less in most series reported in the United States.[53] Higher rates (12 percent) are reported from other countries.[56] About half the infections occur more than 6 months after penetrating keratoplasty.[53,55] Gram-positive bacteria, especially *Staphylococcus aureus*, coagulase-negative staphylococci, and streptococcal species, account for most infections. Of the gram-negative bacteria, *S. marcescens*, *P. aeruginosa*, and *Klebsiella* species are common, particularly in infections associated with extended-wear contact lenses (Figure 35-5). Fungal infections, although less common everywhere than bacterial infections, are more prevalent in warm climates than in colder regions. Common causative organisms include *Candida* and *Aspergillus*.[53] Infections caused by *Mycobacterium*[57,58] and *Acanthamoeba*[59] have also been reported.

Penetrating keratoplasty is occasionally performed for infectious keratitis that is unresponsive to medical therapy or progresses to corneal perforation. Infections caused by bacteria are unlikely to recur if the area of infection has been excised.[60,61] Fungal infections recur more frequently than bacterial infections,[62,63] but penetrating keratoplasty can still be successful in eradicating the infection despite histologic evidence of extension of fungi beyond the surgical margins.[62] Because the predisposing ocular conditions that contributed to the original infection usually do not disappear, bacterial and fungal infections can occur months to years later, usually with a different organism. For this reason, severe ocular surface disease present at the time of penetrating keratoplasty should be surgically corrected if possible. Consideration may be given to covering the graft with a conjunctival flap if the underlying disorder cannot be corrected.[61,64] A partial flap generally does not cause graft rejection and can be compatible with good vision.

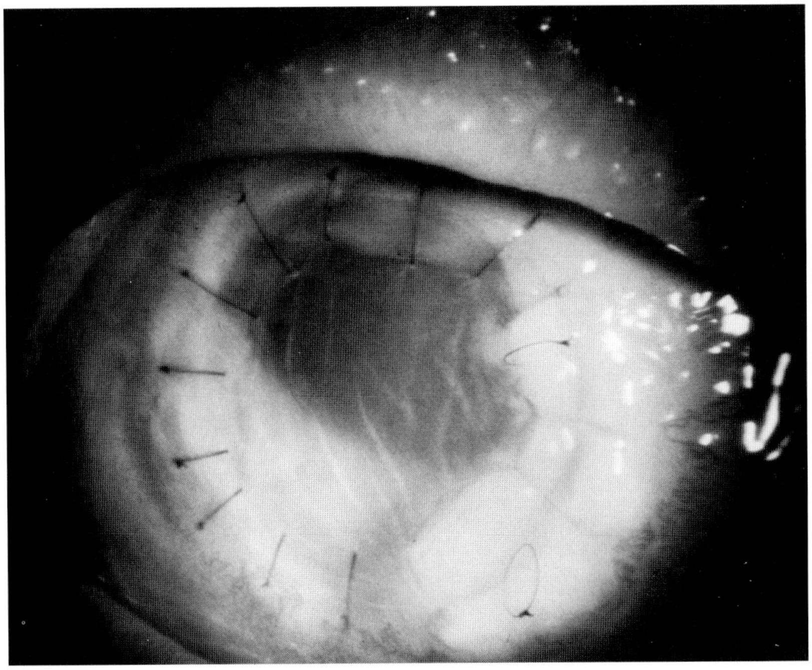

FIGURE 35-5 Bacterial keratitis along the wound 1 month after penetrating keratoplasty. Tissue necrosis has resulted in extrusion of some of the sutures.

In contrast to bacterial and fungal keratitis, *Acanthamoeba* keratitis recurs in approximately 30 percent of grafts.[65] Difficulty in determining the extent of the original infection clinically may be one reason for the high recurrence rate. Recurrence usually manifests as a stromal infiltrate in the peripheral graft, but infection can occur in the epithelium and appear as coarse elevated epithelial lines that can be mistaken for epithelial rejection lines. Medical therapy for *Acanthamoeba* should be continued for several months after penetrating keratoplasty in an attempt to reduce the chance of recurrence.[66] *Acanthamoeba* sometimes starts as a widespread keratitis that later localizes to a central opacity. When the infection appears localized, penetrating keratoplasty is generally effective. Penetrating keratoplasty should not be performed for *Acanthamoeba* keratitis until the infection is under control and the eye is no longer inflamed, if possible.[67]

Diagnosis and treatment of microbial keratitis in a graft are analogous to management of corneal ulcers in general. Corneal scrapings are obtained for smears and cultures, and intensive topical antimicrobial therapy is initiated. Hospitalization is usually necessary. The prognosis for recovery of good visual function is guarded. Many eyes require repeat penetrating keratoplasty, either electively for graft failure or emergently for an unresponsive infection, wound dehiscence, or corneal perforation. Endophthalmitis can develop from a graft infection, especially in the presence of a corneal perforation[53]; however, as in any inflammatory corneal disorder, the presence of a hypopyon in the anterior chamber does not necessarily indicate endophthalmitis.

Preventive measures to help avoid graft infections begin preoperatively with the treatment of dry eyes, exposure, trichiasis, and other eyelid abnormalities. Postoperatively, the recognition and removal of loose, broken, or exposed sutures, vigilant follow-up of patients with epithelial defects, contact lenses, or failed grafts, and careful patient education concerning prompt reporting of symptoms are paramount. Although short-term administration of topical antibiotics in an attempt to prevent infections is warranted for specific conditions, such as an epithelial defect or after suture removal, long-term administration is discouraged. Topical corticosteroids should be tapered to the minimum amount required to maintain graft clarity.[53,55,56]

Infectious Crystalline Keratopathy

Infectious crystalline keratopathy is a unique, indolent corneal infection, occurring mostly in grafts (Figure 35-6). The characteristic crystalline-like infiltrates, typically associated with an overlying epithelial defect, are most commonly caused by colonization of the anterior corneal lamellae with *Streptococcus viridans*.[68-70] Rarely, other organisms, such as *Enterococcus, Peptostreptococcus, Haemophilus aphrophilus, Alternaria, Mycobacterium fortuitum*, and *Candida* species, have been implicated.[70,71] *S. epidermidis* can produce infectious crystalline keratopathy in the posterior stroma.[72] *S. viridans* produces a glycocalyx (biofilm) matrix that is thought to contribute to the crystalline-shaped deposits seen clinically. This

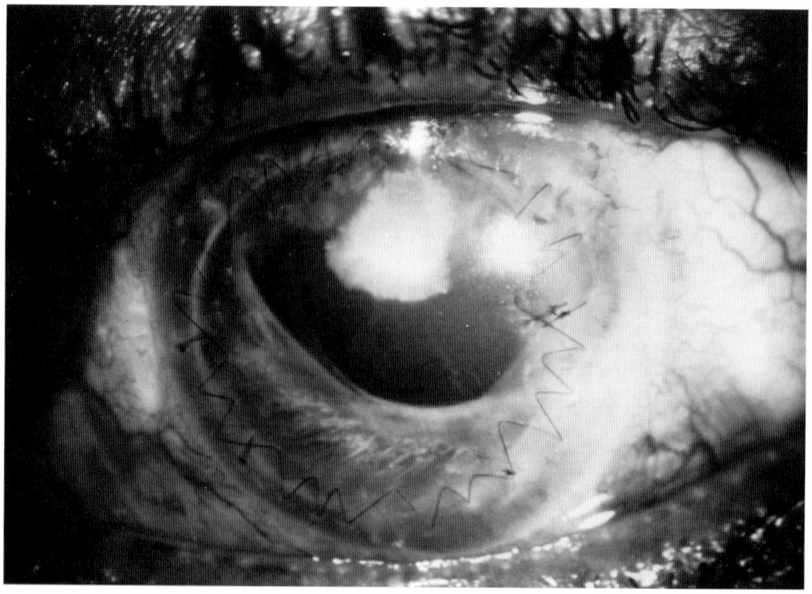

FIGURE 35-6 Infectious crystalline keratopathy.

matrix may also serve to "hide" the bacteria from the immune system, which helps explain the absence of both ocular inflammation and the white cell infiltrate characteristic of these infections.

A culture-proven diagnosis of infectious crystalline keratopathy may be difficult to achieve, especially when the organism is a nutritionally variant strain of *Streptococcus*. Various culture enhancements may be needed, including longer incubation times, pyridoxal hydrochloride supplementation to the media, cross-streaking the media with staphylococci, and incubation in a 5 to 10 percent CO_2 atmosphere.[70] Although in vitro studies show susceptibilities to penicillin G, gentamicin, and cephalothin,[68] *S. viridans* is slow growing, and the response to antibiotic treatment is usually poor. Superficial lamellar keratectomy to remove or debride the infected tissue can be curative; excimer laser ablation has been used successfully to treat a case of very superficial infectious crystalline keratopathy.[73] Often, repeat penetrating keratoplasty is required for definitive therapy; the prognosis is favorable in these cases.[68-70]

Herpes Simplex Keratitis

The reported incidence of recurrent herpes simplex keratitis after penetrating keratoplasty varies depending on the study design, disease definition, and length of follow-up. The recurrence rate is approximately 10 to 18 percent 1 to 3 years postoperatively and increases to approximately 47 percent 15 years postoperatively.[40,74]

A common diagnostic dilemma when caring for patients grafted for herpes simplex keratitis is differentiating recurrent herpetic keratitis from graft rejection. Herpetic keratitis can incite graft rejection and vice versa; thus, the problem can be one or the other, or both concurrently. Theoretically, specific signs are helpful in distinguishing herpetic keratitis from graft rejection. Herpes simplex epithelial keratitis may manifest as a dendritic or geographic ulcer at the graft-recipient junction, in which case the diagnosis is not difficult (Figure 35-7). However, it may also manifest as an ulcer with a less pathognomonic shape, in which case the diagnosis is more difficult, and viral cultures may be helpful. Herpes simplex stromal keratitis usually appears as a localized area of stromal inflammation and edema, with accompanying keratic precipitates and anterior chamber inflammation, and can be difficult, if not impossible, to distinguish from graft rejection.[66,74]

Herpes simplex epithelial keratitis is treated with a topical antiviral agent, such as 1 percent trifluridine eight times a day. Herpes simplex stromal keratitis and corneal graft rejection are treated similarly, with a regimen of topical corticosteroids and an antiviral agent given in equal frequencies. A typical regimen is topical 1 percent prednisolone acetate and 1 percent trifluridine, both administered eight times a day. The frequency is slowly tapered over several weeks, depending on the response. A sub-Tenon's injection of long-acting corticosteroids is contraindicated. Topical antiviral medications are toxic to the corneal epithelium, especially when used for an extended period; conversely, frequent or long-term corticosteroid use without antiviral coverage may promote herpes simplex recurrence.[66]

Routine prophylaxis for herpes simplex infection at the time of penetrating keratoplasty appears prudent, although

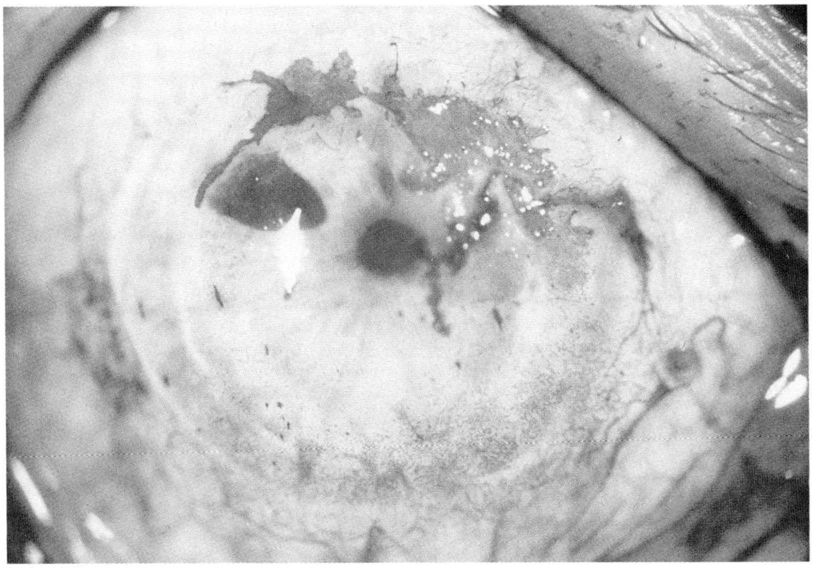

FIGURE 35-7 Rose bengal staining of a geographic ulcer caused by herpes simplex virus after penetrating keratoplasty.

not supported by large controlled studies.[75-78] Topical trifluridine is instilled with a frequency equal to that of topical corticosteroids. Because increased inflammation is expected postoperatively, oral prednisone (60 mg/day) is begun the day before surgery if there are no systemic contraindications, is continued for at least 1 week postoperatively, and is then tapered over the second week. Oral acyclovir (400 mg five times a day) or valacyclovir (500 mg three times a day) is given for 2 weeks postoperatively. In a prospective, randomized trial involving 22 patients, Barney and Foster[76] showed a marked decrease in the rates of recurrent herpes simplex keratitis (0 vs. 44 percent) and graft failure (14 percent vs. 56 percent) at a mean follow-up of 16.5 months in patients who received long-term oral acyclovir. The benefit of postoperative systemic acyclovir has also been demonstrated in a rabbit autokeratoplasty model.[12]

Overall, the prognosis is reasonably good for initial grafts in patients with herpes simplex keratitis. A large, retrospective series that used actuarial analysis showed a greater than 70 percent probability of graft survival at 6 years.[74] Recipient corneal vascularization, active inflammation, multiple inflammatory episodes (recurrent herpes simplex keratitis and/or graft rejection), and repeat grafting increase the risk of graft failure in these patients.[79,80] In addition, these eyes are more susceptible to persistent epithelial defects, as well as bacterial or fungal keratitis, which contribute to graft failure.

Endophthalmitis

Endophthalmitis may occur late in the postoperative course of penetrating keratoplasty. Reported associations include suture removal,[81,82] vitreous incarceration in the keratoplasty wound,[83] and exposed sutures used for transscleral posterior chamber intraocular lens fixation.[84]

Of four reported cases of endophthalmitis following planned suture removal, two showed evidence of anterior wound displacement,[81] and one occurred in a chronically immunosuppressed renal transplant patient whose source of infection appeared to be chronic dacryocystitis.[82] Preventive measures to help avoid infection related to suture removal include strict asepsis and application of topical antibiotics immediately before and for several days after suture removal.

Wound Dehiscence

Dehiscences of penetrating keratoplasty wounds may be divided into three groups: those that occur before suture removal, those that occur immediately after suture removal, and those that are unrelated to suture removal. A dehiscence that occurs before suture removal is usually caused by misplaced, loose, or broken sutures and/or elevated intraocular pressure and is discussed above in the section on early postoperative complications. Careful attention to signs of wound healing, such as vascularization, scarring, and loosening of sutures, helps prevent premature suture removal. However, some wounds that appear healed are unstable. The incidence of wound dehiscence after suture removal may be reduced by the use of an 11-0 suture to support the wound, as in the interrupted 10-0 and running 11-0 suture technique or the double running 10-0 and 11-0 suture technique described in Chapter 34. Following removal of the 10-0 suture(s), the running 11-0 suture is left in place to support the wound for at least 1

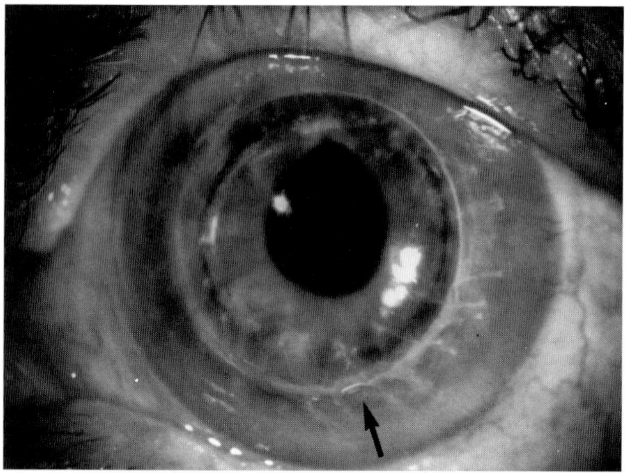

A

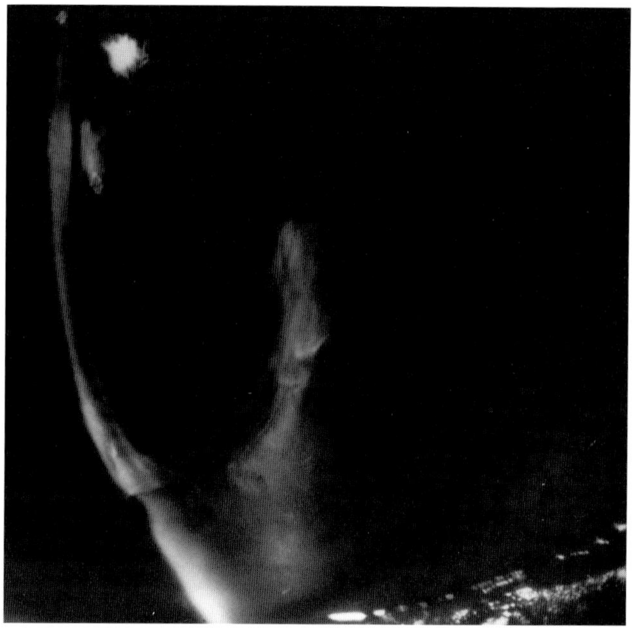

B

FIGURE 35-8 **(A)** Inferior graft override. Note the corneal irregularities inferior to the wound (arrow). **(B)** Slit lamp appearance of the area of graft override. *(continues)*

year unless the suture loosens, breaks, or induces corneal neovascularization, in which case it is removed earlier. Late breakage of nylon sutures is usually caused by degradation of the sutures; therefore, some advocate the use of nondegradable material, such as polyester, for sutures that are intended to remain in place for 1 year or more.[85,86] If the 11-0 suture is inadvertently cut during removal of the 10-0 suture(s), it must be repaired (spliced), because the rate of wound dehiscence in such cases is high, especially when a double running suture technique has been used.[87]

Any time sutures are removed, the patient should be examined within a few days to assess the wound for dehiscence. A wound dehiscence not only threatens the integrity of the eye, but usually induces astigmatism, with the flat axis in the meridian of the dehiscence (Figure 35-8). Placement of sutures across the wound in the area of the dehiscence merely keeps the graft from protruding further. To correctly re-approximate the graft and the recipient cornea, the wound must be opened in the area of the dehiscence. First, 10-0 nylon sutures are placed at either end of the dehiscence; these sutures prevent extension of the dehiscence to the entire wound. The wound between these sutures is opened with a stainless steel blade, the graft is re-approximated to the recipient cornea, and interrupted 10-0 nylon sutures are placed. The entire wound is examined to ensure that the tension caused by placement of these sutures has not caused a dehiscence in another area of the wound.

A penetrating keratoplasty wound never achieves the strength of a normal cornea. Several factors contribute to the persistent weakness of the wound: the use of topical corticosteroids to control inflammation and prevent graft rejection, the use of relatively noninflammatory suture materials (nylon or polyester), and the slow healing response of the recipient cornea. Patients should be made aware that a keratoplasty wound is more vulnerable to trauma than a normal cornea and should be cautioned to avoid environments and activities that place them at risk for trauma.[88–91] The use of protective eyewear, such as polycarbonate spectacle lenses, is advised, especially for monocular patients.

Treatment of a traumatic wound dehiscence involves expeditious closure with interrupted 10-0 nylon sutures under general anesthesia. If the patient has been rendered aphakic by the injury, a scleral support ring is sutured to the eye and an anterior vitrectomy is performed. Cultures are obtained and prophylactic broad-spectrum antibiotics are administered. Postoperatively, the physician should exercise patience in waiting for the graft to clear because a graft with a large endothelial reserve may recover in some cases. Even when graft failure ensues, repeat penetrating keratoplasty has a favorable prognosis if the pos-

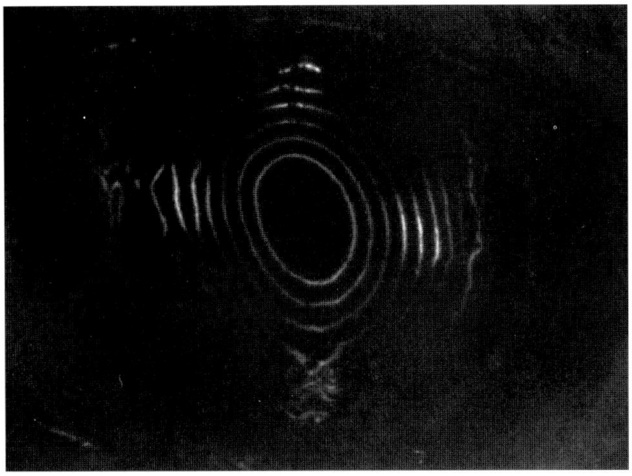

C

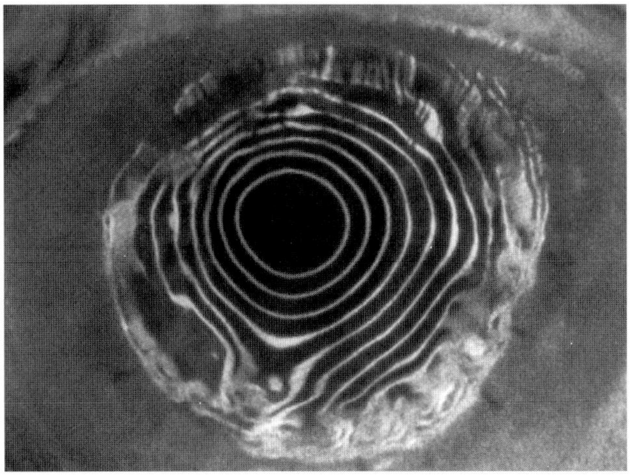

D

FIGURE 35-8 *(continued)* **(C)** Photokeratograph reveals marked flattening in the meridian of the graft override. **(D)** The wound was opened, and the graft was resutured in the proper position. Note that the central mire is more circular. The peripheral mires still show some irregularities in the periphery along the wound.

terior segment is intact. Not surprisingly, the force of the trauma has been found to be the most significant factor affecting the outcome.[88–91]

Corneal Membranes

Stripped Descemet's Membrane

Although a stripped Descemet's membrane is an intraoperative complication of penetrating keratoplasty and, if left in place, causes early problems with the graft, it is discussed here to differentiate it from other causes of corneal membranes.

In markedly edematous corneas, the stroma may be inadvertently separated from Descemet's membrane during removal of the recipient corneal button. This results in a retained Descemet's membrane, which may be difficult to detect intraoperatively. Postoperatively, the membrane appears as a sheet posterior to the graft. Graft failure usually occurs, although there have been reports of creating an opening in the membrane with a neodymium:yttrium-aluminum-garnet (Nd:YAG) laser and salvaging the graft.[92]

Epithelial Ingrowth

Epithelial invasion of the anterior chamber may occur rarely after penetrating keratoplasty. In this condition, corneal or conjunctival epithelium enters the anterior chamber through a poorly healed wound or fistulous tract. The defect may be the result of previous intraocular surgery or trauma[93] or of complications with the keratoplasty wound itself, such as wound dehiscence with iris or vitreous incarceration.[94] Alternatively, epithelial seeding into the anterior chamber may occur by a surgical instrument, full-thickness suture, or traumatic foreign body.[93,95,96]

Proliferation of intraocular epithelium produces an aggressive sheet-like growth over the posterior corneal surface, the anterior chamber structures, and sometimes the posterior segment structures.[97] On the posterior surface of the graft, the lack of cellular contact inhibition in areas of damaged or absent corneal endothelial cells allows formation of a retrocorneal membrane by the invading epithelium.[98] The advancing epithelial edge may resemble an endothelial rejection line (Figure 35-9). Because the tight junctions between epithelial cells create a watertight barrier, corneal edema with loss of clarity may not be seen until the epithelial ingrowth is advanced. Although hypotony may be present initially, epithelial extension over the trabecular meshwork ultimately results in intractable glaucoma, which is frequently the cause of vision loss in these patients. Other signs associated with epithelial ingrowth include pupillary distortion, iritis with large clumps of anterior chamber cells that does not resolve with corticosteroid therapy, and a positive Seidel's test over a leaking wound or fistula. Rarely, an iris inclusion cyst filled with serous fluid or packed with epithelial cells (pearl cyst) may occur.[95,96] The diagnosis of epithelial ingrowth can be differentiated from conditions such as Descemet's membrane detachment, stromal ingrowth, or retrocorneal fibrous membrane by application of argon

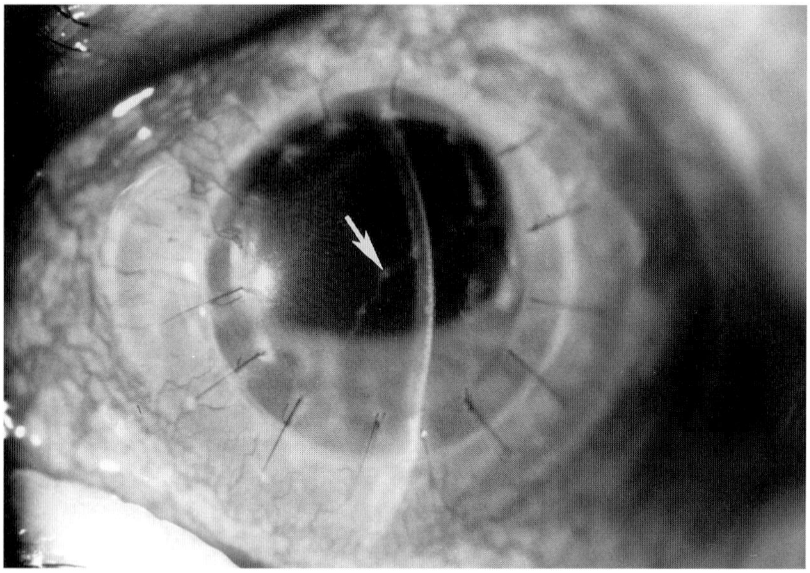

FIGURE 35-9 Epithelial ingrowth advancing across the donor cornea in the direction of the arrow. The slit beam demonstrates that the cornea is not thickened in this region. The intraocular pressure was 60 mmHg.

laser burns to the iris. If epithelium covers the iris surface where the laser burns are applied, a white, fluffy lesion will appear instead of the usual brown spot; this technique can also be used to outline the extent of iris involvement.

Treatment for diffuse epithelial ingrowth is extremely difficult. Radiotherapy, employed in the past, is no longer used because of severe complications. Cryotherapy with air in the anterior chamber to insulate the intraocular contents has been used extensively but risks phthisis. Surgical extirpation of involved ocular structures appears to offer a reasonable chance of preserving vision when performed early in the course of the disorder. In early ingrowth, the abnormal tissue, often with the fistula, can be removed en bloc and replaced with a graft. However, the diagnosis of epithelial ingrowth is often delayed until the ingrowth is too extensive to be amenable to surgical excision. In cases with extensive involvement, defined in one study as greater than 50 percent involvement of the cornea and/or iris surface, prevention of medically uncontrollable glaucoma and palliation of pain by intraocular pressure control using a seton has had reasonable success.[99] The prognosis after removal of an inclusion cyst is favorable if the cyst can be removed in toto while still small.[95,96]

Stromal Ingrowth

Poor posterior wound apposition may result in recipient or donor stromal fibroblasts migrating into the anterior chamber and onto the posterior surface of the graft. Occasionally, the extent of the ingrowth is limited to the peripheral cornea with maintenance of a clear central graft. If the ingrowth is extensive, however, all the endothelium is destroyed and the result is a cloudy and edematous graft. Repeat penetrating keratoplasty with a graft larger than the previous graft is performed to ensure that all of the membrane is removed.

Retrocorneal Fibrous Membrane

A retrocorneal membrane is a sheet of fibrous, collagenous tissue sandwiched between Descemet's membrane and the endothelial cell layer. Clinically, this is usually seen after graft failure caused by rejection but may also be seen in response to other inflammatory events or as a result of contact between the vitreous and the cornea. Histopathologic evidence suggests that the mechanism involves metaplasia of endothelial cells to fibroblast-like cells, with subsequent production of collagenous and Descemet's membrane material.[100] Because the graft is cloudy and edematous, the patient must have repeat penetrating keratoplasty to obtain useful vision.

Glaucoma

Sustained intraocular pressure elevation after penetrating keratoplasty places visual function in double jeopardy due to the potential for both optic nerve and corneal endothelial damage. However, the magnitude and duration of increased intraocular pressure necessary to produce irreversible endothelial damage in human grafts is not known because the experimental evidence is mostly from animal studies. An additional concern with high intraocular pressure after penetrating keratoplasty is the mechanical stress placed on the wound, which can contribute to wound ectasia and dehiscence.

Various studies have confirmed that major risk factors for the development of postkeratoplasty glaucoma are pre-existing glaucoma and aphakia or pseudophakia.[101–104] In a consecutive series of 502 penetrating keratoplasty cases, the incidence of postkeratoplasty glaucoma was 39 percent in aphakic eyes, compared with 17 percent in pseudophakic eyes and 4 percent in phakic eyes.[101] Other reported risk factors include the presence of anterior synechiae with or without other anterior segment abnormalities, and closed-loop anterior chamber intraocular lenses.[40,102] Chronic inflammation is also associated with increased intraocular pressure.

The pathophysiology of postkeratoplasty glaucoma has been the subject of much discussion. Olson and Kaufman[39] suggested that the diameter of the donor corneal button relative to that of the recipient corneal opening is an important determinant of anterior chamber angle distortion and facility of outflow, especially in eyes without lenticular support. Use of a donor corneal button cut with a trephine 0.5 mm larger in diameter than that used to cut the recipient cornea has been shown to reduce the incidence of postkeratoplasty glaucoma in some studies but not in others.[41,42,101,105–107] A tightly sutured wound can contribute to crowding of the anterior chamber angle and thus to increased intraocular pressure. Angle closure from progressive peripheral anterior synechiae can also cause postkeratoplasty glaucoma.

The use of topical corticosteroids can cause intraocular pressure elevation in some patients. The incidence of corticosteroid-induced intraocular pressure elevation is approximately 30 percent in the normal population[108]; the incidence increases in patients with pre-existing open-angle glaucoma, high myopia, diabetes, or a family history of glaucoma. Although corticosteroid-induced intraocular pressure elevation can be seen at any time in the course of therapy, it typically develops after 3 to 8 weeks. Fluorometholone, medrysone, and rimexolone have less intraocular pressure–elevating effects than other corticosteroids and may be used to treat inflammation in patients with a history of corticosteroid-induced intraocular pressure elevation. Periocular injections of long-acting corticosteroids, such as methylprednisolone acetate, should be not be given to individuals predisposed to corticosteroid-induced intraocular pressure elevation because the drugs can cause severe problems with increased intraocular pressure.[109] Corticosteroid-induced glaucoma can usually be managed medically, and the intraocular pressure typically returns to normal once the corticosteroids have been discontinued. Depot corticosteroid material, if present, can be excised if necessary to help control the intraocular pressure elevation, even several months after the injection was given.[109]

The prevention of postkeratoplasty glaucoma begins by controlling any pre-existing glaucoma preoperatively. Usually this can be achieved with glaucoma medications. In cases with medically uncontrollable glaucoma, surgical procedures to lower intraocular pressure are indicated and should probably be performed at the time of penetrating keratoplasty.[110] Combined glaucoma procedures and keratoplasty are successful often enough to be worthwhile. During penetrating keratoplasty, removal of anterior chamber lenses thought to be associated with glaucoma, lysis of anterior synechiae, and placement of iris sutures to create a taut iris diaphragm are measures that may help prevent the development of glaucoma. Inadvertent overtightening of sutures used to close the keratoplasty wound can be avoided by maintaining a consistently deep anterior chamber at all times during suture placement. As mentioned above, use of an oversized donor corneal button may help prevent the development of glaucoma.

Treatment of postkeratoplasty glaucoma involves the use of topical and systemic glaucoma medications, with the topical β-adrenergic antagonists (e.g., timolol) representing a good first choice. However, corneal grafts are more susceptible to punctate epithelial damage associated with timolol and other glaucoma medications than are normal corneas.[111] Topical parasympathomimetic agents should be used prudently in eyes with extensive peripheral anterior synechiae or other severe trabecular damage because these agents may cause a paradoxical elevation of intraocular pressure. These agents lower uveoscleral outflow, which is a major aqueous drainage route in such eyes. In addition, parasympathomimetic agents loosen the tight junctions between vascular endothelial cells and thus break down the blood-ocular barrier. Even weak parasympathomimetic agents have the potential to induce graft rejection.[112]

When medical therapy fails, surgical intervention becomes necessary. Traditional filtering procedures have a high failure rate in postkeratoplasty eyes, similar to the rates in other eyes with previous intraocular surgery and conjunctival scarring.[113] Attempts to maintain a filtering bleb with antimetabolites, such as 5-fluorouracil or mitomycin, may risk graft failure from epithelial or wound toxicity,[114] but if these are carefully used, the procedures can be very effective. Noteworthy are several reports suggesting that performing a trabeculectomy at the time of penetrating keratoplasty can result in good long-term intraocular pressure control,[110,115] and this has also been my experience.

Cyclocryotherapy, in which the ciliary body is destroyed by external application of a cryoprobe, has been widely used to treat postkeratoplasty glaucoma. Although the reported success rates for cyclocryotherapy are high in some series, complications such as severe pain, hemorrhage, chronic inflammation, hypotony, graft failure, and phthisis reduce enthusiasm for this procedure.[36] The technique of using a transscleral Nd:YAG laser for cyclodestruction appears promising; one study of 28 treated eyes showed a 73 percent success rate for lowering intraocular pressure at 2 years, with a relatively low complication rate.[116] The diode laser is easier to use and may be even better.

Argon laser trabeculoplasty has been shown to be effective in the treatment of postkeratoplasty glaucoma.[117] Patients without pre-existing glaucoma appear to respond to argon laser trabeculoplasty better than those with pre-existing glaucoma. Treatment requires an adequate view of the structures of the anterior chamber angle, however, and is therefore limited to patients with a clear graft, minimal wound scarring, and an open anterior chamber angle. Furthermore, the effect of argon laser trabeculoplasty may not be permanent.[118]

Setons may also be used to treat medically uncontrollable glaucoma. Available types of setons include the single-[119,120] and double-plate[121,122] Molteno implant, anterior chamber tube shunt to an encircling band (Schocket procedure),[121,122] and Baerveldt implant.[123] Reported success rates with Molteno implants range from 71 to 91 percent with 1- to 2-year follow-up. The graft failure rate of 26 to 42 percent is similar to that reported for penetrating keratoplasty patients in general undergoing an additional intraocular procedure.[124] These failed grafts may be replaced and can result in an ultimately successful outcome. For uncontrollable glaucoma preoperatively, placement of a seton before penetrating keratoplasty has been suggested.[114,121]

Persistent Mydriasis

After penetrating keratoplasty for keratoconus, an unexplained syndrome of irreversible mydriasis unresponsive to miotics was first recognized by Castroviejo. Urrets-Zavalia was the first to publish a series of cases in which a fixed dilated pupil, iris atrophy, and secondary glaucoma were described as a syndrome.[125] Apparently, up to 10 percent of patients with keratoconus have an iris that may become permanently dilated after postoperative administration of atropine, homatropine, scopolamine, or even phenylephrine.[126] The permanent dilation may be unrelated to the dilating drops, however. A recent study from Israel found no instances of persistent mydriasis in 83 consecutive eyes undergoing penetrating keratoplasty for keratoconus in which 1 percent atropine was routinely given at the end of surgery.[127] Anterior segment fluorescein angiography has demonstrated severe iris ischemia in affected patients,[128] and a possible role for occlusion of iris vessels intraoperatively from pressure of the iris against the edge of the recipient corneal opening or postoperatively from a rise in intraocular pressure has been proposed in the etiology of this syndrome.

Although the existence of Urrets-Zavalia syndrome has been called into question,[127] strong mydriatic agents should probably not be given to keratoconus patients in the immediate postoperative period.

Patients with permanent pupillary dilation may wear a contact lens with a painted iris pattern peripherally and clear optical zone centrally to decrease photophobia.[129]

Cataract

A cataract can cause decreased visual acuity in a patient with a clear corneal graft. The progression of early senescent cataractous lens changes may be accelerated after penetrating keratoplasty.[130] Rarely, poor surgical technique, such as trauma to the anterior lens capsule, excessive manipulation of the iris, or even vigorous irrigation, may damage the lens. Postoperatively, persistent inflammation, hyphema, or hypopyon may cause lens opacities; the mechanism may involve interference with lens metabolism. Postoperative topical medications may cause toxic cataract formation. Examples include anterior capsular vacuoles seen in association with anticholinesterases and posterior subcapsular changes seen with corticosteroids.

Long-term systemic or topical corticosteroid administration is a well-documented cause of cataract formation. The threshold cataractogenic dose for systemic corticosteroids appears to be approximately 10 mg/day of prednisone over 1 or more years in about 30 percent of patients.[131] Topically, a median of 786 drops of 0.1 percent dexamethasone over a median of 10.5 months (average of 2.5 drops per day) was reported to cause lens changes in 28 keratoconus graft patients; the earliest cataract occurred after only 2.5 months and 221 drops (average of 2.9 drops per day).[131] Early in their development, posterior subcapsular cataracts minimally affect visual acuity, and progression can be halted or occasionally reversed by discontinuation of the corticosteroids.[132]

Several measures may be taken to protect the lens. Pilocarpine may be given preoperatively or acetylcholine chloride or carbachol intraoperatively to constrict the pupil and provide a mechanical barrier. Use of a viscoelastic substance not only provides a buffer to trauma, but helps prevent inadvertent contact with the anterior capsule by maintaining a deep anterior chamber. In patients with early senescent lens changes, especially patients older than 50 years, strong consideration should be given to cataract extraction concomitant with penetrating keratoplasty to avoid subjecting the patient (and the graft) to an intraocular procedure in the future, because these cataracts tend to progress after surgery. Postoperative corticosteroids should be tapered to the lowest amount needed to maintain a clear graft. Many keratoconus and other phakic patients can be safely weaned from all corticosteroids within 3 to 6 months after surgery.

Retinal Abnormalities

Retinal Detachment

Retinal detachment after penetrating keratoplasty is a relatively infrequent event but occurs more frequently after this procedure than after extracapsular cataract surgery. In a series of 1,146 cases of penetrating keratoplasty, Musch et al[133] reported an incidence of retinal detachment of 1.9 percent at 6 months, 2.1 percent at 1 year, and 4.7 percent at 43 months. Eyes that had undergone concomitant anterior vitrectomy were four times more likely to develop a retinal detachment than eyes that had not. Forstot et al[48] reported a 2.3 percent incidence of retinal detachment in 610 penetrating keratoplasty cases; all 14 detachments occurred in the group of 261 eyes that had vitreous manipulation, increasing the incidence of retinal detachment in this group to 5.4 percent. A survey of 40,351 Medicare beneficiaries who were admitted to United States hospitals for penetrating keratoplasty between 1984 and 1987 showed a risk of rehospitalization for retinal detachment within 2 years of 1.85 percent.[22] This increased to 2.49 percent for patients who had anterior vitrectomy concomitant with penetrating keratoplasty.

Although the reattachment rate for retinal detachment after cataract surgery is greater than 90 percent, the reattachment rate for retinal detachment after penetrating keratoplasty is 29 to 74 percent.[134] The low reattachment rate parallels the poor visual outcome in patients with retinal detachment after penetrating keratoplasty; less than one-third achieve a final visual acuity of 20/200 or better. The poor visual outcome may be partly explained by pre-existing retinal pathology. However, two other factors are probably significant in these cases: a delay in diagnosis because of the patient's inability to detect a change in an already visually compromised eye, and difficulty in visualizing retinal breaks because of suboptimal optics.

Early diagnosis of a retinal detachment should result in a better outcome. A decrease in visual acuity, even if the visual acuity is initially poor, and an unexplained decrease in intraocular pressure are important signs. Because it may be difficult to detect a small decrease in visual acuity or visual field deficit in a patient in the early postoperative period after penetrating keratoplasty, periodic indirect ophthalmoscopic examinations are advised, especially during the first 6 months. If the retina cannot be seen, B-scan ultrasonography is indicated.[48]

Lessening the risk of developing a postoperative retinal detachment is problematic at the time of penetrating keratoplasty given that vitrectomy is indicated in certain cases. Removal of vitreous with a vitrector set on a high cutting rate and moderate suction instead of with cellulose sponges lessens the risk of retinal traction and tears.

Corneal graft failure is often the result of surgical manipulations and postoperative inflammation associated with retinal reattachment surgery. Endothelial toxicity from prolonged contact with gas (sulfur hexafluoride or perfluropropane) or silicone oil[48,135,136] used for retinal tamponade may cause graft failure. If possible, endothelial contact with these agents should be minimized, but retinal repair considerations take precedence over graft survival because the graft can be replaced at a later date. Pre-existing retinal detachments can be surgically approached by placing a temporary keratoprosthesis to allow visualization of the retina, removing the keratoprosthesis after the retinal surgery is completed, and then placing the graft, as described in Chapter 36.

Macular Edema

Macular edema after penetrating keratoplasty is a frustrating problem for both the surgeon and the patient. The hope raised by a seemingly good result for several months after surgery may be dashed when, unexpectedly, visual acuity decreases or fails to improve despite clearing and thinning of the graft.

In general, the common denominator in the development of macular edema appears to be chronic ocular inflammation, probably mediated by prostaglandins. Macular edema can occur in aphakic or pseudophakic eyes as a result of the surgical manipulation itself. Pathophysiologically, the above conditions lead to abnormal leakage of the perifoveal capillaries. If the edema becomes chronic, intraretinal cyst formation occurs (cystoid degeneration), with destruction of photoreceptors.[137]

The incidence of macular edema from penetrating keratoplasty itself is unknown because an opacified cornea makes it impossible to detect the presence of macular edema preoperatively. Many of the disorders for which penetrating keratoplasty is indicated, such as aphakic or pseudophakic bullous keratopathy, have a high incidence of macular edema. Anterior vitrectomy at the time of penetrating keratoplasty appears to greatly increase the incidence of macular edema. This association has been demonstrated retrospectively as well as prospectively in eyes undergoing combined penetrating keratoplasty and cataract extraction.[138,139]

Attempting to treat macular edema by treating accompanying inflammation with topical, periocular, and/or systemic corticosteroids is traditional but has not definitively been proved beneficial by controlled studies. However, controlled studies have demonstrated the efficacy of several nonsteroidal anti-inflammatory drugs, which inhibit prostaglandin synthesis. Prophylactic administration of indomethacin, either systemically or topically, appears to prevent at least angiographically detectable macular edema after cataract extraction.[140,141] Moreover, a benefit from topical ketorolac administered prophylactically before extracapsular cataract extraction without intraocular lens implantation, as well as therapeutically in chronic aphakic or pseudophakic macular edema following cataract extraction, has been demonstrated.[142,143] Only the latter study, however, showed improved visual acuity with treatment, and neither study showed evidence of a sustained effect. Nonetheless, anecdotal experience with graft patients appears favorable. Although no guidelines exist, I prescribe ketorolac four times a day for a 1 to 2 month trial period for suspected or confirmed macular edema. As with macular edema after cataract surgery, macular edema after penetrating keratoplasty may spontaneously improve or resolve without therapy.[137] Macular edema and visual acuity can continue to improve for at least 18 months after surgery.

Phototoxic Macular Damage

Microscope light-induced retinopathy has been reported after various intraocular procedures, including cataract extraction (with or without intraocular lens implantation), epikeratophakia in phakic eyes, vitrectomy, and combined penetrating keratoplasty, extracapsular cataract extraction, and intraocular lens implantation. Phototoxicity appears to be largely a photochemical process, with some potentiation by heat.[144] Free radical formation by the interaction of light and oxygen may be followed by damage to vulnerable retinal cell mitochondria.[145]

Symptoms include central or paracentral scotomas, which may be associated with decreased visual acuity. Signs include retinal edema in the macular region 1 to 2 days after exposure, followed by gradual hyperpigmentation and pigment clumping of the retinal pigment epithelium weeks to months later. Angiographically, the chronic scar causes choroidal blockage by the pigment, hyperfluorescent window defects, and late hyperfluorescence.[145,146] These changes are similar to those seen in age-related macular degeneration and, also as with age-related macular degeneration, may possibly result in choroidal neovascularization.[144]

The most important risk factor appears to be the length of the operation, especially operating times longer than 100 minutes. Other reported risk factors include diabetes mellitus, hydrochlorothiazide ingestion, and a high proportion of blue wavelength light in the microscope light spectrum. Many simple preventive measures are possible intraoperatively. These include placing an opaque object on the corneal surface, producing pharmacologic pupillary miosis, switching from co-axial to oblique microscope light illumination, tilting the microscope at least 10 degrees off axis, using the lowest possible level of illumination needed, employing a blue light (wavelength less than 515 nm) filter, and keeping the operating time as short as possible.[145]

Corneal Graft Rejection

Penetrating keratoplasty is one of the most successful transplantation procedures, with a 2-year survival rate of more than 90 percent for primary grafts in avascular corneas.[147] With many of the problems of the past having been eliminated by advances in corneal preservation, surgical techniques, and pre- and postoperative care, corneal graft rejection has become the leading cause of secondary graft failure[147] (Figure 35-10). Overall, approximately 25 percent of corneal graft recipients experience at least one episode of rejection, of which approximately 20 percent are irreversible.[148]

Corneal Transplantation Immunology

Although corneal graft rejection results from a complex series of events, many of which are not fully understood, the traditional concept of afferent and efferent arms of the immune response provides a framework for a basic understanding (see Ch. 3). The afferent arm, or sensitization, refers to the presentation of donor corneal antigens to and their recognition by the recipient. The efferent arm refers to the recipient's response to these antigenic stimuli and results in rejection of the donor cornea.

Cell surface glycoproteins known as major histocompatibility antigens, or human leukocyte antigens (HLA antigens), function as the chief mediators of tissue compatibility between the donor and the recipient. These cell surface markers allow the immune system to distinguish cells that are a normal part of the recipient ("self") from those that are not ("nonself"). Other antigens may also contribute to the antigenicity of a corneal graft, including the minor histocompatibility antigens and ABO blood group antigens. Further studies are needed to better define their role in corneal transplantation immunology.[149]

The HLA antigens are coded by multiallelic genes located on the short arm of chromosome 6, which constitutes the major histocompatibility complex. These genetic loci have been designated HLA-A, HLA-B, and HLA-C (class I antigens) and HLA-D/DR (class II antigens). Class I antigens have been found on almost all nucleated cells in the body, including corneal epithelial, stromal, and endothelial cells.

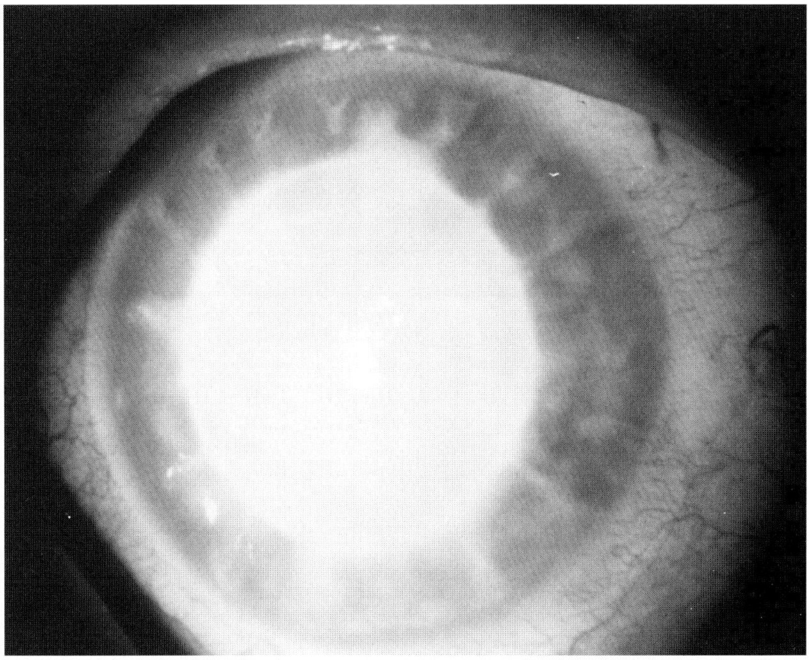

FIGURE 35-10 Totally opaque corneal graft caused by a severe rejection. Note that the recipient cornea is relatively clear.

These antigens interact with a subset of lymphocytes known as cytotoxic T cells, which are primarily responsible for the cellular destruction associated with graft rejection. In contrast, class II antigens are mainly restricted to antigen-presenting cells of the lymphoreticular system, such as B cells, some activated T cells, macrophages and monocytes, and dendritic cells, such as corneal Langerhans cells. The latter are found in highest density within the peripheral corneal epithelium. Under certain stimuli, such as gamma interferon, other corneal cells such as stromal keratocytes and endothelial cells can be induced to express class II antigens. Class II antigens interact with a subset of lymphocytes known as *helper T cells* that respond by secreting a variety of immune stimulators, called *lymphokines*, which perpetuate and accentuate the immune response.

In short, the afferent arm, or sensitization, requires that viable donor cells possessing class II antigens as well as class I antigens and/or minor histocompatibility antigens differing from those of the recipient, come into contact with lymphocyte subpopulations of the recipient capable of generating an immune response. This may be isolated in time from the subsequent efferent or graft rejection arm, which involves sensitized lymphocytes and possibly antibodies coming into contact with and reacting to donor antigen in a cell-mediated-type immune response.

It is widely accepted that corneal graft rejection should be diagnosed only after an initial 10- to 14-day period of postoperative graft clarity. Although this is generally true because of the time required for sensitization to occur, prior sensitization to graft antigens may theoretically result in a hyperacute rejection episode. The 10- to 14-day concept can usually be relied on, however, to differentiate corneal graft rejection from other causes of early graft failure, such as primary donor failure. Conversely, although the highest incidence of rejection occurs within the first year postoperatively, rejection has been reported decades after otherwise successful penetrating keratoplasty.[40]

Clinical Features of Corneal Graft Rejection

By transplanting individual layers of the cornea in rabbits, Khodadoust and Silverstein[150] first demonstrated that the epithelium, stroma, and endothelium could separately undergo immunologic rejection. Clinical correlates of these individual types of rejection have since been documented in humans. In addition, subepithelial infiltrates have been described as a fourth type of rejection.[151] Most rejection episodes do not fall into discrete categories but represent various combinations of the above.[152]

Epithelial Rejection Epithelial rejection appears as an elevated, undulating line that stains with fluorescein or rose bengal (Figure 35-11). The line often starts near a blood vessel at the graft-recipient junction, and represents a zone of donor epithelial destruction by leukocytes. Untreated, the line marches across the surface of the graft over several days to weeks; the area in its wake is replaced by recipient epithelium. In a retrospective study of post-keratoplasty patients followed for a minimum of 1 year, the frequency of epithelial rejection was 10 percent, with an average time to onset of 3 months after surgery.[152]

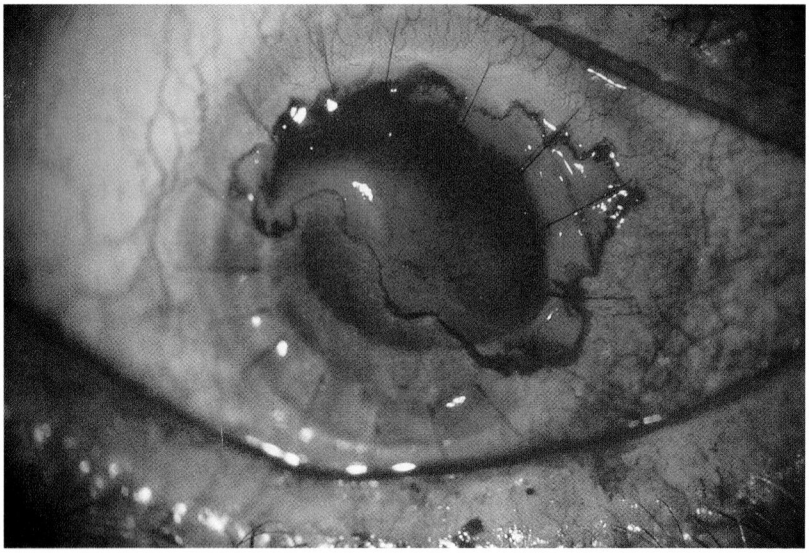

FIGURE 35-11 Rose bengal staining of an epithelial rejection line. (Courtesy of John W. Chandler, M.D., Bellingham, WA.)

Although epithelial rejections are usually asymptomatic and self limited, treatment with topical corticosteroids is indicated because an epithelial rejection may portend a subsequent, more serious endothelial rejection.

Subepithelial Infiltrates Subepithelial infiltrates as a manifestation of corneal graft rejection resemble those seen with epidemic keratoconjunctivitis except that they are confined to the graft (Figure 35-12). The infiltrates are 0.2 to 0.5 mm in diameter, white, and randomly distributed beneath Bowman's layer. The infiltrates are best seen by slit lamp microscopy with broad beam illumination from the side. Mild anterior chamber inflammation may be present. Subepithelial infiltrates usually clear with topical corticosteroid therapy but may leave faint scars. In a retrospective study, the frequency of subepithelial infiltrates was 15 percent, with an average time to onset of 10 months after surgery.[152] As with epithelial rejection, the infiltrates are usually asymptomatic but should be treated with topical corticosteroids because they may be a sign of a more generalized, low-grade immunologic rejection.

Stromal Rejection Stromal rejection as an isolated phenomenon is usually not seen because it is commonly overshadowed by concurrent rejection of the endothelium.

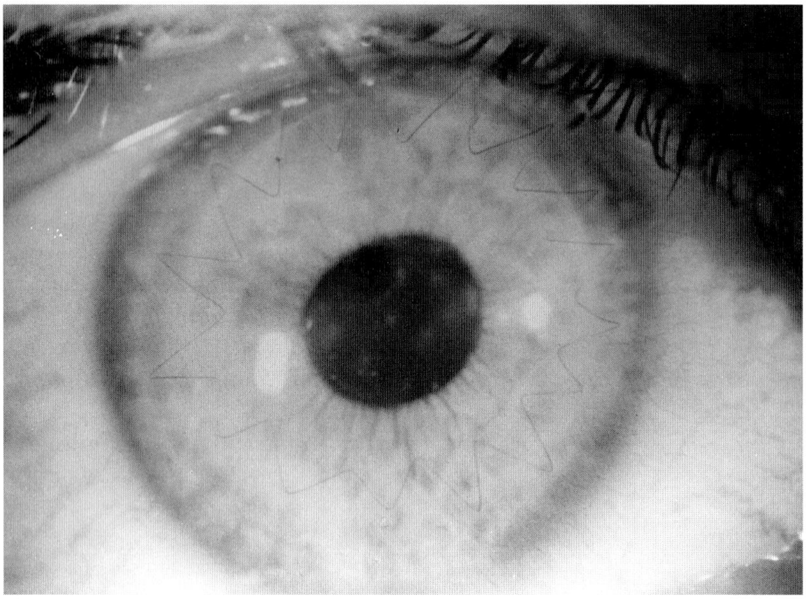

FIGURE 35-12 Subepithelial infiltrates caused by corneal graft rejection.

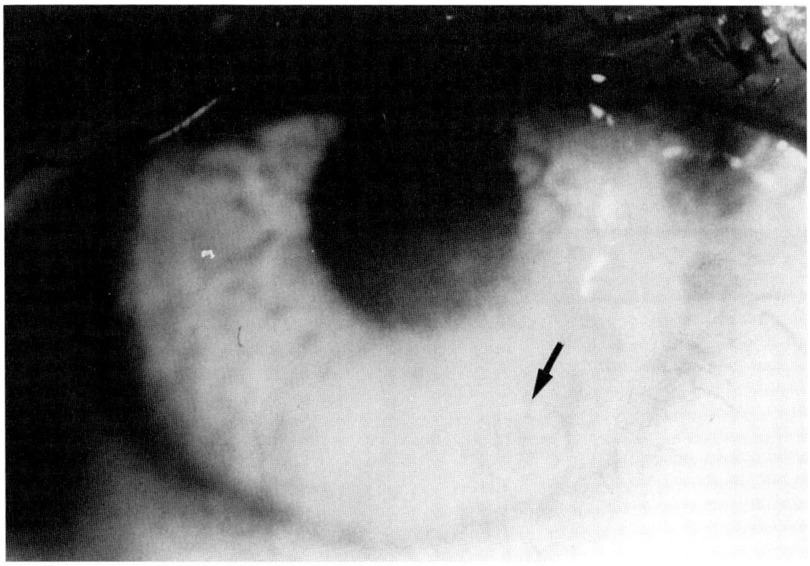

FIGURE 35-13 Stromal rejection. Note the stromal haze adjacent to an area of vascularization (arrow). (Courtesy of John W. Chandler, M.D., Bellingham, WA.)

Nonetheless, isolated stromal rejection has been described as the sudden onset of peripheral, full-thickness corneal haze, usually located near corneal blood vessels, associated with circumcorneal hyperemia[153] (Figure 35-13). Histologically, leukocytes are seen invading the stroma with destruction of the epithelial basement membrane. The reaction may progress centrally if not treated.

Endothelial Rejection Endothelial rejection is the most significant type of corneal graft rejection because it can lead to graft failure. The incidence varies greatly, depending on the patient population and risk factors. Symptoms include decreased visual acuity, which is the most sensitive indicator, redness, pain, photophobia, and tearing.[154] Examination typically reveals a thickened cornea.[155] In some cases, increased corneal thickness is the only sign of rejection. In other cases, the posterior surface of the graft may have either a diffuse scattering of pigmented keratic precipitates or a line of pigmented keratic precipitates (endothelial rejection line or Khodadoust line). An endothelial rejection line usually originates at a vascularized area of the peripheral donor cornea or near a peripheral anterior synechia. If untreated, the endothelial rejection line can march across the graft within days. In general, keratic precipitates represent localized collections of lymphocytes and are associated with destruction of the endothelial cells of the graft. The resultant compromised regulation of corneal hydration is manifested as corneal edema, either diffusely throughout the graft or in the area behind an advancing endothelial rejection line (Figure 35-14). If an adequate view through the edematous graft is possible, mild to moderate anterior chamber inflammation can usually be seen. Elevated intraocular pressure may also be associated with an endothelial rejection.[40,152]

Treatment of Corneal Graft Rejection

Treatment of any allograft rejection is more likely to be successful if the rejection is diagnosed early. Epithelial, subepithelial, and stromal rejections should be treated because they portend a possible endothelial rejection. Topical 1 percent prednisolone acetate or 0.1 percent dexamethasone sodium phosphate eye drops are used at least four times a day and are tapered over 1 month. This contrasts with the more aggressive treatment needed for an endothelial rejection. Although there are no studies proving one treatment regimen superior to others, many clinicians treat an endothelial rejection with topical corticosteroid eye drops every hour while the patient is awake along with 0.05 percent dexamethasone sodium phosphate ointment at bedtime. The corticosteroids are tapered over several weeks to months, depending on the response. In patients with no history of corticosteroid-induced glaucoma or herpes simplex keratitis, a sub-Tenon's injection of methylprednisolone acetate is given. Prednisone at a dosage of 1 mg/kg/day may be given orally in conjunction with the above therapy if the rejection is severe and there are no contraindications. The prednisone is tapered over 1 to 2 weeks. A recent prospective trial demonstrated a lower rate of repeat graft rejection and a higher rate of graft survival in patients with an endothelial rejection treated within 8 days of the onset of rejection with a single intravenous dose of methylprednisolone (500 mg) compared to a tapering dose of oral prednisone (60 to 80 mg); both were added to the same topical corticosteroid treatment regimen.[156] The probability of reversing an endothelial rejection varies from 50 to 91 percent, depending on the severity of the rejection, risk factors, and onset of treatment.[40]

If the signs of an endothelial rejection do not improve within 3 to 4 weeks on maximum topical therapy, further

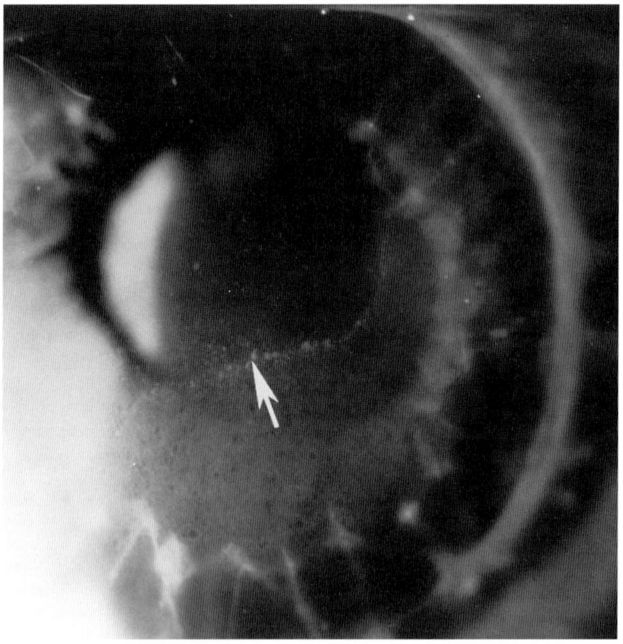

FIGURE 35-14 Endothelial rejection line advancing across the donor cornea in the direction of the arrow. Note the overlying epithelial microcystic edema. (Courtesy of John W. Chandler, M.D., Bellingham, WA.)

treatment is unlikely to help and the graft is pronounced failed. In this case, the topical corticosteroids are tapered to a maintenance dose of one drop two to four times a day until penetrating keratoplasty is repeated. Chronic low-dose topical corticosteroids help prevent corneal neovascularization that would lessen the chance for a successful repeat transplant. If the endothelial rejection responds to treatment and the eye is aphakic or pseudophakic and does not have glaucoma, topical corticosteroids are continued at a dosage of at least one drop per day indefinitely as long as corticosteroid-induced glaucoma does not occur.

Other drugs have been clinically evaluated for the prevention and treatment of allograft rejections in high-risk patients. Systemic antimetabolites, such as azathioprine, are potent immunosuppressive agents but have potentially fatal side effects. Because a corneal graft rejection is not a threat to systemic health, the risks of using these drugs appear to outweigh the benefits.[40] In contrast, cyclosporine[157–161] and the newer drugs FK-506[162] and rapamycin[163] are promising immunosuppressive agents that lack the myelosuppressive hazards of antimetabolites.

Cyclosporine is a neutral, lipophilic, cyclic peptide metabolite of the fungus *Tolypocladium inflatum* Gams. It interferes with the early stage of antigenic sensitization and subsequent proliferation of immunocompetent T cells by, at least in part, preventing the production of lymphokines (e.g., interleukin-2 and gamma interferon) at the DNA/RNA level.[164] Unlike corticosteroids and antimetabolites, which affect almost all elements of the immune system in a shotgun fashion, cyclosporine is mainly T-cell specific. Although cyclosporine has greatly decreased the risk/benefit ratio for treating major organ transplant patients, the toxic effects on the nervous system, liver, and kidneys are a concern.[165]

Because cyclosporine has shown such dramatic success in preventing allograft rejection associated with major organ transplantation, its potential role in high-risk corneal transplantation is currently under investigation. A recent prospective study in high-risk (vascularized) graft patients showed an improved rate of graft survival when oral cyclosporine was added prophylactically to a regimen of topical and/or oral corticosteroids.[166] It was also noted that patients treated for 4 months with oral cyclosporine demonstrated the same improved graft survival as those treated for 1 year. No permanent side effects from the cyclosporine therapy were noted.

In an attempt to avoid the potential systemic toxicity of cyclosporine, topical administration of cyclosporine has stimulated much interest. Because cyclosporine is a high molecular weight, lipid-soluble molecule, the corneal epithelium presents a significant barrier to drug penetration. The vehicle in which the drug is dissolved affects the amount of drug delivered to the cornea and anterior chamber. This fact probably accounts for the variable success rates reported when topical cyclosporine has been tested in animal models of graft rejection.[40] For example, increased cyclosporine levels in rabbit corneas, associated with increased efficacy in preventing graft rejections, were demonstrated with the corneal penetration enhancer Azone.[167] In addition, delivery of cyclosporine to rabbit corneas by collagen shields showed superior efficacy compared to delivery by topical drops containing cyclosporine dissolved in olive oil.[168] Despite the known delivery limitations, however, pilot studies in humans using cyclosporine dissolved in olive or other oils for high-risk grafts have demonstrated promising results. Except for a transient epitheliopathy, no adverse ocular side effects have been reported.[164,169,170] Although a major goal of topical therapy is to avoid systemic dosing, one of these studies showed significant blood levels of cyclosporine after long-term topical administration.[164]

Prevention of Corneal Graft Rejection

Much work has been done in an attempt to identify relevant risk factors for corneal graft rejection. On the basis of previous experimental and/or clinical evidence, probable risk factors include corneal vascularization and previous graft failure. Possible risk factors include young recipient age, excessively large or eccentric grafts, and HLA mismatching. Unlikely risk factors include bilateral grafts, the presence of donor epithelium, donor-recipient sex or race disparity, prior blood transfusion or pregnancy, recent immunization, and corneal preservation methods.[40] Discussion of the more important risk factors follows.

In general, multiple studies support a correlation between the incidence of corneal graft rejection (or graft survival) and the extent of stromal vascularization.[40] Presumably, this correlation is related to enhanced exposure of donor corneal antigens to the systemic circulation and lymphatics. Stromal vessels may develop in a variety of settings, such as previous graft failure, persistent epithelial defect, infection, chemical burn, contact lens wear, and corneal sutures. In contrast with deep corneal vessels, superficial vessels are less likely to incite an immune reaction. Timely removal of sutures and appropriate administration of topical corticosteroids for inflammation are prophylactic measures that help prevent vascularization of the graft.

Use of an argon blue-green or yellow dye laser to photocoagulate stromal vessels, either in the recipient before transplantation or postoperatively in the donor, has been advocated.[171] Although stromal vessels can readily be destroyed with this technique, the vessels usually recur within several weeks, possibly as a result of failure to identify and photocoagulate all small feeder and collateral vessels. Nonetheless, one advantage of photocoagulation of a vascularized recipient cornea just before penetrating keratoplasty is reduction of bleeding during trephination. Further, photocoagulation may be a useful adjunct in the treatment of corneal graft rejection associated with deep stromal vascularization.[171,172]

Although patients with a previous corneal graft failure are considered to be at greater risk of corneal graft rejection than patients who have not had a previous graft failure, the reason is not entirely clear. One possible explanation is sensitization to HLA antigens present in previous grafts. However, because of the large number of HLA antigen types, it is improbable that two grafts will have any HLA types in common. More likely, conditions associated with previous graft failure contribute to higher rejection rates in subsequent grafts. These factors may include inflammation, infection, or, as mentioned above, stromal vascularization.[173]

With major organ transplantation, disparity between donor and recipient HLA antigens is thought to be the predominant basis for allograft rejection, necessitating the routine use of immunosuppressive therapy. Also, it is well known that an accelerated major organ allograft rejection is more likely to occur in the presence of preformed antibodies to HLA donor antigens or ABO blood group incompatibility. Although corneal tissue expresses these antigens, the overall high success rate of corneal transplantation compared with that for other tissues has been attributed to its avascular "immune privilege." However, because vascularized and other high-risk grafts presumably lose this advantage, the possibility that HLA antigen matching may improve corneal graft survival has been the subject of much investigation.[40,173]

Early studies on the effects of matching HLA-A, HLA-B, and HLA-DR antigens on the incidence of immunologic rejection episodes and graft failure resulted in variable conclusions, but the consensus was that HLA antigens are important factors in corneal graft rejection, although the importance of ABO blood group matching was less certain. The findings that formed the basis for this consensus must be viewed with caution, however, because of less-than-ideal study designs and methodologies. Small numbers of patients, retrospective designs, lack of adequate controls, limited or unspecified follow-up, and invalid statistical methods, especially lack of actuarial analysis when variable follow-up time is present, represent some of the difficulties. In addition, a lack of standardization in patient selection and postoperative corticosteroid use complicates comparisons. Because of these limitations, a multicenter, prospective randomized controlled clinical trial, called the *Collaborative Corneal Transplantation Study*, was designed to address the question of whether matching HLA-A, HLA-B and/or HLA-DR antigens, donor-recipient crossmatching, or ABO compatibility affects the outcome of penetrating keratoplasty in high-risk patients. In this study, high-risk patients were defined as those with two or more quadrants of corneal stromal vascularization and/or a history of previous graft rejection. The results showed that matching for HLA-A, HLA-B, or HLA-DR antigens had no effect on overall graft survival, the incidence of irreversible rejection, or the incidence of rejection episodes in high-risk patients.[40,173]

The authors stated reasons why these results may have differed from those of previous studies that showed an influence of HLA type. First, the more intensive postoperative immunosuppression used in the study as well as the extremely diligent follow-up and high patient compliance rate may have negated any effect of HLA matching. This theory is further supported by the unusually low graft failure rate (28 percent) at 2 years from all causes compared to the predicted failure rate (45 percent) from rejection in these high-risk patients. Second, assignment of HLA specificities using current serologic techniques is known to be difficult and subject to error with highly diverse donor and recipient groups, as were present in the study. Third, any unrecognized effect of other antigens, such as those associated with the minor histocompatibility system or other HLA alleles, could not be controlled for.

The Collaborative Corneal Transplantation Study found that among recipients with detectable preoperative lymphocytotoxic antibodies, a positive preoperative donor-recipient crossmatch did not significantly increase the risk of a poor outcome, unlike with major organ transplantation. Induced alloimmunity caused by prior exposure to graft antigens was offered by the authors as a possible explanation.

A final finding of the Collaborative Corneal Transplantation Study was that ABO blood group matching had a beneficial effect on graft outcome. Although the mechanism for this phenomenon remains speculative, evidence suggests that this may be an indirect effect and that the ABO antigens themselves are not the immune system target. Whatever the mechanism, any beneficial effect of ABO matching on graft survival would prove a major public health advantage because donor and recipient matching for ABO compatibility is relatively easy and inexpensive compared to HLA matching. Furthermore, approximately 70 percent of donor and recipient pairs would be compatible by chance alone, thus allowing a plentiful supply of compatible donor tissue.

Recurrence of Recipient Corneal Disorders in Grafts

Visual clouding from a corneal dystrophy is a relatively common indication for penetrating keratoplasty, and additional surgery may be necessary years to decades later because of a recurrence of the dystrophy in the graft. Reis-Bücklers' dystrophy may recur 10 to 15 years after penetrating keratoplasty.[174,175] All three classic stromal dystrophies have been reported to recur, usually within a decade after penetrating keratoplasty, with lattice dystrophy recurring more often than macular or granular dystrophy.[176–178] Reappearance of central crystalline dystrophy has also been reported.[40] In general, the mechanism for these phenomena may involve diffusion of recipient metabolites and/or migration of recipient keratocytes into the graft stroma. This is consistent with the fact that recurrences appear initially in the graft periphery and are more commonly seen in grafts of smaller diameter.[176] Therapy usually involves repeat penetrating keratoplasty, but superficial keratectomy and excimer laser phototherapeutic keratectomy are possible alternatives when recurrences are superficial.[179,180]

Of the posterior corneal dystrophies, recurrent posterior polymorphous dystrophy may cause a membrane-like formation on the posterior surface of the graft within 1 to 2 years after penetrating keratoplasty. The cause may involve resurfacing of Descemet's membrane by abnormal recipient endothelial cells. For two reported cases, eventual regrafting was necessary because of corneal clouding and edema.[181] With Fuchs' endothelial dystrophy, the data suggesting recurrence are less clear. The long-term prognosis for a successful graft in these patients is excellent, however, and any guttae noted in the graft after several years may simply be the result of a latent dystrophy or degeneration in the donor tissue itself.

Astigmatism

A clear graft may be an optical failure if high astigmatism limits visual acuity. Overall, mean postkeratoplasty astigmatism as measured by keratometry averages approximately 4.5 to 5.0 diopters, with approximately 10 percent of grafts having more than 5.0 to 6.0 diopters.[182] High postoperative astigmatism occurs more frequently in eyes with keratoconus, severe scarring, or other conditions with high preoperative toricity or uneven rigidity.

Many of the steps involved in penetrating keratoplasty are thought to influence the final refractive outcome. For example, it has been estimated that pressure on the globe by an eyelid speculum may induce up to 6 diopters of astigmatism.[183] Tight or uneven suturing of the scleral support ring may cause a significant amount of corneal distortion, as evidenced by an oval or peaked recipient corneal opening after trephination.[184] For this reason, some surgeons choose not to use a scleral support ring at all, or to use a ring only for eyes in which there is little or no scleral support, such as aphakic and pediatric eyes.

During trephination, the surgeon must ensure that the trephine is perpendicular to the cornea and guard against inadvertent deformation of the globe. Incision of the recipient cornea with a damaged or dull trephine or with a trephine containing an obturator that compresses a conical or malformed cornea may result in an irregular cut.[185] In keratoconus, use of cautery to shrink the cone before trephination prevents contact between the obturator and the apex of the cone and allows inclusion of more abnormal corneal tissue within the incision. Numerous trephines have been developed in an attempt to produce a more regular incision. Some of these trephines, such as the Barron radial vacuum trephine, fixate the cornea by suction and appear to be superior. Accurate, noncontact trephination with an excimer laser has also been reported.[186] Excision of the recipient corneal button after the trephine incision has been made is a relatively inaccurate procedure and perhaps the major cause of postoperative astigmatism.

In securing the graft, the second suture is crucial because it determines corneal tissue distribution. Failure to place this suture exactly 180 degrees from the first suture in both the donor cornea and recipient corneal rim causes torsion of the graft and postoperative astigmatism. Trephines that mark the recipient cornea and donor cornea for even suture placement, such as the Barron radial vacuum trephine and Barron vacuum donor cornea punch, are available. In addition to being radial, the sutures should be perpendicular to the wound, which provides maximum strength with minimal distortion of the wound.[187]

If the depth of the sutures is not equal in the graft and recipient cornea, the edge of the graft will protrude anteriorly or sink posteriorly when the suture is tightened. Sutures of unequal depth distort the graft and cause misalignment of the anterior surfaces of the graft and recipient cornea; if this misalignment is large, chronic postoperative epithelial defects may occur from uneven tear distribution.

Nonradial sutures can distort the graft and cause astigmatism, as can uneven suture tension. A tight suture causes flattening of the peripheral cornea and steepening of the central cornea in the meridian of the suture. Even when tied with the same tension, long suture bites pull more than short bites.[187]

Intraoperative keratoscopy aids in the evaluation of astigmatism, which can be corrected by replacing one or more interrupted suture(s) or redistributing the tension of a running suture. Before keratoscopy, care is taken to remove all external forces on the eye, such as scleral support rings and eyelid specula. Such suture adjustment appears to reduce postoperative astigmatism in addition to permitting early visual rehabilitation while the sutures are in place.[188]

The influence of graft suturing technique, whether interrupted, single running, double running, or a combination of interrupted and running, has an uncertain correlation with the long-term refractive outcome.[182,189-191] However, early visual rehabilitation while the sutures are still in place is greatly influenced by suture technique.

Although I prefer an adjustable single or double running suture technique, some surgeons advocate the combination of interrupted sutures and a single running suture. Because a running 11-0 nylon or polyester (Mersilene) suture supports the wound, astigmatic error can be reduced early in the healing process by selectively removing one or two interrupted 10-0 nylon sutures at each patient visit.[192] With this method, removal of a tight suture is best guided by a limbus-to-limbus view of the corneal surface, as provided by videokeratography.[193,194] Among the disadvantages of this technique is the increased number of postoperative visits required—a particular burden for patients who must travel some distance to the physician's office.[189] In addition, removal of a tight interrupted suture is an all-or-none phenomenon and has a somewhat unpredictable effect on astigmatism.[190] Finally, problems related to broken sutures, such as irritation, vascularization, microbial keratitis, and graft rejection, may be more likely than with a single or double running suture technique.[189,192]

With double running sutures, early visual rehabilitation is achieved by removal of the 10-0 suture about 3 months after surgery, which improves vision by reducing irregular astigmatism. The amount of regular astigmatism may increase or decrease, however. With the wound secured by the remaining 11-0 suture, a stable refraction is usually achieved 1 month after the 10-0 suture is removed. This is a more practical approach for patients who find it difficult to manage frequent postoperative visits. The lack of control over postoperative astigmatism with this technique is its main disadvantage.[189]

Early significant and titratable reductions in postoperative astigmatism have been achieved with the use of a single running suture technique with intraoperative and/or postoperative adjustment.[195-199] The suture is adjusted by pulling the suture from the flat meridian toward the steep meridian. If necessary, further adjustments can be made on subsequent visits. Usually no extra postoperative visits are required. Suture breakage with subsequent wound dehiscence is a possible complication, and a double running suture with an adjusted 10-0 nylon and an 11-0 polyester suture can be an excellent alternative.

At times, despite all efforts, the surgeon is faced with the need to visually rehabilitate a graft with high residual astigmatism. If spectacles yield good visual acuity, it may be possible to prescribe glasses because graft patients, especially those with keratoconus, are often able to tolerate much larger amounts of spectacle cylinder than are other patients. It is also useful to remember that monocular patients tolerate the meridional magnification produced by highly astigmatic lenses much better than patients with binocular vision. In any event, trial frames can be used to test the patient's ability to tolerate spectacle cylinder.

If glasses do not provide satisfactory acuity or are poorly tolerated, contact lenses are the next option if there are no other contraindications. Although some surgeons prefer to wait 12 to 18 months for wound stabilization before fitting,[200,201] I agree with others[202,203] who fit much earlier in the postoperative course since the presence of sutures (with buried knots) or the use of topical medications is not a contraindication to contact lens wear.[200] In general, a rigid gas-permeable lens should be tried first.[201] If an adequate fit cannot be obtained, other contact lens designs, such as the Soper,[204] Saturn,[204] biaspheric,[205] or piggyback[206] lens, may be tried. Graft patients wearing contact lenses must be monitored closely for complications such as graft neovascularization and infectious keratitis.[207-209] In the absence of other pathology, contact lenses do not appear to increase the incidence of graft rejection.[201]

For patients with high astigmatism who cannot be rehabilitated with spectacles or contact lenses, a variety of surgical options are available. Relaxing incisions,[210-212] arcuate keratotomy,[213] and transverse keratotomy[214] are flattening procedures that are performed in the steep meridian. Compression sutures[215] and wedge resection[212,216,217] are steepening procedures that are performed in the flat meridian. An additive effect may be achieved by combining relaxing incisions with compression sutures.[218] These procedures are discussed in Chapter 38. Another option for the treatment of postkeratoplasty astigmatism is excimer laser photoastigmatic refractive keratectomy, which is discussed in Chapter 42. Photoastigmatic refractive keratectomy, when usable, can often reduce ametropia and permit tolerance of spectacle correction if spectacles cannot be eliminated entirely.

Transmission of Donor Disease

Transmission of disease in donor tissue is discussed in Chapter 33. Most diseases with documented transmission by penetrating keratoplasty fall into the infectious category. Localized bacterial and fungal infections are the most commonly reported, but systemic infections with viral agents represent the greatest hazard. Among the viral diseases transmittable by major organ and/or corneal transplantation are rabies, Creutzfeldt-Jakob disease,[219] and hepatitis B.[220] Viruses known to be transmitted by major organ transplantation but not by corneal transplantation include cytomegalovirus[221,222] and Epstein-Barr virus.[223,224] Human immunodeficiency virus (HIV)[52,220,225] also appears to be in this group, but data are few and potential donors with any risk factors for HIV are excluded. The question of transmission of herpes simplex virus is still unanswered.[12,223] Neurologic diseases for which a viral cause is possible but unproved are exclusions for tissue donation; among these are donor death from a central nervous system disease of unknown etiology, Reyes syndrome, subacute sclerosing panencephalitis, and progressive multifocal leukoencephalopathy.[223]

The only neoplastic disease that has been transmitted via corneal tissue is retinoblastoma.[226] Owing to a possible etiologic link between various viruses and some hematologic cancers, such as blast-form leukemia and Hodgkin's disease, these diseases theoretically pose a higher risk for transmission than other systemic cancers and are therefore considered donor contraindications.[223]

Although unreported, corneal disorders such as anterior and posterior membrane dystrophies, as well as keratoconus, may escape detection and thus may not be excluded from the donor pool. However, with the use of specular microscopy and careful examination of donor tissue, detection and exclusion of at least the major stromal dystrophies or late stages of other disorders before transplantation is likely.[223]

REFERENCES

1. Ingraham HM, Donnenfeld ED, Perry HD: Massive suprachoroidal hemorrhage in penetrating keratoplasty. Am J Ophthalmol 108:670, 1989
2. Price FW Jr, Whitson WE, Ahad KA, Tavakkoli H: Suprachoroidal hemorrhage in penetrating keratoplasty. Ophthalmic Surg 25:521, 1994
3. Reynolds MG, Haimovici R, Flynn HW Jr, et al: Suprachoroidal hemorrhage. Clinical features and results of secondary surgical management. Ophthalmology 100:460, 1993
4. Purcell JJ Jr, Krachmer JH, Doughman DJ, Bourne WM: Expulsive hemorrhage in penetrating keratoplasty. Ophthalmology 89:41, 1982
5. Dohlman C: The function of the corneal epithelium in health and disease. Invest Ophthalmol 10:383, 1971
6. Keates RH, Shriver PA, Gordon J, Shimizu RW: Management of epithelial and wound healing problems after penetrating keratoplasty. Refract Corneal Surg 7:73, 1991
7. Kandarakis AS, Page C, Kaufman HE: The effect of epidermal growth factor on epithelial healing after penetrating keratoplasty in human eyes. Am J Ophthalmol 98:411, 1984
8. Meyer RF, Bobb KC: Corneal epithelium in penetrating keratoplasty. Am J Ophthalmol 90:142, 1980
9. Kim T, Palay DA, Lynn M: Donor factors associated with epithelial defects after penetrating keratoplasty. Cornea 15:451, 1996
10. Beyer CF, Hill JM, Byrd TJ, Kaufman HE: Herpes simplex dendritic keratitis after keratoplasty [letter]. Am J Ophthalmol 112:355, 1991
11. Mannis MJ, Plotnik RD, Schwab IR, Newton R: Herpes simplex dendritic keratitis after keratoplasty. Am J Ophthalmol 111:480, 1991
12. Beyer CF, Byrd TJ, Hill JM, Kaufman HE: Herpes simplex virus and persistent epithelial defects after penetrating keratoplasty. Am J Ophthalmol 109:95, 1990
13. Ruffini JJ, Aquavella JV, LoCascio JA: Effect of collagen shields on corneal epithelialization following penetrating keratoplasty. Ophthalmic Surg 20:21, 1989
14. Groden LR, White W: Porcine collagen corneal shield treatment of persistent epithelial defects following penetrating keratoplasty. CLAO J 16:95, 1990
15. Sugar A, Meyer RF, Bahn CF: A randomized trial of pressure patching for epithelial defects after keratoplasty. Am J Ophthalmol 95:637, 1983
16. Smiddy WE, Hamburg TR, Kracher G, et al: Therapeutic contact lenses. Ophthalmology 97:291, 1990
17. Koenig SB, Harris GJ: Temporary suture tarsorrhaphy after penetrating keratoplasty. Cornea 10:121, 1991

18. Feldman ST: The effect of epidermal growth factor on corneal wound healing: practical considerations for therapeutic use. Refract Corneal Surg 7:232, 1991
19. Pfister RR: Clinical measures to promote corneal epithelial healing. Acta Ophthalmol (Copenh) 202(suppl):73, 1992
20. Turgeon PW, Nauheim RC, Roat MI, et al: Indications for keratoepithelioplasty. Arch Ophthalmol 108:233, 1990
21. Kloess PM, Stulting RD, Waring GO, Wilson LA: Bacterial and fungal endophthalmitis after penetrating keratoplasty. Am J Ophthalmol 115:309, 1993
22. Aiello LP, Javitt JC, Canner JK: National outcome of penetrating keratoplasty. Risks of endophthalmitis and retinal detachment. Arch Ophthalmol 111:509, 1993
23. Guss RB, Koenig S, De La Pena W, et al: Endophthalmitis after penetrating keratoplasty. Am J Ophthalmol 95:651, 1983
24. Leveille AS, McMullan FD, Cavanagh HD: Endophthalmitis following penetrating keratoplasty. Ophthalmology 90:38, 1983
25. Steinemann TL, Kaufman HE, Beuerman RW, et al: Vancomycin-enriched corneal storage medium. Am J Ophthalmol 113:555, 1992
26. Lindquist TD, Roth BP, Fritsche TR: Stability and activity of vancomycin in corneal storage media. Cornea 12:222, 1993
27. Hwang DG, Nakamura T, Trousdale MD, Smith TM: Combination antibiotic supplementation of corneal storage medium. Am J Ophthalmol 115:299, 1993
28. Insler MS, Cavanagh HD, Wilson LA: Gentamicin-resistant *Pseudomonas* endophthalmitis after penetrating keratoplasty. Br J Ophthalmol 69:189, 1985
29. Antonios SR, Cameron JA, Badr IA, et al: Contamination of donor cornea: postpenetrating keratoplasty endophthalmitis. Cornea 10:217, 1991
30. Speaker MG, Menikoff JA: Prophylaxis of endophthalmitis with topical povidone-iodine. Ophthalmology 98:1769, 1991
31. Smolin G, Biswell R: Corneal graft rejection associated with anterior iris adhesion: case report. Ann Ophthalmol 10;1603, 1978
32. Tragakis MP, Brown SI: The significance of anterior synechiae after corneal transplantation. Am J Ophthalmol 74:532, 1972
33. Snyder RW, Sherman MD, Allinson RW: Intracameral tissue plasminogen activator for treatment of excessive fibrin response after penetrating keratoplasty. Am J Ophthalmol 109:483, 1990
34. Heidemann DG, Williams GA, Blumenkranz MS: Tissue plasminogen activator and penetrating keratoplasty. Ophthalmic Surg 21:364, 1990
35. Kaufman HE, West CE, Wood TO, Wind CA: Measurement and control of intraocular pressure in corneal disease. Int Ophthalmol Clin 10:397, 1970
36. Beebe WE: Management of glaucoma in penetrating keratoplasty patients. Refract Corneal Surg 7:67, 1991
37. Alpar JJ: The use of Healon in corneal transplant surgery with and without intraocular lenses. Ophthalmic Surg 15:757, 1974
38. Burke S, Sugar J, Farber MD: Comparison of the effects of two viscoelastic agents, Healon and Viscoat, on postoperative intraocular pressure after penetrating keratoplasty. Ophthalmic Surg 21:821, 1990
39. Olson RJ, Kaufman HE: A mathematical description of causative factors and prevention of elevated intraocular pressure after keratoplasty. Invest Ophthalmol Vis Sci 16:1085, 1977
40. Wilson SE, Kaufman HE: Graft failure after penetrating keratoplasty. Surv Ophthalmol 34:325, 1990
41. Heidemann DG, Sugar A, Meyer RF, Musch DC: Oversized donor grafts in penetrating keratoplasty. A randomized trial. Arch Ophthalmol 103:1807, 1985
42. Bourne WM, Davison JA, O'Fallon WM: The effects of oversize donor buttons on postoperative intraocular pressure and corneal curvature in aphakic penetrating keratoplasty. Ophthalmology 89:242, 1982
43. Lewis RA, Phelps CD: Medical therapy of glaucoma. Ch. 56. In Duane TD, Jaeger EA (eds): Clinical Ophthalmology. Vol. 3. Harper & Row, Philadelphia, 1987
44. Berkowitz RA, Klyce SD, Kaufman HE: Aqueous hyposecretion after penetrating keratoplasty. Ophthalmic Surg 15:323, 1984
45. Ormerod LD, Baerveldt G, Sunalp MA, Riekhof FT: Management of the hypotonous cyclodialysis cleft. Ophthalmology 98:1384, 1991
46. Hay A, Flynn HW Jr, Hoffman JI, Rivera AH: Needle penetration of the globe during retrobulbar and peribulbar injections. Ophthalmology 98:1017, 1991
47. Duker JS, Belmont JB, Benson WE, et al: Inadvertent globe perforation during retrobulbar and peribulbar anesthesia. Patient characteristics, surgical management, and visual outcome. Ophthalmology 98:519, 1991
48. Forstot SL, Binder PS, Fitzgerald C, Kaufman HE: The incidence of retinal detachment after penetrating keratoplasty. Am J Ophthalmol 80:102, 1975
49. Burton TC, Arafat NT, Phelps CD: Intraocular pressure in retinal detachment. Int Ophthalmol 1:147, 1979
50. Wilhelmus KR, Stulting RD, Sugar J, Khan MM: Primary corneal graft failure. A national reporting system. Medical Advisory Board of the Eye Bank Association of America. Arch Ophthalmol 113:1497, 1995
51. Medical Advisory Board: Eye Bank Association of America Medical Standards, October, 1996. Eye Bank Association of America, Washington, DC
52. Wilson S: Corneal preservation. Surv Ophthalmol 33:248, 1989
53. Fong LP, Ormerod LD, Kenyon KR, Foster CS: Microbial keratitis complicating penetrating keratoplasty. Ophthalmology 95:1269, 1988
54. Templeton WC III, Eiferman RA, Snyder JW, et al: *Serratia* keratitis transmitted by contaminated eyedroppers. Am J Ophthalmol 93:723, 1982
55. Bates AK, Kirkness CM, Ficker LA, et al: Microbial keratitis after penetrating keratoplasty. Eye 4:74, 1990
56. al-Hazza SA, Tabbara KF: Bacterial keratitis after penetrating keratoplasty. Ophthalmology 95:1504, 1988

57. Laflamme MY, Poisson M, Chehade N: *Mycobacterium chelonei* keratitis following penetrating keratoplasty. Can J Ophthalmol 22:178, 1987
58. Sossi N, Feldman RM, Feldman ST, et al: *Mycobacterium gordonae* keratitis after penetrating keratoplasty. Arch Ophthalmol 109:1064, 1991
59. Parrish CM, Head WS, O'Day DM, Rowlett W: *Acanthamoeba* keratitis following keratoplasty without other identifiable risk factors. Arch Ophthalmol 109:471, 1991
60. Hill JC: Use of penetrating keratoplasty in acute bacterial keratitis. Br J Ophthalmol 70:502, 1986
61. Kirkness CM, McSteel AD, Rice NS: Penetrating keratoplasty in the management of suppurative keratitis. Dev Ophthalmol 18:172, 1989
62. Sanders N: Penetrating keratoplasty in treatment of fungus keratitis. Am J Ophthalmol 70:24, 1970
63. Kozarsky AM, Stulting RD, Waring GO, et al: Penetrating keratoplasty for exogenous *Paecilomyces* keratitis followed by postoperative endophthalmitis. Am J Ophthalmol 98:552, 1984
64. Kirkness CM, Ficker LA, Steel AD, Rice NS: The role of penetrating keratoplasty in the management of microbial keratitis. Eye 5:425, 1991
65. Peterson RJ, Smith ME, Pepose JS: Recurrent *Acanthamoeba* keratitis following penetrating keratoplasty. Arch Ophthalmol 108:1482, 1990
66. Varley GA, Meisler DM: Complications of penetrating keratoplasty: graft infections. Refract Corneal Surg 7:62, 1991
67. Ficker LA, Kirkness C, Wright P: Prognosis for keratoplasty in *Acanthamoeba* keratitis. Ophthalmology 100:105, 1993
68. Sutton GL, Miller RC, Robinson LP: Infectious crystalline keratopathy. Aust N Z J Ophthalmol 18:151, 1990
69. Pararajasegaram P, Mower G, Barras CW, Coster DJ: An unusual case of crystalline keratopathy. Aust N Z J Ophthalmol 18:155, 1990
70. Ormerod LD, Ruoff KL, Meisler DM, et al: Infectious crystalline keratopathy. Role of nutritionally variant streptococci and other bacterial factors. Ophthalmology 98:159, 1991
71. Lam S, Meisler DM, Krachmer J: Enterococcal infectious crystalline keratopathy. Cornea 12:273, 1993
72. Lubniewski AJ, Houchin KW, Holland EJ: Posterior infectious crystalline keratopathy with *Staphylococcus epidermidis*. Ophthalmology 97:1454, 1990
73. Eiferman RA, Forgey DR, Cook YD: Excimer laser ablation of infectious crystalline keratopathy. Arch Ophthalmol 110:18, 1992
74. Fine M, Cignetti FE: Penetrating keratoplasty in herpes simplex keratitis. Recurrence in grafts. Arch Ophthalmol 95:613, 1977
75. Moyes AL, Sugar A, Musch DC, Barnes RD: Antiviral therapy after penetrating keratoplasty for herpes simplex keratitis. Arch Ophthalmol 112:601, 1994
76. Barney NP, Foster CS: A prospective randomized trial of oral acyclovir after penetrating keratoplasty for herpes simplex keratitis. Cornea 13:232, 1994
77. van Rooij J, Rijneveld WJ, Remeijer LJ, Beekhuis WH: A retrospective study on the effectiveness of oral acyclovir to prevent herpes simplex recurrence in corneal grafts. Eur J Ophthalmol 5:214, 1995
78. Simon AL, Pavan-Langston D: Long-term oral acyclovir therapy. Effect on recurrent infectious herpes simplex keratitis in patients with and without grafts. Ophthalmology 103:1399, 1996
79. Epstein RJ, Seedor JA, Dreizen NG, et al: Penetrating keratoplasty for herpes simplex keratitis and keratoconus. Allograft rejection and survival. Ophthalmology 94:935, 1987
80. Killingsworth DW, Stern GA, Driebe WT, et al: Results of therapeutic penetrating keratoplasty. Ophthalmology 100:534, 1993
81. Forstot SL, Abel R Jr, Binder PS: Bacterial endophthalmitis following suture removal after penetrating keratoplasty. Am J Ophthalmol 80:509, 1975
82. Weiss JL, Nelson JD, Lindstrom RL, Doughman DJ: Bacterial endophthalmitis following penetrating keratoplasty suture removal. Cornea 3:278, 1984
83. Maguire LJ, Franz J, Packer AJ, Kaufman H: Bacterial endophthalmitis associated with vitreous wick after penetrating keratoplasty. Am J Ophthalmol 100:854, 1985
84. Schechter RJ: Suture-wick endophthalmitis with sutured posterior chamber intraocular lenses. J Cataract Refract Surg 16:755, 1990
85. Frueh BE, Feldman ST, Feldman RM: Running nylon suture dissolution after penetrating keratoplasty. Am J Ophthalmol 113:406, 1992
86. Lam S, Tessler HH: Running nylon suture dissolution after penetrating keratoplasty. Am J Ophthalmol 114:240, 1992
87. Olson RJ: Complications associated with running 11-0 nylon suture in penetrating keratoplasty. Ophthalmic Surg 13:558, 1982
88. Farley MK, Pettit TH: Traumatic wound dehiscence after penetrating keratoplasty. Am J Ophthalmol 104:44, 1987
89. Raber IM, Arentsen JJ, Laibson PR: Traumatic wound dehiscence after penetrating keratoplasty. Arch Ophthalmol 98:1407, 1980
90. Topping TM, Stark WJ, Maumenee E, Kenyon KR: Traumatic wound dehiscence following penetrating keratoplasty. Br J Ophthalmol 66:174, 1982
91. Agrawal V, Wagh M, Krishnamachary M, et al: Traumatic wound dehiscence after penetrating keratoplasty. Cornea 14:601, 1995
92. Steinemann TL, Henry K, Brown MF: Nd:YAG laser treatment of retained Descemet's membrane after penetrating keratoplasty. Ophthalmic Surg 26:80, 1995
93. Ferry AP, Madge GE, Mayer W: Epithelialization of the anterior chamber as a complication of penetrating keratoplasty. Ann Ophthalmol 17:414, 1985
94. Leibowitz HM, Elliott JH, Boruchoff SA: Epithelialization of the anterior chamber following penetrating keratoplasty. Arch Ophthalmol 78:613, 1967
95. Claoue C, Lewkowicz-Moss S, Easty D: Epithelial cyst in the anterior chamber after penetrating keratoplasty: a rare complication. Br J Ophthalmol 72:36, 1988

96. Boruchoff SA, Kenyon KR, Foulks GN, Green WR: Epithelial cyst of the iris following penetrating keratoplasty. Br J Ophthalmol 64:440, 1980
97. Kuchle M, Green WR: Epithelial ingrowth: a study of 207 histopathologically proven cases. Ger J Ophthalmol 5:211, 1996
98. Sidrys LA, Demong T: Epithelial downgrowth after penetrating keratoplasty. Can J Ophthalmol 17:29, 1982
99. Fish LA, Heuer DK, Baerveldt G, et al: Molteno implantation for secondary glaucoma associated with advanced epithelial ingrowth. Ophthalmology 97:557, 1990
100. Michels RG, Kenyon KR, Maumenee AE: Retrocorneal fibrous membrane. Invest Ophthalmol 11:822, 1972
101. Foulks GN: Glaucoma associated with penetrating keratoplasty. Ophthalmology 94:871, 1987
102. Kirkness CM, Ficker LA: Risk factors for the development of postkeratoplasty glaucoma. Cornea 11:427, 1992
103. Chien AM, Schmidt CM, Cohen EJ, et al: Glaucoma in the immediate postoperative period after penetrating keratoplasty. Am J Ophthalmol 115:711, 1993
104. Sekhar GC, Vyas P, Nagarajan R, et al: Post-penetrating keratoplasty glaucoma. Indian J Ophthalmol 41:181, 1993
105. Zimmerman T, Olson RJ, Waltman SR, et al: Transplant size and elevated intraocular pressure postkeratoplasty. Arch Ophthalmol 96:2231, 1978
106. Folks G, Perry H, Dohlman C: Oversize corneal donor grafts in penetrating keratoplasty. Ophthalmology 86:490, 1979
107. Perl T, Charlton K, Binder P: Disparate diameter grafting: astigmatism, intraocular pressure, and visual acuity. Ophthalmology 88:774, 1981
108. Motolko MA, Phelps CD: The secondary glaucomas. Ch. 54. In Duane TD, Jaeger EA (eds): Clinical Ophthalmology. Vol. 3. Harper & Row, Philadelphia, 1987
109. Herschler J: Increased intraocular pressure induced by repository corticosteroids. Am J Ophthalmol 82:90, 1976
110. Kirkness CM, Steele AD, Ficker LA, Rice NS: Coexistent corneal disease and glaucoma managed by either drainage surgery and subsequent keratoplasty or combined drainage surgery and penetrating keratoplasty. Br J Ophthalmol 76:146, 1992
111. Wilson RP, Spaeth GL, Poryzees E: The place of timolol in the practice of ophthalmology. Ophthalmology 87:451, 1980
112. Massry GG, Assil KK: Pilocarpine-associated allograft rejection in postkeratoplasty patients. Cornea 14:202, 1995
113. Gilvarry AM, Kirkness CM, Steele AD, et al: The management of post-keratoplasty glaucoma by trabeculectomy. Eye 3:713, 1989
114. Melamed S, Huna R, Avni I: Molteno implant followed by penetrating keratoplasty in corneal graft failure and glaucoma. Ophthalmic Surg 21:670, 1990
115. Insler MS, Cooper HD, Kash PR, Caldwell DR: Penetrating keratoplasty with trabeculectomy. Am J Ophthalmol 100:593, 1985
116. Cohen EJ, Schwartz LW, Luskind RD, et al: Neodymium:YAG laser transscleral cyclophotocoagulation for glaucoma after penetrating keratoplasty. Ophthalmic Surg 20:713, 1989
117. Van Meter WS, Allen RC, Waring GO, Stulting RD: Laser trabeculoplasty for glaucoma in aphakic and pseudophakic eyes after penetrating keratoplasty. Arch Ophthalmol 106:185, 1988
118. Wise JB: Long-term control of adult open angle glaucoma by argon laser treatment. Ophthalmology 88:197, 1981
119. Kirkness CM: Penetrating keratoplasty, glaucoma and silicone drainage tubing. Dev Ophthalmol 14:161, 1987
120. McDonnell PJ, Robin JB, Schanzlin DJ, et al: Molteno implant for control of glaucoma in eyes after penetrating keratoplasty. Ophthalmology 95:364, 1988
121. Beebe WE, Starita RJ, Fellman RL, et al: The use of Molteno implant and anterior chamber tube shunt to encircling band for the treatment of glaucoma in keratoplasty patients. Ophthalmology 97:1414, 1990
122. Sherwood MB, Smith MF, Driebe WT Jr, et al: Drainage tube implants in the treatment of glaucoma following penetrating keratoplasty. Ophthalmic Surg 24:185, 1993
123. Hodkin MJ, Goldblatt WS, Burgoyne CF, et al: Early clinical experience with the Baerveldt implant in complicated glaucomas. Am J Ophthalmol 120:32, 1995
124. Lemp MA, Pfister RR, Dohlman CH: Effect of intraocular surgery on clear corneal grafts. Am J Ophthalmol 70:719, 1970
125. Urrets-Zavalia A: Fixed, dilated pupil, iris atrophy and secondary glaucoma: a distinct clinical entity following penetrating keratoplasty for keratoconus. Am J Ophthalmol 556:257, 1963
126. Gasset AR: Fixed dilated pupil following penetrating keratoplasty in keratoconus (Castroviejo syndrome). Ann Ophthalmol 9:623, 1977
127. Geyer O, Rothkoff L, Lazar M: Atropine in keratoplasty for keratoconus. Cornea 10:372, 1991
128. Tuft SJ, Buckley RJ: Iris ischaemia following penetrating keratoplasty for keratoconus (Urrets-Zavalia syndrome). Cornea 14:618, 1995
129. Nanjiana M: Management of irreversible mydriasis after penetrating keratoplasty. Arch Ophthalmol 95:895, 1977
130. Martin TP, Reed JW, Legault C, et al: Cataract formation and cataract extraction after penetrating keratoplasty. Ophthalmology 101:113, 1994
131. Donshik PC, Cavanagh D, Boruchoff SA, Dohlman CH: Posterior subcapsular cataract induced by topical corticosteroids following keratoplasty for keratoconus. Ann Ophthalmol 13:29, 1981
132. Wood TO, Waltman SR, Kaufman HE: Steroid cataracts following penetrating keratoplasty. Ann Ophthalmol 3:496, 1971
133. Musch DC, Meyer RF, Sugar A, Vine AK: Retinal detachment following penetrating keratoplasty. Arch Ophthalmol 104:617, 1986
134. Sternberg P Jr, Meredith TA, Stewart MA, Kaplan HJ: Retinal detachment in penetrating keratoplasty patients. Am J Ophthalmol 109:148, 1990

135. Bennett SR, Abrams GW: Band keratopathy from emulsified silicone oil. Arch Ophthalmol 108:1387, 1990
136. Beekhuis WH, van Rij G, Zivojnovic R: Silicone oil keratopathy: indications for keratoplasty. Br J Ophthalmol 69:247, 1985
137. Tso MOM: Pathology of cystoid macular edema. Ophthalmology 89:902, 1982
138. Kramer SG: Cystoid macular edema after aphakic penetrating keratoplasty. Ophthalmology 88:782, 1981
139. Nirankari VS, Karesh JW: Cystoid macular edema following penetrating keratoplasty: incidence and prognosis. Ophthalmic Surg 17:404, 1986
140. Jampol LM: Pharmacologic therapy of aphakic cystoid macular edema. A review. Ophthalmology 80:891, 1982
141. Flach AJ: Cyclo-oxygenase inhibitors in ophthalmology. Surv Ophthalmol 36:259, 1992
142. Flach AJ, Stegman RC, Graham J, Kruger LP: Prophylaxis of aphakic cystoid macular edema without corticosteroids. A paired-comparison, placebo-controlled double-masked study. Ophthalmology 97:1253, 1990
143. Flach AJ, Jampol LM, Weinberg D, et al: Improvement in visual acuity in chronic aphakic and pseudophakic cystoid macular edema after treatment with topical 0.5% ketorolac tromethamine. Am J Ophthalmol 112:514, 1991
144. Michels M, Sternberg P: Operating microscope-induced retinal phototoxicity: pathophysiology, clinical manifestations, and prevention. Surv Ophthalmol 34:237, 1990
145. Stamler JF, Blodi CF, Verdier D, Krachmer JH: Microscope light-induced maculopathy in combined penetrating keratoplasty, extracapsular cataract extraction, and intraocular lens implantation. Ophthalmology 95:1142, 1988
146. Cech JM, Choromokos EA, Sanitato JA: Light-induced maculopathy following penetrating keratoplasty and lens implantation. Arch Ophthalmol 105:751, 1987
147. Price FW Jr, Whitson WE, Collins KS, Marks RG: Five-year corneal graft survival. A large, single-center patient cohort. Arch Ophthalmol 111:799, 1993
148. Mader TH, Stulting RD: The high-risk penetrating keratoplasty. Ophthalmol Clin North Am 4:411, 1991
149. Chandler JW: Immunologic considerations in corneal transplantation. p. 725. In Kaufman HE, Barron BA, McDonald MB, Waltman SR (eds): The Cornea. New York, Churchill Livingstone, 1988
150. Khodadoust AA, Silverstein AM: Transplantation and rejection of individual layer of the cornea. Invest Ophthalmol 8:180, 1969
151. Krachmer JH, Alldredge OC: Subepithelial infiltrates: a probable sign of corneal transplant rejection. Arch Ophthalmol 96:2234, 1978
152. Alldredge OC, Krachmer JH: Clinical types of corneal transplant rejection: their manifestations, frequency, preoperative correlates and treatment. Arch Ophthalmol 99:599, 1981
153. Stark WJ: Transplantation immunology of penetrating keratoplasty. Trans Am Ophthalmol Soc 78:1079, 1980
154. Kamp MT, Fink NE, Enger C, et al: Patient-reported symptoms associated with graft reactions in high-risk patients in the collaborative corneal transplantation studies. Collaborative Corneal Transplantation Studies Research Group. Cornea 14:43, 1995
155. McDonnell PJ, Enger C, Stark WJ, Stulting RD, et al: Corneal thickness changes after high-risk penetrating keratoplasty. Collaborative Corneal Transplantation Studies Group. Arch Ophthalmol 111:1374, 1993
156. Hiss JC, Maske R, Watson P: Corticosteroids in corneal graft rejection. Oral versus single pulse therapy. Ophthalmology 98:329, 1991
157. Sundmacher R, Reinhard T, Heering P: Six years' experience with systemic cyclosporin A prophylaxis in high-risk perforating keratoplasty patients. A retrospective study. Ger J Ophthalmol 1:432, 1992
158. Hill JC: Systemic cyclosporine in high-risk keratoplasty. Short- versus long-term therapy. Ophthalmology 101:128, 1994
159. Zhao JC, Jin XY: Local therapy of corneal allograft rejection with cyclosporine. Am J Ophthalmol 119:189, 1995
160. Gebhardt BM, Varnell ED, Kaufman HE: Cyclosporine in collagen particles: corneal penetration and suppression of allograft rejection. J Ocul Pharmacol Ther 11:509, 1995
161. Reinhard T, Sundmacher R, Heering P: Systemic ciclosporin A in high risk keratoplasties. Graefes Arch Clin Exp Ophthalmol 234(suppl 1):S115, 1996
162. Kobayashi C, Kanai A, Nakajima A, Okumura K: Suppression of corneal graft rejection in rabbits by a new immunosuppressive agent, FK-506. Transplant Proc 21:3156, 1989
163. Ohia E, Kulkarni P: Corticosteroids and immunosuppressive agents in rabbit heterolamellar corneal transplant model. Agents Actions 34:165, 1991
164. Belin MW, Bouchard CS, Frantz S, Chmielinska J: Topical cyclosporine in high-risk corneal transplants. Ophthalmology 96:1144, 1989
165. Oates JA, Wood AJJ: Cyclosporin (drug therapy—medical intelligence). N Engl J Med 321:1725, 1989
166. Hill JC: The use of cyclosporine in high-risk keratoplasty. Am J Ophthalmol 107:506, 1989
167. Newton C, Gebhardt BM, Kaufman HE: Topically applied cyclosporine in Azone prolongs corneal allograft survival. Invest Ophthalmol Vis Sci 29:208, 1988
168. Chen YF, Gebhardt BM, Reidy JJ, Kaufman HE: Cyclosporine-containing collagen shields suppress corneal allograft rejection. Am J Ophthalmol 109:132, 1990
169. Goichot-Bonnat L, Chemla P, Pouliquen Y: Cyclosporine A collyre dans la prevention du rejet de greffe de cornee a haut risque. II. Resultats cliniques post-operatoires. J Fr Ophtalmol 10:213, 1987
170. Hoffmann F, Wiederholt M: Topical cyclosporin A in the treatment of corneal graft reaction. Cornea 5:129, 1986
171. Baer JC, Foster CS: Corneal laser photocoagulation for treatment of neovascularization. Efficacy of 577 nm yellow dye laser. Ophthalmology 99:173, 1992
172. Nirankari VS, Baer JC: Corneal argon laser photocoagulation for neovascularization in penetrating keratoplasty. Ophthalmology 93:1304, 1986

173. Collaborative Corneal Transplantation Studies Research Group: The collaborative corneal transplantation studies (CCTS). Effectiveness of histocompatibility matching in high-risk corneal transplantation. Arch Ophthalmol 110:1392, 1992
174. Olson RJ, Kaufman HE: Recurrence of Reis-Bücklers' corneal dystrophy in a graft. Am J Ophthalmol 85:349, 1978
175. Caldwell DR: Post-operative recurrence of Reis-Bücklers' corneal dystrophy. Am J Ophthalmol 85:567, 1978
176. Herman SJ, Hughes WF: Recurrence of hereditary corneal dystrophy following keratoplasty. Am J Ophthalmol 75:689, 1973
177. Akova YA, Kirkness CM, McCartney AC: Recurrent macular corneal dystrophy following penetrating keratoplasty. Eye 4:698, 1990
178. Klintworth GK, Reed J: Recurrence of macular corneal dystrophy within grafts. Am J Ophthalmol 95:60, 1983
179. Talamo JH, Steinert RF, Puliafito CA: Clinical strategies for excimer laser therapeutic keratectomy. Refract Corneal Surg 8:319, 1992
180. McDonnell PJ, Seiler T: Phototherapeutic keratectomy with excimer laser for Reis-Bückler's corneal dystrophy. Refract Corneal Surg 8:306, 1992
181. Boruchoff SA, Weiner MJ, Albert DM: Recurrence of posterior polymorphous corneal dystrophy after penetrating keratoplasty. Am J Ophthalmol 109:323, 1990
182. Swinger CA. Postoperative astigmatism. Surv Ophthalmol 31:219, 1987
183. Olson RJ: Corneal transplantation techniques. p. 743. In Kaufman HE, Barron BA, McDonald MB, Waltman SR (eds): The Cornea. Churchill Livingstone, New York, 1988
184. Olson RJ: The effect of scleral fixation ring placement and trephine tilting on keratoplasty wound size and donor shape. Ophthalmic Surg 12:23, 1981
185. Kaufman HE: Astigmatism after keratoplasty—possible cause and method of prevention. Am J Ophthalmol 94:556, 1982
186. Serdarevic ON, Hanna K Gribomont AC, et al: Excimer laser trephination in penetrating keratoplasty. Morphologic features and wound healing. Ophthalmology 95:493, 1988
187. Eisner G: Eye Surgery. Springer-Verlag, New York, 1980
188. Serdarevic ON, Renard GJ, Pouliquen Y: Randomized clinical trial comparing astigmatism and visual rehabilitation after penetrating keratoplasty with and without intraoperative suture adjustment. Ophthalmology 101:990, 1994
189. Musch DC, Meyer RF, Sugar A, Soong HK: Corneal astigmatism after penetrating keratoplasty. The role of suture technique. Ophthalmology 96:698, 1989
190. Burk LL, Waring GO, Radjee B, Stulting RD: The effect of selective suture removal on astigmatism following penetrating keratoplasty. Ophthalmic Surg 19:849, 1988
191. Musch DC, Meyer RF, Sugar A: The effect of removing running sutures on astigmatism after penetrating keratoplasty. Arch Ophthalmol 106:488, 1988
192. Burk LL, Waring GO, Harris DJ Jr: Simultaneous and sequential selective suture removal to reduce astigmatism after penetrating keratoplasty. Refract Corneal Surg 6;179, 1990
193. Strelow S, Cohen EJ, Leavitt KG, Laibson PR: Corneal topography for selective suture removal after penetrating keratoplasty. Am J Ophthalmol 112:657, 1991
194. Harris DJ Jr, Waring GO, Burk LL: Keratography as a guide to selective suture removal for the reduction of astigmatism after penetrating keratoplasty. Ophthalmology 96:1597, 1989
195. Kaufman HE: Corneal transplant optics and visual disability. Refract Corneal Surg 5:213, 1989
196. Lin DT, Wilson SE, Reidy JJ, et al: An adjustable single running suture technique to reduce postkeratoplasty astigmatism. A preliminary report. Ophthalmology 97:934, 1990
197. McNeill JI, Wessels IF: Adjustment of single continuous suture to control astigmatism after penetrating keratoplasty. Refract Corneal Surg 5:216, 1989
198. Van Meter WS, Gussler JR, Soloman KD, Wood TO: Postkeratoplasty astigmatism control. Single continuous suture adjustment versus selective interrupted suture removal. Ophthalmology 98:177, 1991
199. Nabors G, Vander Zwaag R, Van Meter WS, Wood TO: Suture adjustment for postkeratoplasty astigmatism. Trans Am Ophthalmol Soc 88:289, 1990
200. Smiddy WE, Hamburg TR, Kracher GP, Stark WJ: Visual correction following penetrating keratoplasty. Ophthalmic Surg 23:90, 1992
201. Genvert GI, Cohen EJ, Arentsen JJ, Laibson PR: Fitting gas-permeable contact lenses after penetrating keratoplasty. Am J Ophthalmol 99:511, 1985
202. Mannis MJ, Zadnik K: Fitting gas-permeable contact lenses after penetrating keratoplasty [letter]. Am J Ophthalmol 100:491, 1985
203. Beekhuis WH, van Rij G, Eggink FA, et al: Contact lenses following keratoplasty. CLAO J 17:27, 1991
204. Brightbill FS, Laux DJ: Contact lens fitting. p. 344. In Brightbill FS (ed): Corneal Surgery: Theory, Technique, and Tissue. CV Mosby, St. Louis, 1986
205. Weiner BM, Nirankari VS: A new biaspheric contact lens for severe astigmatism following penetrating keratoplasty. CLAO J 18:29, 1992
206. Caroline PJ, Doughman DJ: A new piggyback lens design for correction of irregular astigmatism—a preliminary report. Contact IOL Med J 5:40, 1979
207. Mannis MJ, Matsumoto ER: Extended-wear aphakic soft contact lenses after penetrating keratoplasty. Arch Ophthalmol 101:1225, 1983
208. Dangel ME, Kracher GP, Stark WJ, et al: Aphakic extended-wear contact lenses after penetrating keratoplasty. Am J Ophthalmol 95:156, 1983
209. Daniel R: Fitting contact lenses after keratoplasty. Br J Ophthalmol 60:263, 1976
210. Troutman RC: Relaxing incisions for astigmatic correction following penetrating keratoplasty. Refract Corneal Surg 5:60, 1989
211. Fronterre A, Portesani GP: Relaxing incisions for postkeratoplasty astigmatism. Cornea 10:305, 1991

212. Krachmer JH, Frenzel RE: Surgical correction of high post keratoplasty astigmatism. Arch Ophthalmol 98:1400, 1980
213. Cohen KL, Tripoli NK, Noecker RJ: Prospective analysis of photokeratoscopy for arcuate keratotomy to reduce postkeratoplasty astigmatism. Refract Corneal Surg 5:388, 1989
214. Saragoussi JJ, Abenhaim A, Waked N, et al: Results of transverse keratotomies for astigmatism after penetrating keratoplasty: a retrospective study of 48 consecutive cases. Refract Corneal Surg 8:33, 1992
215. Limberg MB, Dingeldein SA, Green MT: Corneal compression sutures for the reduction of astigmatism after penetrating keratoplasty. Am J Ophthalmol 108:36, 1989
216. Troutman RC: Microsurgical control of corneal astigmatism in cataract and keratoplasty. Trans Am Acad Ophthalmol Otolaryngol 77:563, 1973
217. Lugo M, Donnenfeld ED, Arentsen JJ: Corneal wedge resection for high astigmatism following penetrating keratoplasty. Ophthalmic Surg 18:650, 1987
218. McCartney DL, Whitney CE, Stark WJ, et al: Refractive keratoplasty for disabling astigmatism after penetrating keratoplasty. Arch Ophthalmol 105:954, 1987
219. Duffy P, Wolf J, Collins G, et al: Possible person-to-person transmission of Creutzfeldt-Jakob disease. N Engl J Med 290:692, 1974
220. Feigenbaum S, Pepose JS: Screening corneal donors for transmissible disease. Arch Ophthalmol 109:941, 1991
221. Pepose JS: The risk of cytomegalovirus transmission by penetrating keratoplasty. Am J Ophthalmol 106:238, 1988
222. Holland EJ, Bennett Sr, Brannian R, et al: The risk of cytomegalovirus transmission by penetrating keratoplasty. Am J Ophthalmol 105:357, 1988
223. O'Day DM: Diseases potentially transmitted through corneal transplantation. Ophthalmology 96:1133, 1989
224. Gottesdiener KM: Transplanted infections: donor-to-host transmission with the allograft. Ann Intern Med 110:1001, 1989
225. Pepose JS, Buerger DG, Paul DA, et al: New developments in serologic screening of corneal donors for HIV-1 and hepatitis B virus infections. Ophthalmology 99:879, 1992
226. Wagoner MD, Dohlman CH, Albert DM, et al: Corneal donor material selection. Ophthalmology 88:139, 1981

36

Prosthokeratoplasty

BRUCE A. BARRON

The success rate of penetrating keratoplasty for some groups of patients is greater than 90 percent.[1] However, there is another group of patients, including those with chemical burns, pemphigoid, Stevens-Johnson syndrome, trachoma, severe dry eyes, and recurrent graft rejections, in whom the potential for successful penetrating keratoplasty is dismal. In this group, the success rate approaches zero.[1] If these patients are to be visually rehabilitated, an alternative to penetrating keratoplasty must be pursued. Such an alternative is prosthokeratoplasty, a procedure in which the cornea is replaced with an artificial cornea (keratoprosthesis). This chapter reviews the background, indications and contraindications, surgical techniques, and results and complications of prosthokeratoplasty. The first part of the chapter discusses permanent prosthokeratoplasty; the second part discusses temporary prosthokeratoplasty.

PERMANENT PROSTHOKERATOPLASTY

Credit for proposing the replacement of an opaque cornea with an artificial cornea is given to de Quengsy, who in 1789 suggested replacing an opaque cornea with a piece of glass.[2-5] Although de Quengsy drew the instruments that might be needed for such a procedure, he did not develop his idea further. During the 1800s, attempts were made at corneal transplantation, but because of the crude surgical techniques and lack of knowledge concerning corneal physiology and immunology, the results were poor. Therefore, other methods of creating a clear corneal window were pursued. The first known attempt at placing a keratoprosthesis in a human eye was made by Nussbaum, who in 1855 inserted a glass crystal into a cornea; it remained in place for 7 months.[3,4,6] Other investigators, including Heusser, von Hippel, Dimmer, and Salzer, implanted various materials such as glass, quartz, and celluloid in the corneas of animals and humans without success.[3,4,7]

With the increasing success of lamellar keratoplasty in the late 1800s and of penetrating keratoplasty in the early 1900s, attention turned to refining these procedures, and there was a loss of interest in artificial corneas. In the early to mid-1900s, several advances were made in the surgical techniques for penetrating keratoplasty that further increased the success of this procedure. However, there remained a group of patients for whom penetrating keratoplasty was not successful. It was for these patients that the concept of an artificial cornea was revived.

Events that occurred during World War II ushered in research that led to the techniques of prosthokeratoplasty described in this chapter. Stone and Herbert[8] observed that fragments of plastic that had become embedded in the eyes of bomber pilots when their cockpit cupolas shattered were well tolerated; this led to investigation of the use of this material (polymethyl methacrylate) for keratoprostheses. (This same observation by others also led to the development of intraocular lenses.[9]) Other materials, including silicone and ceramic, have been investigated, but they do not appear to have any advantages over polymethyl methacrylate.[10-20] Although polymethyl methacrylate is well tolerated by the cornea, extrusion of keratoprostheses, even those made from this material, is still a major problem. Most of the prosthokeratoplasty research over the past 40 years has been directed toward preventing this complication.

Types of Keratoprostheses

Three types of keratoprostheses have been developed over the past 50 years: nonpenetrating (superficial or intralamel-

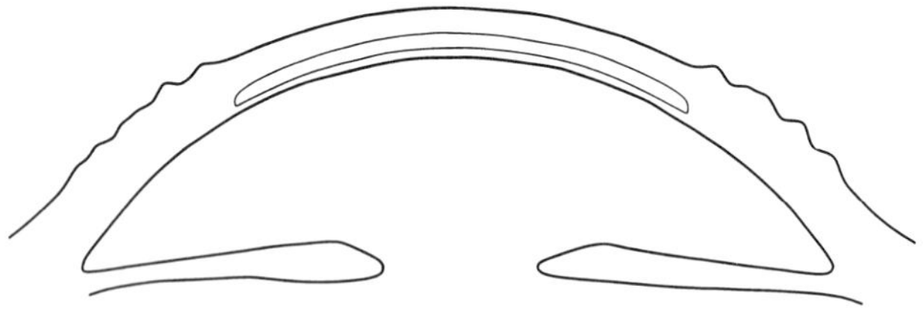

FIGURE 36-1 Intralamellar implant used to treat bullous keratopathy. The cornea anterior to the implant thinned but also frequently opacified and became necrotic.

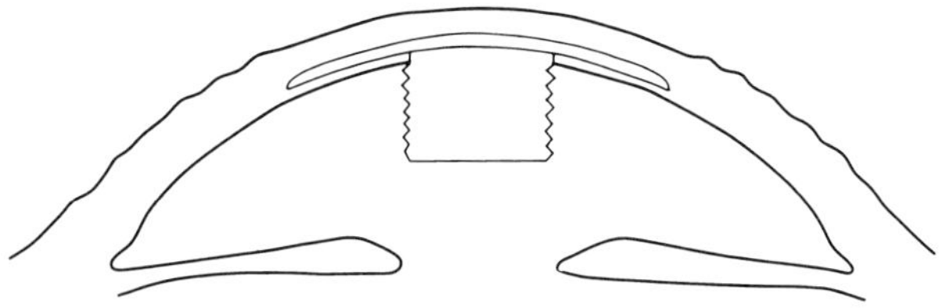

FIGURE 36-2 Posterior penetrating keratoprosthesis used to treat bullous keratopathy. The posterior cylinder was designed to circumvent edematous cornea posterior to the intralamellar implant to improve visual acuity.

lar), penetrating (posterior penetrating or anterior penetrating), and perforating.

Nonpenetrating Keratoprostheses

Although conventional contact lenses may theoretically be considered as superficial keratoprostheses, they are not considered as such in this chapter. The idea of permanently replacing pathologic corneal epithelium with a contact lens bonded with tissue adhesive to the underlying cornea was proposed in 1968,[21] and the first successful use of a methacrylate "epikeratoprosthesis" in a human was reported in the same year.[22] This procedure was theoretically useful in patients with decreased vision caused only by corneal surface abnormalities (e.g., patients with chronic epithelial defects caused by dry eyes). Although the initial results with epikeratoprostheses were encouraging,[23,24] there were complications. Epikeratoprostheses became obsolete with the development of bandage soft contact lenses by Gasset and Kaufman,[25] which are now used to treat many of the disorders for which epikeratoprostheses were originally intended.

Intralamellar keratoprostheses were first designed to be used in a two-stage procedure.[8] In the first stage, a plastic disk was implanted intralamellarly. In the second stage, corneal tissue anterior and posterior to the disk was trephined and removed after sufficient time had elapsed for the periphery of the plastic disk to become firmly fibrosed to the cornea. This two-stage procedure never became clinically popular; however, the first stage of the procedure was used in the 1960s for the treatment of bullous keratopathy[26-30] (Figure 36-1). At that time, the success rate of penetrating keratoplasty for bullous keratopathy was low because the function of the corneal endothelium was poorly understood. It was hypothesized that an intralamellar implant would provide a mechanical barrier to the anterior movement of aqueous humor and cause corneal deturgescence. It was not initially appreciated that this mechanical barrier also prevented necessary nutrients from the aqueous humor from reaching the anterior cornea, which resulted in opacification and necrosis of the cornea anterior to the implant.[26-31] Insertion of the implant as close to Descemet's membrane as possible lessened this complication,[27,28] and "calculated leak" implants were developed.[28-30] These implants had perforations designed to allow enough aqueous humor to leak into the cornea to provide nourishment but not enough to cause edema. Although intralamellar prosthokeratoplasty was successful in controlling bullous keratopathy and in relieving pain in some patients, visual results were usually poor, and anterior and/or posterior corneal opacification and corneal neovascularization were common.[29,30] If the goal was to improve visual acuity, intralamellar implants were useful only in the rare cases in which the cornea was relatively clear. Recognition of the importance of the corneal endothelium, and the subsequent increased success of penetrating keratoplasty for the treatment of bullous keratopathy, made intralamellar implants obsolete for the treatment of this disorder.

Penetrating Keratoprostheses

Penetrating keratoprostheses were developed for use in corneas with partial-thickness opacification. Posterior penetrating keratoprostheses were developed for corneas with posterior opacification in which the anterior cornea was clear[11-13,32,33]; anterior penetrating keratoprostheses were developed for corneas with anterior opacification in which the posterior cornea was clear.[32] Posterior penetrating keratoprostheses were used for the treatment of bullous keratopathy.[11-13] The keratoprosthesis consisted of an intralamellar membrane to anchor the keratoprosthesis and a posterior cylinder (Figure 36-2). As with intralamellar implants, the membrane provided a mechanical barrier to the anterior movement of aqueous humor, which caused deturgescence of the edematous cornea anterior to the membrane. To improve vision, the posterior cylinder penetrated the edematous cornea posterior to the membrane into the

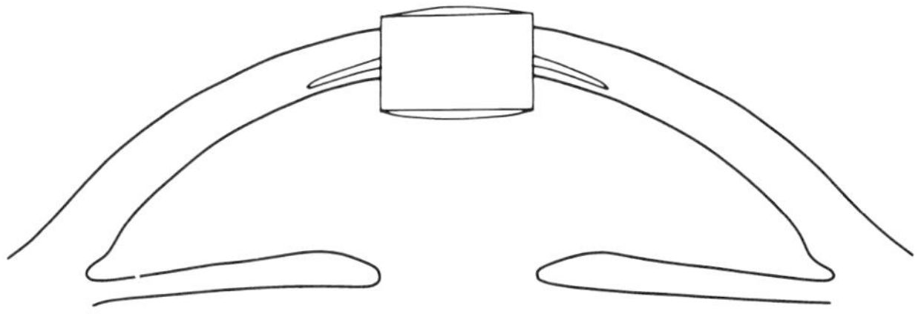

FIGURE 36-3 Perforating keratoprosthesis supported by an intralamellar supporting plate. Extrusion of the keratoprosthesis was common and was caused by necrosis of the cornea anterior to the supporting plate.

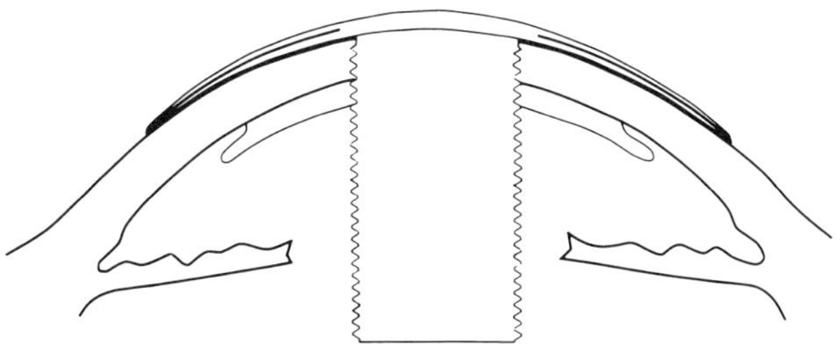

FIGURE 36-4 Nut-and-bolt keratoprosthesis, consisting of a cosmetic contact lens, a perforating optical cylinder, and a retrocorneal supporting plate.

anterior chamber. Although this keratoprosthesis was used in the 1960s, it had many of the same complications as intralamellar implants, including opacification and necrosis of the cornea anterior to the membrane. The increased success of penetrating keratoplasty for the treatment of bullous keratopathy obviated the need for the device. Neither the posterior nor the anterior penetrating keratoprosthesis was very successful because of the tendency of the remaining cornea to opacify, although this opacification could be circumvented by converting the penetrating keratoprosthesis to a perforating keratoprosthesis.[32,33] Choyce's two-piece keratoprosthesis was routinely converted from a posterior penetrating to a perforating keratoprosthesis as part of a multistage procedure.[27–30,34–38] Most corneas in which prosthokeratoplasty is indicated have full-thickness opacities, which make penetrating keratoprostheses unsuitable for visual rehabilitation.

Perforating Keratoprostheses

Perforating keratoprostheses were developed to provide better visual results than nonpenetrating or penetrating keratoprostheses, although the extrusion rate for this type of keratoprosthesis is higher than for the other types. It was discovered early that placement of a polymethyl methacrylate cylinder or collar-button-shaped keratoprosthesis through the cornea resulted in extrusion of the keratoprosthesis.[39,40] Attempts to surround the sides of the cylinder with autologous tissue, such as tooth and bone (osteo-odontokeratoprosthesis),[41–44] cartilage (chondrokeratoprosthesis),[43,44] or nail (onychokeratoprosthesis),[43] and then place it through the cornea also resulted in unacceptable extrusion rates. Therefore, other methods of anchoring the keratoprosthesis to the cornea were explored.

Perforating keratoprostheses have been anchored to the cornea by intralamellar fixation, posterior fixation, or anterior fixation. Intralamellar fixation was accomplished with an intralamellar supporting plate (Figure 36-3). Originally, the supporting plate was made of polymethyl methacrylate.[3] However, this type of keratoprosthesis had the same complication as intralamellar implants: necrosis of the cornea anterior to the supporting plate because of inadequate nutrition.[45] In an attempt to provide more nutrition to the anterior cornea, the plate was reduced in size,[3] fenestrated,[32] and placed as close to Descemet's membrane as possible.[3] Other materials, including Teflon and dacron mesh, were investigated for their ability to provide effective support for the keratoprosthesis and, at the same time, allow diffusion of essential nutrients to the anterior cornea.[45] Even with these modifications, keratoprostheses with these types of supporting plates had unacceptably high extrusion rates.[46]

Posterior fixation was attempted with a nut-and-bolt arrangement.[47] This mushroom-shaped keratoprosthesis consisted of a cosmetic contact lens attached to a threaded optical cylinder that was fixated retrocorneally with a threaded supporting plate (Figure 36-4). It was thought that the contact lens would prevent excessive evaporation from the corneal surface and thus decrease the erosion of corneal tissue surrounding the optical cylinder. This keratoprosthesis frequently extruded because of pressure necrosis caused by the posterior supporting plate,[48] and attention was turned to anterior fixation.

Anterior fixation, which is the method of choice today, involves suturing a supporting plate to the anterior surface of the cornea. This method allows essential nutrients from the aqueous humor to reach all layers of the cornea. However, fixation of a keratoprosthesis to the anterior corneal surface alone results in extrusion of the keratoprosthesis. Various materials, including sclera,[49,50] cornea, fascia lata, temporalis fascia,[51] periosteum,[52] dacron mesh,[53] and eyelid,[52] have been used to reinforce the cornea anterior to the supporting plate in an attempt to prevent extrusion. One type of keratoprosthesis is fixated both posteriorly with a nut-and-bolt arrangement and anteriorly with dacron mesh.[54]

Hernando Cardona (Figure 36-5) has been involved in prosthokeratoplasty research for many years, and he

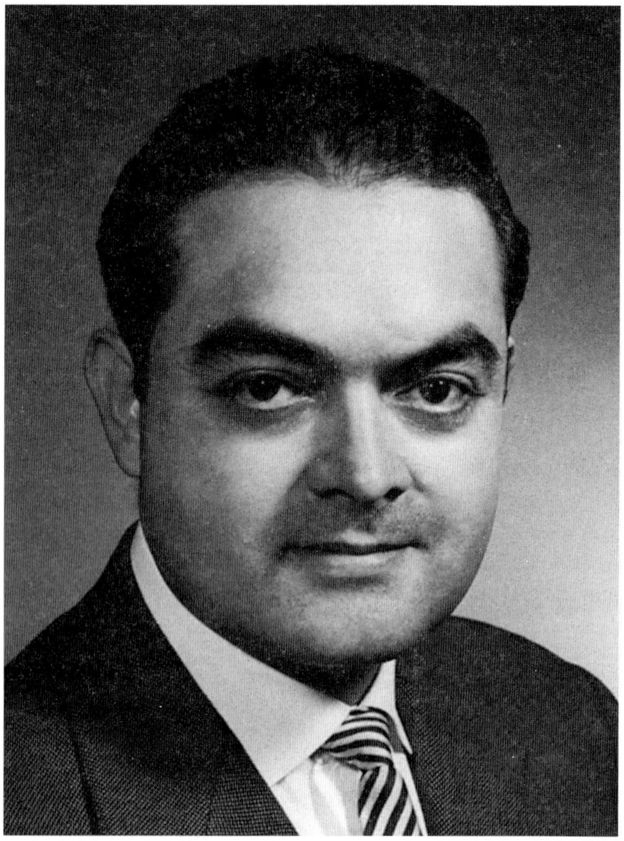

FIGURE 36-5 Hernando Cardona, M.D.

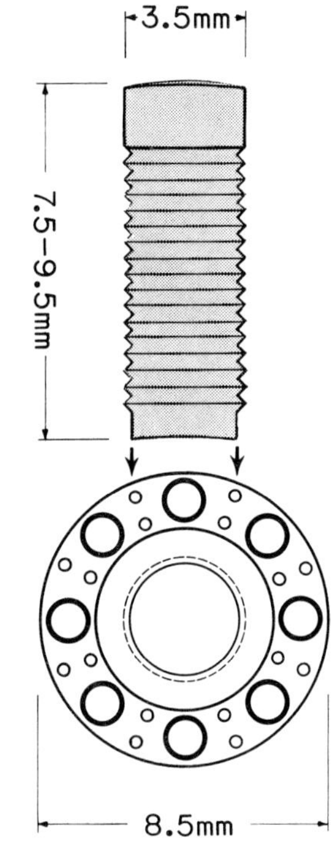

FIGURE 36-6 Cardona through-and-through keratoprosthesis consisting of **(top)** an optical cylinder and **(bottom)** a supporting plate. The optical cylinder is threaded along its length, except for the anterior 1 mm. The supporting plate is 0.3 mm in thickness and has a radius of curvature of 6 mm. The large and small holes in the supporting plate are 1.8 mm and 0.5 mm in diameter, respectively. The center threaded opening is 3.5 mm in diameter.

designed and developed many of the keratoprostheses described in this chapter, including the perforating keratoprosthesis with anterior fixation in use at this time.

The Cardona through-and-through keratoprosthesis consists of two parts: a polymethyl methacrylate optical cylinder and a Teflon supporting plate (Figure 36-6). The optical cylinder is threaded so that its anterior surface can be leveled to the surrounding tissue. Carbon pigment is embedded in the wall of the cylinder to prevent glare. The cylinder is available in lengths from 7.5 to 9.5 mm. If the cylinder is placed through the eyelid, a longer length is preferred, depending on the thickness of the eyelid. The power of the cylinder is calculated by the manufacturer from the axial length measurement of the eye. The cylinder is available with or without a small anterior flange. The supporting plate is perforated with holes that permit suturing of the plate to the cornea and allow tissue to grow through the plate, anchoring it to the cornea. There is a threaded portion in the center of the plate through which the cylinder is screwed. The plate is reinforced intraoperatively with dacron mesh and periosteum. The anterior covering of the periosteum depends on the condition of the eye. In eyes with healthy conjunctiva, the conjunctiva may be used; in eyes with unhealthy conjunctiva, a mucous membrane graft or the eyelid may be used (Figure 36-7).

Indications and Contraindications

Prosthokeratoplasty is indicated in patients with corneal disorders that prevent visual rehabilitation by more conventional means. As aforementioned, these patients include those with chemical burns, ocular pemphigoid, Stevens-Johnson syndrome, trachoma, severe dry eyes, and recurrent graft rejections (Figure 36-8). Although perforating keratoprostheses were used in the past in patients with bullous keratopathy,[55,56] the increased success of penetrating keratoplasty for bullous keratopathy has eliminated this disorder as an indication for prosthokeratoplasty.

Prosthokeratoplasty should not be considered an alternative to penetrating keratoplasty but as a procedure to be used when penetrating keratoplasty has failed or is likely to fail. Although most patients who are candidates for prosthokeratoplasty have had one or more penetrating keratoplasties, a failed corneal graft is not a prerequisite

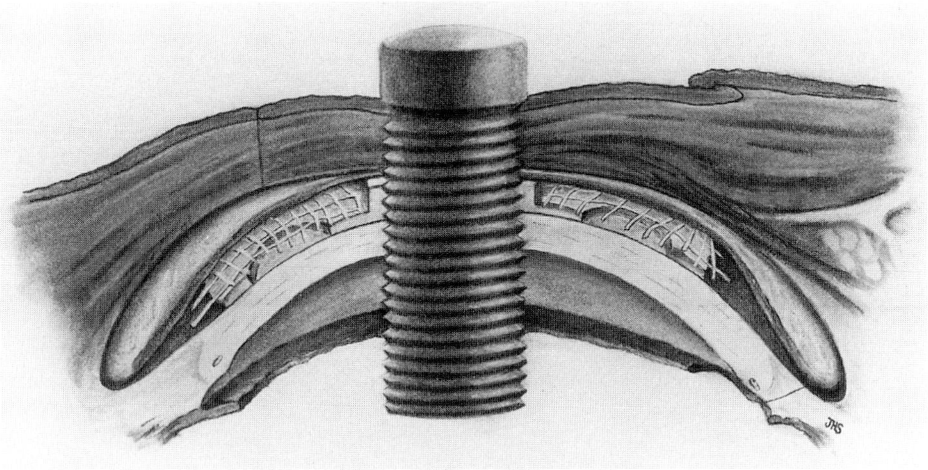

FIGURE 36-7 Cardona through-and-through keratoprosthesis exteriorized through the upper eyelid. The keratoprosthesis is fixated to the cornea anteriorly by a supporting plate, which is covered with dacron mesh, periosteum, and eyelid tissue.

for prosthokeratoplasty. If the corneal disease is such that a corneal graft is likely to fail, there is no need to subject the patient unnecessarily to penetrating keratoplasty before proceeding with prosthokeratoplasty. However, if there is even a small chance that a corneal graft will be successful, penetrating keratoplasty should be performed first.

Prosthokeratoplasty is considered only in patients who have bilateral disabling corneal disease. It is never considered in patients with unilateral corneal disease. Bilateral prosthokeratoplasty is not done if good results have been obtained in one eye. The other eye is reserved for the procedure in the future should the first eye lose vision from long-term complications.

Eyes in which prosthokeratoplasty is considered should have some visual potential, which is often difficult to assess. Minimally, light perception is necessary. Some ophthalmologists have found electroretinography (ERG) and visual evoked response (VER) testing helpful in predicting the visual potential of the eye[6]; however, even if the results of these tests are poor, the patient should be given the benefit of the doubt and the procedure should be attempted if there is no alternative for restoring vision. Before prosthokeratoplasty, ultrasonography is used to evaluate the posterior segment of the eye to rule out retinal detachment and other posterior segment abnormalities.

Intraocular pressure should be under control before prosthokeratoplasty is performed, because it is difficult or impossible to measure after the procedure. If the keratoprosthesis is to be placed through the eyelid, the preoperative intraocular pressure must be normal without

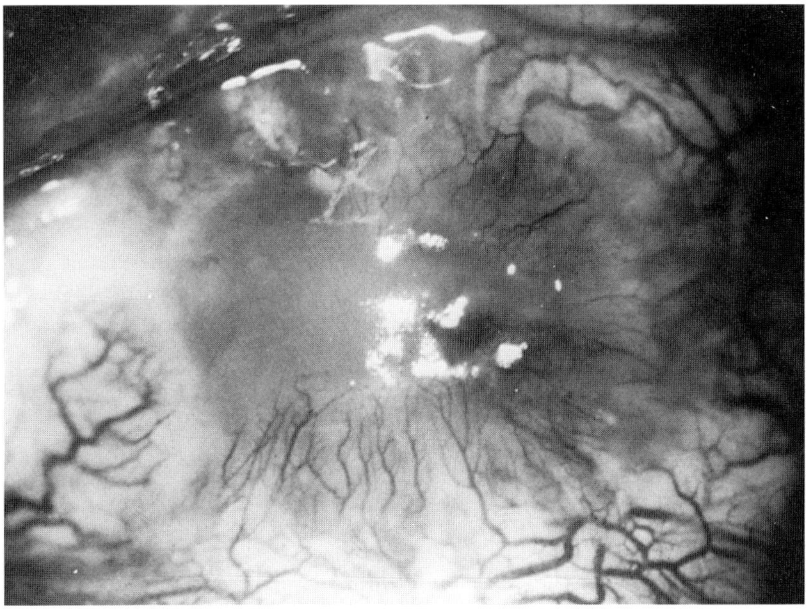

FIGURE 36-8 Cornea after a chemical burn. The prognosis for penetrating keratoplasty is poor.

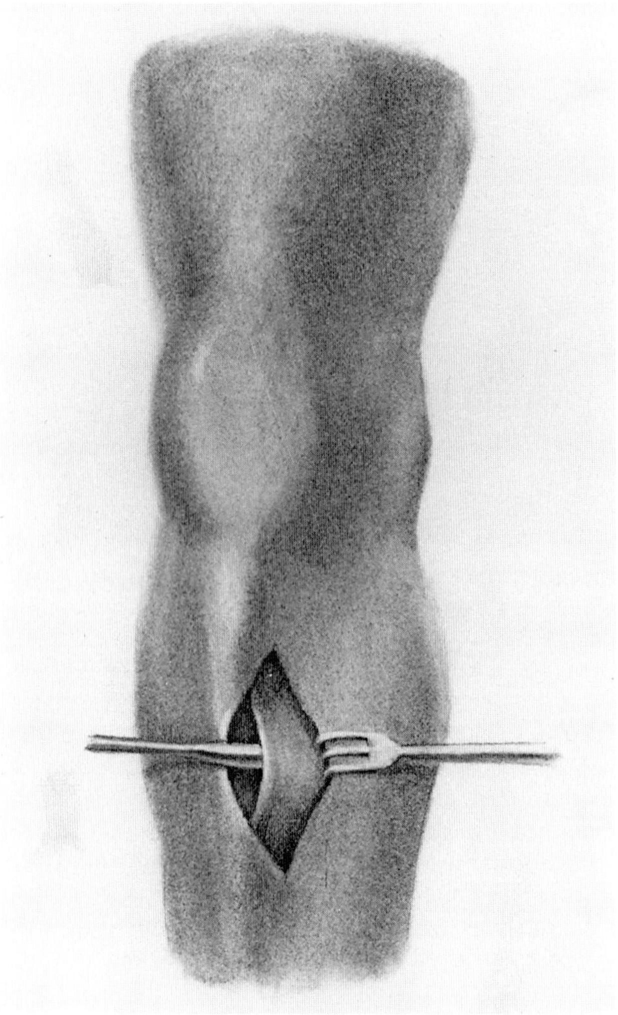

FIGURE 36-9 Elevation of periosteum from the anteromedial surface of the tibia.

the use of topical hypotensive agents because topical medications cannot be given postoperatively.

As outlined above, contraindications to prosthokeratoplasty include functional vision in the other eye, a successful keratoprosthesis in the other eye, no light perception, posterior segment pathology that limits visual potential, and uncontrolled intraocular pressure.

Surgical Techniques

The surgical techniques described below are for the Cardona through-and-through keratoprosthesis reinforced with dacron mesh and periosteum.

Prosthokeratoplasty is usually performed under general anesthesia because the procedure is lengthy and it is necessary to obtain autologous tissue from areas other than the eye. Although fascia lata, temporalis fascia, and periosteum have all been recommended as tissue reinforcements for the keratoprosthesis, pretibial periosteum is probably the easiest for the corneal surgeon to obtain. After the pretibial area is prepared and draped, an incision is made with a #15 Bard-Parker blade along the anterior tibial crest approximately 5 cm inferior to the tibial tuberosity. The incision is deepened until the periosteum is reached. Bleeding is usually minimal and is easily controlled with cautery. The periosteum along the anteromedial tibia is elevated with a periosteal elevator, and a piece of periosteum approximately 2.5 cm by 5 cm is excised and kept moist with saline (Figure 36-9). The subcutaneous tissue is closed with interrupted 3-0 chromic sutures, and the skin is closed with interrupted 6-0 nylon sutures. Antibiotic ointment and a slight pressure dressing are placed over the wound.

The eye is prepared and draped as for any ocular surgery. If the keratoprosthesis is not to be exteriorized through the eyelid, a 360-degree limbal conjunctival peritomy with horizontal relaxing incisions is performed. If the keratoprosthesis is to be exteriorized through the eyelid, all the palpebral and bulbar conjunctiva is removed so that adhesions can form between the eye and eyelids (Figure 36-10). The corneal epithelium is removed with a spatula or #64 Beaver blade, and the anterior corneal, bulbar, and palpebral surfaces are scrubbed with a cellulose sponge saturated with absolute alcohol to kill any remaining epithelial cells. The eye is then irrigated copiously with balanced salt solution. The adhesions that form between the eye and eyelid allow the eye and eyelid to move as a unit, which lessens mechanical forces on the keratoprosthesis and thereby decreases the risk of extrusion. The risk of extrusion is also decreased by excising the tarsal plates and disinserting the horizontal rectus muscles, which allows the keratoprosthesis to be surrounded by pliable tissue and decreases extraocular movements. Some surgeons routinely disinsert the levator palpebrae superioris muscle and excise the orbicularis muscle to decrease movement of the eyelid.[18,20,57] The margins of the upper and lower eyelids are excised to permit adhesions to form between the eyelids and to eliminate eyelash follicles, which improves postoperative hygiene of the keratoprosthesis. Care is taken to avoid excising too much of the eyelid margins; otherwise, the eyelids can be difficult to close at the end of the procedure. The above steps are performed before the eye is entered because there is usually a fair amount of bleeding, which must be controlled before the eye is opened.

The center of the cornea is located and marked by direct visualization, by transillumination, or if necessary, by measurement from the insertions of the rectus muscles. A 3.5-mm trephine is used to outline the central corneal incision (Figure 36-11).

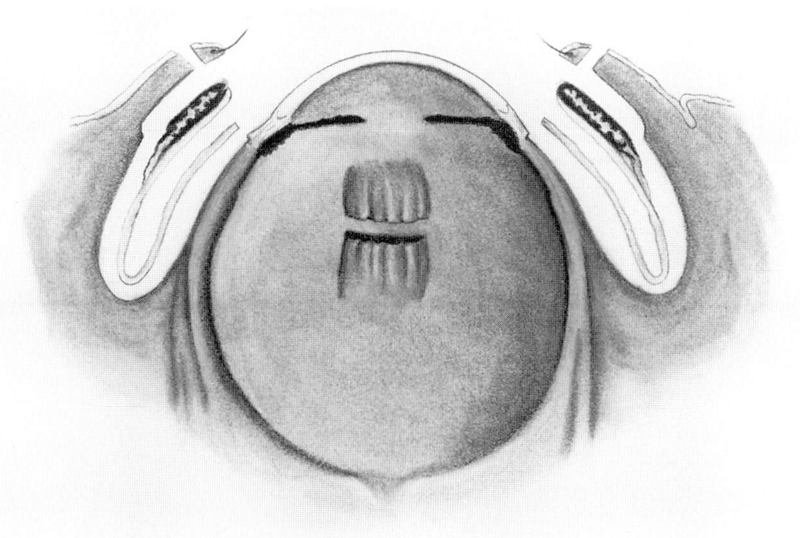

FIGURE 36-10 Schematic cross section of ocular tissues illustrating removal of the conjunctiva, tarsal plates, and eyelid margins. The horizontal rectus muscle has been severed to decrease movement of the eye.

If the eye is phakic, the lens is extracted, whether or not it is cataractous, because a clear lens will become cataractous after placement of the keratoprosthesis. The lens is extracted through a superior limbal incision by an intracapsular technique. If the eye is pseudophakic, the intraocular lens is removed. A deep core vitrectomy is done, and as much iris is removed as possible. The vitrectomy and total iridectomy are performed because of the high incidence of postoperative retroprosthetic membrane formation in eyes that have vitreous and/or iris against the optical cylinder. The superior limbal incision is closed with interrupted 9-0 nylon sutures.

The cornea outlined by the 3.5-mm trephine is excised with Vannas scissors (Figure 36-12). An additional vitrectomy and/or iridectomy is performed through this opening if necessary. Two interrupted 9-0 polypropylene sutures are placed through partial-thickness cornea adjacent and tangential to the corneal opening 180 degrees apart. An estimate is made of the length of optical cylinder that must protrude above the supporting plate to be even with the surrounding tissue at the end of the operation. This length depends on whether the keratoprosthesis is to be exteriorized through the eyelid. The optical cylinder is screwed into the supporting plate to give the estimated length to protrude anteriorly and is screwed into the central opening in the cornea. The ends of each preplaced suture are threaded through two adjacent large holes in the supporting plate and tied (Figure 36-13). To ensure that the cornea is against the posterior surface of the supporting plate, a cyclodialysis spatula inserted through the limbal wound is used to press the cornea anteriorly against the supporting plate. The supporting plate is sutured to the cornea with interrupted 9-0 polypropylene sutures that pass through the large holes in the supporting plate. Additional

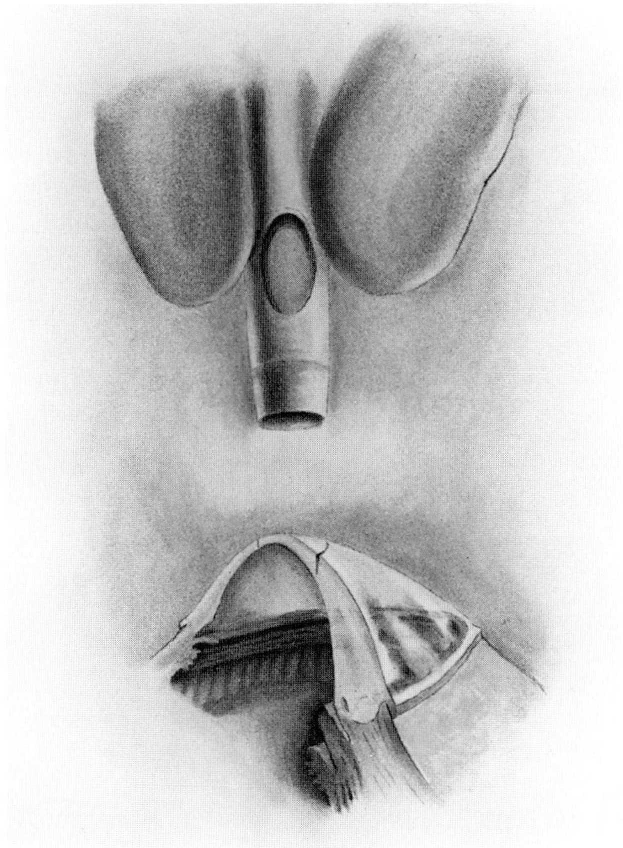

FIGURE 36-11 Partial-thickness trephination of the central cornea with a 3.5-mm trephine.

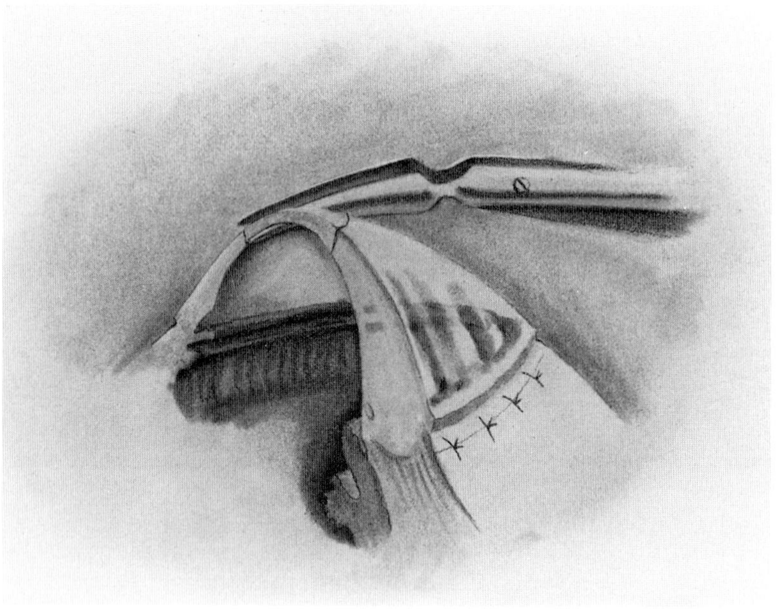

FIGURE 36-12 Removal of the corneal button with Vannas scissors.

sutures are placed through the small peripheral holes and between adjacent large holes (Figure 36-14). The suture ends are trimmed on the knots, which are left unburied if attempts at rotating them into the cornea result in tearing of the tissue. If the cornea is too thin to permit suturing of the supporting plate, a large tectonic lamellar or penetrating graft is placed, the optical cylinder is inserted through a central opening made in the graft, and the supporting plate is sutured to the surface of the graft.

To increase retention of the keratoprosthesis, a circular piece of dacron mesh approximately 20 mm in diameter with a 3.5-mm central opening is placed over the supporting plate and sutured to the superficial sclera with interrupted 9-0 polypropylene sutures (Figure 36-15).

The periosteum is debrided of fat, and a 3.5-mm central opening is made through which the optical cylinder is inserted. The periosteum is placed over the dacron mesh and is sutured to the superficial sclera near the insertions of the rectus muscles with interrupted 8-0 polyglactin sutures. A purse string 9-0 polypropylene suture is placed around the central opening of the periosteum if the periosteum is not snug against the optical cylinder (Figure 36-16).

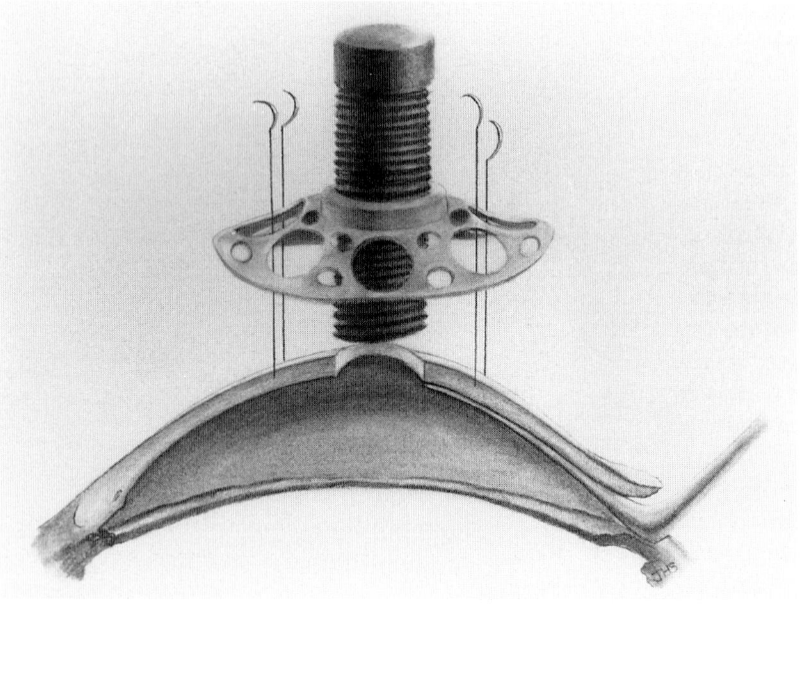

FIGURE 36-13 Insertion of the optical cylinder through the central corneal opening. Preplaced sutures are threaded through holes in the supporting plate. A cyclodialysis spatula has been inserted through the limbal wound to press the cornea anteriorly against the supporting plate.

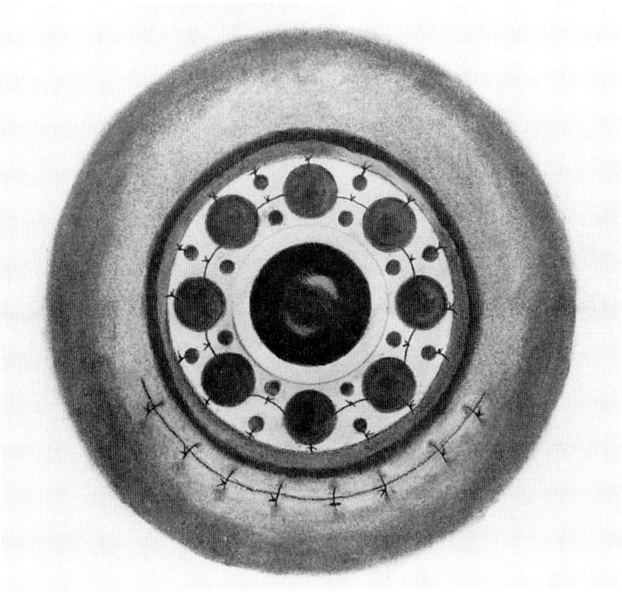

FIGURE 36-14 Supporting plate sutured to the cornea.

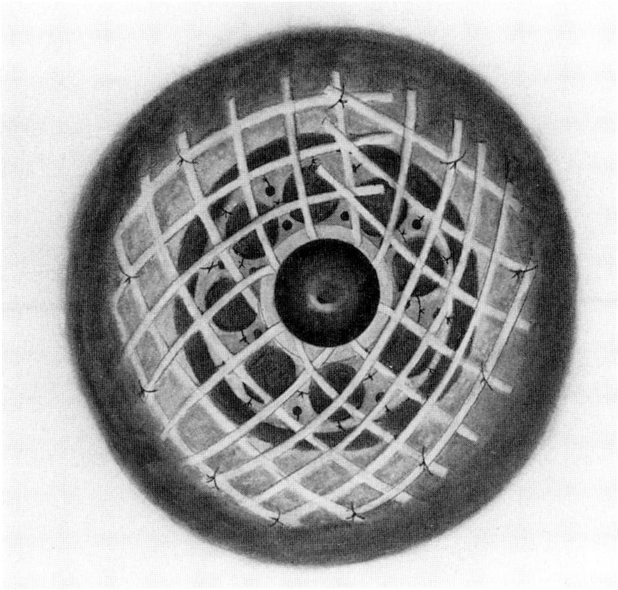

FIGURE 36-15 Dacron mesh covering the supporting plate.

If the keratoprosthesis is not to be exteriorized through the eyelid, the conjunctiva is closed over the periosteum. If the keratoprosthesis is to be exteriorized through the eyelid, the upper eyelid is brought over the keratoprosthesis so that there is no tension on the eyelid. The area of the eyelid overlying the keratoprosthesis is marked, and a 4-mm full-thickness horizontal incision is made through the eyelid at this location. The optical cylinder is inserted through this incision. If the eyelid is too thick for the optical cylinder to be exteriorized, the cylinder may be unscrewed. If the cylinder cannot be safely unscrewed, tissue is excised from the posterior surface of the eyelid. Ideally, the anterior surface of the cylinder should be slightly anterior to the surrounding eyelid tissue. A permanent tarsorrhaphy is performed with 5-0 nylon mattress sutures. Any openings in the eyelid around the optical cylinder are closed with interrupted 6-0 nylon or polyglactin sutures. If cicatricial changes in the upper eyelid prevent it from covering the optical cylinder without tension, the optical cylinder is placed between the eyelids. To prevent postoperative slippage of the optical cylinder into edematous eyelid tissue, a Silastic washer can be placed around the anterior portion of the optical cylinder[58-60] (Figure 36-17). Alternatively, a keratoprosthesis with a small (1.0 to 1.5 mm) flange around the externalized end of the optical cylinder can be used (Figure 36-18).

Periocular antibiotics and corticosteroids are injected, antibiotic ointment is applied, and an eye pad and shield are placed over the eye. On the first postoperative day, the dressing is removed. Antibiotic ointment is placed around the keratoprosthesis and along the tarsorrhaphy four times a day for 2 to 3 weeks and is continued once a day around the keratoprosthesis indefinitely; the ointment is best applied at night so that it does not interfere with vision. Short-term systemic corticosteroids may be necessary to control inflammation. The pretibial skin sutures are removed at 1 week;

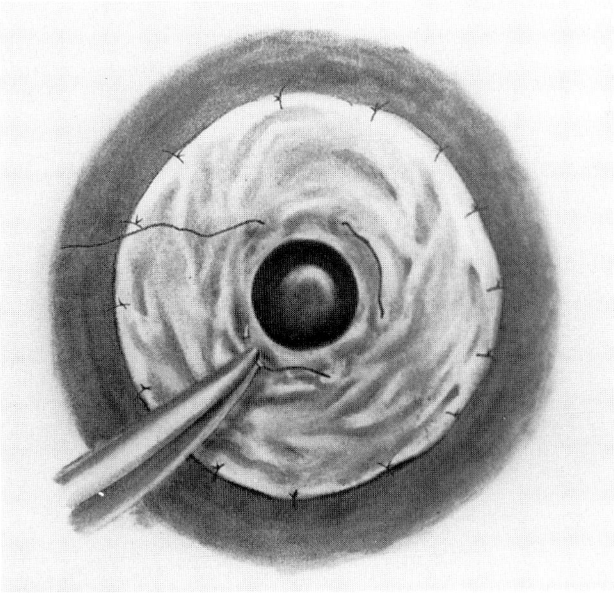

FIGURE 36-16 Periosteum covering the dacron mesh. A purse string suture is placed to approximate the periosteum to the optical cylinder.

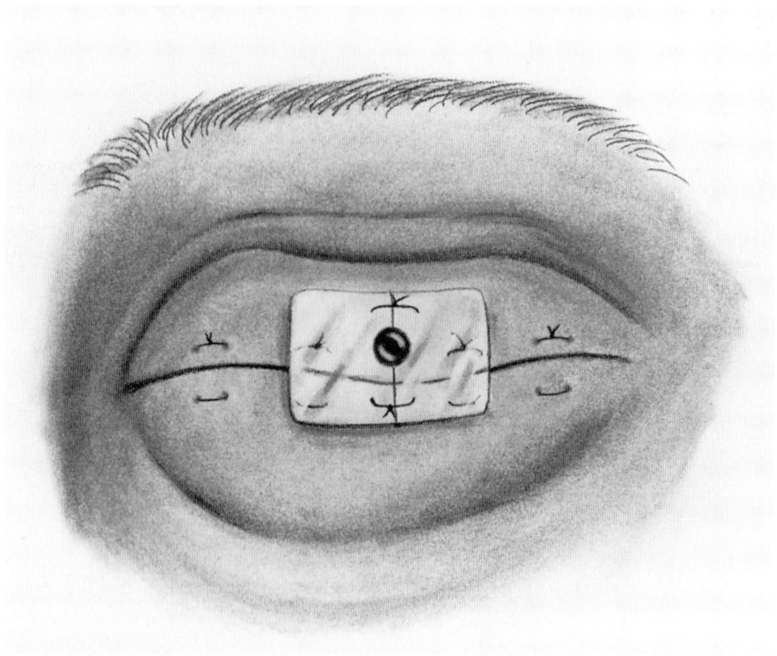

FIGURE 36-17 A Silastic washer is made by punching a 3.5-mm opening in a piece of Silastic with a trephine, cutting the piece in half, and suturing the two halves together. This prevents postoperative slippage of the keratoprosthesis into edematous eyelid tissue. The washer is removed 2 to 3 weeks postoperatively by cutting the sutures.

the Silastic washer and eyelid sutures are removed at 2 to 3 weeks. An optical cylinder exteriorized through the eyelid is cleaned daily with hydrogen peroxide and sterile cotton-tipped applicators. Care is taken to prevent scratching of the anterior surface of the cylinder and to clean the cylinder in a manner so that it does not unscrew.

Results and Complications

The visual results with a keratoprosthesis allow some patients to read but, more important, to become functionally more independent (Figure 36-19). Despite good visual acuity in some patients, however, the visual field is restricted to approximately 30 degrees (Figure 36-20), which limits the types of activities that these patients can safely pursue. Patients should be informed of this preoperatively.

The results and complications of prosthokeratoplasty depend to some extent on the preoperative condition of the eye and on the type of keratoprosthesis used. Eyes with abnormalities limited strictly to the ocular surface tend to do better than eyes with abnormalities involving deeper ocular tissues. Table 36-1 lists reported visual results

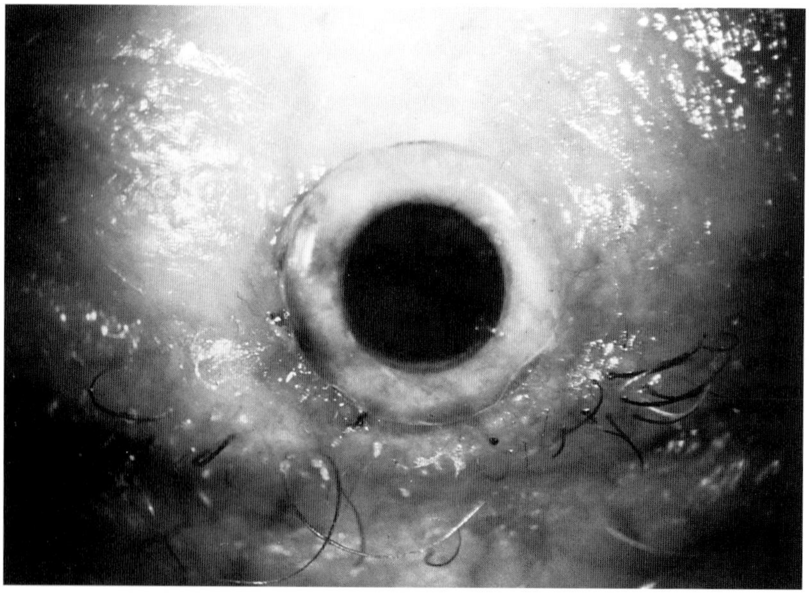

FIGURE 36-18 Postoperative appearance of a Cardona through-and-through keratoprosthesis with an anterior flange. Visual acuity was 20/25.

FIGURE 36-19 (A & B) Postoperative appearance of a Cardona through-and-through keratoprosthesis exteriorized through the upper eyelid. Visual acuity was 20/20.

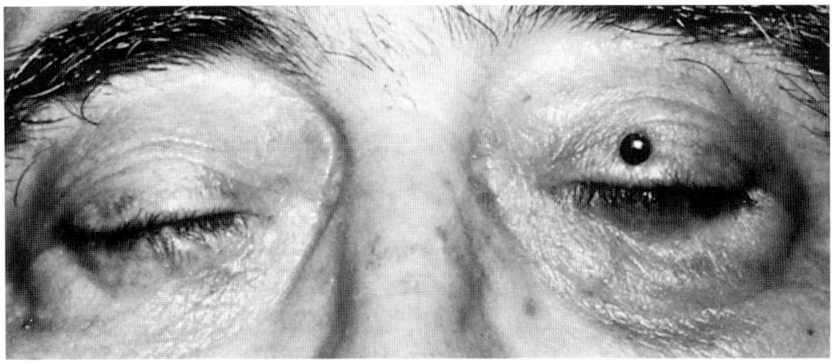

A

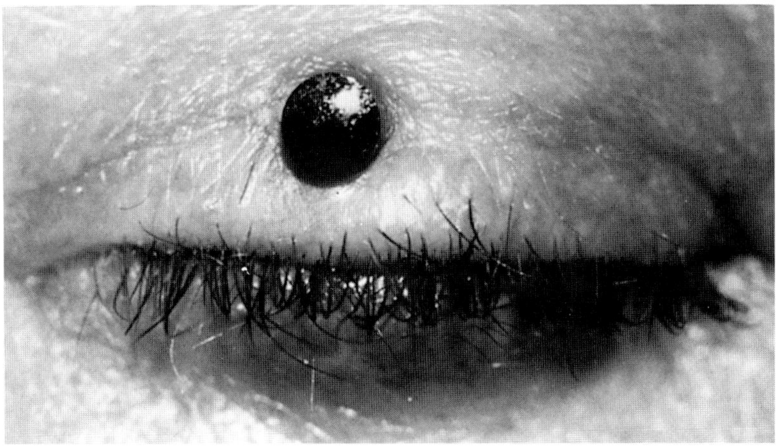

B

			<0	<0	<0	<0			
		<0	<0	6	9	7	<0		
	<0	1	13	12	24	22	15	3	
<0	<0	14	20	23	26	22	20	12	<0
<0	<0	10	24	25	30	28	21	17	<0
<0	<0	14	27	26	32	28	2	18	<0
<0	<0	12	24	21	26	21	20	14	<0
	<0	3	14	22	21	21	16	10	
		<0	<0	6	16	6	<0		
			<0	<0	<0	<0			

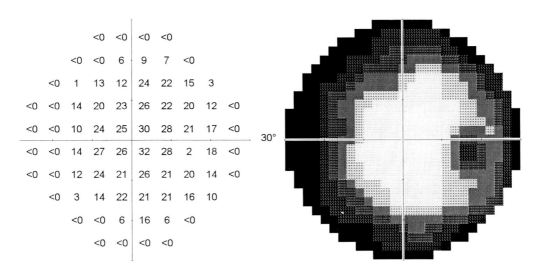

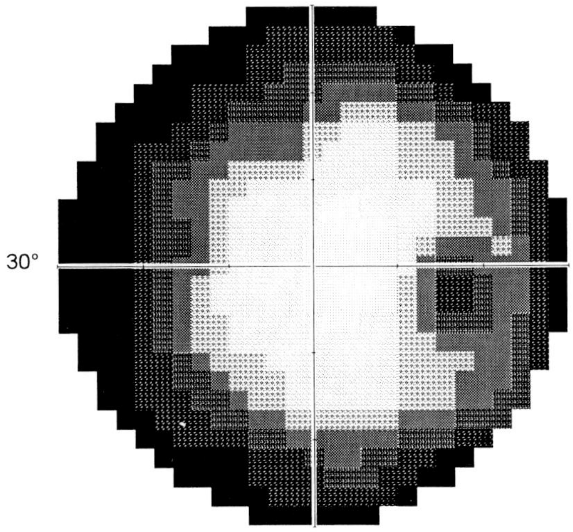

FIGURE 36-20 Results of a Humphrey field analyzer central 30-2 test in a patient with a Cardona keratoprosthesis in the right eye. Visual acuity was 20/25. The numeric grid on the left gives the threshold in decibels for all points tested. The gray scale representation of the visual field is on the right.

TABLE 36-1
Visual Results and Major Complications of Prosthokeratoplasty

		Visual Results			Complications	
Study	*N*	*20/20 to 20/50*	*20/60 to 20/200*	*Less than 20/200*	*Extrusion*	*Retroprosthetic Membrane*
Cardona and DeVoe, 1977[52]	43[a]	7	21	15	0	NR
	24[b]	8	14	2	2	NR
Rao et al, 1979[58]	15	2	3	10	0	1 Early 11 Late
Aquavella et al, 1982[59]	31[b]	5[c]	12	5	0 Intermediate 3 Late	6 12
Cardona, 1983[53]	12	5	5	2	0	NR

Abbreviations: N, number of cases; NR, not reported.
[a] Covered with conjunctiva.
[b] Covered with eyelid.
[c] Visual acuity results on 22 cases only.

and incidences of extrusion and retroprosthetic membrane formation for the Cardona through-and-through keratoprosthesis.[52,53,58,59,61] Other complications of prosthokeratoplasty include glaucoma, vitritis, endophthalmitis, intraocular abscess,[62] orbital cellulitis, retinal detachment, epithelial ingrowth,[63] bone formation in the periosteal graft,[64] and giant papillary conjunctivitis.[65]

One of the most devastating complications of prosthokeratoplasty is extrusion of the keratoprosthesis. Extrusion is more common when the keratoprosthesis is exteriorized through the eyelid.[18] The underlying corneal disorder is usually more severe in these cases, however. Mechanical forces on the keratoprosthesis caused by movement of the eye against the eyelid are probably a significant cause of extrusion.[19] These forces may be decreased by disinsertion of the horizontal rectus muscles and excision of the tarsus and muscular tissue of the eyelid at the time of surgery.[18,20,57] Extrusion may also be caused by the proliferation of fibrous tissue between the cornea and supporting plate of the keratoprosthesis. Extrusion is usually preceded by tissue loss around the keratoprosthesis (Figure 36-21), dislocation of the keratoprosthesis (Figure 36-22), and aqueous humor leakage. Some thinning of tissue surrounding the keratoprosthesis is normal in the immediate postoperative period as edema subsides, but continued thinning is abnormal. Anterior dislocation of the optical cylinder is usually accompanied by a more myopic refraction.

Extrusion of a keratoprosthesis that is not exteriorized through the eyelid is more easily managed than extrusion of a keratoprosthesis that is exteriorized through the eyelid. With the former, the conjunctiva is dissected, another

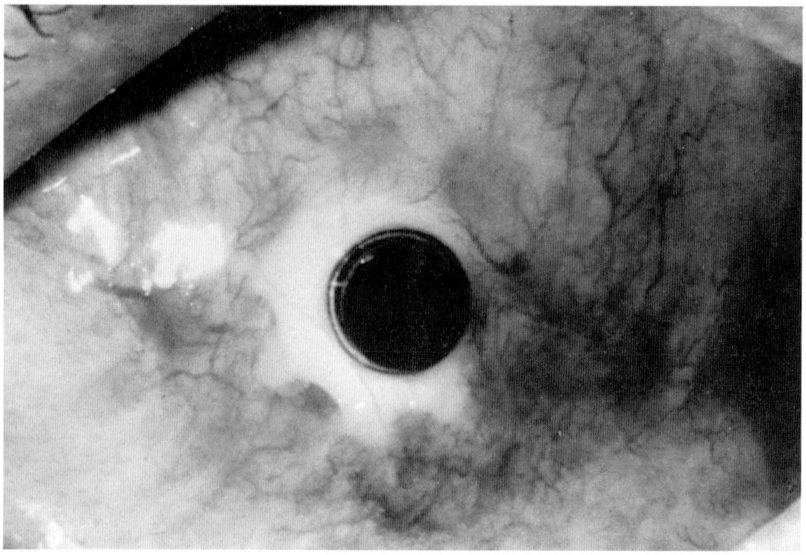

FIGURE 36-21 Tissue loss around a keratoprosthesis that is not exteriorized through the eyelid. Note that the central portion of the supporting plate is visible.

FIGURE 36-22 (A) Front view and (B) side view of an extruding keratoprosthesis that is exteriorized through the upper eyelid. Note the anterior displacement of the optical cylinder and the central cuff of the supporting plate.

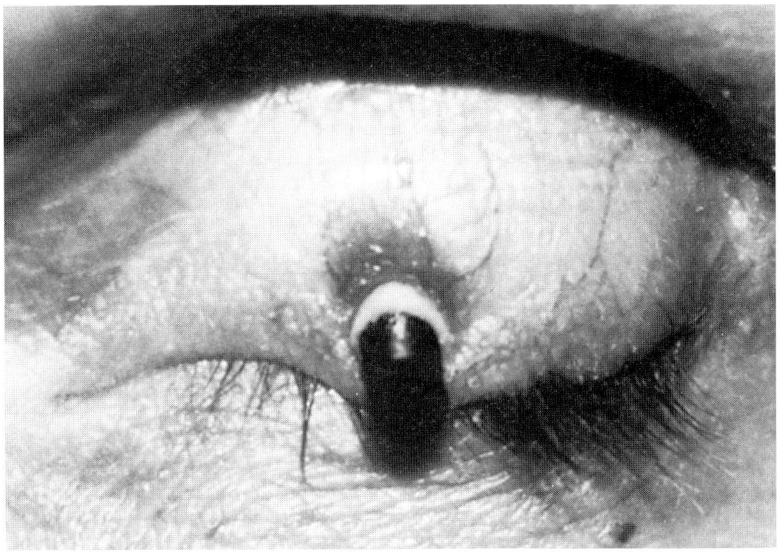

A

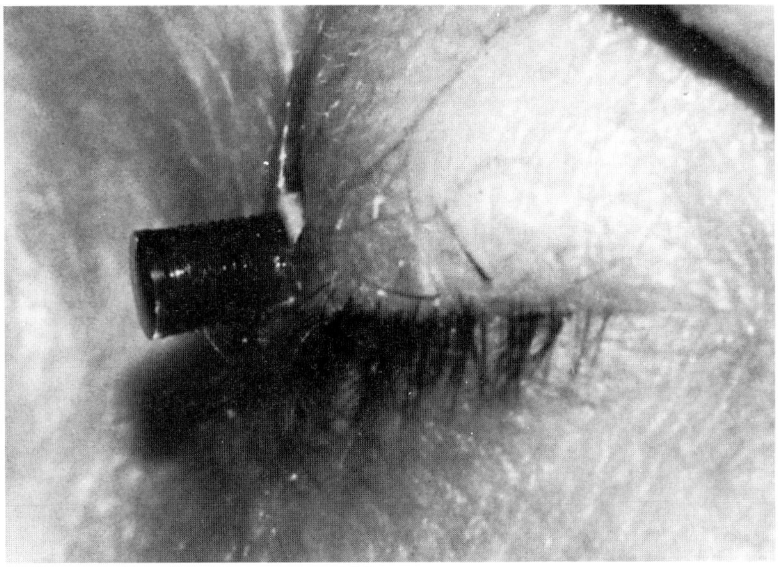

B

layer of supportive tissue, such as periosteum, is placed anterior to the supporting plate, and the conjunctiva is closed around the optical cylinder. If the extrusion cannot be stopped, the entire keratoprosthesis and associated tissue are removed, a large tectonic lamellar or penetrating graft placed, and a new keratoprosthesis inserted through the corneal graft. Management of extrusion of a keratoprosthesis that is exteriorized through the eyelid is difficult because of the firm adhesions between the eyelid, periosteum, dacron mesh, supporting plate, and underlying cornea and sclera. A horizontal incision is made through the eyelid on either side of the optical cylinder, and tissue is dissected down to the dacron mesh. The supporting plate is examined. If the integrity of the eye is intact and the supporting plate is well anchored, periosteum is placed over the dacron mesh and the eyelid is closed. If there is aqueous humor leakage around the keratoprosthesis, the entire keratoprosthesis and associated tissue are removed, a large tectonic lamellar or penetrating graft is placed, and a new keratoprosthesis is inserted through the corneal graft. Extrusion of a keratoprosthesis must be differentiated from pseudoextrusion caused by normal postoperative tissue thinning and from spontaneous unscrewing of the optical cylinder.[66]

Ideally, the anterior surface of the optical cylinder should be slightly anterior to the surrounding tissue. If it is posterior, debris accumulates on the surface, and tis-

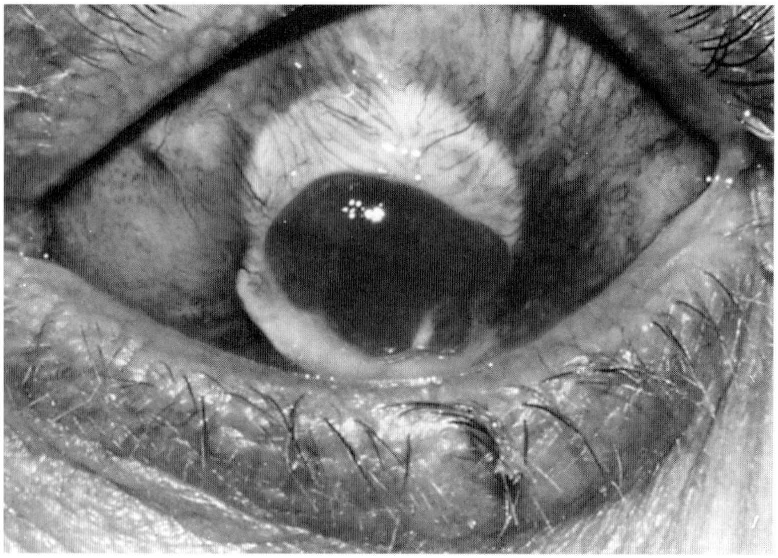

FIGURE 36-23 Growth of conjunctival tissue over the optical cylinder. This is easily treated by excision of the tissue.

sue may grow over the optical cylinder (Figure 36-23). In a keratoprosthesis that is not exteriorized through the eyelid, the anterior surface of the cylinder should not protrude too far because the upper eyelid will hit the cylinder during blinking, causing irritation and unwanted movement of the keratoprosthesis. If the cylinder needs to be screwed farther into the supporting plate, antibiotic is placed around the base of the cylinder, and the cylinder is grasped in a sterile manner and turned clockwise. To minimize the possibility of introducing organisms into the eye, the cylinder should probably be turned no more than two complete revolutions at one time.

Formation of a retroprosthetic membrane is a common complication of prosthokeratoplasty and is a frequent cause of decreased vision. It may result from inflammation and/or vitreous or iris contact with the keratoprosthesis, and is more common if the posterior surface of the optical cylinder is at the same level as the posterior surface of the cornea.[3] Attempts can be made to remove the membrane either anteriorly, by unscrewing the optical cylinder and excising the membrane,[52,58,59] or posteriorly, by inserting a blade posterior to the keratoprosthesis and wiping the membrane away from the posterior surface of the optical cylinder. Treating the membrane with a neodymium:yttrium-aluminum-garnet (Nd:YAG) laser in a manner similar to the treatment of posterior capsular opacification frequently results in nicks in the optical cylinder and is not recommended.[67]

The diagnosis and treatment of glaucoma after prosthokeratoplasty are difficult. Intraocular pressure is estimated by palpation. Observation of the optic nerve for increased cupping, as well as serial visual fields, may aid in the diagnosis. Suspected pressure elevation is treated with an oral hypotensive agent.

Sterile vitritis is a frequent complication of prosthokeratoplasty, occurring in as many as 70 percent of cases.[58] It should be treated with periocular and/or systemic corticosteroids, even though corticosteriods impede wound healing. Any vitritis that occurs in the postoperative period should be considered infectious until proved otherwise and evaluated and treated accordingly.

Infectious endophthalmitis should be evaluated and treated promptly by tapping and culturing the vitreous, injecting antibiotics intravitreally, and giving antibiotics systemically. In severe cases, a pars plana vitrectomy is performed through a skin and scleral incision. Intraocular fiberoptics and indirect ophthalmoscopy facilitate visualization for this complex surgery.

Retinal detachment occurs in as many as 20 percent of prosthokeratoplasty cases.[58] Although the posterior pole can be visualized through the optical cylinder with an ophthalmoscope, the peripheral retina cannot be seen, and ultrasonography must be used to evaluate the peripheral retina. Historically, repair of a retinal detachment occurring in an eye with a keratoprosthesis has not been successful. Scleral buckling procedures are hampered by several factors, and the underlying retinal pathology is not addressed. Inadequate visualization through the keratoprosthesis prevents identification of peripheral retinal breaks, and external drainage of subretinal fluid is difficult. The use of perfluorophenanthrene, a liquid perfluorocarbon derivative, for the repair of retinal detachment in an eye with a keratoprosthesis has been described.[68]

Despite its potential complications, prosthokeratoplasty is a valuable procedure for those patients in whom penetrating keratoplasty is unsuccessful and should be in the corneal surgeon's armamentarium. The procedure can provide patients with several years of vision who would otherwise be blind.

TEMPORARY PROSTHOKERATOPLASTY

Eyes with opaque corneas and posterior segment abnormalities that require a vitrectomy can be managed by removing the cornea and performing an open sky vitrectomy or by replacing the cornea and performing a closed pars plana vitrectomy. A closed pars plana vitrectomy is preferred because intraocular pressure can be maintained and the eye can be manipulated without the risk of prolapsing the intraocular contents. To permit visualization of the posterior segment, the opaque cornea can be replaced with a corneal graft. However, the vitrectomy must usually be postponed until the graft clears. Additionally, the graft may be damaged by the vitrectomy.

In 1981, Landers et al[69] introduced a temporary keratoprosthesis that permits visualization of the posterior segment during pars plana vitrectomy in eyes with opaque corneas. In this procedure, the opaque cornea is removed, the keratoprosthesis is inserted, the pars plana vitrectomy is performed, the keratoprosthesis is removed, and penetrating keratoplasty is performed.

The Landers-Foulks type 2 temporary keratoprosthesis is a clear, threaded polymethyl methacrylate cylinder (Figure 36-24) with concave anterior and posterior surfaces. Anterior struts allow the keratoprosthesis to be sutured to the cornea.

At the beginning of the procedure, a scleral support ring is sutured to the superficial sclera. The recipient cornea is trephined with a trephine 0.2 mm smaller in diameter than the diameter of the keratoprosthesis to be used (i.e., 6.0 mm for the 6.2-mm keratoprosthesis; 7.0 mm for the 7.2-mm keratoprosthesis; 8.0 for the 8.2-mm keratoprosthesis). The recipient corneal button is removed, and the keratoprosthesis is screwed into the corneal opening by applying gentle pressure to the optic with a cotton-tipped applicator and rotating the struts with forceps. The struts are sutured to the cornea with two interrupted 8–0 silk or 9–0 nylon sutures (Figure 36-25). At the completion of the vitrectomy, these sutures are removed and the keratoprosthesis is unscrewed. A penetrating keratoplasty is then done with a donor corneal button 0.5 mm larger than the recipient corneal opening (i.e., 6.5 mm for a 6.0-mm opening; 7.5 mm for a 7.0-mm opening; 8.5 mm for an 8.0-mm opening). If a larger graft is desired, a trephine mark of the desired diameter is made peripheral to the trephine mark used for the keratoprosthesis at the beginning of the procedure before the eye is entered. At

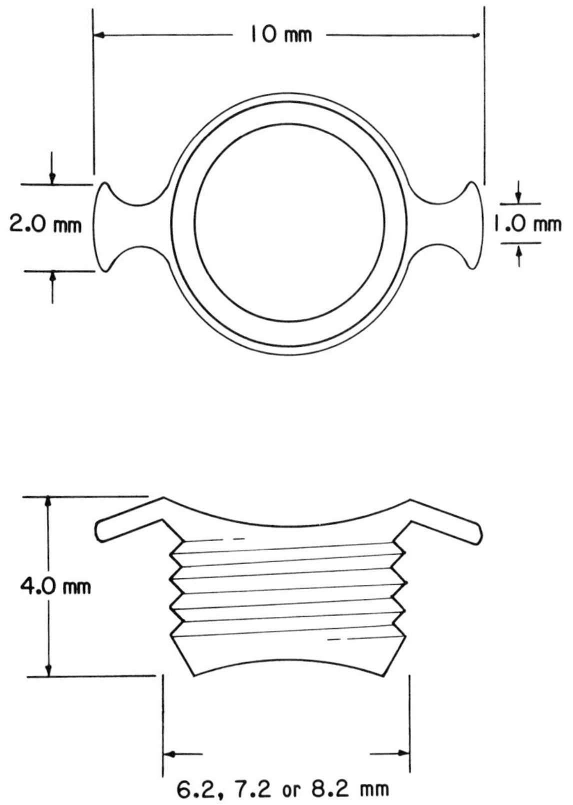

FIGURE 36-24 Landers-Foulks type 2 temporary keratoprosthesis. Top view **(top)** and side view **(bottom)**. The radius of curvature of the anterior and posterior surfaces is 7.8 mm. The refractive power is −85.4 diopters in an aphakic, fluid-filled eye. (Adapted with permission from MB Landers, GN Foulks, DM Landers, et al: Temporary keratoprosthesis for use during pars plana vitrectomy. Am J Ophthalmol 91:615, 1981. Copyright by The Ophthalmic Publishing Company.)

the completion of the vitrectomy, the keratoprosthesis and rim of cornea between the keratoprosthesis and peripheral trephine mark are removed.[70] Interrupted 9–0 nylon sutures are preferred to secure the graft because they provide a strong wound closure that can tolerate final manipulations of the eye, such as scleral depression or air-fluid exchange. The temporary presence of the keratoprosthesis in the recipient corneal opening appears to have no significant effect on wound apposition or healing.

In 1987, Eckardt[71] described a disposable temporary keratoprosthesis (Figure 36-26) made of clear silicone rubber.[72] The optical cylinder is shorter than that of the Landers-Foulks type 2 temporary keratoprosthesis, thereby providing better visualization of the peripheral retina. The Eckardt temporary keratoprosthesis is available with an optical cylinder diameter of 7 mm and is placed in a

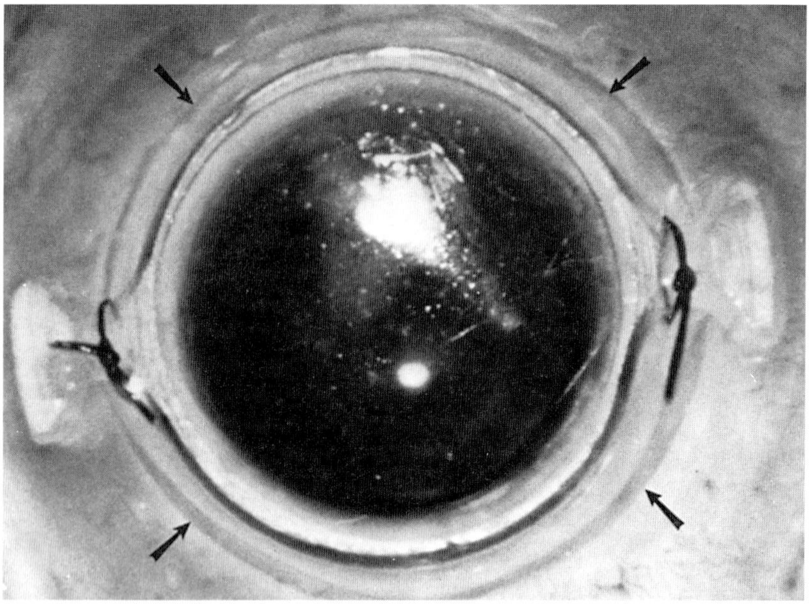

FIGURE 36-25 Landers-Foulks temporary keratoprosthesis sutured to the cornea. Note that a larger trephine mark (arrows) has been made peripheral to the keratoprosthesis because a larger graft was desired.

recipient corneal opening of 6.75 mm. Four to six 8-0 nylon sutures are placed through the peripheral cornea and keratoprosthesis to hold the keratoprosthesis in place.

In 1993, Toth and Landers introduced a wide-field reusable temporary keratoprosthesis made of polymethyl methacrylate to permit visualization of both the central and peripheral retina[73] (Figure 36-27). The Landers wide-field temporary keratoprosthesis has a central peg with a diameter of 6.2 mm, 7.2 mm, or 8.2 mm and a large flange with six suture holes. The recipient cornea is trephined with a trephine 0.2 mm smaller in diameter than the diameter of the keratoprosthesis to be used, and the keratoprosthesis is sutured to the cornea or limbus with interrupted 8-0 or 9-0 nylon sutures.

Although the underlying vitreoretinal abnormalities may limit the visual results, the use of a temporary ker-

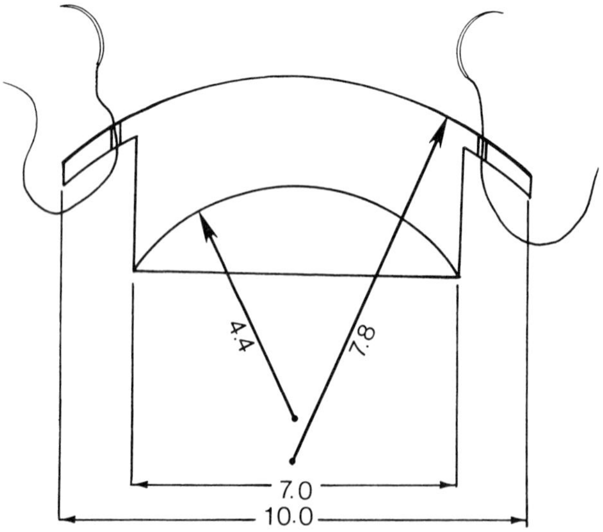

FIGURE 36-26 Eckardt temporary keratoprosthesis. The refractive power is –35 diopters in air. (Adapted with permission from C Eckardt: A new temporary keratoprosthesis for pars plana vitrectomy. Retina 7:34 1987 with permission.)

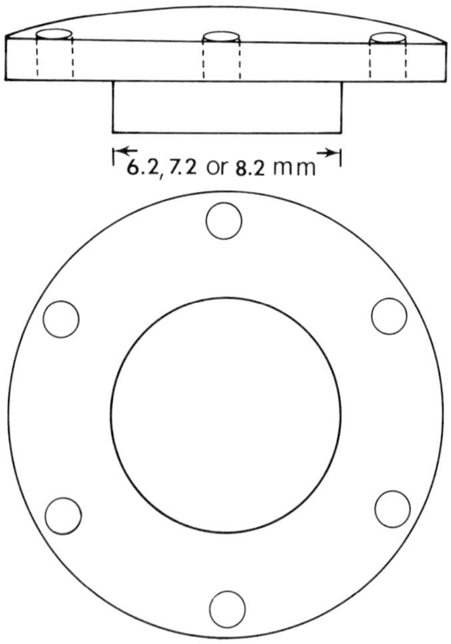

FIGURE 36-27 Landers wide-field temporary keratoprosthesis. Side view **(top)** and top view **(bottom)**.

atoprosthesis permits an attempt at surgical rehabilitation in eyes with vitreoretinal abnormalities and opaque or traumatized corneas.[72,74-76]

REFERENCES

1. Buxton JN, Buxton DF, Westphalen JA: Penetrating keratoplasty. Indications and contraindications. p. 77. In Brightbill FS (ed): Corneal Surgery: Theory, Technique, and Tissue. 2nd Ed. CV Mosby, St. Louis, 1993
2. Mannis MJ, Krachmer JH: Keratoplasty: a historical perspective. Surv Ophthalmol 25:333, 1981
3. Cardona H: Keratoprosthesis. Acrylic optical cylinder with supporting intralamellar plate. Am J Ophthalmol 54:284, 1962
4. Giles CL, Henderson JW: Keratoprosthesis: current status. Am J Med Sci 253:239, 1967
5. Barnham JJ, Roper-Hall MJ: Keratoprosthesis: a long-term review. Br J Ophthalmol 67:468, 1983
6. Polack FM: Keratoprosthesis [editorial]. Invest Ophthalmol 15:593, 1976
7. DeVoe AG: Keratoprosthesis: history, techniques, and indications. Trans Am Acad Ophthalmol Otolaryngol 83:249, 1977
8. Stone W, Herbert E: Experimental study of plastic material as replacement for the cornea. Am J Ophthalmol 36:168, 1953
9. Apple DJ, Mamalis N, Loftfield K, et al: Complications of intraocular lenses. A historical and histopathological review. Surv Ophthalmol 29:1, 1984
10. Cardona H: Plastic keratoprostheses. A description of the plastic material and comparative histologic study of recipient corneas. Am J Ophthalmol 58:247, 1964
11. Brown SI, Dohlman CH: A buried corneal prosthesis. Arch Ophthalmol 70:736, 1963
12. Brown SI, Dohlman CH: A buried corneal implant serving as a barrier to fluid. Arch Ophthalmol 73:635, 1965
13. Dohlman CH, Brown SI: Treatment of corneal edema with a buried implant. Trans Am Acad Ophthalmol Otolaryngol 70:267, 1966
14. Dohlman CH, Refojo MF, Rose J: Synthetic polymers in corneal surgery. I. Glyceryl methacrylate. Arch Ophthalmol 77:252, 1967
15. Ruedemann AD: Silicone keratoprosthesis. Trans Am Ophthalmol Soc 72:329, 1974
16. Lamberts DW, Grandon SC: A new alloplastic material for ophthalmic surgery. Ophthalmic Surg 9:35, 1978
17. Polack FM, Heimke G: Ceramic keratoprostheses. Ophthalmology 87:693, 1980
18. Polack FM: Clinical results with a ceramic keratoprosthesis. Cornea 2:185, 1983
19. Heimke G, Polack FM: Ceramic keratoprosthesis: biomechanics of extrusion in through-the-lid implantation. Cornea 2:197, 1983
20. Kozarsky AM, Knight SH, Waring GO: Clinical results with a ceramic keratoprosthesis placed through the eyelid. Ophthalmology 94:904, 1987
21. Dohlman CH, Refojo MF, Carrol J, Gasset A: Artificial corneal epithelium. Arch Ophthalmol 79:360, 1968
22. Gasset AR, Kaufman HE: Epikeratoprosthesis. Replacement of superficial cornea by methylmethacrylate. Am J Ophthalmol 66:641, 1968
23. Kaufman HE, Gasset AR: Clinical experience with the epikeratoprosthesis. Am J Ophthalmol 67:38, 1969
24. Boruchoff SA: Clinical application of adhesives in corneal surgery. Trans Ophthalmol Soc UK 89:373, 1969
25. Gasset AR, Kaufman HE: Therapeutic uses of hydrophilic contact lenses. Am J Ophthalmol 69:252, 1970
26. Choyce P: Management of endothelial corneal dystrophy with acrylic corneal inlays. Br J Ophthalmol 49:432, 1965
27. Choyce DP: Intra-cameral and intra-corneal implants. A decade of personal experience. Trans Ophthalmol Soc UK 86:507,1966
28. Choyce DP: The present status of intra-cameral and intra-corneal implants. Can J Ophthalmol 3:295, 1968
29. Choyce DP: The present status of keratoprosthesis. Isr J Med Sci 8:1285, 1972
30. Choyce DP: Results of keratoprosthetics in Britain. Ophthalmic Surg 4:23, 1973
31. DeVoe AG: A review of the techniques of keratoprostheses. Surv Ophthalmol 16:170, 1971
32. Stone W Jr, Yasuda H, Refojo MF: A 15-year study of the plastic artificial cornea—basic principles. p. 654. In King JH, McTigue JW (eds): The Cornea. World Congress. Butterworths, Washington, DC, 1965
33. Cardona H: Anterior and posterior mushroom keratoprostheses. An experimental study. Am J Ophthalmol 61:498, 1966
34. Choyce DP: Perforating keratoprosthesis. The Choyce MK II (1967) 2-piece perforating keratoprosthesis. Trans Ophthalmol Soc UK 90:23, 1970
35. Choyce DP: Perforating keratoprosthesis: 60 cases, 1967–72. Trans Ophthalmol Soc UK 92:727, 1972
36. Choyce DP: The Choyce 2-piece perforating keratoprosthesis: seventy cases, 1967–1973. Trans Ophthalmol Soc UK 93:333, 1973
37. Choyce DP: The Choyce 2-piece perforating keratoprosthesis: 107 cases—1967–1976. Ophthalmic Surg 8:117, 1977
38. Choyce DP: Evolution of Choyce 2-piece multistage perforating keratoprosthesis technique: 1967–1978. Ann Ophthalmol 12:740, 1980
39. Györffy I: Acrylic corneal implant in keratoplasty. Am J Ophthalmol 34:757, 1951
40. Dohlman CH, Schneider HA, Doane MG: Prosthokeratoplasty. Am J Ophthalmol 77:694, 1974
41. Strampelli B: Osteo-odonto-keratoprosthesis. Ann Ottal 89:1039, 1963
42. Barraquer J: Keratoplasty and keratoprosthesis. Ann R Coll Surg Engl 40:71, 1967
43. Casey TA: Osteo-odonto-keratoprosthesis. Proc R Soc Med 59:530, 1966

44. Casey TA: Osteo-odontokeratoprosthesis and chondrokeratoprosthesis. Proc R Soc Med 63:313, 1970
45. Cardona H: Keratoprosthesis with a plastic fiber meshwork supporting plate. Report of an experimental and comparative histologic study. Am J Ophthalmol 64:228, 1967
46. DeVoe AG: Current status of the keratoprosthesis. Trans Ophthalmol Soc N Z 25:127, 1973
47. Cardona H: Mushroom transcorneal keratoprosthesis. Bolt and nut. Am J Ophthalmol 68:604, 1969
48. Buxton JN: Keratoprosthesis: personal experiences. Trans Am Acad Ophthalmol Otolaryngol 83:268, 1977
49. Girard LJ, Moore CD, Soper JW, O'Bannon W: Prosthetosclerokeratoplasty—implantation of a keratoprosthesis using full-thickness onlay sclera and sliding conjunctival flap. Trans Am Acad Ophthalmol Otolaryngol 73:936, 1969
50. Girard LJ, Hawkins RS, Nieves R, et al: Keratoprosthesis: a 12-year follow-up. Trans Am Acad Ophthalmol Otolaryngol 83:252, 1977
51. Chilaris G, Liaricos S: Fascia of the temporalis muscle in scleral buckling and keratoprosthesis operations. Am J Ophthalmol 76:35, 1973
52. Cardona H, DeVoe AG: Prosthokeratoplasty. Trans Am Acad Ophthalmol Otolaryngol 83:271, 1977
53. Cardona H: Prosthokeratoplasty. Cornea 2:179, 1983
54. Girard LJ: Keratoprosthesis. Cornea 2:207, 1983
55. Donn A: Aphakic bullous keratopathy treated with prosthokeratoplasty. An analysis of 34 consecutive cases. Arch Ophthalmol 94:270, 1976
56. Donn A: Additional follow-up of 34 cases of prosthokeratoplasty. Trans Am Acad Ophthalmol Otolaryngol 83:281, 1977
57. Aquavella JV: Clinical experience with the Cardona keratoprosthesis. Cornea 2:177, 1983
58. Rao GN, Blatt HL, Aquavella JV: Results of keratoprosthesis. Am J Ophthalmol 88:190, 1979
59. Aquavella JV, Rao GN, Brown AC, Harris JK: Keratoprosthesis: results, complications, and management. Ophthalmology 89:655, 1982
60. Harris JK, Rao GN, Aquavella JV, Lohman LE: Keratoprosthesis: technique and instrumentation. Ann Ophthalmol 16:481, 1984
61. Cardona H: The Cardona keratoprosthesis: 40 years experience. Refract Corneal Surg 7:468, 1991
62. Olson RJ, Kaufman HE: An abscess associated with a through-the-lid keratoprosthesis one year after intraocular lens insertion. Ophthalmic Surg 11:203, 1980
63. Ferry AP, Gordon BL: Epithelialization of the anterior chamber: a complication of prosthokeratoplasty. Arch Ophthalmol 91:281, 1974
64. Carroll CP, Keates RH: Bone formation in a periosteal graft. Arch Ophthalmol 97:916, 1979
65. Srinivasan BD, Jakobiec FA, Iwamoto T, DeVoe G: Giant papillary conjunctivitis with ocular prostheses. Arch Ophthalmol 97:892, 1979
66. Barron BA, Dingeldein S, Kaufman HE: Spontaneous unscrewing of a Cardona keratoprosthesis. Am J Ophthalmol 103:331, 1987
67. Bath PE, McCord RC, Cox KC: Nd:YAG laser discission of retroprosthetic membrane: a preliminary report. Cornea 2:225, 1983
68. Paris CL, Peyman GA, Blinder KJ, et al: Surgical technique for managing rhegmatogenous retinal detachment following prosthokeratoplasty. Retina 11:301, 1991
69. Landers MB, Foulks GN, Landers DM, et al: Temporary keratoprosthesis for use during pars plana vitrectomy. Am J Ophthalmol 91:615, 1981
70. Groden LR, Arentsen JJ: Penetrating keratoplasty following the use of a temporary keratoprosthesis during pars plana vitrectomy. Ophthalmic Surg 15:208, 1984
71. Eckardt C: A new temporary keratoprosthesis for pars plana vitrectomy. Retina 7:34, 1987
72. Gross JG, Feldman S, Freeman WR: Combined penetrating keratoplasty and vitreoretinal surgery with the Eckardt temporary keratoprosthesis. Ophthalmic Surg 21:67, 1990
73. Toth CA, Landers MB III: A new wide-field temporary keratoprosthesis [letter]. Retina 13:353, 1993
74. Koenig SB, McDonald HR, Williams GA, Abrams GW: Penetrating keratoplasty after placement of a temporary keratoprosthesis during pars plana vitrectomy. Am J Ophthalmol 102:45, 1986
75. Mannis MJ, May DR: Use of the temporary keratoprosthesis in the subacute management of massive ocular trauma. Ann Ophthalmol 15:773, 1983
76. Gelender H, Vaiser A, Snyder WB, et al: Temporary keratoprosthesis for combined penetrating keratoplasty, pars plana vitrectomy, and repair of retinal detachment. Ophthalmology 95:897, 1988

37

Radial Keratotomy

George O. Waring III

Radial keratotomy, like most surgical procedures, has evolved and improved as ophthalmologists have defined its role in the management of myopia. This chapter surveys the changes that have occurred in radial keratotomy over the past century and emphasizes some of the current techniques being used to improve its safety, efficacy, predictability, and stability.[1–4] The prevalence of myopia varies widely around the world,[5] so the utility of radial keratotomy will vary as well.

HISTORY OF RADIAL KERATOTOMY

Table 37-1 outlines the history and development of keratotomy for myopia and astigmatism. Interest in keratotomy surgery began in the late 1800s. At that time, corneal astigmatism, including keratoconus, frequently caused functional blindness because neither contact lenses nor penetrating keratoplasty was available.[6] Lans[6] performed experiments in rabbits using keratotomy, keratectomy, and thermal keratoplasty to alter corneal astigmatism. His findings formed the basis for modern radial keratotomy.

In the late 1930s, Sato observed that individuals with keratoconus who developed breaks in Descemet's membrane (corneal hydrops) often experienced corneal flattening and a reduction in both myopia and irregular astigmatism after the breaks healed.[7,8] He developed a technique for making incisions in the posterior cornea to induce flattening in cases of keratoconus and astigmatism. Later, he supplemented this procedure with incisions in the anterior cornea to treat myopia.

After the original observations in human eyes, Sato and Akiyama performed experiments in rabbits, testing at least a dozen different patterns of keratotomy.[7,9–11] They concluded that radial incisions made in the posterior cornea had a greater effect than those made in the anterior cornea and that circumferential incisions were ineffective in flattening the cornea.

When contact lenses became available in Japan in the mid 1950s, Sato stopped performing radial keratotomy to correct myopia. However, the devastating corneal edema that resulted from damage to the corneal endothelium from posterior incisions did not begin to appear until the 1960s, nearly 20 years after the surgery had been performed[12,13] (Figure 37-1).

In the early 1960s, a number of surgeons in the former Soviet Union undertook a series of studies of refractive keratotomy in rabbits. Incisions in the posterior cornea were used originally but were deemed too complicated. In the mid to late 1960s, incisions in the anterior cornea were used. Fyodorov began performing radial keratotomy in humans in about 1974; the first description of his results in humans in the English literature appeared in 1979.[14] Fyodorov and his colleagues made major contributions to radial keratotomy by emphasizing an individualized approach using different variables to customize the procedure for each patient.

In 1978, Bores performed the first radial keratotomy in the United States; he learned the technique from Fyodorov. Radial keratotomy developed in the United States in four stages. From approximately 1978 through 1981, the introductory stage involved refinements of the Russian techniques that used 8 to 32 radial incisions, various patterns of transverse incisions, and optical pachymetry to measure corneal thickness. Publications were limited largely to proceedings of meetings.[15–17]

The second stage began in 1980, when the National Eye Institute funded the Prospective Evaluation of Radial Keratotomy (PERK) study, in which university-based and private practice ophthalmologists cooperated at nine clinical centers. The specially trained surgeons used a single, well-defined operative technique of radial keratotomy on

TABLE 37-1
Highlights in the Development of Keratotomy for Myopia and Astigmatism

Date	*Individual*	*Country*	*Contribution*
1885	H. Schiøtz	Norway	Performed transverse keratotomy for astigmatism
1886–1896	W.H. Bates E. Faber J. Lucciola	United States The Netherlands Italy	Performed transverse keratotomy for astigmatism
1898	L.J. Lans	The Netherlands	Described principles of transverse and radial keratotomy in the laboratory
1939-1955	T. Sato K. Akiyama	Japan	Established principles of transverse and radial keratotomy in rabbits and humans; poor results with posterior keratotomy
1960s	M.P. Pureskin	Former Soviet Union	Confirmed poor results with Sato's posterior keratotomy
1970s	V.S. Beliayev M.K. Tin V.F. Utkin F.S. Yenaleyev	Former Soviet Union	Studied anterior keratotomy with variable numbers of incisions
1972–present	S.V. Fyodorov V.V. Durnev	Former Soviet Union	Included multiple ocular variables, including smaller clear zones, to tailor keratotomy for each patient
1978–1980	L.D. Bores W.D. Myers J. Cowden	United States	Started keratotomy in the United States; added centrifugal and deepening incisions
1980–present	Many individual surgeons	United States	Improved surgical instruments and techniques
1980s	L.A. Ruiz R.L. Lindstrom	Colombia United States	Developed and refined combined radial and transverse keratotomy for myopia and astigmatism
1980–1995	G.O. Waring and the Prospective Evaluation of Radial Keratotomy (PERK) Study	United States	Conducted a monitored, prospective trial of radial keratotomy with 10-year follow-up
1983	S.D. Trokel R. Srinivasan	United States	Described use of excimer laser for refractive keratectomy
1985	M.R. Deitz D.R. Sanders	United States`	Identified hyperopic shift after radial keratotomy
1985	T. Seiler	Germany	Performed excimer laser transverse keratotomy for astigmatism
1989–1994	J.C. Casebeer and the Casebeer-Chiron Study Group	United States	Systematized surgical techniques and nomograms
1993	R.L. Lindstrom	United States	Developed short incisions (mini-RK) to decrease hyperopic shift
1993–present	I.G. Pallikaris S. Slade G. Waring and others	Crete United States	Combined arcuate transverse keratotomy (ARC-T) with excimer laser-assisted in situ keratomileusis (LASIK)

Abbreviation: RK, radial keratotomy.
Source: Adapted with permission from GO Waring: Refractive Keratotomy for Myopia and Astigmatism. Mosby–Year Book, St. Louis, 1992.

435 patients, who were selected and examined according to a detailed protocol.[18] The PERK surgical technique, which involved a nomogram based on refraction, eight centrifugal incisions made with a diamond knife calibrated on a gauge block, and intraoperative ultrasonic pachymetry, is no longer in use. However, the results of the PERK study provide an important baseline against which to assess the improvements that have occurred over the past decade. The results of the PERK study have been published in 36 peer-reviewed articles, including findings at 10 years.[19]

Between approximately 1981 and 1988, a third stage of refinements included the increasing use of four radial incisions, the use of nonintersecting arcuate transverse incisions to correct astigmatism, the observation that centripetal incisions are more effective than centrifugal incisions, and nomograms that included age as a variable. During this period, approximately 300 papers by a variety of surgeons contributed to this progress.

In the fourth stage, the basic approach changed to accommodate the realization that variations in surgical techniques and individual wound healing make the outcome

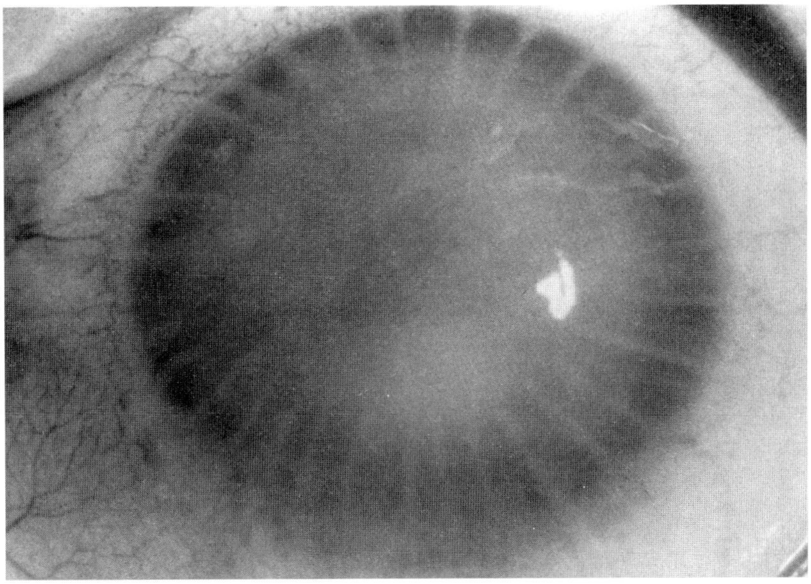

FIGURE 37-1 Cornea after anterior and posterior radial keratotomy of Sato shows extensive edema that occurred because of direct damage to the corneal endothelium by the posterior incisions.

of a single radial keratotomy procedure less than perfectly predictable. The new technique involved intentional undercorrection followed by repeat surgery (enhancements) to achieve the desired result for each patient. New technology included thin (75 to 125 μm), double-edged diamond blades calibrated on a micrometer mounted on a compound microscope. The use of centripetal incisions often produced incisions extending into the central clear zone, a complication that led to the development of bidirectional incisions made with diamond knives partially blunt on one edge. Only a few publications have described these techniques at this writing.[3,20–22]

PRINCIPLES OF RADIAL KERATOTOMY

The following principles of radial keratotomy have been established through laboratory and clinical research[23,24]:

- Approximately 60 percent of the central flattening of the cornea is obtained with the first four incisions,[25] and eight incisions produce approximately 85 percent of the effect achieved with 16 incisions[26–28] (Table 37-2).
- The smaller the diameter of the central clear zone, the greater the amount of central corneal flattening.[29]
- Incisions extending across the limbus into the sclera are no more effective than incisions confined to the cornea,[30] and shorter (2.5 to 3.0 mm) incisions are almost as effective as incisions extending to the limbus.[31]
- Deeper incisions achieve greater flattening of the cornea than do shallower incisions.[32]
- Peripheral deepening incisions do not significantly increase the amount of central corneal flattening[25] (Table 37-3).
- Reoperation that increases the length, depth, or number of incisions increases the effect of the initial surgery.[4]

TABLE 37-2
Change in Corneal Curvature after 4, 8, and 16 Radial Incisions

	Change in Corneal Curvature (Diopters)[a]			
Number of Incisions	*Mean*	*Percentage*[b]	*Standard Error of the Mean*	*Range*
4	5.25	62	0.45	1.50–8.75
8	7.25	85	0.53	3.50–10.25
16	8.50	100	0.50	5.75–10.75

[a] Values recorded as average spherical equivalents rounded to nearest quarter diopter.
[b] Percentage change as related to effects of 16 radial incisions.
Source: Published with permission from JV Jester, T Venet, J Lee, et al: A statistical analysis of radial keratotomy in human cadaver eyes. Am J Ophthalmol 92:172, 1981. Copyright by The Ophthalmic Publishing Company.

TABLE 37-3
Mean Effects of Peripheral Deepening Incisions[a] on Corneal Curvature after 8-Incision Radial Keratotomy

Clear Zone (mm)	*Amount of Additional Corneal Flattening (Diopters)[b]*
3.0	0.06 ± 1.16[c]
4.0	0.27 ± 0.39
5.0	0.35 ± 1.12

[a] Deepening incisions made from a 6.0-mm–diameter zone to the limbus with the blade set at 100 percent of the thinnest corneal thickness measured at the 6.0-mm–diameter zone.
[b] Measured by Terry keratometry.
[c] Mean ± standard deviation.
Source: Adapted with permission from JJ Salz, JJ Rowsey, P Caroline, et al: A study of optical zone size and incision redeepening in experimental radial keratotomy. Arch Ophthalmol 103:590, 1985. Copyright 1985, American Medical Association.

- The same surgical procedure performed by the same surgeon produces a wide range of results (approximately 5 diopters).[27,33,34]
- Radial keratotomy incisions heal normally by histopathologic criteria, but the epithelial plug can persist as long as 4 to 6 years,[27,33] and the healed wounds never regain the strength of normal cornea.

The most important variables that affect the outcome of radial keratotomy are the amount of preoperative myopia, the age of the patient, the diameter of the central clear zone, the depth of the incisions, and the number of incisions. Older patients obtain a greater refractive change (approximately 0.75 to 1.00 diopter per decade), presumably because their corneas heal more slowly and possibly less effectively.

Variables that have minimal or no effect on the outcome include corneal diameter, intraocular pressure, central corneal curvature, sex, ocular rigidity, and corneal thickness (except at the extremes).[35-37] Although intraocular pressure in the normal range usually has little effect on outcome, elevating the pressure to 30 mmHg with topical corticosteroids can temporarily enhance the result of the surgery. However, long-term use of corticosteroids for this purpose should not be considered. Conversely, lowering elevated intraocular pressure with topical timolol has been reported to decrease the effect of radial keratotomy.[38]

PATIENT SELECTION

One reason for renewed interest in radial keratotomy in the 1970s was that individuals whose occupations required good vision without glasses or contact lenses, such as pilots, peace officers, and professional athletes, sought refractive surgery. Early human trials in both the former Soviet Union[14] and the United States[39] emphasized the treatment of this group of patients. However, two early studies of psychological motivations in patients who had radial keratotomy found that occupation was infrequently a factor[40,41] (Table 37-4).

The most common motivation for patients who want radial keratotomy is the desire to see well without contact lenses or spectacles. Bourque et al[40] found that 65 percent of patients entering the PERK study did so to free themselves of dependence on optical correction for good vision. Some expressed the fear of being caught in dangerous situations without their correction or the desire to see well uncorrected in social situations, such as at the beach or while water-skiing. Powers et al[41] confirmed these findings. Both studies found that only a small percentage of patients expressed the need for improved appearance.

Some ophthalmologists have questioned the psychological health of patients who want radial keratotomy, asking "Why would anyone want to undergo eye surgery when spectacles or contact lenses provide good vision?" Bourque and colleagues[40] administered psychological tests to applicants in the PERK study and could not identify psychological abnormalities, such as high propensity for risk taking, depression, or increased use of medical care in the group, compared with a cross-section of normal individuals in the Rand Health Survey.

Radial keratotomy alters the way the eye functions because it changes the way images are focused on the

TABLE 37-4
Single Most Important Reason PERK Patients Reported for Having Surgery

Reasons for Having Surgery	*Percentage of 369 Patients*
Not to be dependent on eyeglasses or contact lenses	65
Occupation	6
To see well all of the time	6
Comfort or convenience of not having to wear eyeglasses or contact lenses	5
Sports	5
Cosmetic purposes	3
To have greater freedom of movement	3
To be more self-confident	1
Other	6

Abbreviation: PERK, Prospective Evaluation of Radial Keratotomy.
Source: Adapted with permission from LB Bourque, R Rubenstein, B Cosand, et al: Psychosocial characteristics of candidates for the Prospective Evaluation of Radial Keratotomy (PERK) study. Arch Ophthalmol 102:1187, 1984. Copyright 1984, American Medical Association.

retina. Because radial keratotomy does not alter the appearance of the patient, it cannot be considered cosmetic surgery, except possibly for those who object to their appearance in glasses. However, radial keratotomy is elective surgery because there is no medical urgency for the operation, and myopia can be managed alternatively with spectacles or contact lenses.

Although criteria for selecting patients may vary from one surgeon to another, some general principles have been established. Because radial keratotomy is an elective operation on an anatomically normal organ, the surgeon bears increased responsibility to inform the patient of the risks and benefits of the operation, and the patient carries increased responsibility to have realistic expectations of the results. Overpromotion of radial keratotomy leads to unrealistic patient expectations and increased numbers of dissatisfied patients postoperatively.[42,43]

Patients who have specific occupational goals should be made aware of the prospective employer's criteria for hiring. For example, the U.S. Air Force will not take into active duty anyone who has had radial keratotomy. A report in a consumer magazine stated that none of the branches of the United States armed forces permits pilots or pilot trainees to undergo radial keratotomy,[44] and more stringent vision testing has been proposed for candidates for other high-risk occupations, such as prospective fire fighters, who have undergone radial keratotomy.[45]

Whether a patient will need glasses or contact lenses postoperatively for distance vision depends on the outcome of the surgery and the patient's criteria for good vision. Many patients elect to use spectacles part-time for special circumstances, such as driving at night. Patients over 40 years of age must realize that they will exchange dependence on spectacles for distance vision for dependence on spectacles for near vision if both eyes are emmetropic after bilateral radial keratotomy. In the PERK study, at 10 years after surgery, 36 percent of patients younger than 40 years of age and 67 percent of patients 40 years of age or older still wore some type of corrective lens, either for distance vision, near vision, or both.[19]

Radial keratotomy is most effective for the correction of 1.50 to 5.00 diopters of myopia. Approximately 50 to 60 percent of patients with a preoperative refraction between -1.50 and -5.00 diopters will achieve an uncorrected postoperative visual acuity of 20/20 or better, and approximately 90 percent will achieve 20/40 or better, but the outcome of surgery for an individual eye is not accurately predictable. Some patients achieve a greater or lesser effect than expected. Patients should be informed of the risk of overcorrection or undercorrection and of the possible need for reoperation.

The patient should have a stable refraction, although if myopia progresses postoperatively, an enhancement procedure can be performed to again reach emmetropia. In general, the patient should be older than 18 years of age; rigid gas-permeable contact lenses should be removed for at least 2 weeks before performing the refraction on which the surgery will be based, although longer periods of time may be necessary for the cornea to stabilize; records of previous refractions should document long-term stability; and there should be no ophthalmoscopic signs of degenerative, pathologic myopia. The level of preoperative best spectacle-corrected visual acuity should be such that the patient has a reasonable chance for achieving useful improvement in uncorrected visual acuity.

There are a number of medical and ophthalmic contraindications to radial keratotomy. Patients with active ocular disease, such as untreated blepharitis or chronic iridocyclitis, should not have radial keratotomy. Patients with a history of herpes simplex keratitis may experience recurrence after surgery and are not candidates for radial keratotomy. Patients with keratoconus should not have radial keratotomy because the outcome of the surgery is unpredictable.[46–49] Subclinical keratoconus can be detected preoperatively by videokeratography (see Ch. 22).[50] Wilson and Klyce[51] evaluated the corneal topography of 53 patients seeking refractive surgery for the correction of myopia and diagnosed keratoconus in three patients (6 percent), an incidence higher than that reported in the general population. They also diagnosed corneal warpage in 38 percent of patients who wore contact lenses.

A certain number of patients who have had radial keratotomy have persistent fluctuating vision, bothersome glare, and ghost images that persist beyond the usual 3 to 6 months postoperatively. While these sequelae may be minor annoyances for most patients, some consider them sufficiently visually disruptive to cause dissatisfaction with the outcome of the surgery. Glare increases when the pupil is large and the patient sees through the paracentral inflection area of corneal curvature and through the central ends of the incisions.[52] A patient with a large pupil who would require a small-diameter optical clear zone for the correction of myopia is not a good candidate for radial keratotomy.

NOMOGRAMS AND PREDICTIVE FORMULAS

To improve the predictability of radial keratotomy, surgeons have sought to identify variables that affect the outcome. They have attempted to relate preoperative variables (i.e., refraction, age, sex, central keratometry readings, intraocular pressure, corneal diameter, and ocular rigidity) and intraoperative variables (i.e., diameter of the optical clear zone, the number of incisions, and the depth of the incisions) in both nomograms and formulas derived from multiple regression analysis.[20,22,35,45,53–55]

To use such nomograms and formulas, the surgeon selects the required preoperative variables and identifies the diameter of the optical clear zone, the number of incisions, and the depth of the incisions. Some programs allow surgeons to enter data from a series of their own cases and then to modify the formula to reflect their own technique. Nomograms and formulas claim to improve the outcome of the surgery and are a convenient, useful guide for making decisions about the surgery. Nevertheless, warnings are in order.

Each formula is based on the experience of one surgeon who used specific surgical techniques. Thus, the surgeon who adopts a particular formula should use surgical techniques similar to the ones on which the formula was based. Few of the formulas currently marketed as software-hardware packages have been published or independently tested.[35,53] Until these two criteria are met, surgeons should view the formulas with caution.

The accuracy called for in some formulas is unrealistic. For example, in one program reviewed by Salz,[55] a 3.0-mm clear zone and eight incisions, used in a 30-year-old man with 5.0 diopters of myopia, are said to reduce myopia by 3.24 diopters if the incisions are 90 percent deep, and by 4.57 diopters if the incisions are 95 percent deep. Using current techniques of radial keratotomy, it is not possible to control incision depth this reliably or to measure the depth of the incisions with an accuracy of 5 percent.

Different programs suggest different surgical protocols for the same theoretical patient. For example, Salz[55] reported the surgery recommended by different programs for a 23-year-old woman with a refraction of −2.50 diopters, an intraocular pressure of 20 mmHg, average central keratometry reading of 44.75 diopters, central corneal thickness of 570 μm, and a corneal diameter of 11.5 mm. For an eight-incision procedure, the recommendations by different programs were: (1) 4.5-mm clear zone, 90 percent depth; (2) 4.0-mm clear zone, 90 percent depth; (3) 3.5-mm clear zone, 90 percent depth; and (4) 3.0-mm clear zone, 80 percent depth. Some programs predict the results of as many as 152 different combinations of clear zone, number of incisions, and incision depth.

The idea that a single formula can serve as a guide to a predictable outcome in radial keratotomy has been abandoned by most surgeons. The current view is that a nomogram serves only as a guide to the initial surgery, which will approximate the desired refractive outcome. Thereafter, a patient may require one or two additional operations to achieve a satisfactory correction.

I currently use a nomogram developed at the Emory Vision Correction Center of the Vision Correction Group, which is designed to achieve either plano or residual myopia after the first operation. It is also designed to use eight incisions in preference to four so that a larger diameter clear zone can be used. The nomogram is based on the amount of refractive myopia and the patient's age but no other patient-related variables. It was derived by regression analysis based on a specific surgical technique used at the Emory Vision Correction Center. The nomogram is reproduced as Table 37-5.

PREOPERATIVE MEDICATIONS

No preoperative medications are required for radial keratotomy. A mild drug for anxiety, such as diazepam (5 or 10 mg), may be given orally to relax the patient, but the patient must remain alert enough to cooperate with marking the center of the entrance pupil. Miotic or mydriatic agents may decrease the accuracy of marking the center of the entrance pupil, and a miotic agent may constrict the pupil unevenly. The miosis induced by the light of the microscope increases patient comfort and helps with the location of the center of the entrance pupil. During reoperation, a dilated pupil increases the visibility of the previous incisions but makes the operation more uncomfortable for the patient. When the pupil is dilated, the protective barrier of the iris over the lens capsule is removed, and corneal perforation carries a greater risk of damage to the lens.

ANESTHESIA

Radial keratotomy can be performed with the use of a topical anesthetic, such as proparacaine (0.5 percent) or tetracaine (0.5 percent). Topical cocaine should be avoided because it damages the epithelium. A few drops of topical anesthetic are sufficient to anesthetize the cornea itself; the conjunctiva is more difficult to anesthetize, particularly at the limbus. Sponges can be soaked in topical anesthetic and applied to the limbus to ensure that the patient will not feel the fixation instrument during the procedure.

The risks of retrobulbar hemorrhage, hypersensitivity reactions to the anesthetic, and inadvertent injection into the longer myopic eye (which has occurred during radial keratotomy[56]) or the optic nerve make intraorbital anesthesia inappropriate for routine use in radial keratotomy. However, uncooperative patients may experience less risk with intraorbital anesthesia, which gives the surgeon more control than topical anesthesia.

TABLE 37-5
Vision Correction Group Radial Keratotomy Nomogram: Diameter of Clear Zone Based on Age and Desired Correction in Diopters[a]

Age (yr)	8 Incisions: Diameter of Clear Zone (mm)								4 Incisions: Diameter of Clear Zone (mm)					
	3.00	3.25	3.50	3.75	4.00	4.25	4.50	4.75	4.00	4.25	4.50	4.75	5.00	5.25
18	4.1	3.6	3.2	2.8	2.5	2.2	1.9	1.7	1.5	1.3	1.1	0.9	0.7	0.5
19	4.2	3.7	3.2	2.8	2.5	2.2	1.9	1.7	1.5	1.3	1.1	0.9	0.7	0.5
20	4.3	3.7	3.3	2.9	2.5	2.2	1.9	1.7	1.5	1.3	1.1	0.9	0.7	0.5
21	4.3	3.8	3.3	2.9	2.6	2.3	2.0	1.8	1.6	1.4	1.2	1.0	0.8	0.5
22	4.4	3.8	3.4	3.0	2.6	2.3	2.0	1.8	1.6	1.4	1.2	1.0	0.8	0.5
23	4.5	3.9	3.4	3.0	2.6	2.3	2.0	1.8	1.6	1.4	1.2	1.0	0.8	0.5
24	4.6	4.0	3.5	3.1	2.7	2.3	2.0	1.8	1.6	1.4	1.2	1.0	0.8	0.5
25	4.7	4.1	3.6	3.1	2.7	2.4	2.1	1.8	1.7	1.4	1.2	1.0	0.8	0.5
26	4.7	4.1	3.6	3.2	2.8	2.4	2.1	1.9	1.7	1.5	1.3	1.1	0.9	0.6
27	4.8	4.2	3.7	3.2	2.8	2.5	2.2	1.9	1.8	1.5	1.3	1.1	0.9	0.6
28	4.9	4.3	3.8	3.3	2.9	2.5	2.2	1.9	1.8	1.5	1.3	1.1	0.9	0.6
29	5.0	4.4	3.8	3.3	2.9	2.5	2.2	1.9	1.8	1.5	1.3	1.1	0.9	0.6
30	5.1	4.5	3.9	3.4	3.0	2.6	2.3	2.0	1.9	1.6	1.4	1.1	0.9	0.6
31	5.3	4.7	3.9	3.4	3.0	2.6	2.3	2.0	1.9	1.6	1.4	1.2	1.0	0.7
32	5.4	4.8	4.0	3.5	3.1	2.7	2.4	2.1	2.0	1.7	1.5	1.2	1.0	0.7
33	5.5	4.9	4.0	3.5	3.1	2.7	2.4	2.1	2.0	1.7	1.5	1.2	1.0	0.7
34	5.6	5.0	4.1	3.6	3.2	2.8	2.4	2.1	2.0	1.8	1.5	1.2	1.0	0.7
35	5.7	5.0	4.2	3.7	3.3	2.8	2.5	2.2	2.1	1.8	1.6	1.3	1.0	0.7
36	5.7	5.1	4.4	3.8	3.3	2.9	2.5	2.2	2.1	1.9	1.6	1.3	1.1	0.8
37	5.8	5.1	4.5	3.9	3.4	2.9	2.6	2.3	2.2	1.9	1.7	1.4	1.1	0.8
38	5.9	5.2	4.6	4.0	3.5	3.0	2.6	2.3	2.2	2.0	1.7	1.4	1.1	0.8
39	6.0	5.3	4.7	4.1	3.6	3.1	2.7	2.3	2.2	2.0	1.7	1.4	1.1	0.8
40	6.1	5.4	4.8	4.2	3.7	3.2	2.7	2.4	2.3	2.0	1.7	1.4	1.1	0.8
41	6.2	5.4	4.8	4.2	3.7	3.2	2.8	2.4	2.3	2.1	1.8	1.5	1.2	0.9
42	6.3	5.5	4.9	4.3	3.8	3.3	2.8	2.5	2.4	2.1	1.8	1.5	1.2	0.9
43	6.4	5.6	5.0	4.4	3.9	3.4	2.9	2.5	2.4	2.1	1.8	1.5	1.2	0.9
44	6.5	5.7	5.1	4.5	3.9	3.4	2.9	2.5	2.4	2.1	1.8	1.5	1.2	0.9
45	6.6	5.8	5.1	4.5	4.0	3.4	3.0	2.6	2.5	2.2	1.8	1.5	1.2	0.9
46	6.6	5.8	5.2	4.6	4.0	3.5	3.0	2.6	2.5	2.2	1.9	1.6	1.3	1.0
47	6.7	5.9	5.2	4.6	4.1	3.5	3.1	2.7	2.6	2.3	1.9	1.6	1.3	1.0
48	6.8	6.0	5.3	4.7	4.1	3.5	3.1	2.7	2.6	2.3	1.9	1.6	1.3	1.0
49	6.9	6.1	5.4	4.8	4.2	3.6	3.2	2.8	2.7	2.3	1.9	1.6	1.3	1.0
50	7.0	6.2	5.5	4.9	4.3	3.7	3.2	2.8	2.7	2.3	1.9	1.6	1.3	1.0
51	7.1	6.2	5.5	4.9	4.3	3.7	3.3	2.9	2.8	2.4	1.9	1.7	1.4	1.0
52	7.2	6.3	5.6	5.0	4.4	3.8	3.3	2.9	2.8	2.4	1.9	1.7	1.4	1.0
53	7.3	6.4	5.7	5.1	4.5	3.9	3.4	3.0	2.9	2.4	1.9	1.7	1.4	1.0
54	7.4	6.5	5.8	5.1	4.5	3.9	3.4	3.0	2.9	2.4	2.0	1.7	1.4	1.0
55	7.5	6.6	5.8	5.2	4.5	3.9	3.4	3.0	2.9	2.5	2.0	1.8	1.4	1.0
56	7.5	6.6	5.9	5.2	4.6	4.0	3.5	3.1	3.0	2.5	2.1	1.8	1.5	1.1
57	7.6	6.7	5.9	5.3	4.6	4.0	3.5	3.1	3.0	2.6	2.1	1.9	1.5	1.1
58	7.7	6.8	6.0	5.3	4.6	4.0	3.5	3.1	3.0	2.6	2.2	1.9	1.5	1.1
59	7.8	6.9	6.1	5.4	4.7	4.1	3.6	3.1	3.1	2.7	2.3	1.9	1.5	1.1
60	7.9	7.0	6.2	5.5	4.8	4.2	3.6	3.2	3.1	2.7	2.3	2.0	1.6	1.2
61	8.0	7.0	6.2	5.5	4.8	4.2	3.7	3.2	3.2	2.8	2.4	2.0	1.6	1.2
62	8.1	7.1	6.3	5.6	4.9	4.3	3.7	3.3	3.2	2.8	2.4	2.1	1.7	1.3
63	8.2	7.2	6.4	5.7	5.0	4.4	3.8	3.3	3.3	2.9	2.5	2.1	1.7	1.3

[a] For use with the Mastel double-cutting blade and guide. Make bidirectional incision centrifugally from clear zone to 8-mm-diameter zone and then centripetally back to clear zone. Blade length varies according to the surgeon's technique—most frequently 90 percent of the inferotemporal paracentral corneal thickness. To use the nomogram, find the patient's age in the first column, then read across to find the largest number that does not exceed the desired correction. Read up to find the recommended central clear zone diameter in millimeters.

SURGICAL TECHNIQUES

Radial keratotomy has progressed from being a complex procedure based on specific nomograms with multiple modifiers to a simpler procedure with fewer modifiers and an emphasis on staged, titratable operations. The goals of radial keratotomy are to avoid overcorrection, leave the patient slightly myopic, and titrate the desired final outcome by means of touch-up/enhancement re-operations. A summary of the development of radial keratotomy surgical techniques is given in Table 37-6.

TABLE 37-6
General Developments in Radial Keratotomy in the United States[a]

	Late 1970s	*PERK Study*	*Mid 1980s*	*1990s*
Range of myopia	-2.00 to -12.00 D	-2.00 to -8.00 D	-1.50 to -6.00 D	-1.00 to -4.00 D
Anesthesia	Retrobulbar	Topical	Topical	Topical
Pupil	Dilated	Natural	Natural	Natural
Central mark	Corneal light reflex	Displaced from light reflex	Center of pupil	Center of pupil
Diameter of clear zone	3–5 mm	3–4 mm	3.0–4.5 mm	3.5–5.5 mm
Clear zone marker	Calipers	Circular marker	Circular marker	Circular marker
Fixation device	Single-tipped forceps	Double-tipped forceps	Double-tipped forceps, compression ring	Forceps or compression ring
Corneal thickness (pachymetry)	Optical	Intraoperative, ultrasonic	Intraoperative, ultrasonic	Intraoperative, ultrasonic
Knife blade	Razor blade	Diamond, angled	Diamond, vertical or angled	Diamond, cutting angled edge, partially blunt vertical edge
Knife handle	Blade breaker	Micrometer	Micrometer	Micrometer
Footplates	Narrow	Broad	Broad	Broad
Gauge block	Grooved edge	Raised edge and cradle	Micrometer microscope	Micrometer microscope
Number of incisions	8–16	8	4–8	4–8
Most important part of incision	Peripheral	Paracentral	Paracentral	Paracentral
Direction of incisions	Centrifugal	Centrifugal	Centripetal or centrifugal	Bidirectional; centrifugal first, centripetal second
Peripheral end of incisions	In sclera	In cornea	In cornea	2 mm inside limbus
Achieved depth of incision	75%	87%	90–95%	90–95%
Incision depth gauge	Yes	No	No	No
Repeat keratotomy	Recut in same scars	Add eight new incisions	Open and deepen or lengthen incisions or add new incisions	Intentional for staged surgery; open and deepen or lengthen incisions or add new incisions
Postoperative patching	Yes	Yes/No	No	No
Major patient characteristics used to determine surgical plan and blade depth	Amount of myopia, corneal thickness, corneal curvature, corneal diameter, ocular rigidity	Amount of myopia, corneal thickness	Amount of myopia, corneal thickness, patient age	Amount of myopia, corneal thickness, patient age

Abbreviations: PERK, Prospective Evaluation of Radial Keratotomy; D, diopters.
[a] Individual surgeons' techniques may vary from these general trends.
Source: Adapted with permission from GO Waring, MJ Lynn, A Nizam, et al: Results of the Prospective Evaluation of Radial Keratotomy (PERK) study five years after surgery. Ophthalmology 98:1164, 1991. Courtesy of Ophthalmology.

Preparation and Draping

Experience has shown that an outpatient location can function adequately for radial keratotomy as long as appropriate attention is paid to clean conditions and sterile technique.

The eyelids are prepped with 10 percent povidone-iodine solution, and a plastic drape is placed over the patient's face. Some patients become claustrophobic beneath the drape; supplemental oxygen delivered through a nasal cannula, a guard to hold the drape off of the face, or a splitting of the drape so that the patient can breathe room air helps to decrease this unpleasant sensation.

A wire eyelid speculum adequately keeps the eyelids open without the crushing effect of a heavier speculum, which can damage the levator aponeurosis and cause postoperative ptosis.[57] Patients should be instructed to try not to forcibly close their eyelids when the speculum is in place.

Marking the Center of the Optical Clear Zone

Because the pupil of the eye determines the image on the retina, it is logical to use the center of the pupil as the center of refractive surgical procedures (see Ch. 46). Uozato and Guyton[58,59] demonstrated the optical basis for using the center of the entrance pupil (the pupillary image one sees when looking at the eye) and defined the errors inherent in using other methods for centering refractive surgical procedures.

Most modern microscopes have an optical centering device, such as a small fiber optic fixation light, on which the patient can fixate (Figure 37-2). If not, a small object can be placed on the objective lens over one of the viewing tubes of the microscope. The patient can fixate on this object and the surgeon can sight monocularly through this side of the microscope; this brings the line of sight of the patient into alignment with the line of sight of the surgeon. The patient should be positioned such that the target is directly above the eye, and the opposite eyelids should be closed.

Because the bright light of the microscope is sometimes uncomfortable for the patient, the microscope light should be at the lowest setting consistent with visibility by the surgeon. As the patient looks at the fixation target, the surgeon marks the center of the entrance pupil by making an impression on the corneal epithelium with a blunt instrument, such as a Sinskey hook. A needle should not be used because it can damage Bowman's layer and create a central scar. Confirmation that this mark is in the correct position can be obtained by having the patient look away and refixate on the target, and by re-marking the center of the entrance pupil. The surface of the cornea is dried with a cellulose sponge to make the marks more easily visible. The two marks should coincide.

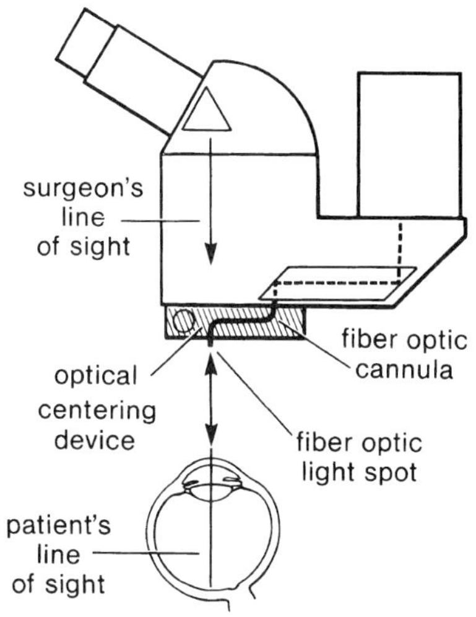

FIGURE 37-2 Example of a patient fixating on the fiber optic fixation light. The surgeon's and patient's lines of sight are aligned. (Reprinted with permission from EB Steinberg, GO Waring: Comparison of two methods of marking the visual axis on the cornea during radial keratotomy. Am J Ophthalmol 96:605, 1983. Copyright by The Ophthalmic Publishing Company.)

Marking the Optical Clear Zone

Fyodorov initially suggested that the diameter of the central clear zone is the most important determinant of the amount of central corneal flattening, with the implication that the paracentral portion of the incisions achieves the greatest flattening effect. This idea was later predicted on a theoretical basis,[28] and confirmed in a mechanical model[26] and in experiments in eye bank eyes.[29] Salz et al[25] showed that with clear zone diameters greater than 5.0 mm, the effect is minimal because the incisions are confined to the peripheral cornea. In cadaver eyes, they found only 2.30 diopters of flattening with a 6.0-mm clear zone, compared to 9.00 diopters of flattening with a 3.0-mm clear zone. A clear-zone diameter smaller than 3.0 mm increases the risk of postoperative glare and irregular astigmatism,[60] and many surgeons use 3.5 mm as the smallest diameter.

The effectiveness of different clear zone diameters depends in part on the uniform depth of the incisions. For example, in the PERK study (in which all eyes had eight incisions with the knife blade set at 100 percent of the thinnest paracentral corneal thickness measurement), the smaller diameter clear zones produced a greater average decrease in myopia.[37]

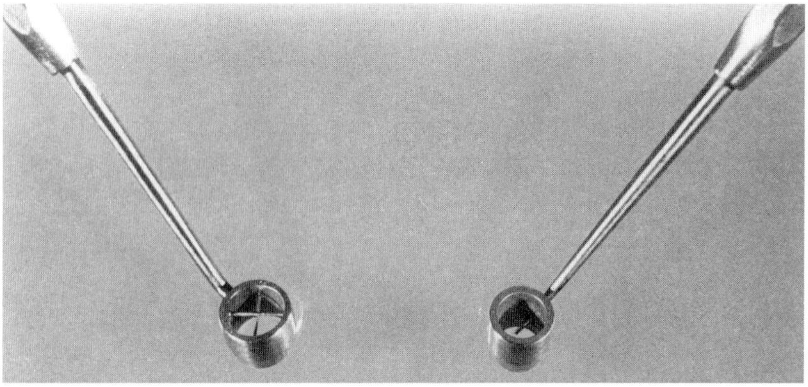

FIGURE 37-3 Two types of central clear zone markers that have a central alignment device. Left, cross hairs. Right, gun-sight style.

A dull, circular clear zone marker of appropriate diameter is used to indent the corneal epithelium, leaving a circular mark that demarcates placement of the central ends of the incisions. While many designs are available, markers with a central alignment device, such as cross hairs, and markers that are about 1 mm tall, work optimally (Figure 37-3).

The corneal surface is dried with a cellulose sponge to reveal the previously made mark over the center of the entrance pupil. The clear zone marker is centered over this mark, oriented perpendicularly on the surface of the cornea,[61] and pressed to slightly indent the epithelium[62] (Figure 37-4). Some surgeons prefer to eliminate marking the center of the clear zone, and they center the marker over the center of the entrance pupil. Proper alignment of the marker is important; if a second mark has to be made, a double set of circles is created, which makes it more difficult for the surgeon to place the knife in the proper paracentral location, so an inked marker is used. After the mark is made, the cornea is moistened with balanced salt solution.

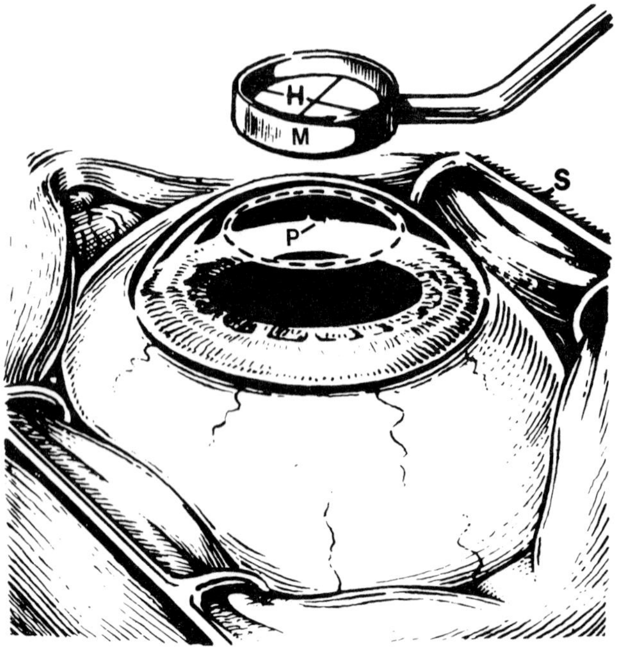

FIGURE 37-4 A clear zone marker (*M*) is used to mark the central clear zone of the cornea (area within the dotted line on the cornea). Cross hairs (*H*) in the marker are used to center this instrument on the center of the entrance pupil (*P*) (*S*, speculum). (Reprinted with permission from GO Waring: Developments in radial keratotomy. Highlights of Ophthalmology Letter 10:1, 1982.)

Measuring the Corneal Thickness

The ultrasonic pachymeter[63] has replaced the optical pachymeter[64] for measuring corneal thickness for radial keratotomy. This device facilitates measurement of corneal thickness because the probe tip can be placed perpendicularly on the cornea at any spot (Figure 37-5). It is easier for paramedical staff to use because it requires only modest training to achieve proficiency, and it is more convenient because it is portable and can be used intraoperatively. The measurement is more precise because it eliminates variation from one observer to another. For accuracy, the proper speed of sound through the cornea (usually 1,640 m/sec) must be set in the pachymeter.

Most of the pachymeters are easy to use and yield minimal interobserver and intersession variations.[65] They require that the tip of the probe be held within 10 degrees of the perpendicular to the cornea before a reading is given. The reading is based on an averaged series of values computed by the instrument. The tip is solid and is 1 to 2 mm in diameter, which allows the user to place it fairly precisely on the cornea. Readings are accurate to 5 to 10 μm.

Commonly, the surgeon places the tip on the cornea and an assistant reads out the numbers. The surgeon selects the most frequent number as the thickness. Some models provide a printout of readings from various locations

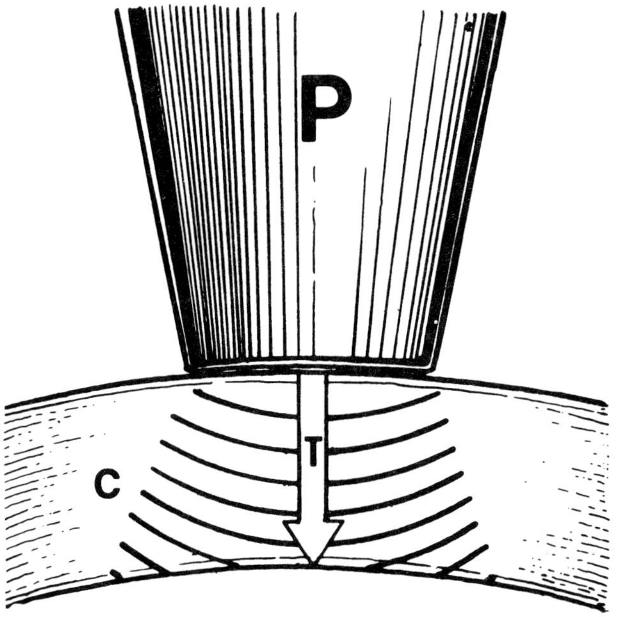

FIGURE 37-5 The ultrasonic pachymeter probe tip (*P*) is placed on the surface of the cornea (*C*). Ultrasonic waves are emitted and detected by the probe. The computation of corneal thickness (*T*) is based on the speed with which sound travels through the cornea. These readings of corneal thickness are used to determine the knife blade length and thus the depth of the incisions in the cornea. (Reprinted with permission from GO Waring: Developments in radial keratotomy. Highlights of Ophthalmology Letter 10:1, 1982.)

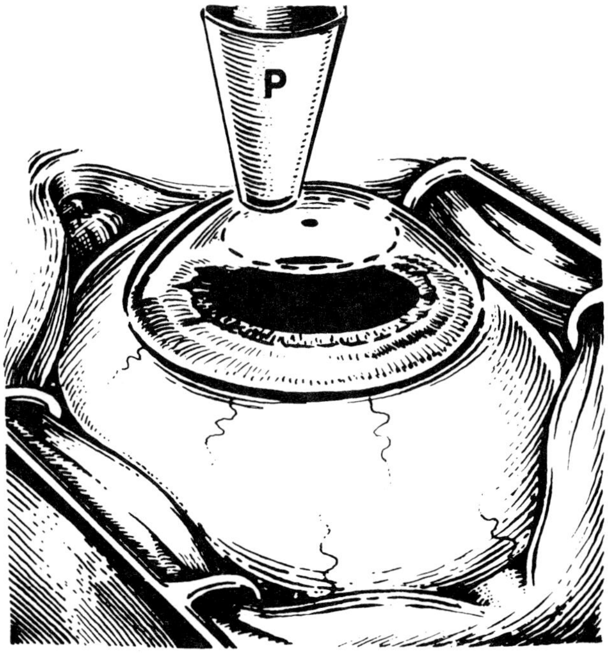

FIGURE 37-6 The paracentral corneal thickness is determined by placing the ultrasonic pachymeter probe tip (*P*) inferotemporally just outside the clear zone mark (dotted line). (Reprinted with permission from GO Waring: Developments in radial keratotomy. Highlights of Ophthalmology Letter 10:1, 1982.)

on the cornea in a preset sequence and calculate the blade length based on given readings.

A comparison of central corneal thickness measurements by ultrasonic pachymetry preoperatively during the clinical examination and intraoperatively after the preparation and draping of the patient showed no clinically significant difference.[66] However, a few patients did show a significant difference, which led to the recommendation that intraoperative pachymetry readings be used as the basis for setting the length of the blade.

The location and number of corneal thickness measurements vary with the surgeon, but most surgeons measure the corneal thickness just peripheral to the clear zone mark inferotemporally, which is the thinnest part of the cornea to be incised (Figure 37-6).

Knives and Calibration Instruments

After the corneal thickness has been measured, the surgeon extends the blade of the radial keratotomy knife a given distance (for example, 100 percent of the thinnest corneal thickness measurement along the clear zone mark) and verifies this distance with a calibration instrument. The assistant keeps the cornea moist with balanced salt solution and shields the eye from the microscope light while this is being done.

Knife Handle

Most micrometer knives used for radial keratotomy consist of a handle, a footplate, and a gem blade that is permanently affixed to the handle (Figure 37-7). The handle has a recess for the blade, which protects it and decreases the chance of damage to the blade when it is not being used. The handle has a micrometer screw mechanism for extending and advancing the blade.

Footplate

The blade extends between two sides of a footplate, the design of which determines how the cutting edge of the blade meets the tissue and how the knife slides across the corneal surface. Footplate designs usually involve flattened block-shaped sides with a blunted leading edge. In some designs, the cutting edge of the blade is recessed between the two sides of the footplate so that the cornea

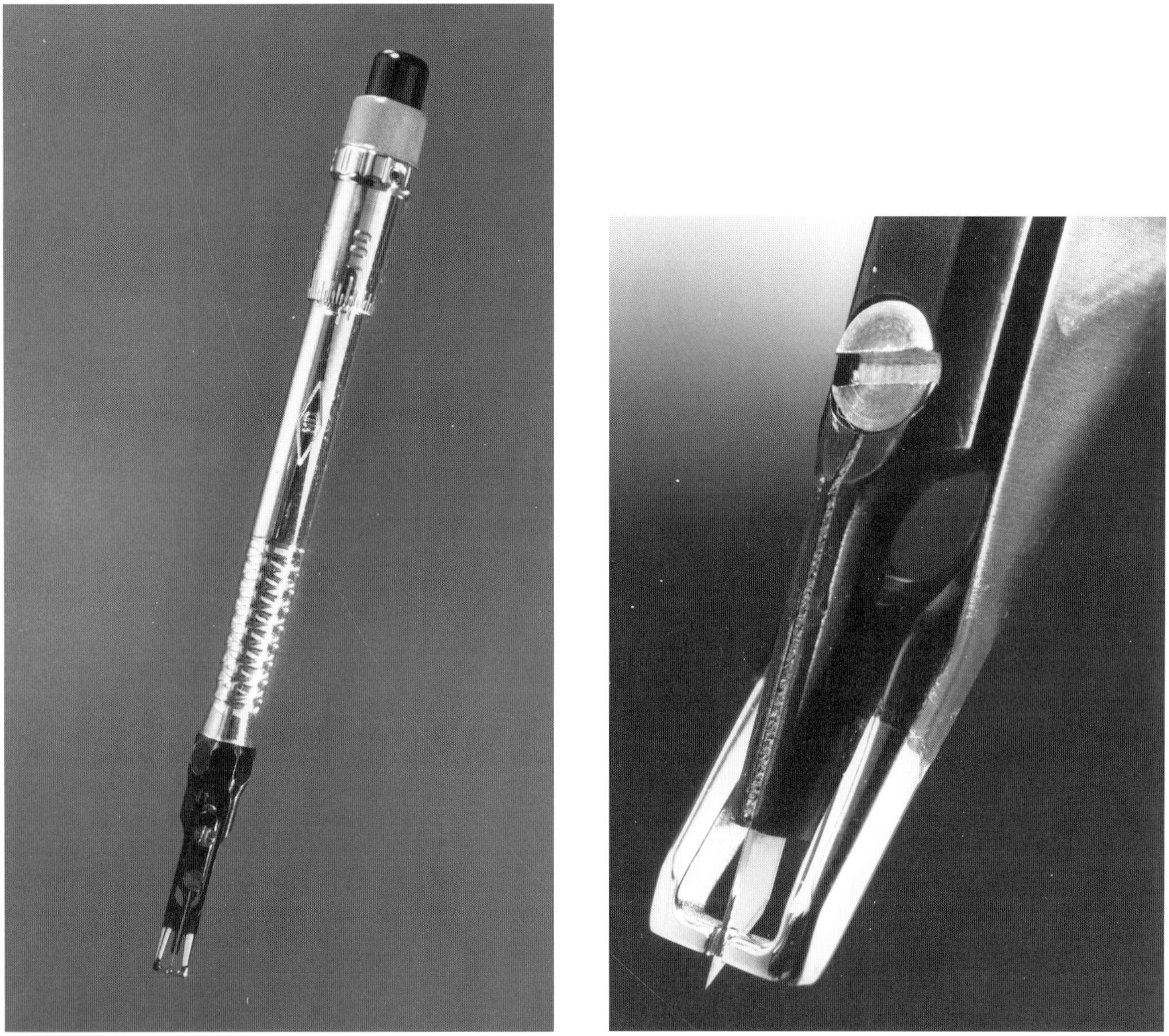

A B

FIGURE 37-7 Example of a radial keratotomy knife. **(A)** The blade is advanced or retracted by turning the micrometer screw mechanism on the handle. **(B)** The diamond blade extends between the sides of the footplate.

is pressed flat just in front of the blade edge. However, some designers think that a completely flat footplate might push tissue away from the cutting edge of the blade and have therefore altered the footplate design so that the knife edge meets the tissue directly, with the flat part of the footplate on either side of the trailing edge of the blade[18] (Figure 37-8).

Wide footplates give more stability and distort the incision less. Footplates designed to allow the surgeon to see the cutting edge of the blade make it possible to stop the incision at a more accurate location. Cutting out the side of the footplate to reveal more of the blade can accomplish this goal. The surface of the footplate must be smooth to avoid causing corneal abrasions as the incisions are made.

Blades

Blades used in radial keratotomy must be sharp and able to make multiple incisions of uniform depth and breadth, producing minimal damage to the corneal tissue, without becoming dull. The exquisite sharpness of the diamond

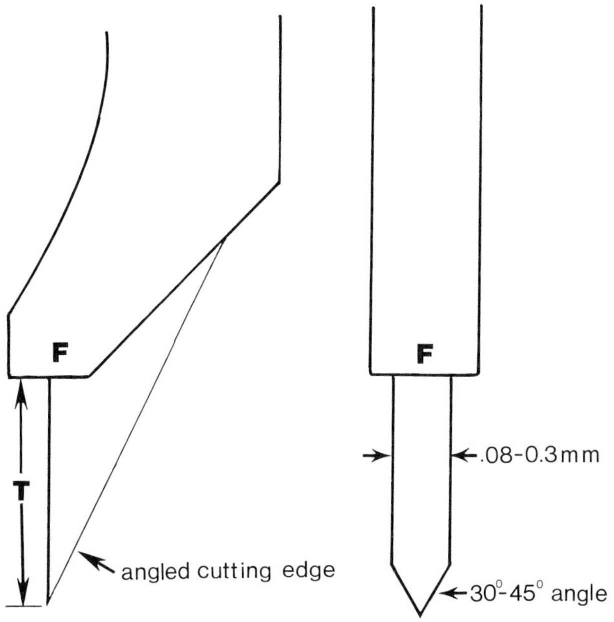

FIGURE 37-8 Schematic diagram of a diamond knife for centrifugal incisions with a footplate (*F*) on either side of the blunt vertical trailing edge of the blade. Left, side view. Right, front view. The length of the blade (*T*), as measured from the footplate to the tip of the blade, is confirmed with a microscope with a micrometer stage.

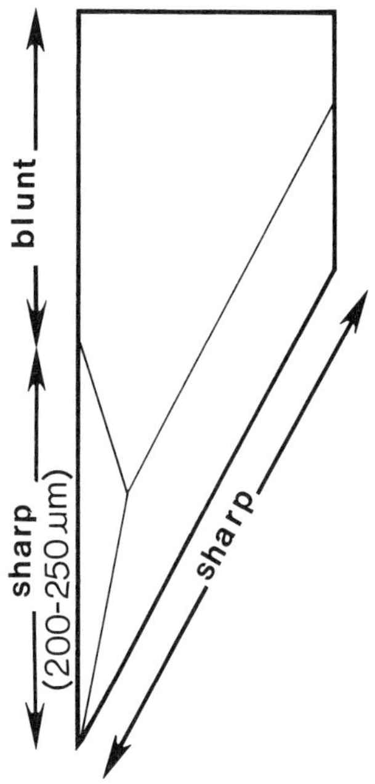

FIGURE 37-9 Schematic diagram of a bidirectional blade depicts cutting edges along the entire angled edge and the distal 200- to 250-μm portion of the vertical edge.

blade that allows it to glide easily through the cornea with minimal force from the surgeon and minimal distortion of the tissue[67] makes it the preferred blade.

Although diamonds are exceedingly hard, they are brittle, so they can be easily damaged or chipped. Thus, only a highly trained person should extend the blade from its protective recess in the handle and clean it with distilled water and a soft cellulose sponge after each use and retract it into the handle. Because a damaged diamond blade must be sent back to the manufacturer for repair, a backup diamond knife should be available. Less expensive ruby and sapphire blades have been marketed for ophthalmic surgery, but they become dull or damaged more quickly than diamond blades.

The configuration of a gem blade determines its cutting characteristics. Most blades measure 1 to 2 mm from front to back and have a side-to-side thickness at the base of 80 to 300 μm. Wider blades track a more stable course through corneal tissue, but they also create more drag. The angle formed by the two sides of the blade as they taper toward the cutting edge is called the *included angle* and varies from 30 to 45 degrees. The amount of angle determines the functional thickness of the blade. A larger included angle creates a greater wedge effect and more tissue drag during the incision. This increased resistance makes the blade feel duller to the surgeon but makes the knife easier to track.

The number and the orientation of the edges are important determinants of the cutting characteristics of the blade. A single-edged blade with a sharp cutting edge and a blunt trailing edge generally tracks through the tissue in a straighter, more stable fashion than does a blade with a double cutting edge. The angle of the cutting edge chosen depends on the technique used by the surgeon. Customarily, an obliquely angled cutting edge is used to cut centrifugally from the clear zone mark to the limbus, whereas a vertically oriented cutting edge is used to cut centripetally from the limbus to the clear zone mark. Blades with an obliquely angled, full cutting edge and a vertically oriented edge consisting of a superficial blunt portion and a deep (200 to 250 μm) cutting portion[20,68,69] (Figure 37-9) have been developed to make a bidirectional incision: first from the clear zone mark to the limbus and second, with the blade kept in the incision, back toward the clear zone mark. During the centripetal portion of the incision, the blunt portion of the vertically oriented edge acts as a guide to keep the blade in the incision and to prevent it from cutting into the clear zone, while the cutting portion recuts

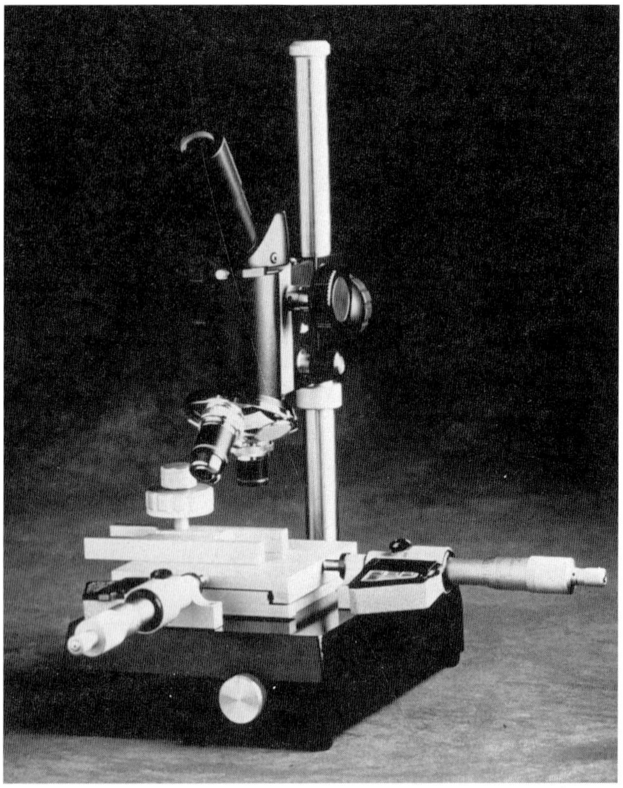

FIGURE 37-10 Commercially available microscope with a micrometer stage used to set the length of the diamond blade. (Exactascope Plus; Courtesy of Sonogage, Inc., Cleveland, OH.)

the bottom of the incision more uniformly and deeply. Commercially available versions of these blades include the Genesis and the Mastel blades.

Calibration Instruments

Regardless of the type of knife handle or blade used, the length of the blade must be verified, because the micrometer screw mechanism in the knife handle may be inaccurate.

Although gauge blocks were used in the past,[18,70] the most reliable way to calibrate the length of the blade at present is to use a bench microscope at a magnification of 150 to 200 × and a micrometer stage marked to permit accurate determination of the length of the blade (Figure 37-10). The knife is mounted on a carrier stage that is moved into position under a microscope. To set the blade, the stage is moved to bring the footplate into view, and the footplate is aligned along the zero baseline of the reticle. The surgeon views the blade against a reticle calibrated in 1- to 10-μm steps and uses the knife handle micrometer to extend the blade to the desired length on

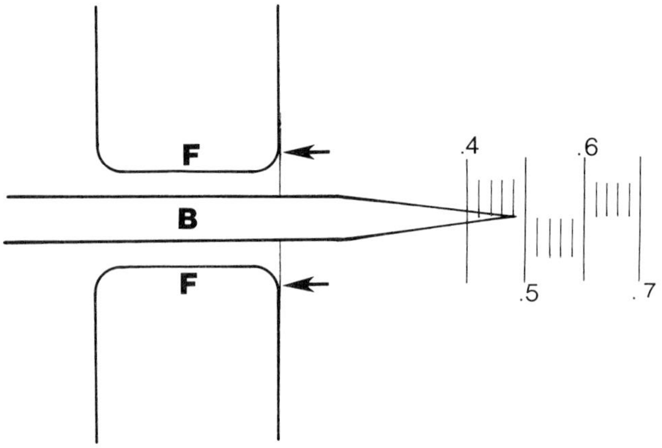

FIGURE 37-11 Schematic diagram of reticle used to set the length of the blade. The footplates (*F*) are aligned along the zero baseline of the reticle (arrows). The blade (*B*) is extended the desired length on the reticle, here 490 μm.

the reticle (Figure 37-11). The use of such an instrument requires orienting the knife so that the footplate and blade are parallel to the surface of the reticle without tilt. Aligning the footplate along the reticle is sometimes difficult, especially if the footplate is curved, so accurate use requires practice. This instrument also allows the surgeon to inspect the sides of the footplate for equal alignment and the blade for chips or damage and for wobble during advancement.

Incision Guides

A radial marker (Figure 37-12) can be used to outline the location of each incision by pressing it onto the cornea and indenting the epithelium. Adding ink to the marker is an unnecessary step.

Although radial keratotomy can be performed effectively freehand, using a guide for the knife usually makes the incisions straighter and possibly more uniformly deep. Radial guides are useful but not essential. The same result

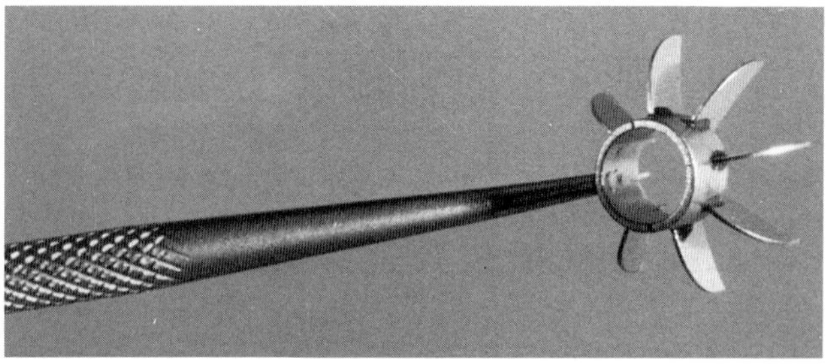

FIGURE 37-12 Central clear zone marker with radial spokes that indent the cornea to serve as a guide for the location of the incisions.

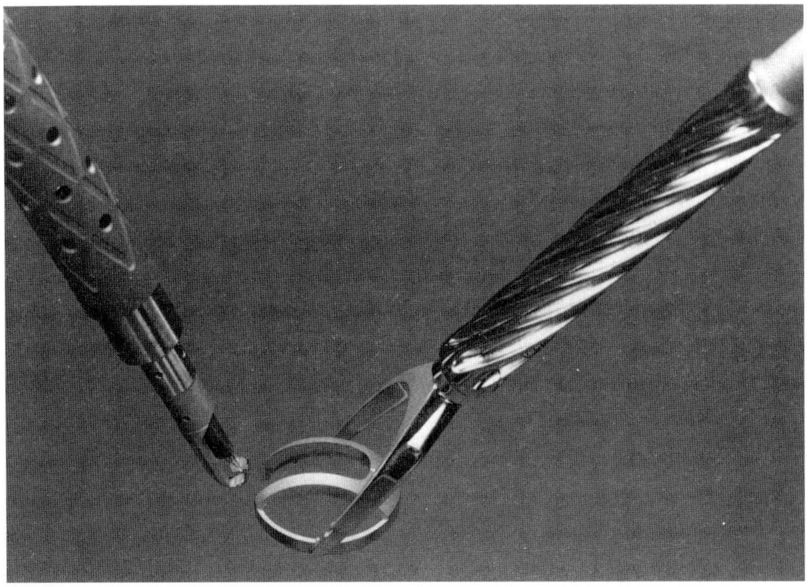

FIGURE 37-13 Mastel Byron radial keratotomy glide (right) and accompanying radial keratotomy knife (left). (Courtesy of Mastel Precision Surgical Instruments, Rapid City, SD.)

is probably achieved if the incisions are spaced equally from one another or, if there is some variance in the spacing, as long as the incisions are radial and not grouped in a single quadrant. The Mastel Byron radial keratotomy glide[71] (Figure 37-13) consists of a circular fixation ring with small teeth and two parallel arches within which the diamond knife footplates fit. The knife is guided by the arches because the footplates fit with fine tolerance into the space between the arches. The glide is repositioned for each incision. The knife made by the manufacturer of the glide must be used. The Krumeich suction bridge[72] combines a suction ring that raises the intraocular pressure with a rotating bridge that arches from limbus to limbus. A specially designed knife with a flat edge that approximates the side of the bridge is used to make the incisions after the pressure is raised; both incisions are made along a single meridian and then the bridge is turned for the next pair of incisions.

Making the Incisions

In the past, when radial keratotomy took longer to perform, the cornea became thinner because of drying from the heat of the microscope light, which increased the chance of perforation.[73] However, excessive wetting of the cornea, particularly after the initial incisions have been made, may induce stromal swelling, resulting in shallower incisions.[74] Most surgeons prefer to keep the cornea moist before making the first incision, dry the corneal surface with a cellulose sponge to reveal the clear zone mark, and make the incisions as rapidly as possible without rewetting the cornea. The fornices should be dried with a cellulose sponge before the first incision is made so that excess fluid (which could be mistaken for aqueous humor) does not flow onto the cornea as the incisions are made.

Pattern of Incisions

Studies have shown that circular incisions steepen the central cornea[75-77] and radial incisions symmetrically placed around a central clear zone flatten the cornea and are the most effective in correcting spherical myopia.

The most effective incision patterns to correct astigmatism are those that place transverse incisions perpendicular to the steepest corneal meridian. Sometimes the transverse incisions are combined with radial incisions (Figure 37-14). When myopia with astigmatism of 1.00 to 3.00 diopters is present, the transverse incisions are placed between the radial incisions without intersecting them, along a zone 6 to 7 mm in diameter. Corneal incisions should not intersect each other. For further discussion of astigmatic keratotomy,[78-86] see Chapter 38.

Number of Incisions

The number of incisions has declined as radial keratotomy has evolved. Sato used up to 80 incisions; surgeons now use eight or four. The use of fewer incisions reflects the observation that most corneal flattening occurs with the first four incisions and that the proportional contribution of additional incisions declines as their number increases.[25] However, eight incisions allow a larger diameter clear zone to be used, which reduces the amount of central corneal distortion. The number of incisions is determined by the amount of myopia, the diameter of the clear zone, and the age of the patient.

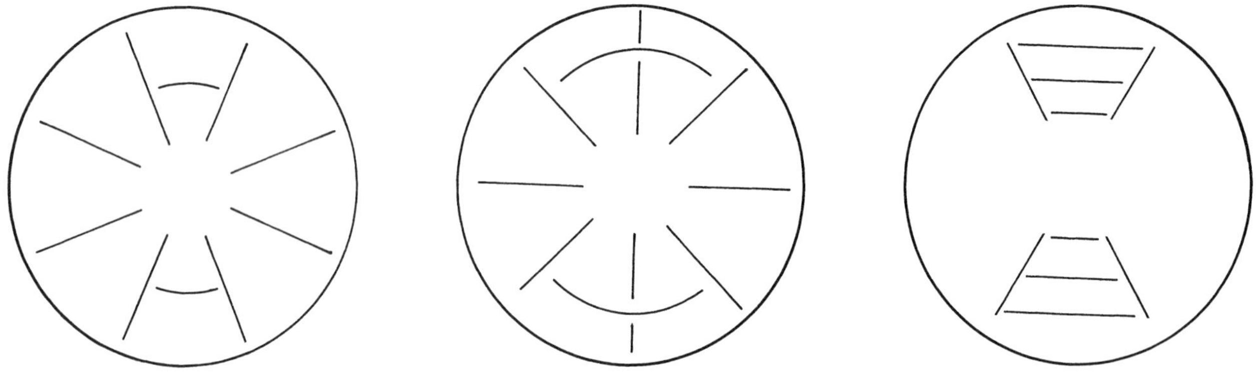

FIGURE 37-14 Selected types of corneal incisions that have been suggested to reduce astigmatism. In all cases, the transverse incisions are made across the steep meridian. **(A)** Arcuate transverse incisions of 20 to 40 degrees between the radial incisions. **(B)** Arcuate transverse incisions of 45 to 80 degrees with interrupted (jump) radial incisions. **(C)** Trapezoidal patterns of incisions for high (5.00 diopters or more) astigmatism.

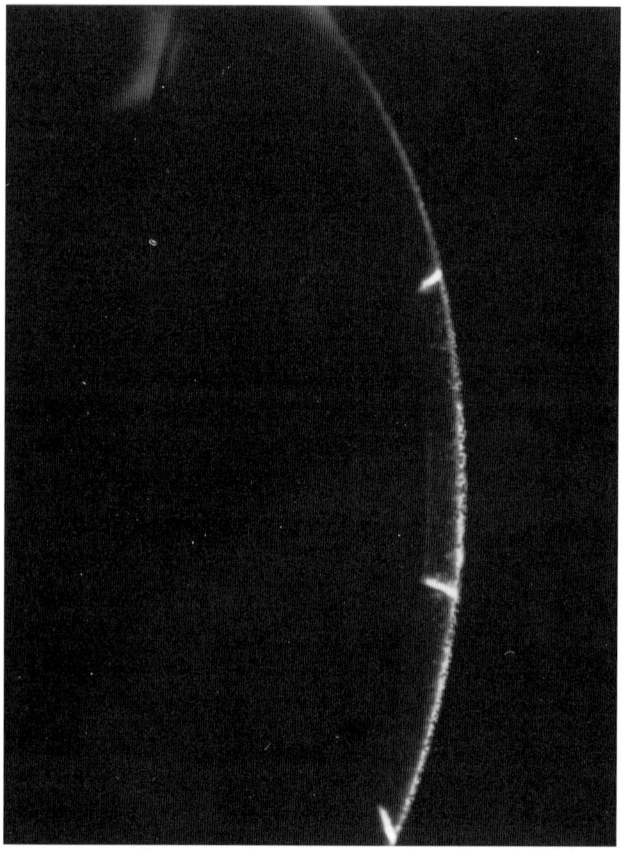

FIGURE 37-15 Variation in incision depth after radial keratotomy. Slit lamp photomicrograph shows the central incision to be about 90 percent of the corneal thickness as desired, but the incision scars above and below this are about 70 percent thickness, illustrating the variation that occurs from incision to incision, even with the same surgeon using the same knife at the same time.

Length of Incisions

Because a circular clear zone centered on the entrance pupil is not concentric with the limbus, individual incisions vary in length. In an attempt to decrease two of the common side effects of radial keratotomy—starburst glare and hyperopic shift—surgeons use shorter incisions with a central clear zone of 3.5 mm or larger and a peripheral diameter of 8 to 9 mm (i.e., making six to eight shorter incisions in preference to making only four longer incisions).[31] Shorter incisions produce approximately 90 percent of the effect of incisions that extend to the limbus.

Depth of Incisions

The depth of the incisions and the diameter of the clear zone are major determinants of the effectiveness of radial keratotomy.[1]

Accurate quantitative data to support the importance of incision depth are difficult to obtain because incision depth is not uniform, either from one end of an incision to the other (the middle part of an incision is usually the deepest) or from one incision to another (incisions made in the same experimental eye by the same surgeon with the same blade length vary in depth from 25 to 100 percent of corneal thickness)[30,33] (Figure 37-15). Factors that contribute to this inconsistency include variations in the surgeon's technique from incision to incision, decreasing intraocular pressure as incisions are made, displacement of tissue by the knife so that the depth of the cut does not correspond to the length of the blade, and variations in thickness in an individual cornea (the peripheral and superior areas are the thickest).

It is difficult to measure the depth of an incision accurately. Intraoperative measurements using calibrated dipsticks are inaccurate because the cornea swells and the dipstick easily pushes the thin posterior stroma posteriorly. Postoperative estimates of the depth of the incision by visual inspection are not precise, although they give a general indication of the depth obtained.[87] Deitz et al[36] increased the accuracy of these measurements by using an optical pachymeter to measure incision depth, a procedure that is difficult and time consuming because microsaccades preclude accurate alignment of the mires with the base of the incision. The difficulty in making incisions of uniform depth is emphasized by the great variability that surgeons use in selecting "fudge factors" to set the blade length, settings that may range from 90 to 115 percent of the central corneal thickness measurement.

Misleading claims of accuracy concerning the depth of radial keratotomy incisions abound in the literature. Formulas and nomograms are proffered that call for an incision depth of "86 percent," and some surgeons claim that their incisions are "95 percent deep," as if they really achieve this uniformly. That the depth of the incision is crucially important there is little doubt; whether a desired depth can be achieved with predictable regularity is a different matter.

Most radial keratotomy surgeons attempt to achieve a uniform incision depth of 90 to 95 percent of corneal thickness. In this technique, incision depth becomes a constant. Obtaining uniformly deep incisions is part of the art of radial keratotomy.

Theoretically, it is desirable to maintain a constant, somewhat elevated intraocular pressure as the incisions are made to help ensure constant depth. As the number of incisions increases, the intraocular pressure falls. When four or eight incisions are made with a diamond knife, intraoperative hypotony is a minor problem, although most surgeons indent the globe with the fixating instrument to raise the intraocular pressure as the incisions are made.

Because the blade does not cut to 100 percent of its length, some surgeons set the blade at 100 to 115 percent of central or paracentral corneal thickness measurements. The actual setting of the blade is based on the surgical technique, the design of the blade, and the direction of the incision. In an incision made by a single pass, the blade cuts closer to Descemet's membrane paracentrally and less close peripherally because the peripheral cornea is about 200 μm thicker than the central cornea. A second pass through the same incision permits the tip of the blade to deepen the incision.[36] Histologic studies demonstrate an inverted Y at the base of some of these incisions, which probably results from the difficulty in reinserting the tip of the blade at the exact apex of the first incision. However, this phenomenon is seldom seen clinically. Bidirectional blades are designed to ensure that the blade stays in the incision as the bottom of the incision is recut,[20,68,70] but the blunt part of the blade can hang up during the centripetal part of the incision.

To obtain an incision that penetrates the cornea to the same percentage depth paracentrally and peripherally, some surgeons have used deepening incisions, in which a second incision is made from the edge of a 6-mm clear zone to the limbus. When making such an incision, the surgeon extends the blade farther than for the first incision by a percentage of corneal thickness, by an arbitrary amount (such as 30 μm), or as indicated by peripheral corneal thickness measurements.[88,89] Peripheral deepening incisions do not significantly increase the effectiveness of radial keratotomy and have been largely abandoned. For example, Salz et al[25] showed that peripheral deepening incisions produce little increased effect in eye bank eyes, presumably because the peripheral part of the incision has less overall effect than the paracentral part.

Direction of Incisions

The depth of an incision is determined in part by the direction in which the surgeon cuts, either centrifugally from the edge of the clear zone to the limbus, centripetally from the limbus to the edge of the clear zone, or bidirectionally[90–93] (Figure 37-16). Freeze fracture electron microscopy of the architecture of centripetal, centrifugal, and bidirectional incisions[93] has shown that an incision made from the limbus to the clear zone is nearly uniformly deep and of maximal depth at the clear zone mark, whereas an incision made from the clear zone toward the limbus is stepped and rounded at the ends and somewhat shallower than the maximal depth at the clear zone mark; a bidirectional incision provides a deeper, more uniform cut.

Centripetal incisions made with a vertical blade are deeper and more uniform than centrifugal incisions made with an oblique blade set to the same length and, therefore, have greater clinical effect.[35,37,79,94,95] Although acceptable results can be achieved with either technique, the surgeon must know the differences between the two techniques and realize that the centrifugal technique requires a longer blade length. Bidirectional blades allow the surgeon first to make a centrifugal incision and then to recut the bottom of the incision centripetally without fear of cutting into the clear zone as long as no centripetal pressure is applied to the knife as it is withdrawn from the cornea after the second pass.

Fixating the Globe

As the incisions are made, the surgeon must hold the globe firmly to ensure a smooth radial course of the knife. If the

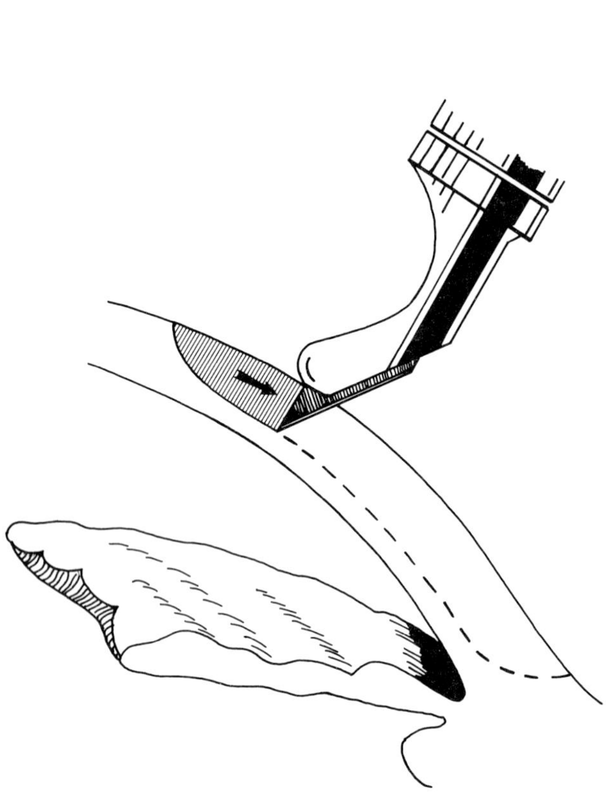

A

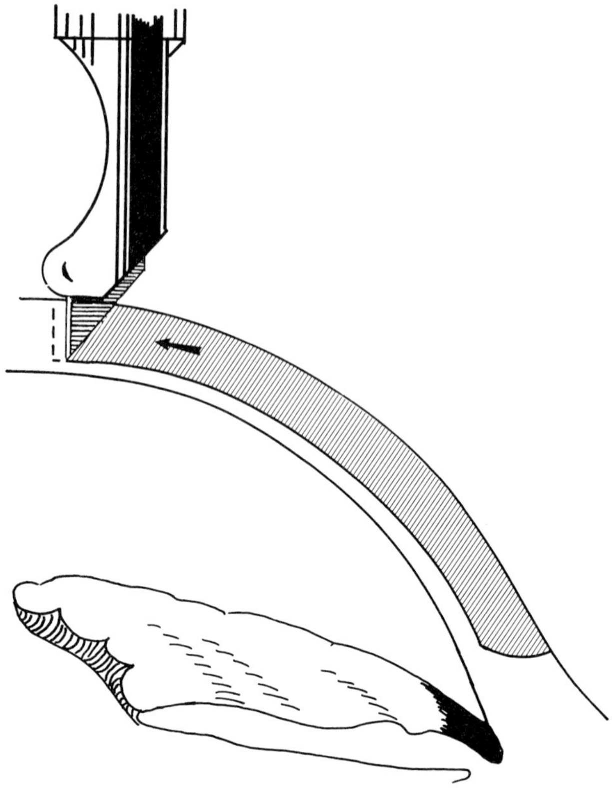

B

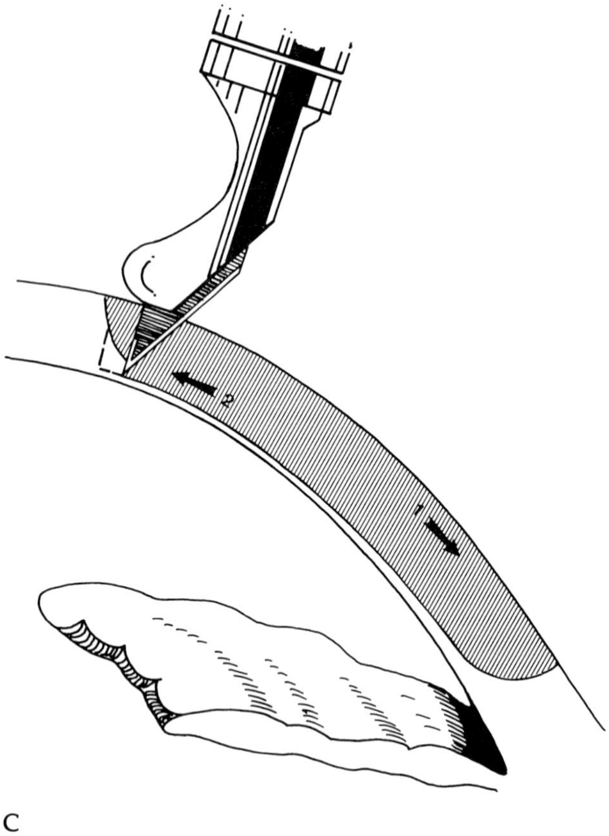

C

FIGURE 37-16 Schematic diagrams of the configurations of incisions created by various radial keratotomy techniques. The hatched areas indicate the portion of the cornea already cut; the dotted lines indicate the future path of the blade. **(A)** Centrifugal incision with a blade with an obliquely angled cutting edge. **(B)** Centripetal incision with a blade with a vertically oriented cutting edge. **(C)** Bidirectional incision with a blade with an obliquely angled, full cutting edge and a vertically oriented edge consisting of a superficial blunt portion and a deep cutting portion.

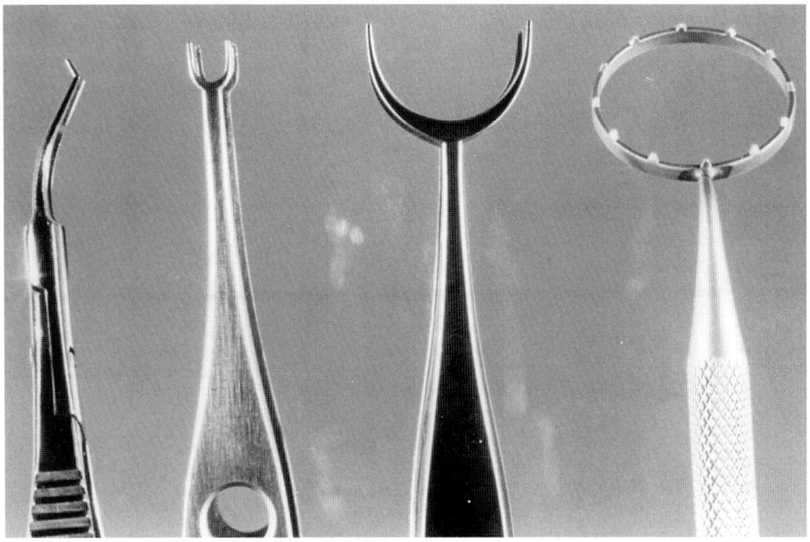

FIGURE 37-17 Different types of fixation instruments used in radial keratotomy. From left to right: single-point fixation forceps, which are less secure because they allow torque around a single point; narrow, double-point fixation forceps; double-point fixation forceps that span the cornea; fixation ring with small, dull teeth that adhere to the conjunctiva and sclera.

globe torques, the knife can stray off course and create an irregular incision that might increase glare, induce astigmatism, or alter the effect of surgery.

Some surgeons simply grasp the limbus with a pair of single-point forceps. However, most surgeons use some type of double-point fixation, with forceps that grasp the limbus with two tips 3 to 7 mm apart or that span the cornea and grasp the limbus at two points 180 degrees apart (Figure 37-17). A circular compression ring 16 mm in diameter that is mounted on a handle fixates the globe by pressing small teeth into the conjunctiva and episclera, which results in good stability as long as the conjunctiva does not slip, but requires slight pressure that may depress the globe into the orbit.[61,65]

Suction rings similar to those used to fixate the globe for keratomileusis can be used to hold the globe just outside the limbus and elevate the intraocular pressure during the incisions.[96,97] Cowden and colleagues[97] reported that using a vacuum suction ring increases the effect of eight-incision radial keratotomy from an average of 5.00 diopters to an average of 6.75 diopters.

Irrigating the Incisions

Irrigating the incisions at the end of the procedure with balanced salt solution decreases the incidence of epithelial inclusions and debris. Care is taken to irrigate the incisions parallel to Descemet's membrane so that Descemet's membrane does not detach.

If the blade nicks a limbal vessel, blood may seep into the incision. Gentle pressure with a cellulose sponge on the bleeding point usually stops the bleeding, and the blood can then be irrigated from the incision.

POSTOPERATIVE CARE

Postoperative use of topical pharmaceutical agents varies among surgeons. Topical antibiotic prophylaxis seems prudent, because bacterial keratitis[98–106] and endophthalmitis[107–109] have been reported after radial keratotomy. Generally, a broad-spectrum antibiotic that does not contain neomycin (to which approximately 10 percent of the population has hypersensitivity reactions) and does not cause epithelial toxicity can be prescribed two to four times daily for 5 days. Cycloplegia is unnecessary. An eye pad is unnecessary; it increases postoperative pain and is cumbersome. The routine use of topical nonsteroidal anti-inflammatory drugs, such as 0.1 percent diclofenac,[110] 0.03 percent flurbiprofen,[111] or 0.5 percent ketorolac, reduces pain and lessens the need for oral analgesics. One drop is given before surgery, immediately after surgery, and four times in the next 24 hours, but not longer. A bandage soft contact lens decreases postoperative pain, especially if there has been disruption of the epithelium adjacent to the incisions.

Systemic analgesia is important because many patients have severe pain for 24 hours after radial keratotomy. Narcotic-based analgesics, such as hydromorphone (2 mg) or oxycodone, may cause gastrointestinal upset that is more bothersome than the eye pain. Oral nonsteroidal anti-inflammatory drugs, such as ketorolac (10 mg), can be effective analgesics.

A short-acting sleeping pill, such as flurazepam (30 mg), can help the patient get through the first night. In general, severe pain is gone within 24 hours after surgery. Patients should be advised of this pain in advance, and radial keratotomy should not be promoted as a "quick-simple-painless" procedure.

In almost all eyes, some of the initial central corneal flattening induced by radial keratotomy is lost as the early corneal edema disappears from the incisions and epithelial plugs occupy the wounds.[112] Thus, if a plano refraction is the desired outcome, a mild overcorrection of 0.25 to 0.50 diopter in the first week after surgery is desirable.

Control of long-term wound healing is difficult and imprecise. Topical corticosteroids retard stromal wound healing, and the use of 1 percent prednisolone acetate four times daily for 30 to 60 days postoperatively was shown to enhance the results of surgery by about 1 diopter.[113] However, a later study of patients undergoing simultaneous bilateral surgery, with one eye treated with dexamethasone twice daily for 3 months, showed no effect on refraction.[114] Currently, a combination antibiotic-corticosteroid drop is used for 5 days; longer term corticosteroids are not used.

To date, although synthesis by recombinant DNA techniques has made growth factors more readily available,[115–117] a practical use for them in the control of healing after radial keratotomy has not been identified.

Unsutured corneal incisions take years to heal and, once healed, are never as strong as the normal cornea. Epithelial plugs may remain in the incisions for many years (Figure 37-18), during which time the remodeling of the stromal scars can be monitored at the slit lamp microscope.[118–122] In the first few weeks after radial keratotomy, the incisions are surrounded by gray, cloudy material, which gradually disappears by 3 months to reveal fine spicules protruding from the sides of the inci-

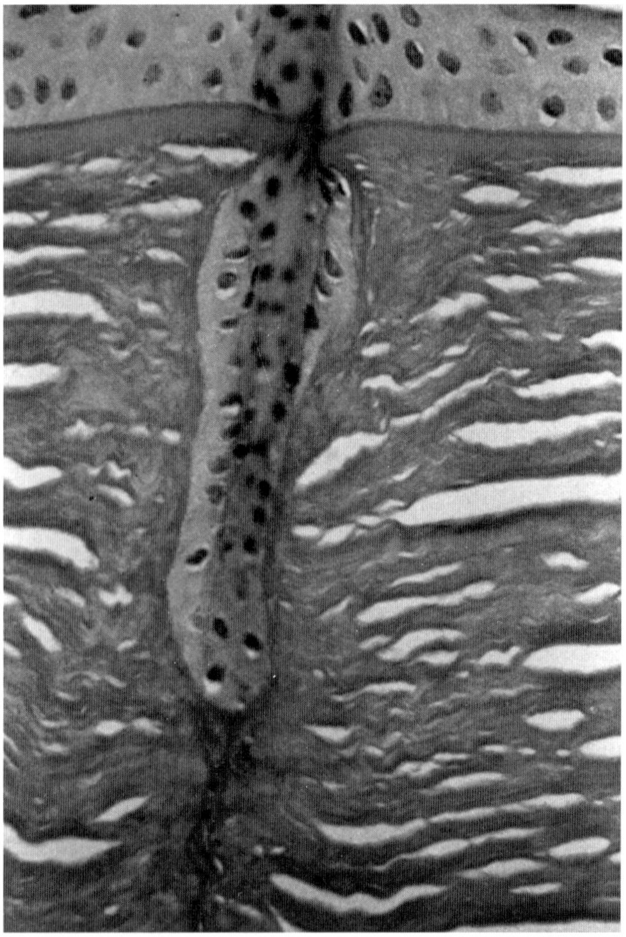

A

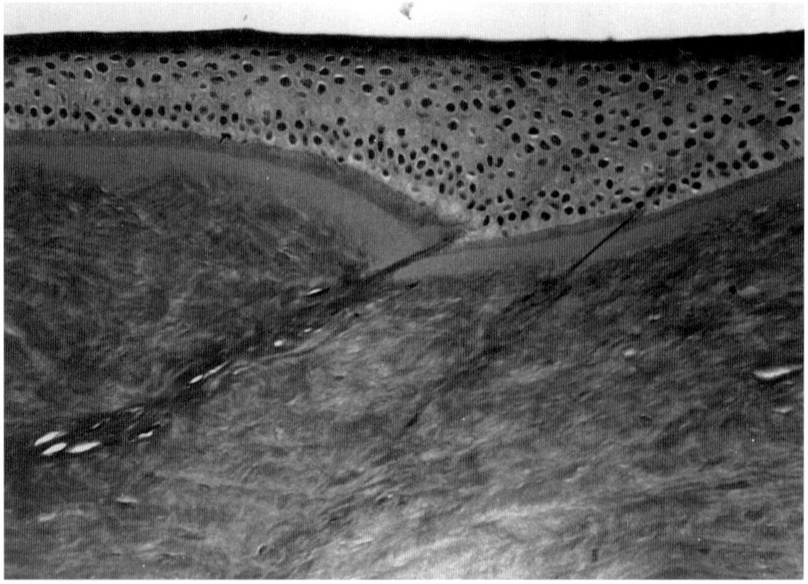

B

FIGURE 37-18 **(A)** Epithelial plug fills the anterior part of the keratotomy wound many months after surgery. (Periodic acid–Schiff, × 100.) **(B)** Cornea 43 months after keratotomy demonstrates epithelial facet over an oblique keratotomy wound, with the hyperplastic epithelium filling in the indentation in the stroma to create a smoother surface. (Periodic acid–Schiff, × 100.) (Reprinted with permission from RA Eiferman, GS Shultz, RE Nordquist, GO Waring III: Corneal wound healing and its pharmacologic modification after refractive keratotomy. p. 749. In GO Waring: Refractive Keratotomy for Myopia and Astigmatism. Mosby–Year Book, St. Louis, 1992. Original courtesy of Perry Binder, M.D.)

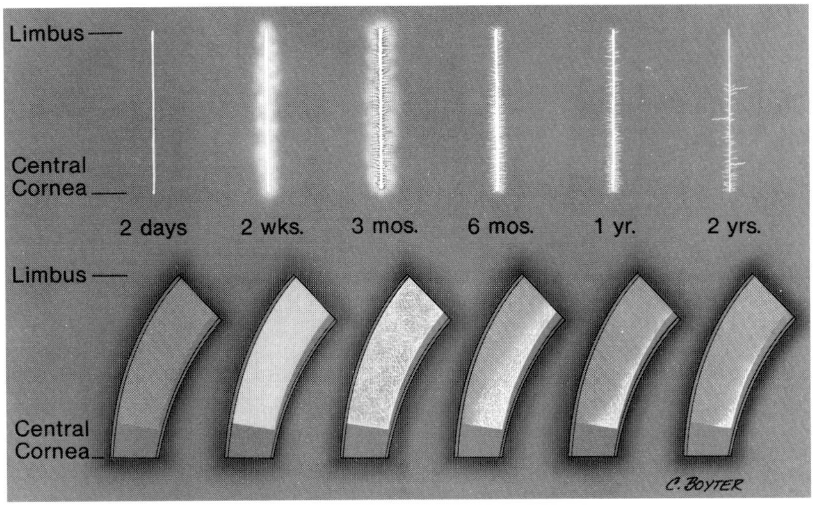

FIGURE 37-19 Natural history of the appearance of incisions 2 days to 2 years after radial keratotomy. At 2 days, the incision is present as a discrete line surrounded by faint edema. By 2 weeks, a diffuse, cloudy, gray haze surrounds both sides of the incision. By about 3 months, fine, discrete spicules appear within the cloudiness. By 6 months, the cloudiness has disappeared and the spicules are more distinct, imparting a feathered appearance to the incision. About this time, spicules begin to disappear from the anterior and paracentral portions of the incision. At 1 year, the density of the spicules has diminished, and they are visible primarily in the deep portion of the incision. By 2 years, only a few discrete spicules extend from the incision, mostly in the deep stroma. (Reprinted with permission from GO Waring, EB Steinberg, LA Wilson: Slit-lamp microscopic appearance of corneal wound healing after radial keratotomy. Am J Ophthalmol 100: 218, 1985. Copyright by The Ophthalmic Publishing Company.)

sions, giving the incisions a feathered appearance. Within the scars, clear zones representing epithelial plugs are often seen. These spicules slowly disappear during the first 2 years after surgery—first from the anterior cornea, then progressively from the more posterior regions—but may persist in the deep stroma for 3 years or more (Figure 37-19). Presumably, this changing appearance reflects the remodeling of the corneal stromal lamellae adjacent to the incisions. It is reasonable to assume that as long as the configuration of the scars continues to change, the shape of the cornea and the refraction may also change. Therefore, it is not surprising that a certain instability in the corneal curvature and ocular refraction occurs after radial keratotomy in the form of morning-to-evening variation and a long-term gradual shift in the hyperopic direction, as discussed below.

RESULTS

Format for Reporting Results

The results of radial keratotomy or any other refractive procedure can be collected in three ways: (1) as part of routine office practice with no attempts at standardization; (2) in an office setting with special attempts to gather data in a systematic manner[36,88,123–126]; and (3) as part of a prospective trial that uses standardized methods of measurement and reporting, such as those used in the PERK study.[18,19,87] Once gathered, the results should be presented in standardized categories to allow for comparison of the findings of different studies.

In establishing standards for efficacy, the current level of comparison is that achieved with spectacles and contact lenses. The commonly used standard of success for refractive surgery, defined as a refraction within ± 1.00 diopter of emmetropia and an uncorrected visual acuity of 20/40 or better, would never be acceptable as the standard for success in the fitting of optical devices. Most myopic patients, particularly those older than 30 years, are unhappy with any postoperative hyperopia and most of those with an uncorrected visual acuity of 20/40 do not function completely independently of optical correction for distance.

Studies of radial keratotomy often report the uncorrected visual acuity and the refractive error separately. In some cases, these two measurements give conflicting evidence regarding the effectiveness of the surgery. For example, a patient with a refraction of –5.00 diopters before surgery who has an uncorrected visual acuity of 20/25 after radial keratotomy would certainly be considered to have a successful result; however, if there was a residual refractive error of –2.00 diopters or +2.00 diopters, both of which are possible with that visual acuity, the procedure would not be considered successful. Nordan et al[127]

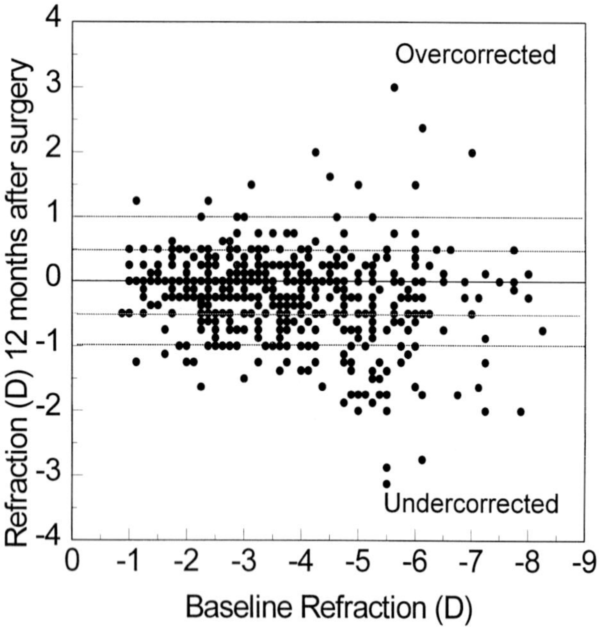

FIGURE 37-20 Scattergram shows the spherical equivalent of the cycloplegic refraction at 1 year after refractive keratotomy in 545 eyes. Enhancement procedures were performed in 39 percent of the eyes. (Adapted from GO Waring III, JC Casebeer, RM Dru, et al: One-year results of a prospective multicenter study of the Casebeer system of refractive keratotomy. Ophthalmology 103:1337, 1996. Courtesy of Ophthalmology.)

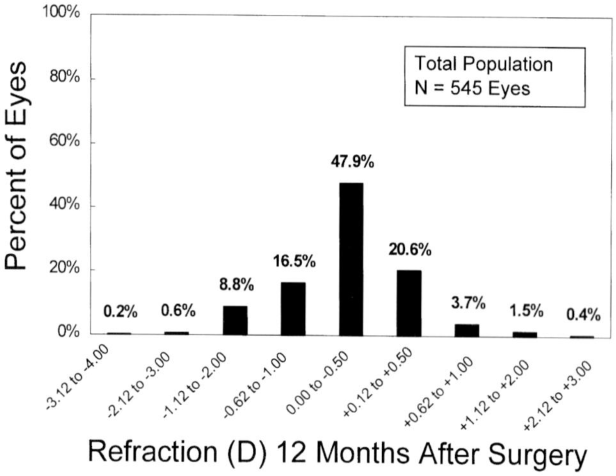

FIGURE 37-21 Histogram demonstrates distribution of spherical equivalent of the cycloplegic refraction at 1 year after refractive keratotomy in 545 eyes. (Adapted from GO Waring, JC Casebeer, RM Dru, et al: One-year results of a prospective multicenter study of the Casebeer system of refractive keratotomy. Ophthalmology 103:1337, 1996. Courtesy of Ophthalmology.)

proposed a simple formula for assessing the effectiveness of refractive surgery that includes both residual refractive error and uncorrected visual acuity. This formula was modified by Lynn and colleagues[128] to create a visual function score that combines refraction and visual acuity results into four subjective categories: excellent, good, fair, and poor. The major effect of using the visual function score instead of simple uncorrected visual acuity or refractive error is to reclassify eyes that have sufficient accommodation to overcome hyperopia. For example, in the PERK study at 4 years,[128] 245 of 385 eyes (64 percent) had an uncorrected visual acuity of 20/25 or better, but 82 percent of these had a hyperopic refractive error that took them out of the excellent visual function score category and put them into the good (37 percent), fair (30 percent), or poor (15 percent) category.

Reports of radial keratotomy studies that average outcomes for groups of patients have little value, because a mean refraction does not reflect overcorrections and undercorrections, which cancel each other. The standard deviation of the mean refractive outcome is useful because it quantifies the spread of the results. A more meaningful representation of results is a scattergram that shows the status of each patient and, in particular, the number of patients who are over- or undercorrected, and to what degree[19,36,87,123–125,129–132] (Figure 37-20). An alternative method of presenting results is the use of tables or histograms that indicate the percentage of eyes within each postoperative range of refraction (Figure 37-21).

Methods of Measuring Results

Refraction

The most precise measurement is the cycloplegic refraction because the patient's accommodation is controlled. A dilated pupil allows more optical aberrations to enter the eye postoperatively, however, making a cycloplegic refraction more difficult. The manifest refraction provides less consistent results, but it indicates the daily functional refraction with fewer optical aberrations. When good fogging technique is used, the manifest and cycloplegic refractions are similar.

Visual Acuity

Visual acuity, with its subjective bias on the part of both examiner and patient, is not as quantifiable as the refraction because it does not correspond exactly to the changes in refractive error and corneal shape. In the PERK study,

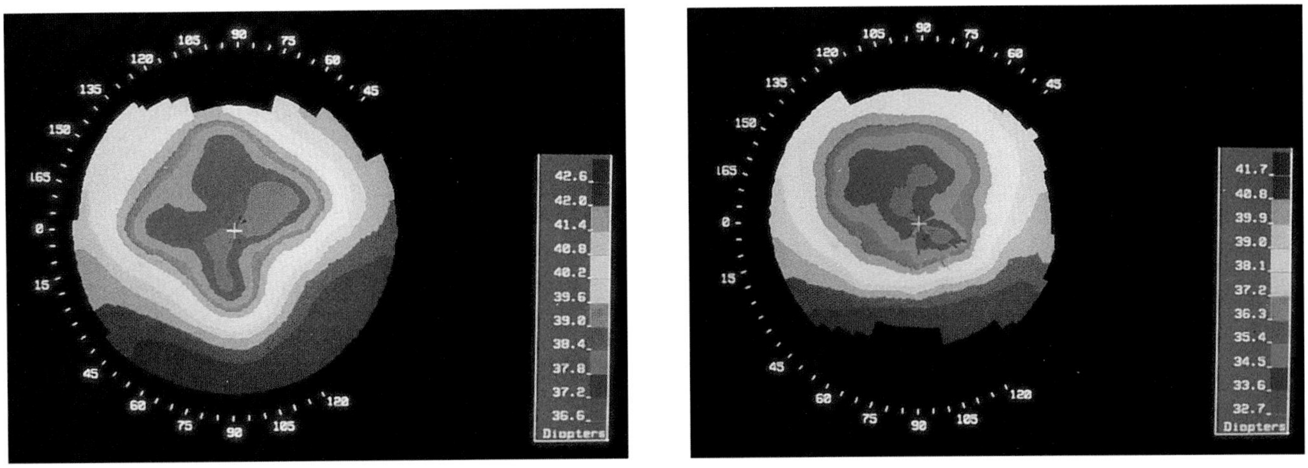

A B

FIGURE 37-22 Videokeratographs showing patterns of power distribution and cross-sectional shape configurations after radial keratotomy. The polygonal pattern is not seen in normal eyes. **(A)** Polygonal pattern, oblate shape; **(B)** round pattern, oblate shape; *(continues)*

95 percent of patients with a postoperative refractive error of −2.00 diopters demonstrated uncorrected visual acuities that ranged from 20/30 to 20/100 using the National Eye Institute's vision charts.[133] The lack of exact correlation between refraction and visual acuity would probably have been even greater in the nonstandardized conditions of office practice.

Contrast Sensitivity

Snellen visual acuity does not provide information about the quality of vision. For example, an individual may read the 20/20 line very briskly or extremely slowly, but the recorded visual acuity is the same. Contrast sensitivity testing is a more sensitive method of determining the visual function of patients after radial keratotomy. In PERK study patients, contrast sensitivity test cards and computer-generated video tests showed no significant decrease in contrast sensitivity compared with normal controls.[87,134]

Keratometry

Central keratometry measures the corneal curvature at two paracentral points approximately 3 mm apart, which represent a minuscule part of the surface of the cornea. Because these two points fall near the edge of the optical clear zone where there is a major change in the corneal curvature after radial keratotomy, the central flattening of the cornea measured by keratometry does not correlate directly with the reduction in myopia measured by refraction. The change in central keratometry measurements is usually less than the change in refraction.[87]

Corneal Topography

Measurement of the shape of the anterior corneal surface is especially important after radial keratotomy because unusual topographic patterns may result, including multifocal optics overlying the pupil. Videokeratoscopes project rings or grids onto the cornea and a video camera captures the image of the mires. Computer software analyzes the pattern of the mires according to optical assumptions and mathematical algorithms and produces color-coded maps of the radius of curvature and dioptric power of the cornea.[135] The methods of analysis of videokeratographs have been well described[136] (see Ch. 46).

The most common topographic pattern after radial keratotomy is a polygonal one, which is not present in normal corneas[137–139] (Figure 37-22). Generally, the number of points in the polygon equals the number of incisions in the cornea—four incisions create a square, eight incisions create an octagon, and so forth. All polygonal patterns are not distinct, however, and some are incomplete or asymmetrical. Bogan et al[138] showed that the mean range of dioptric powers in the 4-mm central area of the cornea was 4.8 ± 4.2 diopters after radial keratotomy, but only 2.0 ± 0.5 diopters in normal corneas. This twofold increase in the power distribution over a standard 4-mm entrance pupil substantiates the concept of a multifocal cornea after radial keratotomy. Analysis of the cross-sectional shape of the corneas showed that approximately 80 percent were flatter centrally than peripherally after radial keratotomy. There was a sharp inflection zone (the paracentral knee) at approximately the 5.5-mm diameter zone.

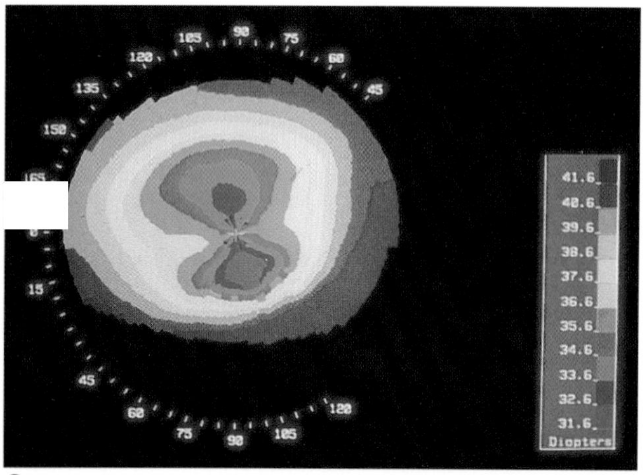

C

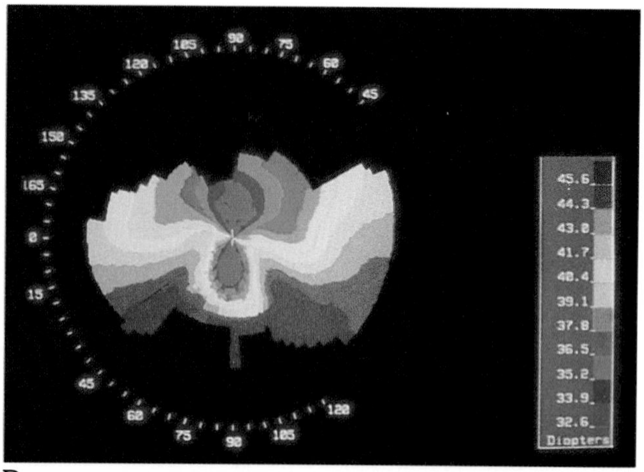

D

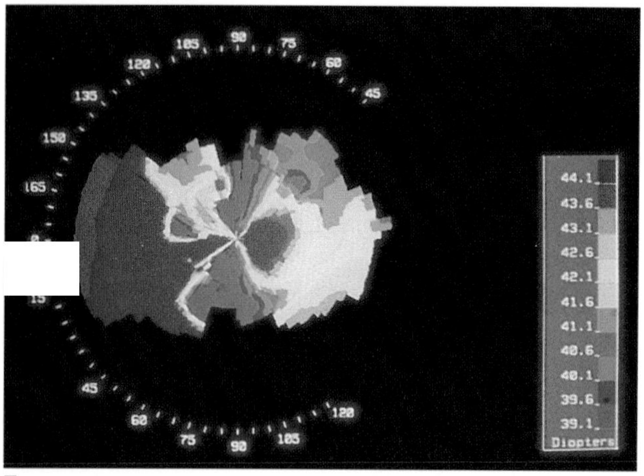

E

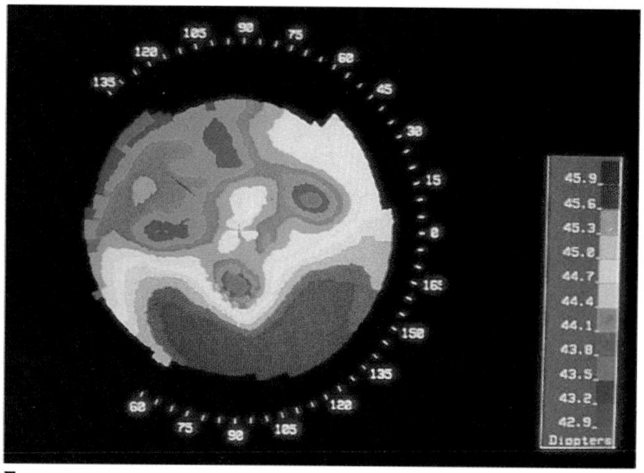

F

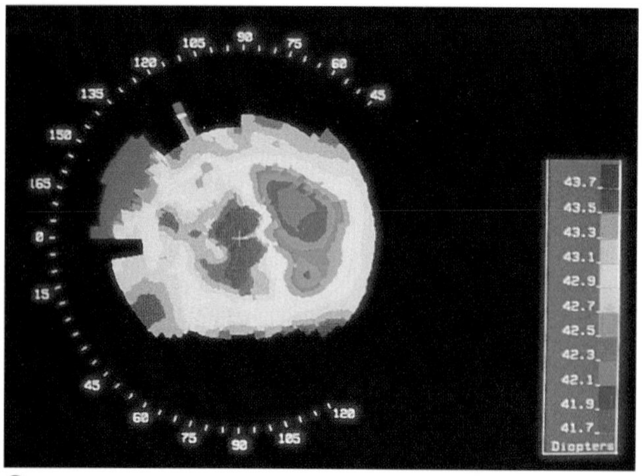

G

FIGURE 37-22 *(continued)* **(C)** symmetrical bow-tie pattern, oblate shape; **(D)** asymmetrical bow-tie pattern, oblate shape; **(E)** bow-tie pattern, mixed prolate/oblate shape; **(F)** polygonal pattern, oblate shape, steep-flat-steep ("nipple") configuration; and **(G)** irregular pattern, irregular shape. (Reprinted with permission from SJ Bogan, RK Maloney, CD Drews, GO Waring: Computer-assisted videokeratography of corneal topography after radial keratotomy. Arch Ophthalmol 109:834, 1991. Copyright 1991, American Medical Association.)

Patient Satisfaction

Although measurement of subjective patient satisfaction is difficult, it is important in clinical practice. One attempt to judge patient satisfaction was the use of a prospectively designed psychometric questionnaire in the PERK study.[40,140,141] In this study,[141] the criteria necessary for patients to be free of distance optical correction were a postoperative refractive error of -0.50 to +0.50 diopter in both eyes and uncorrected visual acuity of 20/20 or better in one eye. The criteria for high patient satisfaction were freedom from distance spectacle lenses and a visual acuity of 20/20 or better in at least one eye (Table 37-7).

In a study of 276 patients having refractive keratotomy with the Casebeer system, Waring et al[22] reported that patient satisfaction was high; 90 percent (247 patients) were very satisfied and 9 percent (25 patients) were moderately satisfied. Ninety-nine percent (271 patients) stated they would have the surgery again.

Efficacy

That radial keratotomy flattens the central cornea and reduces myopia and astigmatism has been known for almost a century.[6] One challenge has been to define the amount of myopia predictably correctable by radial keratotomy. Although some surgeons have claimed good results from surgery performed on patients with 15 diopters of myopia, most report the best outcome in patients with 4 or fewer diopters of myopia, assuming emmetropia is the goal of surgery.[19,36,39,64,87,88,123-132,141,142]

Comparison of the results of radial keratotomy studies is difficult. In most studies, the surgeon used a variety of surgical techniques that changed during the course of the study in an attempt to improve the outcome, making analysis of the effect of specific surgical variables nearly impossible. For example, in seven studies, the percentage of eyes with a refraction between -1.00 and +1.00 diopter at 6 and 12 months after surgery ranged from 39 to 100 percent.[39,129,143-147]

Among published studies, few are directly comparable because of differences in such fundamental aspects as the numbers of incisions used. However, five—the PERK study,[19] Deitz et al,[36] Salz et al,[132] Waring et al (Casebeer-Chiron Study Group),[22] and Verity et al (Refractive Keratoplasty Study Group)[20]—can be examined to depict the improvements and changes that have occurred in radial keratotomy from 1982 through the mid 1990s. The PERK study had a prospective design and used a standardized surgical technique, all eyes receiving eight incisions.[19] The results reflect those achieved in the early 1980s and serve as a benchmark by which to measure progress. The Deitz study[36] represents improvements made by regression equations but also involved eyes in which 8 to 16 incisions were made. In the Salz study,[132] half the eyes received eight incisions and half were treated with only four incisions; this study spans almost a decade and represents the progression and changes in surgery during that time. The Casebeer-Chiron study[22] was a prospective trial by 18 surgeons using four to eight centripetal, single-pass incisions (in 90 percent of the eyes) or bidirectional incisions (in 10 percent of the eyes), and enhancements in approximately one-third of the eyes. The Refractive Keratoplasty Study Group trial[20] involved four to eight bidirectional incisions and a standardized nomogram.

Table 37-8 summarizes the findings of these five studies. The most important advances manifested by the five studies are the reduction in the number of incisions, the reduction in the maximum amount of myopia attempted

TABLE 37-7
PERK Study Patients Free of Distance Correction Lenses 6 Years after Radial Keratotomy

Parameter	*Total No. of Patients Achieving Given Parameter*	*No. of Patients Free of Distance Correction Lenses*
Uncorrected visual acuity in one or both eyes		
20/20 or better	259	198 (76%)
20/25 to 20/40	53	18 (34%)
Residual spherical equivalent refractive error in both eyes		
±0.50 D	72	61 (85%)
±1.00 D	87	34 (39%)

Abbreviations: PERK, Prospective Evaluation of Radial Keratotomy; D, diopters.
Source: Data from LB Bourque, MJ Lynn, GO Waring, et al: Spectacle and contact lens wearing six years after radial keratotomy in the Prospective Evaluation of Radial Keratotomy study. Ophthalmology 101:421, 1994.

TABLE 37-8
Comparison of Five Studies of Radial Keratotomy

	10-Year PERK, 1994[19]	*Deitz et al, 1987*[36]	*Salz et al, 1991*[132]	*Waring et al, 1996*[22]	*Verity et al, 1995*[20]
Dates of surgery	1982–1988	1982–1985	1980–1990	1992–1993	1992–1994
Surgical technique					
Number of incisions (% of eyes)	8 (100)	8 (89) 10–16 (11)	4 (51); 8 (45); 6–12 (4)	4 (28) 8 (72)	2–8
Clear zones in mm (% of eyes)	3.0 (38) 3.5 (32) 4.0 (28) 4.5 (1)	<3.0 (17) 3.00–3.49 (22) 3.50–3.99 (20) ≥4.0 (41)	3.0 (79) 3.5 (15) 4.0 (4) 4.5 (1)	2.75–6.00	3.5–4.0
Percent reoperations	12	0.5	15	39	27
Replicable protocol[a]	Yes	No	No	Yes (90%)	Yes
Population					
Preoperative myopia range (D)	1.50–8.00	1.50–11.90	1.50–11.63	0.88–8.25	1.00–9.50
Follow-up (mean)	10.1 yr	1 yr	NR	1 yr	6.2 mo
Range	4.9–11.8 yr	NR	3 mo–9 yr	9–14 mo	1.5–12 mo
No. of patients	435	NR	135	324	238
No. of eyes	793	972	225	615	375
Eyes reported (%)	88	68	80	89	92
Postoperative refraction (%)					
>1.00 D myopic	17	12	24	9	14
-1.00 to +1.00 D	60	76	73	89	85[b]
>1.00 D hyperopic	23	12	3	2	1
Uncorrected visual acuity (%)					
20/20 or better	53	47	NR	54	NR
20/40 or better	85	88	69	93	95
Best-corrected visual acuity (%)					
Eyes losing ≥2 lines	3	0.5	2	1	0.3
Stability of refraction					
Number of eyes	310	165	100	NR	NR
Follow-up interval	6 mo–10 yr	1–4 yr	3 mo–9 yr	NR	NR
Eyes with hyperopic shift ≥1.00 D (%)	43	31	13	NR	NR
Predictability					
Eyes having ≤2.00 D difference between predicted and actual refractive change (%)	88 (at 5 yr)	94	NR	NR	NR
Results for three baseline refraction groups					
Postoperative refraction ± 1.00 D (%)					
Low: -1.50 to -3.00 D	67	90	97	96	93
Middle: -3.12 to -6.00 D	62	76	81	85	88[c]
High: -6.12 to[d]	54	53	45	76	64[c]
Postoperative uncorrected visual acuity 20/40 or better (%)					
Low: -1.50 to -3.00 D	92	96	100	NR	NR
Middle: -3.12 to -6.00 D	86	89	73	NR	NR
High: -6.12 to[d]	77	77	47	NR	NR

Abbreviations: PERK, Prospective Evaluation of Radial Keratotomy; NR, not reported; D, diopters.
[a] Replicable protocol indicates standardized surgical procedure followed by all surgeons for all patients.
[b] 85 percent ±1 diopter of emmetropia; 92 percent ±1 diopter of planned goal of -0.50 diopter.
[c] Middle defined as 3.25 to 4.25 diopters of myopia; high defined as ≥4.50 diopters of myopia.
[d] Varies from -8.00 to -11.9 diopters.
Source: Adapted with permission from GO Waring, MJ Lynn, A Nizam, et al: Results of the Prospective Evaluation of Radial Keratotomy (PERK) study five years after surgery. Ophthalmology 93:1164, 1991. Courtesy of Ophthalmology.

to be corrected, the use of centripetal and bidirectional incisions, the increasing standardization of nomograms, the increasing number of eyes with refractive outcomes between ±1.00 diopter of emmetropia, the decreasing number of overcorrections, and the increasing number of planned repeat surgeries.

However, can radial keratotomy be called effective if it only partially reduces myopia? For example, if a patient with 9.00 diopters of myopia preoperatively has 3.00 diopters of residual myopia postoperatively, has the surgery been effective? Most patients and ophthalmologists would say no, because the patient still requires full-time optical correction for good distance visual acuity and now has corneal scars. The question is a philosophical one, but the published evidence is clear; successful radial keratotomy is that which frees patients from wearing distance correction the majority of the time and gives 20/20 or better visual acuity in at least one eye. The old standards for success of 20/40 or better uncorrected visual acuity and a refractive error within ±1.00 diopter of emmetropia are unacceptable, both by the profession and by patients.

Predictability of Outcome

The most difficult challenge for the radial keratotomy surgeon is to predict the outcome of the surgery for a single operation in an individual patient. For most patients, the goal is emmetropia or mild residual myopia. However, some patients are called "overresponders" or "underresponders" because of their unpredictable postoperative course. Therefore, surgeons now avoid trying to correct all of the myopia in all patients in a single operation and realize that staged surgery with reoperations (enhancements) is necessary to achieve the desired outcome in the majority of individuals.

The two principal sources of clinical variability are the technique of making the incisions and differences in corneal wound healing among individual patients. Even the best surgeons are unable to make all radial incisions equally deep along the entire length. Furthermore, even if all incisions were identical, it is likely that variations in corneal wound healing would continue to result in unpredictable outcomes for individual patients.

The consistency of a particular technique or series can be expressed as the standard deviation of the refractive outcome. In the Casebeer-Chiron study,[22] the standard deviation was 0.78 diopter (relatively low). The number and percentage of eyes within ±0.50 diopter of the predicted outcome (38 percent of 257 eyes in the PERK study and 68 percent of 378 eyes in the Casebeer-Chiron study), ±1.00 diopter of the predicted outcome, and similar categories will help the clinician understand the predictability of a given series or technique. Predictability can be calculated by measuring the prediction interval or confidence interval, as described elsewhere.[24] In the PERK study at 1 year,[146] the width of the 90 percent prediction interval was 3.42 diopters, which is fairly wide. Other studies have not calculated the prediction interval.

Predictability should be defined as the approximation of the final refractive error (which can probably be measured 3 months after the most recent surgery) and the desired outcome. This is important, because the desired outcome may be residual myopia of 1.00 to 2.00 diopters to achieve monovision or 0.50 diopter to avoid hyperopia. Therefore, unless the desired outcome in all patients in a series is emmetropia, the difference from the desired result should be the basis for calculating predictability.

Stability of Refractive Error

A decrease in myopia occurs in almost all eyes after radial keratotomy.[19,36,87,88,123–126,131,142] During the first few weeks after surgery, most eyes lose some of the effect of the surgery and become more myopic. This phenomenon, commonly referred to as *regression*, is an advantage for those who are overcorrected and a disadvantage for those who are emmetropic or undercorrected. Continued changes in refraction may occur over many years.[19,87,112,142,147] Between 6 months and 10 years after surgery in the PERK study, approximately 54 percent of the eyes remained stable within ±1.00 diopter. The other 46 percent continued to change, with 43 percent showing a shift of 1.00 diopter or more in the hyperopic direction—that is, a continued effect of the operation[19,87] (Figure 37-23). The rate of hyperopic shift was greater from 6 months to 2 years (0.21 diopter/year) than from 2 to 10 years (0.06 diopter/year) (Figure 37-24). Similar results have been reported in a variety of studies with at least 5 years of follow-up[19,88,125,126,131,142] (Table 37-9).

It is unknown what percentage of eyes will experience a hyperopic shift after radial keratotomy. In the PERK study, there was an approximate annual increase of 5 percent. It is unknown what the maximum hyperopic shift can be in eyes that do experience it; in the PERK study, the maximum shift was 6.38 diopters. Regression analysis in the PERK study identified the length of incisions as the only factor correlated with hyperopic shift; longer incisions were associated with a greater hyperopic shift. This led to the use of shorter incisions, sometimes called *mini-RK*, to reduce or prevent this problem. In this procedure, surgeons use a larger diameter clear zone, typically 3.5 mm or greater, and extend incisions only out to an 8.0- or 9.0-mm diameter zone. Of course, this corrects a smaller amount of

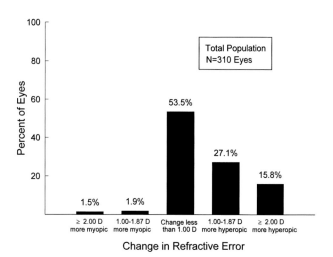

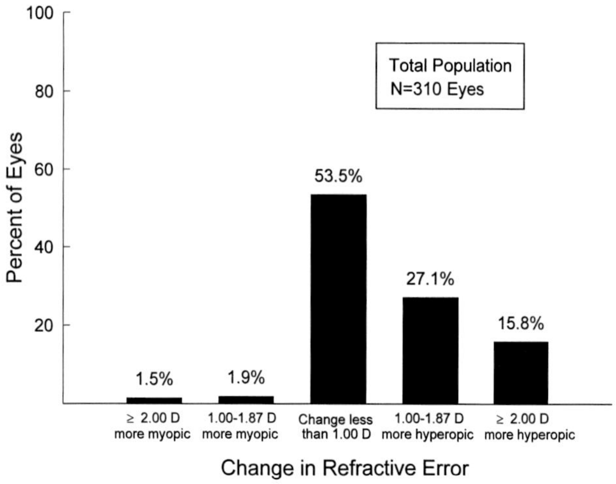

FIGURE 37-23 Bar graph indicates the change in the spherical equivalent of the cycloplegic refraction between 6 months and 10 years after radial keratotomy in the PERK study. Few eyes (3.4 percent) showed a regression of effect. Many eyes (43 percent) showed a hyperopic shift. (Adapted from GO Waring, MJ Lynn, PJ McDonnell, et al: Results of the Prospective Evaluation of Radial Keratotomy [PERK] study 10 years after surgery. Arch Ophthalmol 112:1298, 1994. Copyright 1994, American Medical Association.)

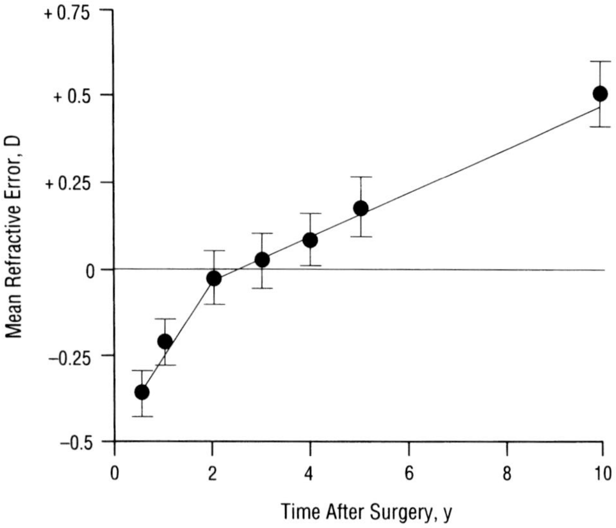

FIGURE 37-24 The mean spherical cycloplegic refractive error at follow-up visits after radial keratotomy for first-operated eyes examined at 10 years that did not undergo reoperation in the PERK study. The mean ± standard error of the mean rate of change before 2 years was 0.21 ± 0.02 diopter per year and after 2 years was 0.06 ± 0.004 diopter per year. Error bars indicate one standard error of the mean. The solid line is the longitudinal piecewise linear regression. (Reprinted with permission from GO Waring, MJ Lynn, PJ McDonnell, et al: Results of the Prospective Evaluation of Radial Keratotomy [PERK] study 10 years after surgery. Arch Ophthalmol 112:1298, 1994. Copyright 1994, American Medical Association.)

myopia. A mean hyperopic shift of 1.00 diopter between 6 months and 3 years after mini-RK in 100 eyes has been reported (R. Lindstrom, personal communication, August, 1996). Other studies have also associated longer incisions with hyperopic shift,[125] but some have not.[124,142] No correlation between any patient variable, such as age or intraocular pressure, and the hyperopic shift was found among the 10-year PERK patients, so there appears to be no basis for identifying patients at risk for this problem before surgery. All studies of stability of refraction are confounded by normal changes in refraction that accompany aging, as described by Ellingsen et al.[148]

Biomechanical reasons for the hyperopic shift are unknown. The avascular cornea heals slowly. A human eye examined histopathologically 17 months after successful radial keratotomy had the epithelial plug still occupying approximately 25 percent of corneal incision depth,[149] and an eye 10 years after radial keratotomy suffered rupture of the wounds after trauma.[150] Such partially healed wounds would be expected to produce a

TABLE 37-9
Hyperopic Shift in Studies of Radial Keratotomy

Study	*Year Published*	*Number of Eyes*	*Follow-Up Interval (yr)*	*Hyperopic Shift ≥1 D (% of Eyes)*
Sawelson and Marks[126]	1995	103	5–10	23
10-year PERK[19]	1994	310	0.5–10	43
Deitz et al[142]	1994	143	1.0–8.5	54
Arrowsmith and Marks[88]	1989	156	1–5	22
Sawelson and Marks[125]	1989	198	1.5–5.0	17
Neumann et al[131]	1984	118	1–5	26

Abbreviation: D, diopters.
Source: Adapted with permission from GO Waring, MJ Lynn, PJ McDonnell, et al: Results of the Prospective Evaluation of Radial Keratotomy (PERK) study 10 years after surgery. Arch Ophthalmol 112:1298, 1994. Copyright 1994, American Medical Association.

change in corneal shape, so the ongoing refractive changes probably represent a continuation of the basic biomechanical change in the cornea that produces the initial central corneal flattening—that is, an increase in the width of the corneal incisions.[46,139,151,152]

COMPLICATIONS

The complications of radial keratotomy have been reviewed in detail by Rashid and Waring.[153,154] There are two types of complications: (1) those that do not decrease corrected visual acuity, and (2) those that decrease or have the potential to decrease corrected visual acuity.

Complications That Do Not Decrease Corrected Visual Acuity

Undercorrection

Undercorrection and overcorrection are the most common complications of radial keratotomy. For most patients, the desirable refractive outcome is mild residual myopia, approximately 0.50 diopter. This outcome (1) allows good uncorrected distance visual acuity because of a slight multifocal effect of the cornea (depending on pupil size), (2) delays the onset of symptomatic presbyopia by creating a more proximate near point, (3) offsets the hyperopic shift, and (4) maintains the myopic state of visual function to which the patient has been accustomed. For patients who are left with an undesirable amount of undercorrection, a second operation can usually be performed, either lengthening or deepening the incisions or adding more incisions. These and other methods for the correction of residual myopia are described below.

Overcorrection

Hyperopia after radial keratotomy is a more disruptive result than residual myopia because it cannot be reduced by further keratotomy surgery. Individuals in their twenties and early thirties who have enough accommodative reserve to overcome the hyperopia may achieve good visual acuity and remain asymptomatic. A postoperative refraction with fogging or cycloplegia is essential in identifying these individuals. These individuals will become symptomatically presbyopic as their accommodative reserve drops, and those with more than 1 diopter of hyperopia will become dependent on an optical correction for good vision both at distance and at near in their fifth decade of life.

Pilocarpine has been reported to be effective in reducing overcorrection after radial keratotomy.[155] Surgical correction of hyperopia after radial keratotomy is described below.

Individuals who are in the range of emmetropia after radial keratotomy will lose their ability to see at near without correction as they become presbyopic. While no data have been published about the effect of radial keratotomy on the onset of presbyopia, it is unlikely that many of these individuals will begrudge the earlier need for reading glasses if they have been able to go without correction for a decade or more before they become presbyopic. That they are no longer able to see at near without correction will not be perceived as a loss, since these individuals will be more like their friends with emmetropia. However, those who are already in the presbyopic age group when they are considering radial keratotomy must be counseled carefully about the instant dependence they will acquire for a reading correction should they become bilaterally emmetropic or hyperopic after surgery.

Asymmetrical Correction

To adequately assess the efficacy of radial keratotomy, the symmetry of outcome should be reported for both eyes in order to identify anisometropia.[156] For example, a 30-year-old patient with a postoperative refraction of -1.00 diopter in one eye and +2.00 diopters in the other eye can see well with each eye, but 3 diopters of anisometropia may create undesirable symptoms. In the 5-year PERK study,[87] the median difference in refraction between the two eyes of 346 patients who had bilateral radial keratotomy was 0.62 diopter, with 12 percent of the eyes having more than 2.00 diopters of anisometropia.

Regular Astigmatism

Up to 2.50 diopters of regular astigmatism may be induced by radial keratotomy in a properly performed case. In the 5-year PERK study,[87] 10 percent of eyes had an increase in refractive astigmatism of 1.00 diopter or more. The factors that induce regular astigmatism are unknown, but asymmetry of the incisions is probably the major cause. Spectacles can correct this astigmatism.

Fluctuating Vision

In the first few months after radial keratotomy, many patients experience fluctuating vision during the day.[157–160] Most patients see better in the morning than in the evening because they are undercorrected and because there is a steepening of the cornea with a concomitant increase in myopia during the day.[160] These changes can be documented in some patients as long as 11 years after surgery.[159]

In the PERK study, approximately half the patients reported fluctuating vision during the day at 1 year after surgery.[157] Of 63 eyes examined 1 year after surgery on two occasions at least 12 hours apart on the same day, 31 percent showed an increase in myopia of 0.50 diopter or more

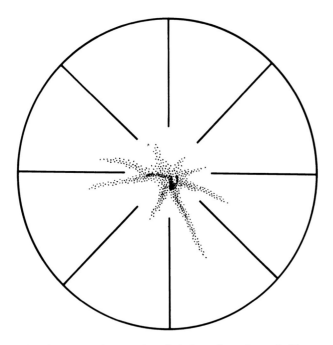

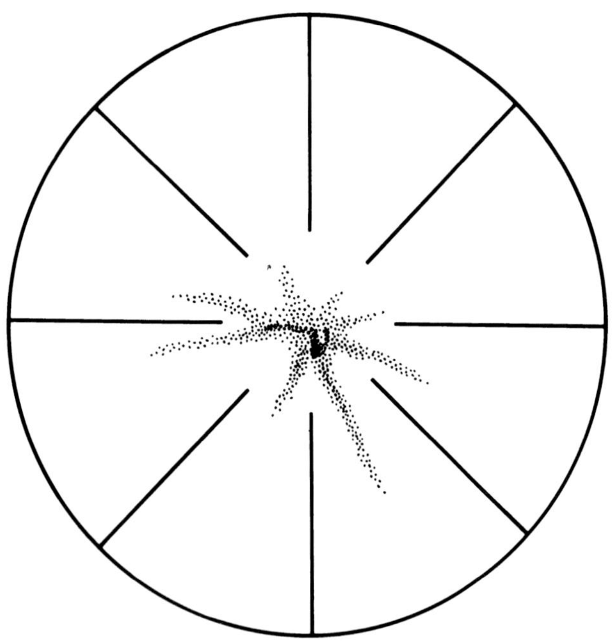

FIGURE 37-25 A corneal epithelial iron line after radial keratotomy located at the junction of the middle and inferior thirds of the cornea shows a stellate configuration in which the inferior branches are usually longer and more prominent than the superior branches. (Reprinted with permission from EB Steinberg, LA Wilson, GO Waring, et al: Stellate iron lines in the corneal epithelium after radial keratotomy. Am J Ophthalmol 98:416, 1984. Copyright by The Ophthalmic Publishing Company.)

between morning and evening, and 2 percent showed a decrease in myopia of 0.50 diopter or more from morning to evening. The unoperated eye of each patient served as a control; 91 percent of these eyes changed by less than 0.50 diopter during the 12-hour period. Of 52 eyes examined 3 years after surgery, 31 percent had a diurnal variation of 0.50 diopter or more in refractive power.[87] Of 71 eyes examined 11 years after surgery, 54 percent had a morning-to-evening change in refractive error of 0.50 diopter or more.[159] A hyperopic shift has also been described at high altitudes in patients who have had radial keratotomy.[161,162]

Nondisabling Glare

Many patients are aware of light scatter from the incisions in the form of a starburst or linear effect around bright lights, but often describe it as resembling the glare associated with contact lenses—a phenomenon that is not very disruptive to vision.

Inclusions in Incisions

Abnormal material may appear in the incisions postoperatively. Most commonly, the epithelium forms persistent, focal inclusions that look like small, pearly nodules in the incision.[163] A large epithelial plug may spread the incision wider, and cleaning out the incision and suturing the wound may decrease an overcorrection.

Epithelial Iron Line

Radial keratotomy induces the formation of a stellate iron line in about 80 percent of eyes.[119] This line consists of a nodular or linear center located at the junction of the middle and inferior thirds of the cornea with arms that radiate for varying distances between the incisions (Figure 37-25). The density varies from being barely perceptible with the slit lamp microscope to a brown-yellow spot visible with a penlight. The extent of the iron line correlates with the amount of corneal flattening achieved by the surgery. The stellate line probably results from subtle surface irregularities caused by the surgery.[119,164]

Problems with Fitting Contact Lenses

Eyes that have undergone radial keratotomy are more difficult to fit with contact lenses than are normal eyes, because the surgery alters corneal topography.[165] Extended-wear soft contact lenses can induce vascularization of the incisions and should be avoided. Daily-wear soft contact lenses can be successfully fitted, but can also cause superficial vascularization. Rigid gas-permeable contact lenses offer the best corrected visual acuity with minimal complications. Whether contact lenses produce a greater incidence of corneal warpage in eyes with radial keratotomy than in normal eyes is unknown; corneal and refractive changes induced by 1 to 5 years of contact lens wear after radial keratotomy have been examined, but the results are ambiguous.[166,167]

Complications That Decrease Corrected Visual Acuity

A major concern about radial keratotomy is that after a properly performed, uncomplicated operation, the eye may not regain the preoperative level of visual acuity with optical correction. Loss or gain of one line of visual acuity on the National Eye Institute charts equals the loss or gain of three letters. This change is within the biological variability of the tests, and therefore a change of two or more lines is the level of clinically meaningful change. In the PERK study at 10 years,[19] 23 of 793 eyes (3 percent) lost two or more lines of best spectacle-corrected visual acuity after radial keratotomy. Of these, 15 eyes (2 percent) had a spectacle-corrected visual acuity of 20/16 to 20/20, five had 20/25, and three had 20/30 (Figure 37-26). More recent studies report a loss of two or more lines of spectacle-corrected visual acuity in approximately 1 percent or fewer eyes (see Table 37-8).

Severe complications that arise from surgical errors or from intraoperative and postoperative occurrences can reduce vision permanently. Because most of these eyes are structurally normal with 20/20 or better spectacle-corrected visual acuity before radial keratotomy, any event that permanently reduces vision is an unacceptable complication, causing great disappointment for both patient and surgeon.

The incidence of severe complications after radial keratotomy is unknown because complications occur sporadically and usually are not reported in the literature.

Irregular Astigmatism

An irregular corneal surface results most commonly from "creative" keratotomy—that is, circular and radial incisions, combined patterns of incisions for astigmatism, multiple reoperations, and incisions that extend too near the visual axis.[168,169] Because a freewheeling approach to radial keratotomy has given way to more refined and careful techniques, this complication is rare. Contact lenses are required to correct the irregular astigmatism.

Disabling Glare

Disabling glare from radial keratotomy incisions is caused by intraocular light scattering and is perceived as unpleasant by the patient. It is more likely to occur when the central clear zone is less than 3 mm in diameter,[60] when the scars are dense, when the pupil is physiologically large, and when the patient is naturally light sensitive. It interferes with the patient's ability to drive at night and to enjoy outdoor activities on hazy or bright days.[168,169]

Disabling glare rarely occurs after an uncomplicated, properly performed radial keratotomy,[36,87,88,123–126] but when it does occur, the only effective treatment is to provide high-quality sunglasses, especially those with an ultraviolet filter. Dilute pilocarpine (0.5 percent) can reduce glare, but patients rarely use it for a long period of time.

Patients with a marked decrease in visual acuity caused by scars from bacterial keratitis, irregular astigmatism, or glare may need penetrating keratoplasty.[168]

Endothelial Damage and Corneal Edema

The majority of Sato's patients developed corneal edema 2 decades or more after the 40 posterior corneal incisions were made.[8,12] This severe complication does not occur after modern radial keratotomy. However, even a properly performed radial keratotomy produces mild damage to the corneal endothelium: cytoplasmic vacuolization, focal areas of endothelial defects, disruption of the endothelial mosaic by breakage of the cell membranes,[27,170–174] and increased endothelial permeability.[118] In extreme cases, severe endothelial cell loss may occur without corneal edema. Salz[169,175] reported a case in which there was a loss of 24 percent of the endothelial cells from the central cornea after repeat radial keratotomy and a case in which there was a 50 percent loss of endothelial cells in a 68-year-old woman after 16-incision radial keratotomy.

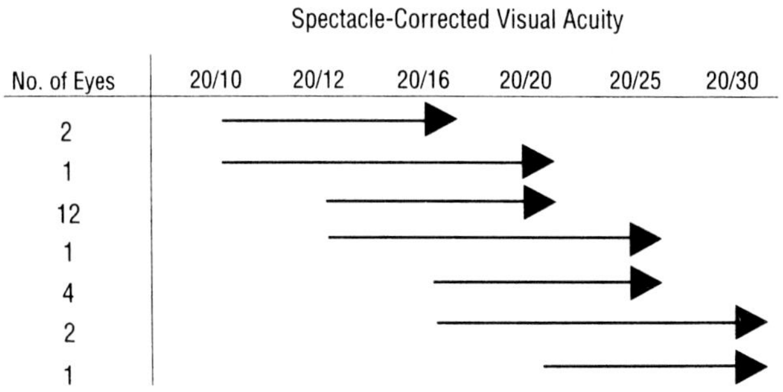

FIGURE 37-26 The spectacle-corrected visual acuity before and after radial keratotomy for 23 eyes that lost two or more Snellen lines of visual acuity in the Prospective Evaluation of Radial Keratotomy study at 10 years. (Reprinted with permission from GO Waring, MJ Lynn, PJ McDonnell, et al: Results of the Prospective Evaluation of Radial Keratotomy [PERK] study 10 years after surgery. Arch Ophthalmol 112:1298, 1994. Copyright 1994, American Medical Association.)

Most studies of endothelial cell damage after radial keratotomy have involved clinical specular microscopy of the central cornea, with reports of 0 to 15 percent cell loss.[176] However, the central measurements were made in the area where no surgery was performed, and mild to moderate damage to the corneal endothelium in the area of the incisions would not be detected by these measurements. Specular microscopy adjacent to or beneath the incisions is more meaningful. Two studies have used this technique.[177,178] In both studies, specular microscopy 6 to 12 months after radial keratotomy showed no decrease in endothelial cell density between or beneath the incisions, compared with the endothelial cell density in the central cornea. Between baseline and 10 years after surgery in the PERK study,[179] there was a 10 to 11 percent decrease in the average cell density in both unoperated eyes and eyes that had undergone radial keratotomy, with no significant changes in the coefficient of variation of cell size or the percent of hexagonal cells. No evidence of endothelial damage from a properly performed radial keratotomy has been published.

Intraoperative Corneal Perforation

Small corneal perforations may occur as the incisions are made, manifesting as a bead of aqueous humor appearing adjacent to the knife. These perforations usually have an uncomplicated course. If the perforation does not leak spontaneously and the anterior chamber remains deep, it is usually possible to complete the operation. A perforation that leaks with external pressure on the cornea can be sealed with a bandage soft contact lens worn for 2 to 5 days. If, however, the perforation leaks spontaneously and the anterior chamber becomes shallow, the perforation must be sutured. Perforations produce scarring at the level of Descemet's membrane and damage to endothelial cells in the area of perforation. All perforations have the potential to cause permanent vision loss because endophthalmitis and epithelial ingrowth may occur.[107,180,181]

The percentage of eyes with corneal perforations was high during the early development of radial keratotomy, reaching 30 percent.[36] As ultrasonic pachymetry and more carefully calibrated diamond knives have become available, this percentage has fallen. Although some surgeons are willing to accept a certain number of corneal perforations as an intrinsic part of radial keratotomy, perforations should be considered an undesirable complication.

Cataract

When a corneal perforation occurs, the blade may lacerate the anterior capsule of the lens, producing a cataract. To restore vision, cataract extraction is required.[182–184]

Endophthalmitis

Endophthalmitis usually develops from invasion of microorganisms through an intraoperative corneal perforation, although it has been reported to occur in cases in which there was no recognizable perforation at the time of surgery.[109] The severity of the infection is proportional to the virulence and the size of the inoculum of the organism. The extent of the invasion may be limited somewhat by the intact lens-iris diaphragm.[107,108]

Microbial Keratitis

Because radial keratotomy breaks the protective epithelial barrier, microorganisms may invade the cornea, especially in eyes in which there is blepharitis or conjunctivitis.[98–106] Beldavs and colleagues[100] reported a patient with chronic blepharitis who had radial keratotomy in both eyes 48 hours apart, and who developed bilateral *Staphylococcus aureus* keratitis within 1 week of surgery. Other organisms reported to cause infectious keratitis after radial keratotomy include *Streptococcus pneumoniae*,[102] *Staphylococcus epidermidis*,[103] *Serratia marcescens*,[106] *Mycobacterium chelonei*,[99] and *Mycobacterium smegmatis*.[105]

Delayed bacterial keratitis can appear 1 to 2 years after surgery. It is attributed to the continued turnover of epithelial cells in the epithelial plug of the wound, which creates attachment sites for the bacteria. Delayed bacterial keratitis is probably more common than acute bacterial keratitis.[185,186]

The outcome has been good in the majority of reported cases of bacterial keratitis after radial keratotomy, largely because the infections occur away from the visual axis in eyes that are otherwise healthy, and patients usually seek aid promptly. However, the results can be devastating if the infection is paracentral, is allowed to progress untreated, or is resistant to management. At least six reports[100–104,106] describe bacterial keratitis developing within 24 hours to 10 days after simultaneous bilateral radial keratotomy; although there is no reason to believe that infection is more common after bilateral than after unilateral surgery, the potential for disastrous consequences from bilateral infection led many of these authors to suggest that simultaneous bilateral surgery should be undertaken with caution, or possibly not at all. Nevertheless, many surgeons perform bilateral simultaneous surgery.

Two cases of fungal keratitis caused by *Candida* species that occurred after radial keratotomy have been described.[187,188] Treatment with topical amphotericin B and oral ketoconazole yielded 20/20 best-corrected visual acuity in one patient.[187] A case of combined *Fusarium* and *Acanthamoeba* keratitis that required therapeutic penetrating keratoplasty has been reported.[189]

Traumatic Rupture of the Globe

Experimental studies of blunt trauma to enucleated animal or human eyes immediately after radial keratotomy demonstrated that the globe ruptures more easily through the incisions,[190,191] and that shorter incisions appear to be capable of withstanding greater pressures than longer incisions.[192] However, these experiments were performed under artificial conditions, with the incisions completely unhealed and the eyeball compressed against a hard surface. Cases of human globes rupturing at radial keratotomy incisions after blunt trauma have occurred (Figure 37-27). The resistance of healed radial keratotomy incisions when struck in the cushioned environment of the orbit remains to be established.

Twenty-eight human eyes that ruptured through refractive corneal incisions have been described.[150] In 26 cases, the interval between the keratotomy procedure and rupture was reported. Three (12 percent) occurred in the immediate 6-week postoperative period, two (8 percent) within 6 months of surgery, and 21 (81 percent) after 6 months. Four eyes ruptured along radial keratotomy incisions more

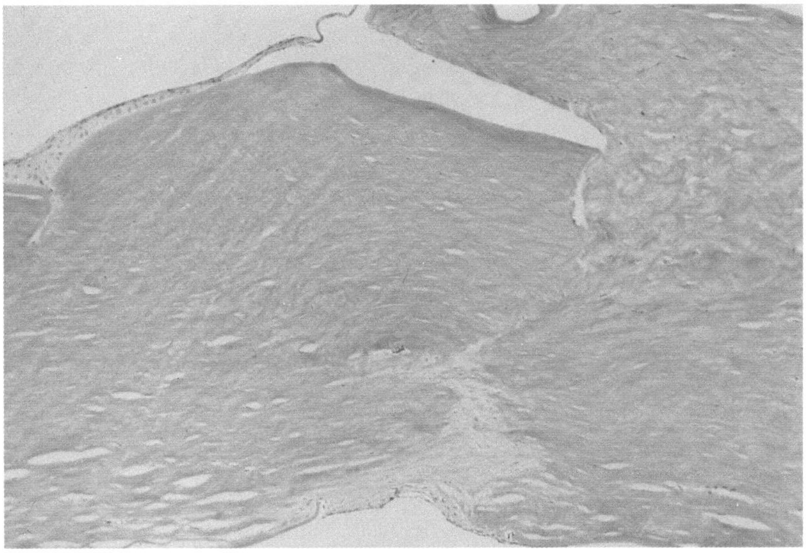

FIGURE 37-27 A light microscopic section through a cornea ruptured through a radial keratotomy scar by blunt trauma during an automobile accident. The cornea was sutured and allowed to heal, and then replaced with a penetrating graft. The wound gapes anteriorly where Bowman's layer was incarcerated during the repair, and a dense sheet of scar tissue is present throughout the thickness of the cornea, with a break in Descemet's membrane posteriorly. (Masson's trichrome, × 25.)

than 5 years after surgery. Twelve eyes ruptured from activities of daily living, seven from assault, five in association with motor vehicle accidents, and four in the course of sports activities. Of the 26 patients who survived their injuries, only one achieved a final best-corrected visual acuity of 20/20; overall, eight had a final visual acuity of 20/40 or better, six had between 20/40 and 20/100, six were legally blind, and six were totally blind in the ruptured eye.

Examples of ocular trauma without rupture of the keratotomy incisions have been also reported.[193–196]

Penetrating keratoplasty wounds never regain the strength of the normal cornea, and such wounds can rupture many years postoperatively.[197] Radial keratotomy wounds, even though they are of only partial thickness, are also not as strong as the normal cornea. Therefore, eyes that suffer severe direct trauma after radial keratotomy are more susceptible to corneal rupture, although such eyes are susceptible to rupture of the globe in any case. Pinheiro et al[192] demonstrated experimentally that corneas with short radial incisions (mini-RK) are less likely to rupture than corneas with incisions that extend to the limbus.

The increased fragility of the cornea after radial keratotomy would appear to be a disadvantage. If trauma that is not severe enough to rupture a normal globe ruptures one that has had radial keratotomy, the disadvantage is clear. On the other hand, trauma severe enough to rupture a normal globe (usually under the rectus muscles, across the limbus, or around the optic nerve) may rupture radial keratotomy scars instead. In such a case, the scars would be an advantage, serving as a release valve and making repair of the globe easier than it would be if the rupture were located posteriorly.

SURGICAL PROCEDURES AFTER RADIAL KERATOTOMY

Incisional Methods for Correction of Residual Myopia

Repeat radial keratotomy may be performed if there is clinically significant residual myopia. Such myopia may occur if the initial operation results in an undercorrection or if the initial operation is part of a staged series of radial keratotomies designed to avoid an overcorrection.

Three variables can be modified in repeat radial keratotomy: the length of the incisions, the depth of the incisions, and the number of incisions.

Increasing the length or depth of the incisions is best accomplished by opening each incision with a dull instrument, such as an intraocular lens hook, because it is difficult to place a second incision in the exact location of the first one. Opening the wound allows the trough of the initial incision to serve as a guide for lengthening or deepening the incision. To lengthen the incision (decrease the diameter of the optical clear zone), the vertical edge of the blade is lowered into the open wound and pushed forward to the edge of the new clear zone mark. As with any centripetal method, this procedure risks cutting into the clear zone. To avoid this risk, some surgeons open the wound, place the knife at the new clear zone mark, and cut in a centrifugal direction to connect the new incision with the old incision. This is facilitated by a knife guide.

If the initial incisions are too shallow on examination with the slit lamp microscope (Figure 37-28), they can be deepened by setting the blade according to the ultrasonic pachym-

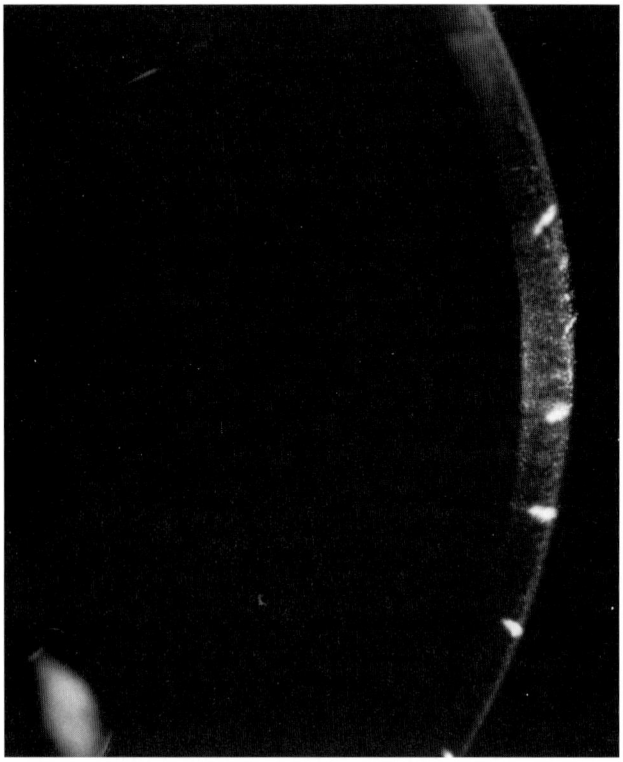

FIGURE 37-28 Shallow incisions after radial keratotomy are shown in this slit lamp photomicrograph. The incisions extend to a depth that is about 30 to 50 percent of the corneal thickness and produce less reduction of myopia than is produced by deep incisions.

etry thickness measurements and the desired depth to be achieved. Without creating pressure on the wound, the surgeon lowers the knife blade into the open wound and slides the blade along the wound to cut the remaining deep stromal tissue. A partially blunt vertical blade (bidirectional blade) allows the surgeon to deepen the incisions by cutting centripetally without the risks of creating a double incision or cutting into the optical clear zone. Franks[198] described a technique of recutting the central 2 mm of each wound that greatly improved his results. In 85 eyes with an initial myopia of less than 6 diopters and a residual refractive error after the first operation of -0.50 to -4.00 diopters, 71 eyes (84 percent) achieved a refraction of 0 to -1.00 diopter after the second procedure. Charlton[199] reported lengthening and deepening incisions in 27 eyes of 20 patients. The residual refractive error after the initial keratotomy surgery was -1.70 diopters; the mean change in refraction was a reduction in myopia of approximately 1.50 diopters. The mean refraction after repeat surgery was -0.18 ±0.57 diopter (range, +1.50 to -1.13 diopters), with 93 percent of the eyes being within 1.00 diopter of emmetropia.

Additional incisions can also be made, particularly in eyes that have an initial four-incision procedure. Cowden and Weber[200] performed an eight-incision repeat radial keratotomy in monkeys 1 year after an initial eight-incision procedure, and obtained an average change in the cycloplegic refraction of +0.50 diopter (range, -0.37 to +1.37 diopters). Villaseñor and Cox[201] performed a second eight-incision radial keratotomy after an initial eight-incision operation in 25 eyes, and found an average change in refraction of +1.00 diopter (range, -1.50 to +3.75 diopters). In the PERK study,[202] 59 eyes underwent repeat eight-incision radial keratotomy. Seventy-seven percent of these eyes had a decrease in myopia of 0.50 diopter or more, 20 percent showed a change of less than 0.50 diopter, and 3 percent demonstrated an increase in myopia.

Adding more incisions is more difficult than making the original incisions. Recentering the clear zone mark requires relocating the center of the entrance pupil and trying to ensure that the new clear zone mark is in the same place as the original one. The original incisions are often difficult to see, especially against a light-colored iris. Dilating the pupil and turning down the intensity of the microscope light can make the original incisions more visible against the red fundus reflex, but this risks damage to the lens should corneal perforation occur. Placing the knife equidistant between the previous incisions and following a radial course between them requires more skill than is required for the initial incisions. A radial keratotomy marker is useful in these cases.

Surgery for residual astigmatism can also be carried out as a secondary procedure, either by deepening or lengthening the original incisions or by adding new incisions. In general, the precept of not crossing incisions should be observed. Therefore, additional transverse incisions should be interrupted if the steep meridian of the astigmatism is in the area of a previously made radial incision (see Ch. 38).

There are many unknowns about repeat operations. Optimal timing has not been established, but the second procedure can be performed as soon as 1 week or as late as several years after the initial surgery. Criteria for reoperations are not well defined. For example, patients whose initial surgery consisted of very deep incisions may have less effect from additional surgery than patients who initially had shallow incisions.[201,202]

In the Casebeer-Chiron study,[22] 39 percent of eyes had repeat operations (enhancement): 43 percent of these had lengthening of the incisions, 40 percent had deepening of the incisions, 21 percent had additional transverse incisions, and 15 percent had additional radial incisions. Fifteen percent of the eyes received more than one enhancement. After each enhancement, approximately 50 to 60 percent of the eyes moved from being undercorrected to within ±0.50 diopter of emmetropia, demonstrating the effectiveness of this staged or titrated approach.

Methods for Correction of Hyperopia

Because radial keratotomy flattens the central cornea by gaping of the incisions and increased volume of the cornea, it can be reversed by closing the incisions with sutures. In this procedure, the incisions are opened, scraped clean of epithelium, and sutured with one or two interrupted sutures placed at approximately the 7-mm diameter zone.[203] Alternatively, one or two continuous purse string sutures can be placed and tightened to steepen the central cornea.[203-207] Damiano et al[204] described a method in which two zone diameters are marked, one at 5 mm and one at 7 mm. The pre-existing radial incisions are opened with an intraocular lens hook to half depth; the needle is placed into the wound at about half depth, passed along the tissue between the two wounds, and brought out in the adjacent wound. Two purse string sutures are placed along the 7- and 5-mm zones. A paracentesis is performed to decompress the anterior chamber, and the sutures are tightened to overcorrect the eye initially. This procedure is followed by some delayed regression of the effect. The authors reported an average corneal steepening of 3.30 diopters (range, 1.00 to 7.50 diopters) in 19 eyes with more than 1 year of follow-up. The long-term stability of refraction after purse string sutures can vary. One report of eight eyes followed for 3 years showed that none of the eyes had a refractive change of more than 1 diopter.[203,208]

Because the intrastromal technique of purse string suturing produced variable effectiveness and stability, Grene developed an over-and-under technique in which the suture bite is taken between the radial incisions and then extends over the top of the radial incision. Theoretically, this would compress the incision better and achieve a greater correction than the completely intrastromal sutures. However, the surface loop can become loose and cause pain and ocular irritation.

Keratomileusis and Epikeratophakia

Radial keratotomy is most effective for myopia of 5 diopters or less. Nevertheless, many patients with high myopia have had radial keratotomy with residual undercorrection. Some of these patients have undergone myopic keratomileusis, with a donor cornea used for the lenticule,[209,210] or keratomileusis in situ.[211] The reported outcomes vary from an overcorrection of +1.75 diopters to an undercorrection of -6.50 diopters.

Excimer laser-assisted in situ keratomileusis (LASIK) can be performed with reasonable predictability, particularly if at least 1 year has passed. The radial wounds do not gape. Because smaller amounts of myopia are generally corrected with this technique (1.00 to 4.00 diopters), the accuracy is reasonably good.

Epikeratophakia after radial keratotomy has been used for large undercorrections[212] and overcorrections[213] that have been stable for 1 year or more.

Excimer Laser Photorefractive Keratectomy

When maximum radial keratotomy has been performed on an eye and there is residual myopia, the patient may request further surgery. Excimer laser photorefractive keratectomy (PRK) is a possible adjunctive procedure, because it works by a different mechanism in a different location on the cornea, but the results of combined radial keratotomy and photorefractive keratectomy have been variable.[214-228] Two unwanted side effects occur frequently enough to make this an undesirable combination: (1) subepithelial haze and scarring occur more frequently, presumably because the photorefractive keratectomy ablation overlies the ends of the radial keratotomy scars, where keratocytes have already been activated by the initial incisions, stimulating them to a more vigorous wound healing response, and (2) irregular astigmatism occurs more frequently, presumably because of the increased subepithelial healing and possibly the combination of the irregularity associated with the incisions plus that induced by the photorefractive keratectomy.

Maloney and colleagues[220,221] reported a 1-year follow-up of 107 eyes that had undergone photorefractive keratectomy after previous refractive surgery or cataract surgery; 90 (84 percent) had had radial keratotomy. Although the mean manifest spherical equivalent refraction fell from -3.7 to -0.6 diopters, 29 percent of eyes lost two or more Snellen lines of spectacle-corrected visual acuity, and central corneal haze was moderate or severe in 8 percent of eyes, leading to the conclusion that photorefractive keratectomy after radial keratotomy is less accurate than photorefractive keratectomy in previously unoperated eyes and is more likely to cause a loss of spectacle-corrected visual acuity. Most of the other studies have reported good results, with few complications, satisfactory uncorrected visual acuities, and little loss of best spectacle-corrected visual acuity. Two studies mentioned a tendency toward overcorrection.[216,222] One study[224] stated that patients with decreased best spectacle-corrected visual acuity after radial keratotomy are less likely to respond well to subsequent photorefractive keratectomy.

Cataract Surgery

Cataract surgery in eyes that have undergone radial keratotomy many years previously will become more common as the population of refractive surgery patients ages. Publications describing cataract surgery with intraocular lens implantation after radial keratotomy cite the problems inherent in calculating the required power of the intraocular lens.[213,229,230]

The major problem in calculating intraocular lens power is that, after radial keratotomy, the cornea has an overall oblate shape that is flatter centrally than paracentrally and peripherally and the central area is not spherical. Thus, standard keratometry, which measures the radius of curvature of the cornea at two points approximately 3 to 4 mm apart, may miss the flattest area of the cornea in the center, causing an overestimation of corneal power and insertion of an intraocular lens of a lower power than is needed, leading to a hyperopic result. Currently, the best way to calculate corneal power for entry into an intraocular lens calculation formula is to use videokeratography and to average the power of the second, third, and fourth rings, assuming they are centered approximately over the entrance pupil. This will give a closer estimate of the central corneal power than keratometry.[231,232]

Penetrating Keratoplasty

Penetrating keratoplasty after radial keratotomy is usually performed because of decreased visual acuity due to irregular astigmatism or central stromal scarring, corneal endothelial decompensation, or scarring from bacterial infection.[99,101,168,233] McNeill[237] described a 56-year-old man who required penetrating keratoplasty for irregular astigmatism and contact lens intolerance 9 years after a 16-incision radial keratotomy with transverse incisions for astigmatism. During keratoplasty surgery, nearly one-third of the peripheral radial keratotomy incisions opened spontaneously, increasing the difficulty of suturing the transplant and demonstrating the long-term instability of the cornea. Placement of an intrastromal purse string suture outside the circumference of the intended trephine cut will hold the radial incisions closed while the host tissue is trephined and the donor tissue is sutured in place.[154,239]

RADIAL KERATOTOMY AFTER OTHER SURGICAL PROCEDURES

Radial keratotomy has been performed in eyes to reduce residual myopia after myopic keratomileusis,[240] epikeratophakia for keratoconus,[241] and penetrating keratoplasty,[242,243] with satisfactory visual outcomes. Because of the complex topographic changes in corneal grafts after penetrating keratoplasty, the results in these cases may be variable and unpredictable.[243] The keratoplasty scar forms a new, functional "limbus," so a larger clear zone and shorter incisions, which may or may not cross the keratoplasty wound, must be used to avoid overcorrection.

Acknowledgments

Parts of this work were supported by PHS grants U01 EY03761 and U10 EY03761 from the National Eye Institute, National Institutes of Health, Bethesda, Maryland. This chapter was adapted in part from Waring GO: The changing status of radial keratotomy for myopia. Part I. J Refract Surg 1:81, 1985 and Part II. J Refract Surg 1:119, 1985.

REFERENCES

1. Waring GO: Refractive Keratotomy for Myopia and Astigmatism. Mosby–Year Book, St. Louis, 1992
2. Thornton SP: Radial and Astigmatic Keratotomy. The American System of Precise, Predictable Refractive Surgery. Slack, Thorofare, NJ, 1994
3. Assil KK, Schanzlin DJ: Radial and Astigmatic Keratotomy. A Complete Handbook for the Successful Practice of Incisional Keratotomy Using the Combined Technique. Poole Press/Slack, Thorofare, NJ, 1994
4. Casebeer C: Casebeer Incisional Keratotomy. Slack, Thorofare, NJ, 1995
5. McCarty CA, Livingston PM, Taylor HR: Prevalence of myopia in adults: implications for refractive surgeons. J Refract Surg 13:229, 1997
6. Lans LJ: Experimentelle Untersuchungen uber Engstehung von Astigmatismus durch nicht-perforirende Corneawunden. Albrecht von Graefes Arch Ophthalmol 45:117, 1898
7. Akiyama K, Shibata H, Kanai A, et al: Development of radial keratotomy in Japan, 1939–1960. p. 179. In Waring GO: Refractive Keratotomy for Myopia and Astigmatism. Mosby–Year Book, St. Louis, 1992
8. Akiyama K, Tanaka M, Kanai A, et al: Problems arising from Sato's radial keratotomy procedure in Japan. CLAO J 10:179, 1984
9. Akiyama K: Study of surgical treatment for myopia. I. Posterior corneal incisions. Nippon Ganka Gakkai Zasshi 56:1142, 1952
10. Akiyama K: Study of surgical treatment for myopia (second report): animal experiment. Nippon Ganka Gakkai Zasshi 59:294, 1955
11. Sato T: Experimental study of posterior half-corneal incisions for myopia. Nippon Ganka Gakkai Zasshi 55:219, 1951
12. Yamaguchi T, Kanai A, Tanaka M, et al: Bullous keratopathy after anterior-posterior radial keratotomy for myopia and myopic astigmatism. Am J Ophthalmol 93:600, 1982

13. Kanai A, Yamaguchi T, Yajima Y, et al: The fine structure of bullous keratopathy after anterioposterior incision of the cornea for myopia. Nippon Ganka Kiyo 30:841, 1979
14. Fyodorov SN, Durnev VV: Operation of dosaged dissection of corneal circular ligament in cases of myopia of mild degree. Ann Ophthalmol 11:1185, 1979
15. Schachar RA, Levy NS, Schachar L (eds): Keratorefraction. LAL Publishing, Denison, TX, 1980
16. Schachar RA, Levy NS, Schachar L (eds): Radial Keratotomy. LAL Publishing, Denison, TX, 1980
17. Schachar RA, Levy NS, Schachar L (eds): Refractive Modulation of the Cornea. LAL Publishing, Denison, TX, 1981
18. Waring GO, Moffitt SD, Gelender H, et al: Rationale for and design of the National Eye Institute Prospective Evaluation of Radial Keratotomy (PERK) study. Ophthalmology 90:40, 1983
19. Waring GO, Lynn MJ, McDonnell PJ, et al: Results of the Prospective Evaluation of Radial Keratotomy (PERK) study 10 years after surgery. Arch Ophthalmol 112:1298, 1994
20. Verity SM, Talamo JH, Chayet A, et al: The combined (Genesis) technique of radial keratotomy. Ophthalmology 102:1908, 1995
21. Werblin TP, Stafford GM: The Casebeer system for predictable keratorefractive surgery. One-year evaluation of 205 consecutive eyes. Ophthalmology 100:1095, 1993
22. Waring GO III, Casebeer JC, Dru RM, et al: One-year results of a prospective multicenter study of the Casebeer system of refractive keratotomy. Ophthalmology 103:1337, 1996
23. Steel DL, Salz JJ: Laboratory evaluation of radial keratotomy. Int Ophthalmol Clin 23:129, 1983
24. Lynn MJ, Waring GO, Kutner MH: Predictability of refractive keratotomy. p. 341. In Waring GO: Refractive Keratotomy for Myopia and Astigmatism. Mosby–Year Book, St. Louis, 1992
25. Salz JJ, Rowsey JJ, Caroline P, et al: A study of optical zone size and incision redeepening in experimental radial keratotomy. Arch Ophthalmol 103:590, 1985
26. Knauss WG, Rapacz P, Sene K, et al: Curvature changes induced by radial keratotomy in solithane model of eye. ARVO abstract. Invest Ophthalmol Vis Sci 20(suppl):69, 1981
27. Jester JJ, Steel D, Salz J, et al: Radial keratotomy in nonhuman primate eyes. Am J Ophthalmol 92:153, 1981
28. Schachar RA, Black TD, Huang T: A physicist's view of radial keratotomy with practical surgical implications. p. 195. In Schachar RA, Levy NS, Schachar L (eds): Keratorefraction. LAL Publishing, Denison, TX, 1980
29. Salz JJ: Clinical results of radial keratotomy in fresh human cadaver eyes. p. 133. In Schachar RA, Levy NS, Schachar L (eds): Keratorefraction. LAL Publishing, Denison, TX, 1980
30. Salz J, Lee J, Jester J, et al: Radial keratotomy in fresh human cadaver eyes. Ophthalmology 88:742, 1981
31. Lindstrom RL: Minimally invasive radial keratotomy: mini-RK. J Cataract Refract Surg 21:27, 1995.
32. Jester JV, Venet T, Lee J, et al: A statistical analysis of radial keratotomy in human cadaver eyes. Am J Ophthalmol 92:172, 1981
33. Steel DL, Jester JV, Salz JJ, et al: Modification of corneal curvature following radial keratotomy in primates. Ophthalmology 88:747, 1981
34. Cowden JW, Cichocki J: Radial keratotomy in monkeys: a one year follow-up report. Ophthalmology 89:684, 1982
35. Arrowsmith PN, Marks RG: Evaluating the predictability of radial keratotomy. Ophthalmology 92:331, 1985
36. Deitz MR, Sanders DR, Raanan MS: A consecutive series (1982–1985) of radial keratotomies performed with the diamond blade. Am J Ophthalmol 103:417, 1987
37. Lynn MJ, Waring GO, Sperduto RD, et al: Factors affecting outcome and predictability of radial keratotomy in the PERK study. Arch Ophthalmol 105:42, 1987
38. Busin M, Suarez H, Bieber S, McDonald MB: Overcorrected visual acuity improved by antiglaucoma medication after radial keratotomy. Am J Ophthalmol 101:372, 1986
39. Nirankari VS, Katzen LE, Richards RD, et al: Prospective clinical study of radial keratotomy. Ophthalmology 89:677, 1982
40. Bourque LB, Rubenstein R, Cosand B, et al: Psychosocial characteristics of candidates for the Prospective Evaluation of Radial Keratotomy (PERK) study. Arch Ophthalmol 102:1187, 1984
41. Powers MK, Meyerowitz BE, Arrowsmith PN, et al: Psychosocial findings in radial keratotomy patients two years after surgery. Ophthalmology 91:1193, 1984
42. Klein PE, Markowitz JA: Patient educational materials for refractive keratotomy. p. 281. In Waring GO: Refractive Keratotomy for Myopia and Astigmatism. Mosby–Year Book, St Louis, 1992
43. Teimeier CG, Abbott RL, Ellis JH: Risk management issues in radial keratotomy surgery. Surv Ophthalmol 39:52, 1994
44. Can surgery free you from glasses? Consumer Reports February:87, 1994
45. Bullimore MA, Sheedy JE, Owen D: Diurnal vision changes in radial keratotomy: implications for visual standards. Refractive Surgery Study Group. Optom Vis Sci 71:516, 1194
46. Binder PS, Nayak SK, Deg JK, et al: An ultrastructural and histochemical study of long-term wound healing after radial keratotomy. Am J Ophthalmol 103:432, 1987
47. Mamalis N, Montgomery S, Anderson C, Miller C: Radial keratotomy in a patient with keratoconus. Refract Corneal Surg 7:374, 1991
48. Ellis W: Radial keratotomy in a patient with keratoconus. J Cataract Refract Surg 18:406, 1992
49. Durand L, Monnot JP, Curillon C, Assi A: Complications of radial keratotomy: eyes with keratoconus and late wound dehiscence. Refract Corneal Surg 8:311, 1992
50. Maguire JL, Bourne WM: Corneal topography of early keratoconus. Am J Ophthalmol 108:107, 1989
51. Wilson SE, Klyce SD: Screening for corneal topographic abnormalities before refractive surgery. Ophthalmology 101:147, 1994
52. Rowsey JJ, Balyeat HD: Preliminary results and complications of radial keratotomy. Am J Ophthalmol 93:437, 1982

53. Thornton SP: Thornton guide for radial keratotomy incisions and optical zone size. J Refract Surg 1:29, 1985
54. Sanders DR, Retzlaff J, Deitz MR: Deitz-Retzlaff-Sanders (DRS) formulas: determination of radial keratotomy surgical parameters. J Refract Surg 1:75, 1985
55. Salz JJ: A consumers' guide to radial keratotomy predictive software. J Refract Surg 1:60, 1985
56. O'Day DM, Feman SS, Elliot JH: Visual impairment following radial keratotomy: a cluster of cases. Ophthalmology 93:319, 1986
57. Linberg JV, McDonald MB, Safir A, Googe JM: Ptosis following radial keratotomy. Ophthalmology 93:1509, 1986
58. Uozato H, Guyton DL: Centering corneal surgical procedures. Am J Ophthalmol 103:264, 1987
59. Uozato H, Guyton DL, Waring GO: Centering corneal surgical procedures. p. 491. In Waring GO: Refractive Keratotomy for Myopia and Astigmatism. Mosby-Year Book, St. Louis, 1992
60. Grimmett MR, Holland EJ: Complications of small clearzone radial keratotomy. Ophthalmology 103:1348, 1996
61. Thornton SP: Surgical armamentarium. p. 89. In Sanders DR, Hofmann RF (eds): Refractive Surgery: A Text of Radial Keratotomy. Slack, Thorofare, NJ, 1985
62. Waring GO: Developments in radial keratotomy. Highlights of Ophthalmology Letter 10:1, 1982.
63. Kremer FB: A new instrument for clinical pachometry. p. 201. In Schachar RA, Levy NS, Schachar L (eds): Radial Keratotomy. LAL Publishing, Denison, TX, 1980
64. Bores LD, Myers W, Cowden J: Radial keratotomy: an analysis of the American experience. Ann Ophthalmol 13:941, 1981
65. Thornton SP, Gardner SK, Waring GO: Surgical instruments used in refractive keratotomy. p. 407. In Waring GO: Refractive Keratotomy for Myopia and Astigmatism. Mosby-Year Book, St. Louis, 1992
66. Villaseñor RA, Santos VR, Cox KC, et al: Comparison of ultrasonic corneal thickness measurements before and during surgery in the Prospective Evaluation of Radial Keratotomy (PERK) study. Ophthalmology 93:327, 1986
67. Galbavy EJ: The use of diamond knives in ocular surgery. Ophthalmic Surg 15:203, 1984
68. Casebeer JC, Shapiro DR: Blade designed for improved safety and accuracy in radial keratotomy. J Cataract Refract Surg 19:314, 1993
69. Parks R, Quantock AJ, Assil KK: Comparison of the standard combined (bidirectional) radial keratotomy technique with the undercut technique in human donor eyes. J Refract Surg 12:77, 1996
70. Lewicky AO: Surgical technique and complications. p. 119. In Sanders DR, Hofmann RF (eds): Refractive Surgery: A Text of Radial Keratotomy. Slack, Thorofare, NJ, 1985
71. Binder PS: Mastel Byron radial keratotomy guide. Refract Corneal Surg 10:656, 1994
72. Krumeich JH, Daniel J, Gast R: The suction bridge for radial keratotomy may avoid late hyperopic shift. J Refract Surg 13:367, 1997
73. Villaseñor RA, Salz J, Steel D, et al: Changes in corneal thickness during radial keratotomy. Ophthalmic Surg 12:341, 1981
74. Bores LD: Historical review and clinical results of radial keratotomy. Int Ophthalmol Clin 23:93, 1983
75. Kiskis AA, Cherry PM: Effects of radial and circular keratotomy in rabbits. Can J Ophthalmol 17:161, 1982
76. Perry LD, Taylor LC: Worsening of myopia following a circular keratotomy. Ophthalmic Surg 13:104, 1982
77. Salz JJ: Keratometric results of radial keratotomy on human cadaver eyes. p. 175. In Schachar RA, Levy NS, Schachar L (eds): Refractive Modulation of the Cornea. LAL Publishing, Denison, TX, 1981
78. Lavery GW, Lindstrom RL: Clinical results of trapezoidal astigmatic keratotomy. J Refract Surg 1:70, 1985
79. Franks JB, Binder PS: Keratotomy procedures for the correction of astigmatism. J Refract Surg 1:11, 1985
80. Fenzl RE: Control of astigmatism using corneal incisions. p. 153. In Sanders DR, Hofmann RF (eds): Refractive Surgery: A Text of Radial Keratotomy. Slack, Thorofare, NJ, 1985
81. Thornton SP, Sanders DR: Graded nonintersecting transverse incisions for correction of idiopathic astigmatism. J Cataract Refract Surg 13:27, 1987
82. Neumann AC, McCarty GR, Sanders DR, Raanan MG: Refractive evaluation of astigmatic keratotomy procedures. J Cataract Refract Surg 15:25, 1989
83. Thornton SP: Astigmatic keratotomy: a review of basic concepts with case reports. J Cataract Refract Surg 16:430, 1990
84. Binder PS, Waring GO: Keratotomy for astigmatism. p. 1085. In Waring GO: Refractive Keratotomy for Myopia and Astigmatism. Mosby-Year Book, St. Louis, 1992
85. Waring GO: Atlas of astigmatic keratotomy. p. 1199. In Waring GO: Refractive Keratotomy for Myopia and Astigmatism. Mosby-Year Book, St. Louis, 1992
86. Price FW, Grene RB, Marks RG, et al: Astigmatism Reduction Clinical Trial: a multicenter progressive evaluation of the predictability of arcuate keratotomy. Evaluation of surgical nomogram predictability. ARC-T Study Group. Arch Ophthalmol 113:277, 1995
87. Waring GO, Lynn MJ, Nizam A, et al: Results of the Prospective Evaluation of Radial Keratotomy (PERK) study five years after surgery. Ophthalmology 98:1164, 1991
88. Arrowsmith PN, Marks RG: Visual, refractive and keratometric results of radial keratotomy: 5-year follow-up. Arch Ophthalmol 170:506, 1989
89. Gills JP: Trephination in combination with radial keratotomy for myopia. p. 91. In Schachar R, Levy NS, Schachar L (eds): Radial Keratotomy. LAL Publishing, Denison, TX, 1980
90. Melles GRJ, Binder PS: Effect of radial keratotomy incision direction on wound depth. Refract Corneal Surg 6:394, 1990
91. Berkeley RG, Sanders DR, Piccolo MG: Effect of incision direction on radial keratotomy outcome. J Cataract Refract Surg 17:819, 1991

92. Melles GR, Wijdh RH, Cost B, et al: Effect of blade configuration, knife action, and intraocular pressure on keratotomy incision depth and shape. Cornea 12:299, 1993
93. Updegraff SA, McDonald MB, Beuerman RW: Freeze-fracture scanning electron microscopy of radial keratotomy incisions. Am J Ophthalmol 3:399, 1994
94. Arrowsmith PN, Sanders DR, Marks RG: Visual, refractive, and keratometric results of radial keratotomy. Arch Ophthalmol 101:873, 1983
95. Flanagan GW, Binder PS: Effect of incision direction on refractive outcome after radial keratotomy. J Cataract Refract Surg 22:915, 1996
96. Gelender H, Parel JM: Vacuum fixation ring for radial keratotomy. Ophthalmic Surg 15:126, 1984
97. Cowden JW, Aguilar J, Seavy DW: Two stage radial keratotomy for the reduction of high myopia vs the suction ring. ARVO abstract. Invest Ophthalmol Vis Sci 26(suppl):202, 1985
98. Wilhelmus KR, Hamburg S: Bacterial keratitis following radial keratotomy. Cornea 2:143, 1983
99. Robin JB, Beatty RF, Dunn S, et al: *Mycobacterium chelonei* keratitis after radial keratotomy. Am J Ophthalmol 102:72, 1986
100. Beldavs RA, Al-Ghamdi S, Wilson LA, et al: Bilateral microbial keratitis after radial keratotomy. Arch Ophthalmol 111:440, 1993
101. Grimmett MR, Holland EJ, Krachmer JH: Therapeutic keratoplasty after radial keratotomy. Am J Ophthalmol 118:108, 1994
102. Leidenix MJ, Lundergan MK, Pfister D, et al: Perforated bacterial corneal ulcer in a radial keratotomy incision secondary to minor trauma. Arch Ophthalmol 112:1513, 1994
103. Leahey AB, Burkholder TO: Infectious keratitis 1 day after radial keratotomy. Arch Ophthalmol 112:1512, 1994
104. Szerenyi K, McDonnell JM, Smith RE, et al: Keratitis as a complication of bilateral, simultaneous radial keratotomy. Am J Ophthalmol 117:462, 1994
105. Lin JC, Sheu MM, Yang IJ: *Mycobacterium smegmatis* keratitis after radial keratotomy—a case report. Kao Hsiung I Hsueh Ko Hseuh Tsa Chih 10:267, 1994
106. Duffey RJ: Bilateral *Serratia marcescens* keratitis after simultaneous bilateral radial keratotomy. Am J Ophthalmol 119:233, 1995
107. Gelender H, Flynn HW, Mandelbaum SH: Bacterial endophthalmitis resulting from radial keratotomy. Am J Ophthalmol 93:323, 1982
108. Rosecan LR: Endophthalmitis and cystoid macular edema after astigmatic keratotomy. Ophthalmic Surg 25:481, 1994
109. McLeod SD, Flowers MD, Lopez PF, et al: Endophthalmitis and orbital cellulitis after radial keratotomy. Ophthalmology 102:1902, 1995
110. Epstein RL, Laurence EP: Effect of topical diclofenac sodium on discomfort after radial keratotomy. J Cataract Refract Surg 20:378, 1994
111. Gwon A, Vaughan ER, Cheetham JK, DeGryse R: Ocufen (flurbiprofen) in the treatment of ocular pain after radial keratotomy. CLAO J 20:131, 1994
112. Waring GO, Lynn MJ, Strahlman ER, et al: Stability of refraction during four years after radial keratotomy in the Prospective Evaluation of Radial Keratotomy study. Am J Ophthalmol 111:133, 1991
113. Hays JC, Rowsey JJ, Balyeat HD: Effect of post-operative steroids on the refractive result of radial keratotomy. ARVO abstract. Invest Ophthalmol Vis Sci 26(suppl):150, 1985
114. Haverbeke L: Assessing the efficacy of topical corticosteroids following radial keratotomy. Refract Corneal Surg 9:379, 1993
115. Schultz GS, Woost PG, Eiferman RA: Modification of corneal wound healing by growth factors. p. 15. In Cavanagh HD (ed): The Cornea: Transactions of the World Congress on the Cornea III. Raven Press, New York, 1988
116. Feldman ST: The effect of epidermal growth factor on corneal wound healing: practical considerations for use. Refract Corneal Surg 7:232, 1991
117. Assil KK, Quantock AJ: Wound healing in response to keratorefractive surgery. Surv Ophthalmol 38:289, 1993
118. Hull DS, Farkas S, Green K, et al: Radial keratotomy and corneal permeability in owl monkeys. Acta Ophthalmol (Copenh) 61:240, 1983
119. Steinberg EB, Wilson LA, Waring GO, et al: Stellate iron lines in the corneal epithelium after radial keratotomy. Am J Ophthalmol 98:416, 1984
120. Fyodorov SN, Sarkizova MB, Kurasova TP: Corneal biomicroscopy following repeated radial keratotomy. Ann Ophthalmol 15:403, 1983
121. Waring GO, Steinberg EB, Wilson LA: Slit-lamp microscopic appearance of corneal wound healing after radial keratotomy. Am J Ophthalmol 100:218, 1985
122. Eiferman RA, Schultz GS, Nordquist RE, Waring GO III: Corneal wound healing and its pharmacologic modification after refractive keratotomy. p. 749. In Waring GO: Refractive Keratotomy for Myopia and Astigmatism. Mosby-Year Book, St. Louis, 1992
123. Deitz MR, Sanders DR: Progressive hyperopia with long-term follow-up of radial keratotomy. Arch Ophthalmol 103:782, 1985
124. Deitz MR, Sanders DR, Raanan MG: Progressive hyperopia in radial keratotomy: long-term follow-up of diamond-knife and metal-blade series. Ophthalmology 93:1284, 1986
125. Sawelson H, Marks RG: Five-year results of radial keratotomy. Refract Corneal Surg 5:8, 1989
126. Sawelson H, Marks RG: Ten-year refractive and visual results of radial keratotomy. Ophthalmology 102:1892, 1995
127. Nordan LT, Bores L, Brint S, et al: Meaningful evaluation of refractive surgery [letter]. J Cataract Refract Surg 14:99, 1988
128. Lynn MJ, Waring GO, Carter JT: Combining refractive error and uncorrected visual acuity to assess the effectiveness of refractive corneal surgery. Refract Corneal Surg 6:103, 1990
129. Kremer FB, Marks RG: Radial keratotomy: prospective evaluation of safety and efficacy. Ophthalmic Surg 14:925, 1983

130. Hoffer KJ, Darin JJ, Pettit TH, et al: Three years' experience with radial keratotomy: the UCLA study. Ophthalmology 90:627, 1983
131. Neumann AC, Osher RH, Fenzl RE: Radial keratotomy: a comprehensive evaluation. Doc Ophthalmol 56:275, 1984
132. Salz JJ, Salz JM, Salz M, Jones D: Ten years experience with a conservative approach to radial keratotomy. Refract Corneal Surg 7:12, 1991
133. Santos VR, Waring GO, Lynn MG, et al: Relationship between refractive error and visual acuity in the Prospective Evaluation of Radial Keratotomy (PERK) study. Arch Ophthalmol 195:86, 1987
134. Ginsburg AP, Waring GO, Steinberg EB, et al: Contrast sensitivity under photopic conditions in the Prospective Evaluation of Radial Keratotomy (PERK) study. Refract Corneal Surg 6:82, 1990
135. Rabinowitz YS, Wilson SE, Klyce SD: Atlas of Corneal Topography. Igaku-Shoin, New York, 1993
136. Klyce SD, Wilson SE: Methods of analysis of corneal topography. Refract Corneal Surg 5:368, 1989
137. Rowsey JJ, Waring GO, Monlux RD, et al: Corneal topography as a predictor of refractive change in the Prospective Evaluation of Radial Keratotomy (PERK) study. Ophthalmic Surg 22:370, 1991
138. Bogan SJ, Maloney RK, Drews CD, Waring GO: Computer-assisted videokeratography of corneal topography after radial keratotomy. Arch Ophthalmol 109:834, 1991
139. Holladay JT, Waring GO: Optics and topography of radial keratotomy. p. 37. In Waring GO: Refractive Keratotomy for Myopia and Astigmatism. Mosby–Year Book, St. Louis, 1992
140. Bourque LB, Cosand BB, Drews C, et al: Reported satisfaction, fluctuation of vision, and glare among patients one year after surgery in the Prospective Evaluation of Radial Keratotomy (PERK) study. Arch Ophthalmol 104:356, 1986
141. Bourque LB, Lynn MJ, Waring GO, et al: Spectacle and contact lens wearing six years after radial keratotomy in the Prospective Evaluation of Radial Keratotomy study. Ophthalmology 101:421, 1994
142. Deitz MR, Sanders DR, Raanan MG, DeLuca M: Long-term (5- to 12-year) follow-up of metal-blade radial keratotomy procedures. Arch Ophthalmol 112:614, 1994
143. Arrowsmith PN, Marks RG: Visual, refractive, and keratometric results of radial keratotomy: one-year follow-up. Arch Ophthalmol 102:1612, 1984
144. Deitz MR, Sanders DR, Marks RG: Radial keratotomy: an overview of the Kansas City Study. Ophthalmology 91:467, 1984
145. Sawelson H, Marks RG: Two year results of radial keratotomy. Arch Ophthalmol 103:505, 1985
146. Waring GO, Lynn MJ, Gelender H, et al: Results of the Prospective Evaluation of Radial Keratotomy (PERK) study one year after radial keratotomy. Ophthalmology 92:177, 1985
147. Fyodorov SN, Agranovsky AA: Long term results of anterior radial keratotomy. J Ocular Ther Surg 1:217, 1982
148. Ellingsen KL, Nizam A, Ellingsen BA, Lynn MJ: Age-related refractive shifts in simple myopia. J Refract Surg 13:223, 1997
149. Ingraham HJ, Guber D, Green WR: Radial keratotomy: clinical pathologic case report. Arch Ophthalmol 103:683, 1985
150. Vinger PF, Mieler WF, Oestreicher JH, Easterbrook M: Ruptured globes following radial and hexagonal keratotomy. Arch Ophthalmol 114:129, 1996.
151. Hanna KD, Jouve FE: Preliminary computer simulation of radial keratotomy. p. 1031. In Waring GO: Refractive Keratotomy for Myopia and Astigmatism. Mosby–Year Book, St. Louis, 1992
152. Binder PS: What we have learned about corneal wound healing from refractive surgery. Refract Corneal Surg 5:98, 1989
153. Rashid ER, Waring GO: Complications of radial and transverse keratotomy. Surv Ophthalmol 34:73, 1989
154. Rashid ER, Waring GO: Complications of refractive keratotomy. p. 863. In Waring GO: Refractive Keratotomy for Myopia and Astigmatism. Mosby–Year Book, St. Louis, 1992
155. Laranjeira E, Buzard KA: Pilocarpine in the management of overcorrection after radial keratotomy. J Refract Surg 12:382, 1996
156. Lynn MJ, Waring GO, Nizam A, et al: Symmetry of refractive and visual acuity outcome in the Prospective Evaluation of Radial Keratotomy (PERK) study. Refract Corneal Surg 5:75, 1989
157. Schanzlin DJ, Cantillo N, Edwards MA, et al: Diurnal change in refraction, corneal curvature, visual acuity, and intraocular pressure after radial keratotomy in the PERK study. Ophthalmology 93:167, 1986
158. Santos VR, Waring GO, Lynn MJ, et al: Morning-to-evening change in refraction, corneal curvature, and visual acuity 2 to 4 years after radial keratotomy in the PERK study. Ophthalmology 95:1487, 1988
159. McDonnell PJ, Nizam A, Lynn MJ, et al: Morning-to-evening change in refraction, corneal curvature, and visual acuity 11 years after radial keratotomy in the Prospective Evaluation of Radial Keratotomy study. Ophthalmology 103:233, 1996
160. Wyzinski P, O'Dell LW: Diurnal cycle of refraction after radial keratotomy. Ophthalmology 94:120, 1987
161. Mader TH, White LJ: Refractive changes at extreme altitude after radial keratotomy. Am J Ophthalmol 119:733, 1995
162. Mader CH, Blanton CL, Gilbert BN, et al: Refractive changes during 72-hour exposure to high altitude after refractive surgery. Ophthalmology 103:1188, 1996
163. Jester JV, Villaseñor RA, Miyashiro J: Epithelial inclusions following radial keratotomy. Arch Ophthalmol 101:611, 1983
164. Davis RM, Lindstrom RL, Doughman DJ, et al: Corneal iron lines after radial keratotomy. ARVO abstract. Invest Ophthalmol Vis Sci 26(suppl):220, 1985
165. Shivitz IA, Arrowsmith PN, Russell BM: Contact lenses in the treatment of patients with overcorrected radial keratotomy. Ophthalmology 94:899, 1987

166. Astin CL: Keratoreformation by contact lenses after radial keratotomy. Ophthalmic Physiol Opt 11:156, 1991
167. Harris WF, Malan DJ, Astin CL: Keratoreformation by contact lenses after radial keratotomy: a re-analysis. Ophthalmic Physiol Opt 12:376, 1992
168. Stainer GA, Shaw EL, Binder PS, et al: Histopathology of a case of radial keratotomy. Arch Ophthalmol 100:1473, 1982
169. Salz JJ: Multiple complications following radial keratotomy in an elderly patient: a case report. Ophthalmic Surg 16:579, 1985
170. Yamaguchi T, Asbell P, Ostrick M, et al: Endothelial damage in monkeys after radial keratotomy performed with a diamond blade. Arch Ophthalmol 102:765, 1984
171. Binder PS, Stainer GA, Zavala EY, et al: Acute morphologic features of radial keratotomy. Arch Ophthalmol 101:1113, 1983
172. Yamaguchi T, Asbell P, Ostrick M, et al: Corticosteroid therapy after anterior radial keratotomy in primates. Am J Ophthalmol 97:215, 1984
173. Yamaguchi T, Kaufman H, Fukushima A, et al: Histologic and electron microscopic assessment of endothelial damage produced by anterior radial keratotomy in the monkey cornea. Am J Ophthalmol 92:313, 1981
174. Yamaguchi T, Asbell P, Ostrick M, et al: Long-term follow-up of primate eyes after anterior radial keratotomy. ARVO abstract. Invest Ophthalmol Vis Sci 26(suppl):150, 1985
175. Salz JJ: Progressive endothelial cell loss following repeat radial keratotomy—a case report. Ophthalmic Surg 13:997, 1982
176. Cross WD, Head WJ: Complications of radial keratotomy. p. 225. In Sanders DR, Hofmann RF: Refractive Surgery: A Text of Radial Keratotomy. Slack, Thorofare, NJ, 1985
177. Asbell PA, Obstbaum S, Justin N: Peripheral endothelial evaluation post radial keratotomy in PERK patients. AAO abstract. Ophthalmology 91(suppl):122, 1984
178. Rich LF, Matsuda M, MacRae S: R.K. and corneal endothelium—a morphometric analysis. ARVO abstract. Invest Ophthalmol Vis Sci 26(suppl):154, 1985
179. Lynn MJ, Geroski DH, Edelhauser HF, et al: The effect of radial keratotomy on the corneal endothelium at 10 years after surgery in the Prospective Evaluation of Radial Keratotomy (PERK) study. ARVO abstract. Invest Ophthalmol Vis Sci 37(suppl):S319, 1996
180. Binder PS: Presumed epithelial ingrowth following radial keratotomy. CLAO J 12:247, 1986
181. MacRae S, Cox W, Bedrossian R, et al: The treatment of persistent wound leak after radial keratotomy. Refract Corneal Surg 9:62, 1993
182. Stark WJ, Martin NF, Maumenee EA: Radial keratotomy II: a risky procedure of unproven long-term success. Surv Ophthalmol 28:101, 106, 1983
183. Baldone JA, Franklin RM: Cataract following radial keratotomy. Ann Ophthalmol 25:416, 1983
184. Gelender H, Gelber EC: Cataract following radial keratotomy. Arch Ophthalmol 101:1229, 1983
185. Mandelbaum S, Waring GO, Forster RK, et al: Late development of ulcerative keratitis in radial keratotomy scars. Arch Ophthalmol 104:1156, 1986
186. Shivitz IA, Arrowsmith PN: Delayed keratitis after radial keratotomy. Arch Ophthalmol 104:1153, 1986
187. Maskin SL, Alfonso E: Fungal keratitis after radial keratotomy. Am J Ophthalmol 114:369, 1992
188. Holgado S, Luna JD, Juàrez CP: Postoperative *Candida* keratitis treated successfully with fluconazole. Ophthalmic Surg 24:132, 1993
189. Gussler JR, Miller D, Jaffe M, Alfonso EC: Infection after radial keratotomy. Am J Ophthalmol 119:798, 1995
190. Larson BC, Kremer FB, Eller AW, et al: Quantitated trauma following radial keratotomy in rabbits. Ophthalmology 90:660, 1983
191. McKnight SJ, Fitz J, Giangiacomo J: Corneal rupture following radial keratotomy in cats subjected to BB gun injury. Ophthalmic Surg 19:165, 1988
192. Pinheiro MN Jr, Bryant MR, Tayyanipour R, et al: Corneal integrity after refractive surgery. Effects of radial keratotomy and mini-radial keratotomy. Ophthalmology 102:297, 1995
193. John ME, Schmitt TE: Traumatic hyphema after radial keratotomy. Ann Ophthalmol 15:930, 1983
194. Spivak L: Case report: radial keratotomy incisions remain intact despite facial trauma from plane crash. J Refract Surg 3:59, 1987
195. Casebeer JC, Shapiro DR, Phillips S: Severe ocular trauma without corneal rupture after radial keratotomy: case reports. J Refract Corneal Surg 10:31, 1994
196. Forstot SL, Damiano RE: Trauma after radial keratotomy. Ophthalmology 95:833, 1988
197. Raber JM, Arentsen JJ, Laibson PR: Traumatic wound dehiscence after penetrating keratoplasty. Arch Ophthalmol 98:1407, 1980
198. Franks S: Radial keratotomy undercorrections: a new approach. J Refract Surg 2:171, 1986
199. Charlton K: Results of two techniques of repeated radial keratotomy. p. 658. In Waring GO: Refractive Keratotomy for Myopia and Astigmatism. Mosby-Year Book, St. Louis, 1992
200. Cowden JW, Weber B: Repeat radial keratotomy in monkeys. Ophthalmology 90:251, 1983
201. Villaseñor RA, Cox KO: Radial keratotomy: reoperations. J Refract Surg 1:34, 1985
202. Cowden JW, Lynn MJ, Waring GO, et al: Repeated radial keratotomy in the Prospective Evaluation of Radial Keratotomy study. Am J Ophthalmol 103:423, 1987
203. Lyle WA, Jin J-C: Circular and interrupted suture technique for correction of hyperopia following radial keratotomy. Refract Corneal Surg 8:80, 1992
204. Damiano RE, Forstot SL, Dukes DK: Surgical correction of hyperopia following radial keratotomy. Refract Corneal Surg 8:75, 1992
205. Lindquist TD, Williams PA, Lindstrom RL: Surgical treatment of overcorrection following radial keratotomy: evaluation of clinical effectiveness. Ophthalmic Surg 22:12, 1991
206. Alió J, Ismail M: Management of radial keratotomy overcorrections by corneal sutures. J Cataract Refract Surg 19:595, 1993

207. Damiano RE, Forstot SL: Correction of radial keratotomy hyperopia [letter]. J Cataract Refract Surg 20:364, 1994
208. Lyle WA, Jin GJC: Long term stability of refraction after intrastromal suture correction of hyperopia following radial keratotomy. J Refract Surg 11:485, 1995
209. Swinger CA, Barker BA: Myopic keratomileusis following radial keratotomy. J Refract Surg 1:53, 1985
210. Nordan LT, Havins WE: Undercorrected radial keratotomy treated with myopic keratomileusis. J Refract Surg 1:56, 1985
211. Polit F, Anwar M, Tabbara K, et al: Subepithelial reticular cicatrization following radial keratotomy in a patient with inactive trachoma. Refract Corneal Surg 8:240, 1992
212. Keates RH, Watson SA, Levy SN: Epikeratophakia following previous refractive keratoplasty surgery: two case reports. J Cataract Refract Surg 12:536, 1986
213. Binder PS, Charlton KH: Surgical procedures performed after refractive surgery. Refract Corneal Surg 8:61, 1992
214. McDonnell PJ, Garbus JJ, Salz JJ: Excimer laser myopic photorefractive keratectomy after undercorrected radial keratotomy. Refract Corneal Surg 7:146, 1991
215. Seiler T, Jean B: Photorefractive keratectomy as a second attempt to correct myopia after radial keratotomy. Refract Corneal Surg 8:211, 1992
216. Georgaras SP, Neos G, Margetis SP, et al: Correction of myopic anisometropia with photorefractive keratectomy in 15 eyes. Refract Corneal Surg 9(suppl):S29, 1993
217. Hahn TW, Kim JH, Lee YC: Excimer laser photorefractive keratectomy to correct residual myopia after radial keratotomy. Refract Corneal Surg 9(suppl):S25, 1993
218. Frangie JP, Park SB, Kim J, et al: Excimer laser keratectomy after radial keratotomy. Am J Ophthalmol 115:634, 1993
219. Durrie DS, Schumer DJ, Cavanaugh TB: Photorefractive keratectomy for residual myopia after previous refractive keratotomy. J Refract Corneal Surg 10(suppl):S235, 1994
220. Maloney RK, Steinert RF, Hersh PS, et al: A multi-center trial of photorefractive keratectomy for residual myopia following previous ocular surgery. AAO abstract. Ophthalmology 101(suppl):74, 1994
221. Maloney RK, Chan W-K, Steinert R, et al: A multicenter trial of photorefractive keratectomy for residual myopia after previous ocular surgery. Ophthalmology 102:1042, 1995
222. Meza J, Perez-Santonja JJ, Moreno E, et al: Photorefractive keratectomy after radial keratotomy. J Cataract Refract Surg 20:485, 1994
223. Ribeiro JC, McDonald MB, Klyce SD: Photorefractive keratectomy after radial keratotomy in a patient with severe myopia. Am J Ophthalmol 118:106, 1994
224. Nordan LT, Binder PS, Kassar BS, et al: Photorefractive keratectomy to treat myopia and astigmatism after radial keratotomy and penetrating keratoplasty. J Cataract Refract Surg 21:268, 1995
225. Ribeiro JC, McDonald MB, Lemos MM, et al: Excimer laser photorefractive keratectomy after radial keratotomy: a multicenter study. J Refract Surg 11:165, 1995
226. Lee YC, Park CK, Sah WJ, et al: Photorefractive keratectomy for undercorrected myopia after radial keratotomy: two-year follow up. J Refract Surg 11(suppl):S274, 1995
227. Bokobza Y, Ancel JM, Aron JJ: Resultats du traitement des sous-corrections de keratotomie radiaire au laser excimer. J Fr Ophtalmol 18:455, 1995
228. Kwitko ML, Gow JA, Bellavance F, et al: Excimer photorefractive keratectomy after undercorrected radial keratotomy. J Refract Surg 11(suppl):S280, 1995
229. Markovits AS: Extracapsular cataract extraction with posterior chamber intraocular lens implantation in a postradial keratotomy patient. Arch Ophthalmol 104:329, 1986
230. Koch DD, Liu JF, Hyde LL, et al: Refractive complications of cataract surgery after radial keratotomy. Am J Ophthalmol 108:676, 1989
231. Hoffer KJ: Intraocular lens power calculation for eyes after refractive keratotomy. J Refract Surg 11:490, 1995
232. Celikkol L, Pavlopoulos G, Weinstein B, et al: Calculation of intraocular lens power after radial keratotomy with computerized videokeratography. Am J Ophthalmol 120:739, 1995
233. Deg JK, Zavala EY, Binder PS: Delayed corneal wound healing following radial keratotomy. Ophthalmology 92:734, 1985
234. Karr DJ, Grutzmacher RD, Reeh MJ: Radial keratotomy complicated by sterile keratitis and corneal perforation. Histopathologic case report and review of complications. Ophthalmology 92:1244, 1985
235. Hersh PS, Kalevar V, Kenyon KR: Penetrating keratoplasty for severe complications of radial keratotomy. Cornea 10:170, 1991
236. Jester JV, Villaseñor RA, Schanzlin DJ, et al: Variations in corneal wound healing after radial keratotomy: possible insights into mechanisms of clinical complications and refractive effects. Cornea 11:191, 1992
237. McNeill JI: Corneal incision dehiscence during penetrating keratoplasty nine years after radial keratotomy. J Cataract Refract Surg 19:542, 1993
238. Parmley V, Ng J, Gee B, et al: Penetrating keratoplasty after radial keratotomy: a report of six cases. Ophthalmology 102:947, 1995
239. McNeill JI, Wilkins DL: A purse-string suture for penetrating keratoplasty following radial keratotomy. Refract Corneal Surg 7:392, 1991
240. Maxwell WA: Myopic keratomileusis: initial results and myopic keratomileusis combined with other procedures. J Cataract Refract Surg 13:518, 1987
241. Casebeer JC, Shapiro DR: Radial keratotomy in intact epikeratoplasty graft. Refract Corneal Surg 9:133, 1993
242. Shapiro MB, Harrison DA: Radial keratotomy for intolerable myopia after penetrating keratoplasty. Am J Ophthalmol 115:327, 1993
243. Gothard TW, Agapitos PJ, Bowers RA, et al: Four incision radial keratotomy for high myopia after penetrating keratoplasty. Refract Corneal Surg 9:51, 1993

38

Astigmatic Keratotomy

David R. Hardten, Y. Ralph Chu, and Richard L. Lindstrom

Astigmatism, like myopia or hyperopia, can decrease visual acuity. Astigmatism is more complex, however, because it has both magnitude and orientation. Thus, it is more difficult to correct with spectacles, contact lenses, or surgery than are spherical refractive errors. The surgical correction of astigmatism was first attempted with astigmatic keratotomy, which is described in this chapter, along with compression sutures and wedge resection. More recently, excimer laser photoastigmatic refractive keratectomy, also called *PARK*, has been used to correct astigmatism (see Ch. 42).

HISTORY OF THE SURGICAL CORRECTION OF ASTIGMATISM

Astigmatic keratotomy appears to have been the first refractive corneal surgical procedure performed by ophthalmologists. In 1885, Schiøtz, a Norwegian ophthalmologist, described a patient who developed 19.50 diopters of astigmatism after cataract surgery.[1] Four months after the cataract surgery, he used a von Graefe knife to make a 3.5-mm penetrating incision at the limbus in the steep meridian, which reduced the astigmatism to 7.00 diopters. Faber, a Dutch ophthalmologist, performed perforating anterior transverse incisions in a 19-year-old patient with 1.50 diopters of idiopathic astigmatism, which reduced the astigmatism to 0.75 diopter and allowed the patient to pursue a career in the Royal Military Academy.[2] Lucciola, of Turin, Italy, was the first ophthalmologist to use nonperforating corneal incisions to correct astigmatism.[3] In 1894, Bates, of New York City, described six patients who developed flattening of the cornea in the meridian that intersected a surgical or traumatic scar.[4] He postulated that corneal incisions made at right angles to the steep meridian might be used to correct astigmatism.

Lans, another Dutch ophthalmologist, performed one of the first systematic studies of refractive surgery while at the University of Leiden in 1896.[5] His doctoral thesis described carefully planned experimentation in rabbits designed to evaluate various patterns of keratotomy, keratectomy, and thermokeratoplasty. These studies defined some basic principles of astigmatic keratotomy. Lans showed that flattening in the meridian perpendicular to a transverse incision is associated with steepening in the orthogonal meridian. He also demonstrated that deeper and longer incisions have a greater effect.

In the 1940s and 1950s, Sato, of Tokyo, Japan, investigated both radial and astigmatic keratotomy.[6–9] He used tangential posterior corneal incisions to decrease astigmatism in 15 eyes an average of 2.50 diopters and also reduced astigmatism an average of 4.20 diopters in 18 eyes with perforating tangential incisions near the limbus.

In the 1970s, a number of surgeons in the former Soviet Union investigated the use of corneal incisions for the correction of myopia and astigmatism. The first major publication in English was by Fyodorov[10] in 1981, in which he discussed the correction of myopic astigmatism using several nonperforating anterior keratotomy patterns.

PRINCIPLES OF ASTIGMATIC KERATOTOMY

The current understanding of astigmatic keratotomy has been developed by many investigators, with the cadaver eye model playing an important role in the evaluation of qualitative and quantitative results.[11–17] Several patterns of corneal incisions have emerged for the correction of astigmatism, including straight transverse incisions, arcuate incisions, and semiradial incisions. There are certain principles of astigmatic keratotomy that apply to all incisional patterns.[18]

Astigmatic keratotomy incisions are placed in the steep meridian, which is the meridian parallel to the axis of plus cylinder and the meridian with the greatest dioptric power. Coupling refers to the relationship between the changes in corneal curvature in the incised meridian and in the unincised meridian 90 degrees away. The coupling ratio, or flattening/steepening ratio, is the amount of flattening in the steep meridian caused by an incision divided by the amount of steepening in the unincised meridian 90 degrees away. When the amount of flattening and steepening are the same, the coupling ratio is 1 and there is no change in the spherical equivalent. The coupling ratio depends on the location, length, and depth of an incision.

Transverse or arcuate incisions have a greater effect when they are closer to the center of the entrance pupil. Most astigmatic keratotomy incisions are placed somewhere between a 5-mm- and an 8-mm-diameter optical zone. Incisions placed more centrally are contraindicated because they can produce irregular astigmatism and glare; incisions placed more peripherally have little effect. Most of the effect of transverse or arcuate incisions is achieved with the first pair of symmetrical incisions (i.e., two incisions that straddle the steep meridian and are 180 degrees from one another). An additional pair of incisions increases the effect 25 to 33 percent. No significant additional effect is achieved by making more than two pairs of incisions. Multiple incisions also increase the instability of the cornea and can result in fluctuation of vision.

Semiradial incisions induce overall corneal flattening at the same time they reduce astigmatism. In general, paired semiradial incisions flatten both the meridian in which they are made and the meridian 90 degrees away, in a ratio of 2:1. Varying the diameter of the optical clear zone affects the degree of myopic correction as well as the degree of astigmatic correction.

Transverse or arcuate incisions should not intersect radial or semiradial incisions. The intersection of two incisions heals poorly and often leads to epithelial inclusion cysts and exaggerated scar formation.[18–20]

PATIENT SELECTION

Astigmatism greater than 1.00 diopter generally requires some form of optical correction for good visual acuity. An astigmatic refractive error of 1.00 to 2.00 diopters reduces uncorrected visual acuity to 20/30 to 20/50, and 2.00 to 3.00 diopters reduces it to 20/70 to 20/100.[21]

Naturally occurring (idiopathic) astigmatism is common. Clinically detectable refractive astigmatism is present in as many as 95 percent of eyes. The incidence of clinically significant astigmatism has been reported to be between 7.5 and 75 percent, depending on the specific study and the definition of clinically significant astigmatism used.[22,23] Approximately 44 percent of the population has more than 0.50 diopter of astigmatism, 10 percent more than 1.00 diopter, and 8 percent 1.50 diopters or more.[22]

Visually significant astigmatism is common after various kinds of ophthalmic surgery, including cataract extraction, lamellar or penetrating keratoplasty, and trabeculectomy. Astigmatism greater than 1.00 diopter occurs often after extracapsular cataract extraction; astigmatism greater than 3.00 diopters is present in as many as 20 percent of cases.[24] High astigmatism after penetrating keratoplasty is even more common. Troutman and Swinger[25] estimated that nearly 10 percent of all clear corneal grafts are complicated by high astigmatism.

Age is an important criterion in screening patients for astigmatic keratotomy. Progression of myopia is greatest during the first and second decades of life; therefore, patients younger than 21 years may not have a stable refraction. Small-diameter optical zones and a larger number of incisions may be required in younger patients, thus increasing the risk of side effects, such as instability of the refractive outcome and fluctuation of vision.

PREOPERATIVE EVALUATION

Careful manifest refraction, keratometry, and videokeratography are performed preoperatively. Patients considering surgical correction of astigmatism must have a stable refraction confirmed by comparison of the preoperative refraction with previous refractions. In most cases, the refractive, keratometric, and topographic cylinder power and axis are similar. In cases of significant disparity, re-measurement and re-evaluation are recommended. Refractive astigmatism may consist of several components, including corneal astigmatism and lenticular astigmatism. Keratometry and videokeratography are better measures of true corneal astigmatism than is refraction. Surgery for naturally occurring and postcataract astigmatism is typically based on the refractive cylinder and axis. For postkeratoplasty astigmatism, keratometric and videokeratographic analysis are generally used in conjunction with the refractive cylinder and axis, because nonorthogonal astigmatism is common in these patients. Videokeratography helps identify patients who would be poor surgical candidates for astigmatic keratotomy because

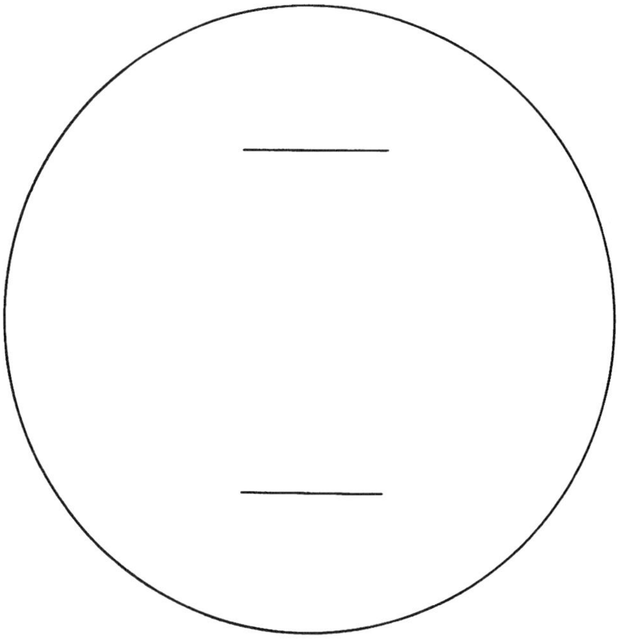

FIGURE 38-1 Transverse incisions.

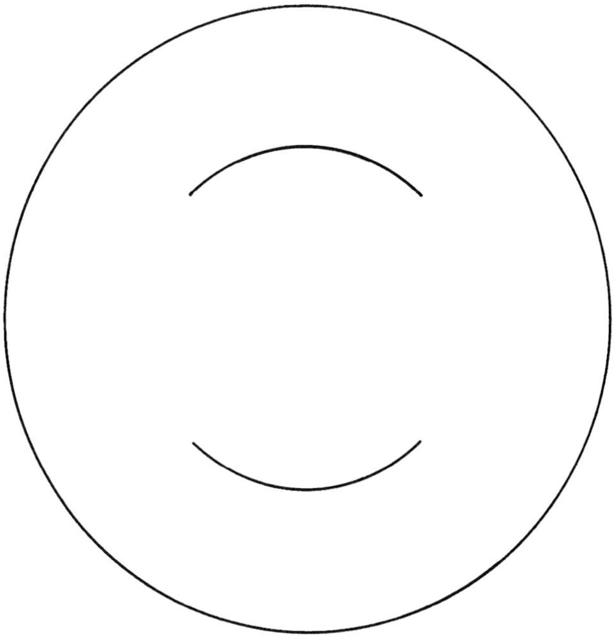

FIGURE 38-2 Arcuate incisions.

of irregular astigmatism, keratoconus, or other corneal abnormalities.

PATIENT PREPARATION

A mild sedative, such as diazepam, is given if needed. No other preoperative medications are required for astigmatic keratotomy. Topical pilocarpine is not recommended because it can skew the position of the pupil and make localization of the center of the true entrance pupil inaccurate.

Some surgeons like to identify the steep meridian preoperatively by placing a drop of topical anesthetic on the eye, having the patient fixate on a distant object, and using a surgical marking pen to mark the limbus in the steep meridian.

The eyelids are prepped with 5 percent povidone-iodine solution. A drape is placed, with care taken to keep the eyelashes out of the way, and an eyelid speculum is inserted. The eye is centered under the operating microscope and is positioned such that the iris plane is perpendicular to the path of the microscope light.

ANESTHESIA

Topical anesthesia is usually sufficient for astigmatic keratotomy. One drop of 0.5 percent proparacaine or tetracaine is applied every 5 minutes for three applications. Peribulbar or retrobulbar anesthesia is usually not necessary and prevents patient fixation, which is useful in proper placement of the incisions. This type of anesthesia is often helpful for wedge resections, however, because the dissection and placement of multiple sutures require good akinesia.

SURGICAL TECHNIQUES

Naturally Occurring Astigmatism

Transverse or Arcuate Incisions

Transverse or arcuate incisions are placed coincident with an optical zone 5 to 8 mm in diameter (Figures 38-1 and 38-2). Incisions placed coincident with a 5-mm optical zone achieve the greatest effect. Incisions should not be placed more centrally because of the risk of encroaching on the visual axis and producing glare. Typically, incisions are placed at a 6- or 7-mm optical zone. Younger patients achieve less effect from a given incision than older patients; therefore, nomograms must be adjusted according to the patient's age. The expected result is decreased by 2 percent per year for patients younger than 30 years and increased by 2 percent per year for patients older than 30 years.

Transverse incisions that are 2 to 5 mm in length (the most commonly used length of transverse incisions) have a coupling ratio of 1 and flatten the steep meridian the same amount as they steepen the flat meridian; therefore, the net effect is no change in the spherical equivalent. Arcuate incisions less than 30 degrees have a coupling ratio greater than 1, those between 30 and 90 degrees (the most commonly used length of arcuate incisions) have a coupling ratio of 1, and those greater than 90 degrees have a coupling ratio less than 1. Arcuate incisions greater than 90 degrees are not recommended because of the risk of late wound dehiscence.

The patient fixates on the operating microscope light or on a fixation light mounted on the microscope. If not done preoperatively, the steep meridian is marked with a surgical marking pen using preoperative landmarks, intraoperative keratometry or keratoscopy, preoperative or intraoperative videokeratography, or a circular protractor that indicates the location of meridians on the surface of the cornea.

If transverse incisions are selected, the area of cornea to be incised can be marked by centering an optical zone marker of the appropriate diameter on the center of the entrance pupil and pressing it on the corneal epithelium. A smaller optical zone marker with a diameter equal to the length of the intended incisions can be inked with gentian violet and placed over the previously made indentation in the corneal epithelium in the steep meridian to delineate the incision length. Alternatively, a transverse marker that has two parallel blades of the appropriate length that are separated by the appropriate distance (5 to 8 mm) can be used if available.

If arcuate incisions are chosen, an optical zone marker of the appropriate diameter is used to outline the optical zone, as described above. We prefer arcuate incisions with an optical zone diameter of 6, 7, or 8 mm for almost all cases. The nomograms for arcuate keratotomy are given in Tables 38-1, 38-2, and 38-3. Nomograms are surgeon dependent, however, and should be adjusted based on individual experience and outcome analysis. A radial marker inked with gentian violet is used to delineate the arc to be incised. A 12-cut marker is used to delineate an arc of 30 degrees, an 8-cut marker is used to delineate an arc of 45 degrees, a 6- or 12-cut marker is used to delineate an arc of 60 degrees, and a 4- or 8-cut marker is used to delineate an arc of 90 degrees. Special arcuate keratotomy markers are available that imprint both the desired optical zone and a graduated scale for the degrees of arc.

The corneal thickness at the optical zone mark in the steep meridian is measured on both sides of the cornea with an intraoperative ultrasonic pachymeter. The blade of a diamond knife is set to 100 percent of the thinnest measurement and is calibrated with a microscope and micrometer stage.

The patient is asked to fixate on the operating microscope light or the fixation light. The blade is inserted into the cornea and, after a pause of a second or two, is slowly and steadily drawn through the cornea. A blade with a vertically oriented cutting edge allows the surgeon good visibility while the incision is being made. A square blade

TABLE 38-1
Nomogram for Arcuate Keratotomy at a 6-mm Optical Zone[a]

	Surgical Option (number and arc length of incisions)					
Patient's Age (yr)	1 × 30 degrees	2 × 30 degrees 1 × 45 degrees	1 × 60 degrees	2 × 45 degrees 1 × 90 degrees	2 × 60 degrees	2 × 90 degrees
20	0.60	1.20	1.80	2.40	3.60	4.80
25	0.68	1.35	2.03	2.70	4.05	5.40
30	0.75	1.50	2.25	3.00	4.50	6.00
35	0.83	1.65	2.48	3.30	4.95	6.60
40	0.90	1.80	2.70	3.60	5.40	7.20
45	0.98	1.95	2.93	3.90	5.85	7.80
50	1.05	2.10	3.15	4.20	6.30	8.40
55	1.13	2.25	3.38	4.50	6.75	9.00
60	1.20	2.40	3.60	4.80	7.20	9.60
65	1.28	2.55	3.83	5.10	7.65	10.20
70	1.35	2.70	4.05	5.40	8.10	10.80
75	1.43	2.85	4.28	5.70	8.55	11.40

[a] To use the table, find the patient's age and then move to the right to find result closest to refractive cylinder without going over. Read up to find the recommended number and arc length of incisions.

TABLE 38-2
Nomogram for Arcuate Keratotomy at a 7-mm Optical Zone[a]

Patient's Age (yr)	Surgical Option (number and arc length of incisions)					
	1 × 30 degrees	2 × 30 degrees 1 × 45 degrees	1 × 60 degrees	2 × 45 degrees 1 × 90 degrees	2 × 60 degrees	2 × 90 degrees
20	0.40	0.80	1.20	1.60	2.40	3.20
25	0.45	0.90	1.35	1.80	2.70	3.60
30	0.50	1.00	1.50	2.00	3.00	4.00
35	0.55	1.10	1.65	2.20	3.30	4.40
40	0.60	1.20	1.80	2.40	3.60	4.80
45	0.65	1.30	1.95	2.60	3.90	5.20
50	0.70	1.40	2.10	2.80	4.20	5.60
55	0.75	1.50	2.25	3.00	4.50	6.00
60	0.80	1.60	2.40	3.20	4.80	6.40
65	0.85	1.70	2.55	3.40	5.10	6.80
70	0.90	1.80	2.70	3.60	5.40	7.20
75	0.95	1.90	2.85	3.80	5.70	7.60

[a] To use the table, find the patient's age and then move to the right to find result closest to refractive cylinder without going over. Read up to find the recommended number and arc length of incisions.

TABLE 38-3
Nomogram for Arcuate Keratotomy at an 8-mm Optical Zone[a]

Patient's Age (yr)	Surgical Option (number and arc length of incisions)					
	1 × 30 degrees	2 × 30 degrees 1 × 45 degrees	1 × 60 degrees	2 × 45 degrees 1 × 90 degrees	2 × 60 degrees	2 × 90 degrees
20	0.20	0.40	0.60	0.80	1.20	1.60
25	0.23	0.45	0.68	0.90	1.35	1.80
30	0.25	0.50	0.75	1.00	1.50	2.00
35	0.28	0.55	0.83	1.10	1.65	2.20
40	0.30	0.60	0.90	1.20	1.80	2.40
45	0.33	0.65	0.98	1.30	1.95	2.60
50	0.35	0.70	1.05	1.40	2.10	2.80
55	0.38	0.75	1.13	1.50	2.25	3.00
60	0.40	0.80	1.20	1.60	2.40	3.20
65	0.43	0.85	1.28	1.70	2.55	3.40
70	0.45	0.90	1.35	1.80	2.70	3.60
75	0.48	0.95	1.43	1.90	2.85	3.80

[a] To use the table, find the patient's age and then move to the right to find result closest to refractive cylinder without going over. Read up to find the recommended number and arc length of incisions.

may track a more stable course through corneal tissue than an angled blade.

One drop each of topical antibiotic solution, corticosteroid, and a nonsteroidal anti-inflammatory drug are applied to the eye. The eye is not routinely patched nor is cycloplegia necessary. The patient is seen 1 day, 1 week, and 1 month postoperatively. Topical antibiotics and corticosteroids are used four times a day for 1 to 2 weeks or until the incisions have re-epithelialized.

The 1-month postoperative result correlates well statistically with the 1-year result. However, additional surgery for undercorrection or overcorrection should not be considered until the refraction and keratometric measurements are stable. If significant undercorrection is noted on the first postoperative day, topical corticosteroids are used four times a day for 1 to 3 months in an attempt to delay wound healing and increase incision gape. Incisions may be reopened and deepened and/or extended if sig-

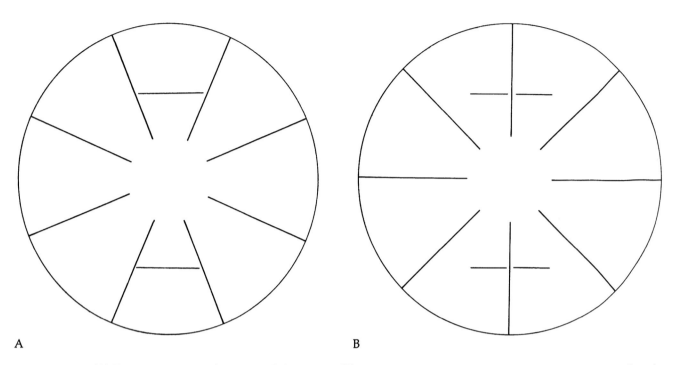

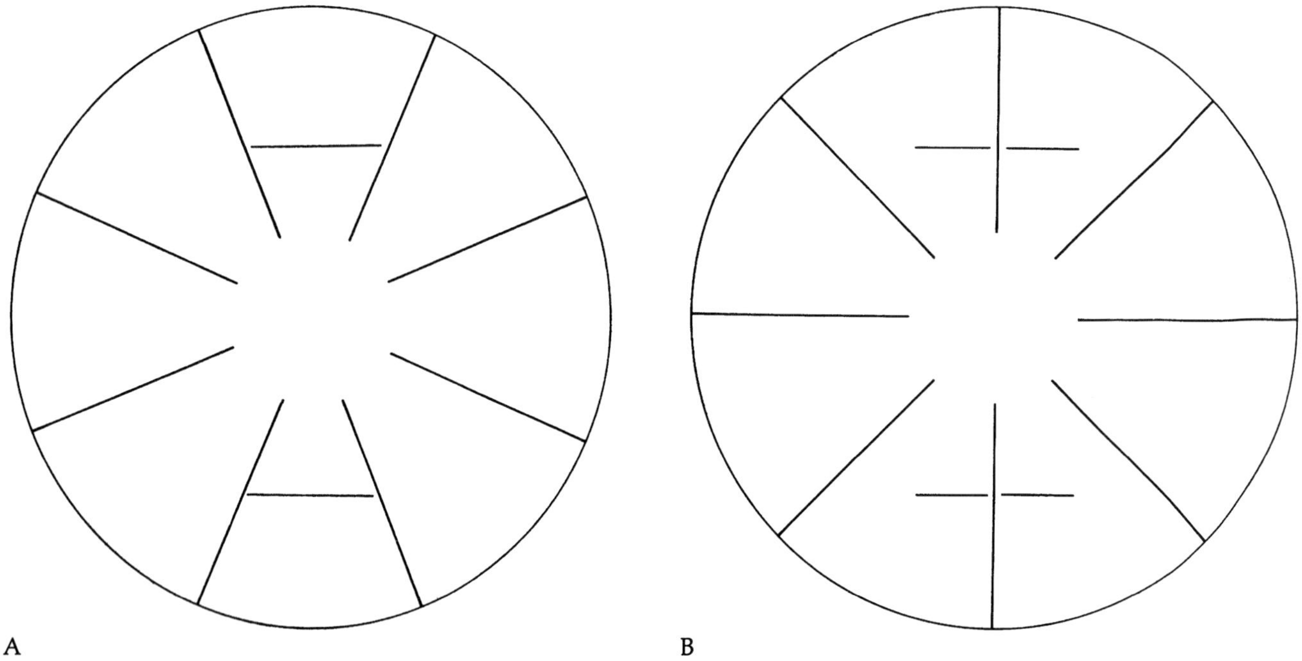

FIGURE 38-3 **(A)** Transverse incisions between radial incisions. **(B)** Transverse incisions straddling radial incisions. Note that the incisions do not intersect.

nificant undercorrection persists after 1 month. In patients with significant overcorrection, topical hypertonic drops, such as 5 percent sodium chloride four times a day for 1 to 3 months, may be useful. If hypertonic agents are not helpful, the incisions may be reopened, irrigated to remove any debris, including epithelial cells, that may be causing the incisions to gape, and sutured with interrupted 11-0 polyester sutures.

Transverse Incisions Combined with Radial Keratotomy Incisions

When transverse incisions are placed in conjunction with radial keratotomy incisions, they may be placed between or straddle the radial incisions (Figure 38-3). Intersecting transverse and radial or semiradial incisions should be avoided because of wound instability and healing problems. Four-incision radial keratotomy cases, if properly planned, allow for placement of transverse incisions in the steep meridian between the radial incisions. In eight-incision radial keratotomy cases, the transverse incisions may either straddle or be placed between the radial incisions. In mini-radial keratotomy, the radial incisions may simply stop short of the transverse incisions. Transverse incisions coupled with radial keratotomy incisions give a substantially greater effect than transverse incisions alone.

Semiradial Incisions

Semiradial incisions are paired incisions usually made from a 3-mm optical zone toward two points that straddle the steep meridian and are separated by 5.5 mm at the limbus (Figure 38-4). These incisions flatten both the meridian in which they are made and the meridian 90 degrees away, in a ratio of 2:1. Therefore, semiradial incisions alone can correct moderate amounts of myopia while also correcting modest amounts of astigmatism. In cadaver eyes, semiradial incisions extending from a 3-mm optical zone corrected 1.4 diopters of astigmatism and 3.9 diopters of myopia, and semiradial incisions extending from a 5-mm optical zone corrected 2.25 diopters of astigmatism and 1.6 diopters of myopia.[15] The effect of refractive keratotomy in cadaver eyes has been shown to be equivalent to the effect achieved in an 80-year-old patient. Thus, the same changes seen in cadaver eyes can be expected in an 80-year-old patient, and roughly 50 percent of this correction can be expected in a 30-year-old patient.

Asymmetrical Radial Incisions

The principles of asymmetrical radial incisions are similar to those of semiradial incisions. By placing the incisions closer together, more flattening is achieved in the steep meridian. When four incisions are used, they are placed 60 degrees apart in the steep meridian rather than symmetrically 90 degrees apart as would be done in a patient with no astigmatism (Figure 38-5A). When six incisions are used, they are grouped together in the steep meridian 45 degrees apart (Figure 38-5B). These incisions reduce both the amount of myopia and the amount of astigmatism by causing greater flattening in the meridian of the incisions than in the meridian 90 degrees away.

Trapezoidal Keratotomy

Semiradial incisions combined with transverse incisions describe the trapezoidal keratotomy procedure popularized by Ruiz.[15] The initial description of this procedure included two sets of semiradial incisions and five pairs of equally spaced transverse incisions (Figure 38-6A). Several studies have shown that the maximum astigmatic correction from trapezoidal keratotomy is obtained with a single pair of transverse incisions placed 5 mm apart between two sets of semiradial incisions extending from a 3-mm optical zone (Figure 38-6B). The multiple pairs of transverse incisions initially described by Ruiz are unnecessary.[14,15,19]

In a clinical study of 64 eyes with naturally occurring astigmatism, Ibrahim et al[26] showed that trapezoidal keratotomy corrects about 5.5 diopters of astigmatism in a 30-year-old patient and up to 11 diopters in an 80-year-old patient. Only 56 percent of the eyes achieved between 80 and 120 percent of the intended correction, and 90 percent achieved between 60 and 150 percent of the intended

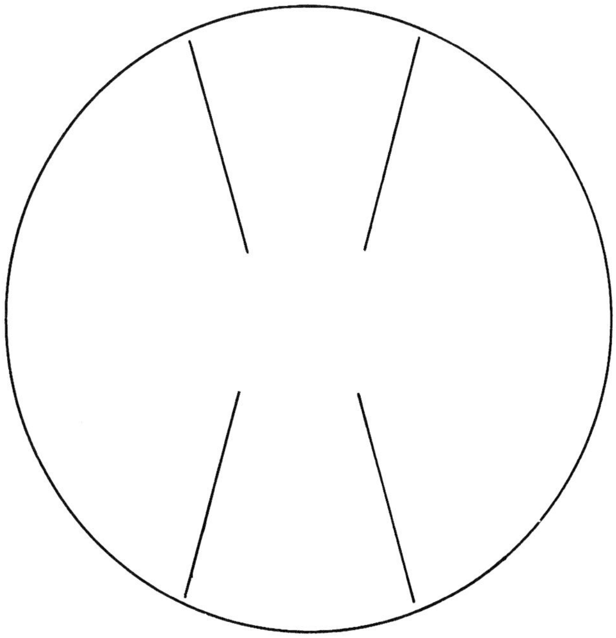

FIGURE 38-4 Semiradial incisions.

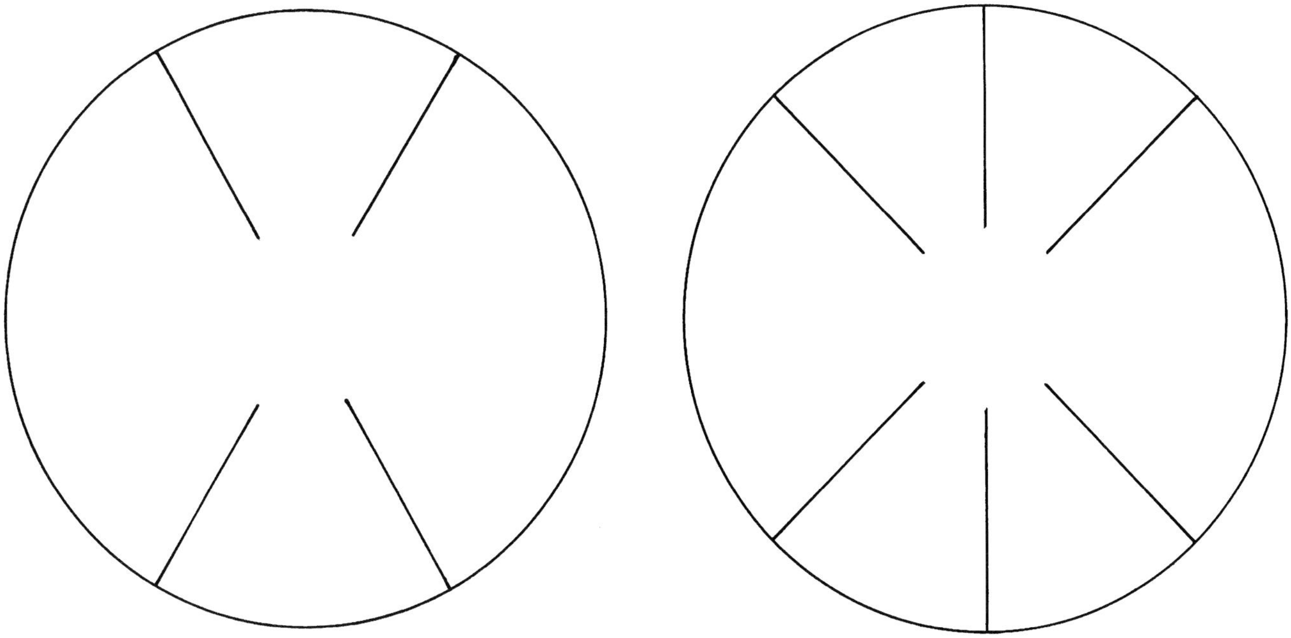

A B

FIGURE 38-5 **(A)** Four radial incisions grouped in the steep meridian. **(B)** Six radial incisions grouped in the steep meridian.

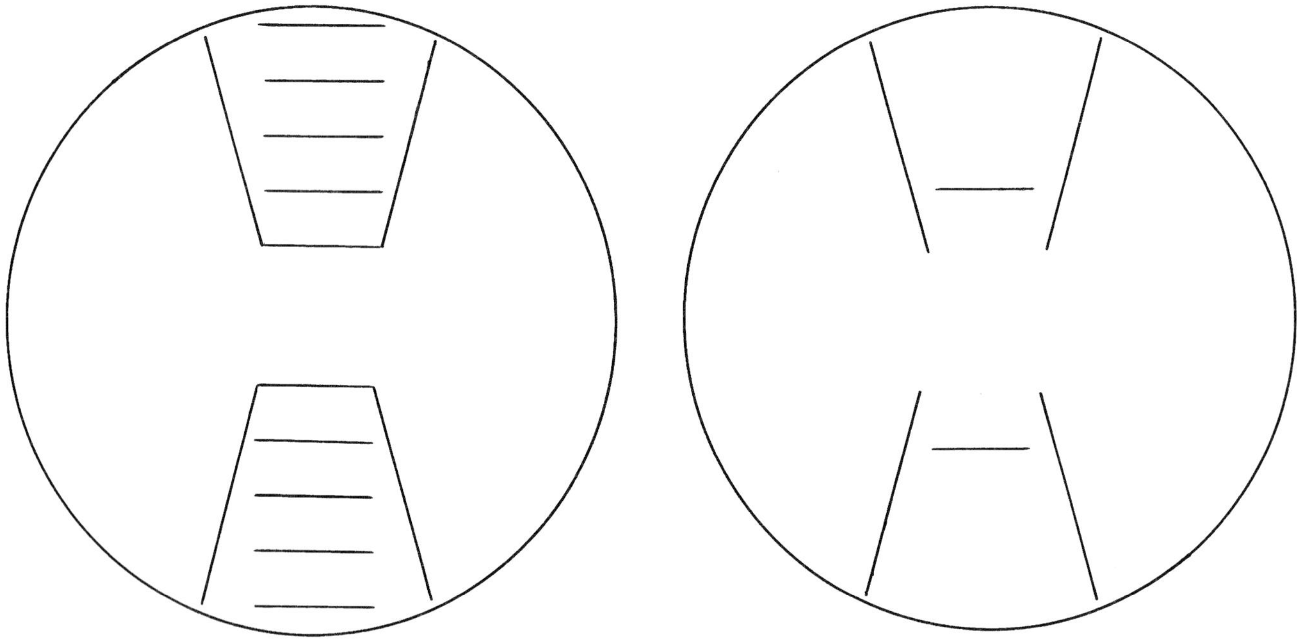

FIGURE 38-6 **(A)** Original trapezoidal keratotomy pattern consisting of five pairs of transverse incisions and two pairs of semiradial incisions. The central transverse incisions connected with the semiradial incisions, which caused problems with healing. **(B)** Trapezoidal keratotomy pattern consisting of one pair of transverse and two pairs of semiradial incisions.

correction, which indicates only fair predictability. Trapezoidal keratotomy is rarely used today.

Postcataract Astigmatism

There is a difference of opinion whether astigmatism caused by wound dehiscence after cataract extraction should be managed surgically by revising the wound or by astigmatic keratotomy. If the wound dehiscence is a structural threat to the eye, wound revision is recommended. If the globe is structurally intact, refractive rehabilitation with reduction of astigmatic anisometropia becomes most important, and astigmatic keratotomy or photoastigmatic refractive keratectomy may be appropriate. The spherical equivalent should be taken into account when considering these procedures; astigmatic keratotomy incisions, unless extremely short or long, are typically neutral as far as the spherical equivalent is concerned, whereas photoastigmatic refractive keratectomy typically induces some hyperopic shift in the refractive error (see Ch. 42).

Postkeratoplasty Astigmatism

Postkeratoplasty astigmatism often necessitates surgical correction because of intolerance to glasses or contact lenses. The surgical correction can be difficult because astigmatism can be irregular and nonorthogonal. Although an ideal goal is to correct all of the astigmatism, a more realistic goal is to reduce the amount of astigmatism so that spectacles or contact lenses can be worn comfortably.

Before any surgical procedures for the correction of postkeratoplasty astigmatism are considered, all sutures should be removed because they can be the cause of the astigmatism. Also, the keratoplasty wound should be inspected for focal abnormalities. Wound dehiscence and graft override cause flattening of the central cornea in that meridian and should be corrected by opening and resuturing the wound in that area (see Ch. 35).

Incisional techniques available for the correction of postkeratoplasty astigmatism include relaxing incisions with or without the use of compression sutures.[25,27–32] Wedge resections can be used for large amounts of astigmatism. Techniques that involve the excimer laser include photoastigmatic refractive keratectomy (see Ch. 42) and laser-assisted in situ keratomileusis (see Ch. 43).

Relaxing Incisions

A cadaver study of the effect of relaxing incisions on corneal topography demonstrated a wide range of effect on corneal astigmatism, ranging from 0.58 diopter of astig-

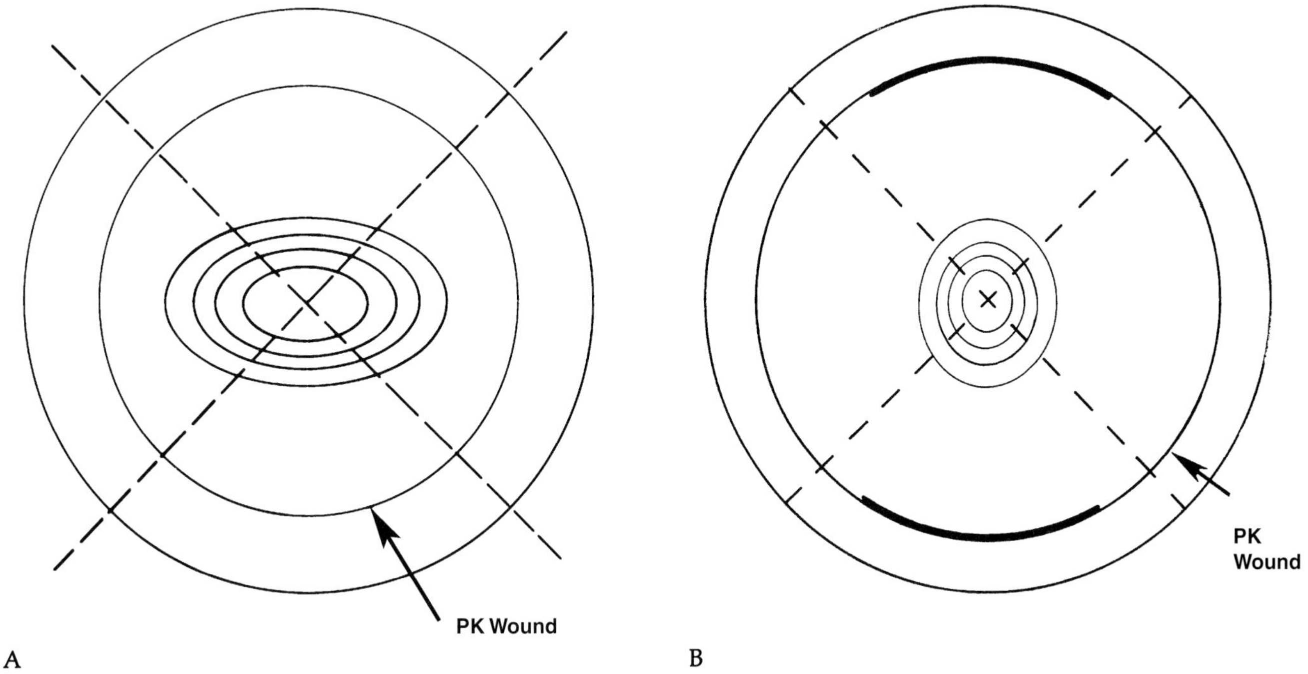

FIGURE 38-7 Arcuate relaxing incisions for symmetrical postkeratoplasty astigmatism. **(A)** Horizontally oval keratoscope mires demonstrate symmetrical steepening in the vertical meridian. **(B)** Two arcuate relaxing incisions made in the penetrating keratoplasty (*PK*) wound straddling the steep meridian result in a reversal of the keratoscope mires.

matic change for a 1-clock-hour incision to 5.93 diopters of change for a 3-clock-hour incision.[32] Two symmetrical relaxing incisions placed 180 degrees apart produced 0.78 diopter of astigmatic change for 1-clock-hour incisions, 4.64 diopters of change for 2-clock-hour incisions, and 13.97 diopters of change for 3-clock-hour incisions. The marked difference between the amount of change for the 2- and 3-clock-hour symmetrical incisions in eye bank eyes indicates a narrow therapeutic zone for relaxing incisions. Clinically, relaxing incisions can result in marked undercorrections and overcorrections when used to treat postkeratoplasty astigmatism. Relaxing incisions effectively flatten the steep meridian and steepen the flat meridian an equal amount. The change in spherical equivalent is therefore negligible.

Relaxing incisions may be made in the keratoplasty wound or 0.5 to 1 mm central to the wound. Although incisions made in the wound often result in wound dehiscence and large changes in astigmatism, they are still commonly used. The technique for relaxing incisions involves dissection of the wound with a stainless steel blade, which is easier to control than a diamond blade. Care is taken because the wound is usually irregular and of variable thickness, and incisions of adequate depth are often difficult to achieve without perforation.

Preoperative measurements of refractive and keratometric astigmatism, videokeratography, and marking of the steep meridian are critical to accurate placement of relaxing incisions. The number of incisions depends on the symmetry of the astigmatism. If the astigmatism is symmetrical, two incisions are made straddling the steep meridian 180 degrees apart (Figure 38-7). If the astigmatism is asymmetrical, one incision is made straddling the steep meridian (Figure 38-8). Another incision in another area may be added if necessary.

The steep meridian is marked preoperatively or intraoperatively with the use of keratometry, keratoscopy, or videokeratography. The cornea is incised with the stainless steel blade, and the incision is progressively deepened and lengthened until the refractive effect is achieved. The length of the incision should never exceed 3 clock hours. Care is taken to avoid perforation; in some cases, blunt dissection with the noncutting edge of the blade is useful.

The use of an intraoperative keratometer, keratoscope, or videokeratoscope such as the PAR system is invaluable for assessing the endpoint (Figure 38-9). A spherical cornea or a 20 percent overcorrection is preferred in most cases in which the incisions are short. A 20 percent undercorrection is preferred in cases in which the incisions are 2 to 3 clock hours in length because longer incisions

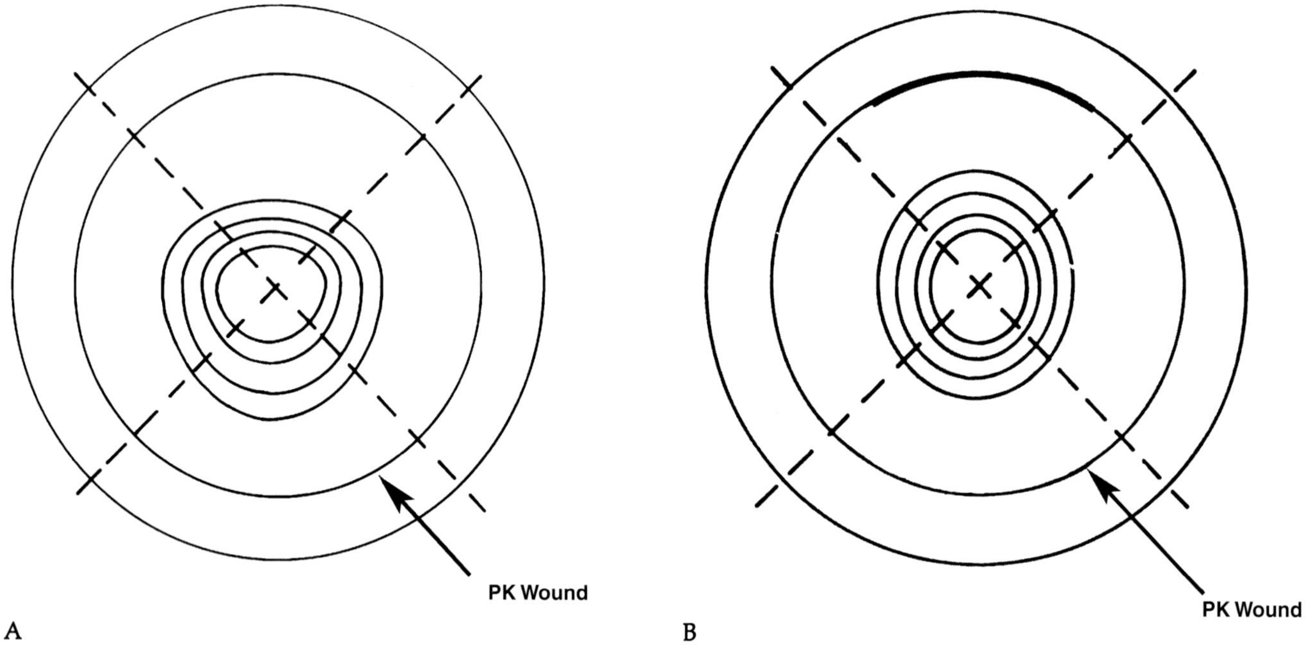

FIGURE 38-8 Arcuate relaxing incisions for asymmetrical postkeratoplasty astigmatism. **(A)** Egg-shaped keratoscope mires demonstrate asymmetrical steepening in the 90-degree meridian. **(B)** One arcuate relaxing incision made in the penetrating keratoplasty (*PK*) wound straddling the 90-degree meridian results in a reversal of the keratoscope mires.

tend to gape progressively as they heal. It is easier to enhance an undercorrection postoperatively by lengthening and/or deepening the original incision than it is to reduce an overcorrection, which requires suturing of the incision.

Compression Sutures

The addition of compression sutures to relaxing incisions can markedly increase the effect of the incisions. Compression sutures are placed across the keratoplasty wound 90 degrees from the relaxing incisions (Figure 38-10). Suture depth should be approximately 80 percent of the corneal thickness. The sutures are tied with a slip knot and the tension is adjusted under intraoperative keratometric or keratoscopic control until an overcorrection of 33 percent is achieved. The sutures are then tied, the ends are trimmed, and the knots are buried.

The recommended suture to use for compression sutures is 11-0 polyester (Mersilene). Nylon is easier to work with but biodegrades with time. Polypropylene is too elastic to maintain strength. Polyester suture is permanent and can be left without the possibility of loss of effect from biodegradation. However, it can cheesewire through the tissue. Sutures of any material may attract blood vessels to the corneal graft, and they also tend to loosen with time.

Wedge Resection

A wedge resection is used for the correction of large amounts of postkeratoplasty astigmatism (Figure 38-11). This procedure is reserved for patients with more than 10 diopters of astigmatism, and is capable of correcting up to 20 diopters of astigmatism. A wedge resection requires a prolonged postoperative rehabilitation because of the need to place multiple sutures, which induce irregular astigmatism. In general, a minimum of 6 months must be allowed for adequate wound healing before selective suture removal. Even so, wedge resection may be preferable to the only alternative—repeat penetrating keratoplasty.

The overall effect of a wedge resection is to steepen the flat meridian approximately twice as much as it flattens the steep meridian. Therefore, the net effect is an increase in myopia or a decrease in hyperopia. For example, if the preoperative refraction is $-6.00 + 12.00 \times 90$, and keratometry readings are 40.00 diopters at 180 degrees by 52.00 diopters at 90 degrees, a perfect result should give postoperative keratometry readings of 48.00 by 48.00 diopters with a refraction of −2.00 diopters. This would result in a 2-diopter myopic shift.

The flat meridian is marked and confirmed with intraoperative keratometry, keratoscopy, or videokeratography. The thickness of the keratoplasty wound is measured with ultrasonic pachymetry, and a diamond

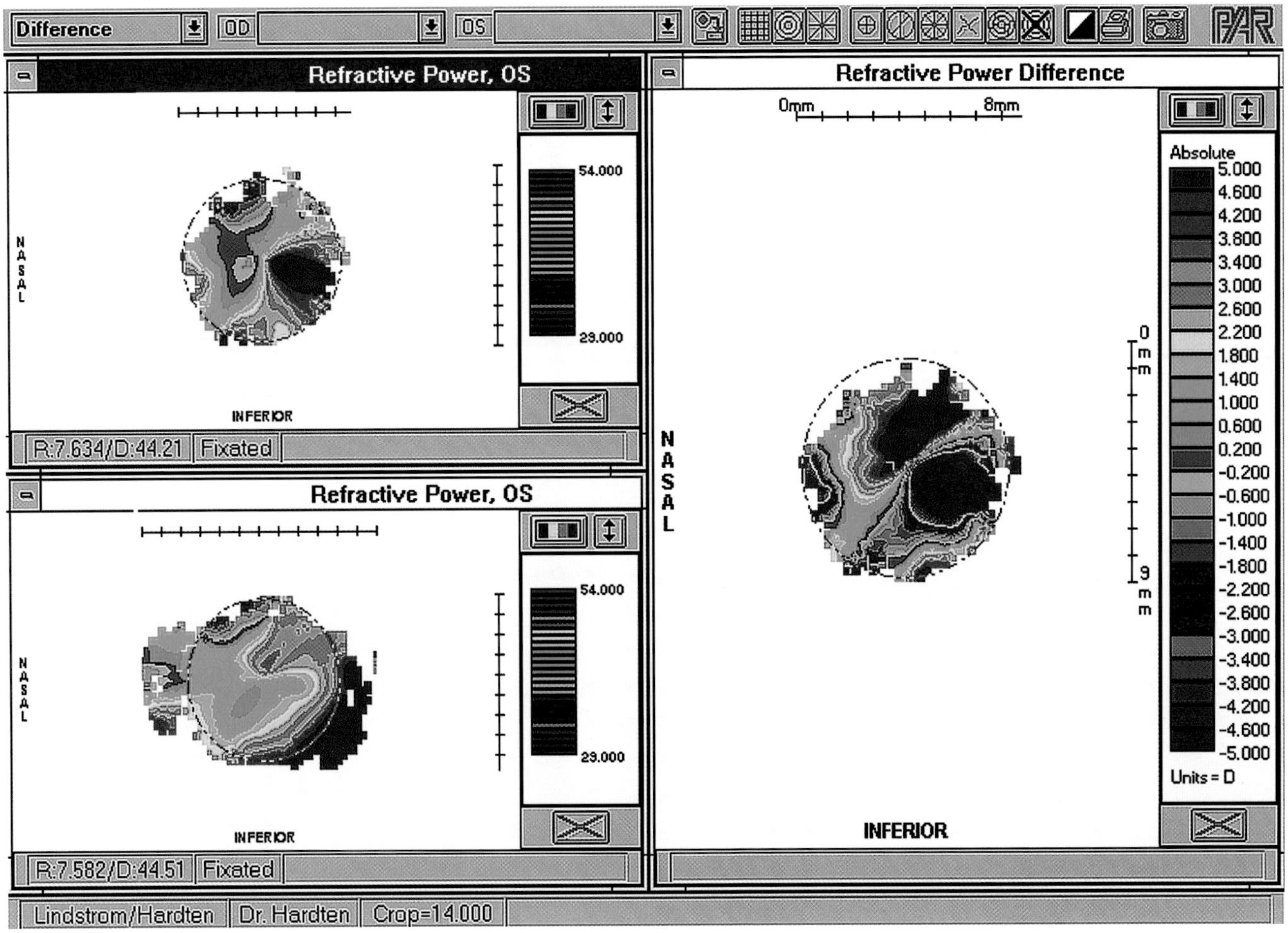

FIGURE 38-9 Intraoperative videokeratographs using the PAR system show the refractive power before (upper left) and after (lower left) astigmatic keratotomy for postkeratoplasty astigmatism. The incision was created in the 5 o'clock meridian, and an improvement in the irregular astigmatism can be seen. The change in refractive power is demonstrated in the refractive power difference map (right).

blade is set at approximately 75 percent of this thickness. The first incision is made concentrically in the keratoplasty wound for 3 clock hours along the flat meridian. A blade with a vertically oriented cutting edge is preferred because it allows better visualization as the incision is made. The placement of the second incision depends on the size of the graft and the character of the recipient bed. For a small graft (7.0-mm diameter or less), the incision is placed peripheral to the wound; for a larger graft or a vascularized bed, placement central to the wound is preferred. The width between the incisions and the amount of tissue resected depend on the desired correction. In general, 1.00 diopter of cylinder reduction is obtained for each 0.1 mm of tissue removed, up to 0.5 mm. Beyond that, the correction obtained doubles. Wedge resections of less than 0.5 mm produce little effect; wedge resections of more than 1.5 mm are not recommended. The two concentric incisions of equal depth are joined at their ends and at the base, and a wedge of tissue is excised.

Five to seven interrupted 10-0 nylon or 11-0 polyester sutures are placed across the wound. Polyester sutures are preferred because the sutures may be left in place indefinitely if the desired effect is achieved. Each suture is placed at 90 percent corneal depth and is tied with a slip-knot. The sutures are then tightened under keratometric or keratoscopic observation until an overcorrection of one-third to one-half of the preoperative cylinder is achieved. For example, if the preoperative cylinder is 12 diopters, the sutures are tightened until a 4- to 6-diopter overcorrection is achieved in the meridian opposite that of the preoperative cylinder. The sutures are then tied, the ends are trimmed, and the knots are buried.

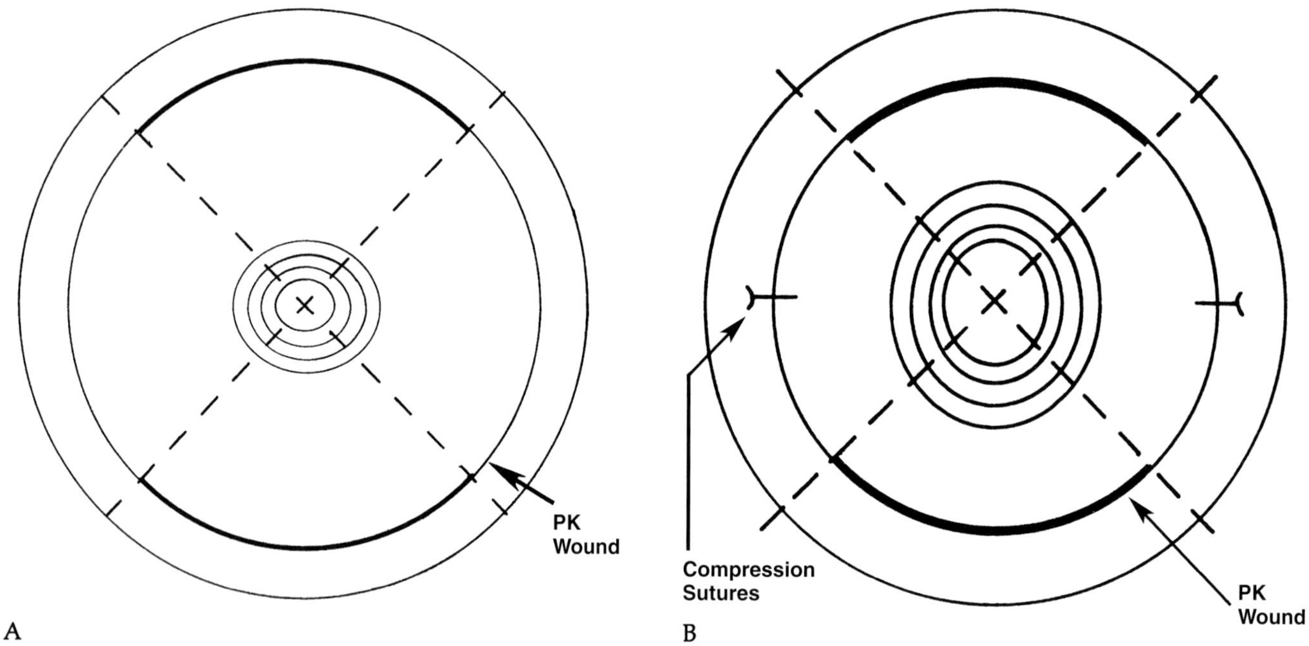

A B

FIGURE 38-10 Arcuate relaxing incisions and compression sutures for postkeratoplasty astigmatism. **(A)** Keratoscope mires demonstrate persistent steepening in the vertical meridian after arcuate relaxing incisions have been made. **(B)** Compression sutures placed across the penetrating keratoplasty (*PK*) wound 90 degrees from the relaxing incisions result in a reversal of the keratoscope mires.

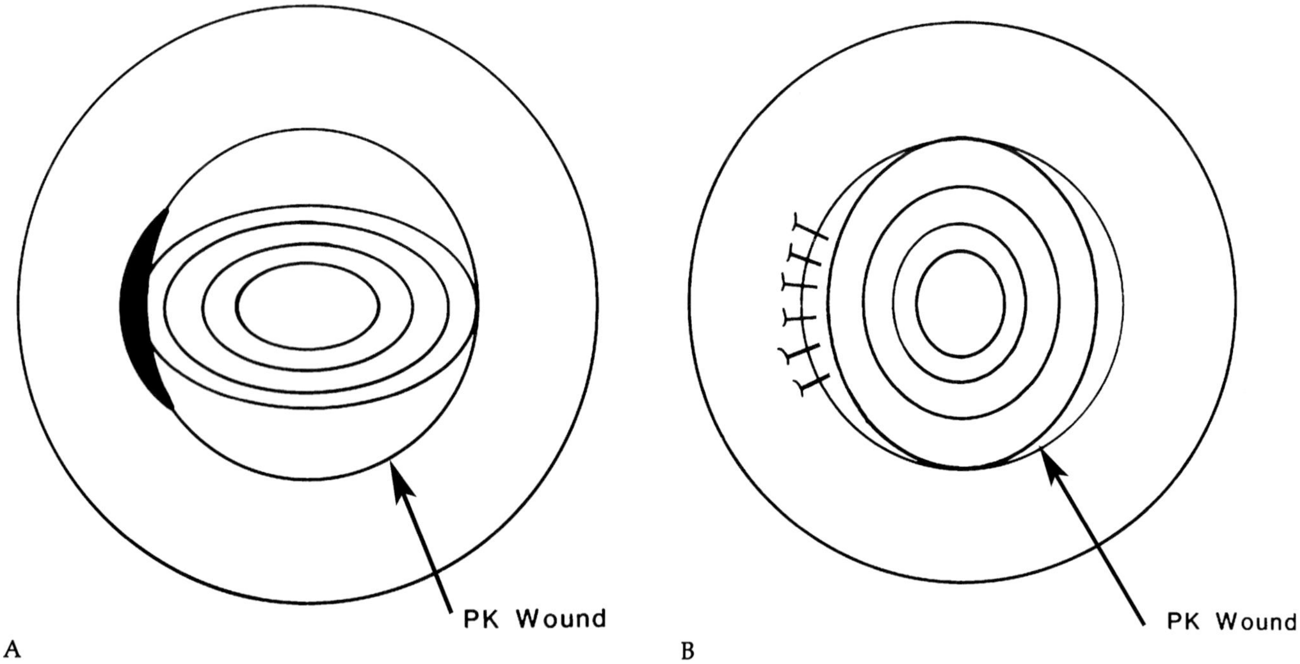

A B

FIGURE 38-11 Wedge resection. **(A)** Horizontally oval keratoscope mires demonstrate significant flattening in the horizontal meridian. The dark area in the penetrating keratoplasty (*PK*) wound indicates the wedge of tissue to be excised. **(B)** After the wedge of tissue has been excised, 10-0 nylon sutures are placed to close the wound.

Postoperative care involves the use of topical antibiotics for 1 week and topical corticosteroids as necessary to maintain graft clarity. Sutures are left in place for a minimum of 8 weeks. Thereafter, one or two sutures may be removed selectively every 3 to 4 weeks in the meridian of the steepest residual astigmatism. Once a satisfactory result is achieved, the remaining sutures may be left in place indefinitely.

COMPLICATIONS

Many of the complications of astigmatic keratotomy are similar to those of radial keratotomy described in Chapter 37.

Undercorrection

Transverse, arcuate, and semiradial incisions share a common problem, namely, some degree of unpredictability. Unpredictability is even greater in eyes that have had prior penetrating keratoplasty because of the variability of wound healing.

Undercorrections are better tolerated than overcorrections, and additional surgery may be performed for undercorrections to achieve the desired result. In cases of undercorrection with residual myopia or astigmatism, the simplest form of management is to use spectacles or contact lenses. Contact lenses can be highly successful when residual refractive errors are present.

Residual refractive errors can also be managed by further refractive surgery. Alternatives include radial and astigmatic keratotomy, photorefractive keratectomy, photoastigmatic refractive keratectomy, and laser-assisted in situ keratomileusis.

Overcorrection

Overcorrections also occur after surgery for astigmatism. In this situation, a shift of 90 degrees is typically seen in the axis of the cylinder. For the management of overcorrections after astigmatic keratotomy, additional incisions can be placed 90 degrees away from the original incisions, or previously placed keratotomy incisions can be bluntly reopened with a Sinskey hook, copiously irrigated with balanced salt solution, and closed with two or three interrupted 11-0 polyester sutures. Polyester sutures can be left in place indefinitely if the desired result is obtained. Control of suture tension with intraoperative keratometry, keratoscopy, or videokeratography, and the use of slip knots is helpful. One should aim for a spherical result to a 30 percent overcorrection with the sutures. Selective suture removal may begin 8 weeks after suture placement, if needed.

Intersecting Incisions

Intersection of keratotomy incisions should be avoided to prevent wound gape and excessive scarring.[20,33] Areas of intersection are frequently characterized by extensive subepithelial opacification and scar formation that spreads out from the wound. Such scars induce irregular astigmatism and also increase light scattering and glare. When two transverse incisions intersect two radial incisions, a block of cornea is created that may actually protrude anteriorly. These types of incisions may take many months to heal and result in variable degrees of corneal opacification.

Corneal Perforation

A microperforation during astigmatic keratotomy can be identified when one or two drops of aqueous humor are noted exuding from the incision. A macroperforation that is large enough to produce shallowing of the anterior chamber requires termination of the procedure and closure of the perforation with sutures. The Prospective Evaluation of Radial Keratotomy (PERK) study reported a 2.3 percent microperforation rate with radial keratotomy.[33] None of these cases required suturing or termination of the surgery. Prolonged dehydration and thinning of the cornea intraoperatively can increase the incidence of corneal perforation.[34] Perforations can induce formation of a scar at the level of Descemet's membrane, damage the corneal endothelium, lead to iridocorneal adhesions, and/or cause laceration of the anterior lens capsule if the incision is continued after perforation in an eye with a shallow anterior chamber.

Endothelial Damage

Keratotomy incisions can cause mild injury to the corneal endothelium.[35,36] After radial keratotomy, central endothelial cell density decreases less than 10 percent; however, a greater degree of endothelial cell injury is noted when corneal perforation occurs during the procedure.[37] Specular microscopic studies have not shown progressive decreases in endothelial cell density or progressive abnormality in endothelial cell morphology in human eyes over the first year after radial keratotomy.[38]

Corneal Scar Formation

Haze or scar formation can occur after any corneal injury, including astigmatic keratotomy. Typically, these scars are not visually significant because of their distance from the central cornea.

Pain

Most patients experience pain, throbbing, or foreign body sensation for 24 to 48 hours after astigmatic keratotomy. Topical nonsteroidal anti-inflammatory drugs and oral analgesics can be helpful in controlling pain. Pain relief by nonsteroidal anti-inflammatory drugs appears to be modulated by reducing prostaglandin E_2 levels.[39] If topical nonsteroidal anti-inflammatory drugs are used without corticosteroid coverage, an increase in polymorphonuclear leukocyte migration into the cornea can occur and cause inflammatory infiltrates. When topical corticosteroids and nonsteroidal anti-inflammatory drugs are used concomitantly, the leukocyte infiltration diminishes. Diclofenac appears to cause greater leukocyte infiltration than ketorolac.[39] The infiltrates are treated by stopping the nonsteroidal anti-inflammatory drug and beginning frequent topical corticosteroids after an infectious cause has been excluded.[40]

Epithelial Inclusion Cysts

Epithelial inclusion cysts in radial keratotomy incisions were seen in 8.6 percent of patients in the PERK study after 1 year, but did not appear to affect the visual results.[33] In the majority of patients, the cysts tend to resolve as collagen remodeling takes place postoperatively.[41]

Epithelial Ingrowth

Epithelial ingrowth has been reported after radial keratotomy.[42] Although it is possible, this complication has not been reported after astigmatic keratotomy. It has been suggested that injection of an irrigating stream through a perforation site should be minimized to avoid the introduction of epithelial cells intraoperatively.[42]

Corneal Iron Deposition

A visually insignificant brown stellate corneal epithelial iron line appears in most eyes after radial keratotomy and may also occur after astigmatic keratotomy. Eighty-one percent of eyes had a stellate epithelial iron line 6 months postoperatively in the PERK study.[43] The iron line appears at the inferior portion of the flattened region of the cornea.

Basement Membrane Changes

Corneal epithelial basement membrane changes, similar to those seen in epithelial basement membrane dystrophy, are often observed after refractive keratotomy.[44] These changes tend to be transient, lasting less than 3 months in the majority of eyes. They are infrequently associated with clinical symptoms or recurrent epithelial erosion.[33]

Infection

Bacterial or fungal keratitis can occur in the immediate postoperative period or can appear several years after refractive keratotomy.[45–47] The incidence appears higher when soft contact lenses, especially extended-wear lenses, are used. In an attempt to prevent this complication, prophylactic topical antibiotics are recommended until re-epithelialization is complete. Causative organisms have included *Pseudomonas*, *Staphylococcus aureus*, and *Staphylococcus epidermidis*. Two cases of *Mycobacterium chelonei* keratitis were reported from the same surgeon's office, in which outpatient radial keratotomy was performed using cold-sterilized instruments.[48]

An unusual complication of refractive keratotomy is the late development of bacterial or fungal ulcerative keratitis.[46–47] All infiltrates were noted to be contiguous with the keratotomy scars. A persistent epithelial plug in the keratotomy wound was implicated in some of these cases.

Infectious keratitis can result in corneal haze, scarring, and a decrease in visual acuity. Appropriate cultures and frequent application of antibiotics are used to diagnose and treat this complication.

Three cases of *S. epidermidis* endophthalmitis occurring 8 to 10 days after refractive keratotomy have been reported.[49,50] All patients had excellent visual outcomes several months postoperatively. In a series of nine cases of endophthalmitis, corneal perforation appeared to be responsible for the introduction of the microorganism into the eye, either during or shortly after the surgical procedure.[49] Thorough preoperative chemical preparation of the eye is imperative, strict adherence to sterile surgical technique is required, and postoperative antibiotics and careful follow-up are recommended. Topical 5 percent povidone-iodine solution has been shown to decrease the incidence of postoperative endophthalmitis and is currently recommended.[51]

Ptosis

Ptosis is a reported complication of radial keratotomy, and could potentially occur after astigmatic keratotomy.[52,53] Because retrobulbar injections and superior rectus bridle sutures were not used in the cases reported, the most likely cause of ptosis was damage to the levator aponeurosis by the eyelid speculum. It has been suggested that a flexible wire speculum might be less likely to induce ptosis than a solid, rigid eyelid speculum.[53]

Traumatic Rupture of Keratotomy Incisions

Any corneal incision results in a scar that does not have the same tensile strength as the original cornea. This is true not only after refractive keratotomy but also after corneal transplantation or accidental trauma.[54] There are several reports of traumatic rupture of keratotomy scars after blunt trauma.[55–57] In a rabbit eye model, Larson et al[58] observed that the blunt force required to rupture the globe after radial keratotomy within 90 days of healing was approximately half that required to rupture control eyes that did not have surgery. In a porcine eye model, Rylander et al[59] demonstrated that ruptures occurred most frequently at the equator in normal, unoperated eyes but through the keratotomy incisions in eyes having previous radial keratotomy.

Visual Aberrations

Glare or starburst caused by scattering of light occurs commonly for a few months after radial keratotomy, but may persist for a year or more.[60] In 9 percent of patients, glare was reported to cause diminished visual acuity, particularly at night or on hazy, bright days.[61,62] With astigmatic keratotomy alone, these complaints are rare.

REFERENCES

1. Schiøtz LJ: Ein Fall von hochgradigem Hornhautstastigmatismus nach Staarextraction: Bessergung auf operativem Wege. Arch Augenheilkd 15:178, 1885
2. Faber E: Operative Behandeling van Astigmatisme. Ned Tijdschr Geeneeskd 2:495, 1895
3. Schimmelpfennig BH, Waring GO III: Development of refractive keratotomy in the nineteenth century. p. 171. In Waring GO: Refractive Keratotomy for Myopia and Astigmatism. Mosby-Year Book, St. Louis, 1992
4. Bates WH: A suggestion of an operation to correct astigmatism. Arch Ophthalmol 23:9, 1894
5. Lans LJ: Experimentelle Untersuchungen uber Entstehung von Astigmatismus durch nich-perforirende Corneawunden. Albrecht von Graefes Arch Ophthalmol 45:117, 1898
6. Sato T: Treatment of conical cornea by incision of Descemet's membrane. Nippon Ganka Gakkai Zasshi 43:541, 1939
7. Sato T: Experimental study on surgical correction of astigmatism. Juntendo Kenkyukaizasshi 589:37, 1943
8. Sato T: Posterior incision of the cornea: surgical treatment for conical cornea and astigmatism. Am J Ophthalmol 33:943, 1950
9. Sato T: Die operative Behandlung des Astigmatismus. Klin Monatsbl Augenheilkd 126:16, 1955
10. Fyodorov SN, Durnev VV: Surgical correction of complicated myopic astigmatism by means of dissection of circular ligament of cornea. Ann Ophthalmol 13:115, 1981
11. Duffey RJ, Jain VN, Tchah H, et al: Paired arcuate keratotomy: a surgical approach to mixed and myopic astigmatism. Arch Ophthalmol 106:1130, 1988
12. Duffey RJ, Tchah H, Lindstrom RL: Spoke keratotomy in the human cadaver eye. J Refract Surg 4:9, 1988
13. Franks JB, Binder PS: Keratotomy procedures for the correction of astigmatism. J Refract Surg 1:11, 1985
14. Lavery GW, Lindstrom RL: Trapezoidal astigmatic keratotomy in human cadaver eyes. J Refract Surg 1:18, 1985
15. Lindquist TD, Rubenstein JB, Rice SW, et al: Trapezoidal astigmatic keratotomy: quantification in human cadaver eyes. Arch Ophthalmol 104:1534, 1986
16. Lindstrom RL: The surgical correction of astigmatism: a clinician's perspective. Refract Corneal Surg 6:441, 1990
17. Salz J, Lee JS, Jester JV, et al: Radial keratotomy in fresh human cadaver eyes. Ophthalmology 88:742, 1981
18. Lindquist TD: Complications of ocular surgery. Int Ophthalmol Clin 32:97, 1992
19. Duke-Elder S, Stewart S, Abrams D: Ophthalmic optics and refraction. p. 274. System of Ophthalmology. Vol 5. CV Mosby, St. Louis, 1970
20. Lindstrom RL, Lindquist RD: Surgical correction of postoperative astigmatism. Cornea 7:138, 1988
21. Donders RL, Moore WD (trans): On the Aromalis of Accommodation and Refraction of the Eye. New Sydenham Society, London, 1864
22. Guyton DL: Prescribing cylinders: the problem of distortion. Surv Ophthalmol 22:177, 1977
23. Jaffe NS, Clayman HM: The pathophysiology of corneal astigmatism after cataract extraction. Ophthalmology 79:615, 1975
24. Troutman RC: Microsurgery of the Anterior Segment of the Eye. CV Mosby, St. Louis, 1987
25. Troutman RC, Swinger C: Relaxing incision for control of postoperative astigmatism following keratoplasty. Ophthalmic Surg 11:117, 1980
26. Ibrahim O, Hussein HA, El-Sahn MF, et al: Trapezoidal keratotomy for the correction of naturally occurring astigmatism. Arch Ophthalmol 109:1374, 1991
27. Barner SS: Surgical treatment of corneal astigmatism. Ophthalmic Surg 7:43, 1976
28. Krachmer JH, Fenzel RE: Surgical correction of high postkeratoplasty astigmatism. Arch Ophthalmol 98:1400, 1980
29. Lavery GW, Lindstrom RL, Hofer LA, Doughman DJ: The surgical management of corneal astigmatism after penetrating keratoplasty. Ophthalmic Surg 16:165, 1985
30. Mandel MR, Shapiro MB, Krachmer JH: Relaxing incisions with augmentation sutures for the correction of postkeratoplasty astigmatism. Am J Ophthalmol 103:441, 1987

31. Sugar J, Kick AK: Relaxing keratotomy for post-keratoplasty high astigmatism. Ophthalmic Surg 14:156, 1983
32. Lundergan MK, Rowsey JJ: Relaxing incisions. Ophthalmology 92:1226, 1985
33. Waring GO III, Lynn MJ, Gelender H, et al: Results of the Prospective Evaluation of Radial Keratotomy (PERK) study one year after surgery. Ophthalmology 90:642, 1983
34. Villaseñor RA, Salz J, Steel D, Krasnow MKA: Changes in corneal thickness during radial keratotomy. Ophthalmic Surg 12:341, 1981
35. Hoffer KJ, Darin JJ, Pettit TH, et al: Three years experience with radial keratotomy: the UCLA study. Ophthalmology 90:627, 1983
36. MacRae SM, Matsuda M, Rich LF: The effects of radial keratotomy on the corneal endothelium. Am J Ophthalmol 100:538, 1985
37. Chiba K, Oak SS, Tsubota K, et al: Morphometric analysis of corneal endothelium following radial keratotomy. J Cataract Refract Surg 13:263, 1987
38. Rowsey JJ, Balyeat HD, Monlux R, et al: Endothelial cell loss after radial keratotomy. Ophthalmology 94:97, 1987
39. Phillips AF, Hayashi S, Seitz B, et al: Effect of diclofenac, ketorolac, and fluorometholone on arachidonic acid metabolites following excimer laser corneal surgery. Arch Ophthalmol 114:1495, 1996
40. Sher NA, Frantz JM, Talley A, et al: Topical diclofenac in the treatment of ocular pain after excimer photorefractive keratectomy. Refract Corneal Surg 9:425, 1993
41. Waring GO III, Lynn MJ, McDonnell PJ, et al: Results of the Prospective Evaluation of Radial Keratotomy (PERK) study 10 years after surgery. Arch Ophthalmol 112:1298, 1994
42. Binder PS: Presumed epithelial ingrowth following radial keratotomy. CLAO J 12:247, 1986
43. Steinberg EB, Wilson LA, Waring GO III, et al: Stellate iron lines in the corneal epithelium after radial keratotomy. Am J Ophthalmol 98:416, 1984
44. Nelson JD, Williams P, Lindstrom RL, Doughman DJ: Map-finger-dot changes in the corneal epithelial basement membrane following radial keratotomy. Ophthalmology 92:199, 1985
45. Cottingham AJ, Berkeley RG, Nordan LT, et al: Bacterial corneal ulcers following keratorefractive surgery: a retrospective study of 14,163 procedures. Presented at the Ocular Microbiology and Immunology Group Meeting. San Francisco, September 28, 1986
46. Mandelbaum S, Waring GO, Forster RK, et al: Late development of ulcerative keratitis in radial keratotomy scars. Arch Ophthalmol 104:1156, 1986
47. Shivitz IA, Arrowsmith PN: Delayed keratitis after radial keratotomy. Arch Ophthalmol 104:1153, 1986
48. Robin JB, Beatty RF, Dunn S, et al: *Mycobacterium chelonei* keratitis after radial keratotomy. Am J Ophthalmol 102:72, 1986
49. Gelender H, Flynn HW, Mandelbaum SH: Bacterial endophthalmitis resulting from radial keratotomy. Am J Ophthalmol 93:323, 1982
50. Manka RL, Gast TJ: Endophthalmitis following Ruiz procedure [letter]. Arch Ophthalmol 108:21, 1990
51. Apt L, Isenberg SJ, Yoshimori R, et al: The effect of povidone-iodine solution applied at the conclusion of ophthalmic surgery. Am J Ophthalmol 119:701, 1995
52. Carroll RP, Lindstrom RL: Blepharoptosis after radial keratotomy. Am J Ophthalmol 102:800, 1986
53. Linberg JV, McDonald M, Safir A, Googe JM: Ptosis following radial keratotomy. Performed using a rigid eyelid speculum. Ophthalmology 93:1509, 1986
54. Maurice DM: The biology of wound healing in the corneal stroma: Castroviejo lecture. Cornea 6:162, 1987
55. Binder PS, Waring GO III, Arrowsmith PN, Wang CL: Traumatic rupture of the cornea after radial keratotomy. Arch Ophthalmol 106:1584, 1988
56. Forstot SL, Damiano RE: Trauma following radial keratotomy. Ophthalmology 94:127, 1987
57. Simmons KB, Linsalata RP: Ruptured globe following blunt trauma after radial keratotomy. Ophthalmology 94:148, 1987
58. Larson BC, Kremer FB, Eller AW, Bernardino VB: Quantitated trauma following radial keratotomy in rabbits. Ophthalmology 90:660, 1983
59. Rylander HG, Welch AJ, Fremming B: The effect of radial keratotomy in the rupture strength of pig eyes. Ophthalmic Surg 14:744, 1983
60. Arrowsmith PN, Marks RG: Visual, refractive and keratometric results of radial keratotomy: a five-year follow-up. Arch Ophthalmol 107:506, 1989
61. Arrowsmith PN, Marks RG: Visual, refractive, and keratometric results of radial keratotomy: a two-year follow-up. Arch Ophthalmol 105:76, 1987
62. Deitz MR, Sanders DR, Marks RG: Radial keratotomy: an overview of the Kansas City study. Ophthalmology 91:467, 1984

39

Epikeratophakia for Aphakia and Myopia

MARGUERITE B. MCDONALD AND KEITH S. MORGAN

Epikeratophakia for aphakia and myopia is a surgical procedure in which a lens made of human corneal tissue is sutured onto the anterior surface of the cornea to change the anterior curvature, and hence, the refractive properties of the cornea (Figure 39-1). The tissue lens consists of Bowman's layer and anterior stroma of a donor cornea that has been frozen and lathed. This chapter describes the history and development of epikeratophakia for the correction of aphakia and myopia, as well as the indications, surgical techniques, postoperative care, and complications associated with this procedure.

HISTORY

Epikeratophakia evolved from keratophakia and keratomileusis,[1] which are lamellar refractive keratoplasty procedures developed by Barraquer in Colombia, South America, more than 30 years ago. Keratophakia was developed originally to treat patients who were unilaterally aphakic and spectacle and contact lens intolerant. At that time, intraocular lenses were in the earliest stages of development and were not yet safe and effective; therefore, secondary intraocular lens implantation was not feasible and there were no other options to restore vision in these functionally blind aphakic eyes. Keratomileusis was developed originally to correct myopia and later adapted for the correction of aphakia.

In the late 1970s, Kaufman went to South America to learn the Barraquer procedures. He was impressed with the ingenuity and technical expertise of Barraquer but thought that there might be a safer, simpler, less expensive, and reversible way to change the anterior corneal curvature to correct refractive errors. If tissue lenses could be made of donor tissue and preserved, the expensive and abstruse technology and equipment needed for their manufacture could be centralized; a central facility could produce tissue lenses to order and ship them to surgeons who were trained to perform the corneal surgery. If a tissue lens could be placed on the anterior surface of the cornea, like a contact lens, instead of on a lamellar bed, the surgery would be less complicated. The surgeon would need only remove the central corneal epithelium of the patient and sew the edge of the tissue lens into a shallow groove made in the peripheral cornea. This would avoid the potential complications of splitting the cornea and provide a reversibility that was not possible with keratophakia and keratomileusis. The tissue lens would be attached to the patient's cornea by only a thin peripheral scar, which would be sufficient to hold it in place. Because scar formation requires a stroma-to-stroma interface and because most of the interface between the patient's cornea and the tissue lens would consist of stroma-to-Bowman's layer, no scarring would occur across the central cornea, and the tissue lens could be removed in the future, if necessary, by breaking the peripheral scar around the circumference of the tissue lens.

Historically, epikeratophakia was performed first in aphakic adult patients who were spectacle and contact lens intolerant and who were not good candidates for secondary intraocular lens implantation.[2–6] Subsequent studies demonstrated that epikeratophakia does not interfere with secondary surgery[7] or the measurement of intraocular pressure,[8] nor does the presence of the extra tissue on the cornea adversely affect the patient's corneal endothelium.[9] Epikeratophakia was next used in aphakic pediatric patients.[10–14] Several years later, epikeratophakia for myopia was developed for spectacle– and contact lens–intolerant patients with severe myopia.[15–17] Epikeratophakia for keratoconus, also called *onlay lamel-*

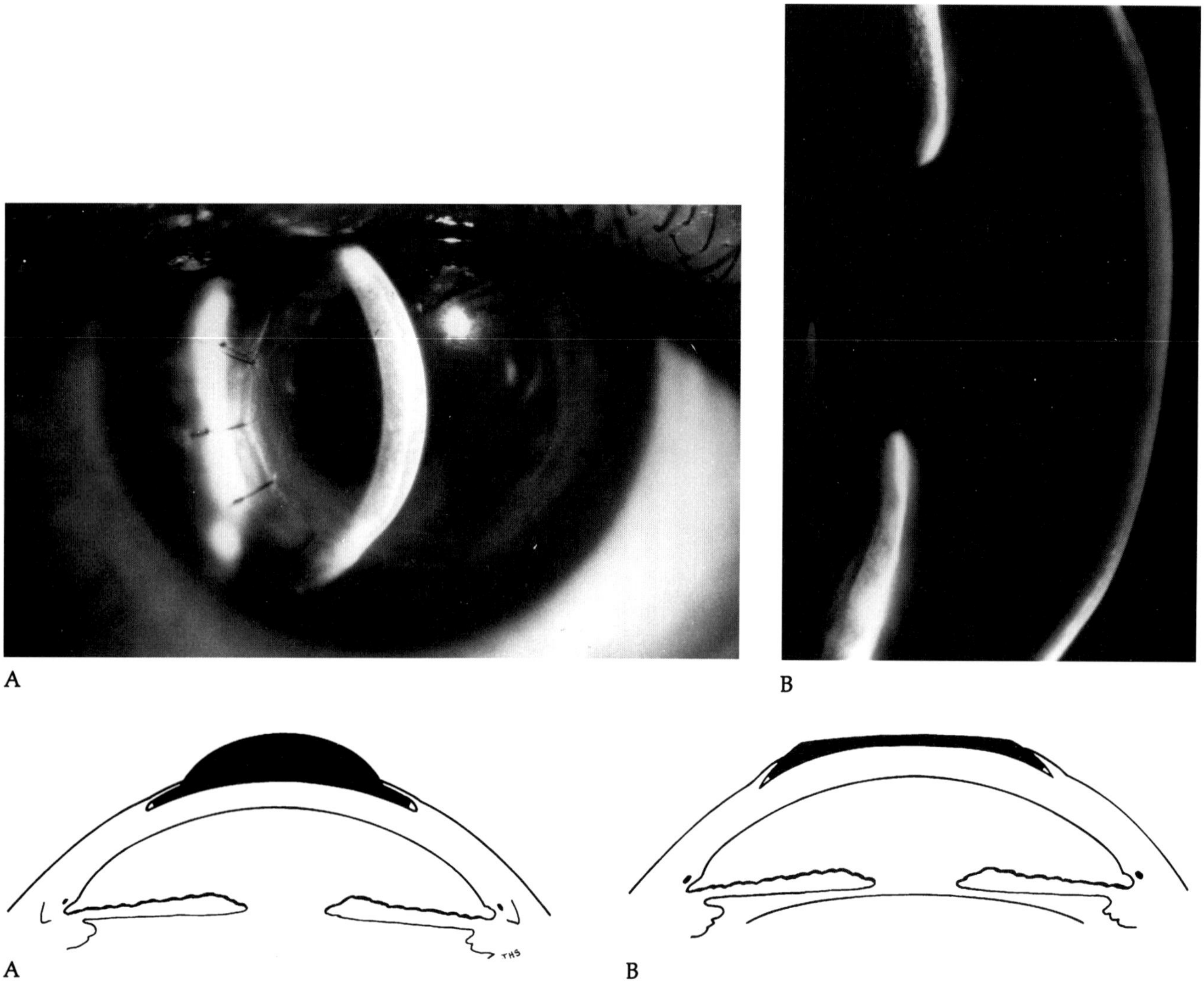

FIGURE 39-1 **(A)** Epikeratophakia for the correction of aphakia. Top: Slit lamp microscopy. Bottom: Diagram. **(B)** Epikeratophakia for the correction of myopia. Top: Slit lamp microscopy. Bottom: Diagram.

lar keratoplasty, was developed after epikeratophakia for aphakia but before epikeratophakia for myopia; it was designed to reinforce the cornea and flatten the cone in contact lens–intolerant keratoconus patients who do not have extensive central scarring[18-20] (see Ch. 32).

In 1986 and 1987, the safety and utility of epikeratophakia were described in a series of nationwide clinical studies involving 234 surgeons and more than 1,200 adult and pediatric patients with aphakia, myopia, or keratoconus.[21-25] Changes in the design and processing of the tissue lens and the surgical procedure continued,[26-32] including the development of the corneal press to reduce stromal hydration before lathing[33,34] and the use of cryoprotectants during freezing of the tissue.[35,36] Over the last 10 years, published results of epikeratophakia for the correction of aphakia[37-45] have been somewhat better than those for the correction of myopia, especially high myopia,[46-50] at least in part because of regression of effect in patients with high myopia. With the emergence of excimer laser photorefractive procedures, tissue additive procedures have become less widely used, especially for the correction of myopia. However, this procedure remains an option for selected patients, as described below.

PATIENT SELECTION AND PREOPERATIVE EVALUATION

Adult Aphakia

Adult candidates for epikeratophakia for aphakia should be spectacle and contact lens intolerant and poor candidates for secondary intraocular lens implantation. Factors to be considered include low endothelial cell density, vitreous in the anterior chamber, distorted anterior chamber architecture from trauma, glaucoma, a functioning filtering bleb that the surgeon does not wish to disturb, previous retinal detachment, and uveitis. Patients older than 80 years should not be routinely considered for epikeratophakia because the tissue lens clears so slowly (6 to 12 months). Patients between 70 and 80 years should be assessed on an individual basis.

Most adult aphakic patients are in the older age group, and many have some external disease, such as blepharitis, dry eyes, or lagophthalmos, that has made them unable to tolerate contact lenses. These external diseases must be diagnosed and treated aggressively before epikeratophakia is performed. In the early years of epikeratophakia, patients with blepharitis, dry eyes, or lagophthalmos were treated medically (and sometimes surgically in the case of lagophthalmos) just before surgery. However, it became apparent that such patients must be treated for at least 2 months before surgery so that the surgeon can establish compliance with medical therapy. All too frequently, patients discontinue therapy for blepharitis or dry eyes immediately after surgery, and the tissue lenses fail as a result of chronic epithelial defects. When patients understand that their external disease will not be eradicated by the surgery and that therapy must be continued indefinitely, surgery can be performed with little risk.

For several years, only unilaterally aphakic patients were considered for epikeratophakia. When the safety and predictability of the procedure were established, patients who had cataracts removed from both eyes became candidates for bilateral epikeratophakia. Bilaterally aphakic patients who are intolerant to contact lenses and are not candidates for intraocular lenses can usually see well with aphakic spectacles in terms of measurable visual acuity, but on a practical level, the magnification and peripheral distortions and scotomata from aphakic spectacles make it difficult for them to function.

Pediatric Aphakia

Epikeratophakia can be performed in children who have congenital or traumatic cataracts.[38,39,45,51–56] Children with cataracts may be considered for epikeratophakia coupled with cataract extraction as a primary procedure if they are too young for intraocular lens implantation and a preoperative trial contact lens fitting is unsuccessful. If it is difficult or impossible to insert and remove the contact lens in the office, it is certain that the parents will have less success at home. Similarly, aphakic children who are spectacle and contact lens intolerant may be candidates for epikeratophakia alone.

Neonates with either unilateral or bilateral cataracts are best managed by prompt cataract extraction coupled with contact lens correction. Most neonates and infants tolerate extended-wear contact lenses well. During the first year of life, the eye undergoes rapid changes in axial length and corneal curvature. During this time, contact lens changes can ensure that the optical correction is appropriate. Often, children begin to dislodge and lose contact lenses around their first birthday. If contact lens loss becomes excessive, epikeratophakia can be used to correct the refractive error. As the eye has already passed through the most rapid period of change in axial length and corneal curvature, the achieved power can be fine tuned with spectacles as the child grows.

Epikeratophakia can be performed in young infants if the parents are unable to manage contact lens care. If epikeratophakia is performed as a primary procedure in short eyes, special formulas are necessary to calculate the desired power.[57] Epikeratophakia can be successful in children younger than 12 months of age; however, normal developmental changes create a myopic shift in the growing eye, and the amount of correction in the tissue lens will no longer be appropriate for the refractive error. As these changes occur, the tissue lens can be removed or exchanged as needed.

Cataract extraction and epikeratophakia can be combined in a single primary procedure. This is especially useful in toddlers with acquired cataracts, for example, children with traumatic cataracts,[52] posterior lenticonus, or subluxated lenses. In these children, the proportions of the eye are nearly those of an adult, and contact lens compliance is poor. If there is a possibility that the child could be contact lens compliant, as determined by an office trial, cataract extraction should be performed initially, and epikeratophakia performed as a secondary procedure if contact lens wear is unsuccessful.

Children who have acquired cataracts with corneal lacerations are excellent candidates for epikeratophakia.[55] In these children, the tissue lens provides support for the weakened and irregular cornea and can lessen irregular and regular astigmatism. The tissue lens also allows corneal sutures to be removed earlier, because it provides mechanical support to the cornea. In children with unilateral corneal lacerations and traumatic cataracts, the keratometry readings from the uninvolved eye may be used to determine the required power of the tissue lens.

Older children (8 to 18 years of age) for whom secondary intraocular lens implantation is contraindicated, such as those with poorly controlled glaucoma or aniridia, seem to be the group in which epikeratophakia has the highest rate of success.[56] In this age group, contact lens compliance, especially with unilateral aphakia, is poor.

Myopia

Candidates for epikeratophakia for myopia should be at least 21 years of age and spectacle and contact lens intolerant, have had stable myopia for at least 1 year before surgery, and have more than 15 diopters of myopia by manifest refraction. Epikeratophakia may be used for any patient with more than 6 diopters of myopia who has had a scleral buckle for a retinal detachment. At this writing, the results of photorefractive keratectomy are poor for the correction of more than 6 diopters of myopia because of haze and regression, and laser-assisted in situ keratomileusis cannot be performed in these patients because the buckle interferes with the placement of the suction ring.

Occasionally, there is an occupational or recreational need for refractive surgery. Patients also request refractive surgery for psychological reasons; for instance, many highly myopic mothers feel more comfortable knowing that they could scoop up their children and exit a burning building without groping for an optical device.

As with aphakic patients, myopic patients frequently have blepharitis, dry eyes, and lagophthalmos, and again, these conditions must be treated for at least 2 months before surgery to establish compliance.

Children with unilateral myopia and anisometropic amblyopia are candidates for epikeratophakia if they are spectacle and contact lens intolerant and young enough to benefit from amblyopia therapy. If the myopia continues to progress after surgery because of an increase in axial length, the tissue lens can be removed or exchanged at a later date to satisfy the increased dioptric requirement.

Ordering the Tissue Lens

Some institutions have the equipment to make tissue lenses in house. Alternatively, tissue lenses may be ordered from Cryo-Optics. The tissue lens is shipped to the surgeon in a vial containing Optisol. Tissue lenses for aphakia and myopia are 8.5 mm in diameter and are available in powers from +5 to +20 diopters and -5 to -20 diopters, respectively. The lens is ordered on the basis of the patient's refraction, corrected to the corneal plane, and the average keratometry measurement. To convert the refraction at the spectacle plane to the refraction at the corneal plane, the vertex distance must be known, and the following formula is used: $P_c = P_s/(1 - vP_s)$, where P_c is the power in diopters at the corneal plane, P_s is the power in diopters at the spectacle plane, and v is the vertex distance in meters. In patients with mild astigmatism (less than 1.5 diopters), the spherical equivalent is used for the spectacle refraction. For children who are undergoing combined cataract extraction and epikeratophakia, the power of the tissue lens is calculated on the basis of axial length and keratometry measurements, using formulas originally designed for the calculation of intraocular lens power for adults.[57,58]

SURGICAL TECHNIQUES

The surgical techniques for epikeratophakia for aphakia and myopia are similar. The center of the entrance pupil is marked with a surgical marking pen containing gentian violet before administration of general or local anesthesia because patient cooperation is required for fixation. For patients who cannot cooperate, topical pilocarpine is administered and the tissue lens is centered on the miotic pupil.

Immediately after the center of the entrance pupil has been marked, the patient is given retrobulbar or general anesthesia. After the eye is prepped and draped, an eyelid speculum is inserted. The choice is one of personal preference; we prefer Jaffe specula. Next, 4-0 silk bridle sutures are placed through the superior and inferior rectus muscles for fixation and to allow movement of the eye.

A blunt spatula, such as the Paton spatula, is used to remove the midperipheral epithelium, leaving a central island containing the centration mark and a 0.5-mm cuff for 360 degrees at the limbus (Figure 39-2). This central island of epithelium is used to center the trephine, as described below, and the limbal cuff of epithelium is essential for epithelialization of the tissue lens. It is important that a blunt spatula be used to remove the epithelium and not something sharper, such as a blade. It is easy to damage Bowman's layer with a blade, creating areas of stroma-to-stroma contact that can result in central scarring between the tissue lens and the underlying cornea, possibly compromising vision and the future reversibility of the procedure.

A 7.0-mm Barron radial vacuum trephine is used to create a shallow peripheral corneal cut. The trephine is described and illustrated in Chapter 34. Before the trephine is used, the blade is observed under the operating microscope and positioned at a level even with the inner wall of the vacuum chamber. The blade is then retracted three quarter-turns from this position so that it will not interfere with the establishment of suction. The cross hairs of

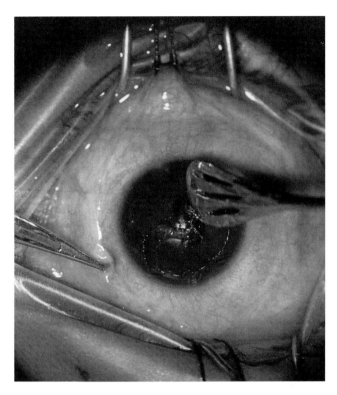

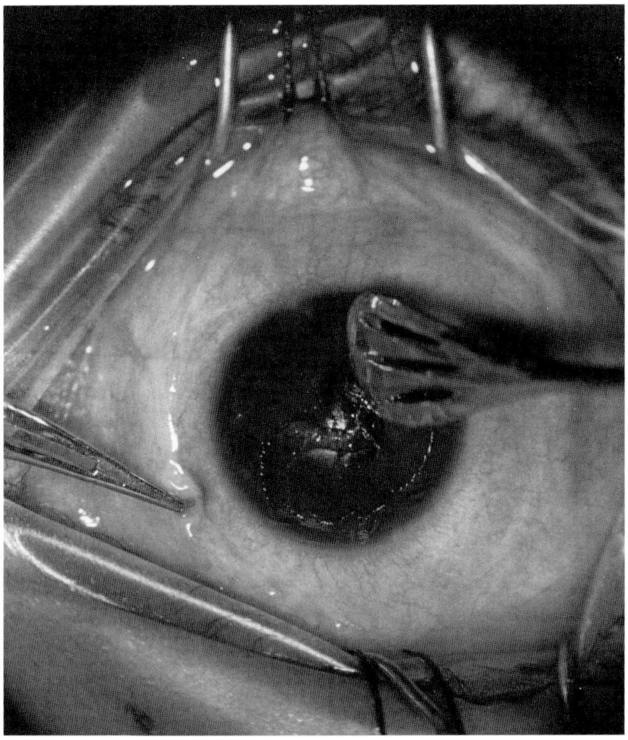

FIGURE 39-2 A Paton spatula is used to remove the mid-peripheral epithelium around the centration mark.

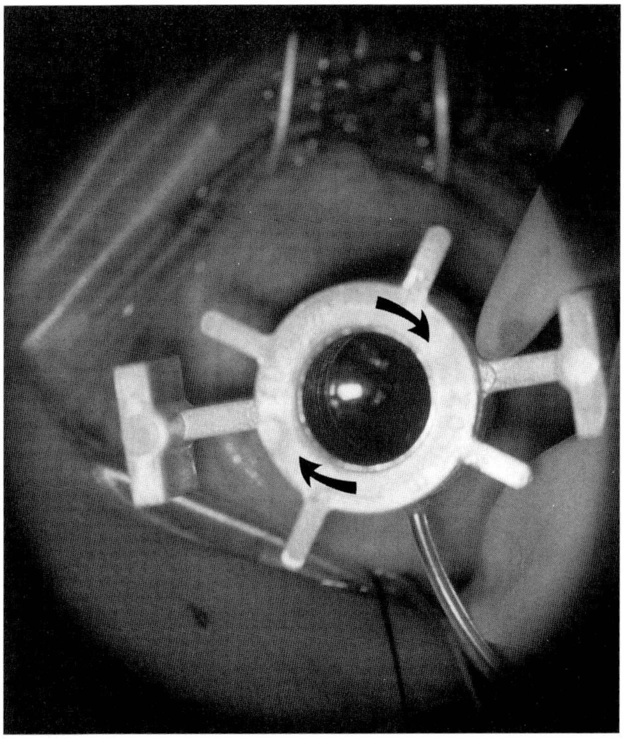

FIGURE 39-3 The spokes of the Barron radial vacuum trephine are turned clockwise to make the initial trephine cut.

the trephine are centered on the centration mark. After the trephine has been centered, the plunger of the 5-ml syringe attached to the trephine is pushed in all the way, and the trephine is pressed gently on the cornea. The plunger is released abruptly to establish suction. The plunger usually stops at the 4-ml mark on the syringe if suction has been obtained. The trephine is gently supported by the struts at the top of the trephine with no upward or downward pressure applied. The plastic spokes on the top of the blade assembly are slowly rotated clockwise five quarter-turns: three quarter-turns to reach the corneal surface, and two quarter-turns to make the cut (Figure 39-3). It is important not to confuse quarter-turns with full-turns, as this may result in a cut that is too deep, or even corneal perforation. The trephine is removed from the eye by pushing in the plunger of the syringe all the way to release suction. The corneal cut created by this method is approximately 0.15 mm deep. The Barron radial vacuum trephine is preferred to a hand-held trephine because it creates a more precise cut of even depth for 360 degrees.

After the trephine cut is made, the island of epithelium containing the centration mark is removed with a blunt spatula. The anterior corneal surface is irrigated with balanced salt solution dispensed from a 20-ml syringe with a 20-μm Millipore filter and cannula; an infant feeding tube attached to suction is used to remove debris and any foreign material floating on the corneal surface and in the fornices (Figure 39-4). It is imperative that epithelium or foreign material not be trapped at the interface between the tissue lens and the recipient cornea to prevent the postoperative formation of cysts or opacities that may interfere with vision. From this point in the surgery, a small plastic disk is placed over the pupil whenever the procedure permits to protect the macula from damage caused by the light from the operating microscope. Additionally, oblique rather than coaxial illumination is used whenever possible to prevent retinal phototoxicity.[59]

In children undergoing combined cataract extraction and epikeratophakia, cataract extraction is performed at this point. A limbal incision is made, the cataractous lens is removed with either a vitrector or an irrigation/aspiration device, and the limbal incision is sutured.

If an annular keratectomy is to be a part of the procedure, it is performed next by removing a 0.5-mm portion of the inner aspect of the trephine cut with Vannas scissors (see Ch. 32). The keratectomy is considered optional in pediatric cases; it is not used in aphakic or myopic adult patients.

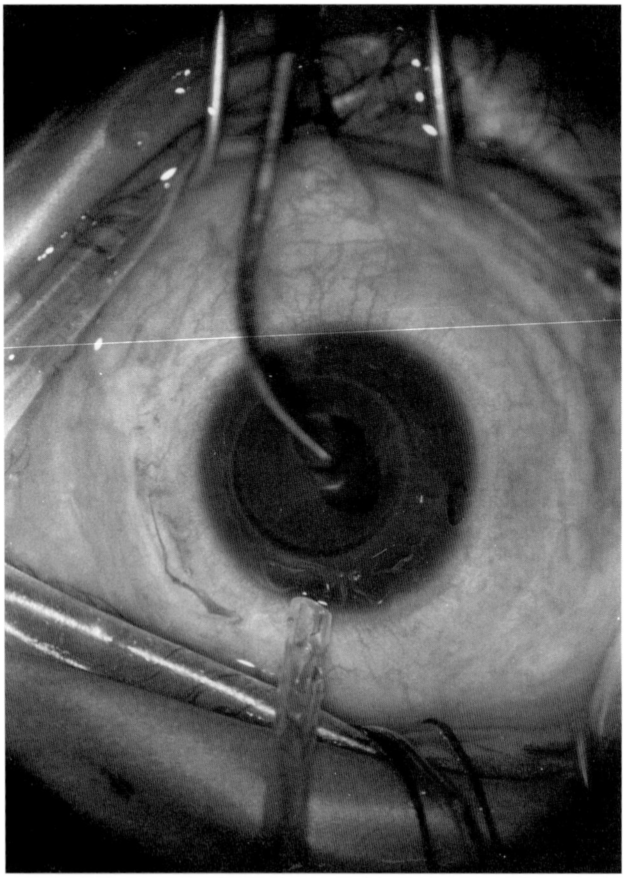

FIGURE 39-4 The surface of the cornea is scrubbed and washed with filtered balanced salt solution and the debris is aspirated with an infant feeding tube.

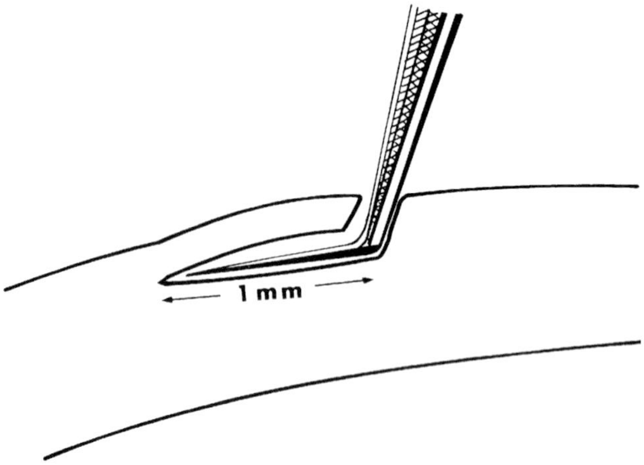

FIGURE 39-5 A peripheral lamellar dissection is created at the base of the trephine cut.

In both adults and children, a peripheral lamellar dissection is performed at the bottom of the trephine cut with an angled lamellar dissector. The peripheral edge of the trephine cut is grasped with a 0.12-mm forceps for stabilization and countertraction, and the instrument is inserted up to the angle and moved around the depth of the trephine cut (Figure 39-5). The dissection extends toward the limbus for 1 mm.

The tissue lens is removed from the vial in which it was shipped and is grasped with a Polack forceps (Figure 39-6). With observation under the highest magnification of the operating microscope, both surfaces of the tissue lens are irrigated with filtered balanced salt solution. While the surgeon gently strokes the surfaces of the tissue lens with the tip of the irrigation cannula, sending a slow stream of balanced salt solution down the surfaces of the tissue lens, the assistant holds the infant feeding tube connected to suction at the other end of the tissue lens so that the

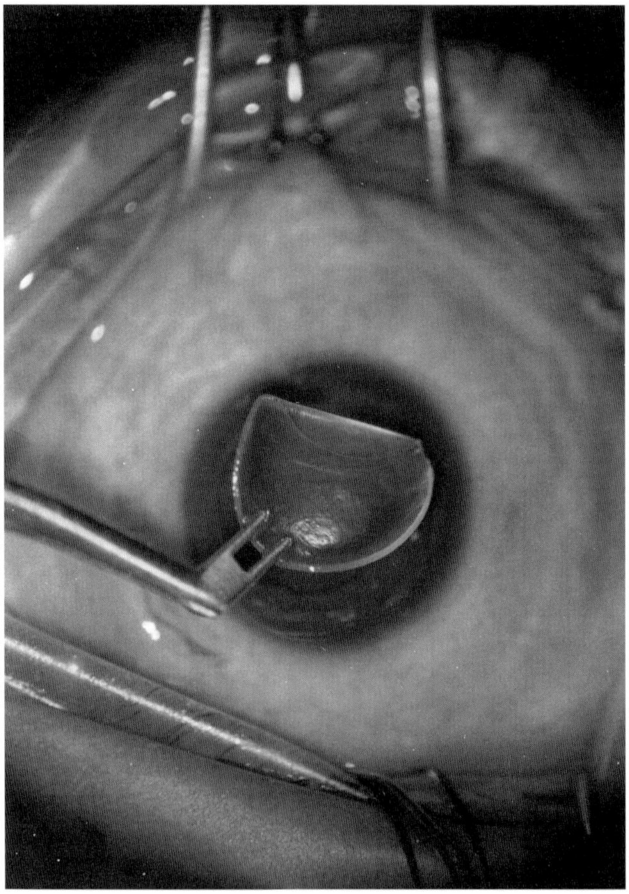

FIGURE 39-6 A Polack forceps is used to grasp the tissue lens and place it on the patient's cornea.

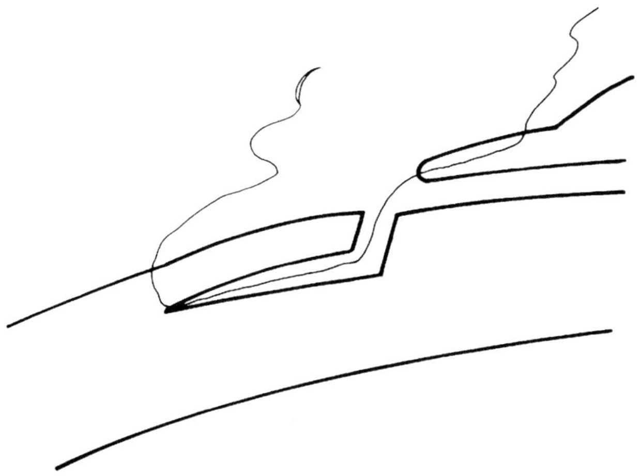

FIGURE 39-7 The first suture is placed 0.75 mm from the edge of the tissue lens, passes through the wing, enters the pocket created by the peripheral lamellar dissection, and exits 1 mm peripheral to the trephine cut.

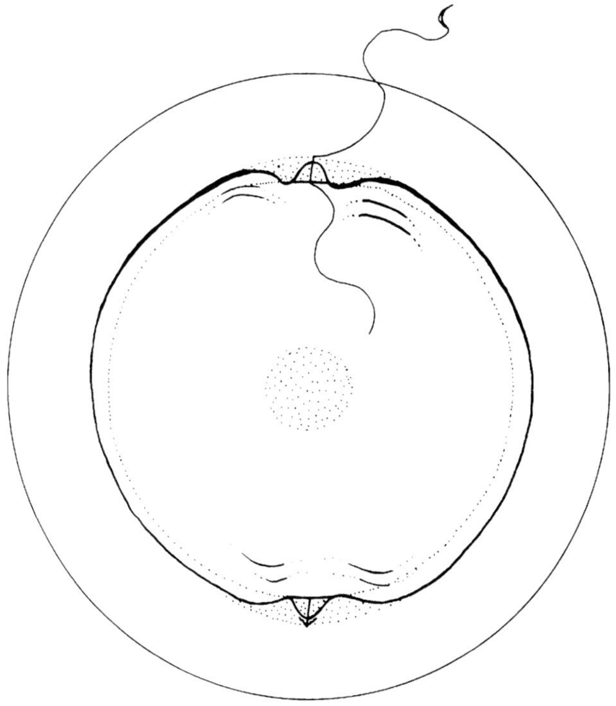

FIGURE 39-8 The second suture is placed 180 degrees from the first suture and should distribute the tissue lens evenly.

stream of fluid carries any foreign material directly into the suction tube.

When all foreign material has been washed from both sides of the tissue lens and Bowman's layer, the tissue lens is placed on the patient's cornea stroma side down. It is not difficult to tell which side of the tissue lens is which: Bowman's layer is shiny and the stroma is dull. Also, the tissue lens assumes a shape much like that of a contact lens, with a convex surface (Bowman's layer) and a concave surface (stroma). Because the diameter of the tissue lens is 8.5 mm and the diameter of the trephine cut is 7.0 mm, the tissue lens appears oversized. The excess tissue is required so that the wing of the tissue lens can be placed beneath the corneal surface without tension, as described below. After the tissue lens is centered, it and the surrounding cornea may be marked for even suture placement by centering a radial marker inked with gentian violet and pressing it on the surface of the tissue lens and surrounding cornea.

Sixteen interrupted 10-0 nylon sutures (16 to 24 sutures in children) are used to attach the tissue lens to the cornea. A Polack forceps is used to grasp the tissue lens for the first suture bite. The needle is placed through the midstroma of the wing. The wing is not merely impaled, which would be technically easier: it is split horizontally by the needle. The first suture is placed superiorly, with a 0.75-mm bite of the wing of the tissue lens and a 1-mm bite of the patient's cornea that passes through the peripheral end of the lamellar keratotomy created by the lamellar dissector (Figure 39-7). This anchors the wing so that it cannot escape the keratotomy and appear above the corneal surface at a later date, causing central corneal flattening in that meridian. The suture is tied with a triple-throw followed by two single-throws.

The next seven sutures are placed in the same fashion. As in penetrating keratoplasty, the second suture is the most important suture and should be placed 180 degrees from the first suture in such a way that the wing of the tissue lens is distributed evenly on both halves of the trephine cut (Figure 39-8). The tissue lens is translucent, and it is easy to see the trephine cut through the tissue. Marking the tissue lens and cornea with gentian violet as described above helps with even placement of the sutures. The sutures are tied so that there are no tension folds across the surface of the tissue lens and no compression of the underlying cornea.

After the first eight sutures have been placed by direct visualization, a Barraquer iris sweep is used to push the wing of the tissue lens below the recipient lip so that it lies in the peripheral lamellar keratotomy created by the lamellar dissector (Figure 39-9). The sutures are rotated so that the suture ends trail behind the knot, forming small arrows pointed toward the limbus (Figure 39-10). To accomplish this, the knots are rotated into the tissue lens and then into the patient's cornea, leaving the suture ends streaming behind. This prevents the knots from becoming impaled like small fishhooks in the peripheral cornea and makes it easy to remove the sutures postoperatively. If a

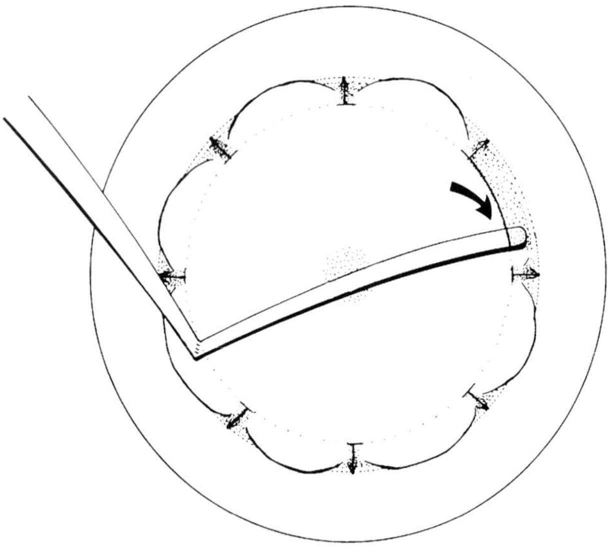

FIGURE 39-9 The edge of the tissue lens is tucked beneath the surface of the cornea after the first eight sutures are placed.

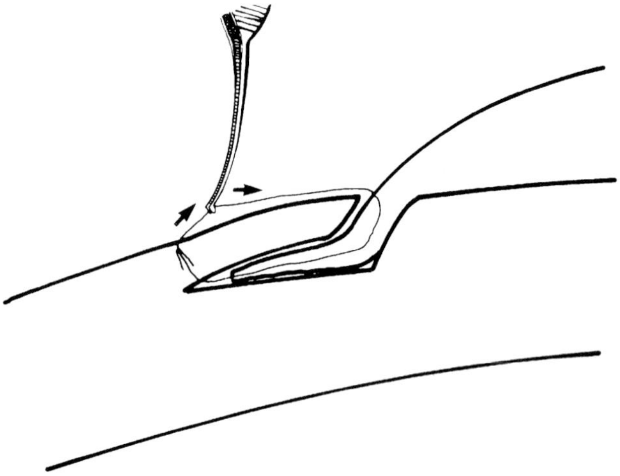

FIGURE 39-10 The sutures are rotated so that the knots lie beneath the surface of the patient's cornea and the suture ends form arrows pointing toward the corneal surface.

knot cannot be rotated into the tissue lens, it is rotated toward the limbus and a small, reverse direction movement is performed to be certain that the suture ends are streaming in the appropriate direction.

After the wing is placed in the lamellar keratotomy, the next eight sutures are placed between the first eight sutures by means of indirect visualization. Because the edge of the wing is now below the surface of the cornea, the surgeon can only guess at the exact location of the needle as it passes through the wing. The needle is placed precisely at the edge of the trephine cut and passed straight down, out, and up for 1 mm (Figure 39-11). This bite should be

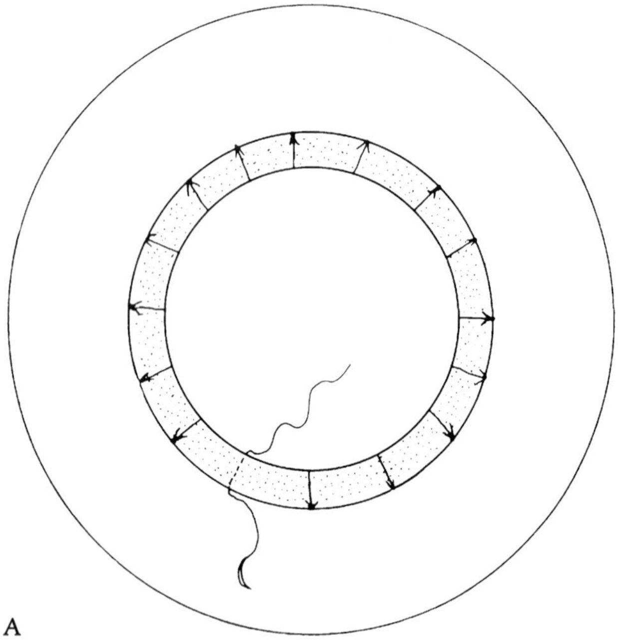

A

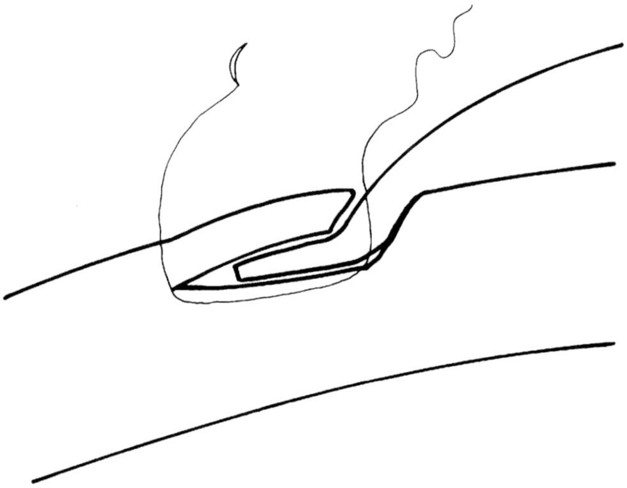

B

FIGURE 39-11 In the placement of the second eight sutures, no attempt is made to split the wing of the tissue lens with the needle. (A) Top view. (B) Side view.

fairly deep, so that the wing is impaled at least once. After the second eight sutures have been placed and tied, the knots are rotated as described above.

After all the sutures have been placed and rotated (Figure 39-12), a surgical keratoscope is used to determine the sphericity of the anterior surface. As much as 15 diopters of astigmatism can easily be induced accidentally, with no folds appearing on the surface of the tissue lens, and no other signs visible to the surgeon. It is important that the eyelid speculum be held up and away from the globe while the eye is checked for sphericity, lest it inadvertently compress the eye and cause distortion. The surface must be irrigated frequently to obtain a clear reflection. With most of the currently available surgical keratoscopes, a slightly oval reflection indicates that there are at least 2 or 3 diopters of corneal astigmatism. A more markedly oval reflection indicates a greater degree of astigmatism, usually caused by tight sutures in the short axis of the oval (Figure 39-13A). Tight sutures are replaced until the reflection from the keratoscope is spherical. (Occasionally, the oval reflection is caused not by tight sutures in the short axis of the oval, but by loose sutures in the long axis of the oval [Figure 39-13B]; these can also be replaced.) Additionally, a hand-held slit beam can be passed at a 45-degree angle over the corneal surface from all four quadrants to detect compression folds in the patient's cornea that are directed toward a tight suture. Nondirectional folds appear at the end of the case because pressure on the eye during epithelial removal and suturing causes hypotony. If the folds all point toward one or two tight sutures, however, the sutures should be replaced. Although these adjustments must be made at the end of a case, when the surgeon may be fatigued, they are well worth the effort, because they go a long way toward eliminating undercorrection and astigmatism, two of the major optical complications of this procedure.

After it has been established that the corneal surface is spherical and the surgeon has rechecked once again that the wing is below the surface of the patient's cornea between the interrupted sutures, gentamicin and 5 percent homatropine drops are instilled and a bandage soft contact lens is placed on the eye. Methylprednisolone acetate (80 mg) and gentamicin (40 mg) are injected sub-Tenon's; no corticosteroids are given to children. The rectus bridle sutures are removed, the eyelid speculum is removed, the eyelids are closed, and a patch and a metal or plastic eye shield are applied.

In adults, a temporary bow-tie tarsorrhaphy may be used instead of the bandage lens and patch. The tarsorrhaphy consists of one to three 5-0 nylon mattress sutures placed through the eyelid margins and tightened until the eyelids blanch. The sutures loosen slightly during the first few hours after they are tied. No bolsters are used. The bow-tie configuration, in which the sutures are not tied in knots but in a bow tie with long ends that are taped on the forehead, permits the tarsorrhaphy to be opened, the eye examined, and the sutures tied again if necessary without having to replace the sutures. The tarsorrhaphy is maintained for 3 weeks, by which time the tissue lens is usually completely re-epithelialized.

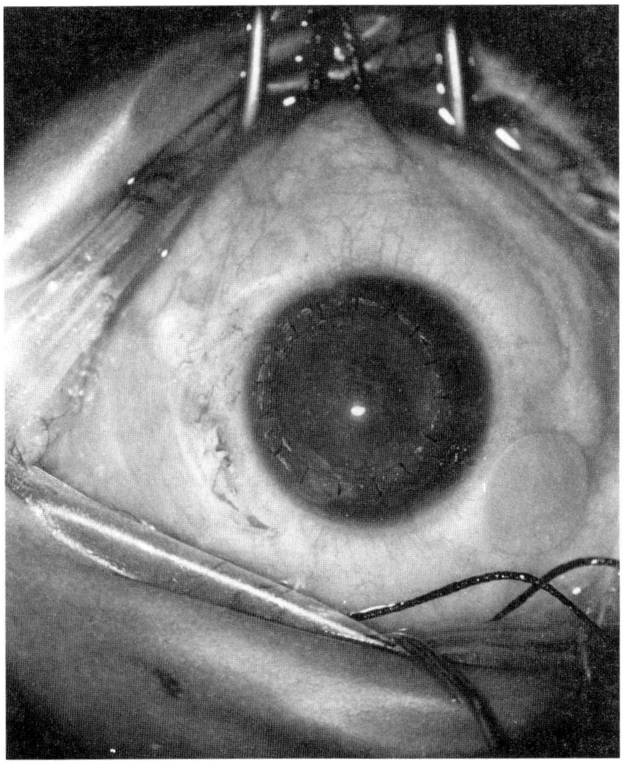

FIGURE 39-12 With all 16 sutures in place, no distortion of the tissue lens is visible. Folds in the patient's cornea are the result of intraoperative hypotony and resolve within a few days. The macula protector has been removed from the visual axis and can be seen in the lower right area of the figure.

POSTOPERATIVE CARE

Epikeratophakia is usually done as outpatient surgery, and patients are discharged in the afternoon on the day of their surgery. Acetaminophen with codeine is prescribed as needed for discomfort. The patient is seen the day after surgery, at which time the eye shield and patch are removed. Approximately 80 percent of patients comfortably wear the bandage lens that was placed at the time of surgery, and the bandage lens allows them to open the eyelids while the epithelium grows over the surface of the tissue lens.

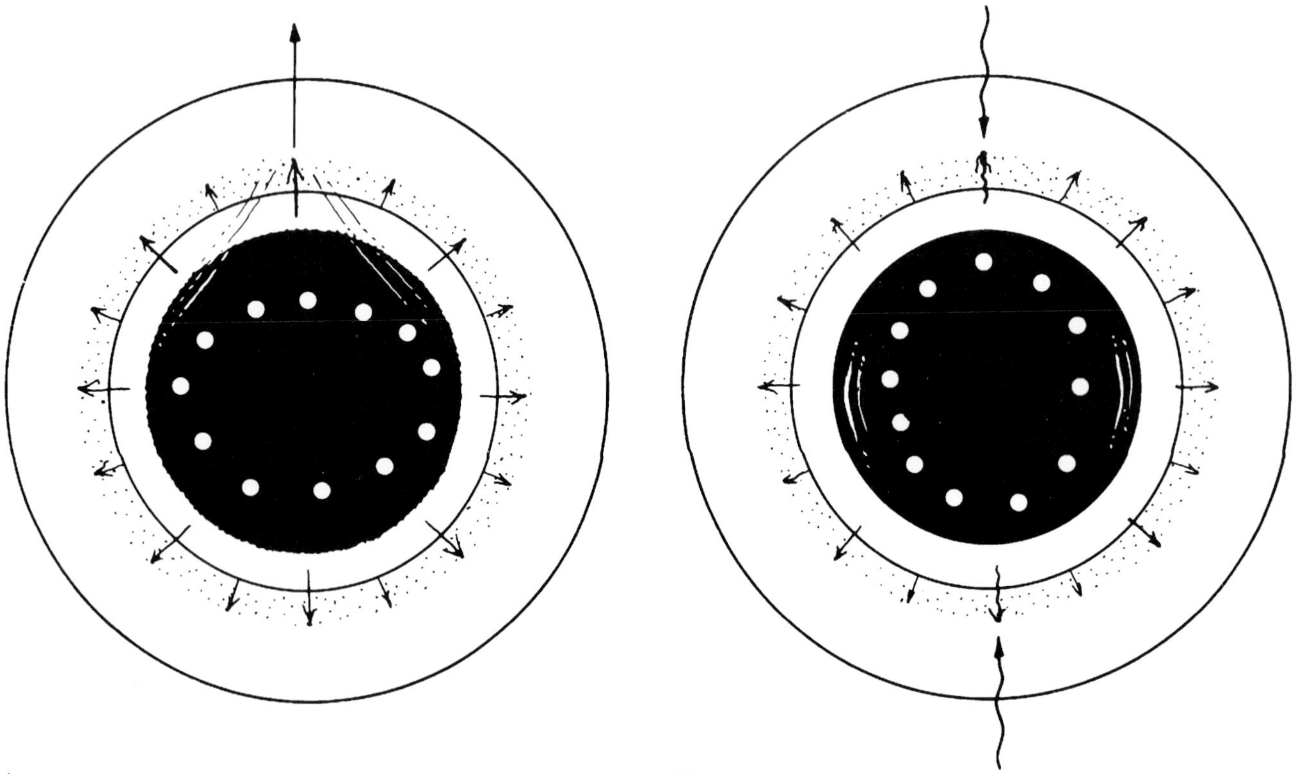

A B

FIGURE 39-13 **(A)** A tight suture steepens the tissue lens in the meridian of the suture, causing the reflection of the lights from the keratoscope to assume an oval shape, with the short axis of the oval in the steep meridian. **(B)** Loose sutures flatten the tissue lens in the meridian of the sutures, producing an oval with the long axis in the flat meridian.

Approximately 20 percent of patients have discomfort caused by a tight bandage lens on the first postoperative day; in these instances, the bandage lens is removed and the eye is patched daily until re-epithelialization is complete. If the bandage lens is tight but the patient is comfortable, the lens is left in place because a tight lens supports re-epithelialization better than a loose one.

After the first postoperative visit, the patient administers homatropine and gentamicin drops to the eye twice a day, uses sunglasses during the day for protection and to decrease photophobia, and sleeps with an eye shield in place at night. The eye is examined every 24 to 48 hours until re-epithelialization is complete. If it is difficult to see the edge of the epithelium through the bandage lens, topical fluorescein may be instilled and a sterile cotton-tipped applicator used to move the lens gently so that fluorescein seeps under the lens and stains the defect. Although fluorescein stains soft contact lenses, the stain does not affect the fit, comfort, or performance of the lens, and the bright yellow color fades within a few hours because of marked tearing during the early postoperative period. This technique allows the surgeon to move the lens and see beneath it without the trauma of lens removal and reinsertion, an act which, in itself, may remove delicate new epithelium. In adult patients, re-epithelialization is usually complete in 4 to 7 days. The bandage lens or patch is removed as soon as re-epithelialization is complete.

For pediatric patients, a bandage lens may be placed on the eye at the end of surgery or, in the case of older children, the eye can be pressure patched until the epithelial cover is complete. Oral amoxicillin is administered (20 mg/kg/day in three divided doses) for 2 to 3 weeks. Young children also wear a clear plastic eye shield with holes through which the parent instills gentamicin and atropine ointments onto the eyelids twice a day. Body heat melts the ointments, which seep into the eye, permitting regular medication without a parent/child battle. In children, the tissue lens often re-epithelializes within 3 to 4 days. The bandage lens may be left in place until the time of an examination under anesthesia (2 to 3 weeks after surgery). At that time, the bandage lens and sutures are removed simultaneously.

In adults, as soon as the patching or bandage lens is discontinued, the homatropine and gentamicin drops are also stopped. Erythromycin ointment or a lubricating ointment without preservatives is used to coat the delicate new epithelium for the next month, starting with four times a day and tapering to no ointment by the end of the month.

A refraction is done as soon as re-epithelialization is complete. Although there is usually a moderate amount of irregular astigmatism caused by the newly formed epithelial surface, this refraction can disclose marked undercorrection and/or astigmatism at a time when suture removal may correct the problem. If the patient is found to be markedly undercorrected, sutures are removed immediately. For example, if an aphakic patient with a preoperative refraction of +12.00 diopters has a refraction of +7.00 diopters during the first week after surgery, at least half of the sutures should be removed and another refraction performed within 24 to 48 hours, followed by removal of the remaining sutures if undercorrection persists.

It is not unusual to have an overcorrection during the first several weeks after surgery when the tissue lens is swollen. In particular, the tissue lens for the correction of myopia tends to provide an interval of overcorrection toward hyperopia that peaks between 2 and 6 months after surgery. Because it is a normal part of the healing process for all tissue lenses to be somewhat swollen for a period of time (which results in an overcorrection), an extreme undercorrection noted during the first week or two is an indication for early suture removal.

Many surgeons do not refract their patients for 1 to 2 months after surgery, by which time the opportunity to correct suturing errors has been lost. Even if the patient has not yet regained best-corrected visual acuity (for instance, if a patient who saw 20/20 preoperatively sees only 20/70 during the first week postoperatively), early refraction is still valuable, because marked undercorrection and astigmatism can be easily treated at this time, avoiding the necessity for relaxing incisions or other secondary surgical interventions at a later date.

If marked undercorrection and astigmatism are not present, and a refraction of plano (or an overcorrection) is found during the first few weeks, the sutures are usually removed 3 weeks after surgery. Loose or neovascularized sutures are removed whenever they are noted—as early as 24 to 48 hours after surgery, if necessary—because loose sutures cause pain, collect mucus, attract blood vessels, promote the formation of sterile abscesses, and increase the risk of infection. Sutures to be removed are cut and pulled out so that the knot emerges from the peripheral corneal side, rather than from the central tissue lens side. Otherwise, an iatrogenic dehiscence of the tissue lens may be created as the knot passes out through the tissue lens and drags the wing of the lens out of the lamellar keratotomy. All sutures are removed within 3 weeks in adult patients and within 2 weeks in children.

The tissue lenses clear more slowly in older patients than in younger patients; most of the adult aphakic patients are in the older age group. The average aphakic patient regains functional vision (20/50 to 20/400) within 1 to 3 weeks after surgery. However, most of these patients require 2 months to achieve a visual acuity within two lines of their preoperative best-corrected visual acuity. The average adult achieves best-corrected visual acuity and final refraction at 2 to 4 months postoperatively, although a few patients (usually the very elderly) require up to 6 months.[23] Occasionally, visual acuity may continue to improve for as long as 12 months postoperatively, but this is unusual. In the average aphakic infant or child, the tissue lens clears rapidly, and patching of the unoperated eye may be undertaken 1 to 2 weeks after suture removal (3 to 4 weeks after surgery) to treat amblyopia. The rapid clearing of the tissue lens in children shortens the period of visual deprivation, which enhances the value of epikeratophakia in the treatment of amblyopia.[24] The results of one study of pediatric epikeratophakia for various indications[45] are shown in Table 39-1 and Table 39-2. One year after surgery, 68 percent of eyes were within 1 diopter of emmetropia and 92 percent were within 3 diopters.

The tissue lenses for myopia, which are thinner than those for aphakia, clear more rapidly even in adults. On the average, a myopic patient with excellent preoperative best-corrected visual acuity can usually see between 20/50 and 20/400 without correction within the first 24 hours postoperatively, although visual acuity fluctuates during the ensuing months.[25] A myopic patient can almost always be refracted to 20/50 or better during the first 2 months, although the refraction may vary from visit to visit. It is typical for a myopic patient to be overcorrected by several diopters; this hyperopia usually peaks between 2 and 4 months, but sometimes as long as 6 months, after surgery; the overcorrection gradually decreases thereafter as the hydration of the tissue lens normalizes.

At any given time during the overcorrected period, however, uncorrected visual acuity is better than would be expected on the basis of refraction. For example, a patient with -15.00 diopters of myopia preoperatively may have a refraction of +3.00 or +4.00 diopters during the second to fourth postoperative month, with an uncorrected visual acuity of 20/50. During this period, the surgeon may be concerned about the hyperopia, but the patient usually has good distance vision and is less concerned. The last visual component to be restored is the ability to read at near. Often, myopic patients see 20/20 uncorrected by 3 or 4 months but may not be able

TABLE 39-1
Long-Term Results of Epikeratophakia in Children[a]

Type of Cataract	*Number of Eyes*	*Mean Age at Refractive Surgery*	*Graft Success (%)*	*Visual Acuity*		
				20/20 to 20/40	*20/50 to 20/200*	*Worse than 20/200*
Congenital cataract, age younger than 12 mo	2	11.0 ± 1.4 mo	50	0	0	1
Congenital cataract, age 12–24 mo	6	17.3 ± 2.7 mo	83	0	2	1
Congenital cataract, age older than 24 mo	6	35.7 ± 7.5 mo	100	0	5	1
Incomplete congenital cataract	13	7.7 ± 2.9 yr	100	5	8	0
Traumatic cataract	15	7.2 ± 4.3 yr	94	4	8	1
Bilateral cataracts	31	48.4 ± 51.4 mo	88	2	11	5
Secondary cataract (uveitis)	9	10.6 ± 24.1 yr	100	2	4	3
TOTAL	82	NR	92	13	38	12

Abbreviation: NR, not reported.
[a] Follow-up ranged from 3 to 5 years. Visual acuity measurements given for 63 children who had successful grafts and who were able to cooperate with evaluation.
Source: Adapted with permission from RJ Uusitalo, HM Uusitalo: Long-term follow-up of pediatric epikeratophakia. J Refract Surg 13:45, 1997.

to read small print with that eye for 6 to 7 months. The reasons for the disparity between distance and near visual acuity are not clear. However, it is a temporary problem, and patients under 40 years of age do well if they are warned in advance that they may need reading glasses for a few months.

TABLE 39-2
Residual Refractive Error in 74 Eyes 1 Year after Pediatric Epikeratophakia

Residual Refractive Error	*Number of Eyes (%)*
Residual Myopia (*diopters*)	
0.00 to −0.50	29 (39.2)
−0.75 to −1.00	7 (9.5)
−1.25 to −2.00	6 (8.1)
−2.25 to −3.00	0 (0)
−3.25 to −6.00	2 (2.7)
−6.25 to −10.00	2 (2.7)
Residual Hyperopia	
+0.25 to +0.50	8 (10.8)
+0.75 to +1.00	6 (8.1)
+1.25 to +2.00	7 (9.5)
+2.25 to +3.00	5 (6.8)
+3.25 to +6.00	2 (2.7)
+6.25 to +10.00	0 (0)

Source: Adapted with permission from RJ Uusitalo, HM Uusitalo: Long-term follow-up of pediatric epikeratophakia. J Refract Surg 13:45, 1997.

COMPLICATIONS

The most common complications of epikeratophakia for aphakia or myopia can be divided into two groups: medical and optical. Most medical complications occur during the first few weeks after surgery. The optical complications, which are nearly always created by surgical error, manifest 4 to 6 months postoperatively.

Medical Complications

Chronic epithelial defects that lead to either scarring or melting of the tissue lens are the most common cause of failure and/or removal of the tissue lens in adult and pediatric aphakic patients. Adult patients often have severe external disease, such as blepharitis, dry eyes, and/or lagophthalmos, which must be looked for, diagnosed, and treated aggressively before surgery. If lagophthalmos is severe, surgery to raise or tighten the lower eyelid may be necessary. Blepharitis and dry eyes must be treated for at least 2 months before surgery to establish that the patient is compliant and that it is understood that his or her external disease is chronic, that it will not disappear after surgery, and that therapy must continue after surgery if surgery is to be successful. Untreated blepharitis can cause marginal ulcers and peripheral vascularization in the tissue lens as easily as it can in an unoperated cornea. If patients with blepharitis and dry eyes are treated aggressively for only 24 to 48 hours before surgery, their eyes can be suitably prepared for surgery, but without continued treatment after surgery, the tissue lens may succumb to the same external forces that afflict the patient's own cornea.

If an adult patient has an epithelial defect of the same size on two consecutive visits during the early postoperative re-epithelialization period, the therapy that was initiated immediately after surgery is altered. For example, if a patient wearing a bandage soft contact lens has a defect that is the same size on two consecutive visits, the lens is removed and the eye is patched. If the defect does not heal with patching, a different type of bandage lens is tried.

If the defect still fails to heal, a temporary bow-tie tarsorrhaphy is performed, as described above. Central "peephole" tarsorrhaphies or lateral tarsorrhaphies are of no use in aiding re-epithelialization. Only complete eyelid closure can promote healing. A patient with a tarsorrhaphy continues to use gentamicin and homatropine drops, but instills them while lying down. The drops are placed over the caruncle, from which they trickle down through the eyelids. The tarsorrhaphy is not opened for 7 days unless the patient complains of pain, discharge, or eyelid swelling, at which time the bow-tie is untied, the eyelids opened, and the eye examined.

If after 7 days the defect has healed, the temporary tarsorrhaphy is taken down. If the defect is the same size or smaller, the sutures are retied. If the defect is larger and the tissue lens is melting, the tarsorrhaphy is taken down and the tissue lens is removed. The temporary tarsorrhaphy may be maintained for a total of 3 weeks (one must remember that chronic defects heal more slowly than normal corneal abrasions). If, however, the defect persists for 21 days after the tarsorrhaphy was performed, even if it is smaller, the tissue lens must be removed.

If a chronic epithelial defect heals in just under 3 weeks, the tissue lens may survive, but there may be residual epithelial or subepithelial haze that decreases vision or causes glare if it is located near the visual axis.

If a chronic epithelial defect in the tissue lens persists for 3 weeks or longer, the tissue lens may melt. A melting tissue lens may appear as homogeneous, gray-white viscous material that can be mistaken for purulence by an inexperienced observer. However, an eye with a melting tissue lens may be less inflamed than an eye with an active infection, and purulence is more opaque than melted cornea. The chalky-white color of purulence and the translucent gray-white appearance of sterile melted corneal tissue are obviously different when viewed side by side, but can be difficult to distinguish when only one of the two is seen.

Epithelium left in the interface during surgery can form cysts, which may be opaque and/or may cause irregular astigmatism. In children, epithelial ingrowth that enlarges and encroaches on the visual axis can be removed successfully by peeling back a small section of the tissue lens and curetting out the epithelial cells.[60] In adults, epithelial inclusion rests usually do not enlarge as they do in children, but they may occasionally enlarge enough to require surgical removal.[61]

Pneumococcal infection after epikeratophakia and temporary tarsorrhaphy in a handicapped pediatric patient,[62] sterile stromal melt of a tissue lens in an elderly man with diabetic retinopathy,[63] and recurrent subepithelial fibrosis in a 29-year-old man necessitating replacement of the tissue lens[64] have been reported.

Optical Complications

Undercorrections and occasional overcorrections are the most common reasons for removal of epikeratophakia tissue lenses for myopia. A few patients who have good dioptric results complain of glare or multiple images, which may also lead to removal of the tissue lens. The cause of these problems is faulty surgical technique.

As described above in the section on postoperative care, tight suturing of a tissue lens for myopia can cause undercorrection. Tight sutures pull the tissue lens taut across the cornea, flattening the anterior surface and pushing the shoulders posteriorly toward the patient's cornea, which then buckles into folds. The combination of flattened shoulders and corneal compression and folds causes undercorrection and glare (Figure 39-14).

If tight sutures are recognized soon after surgery, their removal may reverse the undercorrection. However, if they are not recognized until later, their removal will probably not reverse the undercorrection completely. In this case, a Barron radial vacuum trephine can be used to create a 360-degree relaxing incision.

In general, overcorrection is less common than undercorrection, but it is more common in myopic patients than in aphakic patients. It is the result of the wing not being tucked far enough down into the lamellar keratotomy created by the lamellar dissector. If an overcorrection remains stable for several visits and is still present 6 months after surgery, the tissue lens may be removed entirely, the corneal and tissue lens surfaces irrigated, and the tissue lens resutured more tightly into place. Again, the surgical keratoscope is used to check for large amounts of astigmatism. There is no need to obtain a new tissue lens; the old tissue lens will heal more rapidly after a resuturing procedure because it is already repopulated with keratocytes and covered with epithelium.

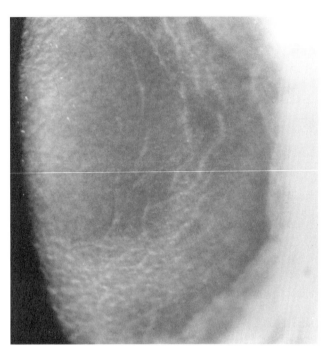

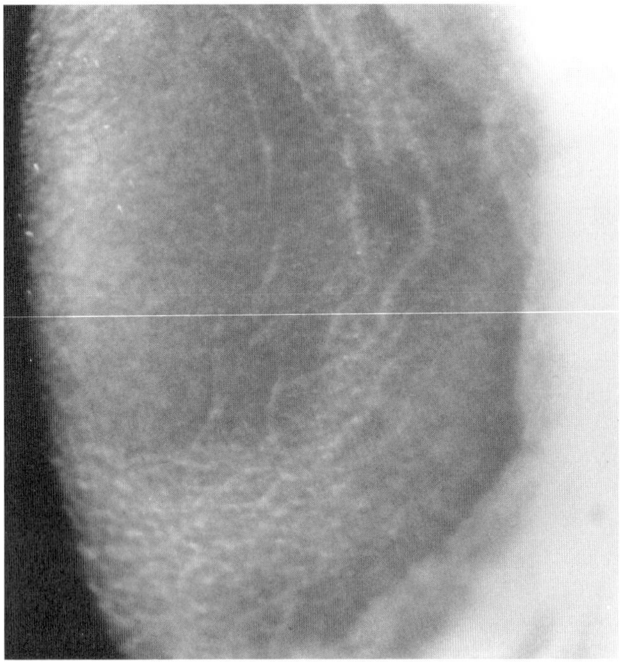

FIGURE 39-14 Compression of the underlying cornea by a tightly sutured tissue lens produces corneal folds that can cause glare.

However, resuturing a lens for overcorrection often causes undercorrection and, therefore, early and frequent refractions and early suture removal for undercorrection are recommended to adjust the refraction toward plano between 1 and 3 weeks after the resuturing procedure.

Another postoperative optical complication is astigmatism, which occurs more frequently if a surgical keratoscope is not used at the end of the case. If astigmatism persists after suture removal, the scar on one or both sides of the steep axis of the tissue lens can be broken for 90 degrees. The epithelium is removed peripheral to the wound in the area where the dehiscence will be done to avoid epithelial ingrowth under the tissue lens.

Separating the tissue lens from the underlying cornea permits the intraocular pressure to push against the patient's cornea and makes the tissue lens more spherical; it is a "one-size-fits-all" procedure for any degree of symptomatic astigmatism. It has been done successfully in cases with more than 10 diopters of astigmatism and in cases with as little as 1 diopter of astigmatism that caused multiple images in one meridian. This procedure can be done in minor surgery on an outpatient basis, and the eye is treated postoperatively as for a corneal abrasion, with dilation, antibiotic drops, and patching until any epithelial defects are healed.

If complications require the removal of a tissue lens, the wound is incised with a stainless steel blade (Figure 39-15A), and the anterior surface of the wing of the tis-

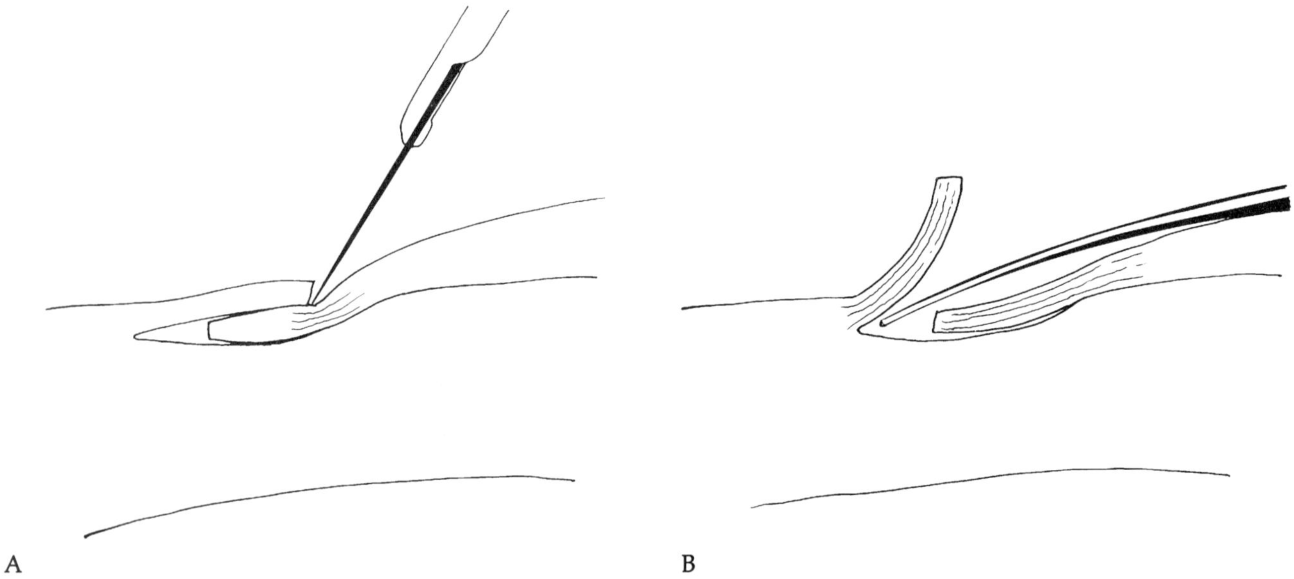

FIGURE 39-15 Removal of the tissue lens. **(A)** The wound edge is identified by gentle dissection with a stainless steel blade. **(B)** The anterior surface (Bowman's layer) of the tissue lens is loosened from the stroma of the patient's cornea with the tip of an iris sweep. *(continues)*

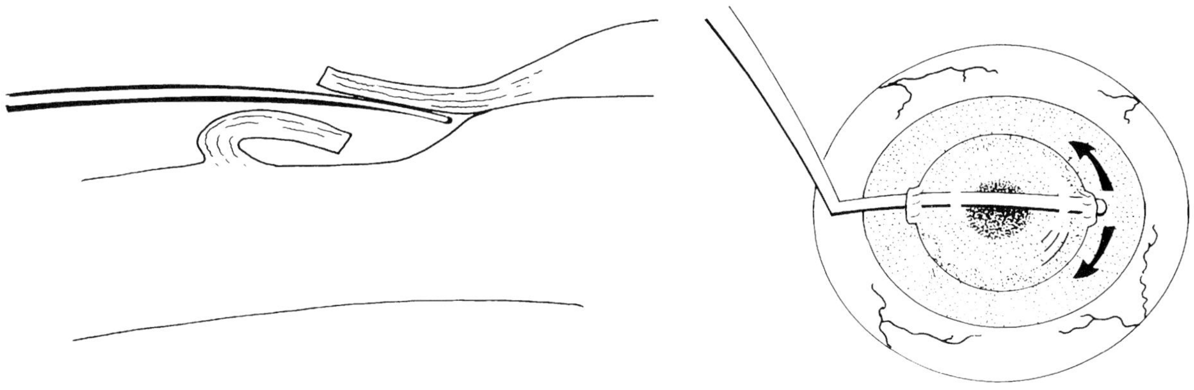

C D

FIGURE 39-15 *(continued)* (C) The posterior surface of the tissue lens is separated from the stromal surface of the peripheral lamellar dissection and the plane between the posterior (stromal) surface of the tissue lens and the anterior surface (Bowman's layer) of the patient's cornea is located with the tip of the iris sweep. (D) After the edge of the tissue lens is loosened in one place, the tip of the iris sweep is passed beneath the tissue lens to the opposite side, and the entire tissue lens is freed by sweeping the instrument back and forth.

sue lens that is tucked into the lamellar dissection is separated from the overlying cornea with an iris sweep (Figure 39-15B). This is easy to do because there is no scarring between Bowman's layer of the tissue lens and the patient's stroma. When the edge of the tissue lens is reached, the iris sweep is passed posteriorly to separate the posterior surface of the tissue lens from the patient's stroma in the area of the lamellar dissection (Figure 39-15C). There is usually a moderate amount of scarring in this area, but the tissues separate easily. In the central cornea, the plane between the posterior surface of the tissue lens and the anterior surface of the patient's cornea (Bowman's layer) is found, and the two are separated by the iris sweep. There is no scarring in this plane. If resistance is met, care is taken to be certain that the iris sweep is not separating the patient's corneal lamellae. The iris sweep is passed across the anterior surface of the patient's cornea to the other side of the wound, where it is pushed through the scar (Figure 39-15D). The tissue lens is removed in toto by passing the iris sweep around the wound for 360 degrees. The eye is treated postoperatively as for a corneal abrasion. In some circumstances, the tissue lens may be replaced with a new lens at the same time.

Photorefractive keratectomy for regression of effect after myopic epikeratophakia in five eyes was not successful.[65] However, photorefractive keratectomy in an aphakic epikeratophakia tissue lens was used successfully to correct a preablation refraction of -13.0 diopters, with no detectable haze 7 months after laser surgery.[66] Whether laser ablation can be used to correct astigmatism after epikeratophakia remains to be evaluated.

REFERENCES

1. Barraquer JI: Keratomileusis and keratophakia. p. 409. In Rycroft PV (ed): Corneoplastic Surgery: Proceedings of the Second International Corneo-Plastic Conference. Pergamon, New York, 1969
2. Kaufman HE: The correction of aphakia. Am J Ophthalmol 89:1, 1980
3. Werblin TP, Kaufman HE, Friedlander MH, Granet N: Epikeratophakia: the surgical correction of aphakia. III. Preliminary results of a prospective clinical trial. Arch Ophthalmol 99:1957, 1981
4. Werblin TP, Kaufman HE, Friedlander MH, et al: A prospective study of the use of hyperopic epikeratophakia grafts for the correction of aphakia in adults. Ophthalmology 88:1137, 1981
5. Werblin TP, Kaufman HE, Friedlander MH, et al: Epikeratophakia—the surgical correction of aphakia. Update 1981. Ophthalmology 89:916, 1982
6. McDonald MB, Koenig SB, Safir A, et al: Epikeratophakia: the surgical correction of aphakia. Update: 1982. Ophthalmology 90:668, 1983
7. Asbell PA, Werblin TP, Loupe DN, et al: Secondary surgical procedures after epikeratophakia. Ophthalmic Surg 13:555, 1982
8. Olson PF, McDonald MB, Werblin TP, Kaufman HE: The measurement of intraocular pressure after epikeratophakia. Arch Ophthalmol 101:1111, 1983
9. Guss RB, Asbell PA, Berkowitz RA, Kaufman HE: Endothelial cell counts after epikeratophakia surgery. Ann Ophthalmol 15:408, 1983
10. Morgan KS, Werblin TP, Asbell PA, et al: The use of epikeratophakia grafts in pediatric monocular aphakia. J Pediatr Ophthalmol Strabismus 18:23, 1981

11. Morgan KS, Werblin TP, Friedlander MH, Kaufman HE: Epikeratophakia in the pediatric patient. A case report. J Ocular Ther Surg 1:198, 1982
12. Morgan KS, Asbell PA, McDonald MB, et al: Preliminary visual results of pediatric epikeratophakia. Arch Ophthalmol 101:1540, 1983
13. Morgan KS, Asbell PA, May JG, et al: Pediatric epikeratophakia. p. 937. In Reinecke RD (ed): Strabismus II: Proceedings of the Fourth Meeting of the International Strabismological Association, October 25-29, Asilomar, CA. Grune & Stratton, Orlando, FL, 1984
14. Morgan KS, Stephenson GS, McDonald MB, Kaufman HE: Epikeratophakia in children. Ophthalmology 91:780, 1984
15. Werblin TP, Klyce SD: Epikeratophakia: the surgical correction of myopia. I. Lathing of corneal tissue. Curr Eye Res 1:591, 1981/1982
16. McDonald MB, Klyce SD, Suarez H, et al: Epikeratophakia for myopia correction. Ophthalmology 92:1417, 1985
17. Suarez E, Arffa RC, Salmeron B, et al: Efficacy of surgical modifications in myopic epikeratophakia. J Refract Surg 1:156, 1985
18. Kaufman HE, Werblin TP: Epikeratophakia for the treatment of keratoconus. Am J Ophthalmol 93:342, 1982
19. McDonald MB, Koenig SB, Safir A, Kaufman HE: Onlay lamellar keratoplasty for the treatment of keratoconus. Br J Ophthalmol 67:615, 1983
20. McDonald MB, Safir A, Waring GO, et al: A preliminary comparative study of epikeratophakia or penetrating keratoplasty for keratoconus. Am J Ophthalmol 103:467, 1987
21. Arffa RC, Busin M, Barron BA, et al: Epikeratophakia with commercially prepared tissue for the correction of aphakia in adults. Arch Ophthalmol 104:1467, 1986
22. McDonald MB, Kaufman HE, Durrie DS, et al: Epikeratophakia for keratoconus. The nationwide study. Arch Ophthalmol 104:1294, 1986
23. McDonald MB, Kaufman HE, Aquavella JV, et al: The nationwide study of epikeratophakia for aphakia in adults. Am J Ophthalmol 103:358, 1987
24. Morgan KS, McDonald MB, Hiles DA, et al: The nationwide study of epikeratophakia for aphakia in children. Am J Ophthalmol 103:366, 1987
25. McDonald MB, Kaufman HE, Aquavella JV, et al: The nationwide study of epikeratophakia for myopia. Am J Ophthalmol 103:375, 1987
26. McDonald MB: The current state of epikeratophakia. p.1. In Jakobiec FA, Sigelman J (eds): Advanced Techniques in Ocular Surgery. WB Saunders, Philadelphia, 1984
27. McDonald MB, Kaufman HE: Refractive keratoplasty. p. 276. In Steele ADMcG, Drews RC (eds): Cataract Surgery (Butterworths International Medical Reviews: Ophthalmology 2). Butterworths, London, 1984
28. McDonald MB, Kaufman HE: Refractive surgery for visual rehabilitation of aphakia. p. 622. In Ginsberg SP (ed): Cataract and Intraocular Lens Surgery: A Compendium of Modern Theories and Techniques. Vol. 2. Aesculapius, Birmingham, AL, 1984
29. McDonald MB, Kaufman HE: Epikeratophakia for aphakia, myopia, and keratoconus in the adult patient. p. 427. In Sanders DR, Hofmann RF, Salz JJ (eds): Refractive Corneal Surgery. Slack, Thorofare, NJ, 1986
30. Morgan KS, Arffa RC, Marvelli TL: Epikeratophakia in the pediatric patient. p. 451. In Sanders DR, Hofmann RF, Salz JJ (eds): Refractive Corneal Surgery. Slack, Thorofare, NJ, 1986
31. McDonald MB, Morgan KS, Kaufman HE: Epikeratophakia: theory, case selection, and major variables in success or failure. p. 498. In Brightbill FS (ed): Corneal Surgery: Theory, Technique, and Tissue. CV Mosby, St. Louis, 1986
32. Arffa RC, McDonald MB, Morgan KS, Kaufman HE: Adult and pediatric epikeratophakia—indications, techniques, and results. p. 230. In Stark JW, Terry AC, Maumenee AE (eds): Anterior Segment Surgery. IOLs, Lasers, and Refractive Surgery. Williams & Wilkins, Baltimore, 1987
33. Safir A, McDonald MB, Klyce SD, et al: The cornea press: restoring donor corneas to normal dimensions and hydration before cryolathing. Ophthalmic Surg 14:327, 1983
34. Safir A, McDonald MB, Friedlander MH, et al: Compensating for thermally caused dimensional changes in the cryolathe. Ophthalmic Surg 15:306, 1984
35. Young RD, Armitage WJ, Bowerman P, et al: Improved preservation of human corneal basement membrane following freezing of donor tissue for epikeratophakia. Br J Ophthalmol 78:863, 1994
36. Cheng HC, Armitage WJ, Yagoubi MI, Easty DL: Viability of keratocytes in epikeratophakia lenticules. Br J Ophthalmol 80:367, 1996
37. Hoyt CS: The optical correction of pediatric aphakia [editorial]. Arch Ophthalmol 104:651, 1986
38. Kelley CG, Keates RH, Lembach RG: Epikeratophakia for pediatric aphakia. Arch Ophthalmol 104:680, 1986
39. Uusitalo RJ, Lehtosalo J: Epikeratophakia in aphakic children. Am J Ophthalmol 103:465, 1987
40. Durrie DS, Habrich DL, Dietze TR: Secondary lens implantation vs epikeratophakia for the treatment of aphakia. Am J Ophthalmol 103:384, 1987
41. Lass JH, Stocker EG, Fritz ME, Collie DM: Epikeratoplasty. The surgical correction of aphakia, myopia, and keratoconus. Ophthalmology 94:912, 1987
42. Francis C, Rootman DS: Epikeratophakia for correction of complicated aphakia. Can J Ophthalmol 29:17:1994
43. Dullaert H, Foets BJ, Missotten L: Epikeratophakia, a valid surgical alternative for the treatment of selected patients with aphakia. Bull Soc Belge Ophtalmol 252:9, 1994
44. Cheng KP, Hiles DA, Biglan AW, et al: Risk factors for complications following pediatric epikeratoplasty. J Cataract Refract Surg 18:270, 1992
45. Uusitalo RJ, Uusitalo HM: Long-term follow-up of pediatric aphakia. J Refract Surg 13:45, 1997
46. Keates RH, Kelley CG: Epikeratophakia for myopia: preliminary considerations. J Refract Surg 1:25, 1985
47. Carney LG, Kelley CG: Visual losses after myopic epikeratoplasty. Arch Ophthalmol 109:499, 1991

48. Kim WJ, Lee JH: Long-term results of myopic epikeratoplasty. J Cataract Refract Surg 19:352, 1993
49. Choi S, Lee JH: Epikeratoplasty for myopia: 2-year results and a proposed nomogram. J Refract Surg 11:497, 1995
50. American Academy of Ophthalmology: Epikeratoplasty. Ophthalmic procedures assessment. Ophthalmology 103:983, 1996
51. Arffa RC, Marvelli TL, Morgan KS: Keratometric and refractive results of pediatric epikeratophakia. Arch Ophthalmol 103:1656, 1985
52. Morgan KS, Marvelli TL, Ellis GS, Arffa RC: Epikeratophakia in children with traumatic cataracts. J Pediatr Ophthalmol Strabismus 23:108, 1986
53. Arffa RC, Marvelli TL, Morgan KS: Long-term follow-up of refractive and keratometric results of pediatric epikeratophakia. Arch Ophthalmol 104:668, 1986
54. Morgan KS, Arffa RC, Marvelli TL, Verity SM: Five year follow-up of epikeratophakia in children. Ophthalmology 93:423, 1986
55. Morgan KS, Stephenson GS: Epikeratophakia in children with corneal lacerations. J Pediatr Ophthalmol Strabismus 22:105, 1985
56. Morgan KS, McDonald MB, Hiles DA, et al: The nationwide study of epikeratophakia for aphakia in older children. Ophthalmology 95:526, 1988
57. Arffa RC, Donzis PB, Morgan KS, Zhou YJ: Prediction of aphakic refractive error in children. Ophthalmic Surg 18:581, 1987
58. Retzlaff J, Sanders D, Kraff M: A Manual of Implant Power Calculations: SRK Formulas. Medford, OR, 1981. Available from authors
59. Brod RD, Barron BA, Suelflow JA, et al: Phototoxic retinal damage during refractive surgery. Am J Ophthalmol 102:211, 1986
60. Morgan KS, Beuerman RW: Interface opacities in epikeratophakia. Arch Ophthalmol 104:1505, 1986
61. Busin M, Cusumano A, Spitznas M: Epithelial interface cysts after epikeratophakia. Ophthalmology 100:1225, 1993
62. Busin M, Cusumano A, Spitznas M: Pneumococcal infection after temporary tarsorrhaphy for epikeratophakia. Refract Corneal Surg 8:375, 1992
63. Bechara SJ, Grossniklaus HE, Waring GO III: Sterile stromal melt of epikeratoplasty lenticule. Arch Ophthalmol 110:1528, 1992
64. Bechara SJ, Grossniklaus HE, Waring GO III: Subepithelial fibrosis after myopic epikeratoplasty: report of a case. Arch Ophthalmol 110:228, 1992
65. Colin J, Sangiuolo R, Malet F, Volant A: Photorefractive keratectomy following undercorrected myopic epikeratoplasties. J Fr Ophtalmol 15:384, 1992
66. Loewenstein A, Lipshitz I, Lazar M: Photorefractive keratectomy for the treatment of myopia after epikeratoplasty: a case report. J Refract Corneal Surg 10(suppl): S285, 1994

40

Principles of Excimer Laser Photoablation

MARGUERITE B. MCDONALD AND DEEPAK CHITKARA

This chapter reviews the principles of the argon-fluoride excimer laser and its interaction with corneal tissue.[1,2]

The use of the excimer laser for the correction of refractive errors, including myopia, astigmatism, and hyperopia, is discussed in Chapters 41, 42, and 43 . Its use for phototherapeutic keratectomy is covered in Chapter 30.

HISTORIC DEVELOPMENT

The term *excimer* is a contraction of the words *excited dimer* and refers to an excited molecular complex of two different elements. In 1975, xenon atoms were shown to react with halogens to form an unstable noble gas–halide compound that rapidly dissociated to the ground state with the release of ultraviolet photons.[3] Subsequently, mixtures of other rare gases and halogens also were found to emit ultraviolet light.[4–7] It was suggested that these emissions had potential as ultraviolet laser systems. In this type of laser, application of a high-voltage discharge (about 30,000 eV) across a chamber containing the rare gas–halide mixture ionizes the mixture, and the excited molecule so produced immediately dissociates to its ground state, releasing a photon of ultraviolet light with a wavelength determined by the mixture.[1] Mixtures of argon-fluoride (ArF), krypton-fluoride (KrF), xenon-chloride (XeCl), and xenon-fluoride (XeF) all have sufficient energies for practical surgical applications, but only the argon-fluoride combination has been found useful for corneal surgery. This mixture emits ultraviolet light with a wavelength of 193.3 nm in pulses of photons that last approximately 10 to 50 ns.

By late 1981, excimer lasers suitable in terms of size and reliability became available for general research.[1] It was at that time that Taboada et al[8] first described the damage done to the rabbit corneal epithelium by the 248-nm krypton-fluoride laser beam and the lack of damage caused by a low-energy argon-fluoride 193-nm beam. In 1983, Srinivasan[9] demonstrated the precision of an 193-nm laser; elegant studies including carving grooves cross-wise in a human hair, as well as studies of the relationship between beam energy and effect on a plastic test specimen, paved the way for biological and medical applications to come.

Trokel performed the first removal of corneal tissue with the 193-nm excimer laser in cadaver animal eyes and showed that tissue ablation is a threshold phenomenon[10] (i.e., a minimum energy is required for each pulse to ablate tissue; below that level, no ablation occurs regardless of the number of pulses[11]). The resulting surface is smooth and uniform to optical standards, with no collateral thermal damage to adjacent unirradiated tissue (Figure 40-1). These observations were confirmed by high-resolution scanning electron microscopy and transmission electron microscopy studies.[12–15]

One of the earliest ideas for use of the excimer laser was to make radial keratotomy–like linear excisions in corneal tissue with the excimer laser.[12,16,17] However, this approach failed to improve the predictability of refractive correction over that achieved with a diamond blade and was abandoned.[18–21]

Wide-area ablation of corneal tissue was first performed in 1984 to excise superficial fungal keratitis in a rabbit cornea.[22] Further studies showed that submicron amounts of corneal tissue could be removed over a relatively wide area, resulting in direct recontouring of the anterior corneal surface.[10,23,24] In 1986, Marshall et al[25] described wide-area ablation with the excimer laser for reshaping the cornea to provide refractive correction, termed *photorefractive keratectomy* or *PRK*. In this procedure, myopia could be corrected by ablating more tissue centrally than

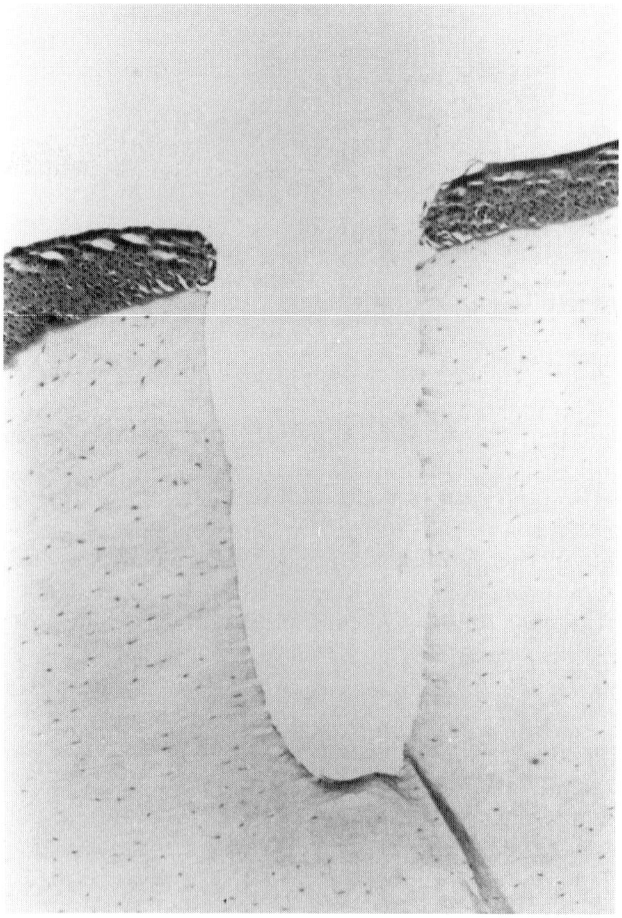

FIGURE 40-1 Histopathologic analysis shows an incisional groove made by the 193-nm argon-fluoride laser. (Courtesy of Stephen L. Trokel, M.D., New York, NY.)

peripherally, effectively flattening the central cornea (Figure 40-2). Hyperopia could be corrected by ablating more tissue peripherally than centrally, thereby effectively steepening the central cornea (Figure 40-3).

In 1988, Munnerlyn et al[26] published equations relating the diameter and depth of ablation to the desired refractive correction. They found that for a given amount of myopic correction, the maximum central depth of the ablation varies directly with the square of the diameter of the ablation zone, as given by the equation

$$t_0 \simeq -S^2 D/8\ (n-1),$$

where t_0 is the maximum central depth of the ablation in μm, S is the diameter of the ablation zone in mm, D is the amount of myopic correction in diopters, and n is the index of refraction of the cornea, which is 1.337 (Figure 40-4). Using Munnerlyn's equations, McDonald et al[27] showed for the first time that a stable refractive change could be created in nonhuman primate corneas by photorefractive keratectomy and that the corneas healed successfully and remained clear.

Also in 1988, the U.S. Food and Drug Administration (FDA) allowed VISX, Inc., in conjunction with the Louisiana State University Eye Center in New Orleans, to begin a Phase I study of photorefractive keratectomy for myopia on nine legally blind eyes.[28,29] The first sighted patient to undergo excimer laser photorefractive keratectomy for myopia was operated on by McDonald et al[28] in June 1988. Histopathology of excimer laser ablation in human eyes was reported by L'Esperance et al[30] in 1988 and McDonald et al[29] in 1990. Over the next few years, more than 2,000 sighted patients in the United States underwent photorefractive keratectomy under the auspices of various FDA study protocols.

In late 1995, the Summit excimer laser was approved for use in performing photorefractive keratectomy for the

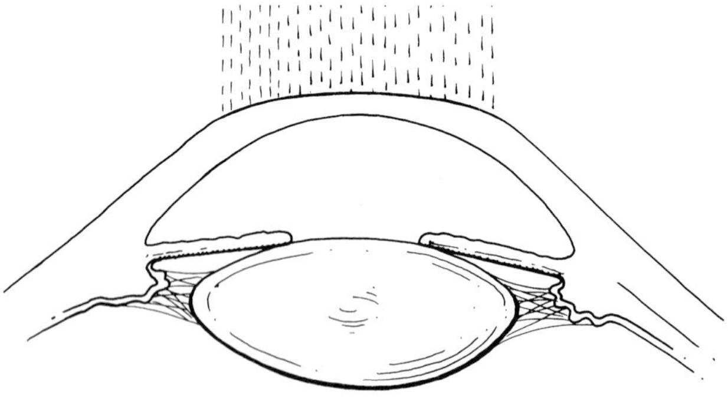

FIGURE 40-2 Photorefractive keratectomy for myopia.

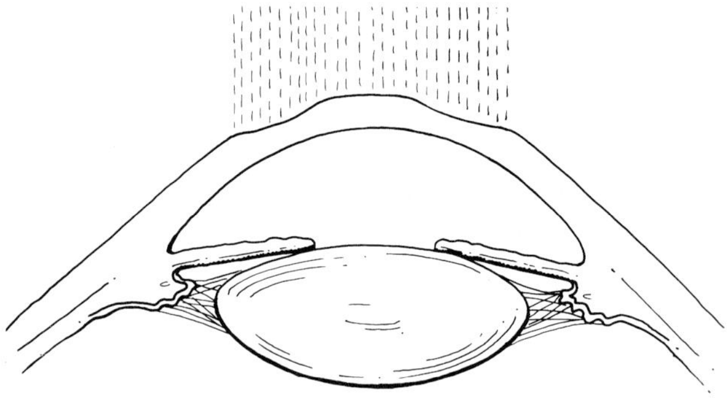

FIGURE 40-3 Photorefractive keratectomy for hyperopia.

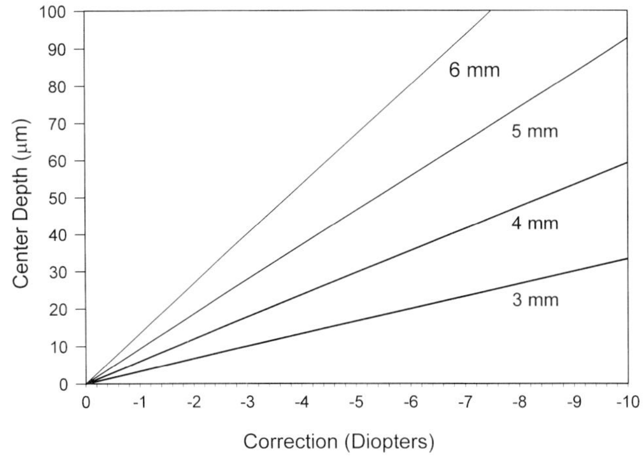

FIGURE 40-4 Depth of cut required for correction of myopia. Each line represents the central depth of cut for a given size treatment zone. For a given dioptric correction, larger diameter treatment zones require deeper ablations. (Reprinted with permission from CR Munnerlyn, SJ Koons, J Marshall: Photorefractive keratectomy: a technique for laser refractive surgery. J Cataract Refract Surg 14:46, 1988. © Journal of Cataract and Refractive Surgery.)

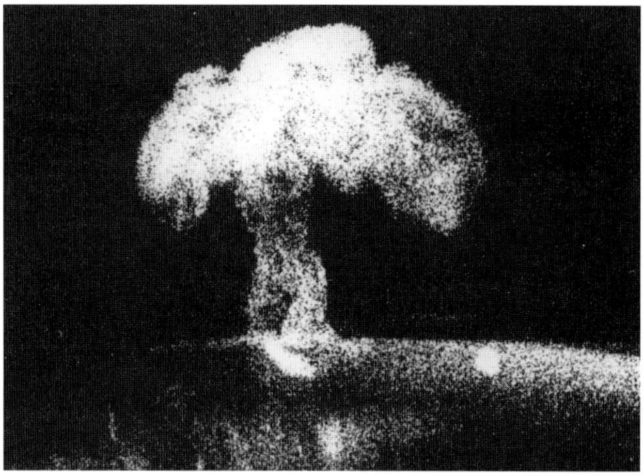

FIGURE 40-5 Ablation plume created at a wavelength of 193 nm and a fluence of 900 mJ/cm^2, shown 50 μs after the excimer pulse. (Reprinted with permission from CA Puliafito, D Stern, RR Krueger, ER Mandel: High-speed photography of excimer laser ablation of the cornea. Arch Ophthalmol 105:1255, 1987. Copyright 1987, American Medical Association.) (Courtesy of Carmen A. Puliafito, M.D., Boston, MA.)

treatment of 1.5 to 7.0 diopters of myopia in patients who are 21 years of age or older and have 1.5 or less diopters of astigmatism. In early 1996, the VISX laser was approved for the treatment of 1 to 6 diopters of myopia in patients who are 18 years of age or older and have 1.0 diopter or less of astigmatism. In early 1997, the VISX laser was approved for the treatment of 0.75 to 4.0 diopters of astigmatism in patients who are 21 years of age or older with up to 6 diopters of spherical myopia at the spectacle plane. (Approval for phototherapeutic keratectomy was granted to both companies before approval for photorefractive keratectomy—in early 1995 for Summit and in late 1995 for VISX.) Currently, these are the only two manufacturers approved by the FDA to market and sell their instruments in the United States. FDA-approved studies of new lasers from these and other companies are currently under way.

Newer lasers have diaphragms that open to control the ablation pattern, but they also have internalized ablation smoothing mechanisms. For instance, the Nidek EC5000 laser has a 7 mm by 2 mm beam that oscillates and rotates as the diaphragm opens, and the Chiron/Technolas Keracor 116 laser also has a beam that oscillates as the diaphragm opens. Other lasers, such as the Autonomous Technologies laser, have a 0.9-mm flying spot aided by an active eye tracker in an effort to make even smoother ablations. The tracking system was designed in anticipation of the ability to make individualized ablations for the correction of irregular astigmatism and spherocylindrical refractive errors guided by real-time corneal topographic evaluation.

MECHANISM OF ACTION

The 193-nm light emitted by the argon-fluoride laser produces its effect by breaking intramolecular bonds. Each photon produced by the laser has an energy of 6.4 eV, which is much greater than the energy required to break the bonds that hold molecules together. Once these bonds are broken, the molecules cannot be reassembled if the photon density exceeds a critical value. This process is called *ablative photodecomposition*, a term that "describes the effect of high energy photon application on material, inducing bond breaking and producing molecular fragments, elementary chemical compounds, bi- and tri-atomic particles, and ions."[31] The large increase in volume accompanied by the extra kinetic energy of the molecular fragments results in formation of a gas heated to 500°K, which is expelled as a plume of particulate matter at a speed of more than 3,000 m/s[32] (Figure 40-5). This gas is composed mainly of small molecular weight materials such as H_3O^- radicals and other simple carbons and hydrocarbons. Droplets or particles created by condensation of these

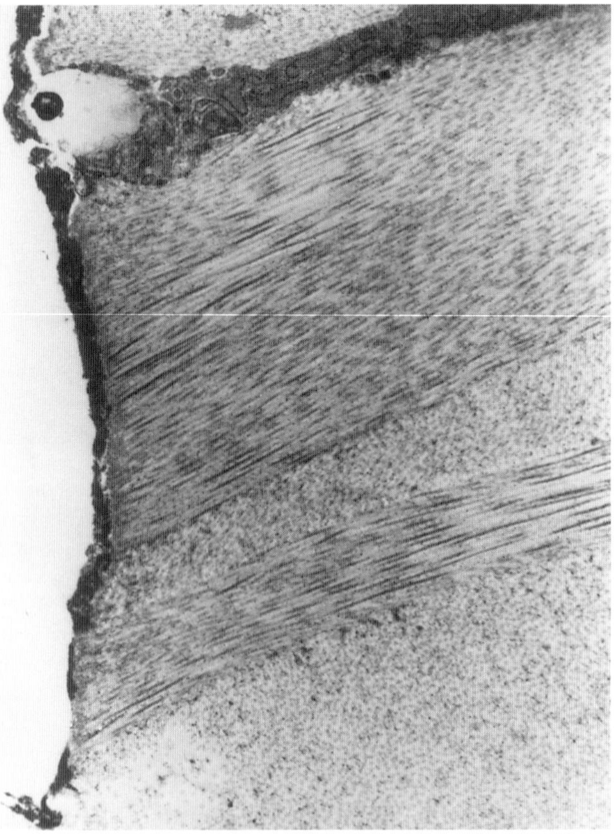

FIGURE 40-6 Transmission electron micrograph shows a pseudomembrane on the ablated surface. Collagen adjacent to the pseudomembrane shows no thermal damage or disruption. (Courtesy of Stephen L. Trokel, M.D., New York, NY.)

gaseous products may be responsible for steep central island formation after laser photoablation.[33]

The recoil caused by high-velocity ejection of the molecular fragments creates a surface wave on the cornea. This, together with an acoustic shock wave created by the impact of the laser pulse, creates an audible snap.[2] Both waves may lead to structural damage to adjacent tissues and the production of surface fluids from within the cornea.

The hot gas condenses on the relatively cold surface of the tissue adjacent to the ablation, creating a thin coating. This so-called *pseudomembrane,* which can be seen by electron microscopy (Figure 40-6), usually disappears within a few days. The pseudomembrane appears to temporarily maintain the integrity of lasered cells at the periphery of the ablation, and its smooth surface may facilitate re-epithelialization of the ablated area. It may also prevent significant stromal swelling that can result from the exposed stroma imbibing fluid from the tear layer. In a dehydrated cornea, the pseudomembrane is irregular in appearance, whereas in a normally hydrated cornea, the pseudomembrane is thin and uniform; it has been suggested that the water helps dissipate any heat generated during the laser procedure.[2]

Significant heat dissipation in the cornea can easily occur with a wide-beam laser operating at the standard repetition rate of 5 to 10 Hz, because the ablation process takes less than 100 ns. In addition, any possible thermal effects are noncumulative, in that each pulse ablates the tissue that was heated by the previous pulse. When wide-beam lasers were used under these conditions in clinical trials, the adjacent stromal tissue increased in temperature by only 5 to 10°C. Hence, the term *cold laser* has been used to describe the excimer laser.

CHARACTERISTICS OF CORNEAL ABLATION

Homogeneity of the laser beam is essential for a smooth ablation. The beam is rectangular as it leaves the laser cavity and may have energy spikes, or hot spots, within it that could cause differential ablation rates. Several methods of beam reshaping have been used, including rotating dove prisms, rotating slit beams, and absorbing cell systems, to compensate for any hot spots and make the beam more homogeneous.

The energy density of the beam is a measure of the amount of laser light energy per unit area and is expressed in mJ/cm^2; it is a function of energy output and beam diameter. The term *fluence* has become common parlance for this parameter and will be used here as well because of its widespread acceptance. It should be noted, however, that fluence is actually a measure of energy per volume, and the proper term for the cross-sectional light per unit area parameter is *irradiance.*[2]

Ablation of corneal tissue with the 193-nm excimer laser occurs at a threshold fluence of approximately 50 mJ/cm^2.[2] As fluence increases above this threshold, each pulse of laser light removes a precise quantity of corneal tissue. The amount of tissue removed per pulse increases as the fluence increases. For example, corneas treated with the Summit laser at 180 mJ/cm^2 have an ablation rate of 0.26 μm per pulse, and corneas treated with the VISX laser at 160 mJ/cm^2 have an ablation rate of 0.25 μm per pulse. More tissue is ablated per pulse when the fluence is high and the beam diameter is large. Consequently, a smaller number of pulses is required for the ablation, and the ablation takes less time, although the repetition rate must be less to allow for thermal relaxation. Such an ablation requires a laser system capable of producing large amounts of energy. These lasers are larger and more costly, use more gas, and more rapidly degrade their optical elements than lasers that produce lower amounts of energy. High fluences and wide beams are associated with larger acoustic shock waves, whereas lower fluences, especially if combined with increased repetition rates, can increase thermal effects unless the beam scans in the appropriate pattern to allow for thermal relaxation of the tissue before the next pass of the beam.

Some laser systems have a more or less homogeneous beam that removes a circular disc of corneal tissue of uniform thickness. Masking the laser beam with a computer-controlled iris diaphragm creates a series of concentric circular beams of increasing or decreasing diameters (depending on whether the diaphragm opens or closes), resulting in ablation of a concave keratectomy. In this way, steps of only 0.1 to 0.4 μm in height are created. Theoretically, the greater the number of steps, the greater the smoothness and the better the optical quality of the healed corneal surface.

A laser with a small-diameter circular beam or a narrow slit beam that moves rapidly across the cornea can also be used to perform wide-area ablations. These lasers produce less power and are smaller and less expensive than their high-powered, broad-beam counterparts. However, because of the rapid movement of these small-diameter beams, the repetition rate must also be correspondingly higher. At these high repetition rates, saccadic eye movements of the patient become increasingly significant and can cause increased surface roughness, resulting in optical haze. Optical eye tracking systems are necessary to overcome this problem.

The ablation rate varies with the level of corneal hydration. Deeper ablations occur when the cornea is dehydrated—that is, more tissue is removed per shot. Under- or overcorrection of 10 to 15 percent or more can result from hyperhydration or dehydration, respectively. Local hydration can be influenced by the amount of time needed to debride the corneal epithelium, the time required to perform the ablation, and the brightness of the operating microscope light. Dry gas blowing across the cornea can dehydrate the cornea and increase the ablation rate.

Corneal scars may have a much lower ablation rate than normal cornea and may even be resistant to ablation. The ablation rate may also be different for the corneal epithelium, Bowman's layer, and stroma, but this is the subject of some debate.[34] Such differences in ablation rate for various types of tissue under various conditions can induce undercorrections of up to 12 percent unless compensated for in advanced algorithms.

As ultraviolet light from the laser strikes the cornea, a photochemical transition causes release of a broad band of ultraviolet light longer in wavelength than that emitted by the laser. This is known as *secondary radiation* or *fluorescence* and can be seen as a faint, bluish light. Only 0.001 percent of incident ultraviolet light from the laser is converted to secondary radiation. The wavelength of laser-induced fluorescence of the epithelium (460 nm) is different from that of the stroma (310 to 320 nm), and the change in color can be used to monitor the removal of epithelium with the laser.[35] The penetration of secondary radiation into the cornea is minimal, because its fluence is less than 5 μJ/cm^2 (which is well below the thresholds for mutagenesis [10 μJ/cm^2] and photokeratitis).

HISTOLOGIC EFFECTS

Epithelium

The epithelial defect created by excimer laser ablation is rapidly covered, initially by epithelial cells sliding over the pseudomembrane that covers the ablated surface. Within the first 3 to 5 days, re-epithelialization is complete and the epithelium is three to five cell layers thick. Over the next 6 months, the epithelium becomes hyperplastic and continues to thicken. Clinically, this hyperplasia is thought to be responsible for at least some of the early regression of the refractive effect. (Although regression can continue for up to 18 months, later changes are more likely to be the result of stromal remodeling.)

Recurrent epithelial erosions after excimer laser ablation are rare, even though normal basement membrane regenerates incompletely.[36] Normal epithelial attachment complexes regenerate within weeks to months after the ablation, however[37] (Figure 40-7).

Bowman's Layer

Bowman's layer does not regenerate after excimer laser ablation. The clinical significance of this is unknown, although it seems evident that this layer is not essential for maintenance of corneal clarity. It has not been determined, however, whether an individual who lacks Bowman's layer is predisposed to rapid stromal involvement if the cornea becomes infected at a later date. It is also notable that with laser-assisted in situ keratomileusis, in which Bowman's layer is preserved, there appears to be less scarring and regression.

Stroma

Stromal changes following ablation evolve over a period of months or even years. Initially, as described above, a thin

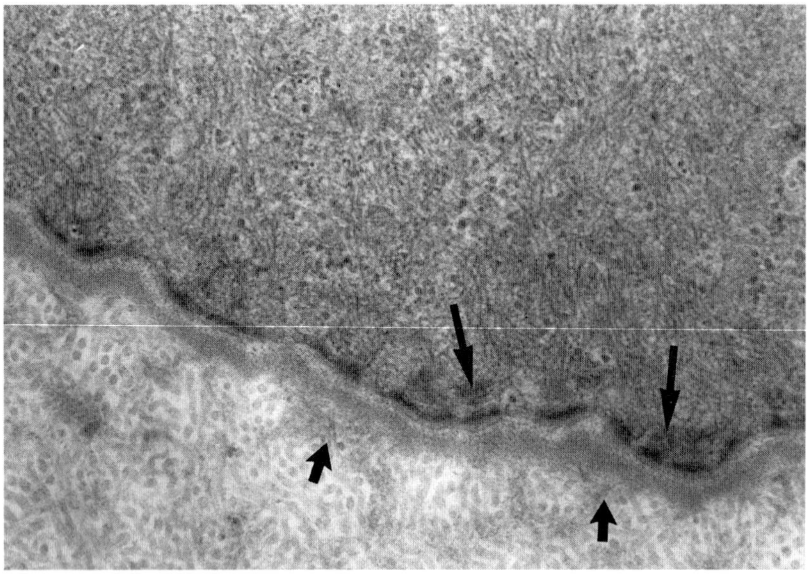

FIGURE 40-7 Transmission electron micrograph of the treated area of a monkey cornea 14 months after excimer laser surgery showing the presence of mature hemidesmosomes (long arrows) and anchoring filaments (short arrows.) (Original magnification × 70,000.) (Reprinted with permission from RW Beuerman, MB McDonald, RS Shofner, et al: Quantitative histological studies of primate corneas after excimer laser photorefractive keratectomy. Arch Ophthalmol 112:1103, 1994. Copyright 1994, American Medical Association.) (Courtesy of Roger W. Beuerman, Ph.D., New Orleans, LA.)

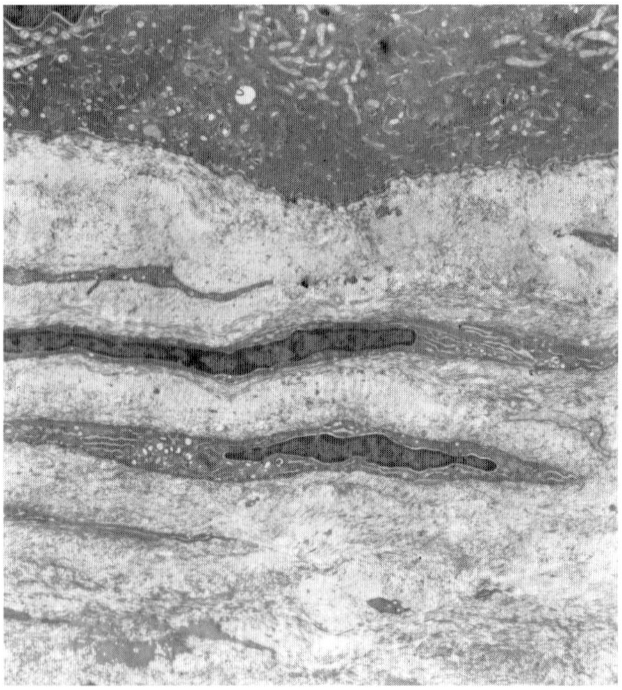

FIGURE 40-8 Monkey cornea with attempted 1.5-diopter correction obtained 14 weeks after excimer laser surgery. The basal lamina is unilaminar. Numerous hemidesmosomes connect the basal cells to the stroma by means of anchoring filaments. Fibroblastic keratocytes are seen in the anterior stroma. (Transmission electron microscopy, original magnification × 4,000.) (Reprinted with permission from MB McDonald, JM Frantz, SD Klyce, et al: One-year refractive results of central photorefractive keratectomy for myopia in the nonhuman primate cornea. Arch Ophthalmol 108:40, 1990. Copyright 1990, American Medical Association.) (Courtesy of Roger W. Beuerman, Ph.D., New Orleans, LA.)

pseudomembrane covers the ablated surface. Within the first 24 hours, inflammatory cells invade the stroma from the tear film. A few days after surgery, the pseudomembrane dissipates and the inflammatory cells and keratocytes disappear from the area beneath the ablation. Thereafter, the stromal keratocytes become fibroblastic, migrate into the zone of the ablation, and begin to produce new collagen and proteoglycans (Figure 40-8). The new collagen and vacuoles containing proteoglycans may be, in part, responsible for the high level of light scatter and corneal haze in the early postoperative period. The activated keratocytes can persist for up to 18 months.[38–44]

Descemet's Membrane

An unusual fibrillar response in the anterior portion of Descemet's membrane has been seen 6 to 15 months after ablation.[38] The nature of this response and its significance are unknown.

Endothelium

Acute endothelial cell loss is minimal unless the ablation approaches Descemet's membrane.[45] When the ablation comes within 40 μm of Descemet's membrane, the damage may be related to acoustic and shock waves. Short-term follow-up of 1 year or less in three studies of photorefractive keratectomy showed minimal endothelial cell loss (up to 3 percent).[46–48]

REFERENCES

1. Trokel S: History and mechanisms of action of excimer laser corneal surgery. p. 1. In Salz JJ, McDonnell PJ, McDonald MB (eds): Corneal Laser Surgery. Mosby–Year Book, St. Louis, 1995
2. Krueger RR, Binder PS, McDonnell PJ: The effects of excimer laser photoablation on the cornea. p. 11. In Salz JJ, McDonnell PJ, McDonald MB (eds): Corneal Laser Surgery. Mosby–Year Book, St. Louis, 1995
3. Velazco JE, Setser DW: Bound-free emission spectra of diatomic xenon halides. J Chem Phys 62:1990, 1975
4. Searles SK, Hart GA: Simulated emission at 281.88 nm from XeBr. Appl Phys Lett 27:243, 1975
5. Ewing JJ, Brau CA: Laser action on the $2\Sigma^+_{1/2} \rightarrow 2\Sigma^+_{1/2}$ bands of K or F and XeCl. Appl Phys Lett 27:350, 1975
6. Brau CA, Ewing JJ: Laser action on XeF. Appl Phys Lett 27:435, 1975
7. Hoffman JM, Hays AK, Tisone GC: High-power UV noble-gas–halide lasers. Appl Phys Lett 28:538, 1976
8. Taboada J, Mikesell GW Jr, Reed RD: Response of the corneal epithelium to KrF excimer laser pulses. Health Phys 40:677, 1981
9. Srinivasan R: Kinetics of the ablative photodecomposition of organic polymers in the far ultraviolet (193 nm). J Vac Sci Technol Bull 4:923, 1983
10. Kreuger RR, Trokel SL: Quantitation of corneal ablation by ultraviolet laser light. Arch Ophthalmol 103:1741, 1985
11. Srinivasan R, Braren B: Excimer laser surgery of the cornea. Am J Ophthalmol 96:710, 1983
12. Marshall J, Trokel S, Rothery S, Schubert H: An ultrastructural study of corneal incisions induced by an excimer laser at 193 nm. Ophthalmology 92:749, 1985
13. Puliafito CA, Steinert RF, Deutsch TF, et al: Excimer laser ablation of the cornea and lens. Experimental studies. Ophthalmology 92:741, 1985
14. Marshall J, Trokel SL, Rothery S, Krueger RR: A comparative study of corneal incisions induced by diamond and steel knives and two ultraviolet radiations from an excimer laser. Br J Ophthalmol 70:482, 1986
15. Kerr-Muir MG, Trokel SL, Marshall J, Rothery S: Ultrastructural comparison of conventional surgical and argon fluoride excimer laser keratectomy. Am J Ophthalmol 103:448, 1987
16. Cotliar AM, Schubert HD, Mandel ER, Trokel SL: Excimer laser radial keratotomy. Ophthalmology 92:206, 1985
17. Loertscher H, Mandelbaum S, Parrish RK II, Parel J-M: Preliminary report on corneal incisions created by a hydrogen fluoride laser. Am J Ophthalmol 102:217, 1986
18. Steinert RF, Puliafito CA: Corneal incision with the excimer laser. p. 401. In Sanders DR, Hofmann RF, Salz JJ (eds): Refractive Corneal Surgery. Slack, Thorofare, NJ, 1986
19. McDonald MB, Beuerman R, Falzoni W, et al: Refractive surgery with the excimer laser. Am J Ophthalmol 103:469, 1987
20. Seiler T, Bende T, Wollensak J, Trokel S: Excimer laser keratectomy for correction of astigmatism. Am J Ophthalmol 105:117, 1988
21. Bansal S, Salz JJ, Tenner A, et al: Clinicopathologic study of healing excimer laser radial excisions. Refract Corneal Surg 6:188, 1990
22. Serdarevic O, Darrell RW, Krueger RR, Trokel SL: Excimer laser therapy for experimental *Candida* keratitis. Am J Ophthalmol 99:534, 1985
23. Srinivasan R: Ablation of polymers and biological tissue by ultraviolet lasers. Science 234:559, 1986
24. Srinivasan R, Sutcliffe E: Dynamics of the ultraviolet laser ablation of corneal tissue. Am J Ophthalmol 103:470, 1987
25. Marshall J, Trokel S, Rothery S, Kruger RR: Photoablative reprofiling of the cornea using an excimer laser: photorefractive keratectomy. Lasers Ophthalmol 1:21, 1986
26. Munnerlyn CR, Koons SJ, Marshall J: Photorefractive keratectomy: a technique for laser refractive surgery. J Cataract Refract Surg 14:46, 1988
27. McDonald MB, Frantz JM, Klyce SD, et al: One-year refractive results of central photorefractive keratectomy for myopia in the nonhuman primate cornea. Arch Ophthalmol 108:40, 1990
28. McDonald MB, Kaufman HE, Frantz JM, et al: Excimer laser ablation in a human eye. Arch Ophthalmol 107:641, 1989
29. McDonald MB, Frantz JM, Klyce SD, et al: Central photorefractive keratectomy for myopia. The blind eye study. Arch Ophthalmol 108:799, 1990
30. L'Esperance FA Jr, Taylor DM, Warner JW: Human excimer laser keratectomy: short-term histopathology. J Refract Surg 4:118, 1988
31. Kermani O, Koort HJ, Roth E, Dardenne MU: Mass spectroscopic analysis of excimer laser ablated material from human corneal tissue. J Cataract Refract Surg 14:638, 1988
32. Puliafito CA, Stern D, Krueger RR, Mandel ER: High-speed photography of excimer laser ablation of the cornea. Arch Ophthalmol 105:1255, 1987
33. Noack J, Tönnies R, Hohla K, et al: Influence of ablation plume dynamics on the formation of central islands in excimer laser photorefractive keratectomy. Ophthalmology 104:823, 1997
34. Seiler T, Kriegerowski M, Schnoy N, Bende T: Ablation rate of human corneal epithelium and Bowman's layer with the excimer laser (193 nm). Refract Corneal Surg 6:99, 1990
35. Phillips AF, McDonnell PJ: Laser-induced fluorescence during photorefractive keratectomy: a method for controlling epithelial removal. Am J Ophthalmol 123:42, 1997
36. Shofner RS, McDonald MB, Beuerman RW, et al: Serial histological studies of monkey corneas after central photorefractive keratectomy (PRK) with the 193 mm excimer laser. ARVO abstract. Invest Ophthalmol Vis Sci 30(suppl):216, 1989

37. Beuerman RW, McDonald MB, Shofner RS, et al: Quantitative histological studies of primate corneas after excimer laser photorefractive keratectomy. Arch Ophthalmol 112:1103, 1994
38. Wu WCS, Stark WJ, Green WR: Corneal wound healing after 193-nm excimer laser keratectomy. Arch Ophthalmol 109:1426, 1991
39. Fantes FE, Hanna KD, Waring GO III, et al: Wound healing after excimer laser keratomileusis (photorefractive keratectomy) in monkeys. Arch Ophthalmol 108:665, 1990
40. Hanna KD, Pouliquen Y, Waring GO III, et al: Corneal stromal wound healing in rabbits after 193-nm excimer laser surface ablation. Arch Ophthalmol 107:895, 1989
41. Binder PS, Anderson JA, Rock ME, Vrabec MP: Human excimer laser keratectomy. Clinical and histopathologic correlations. Ophthalmology 101:979, 1994
42. Lohmann C, Gartry D, Kerr-Muir M, et al: Haze in photorefractive keratectomy: its origins and consequences. Lasers Light Ophthalmol 4:15, 1991
43. Marshall J, Trokel SL, Rothery S, Krueger RR: Long-term healing of the central cornea after photorefractive keratectomy using an excimer laser. Ophthalmology 95:1411, 1988
44. Caubet E: Cause of subepithelial corneal haze over 18 months after photorefractive keratectomy for myopia. Refract Corneal Surg 9(suppl):S65, 1993
45. Zabel R, Tuft S, Marshall J: Excimer laser photorefractive keratectomy: endothelial morphology following area ablation of the cornea. ARVO abstract. Invest Ophthalmol Vis Sci 29(suppl):390, 1988
46. Beldavs RA, Thompson KP, Waring GO III, Reddick DE: Quantitative specular microscopy after PRK. AAO abstract. Ophthalmology 99(suppl):125, 1992
47. Amano S, Shimizu K: Corneal endothelial changes after excimer laser photorefractive keratectomy. Am J Ophthalmol 116:692, 1993
48. Carones F, Brancato R, Venturi E, Morico A: The corneal endothelium after myopic excimer laser photorefractive keratectomy. Arch Ophthalmol 112:920, 1994

41

Photorefractive Keratectomy for Myopia

MARC G. ODRICH AND KENNETH A. GREENBERG

Excimer laser photorefractive keratectomy, or *PRK*, is, like any surgical procedure, constantly evolving. The unique properties of the interaction of 193-nm light with the human cornea were first reported in the late 1970s and early 1980s by Trokel and others.[1-3] In 1988, the equations of Munnerlyn et al[4] described the amount of tissue ablation required to correct various refractive errors. Since then, industry, academia, and ophthalmic surgeons have collaborated in the development and refinement of this technology. At this writing, the U.S. Food and Drug Administration (FDA) has approved the excimer lasers from two manufacturers (VISX, Inc. and Summit Technology) for the correction of myopia, and many other lasers are undergoing FDA evaluation.

There are four basic principles for successful photorefractive keratectomy. These are proper patient selection, proper preoperative evaluation, proper surgical technique, and proper postoperative care. This chapter addresses these principles for the correction of myopia. Photorefractive keratectomy for the correction of astigmatism is discussed in Chapter 42.

PATIENT SELECTION

The importance of identifying the appropriate patient to undergo photorefractive keratectomy cannot be overemphasized. Ultimately, it is the surgeon's responsibility to ensure that a patient is a good candidate for this procedure. Specific visual needs must be discussed at length with each patient, with an understanding of the effects of presbyopia, the possible benefits of monovision, and the concept of "closer is clearer" in the life of the myope.

The amount of myopia (spherical equivalent at the corneal plane) approved by the FDA for correction with photorefractive keratectomy is limited: 1.50 to 7.00 diopters (with no more than 1.50 diopters of astigmatism) in patients 21 years of age or older for the Summit laser and 1.00 to 6.00 diopters (with no more than 1.00 diopter of astigmatism) in patients 18 years of age or older for the VISX laser. (The VISX laser is also approved for the treatment of 0.75 to 4.00 diopters of astigmatism in patients 21 years of age or older who have up to 6.00 diopters of spherical myopia at the spectacle plane.) Stability of refraction, as evidenced by a change of no more than 0.5 diopter in either the spherical or cylindrical component for at least 1 year, must be documented.

Photorefractive keratectomy should not be performed in patients with collagen-vascular disease, other autoimmune diseases, immunodeficiency diseases or syndromes, or any disease likely to affect wound healing. It should also not be performed in women who are pregnant (because of refractive instability) or nursing (because of refractive instability and systemic absorption of the topical corticosteroids given postoperatively). Photorefractive keratectomy should not be performed in patients with a history of keloid formation or signs of keratoconus. Photorefractive keratectomy is not recommended in patients with a history of herpetic eye disease of either simplex or zoster origin. The safety and efficacy of photorefractive keratectomy in patients with glaucoma have not been established.

Patients taking isotretinoin should not undergo photorefractive keratectomy; there have been reports of severe corneal haze formation in patients who have undergone photorefractive keratectomy while on this medication, and some patients on isotretinoin have developed corneal haze even without laser surgery. It is recommended that patients on the antiarrhythmic medication, amiodarone, not undergo photorefractive keratectomy because this drug is associated with the formation of cornea verticillata, and significant loss of best-corrected visual acuity has been observed on closure of the epithelial defect after photorefractive keratectomy. Sumatriptan, which is typically used to treat migraine headaches, has been noted to cause spontaneous epithelial defects in animals; therefore, patients on this medication should probably be counseled against photorefractive keratectomy. Similarly, one should use caution in considering photorefractive keratectomy in patients on antimetabolites or other medications that could affect wound healing.

PREOPERATIVE EVALUATION

A comprehensive ophthalmologic examination is essential preoperatively. The goal of this examination is to identify any conditions that could adversely affect the outcome of photorefractive keratectomy. The examination includes a complete medical and surgical history and a complete listing of all systemic and topical medications and allergies. Some patients seek refractive surgery as an alternative to wearing contact lenses. The cause of contact lens intolerance must be established because this cause may adversely affect the outcome of photorefractive keratectomy.

Current and previous prescriptions for spectacles are helpful in determining the stability of the patient's refraction. Manifest and cycloplegic refractions are essential. The cycloplegic refraction is a confirmatory refraction and can alert the surgeon to any possible unintentional overminusing. If photorefractive keratectomy is performed based on an overminused refraction, the patient will be overcorrected. This may be inconsequential in a 20 year old who has enough accommodative reserve to compensate for the overcorrection but may cause great dissatisfaction in a presbyopic 45 year old who is no longer able to accommodate. Because some older patients retain the capacity to accommodate, however, a cycloplegic refraction is performed routinely, regardless of the patient's age. If the difference between the manifest and cycloplegic refractions is more than 0.50 diopter, the patient should return for a postcycloplegic refraction.

Contact lens wear can cause corneal warpage, as described in Chapter 27. Therefore, polymethyl methacrylate lens wear and rigid gas-permeable lens wear must be discontinued for at least 3 weeks and soft lens wear for at least 2 weeks before the preoperative examination on which the surgical plan will be based. Contact lens wear may then be resumed but must again be discontinued for the same interval before surgery. Patients are often unhappy with these requirements but must be made to realize that failure to follow the instructions can result in an incorrect ablation and an unpredictable result.

Preoperative videokeratography is essential to screen for keratoconus and other corneal abnormalities that make patients unsuitable candidates for photorefractive keratectomy. Videokeratography is especially important in patients who wear contact lenses, which can mask early signs of keratoconus, and in patients with astigmatism or steep corneas. Forme fruste keratoconus cannot be detected easily with any clinical examination except videokeratography.

Eye dominance is determined in all patients and is helpful in planning surgery and exploring monovision as an option in patients with presbyopia. It is useful to know preoperatively if a patient can tolerate the anisometropia that may occur if photorefractive keratectomy is performed on only one eye or if the plan is to correct one eye for distance and the other eye for near. The anisometropia can be simulated preoperatively with the use of contact lenses.

The diameters of the pupils are measured in both bright and dim lights. These measurements are important because a small percentage of young patients will physiologically dilate beyond the planned 6.0-mm-diameter ablation zone; this phenomenon is best detected by placing the patient in a dimly illuminated or dark room for at least 3 minutes to allow for full physiologic (non-pharmacologic) dilation. Age tends to reduce the amount of physiologic dilation. Patients with large pupils are counseled that they may experience visual difficulties such as glare in dim light situations, such as night driving, if they have photorefractive keratectomy.

Careful slit lamp microscopy is performed, with particular emphasis on the signs of chronic blepharitis and dry eyes. Untreated blepharitis or dry eyes can cause difficulties with corneal re-epithelialization postoperatively and result in a poor surgical outcome. Dry eyes are particularly common among laser surgery candidates because this condition can be the cause of the contact lens intolerance that motivates the patient to seek refractive surgery.

Applanation tonometry is required in all patients preoperatively. Any ambiguity regarding the intraocular pressure or health of the optic nerve requires clarification because applanation tonometry in patients after photorefractive keratectomy may be inaccurate.[5,6] This inaccuracy is the result of corneal thinning and the assumptions of the Fick equation, on which the principles of the tonometer are based. If there is concern about a possible glaucomatous process, visual fields are assessed.

Dilated examination of the lens and retina is critical. A patient with a nuclear sclerotic cataract may have an unstable refraction and usually becomes more myopic as the cataract progresses, which can prompt an interest in refractive surgery. Such patients must be identified and are best treated by conventional management of the cataract.

It is important to document posterior pathology preoperatively because myopes tend to have central and peripheral retinal abnormalities that are not cured by refractive surgery. The nature and severity of pre-existing retinal abnormalities must be carefully explained to the patient. The fact that refractive surgery will not reduce the potential for the development or progression of retinal abnormalities in the future, as well as the symptoms and the importance of prompt medical evaluation, should be discussed.

PREOPERATIVE SETUP

All calibration and centering procedures recommended by the manufacturer for a particular laser must be followed exactly to ensure that a beam of known energy and high quality is delivered to the cornea. Typically, this involves ablating a material and measuring the quantity and quality of the ablation. The method by which this calibration is done varies with different laser systems.

Excimer lasers are more sophisticated than other lasers with which ophthalmologists are familiar. As a result, the role of an experienced and well-trained technician in the use of this type of laser is more important than it might be for other types of lasers. Although calibration and operation of the laser system are typically done by the technician, the surgeon is ultimately responsible for ensuring that all calibration and operating parameters are correct, including verification of the data entered into the system before treatment is begun.

PREOPERATIVE MEDICATIONS

No preoperative medications are required for photorefractive keratectomy. Some surgeons prescribe a sedative such as oral diazepam (5 to 10 mg). However, any sedation should be light enough that the patient can cooperate with fixation during the procedure.

There is controversy regarding the use of miotic agents preoperatively. Determination of the center of the entrance pupil is easier when the pupil is small. Therefore, some surgeons instill 1 percent pilocarpine 30 minutes before the procedure. Other surgeons think that miotic agents skew the position of the pupil and prefer to increase the illumination of the microscope to induce physiologic miosis. Mydriatic agents should not be used.

Nonsteroidal anti-inflammatory drugs, both topical and oral, have been used preoperatively to aid in the control of postoperative pain; however, the efficacy of this practice is controversial.

ANESTHESIA

Topical anesthesia is almost always sufficient to keep the patient comfortable during photorefractive keratectomy. Topical proparacaine or tetracaine is usually instilled just before the start of the procedure. Topical anesthetics decrease corneal sensation and the blink reflex, which increases the risk of exposure and corneal desiccation. Corneal dehydration can lead to an increased ablation rate, which can produce an unintentional overcorrection. Therefore, if the anesthetic is administered before the patient is positioned beneath the laser, he or she is instructed to keep both eyes closed as much as possible.

SURGICAL TECHNIQUES

Preparing the Patient

Patients and all operating room personnel are instructed to not wear any cologne or perfume on the day of surgery. Perfume or cologne may reduce the amount of energy delivered to the cornea and make the surgery less predictable. Patients are instructed to wear nonconstricting clothing on the day of surgery and are asked to remove earrings because the vacuum pillow used with some lasers can cause pressure on the ears.

The eyelids of the contralateral eye are patched closed to prevent the patient from cross fixating. The patient is positioned under the laser and a gross alignment is performed, which involves orienting the patient's eye such that the iris plane and the corneal apex are grossly perpendicular to the laser beam. Topical anesthetic is instilled, and an eyelid speculum is placed. The final, precision alignment is then performed. The surgeon places the operating microscope on the highest magnification, focuses on the corneal epithelium or the tear film, and centers the microscope field on the center of the entrance pupil with the patient focusing on the fixation light. The magnification is then reduced so that the entire cornea and some of the limbus are visible.

Locating the Center of the Ablation Zone

Proper centration is crucial in photorefractive keratectomy; otherwise, the ablation will be decentered, leading to postoperative induced astigmatism. As with any refractive surgical procedure, the center of the patient's entrance pupil is used for centering the ablation[7] (see Ch. 46). Only light that passes through the entrance pupil stimulates the rods and cones, and the only area of the cornea that refracts this light is that which overlies the entrance pupil. It is this area that should be ablated.

Neither the reflection of the fixation light nor the reflection of the microscope light should be used as a centering landmark. The corneal light reflex is a virtual image of the light source that is formed by the anterior convex surface of the cornea. The location of this image depends on the location of the light source and the angle at which the rays of light intersect the cornea. As a result, it is a potentially variable point and is unrelated to the area of the cornea that overlies the entrance pupil.

The VISX excimer laser is designed so that the view through the operating microscope, the flashing red fixation light, the laser beam, and the reticule in the ocular are all coaxial. Proper centration involves having the patient fixate on a flashing red fixation light and keeping the patient's entrance pupil centered in the middle of the 4-mm reticule. Constant vigilance is required to maintain this centration.

The Summit excimer laser is equipped with two converging helium:neon (He:Ne) aiming beams. These beams are separated by 180 degrees on the horizontal axis of the laser and, when properly adjusted, are coaxial with the laser beam. The He:Ne beams diverge as they pass through the cornea. Proper centration involves having the patient fixate on a green fixation light in the center of a red fixation ring and keeping the divergent He:Ne beams equidistant from the pupillary border in the horizontal axis. One percent pilocarpine is instilled preoperatively to constrict the pupil to facilitate visualization of the He:Ne beams on the iris.

Removing the Epithelium

There are several methods for removing the corneal epithelium. The key to all methods is to remove the epithelium quickly so that the cornea does not desiccate.

Manual Removal

In this method, the surgeon removes sufficient epithelium to create a denuded area large enough in diameter to accommodate the ablation, while still leaving a peripheral rim of epithelium from which re-epithelialization can proceed postoperatively. A 6.0- to 7.0-mm optical zone marker is centered over the center of the entrance pupil as the patient stares at the fixation light. The marker is then pressed on the corneal epithelium to create a circular impression that demarcates the area of epithelium to be removed. Some surgeons use gentian violet on the optical zone marker so that the mark is more visible. The epithelium within the mark is gently scraped off with a blunt or sharp instrument, such as a Paton spatula or a stainless steel blade (e.g., #15 Bard-Parker blade). Care is taken not to damage Bowman's layer because any indentation in Bowman's layer will be reproduced in the stroma by the ablation. After the epithelium has been removed, the surface of Bowman's layer is wiped with a nonfragmenting methylcellulose sponge (e.g., Merocel surgical spear) saturated with balanced salt solution and squeezed out. The sponge removes any remaining epithelial cell debris from the surface. It also absorbs any excess fluid from the surface or wets the surface if it is dry.

Chemical Removal

Some surgeons instill topical 4 percent cocaine eye drops for anesthesia and also to loosen the epithelium. However, cocaine loosens the entire corneal epithelium, not just the epithelium in the area of the intended ablation. This problem can be minimized by saturating a 6- to 7-mm circular sponge with cocaine and placing it on the area of epithelium to be removed. Other surgeons hold an optical zone marker on the cornea and place 5, 10, 15, or 30 percent ethanol in the marker for up to 30 seconds. After chemical treatment, the epithelium is removed manually as described above. There appear to be no adverse effects from the use of these chemicals.

Removal with a Brush

Some surgeons remove the epithelium with a 7.0-mm–diameter motorized, hand-held brush with nylon bristles (e.g., Amoils Epithelial Remover). The brush removes epithelium rapidly without damaging Bowman's layer. However, centration of the brush can be difficult. Some surgeons believe that this procedure results in more rapid corneal re-epithelialization postoperatively than other methods of epithelial removal.

Laser-Scrape

In this technique, the superficial epithelial cells are ablated with the laser, which is programmed to perform a phototherapeutic keratectomy 6.0 mm in diameter and 40 to 45 μm in depth. Any remaining epithelial basal cells are then removed manually with a blunt instrument (e.g., a Paton or Kimura spatula). This technique has the advantage of allowing the patient to become accustomed to the sights and sounds of the laser before the stroma is ablated. It also allows the surgeon to gauge how well the patient maintains fixation under operative conditions.

Transepithelial Ablation

In transepithelial ablation, the epithelium is ablated with the laser. The entire ablation, both epithelium and stroma, is programmed into the computer and is accomplished by means of one foot-pedal depression, whereas laser-scrape requires a two-part ablation, with one foot-pedal depression for ablating the epithelium and a second depression for ablating the stroma. With transepithelial ablation, the laser is programmed to perform a phototherapeutic keratectomy 6.0 to 6.5 mm in diameter and 50 μm in depth to remove the epithelium. The surgeon observes the faint blue fluorescence characteristic of the epithelial ablation through the microscope, watching carefully for its disappearance as the epithelial ablation is completed and the stromal ablation begins, which usually occurs first in the periphery. The stroma is then ablated with the appropriate algorithm for photorefractive keratectomy. Because the peripheral epithelium is removed first, transepithelial ablation creates an uneven ablation, which can cause topographic abnormalities postoperatively if not compensated or corrected for. Some surgeons increase the correction for myopia 0.50 to 0.75 diopter in patients whose epithelium is removed in this manner to ablate the residual central epithelium that was not ablated initially with the phototherapeutic keratectomy algorithm. Other surgeons have developed their own algorithms for transepithelial ablation.

Ablating the Stroma

After the corneal epithelium with its basement membrane has been removed and the surface of Bowman's layer has been wiped, the centration and focus are checked and the stroma is ablated as quickly as possible, before the cornea begins to desiccate. The most important principle of stromal ablation is to keep the ablation centered over the entrance pupil. The most common error for the beginning surgeon is to create a decentered ablation, which is difficult to correct. The patient is instructed to stare at the fixation light even if it becomes blurred during the ablation. Having the patient maintain fixation is preferable and is more reliable than fixating the eye with a suction ring or other device.

The surgeon keeps one hand or foot on the centering mechanism of the laser and the other hand on the patient's forehead to stabilize the head. Some surgeons position both hands on the sides of the patient's head. During the ablation, the surgeon repeatedly reminds the patient to maintain fixation and constantly monitors the centration of the ablation. If the patient becomes misaligned, the ablation is stopped, the patient is realigned, and the ablation is resumed.

Once the ablation has begun, all operating room personnel are asked not to move because bodies in motion can increase the flow of air over the cornea, which can result in corneal desiccation and an unpredictable ablation. The door to the operating room should remain closed throughout the procedure.

Based on the Munnerlyn lens equations,[4] the relationship between the depth and the diameter of the ablation was recognized by laser manufacturers early in the progress of the clinical studies. Concern regarding the depth of ablation and the amount of tissue to be removed led, initially, to the use of a 4.5- to 5.0-mm–diameter ablation. Patients with this size ablation experienced night vision difficulties (glare), however, which prompted the manufacturers to increase the diameter of the ablation. It became apparent that many of the difficulties were caused by the disparity between physiologic dilation of the pupil to a diameter greater than 6 mm (most commonly in patients younger than 30 years of age) and the less-than-5.0-mm diameter of the ablation. Gradually, the manufacturers adopted a 6.0-mm to 6.5-mm ablation diameter; although increased topographic abnormalities, such as central islands, were and are associated with the larger diameter broad-beam ablations, changes in the laser software can eliminate these unwanted features.

POSTOPERATIVE CARE

As soon as the procedure is completed, a bandage soft contact lens is placed on the cornea in a sterile fashion. A topical antibiotic eye drop, such as ciprofloxacin or ofloxacin, is instilled as a prophylaxis against microbial invasion of the vulnerable, de-epithelialized cornea. The antibiotic is instilled four times a day until re-epithelialization is complete.

A topical cycloplegic agent, such as 2 or 5 percent homatropine, may be used to decrease postoperative photophobia. Some surgeons instill a drop of corticosteroid at the end of the case and instruct the patient to continue this medication four times a day; others prefer to wait until re-epithelialization is complete before initiating topical corticosteroids.

Topical nonsteroidal anti-inflammatory drugs, such as 0.1 percent diclofenac, 0.03 percent flurbiprofen, or 0.5 percent ketorolac, are used primarily to control postoperative pain.[8] Nonsteroidal anti-inflammatory drugs reduce prostaglandin levels and may even have some direct anesthetic effect; however, they have no effect on the leukotriene pathway, which is a mediator of the inflammatory response, and have been implicated in increasing the number of polymorphonuclear leukocytes.[9] There are anecdotal reports of stromal infiltrates in patients who use nonsteroidal anti-inflammatory drugs without concomitant corticosteroids.[10] Therefore, most

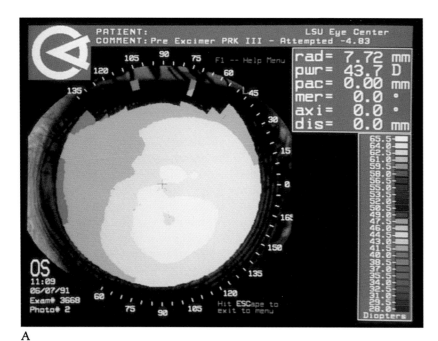

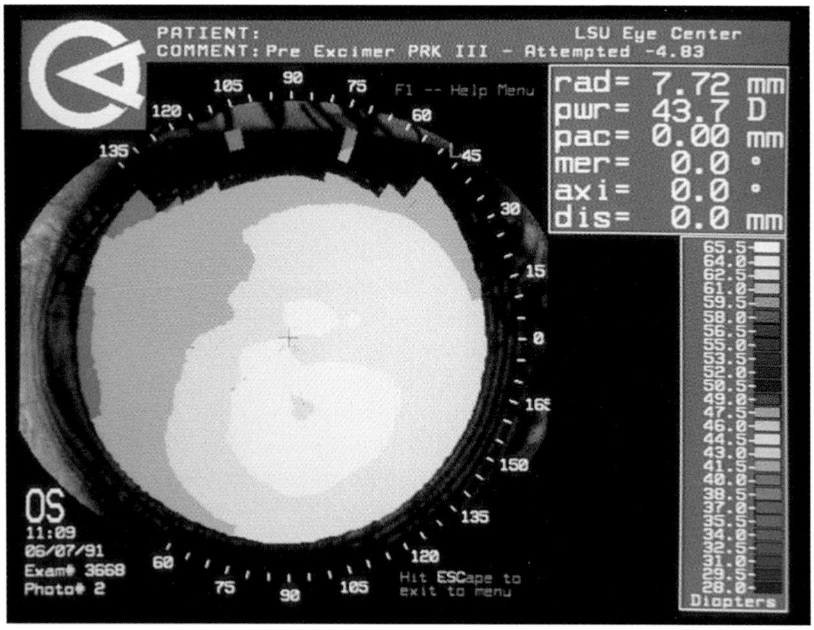

A

FIGURE 41-1 Pre- and postoperative videokeratographs of excimer laser photorefractive keratectomy for myopia. **(A)** Preoperative uncorrected visual acuity was count fingers. Best spectacle-corrected visual acuity was 20/20 with −5.25 +0.25 × 90. *(continues)*

surgeons who prescribe nonsteroidal anti-inflammatory drugs prescribe corticosteroids concomitantly to control or reduce this white cell response. Topical nonsteroidal anti-inflammatory drugs are required only during the first 24 to 48 hours after surgery and should not be used more than four times a day. There is evidence that chronic use impairs epithelial wound healing, and there have been anecdotal reports of corneal melting in patients who use these drugs to excess.

Systemic analgesia is frequently not required if the above regimen is used, but patients are usually given a prescription for acetaminophen with codeine, hydrocodone with acetaminophen, oxycodone with acetaminophen, hydroxyzine pamoate, or a similar analgesic to take as needed for pain.

Patients are seen every 24 to 36 hours until the cornea has re-epithelialized to be certain that no infiltrates or infections have developed. The bandage soft contact lens is left in place until the epithelial defect has closed completely, which typically takes 3 to 4 days. At that time, the bandage lens is removed and the antibiotics are stopped. A bland ophthalmic ointment without preservatives is used liberally to protect the new epithelial surface, which lacks the dense nerve plexus present in an unablated cornea.[11] Aggressive ocular lubrication with nonpreserved artificial tears is recommended for 6 months postoperatively.

Topical corticosteroids are used in a tapering dose for 4 months after surgery. A recommended regimen is fluorometholone four times a day for the first month, three times a day for the second month, twice a day for the third month, and once a day for the fourth month.

After re-epithelialization, patients are typically seen at 1, 3, 6, and 12 months. Each examination should include evaluation of uncorrected and best spectacle-corrected visual acuity, slit lamp microscopy, and measurement of intraocular pressure. Videokeratography should be performed at some time during the first 12 months after surgery (Figure 41-1).

There are two milestones in the visual recovery of patients who have had photorefractive keratectomy. One is the return of preoperative best spectacle-corrected visual acuity, which typically occurs within the first 3 months. The other is refractive stability. Best spectacle-corrected visual acuity almost always recovers before refractive stability is established.

COMPLICATIONS

Loss of Best Spectacle-Corrected Visual Acuity

Loss of best spectacle-corrected visual acuity is one of the most significant complications of any refractive surgical procedure. This loss may be a complication of the procedure itself or may be the result of an unrelated disorder. Possible causes include irregular astigmatism (as can occur with corneal epithelial irregularities or a decentered or irregular ablation), stromal haze, and retinal abnormalities.

FIGURE 41-1 *(continued)* **(B)** One month postoperatively, uncorrected visual acuity was 20/30. Best spectacle-corrected visual acuity was 20/25 with -0.75 +0.25 × 180. Note the well-centered central flattening of the cornea. (Courtesy of Stephen D. Klyce, Ph.D., New Orleans, LA.)

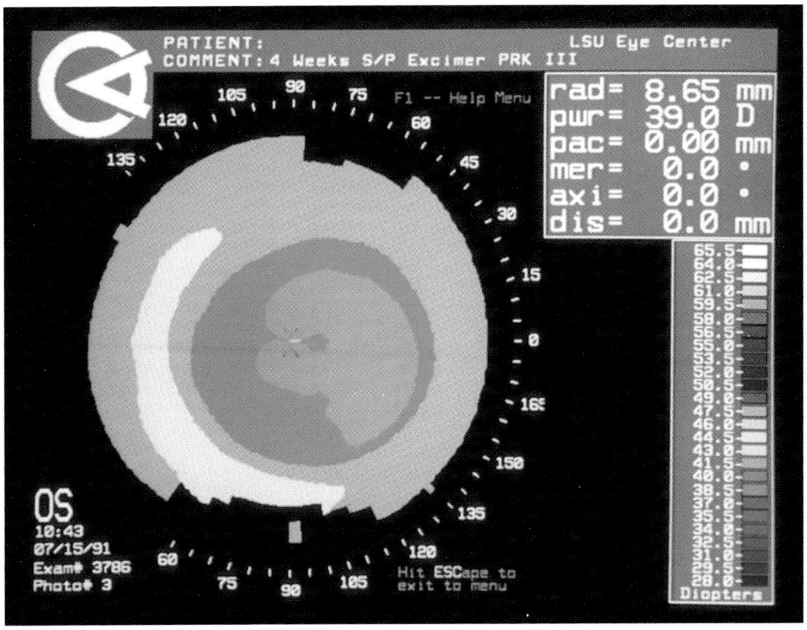

B

Undercorrection

Undercorrection occurs when a patient never attains the refractive goal and is always more myopic (by 0.50 diopter or more) than the intended correction. The most common cause of undercorrection is an ablation based on an incorrect refraction. There is a small group of patients who appear to have steep central corneas with little or no inferior displacement of the steep areas (so they do not fit any formal definition of keratoconus) and who show little or no refractive change after photorefractive keratectomy. It frequently turns out that these patients did not heed the instructions regarding cessation of contact lens wear and continued to wear their lenses until just hours before the initial examination and the surgery. These patients can also be noncompliant with any sort of medication or care regimen, and little can be done to remedy their refractive result if they elect to ignore the surgeon's warnings.

Attempts can be made to treat undercorrections by continuing topical corticosteroids or restarting them if they have been stopped. The mechanism by which topical corticosteroids can ameliorate an undercorrection or a regression is debatable. The most reasonable explanation seems to be corticosteroid-induced inhibition of hyaluronic acid production, which is known to occur in the stroma in both rabbits and humans after excimer laser ablation.[12] Hyaluronic acid causes focal hydration and subsequent steepening. Persistent undercorrections can be treated with a second or even a third laser procedure.

Overcorrection

Overcorrection occurs when a patient is more hyperopic than the intended correction at 1 month or later after surgery. Younger patients can usually compensate for overcorrections by accommodating. Older patients who have lost the ability to accommodate are devastated by this result. Overcorrections can also cause patients who were accustomed preoperatively to seeing objects more clearly by holding them closer to have to move the objects farther away to bring them into focus. Most patients find this change debilitating and unacceptable.

Many surgeons have noticed that patients who are overcorrected by more than 1.00 diopter at 6 weeks postoperatively, and remain so thereafter, often have no corneal haze formation. These patients do not demonstrate the normal healing response to photorefractive keratectomy, which includes a small amount of regression (see below) and a small amount of haze formation. Topical corticosteroids can be stopped in these patients, either abruptly or by a very rapid taper, in an attempt to reverse the overcorrection. Some surgeons debride the corneal epithelium and withhold topical corticosteroids in patients in whom an overcorrection persists and is stable. This debridement has met with variable success. Holmium laser thermokeratoplasty and hyperopic photorefractive keratectomy have been used successfully to treat overcorrections.

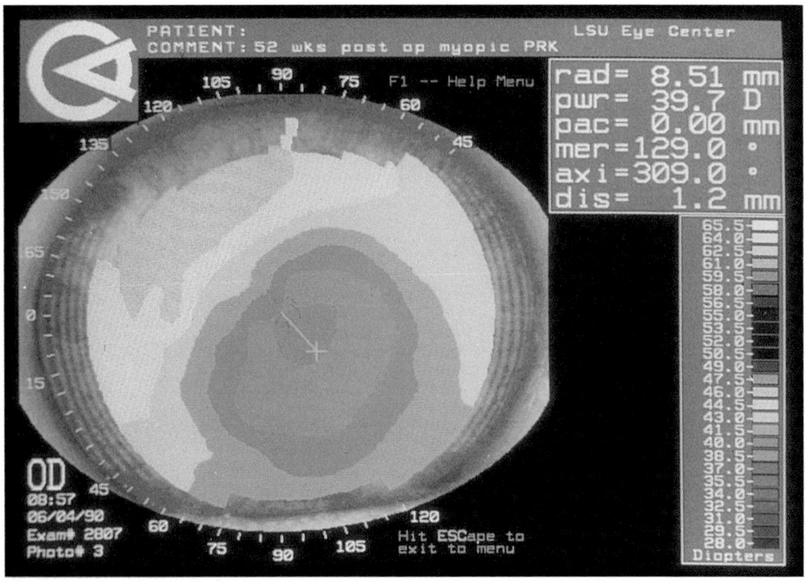

FIGURE 41-2 Decentered ablation after photorefractive keratectomy for myopia. (Courtesy of Stephen D. Klyce, Ph.D., New Orleans, LA.)

Regression

Regression is a loss of refractive effect. One diopter or less of loss of effect is normal in the first 6 weeks of healing, but regression is abnormal if it occurs after the first 6 weeks. Regression that occurs after the first 6 weeks is treated intensively with topical corticosteroids, usually dexamethasone as frequently as every 2 hours for 2 weeks. Treated regressions have been noted to slow, halt, or even reverse, with documented videokeratographic flattening of 1.00 to 3.00 diopters.[12] This flattening occurs because of corneal thinning associated with a reduction in hyaluronic acid and a reduction in hydration, as described above. If topical corticosteroids reduce the regression, they are slowly tapered over at least 4 months. If corticosteroids do not have an effect within 2 weeks, they are rapidly tapered. One must then wait for refractive stability and consider retreatment, if necessary.

Decentration of the Ablation

Decentration of the ablation occurs in less than 1 percent of patients (Figure 41-2). The most common causes of decentration are failure of the patient to fixate properly or continuously, failure of the surgeon to recognize that the patient is not fixating, and failure of the surgeon to keep the laser centered over the entrance pupil. Decentrations less than 1 mm have little refractive impact. Decentrations of more than 1 mm are associated with increased regular and irregular astigmatism. Patients with decentered ablations typically complain of blurred vision, glare, halos, ghosting, or monocular diplopia. It is essential that patients with these complaints be examined thoroughly, particularly with videokeratography. However, not all decentrations seen on videokeratography are true decentrations caused by decentered ablations. Asymmetrical healing and variable videokeratographic alignment (e.g., centering the videokeratographic image on the corneal apex and not the center of the entrance pupil) can cause the cornea to have the appearance of a decentered ablation.

If true decentration is present and is symptomatic, a second ablation can be performed with videokeratographic guidance. The second ablation should have the same diameter as the first ablation and should be displaced an equivalent amount from the center of the entrance pupil in the opposite direction from the displacement of the first ablation. The undercorrection measured by manifest refraction should be corroborated with videokeratographic studies and then may be treated to allow the patient adequate uncorrected visual acuity. A transepithelial phototherapeutic keratectomy is performed initially to remove the epithelium, followed by photorefractive keratectomy of the stroma. Patients with decentered ablations who have been treated in this manner are less symptomatic although there may be residual regular astigmatism postoperatively.

Central Island Formation

A central island is an area of relative central corneal steepening demonstrated on videokeratography (Figure 41-3). A precise quantitative definition is not universally agreed on, but a central island typically consists of an area 2 to 4 mm in diameter with 1.5 to 3.5 diopters of relative corneal steepening.[13-15] Most central islands are

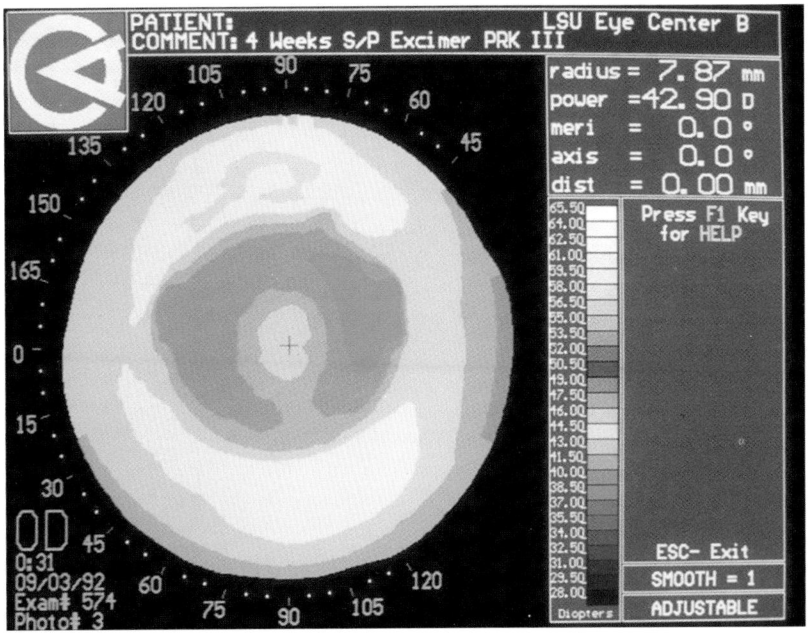

FIGURE 41-3 Central island after photorefractive keratectomy for myopia. (Courtesy of Stephen D. Klyce, Ph.D., New Orleans, LA.)

associated with a 1- to 3-diopter undercorrection and regular astigmatism.

Central islands may cause glare, halos, or other visual disturbances. As stated above, videokeratographic examination is imperative for any patient complaining of these symptoms. Central islands can also cause a one- to two-line loss of best spectacle-corrected visual acuity.

One manufacturer (VISX, Inc.) has incorporated a profile adjustment into its ablation algorithms that redistributes pulses centrally, which has decreased the incidence of central island formation to nearly zero.

Almost all central islands diminish with time without surgical intervention. The disappearance of these islands is largely the result of epithelial remodeling of the surface, although there may be a stromal component as well. In a small percentage of patients, however, the island persists and is symptomatic beyond 6 months. In such patients, the island should be evaluated on at least two different occasions with videokeratography, the size and height quantified, and a refraction done.

Persistent symptomatic islands can be treated with focal photorefractive keratectomy. The laser is first programmed to perform a phototherapeutic keratectomy 40 to 45 μm deep with a beam diameter slightly larger than the diameter of the island. For example, if the diameter of the island is 2.8 mm, an ablation 3.0 to 3.2 mm in diameter is performed. Once the epithelium at the periphery of this area has been ablated, as evidenced by the disappearance of blue fluorescence, the ablation is stopped and the rest of the epithelium overlying the island is removed with a blunt spatula. The diameter and height (in diopters) of the island are then entered into the computer software of the laser, and a photorefractive keratectomy is performed. The advantage of this technique is that only a small amount of central tissue is removed. As discussed in Chapter 40 and illustrated in Figure 40-4, the smaller the ablation zone, the smaller the amount of tissue that needs to be removed to effect a 1-diopter change in the refraction. For example, the depth of ablation required to remove a 2.5-diopter central island 3 mm in diameter is only 7.5 μm, which is in stark contrast to the 30-μm depth needed to achieve the same dioptric change with an ablation 6.0 mm in diameter.

A second method of treating central islands is with the phototherapeutic keratectomy circle mode. The epithelium is removed with a rotating brush or by laser-scrape using a default ablation depth of 40 to 45 μm, watching for the disappearance of the blue fluorescence, and removing the remainder of the epithelium overlying the island with a blunt spatula. An ablation diameter slightly larger than the diameter of the central island as measured on videokeratography is programmed into the laser. For example, a patient who complains of blurred vision with or without image ghosting and has a refraction of -3.00 -0.75×90 and a best spectacle-corrected visual acuity of 20/25 may show a central steepening of 2.5 diopters with a diameter of 2.8 mm in a well-centered ablation bed. A phototherapeutic keratectomy with a diameter of 3.0 mm is programmed into the laser. A transition zone that, in total, is equal to more than 80 percent of the treatment zone is also selected; in this example, a transition zone of 1.4 mm (the total transition zone is $1.4 \text{ mm} \times 2 = 2.8$ mm, because

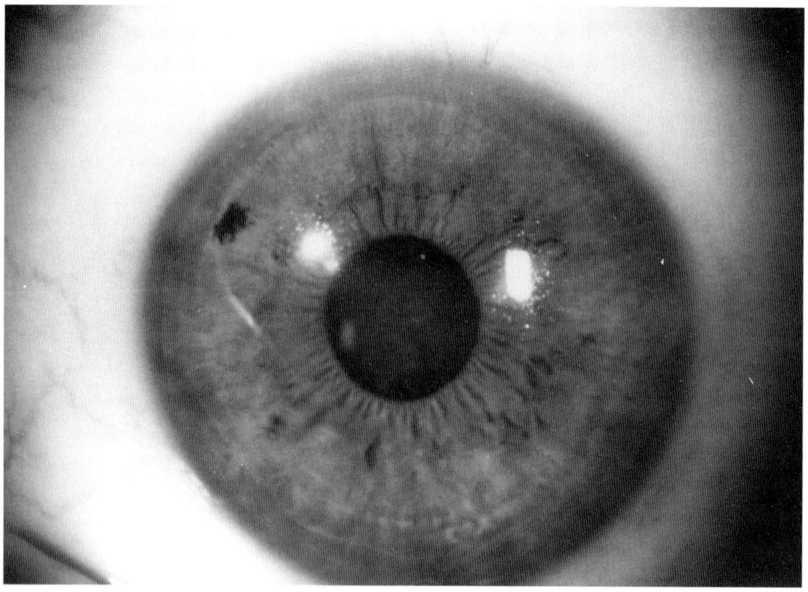

FIGURE 41-4 Grade 0.5 corneal haze 3 months after photorefractive keratectomy for myopia in the patient whose videokeratographs are illustrated in Figure 41-1. At 3 months postoperatively, uncorrected visual acuity was 20/25 +2, and best spectacle-corrected visual acuity was 20/20 -1 with -0.50 sphere.

it is made on both sides of the ablation) would be used, resulting in an ablation diameter of 0.2 mm (3.0 mm − 2.8 mm = 0.2 mm) at the base of the ablation. One should always attempt to undercorrect this problem to avoid hyperopia. In this patient, with 3.375 diopters spherical equivalent myopia by refraction and 2.5 diopters by videokeratography, it is safe to treat 2 diopters. As this is phototherapeutic keratectomy, it is important to recognize that, based on the Munnerlyn formula, which dictates that 1 diopter of correction with a 3.00-mm-diameter ablation requires an ablation depth of 3 μm, 2 diopters of correction will require an ablation depth of 6 μm.

Corneal Haze and Scarring

Haze formation in the superficial stroma is a common finding during the first 4 months after photorefractive keratectomy (Figure 41-4). This haze has been attributed to the deposition of type III collagen by activated keratocytes and fluctuating amounts of sulfated keratan sulfate. The haze has a marbled or reticulated appearance and has been graded in the clinical trials of several laser manufacturers (Table 41-1).[16] It is important to note that if the haze is severe enough to affect the refraction or cause a loss of best spectacle-corrected visual acuity, it is grade 2 or more.

Low grades of corneal haze (grade 1 or less) are an expected part of the healing process in photorefractive keratectomy. If marked haze develops, the potency of the topical corticosteroids is increased by changing from fluorometholone to dexamethasone or prednisolone acetate, and the frequency of administration is increased to four times a day, if necessary. If severe haze develops, either early or late (after 6 months), an aggressive regimen of topical corticosteroids is instituted. There have been anecdotal reports of reduction of corneal haze with a 10- to 14-day course of topical dexamethasone or prednisolone acetate given every 2 to 3 hours during waking hours. If the haze lessens, the corticosteroids are gradually tapered over several months, but if the haze is unresponsive, the corticosteroids are rapidly tapered. Nonsteroidal anti-inflammatory drugs apparently have no effect on corneal haze after photorefractive keratectomy.[17,18] The intraocular pressure and clarity of the lens must be monitored in any patient on chronic corticosteroids.

Given enough time, almost all haze diminishes, even if not treated. Haze that persists and causes loss of best spectacle-corrected visual acuity can be ablated with the laser. Care

TABLE 41-1
Grading of Corneal Haze

Grade	*Description*
0	Clear, possibly with faint haze
0.5	Haze barely detectable
1	Mild haze not affecting refraction
1.5	Haze mildly affecting refraction
2	Moderate haze, refraction possible but difficult
3	Opacity preventing refraction, anterior chamber easily viewed
4	Opacity impairing view of anterior chamber
5	Unable to see anterior chamber

is taken when ablating a cornea with haze after photorefractive keratectomy because the haze itself can lead to an overestimation of the amount of myopia, which can result in an overcorrection.

Corneal Infiltrates

Corneal infiltrates after photorefractive keratectomy may be sterile or infectious. Often the cause is not clear, but any infiltrate should be assumed to be infectious until proved otherwise. The bandage soft contact lens, if present, is removed and cultured, and scrapings are obtained from the infiltrate for smears and cultures as described in Chapter 8. Topical corticosteroids, if used, are temporarily discontinued, and an intensive regimen of topical antibiotics is begun. Topical corticosteroids can usually be restarted after several days of antibiotic treatment.

Sterile infiltrates are typically multiple and subepithelial, and no organisms are seen on Gram staining and nothing grows on the cultures. Sterile infiltrates after photorefractive keratectomy are associated with the use of bandage soft contact lenses and topical nonsteroidal anti-inflammatory drugs.[10] As explained above, nonsteroidal anti-inflammatory drugs suppress the synthesis of prostaglandins by inhibiting cyclooxygenase but leave the leukotriene pathway, which is a mediator of the inflammatory reaction, unchecked. Nonsteroidal anti-inflammatory drugs significantly increase polymorphonuclear leukocyte infiltration, which contributes to the development of the infiltrates.[9] Sterile infiltrates almost always resolve with topical corticosteroid treatment.

Intraocular Pressure Elevation

Intraocular pressure elevation after photorefractive keratectomy appears to be related to the use of topical corticosteroids postoperatively. The reported incidence of elevated intraocular pressure varies from 2.3 to 50 percent and appears to depend on the strength, frequency, and chronicity of corticosteroid use. The incidence is highest 4 to 6 weeks postoperatively, a period that coincides with the most intensive corticosteroid use.[19]

Clinically significant intraocular pressure elevation may be treated with a topical beta-blocker or other topical glaucoma medications, and/or a rapid taper or cessation of the topical corticosteroids. Pilocarpine is avoided because of reported cases of retinal detachment following its use, especially in patients with peripheral retinal disease. To our knowledge, persistent elevation of intraocular pressure has not occurred after photorefractive keratectomy in any patient who has stopped using corticosteroids. In almost all cases, use of the beta-blocker can generally be stopped by 4 weeks after the pressure rise. Patients found to be subject to corticosteroid-induced intraocular pressure elevation should be informed of this tendency and told to report it in the future whenever the possibility of corticosteroid treatment for any condition is considered.

Also, because intraocular pressure measurements after photorefractive keratectomy may be inaccurate,[5,6] there should be a high index of suspicion of glaucoma in any patient who has undergone photorefractive keratectomy and has unusual or glaucomatous optic nerves or visual field loss but apparently normal intraocular pressure measurements.

Pupillary Dilation

Pupillary dilation after photorefractive keratectomy usually occurs within the first month of treatment and resolves after 6 months. In most patients, this correlates with the time of topical corticosteroid use, and pupillary dilation is a reported side effect of topical corticosteroids. No treatment is needed because the dilation is self limited.

Ptosis

Ptosis after photorefractive keratectomy is rare. Although the cause of the ptosis is debated, some surgeons believe it is the result of stretching of Müller's muscle by the eyelid speculum. Topical corticosteroids are known to cause ptosis. To our knowledge, surgical repair has not been required for ptosis after photorefractive keratectomy.

CLINICAL RESULTS

The results of clinical trials with the two excimer lasers approved by the FDA for the correction of mild to moderate myopia with minimal amounts of astigmatism are presented below.

VISX

A prospective, non-randomized, unmasked, multi-center clinical trial was conducted to determine the safety and efficacy of photorefractive keratectomy to treat mild to moderate myopia (up to -6.00 diopters). Safety evaluations were done on a cohort of 909 eyes treated with a 6.0-mm-diameter ablation zone. Efficacy evaluations were done on the 480 eyes of this cohort that had 2 or more years of follow-up.

Patients were evaluated preoperatively, every 24 to 48 hours postoperatively until corneal re-epithelialization occurred, and at 1, 3, 6, 12, 18, and 24 months.

Objective measurements included evaluation of uncorrected and best spectacle-corrected visual acuities, manifest refraction, keratometry, measurement of intraocular pressure, pachymetry, and clinical assessment of the cornea, anterior chamber, lens, vitreous, and retina. Additional measurements performed in subsets of eyes included cycloplegic refraction, glare testing, contrast sensitivity testing, videokeratography, specular microscopy, and assessment of visual fields.

Efficacy, Predictability, and Stability

Of the 480 eyes, preoperative uncorrected visual acuity was 20/40 or better in 0.4 percent of eyes, 20/50 to 20/80 in 5.0 percent, and 20/100 or worse in 94.6 percent. Preoperative best spectacle-corrected visual acuity was 20/20 or better in 97.1 percent, 20/25 to 20/30 in 2.7 percent, and 20/40 in 0.2 percent. Efficacy is demonstrated in Table 41-2, which shows the 2-year postoperative visual results of single laser treatments, stratified by the amount of preoperative myopia. Eyes that underwent retreatment are excluded from these data.

Two years after surgery, uncorrected visual acuity was 20/20 or better in 58.3 percent of eyes, 20/25 or better in 79.8 percent, and 20/40 or better in 93.8 percent. In general, the success rate for each of the efficacy parameters (e.g., percentage of eyes achieving 20/20, 20/25, or 20/40 uncorrected visual acuities) was better in the eyes with smaller amounts of preoperative myopia. Visual recovery was rapid in most cases (Table 41-3); uncorrected visual acuity of 20/40 or better was achieved in 89.6 percent of eyes at 1 month after surgery.

The efficacy and predictability of photorefractive keratectomy in correcting myopia are shown by spherical equivalent manifest refractions measured over time (Table 41-4).

Predictability was good. At any time postoperatively, approximately 90 percent of eyes were within 1.00 diopter

TABLE 41-2

Efficacy of Photorefractive Keratectomy for Myopia in 480 Eyes[a]

	Preoperative Spherical Equivalent					
Parameter Measured	-1.00 to < -2.00 D (n = 37)	-2.00 to < -3.00 D (n = 75)	-3.00 to < -4.00 D (n = 119)	-4.00 to < -5.00 D (n = 128)	-5.00 to -6.00 D (n = 121)	All eyes (n = 480)
Postoperative uncorrected visual acuity (%)						
20/20 or better	70.3	68.0	55.5	60.2	49.6	58.3
20/25 or better	86.5	84.0	77.3	80.5	76.9	79.8
20/40 or better	94.6	96.0	92.4	94.5	92.6	93.8
Postoperative spherical equivalent (%)						
Within ±1.00 D of intended correction	91.7[b]	92.0	93.3	88.3	87.6	90.2[b]
1.00 D or less hyperopic from intended correction (not overcorrected)	100.0[b]	98.7	100.0	99.2	97.5	99.0[b]
1.00 D or less myopic from intended correction (not undercorrected)	91.7[b]	93.3	93.3	89.1	90.1	91.2[b]
More than 1.00 D hyperopic from emmetropia	0.0	0.0	0.0	0.0	0.8	0.2
Preoperative BSCVA of 20/20 or better and postoperative UCVA of 20/25 or better and postoperative SE between -1.0 D and +0.5 D (%)	85.7[b]	82.4[b]	74.8[b]	76.0[b]	75.7[b]	77.4[b,c]

Abbreviations: D, diopter; BSCVA, best spectacle-corrected visual acuity; UCVA, uncorrected visual acuity; SE, spherical equivalent.

[a] All eyes underwent photorefractive keratectomy for myopia with a 6.0-mm-diameter ablation zone. The data are for eyes with 2 or more years of follow-up and initial treatment only.

[b] These values were calculated using an *n* value slightly smaller than the total *n* shown in the column heading due to missing measurements.

[c] Fifteen other eyes had preoperative best spectacle-corrected visual acuity worse than 20/20.

TABLE 41-3
Uncorrected Visual Acuity after Photorefractive Keratectomy for Myopia in 480 Eyes[a]

Uncorrected Visual acuity	*Preoperative (n = 480)*	*1 Month (n = 436)*	*3 Months (n = 415)*	*6 Months (n = 421)*	*12 Months (n = 344)*	*18 Months (n = 294)*	*≥24 Months (n = 480)*
20/20 or better (%)	0.0	32.3	45.1	55.8	63.7	65.6	58.3
20/25 to 20/40 (%)	0.4	57.3	47.5	38.7	31.4	29.6	35.4
20/50 to 20/80 (%)	5.0	9.2	6.7	5.5	4.7	4.4	5.8
20/100 or worse (%)	94.6	1.1	0.7	0.0	0.3	0.3	0.4

[a] All eyes underwent photorefractive keratectomy for myopia with a 6.0-mm-diameter ablation zone. The data are for eyes with 2 or more years of follow-up and initial treatment only.

TABLE 41-4
Efficacy and Predictability of Photorefractive Keratectomy for Myopia in 480 Eyes[a]

Spherical Equivalent	*Preoperative (n = 480)*	*1 Month (n = 434)*	*3 Months (n = 411)*	*6 Months (n = 419)*	*12 Months (n = 342)*	*18 Months (n = 294)*	*≥24 Months (n = 479)*[b]
≥-3.00 D (%)	76.7	0.2	0.5	1.0	0.3	0.3	0.2
-2.00 to <-3.00 D (%)	15.6	0.7	1.7	0.7	0.3	0.7	0.6
-1.00 to <-2.00 D (%)	7.7	6.9	10.0	8.1	12.3	11.2	12.7
-0.50 to +0.50 D (%)	0.0	68.4	69.6	71.6	74.3	72.8	70.8
-1.00 to +1.00 D (%)	0.2	86.9	90.0	92.4	90.4	91.5	90.8
+1.00 to <+2.00 D (%)	0.0	8.5	2.4	1.7	0.9	0.7	0.4
+2.00 to <+3.00 D (%)	0.0	1.6	0.7	0.2	0.3	0.0	0.0
≥+3.00 D (%)	0.0	0.5	0.0	0.0	0.0	0.0	0.0
Within ±0.50 D of intended correction (%)	—	60.1	64.5	68.7	68.1	69.0	64.5
Within ±1.00 D of intended correction (%)	—	83.6	88.1	91.6	91.6	91.8	90.2

Abbreviation: D, diopter.
[a] All eyes underwent photorefractive keratectomy for myopia with a 6.00-mm-diameter ablation zone. The data are for eyes with 2 or more years of follow-up and initial treatment only.
[b] One patient did not stay to have a refractive examination.

of emmetropia, and approximately 90 percent were within 1.00 diopter of the intended correction. There was an initial hyperopic overshoot of 1.00 diopter or more in 10.6 percent of eyes at 1 month; however, this percentage decreased to 1.2 at 1 year and 0.4 at 2 years. Otherwise, refractions remained relatively stable throughout the 2 years of follow-up.

Long-term stability of visual outcome was assessed in 147 eyes for which data were available at the 12-, 18-, and 24-month postoperative examinations (Figure 41-5). This subgroup of eyes was selected to eliminate bias that could result from missed visits during the follow-up period.

Long-term stability of refractive outcome was assessed in 126 eyes for which data were available at the 1-, 3-, 6-, 12-, 18-, and 24-month postoperative examinations (Figure 41-6). Mean refractive error was -4.07 diopters preoperatively, nearly plano (0.08 diopter) at 1 month, and -0.19 diopter at 3 months, after which it remained relatively stable through the 2-year examination. Between 12 and 24 months postoperatively, a myopic shift of 0.5 diopter or more occurred in 17.4 percent of eyes and of 1.0 diopter or more in 2.8 percent of eyes.

Adverse Events

The incidence of adverse events was tabulated at 1, 3 to 6, 12, and 24 or more months postoperatively. The percentage was calculated as the number of occurrences observed at each time period divided by the total number of eyes examined during that time period.

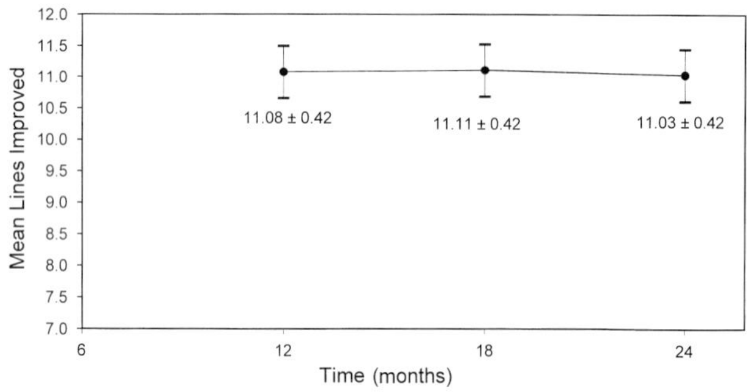

FIGURE 41-5 Number of lines of improvement in uncorrected visual acuity at various times after photorefractive keratectomy for myopia, compared with preoperative uncorrected visual acuity. All 147 cases included had data available for the 12-, 18- and 24-month examinations. Values are means ± standard error of the mean.

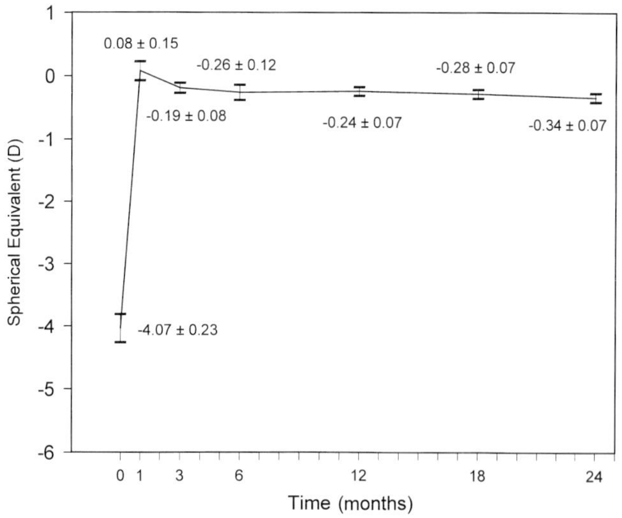

FIGURE 41-6 Spherical equivalent in diopters preoperatively and at various times after photorefractive keratectomy for myopia. All 126 cases included had data for the 1-, 3-, 6-, 12-, 18-, and 24-month examinations. Values are means ± standard error of the mean.

Loss of Best Spectacle-Corrected Visual Acuity The most accurate parameter to assess visual outcome as it pertains to patient safety is the percentage of eyes that lose best spectacle-corrected visual acuity. One of 328 eyes (0.2 percent) lost two or more lines of best spectacle-corrected visual acuity at 2 years postoperatively. Of the eyes with a preoperative best spectacle-corrected visual acuity of 20/20 or better, 1.3 percent had a best spectacle-corrected visual acuity worse than 20/25, and none had a best spectacle-corrected visual acuity worse than 20/40 at 2 or more years postoperatively.

Glare and Other Visual Symptoms The results of glare tests were considered abnormal if there was a loss of best spectacle-corrected visual acuity of two or more lines under moderate glare conditions measured with the Brightness Acuity Tester. Abnormal glare tests were reported in 1.6 percent of eyes at 1 year and in no eyes at 2 or more years.

Subjective evaluations of other visual symptoms were obtained by the use of a patient questionnaire self-administered preoperatively and at 6, 12, 18, and 24 months postoperatively. At 2 or more years postoperatively, 1.3 percent of patients reported significant worsening of double vision, 3.0 percent reported significant worsening of sensitivity to bright lights, and 3.9 percent reported significant worsening of difficulty with night vision compared with preoperative experience.

Overcorrection At 2 or more years postoperatively, 7 of 540 eyes (1.3 percent) were overcorrected by more than 1.00 diopter, and 3 of 540 eyes (0.6 percent) were overcorrected by more than 2 diopters.

Regular Astigmatism Refractive status was assessed at 1, 3, 6, 12, 18, and 24 or more months postoperatively. Between 3.1 percent and 5.4 percent of eyes had an increase of 1.00 diopter or more of refractive cylinder at each of the postoperative time periods. Fewer than 1 percent of the eyes had an increase of 2.00 or more diopters of refractive cylinder at any time postoperatively. No eyes had an increase of 2 or more diopters of refractive cylinder at 1 year or later.

Central Island Formation Videokeratography was performed on a subset of 350 eyes to evaluate surface regularity. The incidence of central islands was 11.8 percent (24 of 203 eyes) at 3 months, 5.9 percent (11 of 185 eyes) at 1 year, and 3.6 percent (2 of 55 eyes) at 2 years. Software refinements further reduced the incidence of central islands to 3.0 percent at 3 months and 0 at 1 year. No clinical correlation was seen between the presence of central islands and outcome data.

Corneal Haze Corneal haze was considered a complication of surgery if recorded as grade 2 or more. (Grade 2 was defined as moderate haze that made refraction possible, but difficult.) Grade 2 or more haze was reported in 1.3 percent of eyes at 3 to 6 months, and in 0.2 percent of eyes at 2 or more years.

Intraocular Pressure Elevation Because the recommended postoperative regimen included the use of topical corticosteroids, intraocular pressure was measured preoperatively and at each postoperative visit starting at 1 month. Intraocular pressure was increased 5 mmHg or more compared with preoperative values in 1.8 to 7.2 percent of eyes at the various examination intervals. Fewer than 1 percent of eyes had an increase of 10 mmHg or more at any time postoperatively.

Lens Abnormalities Fewer than 1 percent of eyes developed new lens abnormalities at any postoperative examination. None of these eyes had a best spectacle-corrected visual acuity worse than 20/25 –1 or loss of two lines of best spectacle-corrected visual acuity at the last examination. Only three eyes (0.6 percent) had lens abnormalities at 2 or more years postoperatively. Seven eyes had lens abnormalities that were not seen on subsequent examination.

Pain Complaints of pain were categorized as none, mild, moderate, or severe. During re-epithelialization, pain was absent in 29.8 percent of eyes and was reported as mild in 39.2 percent, moderate in 23.2 percent, and severe in 6.6 percent.

Other Adverse Events One eye (0.1 percent) had transient corneal edema, and three eyes (0.4 percent) developed a corneal infection, ulcer, or infiltrate. All four events occurred during the first week postoperatively. None of these patients experienced a loss of best spectacle-corrected visual acuity after appropriate treatment. No corneal perforations, intraocular infections, persistent corneal edema, hyphema, hypopyon, or cystoid macular edema were seen.

Effect on Corneal Endothelial Cells Specular microscopy was performed on a subset of 23 eyes. No statistically significant changes in endothelial cell density, coefficient of variation, or percent hexagonality were seen between preoperative and postoperative measurements taken at 6-month intervals during the 2 years of follow up. These results are consistent with published reports that photorefractive keratectomy has no detrimental effects on the human corneal endothelium.[20]

Retreatment

Patients were eligible for retreatment after 6 months of follow-up. Thirty-three eyes (3.6 percent) were retreated. The reasons for retreatment are summarized in Table 41-5 and the results are given in Table 41-6.

The risks of repeat photorefractive keratectomy are the same as those for the original procedure, with the additional caveat that patients who develop corneal haze and an accompanying loss of visual acuity after the first photorefractive keratectomy are similarly prone to develop these complications following retreatment. Surgeons are encouraged to wait for a significant reduction in corneal haze and concomitant refractive stability before considering retreatment. It appears that variation in the healing response is the major cause in the need for retreatment.

Summit Technology

A multicenter clinical study was conducted to determine the safety and efficacy of photorefractive keratectomy to treat mild to moderate myopia (up to 7.00 diopters). A total of 394 eyes of 300 patients were treated with a 6.00-mm-diameter ablation zone. Re-epithelialization was complete in 95.4 percent of eyes within 72 hours, and in all eyes within 1 week.

Efficacy, Predictability, and Stability

Six months after photorefractive keratectomy, uncorrected visual acuity was 20/40 or better in 95 percent of the 394 eyes, and 20/20 or better in 66 percent. One year after surgery, uncorrected visual acuity was 20/40 or better in 98.8 percent of eyes and 20/20 or better in 80.5 percent of eyes.

TABLE 41-5
Reasons for Retreatment after Photorefractive Keratectomy for Myopia

Reason for Retreatment	*Number of Eyes Retreated*	*Percentage of Retreated Eyes (n = 33)*	*Percentage of All Eyes (n = 909)*
Regression[a]	9	27.3	1.0
Undercorrection[b]	12	36.4	1.3
Regression with haze[c]	5	15.2	0.6
Undercorrection with regression and haze	3	9.1	0.3
Other: decentered ablation, haze, induced cylinder	4	12.1	0.4
Total	33	100.0	3.6

Abbreviation: D, diopter.
[a] Regression was defined as a myopic change in spherical equivalent of more than 0.5 D after the intended correction or refractive stability was achieved.
[b] Undercorrection was defined as 0.5 D or more myopic from intended correction through the first 6 months after treatment.
[c] Haze was defined as a grade greater than 1 at any time before retreatment.

TABLE 41-6
Results of Retreatment in 33 Eyes after Photorefractive Keratectomy for Myopia

Parameter Measured	Before First PRK (n = 33)	Before Second PRK (n=33)	After Second PRK (n = 28)[a]
Uncorrected visual acuity (%)			
20/20 or better	0.0	0.0	7.1
20/20 to 20/40	0.0	0.0	71.4
20/50 to 20/80	0.0	84.8	14.3
20/100 or worse	100.0	15.2	7.1
Best spectacle-corrected visual acuity (%)			
Better than 20/20	12.1	6.1	14.8
20/20	81.8	63.6	66.7
20/25	6.1	15.2	14.8
20/30	0.0	12.1	0.0
20/40	0.0	0.0	3.7
20/50	0.0	3.0	0.0
Spherical equivalent refraction (%)			
≥-3.00 D	84.8	6.1	3.6
>-2.00 to -3.00 D	12.1	15.2	3.6
>-1.00 to -2.00 D	3.0	45.5	14.3
-0.50 to +0.50 D	0.0	6.1	50.0
-1.00 to +1.00 D	0.0	30.3	78.6
> +1.00 to +2.00 D	0.0	3.0	0.0
Corneal haze (%)			
0 to 0.5 (trace)	100.0	84.8	92.6
1 to 1.5 (mild)	0.0	9.1	3.7
2 (moderate)	0.0	6.1	0.0
3 (marked)[b]	0.0	0.0	3.7

Abbreviations: PRK, photorefractive keratectomy; D, diopter.
[a] n = 28 for uncorrected visual acuity and spherical equivalent and 27 for best spectacle-corrected visual acuity and corneal haze grading, because of missing data.
[b] No patient was reported to have grade 4 haze.

In terms of predictability and stability, 64.8 percent of eyes were within 0.50 diopter of the intended correction and 89.4 percent were within 1.0 diopter of the intended correction 6 months postoperatively. At 1 year, the percentage of eyes within 0.50 diopter was 51.2 percent and within 1.0 diopter was 86.6 percent.

Adverse Events

Transient complaints reported during the first month after photorefractive keratectomy included pain, foreign body sensation, tearing, photophobia, ghost images, monocular diplopia, and anisocoria. These problems were thought to be related, for the most part, to the epithelial defect created by the procedure.

Loss of Best Spectacle-Corrected Visual Acuity A loss of two or more lines of best spectacle-corrected visual acuity occurred in 6.8 percent of the 394 eyes at 6 months after surgery and in 1.2 percent of eyes at 1 year after surgery. Best spectacle-corrected visual acuity was 20/20 or better in 100 percent of the eyes at 1 year postoperatively.

Glare and Other Visual Symptoms Ten percent of eyes had glare and 10 percent had halos 6 months after photorefractive keratectomy. These percentages were reduced to 2.4 percent each by 1 year.

Corneal Haze A total of 63 percent of eyes had some degree of anterior stromal reticular haze at 6 months after laser surgery; 54 percent had trace haze, 7.3 percent had mild haze, and 2.3 percent had moderate haze. One year postoperatively, 43.9 percent of eyes had haze, graded as trace in all cases.

Intraocular Pressure Elevation Intraocular pressure increased more than 5 mmHg, compared with preoperative values, in 1.8 percent of eyes at 6 months. At 1 year, none of the eyes had elevated intraocular pressure, compared with preoperative measurements.

Other Adverse Events Adverse events reported in fewer than 1 percent of eyes at any time in the course of the clinical study included dryness, foreign body sensation, photophobia, itching, discomfort, difficulty with reading, ghost images, blurred vision, monocular diplopia, corneal epithelial defect, superficial punctate keratitis, microcysts, corneal ulcer, corneal infection, scarring, diffuse nebulae, irregular astigmatism, guttae, iritis, cataract, lens opacity, and ptosis.

One patient developed cystoid macular edema with a macular hole, which was thought not to be related to the laser surgery. Another patient had myopic macular degeneration with peripheral choroidal scarring.

REFERENCES

1. Trokel SL, Srinivasan R, Braren B: Excimer laser surgery of the cornea. Am J Ophthalmol 96:710, 1983
2. Srinivasan R: Kinetics of the ablative photodecomposition of organic polymers in the far ultraviolet (193 nm). J Vac Sci Technol Bull 1:923, 1983
3. Taboada JM, Kessel GW, Reed RD: Response of the corneal epithelium to KrF excimer laser pulses. Health Phys 40:677, 1981
4. Munnerlyn CR, Koons SJ, Marshall J: Photorefractive keratectomy: a technique for laser refractive surgery. J Cataract Refract Surg 14:46, 1988
5. Schipper I, Senn P, Thomann U, Suppiger M: Intraocular pressure after excimer laser photorefractive keratectomy for myopia. J Refract Surg 11:366, 1995
6. Chatterjee A, Shah S, Bessant DA, et al: Reduction in intraocular pressure after excimer laser photorefractive keratectomy: correlation with pretreatment myopia. Ophthalmology 104:355, 1997
7. Uozato H, Guyton DL: Centering corneal surgical procedures. Am J Ophthalmol 103:264, 1987
8. Sher NA, Frantz JM, Talley A, et al: Topical diclofenac in the treatment of ocular pain after excimer photorefractive keratectomy. Refract Corneal Surg 9:425, 1993
9. Phillips AF, Szerenyi K, Campos M, et al: Arachidonic acid metabolites after excimer laser corneal surgery. Arch Ophthalmol 111:1273, 1993
10. Sher NA, Krueger RR, Teal T, et al: Role of topical corticosteroids and nonsteroidal anti-inflammatory drugs in the etiology of stromal infiltrates after excimer photorefractive keratectomy [letter]. J Refract Corneal Surg 10:587, 1994
11. Beuerman RW, McDonald MB, Varnell RJ, Thompson HW: Neurophysiological evaluation of corneal nerves in rabbits following excimer PRK. ARVO abstract. Invest Ophthalmol Vis Sci 34(suppl):704, 1993
12. Fitzsimmons TD, Fagerholm P, Tengroth B: Steroid treatment of myopic regression: acute refractive and topographic changes in excimer photorefractive keratectomy patients. Cornea 12:358, 1993
13. Krueger RR, Saedy NF, McDonnell PJ: Clinical analysis of steep central islands after excimer laser photorefractive keratectomy. Arch Ophthalmol 114:377, 1996
14. Hersh PS, Schwartz-Goldstein BH, The Summit Photorefractive Keratectomy Topography Study Group: Corneal topography of Phase III excimer laser photorefractive keratectomy. Characterization and clinical effects. Ophthalmology 102:963, 1995
15. Johnson DA, Haight DH, Kelly SE, et al: Reproducibility of videokeratographic digital subtraction maps after excimer laser photorefractive keratectomy. Ophthalmology 103:1392, 1996
16. Seiler T, Kahle G, Kriegerowski M: Excimer laser (193 nm) myopic keratomileusis in sighted and blind human eyes. Refract Corneal Surg 6:165, 1990
17. Brancato R, Carones F, Venturi E, Bertuzzi A: Corticosteroids vs diclofenac in the treatment of delayed regression after myopic photorefractive keratectomy. Refract Corneal Surg 9:376, 1993
18. Nassaralla BA, Szerenyi K, Wang XW, et al. Effect of diclofenac on corneal haze after photorefractive keratectomy in rabbits. Ophthalmology 102:469, 1995
19. Segawa K: Ultrastructural changes of the trabecular tissue in the primary open angle glaucoma. Jpn J Ophthalmol 19:317, 1975
20. Carones F, Brancato R, Venturi E, Morico A: The corneal endothelium after myopic excimer laser photorefractive keratectomy. Arch Ophthalmol 112:920, 1994

42

Photoastigmatic Refractive Keratectomy

ALEX POON AND HUGH R. TAYLOR

Astigmatism is an ocular condition in which a point source of light, after passing through the optical system of the eye, is not focused as a point on the retina or in any other plane. It is usually associated with spherical refractive errors. Naturally occurring (idiopathic) astigmatism is common; as many as 95 percent of eyes have some type of measurable astigmatism.[1]

Correction of astigmatism is required for an individual to see well. Optical corrections include spectacles and contact lenses. In patients with large amounts of astigmatism, meridional magnification can cause distortion of images, and spectacles can be intolerable.[2] Hard, rigid gas-permeable, and toric soft contact lenses can all be used to treat astigmatism. Although the risks of contact lens wear are minimal if recommended wear and cleaning regimens are followed, microbial keratitis, corneal vascularization, and other complications can occur and can be catastrophic.[3] Many patients want a method of correction that is more convenient than spectacles or contact lenses. Refractive surgical procedures that correct astigmatism by changing the shape of the cornea have evolved over the past several years. Astigmatic keratotomy is discussed in Chapter 38. Photoastigmatic refractive keratectomy, the correction of astigmatism by changing the anterior corneal curvature using excimer laser photoablation, is the subject of this chapter.

PRINCIPLES OF ASTIGMATISM

Astigmatism occurs when no point focus is formed from a point source of light because of unequal refraction of the light by the optical system of the eye in different meridians (Figure 42-1). Correction of astigmatism requires the elimination of the difference in refractive power between the meridians by external aids, such as spectacles or contact lenses, or by surgically changing the optical components of the eye. Astigmatism may be classified in a number of ways. It is important to identify the type of astigmatism present before considering any corrective treatment.

Regular astigmatism (Figure 42-2) occurs when the steepest and flattest meridians are 90 degrees from each other and the blurred retinal image can be improved with an appropriate cylindrical correction. Oblique astigmatism is a form of regular astigmatism in which the steepest and flattest meridians are more than 10 degrees away from the 90- and 180-degree meridians.

Simple myopic astigmatism occurs when the eye is emmetropic in one meridian and myopic in the other. Compound myopic astigmatism occurs when both the steepest and flattest meridians are focused anterior to the retina. In simple hyperopic astigmatism, the eye is emmetropic in one meridian and hyperopic in the other. Compound hyperopic astigmatism occurs when both meridians are focused posterior to the retina. In mixed astigmatism, one meridian is focused anterior to the retina and the other is focused posterior to the retina.

Irregular astigmatism exists when the amount of astigmatism changes along a given meridian and varies from meridian to meridian (Figure 42-3). It is usually secondary to an irregular corneal surface, and the blurred image cannot be corrected with a cylinder. Hard or rigid gas-permeable contact lenses are used to mask the irregular corneal surface and treat irregular astigmatism.

Idiopathic astigmatism may result from abnormalities in any component of the optical pathway. An abnormality of the anterior corneal surface is the most common cause. In the average cornea, there is a 0.50- to 0.75-diopter difference between the powers of the principal meridians of the anterior surface. In most young individuals, the ver-

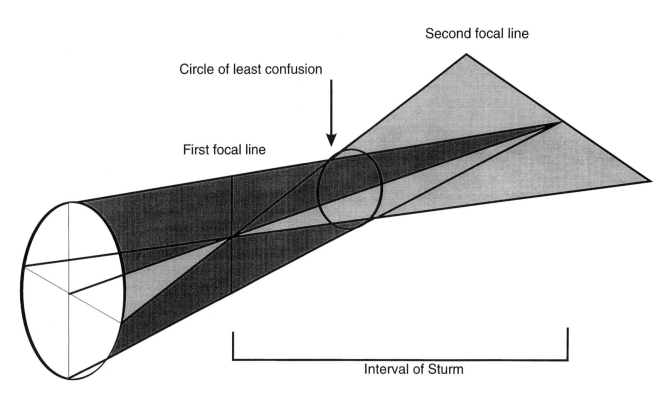

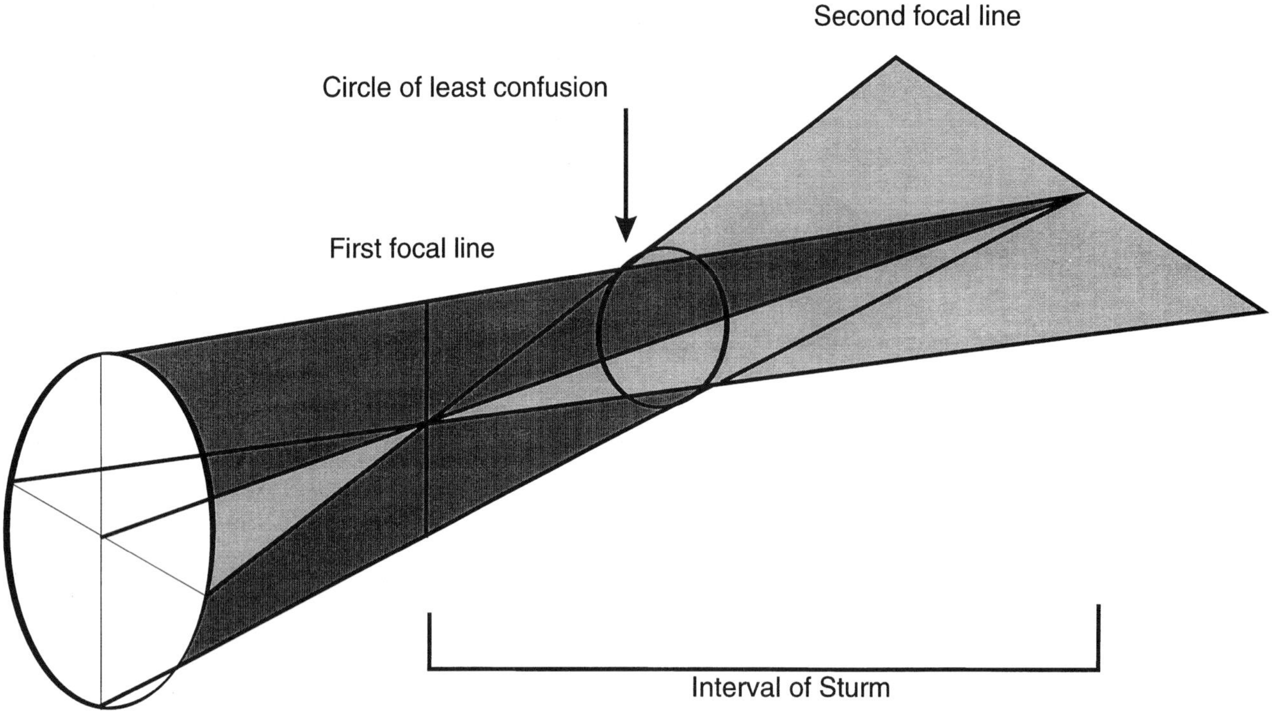

FIGURE 42-1 Schematic diagram of the conoid of Sturm. Astigmatic error produces two focal lines separated by the interval of Sturm. The circle of least confusion is where a point source can be imaged with least blur without astigmatic correction.

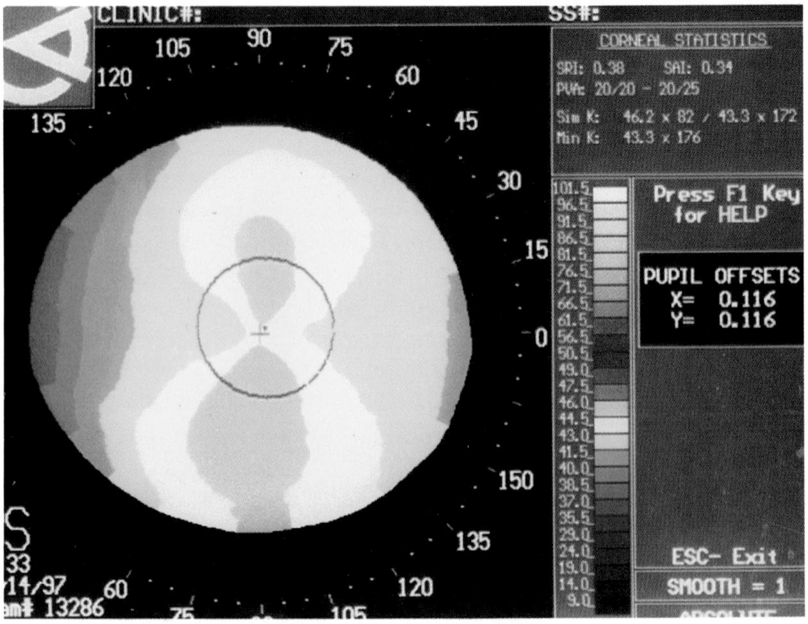

FIGURE 42-2 Videokeratograph illustrating regular with-the-rule astigmatism.

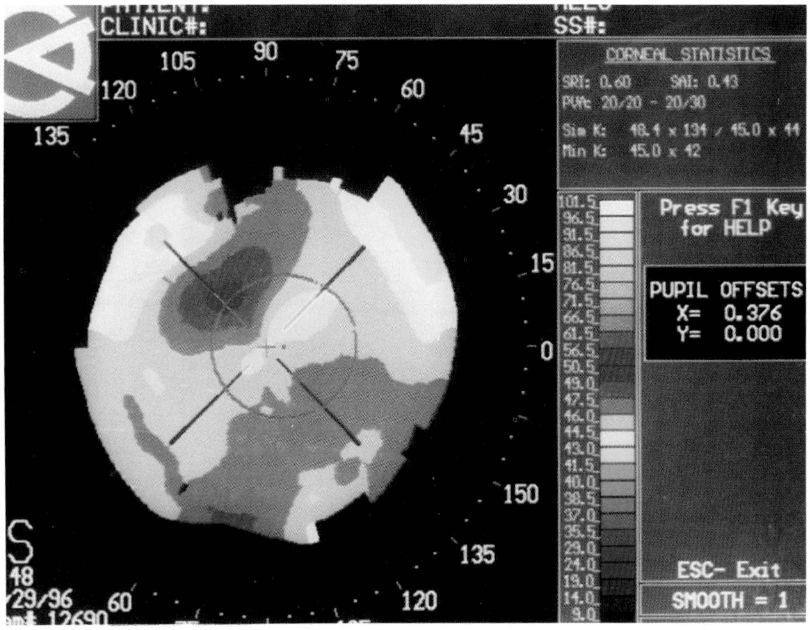

FIGURE 42-3 Videokeratograph illustrating irregular astigmatism.

tical meridian is the steepest meridian, resulting in with-the-rule astigmatism. With age, the vertical meridian flattens and the horizontal meridian steepens, resulting in against-the-rule astigmatism. The posterior corneal surface also contributes to astigmatism. The astigmatic error of the posterior corneal surface is 0.25 to 0.50 diopter, and the principal meridians are usually oriented opposite those of the anterior surface. Thus, astigmatism arising from the posterior surface partially neutralizes that arising from the anterior surface. The crystalline lens has a greater radius of curvature horizontally than vertically. In addition, the cortical lamellae are not always concentric, which means that the refractive index of the lens may be different in different meridians. The absence of a true axis of symmetry within the eye, together with some inherent tilting of the retina, may also be a source of astigmatism.

Astigmatism that is iatrogenic or related to disease states usually is of greater magnitude and more likely to be irregular. Corneal scars, keratoconus, large-incision cataract extraction, and penetrating keratoplasty can all cause astigmatism. A subluxated lens or tilted intraocular lens can also cause astigmatism. As a rule, astigmatism caused by these various conditions is not as easy to correct with refractive surgery as is idiopathic astigmatism. However, astigmatism from large-incision cataract extraction or penetrating keratoplasty is amenable to photoastigmatic refractive keratectomy.

Photorefractive keratectomy for the correction of myopia can induce astigmatism. The amount of surgically induced astigmatism increases with the amount of preoperative myopia and is about 10 percent of the preoperative spherical equivalent. In one report of 155 patients with 1.00 to 15.00 diopters of myopia who underwent photorefractive keratectomy, the average amount of surgically induced astigmatism was 0.50 diopter.[4] Astigmatism after photorefractive keratectomy may be caused by irregular epithelial hyperplasia or by decentration of the ablation.[4] Surgically induced astigmatism can also occur after photoastigmatic refractive keratectomy.

Astigmatism is defined by two components: (1) the power of the cylinder and (2) the axis of the cylinder. Photoastigmatic refractive keratectomy and other refractive surgical procedures for the correction of astigmatism are performed by altering these two components. In the analysis of refractive surgical data, it is inadequate simply to compare the magnitudes of preoperative and postoperative astigmatism without regard to their respective axes. For example, a patient with a preoperative cylinder of 3.00 diopters at 30 degrees has different surgically induced astigmatism if the postoperative cylinder is 0.50 diopter at 30 degrees than if the postoperative cylinder is 0.50 diopter at 100 degrees. To analyze the effect of surgery, one must perform vector analysis, which indicates the change in both the power and the axis of the cylinder. There are several vector analysis formulas that can be used to calculate surgically induced astigmatism from the preoperative and postoperative refractions.[5–8]

HISTORY

Incisional keratotomy to treat astigmatism after cataract extraction was first described by Snellen in 1860, and since

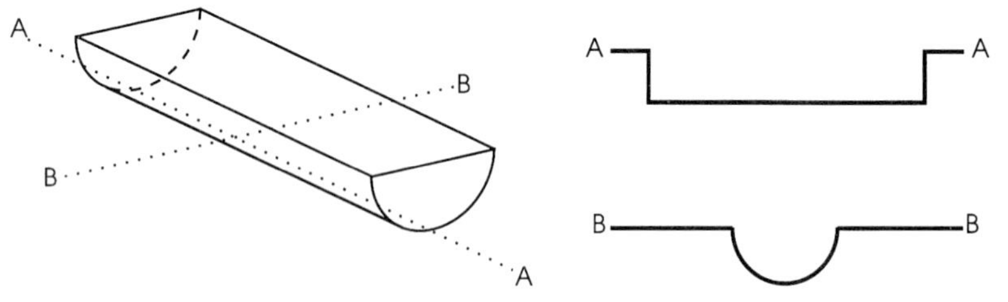

FIGURE 42-4 Schematic diagram of a pure cylindrical ablation for myopic astigmatism. The mechanical axis is identified by the dotted line *A*. Cross section through the mechanical axis *(A)* is identical to phototherapeutic keratectomy, and no refractive change is obtained. Cross section through the meridian perpendicular to the mechanical axis *(B)* is identical to a myopic ablation; flattening occurs in that meridian.

that time, surgeons have used a variety of similar techniques to treat postoperative astigmatism. The development of radial keratotomy by Fyodorov showed that corneal incisions can change the anterior corneal curvature in a somewhat predictable manner.[9] The major disadvantages of incisional keratotomy include a weakened cornea (because of the need to make the depth of the incisions at least 80 percent of the corneal thickness), inaccurate results, and instability of the refractive effect.

Since the late 1980s, considerable work has been done with the argon-fluoride excimer laser to correct refractive errors, including astigmatism. This laser produces pulses of high-energy, short-wavelength (193 nm) ultraviolet radiation. When directed at the cornea, this radiation disrupts intramolecular bonds and ablates the tissue with submicron accuracy with little effect on adjacent tissue. By shaping the beam to ablate more tissue centrally than peripherally, one can make the cornea less steep and the eye less myopic. This procedure is called *photorefractive keratectomy* or *PRK* and has an established role in the treatment of low and moderate myopia, as described in Chapter 41.[10–14] A variant that involves making a greater ablation peripherally than centrally is also being developed to treat hyperopia. By modifying and adding to photorefractive keratectomy techniques, one can ablate a cylindrical or toric shape on the corneal surface to correct astigmatism. The term *photoastigmatic refractive keratectomy* or *PARK* has been coined for this procedure.

LASERS

The excimer laser was initially developed to create radially symmetrical or spherical ablations for the correction of myopia. The problem of astigmatism was addressed by creating cylindrical or toric ablations, first on plastic spheres, then on rabbit corneas, and finally, in 1991, on human eyes.[15] An expanding slit diaphragm was used initially; subsequently other techniques were developed, including scanning beams and various maskings, including ablatable masks. Below is a description of the methodologies used by various excimer lasers for the treatment of astigmatism. At the time of this writing, several lasers were under evaluation by the U.S. Food and Drug Administration (FDA) for the treatment of astigmatism, but only the VISX laser had been approved for this purpose in the United States.

VISX Excimer Laser

The first clinical use of the excimer laser to treat astigmatism was with the expanding slit of the VISX model Twenty/Twenty excimer laser to treat eyes with high astigmatism after penetrating keratoplasty or corneal trauma.[16] This was soon followed by treatment of idiopathic astigmatism associated with myopia.[11,17,18]

Initially, photoastigmatic refractive keratectomy was performed using sequential ablations, in which the cylindrical correction was performed separately, before or after the spherical myopic correction.[11,17,18] In sequential ablations, two separate expanding diaphragms are used one after the other: a slit diaphragm for the cylindrical ablation and a round diaphragm for the spherical ablation. Ablation through the expanding slit diaphragm causes corneal flattening in the meridian perpendicular to the long axis of the slit (Figure 42-4). The long axis of the slit is the mechanical axis and ideally should not undergo refractive changes. With the laser pulsing at a constant rate, the speed of the expansion of the slit diaphragm determines the power of the cylinder induced. The slower the speed, the deeper the central ablation and the higher the power of the cylinder induced. Experience with the VISX laser showed that the early cylindrical corrections, in which the width of the slit equaled the length, were associated with a significant hyperopic shift. Later configurations that reduced the width of the slit to no more than 80 percent of its length were not associated with a hyperopic shift.[11,19]

VISX subsequently developed software that allows myopia and astigmatism to be treated at the same time. The slit diaphragm and the circular diaphragm expand simultaneously to create an elliptical ablation (Figure 42-5). Correction with an elliptical ablation requires that the amount of astigmatism not exceed the amount of

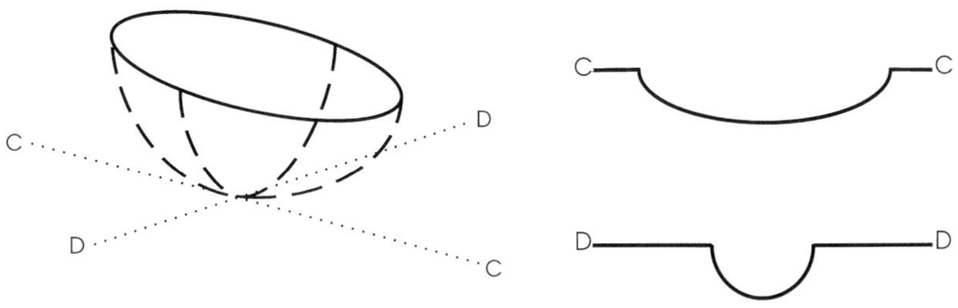

FIGURE 42-5 Schematic diagram of an elliptical ablation for myopic astigmatism shows that the cornea is flattened more in the meridian identified by *D* than in the meridian identified by *C*.

myopia. If the amount of astigmatism exceeds the amount of myopia, sequential ablations must be performed. Early studies in Melbourne, Australia, showed that both sequential and elliptical ablations tended to undercorrect astigmatism, and an increase in the magnitude of treatment by a factor of 1.2 was made and subsequently incorporated into the VISX software.[19]

Summit Excimer Laser

The use of an erodible mask to perform photorefractive keratectomy was introduced in 1989.[20] The mask is a polymethyl methacrylate button bonded to a quartz substrate that is placed between the laser beam and the cornea. The undersurface of the button is flat and the top surface has the curvature change required for the desired refractive correction. The button has an ablation rate similar to that of the corneal stroma. Ablation is performed, and as the thinnest part of the button is completely ablated, the beam starts to ablate the cornea directly underlying that part of the button. Ablation of the entire button effectively translates the curvature of the anterior surface of the button onto the anterior surface of the cornea, resulting in the desired refractive surface (Figure 42-6). Theoretically, this technique has the advantage of being able to correct all kinds of refractive errors because the anterior curvature of the button can be made to have any profile.

Summit excimer lasers initially perform the myopic correction with a diaphragm and then use an ablatable mask for the astigmatic correction in a sequential manner. The original ablatable masks were difficult to center and align because they were held in an eye cup that was positioned manually on the patient's eye.[21-25] To solve this problem, the mask was placed into a cartridge in the optical rail of the excimer laser path.[26] At the time of this writing, toric masks that can correct both myopia and astigmatism at the same time were being evaluated.

Aesculap-Meditec Excimer Laser

The Aesculap-Meditec MEL 60 excimer laser uses a scanning slit beam and a rotating mask. The scanning beam moves uniformly over a circular area. Without a mask, a uniform ablation of 1 μm is achieved with each scanning process. Myopia and astigmatism are corrected by the use of a rotating metal mask with an appropriate hourglass-shaped opening[27] (Figure 42-7). The mask is secured to the eye by a suction ring. When the mask is rotated in equidistant angular steps over 360 degrees, a radially symmetrical ablation is achieved that corrects myopia. By varying the angular steps between scans, the ablation can be made deeper in one meridian than in the other meridians, thus achieving astigmatic correction.

Early attempts to correct hyperopic astigmatism with this laser have been reported.[28] The mask for hyperopic correction has a 9-mm-diameter aperture in a rotating template (Figure 42-8). The central cornea is steepened in the 6-mm-diameter treatment area; there is a transition zone between 6 and 9 mm. The central 0.3 to 0.5 mm of cornea is not ablated. As with the treatment of myopic astigmatism, the treatment of hyperopic astigmatism involves uneven rotation of the mask so that the ablation is deeper in one meridian than in the others.

Schwind Excimer Laser

The Schwind excimer laser originally used a revolving steel band with several apertures through which the laser beam passed.[29] Myopic ablations were created by the laser beam passing through round apertures of increasing sizes. Initially, toric ablations were created with the use of oval apertures aligned in the correct axis. Early reports were encouraging,[29] but further results have not been published. Subsequently, the steel band was replaced by a fractile mask because of patent issues.

Scanning Lasers

The Chiron/Technolas Keracor 117, Nidek EC-5000, and LaserSight Laser-Scan 2000 excimer lasers employ a scanning mechanism for photoablation. The smaller beam of scanning lasers allows for a smaller and cheaper system, but the ablation generally requires more time. The Nidek EC-5000 has a linear laser beam that sweeps the

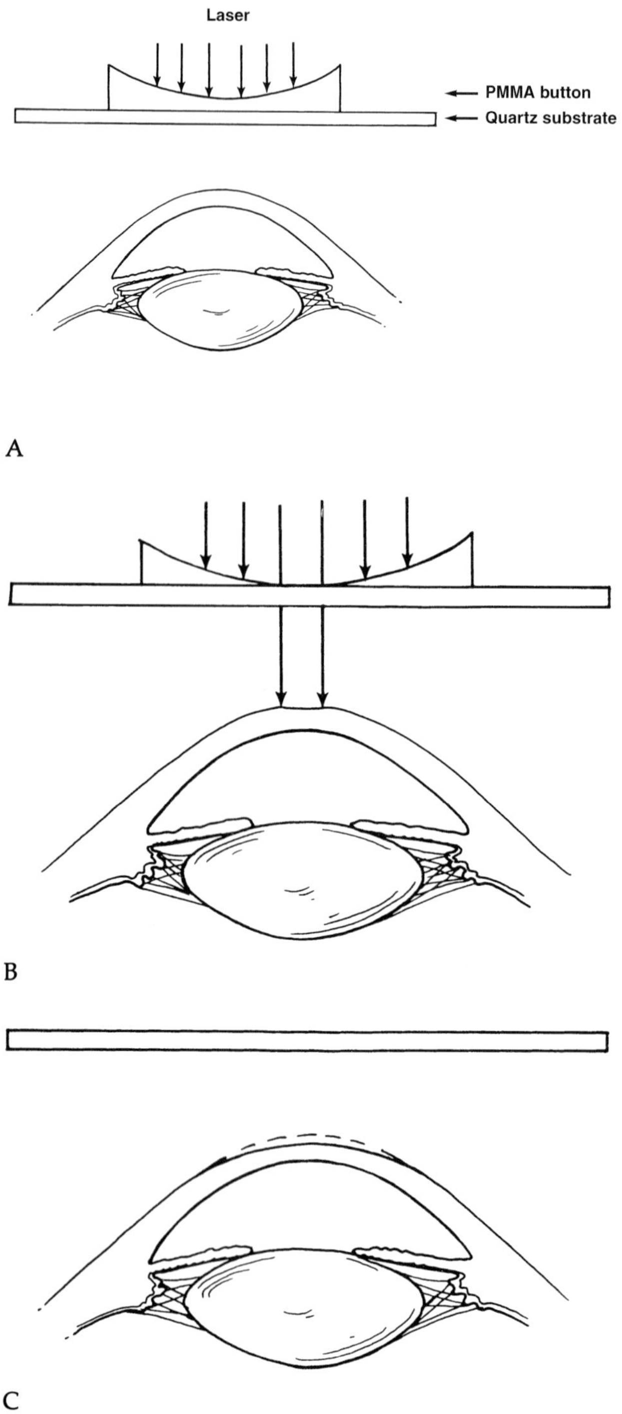

FIGURE 42-6 (A) Schematic diagram shows a mask placed between the laser and the eye. (B) The laser ablates through the thinnest part of the mask first and then begins ablating corneal tissue. (C) The shape of the anterior surface of the mask is summated on the anterior corneal surface. PMMA, polymethyl methacrylate.

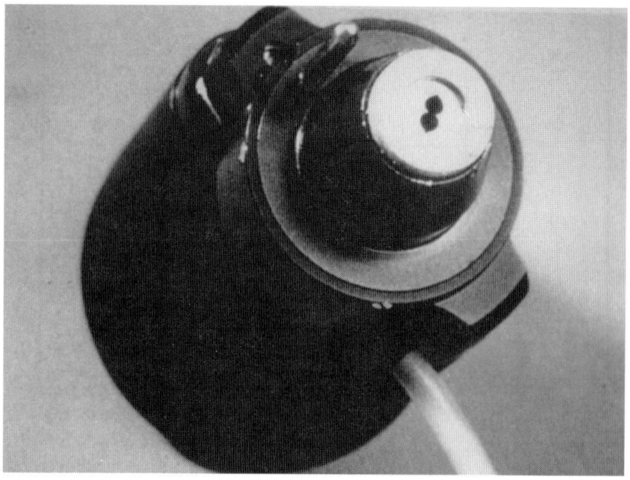

FIGURE 42-7 Meditec rotating mask used for the treatment of myopia and myopic astigmatism. The mask has an hourglass-shaped opening. (Reprinted with permission from D Dausch, R Klein, M Landesz, E Schröeder: Photorefractive keratectomy to correct astigmatism with myopia or hyperopia. J Cataract Refract Surg 20[suppl]:252, 1994. © Journal of Cataract and Refractive Surgery.)

corneal surface in six directions (Figure 42-9). Astigmatic correction is achieved by programming the scanning laser to ablate in one meridian for a longer period of time. Myopic astigmatism and hyperopic astigmatism can be treated with this technique.

The longer treatment time required for scanning lasers allows more opportunity for loss of patient fixation or centration. Therefore, some companies have developed scanning lasers with some type of tracking mechanism, such as the Autonomous Technologies T-PRK excimer laser and the Chiron/Technolas Keracor 116 excimer laser.

PATIENT SELECTION

It is important that patients considering photoastigmatic refractive keratectomy be properly evaluated and counseled and that the options for correction of astigmatism be discussed. It seems reasonable to treat astigmatism of 1.00 diopter or more, in that 1.00 diopter of astigmatism by itself can decrease visual acuity by one or two lines, depending on the axis of the cylinder.[30,31]

In general, the selection criteria for photoastigmatic refractive keratectomy are similar to those for photorefractive keratectomy described in Chapter 41. Patients should be at least 18 years of age. Best-corrected visual acuity should be 20/40 or better in both eyes. Keratometry and refraction should be stable, with 1.00 to 6.00 diopters of astigmatism and no more than 15.00 diopters of myopia at the corneal plane. (In the United States, the VISX laser is approved for the correction of 0.75 to 4.00 diopters of astigmatism at the spectacle plane in patients 21 years of age or older with 6.00 diopters or less of spherical myopia at the spectacle plane.) Soft contact lenses should be removed at least 1 week and hard contact lenses at least 1 month before the patient is evaluated for photoastigmatic keratectomy.

Although idiopathic regular astigmatism can be corrected with spectacles or contact lenses, photoastigmatic refractive keratectomy is well suited to individuals who are unable to tolerate these optical aids or who have occupational or recreational needs that preclude their use. Irregular astigmatism is more difficult to treat with photoastigmatic refractive keratectomy, and a trial of hard or rigid gas-permeable contact lens wear is recommended.

Most patients seeking excimer laser surgery for the correction of myopia have concomitant astigmatism. Patients with mild myopia (less than 5.00 diopters) have an average of 1.00 diopter of astigmatism, those with moderate myopia (between 5.00 and 10.00 diopters) an average of 1.20 diopters, and those with severe myopia (more than 10.00 diopters) an average of 1.39 diopters. Astigmatism associated with myopia should be treated at the same time as the myopia to achieve optimal uncorrected visual acuity postoperatively.[32]

Keratoconus has traditionally been regarded as a contraindication to both photorefractive keratectomy and photoastigmatic refractive keratectomy because of the instability of refraction and the likelihood of progression after treatment. Most patients with keratoconus who have no apical scarring obtain functional vision with hard or rigid gas-permeable contact lenses. However, contact lenses become increasingly difficulty to fit as the cornea becomes more conical. By reshaping the anterior corneal surface, contact lens fitting may be facilitated. In certain patients in whom keratoconus has progressed to a stage at which contact lenses can no longer be worn and penetrating keratoplasty would be required for visual rehabilitation, the anterior corneal surface can be reshaped with the excimer laser to aid contact lens fitting, improve visual acuity, and delay penetrating keratoplasty, if only temporarily. For these patients, nothing is lost if the laser treatment is unsuccessful.

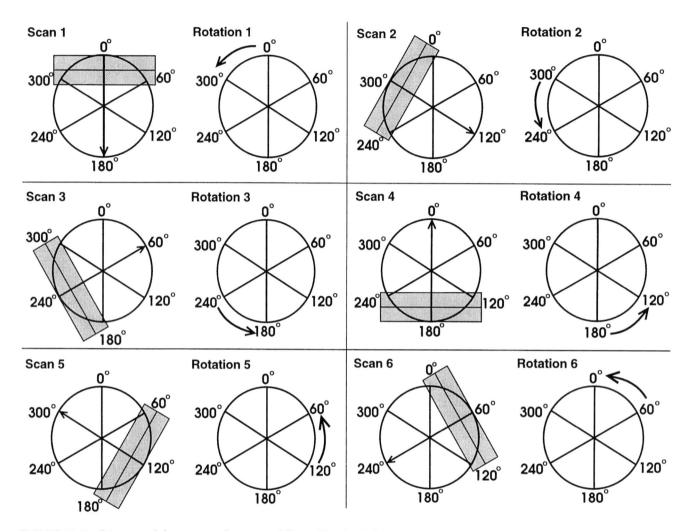

FIGURE 42-8 Meditec rotating mask used for the treatment of hyperopia and hyperopic astigmatism.

PREOPERATIVE EVALUATION

Patients who have decided to undergo photoastigmatic refractive keratectomy should have a thorough ophthalmologic examination. Uncorrected and best spectacle-corrected visual acuities for distance and near are measured, and manifest refractions for distance and near are performed. Assessment of near vision is especially important in myopic patients who are approaching presbyopia but who have not yet begun to wear spectacles for near. Patients who do not have a best spectacle-corrected visual acuity of 20/20 must be evaluated for the cause. Slit lamp and funduscopic examinations are performed to detect the presence of active ocular disease, including blepharitis, dry eyes, ocular surface disorders, ectatic corneal degenerations, glaucoma, cataracts, and/or retinal disease.

Although keratometry is usually performed, more information is provided by videokeratography. Videokeratography provides data for a larger area of the cornea

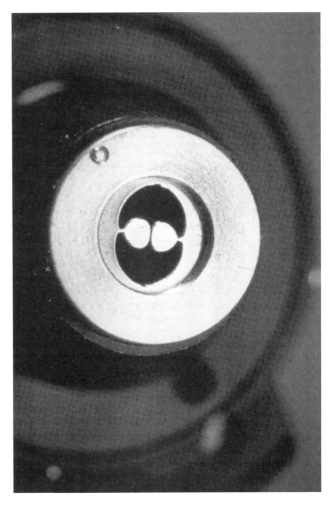

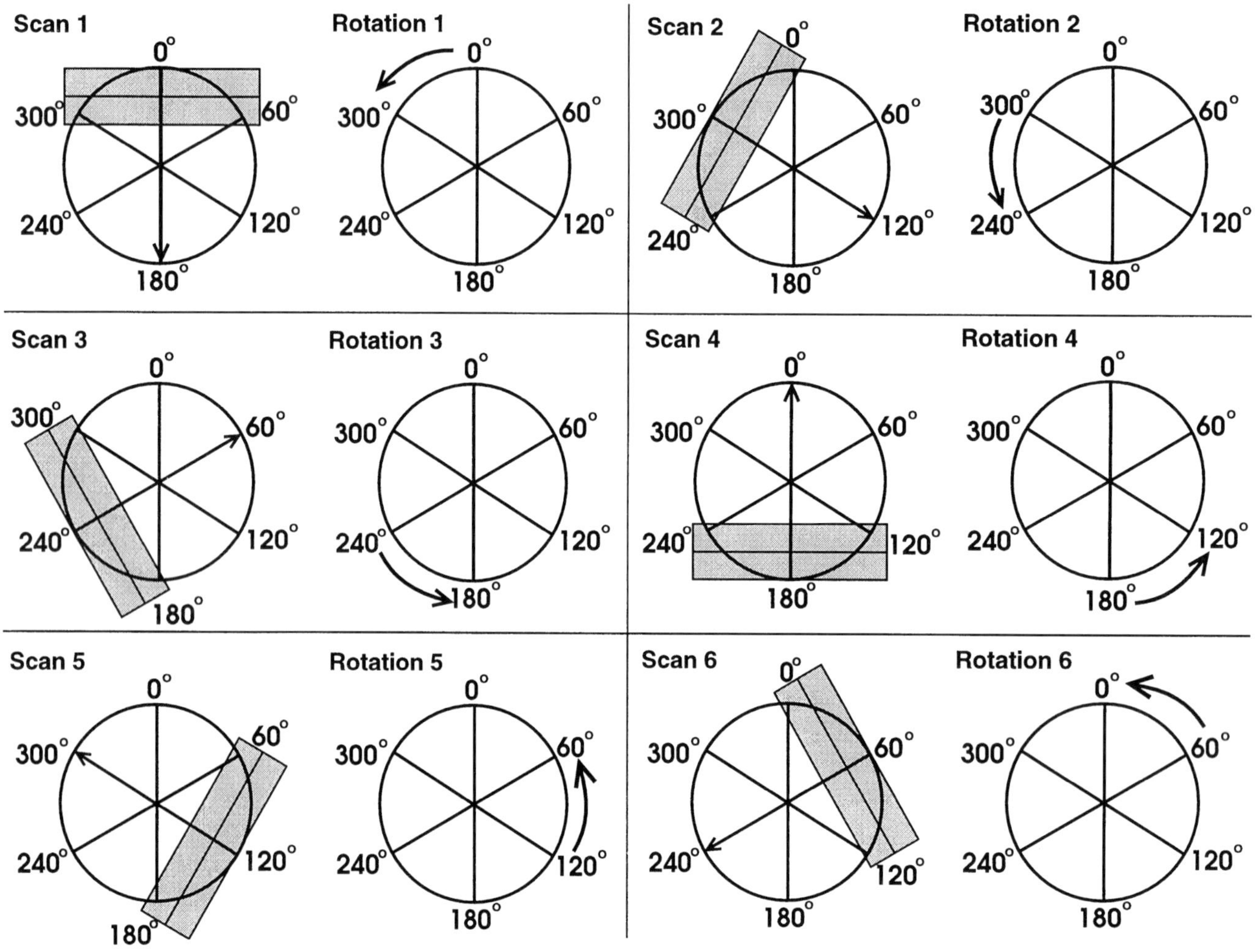

FIGURE 42-9 Diagram of the pattern of scanning followed by the Nidek EC-5000 scanning excimer laser. The slit scans over the whole cornea back and forth once starting from the 12 o'clock position. It then rotates 60 degrees counterclockwise, scans in a similar fashion, and rotates another 60 degrees. In total, six series of scans are performed to cover a full circle. Astigmatism is corrected by manipulating the time spent ablating in one meridian compared with another.

and presents that data in a color-coded map of corneal surface powers (see Ch. 46). Videokeratography has become invaluable in distinguishing between regular and irregular astigmatism and in identifying early keratoconus. Controversy exists whether the older Placido-disk based videokeratoscopes, which measure dioptric power by projecting mires on the anterior corneal surface, or newer systems that measure corneal elevation provide more useful information for photorefractive keratectomy.[33-35] At the time of this writing, more of the Placido-disk-based videokeratoscopes were in use, and their reliability and consistency had already been established.

Subtraction or difference maps that display the dioptric change in corneal power between two maps of the same cornea taken at different times are available in most videokeratography systems. This analysis allows comparison of the changes in corneal topography over time, and is invaluable in assessing the effect and stability of refractive surgery.

Most surgeons perform photoastigmatic refractive keratectomy based on the cylinder component of the manifest refraction. However, refractive astigmatism usually differs from keratometric or videokeratographic astigmatism. In the past, ablations for astigmatism have been based on the refraction. If there is a disparity between refractive and corneal astigmatism, the resulting cornea will be nonspherical, even when the postoperative refraction is plano. It has been suggested that this may cause aberrations and degradation of vision.[36] Visual outcome may be improved by taking into account both refractive and corneal astigmatism. Alpins[36] suggested basing treatment on a compromise between refractive and corneal astigmatism to optimize visual outcome. To our knowledge, no published studies have compared the results of photoastigmatic refractive keratectomy based on refraction, videokeratography, and/or a compromise between the two.

SURGICAL TECHNIQUES

The amount of astigmatism to be corrected is based on the manifest refraction, expressed in negative-cylinder form, converted to the corneal plane. With the VISX laser, astigmatism and myopia are treated simultaneously with an elliptical ablation unless the magnitude of the cylinder exceeds the magnitude of the sphere, in which case sequential ablations are performed.

Irregular astigmatism can be treated by using a combination of phototherapeutic keratectomy and photorefractive keratectomy (see Ch. 30). Corneal topography is used to guide treatment. Steep areas seen on topographic maps are treated using phototherapeutic keratectomy, in which the depth of ablation is constant for the area treated. Multiple phototherapeutic keratectomies are performed to ablate all steep areas, followed by a central spherical ablation to correct any residual myopia.[20] In the future, videokeratography used in conjunction with a scanning or flying spot laser may provide more accurate treatment of irregular astigmatism.

The treatment itself is similar to photorefractive keratectomy, as described in Chapter 41. The alignment of the eye and the laser is especially important. Some suggest that the patient's cornea be marked at the 90- and 180-degree meridians to help align the cornea with the laser. We tested a more rigorous alignment system, in which the patient verified the axis after being positioned under the laser immediately before treatment.[37] In a prospective randomized study,[37] however, this system did not improve the correction of astigmatism. Much of the putative axis misalignment seen postoperatively may be the result of variations in epithelial healing and irregular epithelial hyperplasia. Therefore, it is probably not necessary to do more to align the axis intraoperatively other than to ensure that the patient is correctly placed under the laser with the head and body straight.

POSTOPERATIVE CARE

Postoperative management after photoastigmatic refractive keratectomy is similar to that for photorefractive keratectomy. Patients are examined every 24 to 48 hours until the cornea has re-epithelialized. Patients can then be examined 1 week and 1, 3, 6, and 12 months postoperatively. Refraction, uncorrected and best spectacle-corrected visual acuities, corneal haze, and intraocular pressure are evaluated, and videokeratography is performed at each visit (Figure 42-10).

RESULTS

Myopic Astigmatism

Table 42-1 summarizes the major reports on photoastigmatic refractive keratectomy.[4,11,17,22,24–27,29,38–47] It is difficult to compare the results from the various studies because of different patient profiles and different ways in which data are presented. Some studies used vector analysis to determine the treatment outcome. Several simply calculated the surgical effect arithmetically, however. Although this latter method may give an idea of the effect of treatment in an individual patient, it is not adequate for the determination of trends or the mean of a series of patients. Vector analysis is essential to judge the success of photoastigmatic refractive keratectomy and to compare one technique with another.

The results of photoastigmatic refractive keratectomy are encouraging, with most large studies reporting a greater than 60 percent reduction in astigmatism, and a 70 to 80 percent chance of obtaining an uncorrected visual acuity of 20/40 or better. With the VISX Twenty/Twenty excimer laser, we found undercorrection in the early cases but a subsequent increase in the magnitude of treatment by a factor of 1.2 resulted in improvement from 78 percent of the intended correction to 90 percent.

The Melbourne Group[4] found that with the VISX Twenty/Twenty excimer laser, patients with mild myopia (less than 5.00 diopters) did better in terms of reduction of astigmatism than patients with higher amounts of myopia; the efficacy of the astigmatic correction was reduced for patients with moderate myopia (5.00 to 10.00 diopters) and those with severe myopia (more than 10.00 diopters).[4] In contrast, using the Summit ablatable masks, Danjoux et al[26] found that patients with more than 6 diopters of myopia had a higher astigmatism correction index (surgically induced astigmatism/target-induced astigmatism × 100) than patients with lower amounts of myopia, and Niles et al[25] observed little difference between patients with less than 8.00 diopters of myopia and those with more than 8.00 diopters of myopia, although uncorrected visual acuity was worse in the high myopia group. Other studies have supported the idea that postoperative visual acuity depends to a greater extent on the preoperative sphere than on the cylinder[14,40]; the photorefractive

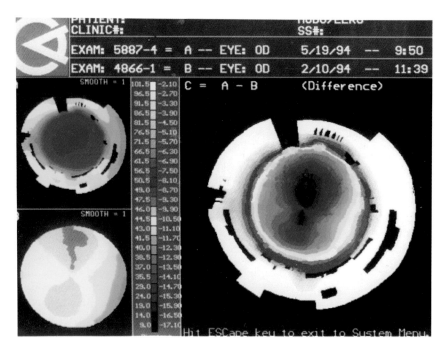

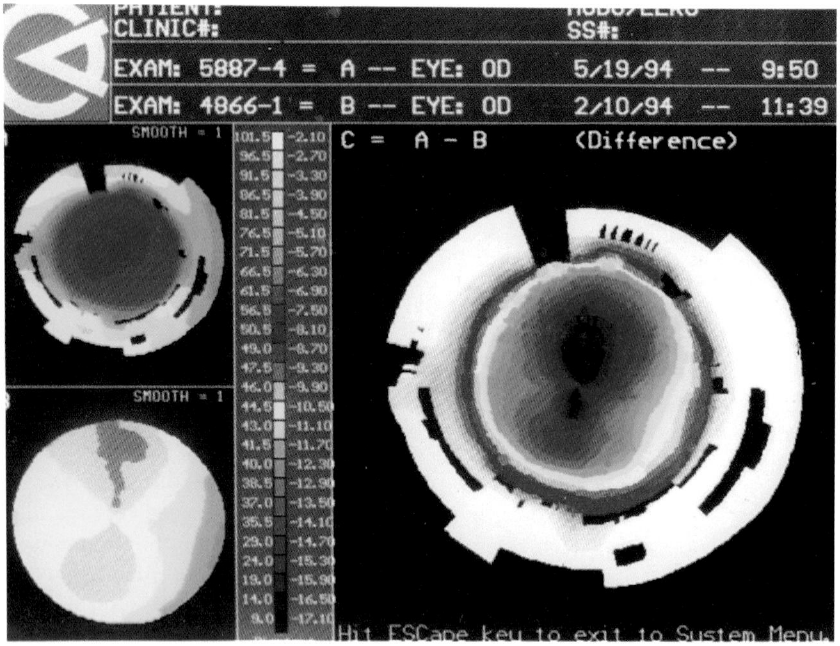

FIGURE 42-10 Videokeratographs of a patient who underwent photoastigmatic refractive keratectomy. Preoperative refraction was -14.00 -2.25 × 172. **(A)** Postoperative videokeratograph shows a well-centered ablation. **(B)** Preoperative videokeratograph illustrates the astigmatic component. **(C)** Videokeratograph showing the difference between A and B.

keratectomy data for spherical myopia are also consistent with this concept.

Some investigators compared photoastigmatic refractive keratectomy between patients with different levels of astigmatism. Danjoux et al[26] reported that the astigmatic correction index was better for low (less than 1.50 diopters) and moderate (1.51 to 3.00 diopters) astigmatism than for high (more than 3.01 diopters) astigmatism. However, Kremer et al[11] found that the correction of astigmatism was most accurate for those with higher amounts of astigmatism. Again, the difference between studies can be attributed to the different lasers used and the differing methods of data analysis.

In early studies in which sequential photoastigmatic refractive keratectomy ablations were performed with the VISX Twenty/Twenty excimer laser, the spherical ablation was adjusted to compensate for the hyperopic shift from the cylindrical ablation. The need for this adjustment in sequential ablations was practically eliminated by decreasing the width of the cylindrical ablation from 6 mm to 4.5 mm; the adjustment was not needed at all for elliptical ablations that corrected astigmatism and myopia simultaneously. The Melbourne group found an overcorrection of 1.00 diopter or more in only 2.2 percent of eyes undergoing photorefractive keratectomy and photoastigmatic refractive keratectomy.[48]

In most reports, apparent axis misalignment appears to be significant. Misalignment causes undercorrection of cylinder and induces cylinder in a new axis.[49] Theories put forth for the misalignment include incorrect preoperative refraction, misalignment of the patient's head with the laser beam, and involuntary cyclotorsion or other movement of the eye during treatment. The accuracy of astigmatic correction appeared to be less for astigmatism of less than 1.00 diopter.[4] This finding was consistent for all levels of myopia. As mentioned above, we found no advantage in using an in situ axis alignment system.[37]

Regression after photoastigmatic keratectomy appears to follow the same pattern as regression after photorefractive keratectomy—that is, greater for higher amounts of refractive error. In one study, among patients treated with photoastigmatic refractive keratectomy, the mean postoperative spherical equivalent for patients with mild myopia (less than 5.00 diopters) was $+0.05 \pm 0.62$ diopter at 1 month and -0.59 ± 0.61 diopter at 12 months.[10] Patients with moderate myopia (5.00 to 10.00 diopters) regressed from $+0.50 \pm 1.17$ diopter at 1 month to -1.09 ± 1.07 diopters at 12 months, whereas those with severe myopia regressed the most, with a mean postoperative spherical equivalent of -0.38 ± 1.11 diopter at 1 month and -2.61 ± 1.92 diopters at 12 months. At this writing, we know of no publications that report more than 2 years of follow-up after astigmatic correction.

Hyperopic Astigmatism

The Aesculap-Meditec excimer laser can treat hyperopic astigmatism with a rotating non-ablatable mask.[28]

TABLE 42-1
Results of 19 Studies of Photoastigmatic Refractive Keratectomy

				Postoperative			
Study	*Laser (model)*	*Number of Eyes*	*Follow-Up (mo)*	*Refraction (within 1 D of intended correction) (%)*	*Uncorrected Visual Acuity (20/40 or better) (%)*	*Correction of Astigmatism (percent of intended correction achieved)*	*Axis Error*
Tabin et al (Melbourne Group), 1996[4]	VISX (Twenty/Twenty)	333	12	72	71	90[a]	55% less than 10 degrees
Kremer et al, 1996[11]	VISX (Twenty/Twenty)	92	12	≈70	80.4 (20/35 or better)	47.6 (low)[b] 68.4 (moderate) 80.7 (high)	38.3% less than 5 degrees
Pender, 1994[17]	VISX (Twenty/Twenty)	8	12–18	50	62.5	59[c]	50% less than 10 degrees[c]
Spigelman et al, 1994[38]	VISX (Twenty/Twenty)	70	6	NR	71	NR	NR
Kim et al, 1994[39]	VISX (Twenty/Twenty)	168	6	NR	91	56[c]	46% less than 10 degrees[c]
Horgan and Pearson, 1996[40]	VISX (Twenty/Twenty)	51	6	−1.12 (mean SE)	91 (20/30 or better)	24 (low)[d] 66.3 (moderate) 40.6 (high) overall: 79% within 0.50 D of intended correction	34% less than 20 degrees
Alió et al, 1995[41]	VISX (Twenty/Twenty)	46	12	NR	20/25 (mean)	−0.50 ± 0.20 D cylinder (mean)	100% less than 5 degrees
Cherry et al, 1994[22]	Summit, with eyecup	34	3	44	NR	50[c]	68% less than 10 degrees[c]
Hersh and Patel, 1994[24]	Summit, with eyecup	10	2–4	50	63	Mean decrease in cylinder of 0.62 D[c]	NR
Brancato et al, 1996[42]	Summit, with ablatable mask	124	12	88	NR	94[c]	NR
Danjoux et al, in press[26]	Summit, with ablatable mask	59	12	−0.02 ± −0.67 (mean SE ± 1 SD)	79.1	69	−2.35 (mean)
Niles et al, 1996[25]	Summit (Omnimed), with Emphasis mask	25	6	NR	76	73.1	NR
Tasindi et al, 1996[43]	Meditec	46	12	73.9	91.3	67.4% within 0.50 D of intended correction	NR
Zadok et al, 1996[44]	Meditec	128	12–18	NR	79.7	77.3% achieved complete reduction of cylinder	NR

TABLE 42-1 *(continued)*

Study	Laser (model)	Number of Eyes	Follow-Up (mo)	Postoperative: Refraction (within 1 D of intended correction) (%)	Postoperative: Uncorrected Visual Acuity (20/40 or better) (%)	Correction of Astigmatism (percent of intended correction achieved)	Axis Error
Dausch et al, 1994[27]	Meditec (MEL 60)	29	3	84.6	54.1	83.3% within 0.50 D of intended correction	Mean shift 2.0 ± 13.3 degrees
Förster et al, 1995[29]	Schwind	2	6	100	50	80[c]	50% less than 10 degrees
Vidaurri-Leal et al, 1996[45]	Coherent-Schwind (Keratom)	38	1–6	71	77	NR	NR
Colin et al, 1996[46]	Technolas	38	12	NR	NR	45[c]	NR
Williams et al, 1996[47]	Novatec	10	3	90	100	71[c]	NR

Abbreviations: D, diopters; NR, not reported; SE, spherical equivalent; SD, standard deviation.
[a] 1.2 adjustment factor used.
[b] High cylinder = -2.75 to -5.0 D; moderate = -1.25 to -2.50 D; low = -0.5 to -1.00 D.
[c] No vector analysis used or not mentioned.
[d] High cylinder = >-2.25 D; moderate = -1.25 to -2.00 D; low = -0.25 to -1.00 D.

Results from patients with a stable refraction of less than 6.50 diopters of cylinder and less than 8.00 diopters of hyperopia showed that at 18 months, 82 percent of 17 treated eyes were within 1.00 diopter of the intended correction, and 93 percent had an uncorrected visual acuity of 20/40 or better. Mean refractive cylinder decreased from -2.33 ± 1.32 diopters preoperatively to -0.44 ± 0.67 diopters at 18 months, and 76 percent of the eyes had cylinder of 1.00 diopter or less. After 12 months, 75 percent of eyes had no astigmatism; those that did had a postoperative cylinder axis within 10 degrees of the preoperative axis. At 18 months, 93 percent of patients had an uncorrected visual acuity of 20/40 or better.

Treatment of hyperopic astigmatism can be achieved with lasers that use ablatable masks,[28] as well as with scanning lasers. However, there are as yet no published results of the treatment of hyperopic astigmatism with scanning lasers.

Mixed Astigmatism

The treatment of mixed astigmatism is more complicated than the treatment of myopic or hyperopic astigmatism. In the study by Dausch et al,[28] myopic cylinder was treated first, then the spherical hyperopia was corrected. In 11 eyes with 18 months of follow-up, mean refractive cylinder decreased from -4.75 ± 1.17 diopters preoperatively to -0.89 ± 0.60 diopters, 63 percent of eyes had 1.00 diopter or less of cylinder, and 82 percent of eyes had an uncorrected visual acuity of 20/40 or better.

Keratoconus

We recently reviewed the 6-month postoperative results of photoastigmatic refractive keratectomy in 13 patients with keratoconus. These patients had nonprogressive keratoconus, were contact lens intolerant, and had insignificant apical scarring. It was required that the cornea be of adequate thickness preoperatively so that after the ablation, a thickness of 300 μm remained. Overall, 63 percent experienced improvement in uncorrected visual acuity and 88 percent had improvement in best spectacle-corrected visual acuity at 6 months. Fifty percent of the laser-treated patients gained two lines of best-corrected visual acuity. The mean haze score 6 months after ablation was 1.44 (Figure 42-11).

Postsurgical and Irregular Astigmatism

Several studies have evaluated the efficacy of photoastigmatic refractive keratectomy in reducing astigma-

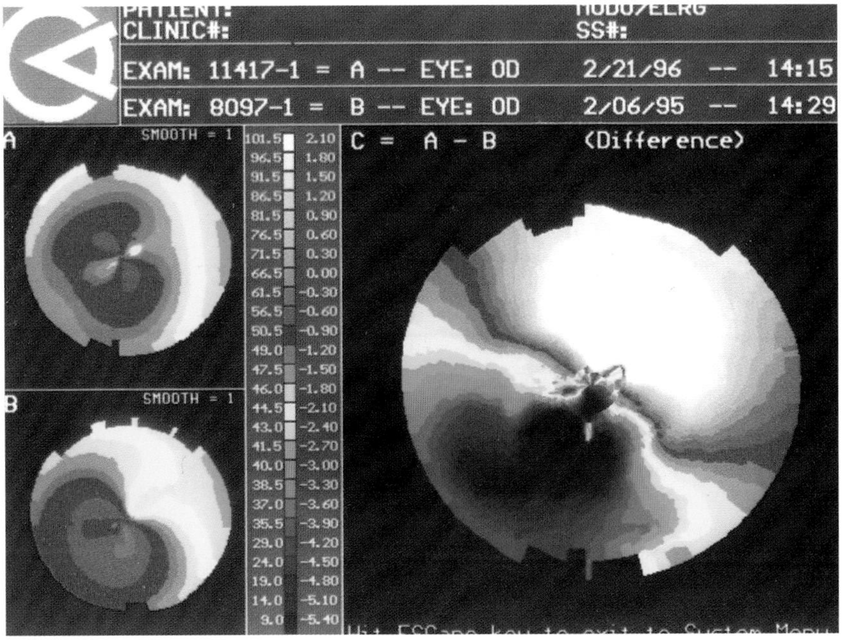

FIGURE 42-11 Videokeratographs of a patient with keratoconus who underwent photoastigmatic refractive keratectomy. Preoperatively, uncorrected visual acuity was 20/120 and best spectacle-corrected visual acuity was 20/40. Manifest refraction was plano −7.00 × 45. Six months postoperatively, uncorrected visual acuity was 20/60 and best spectacle-corrected visual acuity was 20/40, with a refraction of −0.50 −2.00 × 10. The postoperative videokeratograph is shown in **A**, the preoperative videokeratograph in **B**, and the difference map in **C**.

tism after penetrating keratoplasty[32,50,51]; the average reduction in refractive astigmatism ranged from 48 percent to 81 percent. Although uncorrected visual acuity improved in 50 percent of patients, only 15 percent had an uncorrected visual acuity of 20/40 or better. In addition, a decrease of two lines of best spectacle-corrected visual acuity occurred in 20 percent of eyes. Possible causes of the decrease in best spectacle-corrected visual acuity include the development of postoperative corneal haze and scarring, decentration of the ablation, and most important, inadequately treated irregular astigmatism. Some have suggested that the healing response in a corneal graft is different from that of a normal cornea, which could account for the less favorable outcome.[50]

Patients who underwent excimer laser treatment of astigmatism after cataract extraction fared better than those who had laser surgery after penetrating keratoplasty, but it should be noted that cataract patients generally have less myopia and astigmatism to correct. Postoperatively, 43 percent had an uncorrected visual acuity of 20/40 or better, and 92 percent were within 2.00 diopters of the intended correction.[4]

Irregular astigmatism is a common problem encountered by ophthalmologists. It usually occurs after trauma, infection, penetrating keratoplasty, pterygium excision, cataract extraction, and other surgical procedures. Idiopathic irregular corneal astigmatism is a less common entity. Initial results of the treatment of irregular astigmatism with a combination of multiple phototherapeutic keratectomies to flatten localized steep areas and photorefractive keratectomy to correct myopia are encouraging. A more integrated approach involving a videokeratoscope linked to a computer that can generate a unique treatment algorithm for each patient may lead to better results in the future.

COMPLICATIONS

Complications of photoastigmatic refractive keratectomy are similar to those of photorefractive keratectomy. It has been reported that photoastigmatic refractive keratectomy and photorefractive keratectomy used in the treatment of myopic astigmatism and myopia up to −7.50 diopters are associated with a 4 percent or less risk of significant complications affecting vision at 1 year.[52]

The complications reported for 333 photoastigmatic refractive keratectomy and 155 photorefractive keratectomy patients in the Melbourne excimer laser study group included 2.1 percent with a haze score of 2 or more at 1 year and 4.5 percent with intraocular pressure elevation.[4] Loss of two lines of best-corrected visual acuity occurred in 6.1 percent of patients. Other complications are rare.[4,11,17,25,27,28,40]

With hyperopic astigmatic correction, best-corrected visual acuity may be reduced in 13 to 18 percent of patients.[28] Central haze is not a problem because the ablation is mainly paracentral, although haze may develop at the border of the ablated zone and the central cornea.

Acknowledgments

We would like to thank Dr. Noel Alpins for providing information on his method of vector analysis and treatment of astigmatism.

REFERENCES

1. Agapitos PJ, Lindstrom RL: Astigmatic keratotomy. Ophthalmol Clin North Am 5:709, 1992
2. Katz M: The human eye as an optical system. p. 43. In Tasman W, Jaegar EA (eds): Duane's Clinical Ophthalmology. Lippincott-Raven, Philadelphia, 1995
3. Dart JK: Disease and risks associated with contact lenses. Br J Ophthalmol 77:49, 1993
4. Tabin GC, Alpins N, Aldred GF, et al: Astigmatic change 1 year after excimer laser treatment of myopia and myopic astigmatism. Melbourne Excimer Laser Group. J Cataract Refract Surg 22:924, 1996
5. Naylor EJ: Astigmatic difference in refractive errors. Br J Ophthalmol 55:422, 1968
6. Naeser K, Behrens JK, Naeser EV: Quantitative assessment of corneal astigmatic surgery: expanding the polar values concept. J Cataract Refract Surg 20:162, 1994
7. Olsen T, Dam-Johansen M: Evaluating surgically induced astigmatism. J Cataract Refract Surg 20:517, 1994
8. Jaffe NS, Clayman HM: The pathophysiology of corneal astigmatism after cataract extraction. Trans Am Acad Ophthalmol Otolaryngol 79:615, 1975
9. Hofmann RF: The surgical correction of idiopathic astigmatism. p. 243. In Sanders DR, Hofmann RF, Salz JJ (eds): Refractive Corneal Surgery. Slack, Thorofare, NJ, 1986
10. Snibson GR, Carson CA, Aldred GF, Taylor HR: One-year evaluation of excimer laser photorefractive keratectomy for myopia and myopic astigmatism. Melbourne Excimer Laser Group. Arch Ophthalmol 113:994, 1995
11. Kremer I, Gabbay U, Blumenthal M: One-year follow-up results of photorefractive keratectomy for low, moderate, and high primary astigmatism. Ophthalmology 103:741, 1996
12. Epstein D, Frueh BE: Indications, results and complications of refractive corneal surgery with lasers. Curr Opin Ophthalmol 6:73, 1995
13. Tengroth B, Epstein D, Fagerholm P, et al: Excimer laser photorefractive keratectomy for myopia: clinical results in sighted eyes. Ophthalmology 100:739, 1993
14. McCarty CA, Aldred GF, Taylor HR: Comparison of results of excimer laser correction of all degrees of myopia at 12 months postoperatively. Melbourne Excimer Laser Group. Am J Ophthalmol 121:372, 1996
15. McDonnell PJ, Moreira H, Garbus J, et al: Photorefractive keratectomy to create toric ablations for correction of astigmatism. Arch Ophthalmol 109:710, 1991
16. McDonnell PJ, Moreira H, Clapham TN, et al: Photorefractive keratectomy for astigmatism: initial clinical results. Arch Ophthalmol 109:1370, 1991
17. Pender PM: Photorefractive keratectomy for myopic astigmatism: phase IIA of the Federal Drug Administration study (12 to 18 months follow-up). Excimer Laser Study Group. J Cataract Refract Surg 20(suppl):262, 1994
18. Taylor HR, Guest CS, Kelly P, et al: Comparison of excimer laser treatment of astigmatism and myopia. Arch Ophthalmol 111:1621,1993
19. Taylor HR, Kelly P, Alpins N: Excimer laser correction of myopic astigmatism. J Cataract Refract Surg 20(suppl):243, 1994
20. Gobbi PG, Carones F, Scagliotti F, et al: A simplified method to perform photorefractive keratectomy using an erodible mask. J Refract Corneal Surg 10(suppl 2):S247, 1994
21. Maloney RK, Friedman N, Harmon T, et al: A prototype erodible mask delivery system for the excimer laser. Ophthalmology 100:542, 1993
22. Cherry PMH, Tutton MK, Bell A, et al: Treatment of myopic astigmatism with photorefractive keratectomy using an erodible mask. J Refract Corneal Surg 10(suppl 2):S239, 1994
23. Friedman MD, Bittenson S, Brodsky L, et al: OmniMed II: a new system for use with the Emphasis erodible mask. J Refract Corneal Surg 10(suppl 2):S267, 1994
24. Hersh PS, Patel R: Correction of myopia and astigmatism using an ablatable mask. J Refract Corneal Surg 10(suppl 2):S250, 1994
25. Niles C, Culp B, Teal P: Excimer laser photorefractive keratectomy using an erodible mask to treat myopic astigmatism. J Cataract Refract Surg 22:436, 1996
26. Danjoux JP, Lawless MA, Rogers C: Treatment of myopic astigmatism with the Summit Apex Plus excimer laser. J Cataract Refract Surg, in press
27. Dausch D, Klein R, Landesz M, Schröeder E: Photorefractive keratectomy to correct astigmatism with myopia or hyperopia. J Cataract Refract Surg 20(suppl):252, 1994
28. Dausch DGJ, Klein RJ, Schröder E, Niemczyk S: Photorefractive keratectomy for hyperopic and mixed astigmatism. J Refract Surg 12:684, 1996
29. Förster W, Beck R, Borrmann A, Busse H: Correcting myopic astigmatism with an areal 193 nm excimer laser ablation. J Cataract Refract Surg 21:278, 1995
30. Bennett AG, Rabbetts RB: Clinical Visual Optics. Butterworths, London, 1989
31. Taylor HR: Comparison of excimer laser treatment of astigmatism and myopia. In reply [correspondence]. Arch Ophthalmol 112:1509, 1994
32. Alpins NA, Tabin GC, Taylor HR: Photoastigmatic refractive keratectomy (PARK). p. 243. In McGhee CNJ, Taylor HR, Gartry DS, Trokel SL (eds): Excimer Lasers in Ophthalmology: Principles and Practice. Martin Dunitz Ltd, London, 1997
33. Belin MW, Ratliff CD: Evaluating data acquisition and smoothing functions of currently available videokeratoscopes. J Cataract Refract Surg 22:421, 1996
34. Maguire LJ: Computer corneal analysis. Focal Points in Ophthalmology 14(5):1, 1996

35. McGhee CNJ, Weed KH: Computerized videokeratography in clinical practice. p. 97. In McGhee CNJ, Taylor HR, Gartry DS, Trokel SL (eds): Excimer Lasers in Ophthalmology: Principles and Practice. Martin Dunitz Ltd, London, 1997
36. Alpins NA: New method of targeting vectors to treat astigmatism. J Cataract Refract Surg 23:65, 1997
37. Vajpayee RB, Aldred GF, McCarty CA, Taylor HR: Evaluations of axis alignment system for correction of myopic astigmatism with the excimer laser. Ophthalmology, in press
38. Spigelman AV, Albert WC, Cozean CH, et al: Treatment of myopic astigmatism with the 193 nm excimer laser utilizing aperture elements. J Cataract Refract Surg 20(suppl):258, 1994
39. Kim YJ, Sohn J, Tchah H, Lee CO: Photoastigmatic refractive keratectomy in 168 eyes: six-month results. J Cataract Refract Surg 20:387, 1994
40. Horgan SE, Pearson RV: The early results of excimer laser photorefractive keratectomy for compound myopic astigmatism. Eur J Ophthalmol 6:113, 1996
41. Alió JL, Artola A, Ayala M, Claramonte P: Correcting simple myopic astigmatism with the excimer laser. J Cataract Refract Surg 21:512, 1995
42. Brancato R, Carones F, Venturi E, et al: Accuracy of the erodible mask in-the-rail excimer laser delivery system in compound astigmatic correction. AAO abstract. Ophthalmology 103(suppl):S158, 1996
43. Tasindi E, Talu H, Ciftci F, Acar S: Excimer laser photorefractive keratectomy (PRK) in myopic astigmatism. Eur J Ophthalmol 6:121, 1996
44. Zadok D, Haviv D, Hefetz L, et al: Excimer laser photoastigmatic keratectomy (PARK)—18 month's follow-up. AAO abstract. Ophthalmology 103(suppl):S185, 1996
45. Vidaurri-Leal J, Helena MC, Talamo JH, et al: Excimer photorefractive keratectomy for low myopia and astigmatism with the Coherent-Schwind Keratom. J Cataract Refract Surg 22:1052, 1996
46. Colin J, Cochener B, le Floch G: Excimer laser treatment of astigmatism. AAO abstract. Ophthalmology 103(suppl):S129, 1996
47. Williams EJ, Chayet AS, Tong S: Toric PRK using the Novatec solid-state laser with scanning delivery system and active eye tracker—three month results. AAO abstract. Ophthalmology 103(suppl):S84, 1996
48. Vajpayee RB, McCarty CA, Aldred G, Taylor HR: Overcorrection after excimer laser treatment of myopia and myopic astigmatism. Arch Ophthalmol 114:252, 1996
49. Stevens JD: Astigmatic excimer laser treatment: theoretical effects of axis misalignment. Eur Implant Ref Surg 6:310, 1994
50. Lazzaro DR, Haight DH, Belmont SC, et al: Excimer laser keratectomy for astigmatism occurring after penetrating keratoplasty. Ophthalmology 103:458, 1996
51. Amm M, Duncker GI, Schröder E: Excimer laser correction of high astigmatism after keratoplasty. J Cataract Refract Surg 22:313, 1996
52. McGhee CNJ, Ellerton CR: Complications of excimer laser photorefractive surgery. p. 379. In McGhee CNJ, Taylor HR, Gartry DS, Trokel SL (eds): Excimer Lasers in Ophthalmology: Principles and Practice. Martin Dunitz Ltd, London, 1997

43

Laser-Assisted In Situ Keratomileusis

STEPHEN G. SLADE, JEFFERY MACHAT,
AND JOHN F. DOANE

Laser-assisted in situ keratomileusis, also known as *LASIK*, is a refractive lamellar surgical procedure that alters the anterior curvature of the cornea by removing stroma from within the cornea, leaving Bowman's layer and the epithelium virtually intact (Figure 43-1). The technique involves creating an anterior corneal flap with a microkeratome, ablating the underlying stromal bed with an excimer laser, and replacing the flap. The flap helps to mask any stromal irregularities created by the ablation and to protect the ablated surface from many of the wound healing mechanisms operative in excimer laser photorefractive keratectomy, in which the ablated surface is exposed. Laser-assisted in situ keratomileusis potentially offers a more rapid, easier recovery and fewer postoperative visits and medications, and in patients with large refractive errors, perhaps greater accuracy of correction compared with other refractive surgical procedures. Other advantages of laser-assisted in situ keratomileusis include the stability of postoperative results, the ease of retreating any residual postoperative refractive error, and applicability to a wide range of refractive errors. Disadvantages include a considerable learning curve; potential complications with the microkeratome; and the inability to correct very large amounts of myopia, because the need for a flap, which is 160 μm thick, requires that the ablation start deep in the cornea.

HISTORY

Lamellar refractive surgery developed from the concepts and work of Barraquer in Bagotá, Colombia.[1-3] In the original keratomileusis procedure for myopia (Figure 43-2), a disk approximately 300 μm thick was dissected from the anterior cornea in a freehand fashion with a Paufique knife or corneal dissector. The tissue was then transported across Bagotá to a separate facility, where the epithelial surface was glued onto a contact lens lathe and the stromal surface was carved and reshaped to thin the center of the disk, creating a concave lens. This lens was then transported back across Bagotá, where it was repositioned on the patient's cornea. Two interrupted sutures were placed, and a conjunctival flap was dissected, inverted, and laid over the cornea. The patient's eyelids were then sewn shut to encourage healing.

Barraquer's results with this procedure were promising. Overall, 80 percent of the patients showed improvement in uncorrected visual acuity.[4-6] Few significant complications were encountered; in the first 200 cases, reported problems included epithelium in the peripheral interface, irregular astigmatism, and two infections. Barraquer later introduced the use of a microkeratome to remove the corneal disk and added freezing circuits to the lathe to create a cryolathe that could more accurately shape the corneal tissue.

Swinger, Nordan, and Troutman introduced keratomileusis in the United States in the late 1970s.[7] Good results were obtained initially by several investigators; however, the technique never gained widespread acceptance.[7-14] The main difficulties with keratomileusis were the learning curve for performing the keratectomy and the complexity of the cryolathe. The depth of the keratectomy was determined, in part, by the speed at which the hand-driven microkeratome passed across the cornea, and any irregularity in this cut manifested as irregular astigmatism of the anterior corneal surface.

Several attempts were made to improve and simplify lamellar refractive keratoplasty so that it could be used by more ophthalmologists. Kaufman and Werblin developed epikeratophakia (Figure 43-3), which eliminated the

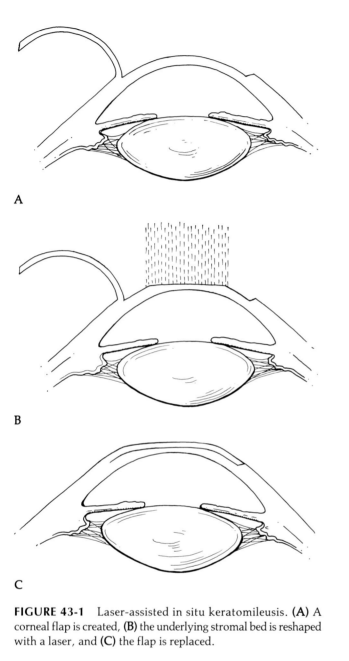

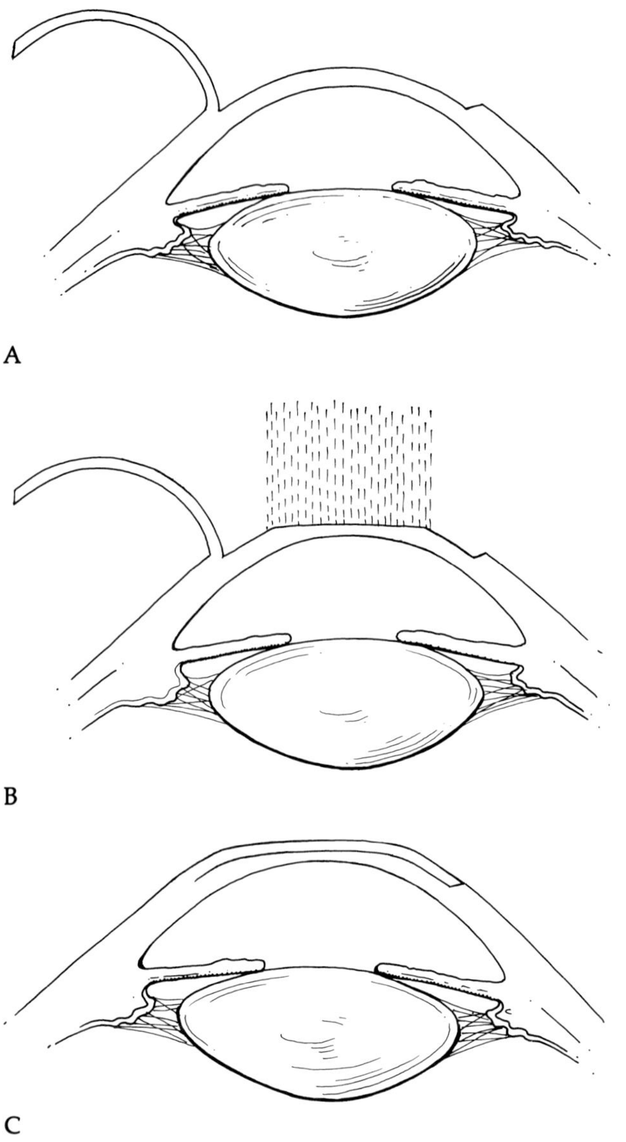

FIGURE 43-1 Laser-assisted in situ keratomileusis. **(A)** A corneal flap is created, **(B)** the underlying stromal bed is reshaped with a laser, and **(C)** the flap is replaced.

need for the surgeon to own a cryolathe or operate a microkeratome[15–22] (see Ch. 39). Barraquer, Krumeich, and Swinger eliminated the need for a cryolathe by performing keratomileusis with a nonfreeze technique.[23,24] A disk of anterior cornea was cut with a microkeratome, placed epithelial surface down on a specially formed suction die, reshaped from the stromal surface with a microkeratome, and replaced on the patient's cornea. This procedure was never widely used because of its complexity.

The concepts of not needing to freeze the corneal tissue for reshaping and using a microkeratome to make the refractive cut led Barraquer and Ruiz to develop in situ keratomileusis, a procedure that alters the anterior corneal curvature by cutting a lamellar disk of anterior cornea as a cap or hinged flap, performing a refractive cut on the exposed stromal bed, and then replacing the cap or flap (Figures 43-4 and 43-5).

In situ keratomileusis is limited by the accuracy of the microkeratome because the thickness of the refractive cut is responsible for the power correction. As mentioned above, the thickness of a keratectomy depends, in part, on the speed of the microkeratome. (In standard ker-

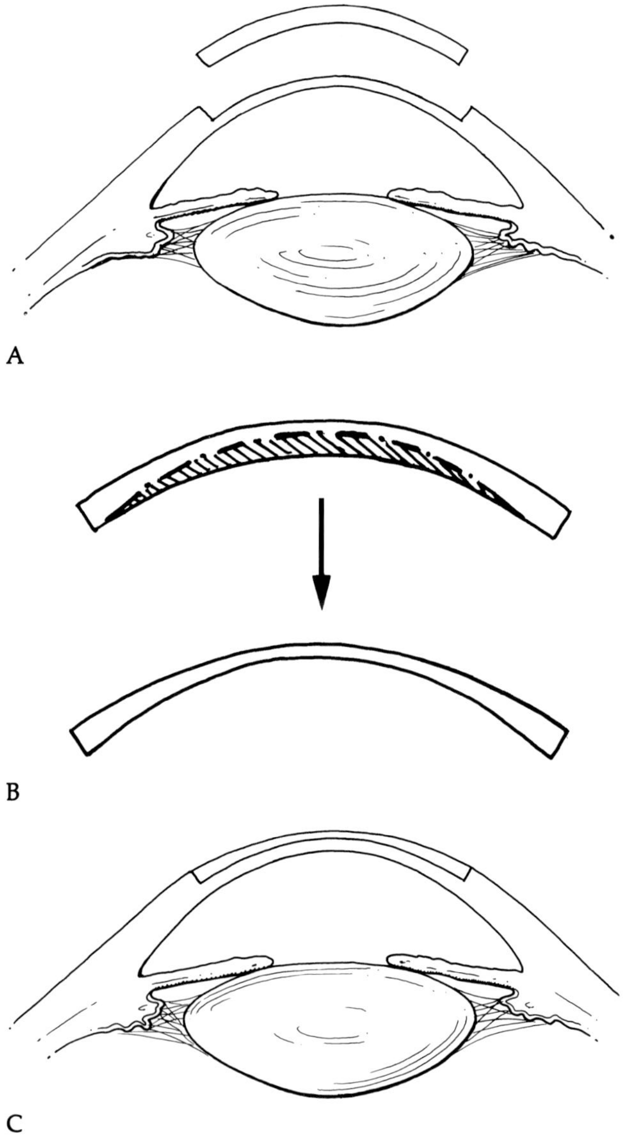

FIGURE 43-2 Keratomileusis. **(A)** An anterior corneal disk is removed, **(B)** reshaped with a lathe, and **(C)** replaced to change the anterior corneal curvature.

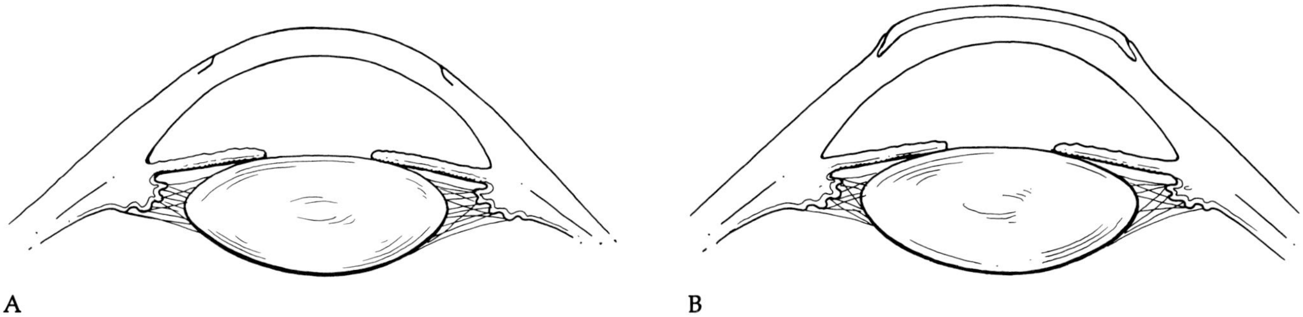

FIGURE 43-3 Epikeratophakia. **(A)** A peripheral circular keratotomy and lamellar dissection are performed, and **(B)** a lens made of human corneal tissue is placed to change the anterior corneal curvature.

atomileusis, in which the thickness of the resected tissue does not determine the power correction, this relationship is not as critical.) Early published series of in situ keratomileusis in which a standard manual microkeratome was used showed a wide range of results.[25,26] Typically, uncorrected visual acuity improved, but best spectacle-corrected visual acuity often diminished because of irregular astigmatism. To improve this procedure, surgeons tried to develop a microkeratome that would be accurate, consistent, and safe.[27] The microkeratome most commonly used today was developed by Ruiz in the late 1980s (Figure 43-6). It has an automated, geared device that controls the speed of the microkeratome as it passes across the cornea so that a more consistent cut is possible. In situ keratomileusis with this microkeratome has become known as *automated lamellar keratoplasty* or *ALK*.

Automated lamellar keratoplasty proved useful for patients with high myopia but was limited by the inaccuracy of the microkeratome.[28,29] (It is beyond the limits of a mechanical device to remove corneal tissue with single-micron accuracy.) Also, the microkeratome cannot create a lenticular or astigmatic cut. These problems led Buratto and others to explore new ways to make the critical refractive cut; in the late 1980s, they began using the excimer laser for this purpose.[30-36] Buratto et al[35] reported good results in 30 eyes of 22 patients in which an excimer laser was used to ablate either the undersurface of a 300-μm-thick corneal cap or the stromal bed after a free corneal cap had been removed. Brint and Slade[37] were the first to use the current technique of laser-assisted in situ keratomileusis in which, under topical anesthesia, a corneal flap is cut with a geared microkeratome, the stromal bed beneath the flap is ablated with an excimer laser, and the flap is repositioned without the use of sutures.

The excimer laser has the accuracy to remove corneal tissue precisely and the ability to make a lenticular rather than a lamellar cut. It is also able to correct astigmatism. Although laser-assisted in situ keratomileusis is still in the

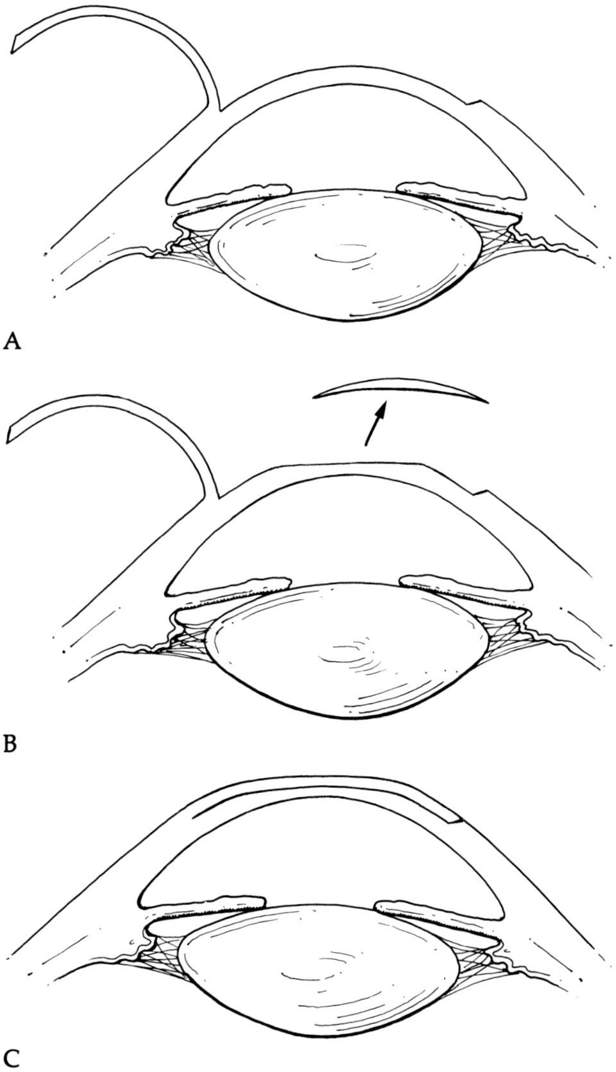

FIGURE 43-4 In situ keratomileusis or automated lamellar keratoplasty. **(A)** A corneal cap or flap, as shown, is created, **(B)** the underlying stromal bed is reshaped with a microkeratome, and **(C)** the cap or flap is replaced.

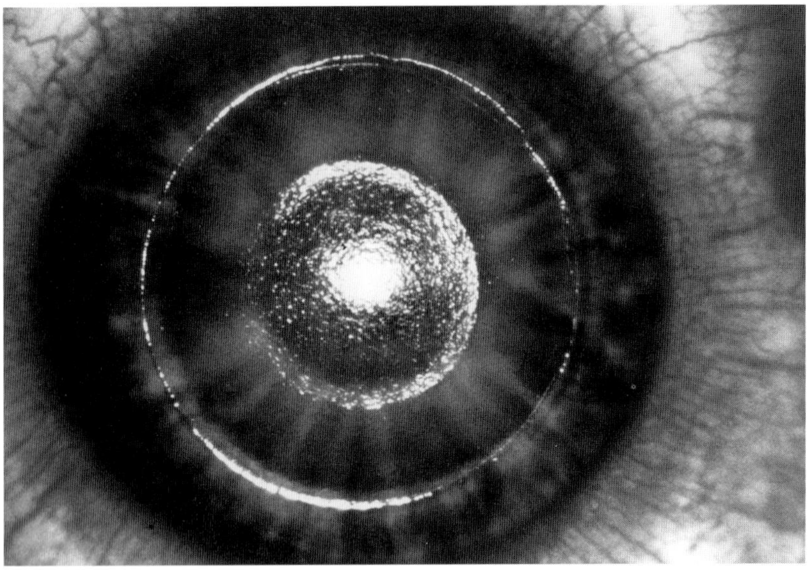

FIGURE 43-5 Automated lamellar keratoplasty (ALK) bed showing two cuts. The large cut creates a free cap, which is replaced at the end of the procedure. The small cut is the refractive cut, the depth and diameter of which determine the power of the correction.

early stages of development at this writing, it has stimulated much interest and gained considerable acceptance among refractive surgeons.

PATIENT SELECTION

Refractive surgery patients in general should be at least 18 years of age because of the need for informed consent as well as the requirement for stability of refractive error. For each patient, laser-assisted in situ keratomileusis should be compared with other refractive surgical procedures, such as excimer laser photorefractive keratectomy and radial keratotomy, and the best procedure chosen for the patient's needs and refractive error. Also, it cannot be overemphasized that it is essential to follow good practice with regard to patient education and informed consent, to prevent unrealistic patient expectations.

Laser-assisted in situ keratomileusis may be considered for the correction of 0.5 to 15 diopters of myopia or 0.5 to 5 diopters of hyperopia. Up to 8 diopters of astigmatism may also be corrected. These ranges are not absolute indications for the procedure, however. Although patients with high myopia obtain slightly better results with laser-assisted in situ keratomileusis than with photorefractive keratectomy or radial keratotomy, patients with less than 6 diopters of myopia obtain similar results with all three procedures. The treatment of hyperopia is more limited. Patients with more than 6 diopters of hyperopia lose more lines of best spectacle-corrected visual acuity and have a longer recovery time than patients with lower amounts of hyperopia.

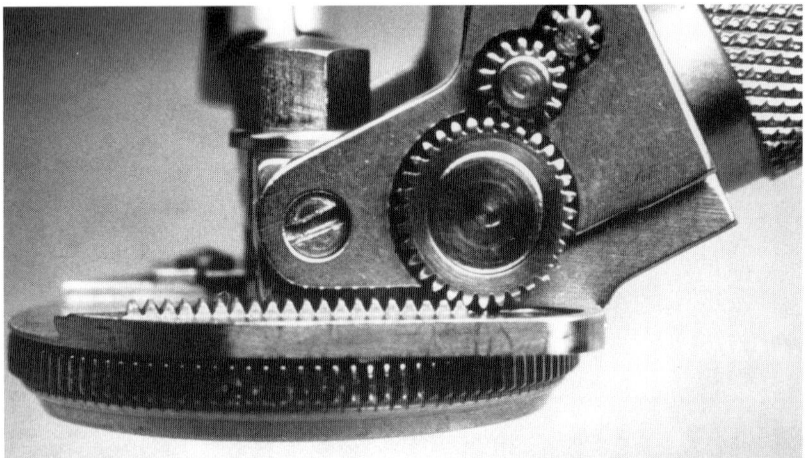

FIGURE 43-6 Automatic Corneal Shaper consisting of an automated microkeratome and pneumatic fixation ring. The geared mechanism allows the surgeon to make a smooth cut without having to control the speed of the microkeratome.

The lower limit of myopia or hyperopia treatable with laser-assisted in situ keratomileusis is usually determined by the surgeon's comfort with the microkeratome. Although a keratectomy is no more risky in a patient with 2 diopters of myopia than in a patient with 12 diopters of myopia, photorefractive keratectomy offers the same accuracy in patients with low or moderate myopia without the use of the microkeratome, and is, therefore, a reasonable alternative. In patients with smaller refractive errors, the surgeon must weigh the advantages of the faster, easier recovery and fewer but potentially more serious complications of laser-assisted in situ keratomileusis against the relative safety but slower recovery associated with photorefractive keratectomy. Photorefractive keratectomy is the clear choice for patients with anterior stromal opacities or recurrent epithelial erosions, who would benefit from the phototherapeutic keratectomy aspect of the procedure.

PREOPERATIVE EVALUATION AND SURGICAL PLANNING

Evaluation of a prospective candidate for laser-assisted in situ keratomileusis includes screening for keratoconus, epithelial basement membrane disease, and active corneal disease or infection. Refractive lamellar keratoplasty in a patient with keratoconus is controversial because thinning an already thinned cornea could hasten the progression of the ectasia. A history of recurrent erosions is considered a relative contraindication because the microkeratome is likely to rub off any loose epithelium during the keratectomy, and an epithelial defect can jeopardize the sealing of the flap and lead to stromal melt or epithelial ingrowth beneath the flap. All patients should be screened for retinal disease and treated, if necessary, before surgery. The pneumatic fixation ring raises the intraocular pressure above 65 mmHg, which should be taken into consideration in older patients with fragile retinal vessels.

The patient must be sufficiently cooperative for topical anesthesia, and there should be adequate exposure of the globe to accommodate the pneumatic fixation ring and microkeratome.

Several preoperative measurements are critical. The refractive state of the eye must be known with as much accuracy as possible, and the refraction should be checked and rechecked. A patient wearing contact lenses, hard or soft, must discontinue lens wear long enough for the cornea to stabilize and for any contact lens–induced corneal warpage or astigmatism to resolve. This may take weeks or months for long-term wearers of hard lenses.

Astigmatism must be properly diagnosed, and any irregular astigmatism must be identified. In patients with reduced preoperative best-corrected visual acuity, corneal pathology and opacities must also be ruled out. Refraction, keratometry, and videokeratography are important components in the evaluation of astigmatism. The cylinder axis found on refraction should correlate with the axis found on keratometry and videokeratography. The refractive astigmatism must be corneal and not lenticular, because treatment of lenticular astigmatism with corneal ablation may create a crossed cylinder in the eye (i.e., a cornea with cylinder in one axis to correct a lens with cylinder in the opposite axis) and make things worse, especially if, in later years, the patient develops a cataract and the lenticular component of the astigmatism is removed.

It is necessary to know the corneal thickness, particularly in a patient with high myopia who would require a deep ablation. When planning the procedure, three thickness measurements must be considered: the thickness of the flap, the depth of the ablation, and the thickness of the corneal bed after the ablation. The thicker the flap, the less likely it is that irregular astigmatism will develop postoperatively; however, a thicker flap will also result in less corneal thickness remaining for the ablation. A 160-μm-thick flap appears ideal. With an optical zone diameter of 6 mm, each diopter of correction of myopia requires ablation of approximately 14 μm of corneal depth. The thickness of the corneal bed after the ablation should be no less than 200 μm to prevent corneal ectasia and to separate the ablation from the corneal endothelium. For example, if the central corneal thickness preoperatively is 500 μm, then creating a 160-μm flap leaves 340 μm of cornea to be ablated. Of this, the maximum amount of cornea that may be ablated is 140 μm, which is enough to correct about 10 diopters of myopia with a single-zone ablation.

A single-zone ablation can be used for the correction of no more than 12 to 15 diopters of myopia, depending on corneal thickness, because of the need to leave at least a 200-μm-thick corneal bed after the ablation. Multizone ablation can correct greater amounts of myopia—up to approximately 20 diopters—and requires removal of less tissue than an equivalent 6-mm-diameter single-zone ablation, but the optical zone is smaller and some visual quality is sacrificed, especially in low-light situations.

It is important to consider the corneal curvature preoperatively. If the corneal curvature is less than 38 diopters, less cornea is exposed to the microkeratome and a free corneal cap may be produced instead of a flap.

The desired amount of correction of the spherical component of the refractive error must be decided. Correction of the dominant eye for distance and the nondominant eye for near should be considered, where appropriate.

The treatment plan for astigmatism varies depending on the type of astigmatism. The component of decreased vision attributable to only the spherical error should be identified; if correction of only the spherical error is sufficient, consideration should be given to leaving the astigmatism alone. In general, with-the-rule astigmatism (steep at 90 degrees) should be slightly undercorrected and against-the-rule astigmatism (steep at 180 degrees) slightly overcorrected. Patients who have with-the-rule astigmatism often have a better range and depth of vision than patients who have a spherical refractive error. If the fellow eye has astigmatism, especially oblique astigmatism, that the patient does not plan to have treated, the matching oblique astigmatism should be left alone.

The effect that treating the cylinder has on the spherical component of the refraction should be considered. Many lasers create a hyperopic shift when used to treat astigmatism. This would be undesirable in a patient with a hyperopic spherical component. In this case, an astigmatic keratotomy that has a coupling ratio that reduces hyperopia might be more appropriate. Alternatively, a scanning laser that has the ability to treat hyperopia and astigmatism could be used, if available.

The correct nomogram must be used. Lasers come with algorithms, not nomograms. Algorithms do not vary according to surgical technique, the environment of the room, or the state of the lenses and gas in the laser, whereas nomograms can take these variables into account. In laser-assisted in situ keratomileusis, the surgeon must develop his or her own nomogram, or changes to the laser software, based on the conditions under which he or she actually performs the procedure.

SURGICAL TECHNIQUES

Over the past few years, many new developments in laser-assisted in situ keratomileusis have increased the ease of the procedure and improved the results. These advancements include the use of topical anesthesia, sutureless fixation of the corneal flap, and improvements in the design and function of the excimer laser.

Preoperative Setup

The success of laser-assisted in situ keratomileusis depends on appropriate evaluation and counseling of the patient as described above, pretesting of the laser, and proper setup of the microkeratome. An environment in which the surgical team watches, checks, and questions each other during the setup procedure is encouraged. The humidity, temperature, and air flow of the operating room are checked. The excimer laser is turned on and tested before the patient is brought into the room. The fluence is checked for the cutting rate and the beam pattern. A 160-μm plate and new blade are placed into the microkeratome after the entire system has been tested.

Anesthesia, Preparation, and Draping

Mild sedation with oral diazepam (5 or 10 mg) is encouraged but the patient must be alert enough to fixate. Pilocarpine can artificially skew the position of the pupil and is not recommended. Topical proparacaine is instilled for anesthesia. A minimal amount should be used to avoid softening the epithelium; one drop before the surgical preparation and one drop before the keratectomy is usually adequate.

The patient is brought into the room. The refraction is programmed into the laser, and the number of pulses is planned and recorded. A surgical skin prep is performed and the patient is draped with a drape that has a central opening. Care is taken to drape the eyelashes out of the way. An eyelid speculum that provides maximum exposure of the cornea is placed.

Keratectomy

We recommend using a corneal marker that creates a pararadial line to ensure proper orientation of a free cap, if one is created (Figure 43-7). Corneal markers are not reliable for precise alignment of a flap because they mark the epithelium, not the stroma, and pressure from the microkeratome can displace the epithelium, resulting in misalignment of the tissue even when the marks are matched.

Once good exposure has been obtained with a suitable eyelid speculum and any conjunctival chemosis has been milked away, the pneumatic fixation ring specific for laser-assisted in situ keratomileusis is placed on the eye. This ring fixates the eye, provides a track for the microkeratome, and raises the intraocular pressure. Fixation should not be tested by pulling up on the ring because this could break suction. If there is any break in suction or the ring is removed, suction will be more difficult to obtain the second time.

An intraocular pressure of 65 mmHg or higher is essential for a smooth, even keratectomy and must be verified immediately before the keratectomy is performed. Although there are many cues to the achievement of high pressure, such as dilation of the pupil, the sound of the suction pump, and the rigidity of the cornea to the touch, the pressure is best verified with a Barraquer tonometer (Figure 43-8). This instrument consists of a conical lens with a convex upper surface that acts as a magnifying glass and a flat undersurface that is marked with a cir-

FIGURE 43-7 **(A)** Corneal marker marking the cornea. **(B)** The pararadial line helps orient the corneal flap in case a free cap is produced.

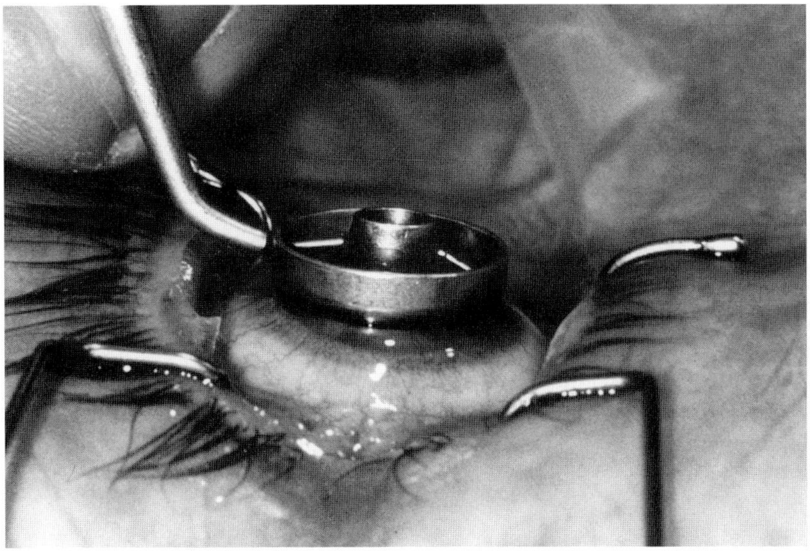

A

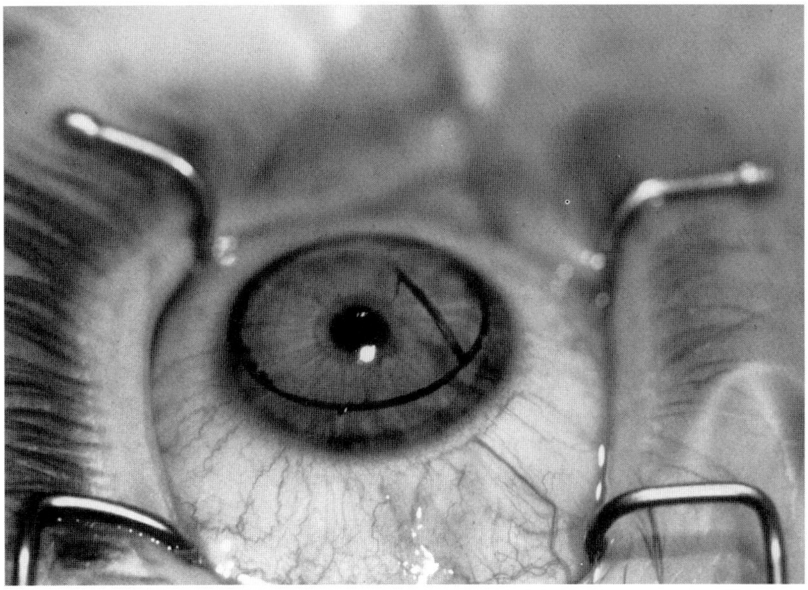

B

cle. The tonometer is held by an external ring and is placed on a dry cornea. An applanation smaller than the circle marked on the undersurface of the tonometer indicates that the intraocular pressure is higher than 65 mmHg. If the applanation is larger than the circle, the intraocular pressure is too low.

After fixation has been obtained and a high intraocular pressure has been confirmed, the eye is wiped with a cellulose sponge soaked in balanced salt solution, or a drop of balanced salt solution is placed on the cornea to wet and lubricate it. The automated microkeratome is placed temporally into the dovetail groove on the fixation ring to lock it into position (Figure 43-9). A foot pedal is used to turn on the microkeratome, which then passes across the cornea until the stopper mechanism is reached, ending the passage and creating the flap. The microkeratome is then reversed off the cornea by means of the foot pedal. Suction is broken, and the fixation ring is removed from the eye.

Laser Ablation

After the keratectomy has been completed, the surgeon may pause, recheck the laser, reassure the patient, and position

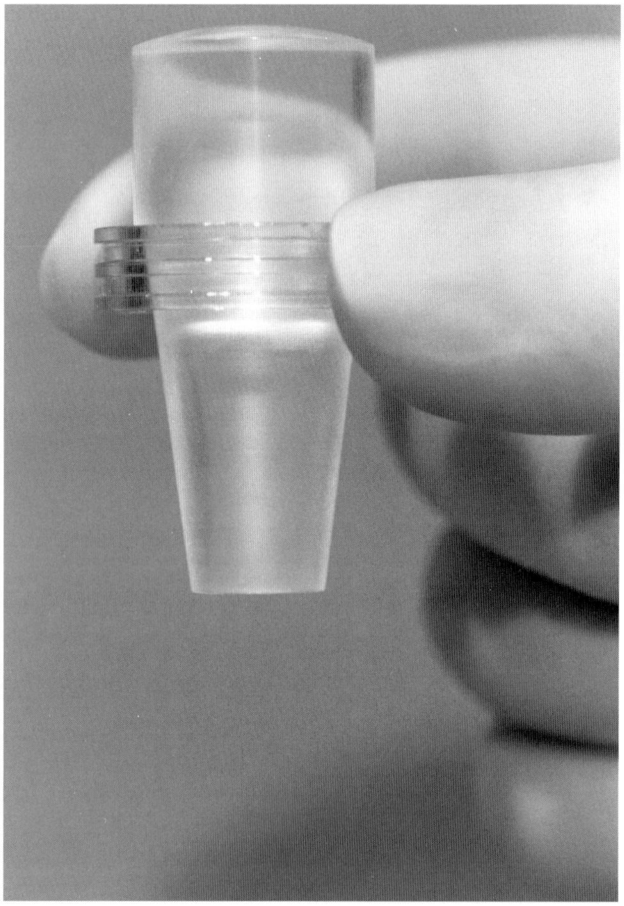

FIGURE 43-8 Barraquer tonometer.

the patient's head. The time between lifting the flap, exposing the stromal bed, and starting the ablation should be kept constant from case to case in an attempt to control the hydration rate of the stroma (Figure 43-10). The cornea is positioned such that the ablation is centered over the center of the entrance pupil as the patient fixates on the fixation light of the laser. It is important to ensure that the excimer beam is properly focused and that it strikes the cornea in a perpendicular manner to prevent an irregular ablation. During the ablation, the cornea is observed to maintain centration and the patient is reminded to maintain fixation. The hydration status of the cornea is also watched and the stromal bed is wiped with a blunt instrument during a pause in the ablation if the hydration is uneven.

Repositioning the Flap

After the ablation, the flap and the stromal bed are moistened with balanced salt solution. Care is taken not to irrigate too extensively at this stage because meibomian secretions and debris in the cul-de-sac can be washed onto the exposed stromal bed. A blunt instrument is used to reposition the flap. A special curved cannula (Slade LASIK cannula) is valuable to irrigate beneath the flap to remove debris and prevent contaminants in the cul-de-sac from being washed up into the interface (Figure 43-11). After the flap has been repositioned, the edge of the flap is checked to make sure it is even as an indication of the stromal alignment, the surface of the flap is examined to be certain there are no wrinkles or striae, and the interface is inspected to locate and remove any visible debris. After 2 to 3 minutes, the adhesion of the flap is evaluated by depressing the peripheral host cornea and watch-

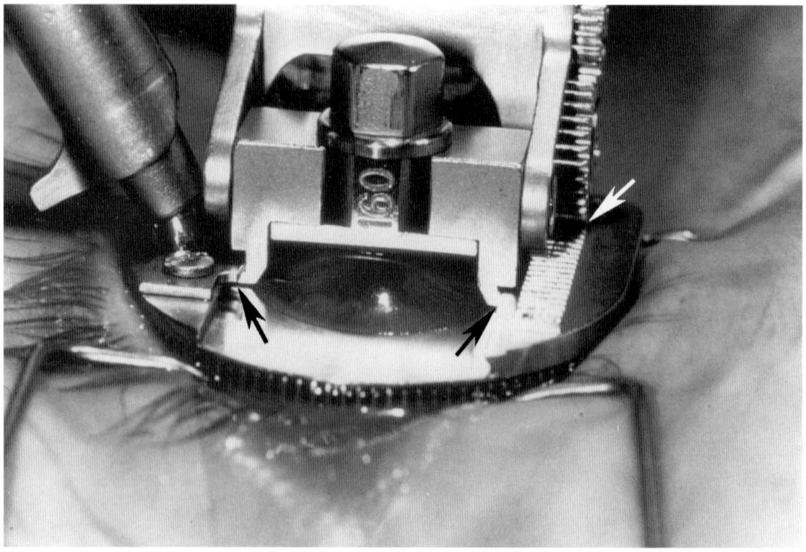

FIGURE 43-9 View (from nasal aspect) of the microkeratome locked into position in the pneumatic fixation ring (black arrows). The lower gear of the microkeratome has teeth that fit into teeth on the ring (white arrow).

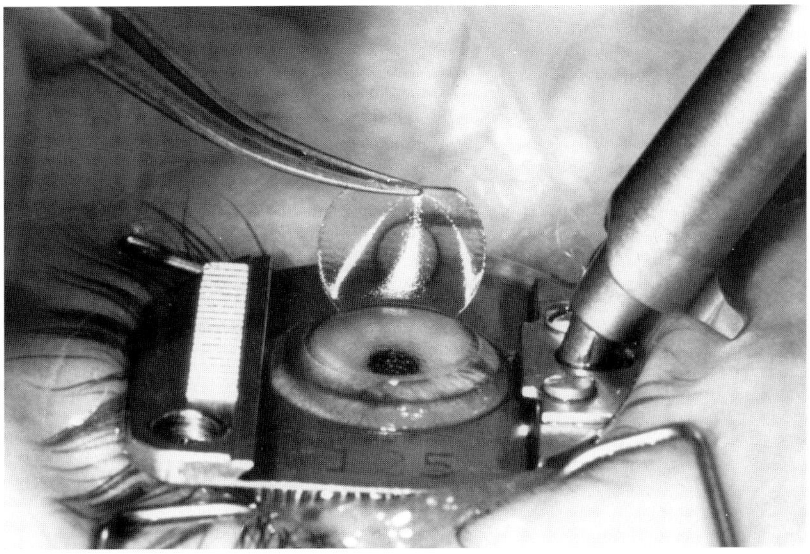

FIGURE 43-10 View (from temporal aspect) of the corneal flap.

ing to ensure that the resulting striae radiate into the flap (Figure 43-12). When adhesion is achieved, antibiotics and corticosteroids and/or a nonsteroidal anti-inflammatory drug are placed on the eye. A clear shield is taped over the eye. The patient is instructed to wear the shield until the first return visit, which is scheduled for the day after surgery.

Technique for Treatment of Astigmatism

Laser Ablation

The following steps may be added to combine excimer laser treatment of astigmatism with the laser treatment of the spherical component of the refraction.

The cylinder axis may be marked at the slit lamp microscope immediately before surgery or in the operating room. Alternatively, the surgeon may use a landmark on the surface of the eye, such as a scleral vessel. Small conjunctival vessels may be obscured by the edema caused by the fixation ring or by hyperemia and should not be used for this purpose. Iris landmarks are difficult to see through the bed of the keratectomy and should also not be used. We prefer to place a reference mark on the patient's eye just before the patient lies down. After a drop of topical anesthetic has been placed on the eye, the patient is instructed to look at a distant point, and a surgical marking pen is used to place a small dot at the limbus at the 6 o'clock position. Care is taken to avoid disrupting the corneal epithelium. The mark is used during the ablation by aligning it with the microscope reticule. If an epithelial abrasion results from the mark, the patient should be warned of the greater likelihood of pain for the first few hours postoperatively.

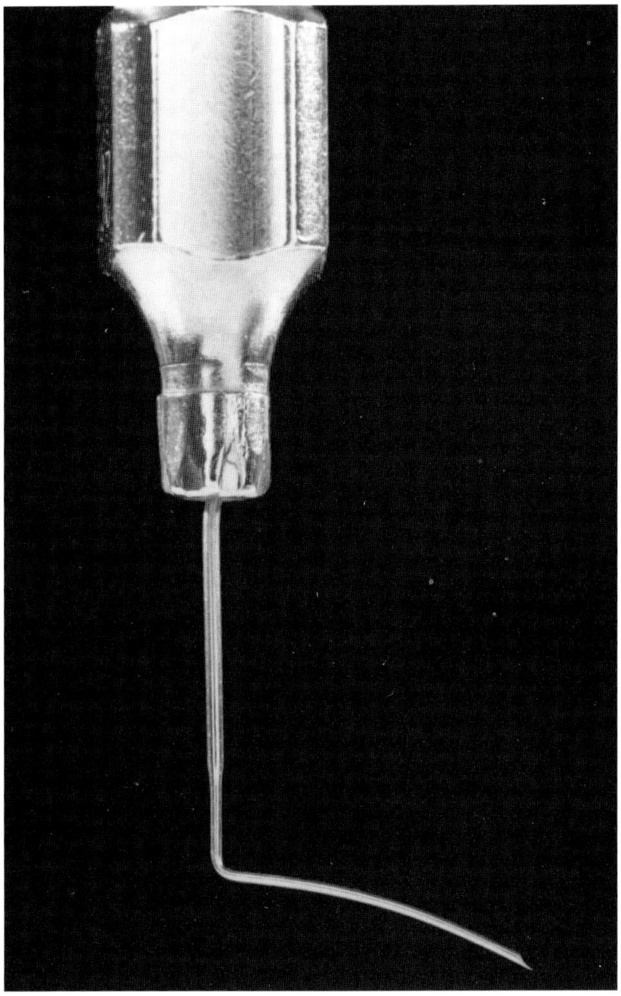

FIGURE 43-11 Slade LASIK cannula.

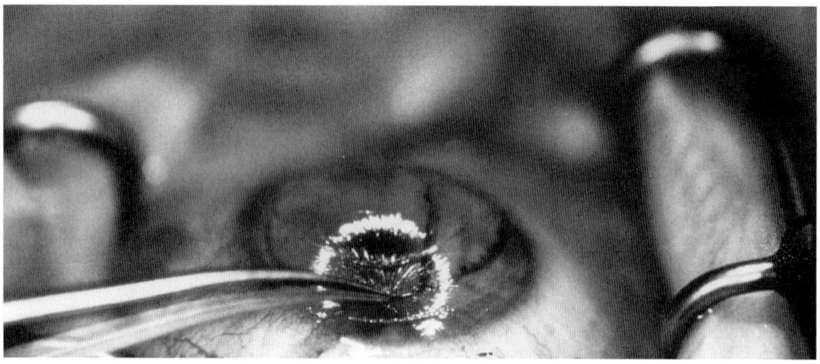

FIGURE 43-12 Corneal striae produced by depression of the peripheral cornea with a forceps. The striae radiate into the flap, indicating that the flap is adherent to the stromal bed.

The keratectomy is performed in the usual fashion but is located such that the flap will be out of the path of the laser, if possible. For most patients who have with-the-rule astigmatism, a flap with the hinge located superiorly is best. If the hinge is located nasally, the flap should be decentered enough nasally to allow space for the ablation.

The ablation is performed with care to protect the undersurface of the flap from the ablation in large-dimension scanning techniques. The accumulation of fluid during the ablation must be monitored to avoid puddles that would mask parts of the bed and cause an irregular ablation. The flap is replaced in the usual manner, and the procedure is completed in the standard fashion.

Incisional Keratotomy

If laser-assisted in situ keratomileusis is to be combined with incisional keratotomy, the cylinder axis is marked as described above and the ablation to correct the spherical component of the refraction is performed in the usual fashion. The ablation is performed first, before the keratotomy, because measuring the corneal thickness and making the incision(s) can indent the cornea and create an irregular surface that could result in irregular astigmatism when the cornea is ablated.

The length of the diamond blade is preset to the preoperative corneal thickness minus 160 μm. After the ablation, the corneal thickness is measured directly at the site of the planned keratotomy, and the blade is adjusted accordingly. Arcuate incisions are placed at a 7-mm optical zone. Incisions placed more centrally increase the effect but can induce irregular astigmatism. The flap is replaced in the usual manner.

Alternatively, the surgeon may wait until after the laser surgery to see if the astigmatism has changed. This is a good idea if the amount of preoperative astigmatism is small. Also, the ablation itself can induce or alter pre-existing astigmatism. If the incisions are made within a few months, they are placed peripheral to the flap at an 8-mm or greater optical zone, depending on the diameter of the flap. If 4 or more months have passed, the flap can usually be safely cut, so the incisions are placed at the 7-mm optical zone.

Retreatment

One of the advantages of laser-assisted in situ keratomileusis is the relative ease of retreatment. In general, before an attempt is made to treat an undercorrection, the postoperative refraction should be stable, which usually is achieved by 3 months after surgery. Some surgeons may wait 4 to 6 months, however, whereas others prefer to retreat as soon as a significant undercorrection is identified. Typically in this procedure, the flap is lifted and additional ablation is done on the stromal bed, although some surgeons prefer to create an entirely new flap with the microkeratome and ablate the underlying bed as if the patient had not had a previous keratectomy. Other surgical possibilities include radial or astigmatic keratotomy. Treating a laser-assisted in situ keratomileusis flap with photorefractive keratectomy has not proven useful because the flap is much more likely to develop haze than is an untreated cornea. However, laser-assisted in situ keratomileusis can be used successfully to retreat patients who have had previous corneal surgery, including photorefractive keratectomy, automated lamellar keratoplasty, radial keratotomy, laser-assisted in situ keratomileusis, and penetrating keratoplasty (Figure 43-13).

Alternative Techniques

There is some disagreement over which technique is better: performing the ablation on a free corneal cap (Buratto technique) or on the underlying stromal bed. Ablation of the cap has the advantage of perfect centration and a nonmoving target. In this procedure, a 300-μm–thick cap is removed, placed stromal-side up, and ablated. Care is taken to position the cap perpendicularly to the laser beam. A further advantage is that, in the event of a severe problem, the damaged cap can be replaced with an ablated piece of donor corneal tissue. This may also be done if, for some

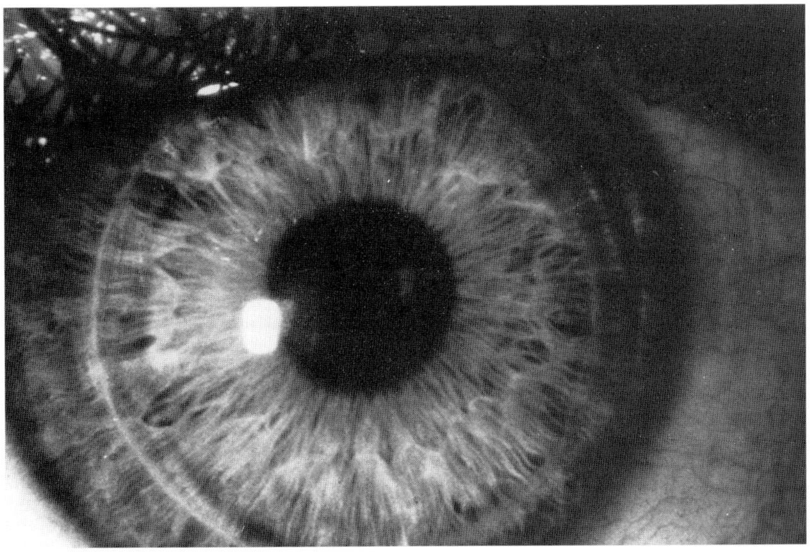

FIGURE 43-13 Clear corneal graft 1 day after laser-assisted in situ keratomileusis for postkeratoplasty myopia.

reason, the cap is lost. Another inherent advantage of ablation of the cap involves centration. If the cornea is marked at the center of the entrance pupil with a surgical marking pen before the keratectomy, the ablation can be centered on this mark, even though the keratectomy may have been slightly decentered. A poorly centered corneal stromal ablation is remedied only with great difficulty.

POSTOPERATIVE CARE

The simplicity of the postoperative care of a patient who has had laser-assisted in situ keratomileusis is a major advantage of the procedure.

Examination on the first postoperative day is critical. If the eye is satisfactory at that time, few problems are likely to occur later. The position of the corneal flap or cap is evaluated, and any corneal edema or debris in the interface is noted. The flap should be attached and difficult to discern (Figure 43-14). The corneal epithelium should be intact, and there should be no fluorescein staining of the cornea. Uncorrected visual acuity is usually good—approximately 20/30 or 20/40 in patients with low to moderate myopia. Final visual recovery may take several weeks and may be delayed significantly longer if there is irregular astigmatism. If there is edema, decreased vision, or discomfort, the eye must be further evaluated and treated.

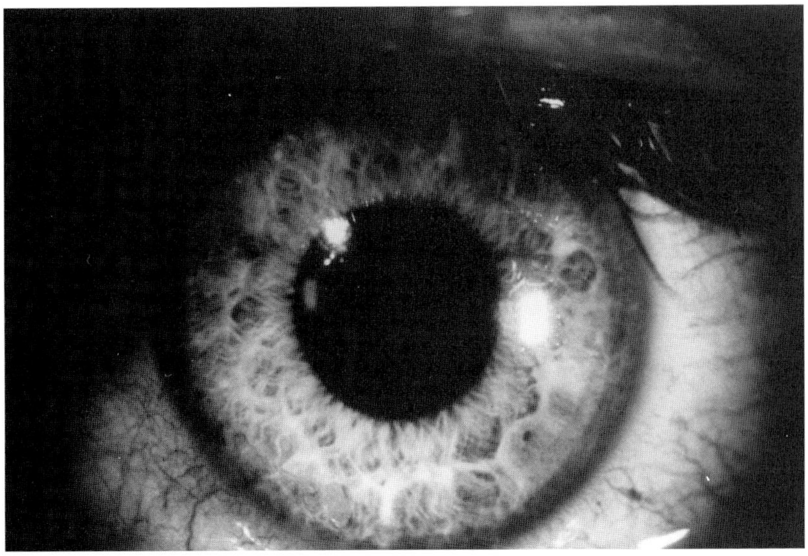

FIGURE 43-14 Cornea 1 hour after laser-assisted in situ keratomileusis demonstrating the rapid return to normal clarity.

Postoperative medications include a topical antibiotic eye drop, such as an aminoglycoside or fluoroquinolone, for the first 5 days. Topical corticosteroids are not necessary but may be added to increase patient comfort. We use a combination antibiotic-corticosteroid eye drop four times a day for 5 days. Artificial tears are often helpful on an as-needed basis for the first few days. There may be a foreign body sensation immediately after surgery, but generally there is no pain and the patient should be comfortable. If there is pain, it usually lasts only for the first few hours after the procedure until the epithelium covers the edges of the flap. Systemic analgesia is typically not necessary, but a nonsteroidal anti-inflammatory drug may be given for use on the first postoperative day.

The patient should be told to avoid any activity in which the eye could be traumatized. Contact sports should be avoided, but the patient can jog, swim, and resume normal activity, including taking a shower, on the day after surgery.

COMPLICATIONS

Complications of laser-assisted in situ keratomileusis include all of the complications of eye surgery in general, such as infection, as well as specific complications, such as irregular astigmatism and epithelialization of the stromal interface. Postoperative visual complaints are similar to those encountered in other refractive surgical procedures and include glare, halos, and decreased contrast sensitivity. Unusual and vision-threatening complications, such as vascular occlusion, macular hemorrhage, perforated globe, and microbial infection, can occur with any of the lamellar refractive surgical procedures.

Complications Related to Preoperative Factors

Complications resulting from pre-existing conditions or improper preoperative evaluation are largely preventable. A thorough patient history and examination will alert the surgeon to potential complications, such as recurrent erosions. If the refraction is unstable, if there is evidence of keratoconus, or if the cornea is too thin, laser-assisted in situ keratomileusis should not be considered.

Laser-Related Complications

There is a great deal of technology involved in laser-assisted in situ keratomileusis, including the laser, the microkeratome, and the examination instruments. All must be compulsively checked and rechecked before use.

Laser-related complications are myriad. The laser is not a static, but a fluctuating instrument. The power varies from case to case depending on the level of contaminants built up in the gas over the life of a single fill, the lenses continually degrade over hundreds of cases, and the overall performance varies with the temperature, humidity, and air purity of the room. The fluence, or "cutting rate," of the laser must be known before and after each case. Likewise, the beam profile or homogeneity must be known before each case. Fluence plates are available to test these parameters. An improper fluence will result in an undercorrection or overcorrection, and poor homogeneity can cause an irregular ablation. The alignment of the beam must be checked as well.

Central Island

A central island is one of the most common irregular ablations encountered and consists of a small steep area in the central cornea (Figure 43-15). In most cases, it can be demonstrated by videokeratography within 1 hour after surgery and usually regresses over time. A central island can occur as a result of a cooler central beam, irregular hydration during the ablation with a central accumulation of fluid that masks the central stroma, or delayed clearance of ablation debris from the central cornea that masks the central stroma. Scanning lasers largely avoid the problem of central islands.

Typically, a patient with a central island complains of visual disturbances, has a best spectacle-corrected visual acuity of 20/30 to 20/40, and has a few diopters of residual myopia. The diagnosis is made by videokeratography. One aid to diagnosis is to examine the preoperative videokeratograph, because many corneas have the appearance of a central island preoperatively that will still be present after the ablation.

Central islands are best avoided but are treatable. They occur more frequently when there is a large single treatment zone and can be prevented by increased wiping of the central cornea to dry the stroma or by additional ablation of the central 2.5 mm of the cornea. If a central island occurs and causes symptoms, it can be treated by lifting the flap and ablating a 2.7-mm–diameter central zone.

Overcorrection

In the past, overcorrection has been the most difficult to manage refractive complication of refractive surgical procedures. A myopic patient who would have been merely disappointed with some residual postoperative myopia after radial keratotomy was generally extremely unhappy with any postoperative hyperopia. For most refractive

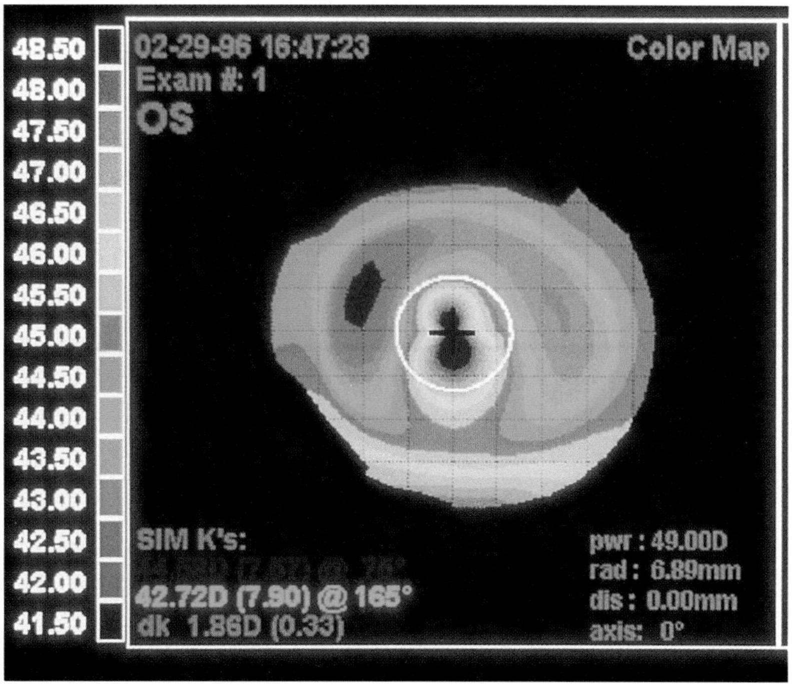

FIGURE 43-15 Videokeratograph of a cornea 1 hour after laser-assisted in situ keratomileusis demonstrating a central island.

surgical procedures, undercorrections could be treated with additional surgery, but overcorrections could not.

After laser-assisted in situ keratomileusis, approximately 10 to 20 percent of any overcorrection may disappear with time because of the slight regression of effect seen in most patients. If an overcorrection persists, keratometry, videokeratography, and pachymetry should be done, compared with preoperative measurements, and correlated with the postoperative refraction. If they do not correlate with the postoperative refraction, the patient may have irregular astigmatism and desire more plus power to make the image larger. The treatment should be reviewed to see if the correct ablation was done. Typing errors can occur during the entry of patient data into the computer of the laser.

If treatment of an overcorrection is necessary, the best choice is hyperopic laser-assisted in situ keratomileusis. During the first few months, the original flap may be lifted, with care taken to create a clean cleavage of the epithelium at the keratectomy site. After 3 or 4 months, a new keratectomy may be performed. Some surgeons prefer to lift the original flap even years after it was created, however.

Undercorrection

Undercorrections are more easily dealt with than overcorrections. A printout of the laser treatment for the case should be reviewed in an attempt to determine the cause of the undercorrection. The postoperative refraction should be stable before an attempt is made to treat an undercorrection. The flap may be lifted or a new keratectomy performed as described above and the stromal bed ablated again. We use the same nomogram for a retreatment as was used for the initial treatment. Photorefractive keratectomy should not be performed on the anterior surface of the flap. Radial keratotomy may be considered for small undercorrections after 3 months.

Microkeratome-Related Complications

Perhaps the most difficult complications of laser-assisted in situ keratomileusis are those resulting from an improper keratectomy. Although lamellar surgical procedures appear to be devoid of the complications associated with intraocular surgery, they are critically dependent on proper use of the microkeratome. It takes only 3 seconds for the microkeratome to make the cut, and very little can be done during this time to correct a problem, even if one is recognized. Preoperative inspection, proper assembly, and thorough testing of the microkeratome are critical, as are the education and skill of the surgeon. Careful attention to minute detail is essential while this instrument is in use. Appropriate placement of the fixation ring, consistent suction throughout the procedure, and the smooth movement of the microkeratome across the cornea are all essential elements of a successful lamellar resection.

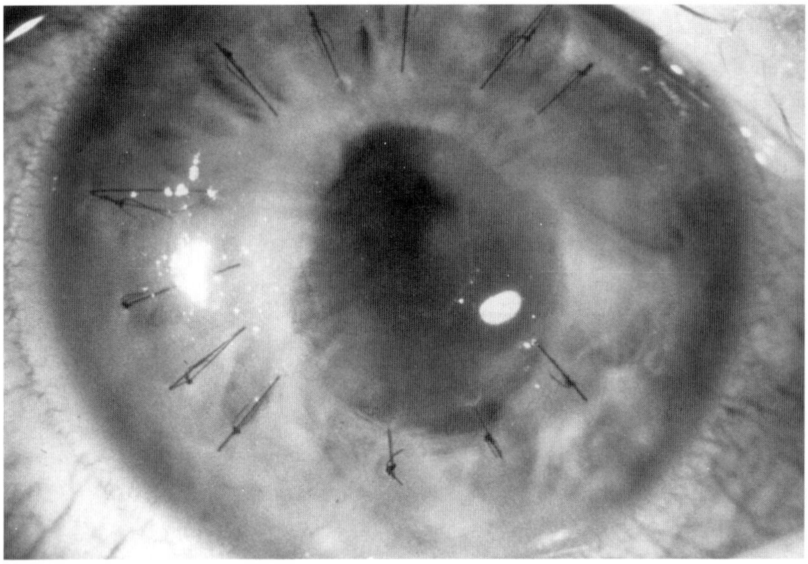

FIGURE 43-16 Sutured corneal perforation caused by an incorrectly assembled microkeratome. (Courtesy of Alan Sugar, M.D., Ann Arbor, MI.)

Irregular Astigmatism

The most common significant problem with any lamellar refractive surgical procedure is irregular astigmatism, which is caused by microscopic roughness or irregularity of the surface of the cornea. Irregular astigmatism can be diagnosed by irregular mires on keratometry or by videokeratography. Irregular astigmatism as a cause of decreased visual acuity is confirmed by improvement with placement of a hard contact lens. In many patients, irregular astigmatism diminishes during the first year and, in some, it continues to decrease throughout the second year after surgery. When visual acuity does not improve and the patient is unable to wear a contact lens, a thick homoplastic lamellar graft is the only treatment option. One of the advantages of laser-assisted in situ keratomileusis is that no matter how irregular the keratectomy, when the flap is replaced it always matches the underlying bed.

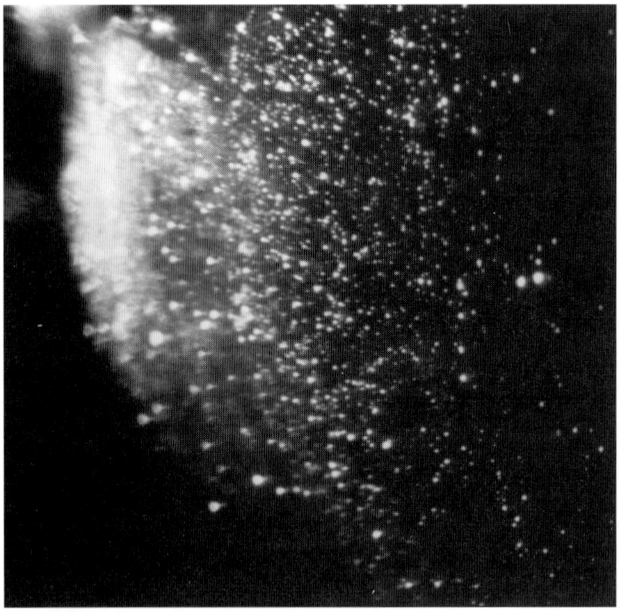

FIGURE 43-17 High magnification view of talc in the interface after laser-assisted in situ keratomileusis.

Improper Keratectomy

Other microtome-related complications include a poor keratectomy caused by a used, dirty, or damaged blade. Poor suction can result in an incomplete keratectomy, a poor flap, or a free cap. A free cap should not present a major problem or preclude the ablation. The cap is simply removed from the microkeratome, placed in an antidesiccation chamber, and replaced after the ablation. The eyelids are taped shut at the end of the procedure and carefully opened by the surgeon the next day.

The use of an improper microkeratome plate, an improperly positioned plate, or no plate at all can result in disaster, with entry into the anterior chamber (Figure 43-16).

Surgeon-Related Complications

Complications specific to the surgeon's technique include interface contamination, decentration of the ablation, and improper positioning of the flap.

Interface Opacities

Many materials can inadvertently come to rest in the interface, including blood, talc, stainless steel blade dust, fibers, and meibomian secretions (Figure 43-17).

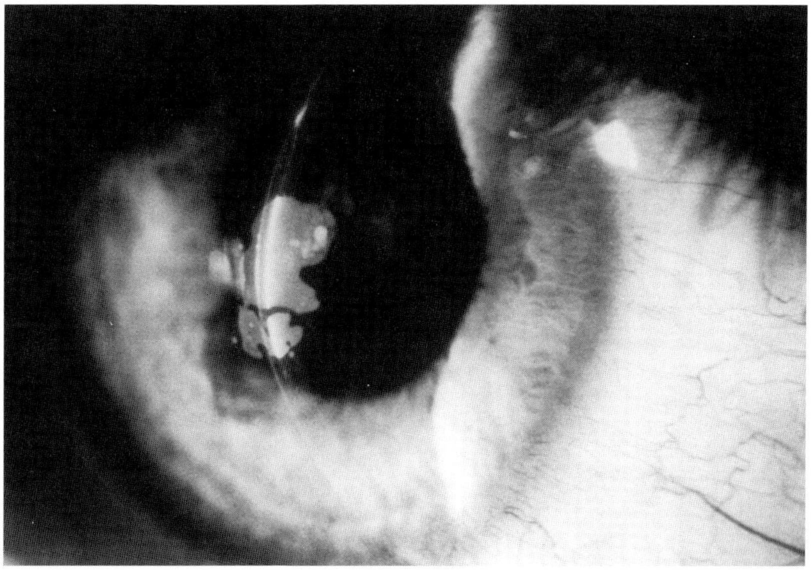

FIGURE 43-18 Epithelium in the interface after laser-assisted in situ keratomileusis.

Most do not cause any visual disturbance. Good technique and proper irrigation prevent most of these problems. No lubricating oil or instrument milk should be used on the microkeratome because they can contaminate the interface.

The only major interface problem is epithelium (Figure 43-18), which may be introduced in three ways: implantation during the procedure, ingrowth from the keratectomy edge, or ingrowth from intrastromal epithelial plugs in patients who have had previous keratotomies (e.g., radial keratotomy). Epithelium in the interface can be ignored unless it is growing, causing stromal melting, obscuring the visual axis, or causing astigmatism. Epithelium can be removed by lifting the flap, scraping the cells off the bed and undersurface of the flap, prophylactically ablating these surfaces with a few laser shots, and replacing the flap.

Decentration of the Flap

In laser-assisted in situ keratomileusis, the flap may be decentered with no visual consequences. Often the flap is intentionally displaced nasally to provide more room for the ablation or inferiorly to avoid an area of vessels from a superior pannus.

Decentration of the Ablation

Centration of the ablation is separate from centration of the flap and depends on the technique of the surgeon and the alignment of the laser. Decentration of the ablation may be minimized by making sure the patient is fixating, carefully checking the position beam, and monitoring the ablation. If decentration occurs, the best approach to correction is the use of a scanning laser (Figure 43-19).

Displacement of the Flap

Displacement of the flap can vary from subtle wrinkles to a flap that is completely separated from the cornea. Striae that cause irregular astigmatism and decreased visual acuity should be treated as soon as possible by lifting the flap and repositioning it. In the case of a loose flap, the epithelium is cleaned off the bed and the flap is repositioned. If the flap is not attached firmly in place the next day, it should be repositioned and sutured with an antitorque suture. If the flap is lost, the eye should be treated as if the patient had undergone photorefractive keratectomy, with the expectation of increased risk of haze. If significant haze develops despite topical corticosteroids, a thick homoplastic lamellar graft may be done.

Complications Related to Postoperative Factors

If an intralamellar infection develops after laser-assisted in situ keratomileusis, it must be treated aggressively (Figure 43-20). The flap should be lifted, the area first cultured and then irrigated with a bactericidal solution, and the patient started on fortified topical antibiotics. The flap may have to be removed if the infection is not controlled.

CLINICAL RESULTS

Myopia

Buratto et al[38] reported the first large series of cases of laser-assisted keratomileusis for the correction of myopia.

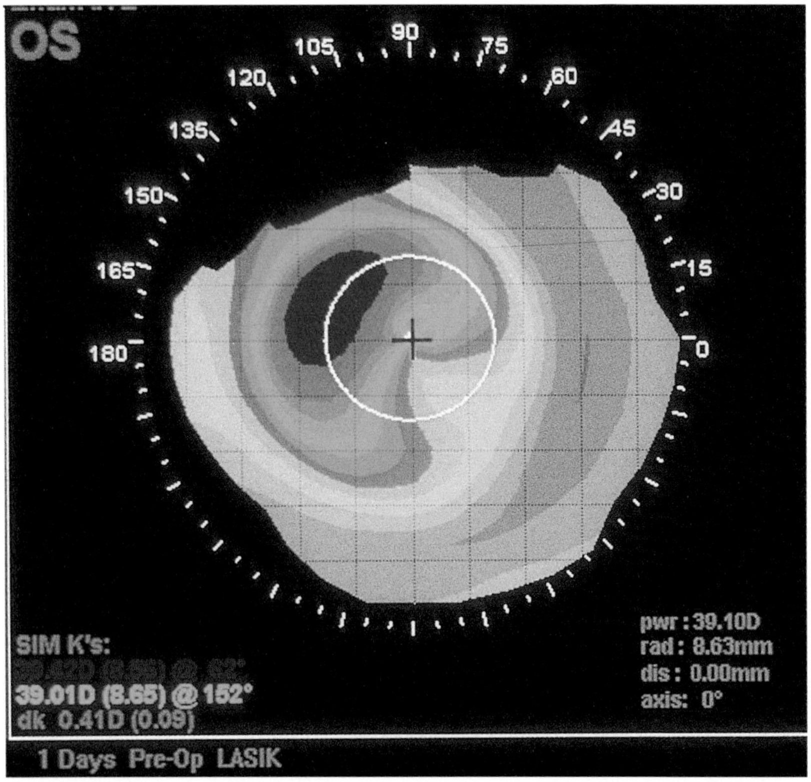

A

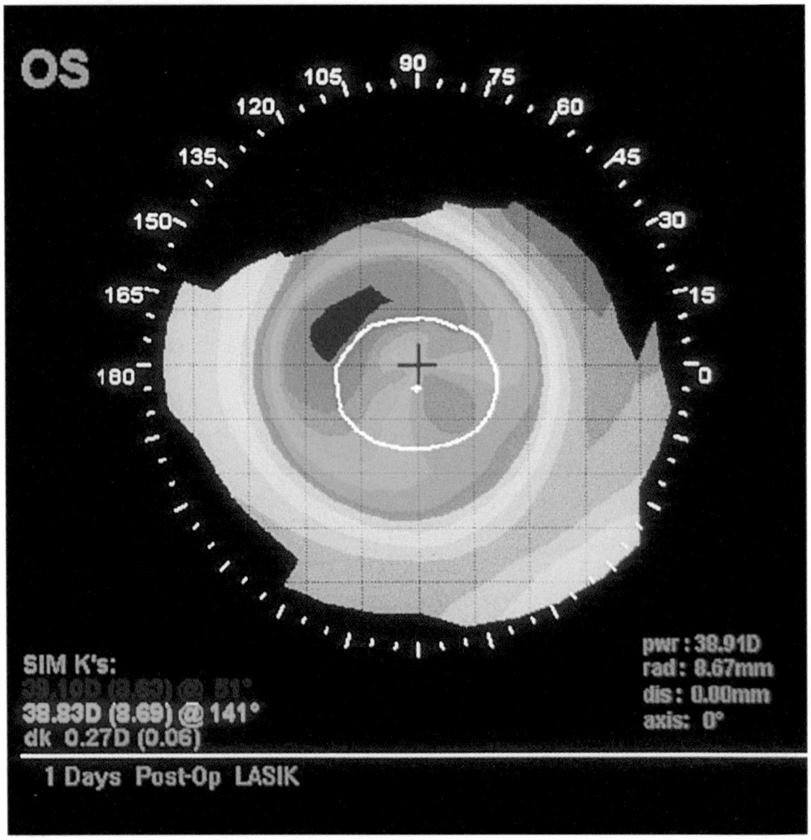

B

FIGURE 43-19 An irregular ablation that resulted in a central peninsula is shown **(A)** before and **(B)** after treatment with a scanning laser. Uncorrected visual acuity increased from 20/50 with poor quality to 20/30 with acceptable quality.

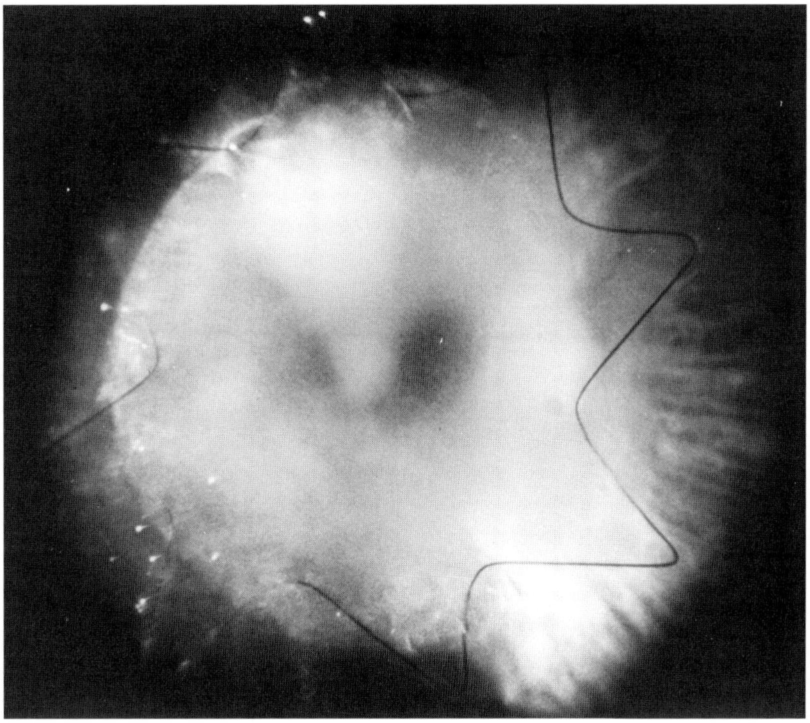

FIGURE 43-20 Infection in the interface after automated lamellar keratoplasty.

Since then, most studies have shown that accuracy (defined as the likelihood of a postoperative refraction within 1.0 diopter of the intended correction) is greater for the correction of low amounts of myopia than for the correction of high amounts of myopia. In some studies,[39,40] ranges of postoperative astigmatism and residual refractive error as large as 6 to 10 diopters have been reported. Complication rates similar to those seen with other forms of refractive lamellar surgery have been described.[39]

In 1991, Brint, Slade, and others[37] initiated the Summit Technology multicenter Phase I study of excimer laser-assisted in situ keratomileusis for the treatment of myopia; this was the first FDA-approved study of this procedure in the United States. The microkeratome used was the Chiron Automatic Corneal Shaper. The range of corrections attempted was 6 to 25 diopters of myopia. Photoablation was performed on the undersurface of a 300-μm-thick corneal cap in 53 eyes and on the underlying stromal bed after a 160-μm-thick corneal cap was resected in four eyes. At first, the caps were sutured; later in the study they were not. In most eyes, epithelialization was complete the morning after surgery.

Results at 6 months showed that 66 percent of eyes had 20/40 or better uncorrected visual acuity, and 46 percent were within 1 diopter of the intended correction. No change in mean refractive cylinder was observed, but 21 percent of patients had induced irregular astigmatism. Complications included two corneal caps perforated during laser ablation. In one case, the cap was replaced with an ablated homoplastic lenticle that proved to have an inadequate correction, such that the patient remained highly myopic. One patient from the "no suturing" group required repositioning of the cap 3 days postoperatively. One procedure was interrupted because the laser stopped firing during the procedure. Additional complications included one patient with mild wrinkling of Bowman's layer, one patient with mild irregularity and mild opacification of Bowman's layer, and eight patients with mild interface debris. One patient complained of seeing ghost images that were graded as mild, and one patient experienced marked halos.

A later study by Fiander and Tayfour[41] demonstrated that the algorithms used for photorefractive keratectomy may not be directly applicable to laser-assisted in situ keratomileusis. The authors noted overcorrection in patients with all degrees of preoperative myopia. Notably, the overcorrection appeared to be a predictable fixed percentage based on the amount of preoperative refractive error.

A variety of clinical studies involving patients with 0.25 to 29 diopters of myopia have been published or reported (Table 43-1),[39-45] but comparisons are difficult because instrumentation, nomograms, and techniques, as well as patient groupings and reporting formats, vary widely from study to study. Two studies[41,44] that used the Sum-

TABLE 43-1
Comparison of Seven Studies of Laser-Assisted In Situ Keratomileusis (LASIK)

Study Parameter	Fiander and Tayfour, 1995[41]	Gomes, 1995[40]	Kremer and Dufek, 1995[42]	Güell and Muller, 1996[43]	Knorz et al, 1996[39]	Salah et al, 1996[44]	Ruiz et al, submitted[45]
Number of eyes	124	42	31	43	51	88	130[a]
Length of follow-up (mo)	3–11	1–12	6	6	4–6	5.2 (mean)	12
Preoperative spherical equivalent (D)							
Mean	–7.65	NR	–6.25	NR	–14.80	–8.24	–3.61
Standard deviation	NR	NR	NR	NR	± 7.28	NR	± 2.95
Range	–3.75 to –27.0	–12.50 to –29.0	–3.5 to –11.75	–7.0 to –18.50	–6.0 to –29.0	–2.0 to –20.0	–0.25 to –18.25
Preoperative cylinder (D)							
Mean	0.88	NR	NR	NR	NR	NR	1.15
Standard deviation	NR	NR	NR	NR	NR	NR	± 1.31
Range	0 to 2.00	NR	0.25 to 2.75	NR	NR	NR	0 to 8.0
Postoperative spherical equivalent (D)							
Mean	+0.27	NR	–0.5	NR	–1.90	+0.22	–0.22
Standard deviation	NR	NR	NR	NR	± 2.75	± 1.42	± 0.32
Range	–2.75 to +4.0	–4.75 to +4.75	–3.5 to +2.0	–5.25 to 0	–9.50 to +2.25	NR	–2.5 to +1.5
Postoperative cylinder (D)							
Mean	1.24	NR	0.64	NR	NR	NR	0.35
Standard deviation	NR	NR	NR	NR	NR	NR	± 0.4
Range	0 to 4	NR	0.25 to 3.5	NR	NR	NR	0 to 2
Postoperative uncorrected visual acuity (%)							
20/20 or better	NR	NR	NR	NR	8	36	67
20/25 or better	50	NR	NR	NR	NR	NR	85
20/40 or better	81	NR	81	37	29	71	93
Accuracy of correction (%)							
Within ±1.00 D of intended	74	50	74	63	47	73	98
Within ±0.50 D of intended	NR	31	NR	33	37	NR	90
Change in best-corrected visual acuity (%)							
Lost 2 or more lines	0	NR	0	0	12	3.4	0
Gained 2 or more lines	NR	NR	NR	NR	NR	NR	17.1
Laser	Summit OmniMed	NR	Custom	Chiron/ Technolas Keracor 116	Chiron/ Technolas Keracor 116	Summit OmniMed	Chiron/ Technolas Keracor 116
Microkeratome	Chiron ACS	Freehand	NR	Chiron ACS	Chiron ACS	Chiron ACS	Chiron ACS
Nomogram	Personalized	Single-zone 5.0 mm or two-zone 4.5 and 5.0 mm	Personalized	Personalized, modified	Single-zone 4.0 to 5.0 mm or multizone 3.0 to 6.0 mm with pretreatment	PRK or MKM program or Salah LASIK nomogram, version 1993	Ruiz

Abbreviations: NR, not reported; D, diopters; ACS, Automatic Corneal Shaper; PRK, photorefractive keratectomy; MKM, myopic keratomileusis.
[a] Of the 171 patients in the study, 130 had complete examinations for 1 year after surgery.

mit OmniMed laser noted a tendency toward overcorrection, which was greater with increasing amounts of preoperative myopia. One group of authors[39] who used the Chiron/Technolas Keracor 116 laser in the multizone mode found that most eyes were undercorrected, whereas another study[43] using the same laser in the same mode reported acceptable predictability with correction of refractive errors up to -12 diopters. A third group[45] that used the Chiron laser for the treatment of both myopia and astigmatism in 130 patients reported excellent visual results and predictability; it should be noted, however, that most of their patients had mild myopia (mean preoperative spherical equivalent of -3.61 ± 2.95 diopters), a population more likely to achieve predictable results and less likely to have degenerative myopic maculopathy than the patients in the other studies, most of whom had moderate to severe myopia.

Complications other than under- or overcorrection reported in these studies included decentration of the ablation[40,41] causing induced cylinder greater than 2.00 diopters in 2 of 124 patients,[41] loss of two lines of best spectacle-corrected visual acuity caused by irregular astigmatism[39,44] or prominent central islands,[39] loss of best spectacle-corrected visual acuity because of progression of myopic maculopathy,[43,44] transient halos and impaired night vision,[42,43] transient foreign body sensation,[42] interface debris,[45] epithelial implantation and ingrowth with no visual consequences,[43,45] folds in Bowman's layer not encroaching on the visual axis,[45] vitreous hemorrhage,[40] and retinal detachment.[40] Two studies reported inadvertent severing of the flap during the procedure, with no postoperative consequences.[43,44] One study reported two eyes with peripheral keratectomy edge haze[45]; no study reported significant postoperative corneal haze affecting visual acuity.

One of the few randomized prospective comparisons between photorefractive keratectomy and laser-assisted in situ keratomileusis was the Chiron-sponsored clinical trial, which began in November, 1994. In this study, 259 eyes with a spherical equivalent refraction of -4 to -10 diopters and less than 1 diopter of cylinder were randomized to either photorefractive keratectomy (122 eyes) or laser-assisted in situ keratomileusis (137 eyes). The study data indicated that the results of laser-assisted in situ keratomileusis are better than those of photorefractive keratectomy in the early period after surgery, but that the results of the two procedures become essentially equal later in the postoperative period. On the first postoperative day, 68 percent of the eyes that underwent laser-assisted in situ keratomileusis had an uncorrected visual acuity of 20/40 or better, compared with only 14 percent of the eyes that underwent photorefractive keratectomy. By 3 months, however, 80 percent of the eyes in both groups had an uncorrected visual acuity of 20/40 or better. At 1 month, 8 percent of the photorefractive keratectomy eyes had lost more than two lines of best spectacle-corrected visual acuity, compared with 1 percent of the laser-assisted in situ keratomileusis eyes. By 12 months, however, none of the photorefractive keratectomy eyes and only one of the laser-assisted in situ keratomileusis eyes lost more than two lines of best spectacle-corrected visual acuity.

Astigmatism

Variable spot scanning for the treatment of astigmatism associated with myopia was reported by Ruiz et al.[45] A total of 91 of the 171 eyes had preoperative astigmatism ranging from 1.00 to 8.00 diopters (mean 1.31 diopters); 56 eyes in this group had 12 or more months of follow-up. At 1 year, mean astigmatism in these eyes was reduced to 0.35 diopter; 94 percent had uncorrected visual acuity of 20/40 or better, and 65 percent had uncorrected visual acuity of 20/20 or better. No eyes lost two or more lines of best spectacle-corrected visual acuity at 1 year after surgery.

Hyperopia

Laser-assisted in situ keratomileusis for the treatment of hyperopia involves removing tissue in a peripheral trench to steepen the central corneal curvature. Because the ablation for hyperopia is necessarily deeper and steeper than the ablation for a similar amount of myopia, one advantage of laser-assisted in situ keratomileusis over photorefractive keratectomy for hyperopia may be reduced scarring. Early results are promising, although these patients seem to lose more lines of best spectacle-corrected visual acuity than patients with similar amounts of myopia, possibly as a result of decentration of the ablation and induced irregular astigmatism. A scanning technique in which the beam is directed by movable mirrors (PLANO-SCAN) is being tested for the correction of astigmatism associated with hyperopia; results in 18 eyes at 1 month showed moderate undercorrection across the entire range of up to 4 diopters of attempted correction.

FOR THE FUTURE

No peer-reviewed article has yet been published that reports short-term or long-term results for any refractive surgical technique that match the results of spectacles or contact lenses with regard to efficacy and safety for any level of refractive disorder. Thus, the ultimate goal of refractive surgery in general and laser-assisted in situ keratomileusis in particular may very well be to produce a correction that is adjustable, reversible, and quantitatively and qualitatively equal to or better than that possible with spectacles or contact lenses.

Future advancements in laser correction of refractive errors depend on the design of increasingly sophisticated lasers and methods of measuring the cornea, as well as the ability to link the two to produce a real-time feedback loop that monitors the progress of the ablation and directs the laser accordingly. A laser with this type of guidance system should be capable of producing any ablation pattern without the constraints associated with current circular diaphragm-controlled broad-beam lasers. Thus, these lasers would provide an efficient system for the treatment of regular astigmatism and could also be used to treat irregular astigmatism and decentered ablations.

Laser-assisted in situ keratomileusis is a part of the continuum of refractive procedures first initiated by Barraquer 50 years ago. It offers a nonfreeze, nonsuture, minimally invasive procedure that can be performed under topical anesthesia. Visual recovery is rapid and irregular astigmatism rates are low. Patient comfort is excellent. One of the main advantages is the ability to minimize the wound healing response by providing a virtual "intrastromal ablation" at a time when the dream of true intrastromal ablation remains distant. Enthusiasm for early results must be tempered, however, by the fact that long-term results are not yet available. For the surgeon, the capital expenditure involved—for both a microkeratome and an excimer laser—requires a significant financial commitment. Also, this is a skill-intensive procedure, and the operative risks are not negligible. Nevertheless, laser-assisted in situ keratomileusis appears to represent a step forward in terms of efficacy, predictability, and stability, and future long-term follow-up studies and new controlled studies will continue to define these parameters, as well as safety and patient satisfaction.

REFERENCES

1. Barraquer JI: Queratoplastia refractiva. Estudios Inform Oftal Inst Barraquer 10:2, 1949
2. Barraquer JI: Results of hypermetropic keratomileusis, 1980–1981. Int Ophthalmol Clin 23(3):25, 1983
3. Barraquer JI: Results of myopic keratomileusis. J Refract Surg 3:98, 1987
4. Barraquer JI : Keratomileusis for myopia and aphakia. Ophthalmology 88:701, 1981
5. Barraquer JI: Method for cutting lamellar grafts in frozen corneas: new orientations for refractive surgery. Arch Soc Am Ophthalmol 1:237, 1958
6. Barraquer JI. Keratomileusis. Int Surg 48:103, 1967
7. Troutman RC, Swinger CA: Refractive keratoplasty: keratophakia and keratomileusis. Trans Am Ophthalmol Soc 76:329, 1978
8. Taylor DM, Stern AL, Romanchuk KG: Keratophakia. Clinical evaluation. Ophthalmology 88:1141, 1981
9. Friedlander MH, Werblin TP, Kaufman HE, Granet NS: Clinical results of keratophakia and keratomileusis. Ophthalmology 88:716, 1981
10. Swinger CA, Barker BA: Prospective evaluation of myopic keratomileusis. Ophthalmology 91:785, 1984
11. Nordan LT, Fallor MK: Myopic keratomileusis: 74 consecutive non-amblyopic cases with one year of follow-up. J Refract Surg 2:124, 1986
12. Maguire LJ, Klyce SD, Sawelson H, et al: Visual distortion after myopic keratomileusis. Computer analysis of keratoscope photographs. Ophthalmic Surg 18:352, 1987
13. Nordan LT: Keratomileusis. Int Ophthalmol Clin 31(4):7, 1991
14. Barraquer C, Gutierrez A, Espinosa A: Myopic keratomileusis. Short term results. Refract Corneal Surg 5:307, 1989
15. Kaufman HE: The correction of aphakia. Am J Ophthalmol 89:1, 1980
16. Werblin TP, Klyce SD: Epikeratophakia: the surgical correction of aphakia. I. Lathing of corneal tissue. Curr Eye Res 1:123,1981
17. Werblin TP, Klyce SD: Epikeratophakia: the surgical correction of myopia: I. Lathing of corneal tissue. Curr Eye Res 1:591, 1981/1982
18. Werblin TP: Epikeratophakia. Techniques, complications and clinical results. Int Ophthalmol Clin 23(3):45, 1983
19. McDonald MB, Kaufman HE, Aquavella JV, et al: The nationwide study of epikeratophakia for myopia in adults. Am J Ophthalmol 103:375, 1987
20. Reidy JJ, McDonald MB, Klyce SD: The corneal topography of epikeratophakia. Refract Corneal Surg 6:26, 1990
21. Goosey JD, Prager TC, Goosey CB, et al: Stability of refraction during two years after myopic epikeratoplasty. Refract Corneal Surg 6:4, 1990
22. Goosey JD, Prager TC, Marvelli TL, et al: Epikeratophakia without annular keratectomy. Ann Ophthalmol 19:388, 1987
23. Swinger CA, Krumeich J, Cassiday D: Planar lamellar refractive keratoplasty. J Refract Surg 2:17, 1986
24. Zavala EY, Krumeich J, Binder PS: Laboratory evaluation of freeze vs nonfreeze lamellar refractive keratoplasty. Arch Ophthalmol 105:1125, 1987
25. Bas AM, Nano HD: In situ myopic keratomileusis results in 30 eyes at 15 months. Refract Corneal Surg 7:223, 1991
26. Arenas-Archila E, Sanchez-Thorin JC, Naranjo-Uribe JP, Hernandez-Lozano A: Myopic keratomileusis in situ: a preliminary report. J Cataract Refract Surg 17:424, 1991
27. Hofmann RF, Bechara SJ: An independent evaluation of second generation suction microkeratomes. Refract Corneal Surg 8:348, 1992
28. Colin J, Mimouni F, Robinet A: The surgical treatment of high myopia. Comparison of epikeratoplasty, ker-

atomileusis and minus power anterior chamber lenses. Refract Corneal Surg 6:245, 1990
29. Slade SG, Rozakis, G, Dulaney, D, et al: Prospective evaluation of keratomileusis in situ. Submitted
30. Altmann J, Grabner G, Husinsky W, et al: Corneal lathing using the excimer laser and a computer-controlled positioning system: Part I—Lathing of epikeratoplasty lenticules. Refract Corneal Surg 7:377, 1991
31. Buratto L, Ferrari M : Retrospective comparison of freeze and non-freeze myopic epikeratophakia. Refract Corneal Surg 5:94, 1989
32. Peyman GA, Badaro RM, Khoobehi B: Corneal ablation in rabbits using an infrared (2.9-μm) erbium:YAG laser. Ophthalmology 96:1160, 1989
33. Pallikaris IG, Papatzanaki ME, Stathi EZ, et al: Laser in situ keratomileusis. Lasers Surg Med 10:463, 1990
34. Marshall J, Trokel SL, Rothery S, Krueger RR: Long term healing of the central cornea after photorefractive keratectomy using an excimer laser. Ophthalmology 95:1411, 1988
35. Buratto L, Ferrari M, Rama P: Excimer laser intrastromal keratomileusis. Am J Ophthalmol 113:291, 1992
36. Hagen KB, Kim EK, Waring GO III: Comparison of excimer laser and microkeratome myopic keratomileusis in human cadaver eyes. Refract Corneal Surg 9:36, 1993
37. Brint SF, Ostrick DM, Fisher C, et al: Six-month results of the multicenter phase I study of excimer laser myopic keratomileusis. J Cataract Refract Surg 20:610, 1994
38. Buratto L, Ferrari M, Genisi C: Myopic keratomileusis with the excimer laser: one-year follow up. Refract Corneal Surg 9:12, 1993
39. Knorz MC, Liermann A, Seiberth V, et al: Laser in situ keratomileusis to correct myopia of -6.00 to -29.00 diopters. J Refract Surg 12:575, 1996
40. Gomes M: Laser in situ keratomileusis for myopia using manual dissection. J Refract Surg 11(suppl):S239, 1995
41. Fiander DC, Tayfour F: Excimer laser in situ keratomileusis in 124 myopic eyes. J Refract Surg 11(suppl):S234, 1995
42. Kremer FB, Dufek M: Excimer laser in situ keratomileusis. J Refract Surg 11(suppl):S244, 1995
43. Güell JL, Muller A: Laser in situ keratomileusis (LASIK) for myopia from -7 to -18 diopters. J Refract Surg 12:222, 1996
44. Salah T, Waring GO III, El Maghraby A, et al: Excimer laser in situ keratomileusis under a corneal flap for myopia of 2 to 20 diopters. Am J Ophthalmol 121:143, 1996
45. Ruiz LA, Slade SG, Updegraff SA, et al: A single center study to evaluate the efficacy, safety and stability of laser in situ keratomileusis for low, moderate, and high myopia with and without astigmatism. Submitted

44

Intrastromal Corneal Ring

PENNY A. ASBELL

The field of refractive surgery is undergoing fundamental changes that may alter the way refractive errors are corrected surgically. As advances in technology have occurred, there has been increasing consumer interest in, as well as increased expectations for, refractive surgery as an alternative to spectacles and contact lenses. For every refractive surgical procedure, patients and eye care professionals alike are interested in efficacy, predictability, safety, reversibility, and the ability to correct different types of refractive errors. This chapter discusses a new refractive surgical procedure in which implantation of a polymethyl methacrylate ring or ring segments in the peripheral corneal stroma is used to correct myopia.

HISTORY

The intrastromal corneal ring was developed in the 1980s, and animal studies were begun in 1985. In early 1991, rings were implanted in corneas of nonfunctional human eyes as part of a study conducted in Brazil. Shortly thereafter, a similar study was done in the United States. Implantation of the rings in corneas of sighted eyes was initiated in Brazil in late 1991, and implantation in corneas of sighted eyes in the United States was implemented in 1993 as part of a U. S. Food and Drug Administration (FDA)–regulated Phase II study. Implantation of the rings in contralateral eyes was permitted starting in 1994. In May 1995, implantation of intrastromal corneal ring segments was introduced into Phase II clinical studies in the United States, and implantation of the ring segments in contralateral eyes began in November 1995.

DEVICE DESCRIPTION

The Kera-Vision intrastromal corneal ring, or ICR, is an investigational device designed to correct mild to moderate myopia by flattening the anterior corneal curvature without encroaching on the visual axis. The device is an open-ended polymethyl methacrylate ring with an outer diameter of 8.1 mm and an inner diameter of 6.77 mm (Figure 44-1). It is inserted through a peripheral radial incision made with a diamond knife at two-thirds corneal depth into a 360-degree peripheral intrastromal channel created with specially designed instruments (Figure 44-2). Changes in the anterior corneal curvature are achieved by using rings of different thicknesses; thicker rings cause more corneal flattening than thinner rings. Rings with thicknesses of 0.25, 0.30, 0.35, 0.40, and 0.45 mm have been evaluated.

The intrastromal corneal ring segments, or ICRS, are a recent design modification of the intrastromal corneal ring that splits the ring into two segments, each having an arc length of 150 degrees (Figure 44-3). Like the intrastromal corneal ring, the ring segments flatten the anterior corneal curvature with no invasion of the visual axis. One advantage of the ring segments is that the implantation technique is simpler than that required for the ring. Additionally, the ring segments do not have to be positioned near the radial corneal incision, which minimizes the potential for the kinds of incision-related complications that were encountered in some cases with the ring.

PATIENT SELECTION

Both the intrastromal corneal ring and the intrastromal corneal ring segments are designed to correct mild to mod-

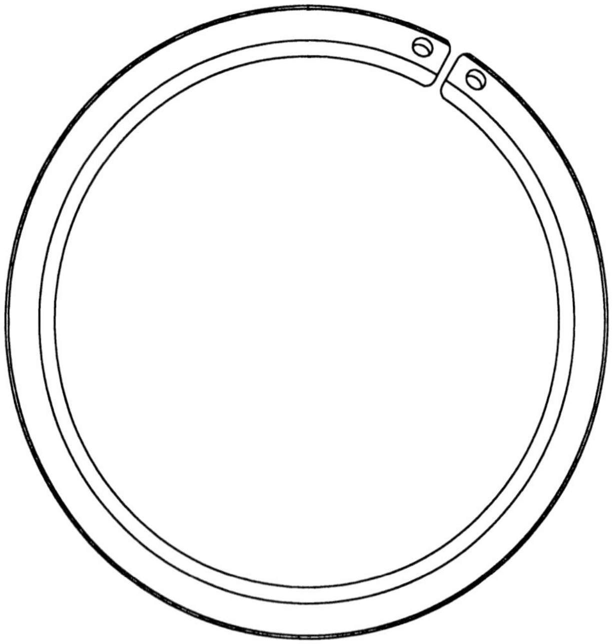

FIGURE 44-1 Intrastromal corneal ring.

erate myopia (1.0 to 5.0 diopters) by means of a potentially adjustable, reversible procedure that does not appear to significantly alter the natural aspheric shape of the central 6-mm-diameter region of the cornea. Nomograms relating ring thicknesses to predicted corrections are given in Tables 44-1 and 44-2.

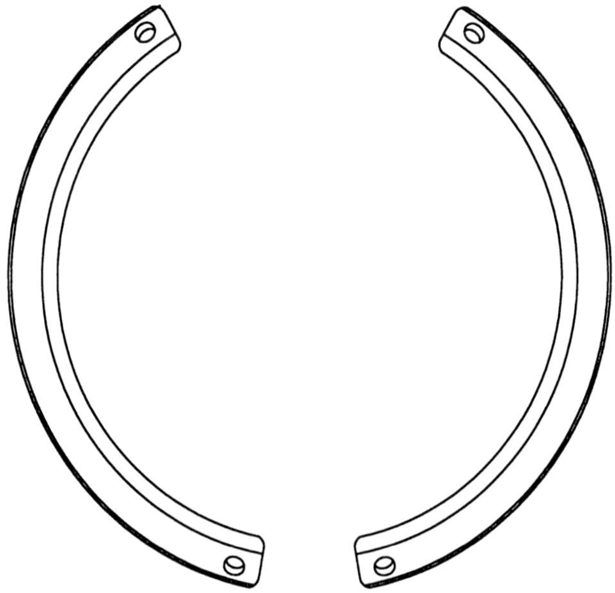

FIGURE 44-3 Intrastromal corneal ring segments.

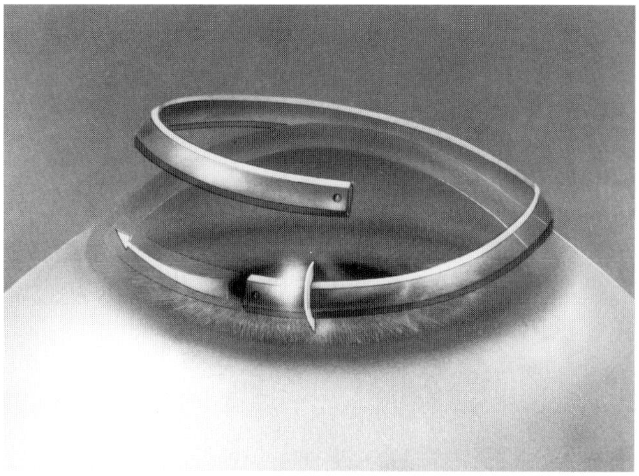

FIGURE 44-2 Insertion of an intrastromal corneal ring through a peripheral radial incision into an intrastromal channel.

PREOPERATIVE EVALUATION

Under the FDA Phase II study protocol, the preoperative evaluation should be done no more than 1 month before surgery. The patient's medical history is reviewed, and a complete ophthalmologic examination of both eyes is performed, including the following evaluations: uncorrected and best spectacle-corrected visual acuities using standardized visual acuity charts and lighting, manifest refraction, cycloplegic refraction, near visual acuity, glare testing, contrast sensitivity testing, keratometry, videokeratography, slit lamp examination, ophthalmoscopy, tonometry, ultrasonic pachymetry of both the central and peripheral cornea, esthesiometry, automated visual field testing, A-scan ultrasonography, photography, and specular microscopy.

SURGICAL TECHNIQUES

The surgical techniques for implanting the intrastromal corneal ring and the intrastromal corneal ring segments are similar. In this section, the surgical technique for implanting the intrastromal corneal ring segments is described and variations relating to implantation of the intrastromal corneal ring are noted.

Implantation of the intrastromal corneal ring segments can be done with local anesthesia alone, topical anesthesia alone, topical anesthesia in conjunction with mild, short-acting sedation, or topical anesthesia with intravenous conscious sedation.

Povidone-iodine solution (2.5 percent) is applied to the cul-de-sac, left for 2 minutes, and rinsed away with ster-

TABLE 44-1
Predicted Correction for the Intrastromal Corneal Ring by Thickness and Type of Incision

	Predicted Correction (Diopters)	
Thickness of Ring (mm)	Radial Incision	Circumferential Incision
0.25	-1.50	-0.50
0.30	-2.50	-1.50
0.35	-3.50	-2.50
0.40	-4.50	-3.50
0.45	-5.50	-4.50

TABLE 44-2
Predicted Correction for the Intrastromal Corneal Ring Segments by Thickness

Thickness of Ring (mm)	Predicted Correction (Diopters)[a]
0.25	-1.00
0.30	-2.00
0.35	-3.00
0.40	-4.00
0.45	-5.00

[a]Radial incision.

ile balanced salt solution. Patients are prepped and draped as for any anterior segment surgery.

An 11-mm optical zone marker with cross hairs is centered over the geometric center of the cornea and is pressed on the anterior corneal surface so that the cross hairs make an indentation mark at the center of the cornea. This mark may be enhanced with a surgical marking pen. An incision and placement marker is inked with gentian violet and is used to mark the epithelium where the ring segments are to be placed at an 8-mm-diameter optical zone and where the superior 2-mm radial incision is to be made (Figure 44-4). The corneal thickness at the center of the radial mark is measured by ultrasonic pachymetry, and a diamond knife set to 68 percent of this measurement is used to make a 2-mm radial incision. The corneal tissue at the base of the incision is separated laterally with a modified stromal spreader to prepare a corneal pocket on each side of the incision. A vacuum centering guide is positioned around the center corneal mark. This device fixates the eye by vacuum and provides a guide for the dissector. The dissector is inserted into the radial incision, and blunt dissection of the cornea at two-thirds depth is performed in the clockwise and counterclockwise directions to create two stromal channels. The vacuum is released and the vacuum centering guide is removed.

The intrastromal corneal ring segments are inserted through the radial incision into the stromal channels with specially designed forceps (Figure 44-5). The segments are positioned with a Sinskey hook nasally and temporally, such that the superior ends are approximately 3 mm apart and symmetrically positioned around the radial incision. Care is taken that neither segment lies directly beneath the incision (Figure 44-6). The incision is closed with two interrupted 10-0 nylon sutures.

The same technique is used for implanting the intrastromal corneal ring. In this case, however, the cornea is dissected clockwise and counterclockwise to create one complete circular channel. If the dissections create two nonconnecting channels, a channel connecting instrument is inserted into the deeper channel and used to dissect anteriorly into the more superficial channel, thus connecting the two channels. The intrastromal corneal ring is rotated manually into the channel until the ends of the ring meet at the incision. Before the ring is inserted, a 10-0 polypropylene suture is threaded through the positioning hole in the trailing end of the ring. Once the ring is in place, the suture is threaded through the other positioning hole and tied. The suture ends are trimmed, and the knot is buried in one of the positioning holes. The ring juncture is rotated

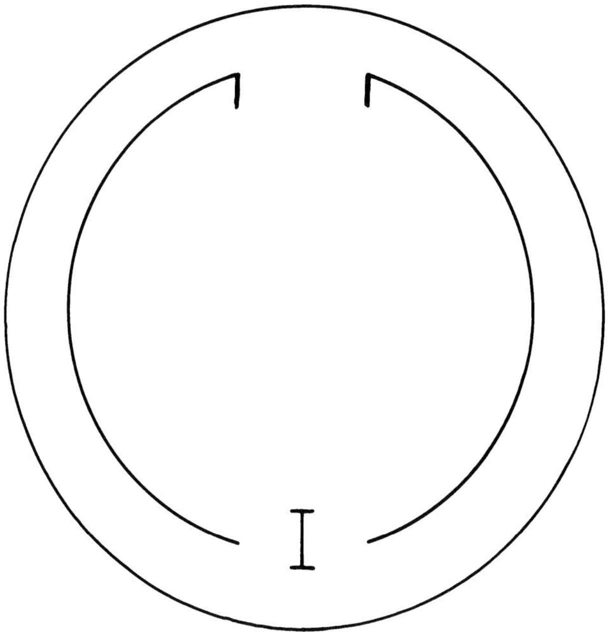

FIGURE 44-4 Cornea marked with the incision and placement marker. The 2-mm radial mark indicates where to make the incision. The two 150-degree arcuate marks are at an 8-mm optical zone and indicate where to place the ring segments.

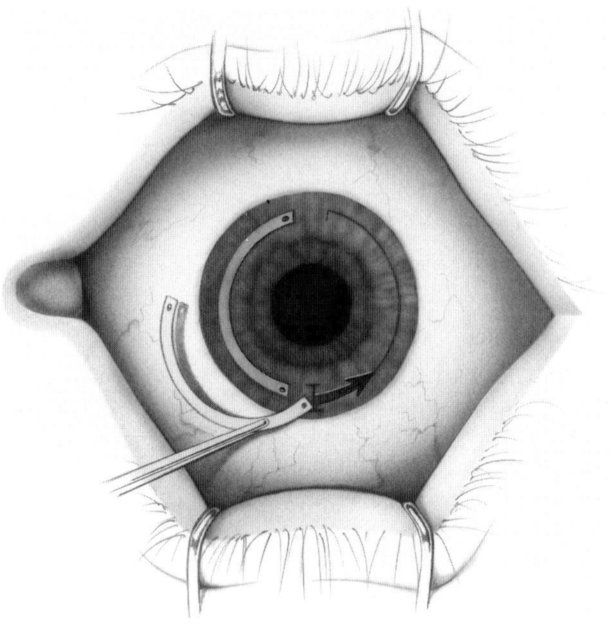

FIGURE 44-5 Insertion of intrastromal corneal ring segments through a peripheral radial incision into intrastromal channels.

1 to 2 clock hours away from the incision site, and the incision is closed with interrupted 10-0 nylon sutures.

POSTOPERATIVE CARE

After the procedure, a combination antibiotic-corticosteroid ointment or solution is applied, and an eye patch and shield are placed. To keep the patient from rubbing the eye during the healing process, the shield should be worn at night for 3 to 6 weeks, until the sutures have been removed. Analgesics may be used for postoperative discomfort.

A combination antibiotic-corticosteroid solution is used four times a day for the first postoperative week, after which it is discontinued and a 3-week course of topical corticosteroids is prescribed, starting with one drop four times a day for the second postoperative week and tapering thereafter. If the epithelium has not healed at the end of 1 week, the combination antibiotic-corticosteroid solution is continued until re-epithelialization is complete. All postoperative medications are discontinued by 1 month after surgery.

Sutures are removed 4 to 6 weeks postoperatively if the incision is healed. If not, the sutures are left in place until healing is adequate. Sutures may be removed earlier if they loosen or cause superficial neovascularization. If sutures are tight and induce 1.0 diopter or more of astigmatism, they may be removed as early as 2 weeks after the procedure, provided the incision has healed properly.

COMPLICATIONS

Intrastromal Corneal Ring

Complications observed to date among the 90 patients in the FDA Phase II study of the intrastromal corneal ring include localized incision-related complications involving epithelial defects beyond the typical postoperative healing period of 3 to 7 days, epithelial plug formation, and wound dehiscence; superficial neovascularization;

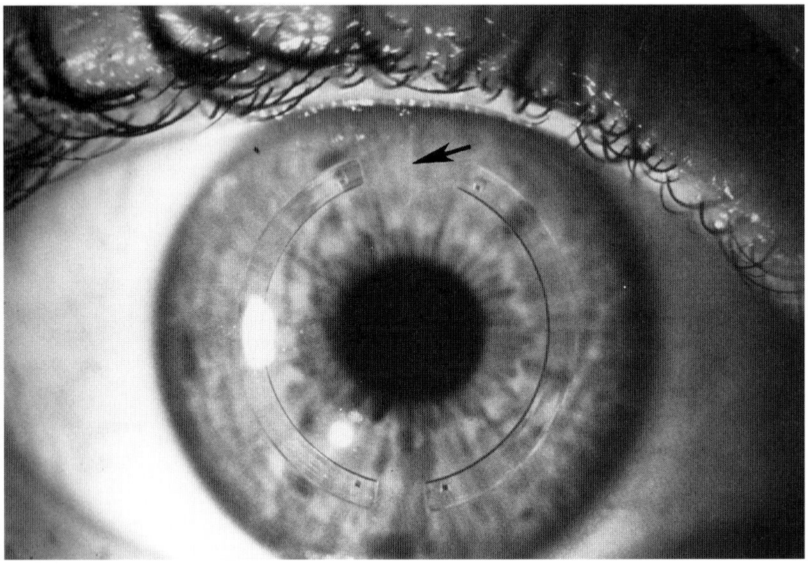

FIGURE 44-6 Clinical appearance of intrastromal corneal ring segments. The peripheral radial incision through which the segments were inserted is seen superiorly as a faint vertical scar (arrow).

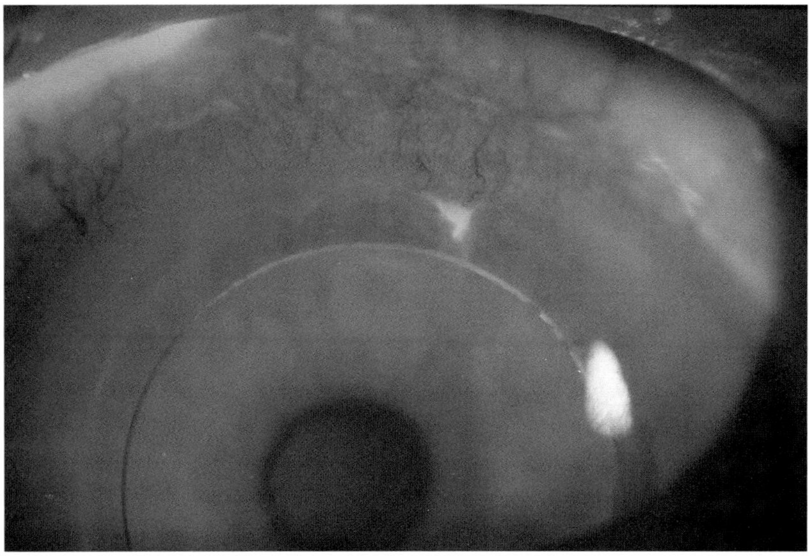

FIGURE 44-7 Fluorescein staining of an area of epithelial breakdown over an intrastromal corneal ring inserted through a circumferential incision. The ring was explanted and the epithelium healed.

surgically induced astigmatism; and a transient reduction in corneal sensation.

When it was recognized that problems with healing of the radial incision were related to incomplete apposition of the edges of the incision at the time of surgery or to premature removal of sutures, emphasis was placed on complete apposition of the edges of the incision and leaving the sutures in place for a longer period of time. To further minimize incision-related complications, the incision was modified to a 3- to 5-mm circumferential incision placed peripheral to the intended location of the outer edge of the ring. However, the formation of small fistulas was encountered in some cases in which a circumferential incision was used (Figure 44-7). Corneal neovascularization, both superficial and deep, was observed in cases in which either the radial or the circumferential incision was made too close to the limbus.

Other observations included haze in the intrastromal channel around the ring and deposits in the intrastromal channel (Figure 44-8) and within the positioning holes of the ring. The haze appeared to be nonprogressive, clinically inconsequential, and not vision-threatening, and dissipated with time.[1-3] The deposits remained localized and had no apparent visual consequences. Histologic examination of intrastromal corneal rings explanted from nonfunctional eyes in the Phase I study showed that the

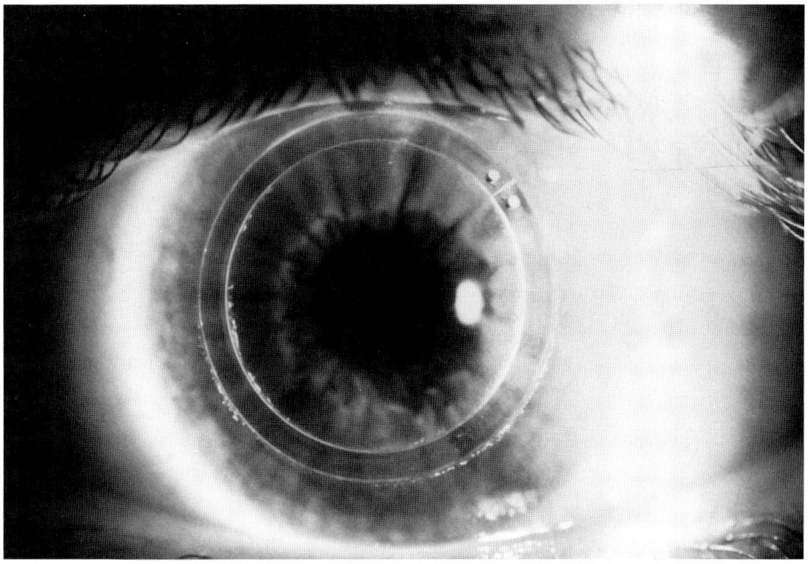

FIGURE 44-8 Deposits in the channel surrounding an intrastromal corneal ring.

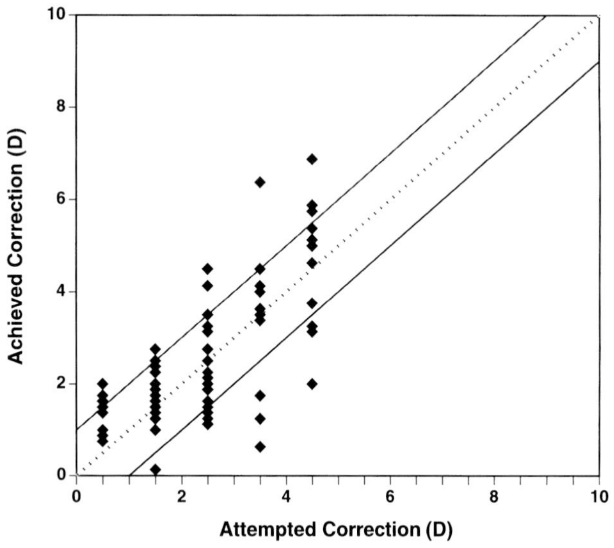

FIGURE 44-9 Scattergram of the attempted versus the achieved correction in 81 patients 1 year after implantation of an intrastromal corneal ring. The corrections are expressed as the spherical equivalent of the manifest refraction in diopters (*D*).

deposits in the positioning holes consisted of keratocytes surrounded by concentric layers of newly synthesized collagen and proteoglycan.[4]

Iron lines similar to those noted after other refractive surgical procedures were observed in the corneal epithelium. The lines were superficial and followed the inner circumference of the ring.[5] They probably developed as a consequence of changes in the topography of the epithelial surface, and did not appear to be clinically significant.[6–8]

Twelve of the 90 implanted intrastromal corneal rings were removed by approximately 2 years after surgery. Six were removed because of patient dissatisfaction with the refractive outcome, five because of incision-related complications, and one because of photophobia. After ring removal, all patients had a best spectacle-corrected visual acuity of 20/20 or better, were within one line of their preoperative best spectacle-corrected visual acuity, and were within 1.0 diopter of their preoperative manifest refraction. Corneal curvatures, as measured by keratometry, also returned to preoperative baseline values. These results indicate that the refractive effect of the intrastromal corneal ring is reversible when the ring is removed.[9] Histologic examination of a cornea from a nonfunctional eye 8 months after removal of an intrastromal corneal ring showed minimal disruption of the corneal stroma.[10]

Intrastromal Corneal Ring Segments

Many of the complications associated with the intrastromal corneal ring were not seen in a series of 77 patients in the FDA Phase II study of the intrastromal corneal ring segments at postoperative month 3. Observations similar to those encountered with the ring included channel haze and deposits in the intrastromal channels and in the placement holes at the end of the ring segments. In 11 cases, epithelial inclusion cysts in the incision were noted. There were no cases of corneal neovascularization, corneal melting, stromal thinning, or fistula formation. Suture-induced astigmatism of 1.00 diopter or more was observed in approximately 20 percent of cases, but diminished over time. The affected patients had good uncorrected visual acuities; 14 of the 15 patients (93 percent) saw 20/40 or better. No incision-related complications occurred in patients receiving the intrastromal corneal ring segments.

Four of the 77 intrastromal corneal ring segments implanted as part of the FDA Phase II study were removed by postoperative month 6. Two were removed because of patient dissatisfaction with the refractive result, one because of infiltrates in the stromal channel that were potentially of microbial origin (*Staphylococcus epidermidis* was cultured from the explanted segments), and one because of posterior migration of a segment secondary to an unrecognized microperforation at the time of surgery that was probably caused by incorrect setting of the blade. The ring segments were easily removed, and all four patients returned to their preoperative refractive status, which suggests that the refractive effect of the intrastromal corneal ring segments is reversible.

RESULTS

Preliminary findings indicate that the intrastromal corneal ring and intrastromal corneal ring segments are effective in decreasing low to moderate degrees of myopia and that the refractive results appear to be predictable and stable. Both of these devices are compatible with excellent visual acuity and satisfactory visual function.

The 1-year results from the FDA Phase II study of the intrastromal corneal ring showed that the ring had been explanted in nine patients. For the remaining 81 patients, uncorrected visual acuity was 20/40 or better in 88 percent, 20/50 to 20/63 in 10 percent, and 20/80 to 20/100 in 2 percent. Seventy-three percent were within 1 diopter of the intended correction (Figure 44-9). The postoperative refraction appeared stable (Figure 44-10). Four patients lost two lines of best spectacle-corrected visual acuity. Of these, two patients had a postoperative best spectacle-

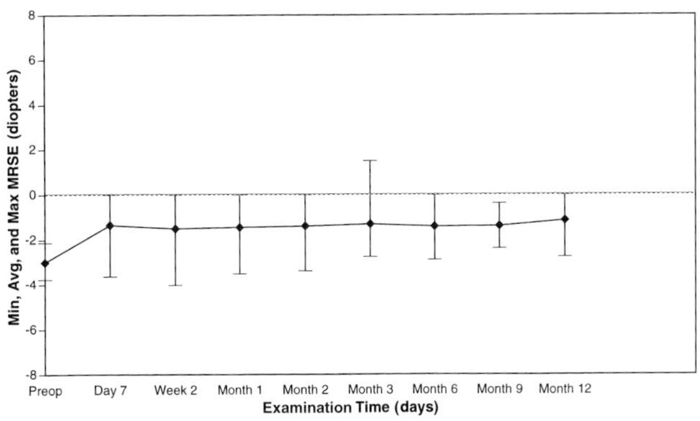

FIGURE 44-10 The mean spherical equivalent of the manifest refraction (*MRSE*) over time in 28 patients after implantation of a 0.30-mm thick intrastromal corneal ring.

corrected visual acuity of 20/20 and two had 20/25. No patient lost more than two lines of best spectacle-corrected visual acuity. Subjective responses from the patients showed that 84 percent would consider having this procedure in the fellow eye.

Six-month results from the FDA Phase II study of the intrastromal corneal ring segments were available for 68 of the 77 patients; the ring had been explanted in four patients, and 6-month data were not available for five patients. Uncorrected visual acuity was 20/25 or better in 81 percent of eyes and 20/40 or better in 94 percent. Seventy-seven percent were within 1 diopter of the intended correction (Figure 44-11). Postoperative refractions appeared stable (Figure 44-12). Four patients lost two lines of best spectacle-corrected visual acuity. Of these, three patients had a postoperative best spectacle-corrected visual acuity of 20/20, and one patient had 20/25. No patient lost more than two lines of best spectacle-corrected visual acuity. Ninety-seven percent of the patients in this study said they would consider having the procedure in the other eye.

As the field of refractive surgery advances, patients and professionals are no longer satisfied only with obtaining good uncorrected visual acuity, as tested by Snellen charts. Quality vision is demanded as well, although it is more difficult to evaluate and assess objectively. In the FDA Phase II studies, contrast sensitivity with and without a glare source is being evaluated. Preliminary evaluation of 46 patients implanted with the intrastromal corneal ring showed no statistically significant change in contrast sensitivity, with or without glare, between the preoperative and 12-month postoperative examinations at any of the five spatial frequencies tested.[11] Similarly, an assessment of 98 patients with intrastromal corneal ring segments showed no functionally significant difference in

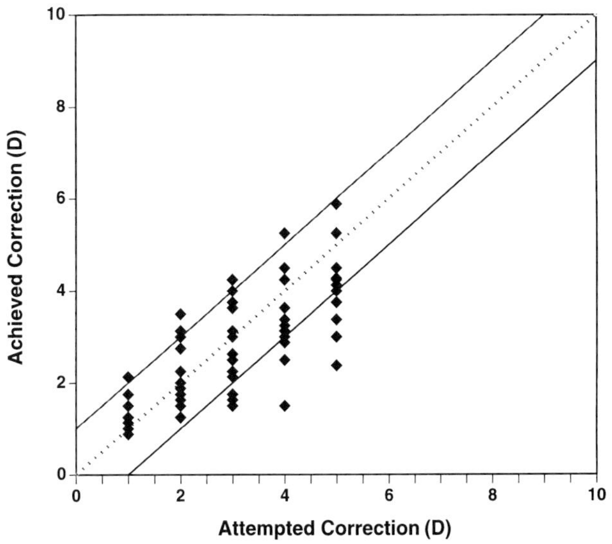

FIGURE 44-11 Scattergram of attempted versus achieved correction in 68 patients 6 months after implantation of intrastromal corneal ring segments. The corrections are expressed as the spherical equivalent of the cycloplegic refraction in diopters (*D*).

contrast sensitivity, with or without glare, between the preoperative and 3-month postoperative evaluations.

Corneal topographic studies demonstrated that the normal positive asphericity of the cornea is maintained after placement of the intrastromal corneal ring or ring segments, which may be a factor in achieving quality vision with minimal optical distortion. There is a general flattening of the central cornea, but, unlike other refractive surgical procedures for myopia, implantation of an intrastromal corneal ring or ring segments maintains the

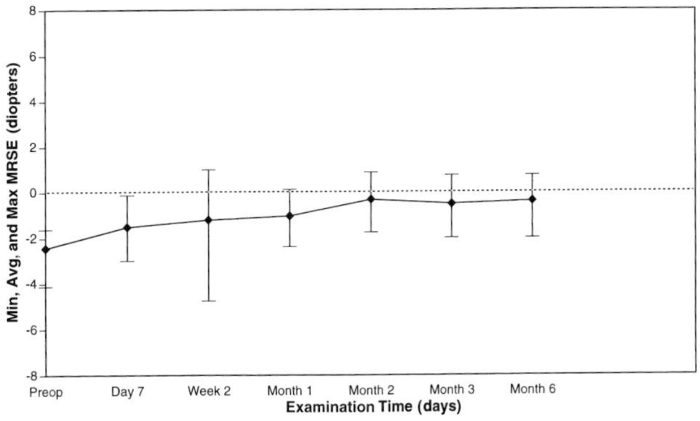

FIGURE 44-12 The mean spherical equivalent of the manifest refraction (*MRSE*) over time in 14 patients after implantation of 0.30-mm-thick intrastromal corneal ring segments.

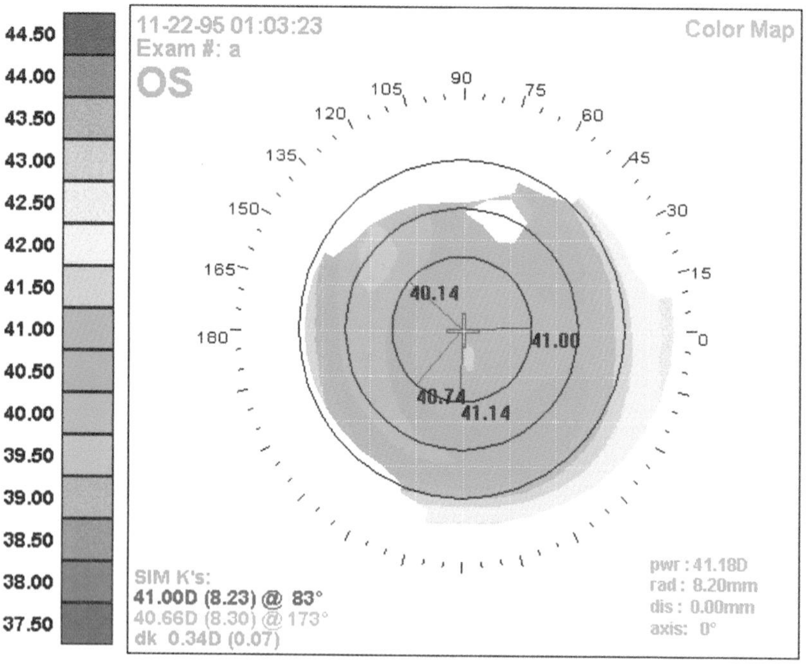

FIGURE 44-13 Videokeratograph demonstrating prolate asphericity of the cornea after implantation of intrastromal corneal ring segments.

natural, prolate asphericity of the cornea (Figure 44-13). Radial keratotomy, photorefractive keratectomy, automated lamellar keratoplasty, and laser-assisted in situ keratomileusis have all been shown to flatten the central cornea in a way that results in a negative asphericity, which may create visual distortions affecting the quality of vision.

Based on the results from the FDA Phase II studies on the efficacy and safety of the intrastromal corneal ring and ring segments, the clinical studies have been expanded. In late 1996, the FDA Phase III study was initiated to continue to evaluate the safety and efficacy of the ring segments. In addition, the concept of the intrastromal ring and ring segments is being developed for evaluation in the treatment of other types of refractive errors, including higher myopia, hyperopia, and astigmatism.

REFERENCES

1. Nosé W, Neves RA, Schanzlin DJ, Belfort R Jr: The intrastromal corneal ring—one-year results of first implants in humans. A preliminary nonfunctional eye study. Refract Corneal Surg 9:452, 1993
2. Assil KK, Barrett AM, Fouraker BD, Schanzlin DJ: One-year results of the intrastromal corneal ring in nonfunctional human eyes. Arch Ophthalmol 113:159, 1995
3. Nosé W, Neves RA, Burres TE, et al: Intrastromal corneal ring: 12-month sighted myopic eyes. J Refract Surg 12:20, 1996
4. Quantock AJ, Assil KK, Schanzlin DJ: Electron microscopic evaluation of intrastromal corneal rings explanted from nonfunctional human eyes. J Refract Corneal Surg 10:142, 1994
5. Assil KK, Quantock AJ, Barrett AM, Schanzlin DJ: Corneal iron lines associated with the intrastromal corneal ring. Am J Ophthalmol 116:350, 1993
6. Steinberg EB, Wilson LA, Waring GO III, et al: Stellate iron lines in the corneal epithelium after radial keratotomy. Am J Ophthalmol 98:416, 1984
7. Mannis MJ: Iron deposition in the corneal graft. Another corneal iron line. Arch Ophthalmol 101:1858, 1983
8. Koenig SB, McDonald MB, Yamaguchi T, et al: Corneal iron lines after refractive keratoplasty. Arch Ophthalmol 101:1862, 1983
9. Durrie DS, Asbell PA, Burris JE, Schanzlin DJ: Reversible refractive effect: data from the Phase II study of the 360 degree ICR in myopic eyes. American Society of Cataract and Refractive Surgery Annual Meeting, Seattle, Washington, June 1–5, 1996
10. Quantock AJ, Kincaid MC, Schanzlin DJ: Stromal healing following explantation of an ICR (intrastromal corneal ring) from a nonfunctional human eye. Arch Ophthalmol 113:208, 1995
11. Ginsburg AP, Asbell PA, Durrie DS, Schanzlin DJ: The ICR (intrastromal corneal ring): preliminary contrast sensitivity and glare testing results. AAO abstract. Ophthalmology 102(suppl):155, 1995

45

Phakic Intraocular Lenses

STEPHEN C. KAUFMAN

Spectacles and contact lenses provide refractive correction for individuals with myopia or hyperopia, but the quality of vision progressively degrades as the amount of refractive correction required increases. In patients with moderate to severe myopia, spectacles produce peripheral distortion and minify the image on the retina. Patients with hyperopia have a unique disadvantage in that, without a refractive correction, objects at neither near nor far are in focus. As with myopia, distortion induced by spectacles for hyperopia increases as the hyperopia increases. Contact lenses can correct relatively large refractive errors while reducing or eliminating the visual distortion that is common with spectacles. Contact lens wear is not without risks, however, and some patients are unable to wear contact lenses.

Thus, individuals with large refractive errors may be severely visually handicapped with no satisfactory means of correction. Although recent developments in refractive surgery may provide safe and effective approaches to the treatment of mild to moderate myopia, there are currently no large-scale, long-term studies that unequivocally support the use of radial keratotomy, photorefractive keratectomy, laser-assisted in situ keratomileusis, or automated lamellar keratoplasty for the correction of high myopia. The surgical options for hyperopia are even more limited.

An alternative capable of correcting high myopia or hyperopia is the intraocular lens. Once a patient requires removal of a cataractous lens, placement of an intraocular lens generally provides good vision, but the problems associated with aphakia make removal of a healthy crystalline lens for the correction of high myopia problematic.[1] Studies in Europe over the past 40 years and recently in the United States have focused on supplementing the refraction of the eye with an intraocular lens without removing the crystalline lens. This chapter describes the use of intraocular lenses for refractive correction in phakic patients.

HISTORY

More than 40 years ago, Barraquer and others conceived the idea of using an anterior chamber intraocular lens to correct myopia in a phakic patient. Many different types of anterior chamber lenses have since been devised for this purpose, but most of the early lenses required complicated surgical techniques for implantation and were found to damage the corneal endothelium, induce uveitis, damage the iris, dislocate, and cause cataracts postoperatively.

One design, developed in 1977 by Worst in The Netherlands, was based on the concept of iris fixation. This lens, originally known as the *Worst lens*, has undergone a number of modifications and is now known as the *Worst-Fechner iris-claw* or *lobster-claw lens*. The name is derived from the two pairs of pincer-like structures that are used to anchor the lens to the peripheral iris (Figure 45-1). This lens was produced in powers that ranged from –7.00 to –28.00 diopters, and in plus powers as well.

In 1987, clinical studies of a new phakic anterior chamber lens for high myopia were begun by Baikoff in France. The lens design was based on that of the Kelman Multiflex anterior chamber intraocular lens, which at that time had been in use for more than 15 years and had been shown to be a safe anterior chamber lens.[2] Like the Kelman lens, the Baikoff lens was an open loop, 4-point fixation lens made of polymethyl methacrylate (Figure 45-2).

Visual results with this lens were excellent. However, endothelial cell damage in the midperipheral cornea became apparent 2 years after implantation,[3] which led to a design modification that decreased the anterior vault from 25

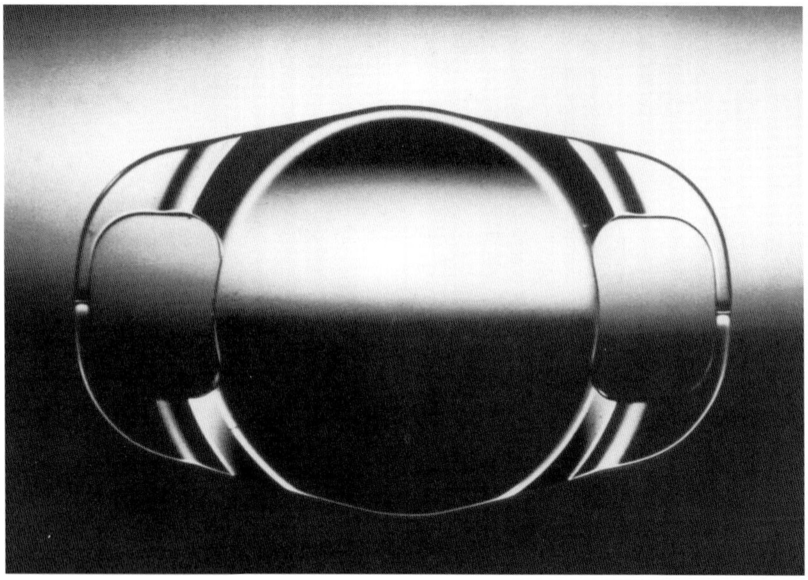

FIGURE 45-1 The iris-fixated Worst-Fechner lobster-claw anterior chamber phakic intraocular lens. (Courtesy of Professor Dr. Jan G.F. Worst, Haren, The Netherlands.)

degrees to 20 degrees and reduced the diameter of the optic by 0.5 mm. These changes to the portion of the lens closest to the endothelium increased the distance between the corneal endothelial surface and the periphery of the lens optic. The new lens was designated the *Baikoff ZB5M* and was produced by Domilens in powers ranging from -8.00 to -30.00 diopters. Although hundreds of Baikoff ZB5M lenses have been implanted throughout the world, at this writing the only clinical study of this lens in the United States was conducted at the Louisiana State University (LSU) Eye Center in New Orleans, beginning in 1991.

A number of new intraocular lenses are being developed for the correction of high myopia and hyperopia in phakic patients. Some of these lenses, such as those from Chiron-Domilens and Ophthalmic Innovations International are based on the Kelman Multiflex design. Some, such as those from Chiron-Adatomed and Staar Surgical Company, are intraocular contact lens–type designs that are placed between the iris and the crystalline lens. Some of these lenses are being marketed in Europe, and some are undergoing clinical investigation in the United States, but none is commercially available in this country at this writing.

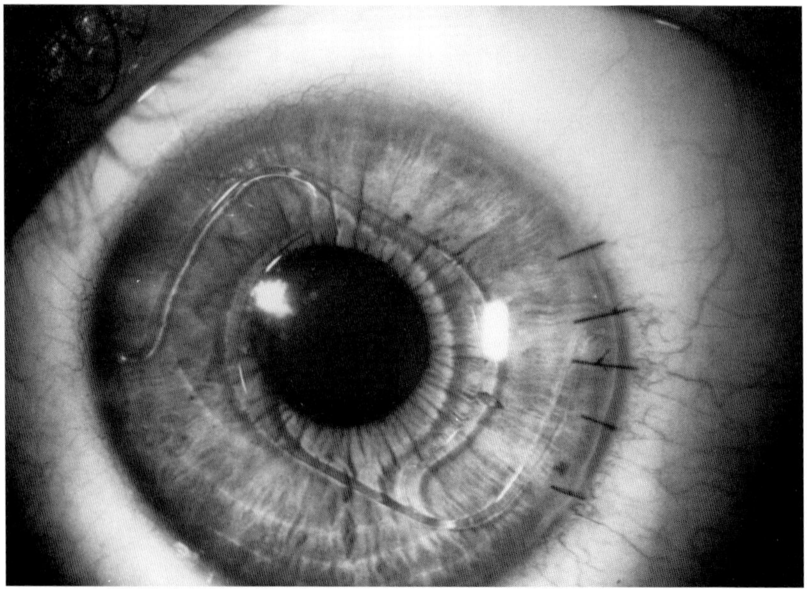

FIGURE 45-2 The Baikoff ZB5M anterior chamber phakic intraocular lens.

PATIENT SELECTION

Spectacles or contact lenses should be tried first for all patients with refractive errors. If spectacle correction is unsatisfactory and intolerance precludes the use of contact lenses, surgical alternatives may be considered.

Patient selection for the surgical correction of refractive errors is based on the degree of myopia, as well as life-style factors such as occupation and leisure activities. Photorefractive keratectomy appears to be highly accurate for the correction of 6.00 diopters or less of myopia (see Ch. 41). For moderate to high myopia, laser-assisted in situ keratomileusis is an option (see Ch. 43). Patients with hyperopia are at a disadvantage because virtually all refractive surgical procedures are designed to treat myopia. Procedures under investigation for the correction of hyperopia include adaptation of procedures for myopia, such as excimer laser surgery and implantable stromal rings, but all of these modalities are investigational at this writing.

Phakic anterior chamber intraocular lenses can correct virtually any degree of myopia; lenses have been made in powers from -7.00 to -30.00 diopters. However, all of the currently available lenses produce glare in dim light and are not recommended for persons who must drive at night. Occupations, sports, or hobbies associated with the risk of ocular trauma are contraindications. Organic exclusionary criteria include corneal abnormalities (especially endothelial disorders), abnormal or shallow anterior chamber, iris abnormalities (notably iris atrophy or rubeosis), abnormal anterior chamber angle, ocular hypertension, cataract, and retinal abnormalities that might increase the risk of retinal detachment.

PREOPERATIVE EVALUATION AND TREATMENT

Manifest and cycloplegic refractions are performed, and stability of the refraction is confirmed by comparing the results to previous refractions. A complete ophthalmologic examination is performed, with emphasis on excluding the presence of any of the disorders outlined in the previous section. Any retinal abnormalities should be treated. The axial length is measured with A-scan ultrasonography. Selection of the power of the lens required is based on nomograms for each type of lens that take into account the axial length and the amount of myopia. Determination of central and midperipheral endothelial cell densities is essential.

For the Baikoff ZB5M lens, selection of the correct diameter requires a relatively accurate approximation of anterior chamber diameter. Generally, the white-to-white corneal diameter is measured and 1 mm is added. This method is adequate for most individuals; however, it occasionally results in an over- or underestimation of the anterior chamber diameter. If the lens is too short, the lens may spin within the anterior chamber. If the lens is too long, the anterior chamber angle and iris are distorted, which may cause inflammation or an elliptical pupil.

Because of the unique vault of the lens optic, a peripheral iridotomy may not be required. Nevertheless, all of the lens manufacturers recommend performing one or more argon or neodymium:yttrium-aluminum-garnet (Nd:YAG) laser peripheral iridotomies 90 degrees from the future location of the lens haptics at least 1 week before the lens is implanted.

ANESTHESIA

In the first phase of the Baikoff ZB5M lens study at the LSU Eye Center, patients underwent general anesthesia. It soon became apparent that the procedure could be performed safely under local anesthesia in cooperative patients, however, and implantation of the lens in the second eyes of this study group was performed under local anesthesia. Implantation of the Worst-Fechner lobster-claw lens or the intraocular contact lens can also be done under local anesthesia.

SURGICAL TECHNIQUES

A miotic agent is generally used preoperatively or intraoperatively to protect the crystalline lens, except in patients in whom a contact lens-type intraocular lens is to be placed between the iris and the crystalline lens, in which case the pupil is dilated. Because of the design of the various lenses, only the Worst-Fechner lobster-claw lens can be positioned over an eccentric pupil.

Baikoff ZB5M Anterior Chamber Intraocular Lens

The patient is prepared and brought into the operating room in the same manner as for cataract surgery. A temporal incision provides unobstructed access for lens

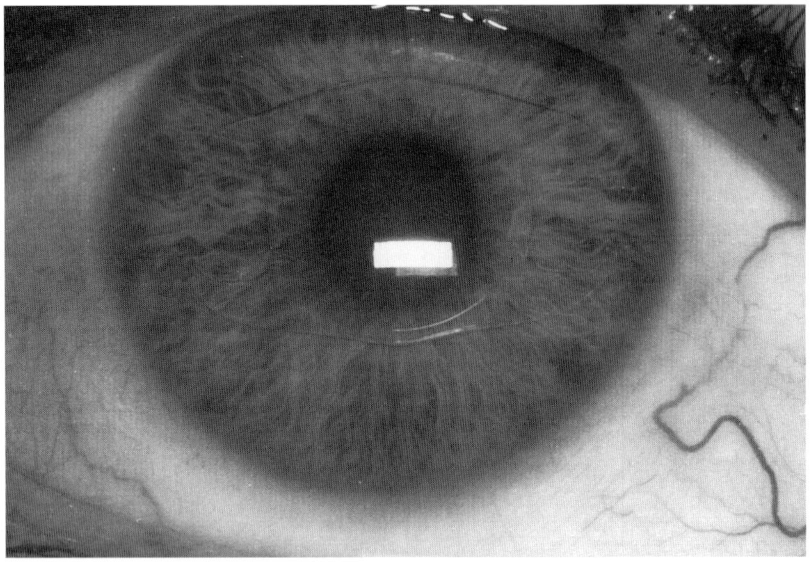

FIGURE 45-3 The Worst-Fechner lobster-claw lens permits the surgeon to center the lens over the pupil. (Courtesy of Professor Dr. Jan G.F. Worst, Haren, The Netherlands.)

implantation and induces minimal postoperative astigmatism. The incision may be made in another area in an attempt to correct a moderate amount of pre-existing astigmatism. However, unobstructed access to the incision site is of the utmost importance to avoid trauma to the crystalline lens or iris when the intraocular lens is inserted. To this end, a peripheral, 6-mm, clear corneal incision is constructed in a biplane fashion. A viscoelastic substance is injected into the anterior chamber to protect the corneal endothelium and the crystalline lens. At this point, some surgeons prefer to use a lens glide; however, it is not difficult to insert the lens without this device.

The surgeon grasps the optic with the lens inserter in one hand and opens the incision with a 0.12-mm forceps in the other hand. Care is taken to guide the leading footplates directly into the anterior chamber angle that is 180 degrees away from the incision. The lens should not be allowed to touch the endothelium or the crystalline lens or slide against the iris. While the lens forceps are holding the leading footplates in the angle, the trailing haptic is grasped with a second pair of forceps and pressure is applied toward the leading haptic. This maneuver permits removal of the lens forceps without allowing the leading footplates to back up and cause iris tuck. The trailing haptic is then placed into the angle immediately adjacent to the incision.

The iris is checked; if the pupil is oval or distorted, the lens is removed and reinserted. If the pupil remains irregular, a shorter lens is probably needed.

After the lens is inserted, the viscoelastic substance is removed from the anterior chamber and the incision is closed with interrupted 10-0 nylon sutures. The intraocular pressure is normalized with balanced salt solution, if necessary, and the incision is checked to be certain there are no leaks.

Worst-Fechner Anterior Chamber Lobster-Claw Lens

A variety of methods have been used for implantation of the Worst-Fechner lobster-claw lens. The most straightforward method involves making paracentesis sites near the 3 o'clock and 9 o'clock positions at the limbus. Next, a 6-mm limbal or very peripheral clear corneal incision is made superiorly. A viscoelastic substance is injected into the anterior chamber and a peripheral iridectomy is performed if a laser peripheral iridotomy was not performed preoperatively. The lens is inserted through the incision, with care taken to prevent endothelial cell damage. Additional viscoelastic substance can be injected if needed.

After the lens is inserted, it is rotated into a horizontal position. One of the lens haptics is grasped with fixation forceps that are inserted into the anterior chamber through the incision. A second pair of forceps or a specialized iris incarceration instrument is introduced through the nearest paracentesis site and is used to pull a portion of the iris through the lobster-claw haptic. This procedure is repeated for the opposite haptic. The viscoelastic substance is removed from the eye and the incision is closed with interrupted 10-0 nylon sutures. The intraocular pressure is normalized and wound integrity is verified (Figure 45-3).

Staar Posterior Chamber Intraocular Contact Lens

The Staar posterior chamber phakic intraocular contact lens is inserted through a 4-mm or shorter clear corneal incision by means of a lens injector device. The lens unfolds in the anterior chamber. The periphery of the plate haptic is tucked behind the already dilated iris. After lens placement is checked, an intraocular miotic agent is used to constrict the pupil.

POSTOPERATIVE CARE

Regardless of the type of lens inserted, antibiotic and corticosteroid drops are instilled in the eye or over a collagen shield, the eye is patched, and a Fox shield is placed at the end of the procedure. On the first postoperative day, the patch is removed and the eye is examined. The position and shape of the pupil and the appearance of the wound are noted. If significant pupillary abnormalities are present, the lens should be removed and replaced. Lens centration is documented.

Broad-spectrum topical antibiotic and corticosteroid eye drops are applied four times a day. Usually, the antibiotic drops are discontinued after 2 weeks. The corticosteroids may be continued for 2 to 3 weeks and then tapered or may be required for up to 8 weeks depending on anterior chamber inflammation and patient symptoms, including photophobia.

Patients are instructed not to rub their eyes. Most patients can return to nonstrenuous activities within a few days after surgery.

RESULTS

Garcia et al[4] showed that visual acuity in eyes with phakic intraocular lenses was better than that obtained with spectacles or contact lenses because of the larger retinal image provided by the intraocular lens.

In the LSU study of the Baikoff ZB5M lens, there were five patients, all women, all with preoperative uncorrected visual acuities of 20/800. Lenses were implanted in one eye of each patient, and if the patient requested it, in the second eye 1 year later. All patients elected to have implantation in the second eye, for a total of 10 eyes in the study. Two years postoperatively, uncorrected visual acuity was better than 20/40 in all 10 eyes and 20/25 or better in four eyes. Mean preoperative refractive error was -9.00 diopters; 2 years postoperatively, mean refractive error was -0.875 diopters. No patients were hyperopic after surgery. One patient required an astigmatic keratotomy to correct pre-existing astigmatism. Studies by Baikoff and his colleagues showed that 80 to 90 percent of their patients with a mean preoperative refractive error of -14.94 diopters were within 2 diopters of the intended correction and 50 to 60 percent were within 1 diopter of the intended correction.[5,6]

A study of the Worst-Fechner lobster-claw lens reported that 74 percent of 26 eyes with a mean preoperative refractive error of -14.7 diopters were within 1 diopter of emmetropia after surgery.[7] Thirty-seven percent had an uncorrected visual acuity of 20/40 or better, and 80 percent had a best-corrected visual acuity of 20/40 or better postoperatively.

In a small study of the Staar intraocular contact lens by Assetto et al,[8] 75 percent of 15 eyes with a mean preoperative refractive error of -15.3 diopters had less than 2 diopters of residual myopia and 31 percent had less than 1 diopter of residual myopia after surgery. No patient was hyperopic postoperatively. The first three lenses implanted were removed and replaced because of incorrect power calculations. Akers[9] recently presented preliminary data on a clinical study of the Staar intraocular contact lens in 19 patients. One surgical and two postoperative complications were reported. The postoperative complications consisted of one case of endophthalmitis and one of pupillary block. The surgical complication resulted from the insertion of the lens upside down; the lens was removed and replaced in the proper orientation with no visual or other consequences.

Preliminary findings from European studies of the Chiron-Adatomed posterior chamber phakic intraocular lens describe a high percentage of cases with iris pigment deposits on the anterior surface, which usually disappeared within approximately 3 months.[10]

COMPLICATIONS

Complications are a serious consideration in the implantation of a phakic intraocular lens because the majority of candidates for this procedure can be corrected at least to some extent with spectacles or contact lenses. Despite the fact that an individual may obtain better corrected visual acuity with a phakic intraocular lens than with spectacles or a contact lens, complications must be minimized or eliminated before any of these lenses are approved for use in the United States.

Endothelial Cell Damage

A number of investigators have pointed out that corneal endothelial cell loss after intraocular lens implantation may not be immediately evident and pseudophakic bullous keratopathy may not appear until 13 to 34 months postoperatively.[11-14] With more than 4 years of follow-up in the LSU study of the Baikoff ZB5M lens, however, no significant long-term endothelial cell loss has been seen. The initial postoperative endothelial cell loss of 300 to 500 cells/mm^2 was similar to the 300 cells/mm^2 loss reported by Perez-Santonja et al[15] for both the Baikoff ZB5M lens and the Worst-Fechner lobster-claw lens. In their study,[15] both lens groups showed endothelial cell losses of approximately 11 percent at 6 months; after 24 months, losses were 12.3 percent in the Baikoff ZB5M lens group and 17.6 percent in the Worst-Fechner lens group.

Anterior Chamber Inflammation

In the LSU study of the Baikoff ZB5M lens, 5 of the 10 eyes required topical corticosteroids for up to 8 weeks. After 8 weeks, no inflammation was detected and the patients were asymptomatic.

Anterior chamber inflammation is a concern with the Worst-Fechner lobster-claw lens because placement of the lens depends on incarceration of the iris between the claws of the haptics. Early studies by Fechner's group[16] suggested a high incidence of iritis with this lens; subsequently, however, measurement of inflammation by means of a laser cell-flare meter found no significant inflammation during a 13-month follow-up period.[17] A study by Perez-Santonja et al[18] detected significant signs of chronic inflammation by means of fluorophotometry and lens transmittance, although no clinical signs of inflammation were seen.

Intraocular Pressure Elevation

Because the Baikoff ZB5M lens is supported by footplates that rest in the anterior chamber angle, damage to the aqueous filtration system is a concern. None of the patients in the LSU study of this lens showed significant increases or decreases in intraocular pressure. In Baikoff's initial studies using the earlier design, hypotony was noted in 22 percent of the patients.[19]

Glaucoma would be an unexpected complication of the Worst-Fechner lobster-claw lens because it is iris fixated. In an early report of patients undergoing implantation of the lobster-claw lens who received 100 mg of prednisone orally and 250 mg of prednisone intravenously immediately before surgery, 100 mg of prednisone orally on postoperative day 1, and 50 mg of prednisone orally and topical prednisolone postoperatively thereafter to reduce inflammation,[16] 10 of 62 eyes developed corticosteroid-induced glaucoma, which resolved after the corticosteroids were discontinued. A later expanded publication concerning this study[20] documented 20 cases of postoperative glaucoma in 125 eyes. Seventeen of these cases were corticosteroid related, one resulted from incomplete removal of the viscoelastic substance, and two were caused by postoperative intraocular inflammation.

One case of ischemic optic neuropathy was reported in an eye with a Worst-Fechner lobster-claw lens.[21] The authors hypothesized that the increased intraocular pressure after lens implantation, in combination with the patient's systemic hypotension, combined to cause ischemic optic neuropathy.

Pupillary Block

Pupillary block with subsequent increased intraocular pressure results from a blockage of the normal aqueous pathway between the iris and the optic of the lens. The Worst-Fechner lobster-claw lens lies closer to the iris, which may increase the risk of pupillary block, compared with the Baikoff ZB5M lens. Both lens manufacturers recommend performing a peripheral iridotomy 1 week before lens insertion to prevent this complication, as described above. Akers[9] reported one case of pupillary block among 19 patients with the Staar intraocular contact lens. If pupillary block occurs, a peripheral iridotomy should be performed.

Elliptical Pupil

Elliptical pupils developed in three eyes in the LSU study of the Baikoff ZB5M lens. Although no pupillary distortion was evident immediately postoperatively, the pupils in these three eyes became increasingly elliptical along the axis of the haptics in the 6 months after lens implantation (Figure 45-4). Gonioscopy revealed that the lens footplates were well positioned and no iris tuck was present. Two of these eyes were in the same patient, despite the fact that the calculated size of the lens was reduced by 1 mm in the second eye.

None of the lenses inserted in the LSU study spun in the anterior chamber and none exhibited an increased anterior vault, suggesting that estimates of anterior chamber diameter were reasonably accurate. Nevertheless, the cause of the pupillary distortion was thought to be due to a lens that was too large. As the haptics exerted lateral force on the footplates, the force was redirected posteriorly by the semirigid sclera. The rigidity of the iris and structures within the angle was insufficient to counteract the posterior forces produced by the footplates of the lens. Therefore, as the footplates slowly crept peripherally and posteriorly, the iris was secondarily stretched in the axis of the footplates. Saragoussi et al[22] used ultra-

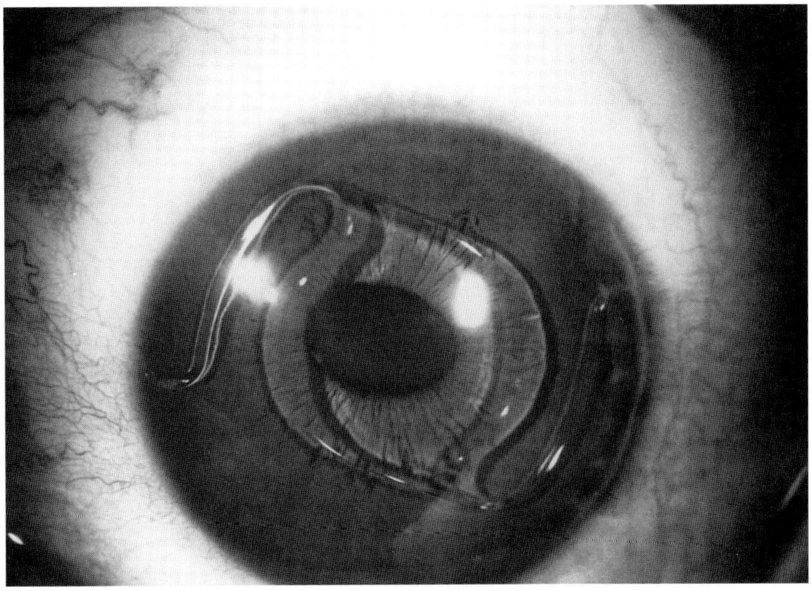

FIGURE 45-4 An elliptical pupil in an eye with a Baikoff ZB5M lens, 3 months after implantation.

sonic biomicroscopy to document the posterior displacement of the haptics in six patients with the Baikoff ZB5M lens. Four of these patients developed elliptical pupils. Apple and coworkers[23,24] suggested that the distorted pupil seen with this type of anterior chamber lens is caused by the development of a retractable fibrous membrane. It remains unclear, however, whether the fibrous membrane is the primary cause of the pupillary distortion or whether the primary cause is the iris and angle trauma caused by the extreme forces exerted by the haptics of these lenses. This phenomenon had no effect on visual acuity. It has not been reported in association with the iris-fixated lobster-claw lens design.

Intraocular Lens Decentration

Because the haptics of the Baikoff ZB5M lens are of equal length and must be placed 180 degrees apart to provide equal pressure on the footplates, the optic is centered within the anterior chamber. This geometric center typically does not coincide with the center of the pupil, so decentration of the optic with respect to the visual axis is unavoidable. Based on our observations, the optic is decentered no more than 0.75 mm from the center of the pupil. Normally, this small degree of decentration would not be a concern; however, because of the small diameter of the optic and the abrupt blending of the lens edge, small discrepancies in centration of the optic over the pupil can result in an increased incidence of glare and halos in dim light.

In that the Worst-Fechner lobster-claw lens is iris-fixated, the surgeon can position the optic over the pupil during lens insertion. Despite this seeming advantage, however, a small study of patients with the Worst-Fechner lens revealed that the mean lens decentration was 0.5 mm from the pupillary center.[25] Additionally, in Fechner's original study,[20] three of 62 lenses required recentering.

Glare and Halos

The most common and consistent complaints of patients with phakic anterior chamber intraocular lenses are glare and halos. These visual disturbances occur primarily at night when the pupil is dilated. In the LSU study of the Baikoff ZB5M lens, three of the five patients noted glare and halos with their first implant. Nevertheless, all three elected to have a lens placed in the second eye because they thought that the visual disturbances were far outweighed by the refractive correction and quality of vision supplied by the lenses. The patient who developed bilateral elliptical pupils did not complain of glare. Approximately 25 to 35 percent of patients with aphakic anterior chamber intraocular lenses complain of glare and halos, regardless of the type of anterior chamber intraocular lens implanted.[7,19,26,27]

Although Landesz et al[7] reported that the severity of the halos and glare diminished gradually over a 6-month period in the majority of patients with the Worst-Fechner lobster claw lens, this was not the case for the LSU patients with the Baikoff ZB5M lens. The glare persisted, unchanged, in all three patients up to 5 years after implantation. Initially, these patients were given 1 percent pilocarpine with instructions to apply the drops once in the evening. Although none of them experienced the brow ache that is occasionally associated with pilocarpine, they all complained of "dim vision" and all chose to discontinue the use of the drug.

To examine the complaints of glare and halos, a study was undertaken to compare the degree of visual disability in the Baikoff ZB5M lens patients with the typical amount of visual disturbance experienced by highly myopic patients wearing spectacles or contact lenses. Patients similar to the five phakic intraocular lens patients in terms of degrees of myopia but who wore glasses, rigid gas-permeable contact lenses, or soft contact lenses were recruited. Four tests comparing glare and contrast sensitivity were used: (1) the MCT 8000; (2) the Regan low contrast acuity test; (3) the Pelli-Robson contrast sensitivity test; and (4) the Brightness Acuity Tester. The MCT 8000 nighttime glare and contrast sensitivity test revealed a significant decrease in visual acuity in the Baikoff ZB5M intraocular lens group, compared with the control group, providing an objective measure of the patients' subjective visual complaints.

None of the three patients who complained of glare and halos elected to have the phakic anterior chamber intraocular lens removed when this option was offered, and all five patients involved in the study stated that they would repeat the procedure if offered the choice again.

Cataract

Cataract formation is always a consideration with the implantation of an intraocular device in a phakic patient. None of the eyes with Baikoff ZB5M lenses in the LSU study developed cataracts, and to my knowledge, no cataracts have been reported with this lens in any published study. Izac[28] recently reported cataract formation in two eyes with Worst-Fechner lobster-claw lenses.

Retinal Detachment

None of the five patients in the LSU study of the Baikoff ZB5M lens developed a retinal detachment. Alió et al[29] described three cases of retinal detachment with the Baikoff ZB5M lens in highly myopic patients with axial lengths of 28.8 to 29.0 mm. Retinal detachments were also noted by Choyce[26] in 3 of 74 eyes with Baikoff ZB5M lenses and preoperative refractions that ranged from −20.00 to −30.00 diopters. One case of retinal detachment was reported in a highly myopic patient with the Worst-Fechner lobster-claw lens.[20]

It is unclear whether placement of an anterior chamber phakic intraocular lens increases the risk of retinal detachment. This complication should always be considered, however, and the possibility of increased risk presented clearly to the patient. The risk may be further increased if pilocarpine is given to reduce glare.

REFERENCES

1. Colin J, Robinet A: Clear lensectomy and implantation of a low-power posterior chamber intraocular lens for correction of high myopia. A four-year follow-up. Ophthalmology 104:73, 1997
2. Auffarth GU, Wesendahl TA, Brown SJ, Apple DJ: Are there acceptable anterior chamber intraocular lenses for clinical use in the 1990's? An analysis of 4,104 explanted anterior chamber intraocular lenses. Ophthalmology 100:1913, 1994
3. Saragoussi JJ, Cotinat J, Renard G, et al: Damage to the corneal endothelium by minus power anterior chamber intraocular lenses. Refract Corneal Surg 7:282, 1991
4. Garcia M, Gonzalez C, Pascual I, Fimia A: Magnification in visual acuity in highly myopic phakic eyes corrected with an anterior chamber intraocular lens versus by other methods. J Cataract Refract Surg 22:14, 1996
5. Joly P, Baikoff G, Bonnet P: Mise en place d'un implant négatif de chambre antérieure chez des sujects phakes. Bull Soc Ophtalmol Fr 5:727, 1989
6. Baikoff G: Phakic anterior chamber I.O.L. Int Ophthalmol Clin 31:75:1991
7. Landesz M, Worst J, Siertsema J, Van Rij G: Correction of high myopia with the Worst myopia claw intraocular lens. J Refract Surg 11:16, 1995
8. Assetto V, Benedetti S, Pesando P: Collamer intraocular contact lens to correct myopia. J Cataract Refract Surg 22:551, 1996
9. Akers A: The Staar intraocular contact lens. Annual meeting of The International Intra-Ocular Implant Club. Casa de Campo, Dominican Republic, February, 1997
10. Marinho A, Peña Ferreira A, Pinto R, et al: Posterior chamber IOL for high myopia in phakic eyes II (clinical results—one year follow-up). Symposium on Cataract, IOL, and Refractive Surgery. Annual meeting of the American Society for Cataract and Refractive Surgery (ASCRS), San Diego, CA, April, 1995
11. Wilson S: The correction of myopia by lens implantation into phakic eyes. Am J Ophthalmol 108:465, 1989
12. Cohen E, Brady S, Leavitt K, et al: Pseudophakic bullous keratopathy. Am J Ophthalmol 106:264, 1989
13. Meyer R, Sugar A: Penetrating keratoplasty in pseudophakic bullous keratopathy. Am J Ophthalmol 90:677, 1980
14. Waring G, Stulting R, Street D: Penetrating keratoplasty for pseudophakic corneal edema with exchange of intraocular lenses. Arch Ophthalmol 105:58, 1987
15. Perez-Santonja J, Iradier M, Sanz-Iglesias L, et al: Endothelial changes in phakic eyes with anterior chamber intraocular lenses to correct high myopia. J Cataract Refract Surg 22:1017, 1996
16. Fechner P, Van der Heijde G, Worst J: The correction of myopia by lens implantation into phakic eyes. Am J Ophthalmol 107:659, 1989
17. Fechner P: Intraocular lenses for the correction of myopia in phakic eyes. Short-term success and long-term caution. Refract Corneal Surg 6:242, 1990

18. Perez-Santonja JJ, Hernandez JL, Benitez del Castillo JM: Fluorophotometry in myopic phakic eyes with anterior chamber intraocular lenses to correct severe myopia. Am J Ophthalmol 118:316, 1994
19. Baikoff GD: Refractive phakic intraocular lenses. p. 435. In Elander R, Rich LF, Robin JB (eds). Principles and Practice of Refractive Surgery. WB Saunders, Philadelphia, 1997
20. Fechner P, Strobel J, Wichmann W: Correction of myopia by implantation of a concave Worst-iris-claw lens into phakic eyes. Refract Corneal Surg 7:286, 1991
21. Perez-Santonja J, Bueno J, Meza J, et al: Ischemic optic neuropathy after intraocular lens implantation to correct high myopia in a phakic patient. J Cataract Refract Surg 19:651, 1993
22. Saragoussi J-J, Puech M, Assouline M, et al: Ultrasound biomicroscopy of Baikoff anterior chamber phakic intraocular lenses. J Refract Surg 13:135, 1997
23. Apple DJ, Brems RN, Park RB, et al: Anterior chamber lenses. Part I: complications and pathology and a review of designs. J Cataract Refract Surg 13:157, 1987
24. Apple DJ, Hansen SO, Richards SC, et al: Anterior chamber lenses. Part II: a laboratory study. J Cataract Refract Surg 13:175, 1987
25. Perez-Torregrosa V, Menezo J, Harto M, et al: Digital system measurement of decentration of Worst-Fechner iris claw myopia intraocular lens. J Refract Surg 11:26, 1995
26. Choyce DP: Treatment of myopia with minus-optic anterior chamber lenses in phakic eyes. Symposium on Cataract, IOL, and Refractive Surgery. Annual meeting of the American Society for Cataract and Refractive Surgery (ASCRS), San Diego, CA, April, 1995
27. Baikoff G, Joly P: Comparison of minus power IOLs and myopic epikeratoplasty in phakic eyes. Refract Corneal Surg 6:252, 1990
28. Izac D: Worst myopia claw IOL implantation into the phakic eye. Annual meeting of The International Intra-Ocular Implant Club. Casa de Campo, Dominican Republic, February, 1997
29. Alió J, Ruiz-Moreno J, Artola A: Retinal detachment as a potential hazard in the surgical correction of severe myopia with phakic anterior chamber lenses. Am J Ophthalmol 115:145, 1993

46

Corneal Topography

Stephen D. Klyce, Naoyuki Maeda, and Thomas J. Byrd

The increasing popularity, as well as the variety, of refractive surgical procedures has been a driving force behind the need for a better understanding of corneal topography. Corneal topographic analysis can evaluate the effects and stability of procedures that change the contour of the cornea and is also useful in the diagnosis and management of corneal pathology.

The cornea, or more accurately, the air/tear film interface, provides approximately two-thirds of the refractive power of the eye, and the curvature of the anterior corneal surface and the uniformity of this curvature are important determinants of optical quality. Most current methods of topographic analysis actually measure the surface of the tear film, not the surface of the cornea. In this chapter, the term *corneal topography* refers to the topography of the anterior corneal surface and its associated tear film.

This chapter presents a review of corneal topography, a brief history of various methods of corneal topographic analysis, a description of videokeratography, and clinical examples of videokeratography that illustrate its use in the diagnosis and management of corneal and refractive disorders.

CORNEAL GEOGRAPHY

The corneal surface can be divided into four anatomic zones: the central zone, the paracentral zone, the peripheral zone, and the limbal zone.[1] The central zone is approximately 4 mm in diameter and overlies the entrance pupil; it determines high-resolution image formation on the fovea. The cornea is relatively spherical in the central zone. Surrounding the central zone is the paracentral zone, where the cornea begins to flatten. The topography of the paracentral zone gains optical importance under dim illumination when the pupil dilates. Knowledge of the shape of the cornea in this zone also facilitates contact lens fitting. The peripheral zone is the area where the cornea flattens the most and becomes more aspherical. The cornea is flattest in the limbal zone. Dimensional changes in the limbal zone as a result of surgery can affect the shape of the more central areas of the cornea.

The geometric center of the cornea can be located by estimation or by mathematically calculating the center of the noncircular limbal zone outline. In refractive surgery, the geometric center of the cornea is of limited use. More relevant is the intersection of the cornea and the line of sight. The line of sight is the line connecting a fixation point with the center of the entrance pupil (Figure 46-1). The entrance pupil is the pupillary image one sees when looking at the eye. It is approximately 0.5 mm closer to the cornea and about 14 percent larger than the real pupil.[2] With the best optics for the eye as the sole consideration, refractive surgical procedures should be centered on the point where the line of sight intersects the cornea.[2] This point can be located by having the patient fixate on a target coincident with the line of sight of the observing surgeon and marking the cornea at the center of the patient's entrance pupil.[2,3]

The vertex normal is the line that connects a fixation point and its perpendicular intersection with the anterior corneal surface. The corneal vertex is the point through which the vertex normal passes and is usually somewhat inferonasal to the point where the line of sight intersects the cornea. The vertex normal is important in corneal topographic analysis because all keratoscopes use it as the center of the mire images.

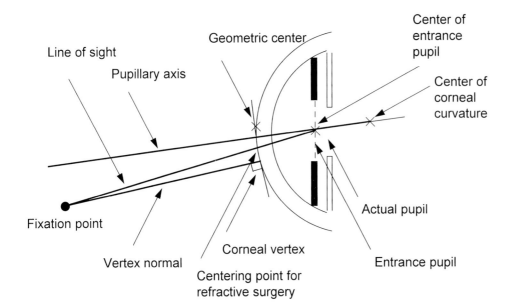

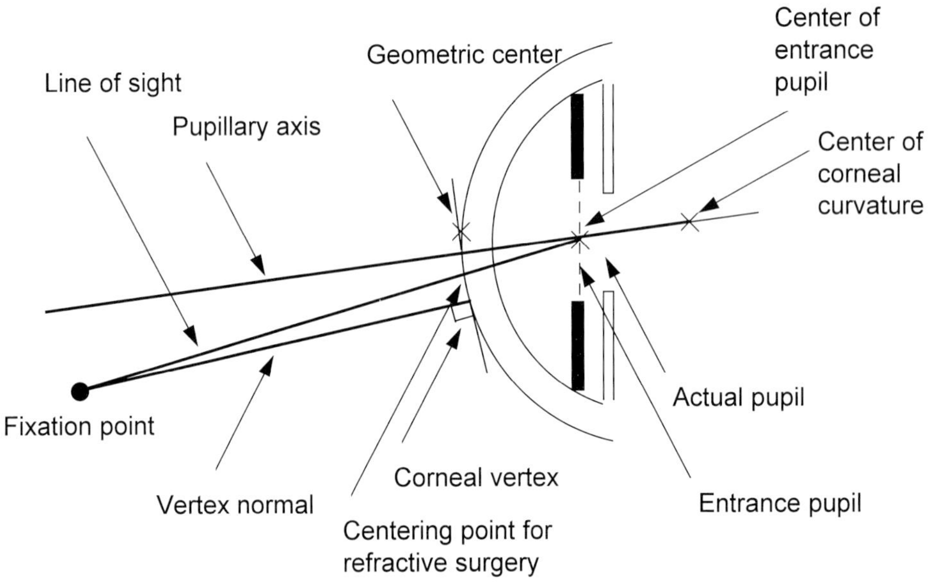

FIGURE 46-1 Schematic representation of optical geometry of the cornea.

The pupillary axis is the line connecting the center of the entrance pupil and the center of curvature of the anterior corneal surface. Although the pupillary axis can be located clinically, it does not coincide with the line of sight; the pupillary axis usually passes through the cornea temporal to the line of sight. The intersection of the cornea and the pupillary axis should not be used to center refractive surgical procedures.

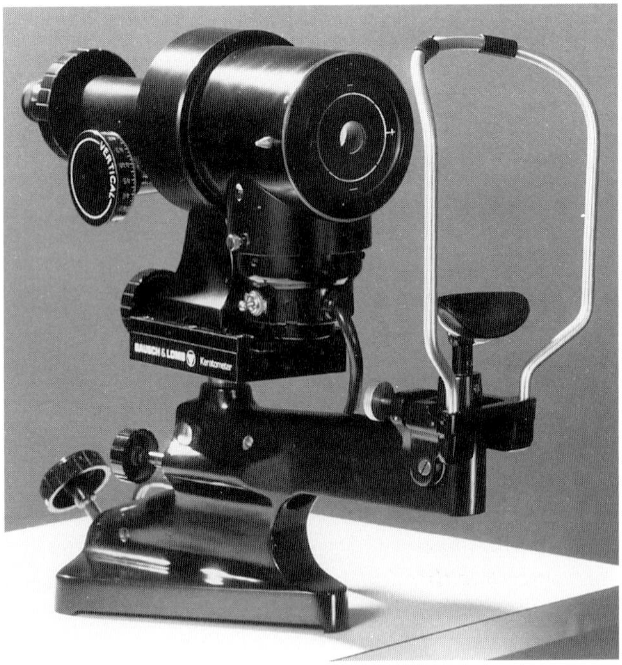

FIGURE 46-2 Bausch & Lomb keratometer.

METHODS OF TOPOGRAPHIC ANALYSIS

Keratometry

In 1728, Pourfour de Petit invented the ophthalmometer, a device used to measure the dimensions of the eye. Helmholtz[4] and Javal[5] refined the instrument so that it specifically measured the anterior corneal curvature. Although the term *ophthalmometer* is still used in many parts of the world, ophthalmologists in some countries, including those in the United States, use the term *keratometer,* which is a trade name of Bausch & Lomb, Inc. (Figure 46-2).

The principle of keratometry is fundamental to corneal topographic analysis. Keratometry uses the measured distance between two pairs of fixed points reflected from the anterior corneal surface along orthogonal meridians to describe the central corneal shape. The points are on the paracentral cornea and are separated by approximately 3 mm. The keratometer projects an illuminated target onto the corneal surface from a fixed distance that is determined by focus and alignment. The maximum and minimum diameters of the reflected images are determined by comparison with the diameters measured on calibration spheres. These measurements provide the radius of curvature of the central cornea as well as the amount and axis of astigmatism if present.

Keratometry is a reasonably accurate[6] and reliable tool for measuring corneal contours. It is routinely used to fit contact lenses and to calculate, preoperatively, the power of an intraocular lens required to visually rehabilitate an aphakic eye. Keratometry provides limited

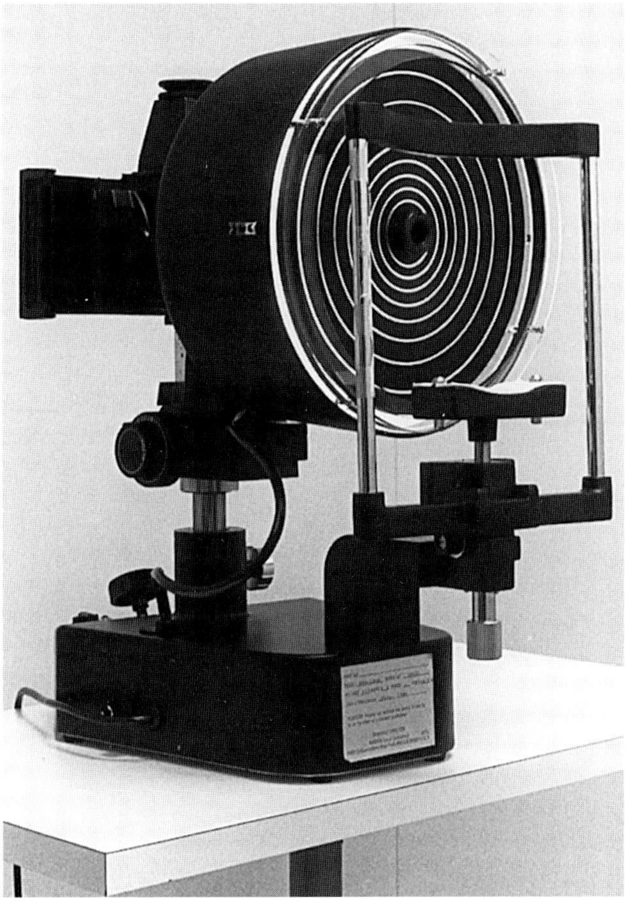

FIGURE 46-3 Nidek photokeratoscope.

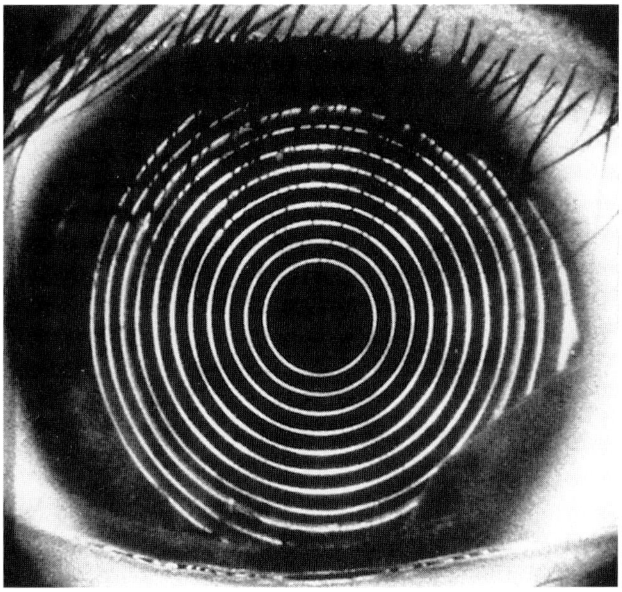

FIGURE 46-4 Photokeratograph of a normal cornea. The mires are evenly spaced and circular. There is eclipse of the peripheral mires from the nose inferonasally and from the eyelashes superiorly.

information, however; no data are obtained from the central or peripheral cornea. In addition, keratometry assumes that the cornea is a sphere (or spherocylinder in the case of an astigmatic cornea). Corneas with irregular astigmatism and corneas subjected to refractive surgery have shapes that deviate markedly from a spherocylinder; even normal corneas are often aspherical and asymmetrical.[7] Therefore, keratometry cannot be used to accurately evaluate corneas that differ noticeably from a sphere or spherocylinder.

Keratoscopy

A keratoscope is an instrument that projects multiple concentric rings called mires on the anterior corneal surface. Although technically the term *mire* refers to the image projected from the instrument, it is used in this chapter to refer both to the projected image and to the image reflected from the cornea. Keratoscopy is the direct visual inspection of the mires. Topographic information from a large area of the cornea and a variety of abnormalities of corneal shape can be recognized by keratoscopy. A camera can be added to photograph the mires, turning the keratoscope into a photokeratoscope (Figure 46-3). The photographs obtained are called *photokeratographs*.

The diameter, spacing, and width of the mires are influenced by corneal power. A photokeratograph of a normal cornea is shown in Figure 46-4. The circular shape of the central mires, their concentric nature, and their width produce a uniform spacing along every meridian, which is characteristic of corneas with uniform power distribution and no evidence of marked astigmatism. Small-diameter, closely spaced, and narrow mires are seen in corneas that have high power (steep regions or short radius of curvature) (Figure 46-5). Large-diameter, widely spaced, and broadened mires are seen in corneas that have low power (flat regions or long radius of curvature) (Figure 46-6).

Elliptical distortion of the mires is the hallmark of regular astigmatism, with the short axis of the ellipse falling on the steepest (highest power) meridian and the long axis of the ellipse falling on the flattest (lowest power) meridian (Figure 46-7). Irregular spacing between mires and tortuosity of mires are characteristic of irregular astigmatism and can occur in ectatic corneal degenerations. In moderately advanced keratoconus (Figure 46-8), the central mires have smaller-than-normal diameters (indicating a

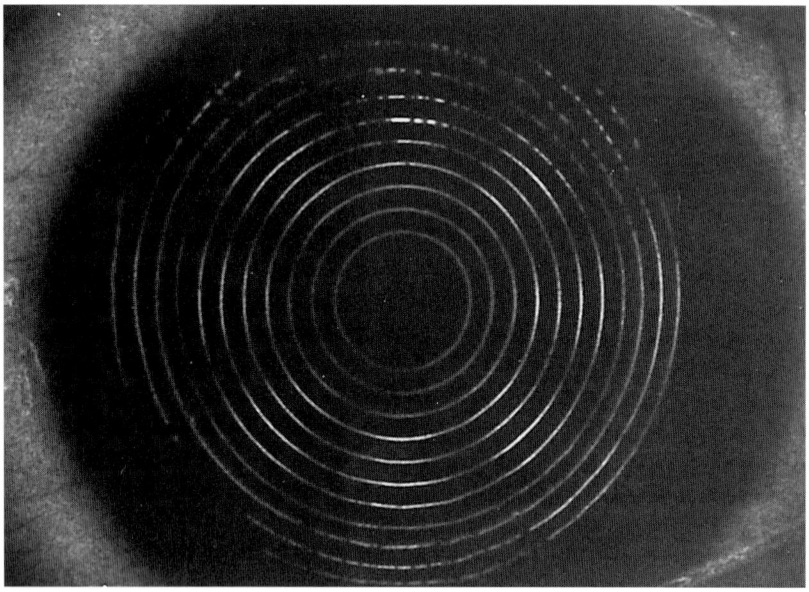

FIGURE 46-5 Photokeratograph of a cornea with a central keratometry reading of 46.12 by 46.12 diopters. Note the small diameter of the central mire.

high power), they begin to take on a teardrop shape, and they are no longer concentric. The spacing between the mires is not uniform, especially in the paracentral inferior regions of the cornea, where they become quite narrow. Irregular astigmatism can also be caused by corneal scars (Figure 46-9) or dry eyes (Figure 46-10). In stromal scarring, the regional changes in stromal architecture can alter corneal shape some distance away. Tear film breakup causes irregular astigmatism that can greatly diminish spectacle visual acuity. Such irregularities are usually confined to the tear film and epithelial surface.

Although visual inspection of a photokeratograph allows identification of a variety of corneal shape anomalies,[8] regular astigmatism of less than 3 diopters cannot be detected by visual inspection. When the central cornea is steep, as occurs in epikeratophakia for aphakia or keratomileusis for hyperopia, even larger amounts of astigmatism cannot be detected by visual inspection because the mires are so close to each other. Additionally, visually debilitating amounts of corneal asphericity (changes in corneal power from the center to the periphery) can go undetected by visual inspection.[9]

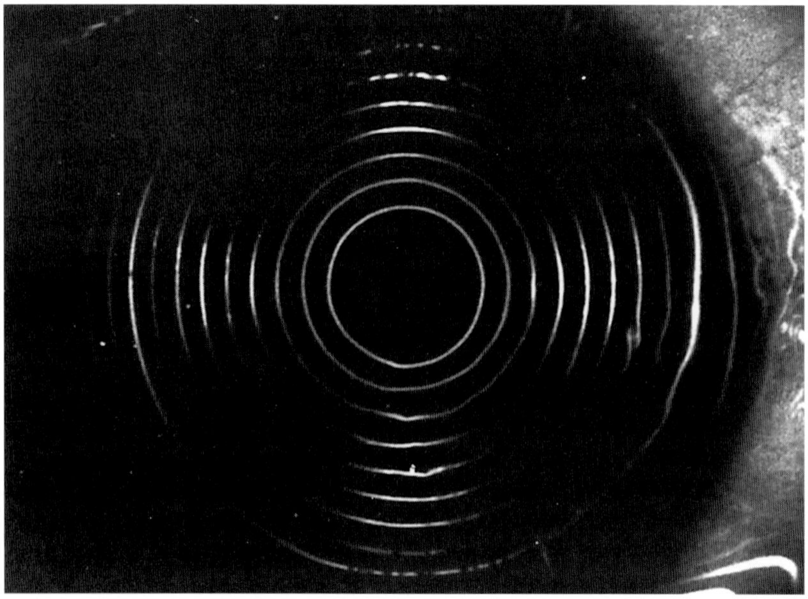

FIGURE 46-6 Photokeratograph of a cornea with a central keratometry reading of 40.5 by 40.5 diopters. Note the large diameter of the central mire. The irregularity of the inferior peripheral mires is caused by pooling of the tears.

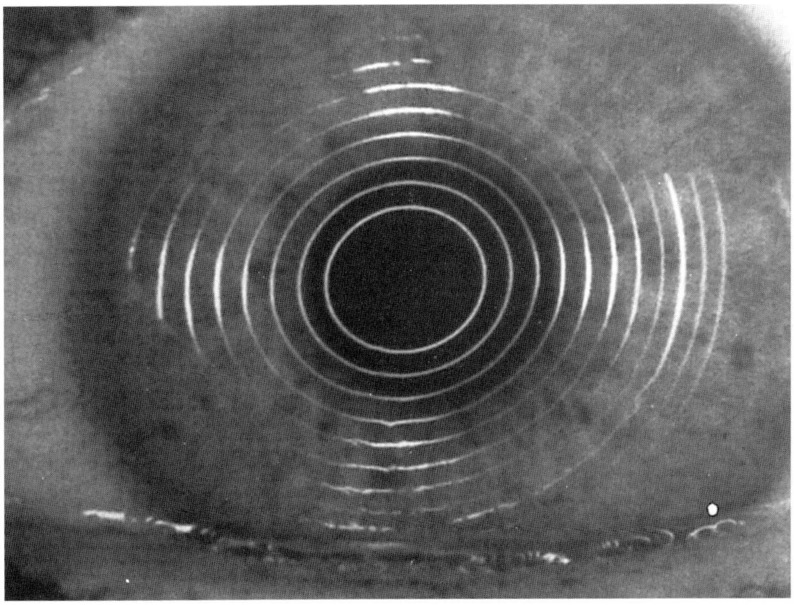

FIGURE 46-7 Photokeratograph of a cornea with moderately high regular astigmatism. Note the elliptical shape of the central mire and the symmetry along the long and short axes. The central keratometry reading is 39.25 by 45.50 diopters at 100 degrees. The central mire is longest along the 10-degree meridian and shortest along the 100-degree meridian. The distortion of the inferior mires is caused by pooling of the tears.

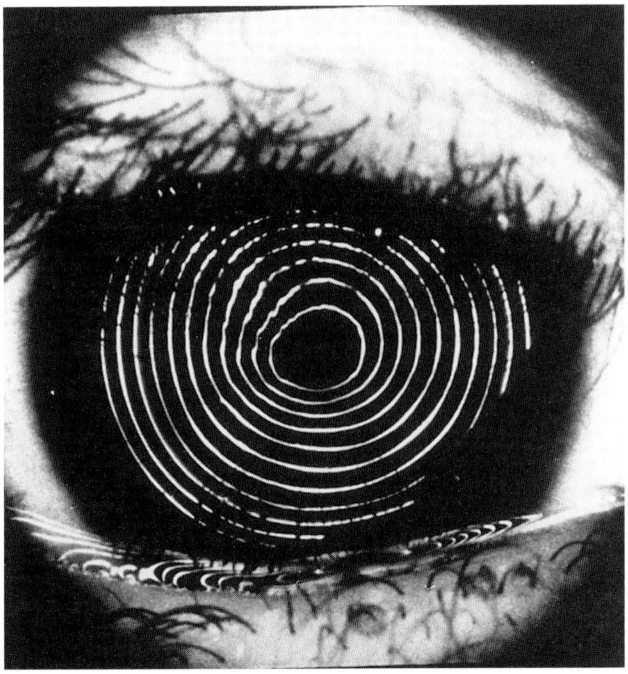

FIGURE 46-8 Photokeratograph of a cornea with moderately advanced keratoconus. Note the small diameter of the central mire (indicating a high central corneal power), the egg-shaped central mire (indicating asymmetrical astigmatism), and the irregular spacing between the mires.

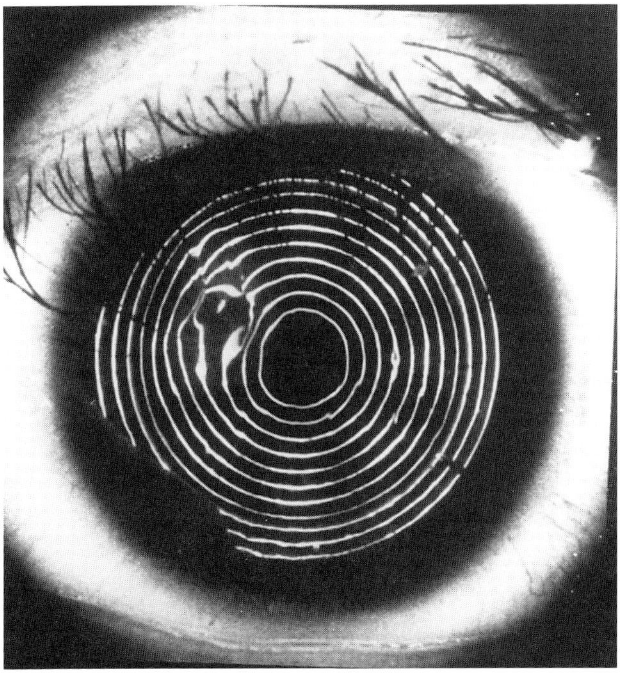

FIGURE 46-9 Photokeratograph of a cornea after herpetic stromal keratitis. The irregularity of the mires in the superonasal paracentral cornea indicates the region where scarring occurred. The paracentral scar has affected the shape of the central mire, which shows the presence of irregular astigmatism.

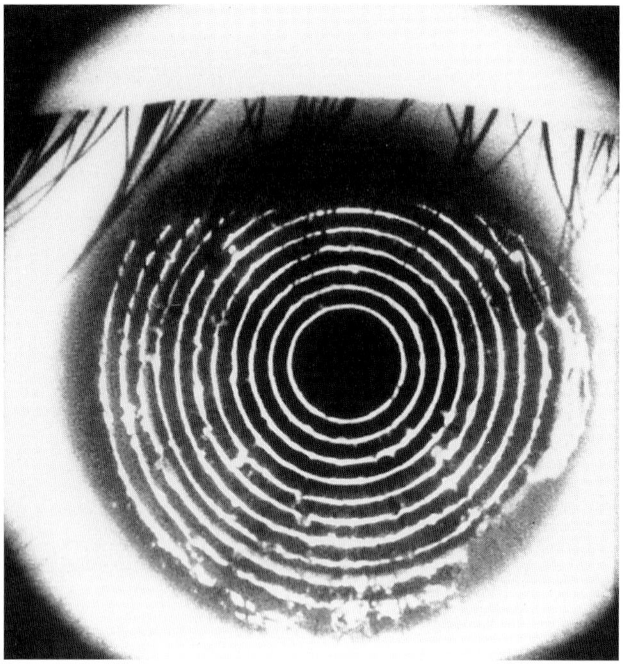

FIGURE 46-10 Photokeratograph of a cornea in a dry eye patient. Note that irregular astigmatism can increase to the point where individual mires break up and occasionally coalesce into one another.

Videokeratography

Instrumentation

The advent of widespread refractive surgery and the development of new contact lens designs led to the development of more precise and sensitive methods to measure and display corneal topography. Automated analysis of corneal topography uses computers to map the cornea, digitize the position of the mires,[8,10] derive and implement the necessary mathematical relationships for the three-dimensional reconstruction of corneal shape,[11-13] and present the data representing the corneal shape in a way that maximizes clinical use.[14-16] The systems that perform this analysis incorporate a video camera for data collection and are called *videokeratoscopes*.

The first videokeratoscope available for routine clinical use, the Computed Anatomy TMS-1, uses a collimating cone to project 25 or 30 rings on the cornea. The cone fits inside the orbital rim and permits data to be collected from the entire corneal surface. This adaptation overcomes a major limitation of keratoscopes that use large-diameter Placido disk targets: limited coverage of the paracentral and peripheral cornea because of shadows created by the ridge of the brow and the nose.

Movement artifact is minimized with the use of a video camera, which can gather the necessary data in 30 msec. Because multiple rings are used, information density is high, yielding as many as 8,000 data points[14]; the separation between mires averages 0.17 mm on the corneal surface. With this system, the smallest mire leaves only a 0.45-mm diameter of central cornea unexplored. With the 25-ring cone, a 9-mm diameter of the cornea is analyzed; the 30-ring cone, designed primarily for contact lens work, can evaluate up to a 10.5-mm diameter of the cornea.

Since the introduction of the TMS-1, a variety of other videokeratoscopes have been marketed. Some are Placido disk–based devices that project mires onto the corneal surface and detect the positions of these mires automatically. These instruments differ in their focusing methods, Placido disk arrangements, reconstruction algorithms (usually proprietary), and presentation schemes.

Presentation

Presentation schemes of early automated topographic analysis systems included numerical power plots[8] and wire models.[10,17,18] These techniques provided more detailed information than simple keratometry, but did not make shape trends readily apparent.

The Louisiana State University color-coded map of corneal surface powers is the mode of presentation used by modern videokeratoscopes. The maps produced by videokeratoscopes are called *videokeratographs*, and the procedure is called *videokeratography*. These maps display corneal surface power distribution, permit rapid recognition of corneal shape through pattern recognition, and reveal the presence of abnormal powers in the cornea by means of spectral analysis. In these maps, greens and yellows represent powers characteristic of those found in the normal cornea. Cool colors (violets, blues) represent lower powers; warm colors (oranges, reds) represent higher powers.[19]

The amount of information displayed by the videokeratograph is determined in part by the topographic scale. The absolute scale, or international standard scale,[7] was developed for clinical presentation of corneal surface shape distortions to make only clinically relevant information obvious. This information is obtained when the interval between the contours of the power plot is set to 1.5 diopters. To cover the entire range of powers that could be encountered in a given cornea, the lower and higher ends of the scale were originally assigned power intervals of 5.0 diopters. Another scale uses intervals of 1.5 diopters over the entire range, which is reduced to 28.0 to 65.5 diopters.[20] A scale that uses

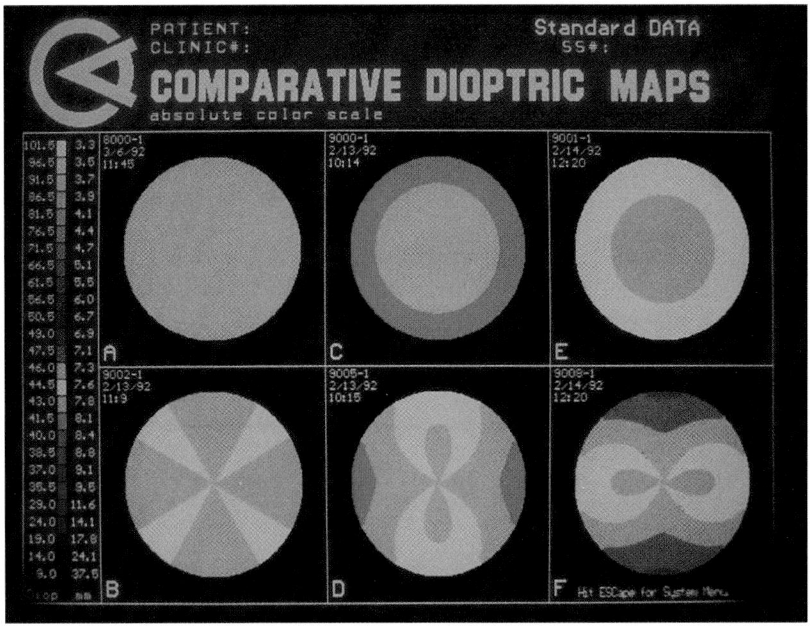

FIGURE 46-11 Theoretical surfaces used to understand the color-coded contour map. Note the use of the absolute scale. **(A)** The uniform color-coded map of a 43.0-diopter calibration sphere. **(B)** Topography of a pure spherocylinder. The steep meridian (warmer colors) is at 90 degrees. This map is radially symmetrical, with the color patterns having a fan shape. **(C)** Topographic map of a prolate ellipse that is steeper centrally than peripherally. **(D)** Map of a simulated cornea with pure with-the-rule astigmatism and peripheral flattening. This map closely mimics many corneas with natural astigmatism exhibiting the normal, or positive, bowtie pattern. **(E)** Map of an oblate ellipse that is flatter centrally than peripherally. **(F)** Map of a simulated cornea that has with-the-rule astigmatism and peripheral steepening. This map shows a horizontally aligned bowtie pattern; this abnormal, or negative, bowtie is represented by a cooler color.

intervals of 1.0 diopter, starting at 32.0 diopters, has also been recommended. All these scales are fixed and, when used consistently, facilitate the learning of corneal topographic analysis.

Another approach to color-coded mapping is the adaptive color scale,[14] which expands or contracts its range according to the range of powers present in a given cornea. Although this scale offers the advantage of great topographic detail, the meanings discussed above for color are lost, normal corneas are made to look abnormal, and abnormal corneas can be made to appear closer to normal.

Videokeratographs of several artificial surfaces, including a calibration sphere and several types of ellipses, are illustrated in Figure 46-11. A sphere is characterized by a single color because the radius of curvature, and hence the surface power, is uniform. Prolate shapes (steeper in the center) and oblate shapes (steeper in the periphery) display concentric circular color patterns. The normal cornea has a prolate shape.

Other methods used to calculate corneal surface powers include spherically based algorithms, axial methods, the instantaneous radius of curvature, and refractive power. Spherically based algorithms generally provide color-coded contour maps that are the most useful in diagnosis, inasmuch as the color patterns for normal corneas are uncomplicated and easily interpretable.

Quantitative Descriptors of Corneal Topography

Although videokeratography provides a great deal of qualitative information about a patient's corneal topography through pattern recognition and color cuing, this information alone is not suitable for evaluating clinical trial data collected from a large group of patients over multiple visits and from multiple centers. The statistical analysis of topographic data essential to a scientific study can be obtained from numerical indices derived from raw topographic data. In turn, these indices provide quantitative reference points to guide and assess the effects of therapy.

Such quantitative indices have been developed for the TMS-1 videokeratoscope. The simulated keratometry (SimK) values[21,22] provide information analogous to values obtained by a keratometer and eliminate the need to obtain separate keratometry measurements. The spherocylindrical simulated keratometry values are obtained from data points on mires 7, 8, and 9 of the TMS-1 videokeratoscope and provide the power and location of the steepest meridian and the power of the meridian 90 degrees away. The power and axis of the actual flattest meridian (MinK), regardless of the angle between the steepest and flattest meridians, are also provided. Good correlation has been demonstrated between these values and refractive cylinder.[23]

The surface asymmetry index (SAI)[21,24] is a centrally weighted summation of differences in corneal power between corresponding points 180 degrees apart on 128 equally spaced meridians crossing all the mires in the TMS-1 videokeratoscope. Theoretically, the surface asymmetry index value is zero for a perfect sphere, for a surface with perfectly spherocylindrical regular astigmatism, and for any surface with a power that is radially symmetrical. The higher the surface asymmetry index, the more asymmetrical the surface. The surface asymmetry index can quantify changes in asymmetrical corneal irregularities that occur after penetrating keratoplasty[25] and in eyes with contact lens–induced corneal warpage.[26] The surface asymmetry index is sensitive to paracentral keratoconus and forms part of the basis for an automatic keratoconus pattern detection scheme.[27]

The surface regularity index (SRI)[22,28] reflects local power fluctuations along each of the 10 central mires of the TMS-1 system. The surface regularity index correlates with localized surface regularity within the central area of the cornea that corresponds approximately to the area of the entrance pupil. One study[28] showed a high correlation between the surface regularity index and best spectacle-corrected visual acuity. The surface regularity index can predict the optical performance of a given patient with an otherwise normal eye based on the corneal topography.

Camp and co-workers[29] developed a program that uses corneal topographic data and a ray tracing method to simulate the patient's vision. The corneal surface is modeled by a topographic analysis system, and refraction is simulated by computerized ray tracing analysis. The computer program uses the corneal surface as a lens and refracts a variety of objects, displaying the resulting images on a video monitor to evaluate the effect of corneal topography on optical performance. The procedure shows the clinician the degree of image degradation that occurs in eyes with irregular astigmatism or that have undergone refractive surgery.[30] Although the information produced is subjective, this approach is useful as a teaching tool and as a way to evaluate the correspondence between specific topographies and corneal optical quality.

Other Potential Methods of Topographic Analysis

At least two other technological approaches have been developed in an attempt to measure corneal shape at resolutions both lower and potentially higher than can be accomplished with keratoscopy.

Interferometry has the potential to measure corneal shape at higher resolution. Studies[31–34] indicate that Moire fringes, holography, and similar approaches may be able to detect subtle alterations in corneal topography. However, the applicability of interferometry to the analysis of the range of topographic distortion found in the normal cornea is limited, because it compares small differences between two surfaces.

Rasterstereography uses a projected grid of light to illuminate fluorescein-dyed tears on the ocular surface. The fluorescein pattern is then photographed at a defined angle, and the surface topography is determined directly by the distortion of the projected grid.[18,35,36] Because a reflective surface is not essential, rasterstereography could prove useful in the imaging of highly irregular, de-epithelialized, or ulcerated corneas. However, rasterstereography is inherently less sensitive than keratoscopy in its ability to detect subtle topographic changes, because rasterstereography uses a projected technique that visualizes the surface directly rather than a reflection technique that amplifies topographic distortions. To date, neither interferometry nor rasterstereography has achieved notable success in clinical applications.[37]

The analysis of slit images can also be used to assess corneal topography, and in theory could yield not only curvature information relative to the corneal surface, but also curvature information from the endothelial surface of the cornea. The advantage would be that true corneal power could be calculated from individual corneas, incorporating both anterior and posterior surface curvatures and corneal thickness in the calculation. Videokeratoscopes, on the other hand, use the reflection of mires only from the surface of the tear film and assume a standard corneal thickness and internal surface curvature in the presentation of corneal power. The original corneal modeling system, the Computed Anatomy CMS, was the first device to use slit imagery to measure the curvature of the endothelial surface; that curvature information was combined with Placido disk-based information from the anterior surface to construct an optical model for the entire cornea. However, this concept never achieved wide commercial acceptance. More recently, one company has devised a system (Orbscan Topography-Pachymetry System) that measures anterior and posterior corneal surface curvatures as well as corneal thickness with a scanning slit device. This device shows potential, but its clinical utility and accuracy must await the appearance of validation studies in the peer-reviewed literature.

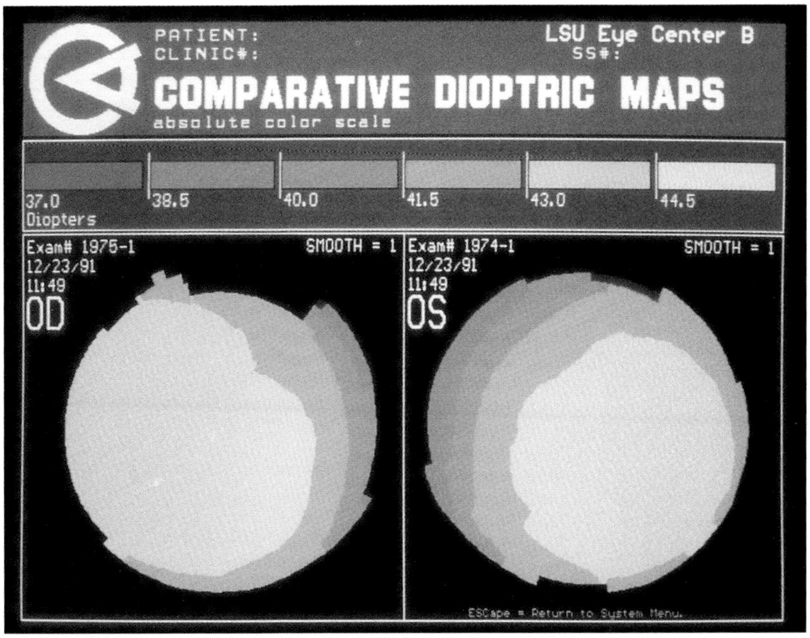

FIGURE 46-12 Color-coded maps of the normal corneas of an individual. Note that the color-coded maps of both eyes show a uniform, spherical shape in the center, and have radial symmetry, peripheral flattening, and nonsuperimposable mirror image symmetry.

CLINICAL APPLICATIONS OF VIDEOKERATOGRAPHY

Normal Cornea

The topography of the normal cornea has essentially four distinguishing characteristics[46,39] (Figure 46-12). First, the normal cornea flattens progressively from the center to the periphery by 2 to 4 diopters, with the nasal hemimeridians flattening more than the temporal hemimeridians. This aspherical feature corrects to some degree for spherical aberration in the eye. Second, each cornea has variations in topographic pattern that are generally unique to the individual. For this reason, corneas are not well described by elliptical approximation. Third, the two corneas of one individual normally exhibit nonsuperimposable mirror-image symmetry (enantiomorphism), which can be helpful when diagnosing unilateral disease. Finally, the normal cornea exhibits relative smoothness and absence of significant irregular astigmatism.

Naturally occurring corneal topographic patterns are classified by shape as round (23 percent), oval (21 percent), symmetrical bowtie (18 percent), asymmetrical bowtie (32 percent), or irregular (7 percent).[40] Although this classification is somewhat arbitrary and includes naturally occurring anomalies of corneal shape, such as bowtie and irregular patterns, it does describe the range of normalcy in which good vision can be obtained.

Regular Astigmatism

The most common naturally occurring deviation from the optically adequate normal cornea is regular astigmatism (Figure 46-13). Regular astigmatism is usually with the rule, with the steep meridian at 90 degrees, but oblique and against-the-rule astigmatisms are encountered as well. Regular astigmatism can be recognized on the videokeratograph as a symmetrical bowtie-shaped pattern of high power.

Irregular Astigmatism

Irregular astigmatism has a variety of causes and a variety of appearances on videokeratography. Generally, every deviation from a pure ellipsoidal shape is called *irregular astigmatism*. Irregular astigmatism can be devastating to vision when it occurs centrally within the pupillary area; it can be present even on a surface that clinically appears relatively smooth. Functionally, irregular astigmatism is that component of astigmatism that cannot be corrected with spectacles. Common causes of irregular astigmatism include dry eyes, corneal scars, ectatic corneal degenerations, pterygium, contact lens warpage or overwear, trauma, and surgery, including cataract surgery, penetrating keratoplasty, and refractive surgery.

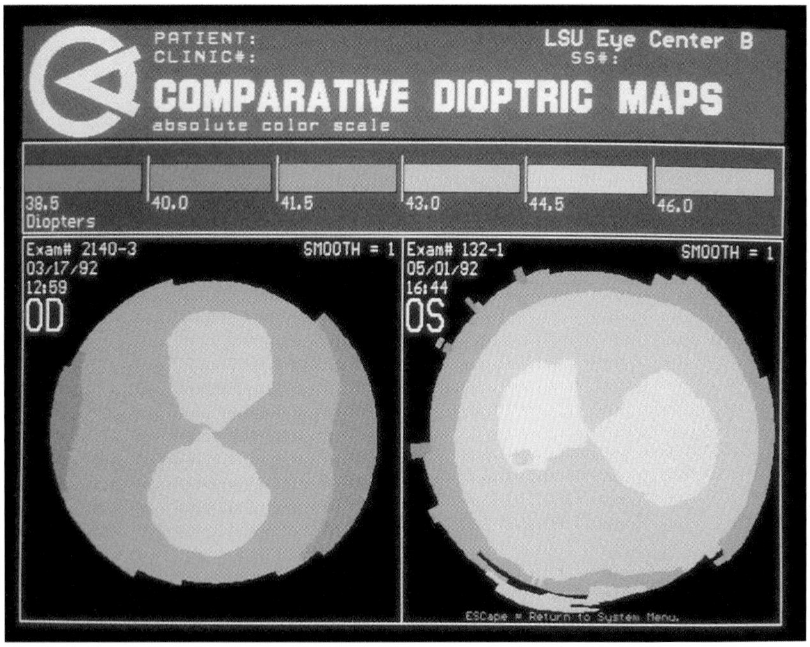

FIGURE 46-13 Color-coded maps of regular astigmatism. Left map shows with-the-rule astigmatism, which is indicated by the vertically oriented bowtie pattern. Right map shows against-the-rule astigmatism indicated by the horizontally oriented bowtie pattern. The maps indicate that both corneas have radial symmetry and peripheral flattening.

Corneal Ectasia

An important application of videokeratography is the screening of candidates for refractive surgery. Patients with irregular astigmatism caused by corneal ectasia do not achieve good vision with spectacles and tend to opt for contact lenses and to seek refractive surgery. It is important to identify these patients. Topographic screening is essential before any anticipated refractive surgical procedure because, at present, all refractive surgical procedures are based on the configuration of a normal, healthy cornea. Early detection of keratoconus can save the patient from an incisional or photoablative refractive surgical procedure that likely will not achieve the desired visual outcome.

Keratoconus

Keratoconus is the most frequently encountered ectatic corneal disorder. Its advanced stage is characterized by pronounced localized stromal thinning with a conical protrusion of the central cornea, causing irregular astigmatism and high myopia. The advanced stage of keratoconus is easily diagnosed on slit lamp examination; a Fleischer's ring, stromal thinning, and Vogt's striae are visible. Mild keratoconus cannot be detected easily with any clinical examination except videokeratography[41–43] (Figure 46-14). Videokeratography alone is not sufficient for the diagnosis of keratoconus, however, because other conditions, such as corneal warpage from contact lens wear, can produce videokeratographs that mimic mild keratoconus.

Keratoconus often appears on videokeratography as a high central corneal power, an inferior cornea that is steeper than the superior cornea, a large difference between the power of the corneal apex and that of the periphery, and often a disparity in the central power between the two corneas of a given patient.[43] Wilson and co-workers[44] demonstrated that approximately 73 percent of keratoconus patients have peripheral cones with steepening that extends to the limbus but is usually restricted to one or two quadrants (Figure 46-15). The remaining 25 percent of patients have steepening restricted to the central cornea (Figure 46-16). A large disparity was found between the two corneas of individual patients in terms of the power at the apex of the cone and the total corneal cylinder. Of great importance in the detection of keratoconus was the finding that cones are not always centered inferiorly; in fact, cone apexes were observed not only centrally but also in the superior paralimbal cornea.

Videokeratography performed on family members of patients with keratoconus has detected subtle corneal shape abnormalities that appear to represent a variable expression of an autosomal dominant gene that contributes to the development of keratoconus.[45] Keratoconus is discussed further in Chapter 22.

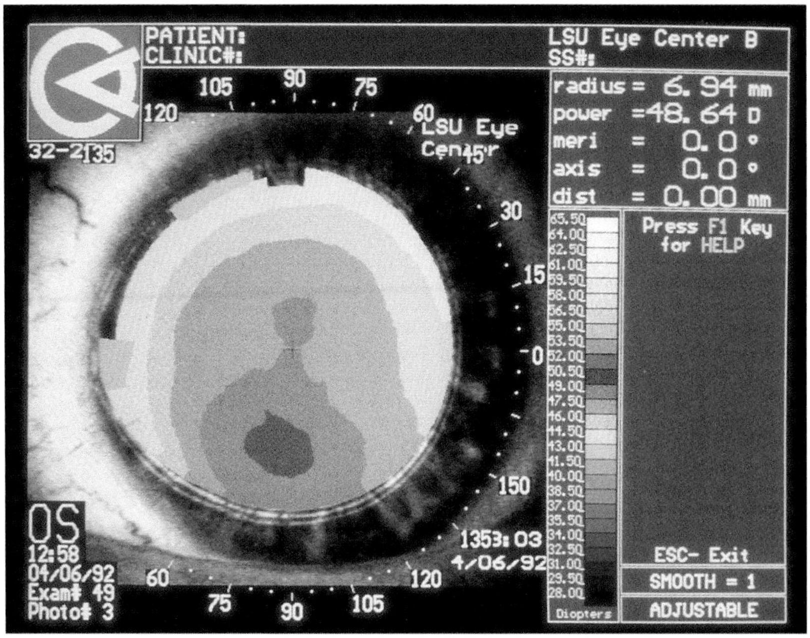

FIGURE 46-14 Color-coded map of a cornea with an early, or preclinical, keratoconus-like pattern. Note the localized inferior region of high power and the asymmetry between the superior and inferior cornea. In this early stage, there are usually no clinical signs.

Pellucid Marginal Degeneration

Pellucid marginal degeneration is characterized by a narrow band of corneal thinning located 1 to 2 mm from the inferior limbus. Topographic analysis shows marked flattening of the central cornea along the vertical axis, with severe against-the-rule astigmatism, and marked steepening of the inferior peripheral cornea[8] (Figure 46-17). Inferior steepening can also extend into the midperipheral oblique corneal quadrants; the axes of marked corneal cylinders in these corneas are not usually orthogonal.[46] Based on these topographic findings, diagnosis of pellucid marginal degeneration can be made even in patients without the classic slit lamp findings of the disorder.[46] Pellucid marginal degeneration is discussed further in Chapter 22.

Terrien's Marginal Degeneration

Terrien's marginal degeneration is a slowly progressive, peripheral corneal thinning disorder that preferentially affects the superior and inferior cornea, although it may occur anywhere around the limbus. Topographic analy-

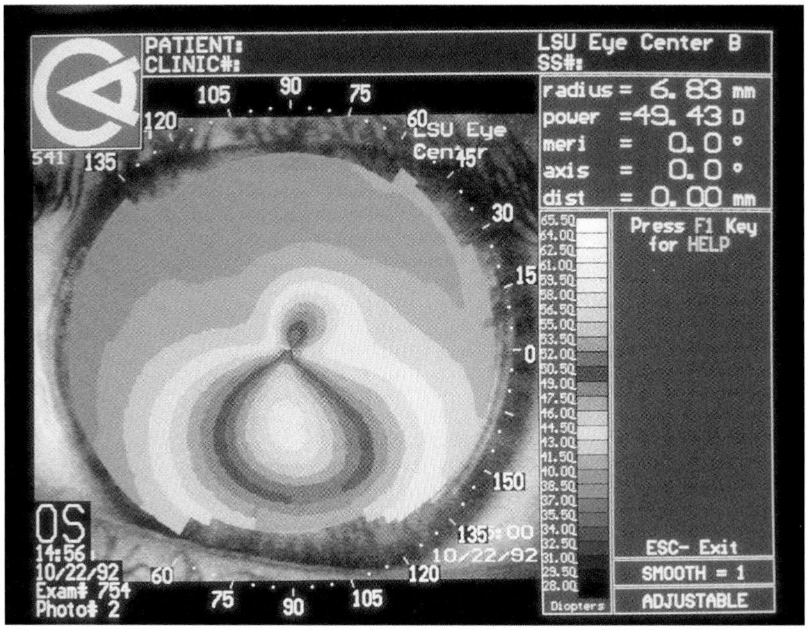

FIGURE 46-15 Color-coded map of peripheral keratoconus. Note the inferior steepening.

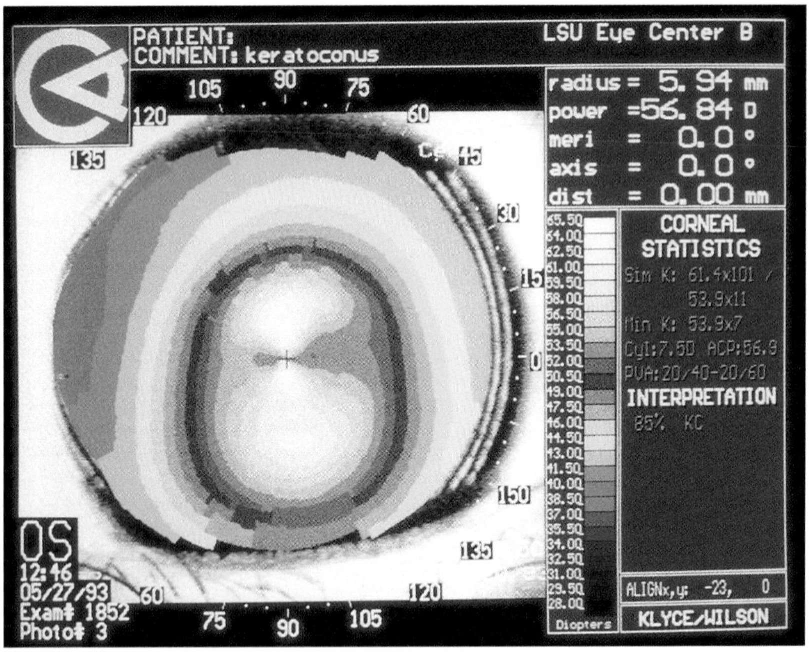

FIGURE 46-16 Color-coded map of central keratoconus. (Courtesy of Leo J. Maguire, M.D., Rochester, MN.)

sis demonstrates flattening over the areas of thinning.[47] When the thinning is restricted to the superior and inferior margins of the cornea, a relative steepening of the cornea is observed approximately 90 degrees away from the midpoint of the thinned area. This steepening results in high against-the-rule or oblique astigmatism. If the area of thinning is either small or completely circumferential, the central cornea may remain relatively spherical. These topographic changes are not specific for Terrien's marginal degeneration. Their origin may be attributed to asymmetrical weakening of the cornea and the effect of intraocular pressure. Although the cornea is essentially inelastic, a weakened segment of stroma can permit regional arcuate flexure caused by intraocular pressure, producing the type of distortions seen in this and other forms of corneal ectatic disorders. Terrien's marginal degeneration is discussed further in Chapter 20.

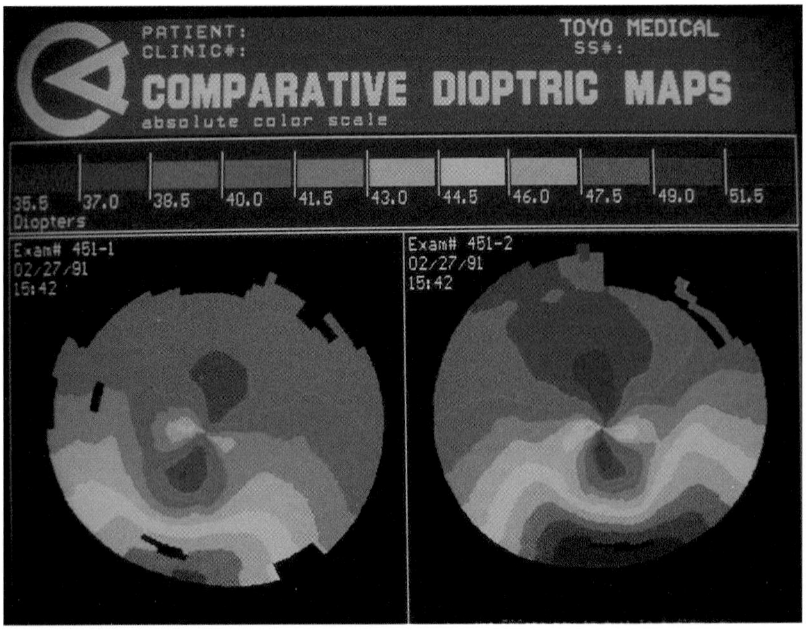

FIGURE 46-17 Color-coded maps of pellucid marginal degeneration. Both corneas have severe against-the-rule astigmatism and crescent-shaped areas of high power inferiorly.

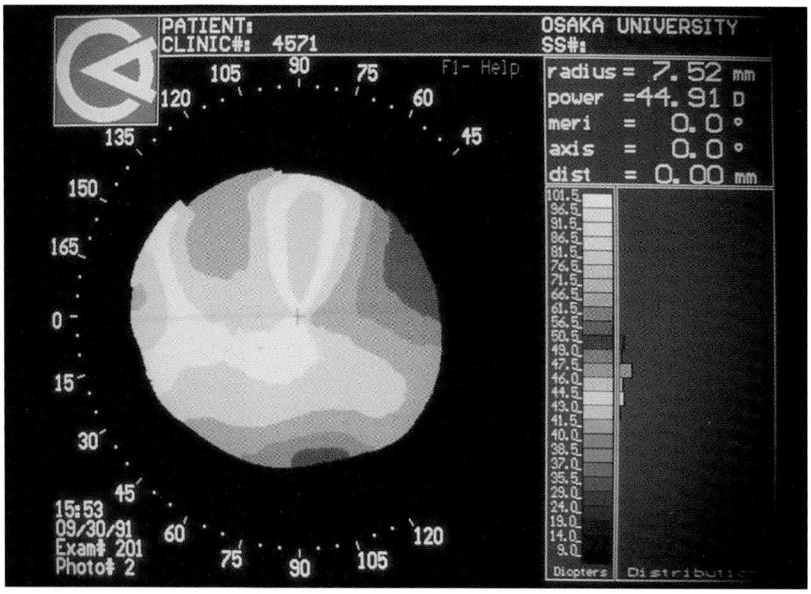

FIGURE 46-18 Color-coded map of a penetrating keratoplasty graft. Note the irregular astigmatism with asymmetry of the power and angle between the two major hemimeridians and the high power areas near the host/graft junction.

Penetrating Keratoplasty

Although penetrating keratoplasty is highly successful in providing a transparent replacement for diseased corneal tissue, refractive results with the procedure may be less than optimal. Corneal surgeons have reduced post-keratoplasty astigmatism from two-digit values to less than the 4-diopter current average. This amount of regular astigmatism can be tolerated and effectively corrected with spectacles. However, irregular astigmatism associated with penetrating keratoplasty cannot be corrected with spectacles and is often more devastating to visual acuity than is regular astigmatism. Videokeratography of the graft is often characterized by a large amount of broadly based irregular astigmatism manifested by separation of the hemimeridians of highest and lowest power by an angle other than 90 degrees, asymmetry of power between the two major hemimeridians, and areas of high power near the wound[48,49] (Figure 46-18).

Relaxing incisions are sometimes used to reduce post-keratoplasty astigmatism. In the past, incisions were made using keratometry or keratoscopy for guidance. These methods could not always detect irregular or asymmetrical astigmatism, and consequently, irregular astigmatism persisted.[48] Videokeratographic determination of the location and extent of steep areas may be more useful to increase the effectiveness of relaxing incisions.[48,49] Many have found videokeratography useful to guide and/or assess other methods of correcting postkeratoplasty astigmatism, such as selective suture removal,[50] adjustment of running sutures[51] (Figure 46-19), and postkeratoplasty orthokeratology (use of a rigid contact lens in the early postoperative period to attempt to mold the cornea into a more spherical shape as the wound heals).

Refractive Surgery

The goal of refractive surgery is to produce a predictable and permanent change in the curvature of the anterior corneal surface over a broad central area. Although penetrating and lamellar keratoplasty, cataract extraction, and excimer laser phototherapeutic keratectomy are seldom performed for purely refractive indications, these procedures can induce significant changes in refraction.[8] Although the overall or integrated refractive change induced by corneal surgery can be evaluated with traditional methods, corneal topographic analysis is necessary to evaluate specific surface anomalies that often accompany corneal surgery.

Radial Keratotomy

During radial keratotomy, the surgeon makes a series of symmetrical radial incisions around a central clear zone, which results in central flattening of the cornea.[52] The effect increases with more and/or deeper incisions and with incisions that extend centrally to encroach on the line of sight.[53] Topographic analysis has demonstrated that radial keratotomy causes the expected reversal of the usual pattern of gradual corneal flattening from the center to the periphery.[54-56] Many corneas (59 percent) that undergo radial keratotomy exhibit a polygonal topographic pattern not seen

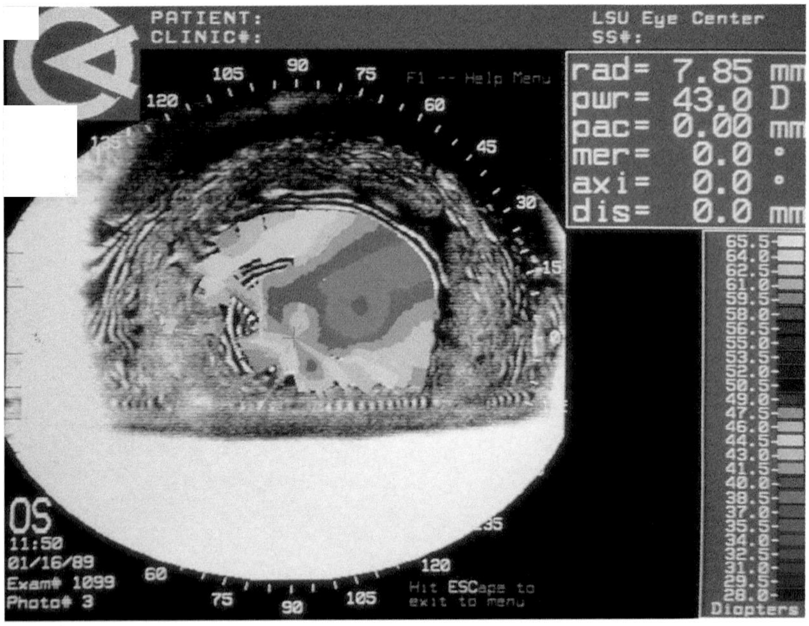

A

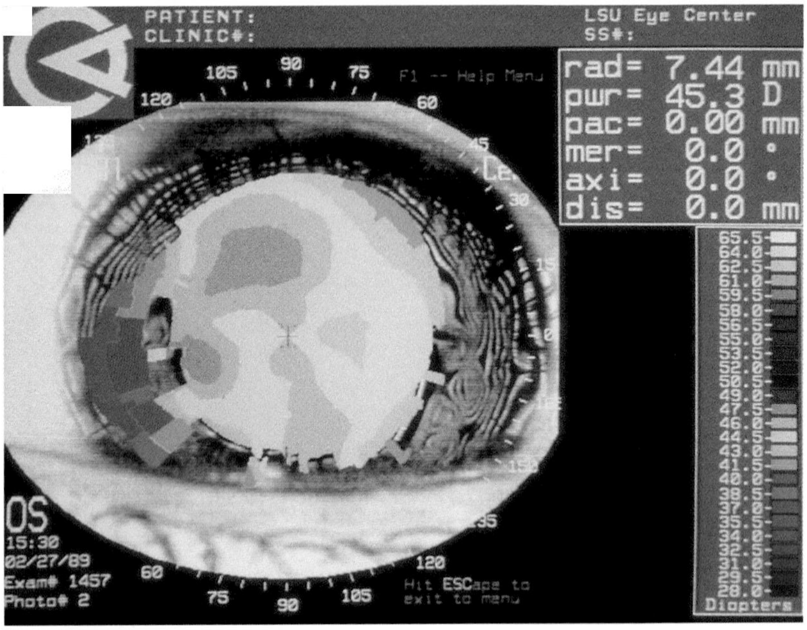

B

FIGURE 46-19 Color-coded maps of postkeratoplasty suture adjustment. **(A)** The map shows the cornea before suture adjustment, with severe regular astigmatism (6.8 diopters) and irregular astigmatism. **(B)** The map shows the cornea 1 month after suture adjustment, with a marked decrease in astigmatism. (Reprinted with permission from Lin DTC, Wilson SE, Reidy JJ, et al: An adjustable single running suture technique to reduce postkeratoplasty astigmatism: a preliminary report. Ophthalmology 97:934, 1990. Courtesy of Ophthalmology.)

in normal corneas (Figure 46-20). Although the central corneal zone usually exhibits less irregular astigmatism after radial keratotomy than after tissue onlay procedures, a degree of nonuniformity in power distribution in the central cornea is typical.[19]

McDonnell and co-workers[57] suggest that such nonuniformity could work to the presbyopic patient's advantage. They observed several patients with excellent postoperative uncorrected acuities inconsistent with their spherical equivalents due to the presence of multifocal zones. These patients also demonstrated excellent uncorrected far and near vision in the same eyes. As with multifocal intraocular lenses and multifocal contact lenses, however, there can be significant tradeoffs to simultaneous multiple foci, particularly when there are more than two foci or when the foci are not sharply defined. The disadvantages include a reduction in contrast sensitivity and uncomfortable or disturbing optical phenomena, such

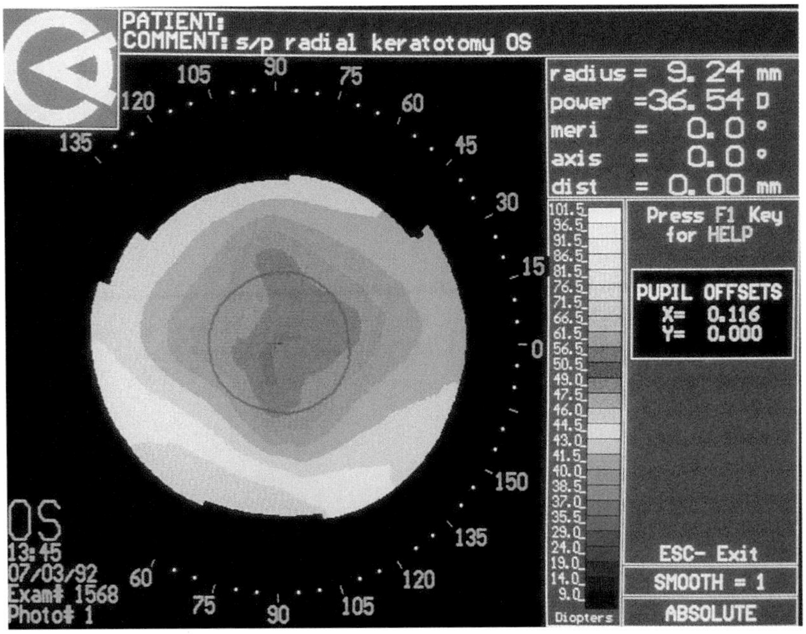

FIGURE 46-20 Color-coded map of a four-incision radial keratotomy. Note the central flattening of the cornea with the polygonal shape corresponding to the four incisions.

as blur or diplopia. In addition, patients in whom the multifocal lens effect is extreme (variations in central corneal power of more than 15 diopters) may experience severe vision loss.[58]

Diurnal fluctuation in visual acuity is a frequent complaint after radial keratotomy, although in some cases the fluctuation appears to diminish with time. Topographic analysis has demonstrated that patients complaining of diurnal fluctuation are more likely to have dumbbell-shaped or split treated zones than round or band-like zones.[55]

Excimer Laser Photorefractive Keratectomy

Photorefractive keratectomy (PRK) with the 193-nm argon-fluoride excimer laser alters the anterior corneal curvature through selective removal of tissue by photoablation. Videokeratographs of corneas after photorefractive keratectomy for myopia (Figure 42-21) indicate

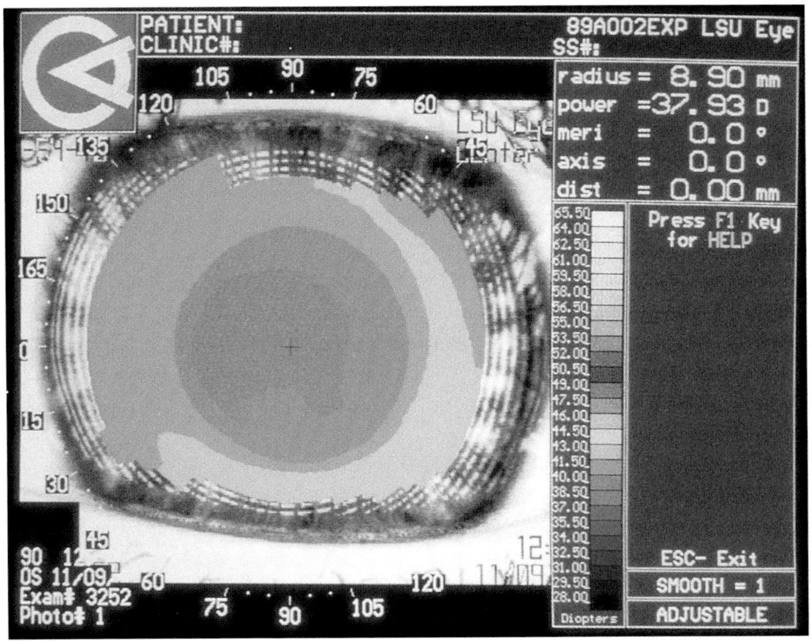

FIGURE 46-21 Color-coded map of excimer laser photorefractive keratectomy for the correction of myopia. Note that the central flattening of the treated zone is uniform and there is a smooth transition between this zone and the periphery.

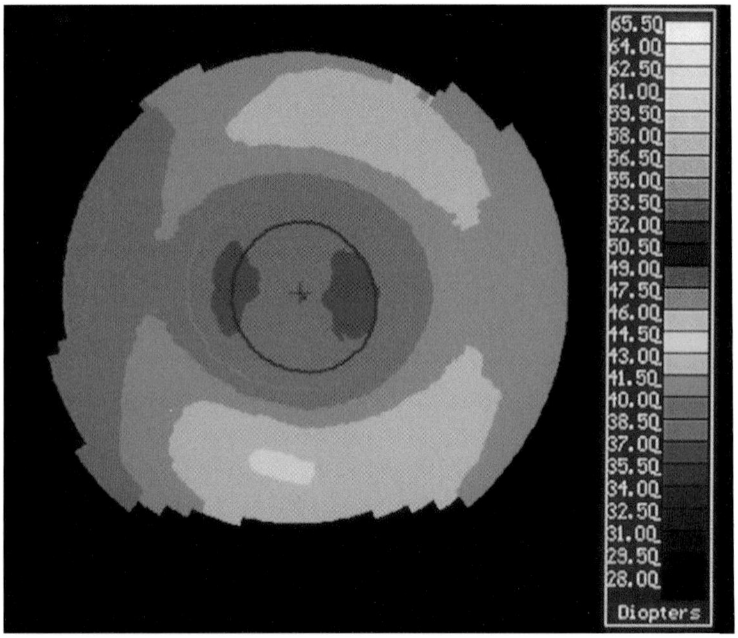

FIGURE 46-22 Laser-assisted in situ keratomileusis 1 month postoperatively. Although the optical zone is somewhat small (4.5 to 5.0 mm) the central topography shows good uniformity.

a nearly circular zone of uniformly reduced central cornea power corresponding to the area of ablation.[59,60] There is a smooth transition of power from the ablated zone to the peripheral cornea.[61] Topographic analysis shows that photorefractive keratectomy has a level of precision greater than that achieved with other refractive surgical procedures. By using computer-assisted corneal topographic analysis to determine the average power of the ablated zone, a greater change was detected than could be identified by keratometric measurements alone.

Maloney[3] reviewed the principles involved in locating the zone to be ablated in photorefractive keratectomy, re-emphasizing the need to center the procedure over the center of the patient's entrance pupil.[2] The size and centration of the ablated zone can be appreciated and measured only with videokeratography.[61,62] Centration errors of 1 mm or more are not uncommon despite meticulous centration procedures used during photorefractive keratectomy, although on average, ablation zone centers differ by less than 0.50 mm from the center of the entrance pupil. It is important that ablated zones be large enough in diameter to compensate for the inherent error in centration that exists with all refractive surgical procedures.

Laser-Assisted In Situ Keratomileusis

Laser-assisted in situ keratomileusis (LASIK), which was introduced by Pallikaris,[63,64] has been used to extend the range of myopic correction by the excimer laser. Radial keratotomy and photorefractive keratectomy appear most effective for the correction of 6 diopters or less of myopia, whereas laser-assisted in situ keratomileusis appears effective for the correction of low, moderate, and high myopia. Although published reports of long-term follow-up for laser-assisted in situ keratomileusis are not available at this writing, the larger treatment range and rapid visual recovery are distinct advantages of this procedure over other refractive surgical procedures. A topographic example of a cornea after laser-assisted in situ keratomileusis is shown in Figure 46-22. Because the procedure relies on a microkeratome for the creation of a corneal flap, irregular astigmatism can be a confounding complication (Figure 46-23).

Epikeratophakia

Epikeratophakia involves placement of a lathe-cut tissue lens of donor corneal stroma and Bowman's layer on the surface of the recipient Bowman's layer to change the anterior corneal curvature, and hence, the refractive power of the eye. This procedure is performed for myopia, hyperopia, and keratoconus. As with many other refractive surgical procedures, keratometry does not accurately reflect the change in refraction produced by epikeratophakia,[65] primarily because the keratometer does not take readings from the center of the cornea.

Each epikeratophakia procedure has characteristic topographic features.[66] Central corneal steepening is achieved with aphakic epikeratophakia, but even with patients who achieve excellent uncorrected visual acuity, irregular astigmatism and a 4- to 6.5-diopter range of power distribution has been demonstrated centrally[67] (Figure 46-24).

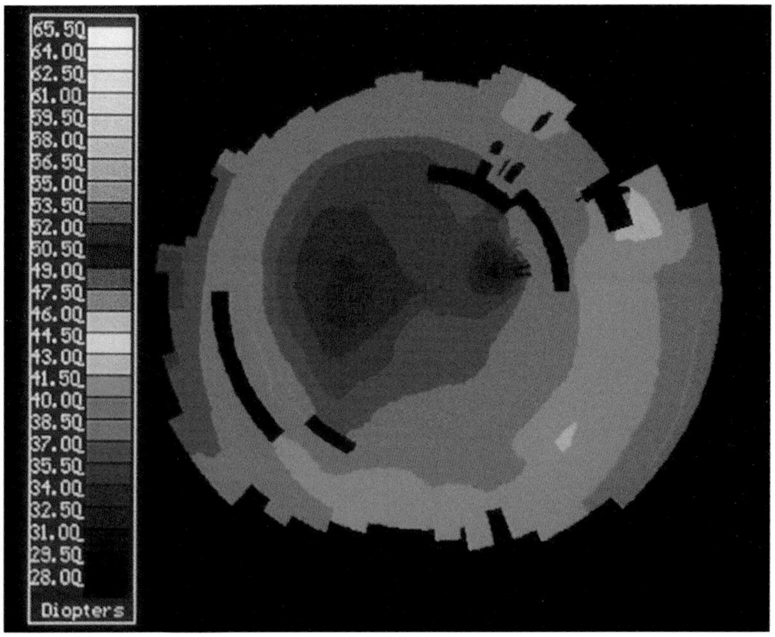

FIGURE 46-23 A significant amount of irregular astigmatism occurred in this eye after laser-assisted in situ keratomileusis with a loss of two lines of best-corrected visual acuity. It is not possible to determine from this topographic analysis whether the source of the astigmatism was a nonuniform laser beam or suboptimal microkeratome performance.

Epikeratophakia for myopia was the first refractive surgical procedure in which videokeratography was used to improve results. Early cases were analyzed and found to have a central treated zone smaller in diameter than predicted. Outside the treated zone, the power of the tissue lens surface increased steadily, indicating a progressive steepening of the cornea as the tissue lens/host interface was approached. In some cases, decentration was also readily apparent.[68] With the feedback provided by videokeratography, the treated zone was enlarged by modifying the surgical attachment and tissue lens design parameters, and better methods were established for improving centration.

In epikeratophakia for keratoconus, a 9-mm tissue lens is placed on an 8.5-mm bed to flatten the cone. This procedure decreases both the anterior and posterior corneal curvatures. Corneal topographic analysis shows diffuse flattening, with a large treated zone.[69] Preoperative videokeratography is used to identify the full topographic extent of the cone and to indicate the need for purposeful decentration of the tissue lens to provide a maximal flattening effect.[66]

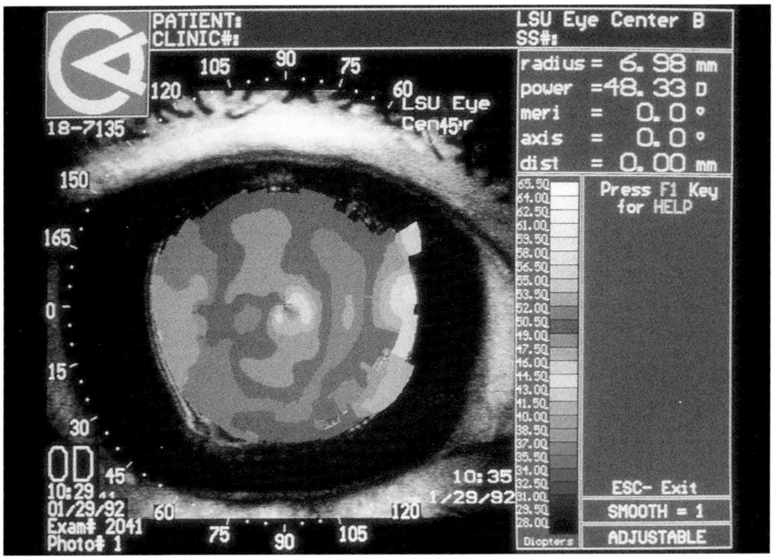

FIGURE 46-24 Color-coded map of epikeratophakia for aphakia. The central corneal power is 48.33 diopters, with irregularity in the refractive power distribution.

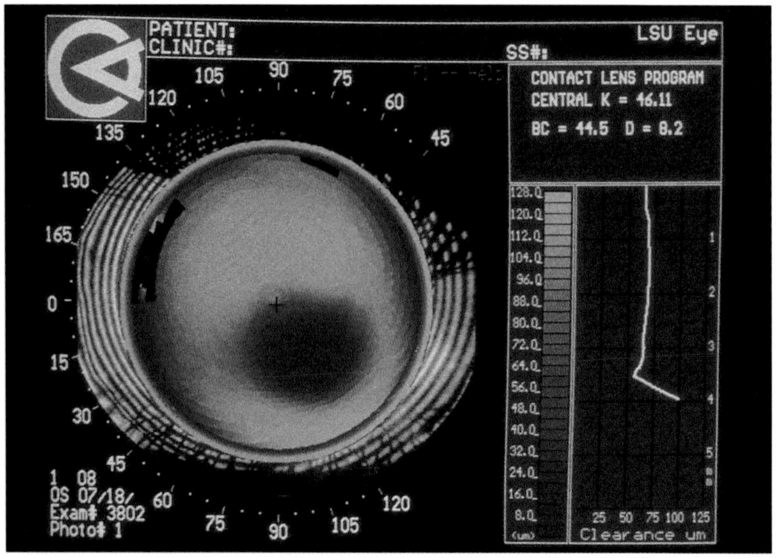

FIGURE 46-25 Simulated contact lens fluorescein pattern in a keratoconus cornea. Modern algorithms permit the simulation of the contact lens fluorescein pattern to help evaluate lens designs and perhaps create new designs that will better serve the needs of unusually shaped corneas, such as occur in keratoconus.

In cases in which high postoperative astigmatism ensues after epikeratophakia procedures, videokeratography can help in planning the appropriate surgical intervention.[66]

Contact Lenses

Contact lens fitting can be a time-consuming, trial-and-error process, particularly in patients with the irregular astigmatism that occurs with keratoconus, penetrating keratoplasty, and refractive surgery. Although many patients with advanced keratoconus can delay penetrating keratoplasty with careful refitting of contact lenses,[70] many practitioners lack the skill and experience necessary to fit these difficult cones. Use of videokeratography to define the location, extent, and power of the cone can assist in contact lens selection.[71] Alternatively, because corneal topographic analysis reconstructs the corneal surface, it has been used to simulate the clinical fluorescein test used to fit contact lenses[72] (Figure 46-25). In this way, rigid contact lens fitting may be facilitated, particularly for difficult cases.

Contact lens-induced corneal warpage can be seen in both soft and rigid contact lens wearers and has also been associated with annular tinted soft lenses[73] (see Ch. 27). Signs of corneal warpage include spectacle blur after lens removal, loss of best-corrected spectacle visual acuity, and distortion of keratometer or keratoscope mires. Wilson and co-workers[23,26] provided a detailed discussion of the topographic alterations associated with contact lens warpage. Central irregular astigmatism, loss of radial symmetry, and frequent reversal of the normal topographic pattern of progressive flattening from the center to the periphery were noted. In some cases, those changes correlated with the resting position of the contact lens (Figure 46-26). The topographic change caused by the superior resting position of a rigid contact lens is similar to that noted in early keratoconus and is called *pseudokeratoconus*. Although 4 to 6 weeks out of lenses appears to be enough time to resolve warpage caused by soft lenses, corneal topography can take up to 5 months to stabilize after discontinuation of rigid lenses. Corneal warpage is seemingly permanent in some cases; when warpage consists of significant radially asymmetrical astigmatism, a permanent reduction in best spectacle-corrected visual acuity can be anticipated.

Because contact lens warpage can produce a pattern identical to that of early keratoconus (pseudokeratoconus), it is important to be able to distinguish between the two, particularly when screening patients for refractive surgery. Generally, discontinuation of contact lens wear until a stable topography is achieved is the preferred method for differential diagnosis. If the keratoconic pattern transforms into a bowtie pattern and stabilizes, then contact lens warpage is the likely cause of the pattern. If the keratoconic pattern persists, the diagnosis is less certain: the patient has either a permanently warped cornea or keratoconus. The patient should discontinue use of contact lenses for 6 months and return for repeat topographic analysis. Often when keratoconus is associated with lens wear, the keratoconic pattern becomes more pronounced soon after cessation of lens wear because

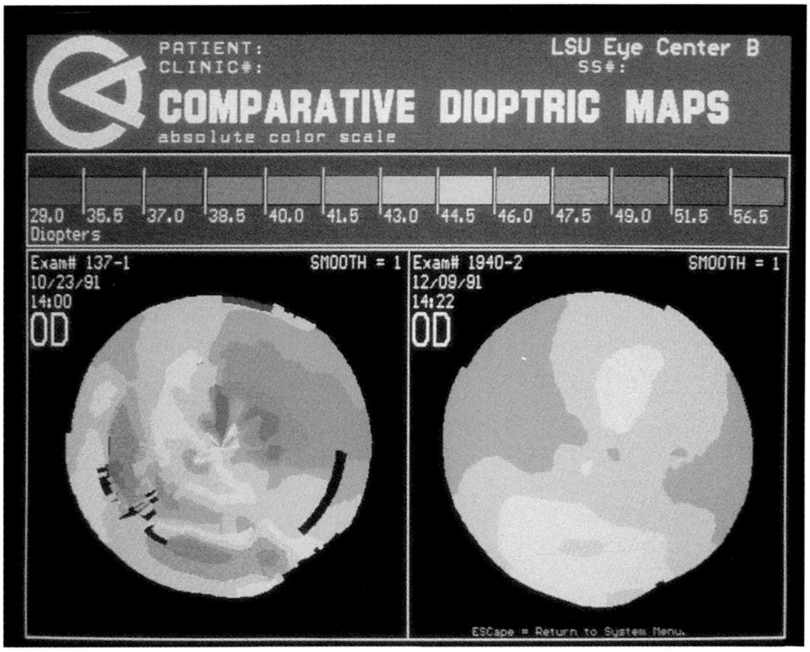

FIGURE 46-26 Color-coded maps of contact lens-induced corneal warpage. The left map illustrates a cornea warped from a decentered rigid gas-permeable contact lens. There is central irregular astigmatism, superonasal flattening underlying the decentered contact lens, flattening along the contact lens margin, and peripheral steepening on the side opposite the decentration. The right map illustrates the improved topography 6 weeks after changing to a smaller-diameter lens. Note the presence of a keratoconus pattern that could represent pseudokeratoconus (contact lens warpage) or true keratoconus. Differentiation would require cessation of lens wear and re-examination with videokeratography.

contact lenses tend to flatten certain types of cones. If the patient cannot discontinue wearing contact lenses, fitting the patient with a lens that rides centrally in its primary position may reverse pseudokeratoconus. Finally, if keratoconus is suspected, the topographic pattern of the other eye should be studied. With contact lens-induced warpage, the effects often are very similar bilaterally. Conversely, keratoconus is usually more advanced in one eye than in the other.

REFERENCES

1. Waring GO: Making sense of keratospeak II: proposed conventional terminology for corneal topography. Refract Corneal Surg 5:362, 1989
2. Uozato H, Guyton DL: Centering corneal surgical procedures. Am J Ophthalmol 103:264, 1987
3. Maloney RK: Corneal topography and optical zone location in photorefractive keratectomy. Refract Corneal Surg 6:363, 1990
4. Helmholtz H: Treatise on Physiologic Optic. Translated from the third German edition. Southall JP (ed). Banta, Menasha, WI, 1924
5. Javal E: Troisème contribution a l'ophthalmométrie: description de quelques images keratoscopies. Ann Ocul (Paris) 89:5, 1883
6. Zadnik K, Mutti DO, Adams AJ: The repeatability of measurement of the ocular components. Invest Ophthalmol Vis Sci 33:2325, 1992
7. Klyce SD, Dingeldein SA: Corneal topography. p. 61. In Masters B (ed): Noninvasive Diagnostic Techniques in Ophthalmology. Springer-Verlag, New York, 1990
8. Rowsey JJ, Reynolds AE, Brown R: Corneal topography. Corneascope. Arch Ophthalmol 99:1093, 1981
9. Maguire LJ, Klyce SD, Sawelson H, et al: Visual distortion after myopic keratomileusis: computer analysis of keratoscope photographs. Ophthalmic Surg 18:352, 1987
10. Klyce SD: Computer-assisted corneal topography: high-resolution graphic presentation and analysis of keratoscopy. Invest Ophthalmol Vis Sci 25:1426, 1984
11. Reynolds AE: Corneal topography as found by photo-electric keratoscopy. Contacto 3:229, 1959
12. Clark BAJ: Conventional keratoscopy—a critical review. Aust J Optom 56:140, 1973
13. Doss JD, Hutson RL, Rowsey JJ, Brown DR: Method for calculation of corneal profile and power distribution. Arch Ophthalmol 99:1261, 1981
14. Gormley DJ, Gersten M, Koplin RS, Lubkin V: Corneal modeling. Cornea 7:30, 1988
15. El Hage SG: A computerized corneal topographer for use in refractive surgery. Refract Corneal Surg 5:418, 1989
16. Koch DD, Foulks GN, Moran CT, Wakil JS: The corneal EyeSys system: Accuracy, analysis and reproducibility of first-generation prototype. Refract Corneal Surg 5:424, 1989
17. Itoi M, Maruyama Y: A new photokeratometry system. J Jpn Contact Lens Soc 20:119, 1978
18. Warnicki JW, Rehkopf PG, Curtin SA, et al: Corneal topography using computer analyzed rasterstereographic images. Appl Optics 27:1135, 1988

19. Maguire LJ, Singer DE, Klyce SD: Graphic presentation of computer-analyzed keratoscope photographs. Arch Ophthalmol 105:223, 1987
20. Wilson SE, Klyce SD, Husseini ZM: Standardized color-coded maps for corneal topography. Ophthalmology 100:1723, 1993
21. Dingeldein SA, Klyce SD, Wilson SE: Quantitative descriptors of corneal shape derived from computer-assisted analysis of photokeratographs. Refract Corneal Surg 5:372, 1989
22. Wilson SE, Wang JY, Klyce SD: Quantification and mathematical analysis of photokeratoscopic images. p. 1. In Schanzlin DJ, Robin JB (eds): Corneal Topography. Measuring and Modifying the Cornea. Springer-Verlag, New York, 1992
23. Wilson SE, Lin DTC, Klyce SD, et al: Rigid contact lens decentration: a risk factor for corneal warpage. CLAO J 16:177, 1990
24. Wilson SE, Klyce SD: Advances in the analysis of corneal topography. Surv Ophthalmol 35:269, 1991
25. Lin DTC, Wilson SE, Reidy JJ, et al: Topographic changes that occur with 10-0 running suture removal following penetrating keratoplasty. Refract Corneal Surg 6:21, 1990
26. Wilson SE, Lin DTC, Klyce SD, et al: Topographic changes in contact lens-induced corneal warpage. Ophthalmology 97:734, 1990
27. Maeda N, Klyce SD, Dehkhoda MT, Smolek MK: Automated keratoconus detection with corneal topography analysis. Abstracts of the 1992 Annual Scientific Meeting of the Castroviejo Cornea Society, Dallas, TX
28. Wilson SE, Klyce SD: Quantitative descriptors of corneal topography: a clinical study. Arch Ophthalmol 109:349, 1991
29. Camp JJ, Maguire LJ, Cameron BM, Robb RA: A computer model for the evaluation of the effect of corneal topography on optical performance. Am J Ophthalmol 109:379, 1990
30. Maguire LJ, Zabel RW, Parker P, Lindstrom RL: Topography and raytracing analysis of patients with excellent visual acuity 3 months after excimer laser photorefractive keratectomy for myopia. Refract Corneal Surg 7:122, 1991
31. Politch J: Optical and long wave holography: potential applications in ophthalmology. Doc Ophthalmol 42:165, 1977
32. Smith TW: Corneal topography. Doc Ophthalmol 43:249, 1977
33. Baker PC: Holographic contour analysis of the cornea. p. 82. In Masters BR (ed): Noninvasive Diagnostic Techniques in Ophthalmology. Springer-Verlag, New York, 1990
34. Smolek MK: Analysis of bovine ocular distension via real-time holographic interferometry. Doctoral dissertation. Indiana State University Graduate School, Bloomington, IN. Microfilms International Publishers, Ann Arbor, MI, 1986
35. Arffa RC, Warnicki JW, Rehkopf PG: Corneal topography using rasterstereography. Refract Corneal Surg 5:414, 1989
36. Belin MW, Litoff D, Strods SJ, et al: The PAR technology corneal topography system. Refract Corneal Surg 8:88, 1992
37. Klyce SD, Wilson SE: Methods of analysis of corneal topography. Refract Corneal Surg 5:368, 1989
46. Edmund C, Sjontoft E: The central-peripheral radius of the normal corneal curvature. A photokeratoscopic study. Acta Ophthalmol (Copenh) 63:670, 1985
39. Dingeldein SA, Klyce SD: The topography of normal corneas. Arch Ophthalmol 107:512, 1989
40. Bogan SJ, Waring GO, Ibrahim O, et al: Classification of normal corneal topography based on computer-assisted videokeratography. Arch Ophthalmol 108:945, 1990
41. Maguire LJ, Lowry JC: Identifying progression of subclinical keratoconus by serial topography analysis. Am J Ophthalmol 112:41, 1991
42. Maguire LJ, Bourne WM: Corneal topography of early keratoconus. Am J Ophthalmol 108:107, 1989
43. Rabinowitz YS, McDonnell PJ: Computer-assisted corneal topography in keratoconus. Refract Corneal Surg 5:400, 1989
44. Wilson SE, Lin DTC, Klyce SD: Corneal topography of keratoconus. Cornea 10:2, 1991
45. Rabinowitz YS, Garbus J, McDonnell PJ: Computer-assisted corneal topography in family members of patients with keratoconus. Arch Ophthalmol 108:365, 1990
46. Maguire LJ, Klyce SD, McDonald MB, Kaufman HE: Corneal topography of pellucid marginal degeneration. Ophthalmology 94:519, 1987
47. Wilson SE, Lin DTC, Klyce SD, Insler MS: Terrien's marginal degeneration: corneal topography. Refract Corneal Surg 6:15, 1990
48. Maguire LJ, Bourne WM: Corneal topography of transverse keratotomies for astigmatism after penetrating keratoplasty. Am J Ophthalmol 107:323, 1989
49. Frangieh GT, Kwitko S, McDonnell PJ: Prospective corneal topographic analysis in surgery for postkeratoplasty astigmatism. Arch Ophthalmol 109:506, 1991
50. Strelow S, Cohen EJ, Leavitt KG, Laibson PR: Corneal topography for selective suture removal after penetrating keratoplasty. Am J Ophthalmol 112:657, 1991
51. Lin DTC, Wilson SE, Reidy JJ, et al: An adjustable single running suture technique to reduce postkeratoplasty astigmatism: a preliminary report. Ophthalmology 97:934, 1990
52. Villaseñor RA, Itoi M, Harris DF, Robin JB: Corneal topography and refractive surgery. Cornea 2:323, 1983
53. Rowsey JJ: Ten caveats in keratorefractive surgery. Ophthalmology 90:148, 1983
54. Fleming JF: Corneal topography and radial keratotomy. J Refract Surg 2:249, 1986
55. McDonnell PJ, McClusky DJ, Garbus JJ: Corneal topography and fluctuating visual acuity after radial keratotomy. Ophthalmology 96:665, 1989
56. Bogan SJ, Maloney RK, Drews CD, Waring GO: Computer-assisted videokeratography of corneal topography after radial keratotomy. Arch Ophthalmol 109:834, 1991

57. McDonnell PJ, Garbus J, Lopez PF: Topographic analysis and visual acuity after radial keratotomy. Am J Ophthalmol 106:692, 1988
58. Maguire LJ, Bourne WM: A multifocal lens effect as a complication of radial keratotomy. Refract Corneal Surg 5:394, 1989
59. McDonald MB, Franz JM, Klyce SD, et al: Central photorefractive keratectomy for myopia. The blind eye study. Arch Ophthalmol 108:799, 1990
60. Sher NA, Barak M, Daya S, et al: Excimer laser photorefractive keratectomy in high myopia. Arch Ophthalmol 110:935, 1992
61. Wilson SE, Klyce SD, McDonald MB, et al: Changes in corneal topography after excimer laser photorefractive keratectomy for myopia. Ophthalmology 98:1346, 1991
62. Klyce SD: Corneal topography and mapping. p. 19. In Thompson FB, McDonnell PJ (eds): Color Atlas/Text of Excimer Laser Surgery. The Cornea. Igaku-Shoin, New York, 1992
63. Pallikaris IG, Papatzanaki ME, Stathi EZ, et al: Laser in situ keratomileusis. Lasers Surg Med 10:463, 1990
64. Pallikaris IG, Papatzanaki ME, Siganos DS, Tsilimbiaris MK: A corneal flap technique for laser in situ keratomileusis: human studies. Arch Ophthalmol 109:1699,1991
65. Arffa RC, Klyce SD, Busin M: Keratometry in epikeratophakia. J Refract Surg 2:61, 1986
66. Reidy JJ, McDonald MB, Klyce SD: The corneal topography of epikeratophakia. Refract Corneal Surg 6:26, 1990
67. Maguire LJ: Corneal topography of patients with excellent Snellen visual acuity after epikeratophakia for aphakia. Am J Ophthalmol 109:162, 1990
68. Maguire LJ, Klyce SD, Singer DE, et al: Corneal topography in myopic patients undergoing epikeratophakia. Am J Ophthalmol 103:404, 1987
69. Uusitalo RJ, Lehtosalo J, Klyce SD: One-year follow-up of epikeratophakia after keratoconus. Graefes Arch Clin Exp Ophthalmol 227:401, 1989
70. Belin MW, Fowler WC, Chambers WA: Keratoconus. Evaluation of recent trends in the surgical and nonsurgical correction of keratoconus. Ophthalmology 95:335, 1988
71. Rabinowitz Y, Garbus JJ, Garbus C, McDonnell PJ: Contact lens selection for keratoconus using a computer-assisted videokeratoscope. CLAO J 17:88, 1991
72. Klyce SD, Estopinal HA, Gersten M, et al: Fluorescein exam simulation for contact lens fitting. ARVO abstract. Invest Ophthalmol Vis Sci 33(suppl):697, 1992
73. Schanzer MC, Mehta RS, Arnold TP, et al: Irregular astigmatism induced by annular tinted contact lenses. CLAO J 15:207, 1989

Index

Note: Page numbers followed by *f* indicate figures; page numbers followed by *t* indicate tables.